ACCCN's
Critical Care Nursing

3e

ACCCN's
Critical Care Nursing

3e

Leanne Aitken

RN, PhD, BHSc(Nurs)Hons, GCertMgt, GDipScMed(ClinEpi), FACCCN,
FACN, FAAN, Life Member – ACCCN
Professor of Critical Care Nursing, School of Nursing and Midwifery
and NHMRC Centre of Research Excellence in Nursing (NCREN),
Menzies Health Institute Queensland, Griffith University, Qld, Australia
Intensive Care Unit, Princess Alexandra Hospital, Qld, Australia
Professor of Nursing, School of Health Sciences,
City University London, UK

Andrea Marshall

RN, PhD, MN(Research), BN, Grad Cert Ed Studies (Higher Ed),
IC Cert, FACCCN, FACN, Life Member – ACCCN
Professor of Acute and Complex Care Nursing, School of Nursing and
Midwifery and NHMRC Centre of Research Excellence in Nursing (NCREN),
Menzies Health Institute Queensland, Griffith University, Qld, Australia
Intensive Care Unit, Gold Coast Hospital and Health Service, Qld, Australia

Wendy Chaboyer

RN, PhD, MN, BSc(Nu)Hons, Crit Care Cert, FACCCN,
Life Member – ACCCN
Professor and Director, NHMRC Centre of Research Excellence
in Nursing (NCREN), Menzies Health Institute Queensland,
Griffith University, Qld, Australia
Professor, Institute of Health and Care Sciences,
University of Gothenburg, Sweden

ELSEVIER

ELSEVIER

Elsevier Australia. ACN 001 002 357
(a division of Reed International Books Australia Pty Ltd)
Tower 1, 475 Victoria Avenue, Chatswood, NSW 2067

National Library of Australia Cataloguing-in-Publication Data

ACCCN's critical care nursing / [editors] Leanne Aitken,
Andrea Marshall & Wendy Chaboyer.

3rd edition.

9780729542005 (paperback)

Intensive care nursing--Australia.

Aitken, Leanne, editor.
Marshall, Andrea, editor.
Chaboyer, Wendy, editor.

616.028

Senior Content Strategist: Libby Houston
Content Development Specialist: Martina Vascotto
Project Manager: Devendran Kannan
Edited by Linda Littlemore
Proofread by Laura Davies
Design by Natalie Bowra
Permissions by Sarah Thomas & Anita Mercy Vethakkan
Index by Robert Swanson
Typeset by Midland Typesetters, Australia
Printed in China by 1010 Printing International Limited

Contents

Foreword

Ruth M Kleinpell

Advances in critical care treatments, procedures and technologies mandate that critical care nurses maintain current knowledge of disease states, management principles for acute and critical illness and best care principles including clinical practice guidelines. As a specialty area of nursing practice, critical care nursing is focused on the care of patients who are experiencing life-threatening illness. Globally, critical care nurses provide care to ensure that critically ill patients and their families receive optimal care.

This third edition of the Australian College of Critical Care Nurses' (ACCCN's) *Critical Care Nursing* is a valuable resource for critical care nursing. The editors, who are acknowledged expert practitioners, educators and researchers in critical care nursing, have organised the book into topics covering essential concepts in critical care. The book content addresses aspects of critical care nursing practice, quality and safety concepts, ethical issues, pathophysiology and management of a variety of critical illness states, recovery and rehabilitation after critical illness, psychological care and family-centred care concepts, among other topics. The chapters are written by established experts in the field of critical care and provide a comprehensive overview of critical care nursing principles of practice. The book provides up-to-date information on evidence-based practices and the chapters incorporate a variety of educational resources including website links, case studies, practice tips and appendices addressing practice standards for critical care nursing,

laboratory analysis application and a comprehensive glossary of terms.

ACCCN's *Critical Care Nursing* is an outstanding resource for critical care nurses, regardless of the practice setting. In seeking to provide complex high intensity care, therapies and interventions, critical care nurses will find that this third edition of the book reviews essential content related to critical care nursing knowledge and skills to provide care to acute and critically ill patients and their families.

Critical care nursing is one of the largest specialty areas of nursing practise as, internationally, more than 600,000 critical care nurses practise in high acuity, acute care or critical care. It is well established that maintaining knowledge of current practice, evidence-based care and integrating research in clinical practice for critical care patients are essential components of critical care nursing. This third edition of ACCCN's *Critical Care Nursing* provides a comprehensive expert resource for critical care nurses to enable them to further develop their knowledge and enhance their clinical nursing expertise.

Ruth **Kleinpell** PhD RN FAAN FCCM
Director, Center for Clinical Research & Scholarship
Rush University Medical Center
Professor, Rush University College of Nursing
Nurse Practitioner, Rush Lincoln Park Urgent Care,
Chicago, Illinois USA
President, World Federation of Critical Care Nurses
(http:www.wfccn.org)

Foreword

Doug Elliott

It is a great privilege and with a sense of pride that I write these comments for this 3rd edition of *ACCCN's Critical Care Nursing*. As lead editor of the previous two editions, publication of this revision confirms our initial thoughts that there was a clear disciplinary need and reader demand for an original text from this area of the world, and that our community contained a critical mass of scholarly writers able to deliver a comprehensive text on critical care nursing. An ensuing strong and enduring collaborative relationship between the College, the Publisher and the Editors has resulted in this robust legacy of knowledge for our specialty.

Critical care continues to be a dynamic and evolving clinical specialty, and maintaining currency of knowledge can be a challenge for nurse clinicians and students. This edition reflects the current evidence base for critical care nursing, tailored for practice in the Australian, New Zealand and Asia–Pacific region. The text continues a strong focus of application of research findings to practice,

with pedagogical features including summary tables, illustrative figures, case studies and research vignettes to support active and reflective learning.

The editors, all leading experts in their specialty fields, have assembled a strong and varied set of chapter authors from both clinical and academic settings, mostly from Australia, but also some notable contributions from key international experts. The resulting collection of 29 chapters provides a comprehensive resource for critical care nurses and students seeking to maintain or develop their knowledge and skillset in the holistic care of critically ill patients.

Doug **Elliott** RN, PhD, MAppSc (Nurs),
BAppSc (Nurs), ICCert
Professor of Nursing
Faculty of Health
University of Technology Sydney
Past Co-Editor
ACCCN's Critical Care Nursing (2007, 2012)

Preface

Critical care as a clinical specialty is over half a century old. With every successive decade, advances in the education and practices of critical care nurses have been made. Today, critical care nurses are some of the most knowledgeable and highly skilled nurses in the world, and ongoing professional development and education are fundamental elements in ensuring we deliver the highest quality care to our patients and their families.

This book is intended to encourage and challenge nurses to further develop their critical care nursing practice. Our vision for the first edition was for an original text from Australasian authors, not an adaptation of texts produced in other parts of the world.

As international interest in our text has grown, we have expanded its content to reflect the universal core elements of critical care nursing practice while still retaining specific information that captures the unique elements of contemporary critical care nursing in Australia, New Zealand and other similar practice environments such as the United Kingdom and some parts of Europe and Asia.

This third edition of *ACCCN's Critical Care Nursing* has 29 chapters that reflect the collective talent and expertise of 54 contributors – a strong mix of academics and clinicians with a passion for critical care nursing – in showcasing the practice of critical care nursing in Australia, New Zealand, Asia and the Pacific. We also engaged contributors beyond Australasia to reflect global practices and to extend the applicability of our text to a wider geographical audience. All contributors were carefully chosen for their current knowledge, clinical expertise and strong professional reputations.

The book has been developed primarily for use by practising critical care clinicians, managers, researchers and graduate students undertaking a specialty critical care qualification. In addition, senior undergraduate students studying high acuity nursing subjects will find this book a valuable reference tool, although it goes beyond the learning needs of these students. The aim of the book is to be a comprehensive resource, as well as a portal to an array of other important resources, for critical care nurses. The nature and timeline of book publishing dictate that the information contained in this book reflects a snapshot in time of our knowledge and understanding of the complex world of critical care nursing. We therefore encourage our readers to continue to also search for the most contemporary sources of knowledge to guide their clinical practice. A range of website links have been included in each chapter to facilitate this process.

This third edition is divided into three broad sections: the scope of critical care nursing, core components of critical care nursing and specialty aspects of critical care nursing. Inclusion of new chapters and significant revisions to existing chapters were based on our reflections and suggestions from colleagues and reviewers as well as on evolving and emerging practices in critical care.

Section 1 introduces a broad range of professional issues related to practice that are relevant across critical care. Initial chapters provide contemporary information on the scope of practice, systems and resources and ethical issues, with expanded information on quality and safety, and recovery and rehabilitation in critical care.

Content presented in Section 2 is relevant to the majority of critical care nurses, with a focus on concepts that underpin practice such as essential physical, psychological, social and cultural care. Remaining chapters in this section present a systems approach in supporting physiological function for a critically ill individual. This edition now has multiple linked chapters for some of the major physiological systems – four chapters for cardiovascular, three for respiratory and two for neurological. In this third edition we have a stronger emphasis on nutrition assessment and therapeutic management, with this topic now having a dedicated chapter. Chapters on support of renal function; gastrointestinal, metabolic and liver alterations; management of shock; and multi-organ dysfunction complete this section.

Section 3 presents specific clinical conditions such as emergency presentations, trauma, resuscitation, paediatric considerations, pregnancy and postpartum considerations and organ donation, by building on the principles outlined in Section 2. To this section we have added a specific chapter on postanaesthesia recovery to acknowledge the importance of this work, which might occur in some critical care areas, particularly after hours. This section enables readers to explore some of the more complex or unique aspects of specialty critical care nursing practice.

Chapters have been organised in a consistent format to facilitate identification of relevant material. Where appropriate, each chapter commences with an overview of the relevant anatomy and physiology and the epidemiology of the clinical states internationally and then in the Australian and New Zealand setting. Nursing care of the patient, delivered independently or provided collaboratively with other members of the healthcare team, is then presented. Pedagogical features include a case study that elaborates relevant care issues and a critique of a research publication that explores a related topic. Tables, figures and practice tips have been used extensively throughout each chapter to identify areas of care that are particularly pertinent for readers. Each chapter also has specific learning activities and model responses to these questions to further support learning can be found online. It is not our intention that readers progress sequentially through the book, but rather explore chapters or sections that are relevant for different episodes of learning or practice.

The delivery of effective, high-quality critical care nursing practice is a challenge in contemporary health care. We trust that this book will be a valuable resource in supporting your care of critically ill patients and their loved ones.

Leanne **Aitken**
Andrea **Marshall**
Wendy **Chaboyer**

About the
Australian College of Critical Care Nurses (ACCCN)

The Australian College of Critical Care Nurses, with over 2400 members, is the peak professional organisation representing critical care nurses in Australia. Membership types include standard members, international members, associate members, life members, honorary members and corporate members. All individual members are eligible and are encouraged to participate in the activities of the College and receive the College journal and *Critical Times* publication, in addition to discounts for ACCCN conference registration and for ACCCN publications. Life and honorary memberships are awarded to individuals in recognition of their outstanding contribution to ACCCN and/or to critical care nursing excellence in Australia.

ACCCN is a company limited by guarantee and has branches in each state of Australia, with two members from each state branch management committee forming the ACCCN National Board of Directors. Each committee facilitates the activities of the College at a local/state level and provides local and, at times, national representation. The ACCCN Editorial Committee and Editorial Board, under the leadership of the editor of the *Australian Critical Care (ACC)* journal, are responsible for College publications including the journal *Australian Critical Care* and the digital newspaper *Critical Times*.

There are a number of national advisory panels and special interest groups dedicated to providing the organisation with expert opinion on issues relating to critical care nursing. These include:

Resuscitation Advisory Panel, which consists of 12 members representing each branch of the ACCCN, plus a paediatric nurse representative. It has developed a complete suite of contemporary advanced life support and resuscitation educational materials and offers its ACCCN National ALS Courses throughout Australia

Research Advisory Panel which, in addition to providing expert advice to ACCCN, is responsible for evaluating and making recommendations on research strategy and grant submissions to ACCCN, and for evaluating abstracts submitted to the ANZICS/ACCCN Annual Scientific Meeting on Intensive Care

Education Advisory Panel, which advises ACCCN on all matters relating to education specific to critical care nursing. This panel has developed a position paper on critical care nursing education and written submissions on behalf of ACCCN to national reviews of nursing education

Workforce Advisory Panel, which has represented ACCCN on a number of national health workforce and nursing committees. The panel has also developed position statements on nurse staffing for intensive care and high-dependency units in Australia, and annually reviews the dataset design for national workforce data collection in conjunction with ANZICS

Organ and Tissue Donation and Transplantation Advisory Panel, which advises the board and developed a position statement on organ donation and transplantation as it relates to intensive care. It disseminates related information to critical care nurses regarding the promotion and national reform objectives of organ and tissue donation in Australia

Quality Advisory Panel, which provides expert knowledge, advice and information to ACCCN on matters relevant to critical care nursing practice relating specifically to patient management

Paediatric Advisory Panel, which provides expert knowledge, advice and information to ACCCN on matters relevant to paediatric critical care nursing in addition to recommending content and speakers for the annual ACCCN conferences

The ICU Liaison Special Interest Group, which is a collective group of ACCCN members who have an interest in ICU liaison/outreach and work together to discuss matters relevant to this area of increasing critical care nursing focus.

In addition to branch educational events and symposiums, ACCCN conducts three national conferences each year: ACCCN Institute of Continuing Education (ICE) and, in conjunction with our medical colleagues from The Australian and New Zealand Intensive Care

Society (ANZICS), the ANZICS/ACCCN Annual Scientific Meeting on Intensive Care and the Australian and New Zealand Paediatric and Neonatal Intensive Care Conference.

ACCCN has a representative on the Australian Resuscitation Council (ARC), and has representation at a federal government advisory level through the Nursing and Midwifery Stakeholder Reference Group (NMSRG) chaired by the Chief Nurse of Australia, and is also a member of the Coalition of National Nursing Organisations (CoNNO). The founding Chairperson of the World Federation of Critical Care Nurses (WFCCN) continues to represent ACCCN on the WFCCN Council, and the College also has representatives on the World Federation of Paediatric Intensive and Critical Care Societies, and is a member of the Intensive Care Foundation.

More information can be found on the ACCCN website: www.acccn.com.au.

About the editors

Leanne Aitken is Professor of Critical Care Nursing at Griffith University and Princess Alexandra Hospital, Queensland, Australia, and also Professor of Nursing at City University London, United Kingdom. She has had a long career in critical care nursing, including practice, education and research roles. In all her roles, Leanne has been inspired by a sense of enquiry, pride in the value of expert nursing and a belief that improvement in practice and resultant patient outcomes is always possible. Research interests include developing and refining interventions to improve long-term recovery of critically ill and injured patients, decision-making practices of critical care nurses and a range of clinical practice issues within critical care and trauma.

Leanne has been active in ACCCN for more than 25 years and was made a Life Member of the College in 2006 after having held positions on state and national boards, coordinated the Advanced Life Support course in Western Australia in its early years, chaired the Education Advisory Panel and been an Associate Editor with *Australian Critical Care*. In addition, she is a peer reviewer for a number of national and international journals and reviews grant applications for a range of organisations within Australia and overseas; she was the immediate past Co-Chair of the Scientific Review Committee of the Intensive Care Foundation. Leanne is an Ambassador for the World Federation of Critical Care Nurses and is the representative on a number of sepsis-related working groups including an international group that authored a companion paper to the Surviving Sepsis Campaign guidelines to summarise the evidence underpinning nursing care of the septic patient, the revision of the Surviving Sepsis Campaign guidelines and the Global Sepsis Alliance.

Andrea Marshall is Professor of Acute and Complex Care Nursing at Griffith University and Gold Coast Health, Queensland. She has been working in critical care as a clinician, educator and researcher for more than two decades. Andrea has a strong interdisciplinary focus on research and in particular how the best evidence is translated into clinical practice to optimise outcomes for critically ill patients and their families. As a previous NHMRC Translating Research into Practice (TRIP) Fellow, she is strongly committed to developing and testing strategies for the effective implementation of research into clinical practice. Her program of research also focuses on improving nutrition delivery to acute and critically ill patients during hospitalisation and following discharge.

Andrea has been Editor with *Australian Critical Care* since 2003. She is an active member of the Australian College of Critical Care Nurses and has previously held executive positions with the New South Wales Branch of the College as well as being a longstanding member of both the Education Advisory and Research Advisory Panels. In 2014 her contribution to the College was recognised with Life Membership. She is an active reviewer for several funding bodies including the NHMRC and Intensive Care Foundation and contributes to the peer review process for over 10 international journals, many of which have an interdisciplinary focus.

Wendy Chaboyer is Professor of Nursing at Griffith University and the Director of the Centre of Research Excellence in Nursing Interventions for Hospitalised Patients, funded by the National Health and Medical Research Council (NHMRC) (2010–2015). Wendy has 30 years of experience in the critical care area, as a clinician, educator and researcher, and she is passionate about the contribution nurses can make to the hospital experience for patients and their families. Her early research examined ICU patients' experiences and the role nurses can play to assist in their transition from ICU to the ward. She has subsequently focused on patient safety, undertaking research into adverse events after ICU, clinical handover and 'transforming care at the bedside'. Three recent areas of work have been in relation to patient participation in care, pressure injury (ulcer) prevention and surgical dressings to prevent surgical site infections.

Wendy has been active in ACCCN since her arrival in Australia in the early 1990s and was awarded Life Membership in 2006. She has been a National Board member and member of the Queensland Branch Management Committee. Wendy is a past Chair of the Research Advisory Panel and past Chair of the Quality Advisory Panel of the ACCCN. She played a role in the formation of the World Federation of Critical Care Nurses and continues to support their activities. Wendy reviews for a number of journals and funding bodies such as the NHMRC and the Australian Research Council.

List of contributors

Leanne Aitken RN, PhD, BHSc(Nurs)Hons, GCertMgt, GDipScMed(ClinEpi), FACCCN, FACN, FAAN, Life Member – ACCCN
Professor of Critical Care Nursing, School of Nursing and Midwifery and NHMRC Centre of Research Excellence in Nursing (NCREN), Menzies Health Institute Queensland, Griffith University, Qld, Australia
Intensive Care Unit, Princess Alexandra Hospital, Qld, Australia
Professor of Nursing, School of Health Sciences, City University London, UK

Robyn Aitken RN, Cert Anaes/Rec, BEdSt, MEdSt, PhD
Acting Chief Nursing and Midwifery Officer, Northern Territory Department of Health, NT, Australia
Professorial Fellow, Charles Darwin University, NT, and Flinders University, SA, Australia

Ian Baldwin RN, PhD
Clinical Educator Intensive Care Unit and Adjunct Professor, RMIT and Deakin University, Vic, Australia
Clinical Educator, Austin Health, Vic, Australia

Catherine Bell RN, MN (Crit Care)
Intensive Care Clinical Nurse Consultant – Trauma, Alfred Hospital, Vic, Australia

Bronagh Blackwood RGN, RNT, PhD
Senior Lecturer, School of Medicine, Dentistry and Biomedical Sciences, Queen's University, Belfast, Northern Ireland, UK

Tom Buckley RN, BHSc(Hons), MN (Research), GCertHPol, Cert ICU, PhD
Coordinator Master of Nursing (Clinical Nursing & Nurse Practitioner)/Senior Lecturer, Sydney Nursing School, The University of Sydney, NSW, Australia

Rand Butcher RN, MClinSc (Intensive Care Nursing), GradDipN (Nurse Education), BHlthSci (Nursing)
Critical Care Clinical Nurse Consultant, Northern New South Wales Local Health District
Adjunct Lecturer, School of Nursing and Midwifery, Griffith University, Qld, Australia

Wendy Chaboyer RN, PhD, MN, BSc(Nu)Hons, Crit Care Cert, FACCCN, Life Member – ACCCN
Professor and Director, NHMRC Centre of Research Excellence in Nursing (NCREN), Menzies Health Institute Queensland, Griffith University, Qld, Australia
Professor, Institute of Health and Care Sciences, University of Gothenburg, Sweden

Diane Chamberlain RN, BNBSc, MN(Critical Care), MPH, PhD
Senior Lecturer, Flinders University, SA, Australia
National President – ACCCN

Maureen Coombs RN, PhD, MBE
Professor in Clinical Nursing (Critical Care), Graduate School of Nursing Midwifery and Health, Victoria University of Wellington, New Zealand
Capital and Coast District Health Board, Wellington, New Zealand

Karena Conroy BSocSci(Hons), PhD
Researcher, Intensive Care Co-ordination & Monitoring Unit, Agency for Clinical Innovation, NSW, Australia
Honorary Associate, Faculty of Health, University of Technology, Sydney, NSW, Australia

Fiona Coyer RN, PGCEA, MSc Nursing, PhD
Professor of Nursing, Queensland University of Technology and Metro North Hospital and Health Service, Qld, Australia

Julia Crilly RN, MEmergN (Hons), PhD
Associate Professor, Emergency Care, Griffith University, and Gold Coast Hospital and Health Service, Qld, Australia

Judy Currey RN, BN, BN(Hons), CritCareCert, GCertHE, GCertSc(App Stats), PhD
Associate Professor in Nursing, Director of Postgraduate Studies, Deakin University, Vic, Australia

Jennifer Dennett RN, MN, BAppSc (Nursing), CritCareCert, Dip Management, MRCNA
Nurse Unit Manager, Critical Care, Oncology, Cardiology, Renal Dialysis, Central Gippsland Health Service, Vic, Australia

Malcolm James Dennis RN, CritCareCert, BEd, IBHRE-CCDS
Technical Field Expert, Cardiac Rhythm Management Division, St Jude Medical, Vic, Australia

Andrea Driscoll NP, CCC, MEd, MN, PhD, FAHA, FCSANZ, FACNP
Associate Professor, School of Nursing and Midwifery, Faculty of Health, Deakin University, Vic, Australia
Heart Foundation Fellow

Trudy Dwyer RN, Nurs Cert, BHScN, ICU Cert, GD FlexLng, MClincEd, PhD
Associate Professor, Central Queensland University, Qld, Australia

Rosalind Elliott RN, PhD
Lecturer, Faculty of Health, University of Technology, Sydney, NSW, Australia

Paula Foran RN, PhD, Master Professional Education &Training, Grad Dip Adult Education & Training, Cert Anaesthesia & Post Anaesthesia Nursing
Honorary Conjoint Senior Clinical Lecturer, School of Nursing and Midwifery, Deakin University, and South West Healthcare, Vic, Australia

Deborah Friel BHSc, GC CritCare, GC ClinNr, GC Mmnt, GCTE
Lecturer, School of Nursing and Midwifery, Central Queensland University, Qld, Australia

Robyn Gallagher RN, MN, BA, PhD
Professor of Nursing, Charles Perkins Centre, Sydney Nursing School, The University of Sydney, NSW, Australia

David Glanville RN, BNsg, GDipNsg(CritCare), MN
Nurse Educator (Critical Care), Epworth Freemasons Hospital, Vic, Australia

Christopher J Gordon RN, BN, MExSc, PhD
Senior Lecturer, Sydney Nursing School, The University of Sydney, NSW, Australia

Sher Michael Graan RN, BHS-Nursing, Post Grad Dip Crit Care, MN
Clinical Instructor, King Faisal Specialist Hospital and Research Center (Magnet Accredited), Saudi Arabia

Bernadette Grealy RN, RM, GradCertCritCare, DipAScN, BN, MN, Life Member – ACCCN
Nursing Director, Intensive Care Services & Hyperbaric Medicine, Central Adelaide Local Health Network, SA, Australia

Carol Grech RN, PhD
Head, School of Nursing and Midwifery, University of South Australia, SA, Australia

Melanie Greenwood MN, Graduate Certificate in UniLearn & Teach, Intensive Care Cert, Neuroscience Cert
Senior Lecturer, School of Health Sciences, University of Tasmania, Tas, Australia

Janice Gullick RN, PhD, MArt, BFA, Cardiothoracic Cert, FACN
Director, Postgraduate Advanced Studies, and Coordinator, Master of Intensive Care & Emergency Nursing, Sydney Nursing School, The University of Sydney, NSW, Australia

Denise Harris RN, BHSc(Nurs), GradDipHlthAdmin&InfoSys, MN(Res), ICCert
Assistant Director of Clinical Services – Cardiac Services & Critical Care, Pindara Private Hospital, Qld, Australia

Ian Jacobs RN, PhD, BAppSc, DipEd, FCNA, FANZCP, FERC, FAHA
Clinical Services Director, St John Ambulance (Western Australia)
Professor of Resuscitation and Pre-Hospital Care and Director, Prehospital Resuscitation & Emergency Care Research Unit, Curtin University, WA, Australia

David Johnson RN, Grad Dip (Acute Care Nurs), MHealth Sci Ed, A&E Cert, MCN
Director of Nursing, Caloundra Health Service, Sunshine Coast Hospital and Health Service, Queensland Health, Qld, Australia

Alison Juers RN, BN (Dist), MN (Crit Care)
Intensive Care Nurse Educator, Brisbane Private Hospital, Qld, Australia

Tina Kendrick RN, PIC Cert, BNurs (Hons), MNurs, FACCN, FACN
Clinical Nurse Consultant – Paediatrics
Newborn and Paediatric Emergency Transport Service (NETS), NSW, Australia

Emma Kingwell RN, RM BSc, GradCert CritCare Nsg, PGDip (Mid), MPhil (Nsg and Mid)
Nurse and Midwifery Educator, King Edward Hospital for Women, WA, Australia

Ruth Kleinpell RN, PhD, FAAN, FCCM
Director, Center for Clinical Research and Scholarship, Rush University Medical Center, and Professor, Rush University College of Nursing, Chicago, IL, USA

Leila Kuzmiuk RN, BN CPIT, DipAdvClinNursing, MN, Grad Cert Hlth ServMgt
Nurse Educator, Intensive Care Services, John Hunter Hospital, New England Health, NSW, Australia

Gavin D Leslie RN, PhD, BAppSc, Post Grad Dip (Clin Nurs) FCNA, FACCCN
Professor, Critical Care Nursing, School of Nursing, Midwifery & Paramedicine, Curtin University, WA, Australia

Frances Lin RN, BMN, MN(Hons), PhD
Senior Lecturer, School of Nursing and Midwifery, Griffith University, Qld, Australia

Andrea Marshall RN, PhD, MN(Research), BN, Grad Cert Ed Studies (Higher Ed), IC Cert, FACCCN, FACN, Life Member – ACCCN
Professor of Acute and Complex Care Nursing, School of Nursing and Midwifery and NHMRC Centre of Research Excellence in Nursing (NCREN), Menzies Health Institute Queensland, Griffith University, Qld, Australia
Intensive Care Unit, Gold Coast Hospital and Health Service, Qld, Australia

Elaine McGloin Cert Crit Care
Clinical Nurse Consultant, Intensive Care Services, Royal
Prince Alfred Hospital, NSW, Australia

Marion Mitchell RN, Grad Cert (Higher Ed), PhD,
FACCN, Centaur Fellow
Associate Professor Critical Care, School of Nursing and
Midwifery, Menzies Health Institute Queensland, Griffith
University, Qld, Australia
Princess Alexandra Hospital, Qld, Australia

Margherita Murgo BN, MN(Crit Care), Dip Project Mgt
Project Officer (Delegation and Escalation Project),
Clinical Excellence Commission, NSW, Australia

Wendy Pollock RN, RM, GCALL, Grad Dip Crit Care
Nsg, Grad Dip Ed, PhD
Director, Maternal Critical Care, and Honorary Senior
Fellow, The University of Melbourne, Vic, Australia
Honorary Research Fellow, La Trobe University, Vic,
Australia

Anne-Sylvie Ramelet RN, PhD, RSCN, ICU Cert
Professor of Nursing and Director, Institute of Higher
Education and Research in Healthcare, University of
Lausanne, Switzerland

Janice Rattray MN, PhD, DipN, RGN, SCM
Reader in Acute and Critical Care Nursing, School of
Nursing and Health Sciences, University of Dundee,
Scotland, UK

Mona Ringdal RN, MN, PhD
Senior Lecturer, Director of Postgraduate Nursing
and Master Programme, Institute of Health and
Care Sciences, Sahlgrenska Academy, University of
Gothenburg, Sweden

Louise Rose BN, ICU Cert, Adult Ed Cert, MN, PhD
TD Nursing Professor in Critical Care Research,
Sunnybrook Health Sciences Centre
Associate Professor, Lawrence S. Bloomberg Faculty of
Nursing, University of Toronto, Canada
Adjunct Scientist, Institute for Clinical Evaluative Sciences
CIHR New Investigator
Director of Research, Provincial Centre of Weaning
Excellence, Toronto East General Hospital
Adjunct Scientist, Mount Sinai Hospital, Li Ka Shing
Institute, St Michael's Hospital, West Park Healthcare Centre

Kerstin Prignitz Sluys PhD, APRN
Associate Professor, Red Cross University College,
Affiliated Researcher, Karolinska Institutet, Stockholm,
Sweden

Ged Williams RN, RM, Crit Care Cert, MHA, LLM,
FACHSM, FACN, FAAN
Nursing and Allied Health Consultant, Abu Dhabi Health
Service, United Arab Emirates
Founding President, World Federation of Critical Care
Nurses

Teresa Williams RN, ICU Cert, BNurs, MHlthSci(Res),
GDClinEpi, PhD
Senior Research Fellow, Prehospital Resuscitation and
Emergency Care, School of Nursing Midwifery and
Paramedicine, Curtin University, WA, Australia

Denise Wilson RN, PhD, FCNA(NZ)
Professor of Māori Health, Auckland University of
Technology, New Zealand

Sharon M Wetzig BN, Grad Cert Nsg (Crit Care), MEd
Education Consultant, Carramar Education, Qld, Australia

List of reviewers

Jan Alderman RN, BNs, Grad Dip Anaesthetics and Recovery Nursing, Masters/PhD candidate in Clinical Science
Course Co-ordinator, Lecturer, School of Nursing, University of Adelaide, SA, Australia

Sally Bristow RN, BN, Grad Dip Mid, RM, MN
Nursing Academic, University of New England, NSW, Australia

Elyse Coffey BNurs, GDipNur(periop), MNurs
Associate Lecturer, Deakin University, Vic, Australia
Clinical Nurse Specialist, Alfred Hospital, Vic, Australia

Rachel Cross RN, BN, GradCertEmergNurse, MNP
Lecturer Practitioner, La Trobe University School of Nursing and Midwifery/Emergency and Trauma Centre, Alfred Hospital, Vic, Australia

Lori Delaney RN, B Nurs, GC Ed, GDCC, MN, JBICF
Assistant Professor in Clinical Nursing, University of Canberra, ACT, Australia
PhD scholar, College of Medicine, Australia National University, ACT, Australia

Janice Elliott RN, BNsg, Grad Dip (Emerge Nursing), Master of Nursing Science
Registered Nurse, Royal Adelaide Hospital Emergency Department, SA, Australia
Clinical Title Holder, School of Nursing, University of Adelaide, SA, Australia

Beverley Ewens RN, BSc(Hons), PG Dip Critical Care, PhD candidate
Lecturer, School of Nursing and Midwifery, Edith Cowan University, WA, Australia

Steven A Frost RN, ICU Cert, MPH, PhD
Lecturer, Intensive Care, Liverpool Hospital and University of Western Sydney, NSW, Australia

Emily Susannah Kavanagh BN, GradCert Crit Care
Donation Specialist Nurse, Tamworth Rural Referral Hospital, NSW, Australia

Elizabeth Kraft RN, BN, GradDip (Anaes & Rec), MN, MACN
Clinical Service Coordinator, Day Surgery Unit/Surgical Admission Suite/Day Surgery Overnight, Royal Adelaide Hospital, SA, Australia

Renee McGill RN, MN (Education), Grad Cert Crit Care, BSci (Nurs)
Simulation Lead, Lecturer in Nursing, School of Nursing, Midwifery and Indigenous Health, Faculty of Science, Charles Sturt University, NSW, Australia

Gayle McKenzie RN, MEd, GradDip AdvNsg Crit Care, GradCert AdvNsg Clin Ed, BSocSc
Lecturer in Acute Nursing, La Trobe University, Alfred Clinical School, Vic, Australia

Stephen McNally RN(Emergency), PhD
Director of Academic Programs (Undergraduate), University of Western Sydney, NSW, Australia

Claire Minton RN, MN, PhD candidate
Lecturer, School of Nursing, Massey University, New Zealand

Jonathan Mould RN, PhD
Lecturer, School of Nursing and Midwifery, Curtin University, WA, Australia

Holly Northam RN, RM, Masters of Crit Care Nurs, MACN, Churchill Fellow
Assistant Professor in Critical Care Nursing, University of Canberra, ACT, Australia

Darrin Penola RN, MN (Crit Care)
Clinical Nurse Consultant, Thoracic Medicine, St Vincent's Hospital, NSW, Australia

Ron Picard RN, MHSc, CCN
Nursing Lecturer, La Trobe Rural Health School, Vic, Australia

Natashia Scully BA, BN GradCertTertiaryEd, PostGradDipNSc, MPH, MACN
Lecturer in Nursing, University of New England, NSW, Australia

Peita Sims RN, BAppSc (HealthProm), BNurs, Grad Dip (Crit Care)
ICU Liaison Nurse, Epworth Healthcare, Vic, Australia

Kerry Southerland RN, ICU cert, BAppSc (Nursing), MClinNurs (Crit Care), GradCertTertTeach
Lecturer, School of Nursing & Midwifery, Curtin University, WA, Australia

Jane Zeng CNE, ADNP
Post Graduate Subject Coordinator, University of Melbourne, Vic, Australia
Clinical Nurse Educator – ICU, Western Health, Vic, Australia

Acknowledgements

A project of this nature and scope requires many talented and committed people to see it to completion. The decision to publish this third edition was supported enthusiastically by the Board of the Australian College of Critical Care Nurses (ACCCN) and Elsevier Australia. To our chapter contributors for this edition, both those returning from the previous editions and our new collaborators – thank you for accepting our offer to write, for having the courage and confidence in yourselves and us to be involved in the text and for being committed in meeting writing deadlines while developing the depth and quality of content that we had planned. We also acknowledge the work of chapter contributors from our previous editions – Harriet Adamson, Susan Bailey, Julie Benbenishty, Martin Boyle, Wendy Corkhill, Sidney Cuthbertson, Suzana Dimovski, Bruce Dowd, Ruth Endacott, Claire Fitzpatrick, Paul Fulbrook, Gabrielle Hanlon, Michelle Kelly, Bridie Kent, Anne Morrison, Maria Murphy, Louise Niggemeyer, Amanda Rischbieth, Wendy Swope, Paul Thurman, Jane Treloggen and Vicki Wade.

The Editors would like to specifically acknowledge the contribution of Professor Ian Jacobs, who co-authored Chapter 25, *Resuscitation*, prior to his unexpected death. Ian was an internationally renowned specialist in resuscitation and prehospital care and has made a sustained contribution to teaching, research and policy in the field. One of his earliest associations with ACCCN was as convenor of the Advanced Life Support course in Western Australia in the early 1990s. Ian was the Chairperson of the Australian Resuscitation Council and Co-Chair of the International Liaison Committee on Resuscitation.

Continued encouragement and support from the Board and members of ACCCN, for having the belief in us as editors and authors to uphold the values of the College, is much appreciated. We also acknowledge support from the staff at Elsevier Australia, our publishing partner. Thanks to our Senior Content Strategist, Libby Houston, for guiding this major project; our Content Development Specialist, Martina Vascotto; and to Linda Littlemore, our editor. In Publishing Services, Devendran Kannan, thanks for your work with production. To others who produced the high quality figures, developed and executed the marketing plan and undertook myriad other activities, without which a text such as this would never come to fruition, thank you. We acknowledge our external reviewers who devoted their time to provide insightful suggestions in improving the text and contributed to the quality of the finished product.

To Doug Elliott, thank you for your original vision for this text, for having the courage and commitment to make it happen and for your support, albeit from a distance, for continuing the journey.

Finally, and most importantly, to our respective loved ones – Steve; David, Abi and Hannah; and Michael – thanks for your belief in us, and your understanding and commitment in supporting our careers.

Leanne **Aitken**
Andrea **Marshall**
Wendy **Chaboyer**

Detailed contents

Abbreviations

AACN	American Association of Critical-Care Nurses
ABG	arterial blood gas
A/C	assist control ventilation
ACCCN	Australian College of Critical Care Nurses
ACCESS	assistance, coordination, contingency, education, supervision, support
ACEI	angiotensin-converting enzyme inhibitor
ACh	acetylcholine
ACS	acute coronary syndrome
ACT	activated clotting time
ADAPT	Australasian Donation Awareness Program
ADL	activities of daily living
AED	automatic external defibrillator
AF	atrial fibrillation
AFE	amniotic fluid embolism
AIVR	accelerated idioventricular rhythm
AKI	acute kidney injury
ALF	acute liver failure
ALI	acute lung injury
ALS	advanced life support
ALT	alanine amino transferase
AMI	acute myocardial infarction
ANP	atrial natriuretic peptide
ANS	autonomic nervous system
ANZBA	Australia and New Zealand Burns Association
ANZICS	Australian and New Zealand Intensive Care Society
AoCLF	acute on chronic liver failure
APACHE	Acute Physiology And Chronic Health Evaluation (score)
APC	activated protein C
APH	antepartum haemorrhage
APRV	airway pressure release ventilation
APTT	activated partial thromboplastin time
ARC	Australian Resuscitation Council
ARDS	adult respiratory distress syndrome
ARB	angiotensin receptor blocker
ARF	acute renal failure
aSAH	aneurysmal subarachnoid haemorrhage
AST	aspartate aminotransferase
ATN	acute tubular necrosis
ATP	adenosine triphosphate
ATP	anti-tachycardia pacing
ATS	Australasian Triage Scale
AV	arteriovenous
AV	atrioventricular
AV	atrioventricular node

AVNRT	atrioventricular nodal reentry tachycardia
BACCN	British Association of Critical Care Nurses
BBB	blood–brain barrier
BE	base excess
BiPAP	bi-phasic positive airways pressure
BLS	basic life support
BMI	body mass index
BNP	B-type natriuretic peptide
BP	blood pressure
BPS	Behavioural Pain Scale
BSLTx	bilateral sequential lung transplantation
BTF	Brain Trauma Foundation
CABG	coronary artery bypass graft
CAM-ICU	Confusion Assessment Method for the Intensive Care Unit
CAP	community acquired pneumonia
CAUTI	catheter-associated urinary tract infection
CAV	cardiac allograph vasculopathy
CAVH	continuous arteriovenous haemofiltration
CBF	cerebral blood flow
CRRT	continuous renal replacement therapy
CCU	coronary/cardiac care unit
CHD	coronary heart disease
CHF	chronic heart failure
CI	cardiac index
CIM	critical illness myopathy
CINM	critical illness neuromyopathy
CIP	critical illness polyneuropathy
CLAB	central line-associated bacteraemia
CLABSI	central line associated blood stream infection
CMV	cytomegalovirus
CNC	clinical nurse consultant
CNE	clinical nurse educator
CNM	clinical nurse manager
CNS	central nervous system
CO	cardiac output
CO_2	carbon dioxide
COPD	chronic obstructive pulmonary disease
COPE	Committee of Publication Ethics
CPAP	continuous positive airway pressure
CPB	cardiopulmonary bypass
CPG	clinical practice guidelines
CPOE	computerised provider order entry
CPOT	Critical-care Pain Observation Tool
CPP	cerebral perfusion pressure
CPR	cardiopulmonary resuscitation
CRT	cardiac resynchronisation therapy
CSF	cerebral spinal fluid
CT	computerised tomography

CTAS	Canadian Triage and Acuity Scale	**H$^+$**	hydrogen ion
CTG	cardiotocograph	**H$_2$CO$_3$**	carbonic acid
CVAD	central venous access device	**H$_2$RA**	histamine 2 receptor antagonist
CVC	central venous catheter	**HADS**	Hospital Anxiety and Depression Scale
CVP	central venous pressure	**HAI**	hospital-acquired infection
CVR	cerebrovascular resistance	**Hb**	haemoglobin
CVVH	continuous venovenous haemofiltration	**HCM**	hypertrophic cardiomyopathy
CVVHDf	continuous venovenous haemodiafiltration	**HCO$_3^-$**	bicarbonate ion
CX	circumflex coronary artery	**HD**	haemodialysis
CXR	chest X-ray	**HDU**	high dependency unit
DCD	donation after cardiac death	**HELLP**	haemolysis, elevated liver enzymes and low platelets
DCM	dilated cardiomyopathy		
DCS	damage-control surgery	**HFO**	high flow oxygen
DIC	disseminated intravascular coagulation	**HFOV**	high frequency oscillation ventilation
DKA	diabetic ketoacidosis	**HFpEF**	heart failure with preserved ejection fraction
DNA	deoxyribonucleic acid		
DNAR	do not attempt resuscitation	**HFrEF**	heart failure with reduced ejection fraction
DPL	diagnostic peritoneal lavage	**HHS**	hyperosmolar hyperglycaemic state
DTS	Davidson Trauma Scale	**Hib**	*Haemophilus influenzae* type b
DVT	deep vein thrombosis	**HIV**	human immunodeficiency virus
EBN	evidence-based nursing	**HLA**	human leukocyte antigen
EC	extracorporeal circuit	**HME**	heat and moisture exchanger
ECG	electrocardiography	**HR**	heart rate
ECMO	extracorporeal membrane oxygenation	**HRC**	Health Research Council
ED	emergency department	**HRECs**	Human Research Ethics Committees
EEG	electroencephalogram/ electroencephalography	**HRQOL**	health related quality of life
		HRS	hepatorenal syndrome
EGDT	early goal-directed therapy	**HSV**	herpes simplex virus
EMSB	early management of severe burns	**IABP**	intra-aortic balloon pump
EN	enteral nutrition	**IAH**	intra-abdominal hypertension
EPAP	expiratory positive airway pressure	**IAP**	intra-abdominal pressure
EPUAP	European Pressure Ulcer Advisory Panel	**ICC**	intercostal catheter
ESI	emergency severity index	**ICD**	implantable cardioverter defibrillator
ET	endothelin	**ICDSC**	Intensive Care Delirium Screening Checklist
ETCO$_2$	end-tidal carbon dioxide	**ICH**	intracerebral haemorrhage
ETT	endotracheal tube	**ICN**	International Council of Nurses
EVD	external ventricular drain	**ICP**	intracranial pressure
EVLW	extravascular lung water	**ICS**	Intensive Care Society (UK)
EVLWI	extravascular lung water index	**ICU**	intensive care unit
F	frequency	**ICU-AW**	intensive care unit acquired weakness
FAST	focused assessment with sonography in trauma	**I:E**	inspiratory/expiratory ratio
		IES	Impact of Event Scale
FBC	full blood count	**IL**	interleukin
FES	fat embolism syndrome	**ILCOR**	International Liaison Committee on Resuscitation
FiO$_2$	fraction of inspired oxygen		
FOUR	Full Outline of Unresponsiveness scale	**IM**	intramuscular
FTE	full time equivalent (staff)	**IMA**	internal mammary artery
f/V$_T$	frequency/tidal volume	**INR**	international normalised ratio
GABA	gamma-aminobutyric acid	**IPAP**	inspiratory positive airway pressure
GBS	Guillain–Barré syndrome	**ITBV**	intrathoracic blood volume
GCS	Glasgow Coma Scale	**ITBVI**	intrathoracic blood volume index
GEDV	global end-diastolic volume	**IV**	intravenous
GEDVI	global end-diastolic volume index	**IVC**	inferior vena cava
GFR	glomerular filtration rate	**JVP**	jugular venous pressure
GTN	glyceryl trinitrate	**kPa**	kilopascals

LAD	left anterior descending
LAP	left atrial pressure
LBBB	left bundle branch block
LMA	laryngeal mask airway
LOS	length of stay
LV	left ventricle
LVAD	left ventricular assist device
LVEDV	left ventricular end-diastolic volume (preload)
LVEF	left ventricular ejection fraction
LVF	left ventricular failure
LVSWI	left ventricular stroke work index
MAP	mean arterial pressure
MEDSAFE	Medical Devices Safety Authority (New Zealand)
MELD	model of end-stage liver disease
MERS-CoV	Middle East respiratory syndrome coronavirus
MET	medical emergency team
MI	myocardial infarction
MIDCABG	minimally invasive direct coronary artery bypass grafting
MMSE	Mini-Mental Status Examination
MODS	multiple organ dysfunction syndrome
MRC	Medical Research Council
MRI	magnetic resonance imaging
MRO	multi-resistant organism
MRSA	methicillin-resistant *Staphylococcus aureus*
MTS	Manchester Triage Scale
MV	mechanical ventilation
NAS	Nursing Activities Score
NEMS	Nine Equivalents of nursing Manpower use Score
NETS	newborn emergency transfer service
NEXUS	National Emergency X-radiography Utilization Study
NFkB	nuclear factor kappa B
NHMRC	National Health and Medical Research Council
NHS	National Health Service (UK)
NICE	National Institute for Health and Care Excellence
NIPPV	non-invasive positive pressure ventilation
NIPSV	non-invasive pressure support ventilation
NIV	non-invasive ventilation
NO	nitric oxide
NOC	Nurses' Observation Checklist
NPC	nurse practice coordinator
NPUAP	National Pressure Ulcer Advisory Panel
NSAID	non-steroidal anti-inflammatory drug
NTS	non-technical skills
NUM	nursing unit manager
NUTRIC	NUTritional RIsk in the Critically ill score
NYHA	New York Heart Association
O_2	oxygen
OHCA	out-of-hospital cardiac arrest
OPCAB	off pump coronary artery bypass
ORIF	open reduction internal fixation
Pa	arterial pressure
P_A	alveolar pressure
PAC	pulmonary artery catheter
P_aCO_2	partial pressure of carbon dioxide in arterial blood
PACU	post-anaesthesia care unit
PaO_2	partial pressure of oxygen in arterial blood
PAP	pulmonary artery pressure
Paw	airway pressure
$PbtO_2$	brain tissue oxygenation
PCA	patient-controlled analgesia
PCI	percutaneous coronary intervention
PCP	phencyclidine
PCV	pressure controlled ventilation
PCWP	pulmonary capillary wedge pressure
PD	peritoneal dialysis
PDH	pulmonary dynamic hyperinflation
PE	pulmonary embolism
PEA	pulseless electrical activity
PEEP	positive end-expiratory pressure
PELD	paediatric end-stage liver disease
$PetCO_2$	partial pressure of end-tidal carbon dioxide
PGD	primary graft dysfunction
pH	acid–alkaline logarithmic scale
PI	pressure injury
PiCCO	pulse induced contour cardiac output
PICS	post-intensive care syndrome
PICU	paediatric intensive care unit
P_{insp}	inspiratory pressure
PN	parenteral nutrition
PNS	peripheral nervous system
PPE	personal protective equipment
PPH	postpartum haemorrhage
PPI	proton pump inhibitors
PR	pulse rate
pRIFLE	paediatric risk, injury, failure, loss and end-stage kidney disease criteria
PSG	polysomnography
PSV	pressure support ventilation
PT	prothrombin
PTA	post-traumatic amnesia
PTCA	percutaneous transluminal coronary angioplasty
PTSD	post-traumatic stress disorder
PTSS	post-traumatic stress symptoms
PTT	partial thromboplastin time
PV	per vagina
Pv	venous pressure
PVR	pulmonary vascular resistance
R	respiration
RAAS	renin–angiotensin–aldosterone system
RAP	right atrial pressure

RBANS	Repeatable Battery for the Assessment of Neuropsychological Status		**SpO$_2$**	saturation of oxygen in peripheral tissues
RBC	red blood cells		**STEMI**	ST-elevation myocardial infarction
RCA	right coronary artery		**SV**	stroke volume
RCM	restrictive cardiomyopathy		**SVG**	saphenous vein graft
RCSQ	Richards–Campbell Sleep Questionnaire		**SvO$_2$**	saturation of oxygen in venous system
RCT	randomised controlled trial		**SVR**	systemic vascular resistance
RDC	regional donor coordinator		**SVT**	supraventricular tachycardia
REE	resting energy expenditure		**SWS**	slow wave sleep
REM	rapid eye movement		**T$_3$**	triiodothyronine
RICA	right internal carotid artery		**TAD**	thoracic aortic dissection
ROSC	return of spontaneous circulation		**TBI**	traumatic brain injury
RR	respiratory rate		**TBSA**	total body surface area
RRS	rapid response system		**TEG**	thromboelastograph
RRT	renal replacement therapy		**TGA**	Therapeutic Goods Administration
RSV	respiratory syncytial virus		**TIMI**	thrombolysis in myocardial infarction
RV	right ventricular		**TIPS**	transjugular intrahepatic portosystemic shunt/stent
RVEDV	right ventricular end-diastolic volume		**TISS**	Therapeutic Intervention Scoring System
RVEDVI	right ventricular end-diastolic volume index		**TNFa**	tumour necrosis factor alpha
RVEF	right ventricular ejection fraction		**TOE**	transoesophageal echocardiography
RVF	right ventricular failure		**TSANZ**	Transplant Society of Australia and New Zealand
SA	sinoatrial node		**TST**	total sleep time
SAH	subarachnoid haemorrhage		**UO**	urine output
SaO$_2$	saturation of oxygen in arterial blood		**URTI**	upper respiratory tract infection
SAPS	Simplified Acute Physiology Score		**VAD**	ventricular assist device
SARS	severe acute respiratory syndrome		**VAE**	ventilator-associated event
SBP	systolic blood pressure		**VAP**	ventilator-associated pneumonia
SBT	spontaneous breathing trial		**VAS**	visual analogue scale
SCA	sudden cardiac arrest		**VATS**	video-assisted thoroscopic surgery
SCI	spinal cord injury		**VCV**	volume controlled ventilation
SCUF	slow continuous ultrafiltration		**VE**	expired minute volume
SE	status epilepticus		**VF**	ventricular fibrillation
SICQ	Sleep in Intensive Care Questionnaire		**V/Q**	ventilation/perfusion
SIMV	synchronised intermittent mandatory ventilation		**VRE**	vancomycin-resistant enterococci
SIRS	systemic inflammatory response syndrome		**V$_T$**	tidal volume
SjO$_2$	jugular venous oxygen saturation		**VT**	ventricular tachycardia
SLED	slow low efficiency dialysis		**VTE**	venous thromboembolism
SLTx	single lung transplantation		**WCC**	white cell count
SNS	sympathetic nervous system		**WFCCN**	World Federation of Critical Care Nurses
SOFA	sequential organ failure assessment		**WHO**	World Health Organization
SOMANZ	Society of Obstetric Medicine of Australia and New Zealand		**WPW**	Wolff–Parkinson–White (syndrome)

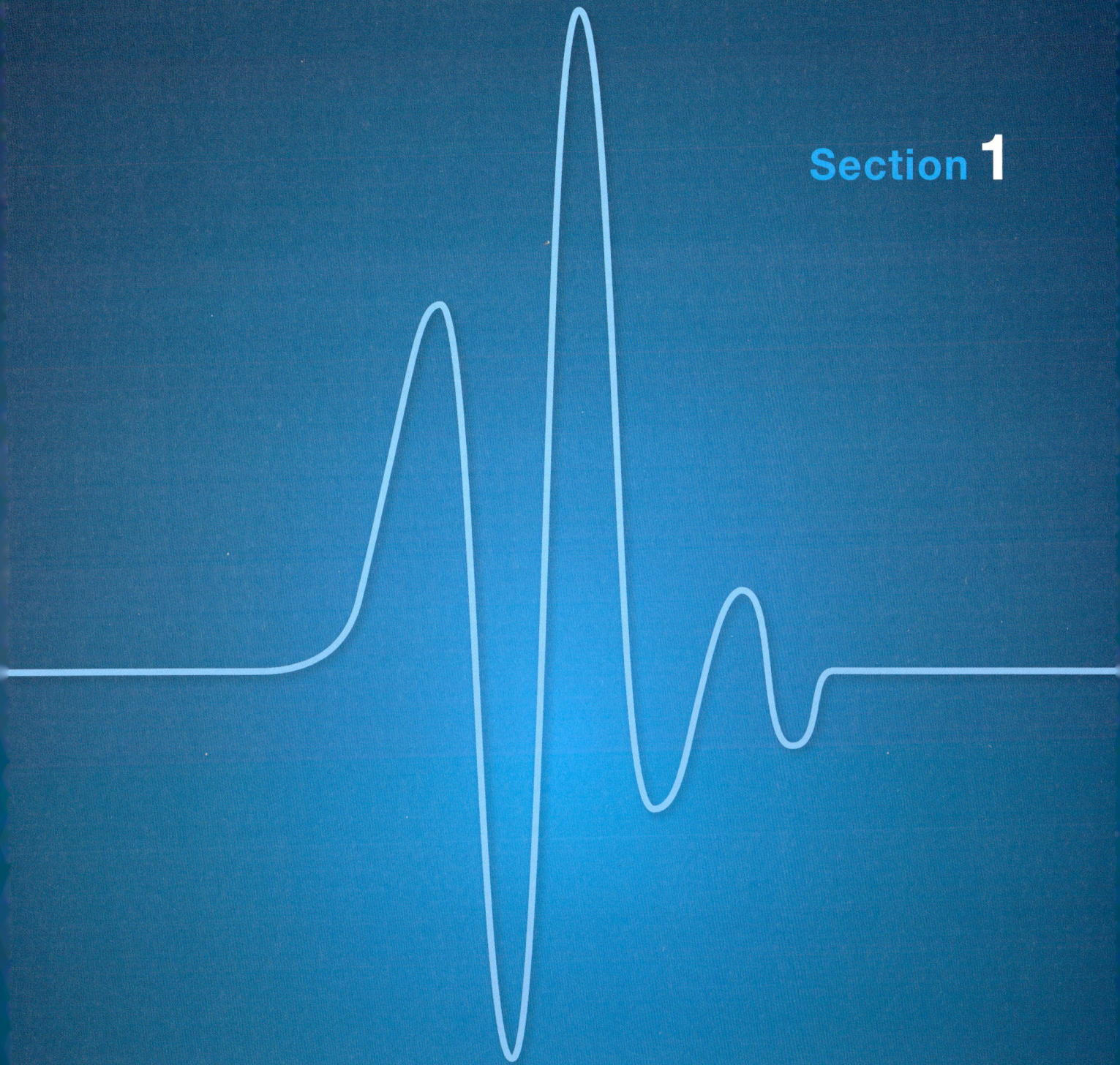

Scope of critical care

Chapter 1

Scope of critical care practice

Leanne Aitken, Wendy Chaboyer, Andrea Marshall

KEY WORDS

clinical leadership

critical care
nursing

roles of critical
care nurses

Learning objectives

After reading this chapter, you should be able to:

- describe the history and development of critical care nursing practice, education and professional activities

- discuss the influences on the development of critical care nursing as a discipline and the professional development of individual nurses

- outline the various roles available to nurses within critical care areas or in outreach services

- consider processes in the work and professional environment that are influenced by local leadership styles.

Introduction

For over 50 years critical care services have been supporting the sickest of patients and today they are available in most countries in the world.[1] Although the focus was originally at local, regional and national levels, there is now an imperative for a strong international focus for the delivery of critical care services. International collaborations are necessary for responding to events that result in a sudden increased need for critical care services, such as the recent influenza pandemic.[2]

There is unprecedented demand for critical care services globally. Increasing population sizes and extended life expectancies mean that the projected need for critical care beds will continue to increase.[3] In Australia and New Zealand, there are approximately 124,000 admissions to 141 general intensive care units (ICUs) per year; this includes 6000 patient readmissions during the same hospital episode.[4] Patients admitted to coronary care, paediatric or other specialty units not classified as a general ICU are not included in these figures, so the overall clinical activity for 'critical care' is much higher (e.g. there were also 10,000 paediatric admissions to PICUs).[4] Importantly, critical care treatment is a high-expense component of hospital care; one conservative estimate of the cost exceeded A$2600 per day, with more than two-thirds going to staff costs, one-fifth to clinical consumables and the rest to clinical support and capital expenditure.[5] In European countries a direct cost analysis suggests the costs per ICU day range from €1168 to €2025,[6] while in developing countries such as India the cost is substantially less (approximately US$200 per day)[7] although this continues to represent a substantial cost relative to the cost of living. The cost of critical care is, however, difficult to determine because there is no internationally agreed methodology, there is a wide variation in resource consumption by patients in different settings, and there are different models of care.[8,9]

This chapter provides a context for subsequent chapters, outlining some key principles and concepts for studying and practising nursing in a range of critical care areas. Development of the specialty is discussed, along with the professional development and evolving roles of critical care nurses in contemporary health care. The scope of critical care nursing is described including advanced practice roles and, specifically, the nurse practitioner role. Leadership, as it pertains to the practice and development of critical care nursing, is also reviewed.

Critical care nursing

Critical care as a specialty in nursing has developed over the last 30 years.[10,11] Importantly, the development of the specialty has occurred in concert with the development of intensive care medicine as a defined clinical specialty. Critical care nursing is defined by the World Federation of Critical Care Nurses as:

> Specialised nursing care of critically ill patients who have manifest or potential disturbances of vital organ functions. Critical care nursing means assisting, supporting and restoring the patient towards health, or to ease the patient's pain and to prepare them for a dignified death. The aim of critical care nursing is to establish a therapeutic relationship with patients and their relatives and to empower the individuals' physical, psychological, sociological, cultural and spiritual capabilities by preventive, curative and rehabilitative interventions.[12]

Critically ill patients are those at high risk of actual or potential life-threatening health problems.[13] Care of the critically ill can occur in a number of different locations in hospitals. Critical care is generally considered a broad term, incorporating subspecialty areas of emergency, coronary care, high-dependency, cardiothoracic, paediatric and general intensive care units.[14]

Development of the critical care body of knowledge

Critical care as a specialty emerged in the 1950s and 1960s in Australasia, North America, Europe and South Africa.[10,15–18] During these early stages, critical care consisted primarily of coronary care units for the care of cardiology patients, cardiothoracic units for the care of postoperative patients and general intensive care units for the care of patients with respiratory compromise. Later developments in renal, metabolic and neurological management led to the principles and context of critical care that exist today.

Development of critical care nursing was characterised by a number of features,[10] including:

- the development of a new, comprehensive partnership between nursing and medical clinicians
- the collective experience of a steep learning curve for nursing and medical staff
- the courage to work in an unfamiliar setting, caring for patients who are extremely sick – a role that required the development of higher levels of competence and practice
- a high demand for education specific to critical care practice, which was initially difficult to meet owing to the absence of experienced nurses in the specialty
- the development of technologies such as mechanical ventilators, cardiac monitors, pacemakers, defibrillators, dialysers, intra-aortic balloon pumps and cardiac assist devices, which prompted development of additional knowledge and skills.

There was also recognition that improving patient outcomes through optimal use of these technologies was linked to nurses' skills and staffing levels.[19] The role of adequately educated and experienced nurses in these units was recognised as essential from an early stage,[15] and led to the development of the nursing specialty of critical care. Although not initially accepted, nursing expertise, ability to observe patients and appropriate nursing intensity are now considered essential elements of critical care.[19,20]

As the practice of critical care nursing evolved, so did the associated areas of critical care nursing education and specialty professional organisations, of which there are at least 37 organisations across six continents.[21] The combination of adequate nurse staffing, observation of the patient and the expertise of nurses to consider the complete needs of patients and their families is essential to optimise the outcomes of critical care. As critical care continues to evolve, the challenge remains to combine excellence in nursing care with judicious use of technology to optimise patient and family outcomes.

Research

The development of a body of knowledge is a key characteristic of both professions[22] and specialties within professions. One criterion for a specialty identified over two decades ago by the International Council of Nurses (ICN)[23] is that it is based on a core body of nursing knowledge that is being continually expanded and refined by research. Importantly, the ICN acknowledges that mechanisms are needed to support, review and disseminate research.

Research is fundamental to the development of nursing knowledge and practice. Research is a systematic inquiry using structured methods to understand an issue, solve a problem or refine existing knowledge. Qualitative research involves in-depth examination of a phenomenon of interest, typically using interviews, observation or document analysis to build knowledge and enable depth of understanding. Qualitative data analysis is in narrative (text) form and involves some form of content or thematic analysis, with findings generally reported as narrative (where words rather than numbers describe the research findings). In contrast, quantitative research involves the measurement (in numeric form) of variables and the use of statistics to test hypotheses. Results of quantitative research are often reported in tables and figures, identifying statistically significant findings. One particular type of quantitative research, the clinical trial (randomised controlled trial, or RCT), is used to test the effect of a new nursing intervention on patient outcomes. In essence, clinical trials involve:

1 randomly allocating patients to receive either a new intervention (the experimental or intervention group) or an alternative or standard intervention (the control group)

2 delivering the intervention or alternative treatment

3 measuring an a priori identified patient outcome.[24]

Statistical analyses are used to determine whether the new intervention is better for patients than the alternative treatment.

Mixed methods research has now emerged as an approach that integrates data from qualitative and quantitative research at some stage in the research process.[25] In mixed methods approaches, researchers decide on both the priority and sequence of qualitative and quantitative

methods. In terms of priority, equal status may be given to both approaches. Priority is indicated by using capital letters for the dominant approach, followed by the symbols + and → to indicate either concurrent or sequential data collection, for example:

- QUAL + QUANT: both approaches are given equal status and data collection occurs concurrently.
- QUAL + quant: qualitative methods are the dominant approach and data collection occurs concurrently.
- QUAL → quant: the qualitative study is given priority and qualitative data collection will occur before quantitative data collection.

Irrespective of which type of research design is used, there are a number of common steps in the research process (Table 1.1), consisting of three phases: planning for the research, undertaking the research and analysing and reporting on the research findings.

Clinical research and the related activities of unit-based quality improvement are integral components in the practice, education and research triad.[27] Partnerships between clinicians and academics, and the implementation of clinical academic positions, including at the professorial level,[28] provide the necessary infrastructure and organisation for sustainable clinical nursing and multidisciplinary research.

TABLE 1.1

Steps in the research process

STEP	DESCRIPTION
Identify a clinical problem or issue	Clinical experience and practice audits are two ways that clinical issues or problems are identified
Review the literature	A comprehensive literature review is vital to ensure that the issue or problem has not yet been solved and that the proposed research builds on what is already known, and extends it to fill a gap in knowledge
Develop a clear research question	A precise question may follow either of two approaches: PICO (population, intervention, comparator, outcome), SPIDER (sample, phenomenon of interest, design, evaluation, research type)[26]
Write a research proposal	Write a clear description of the proposed research design and sample and a plan for data collection and analysis. Ethical considerations and the required resources (i.e. budget and personnel) for the research are identified
Secure resources	Resources such as funding for supplies and research staff, institutional support and access to experienced researchers are needed to ensure a study can be completed. Plans for how to access the relevant type and number of study participants are also considered
Obtain ethics approvals	Approval of the proposed research by a human research ethics committee (HREC) is required before the study can commence
Conduct the research	Adequate time for recruitment of participants, data collection and analysis are crucial to ensure that valid and relevant results are obtained
Disseminate the research findings	Discussion of the results and implications for practice with clinicians within the study site should occur as soon as possible. Distribution of a brief summary of the results is also frequently provided to study participants. Conference presentations and journal publications are two additional ways that research findings are disseminated and are vital to ensure that both nursing practice and nursing knowledge continue to be developed

FIGURE 1.1 Example of a critical care nursing research program.

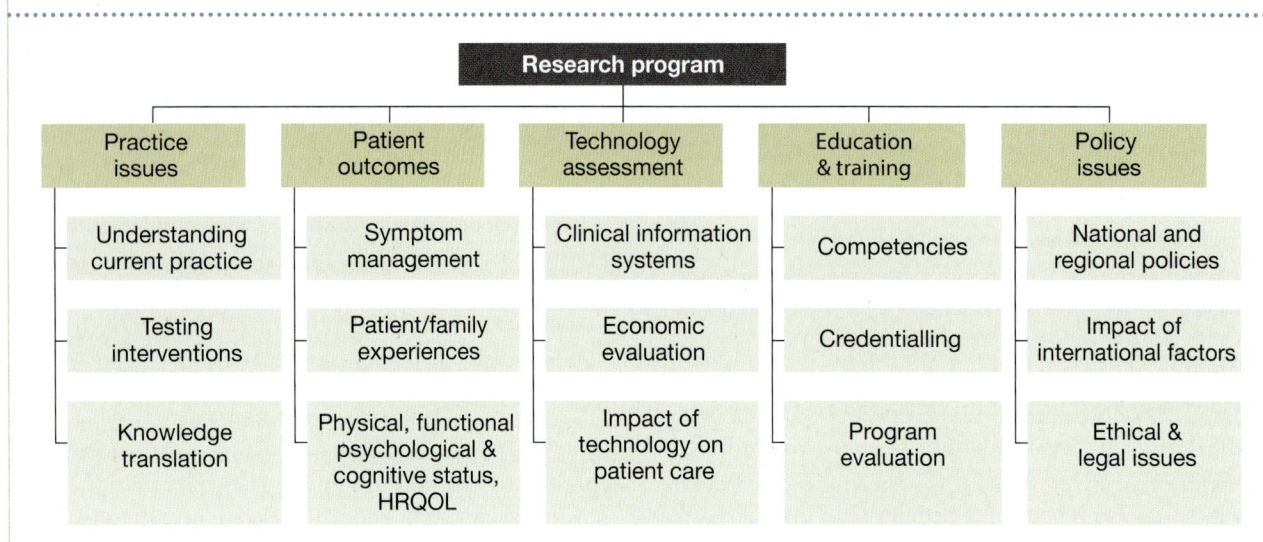

A strong research culture is evident in critical care nursing, transcending geographical, epistemological and disciplinary boundaries to focus on the core business of improving care for critically ill patients. Our collective aim is to develop a sustainable research culture that incorporates strategies that facilitate communication, cooperation, collaboration and coordination both between researchers with common interests and with clinicians who seek to use research findings in their practice. A sample of a guiding structure for a coherent research program that highlights the major issues affecting critical care nursing practice is illustrated in Figure 1.1, with identified themes and topic exemplars.

A number of resources are available to critical care nurses interested in undertaking research. For example, a number of critical care nursing professional organisations provide funding for research on a competitive basis. Funding is also available to critical care nurses through other critical care organisations not specific to nursing, such as the Intensive Care Foundation in Australia. Additionally, many regions have clinical trials groups that hold regular meetings where potential research can be discussed and research proposals refined. There is great value in receiving a critical review of proposed research before the study is undertaken, as assessors' comments help to refine the research plan.

Over the years, various groups have identified priorities for critical care research.[29,30] A review of this literature identified the following research priorities: nutrition support, infection control, other patient care issues, nursing roles, staffing and end-of-life decision making,[31] although these priorities are likely to change based on scientific advances and societal priorities.

While not all nurses are expected to conduct research, it is a professional responsibility to use research in practice.[32] Chapter 3 provides a detailed description of research utilisation approaches, with a description of evidence-based practice and the use of evidence-based clinical practice guidelines. In addition, each chapter in this text contains a research critique to assist nurses in developing critical appraisal skills, which will help to determine whether research evidence should change practice.

Education

Appropriate preparation of specialist critical care nurses is a vital component in providing quality care to patients and their families.[12] A central tenet within this framework of preparation is the formalised education of nurses to practise in critical care areas.[33] Formal education – in conjunction with experiential learning, continuing professional development and training and reflective clinical practice – is required to develop competence in critical care nursing. The knowledge, skills and attitude necessary for quality critical care nursing practice have been articulated in competency statements[34-36] and within certification processes that recognise the knowledge and expertise of critical care nurses.[37]

Critical care nursing education developed in unison with the advent of specialist critical care units. Initially, this consisted of ad hoc training developed and delivered in the work setting, with nurses and medical officers learning together. For example, medical staff brought expertise in physiology, pathophysiology and interpretation of electrocardiographic rhythm strips, while nurses brought expertise in patient care and how patients behaved and responded to treatment.[19,38] Training was, however, fragmented and 'fitted in' around ward staffing needs. Post-registration critical care nursing courses were subsequently developed from the early 1960s in both Australasia and the UK.[10,15] Courses ranged in length from 6 to 12 months and generally incorporated employment as well as specific days for lectures and class work. Given the specific nature of these courses developed to meet the local needs of individual hospitals and regions, differences in content and practice developed between hospitals, regions and countries.[39-41]

During the 1990s the majority of these hospital-based courses in Australasia were discontinued as universities developed postgraduate curricula to extend the knowledge and skills gained in pre-registration undergraduate courses. A similar move to the tertiary sector occurred in the UK and much of Europe during the 1990s and the following decade. A significant proportion of critical care nurses now undertake specialty education in the tertiary sector, often in a collaborative relationship with one or more hospitals.[10] One early study of students enrolled in university-based critical care courses in Australia[42] identified a number of burdens (workload, financial, study–work conflicts), but also a number of benefits (e.g. better job prospects, job security).

Internationally, there are a number of different ways in which critical care nurses receive education specific to their practice.[43] Within Australia and New Zealand, most tertiary institutions currently offer postgraduate critical care nursing education at a Graduate Certificate or Graduate Diploma level as preparation for specialty practice, although this is often provided as a Master's degree.[44] In the UK, similar provisions for postgraduate critical care nursing education at multiple levels are available, although some universities also offer critical care specialisation at the undergraduate level (for example, City University London). Education throughout Europe has undergone significant change in the past 10 years as the framework articulated under the Bologna Process has been implemented.[45] In relation to critical care nursing, this has led to the expansion of programs, primarily at the postgraduate level, for specialist nursing education. Critical care nursing education in the USA maintains a slightly different focus, with most postgraduate studies being generic in nature, including a focus on advanced practice roles such as clinical nurse specialists and nurse practitioners, while specialty education for critical care nurses is undertaken as continuing education.[46] Employment in critical care, with associated assessment of clinical competence, remains an essential component of many university-based critical care nursing courses.[44,47] The diversity of critical care programs internationally means that there is likely significant variability in programs and

outcomes. Recent work in Australia has been completed to develop critical care nurse education practice standards that can assist in achieving consistent graduate practice outcomes and can inform professional health workforce standards.[48]

Both the impact of post-registration education on practice and the most appropriate level of education that is required to underpin specialty practice remain controversial, with no universal acceptance internationally.[43,49–52] Globally, the Declaration of Madrid, which was endorsed by the World Federation of Critical Care Nurses, provides a baseline for critical care nursing education (see the website, www.wfccn.org, for the position statement).[12]

A range of factors continue to influence critical care nursing education provision, including government policies at national and state levels, funding mechanisms and resource implications for organisations and individual students, education provider and healthcare sector partnership arrangements, and tensions between workforce and professional development needs.[53] Recruitment, orientation, training and education of critical care nurses can be viewed as a continuum of learning, experience and professional development.[12] The relationships between the various components related to practice, training and education are illustrated in Figure 1.2, on a continuum from 'beginner' to 'expert' and incorporating increasing complexities of competency. Assessing the level of competency of a critical care nurse is challenging[54] although ways of measuring competency are being explored.[55] All elements comprising the notion of competence are equally important in promoting quality critical care nursing practice.

Practice- or skills-based continuing education sessions support clinical practice at the unit level.[56] (Orientation and continuing education issues are discussed further in the context of staffing levels and skills mix in Chapter 2.) Many countries now incorporate requirements for continuing professional development into their annual licensing processes. Specific requirements include elements such as minimum hours of required professional development and/or ongoing demonstration of competence against predefined competency standards.[57,58]

FIGURE 1.2 Critical care nursing practice: training and education continuum.

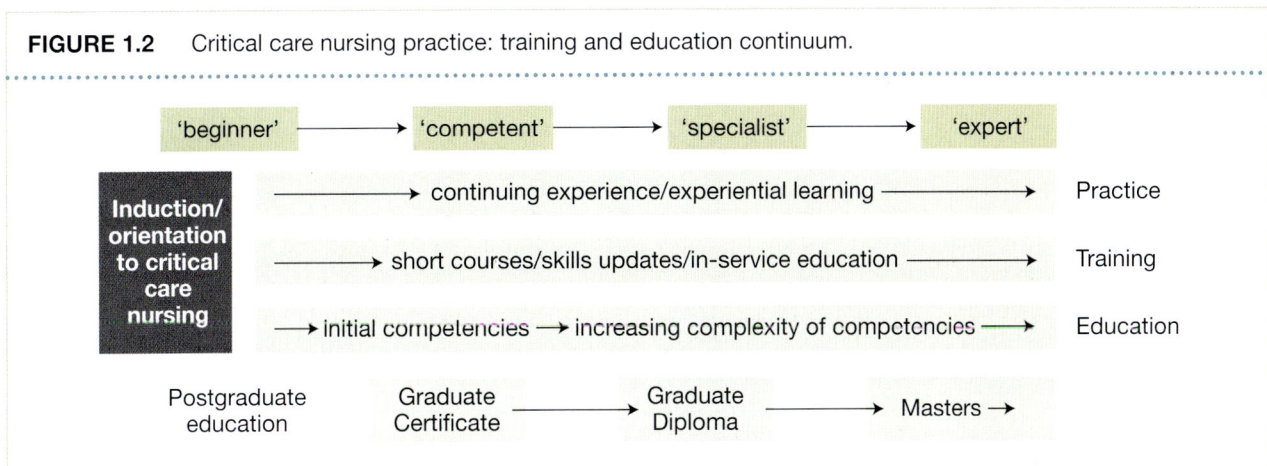

Specialist critical care competencies

Critical care nursing involves a range of skills, classified as psychomotor (or technical), cognitive or interpersonal. Performance of specific skills requires special training and practice to enable proficiency. Clinical competence is a combination of skills, behaviours and knowledge, demonstrated by performance within a practice situation[59] and specific to the context in which it is demonstrated.[55] A nurse who learns a skill and is assessed as performing that skill within the clinical environment is deemed competent. The Australian College of Critical Care Nurses developed a revised set of practice standards for specialist critical care practice which comprises 15 practice standards grouped into four domains: professional practice, provision and cordination of care, critical thinking and analysis, and collaboration and leadership[34] (refer to *Appendix A* and to the ACCCN website, listed in *Online resources* at the end of this chapter). These revised standards were developed over 2013–2015 through a two-phase process. Focus groups were held to identify main themes that informed development of draft standards that were refined during a Delphi process involving a national panel of critical care nurses. Other competency domains and assessment tools have also been developed.[55,60] Although articulated slightly differently, the American Association of Critical-Care Nurses (AACN) provides 'Standards of Practice and Performance for the Acute and Critical Care Clinical Nurse Specialist',[60] which outlines six standards of practice (assessment, diagnosis, outcome identification, planning, implementation and evaluation) and eight standards of professional performance (quality of care, individual practice evaluation, education, collegiality, ethics, collaboration, research and resource utilisation) (see *Online resources*).

Professional organisations

Professional leadership of critical care nursing has undergone considerable development in the past three decades. Within Australia, the ACCCN (formerly the Confederation of Australian Critical Care Nurses) was formed from a number of preceding state-based specialty nursing bodies (e.g. the Australian Society of Critical Care Nurses, the Clinical Nurse Specialists Association) that had provided professional leadership for critical care nurses since the early 1970s. In New Zealand, the professional interests of critical care nurses are represented by the New Zealand Nurses Organisation, Critical Care Nurses Section, as well as affiliation with the ACCCN. The ACCCN has strong professional relationships with other national peak nursing bodies, the Australian and New Zealand Intensive Care Society (ANZICS), government agencies and individuals, and healthcare companies.

Professional organisations representing critical care nurses were formed as early as the 1960s in the USA with the formation of the AACN.[37] Other organisations have developed around the world, such as the British Association of Critical Care Nurses (BACCN), and critical care nursing bodies now operate in all six continents.

In 2001 the inaugural meeting of the World Federation of Critical Care Nurses (WFCCN) was formed to provide professional leadership at an international level.[21,61] The ACCCN is a foundation member of the WFCCN and a member association of the World Federation of Societies of Intensive Care and Critical Care Medicine, and maintains a representative on the councils of both these international bodies. (See the ACCCN website, listed in *Online resources*, for further details about professional activities.)

Critical care nursing roles

As critical care nursing has developed, so too has the range of roles performed by critical care nurses. Much of this textbook describes the specialty practice and roles in critical care nursing. Critical care nursing is an example of 'horizontal' specialisation within nursing with other specialties such as oncology and aged care, whereas advanced practice nursing can be considered 'vertical' specialisation within the specialty of critical care. This section focuses on advanced practice roles in critical care. The term advanced practice may be viewed as an umbrella, describing a number of related roles including nurse practitioners. The ICU liaison nurse and the ICU outreach nurse are examples of advanced practice nursing roles. Some advanced practice nurses may also be legally recognised as nurse practitioners, as some ICU liaison nurses are. In this section we describe the ICU liaison nurse role, also described as the ICU outreach nurse in some settings, as an example of advanced practice nursing roles. Information on nurse practitioners is then provided.

Advanced practice nursing roles

There is potentially a huge range of advanced practice nursing roles that may be enacted in critical care. For example, critical care nurses could choose to develop advanced knowledge and skills in the areas of palliative care, transport/retrieval or care of the elderly patient. Collectively, what is common is the need to develop advanced knowledge and skills in the particular area of expertise. Interestingly, it also seems that these roles may emerge as a means of overcoming service gaps. The ICU liaison nurse is described as an example of an advanced practice role. The ICU liaison nurse role, which emerged in the late 1990s in Australia, is similar to the critical care outreach role developed around the same time in the UK.[62] These roles include activities such as following up patients discharged from the ICU and providing expert advice for ward patients with complex care needs, including those experiencing clinical deterioration. Early research showed that Australian ICU liaison nurses focused on staff education and support, ward liaison, patient care and support and family education and support.[63] A comparison of the UK outreach services and the Australian liaison nurse services found many similarities between the two roles.[62] More contemporary research showed that liaison nurse services operated in 27% of public Australian ICUs.[64] This survey also identified that ICU liaison nurses were involved in activities related to education, collaboration (including consultation), expert practice and research/quality.[64] Most of the liaison nurses were classified as clinical nurse consultants or clinical nurse specialists.[64] In those hospitals that had the service, 55% of the liaison nurses were part of the rapid response team.[64] A recent Argentinian study of the activities undertaken by ICU liaison nurses in the first year of the service showed that 98% of the 387 patients they saw had been discharged from the ICU.[65] The service was provided 24 hours per day, 7 days per week.[65] Of the 5973 patient care activities performed during the year, over 95% were related to patient assessment, with various other activities such as patient and family education and support, airway management and patient safety activities making up the other 15%.[65] In terms of the 1709 staff education activities undertaken during the first year, 33% were related to patient safety such as skin care, infection and falls prevention, 20% and 17% of the other educational activities were related to nursing assessment and airway management, respectively.[65] A 2014 meta-analysis of the effect of the ICU liaison nurse on ICU readmissions showed a positive effect with a risk ratio of 0.91 (95% confidence intervals 0.75–0.99).[66] Thus, it appears that the evidence base for this advanced practice nursing role is growing.

Nurse practitioners

The International Council of Nursing (ICN) defines the nurse practitioner/advanced practice roles as a 'registered nurse who has acquired the expert knowledge base, complex decision-making skills and clinical competencies for expanded practice, the characteristics of which are shaped by the context and/or country in which she/he is credentialed to practice'.[67] The ICN notes that the education of nurse practitioners/advanced practice nurses is at an advanced level and is accredited or approved, with some form of licensure, registration, certification or credentialing. This description of nurse practitioners/advanced practice nurses should not be confused with specialist critical care nurses who are credentialed. In some countries, including Australia, the nurse practitioner role is legislated and is distinct from other advanced practice roles such as clinical nurse consultants or specialists.

The ICN[67] describes the nature of practice of nurse practitioners/advanced practice nurses as including a high degree of autonomy and independent practice. While the ICN acknowledges country specific regulation, it suggests nurse practitioners/advanced practice nurses will be able to diagnose, prescribe medications and treatments, refer clients to other health professionals and admit patients to hospital. Skills such as advanced health assessment and decision making are required. There are a number of nurse practitioner/advanced practice nursing roles in critical care. A review described three nurse practitioner roles: 1) adult, 2) paediatric and 3) neonatal.[68] The author described aspects of the role including direct patient management, assessment, diagnosis, monitoring and procedural activities.[68] Retrieval and trauma nurse practitioners have

also emerged.[68,69] As part of her review, Fry[68] described the historical developments of the nurse practitioner role in critical care. She noted that the role was established in the United States in the 1960s, in the United Kingdom in the 1980s, in Canada and New Zealand in around 2000 and to some extent in Australia in 1995, although formal recognition of the nurse practitioner role did not occur in Australia until somewhat later.[68]

There is a growing body of research on the nurse practitioner/advanced practice nursing roles. While a comprehensive review of this work is beyond the scope of this text, several recent studies are described. One study described the activities undertaken by 30 Australian nurse practitioners in 2008/09.[70] The sample included eight emergency, three cardiac, two neonatal and one paediatric nurse practitioners. The five most frequent activities were: meetings and administration, coordination of care, documentation, performing procedures and history taking.[70] A more recent Australian study conducted in 2010 examined prescribing practices specifically.[71] The sample of 209 nurse practitioners included 66 emergency care (adult) and 12 paediatric/neonatal nurse practitioners. In total, 78% of the nurses reported prescribing medications.[71] The five most frequent medications prescribed were: anti-infectives, analgesics, psychotropics and cardiovascular and musculoskeletal drugs.[71] In Taiwan, 374 of 582 invited nurse practitioners (response rate 64%) completed a survey of the competencies they required and possessed.[72] The competencies assessed included direct care, medical assistance, communication and coordination, practical guidance, clinical research, professional consultation, ethical decision making, leadership and reform and cultural competency.[72] The scores for all required competencies were consistently higher than the scores for actual competencies. Chang and colleagues[72] noted that, in Taiwan, the nurse practitioner role was actually more similar to the physician assistant role as it predominantly involved medical assistance. Finally, a recent Canadian study examined perceptions of team effectiveness in two cardiology services using the case study methodology.[73] There were 59 participants in the study who were described as those within nursing (n = 28), 'interprofessionals' outside of nursing (n = 19) and managers (n = 12). Participants perceived the nurse practitioners improved team effectiveness in a number of ways including: decision making, communication, cohesion, care coordination, problem solving and providing a focus on patients and families.[73] Thus, the various roles and opportunities for nurse practitioners in the critical care environment appear to be growing.

Leadership in critical care nursing

Effective leadership within critical care nursing is essential at several organisational levels, including the unit and hospital levels, as well as within the specialty on a broader professional scale. The leadership required at any given time and in any specific setting is a reflection of the surrounding environment. Regardless of the setting, effective leadership involves having and communicating a clear vision, motivating a team to achieve a common goal, communicating effectively with others, role modelling, creating and sustaining the critical elements of a healthy work environment and implementing change and innovation.[74-77] Leadership at the unit and hospital levels is essential to ensure excellence in practice, as well as adequate clinical governance. In addition to the generic strategies described above, it is essential for leaders in critical care units and hospitals to demonstrate a patient focus, establish and maintain standards of practice and collaborate with other members of the multidisciplinary healthcare team.[74]

Leadership is essential to achieve growth and development in our specialty and is demonstrated through such activities as conducting research, producing publications, making conference presentations, representation on relevant government and healthcare councils and committees and participation in organisations such as the ACCCN, BACCN, AACN, European federation of Critical Care Nursing associations (EfCCNa) and the WFCCN. As outlined earlier in this chapter, we have seen the field of critical care grow from early ideas and makeshift units to a well-developed and highly organised international specialty in the course of a generation. Such development would not have been possible without the vision, enthusiasm and commitment of many critical care leaders throughout the world.

Leadership styles vary and are influenced by the mission and values of the organisation as well as the values and beliefs of individual leaders. These styles of leadership are described in many different ways, sometimes by using theoretical underpinnings such as 'transactional' and 'transformational' and sometimes by using leadership values and characteristics. Regardless of the terminology in use, some common principles can be expressed. Desired leadership characteristics include the ability to:

- articulate a personal vision and expectations
- act as a catalyst for change
- establish and implement organisational standards
- model effective leadership behaviours through both change processes and stable contexts
- monitor practice in relation to standards and take corrective action when necessary
- recognise the characteristics and strengths of individuals, and stimulate individual development and commitment
- empower staff to act independently and interdependently
- inspire team members to achieve excellence.[78-83]

Personal characteristics of an effective leader, regardless of the style, include honesty, integrity, justice, commitment, credibility, courage and wisdom, as well as the ability to develop an open, trusting environment and be approachable and supportive.[83,84] Effective leaders inspire their team members to take the extra step towards achieving the goals articulated by the leader and to feel that they are valued, independent, responsible and autonomous individuals within the organisation.[83] Members of teams with effective leaders are not satisfied with maintaining the status quo, but believe in the vision and goals articulated by the leader and are prepared to work towards achieving a higher standard of practice.

Although all leaders share common characteristics, some elements vary according to leadership style. Different styles – for example, transactional, transformational, authoritative or laissez faire – incorporate different characteristics and activities. Having leaders with different styles ensures that there is leadership for all stages of an organisation's operation or a profession's development. A combination of leadership styles also helps to overcome team member preferences and problems experienced when a particularly visionary leader leaves. The challenges often associated with the departure of a leader from a healthcare organisation are generally reduced in the clinical critical care environment, where a nursing leader is usually part of a multidisciplinary team, with resultant shared values and objectives.

Clinical leadership

Effective critical care nurses demonstrate leadership characteristics regardless of their role or level of practice; such leadership is an essential component of any effective team.[85] Leadership in the clinical environment incorporates the general characteristics listed above, but has the added challenges of working within the boundaries created by the requirements of providing safe patient care 24 hours a day, 7 days a week. It is therefore essential that clinical leaders work within an effective interdisciplinary model, so that all aspects of patient care and family support, as well as the needs of all staff, are met.[85] Effective clinical leadership of critical care is essential in achieving:

- effective and safe patient care
- high quality, evidence-based health care
- satisfied patients and family members
- satisfied staff, with a high level of retention
- development of staff through an effective coaching and mentoring process.[86-88]

Effective clinical leaders build cohesive and adaptive work teams,[82] and improve interdisciplinary collaboration.[89] They also promote the intellectual stimulation of individual staff members, which encourages the analysis and exploration of practice that is essential for evidence-based nursing.[83] Clinical leadership is particularly important in contemporary critical care environments in times of dynamic change and development. We are currently witnessing significant changes in the organisation and delivery of care, with the development of new roles such as the nurse practitioner (see this chapter) and liaison nurse (see Chapter 3), the introduction of services such as rapid response systems, including medical emergency teams (see Chapter 3) and the extension of activities across the care continuum (see Chapter 4). Effective clinical leadership ensures that:

- critical care personnel are aware of, and willing to fulfil, their changing roles
- personnel in other areas of the hospital or outside the hospital recognise the benefits and limitations of developments, are not threatened by the developments and are enthusiastic to use the new or refined services provided by critical care
- patients receive optimal quality of care.

The need to provide educational opportunities to develop effective clinical leadership skills is recognised.[78] Although not numerous in number or variety, programs are beginning to be available internationally that are designed to develop clinical leaders, both within the clinical environment and in partnership with higher education institutions.[77,90,91] Factors that influence leadership ability include the external and internal environment, demographic characteristics such as age, experience, understanding, stage of personal development including self-awareness capability and communication skills.[78,80,90] In relation to clinical leadership, at least some of the development of these factors must be in a clinical setting, so the development of clinical leaders should be based in that environment. Development programs based on mentorship, with strong academic support, are superbly suited to developing those that demonstrate potential for such capabilities.[78,91]

Mentorship has received significant attention in the healthcare literature and has been specifically identified as a strategy for clinical leadership development.[92–94] Although many different definitions of mentoring exist, common principles include a relationship between two people with the primary purpose of one person in the relationship developing new skills related to their career.[95] A related process might also be referred to as coaching.[96,97] Mentoring programs can be either formal or informal and either internal or external to the work setting. Mentorship involves a variety of activities directed towards facilitating new learning experiences for the mentee, guiding professional development and career decisions, providing emotional and psychological support and assisting the mentee in the socialisation process both within and outside the work organisation to build professional networks.[93,95,97] Role modelling of occupational and professional skills and characteristics is an important component of mentoring that helps develop future clinical leaders.[93]

Summary

This chapter has provided a context for subsequent chapters, outlining some key issues, principles and concepts for practising and studying nursing in a range of critical care areas. Critical care nursing now encompasses a broad and ever-expanding scope of practice. The previous focus on patients in ICU only has given way to a broader concept of caring for an individual located in a variety of clinical locations across a continuum of critical illness.

The discipline of critical care nursing, in collaboration with multidisciplinary colleagues, continues to develop to meet the expanding challenges of clinical practice in today's healthcare environment. Critical care clinicians also continue their professional development individually, focusing on clinical practice development, education and training and on quality improvement and research activities, to facilitate quality patient and family care during a time of acute physiological derangement and emotional turmoil. The principles of decision making and clinical leadership at all levels of practice serve to enhance patient safety in the critical care environment.

Case study

James is a 54-year-old male who is 5 days post an Ivor Lewis oesophagectomy for cancer; his post-operative progress to this point has followed a routine course. The ICU outreach nurse's first contact with this patient is a direct referral from the primary care nurse on the ward who is concerned with his tachypnoea, tachycardia and low grade temperature. James is reviewed by the ICU outreach nurse in regard to the following:

- physical assessment
- review of clinical course/notes and observation charts
- review of radiological and pathological investigations
- discussion of concerns with the primary care nurse.

During this assessment James is noted to have a low grade temperature (37.7° C) with two documented episodes of elevated temperature over the last 8 hours and increasing heart rate (HR) of 115 beats/min

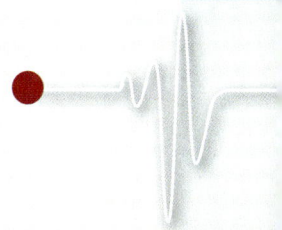

and respiratory rate (RR) of 26 breaths/min. On auscultation of the patient's chest he was found to have decreased air entry to both lung bases and coarse crackles in the right middle lobe. James had dry mucous membranes, reported thirst and denied pain. He had not had a chest X-ray (CXR) in the previous 24 hours and had a rising white cell count (WCC) on his full blood count (FBC) over the last 48 hours.

Advanced assessment skills: ICU outreach nursing requires an advanced level of nursing assessment skills. Outreach nurses must have the ability to effectively undertake a physical assessment and integrate these findings with other available assessment data such as radiological and pathological investigations to rapidly build a clear picture of why the patient is clinically deteriorating. This integration of assessment findings enables appropriate decisions around escalation of patient care to be made.

Progress: findings of this assessment were discussed with the resident medical officer and subsequently the registrar of the treating team, with a provisional diagnosis of sepsis made. A CXR, septic screen, increased intravenous fluids and broad spectrum intravenous antibiotics were ordered. In discussion with the primary care nurse, observations were increased to 2nd hourly and a strict fluid balance commenced. James was placed on the list for review by the outreach nurse during the next shift.

Subsequently, the ICU outreach nurse came into contact with James prior to this review as part of the rapid response team (RRT) call. James had further respiratory deterioration. He had a RR of 30 breaths/min, SpO_2 of 92% on a non-rebreathing mask at 15 L/min of oxygen and was using his accessory muscles to a moderate degree. As a member of the RRT (airway nurse) the outreach nurse discussed the indications and possible benefits of high flow oxygen (HFO) for this patient. The outreach nurse set up and implemented this therapy and provided bedside education for the ward nursing staff. In discussion with the nurse in charge of the ward, a 1:1 registered nurse special for James was arranged, and a plan for management of any deterioration was developed with the nursing and medical staff. James was also referred to the on-call physiotherapist to ensure ongoing chest physiotherapy overnight.

James was reviewed by the outreach nurse 4 hours after the RRT call, and he appeared fatigued but was maintaining his SpO_2 at ≥95% on 30 L/min of 45% HFO. The medical staff were again contacted and, after consultation, an arterial blood gas was taken, processed and interpreted. With further medical and nursing team consultation James' oxygen flow was increased to 40 L/min to assist with the work of breathing; concurrently, the observation frequency was increased to hourly. Progress included the following:

- James was reviewed 2 hours later; his work of breathing had decreased, and he had tolerated physiotherapy well and was clearing secretions effectively.

- James was reviewed on the next outreach nurse shift. His clinical condition continued to improve. The outreach nurse provided education to the nursing and junior medical staff regarding the indications, process and rationale for weaning of HFO. Discussion occurred with the nurse in charge of the ward and 1:1 nursing special was ceased for James as the primary care nurse felt he could be closely monitored with normal staffing levels at this time.

- James was reviewed on the following shift. On clinical assessment air entry had improved, he had a decreasing sputum load and observations were RR 20 breaths/min, HR 95 beats/min, SpO_2 ≥95% on 25% HFO at 30 L/min, BP 130/90 mmHg and urine output 30–80 mL/h. The primary care nurse was satisfied with the clinical plan for James and it was mutually agreed to remove the patient from the outreach nurse review service.

DISCUSSION
Effective communication skills

ICU outreach nursing requires exemplary communication skills. The outreach nurse must be able to effectively liaise with the ward nursing staff and clearly present their assessment findings and recommendations for management to the multidisciplinary team. In this instance:

- education was provided to ward nursing staff regarding the use of HFO and associated care
- a clear plan was developed to manage any further deterioration
- in conjunction with the nurse in charge of the ward the outreach nurse assisted in facilitating a 1:1 nursing ratio for this patient to ensure close monitoring of the patient's condition and safe staffing levels for other patients on the ward.

Leadership and corporate knowledge

Outreach nurses strive to create an inclusive culture wherein they provide the support for ward-based nursing teams to manage deteriorating patients. Their role is not to intervene or take over the care of the patient, but to provide appropriate support, education and potential care strategies. Achieving this goal requires tact, diplomacy and emotional intelligence as well as knowledge of the facilities and services available in the organisation in which they work. An understanding of the corporate/operational knowledge, both explicit and tacit in each ward, can provide great advantage in overcoming the challenges of effectively managing the deteriorating patient, such as staffing and ward specific protocols and practices. This knowledge contributes to the development of effective plans to manage deteriorating patients in each of the specific clinical settings.

CASE STUDY QUESTIONS

1 During an episode of patient deterioration urgent treatment may be required and, consequently, there may be limited opportunity for learning by the ward nursing staff caring for the deteriorating patient. What strategies might you use to optimise learning in this scenario?

2 As an ICU outreach nurse (or other consultant who provides support on multiple wards), you notice that the ward-based nursing staff appear reticent to report problems or access support through the ward hierarchy. You broach this subject with several nurses and they indicate they feel powerless and are afraid of the senior staff in both the nursing and medical professions. How would you support the nursing staff in this environment?

The authors thank Shannon Crouch and Amanda Vaux, CNCs Outreach, Princess Alexandra Hospital, for developing this *Case study*.

RESEARCH VIGNETTE

Lakanmaa RL, Suominen T, Perttila J, Ritmala-Castren M, Vahlbert T, Leino-Kilpi H. Graduating nursing students' basic competence in intensive and critical care nursing. J Clin Nurs 2014;23:645–53

Abstract

Aims and objectives: To describe and evaluate the basic competence of graduating nursing students in intensive and critical care nursing.

Background: Intensive and critical care nursing is focused on severely ill patients who benefit from the attention of skilled personnel. More intensive and critical care nurses are needed in Europe. Critical care nursing education is general post-qualification education that builds upon initial generalist nursing education. However, in Europe, new graduates practise in intensive care units. Empirical research on nursing students' competence in intensive and critical care nursing is scarce.

Design: A cross-sectional survey design.

Methods: A basic competence scale (Intensive and Critical Care Nursing Competence Scale, version 1) and a knowledge test (Basic Knowledge Assessment Tool, version 7) were employed among graduating nursing students (n = 139).

Results: Sixty-nine percent of the students self-rated their basic competence as good. No association between self-assessed Intensive and Critical Care Nursing-1 and the results of the Basic Knowledge Assessment Tool-7 was found. The strongest factor explaining the students' conception of their competence was their experience of autonomy in nursing after graduation.

Conclusion: The students seem to trust their basic competence as they approach graduation. However, a knowledge test or other objective method of evaluation should be used together with a competence scale based on self-evaluation.

Relevance to clinical practice: In nursing education and in clinical practice, for example, during orientation programmes, it is important not only to teach broad basic skills and knowledge of intensive and critical care nursing, but also to develop self-evaluation skills through the use of special instruments constructed for this purpose.

Critique

This interesting study focused on Finnish nursing students' perceptions of their competence. As described by the authors, in Finland basic nursing education is provided by polytechnics (also described as universities of applied sciences). There is no graduate specialty education, thus intensive and critical care nursing is taught in the undergraduate program. Therefore, the students recruited to the study were students in the last semester of their undergraduate education. The sample was drawn from four polytechnics, each of which was located near a university hospital. All nurses in their final semester of education were invited to participate in a survey. A total of 139 nurses completed it, for a response rate of 59%. The fact that four sites were sampled and the response rate was reasonably good suggests the findings may be generalisable to other similar settings.

The survey was comprised of demographic data and two instruments, the Intensive and Critical Care Nursing Competence Scale (ICCN-CS-1), which was developed by the Finnish authors, and the Basic Knowledge Assessment Tool version 7 (BKAT-7), which had previously been developed in the USA. The BKAT-7 has 100 items and has been extensively used and has been translated into several languages. In this study, it was used to test the criterion validity of the ICCN-CS-1. That is, participants who score high on the ICCN-CS-1 knowledge base questions should also score high on the BKAT-7 if the ICCN-CS-1 is a valid measuring instrument. The ICCN-CS-1 was developed using a standard process of reviewing the literature, and employing a Delphi study. The ICCN-CS-1 is a 108-item instrument comprised of two main sections, clinical competence and professional competence, both of which have items related to knowledge, skills and attitudes/values. The reliability of the ICCN-CS-1 was good with Cronbach's alphas of 0.87–0.98, although the highest alpha suggests there may be more items than needed. Total scores on the ICCN-CS-1 were calculated by adding the individual item scores together for the total instrument, for the two sections of clinical and professional competence and also for the groupings of items within each of these sections and for the classification as knowledge, skills and attitude/values. Then, score ranges were classified as excellent, good, moderate or poor competence.

Participants were given 90 minutes to complete the survey. It is not clear why this amount of time was allowed or if the timing may have affected the responses. However, the authors note they completed a pilot study, which suggested that this time may be feasible. Returned surveys implied consent; ethics approval was gained from the relevant ethics committees and permission to use the BKAT-7 was also obtained.

The researchers report that in terms of self-rated 'basic' competence (i.e. overall competence instrument score), 25% rated it as excellent, 69% rated it as good and 6% rated it as moderate. In fact, mean scores for clinical and professional competence were similar at 3.70 ($\pm$ 0.55) and 3.75 ($\pm$ 0.47). When considering these same items in relation to knowledge, skill and attitude/values, both knowledge and skills at 3.28 ($\pm$ 0.62) and 3.20 ($\pm$ 0.67) appeared to be lower than attitudes/values at 4.68 ($\pm$ 0.36). The researchers report there was no association between the ICCN-CS-1 and the BKAT-7 suggesting that criterion validity of the ICCN-CS-1 was not supported. Yet, they report the level of significance (i.e. p-value) for the correlation was 0.012, which is statistically significant. Perhaps because the Pearson's correlation was only 0.21, they believed that the finding was not clinically meaningful but this is different to whether there was a statistically significant correlation (which there was based on the results presented). In the discussion the researchers explained potential reasons for the finding that participants scored very low on the BKAT-7 instrument.

The discussion was thoughtful and well written. The relevance to clinical practice was briefly mentioned and suggestions for future work were woven into the discussion. Limitations of the research were also identified. Although the paper was reasonably clear, it took time to understand the ICCN-CS-1 in terms of the sections, the subsections and how items were also classified as knowledge, skills and attitudes/values. It also took time to understand how the instrument was scored. Overall though, this was an interesting study undertaken by a reasonably large team of researchers led by a nurse, who was doing this study as part of her PhD.

Learning activities

1 Consider the leaders to whom you are exposed in your work environment and identify the characteristics they display that influence patient care. Reflect on whether these are characteristics that you possess or how you might develop them.

2 All registered nurses are expected to demonstrate leadership in clinical practice. Reflect on what leadership activities you undertake as part of your role. What strategies could you use to evaluate and further develop your leadership skills?

3 A colleague who has been working in ICU for the past 3 years indicates that they are interested in moving beyond a role in direct patient care and would like to eventually move into a clinical leadership position. What strategies might you suggest they investigate to position them well for the future?

4 Consider the role that you have within critical care and examine the influence that research has on that role. How might you use research to inform your practice more effectively? Are there strategies that you could implement to influence the research that is undertaken so that it meets your needs?

5 Reflect on your practice and experience over the past year. What professional development activities have you undertaken and what new knowledge and skills have you developed?

Online resources

American Association of Critical-Care Nurses, www.aacn.org

Annual Scientific Meeting on Intensive Care, www.intensivecareasm.com.au

ANZICS Clinical Trials Group, www.anzics.com.au/clinical-trials-group

Australia and New Zealand Intensive Care Society, www.anzics.com.au

Australian College of Critical Care Nurses, www.acccn.com.au

British Association of Critical Care Nurses, www.baccn.org.uk

Canadian Critical Care Trials Group, www.ccctg.ca/Home.aspx

College of Intensive Care Medicine (CICM), www.cicm.org.au

European Society of Intensive Care Medicine, www.esicm.org

Intensive Care Foundation (Australia and New Zealand), www.intensivecarefoundation.org.au

Intensive Care National Audit and Research Centre, www.icnarc.org

King's College, London, www.kcl.ac.uk/schools/nursing

NHS Leadership Academy, The Healthcare Leadership Model, www.leadershipacademy.nhs.uk/discover/leadershipmodel

Royal College of Nursing (UK) Critical Care and In-Flight Nursing Forum community, www.rcn.org.uk/development/communities/rcn_forum_communities/critical_inflight

Scottish Intensive Care Society, www.scottishintensivecare.org.uk/sics/research/index.htm

World Federation of Critical Care Nurses, http://en.wfccn.org

Further reading

Andrew S, Halcomb EJ. Mixed methods research for nursing and the health sciences. Oxford: Wiley-Blackwell; 2009.

Scholes J. Developing expertise in critical care nursing. Oxford: Blackwell Publishing; 2006.

Swanwick T, McKimm J. ABC of clinical leadership. London: BMJ Books; 2010.

References

1 Murthy S, Wunsch H. Clinical review: international comparisons in critical care – lessons learned. Crit Care 2012;16(2):218.

2 Sprung CL, Zimmerman JL, Christian MD, Joynt GM, Hick JL, Taylor B et al. Recommendations for intensive care unit and hospital preparations for an influenza epidemic or mass disaster: summary report of the European Society of Intensive Care Medicine's Task Force for intensive care unit triage during an influenza epidemic or mass disaster. Intensive Care Med 2010;36(3):428–43.

3 Rhodes A, Moreno RP. Intensive care provision: a global problem. Revista brasileira de terapia intensiva 2012;24(4):322–5.

4 Australian and New Zealand Intensive Care Society (ANZICS). Centre for Outcome and Resource Evaluation Annual Report 2011–2013. Melbourne: ANZICS, 2013.

5 Rechner IJ, Lipman J. The costs of caring for patients in a tertiary referral Australian Intensive Care Unit. Anaesth Intensive Care 2005;33(4): 477–82. Epub 2005/08/27.

6 Tan SS, Bakker J, Hoogendoorn ME, Kapila A, Martin J, Pezzi A et al. Direct cost analysis of intensive care unit stay in four European countries: applying a standardized costing methodology. Value Health 2012;15(1):81–6. Epub 2012/01/24.

7 Shweta K, Kumar S, Gupta AK, Jindal SK, Kumar A. Economic analysis of costs associated with a Respiratory Intensive Care Unit in a tertiary care teaching hospital in Northern India. Indian Journal of Critical Care Medicine : peer-reviewed, official publication of Indian Society of Critical Care Medicine. 2013;17(2):76–81. Epub 2013/08/29.

8 Prin M, Wunsch H. International comparisons of intensive care: informing outcomes and improving standards. Curr Opin Crit Care 2012;18(6):700–6.

9 Seidel J, Whiting PC, Edbrooke DL. The costs of intensive care. Contin Educ Anaesth Crit Care Pain 2006;6(4):160–63.

10 Wiles V, Daffurn K. There's a bird in my hand and a bear by the bed – I must be in ICU. The pivotal years of Australian critical care nursing. Melbourne: Australian College of Critical Care Nurses Ltd; 2002.

11 Hilberman M. The evolution of intensive care units. Crit Care Med 1975;3(4):159–65.

12 World Federation of Critical Care Nurses. Constitution of the World Federation of Critical Care Nurses. World Federation of Critical Care Nurses; 2006 [cited 2014 21 May].

13 American Association of Critical-Care Nurses. Critical Care Nursing Fact Sheet. Aliso Viejo: American Association of Critical Care Nurses; 2005 [cited 2005 7 October].

14 Australian College of Critical Care Nurses. Australian College of Critical Care Nurses Website. Melbourne: Australian College of Critical Care Nurses; 2005 [cited 2005 7 October].

15 Gordon IJ, Jones ES. The evolution and nursing history of a general intensive care unit (1962–1983). Intensive Crit Care Nurs 1998;14(5):252–7.

16 Prien T, Meyer J, Lawin P. Development of intensive care medicine in Germany. J Clin Anesth 1991;3(3):253–8.

17 Scribante J, Schmollgruber S, Nel E. Perspectives on critical care nursing: South Africa. Connect: The World of Critical Care Nursing 2005;3(4):111–5.

18 Grenvik A, Pinsky MR. Evolution of the intensive care unit as a clinical center and critical care medicine as a discipline. Crit Care Clin 2009;25(1):239–50, x. Epub 2009/03/10.

19 Fairman J, Lynaugh JE. Critical care nursing: A history. Philadelphia: University of Pennsylvania Press; 1998.

20 Scholes J. Developing expertise in critical care nursing. Oxford: Blackwell Publishing; 2006.

21 World Federation of Critical Care Nurses. World Federation of Critical Care Nurses Website. World Federation of Critical Care Nurses; 2014 [cited 2014 19 May].

22 Morris PWG, Crawford L, Hodgson D, Shepherd MM, Thomas J. Exploring the role of formal bodies of knowledge in defining a profession – the case of project management. International Journal of Project Management 2006;24(8):710–21.

23 International Council of Nurses (ICN). Guidelines on Specialisation in Nursing. Geneva: International Council of Nurses; 1992.

24 Polit DF, Tatano Beck C. Nursing research: Generating and assessing evidence for nursing practice. Philadelphia: Wolters Kluwer; 2012.

25 Bergman MM, editor. Advances in mixed methods research: Theories and applications. Los Angeles: Sage; 2008.

26 Cooke A, Smith D, Booth A. Beyond PICO: the SPIDER tool for qualitative evidence synthesis. Qual Health Res 2012;22(10):1435–43. Epub 2012/07/26.

27 Elliott D. Making research connections to improve clinical practice [editorial]. Aust Crit Care 2000;13:2–3.

28 Wallis M, Chaboyer W. Building the clinical bridge: an Australian success. Nursing Research and Practice 2012;2012:579072.

29 Deutschman CS, Ahrens T, Cairns CB, Sessler CN, Parsons PE, Critical Care Societies Collaborative UTFoCCR. Multisociety task force for critical care research: key issues and recommendations. Am J Crit Care 2012;21(1):15–23.

30 Wilson S, Ramelet AS, Zuiderduyn S. Research priorities for nursing care of infants, children and adolescents: a West Australian Delphi study. J Clin Nurs 2010;19(13–14):1919–28.

31 Marshall A. Research priorities for Australian critical care nurses: do we need them? Aust Crit Care 2004;17(4):142–4, 6, 8–50. Epub 2007/11/28.

32 Swenson-Britt E, Reineck C. Research education for clinical nurses: a pilot study to determine research self-efficacy in critical care nurses. J Contin Educ Nurs 2009;40(10):454–61. Epub 2009/10/17.

33 Australian College of Critical Care Nurses (ACCCN). Position Statement on the Provision of Critical Care Nursing Education. Melbourne: ACCCN, 2006.

34 Australian College of Critical Care Nurses. Competency standards for specialist critical care nurses, 3rd ed. Melbourne: Australian College of Critical Care Nurses; 2015.

35 Aari RL, Tarja S, Helena LK. Competence in intensive and critical care nursing: a literature review. Intensive Crit Care Nurs 2008;24(2):78–89. Epub 2008/01/22.

36 Bench S, Crowe D, Day T, Jones M, Wilebore S. Developing a competency framework for critical care to match patient need. Intensive Crit Care Nurs 2003;19(3):136–42.

37 American Association of Critical-Care Nurses. American Association of Critical-Care Nurses Website. Aliso Viejo: American Association of Critical-Care Nurses; 2014 [cited 2014 22 September].

38 Coghlan J. Critical care nursing in Australia. Intensive Care Nurs 1986;2(1):3–7.

39 Armstrong DJ, Adam J. The impact of a postgraduate critical care course on nursing practice. Nurse Education in Practice 2002;2(3):169–75.

40 Badir A. A review of international critical care education requirements and comparisons with Turkey. Connect: The World of Critical Care Nursing 2004;3(2):48–51.

41 Baktoft B, Drigo E, Hohl ML, Klancar S, Tseroni M, Putzai P. A survey of critical care nursing education in Europe. Connect: The World of Critical Care Nursing. 2003;2(3):85–7.

42 Chaboyer W, Dunn SV, Theobald K, Aitken L, Perrott J. Critical care education: an examination of students' perspectives. Nurse Educ Today 2001;21(7):526–33.

43 Gill FJ, Leslie GD, Grech C, Latour JM. A review of critical care nursing staffing, education and practice standards. Aust Crit Care 2012;25(4):224–37.

44 Aitken LM, Currey J, Marshall A, Elliott D. The diversity of critical care nursing education in Australian universities. Aust Crit Care 2006;19(2):46–52.

45 European Commission – Education and Training. The Bologna process – Towards the European higher education area. Brussels: European Commission; 2010.

46 Skees J. Continuing education: a bridge to excellence in critical care nursing. Crit Care Nurs Quarterly 2010;33(2):104–16. Epub 2010/03/18.

47 Hanley E, Higgins A. Assessment of clinical practice in intensive care: a review of the literature. Intensive Crit Care Nurs 2005;21(5):268–75. Epub 2005/09/27.

48 Gill FJ, Leslie GD, Grech C, Boldy D, Latour JM. Development of Australian clinical practice outcome standards for graduates of critical care nurse education. J Clin Nurs 2014. Epub 2014/05/13.

49 Hardcastle JE. 'Back to the bedside': graduate level education in critical care. Nurse Educ Pract 2008;8(1):46–53.

50 Rose L, Goldsworthy S, O'Brien-Pallas L, Nelson S. Critical care nursing education and practice in Canada and Australia: a comparative review. Int J Nurs Stud 2008;45(7):1103–9.

51 Gijbels H, O'Connell R, Dalton-O'Connor C, O'Donovan M. A systematic review evaluating the impact of post-registration nursing and midwifery education on practice. Nurse Educ Pract 2010;10(2):64–9.

52 Pirret A. Master's level critical care nursing education: a time for review and debate. Intensive Crit Care Nurs 2007;23(4):183–6.

53 Underwood M, Elliott D, Aitken L, Austen D, Currey J, Field T et al. Position statement on postgraduate critical care nursing education – October 1999. Aust Crit Care 1999;12(4):160–4.

54 Fisher MJ, Marshall AP, Kendrick TS. Competency standards for critical care nurses: do they measure up? Aust J Adv Nurs 2005;22(4):32–40.

55 Lakanmaa RL, Suominen T, Perttila J, Ritmala-Castren M, Vahlberg T, Leino-Kilpi H. Basic competence in intensive and critical care nursing: development and psychometric testing of a competence scale. J Clin Nurs 2014;23(5–6):799–810.

56 Nalle MA, Brown ML, Herrin DM. The Nursing Continuing Education Consortium: a collaborative model for education and practice. Nursing Administration Quarterly 2001;26(1):60–6.

57 Cowan DT, Norman I, Coopamah VP. Competence in nursing practice: a controversial concept – a focused review of literature. Nurse Educ Today 2005;25(5):355–62.

58 Boyle M, Butcher R, Kenney C. Study to validate the outcome goal, competencies and educational objectives for use in intensive care orientation programs. Aust Crit Care 1998;11(1):20–4.

59 Numminen O, Meretoja R, Isoaho H, Leino-Kilpi H. Professional competence of practising nurses. J Clin Nurs 2013;22(9–10):1411–23.

60 American Association of Critical-Care Nurses (AACN). Scope of Practice and Standards of Professional Performance for the Acute and Critical Care Clinical Nurse Specialist. Aliso Viejo, California: American Association of Critical-Care Nurses; 2002.

61 Williams G, Chaboyer W, Thornsteindottir R, Fulbrook P, Shelton C, Wojner A et al. Worldwide overview of critical care nursing organizations and their activities. Int Nurs Rev 2001;48(4):208–17. Epub 2002/01/05.

62 Endacott R, Chaboyer W. The nursing role in ICU outreach: an international exploratory study. Nursing in Critical Care 2006;11(2):94–102. Epub 2006/03/25.

63 Chaboyer W, Foster MM, Foster M, Kendall E. The Intensive Care Unit liaison nurse: towards a clear role descrption. Intensive and Critical Care Nurses 2004;20:77–86.

64 Eliott S, Chaboyer W, Ernest D, Doric A, Endacott R. A national survey of Australian Intensive Care Unit (ICU) Liaison Nurse (LN) services. Australian Critical Care 2012;25(4):253–62.

65 Alberto L, Zotarez H, Canete AA, Niklas JE, Enriquez JM, Geronimo MR et al. A description of the ICU liaison nurse role in Argentina. Intensive Crit Care Nurs 2014;30(1):31–7.

66 Niven DJ, Bastos JF, Stelfox HT. Critical care transition programs and the risk of readmission or death after discharge from an ICU: a systematic review and meta-analysis. Crit Care Med 2014;42(1):179–87. Epub 2013/08/31.

67 ICN Nurse Practitioner/Advanced Practice Nursing Network. Definition and characteristics of the role – Nurse practitioner and advanced practice roles. Geneva: International Council of Nurses (ICN), <http://www.international.aanp.org/Practice?APNRoles>; 2014 [accessed 22.09.14].

68 Fry M. Literature review of the impact of nurse practitioners in critical care services. Nursing in Critical Care 2011;16(2):58–66.

69 Herring S. Retrieval nurse practitioners: the role and the challenges. Australian Critical Care 2013;26(3):102–3.

70 Gardner G, Gardner A, Middleton S, Della P, Kain V, Doubrovsky A. The work of nurse practitioners. J Adv Nurs 2010;66(10):2160–9. Epub 2010/07/20.

71 Buckley T, Cashin A, Stuart M, Browne G, Dunn SV. Nurse practitioner prescribing practices: the most frequently prescribed medications. J Clin Nurs 2013;22(13–14):2053–63.

72 Chang IW, Shyu Y-I, Tsay P-K, Tang W-R. Comparison of nurse practitioners' perceptions of required competencies and self-evaluated competencies in Taiwan. Journal of Clinical Nursing 2012;21(17–18):2679–89.

73 Kilpatrick K. How do nurse practitioners in acute care affect perceptions of team effectiveness? J Clin Nurs 2013;22(17–18):2636–47. Epub 2013/03/29.

74 Davidson PM, Elliott D, Daly J. Clinical leadership in contemporary clinical practice: implications for nursing in Australia. J Nurs Manag 2006;14(3):180–7.

75 Shirey MR. Authentic leaders creating healthy work environments for nursing practice. Am J Crit Care 2006;15(3):256–67.

76 Shirey MR, Fisher ML. Leadership agenda for change toward healthy work environments in acute and critical care. Critical care nurse 2008;28(5):66–79. Epub 2008/10/02.

77 Crofts L. A leadership programme for critical care. Intensive Crit Care Nurs 2006;22(4):220–7.

78 Cook MJ. The renaissance of clinical leadership. Int Nurs Rev 2001;48(1):38–46.

79 De Geest S, Claessens P, Longerich H, Schubert M. Transformational leadership: worthwhile the investment! Eur J Cardiovasc Nurs 2003;2(1):3–5.

80 Manojlovich M. The effect of nursing leadership on hospital nurses' professional practice behaviors. J Nurs Adm 2005;35(7-8):366–74.

81 Murphy L. Transformational leadership: a cascading chain reaction. J Nurs Manag 2005;13(2):128–36.

82 Ohman KA. Nurse manager leadership. J Nurs Adm 1999;29(12):16, 21.

83 Ohman KA. The transformational leadership of critical care nurse-managers. Dimens Crit Care Nurs 2000;19(1):46–54.

84 Stanley D. Clinical leadership characteristics confirmed. Journal of Research in Nursing 2014;19(2):118–28

85 Richardson J, West MA, Cuthbertson BH. Team working in intensive care: current evidence and future endeavors. Curr Opin Crit Care 2010;16(6):643–8. Epub 2010/08/26.

86 Bender M, Connelly CD, Glaser D, Brown C. Clinical nurse leader impact on microsystem care quality. Nurs Res 2012;61(5):326–32. Epub 2012/09/01.

87 Eggenberger T. Exploring the charge nurse role: holding the frontline. J Nurs Adm 2012;42(11):502–6. Epub 2012/10/27.

88 Tregunno D, Jeffs L, Hall LM, Baker R, Doran D, Bassett SB. On the ball: leadership for patient safety and learning in critical care. J Nurs Adm 2009;39(7–8):334–9.

89 Bender M, Connelly CD, Brown C. Interdisciplinary collaboration: the role of the clinical nurse leader. J Nurs Manag 2013;21(1):165–74. Epub 2013/01/24.

90 Dierckx de Casterle B, Willemse A, Verschueren M, Milisen K. Impact of clinical leadership development on the clinical leader, nursing team and care-giving process: a case study. J Nurs Manag 2008;16(6):753–63.

91 Omoike O, Stratton KM, Brooks BA, Ohlson S, Storfjell JL. Advancing nursing leadership: a model for program implementation and measurement. Nurs Adm Q 2011;35(4):323–32. Epub 2011/09/09.

92 McCloughen A, O'Brien L, Jackson D. Esteemed connection: creating a mentoring relationship for nurse leadership. Nurs Inq 2009;16(4):326–36.

93 Taylor CA, Taylor JC, Stoller JK. The influence of mentorship and role modeling on developing physician-leaders: views of aspiring and established physician-leaders. J Gen Intern Med 2009;24(10):1130–4.

94 Williams AK, Parker VT, Milson-Hawke S, Cairney K, Peek C. Preparing clinical nurse leaders in a regional Australian teaching hospital. J Contin Educ Nurs 2009;40(12):571–6.

95 Redman RW. Leadership succession planning: an evidence-based approach for managing the future. J Nurs Adm 2006;36(6):292–7.

96 Hancock B. Developing new nursing leaders. Am J Nurs 2014;114(6):59–62. Epub 2014/05/30.

97 McNamara MS, Fealy GM, Casey M, O'Connor T, Patton D, Doyle L et al. Mentoring, coaching and action learning: interventions in a national clinical leadership development programme. J Clin Nurs 2014;23(17–18):2533–41. Epub 2014/01/08.

Chapter 2

Systems and resources

Denise Harris, Ged Williams

Learning objectives

After reading this chapter, you should be able to:

- describe historical influences on the development of critical care and the way this resource is currently viewed and used
- explain the organisational arrangements and interfaces that may be established to govern a critical care unit
- identify resources and supports that assist in the governance and management of a critical care unit
- describe considerations in planning for the physical design and equipment requirements of a critical care unit
- describe the human resource requirements, supports and training necessary to ensure a safe and appropriate workforce
- explain common risks and the appropriate strategies, policies and contingencies necessary to support staff and patient safety
- discuss leadership and management principles that influence the quality, efficacy and appropriateness of the critical care unit
- discuss critical care considerations in responding to the threat of a pandemic.

Introduction

In 1966 Dr B Galbally, a hospital resuscitation officer at St Vincent's Hospital, Melbourne, published the first article on the planning and organisation of an intensive care unit (ICU) in Australia.[1] He identified that critically ill patients who have a reasonable chance of recovery require life-saving treatments and constant nursing and medical care, but that this intensity of service delivery 'does not necessarily continue until the patient dies, and it should not continue after the patient is considered no longer recoverable'.[1]

The need for prudent and rational allocation of limited financial and human resources was as important in the 1960s as it is today. This chapter explores the influences on the development of critical care and the way this resource is currently viewed and used; describes various organisational, staffing and training arrangements that need to be in place; considers the planning, design and equipment needs of a critical care unit; covers other aspects of resource management including the budget and financial modelling; and finishes with a description of how critical care staff may respond to a pandemic or other acute and dramatic demands on resources. First, however, important ethical decisions in managing the resources of a critical care unit are discussed below.

> **Practice tip**
>
> Ethical decision making in terms of managing resources at the unit level is as critical as ethical decision making at the individual patient level in terms of access to scarce critical care resources. Open and transparent decision making is imperative.

Ethical allocation and utilisation of resources

In management, as in clinical practice, careful consideration of the pros and cons of various decisions must be made on a daily basis. The interests of the individual patient, extended family, treating team, the organisation and the broader community are rarely congruent, nor are they usually consistent. Decisions surrounding the provision of critical care services are often governed by a compromise between conflicting interests and ethical theories. Two main perspectives on ethical decision making, *deontological* and *utilitarian*, are explored briefly.[2]

The *deontological* principle suggests that a person has a fundamental duty to act in a certain way – for example, to provide full, active medical treatment to all persons. The rule of rescue, or the innate desire to do something – anything – to help those in dire need, may be a corollary to the deontological principle. These two concepts, the duty to act and the rule of rescue, tend to sit well with many trained and skilled clinicians and the Hippocratic Oath. In critical care there are some families and some clinicians who, for personal and/or religious reasons, take a strong stand and demand treatments and actions based on a deontological view (i.e. the fundamental belief that a certain action is the only one that should be considered in a given situation).

At the other extreme is the *utilitarian* view, which suggests an action is right only if it achieves the greatest good for the greatest number of people. This concept tends to sit well with pragmatic managers and policy makers. An example of a utilitarian view might be to ration funding allocated to heart transplantation and to utilise any saved money for prevention and awareness campaigns. A heart disease prevention campaign lends a greater benefit to a greater number in the population than does one transplant procedure.

The appropriate provision and allocation of critical care services and resources tend to sit somewhere between these two extreme positions. This dilemma is true of all health services, but critical care, because of its high-technology, high-cost, low-volume outputs, is under particular scrutiny to justify its resource usage within a healthcare system. Therefore, not only do critical care managers need to be prudent, responsible and efficient guardians of this precious resource, they need to be seen as such if they are to retain the confidence of, and legitimacy with, the broader community values of the day.

Historical influences

Developing larger and more sophisticated services such as ICUs can attract media and public attention. The 1960s and early 1970s saw the development of the first critical care units in many parts of the developed world. If a hospital was to be relevant, it had to have one. In fact, what distinguished a tertiary referral teaching hospital from other hospitals was at its fundamental conclusion, the existence of a critical care unit.[3] Over time, practical reasons for establishing critical care units have led to their spread to most acute hospitals with more than 100 beds. Reasons for the proliferation of critical care services include, but are not limited to:

- economies of scale by cohorting critically ill patients to one area
- development of expertise in doctors and nurses who specialise in the care and treatment of critically ill patients
- an ever-growing body of research demonstrating that critically ill patient outcomes are better if patients are cared for in a specifically equipped and staffed critical care unit.[4]

Funding for critical care services has evolved over time to be somewhat separate from mainstream patient funding, owing to the unique requirements of critical care units. Critical care is unique because patients are at the severe end of the disease spectrum. For instance, the funding provided for a patient admitted for chronic obstructive airway disease in an ICU on a ventilator is very different from that provided for a patient with the same diagnosis, but treated in a medical ward only. Each country/jurisdictional health department tends to create its own unique approach to funding ICU services. For instance, the Research and Development Corporation study[4] examined funding methods in many countries and concluded that there was no obvious example of 'best practice' or a dominant approach used by a majority of systems. Each approach had advantages and disadvantages, particularly in relation to the financial risk involved in providing intensive care. Although the risk of underfunding intensive care may be highest in systems that apply Diagnosis Related Groups (DRGs) to the entire episode of hospital care, including intensive care, concerns about potential underfunding were voiced in all systems reviewed. Arrangements for additional funding in the form of co-payments or surcharges may reduce the risk of underfunding. However, these approaches also face the difficulty of determining the appropriate level to be paid.[4]

Australia has established the Independent Hospital Pricing Authority whose task it has been to harmonise the variations in funding processes across all states and territories and to establish a common, consistent and transparent funding process to be agreed by all.[5] But agreement on a common funding model for intensive care services has been difficult.

The Independent Hospital Pricing Authority determined they would develop a list of ICUs that will be eligible to receive an ICU adjustment based on a measure of the size of the ICU and the overall complexity of the mix of patients within each ICU, but would continue working with stakeholders and jurisdictions to explore alternative patient-based mechanisms for determining the ICU adjustment for future years during 2014.[6] The current Australian National Efficient Price Determination for 2014 used a total sample of 56,835 separations with ICU hours and costs from establishments with eligible ICUs/PICUs.

The weighted mean of the hourly ICU costs taken across states was used to derive a national ICU rate of $190.[7] Eligible ICUs and PICUs are those belonging to hospitals that report more than 24,000 ICU hours with more than 20% of those hours reported to involve the use of mechanical ventilation. The specified hospitals with eligible ICUs and/or PICUs number a total of 71 (NSW 25, Qld 17, Vic 15, SA 5, WA 4, Tas 2, NT 2, ACT 1).[7] Although the Independent Hospital Pricing Authority outcome may appear to be a complex compromise, it is in fact a significant step forward to have a single funding model across the country, albeit at the strategic level. Future work by Independent Hospital Pricing Authority and others hopes to further refine the precise patient-based measures that can align critical care activity with funding more accurately with the ultimate ideal being that the measures will also align with quality performance and outcomes.

At the hospital level, most critical care units have capped and finite budgets that are linked to 'open beds' – that is, beds that are equipped, staffed and ready to be occupied by a patient, regardless of whether they are actually occupied.[8] This is one crude yet common way that hospitals can control costs emanating from the critical care unit. The other method is to limit the number of trained and experienced nurses available to the specialty; consequently, a shortage of qualified critical care nurses results in a shortage of critical care beds, resulting in a rationing of the service available. The capping of beds and qualified critical care nurse positions can be convenient mechanisms to limit access and utilisation of this expensive service – critical care.

Practice tip

The capping of beds and qualified critical care nurse positions can be convenient mechanisms to limit access and utilisation of this expensive service – critical care.

Funding based on achieving positive patient outcomes would be ideal, as it would ensure that critical care units were using their resources only for those patients who were most likely to achieve positive outcomes in terms of morbidity and mortality. However, funding based only on health outcomes does raise the risk of encouraging clinicians to 'cherrypick' only the most 'profitable' or 'successful' patient groups at the expense of others. In private (for-profit) hospitals or countries with very poor health systems, cherrypicking only those patients for whom a successful outcome is guaranteed is likely to be more common, whereas in the public hospitals of most Western countries an educated assessment is often applied to the decision as to whether a patient should enter the critical care unit or not.

It is vital to note the very important role played by rural and isolated health services and, in particular, critical care units and outreach services in these regions. Many of the contemporary activity-based funding formulas are difficult to apply to these settings. There are diseconomies of scale in such settings as a result of small bed numbers, limited but highly skilled nurses and doctors and unpredictable peaks and troughs in demand, which make workforce planning and the management of call-in/overtime and fatigue problems difficult for small teams to manage. The professional isolation and limited access to education, training and peer support can also create morale problems for some members of the team. Furthermore, the diseconomies and isolation require empathetic funding processes to recognise the difficulties unique to regional and isolated critical care services. If such units are to remain viable and capable of delivering levels of safe and effective care equivalent to those expected in larger metropolitan hospitals, additional funding and support is required to compensate for the cost and tyranny of distance.

Economic considerations and principles

One early comprehensive study of costs found that 8% of patients admitted to the ICU consumed 50% of resources but had a mortality rate of 70%, while 41% of patients received no acute interventions and consumed only 10% of resources.[9] More recent studies show that, although critical care services are increasingly being provided to patients who are older and with a higher severity of acute and chronic illnesses, long-term survival outcome has improved with time, suggesting that critical care services may still be cost-effective despite the changes in case-mix.[10–12]

Some authors provide scenarios as examples of poor economic decision making in critical care and argue for less extreme variances in the types of patient ICUs choose to treat in order to reduce the burden of cost on the health dollar.[13,14] Others have suggested that if all health care provided were appropriate, rationing would not be required.[15] Defining what is 'appropriate' can be subjective, although not always. The Research and Development

TABLE 2.1

Approaches to assessing treatment options

APPROACH	DESCRIPTION
Benefit–risk approach	The benefit of treatment and the inherent risks to the patient are assessed to inform a decision; this approach excludes monetary costs
Benefit–cost approach	Evaluate the benefit and cost of the decision to proceed; this approach incorporates cost to patient and society
Implicit approach	The medical practitioner provides the service and judges its appropriateness

Adapted from Ettelt S, Nolte E. Funding intensive care – approaches in systems using diagnosis-related groups. Cambridge: Rand Europe, <http://www.rand.org/content/dam/rand/pubs/technical_reports/2010/RAND_ TR792.pdf>; 2010 [accessed 29.07.14], with permission.

Corporation group[4,16] suggests that there are at least three approaches that can be used to assess appropriateness of care (Table 2.1). These include the benefit–risk, benefit–cost and implicit approaches.

The first two approaches are considered to be explicit approaches, while the third tends to be implicit. However, all approaches have a subjective element. Although the implicit approach is considered to be subjective in nature, the medical practitioner must contemplate benefit–risk and benefit–cost considerations but should also involve the patient/family in the contemplation and ultimate decision. Similar discussions have been advocated by the Taskforce on Values, Ethics and Rationing in Critical Care who suggest rationing is not only unavoidable but essential to ensuring the ethical distribution of medical goods and services.[17]

What is best for the patient is not just the opinion of the treating doctor and needs to be considered in much broader terms such as the patient's previous expressed wishes and the family's opinion as de facto patient representatives. The quality of the decision and the quality of the expected outcome require many competing considerations.

Practice tip

What is best for the patient is not just the opinion of the treating doctor and needs to be considered in much broader terms such as the patient's previous expressed wishes and the family's opinion as de facto patient representatives.

Proponents of the 'quality' agenda in health care have argued for 'best practice' and 'best outcomes' in the provision of health services, although it may be more pragmatic to consider 'value' when discussing what is and what is not an appropriate decision in critical care. The following equation expresses the concept 'value' simply:

$$\text{Value} = \frac{\text{Quality}}{\text{Cost}} = \frac{\text{Benefit} \times \text{Sustainability}}{\text{Price} \times \text{Suffering}}$$

The quality of the outcome is a function of the benefit to be achieved and the sustainability of the benefit. The benefit of critical care is associated with such factors as survival, longevity and improved quality of life (e.g. greater functioning capacity and less pain and anxiety). The benefit is enhanced by sustainability: the longer the benefit is maintained, the better it is.[18]

Cost is separated into two components, monetary (price) and non-monetary (suffering). Non-monetary costs include such considerations as morbidity, mortality, pain and anxiety in the individual, or broader societal costs and suffering (e.g. opportunity costs to others who might have used the resources but for the current occupants, and what other health services might have been provided but for the cost of this service).[18]

Ethico-economic analyses of services such as critical care and expensive treatments such as organ transplantation are the new consideration of this century and are as important to good governance as are discussions of medico-legal considerations. Sound ethical principles to inform and guide human and material resource management and budgets ought to prevail in the management of limited health resources.[2]

Budget and finance

This section provides information on types of budget, the budgeting process and how to analyse costs and expenditures to ensure that resources are utilised appropriately and in line with the service management plan, that is the operational and service goals of the critical care team expected by the hospital and broader community. As noted by one author, 'Nothing is so terrifying for clinicians accustomed to daily issues of life and death as to be given responsibility for the financial affairs of their hospital division!'.[15] Yet, in essence, developing and managing a budget for a critical care unit follows many of the same principles as managing a family budget. Consideration of value for money, prioritising needs and wants and living within a relatively fixed income is common to all. This section in no way undermines the skill and precision provided by the accounting profession, nor will it enable clinicians to usurp the role of hospital business managers. Rather, the aim is to provide the requisite knowledge to empower clinicians to manage the key components of budget development and budget setting, and to know what questions to ask when confronted by this most daunting responsibility of managing a service budget.

> **Practice tip**
>
> Nothing is so terrifying for clinicians accustomed to daily issues of life and death as to be given responsibility for the financial affairs of their hospital division!

Types of budget

There are essentially three types of budget that a manager must consider: personnel, operational and capital. Within these budget types, there are two basic cost types: fixed and variable. Fixed costs are those essential to the service and are relatively constant, regardless of the fluctuations in workload or throughput (e.g. nurse unit manager salary, security, ventilators). Variable costs change with changing throughput (e.g. nurse agency or consumables usage), especially if used in response to influx of demand and resulting consumables such as linen, dressings and drugs.

Personnel budget

Health care is a labour-intensive service, and critical care epitomises this fact with personnel costs being the most expensive component of the unit's budget. The staffing requirement for critical care generally follows a formula of x nurses per open (funded) bed. This figure is expressed in full-time equivalents (FTEs), i.e. the equivalent of a person working a 40-hour week if the standard full-time working week is 40 hours. This may equate to 5×8-hour shifts per week or 20×12-hour shifts in a 6-week period.

Personnel costs include productive and non-productive hours. Productive hours are those utilised to provide direct work. A manager will determine the minimum or optimum number of nurses to be rostered per shift and then calculate the nursing hours per day, multiplied by the hourly rate of pay and any penalties that are to be attributed to work done during the after-business-hours period. Non-productive hours include sick leave, holiday leave, education hours, maternity leave and any other paid time away from the actual job that staff are employed to do.

Personnel budgets tend to be fixed costs, in that the majority of staff are employed permanently, based on an expected or forecast demand. Prudent managers tend to employ 5–10% less than the actual forecast demand and use casual staff to 'flex-up' the available FTE staff establishment in periods of increasing demand, hence contributing a small but variable component to the personnel budget.[19]

Operational budget

All other non-personnel costs (except major capital equipment) tend to be allocated to the operational budget. This includes fixed costs such as minor equipment, maintenance contracts, utility costs (e.g. electricity) and variable costs that fluctuate with patient type and number (e.g. pharmaceuticals, meals, consumable supplies such as gloves and dressings, laundry).

Compared with personnel costs, operational costs in critical care tend to be relatively small, but they can be managed and rationed with the help of good information and cooperation. For example, there is a range of dressing materials available on the market, and a simple dressing that requires less expensive materials should always be used unless a more expensive product is indicated and a protocol exists to inform staff of this clinical need.

> **Practice tip**
>
> Compared with personnel costs, operational costs in critical care tend to be relatively small and can be managed and rationed with the help of good information and cooperation.

Fixed costs can also be turned into variable costs and hence encourage efficient usage. For example, pressure-reduction mattresses, traditionally purchased as a fixed asset with variable (and unpredictable) repair and maintenance costs, can now be leased on a per-day or per-week basis, with no need for storage, cleaning or maintenance costs. Further, critical care managers can work with other hospital managers to create 'purchasing power' by cooperating to standardise the range of products used to obtain a better price for a product that will benefit all users.

Capital budget

Capital budget items are generally expensive and/or large fixed assets that are considered long-term investments, such as building extensions, renovations and large equipment purchases. Capital budget items tend to be considered as assets that are depreciated over time. Most hospitals consider these items as a global asset – that is, as a group of investment items and activities for the hospital – rather than attributing these costs to an individual unit or department.

To request a capital budget item, a written proposal is generally required describing the item, its expected benefits, whether it replaces an existing item's service or function, the cost, possible revenue and cost-mitigating benefits. This analysis does not always have to demonstrate a profit, although the value and benefit of the service would need to be established.

Budget process

The budget includes three fundamental steps: 1) budget preparation and approval, 2) budget analysis and reporting and 3) budget control and action.

> **Practice tip**
>
> The budget includes three fundamental steps: 1) budget preparation and approval, 2) budget analysis and reporting and 3) budget control and action.

Budget preparation and approval

A budget plan essentially runs in parallel with a unit or service management plan, forecasting likely activity and resulting financial costs. In most circumstances the preceding year's activity and costs are a good benchmark on which to base the next year's budget. However, hospital expectations in terms of new services, greater patient throughput or changes to staff salary entitlements will need to be factored into the new budget.

The budget period is generally a financial year, but developing monthly budgets (cash flowing) to coincide with predictable variations allows for a more realistic representation of how costs are incurred and paid throughout the financial year period. If the budget plan is well constructed, one always hopes and expects the final budget allocation (i.e. the approved budget) to be close to achievable.

Budget analysis and reporting

Most critical care managers analyse their expenditure against budget projections on a monthly basis, to identify variances from planned expenditure. Information should not merely be financial: a breakdown of the monthly and year-to-date expenditures for personnel (productive and non-productive), and operational (fixed and variable) costs, should be matched against other known measurable indicators of activity or productivity (e.g. patient bed-days, patient diagnosis types/groups and staffing hours, including overtime and other special payments).[15]

One common management maxim is: if it cannot be measured, then it cannot be controlled. Clinical managers therefore need to work closely with finance managers to develop consistent data measurements and reports to inform themselves and staff about where they should focus their efforts to achieve the approved budget target.

Budget control and action

When signs of poor performance or financial overrun are evident, managers cannot merely analyse the financial reports, hoping that things will sort themselves out. Every variance of a sizeable amount requires an explanation. Some will be obvious: an outbreak of community influenza among staff will increase sick leave and casual staff costs for a period of time. Other overruns can be insidious but no less important: overtime payments, although sometimes unavoidable, can also reflect poor time management or a culture of some staff wanting to boost their income surreptitiously.[19]

An effective method of controlling the budget is to actively engage staff in the process of managing costs. Managers can explain to staff how the budget has been developed and how their performance against budget is progressing, and identify areas for potential improvement. Seeking ideas from staff on how to improve efficiency and productivity and giving them some responsibility for the budget performance can encourage an esprit de corps and improvements from the whole team that a single manager cannot achieve alone.[20]

Developing a business case

The most common reason for writing a business case is to justify the resources and capital expenditure to gain the support and/or approval for a change in service provision and/or purchase of a significant new piece of equipment/technology. This section provides an overview of a business case and a format for its presentation. The business case can be an invaluable tool in the strategic decision-making process, particularly in an environment of constrained resources.[21]

A business case is a management tool that is used in the process of meeting the overall strategic plan of an organisation. Within a setting such as health care, the business case is required to outline clearly the clinical need and implications to be understood by leaders. Financial imperatives, such as return on investment, must also be defined and identified.[22,23] A business case is a document in which all the facts relevant to the case are documented and linked cohesively. Various templates are available (see *Online resources*) to assist with the layout. Key questions are generally the starting point for the response to a business case: why, what, when, where and how, with each question's response adding additional information to the process (Table 2.2). Business cases can vary in length from many pages to just a couple. Most organisations will have standardised headings and formats for the presentation of these documents. If the document is lengthy inclusion of an executive summary is recommended to summarise the salient points of the business case (Box 2.1).

> **Practice tip**
>
> A business case is a management tool that is used in the process of meeting the overall strategic plan of an organisation.

BOX 2.1

Business case: Sample headings

Title

Purpose

Background

Key issues

Cost–benefit analysis

Recommendations

Risk assessment

In summary, the business case is an important tool that is increasingly required at all levels of an organisation to clearly define a proposed service change or equipment purchase. This document should include clear goals and outcomes, a cost–benefit analysis, quality and safety considerations and timelines for achievement of the solution.

> **TABLE 2.2**
> Key questions in writing a business case
>
> | QUESTION | EXAMPLE |
> | --- | --- |
> | **Why?** | Consider the background to the project, and why it is needed, including PEST (political, economic, sociological, technological) and SWOT (strengths, weaknesses, opportunities and threats) analysis |
> | **What?** | Clearly identify and define the project and the purpose of the business case and outline the solution. Clearly defined goals, outcomes and measurable benefits should be documented |
> | **What if?** | Make a risk assessment of the current situation, including any controls currently in place to address/mitigate the issue, and a risk assessment following the implementation of the proposed solution |
> | **When?** | Determine the timelines for the implementation and achievement of the project/solution |
> | **Where?** | Consider the context within which the project will be undertaken, if not already included in the background material |
> | **How?** | Determine how much money, people and equipment, for example, will be required to achieve the benefits. A clear cost–benefit analysis should be included in response to this question |

Critical care environment

A critical care unit is a distinct unit within a hospital that has easy access to the emergency department, operating theatre and medical imaging. It provides care to patients with a life-threatening illness or injury and concentrates the clinical expertise and technological and therapeutic resources required. The College of Intensive Care Medicine (CICM)[24] and the Intensive Care Society[25] define three levels of intensive care to support the role delineation of a particular hospital, dependent upon staffing expertise, facilities and support services. Critical care facilities vary in nature and extent between hospitals and are dependent on the operational policies of each individual facility. In smaller facilities, the broad spectrum of critical care may be provided in combined units (intensive care, high-dependency [HDU], coronary care unit [CCU]) to improve flexibility and aid the efficient use of available resources.[26] While there are no national guidelines for defining standards of workforce and facility expectations with respect to CCUs, some state health services have developed their own to try and encourage consistent standards of practice across CCUs.

Environmental design

The functional, organisational and unit designs are governed by available finances, an operational brief and the building and design standards of the state or country in which the hospital is located. A critical care unit should have access to minimum support facilities, which include staff station, clean utility, dirty utility, store room(s), education and teaching space, staff amenities, patients' ensuites, patients' bathroom, linen storage, disposal room, pathology area and offices. Most notably, the actual bed space/care area for patients needs to be well designed.[26,27]

The design of the patient's bed-space has received considerable attention in recent years. Most governments have developed minimum guidelines to assist in the design

process. Each bed space should be a minimum of 20–25 square metres and provide for visual privacy from casual observation. At least one hand basin per single room or per two beds should be provided to meet minimum infection control guidelines.[26,27] Each bed space should have piped medical gases (oxygen and air), suction, adequate electrical outlets (essential and non-essential), data points and task lighting sufficient for use during the performance of bedside procedures. Further detailed descriptions are available in various health department documents.[26,27]

Equipment

Since the advent of critical care units, healthcare delivery has become increasingly dependent on medical technology to deliver that care. Equipment can be categorised into several funding groups: capital expenditure (generally in excess of A$10,000 or £5,000), equipment expenditure (all equipment less than A$10,000 or £5,000) and the disposable products and devices required to support the use of equipment. This section examines how to evaluate, procure and maintain that equipment.

Initial set-up requirements

Critical care units require baseline equipment that allows the unit to deliver safe and effective patient care. The list of specific equipment required by each individual unit will be governed by the scope of that unit's function. For example, a unit that provides care to patients after neurosurgery will require the ability to monitor intracranial pressure. Table 2.3 lists the basic equipment requirements for a critical care unit. Information technology and communications options and requirements are growing rapidly in health and in particular in the critical care environment. The rapid pace of innovation and change in this area requires managers to think carefully when setting up information technology infrastructure and to be careful not to over capitalise on technology that might not be

---

TABLE 2.3
Basic equipment requirements

MONITORING	THERAPEUTIC
Monitors (including central station)	Ventilators (invasive and non-invasive)
End-tidal CO_2 monitoring	Infusion pumps
Arterial blood gas analyser (± electrolytes)	Syringe drivers
Invasive monitoring	CVVHDF
• arterial	EDD-f
• central venous pressure	Resuscitators
• intracranial pressure	Temporary pacemaker
• pulse-induced contour cardiac output pulmonary artery	Defibrillator
Access to image intensifier	Suctioning apparatus
Ultrasound	
Access to CT/MRI	

CT = computerised tomography; CVVHDF = continuous veno-venous haemodiafiltration; EDD-f = extended daily dialysis filtration; MRI = magnetic resonance imaging.

BOX 2.2

Example criteria for product evaluation

- Safety
- Performance
- Quality
- Use
  - purpose
  - ease of
- Cost–benefit analysis
  - include disposables
- Cleaning
  - central sterilising supply unit
  - infection control
- Regulatory control
  - Therapeutic Goods Administration
  - Standards
- Adaptability to future technological advancements
- Service agreements
- Training requirements

Adapted from:

Association of Operating Room Nurses. Recommended practices for product selection in perioperative practice settings. AORN J 2004;79:678–82, with permission.

Elliott D, Hollins B. Product evaluation: theoretical and practical considerations. Aust Crit Care 1995;8(2):14–9, with permission.

---

easily upgradeable when new and more efficient or more effective substitutes come on to the market. Envisioning what might be available in the future is difficult but it is important to consider such matters carefully to avoid very expensive upgrades in the future.[28] Further information on information and communication technology can be found in Chapter 3.

Practice tip

Envisioning what might be available in the future is difficult but it is important to consider such matters carefully to avoid very expensive upgrades in the future.

Purchasing

The procurement of any equipment or medical device requires a rigorous process of selection and evaluation. This process should be designed to select functional, reliable products that are safe, cost-effective and environmentally conscious and that promote quality of care while avoiding duplication or rapid obsolescence.[29] In most healthcare facilities, a product evaluation committee exists to support this process, but if this is not the case it is strongly recommended that a multidisciplinary committee be set up, particularly when considering the purchase of equipment requiring capital expenditure.[30]

The product evaluation committee should include members who have an interest in the equipment being considered and should comprise, for example, biomedical engineers and representatives from the central sterile supply unit administration, infection control, end users and other departments that may have similar needs. Once a product evaluation committee has been established, clear,

objective criteria for the evaluation of the product should be determined (Box 2.2). Ideally, the committee will screen products and medical devices before a clinical evaluation is conducted to establish its viability, thus avoiding any unnecessary expenditure in time and money.[29]

The decision to purchase or lease equipment will, to some extent, be governed by the purchasing strategy approved by the hospital or health authority. The advantages of leasing equipment include the capital expenditure being defrayed over the life of the lease (usually 36 months), with ongoing servicing and product upgrades built into the lease agreement and price structure. Any final presentation from the product evaluation committee should therefore include a recommendation to purchase or lease, based on a cost–benefit analysis of the ongoing expenditure required to maintain the equipment.

Replacement and maintenance

The process for replacement of equipment is closely aligned with the process for the purchase of new equipment. The stimulus for the process to begin, however, can be either the condemning of equipment by biomedical engineers or the planned replacement of equipment nearing the end of its life cycle. In general, most capital equipment is deemed to have a life cycle of 5 years. This time frame takes into account both the longevity of the physical equipment and its technology.

Ongoing maintenance of equipment is an important part of facilitating safety in the unit. Maintenance may be provided in-house by individual facility biomedical departments or as part of a service contract arrangement with the vendor company. The provision of a maintenance/service plan should be clearly identified during the procurement phase of the equipment's purchase process. Although equipment maintenance is not the direct responsibility of the nurses in charge of the unit, they should be aware of the scheduled maintenance plan for all equipment and ensure that timely maintenance is undertaken.

Routine ongoing care of equipment is outlined in the product information and user manuals that accompany devices. This documentation clearly outlines routine care required for cleaning, storage and maintenance. All staff involved in the maintenance of clinical equipment should be trained and competent to carry it out. As specialist equipment is a fundamental element of critical care, effective resourcing includes consideration of the purchase, set-up, maintenance and replacement of equipment. Equipment is therefore an important aspect of the budget process.

> ### Practice tip
>
> The provision of a maintenance/service plan should be clearly identified during the procurement phase of the equipment's purchase process.

Staff

Staffing critical care units is an important human resource consideration. The focus of this section is on nursing staff, although the important role that medical staff and other ancillary health personnel provide is acknowledged. Nurses' salaries consume a considerable portion of any unit budget and, owing to the constant presence of nurses at the bedside, appropriate staffing plays a significant role in the quality and safety of care delivered. Nurse staffing levels influence patient outcomes both directly, through the initiation of appropriate nursing care strategies, and indirectly, by mediating and implementing the care strategies of other members of the multidisciplinary healthcare team.[31] Therefore, ensuring an appropriate skill mix is an important aspect of unit management. This section considers how appropriate staffing levels are determined and the factors, such as nurse-to-patient ratios and skill mix, which influence them.

Staffing roles

There are a number of different nursing roles in the ICU nursing team, and various guidelines determine the requirements of these roles. Various critical care nursing organisations have position statements surrounding the critical care workforce and staffing.[32–34] A designated nursing manager (nursing unit manager/nurse practice coordinator/clinical nurse manager, or equivalent title) is required for each unit to direct and guide clinical practice. The nurse manager must possess a post-registration qualification in critical care or in the clinical specialty of the unit.[24,25,32–34] A clinical nurse educator (CNE) should be available in each unit. The ACCCN recommends a minimum ratio of one full-time equivalent (FTE) CNE for every 50 nurses on the roster, to provide unit-based education and staff development.[32] Registered nurses within the unit are generally nurses with formal critical care postgraduate qualifications and varying levels of critical care experience. Although no specific staffing references are made for CCUs it is recommended they align to the standards established in other critical care areas until such time as specific CCU staffing guidelines have been developed in Australia.

In many developed economies, specialist critical care nurse education has moved into the tertiary education sector. Prior to this, and still in many other countries, critical care education has taken the form of hospital-based certificates.[35] Since this move, postgraduate, university-based programs at the graduate certificate or postgraduate diploma level are now available, although some hospital-based courses that articulate to formal university programs may also be accessible. Some critical care nursing organisations have developed position statements on the provision of critical care nursing education.[36–38] Various support staff are also required to ensure the efficient functioning of the department, including, but not limited to, administrative/clerical staff, domestic/ward assistant staff and biomedical engineering staff.

Staffing levels

A staff establishment refers to the number of nurses required to provide safe, efficient, quality care to patients. Staffing levels are influenced by many factors, including the economic, political and individual characteristics of the unit in question. Other factors, such as the population served, the services provided by the hospital and by its neighbouring hospitals and the subspecialties of medical staff working at each hospital also influence staffing. Specific issues to be considered include nurse-to-patient ratios, nursing competencies and skill mix.

The starting point for most units in the establishment of minimum, or base, staffing levels is the patient census approach. This approach uses the number and classification (ICU, HDU or CCU) of patients within the unit to determine the number of nurses required to be rostered on duty on any given shift. In many countries a registered nurse-to-patient ratio of 1:1 for ICU patients and 1:2 for high-dependency unit (HDU) patients has been accepted for many years.[32–34] Other countries, such as the USA, have lower nurse staffing levels, but in those countries nursing staff is augmented by other types of clinical or support staff, such as dialysis and respiratory technicians.[39] The limitations of this staffing approach are discussed later in this chapter. Once the base staffing numbers per shift have been established, the unit manager is required to calculate the number of FTEs that are required to implement the roster. One FTE is equivalent to the number of hours worked in one week by a full-time employee.

The development of the nursing establishment is dependent on many factors. Historical data from previous years of patient throughput and patient acuity assist in the determination of future requirements. It is often helpful for new units to contact a unit of similar size and service profile to ascertain their experiences.

Nurse-to-patient ratios

Nurse-to-patient ratios refer to the number of nursing hours required to care for a patient with a particular set of needs. In ICUs identified as combined units incorporating intensive care, coronary care and high-dependency patients,[40] different nurse-to-patient ratios are required for these often diverse groups of patients. It is important to note that nurse-to-patient ratios may be provided merely as a guide to staffing levels, and implementation should depend on patient acuity, local knowledge and expertise.

Australia and New Zealand have several documents that guide nurse-to-patient ratios (Table 2.4). The WFCCN states that critically ill patients require one registered nurse to be allocated at all times.[34] The College of Intensive Care Medicine and Intensive Care Society in the United Kingdom also identified the need for a minimum nurse-to-patient ratio of 1:1 for intensive care patients and 1:2 for high-dependency patients.[24,25]

> ### Practice tip
>
> The WFCCN states that critically ill patients require one registered nurse to be allocated at all times.

TABLE 2.4

Documents that guide the nurse-to-patient ratios in critical care

DOCUMENT	RECOMMENDATIONS
ACCCN: Position statement on intensive care nurse staffing[32]	• ICU patients (clinically determined) should have a 1:1 nurse-to-patient ratio • HDU patients (clinically determined) should have a 1:2 nurse-to-patient ratio
ACCCN: Position statement on the healthcare workers other than division 1 registered nurses in intensive care[58]	• All intensive care patients must have a registered nurse (division 1) allocated exclusively to their care • High-dependency or step-down patients (in intensive care) who require a nurse-to-patient ratio of 1:2 should have a registered nurse (division 1) allocated exclusively to their care • Enrolled nurses (division 2) and unlicensed assistive personnel may be allocated roles to assist the registered nurse, but any activities that involve direct contact with the patient must always be performed in the immediate presence of the registered nurse (division 1)
New Zealand Nursing Organisation, Critical Care Section: Philosophy and Standards for Nursing Practice in Critical Care[41]	• The critically ill and/or ventilated patient will require a minimum 1:1 nurse-to-patient ratio • At times, patients in the critical care unit may have higher or lower nursing acuity; the critical care nurse in charge of the shift determines any variation from the 1:1 ratio, taking into account context, skill mix and complexity
WFCCN: Declaration of Buenos Aires, Position Statement on the Provision of Critical Care Nursing Workforce[34]	• Critically ill patients (clinically determined) require one registered nurse at all times • High-dependency patients (clinically determined) in a critical care unit require no less than one nurse for two patients at all times
College of Intensive Care Medicine (CICM): Minimum Standards for Intensive Care Units[24]	• A minimum of 1:1 nursing is required for ventilated and other similarly critically ill patients, and nursing staff must be available to greater than a 1:1 ratio for patients requiring complex management (e.g. ventricular assist device) • The majority of nursing staff should have a post-registration qualification in intensive care or in the specialty of the unit • All nursing staff in the unit responsible for direct patient care should be registered nurses
College of Intensive Care Medicine (CICM): Recommendations on Standards for High-Dependency Units Seeking Accreditation for Training in Intensive Care Medicine[102]	• The ratio of nursing staff to patients should be 1:2 • All nursing staff in the HDU responsible for direct patient care should be registered nurses, and the majority of all senior nurses should have a post-registration qualification in intensive care or high-dependency nursing • A minimum of two registered nurses should be present in the unit at all times when a patient is present

ACCCN = Australian College of Critical Care Nurses; WFCCN = World Federation of Critical Care Nurses.

The ACCCN,[32] British Association of Critical Care Nurses[33] and the Critical Care Nurses Section – New Zealand Nurses Organisation[41,42] have outlined the appropriate nurse staffing standards for ICUs within the context of accepted minimum national standards and evidence that supports best practice. The WFCCN statement identifies key principles to meet the expected standards of critical care nursing (Table 2.5).

These recommendations serve merely to guide nurse-to-patient ratios, as extraneous factors such as the clinical practice setting, patient acuity and the knowledge and expertise of available staff will influence final staffing patterns that may be adapted to suit the requirements of individual countries or units. In particular, patient dependency scoring tools are designed to guide these staffing decisions and are discussed below.

Patient dependency

Patient dependency refers to an approach to quantify the care needs of individual patients, so as to match these needs to the nursing staff workload and skill mix.[43] For many years, patient census was the commonest method for determining the nursing workload within an ICU. That is, the number of patients dictated the number of nurses required to care for them, based on the accepted nurse-to-patient ratios of 1:1 for ICU patients and 1:2 for HDU patients. This reflects the unit-based workload, and is also the common funding approach for ICU bed-day costs.

The nursing workload at the individual patient level, however, is also reflective of patient acuity, the complexity of care required and both the physical and the psychological status of the patient.[43] Strict adherence to the patient census model leads to the inflexibility of matching

TABLE 2.5

Ten key points of intensive care nursing staffing

POINT	DESCRIPTION
1 ICU patients (clinically determined)	Require a standard nurse-to-patient ratio of at least 1:1
2 High-dependency patients (clinically determined)	Require a standard nurse-to-patient ratio of at least 1:2
3 Clinical coordinator (team leader)	There must be a designated critical-care-qualified senior nurse per shift who is supernumerary and whose primary role is responsibility for the logistical management of patients, staff, service provision and resource utilisation during a shift
4 ACCESS nurses	These are nurses in addition to the bedside nurses, clinical coordinator, unit manager, educators and non-nursing support staff. They provide **A**ssistance, **C**oordination, **C**ontingency, **E**ducation, **S**upervision and **S**upport
5 Nursing manager	At least one designated nursing manager (NUM/CNC/NPC/CNM or equivalent) who is formally recognised as the unit nurse leader is required per ICU
6 Clinical nurse educator	At least one designated CNE should be available in each unit. The recommended ratio is one FTE CNE for every 50 nurses on the ICU roster
7 Clinical nurse consultants	Provide global critical care resources, education and leadership to specific units, to hospital and area-wide services and to the tertiary education sector
8 Critical care nurses	The ACCCN recommends an optimum specialty qualified critical care nurse proportion of 75%
9 Resources	These are allocated to support nursing time and costs associated with quality assurance activities, nursing and multidisciplinary research, and conference attendance
10 Support staff	ICUs are provided with adequate administrative staff, ward assistants, manual handling assistance/equipment, cleaning and other support staff to ensure that such tasks are not the responsibility of nursing personnel

ACCCN = Australian College of Critical Care Nurses; CNC = clinical nurse consultant; CNE = clinical nurse educator; CNM = clinical nurse manager; FTE = full-time equivalent; NPC = nurse practice coordinator; NUM = nursing unit manager.

Adapted from Australian College of Critical Care Nurses. ICU Staffing Position Statement (2003) on Intensive Care Nursing Staffing. Melbourne: ACCCN, <http://www.acccn.com.au/documents/item/20>; 2003 [accessed 29.07.14], with permission.

nursing resources to demand. For example, some ICU patients receive care that is so complex that more than one nurse is required, and an HDU patient may require less medical care than an ICU patient, but conversely may require more than 1:2 nursing care level secondary to such factors as physical care requirements, patient confusion, anxiety, pain or hallucinations.[43] A patient census approach therefore does not allow for the varying nursing hours required for individual patients over a shift, nor does it allow for unpredicted peaks and troughs in activity, such as multiple admissions or multiple discharges.

There are many varied patient dependency/classification tools available, with their prime purpose being to classify patients into groups requiring similar nursing care and to attribute a numerical score that indicates the amount of nursing care required. Patients may also be classified according to the severity of their illness. The therapeutic intervention scoring system (TISS) was developed to determine severity of illness, to establish nurse-to-patient ratios and to assess current bed utilisation.[44] This system attributes a score to each procedure/intervention performed on a patient, with the premise that the greater the number of procedures performed, the higher the score, the higher the severity of illness, the higher the intensity of nursing care required.[43] Since its development in the mid-1970s, TISS has undergone multiple revisions, but this scoring system, like the Acute Physiologic and Chronic Health Evaluation (APACHE)[45] and Simplified Acute Physiology Score (SAPS),[46] still captures the therapeutic requirements of the patient. It does not, however, capture the entirety of the nursing role. Therefore, while these scoring systems may provide valuable information on the acuity of the patients within the ICU, it must be remembered that they are not accurate indicators of total nursing workload. Other specific nursing measures have been developed, but have not gained universal clinical acceptance or application.

Skill mix

Skill mix refers to the ratio of caregivers with varying levels of skill, training and experience in a clinical unit. In critical care, skill mix also refers to the proportion of registered nurses possessing a formal specialist critical care qualification. The ACCCN recommends an optimum qualified critical care nurse to unqualified critical care nurse ratio of 75%.[32] In Australia and New Zealand, approximately 50% of the nurses employed in critical care units currently have some form of critical care qualification.[40]

Practice tip

The ACCCN recommends an optimum qualified critical care nurse to unqualified critical care nurse ratio of 75%.

Debate continues in an attempt to determine the optimum skill mix required to provide safe, effective nursing care to patients.[47–51] Much of the research fuelling this debate has been undertaken in the general ward setting, and still predominantly in the USA. However, it has provided the starting point for specialty fields of nursing to begin to examine this issue. The use of nurses other than registered nurses in the critical care setting has been discussed as one potential solution to the current critical care nursing shortage.[52]

Published research on skill mix has examined the substitution of one grade of staff with a lesser skilled, trained or experienced grade of staff and has utilised adverse events as the outcome measure. A significant proportion of research suggests that a rich registered nurse skill mix reduces the occurrence of adverse events.[48,53,54] A comprehensive review of hospital nurse staffing and patient outcomes noted that existing research findings with regard to staffing levels and patient outcomes should be used to better understand the effects of skill mix dilution, and justify the need for greater numbers of skilled professionals at the bedside.[55]

While there has not been a formal examination of skill mix in the critical care setting in Australia and New Zealand, two older publications[56,57] informing this debate emerged from the Australian Incident Monitoring Study – ICU (AIMS–ICU). Of note, 81% of the reported adverse events resulted from inappropriate numbers of nursing staff or inappropriate skill mix.[56] Furthermore, nursing care without expertise could be considered a potentially harmful intrusion for the patient, as the rate of errors by experienced critical care nurses was likely to rise during periods of staffing shortages, when inexperienced nurses required supervision and assistance.[31,56] These important findings provide some insight into the issues surrounding skill mix.

Professional organisations have developed position statements on the use of staff other than registered nurses in the critical care environment.[32,58] The British Association of Critical Care Nurses asserts that healthcare assistants employed in a critical care setting must undertake only direct patient care activities for which they have received training and for which they have been assessed competent under the supervision of a registered nurse.[33]

Staffing levels and skill mix within critical care units should therefore be based on individual unit needs (e.g. unit size and location) and patient clinical presentations/acuity, and be guided by the best available evidence to ensure safe, quality care for their patients within the context of national standards, expectations and resources.

Rostering

Once the nursing establishment for a unit is determined and skill mix considered, the rostering format is decided. In times of nursing shortages, one of the factors identified as affecting the retention of staff is the ability to provide flexibility in rostering practices. To some extent, rostering practices are governed by government, hospital and industrial policies and these should be considered when deciding the roster format for individual units.

The traditional shift patterns are based on 3×8-hour shifts per day (Figure 2.1). With the increased demand for flexible rosters has come the introduction of additional shift lengths, most notably the 12-hour shift. The implementation of a 12-hour roster requires careful consideration of its risks and benefits, with full consultation of all parties, unit staff, hospital management and the relevant nurses' union. Perceived benefits of working a 12-hour roster include improvement in personal/social life, enhanced work satisfaction and improved patient care continuity. Perceived risks, such as an alteration in the level of sick-leave hours, decreased reaction times and reduced alertness during the longer shift, have not been found to be significant.[59] A reported disadvantage of 12-hour shifts is the loss of the shift overlap time, which has traditionally been used for providing in-unit educational sessions. A consideration, therefore, for units proposing the implementation of a 12-hour shift pattern is to build formal staff education sessions into the proposal.

Education and training

During the latter half of the 20th century specialist critical care nursing education made the transition from hospital-based courses in to the tertiary education sector. Although some hospitals maintain in-house critical care courses, these are generally designed to meet the tertiary requirements of postgraduate education and to articulate with higher level university programs.

Some organisations, both private and public, continue to offer a variety of short continuing education courses as well, generally at a fairly basic level of knowledge and skills, which play a role in providing an introduction for a novice practitioner.[36] Position statements on the preparation and education of critical care nurses are available[36,37,60] that present frameworks to ensure that the curricula of courses provide adequate content to prepare nurses for this specialist nursing role.

Nursing has always been a profession that has required currency of knowledge and clinical skills through continuing education input, because of the rapidly changing knowledge base and innovative treatment regimens. These changes are occurring at an increasingly rapid rate, particularly in critical care. The need for critical care nurses to maintain current, up-to-date knowledge across a broad range of clinical states has therefore never been more important. Specific issues related to orientation and continuing education programs are briefly discussed below.

Orientation

The term orientation reflects a range of activities, from a comprehensive unit-based program, attendance at a hospital induction program covering the mandatory educational requirements of that facility, through to familiarisation with the layout of a department. The aim of an orientation program is the development of safe and effective practitioners.[61]

Unit-specific orientation should be a formal, structured program of assessment, demonstration of competence and identification of ongoing educational needs, and should

---

FIGURE 2.1   Calculating staff requirements.

The following example is for a 6-bed intensive care unit. A roster has been determined to employ 6 nurses using a 3-shift/day approach (morning, evening, night [10 h]). A 2-hour morning (a.m.) to afternoon (p.m.) shift handover period and a 30-minute afternoon to night (ND) shift handover period are included. Local shift times and practices can be substituted.

Step 1 Calculate the number of working hours needed:

a.m. shift	0700 to 1530	= 7.6 h $\times$ 6 nurses $\times$ 7 days	319.2 h
p.m. shift	1330 to 2200	= 7.6 h $\times$ 6 nurses $\times$ 7 days	319.2 h
Night shift	2130 to 0730	= 10 h $\times$ 6 nurses $\times$ 7 days	420 h
Total			1058.4 h

These initial figures do not include sick leave or annual leave. An additional adjustment is therefore required to factor in paid, unpaid, sick and study leave. A 22% 'leave allowance' is included to accommodate these aspects. A locally derived figure may be substituted here, usually available from the finance or personnel department.

Step 2 Add the leave allowance:
1058.4 h $\times$ 1.22 (leave allowance) = 1291.2 h/38 h (1 FTE) = 33.9 FTEs

With a staffing pattern of 6 staff per shift, this unit requires an establishment of 33.9 full-time equivalents (FTEs) to meet the needs of this roster. This figure does not include positions such as the nurse unit manager, team leader/shift coordinator and clinical nurse educator, as outlined in the ACCCN guidelines[32] and Table 2.7.

be developed to meet the needs of all staff who are new to the unit. Competency-based orientation is learner-focused and based on the achievement of core skills that reflect unit needs and enable new employees to function in their role at the completion of the orientation period.[62] A number of countries have developed core competency standards for specialist critical care nurses[42,63,64] that may be used as a framework on which to build competency-based orientation programs.

> **Practice tip**
>
> Unit-specific orientation should be a formal, structured program of assessment, demonstration of competence and identification of ongoing educational needs, and should be developed to meet the needs of all staff who are new to the unit.

Continuing education

In 2003, both the Royal College of Nursing Australia and the College of Nursing implemented systems of formally recognising professional development, with the awarding of continuing education points. While professional development has always been a requirement of continuing practice, this process is becoming more formalised. On 1 July 2010 the Australian Health Practitioner Regulation Agency came into being as a national health practitioner body. With this, a formal requirement for continuing education or professional development was mandated. The Nursing and Midwifery Board of Australia, a subgroup of the above agency, clearly identifies the standard for continuing professional development of nurses and midwives.[65] In New Zealand there is an expectation that a minimum of 60 hours professional development and 450 hours of clinical practice will be undertaken over a three-year period for the purposes of registration renewal.[66] Conversely, North American nursing associations have for many years had formal programs for recognising continuing education and awarding continuing education points. These continuing education points have often been required to support continued registration. This concept has subsequently been implemented in the UK and Europe.[67]

Risk management

Managing risk is a high priority in health, and critical care is an important risk-laden environment in which the manager needs to be on the lookout for potential error, harm and medico-legal vulnerability. The Sentinel Events Evaluation study[68] has given an indication of this risk for critical care patients. It was a 24-hour observational study of 1913 patients in 205 ICUs worldwide, which identified 584 errors causing harm or potential harm to 391 patients. The Sentinel Events Evaluation study authors concluded there was an urgent need for development and implementation of strategies for prevention and early detection of errors.[68] A second study by the same team specifically targeted errors in administration of parenteral

drugs in ICUs.[69] In this study 1328 patients in 113 ICUs worldwide were studied for 24 hours; 861 errors affecting 441 patients occurred, or 74.5 parenteral drug administration errors per 100 patient days. The authors concluded that organisational factors such as error reporting systems and routine checks can reduce the risk of such errors.[69]

What is more alarming is that many health practitioners do not acknowledge their own vulnerability to error. One study asked airline flight crews (30,000) and health professionals (1033 ICU/operating room doctors and nurses, of whom 446 were nurses) from five different countries a simple question, 'Does fatigue affect your (work) performance?', with fascinating results.[70] Of those responding, the following replied in the affirmative to the question: pilots and flight crew, 74%; anaesthetists, 53%; surgeons, 30% (a figure for nurses' responses to this question was not provided in the study). The study also found that only 33% of hospital staff thought errors were handled appropriately in their hospital and that over 50% of ICU staff found it hard to discuss errors.[70] Chapter 3 provides more information in this area including a description of non-technical skills and how training can help make critical care units safer for patients and staff, as well as key governance and management responsibilities in all aspects of the health system.

> **Practice tip**
>
> It is alarming that many health practitioners do not acknowledge their own vulnerability to error.

Managerial activities that affect quality, safety and risk performance have also been systematically reviewed highlighting the need to establish goals and strategy to improve care, setting the quality agenda, engaging in quality, promoting a quality improvement culture, managing resisters and procurement of organisational resources for quality.[71] In addition, such activities advocate for positive actions such as establishment of a Board quality committee, with a specific item on quality at the Board meeting, a quality performance measurement report and a dashboard with national quality and safety benchmarks, performance evaluation attached to quality and safety and an infrastructure for staff–manager interactions on quality strategies.[71] Such activities are equally pertinent at the ICU management level.

Governance and management of the critical care environment require a multidisciplinary team of senior clinician managers who understand both the clinical risks and the quality cycles of the environment as well as the executive requirements for financial and organisational viability. An astute and careful balance between good clinical governance (patient care and clinician practices) and good corporate governance (hotel, finance, IT and other support services) is required to ensure sustainable and appropriate health care for all users. The take-home message in all this is that managers in hospitals manage enormous risks with patients, staff and visitors but often do not appreciate their own level of vulnerability to error and risk. Yet claims of negligence and charges of incompetence can be as threatening to the manager as they are to the clinician.

Negligence

Negligence is a legal term that can be proven only in a court. In tort law four aspects to the charge of negligence were generally accepted:

1 The provider owed a duty of care to the recipient.
2 The provider failed to meet that duty, resulting in a breach of care.
3 The recipient sustained damages (loss) as a result.
4 The breach by the provider caused the recipient to suffer reasonably foreseeable damages.[72]

Since the introduction of civil liability legislation in most states and territories of Australia, courts use a multi-factorial assessment of all the facts to determine the level of liability or otherwise of the defendant. In relation to defences, while on the surface the legislation appears to place limits on the liability of health professionals, in practice it appears to have not made much difference to the outcome of whether there is a negligence action. The greatest impact has been on the quantum of damages. Therefore, the result is that health professionals are held liable for negligence but the damages are reduced because of statutory limits like thresholds and caps.[73]

Critical to reducing liability in this area is the need for health services and managers to have in place current policies, procedures and supervision processes to ensure contemporary and safe practices among its workforce.

The role of leadership and management

Managers must also be leaders, and the need to have good leaders and managers is as relevant to critical care as it is to any other business or clinical entity. Seminal research studies on organisational structures in ICUs across the USA in the 1980s[74] and 1990s[75] demonstrated the important role leadership plays in patient care and risk management in the ICU. Using APACHE scoring, organisational efficiency and risk-adjusted survival were measured. High-performing ICUs demonstrated that actual survival rates exceeded predicted survival rates.[74,75]

Further investigation and analysis of the higher-performing units noted that these units had well-defined protocols, a medical director to coordinate activities, well-educated nurses and collaboration between nurses and doctors.[74,75] Clear and accessible policies and procedures to guide staff practice in the ICU setting were also highlighted. These policies and procedures need to be in written form, simple to read and in a consistent format, evidence-based, easy to understand and easy to apply. Box 2.3 shows a possible format for clinical policies and protocols.

The latter study by Zimmerman et al[75] showed similar characteristics: they had a patient-centred culture, strong

BOX 2.3

Sample headings to define a policy

- Policy
- Rationale
- Procedure
- Statistical reports (e.g. to measure compliance with or outcome of policy)
- Other information
- Contact person
- References
- Filing instructions
- Date of issue
- Date for review
- Signature and designation of authorising officer

medical and nursing leadership, effective communication and coordination and open and collaborative problem solving and conflict management. One cannot underestimate the value of strong, dedicated and collaborative leadership from managers as the key to organisational success in the critical care setting. These factors are as pertinent now as they were when first studied over 30 years ago and remind us of the important role of leadership in ensuring the safety of patients, visitors and staff alike in this complex health setting.[76,77] Chapter 1 contains a discussion about leadership.

Managing injury: Staff, patient or visitor

When staff members are injured, the response must be swift and deliberate. Injury can come in many forms, involving physical injuries or biological exposures, for example. More often, the problems are grievances, such as missing out on an opportunity afforded to others (e.g. a promotion), feeling marginalised by others or not getting a preferred roster.

For patients, an injury can be physical, such as a drug error or an iatrogenic infection; however, the injury can also be non-physical and can affect patients, visitors and staff members, as with complaints about lack of timely information, misinformation or rudeness of staff. In all circumstances a manager needs to intervene proactively to minimise or contain the negativity or harm felt by the 'victim'. Regardless of the cause of the injury, the principles governing good risk management are common to many situations and are summarised in Box 2.4.

If an incident does occur, it is always prudent to document the event as soon as possible afterwards and when it is safe to do so. The clinician who discovers and follows up an incident must document the event, asking the questions that a manager, family member, police officer, lawyer or judge might wish to ask. The written account provided soon after the event or incident by a person closely involved in or witness to it will form a very important testimonial in any subsequent investigation. Key points to document are identified in Table 2.6.

BOX 2.4

Defensive principles to minimise risk after an incident (patient or staff)

- Those persons encouraged to participate in decision making are more inclined to 'own' the decisions made; therefore, involve them in deciding how the issue is to be tackled and help to make the expectations realistic.
- Education of the person in the various aspects of the incident/activity will reduce fear and anxiety.
- Explain the range of possible outcomes and where the affected person is currently situated on that continuum.
- Provide frequent and accurate updates on the person's situation and what is being done to improve that situation.
- Maintain a consistent approach and as far as possible the same person should provide such information/feedback.

Adapted from Williams G. Quality management in intensive care. In: Gullo A, ed. Anesthesia, pain, intensive care and emergency medicine. Berlin: Springer-Verlag; 2003: pp. 1239–50, with permission.

Practice tip

If an incident does occur, it is always prudent to document the event as soon as possible afterwards and when it is safe to do so.

Contemporary wisdom in modern health agencies advocates open disclosure: telling the truth to the patient or family about why and how an adverse event has occurred.[78,79] This practice may be contrary to informed legal advice and may not preclude legal action against the staff or institution.[80–82] However, openly informing the patient/family of what has occurred can regain trust and respect, and may help to resolve anger and frustration. The open disclosure process can also provide learning and education on how such events can be prevented in the future, a right for which many consumer advocates are now lobbying.[83]

The process of root cause analysis can also assist the team to explore in detail the sequence of events and system failures that precipitated an incident and help to inform future system reforms to minimise harm. An root cause analysis is a generic method of 'drilling down' to identify hospital system deficiencies that may not immediately be apparent, and that may have contributed to the occurrence of a 'sentinel event'. The general characteristics of an root cause analysis are that it:[84]

- focuses on systems and processes, not individual performance
- includes a review of the relevant literature
- examines the event extensively for underlying contributing causes
- enables procedure and system modifications.

Despite more than two decades of human error studies in health and critical care specifically, the incidence of error, omission and patient harm does not appear to be improving at the rate hoped.[68,69]

TABLE 2.6

Key points when documenting an incident in a patient's file notes

QUESTION	EXPLANATION
Where did the incident occur?	For example, bedside, toilet, drug room
Were there any pre-event circumstances of significance?	For example, short-staffed, no written protocol
Who witnessed the event?	Including staff, patient, visitors
What was done to minimise negative effects?	For example, extra staff brought to assist, slip wiped up, sign placed on front of patient chart warning of reaction/sensitivity etc
Who in authority was notified of the incident?	Involving a senior, experienced manager/authority should help expedite immediate and effective action
Who informed the victim of the event? What was the victim told? What was the response?	Clear, concise and non-judgemental explanations to the victim or representative are necessary as soon as possible, preferably from a credible authority (manager/director)
What follow-up support, counselling and revision occurred?	This is important for both victim and perpetrator; ascertain when counselling occurred and who provided it
What review systems were commenced to limit recurrence of the event?	Magistrates and coroners in particular want to know what system changes have occurred to limit the recurrence of the event

Adapted from Williams G. Quality management in intensive care. In: Gullo A, ed. Anesthesia, pain, intensive care and emergency medicine. Berlin: Springer-Verlag; 2003: pp. 1239–50, with permission.

Measures of nursing workload or activity

Several workload measures have been developed in an attempt to capture the complexity and diversity of critical care nursing practice (see Table 2.7 for common instruments).[44,85,86] Some hospitals use an electronic care plan with activity timings to calculate nursing time and workload. An Australian instrument, the critical care patient dependency tool,[87] was developed to measure nursing costs in the ICU and is still used in some units to document workload,[88] although no further validation studies have been published since the original research in 1993. The most common instruments used in clinical practice and research are variants of the TISS and the Nursing Activities Score (NAS) (see Tables 2.7 and 2.8).

The TISS was initially developed to measure severity of illness and related therapeutic activities, but has been widely used as a proxy measure of nursing workload in the ICU. One of the primary uses was to aid quantitative comparison between patients in order to allocate resources, with ongoing daily measurements giving an indication of patients' progress.[89] The original TISS had a number of areas for scoring, including patient care and monitoring,

procedures, infusions and medications and cardiopulmonary support. Points assigned to specific interventions ranged from 1 to 4 for a 24-hour period. A higher score signified a greater therapeutic effort. Several revisions and variants of TISS have been developed in Europe, including TISS-28[44] and the nine equivalents of nursing manpower use score (NEMS).[90]

TISS-28 was refined to be a more user-friendly instrument, with similar precision to measure nursing workload, staffing requirements and costing, and to differentiate between ICU and HDU patients.[87] This simplified version of 28 items is divided into basic activities (including monitoring and medications), ventilatory support, cardiovascular support, renal support, neurological support, metabolic support and specific interventions. The score range is from 1 to 8 for each activity, with an ICU-type patient expected to score over 40 points. It was estimated that a critical care nurse was able to provide 46 TISS-28 points per shift, with a score <10 signifying a ward patient, 10–19 an HDU-type patient and >20 an HDU/ICU level.[44] Most studies report mean daily TISS scores from 21 (±12)[91] to 36 (range 29–49).[92] Such diversity in scores reflects a range in acuity of patients. TISS was not, however, developed as a predictive tool – rather as a record of the level of nursing intervention

TABLE 2.7
Common ICU nursing workload instruments

INSTRUMENT	COMPONENTS	SCORING/INTERPRETATION
TISS 1983[103] (USA)	5788/7684 nursing activities related to therapeutic interventions; 0–4 points per variable	Most ICU patients: 10–60 points Acuity: class IV (≥40 points); III (20–39); II (10–19); I (<10)
Intensive Care Society 2013 (UK)	4 levels of care, with qualitative assessment of organ systems	0 = routine ward care 1 = ward care supported by critical care team 2 = support and monitoring of single organ dysfunction/failure 3 = complex support and monitoring of multiple organ dysfunction/failure
TISS-28 1996[44] (Europe)	28 in 7 categories; points vary per item (0–8)	46 points = 1:1 nursing/shift 23 points = HDU patient (1:2 staff-to-patient ratio)
NEMS 1997[86] (Europe)	9 categories with varied points per item (3–12): basic monitoring, intravenous medication, mechanical ventilation, supplementary ventilatory care, single/multiple vasoactive medications, dialysis, interventions in/outside ICU	Equivalent scores to TISS-28; lack of discrimination limits use in predicting or calculating workload at the individual patient level
Critical Care Patient Dependency Tool 1996[87] (Australia)	7 categories scored 1–4 points: (a) hygiene, mobility, wound care; (b) fluid therapy, intake and output, elimination; (c) drugs, nutrition; (d) respiratory care; (e) observations, monitoring, emergency treatment; (f) mental health care, support; (g) admission, discharge, escort	4 levels of nursing time per shift: A = ≤10 points = <8 hours B = 11–15 points = 8 hours (1:1 ratio) C = 16–21 points = 9–16 hours D = >22 points = >16 hours (2:1 ratio)
NAS 2003[85] (Europe/multinational validation)	23 items (5 with sub-items); varied points per item (1.3–32) (see Table 2.8 for details)	Measures calculated percentage of nursing time (in 24 hours) on patient-level activities; 100% = 1 nurse per shift

TABLE 2.8
Nursing Activities Scale

NURSING ACTIVITIES SCORE	POINTS
NURSING ACTIVITIES	
1 Monitoring and titration	
a Hourly vital signs, regular registration and calculation of fluid balance	4.5
b Present at bedside and continuous observation or active for ≥2 h in a shift, for reasons of safety, severity, or therapy (e.g. non-invasive mechanical ventilation, weaning procedures, restlessness, mental disorientation, prone position, donation preparation and administration of fluids or medication, assisting specific procedure)	12.1
c Present at bedside and active for 4 h or more in any shift for reasons of safety, severity, or therapy (see 1b)	19.6
2 Laboratory, biomedical and microbiological investigations	4.3
3 Medication, vasoactive drugs excluded	5.6
4 Hygiene procedures	
a Performing hygiene procedures such as dressing of wounds and intravascular catheters, changing linen, washing patient, incontinence, vomiting, burns, leaking wounds, complex surgical dressing with irrigation or special procedures (e.g. barrier nursing, cross-infection-related, room cleaning after infections, staff hygiene)	4.1
b Performance of hygiene procedures took >2 h in any shift	16.5
c Performance of hygiene procedures took >4 h in any shift	20.0
5 Care of drains, all (except gastric tube)	1.8
6 Mobilisation and positioning, including procedures such as turning the patient, mobilisation of the patient, moving from bed to a chair and team lifting (e.g. immobile patient, traction, prone position)	
a Performing procedure(s) up to 3 times per 24 h	5.5
b Performing procedure(s) more frequently than 3 times per 24 h, or with two nurses	12.4
c Performing procedure with three or more nurses, any frequency	17.0
7 Support and care of relatives and patient, including procedures such as telephone calls, interviews, counselling; often the support and care of either relatives or patient allows staff to continue with other nursing activities	
a Support and care of either relatives or patient requiring full dedication for about 1 h in any shift such as to explain clinical condition, dealing with pain and distress and difficult family circumstances	4.0
b Support and care of either relatives or patient requiring full dedication for 3 h or more in any shift, such as death, demanding circumstances (e.g. large number of relatives, language problems, hostile relatives)	32.0
8 Administration and managerial tasks	
a Performing routine tasks such as: processing of clinical data, ordering examinations, professional exchange of information (e.g. ward rounds)	4.2
b Performing administrative and managerial tasks requiring full dedication for about 2 h in any shift such as research activities, protocols in use, admission and discharge procedures	23.2
c Performing administrative and managerial tasks requiring full dedication for about 4 h or more of the time in any shift such as a death and organ donation procedures, coordination with other disciplines	30.0
VENTILATORY SUPPORT	
9 Respiratory support: any form of mechanical ventilation/assisted ventilation with or without PEEP, spontaneous breathing with or without PEEP, with or without endotracheal tube supplementary oxygen by any method	1.4
10 Care of artificial airways: endotracheal or tracheostomy cannula	1.8
11 Treatment for improving lung function: thorax physiotherapy, incentive spirometry, inhalation therapy, intratracheal suctioning	4.4
CARDIOVASCULAR SUPPORT	
12 Vasoactive medication, disregard type and dose	1.2
13 Intravenous replacement of large fluid losses, fluid administration >83 L/m/day	2.5
14 Left atrium monitoring: pulmonary artery catheter with or without cardiac output	1.7
15 Cardiopulmonary resuscitation after arrest, in past period of 24 h	7.1

NURSING ACTIVITIES SCORE	POINTS
RENAL SUPPORT	
16 Haemofiltration techniques, dialysis techniques	7.7
17 Quantitative urine output measurement (e.g. by indwelling catheter)	7.0
NEUROLOGICAL SUPPORT	
18 Measurement of intracranial pressure	1.6
METABOLIC SUPPORT	
19 Treatment of complicated metabolic acidosis/alkalosis	1.3
20 Intravenous hyperalimentation	2.8
21 Enteral feeding through gastric tube or other gastrointestinal route	1.3
SPECIFIC INTERVENTIONS	
22 Specific intervention in the ICU: endotracheal intubation, insertion of pacemaker, cardioversion, endoscopies, emergency surgery in the previous 24 h, gastric lavage; routine interventions without direct consequences to the clinical condition of the patient (e.g. X-ray, ECG, echo, dressings, insertion of CVC or arterial catheters) not included	2.8
23 Specific interventions outside the ICU; surgery or diagnostics procedures	1.9
TOTAL NURSE ACTIVITIES SCORE	

Adapted from Miranda DR, Nap R, de Rijk A, Schaufeli W, Iapichino G, System TWGTIS. Nursing activities score. Crit Care Med 2003;31(2):374–82, with permission.

required. One study noted that patients with longer ICU stays and worse quality of life outcomes did not have the increase in resource consumption that would have been predicted, as reflected by their TISS.[91] A number of direct-care nursing activities were not captured by TISS-28 (e.g. hygiene, activity/movement, information and emotional support), and a revised instrument, the nursing activities score, was developed to address those limitations.[85] In this study, the NAS explains 81% of nursing time, whereas the earlier TISS-28 explains only 43%; thus the NAS has become more widely used and appears simpler with only 23 measurable items.[93,94]

Management of pandemics

Planning for the impact, or potential impact, of a pandemic is required at the organisational and operational levels, as is the identification of its direct clinical implications. This section highlights the areas to be considered at the organisational level when assessing the response of an individual facility to such an event.

Intensive care beds and their associated resources (equipment and staffing) are finite resources and an organisational response is required to maximise potential ICU capacity. Lessons can be learnt from the global H1N1 pandemic in 2009. The knowledge gained from this experience clearly identifies the need to plan for the potential increased demand on critical care services.[95] While it is beyond the scope of this chapter to cover this subject comprehensively, the aim is to outline briefly the areas for further examination, touching on the concept of the

development of a surge plan. Chapter 14 contains a description of critical care responses to respiratory pandemics.

In earlier experience[95–101] the key role that critical care units have to play in an organised response to a pandemic, particularly an airborne one such as influenza, has been demonstrated, as has the reality that critical care units have been more severely affected than other clinical areas of a hospital. Demand for these services will, at these times, exceed normal supply.

Development of a surge plan

Hota et al[95] describe the preparations for a surge to service under the three headings 'Staff', 'Stuff' and 'Space'. The resources required will be examined under these headings.

Staff

The ability to provide additional staff for a potentially expanded critical care bed base should examine the following:

- staff with critical care skills who do not currently work in this area
- staff from other areas with critical care-based skills, such as recovery, anaesthetics, coronary care
- provision of training and education to support less experienced staff
- development of critical care nursing teams in which critical care expertise is spread across the teams to manage the patient load appropriately, i.e. in satellite units
- planning for critical care staff sick leave
- provision to redeploy pregnant staff

- provision of training and education for all staff to avoid panic and concern, for example, domestic and catering staff.

Stuff

The ability to manage supplies at times of uncertain demand is a key element for examination, as is the knowledge and understanding of the processes for accessing additional equipment such as ventilators and medications from state emergency stockpiles, for example:

- Ensure supplies of appropriate personal protective equipment.
- Develop plans/policies for the rational use of personal protective equipment.
- Ensure supplies, and access to supplies, of required medications.
- Plan the ability to boost ventilator capacity, such as with increased use of BiPAP or accessing the state emergency stockpile.

Space

This would examine and plan for strategies to functionally increase the available critical care bed capacity, as follows:

- Defer elective surgery.
- Explore the ability of local private hospitals to assist with service provision for non-deferrable surgical cases.

- Identify alternative clinical areas within the hospital that may provide additional critical care beds as a satellite unit, such as recovery and coronary care.
- Triage access to limited ventilation and/or critical care resources.[98,101]

Critical care surge plan

Templates to assist in the development of a critical care surge plan are available.[96] The following example is formatted in a graduated approach and is shown as a percentage (%) of current unit capacity:

- pre-surge
- minor surge: 5–10%
- moderate surge: 11–20%
- major surge: 21–50%
- large scale emergency >50%

The use of such a template, which can be populated with locally appropriate definitions and information, can provide the basis for a comprehensive unit/facility specific response to the requirement for a graduated response to a pandemic. Planning for events such as a pandemic requires a coordinated, collaborative approach from all members of the healthcare team, resulting in scalable, flexible plans that are underpinned by the normal management structure and ensure effective lines of communication.[100]

Summary

The management of all resources in the critical care unit is key to meeting the needs of the patients in a safe, ethical, timely and cost-effective manner. Many factors influence not only the resources available but also how these resources are allocated. Managers of critical care units are required to be knowledgeable in the design and equipping of units; human resource management, including the make-up of the nursing workforce; and the fundamentals of the budget – how it is determined, monitored and managed. Understanding the principles of risk management and tools such as those that measure nursing workload help nurse managers in their planning and decision making. Having good structures and processes in place facilitates the delivery of care during times of crisis, such as what is experienced when pandemics occur.

Case study

The Royal Hospital is a 250-bed, non-metropolitan, general teaching public hospital that is planning to expand its intensive care unit from 7 to 10 beds. Your task as the nursing unit manager is to plan what additional nursing resources are required to make this a functional unit once it is fully commissioned. The hospital is geographically located close to a 300-bed private hospital and 5 kilometres from a large regional airport that receives direct flights from Asia. This hospital also has a separate 5-bed CCU and 12-bed post anaesthetic care unit (PACU).

Among other things you must consider certain tasks and make recommendations to the Director of Nursing of The Royal Hospital (see the *Case study* question). Utilise information contained in this chapter to inform your work and recommendations.

CASE STUDY QUESTION

1 Calculate the additional staffing numbers in FTEs that you will require to staff the increase in beds. Determine the estimated cost of these additional staff, including a breakdown of both productive and non-productive FTEs required.

RESEARCH VIGNETTE

Lucchini A, De Felippis C, Elli S, Schifano L, Rolla F, Pegoraro F, Funagalli R.
Nursing activities score (NAS): 5 years of experience in the intensive care units of an Italian hospital.
Intensive Crit Care Nurs 2014;30:152–158

Abstract

Objective: To retrospectively analyse the application of the Nursing Activities Score (NAS) in an intensive care department from January 2006 to December 2011.

Method: The sample consists of 5856 patients in three intensive care units (GICU: General Intensive Care Unit, Neuro ICU: Neurological Intensive Care Unit, CICU: Cardiothoracic Intensive Care Unit) of an Italian University Hospital.

The NAS was calculated for each patient every 24 hours. In patients admitted to general ICU, the following scores were also recorded along with the NAS: SAPS 2 and SAPS 3 (Simplified Acute Physiology Score), RASS (Richmond Agitation Sedation Scale) and Braden.

Results: The mean NAS for all patients was 65.97% (standard deviation [SD] $\pm$2.53), GICU 72.55% (SD $\pm$16.28), Neuro ICU 59.33% (SD $\pm$16.54), CICU 63.51% (SD $\pm$14.69). The average length of hospital stay (LOS) was 4.82 (SD $\pm$8.68). The NAS was high in patients with increasing LOS ($p<0.003$) whilst there were no significant differences for age groups except for children 0–10 years ($p<0.002$). The correlation of NAS and SAPS 2 was $r=0.24$ ($p=0.001$), NAS and SAPS 3 was $r = -0.26$ ($p=0.77$), NAS and RASS was $r = -0.23$ ($p=0.001$), NAS and Braden was $r = 0.22$ ($p=0.001$).

Conclusions: This study described the daily use of the NAS for the determination of nursing workload and defines the staff required.

Critique

This study was a retrospective, single centre, observational study designed to primarily examine the mean NAS score level of admitted patients and compare that data to the nursing workforce that had actually been rostered. Secondary objectives were to examine the differences in NAS scores and therefore nursing workloads between various units and to determine if there was a relationship between mean NAS scores and other variables, namely level of sedation, SAPS2, SAPS3 and risk of pressure ulcer development.

The chosen methodology was suitable and data collection and analysis were appropriate, although there are recognised limitations of using retrospective data for research purposes. Ethics approval was gained from the hospital ethics committee. Descriptive statistics (measures of central tendency such as mean, median and deviance from the mean) have been used to compare the patient populations in the various units, and Spearman's correlation, a technique that permits analysis of ordinal level data, was used to examine the relationships between NAS and SAPS2, SAPS3, RASS and Braden scores.

The findings of this study were that patients cared for in the GICU had a statistically significant higher median NAS score (72.55; $p<0.001$) than those in the other two units; patients with an increased length of stay demonstrated a statistically significant higher median NAS score ($p<0.003$). The study investigators also identified 15 diagnoses in this patient population and the only illness that was predictive of a statistically significant higher median NAS score was patients on extracorporeal membrane oxygenation. No relationship was found between the NAS and the other variables examined.

The authors acknowledged the limitations of a single site study, meaning the findings may not reflect other settings. They also identified that the sample (5856 patients) was not equally distributed across all units studied and that, while the GICU showed a higher median NAS score than the other two units, this may have been due to this patient group being more heterogeneous than the other two groups. Finally, as a retrospective study, the findings may not reflect current practice.

Learning activities

1   Identify the three approaches suggested by the Research and Development Corporation to economic decision making in the ICU when assessing treatment options.

2   Identify the three fundamental steps in the budget process.

3   List the main nursing activities identified in the Nursing Activity Scale 2003.

4   List the criteria that should be included in the evaluation of a new product.

5   In preparation for writing a critical care surge plan, calculate the surge capacity required for a 10- and 25-bed capacity ICU.

Online resources

Ettelt S, Nolte E. Funding intensive care: approaches in systems using diagnosis-related groups, www.rand.org/pubs/technical_reports/2010/RAND_TR792.pdf

Guidance on completing a business case, Mersey Care NHS Trust, UK, www.merseycare.nhs.uk/Library/What_we_do/Corporate_Services/Service_Development_Delivery/Document_Library/Business%20Case%20Guidance.pdf

Medical Algorithms Project website, www.medal.org/visitor/login.aspx

Tasmanian Government business case (small) template and guide, www.egovernment.tas.gov.au/__data/assets/word_doc/0013/15520/pman-temp-open-sml-proj-bus-case.doc

University of Queensland ITS business case guide and template, www.its.uq.edu.au/docs/Business_Case.doc

Further reading

Durbin CG. Team model: advocating for the optimal method of care delivery in the intensive care unit. Crit Care Med 2006;34(3Suppl):S12–S17.

Grover A. Critical care workforce: a policy perspective. Crit Care Med 2006;34(3Suppl):S7–11.

Kirchhoff KT, Dahl N. American Association of Critical-Care Nurses' national survey of facilities and units providing critical care. Am J Crit Care 2006;15:13–28.

Narasimhan M, Eisen LA, Mahoney CD et al. Improving nurse–physician communication and satisfaction in the intensive care unit with a daily goals worksheet. Am J Crit Care 2006;15(2):217–22.

Parker MM. Critical care disaster management. Crit Care Med 2006;34(3Suppl):S52–55.

Redden PH, Evans J. It takes teamwork… The role of nurses in ICU design. Crit Care Nurs Q 2014;37(1):41–52.

Robnett MK. Critical care nursing: workforce issues and potential solutions. Crit Care Med 2006;34(3Suppl):S25–31.

Valentin A, Ferdinande P. Recommendations on basic requirements for intensive care units: structural and organizational aspects. Inten Care Med 2011;37(10):1575–1587.

References

1   Galbally B. The planning and organization of an intensive care unit. Med J Aust 1966;1(15):622–4.

2   Johnston MJ. Bioethics: A nursing perspective. Chatswood, NSW, Australia: Elsevier; 2009.

3   Wiles V, Daffurn K. There is a bird in my hand and a bear by the bed – I must be in ICU. Sydney: Australian College of Critical Care Nurses; 2002.

4   Ettelt S, Nolte E. Funding Intensive Care – approaches in systems using diagnosis-related groups. Cambridge: Rand Europe, <http://www.rand.org/content/dam/rand/pubs/technical_reports/2010/RAND_TR792.pdf>; 2010 [accessed 29.07.14].

5   Independent Hospital Pricing Authority. The Pricing Framework for Australian Hospitals Services 2014–15. Australia: Commonwealth of Australia, <http://www.ihpa.gov.au/internet/ihpa/publishing.nsf/Content/ CA25794400122452CA257C1B0001F452/$File/Pricing-Framework-Aust-PublicHospitalServices-2014-15.pdf>; 2013 [accessed 29.07.14].

6   Independent Hospital Pricing Authority. National Pricing Model, Technical Specifications, 2014–15. Australia: Commonwealth of Australia, <http://www.ihpa.gov.au/internet/ihpa/publishing.nsf/Content/ CA25794400122452CA257C8A001918C9/$File/07Technical Specifications 2014-15.pdf>; 2014 [accessed 29.07.14].

7 Independent Hospital Pricing Authority. National Efficient Price Determination 2014–15. Australia: Commonwealth of Australia, <http://www. ihpa.gov.au/internet/ihpa/publishing.nsf/Content/CA25794400122452CA257C8400185FBC/ $File/National Efficient Price Determination 2014-15.pdf>; 2014 [accessed 29.07.14].

8 Australian Health Workforce Advisory Committee. The critical care nurse workforce in Australia. Australia: AHWAC, <http://www.ahwo.gov.au/ documents/Publications/2002/The critical care nurse workforce in Australia.pdf>; 2002 [accessed 29.07.14].

9 Oye RK, Bellamy PE. Patterns of resource consumption in medical intensive care. Chest 1991;99(3):685–9.

10 Crozier TM, Pilcher DV, Bailey MJ, George C, Hart GK. Long-stay patients in Australian and New Zealand intensive care units: demographics and outcomes. Crit Care Resusc 2007;9(4):327–33.

11 Williams TA, Ho KM, Dobb GJ, Finn JC, Knuiman MW, Webb SA. Changes in case-mix and outcomes of critically ill patients in an Australian tertiary intensive care unit. Anaesth Intensive Care 2010 Jul;38(4):703–9.

12 Duke GJ, Barker A, Knott CI, Santamaria JD. Outcomes of older people receiving intensive care in Victoria. Med J Aust 2014;200(6):323–6.

13 Paz HL, Garland A, Weinar M, Crilley P, Brodsky I. Effect of clinical outcomes data on intensive care unit utilization by bone marrow transplant patients. Crit Care Med 1998;26(1):66–70.

14 Goldhill DR, Sumner A. Outcome of intensive care patients in a group of British intensive care units. Crit Care Med 1998;26(8):1337–45.

15 Lawson JS, Rotem A, Bates PW. From clinician to manager. Sydney: McGraw-Hill; 1996.

16 Strosberg MA, Wiener JM, Baker R, Fein IA, eds. Rationing America's medical care: the Oregon plan and beyond. Washington DC: The Brookings Institute Press; 1992.

17 Truog RD, Brock DW, Cook DJ, Danis M, Luce JM, Rubenfeld GD et al. Rationing in the intensive care unit. Crit Care Med 2006;34(4):958–63; quiz 71.

18 Williams G. Quality management in intensive care. In: Gullo A, ed. Anesthesia, pain, intensive care and emergency medicine. Berlin: Springer-Verlag; 2003: pp. 1239–50.

19 Gan R. Budgeting. In: Crowther A, ed. Nurse managers: a guide to practice. Sydney: Ausmed; 2004.

20 Donahue L, Rader S, Triolo PK. Nurturing innovation in the critical care environment: transforming care at the bedside. Crit Care Nurs Clin North Am 2008;20(4):465–9.

21 Capezio P. Manager's guide to business planning. Madison: McGraw-Hill; 2010.

22 Weaver DJ, Sorrells-Jones J. The business case as a strategic tool for change. J Nurs Adm 2007;37(9):414–9.

23 Paley N. Successful business planning – energizing your company's potential. London: Thorogood; 2004.

24 College of Intensive Care Medicine (CICM). Minimum standards for intensive care units. Australia.: CICM, <http://www.cicm.org.au/cms_files/ IC-01 Minimum Standards For Intensive Care Units - Current September 2011.pdf>; 2011 [accessed 29.07.14].

25 The Faculty of Intensive Care Medicine/Intensive Care Society. Core Standards for Intensive Care Units, <http://www.ics.ac.uk/ics-homepage/ guidelines-standards/>; [accessed 29.07.14].

26 Australian Health Infrastructure Alliance. Australasian health facility guidelines: Part B – Health Facility Briefing and Planning 360-Intensive Care-General. North Sydney: AHIA, <http://healthfacilityguidelines.com.au/AusHFG_ Documents/Guidelines/%5BB-0360%5D Intensive Care-General.pdf>; 2014 [accessed 29.07.14].

27 Department of Health. Health Building Note 04-02 – Critical Care Units. New Zealand: Crown, <http://www.dhsspsni.gov.uk/hbn_04-02_critical_ care_units_final.pdf>; 2013 [29.07.14].

28 Mahbub R. Technology and the future of intensive care unit design. Crit Care Nurs Q 2011;34(4):332–3.

29 Association of Operating Room Nurses. Recommended practices for product selection in perioperative practice settings. AORN J 2004;79:678–82.

30 Elliott D, Hollins B. Product evaluation: theoretical and practical considerations. Aust Crit Care 1995;8(2):14–9.

31 Kelly DM, Kutney-Lee A, McHugh MD, Sloane DM, Aiken LH. Impact of critical care nursing on 30-day mortality of mechanically ventilated older adults. Crit Care Med 2014;42(5):1089–95.

32 Australian College of Critical Care Nurses. ICU Staffing Position Statement (2003) on Intensive Care Nursing Staffing. Melbourne: ACCCN, <http://www.acccn.com.au/documents/item/20>; 2003 [accessed 29.07.14].

33 British Association of Critical Care Nurses. Standards for Nurse Staffing in Critical Care. BACCN, <http://www.baccn.org.uk/about/downloads/ BACCN_Staffing_Standards.pdf>; 2009.

34 World Federation of Critical Care Nurses. Declaration of Buenos Aires: Position statement on the provision of critical care nursing workforce, <http://wfccn.org/publications/workforce>; 2005 [accessed 29.07.14].

35 Williams G, Schmollgruber S, Alberto L. Consensus forum: worldwide guidelines on the critical care nursing workforce and education standards. Crit Care Clin 2006;22(3):393–406, vii.

36 Australian College of Critical Care Nurses. Position statement on the provision of critical care nursing education. Melbourne: ACCCN, <http://www.acccn.com.au/documents/item/19>; 2006 [accessed 29.07.14].

37 World Federation of Critical Care Nurses. Declaration of Madrid: Position statement on the provision of critical care nursing education, <http://wfccn.org/publications/education>; 2005 [accessed 29.07.14].

38 Valentin A, Ferdinande P. Esicm Working Group on Quality Improvement. Recommendations on basic requirements for intensive care units: structural and organizational aspects. Intensive Care Med 2011;37(10):1575–87.

39 Haupt MT, Bekes CE, Brilli RJ, Carl LC, Gray AW, Jastremski MS, et al. Guidelines on critical care services and personnel: recommendations based on a system of categorization of three levels of care. Crit Care Med 2003;31(11):2677–83.

40 Carter R, Hicks P. Intensive Care Resources and Activity in Australia and New Zealand – Activity Report 2010–2011. Australia: ANZICS, <http://www.anzics.com.au/core/reports>; 2012 [accessed 29.07.14].

41 Critical Care Nurses' Section: New Zealand Nurses Organisation. Minimum Guidelines for Intensive Care Nurse Staffing in New Zealand. Wellington: NZNO, <http://www.nzno.org.nz/Portals/0/CCNS Min guidelines for Intensive Care Oct 05.pdf>; 2005 [accessed 29.07.14].

42 Critical Care Nurses' Section: New Zealand Nurses Organisation. New Zealand standards for critical care nursing practice. Wellington: NZNO, <http://www.nzno.org.nz/Portals/0/publications/New Zealand standards for critical care nursing practice, 2014.pdf>; 2014 [accessed 29.07.14].

43 Adomat R, Hewison A. Assessing patient category/dependence systems for determining the nurse/patient ratio in ICU and HDU: a review of approaches. J Nurs Manag 2004;12(5):299–308.

44 Miranda DR, de Rijk A, Schaufeli W. Simplified Therapeutic Intervention Scoring System: the TISS-28 items – results from a multicenter study. Crit Care Med 1996;24(1):64–73.

45 Knaus WA, Draper EA, Wagner DP, Zimmerman JE. APACHE II: a severity of disease classification system. Crit Care Med 1985;13(10):818–29.

46 Le Gall JR, Loirat P, Alperovitch P, Glaser P, Granthil C, Mathieu D et al. A simplified acute physiology score for ICU patients. Crit Care Med 1984;12:975–7.

47 Cho SH, Hwang JH, Kim J. Nurse staffing and patient mortality in intensive care units. Nursing Res 2008;57(5):322–30.

48 Duffield C, Roche M, Diers D, Catling-Paull C, Blay N. Staffing, skill mix and the model of care. J Clin Nurs 2010;19(15-16):2242–51.

49 Numata Y, Schulzer M, van der Wal R, Globerman J, Semeniuk P, Balka E et al. Nurse staffing levels and hospital mortality in critical care settings: literature review and meta-analysis. J Adv Nurs 2006;55(4):435–48.

50 Robinson S, Griffiths P, Maben J. Calculating skill mix: implications for patient outcomes and costs. Nursing Management 2009;16(8):22–3.

51 Flynn M, McKeown M. Nurse staffing levels revisited: a consideration of key issues in nurse staffing levels and skill mix research. J Nurs Manag 2009;17(6):759–66.

52 Heinz D. Hospital nurse staffing and patient outcomes: a review of current literature. Dimens Crit Care Nurs 2004;23(1):44–50.

53 Cho E, Sloane DM, Kim EY, Kim S, Choi M, Yoo IY et al. Effects of nurse staffing, work environments, and education on patient mortality: an observational study. Int J Nurs Stud 2014;52(11):975–81.

54 Aiken LH, Sloane DM, Bruyneel L, Van den Heede K, Griffiths P, Busse R et al. Nurse staffing and education and hospital mortality in nine European countries: a retrospective observational study. Lancet 2014;383(9931):1824–30.

55 Duffield C, Roche M, O'Brien-Pallas L, Diers D, Aisbett C, King M et al. Glueing it together: nurses, their work environment and patient safety. Sydney: University of Technology Sydney, <http://www.health.nsw.gov.au/pubs/2007/pdf/nwr_report.pdf>; 2007.

56 Beckmann U, Baldwin I, Durie M, Morrison A, Shaw L. Problems associated with nursing staff shortage: an analysis of the first 3600 incident reports submitted to the Australian Incident Monitoring Study (AIMS-ICU). Anaesth Intensive Care 1998;26(4):396–400.

57 Morrison AL, Beckmann U, Durie M, Carless R, Gillies DM. The effects of nursing staff inexperience (NSI) on the occurrence of adverse patient experiences in ICUs. Aust Crit Care 2001;14(3):116–21.

58 Australian College of Critical Care Nurses. Position statement on the use of healthcare workers other than division 1 registered nurses in intensive care. Melbourne: ACCCN, <http://www.acccn.com.au/documents/item/21>; 2006 [accessed 29.07.14].

59 Campolo M, Pugh J, Thompson L, Wallace M. Pioneering the 12-hour shift in Australia – implementation and limitations. Aust Crit Care 1998;11(4):112–5.

60 Critical Care Nurses' Section: New Zealand Nurses Organisation. Critical Care Nurses' Section Position Statement (2010) on the Provision of Critical Care Nursing Education. Wellington: NZNO, <http://www.nzno.org.nz/Portals/0/Docs/Groups/ Critical Care Nurses/CCNS Position Statement on the Provision of Crticial Care Nursing Education 2010.pdf>; 2010 [accessed 29.07.14].

61 Boyle M, Butcher R, Kenney C. Study to validate the outcome goal, competencies and educational objectives for use in intensive care orientation programs. Aust Crit Care 1998;11(1):20–4.

62 Harper JP. Preceptors' perceptions of a competency-based orientation. J Nurses Staff Dev 2002;18(4):198–202.

63 American Association of Critical Care Nurses. Institute for Credentialing Excellence (ICE) and National Commission for Certifying Agencies (NCCA). AACN, <http://www.aacn.org/wd/certifications/content/ncca.pcms?menu=certification>; 2014 [accessed 29.07.14].

64 Canadian Association of Critical Care Nurses. CNCC-C and CNCCP-C Certification Canada: CACCN, <http://www.caccn.ca/en/resources/cnccc_and_cnccpc_certification/>; 2014 [accessed 29.07.14].

65 Nursing and Midwifery Board of Australia. Nursing and midwifery continuing professional development registration standard, <http://www.nmc-uk.org/Registration/Staying-on-the-register/Meeting-the-Prep-standards/>; 2010 [accessed 29.07.14].

66 Nursing Council of New Zealand. Guidelines for competence assessment. Wellington: NZNO, <http://www.nursingcouncil.org.nz/Nurses/Continuing-competence/Competence-assessment>; 2008 [accessed 29.07.14].

67 Nursing and Midwifery Council. Meeting the PREP requirements, <http://www.nmc-uk.org/Registration/Staying-on-the-register/Meeting-the-Prep-standards/>; 2010 [accessed 29.07.14].

68 Valentin A, Capuzzo M, Guidet B, Moreno R, Dolanski L, Bauer P et al. Patient safety in intensive care: results from the multinational Sentinel Events Evaluation (SEE) study. Intensive Care Med 2006;32(10):1591–8.

69 Valentin A, Capuzzo M, Guidet B, Moreno R, Metnitz B, Bauer P et al. Errors in administration of parenteral drugs in intensive care units: multinational prospective study. Br Med J 2009;338:b814.

70 Sexton JB, Thomas EJ, Helmreich RL. Error, stress, and teamwork in medicine and aviation: cross sectional surveys. Br Med J 2000;320 (7237):745–9.

71 Parand A, Dopson S, Renz A, Vincent C. The role of hospital managers in quality and patient safety: a systematic review. BMJ Open. 2014;4(9):e005055.

72 MacFarlane PJM. Queensland health law book. 10th ed. Brisbane: Federation Press; 2000.

73 Yule J. Defences in medical negligence: to what extent has tort law reform in Australia limited the liability of health professionals? JALTA 2011;4(1&2):53–63.

74 Knaus WA, Draper EA, Wagner DP, Zimmerman JE. An evaluation of outcome from intensive care in major medical centers. Ann Intern Med 1986;104(3):410–8.

75 Zimmerman JE, Shortell SM, Rousseau DM, Duffy J, Gillies RR, Knaus WA et al. Improving intensive care: observations based on organizational case studies in nine intensive care units: a prospective, multicenter study. Crit Care Med 1993 Oct;21(10):1443–51.

76 Curtis JR, Cook DJ, Wall RJ, Angus DC, Bion J, Kacmarek R et al. Intensive care unit quality improvement: a "how-to" guide for the interdisciplinary team. Crit Care Med 2006;34(1):211–8.

77 Thomas EJ, Sexton JB, Helmreich RL. Discrepant attitudes about teamwork among critical care nurses and physicians. Crit Care Med 2003;31(3):956–9.

78 Australian Commission on Safety and Quality in Healthcare. Australian Open Disclosure Framework. Sydney: Commonwealth of Australia, <http://www.safetyandquality.gov.au/wp-content/uploads/2013/03/Australian-Open-Disclosure-Framework-Feb-2014.pdf>; 2013 [accessed 29.07.14].

79 Iedema RA, Mallock NA, Sorensen RJ, Manias E, Tuckett AG, Williams AF et al. The National Open Disclosure Pilot: evaluation of a policy implementation initiative. Med J Aust 2008;188(7):397–400.

80 Gold M. Is honesty always the best policy? Ethical aspects of truth telling. Intern Med J 2004;34(9-10):578–80.

81 Madden B, Cockburn T. Bundaberg and beyond: duty to disclose adverse events to patients. J Law Med 2007;14(4):501–27.

82 Johnstone M. Clinical risk management and the ethics of open disclosure. Part I. Benefits and risks to patient safety. AENJ 2008;11(2):88–94.

83 Harrison R, Birks Y, Hall J, Bosanquet K, Harden M, Iedema R. The contribution of nurses to incident disclosure: a narrative review. Int J Nurs Stud 2014;51(2):334–45.

84 Department of Human Services Victoria. Clinical risk management, root cause analysis, <http://www.health.vic.gov.au/clinrisk/investigation/root-cause-analysis.htm>; 2014 [accessed 29.07.14].

85 Miranda DR, Nap R, de Rijk A, Schaufeli W, Iapichino G, System TWGTIS. Nursing activities score. Crit Care Med 2003;31(2):374–82.

86 Miranda DR MR, Iapichino G. Nine equivalents of nursing manpower use score (NEMS). Intensive Care Med 1997;23:760–65.

87 Ferguson L, Harris-Ingall A, Hathaway V. NSW critical care nursing costing study. Sydney: Sydney Metropolitan Hospitals Consortium; 1996.

88 Donoghue J, Decker V, Mitten-Lewis S, Blay N. Critical care dependency tool: monitoring the changes. Aust Crit Care 2001;14(2):56–63.

89 Miranda DR MR, Iapichino G. The Therapeutic Intervention Scoring System: one single tool for the evaluation of workload, the work process and management? Intensive Care Med 1997;23:615–17.

90 Rothen HU, Kung V, Ryser DH, Zurcher R, Regli B. Validation of "nine equivalents of nursing manpower use score" on an independent data sample. Intensive Care Med 1999 Jun;25(6):606–11.

91 Rivera-Fernandez R, Sanchez-Cruz JJ, Abizanda-Campos R, Vazquez-Mata G. Quality of life before intensive care unit admission and its influence on resource utilization and mortality rate. Crit Care Med 2001;29(9):1701–9.

92 Jones C, Skirrow P, Griffiths RD, Humphris GH, Ingleby S, Eddleston J et al. Rehabilitation after critical illness: a randomized, controlled trial. Crit Care Med 2003;31(10):2456–61.

93 Debergh DP, Myny D, Van Herzeele I, Van Maele G, Reis Miranda D, Colardyn F. Measuring the nursing workload per shift in the ICU. Intensive Care Med 2012;38(9):1438–44.

94 Padilha KG, de Sousa RM, Queijo AF, Mendes AM, Reis Miranda D. Nursing Activities Score in the intensive care unit: analysis of the related factors. Intensive Crit Care Nurs 2008;24(3):197–204.

95 Hota S, Fried E, Burry L, Stewart TE, Christian MD. Preparing your intensive care unit for the second wave of H1N1 and future surges. Crit Care Med 2010;38(4 Suppl):e110–9.

96 Daugherty EL, Branson RD, Deveraux A, Rubinson L. Infection control in mass respiratory failure: preparing to respond to H1N1. Crit Care Med 2010;38(4 Suppl):e103–9.

97 Funk DJ, Siddiqui F, Wiebe K, Miller RR, 3rd, Bautista E, Jimenez E et al. Practical lessons from the first outbreaks: clinical presentation, obstacles, and management strategies for severe pandemic (pH1N1) 2009 influenza pneumonitis. Crit Care Med 2010;38(4 Suppl):e30–7.

98 Hick JL, O'Laughlin DT. Concept of operations for triage of mechanical ventilation in an epidemic. Acad Emerg Med 2006;13(2):223–9.

99 New South Wales Health. Influenza guidelines for the intensive care unit GL2010_007. Sydney: NSW Health, <http://www0.health.nsw.gov.au/policies/gl/2010/pdf/GL2010_007.pdf>; 2010 [accessed 29.07.14].

100 World Health Organization. Pandemic influenza risk management – interim guidance. Geneva: WHO, <http://www.who.int/influenza/preparedness/pandemic/influenza_risk_management/en/>; 2013.

101 New South Wales Health. Influenza pandemic – providing critical care: PD2010_28. Sydney: NSW Health, <http://www0.health.nsw.gov.au/policies/pd/2010/PD2010_028.html>; 2010 [accessed 20.07.14].

102 College of Intensive Care Medicine (CICM). Guidelines for intensive care units seeking accreditation for training in intensive care medicine (CICM). <http://www.cicm.org.au/cms_files/IC-3 Guidelines for Intensive Care Units Seeking Accreditation for Training in Intensive Care Medicine.pdf>; 2010 [accessed 29.07.14].

103 Keene AR, Cullen DJ. Therapeutic Intervention Scoring System: update 1983. Crit Care Med 1983;11(1):1–3.

Chapter 3

Quality and safety

Wendy Chaboyer, Karena Conroy

Learning objectives

After reading this chapter, you should be able to:

- describe the contribution that evidence-based nursing can make to critical care nursing practice
- identify the steps in developing clinical practice guidelines
- explain the role care bundles and checklists have in promoting quality and safety in critical care nursing practice
- discuss rapid response systems used to respond to deteriorating patients
- describe the use of information and communication technologies in critical care
- identify techniques used to understand situations that place patients at risk of adverse events in critical care
- identify strategies to improve the safety culture in critical care.

Introduction

Today's critical care units are both busy and complex, where nurses, doctors and other health professionals use their knowledge, skills and technology to provide patient care. In fact, this complexity makes errors a common occurrence; one large international study in 205 intensive care units (ICU) showed that 39 serious adverse events occurred per 100 patient days.[1] The Institute of Medicine in the USA defines quality of health care as 'the degree to which health services for individuals and populations increase the likelihood of desired health outcomes and are consistent with current professional knowledge'.[2] Critical care nurses are well known for their skills in patient assessment. In fact, this ongoing surveillance of patient condition means that nurses are ideally positioned to prevent, discover and correct healthcare errors.[3] Thus, nurses play a key role in improving quality and safety in health care. This chapter provides a review of quality and safety in critical care. First, an overview of evidence-based nursing and clinical practice guidelines is given to provide a foundation to consider quality and safety. Next, quality and safety monitoring are considered. Included in this section are the topics of care bundles, checklists and information and communication technologies. Finally, patient safety, including safety culture, rapid response systems and non-technical skills, is described. In Chapter 2 risk management, clinical governance and the role of clinical leaders and managers in delivering critical care services were addressed; this information is complementary to what is discussed in Chapter 3.

Evidence-based nursing

Evidence-based nursing (EBN) is the 'application of valid, relevant, research-based information in nurse decision-making.'[4] Research evidence, however, is only one of four considerations in making a clinical decision. Three other considerations include: 1) knowledge of patients' conditions (i.e. preferences and symptoms); 2) the nurses' clinical expertise and judgment; and 3) the context in which the decision is taking place (i.e. setting, resources). Figure 3.1 provides a schematic representation of EBN, using an example of a decision about weaning a patient from a mechanical ventilator.

EBN has emerged as a way to improve nursing practice by considering the care that nurses give to patients, and whether this care results in the best possible outcomes for patients. It has been viewed as both an attitude and a process. As an attitude, it is a way of approaching practice that is critical and questioning. As a process, a number of steps in EBN have been described. Figure 3.2 identifies these steps, with more details about each step being provided below.

Translate a clinical query into a structured question

In situations where nurses have to make clinical decisions, it is important for them to carefully consider the issue or problem they are facing as it influences what research evidence should be used to make decisions. Thus, the first step in the EBN process is translating a clinical query into a well-defined, answerable, structured question. A well-recognised approach is the **p**opulation, **i**ntervention,

FIGURE 3.2 Steps in the EBN process.

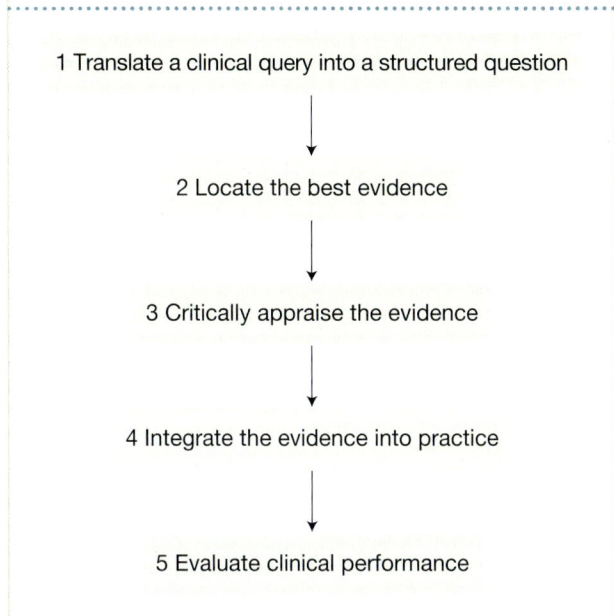

1 Translate a clinical query into a structured question

2 Locate the best evidence

3 Critically appraise the evidence

4 Integrate the evidence into practice

5 Evaluate clinical performance

comparison, **o**utcome format, more often referred to as PICO. The population reflects the patient group or clinical scenario of concern. The intervention is one option for the particular nursing practice. The comparison is the current practice, or the second option for practice. Finally, the outcome is the effect that the nurse is hoping to achieve, which should reflect a patient outcome. Another schema, SPIDER (**s**ample, **p**henomenon of **i**nterest, **d**esign, **e**valuation, **r**esearch type), can be used for questions that are not about the effect of an intervention on an outcome.[5] Table 3.1 provides three examples of PICO questions relevant to critical care nursing.

FIGURE 3.1 Schematic representation of evidence-based nursing including an example of weaning from mechanical ventilation.

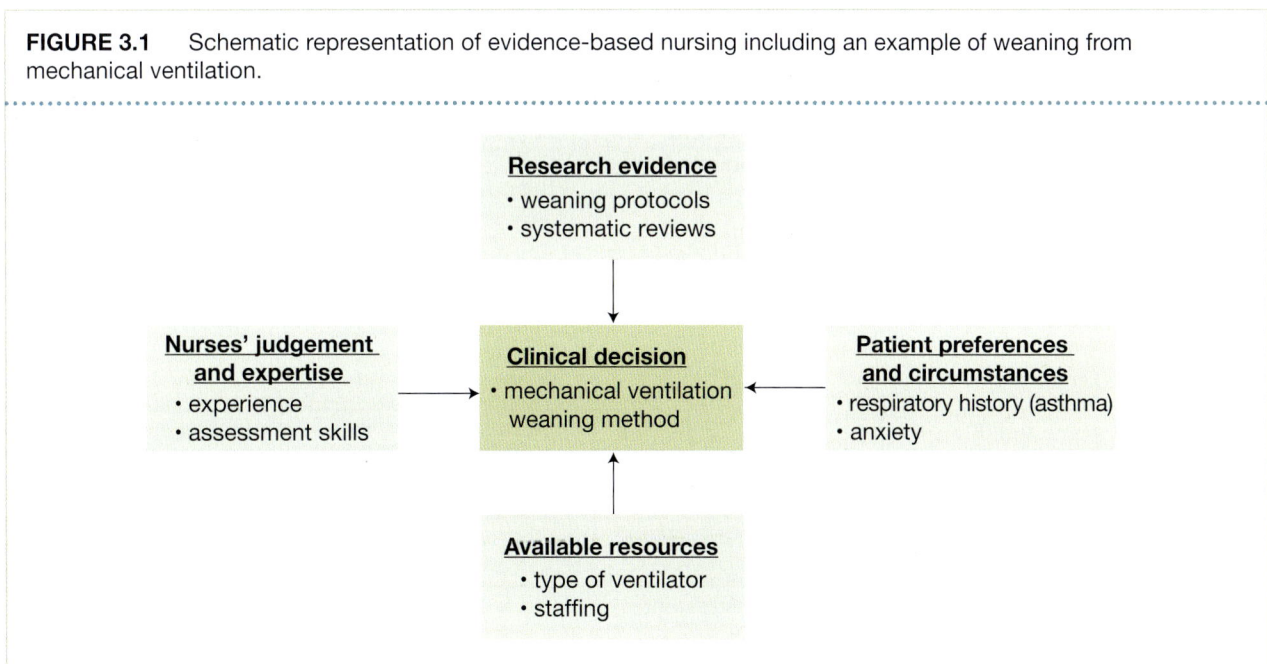

Research evidence
• weaning protocols
• systematic reviews

Nurses' judgement and expertise
• experience
• assessment skills

Clinical decision
• mechanical ventilation weaning method

Patient preferences and circumstances
• respiratory history (asthma)
• anxiety

Available resources
• type of ventilator
• staffing

TABLE 3.1

Examples of clinical questions using the PICO format

EXAMPLE	P – POPULATION	I – INTERVENTION	C – COMPARISON	O – OUTCOME
1	Postoperative cardiac surgery patients	Knee-length graduated compression stockings	Thigh-length graduated compression stockings	Prevention of deep vein thrombosis
2	Mechanically ventilated patients	Nurse-led weaning protocols	Standard practice (doctor-driven)	Extubation
3	Intubated patients	Brushing teeth with a toothbrush and toothpaste	Normal saline mouth rinse	Ventilator-associated pneumonia

Locate the best evidence

After well-defined, answerable, structured questions have been developed, nurses can turn to reviewing the literature to find the answers. First, the evidence has to be located, which involves searching library databases. Some of the databases generally searched include Ovid CINAHL, PubMed and the Cochrane Library. Articles that relate to the question then have to be retrieved. These articles may be reports about primary research (i.e. written by the person conducting the research), systematic reviews of existing research or clinical practice guidelines that have been developed from primary research and systematic reviews.

Critically appraise the evidence

Once the various sources of evidence have been retrieved, they are then assessed for their quality and relevance to the clinical question. In Australia, the National Health and Medical Research Council (NHMRC)[6] has described strategies to assess the body of research evidence, which provide a useful framework to consider research evidence for improving nursing interventions, and identify three questions to ask regarding potential interventions:

1 Is there a real effect?

2 Is the size of the effect clinically important?

3 Is the evidence relevant to practice?

This first question regarding the real effect relates to the strength of the research that has been conducted. The strength of the research has three dimensions: level of evidence, quality of the individual studies and their statistical precision (denoted by P values or confidence intervals). The second question focuses on whether meaningful improvements to patient care and outcome will result if the research findings are applied in practice. It also considers how the intervention compares with current practices in terms of patient care and outcomes. That is, if the research is dated and clinical practice has evolved, the findings of the dated research may be less relevant to current practice.

The third question conveys the notion that potential benefits or outcomes of the intervention must be both important to the patient and able to be replicated in other settings. The NHMRC[6,7] identifies three types of outcome, surrogate, clinical and patient-relevant, which are not mutually exclusive (see Table 3.2). Surrogate outcomes are often used in critical care where measurement of the actual physiological change (e.g. oxygen-carrying capacity of the blood) is replaced by a more accessible, and equally acceptable, parameter (e.g. oxygen saturation). Clinical outcomes are those of direct relevance to clinical practice, and patient-relevant outcomes are those likely to be articulated as significant by the patient/carer. When assessing research evidence, the type of outcome used in the research should be considered.

Recognising the contribution of a variety of research questions beyond intervention-type questions, the NHMRC has extended its framework for assessing research quality, to support the development of clinical practice guidelines (CPG).[7] This extension asks the questions:

1 What is the evidence base (number of studies and quality, levels of evidence)?

2 How consistent are the study findings?

TABLE 3.2

Types of outcome

OUTCOME	DEFINITION	ICU EXAMPLE
Surrogate	Some physical sign or measurement substituted for a clinically meaningful outcome	• Oxygen saturation • Vital capacity
Clinical	Outcome defined on the basis of the problem	• Ventilator days • Hospital readmission
Patient-relevant	Outcomes that are important to the patient	• Functional ability • Quality of life

3 What is the proposed clinical impact of the evidence?

4 How generalisable is the evidence?

5 How applicable is the evidence to the context?

Assessing research results involves an understanding of the quality of evidence for a particular nursing practice.

Integrate the evidence into practice

When good quality evidence for a particular practice is identified, it is important to then consider this evidence alongside nurses' expertise, patient preferences and available resources. In essence, evidence may suggest that a particular practice achieves the best patient outcomes, but if the nurse does not have the skills needed to implement the practice, the resources are not available, either the patient does not want the intervention or their situation is such that the intervention may not be appropriate for them, this practice should not be implemented. However, in many situations the practice will be applicable to the patient and nurses will have the skills and the resources to implement the practice. At times, implementing this new practice may take the form of developing a CPG or protocol for a particular nursing activity. CPGs are described in the next section.

Evaluate clinical performance

Once a new practice has been implemented, it is important for nurses to assess whether it is having the desired effect. At the individual patient level, this often involves assessing the patient whereas, at the unit level, it may involve either a practice audit or research. Practice audits often involve reviewing patient charts to determine both the extent to which the new practice has been implemented and related patient outcomes. Research may seek to understand similar things, but generally takes a more formal approach, addressing issues such as appropriate study designs, ethics approvals etc.

Practice tip

Audit and feedback can be used to support and reinforce practice improvements.

Clinical practice guidelines

The development and use of CPGs is one strategy to implement EBN and improve healthcare.[8,9] CPGs are statements about appropriate health care for specific clinical circumstances that assist practitioners in their day-to-day practice.[9,10] They are systematically developed to assist clinicians, consumers and policy makers in healthcare decisions and provide critical summaries of available evidence on a particular topic.[11] Other terms used synonymously with CPGs include protocols and algorithms. There are a number of benefits of using CPGs. They are seen to be central to quality patient care because, in essence, they standardise care.[11] They can guide decisions and can be used to both justify and legitimise activities and practices.[12] However, limitations have also been identified. Poorly developed guidelines may not

improve care and may actually result in substandard care.[11,12] In the critical care area, the Intensive Care Coordination and Monitoring Unit of the New South Wales Department of Health has led the development of CPGs associated with a number of common nursing interventions that are available online including: 1) eye care; 2) oral care; 3) pressure injury prevention; 4) physical activity and movement; 5) temperature measurement; 6) arterial line care; 7) central venous access device care; 8) suctioning an artificial airway; 9) tracheal tube stabilisation; 10) tracheostomy care; and 11) non-invasive ventilation.[12]

Clinical audits are often used to establish the need to develop new CPGs and protocols at the local unit level. Clinical audits generally involve chart reviews, but may also use direct observation or surveys of practice. Clinical audits often reveal variations in practice that are without adequate justification.

Developing, implementing and evaluating clinical practice guidelines

A number of steps are undertaken when developing clinical practice guidelines. Table 3.3 provides an overview of these steps, which has been adapted from Miller and Kearney's work.[11] Other organisations such as the NHMRC also provide detailed descriptions for various aspects of the CPG development and reporting process.[13,14]

While research, systematic review and expert opinion form the foundation for CPGs, the quality of evidence must be assessed and overall summaries of the knowledge to date are essential. These summaries are then used to develop the guidelines, which generally include a series of statements about the care to be provided and a rationale for this care.

Once the guidelines are developed, a group of experts and users should assess the guidelines for accuracy, clinical utility and comprehension. International experts developed and have subsequently revised a 23-item appraisal instrument, termed the Appraisal of Guidelines for Research and Evaluation II (AGREE II), that assesses six domains: 1) scope and purpose of the CPG (3 items); 2) stakeholder involvement in CPG development (3 items); 3) rigour of development (8 items); 4) clarity and presentation (3 items); 5) applicability (4 items); and 6) editorial independence (2 items).[15] Instruments such as AGREE II can be used to assess the quality of CPG.

Based on the assessment of the CPG, revisions may be required. Next, strategies for disseminating and implementing the guidelines should be developed. Importantly, simply publishing and circulating CPGs will have a limited impact on clinical practice, so specific activities must be undertaken to promote CPG adherence.[16] The following seven strategies have been shown to be moderately effective in promoting guideline adherence: 1) interactive small group sessions, 2) educational outreach visits, 3) reminders, 4) computerised decision support, 5) introduction of computers in practice, 6) mass media campaigns and 7) combined interventions.[9,17] A Canadian study identified the following factors as important for adherence

TABLE 3.3

Steps in developing clinical practice guidelines

STEP	DESCRIPTION
Find the evidence	After deciding on what is considered evidence, databases such as CINAHL and PubMed must be searched to find relevant studies and expert opinions
Evaluate the evidence	Relevant studies and expert opinion papers must be critically appraised for their strengths and weaknesses. This may or may not incorporate a systematic review
Synthesise the evidence	General summary statements about the state of knowledge on a particular topic are developed
Design the guidelines	Written summaries, algorithms and/or summary sheets will be developed that include statements about appropriate healthcare practices and their rationale
Appraise the guidelines	Validity, reliability, clinical applicability, flexibility and clarity are some criteria that can be used to assess the guidelines
Disseminate and implement the guidelines	Specific strategies such as seminars and patient chart reminders must be developed to increase awareness, acceptance and implementation of the guidelines
Review and reassess the guidelines	Clinical audits and research may be used to regularly evaluate the impact the guidelines have had on patient care and outcomes

Adapted from Miller M, Kearney N. Guidelines for clinical practice: development, dissemination and implementation. Int J Nurs Stud 2004; 41:813–21, with permission.

to CPGs: characteristics of the CPG, implementation process, institutional characteristics, provider intent and patient characteristics.[16] Finally, a process for regularly evaluating and updating the guidelines must be developed, which may involve quality improvement activities or clinical research. In summary, by developing, using and evaluating CPGs, nurses may improve patient care and outcomes. Additionally, use of CPGs should ensure that nursing practice is based on the best available evidence.

Quality and safety monitoring

This section discusses unit-level measures used to evaluate the quality and safety of care for critically ill patients. Quality and safety in health care is commonly described in terms of Donabedian's approach[18] with three major domains:

1 structure – the way the healthcare setting and/or system is organised to deliver care (e.g. staffing, beds, equipment)

2 process – the practices involved in the delivery of care (e.g. pressure ulcer prevention strategies)

3 outcomes – the results of care in terms of recovery, restoration of function and/or survival (e.g. mortality, health-related quality of life).

A fourth domain of culture or context has been suggested, specifically for patient safety models, to evaluate the context in which care is delivered.[19] The contemporary model for healthcare improvement recognises that the resources (structure) and activities carried out (processes) must be addressed within a given context (culture) to improve the quality of care (outcome). The overall aim of quality improvement is to provide safe, effective, patient-centred, timely, efficient and equitable health care.[20] Quality improvement activities identify and address

gaps between knowledge and practice. Importantly, these activities need to reflect the most recent and robust clinical evidence to improve patient care and reduce harm. Various activities have been used in the ICU setting to translate research findings into improved clinical practice.[21,22]

The most common approach used for rapid improvement in health care is the **p**lan–**d**o–**s**tudy–**a**ct (PDSA)[23] method where four essential steps are carried out in a continuous fashion to ensure processes are continually improved:

1 Plan – identify a goal, specify aims and objectives to improve an area of clinical practice, and how that might be achieved (i.e. how to test the intervention).

2 Do – implement the plan of action, collect relevant information that will inform whether the intervention was successful and in what way, taking note of problems and unexpected observations that arise.

3 Study – evaluate the results of the intervention, particularly its impact on practice improvement, noting any strengths and limitations of the intervention.

4 Act – determine whether the intervention should be adopted, abandoned or adapted for further rapid cycle testing recommencing at the plan phase.

Quality monitoring includes measurement of, and response to, the incidence and patterns of adverse events (AEs). The rate of AEs varies greatly; retrospective studies from various countries have revealed that AEs occur in 4–17% of hospitalisations.[24–28] One systematic review of eight large international studies, representing a total of almost 75,000 patients, found a median incidence of adverse events to be 9%.[29] Patients who have an ICU stay may be at an even greater risk. In an international study encompassing 29 countries, serious adverse events were shown to occur in ICUs at a rate of 39 events per

100 patient days with those related to indwelling lines, prescription or administration of medications, equipment failure (e.g. infusion devices, ventilators) and airway (e.g. unplanned extubation) the most frequently reported.[1] Similar categories were also reported as highly prevalent in a more recent study in the United Kingdom;[30] however, there was also a high rate of incidents related to patient transfers, pressure sores and infection control issues.

A number of methods for reporting adverse events such as direct observation, chart audit and self or facilitated reporting can be used; each has its strengths and limitations.[31] Direct observation methods have been identified as being the most reliable method of detection.[32] Trained observers report more unintended events but this method is expensive, labour intensive and vulnerable to the Hawthorne effect.[33] Both chart audits and incident reporting only reflect what is charted or reported, but even when chart audit, incident reporting, general practitioner reporting and external sources such as coronial review are used together, some adverse events will still be missed.[34,35] Voluntary or facilitated reporting, such as the Intensive Care Unit Safety Reporting System[36] and the Australian Incident Monitoring Study in Intensive Care,[37] are routinely used surveillance methods in many countries.

Medication administration is the most common intervention in health care, but the medication management process in the acute hospital setting is complex, and creates risk for patients. As a result, medication-related events are one of the most common adverse events for critically ill patients.[1] A Japanese study of adverse drug events in 459 patients found 99 adverse events occurred in 70 patients (i.e. 15% of patients).[38] Although the rates of medication errors and adverse drug events vary greatly between settings despite geographical location, they are common in critical care units,[32,39] with higher rates of harmful errors than non-ICU settings, and those errors are more likely to be associated with requiring life-sustaining intervention, permanent harm or death.[40]

In order to measure medication safety – either by error or adverse event – the following definitions are typically applied:

- error is a failure in clinical management, resulting in potential harm to the patient
- adverse events relate to actual patient harm (injury).[41]

Issues of measurement impact on reported error/adverse event rates and their interpretation. The way in which medication errors, for example, are calculated requires careful consideration of both the numerator (e.g. count of any error in the medication process) and the denominator (this could be the number of patients, patient days, medication days, administered doses – depending on the aim or purpose of the measure).[39]

The true incidence of both errors and adverse events has been found to be higher than what was reported[34,35,42,43] and, in the absence of evidence to the contrary, this is likely to have remained unchanged. Fortunately, most healthcare errors do not result in patient harm because of safety-net processes.[40,44] Despite this, it has been estimated that one potentially serious intravenous drug error occurs every day in a 400-bed hospital,[42] and in Australia, the rates of medication incidents range from 14% to 27% of all reported incidents, second only to falls in acute care settings.[45] Such errors can lead to costly additional treatments and prolonged hospital stays as well as other implications for patients, families and healthcare providers.[39] Approximately 5% of medication errors relate to infusion pumps. These pumps are used to administer high-impact medications, such as inotropes, heparin or antineoplastics.[46] Medication errors reported from a database contributed by 537 hospitals with ICUs were made during the administration phase of medication use, and were commonly errors of omission, caused by improper dose or quantity and incorrect administration technique.[40] The leading sources of errors that caused harm in ICUs were knowledge and performance deficits (57%), not following procedure or protocol (26%), communication (15%) and dispensing device errors (14%).[40] In response to the body of evidence pertaining to medication error, a number of strategies have been instituted; for example, in Australia under the auspices of the National Medicines Policy, the quality use of medicines map is a searchable online database of related projects to assist health practitioners and researchers plan and carry out their work, and help policy makers evaluate quality use of medicines activity for potential use in policy development.

Practice tip

Given the high frequency and consequences of medication errors, it is important to be cognisant of the potential for error and the strategies that can be used to prevent such errors, such as limiting interruptions.

It is important to evaluate interventions that can reduce the incidence and impact of adverse intravenous drug events, particularly in critical care settings.[47,48] Evidence suggests that nurses who are interrupted while administering medications may have an increased risk of making medication errors,[49] prompting calls for all healthcare workers to make concerted efforts to reduce interruptions to clinical tasks.[50] Other activities examining quality of care include the analysis of incident reports that use the World Health Organization's International Classification for Patient Safety[51] and measuring and evaluating quality indicators such as the Australian Council on Healthcare Standards (ACHS) indicators for intensive care that include:

- inability to admit a patient to the ICU due to inadequate resources
- deferral or cancellation of elective surgery due to unavailability of an ICU bed
- transfer of patients to another facility due to unavailability of an ICU bed
- delays on discharging patients from the ICU of more than 6 hours

- discharge of patients from the ICU after hours (i.e. between 6 p.m. and 6 a.m.)
- recognising and responding to clinical deterioration within 72 hours of being discharged from ICU
- appropriate treatment of patients for venous thromboembolism prophylaxis within 24 hours of admission to the ICU
- ICU central line–associated bloodstream infection rates
- use of patient assessment systems (participation in national databases and surveys).[52]

Similar activities are evident internationally, where concepts of 'safety science' (error reduction and recovery) have been applied to critical care practice.[53,54] Examples include the Safer Patients Initiative to implement interventions to improve delivery of care to ventilated patients[55] and multi-faceted collaborative projects to reduce catheter-related bloodstream infections in a large number of ICUs.[56,57] Process indicators of quality care have been developed, including care related to the prevention of ventilator-associated pneumonia (VAP) and central venous catheter management. Table 3.4 outlines process indicators with good clinical evidence and/or strong

TABLE 3.4

Evidence-based process indicators

PROCESS	AIM	MEASURE	CALCULATION METHOD
Glycaemic control	Encourage normo-glycaemia	Percent of blood sugars in the 6–10 mmol/L range	No. of glucose values within range / Total no. glucose tests × 100
Glycaemic control	Decrease hypo-glycaemia	Percent of blood sugars ≤2.2 mmol/L	No. of glucose values ≤2.2 mmol/L / Total no. glucose values collected × 100
Glycaemic control	Decrease hyper-glycaemia	Percent of blood sugars >10 mmol/L	No. of glucose values >10 mmol/L / Total no. glucose tests × 100
Pressure ulcer prevention	Increase full preventative care	Percent of patients at risk for pressure ulcers who receive all of the following: • Daily inspection of skin for pressure ulcers • Proper management of moisture including cleaning and moisturising skin • Optimisation of nutrition • Repositioning every 2 hours • Use of pressure-relieving surfaces	No. of patients at risk for pressure ulcers who receive all care components / Total no. patients identified at risk for pressure ulcers
Pressure ulcer prevention	Reduce incidence of pressure ulcers	Pressure ulcer incidence per 100 admissions	No. of pressure ulcers developed in ICU / Total no. of ICU admissions × 100
Pressure ulcer prevention	Increase pressure ulcer admission assessment	Percent of patients who receive the following on admission to ICU: • Assessment of pressure ulcer risk using validated risk assessment tool • Skin assessment to identify existing pressure ulcers	No. of patients for whom all components of proper pressure ulcer admission assessment were performed and documented / Total no. of patients admitted to ICU
Pressure ulcer prevention	Increase pressure ulcer risk re-assessment	Percent of patients for whom pressure ulcer risk re-assessment was performed using a validated risk assessment tool at least daily and documented	No. of patients received pressure ulcer risk re-assessment / Total no. ICU patients × 100. Exclude patients in ICU <24 hours
Central line-associated bloodstream infections (CLABSI)	Decrease CLABSI rate	CLABSI rate per 1000 central line-days	No. of confirmed cases of CLABSI / Total no. of central line-days × 1000
Ventilator-associated pneumonia (VAP)	Decrease VAP rate	VAP rate per 1000 ventilator days	No. of confirmed cases of VAP / Total no. of ventilator days × 1000

Adapted from:

Australian Commission on Safety and Quality in Health Care (ACSQHC). National Safety and Quality Health Service Standards. Sydney: ACSQHC, <http://www.safetyandquality.gov.au/our-work/healthcare-associated-infection/national-hai-surveillance-initiative/national-definition-and-calculation-of-central-line-associated-blood-stream-infection/>; 2011 [accessed 03.09.14], with permission

Institute for Healthcare Improvement, <http://www.ihi.org/resources/Pages/Measures/ EvaluationofGlycemicControl.aspx>; [accessed 03.09.14], with permission.

recommendations provided by professional bodies, such as the Institute for Healthcare Improvement (USA-based with multinational scope) and the Australian Commission on Safety and Quality in Health Care.

Practice tip

Adhering to the practices included in a ventilator care bundle (where appropriate), may lead to improved patient and service efficiency outcomes.

A range of clinical support tools has been developed that are used to measure compliance with these best-practice clinical standards. Daily goals forms, for example, have been used to aid communication between clinicians during and after multidisciplinary ward rounds and ensure that all staff are aware of what care the patient should be receiving and what the clinical plan is.[58,59] A popular mnemonic developed for use by ICU clinicians during patient assessment is 'FASTHUG' which stands for **f**eeding, **a**nalgesia, **s**edation, **t**hromboembolism prophylaxis, **h**ead-of-bed elevation, stress **u**lcer prevention and **g**lucose management.[60] Along with care bundles and checklists (detailed below) these tools facilitate standardised care and improve communication between clinicians.[61]

Care bundles

One quality improvement approach to the optimal use of best practice guidelines at the bedside is the development of 'care bundles'. A care bundle is a set of evidence-based interventions or processes of care, applied to selected patients in order to standardise and ensure appropriate delivery of care. A number of bundles have been developed for critical care by the Institute for Healthcare Improvement (IHI) (see Table 3.5). Studies examining the process of care delivery in critical care units using the ventilator care bundle revealed that increased bundle compliance was associated with decreased ICU length of stay, reduced ventilator days and increased ICU patient throughput,[62] in addition to decreased rates of ventilator-associated pneumonia.[62-66]

Other quality improvement studies have targeted similar processes of care without taking the bundled approach. One multicenter, cluster-randomised trial involving 15 ICUs in Canada[22] evaluated the effectiveness of a multifaceted quality improvement program (videoconference-based forums that included audit and

TABLE 3.5

Institute for Healthcare Improvement care bundles

BUNDLE NAME	AIM	BUNDLE COMPONENTS
Central line	Prevent central line-associated bacteraemia	• Hand hygiene • Maximal barrier precautions • Chlorhexidine skin antisepsis • Optimal catheter site selection with avoidance of the femoral vein for central venous access in adult patients • Daily review of line necessity with prompt removal of unnecessary lines
Ventilator care	Prevent ventilator-associated pneumonia	• Elevating the head of the patient's bed to 30–45° • Daily assessment of the patient's readiness to extubate or wean from the ventilator • Daily 'sedation vacations' or gradually lightening sedative use each day • Delivering both PUD and DVT prophylaxis • Daily oral care with chlorhexidine
Severe sepsis 3-hour resuscitation	Reduce mortality due to severe sepsis	• Serum lactate measured • Blood cultures obtained prior to antibiotic administration • Administer broad-spectrum antibiotics • Administer crystalloid 30 mL/kg for hypotension or lactate ≥4 mmol/L

6-hour septic shock	Reduce mortality due to severe sepsis	• Apply vasopressors (for hypotension that does not respond to initial fluid resuscitation) to maintain a MAP ≥65 mmHg
		• In the event of persistent arterial hypotension despite volume resuscitation (septic shock) or initial lactate ≥4 mmol/L (36 mg/dL):
		  ○ Measure CVP
		  ○ Measure $ScvO_2$
		  ○ Re-measure lactate if initial lactate was elevated

CVP = central venous pressure; DVT = deep vein thrombosis; MAP = mean arterial pressure; PUD = peptic ulcer disease; $ScvO_2$ = central venous oxygen saturation.

Adapted from Institute for Healthcare Improvement. How-to-guide: Prevent ventilator-associated pneumonia. Cambridge, MA, <http://www.ihi.org/knowledge/Pages/Tools/HowtoGuidePreventVAP.asp>; 2012 [accessed 03.09.14], with permission.

feedback, expert-led educational sessions, dissemination of algorithms) to improve delivery of six evidence-based practices: 1) prevention of ventilator-associated pneumonia via semi-recumbent positioning, 2) thromboembolism prophylaxis, 3) daily spontaneous breathing trials, 4) prevention of central line-associated blood stream infection (CLABSI) via use of a sterile insertion checklist, 5) early enteral feeding and 6) decubitus ulcer prevention via use of the Braden scale. Results showed that adoption of the targeted practices was greater in intervention than control ICUs, and improvement was greatest for CLABSI prevention and semi-recumbent positioning. Importantly, the authors noted that the effect of their intervention was greatest for ICUs with low baseline adherence to certain practices, suggesting that efforts should be directed specifically to where delivery of care is lacking.

Checklists

Checklists have the potential to prevent omissions in care by serving as reminders to healthcare providers for the delivery of appropriate quality care for every patient, every time, in complex clinical environments. A checklist typically contains a list of action items or criteria arranged in a systematic way, allowing the person completing it to record the presence or absence of individual items to ascertain that all are considered or completed.[67]

In critical care settings, checklists have been used to facilitate staff training, detect errors, check compliance with safety standards and evidence-based processes of care (such as those outlined previously), increase knowledge of patient-centred goals and prompt clinicians to review certain practices on morning rounds in the ICU. Reviews of studies that have evaluated the use of checklists noted a number of benefits such as improved understanding of patient therapy goals, improved compliance with safety standards and evidence-based care and detection of patient safety errors and omissions in care, and found they were useful in preparing for a procedure and were not time-consuming or labour intensive.[68,69]

Some of these studies suggested that checklists also contributed to improved outcomes such as reduced length of stay, ventilator days, unit mortality;[70] reduced CLABSI;[71] and reduced mean monthly rates of ventilator-associated pneumonia.[72] Another study has also suggested decreased infection rates (for CLABSI, ventilator-associated pneumonia, urinary tract infections) in a trauma ICU.[73] However, the lack of methodological rigour in these studies prevents inferring causal links between checklist use and improved outcomes.[69] When used in isolation, checklists may not be sufficient to improve care. One study testing the utility of checklists for use on the daily ward round in an ICU demonstrated improvements in both processes and outcomes of care only when clinicians were prompted by a non-care-providing resident physician after an aspect of care covered by the checklist was omitted or overlooked.[74] Careful consideration of both checklist design and implementation is required when planning to incorporate checklists into the clinical setting.[67]

> **Practice tip**
>
> When developed in line with published guidelines, checklists may improve practice delivery by serving as an aide-mémoire.

Information and communication technologies

Health departments continue to develop systems and processes that will result in a complete electronic medical record. Critical care in particular is at the forefront of these developments, with bedside clinical information systems, order-entry strategies, decision support, handheld technologies and telehealth initiatives continuing to evolve and influence practice. This section examines the current and future impacts that these technologies will have on patient care and safety, and on clinician workflows and practices, as clinical information fully assimilates with evidence-based practice and clinical decision support systems.

Clinical information systems

Clinical information systems may enable improved data collection, storage, retrieval and reporting of patient-based information; and facilitate unit-based outcomes research and quality improvement activities.[75] Computerisation of monitoring and therapeutic activities for critically ill patients began in the 1960s, and has evolved to encompass all aspects of patient care such as cardiorespiratory monitoring, mechanical ventilation, fluid and medication delivery, imaging and results of diagnostic testing.[76,77] Patient-based bedside clinical information systems offer increasingly sophisticated functionality and device interfaces,[78] enabling real-time data capture, trending and reporting[76] and linkage to relational databases.[79,80]

The introduction of intravenous 'smart pump' technology is one application aimed at reducing adverse drug events and improving patient care by supporting evidence-based guidelines for medication management.[81] The operator-error prevention software is based on a device-based drug library with institution-established concentrations/dosage limits incorporated in the function of the pump. Resulting software functions include clinician alerts (for keystroke errors)[46] and transaction log data (post-incident analysis).[81,82] Medication errors and adverse drug events can be detected by this software. One Australian study has revealed significant reductions in medication administration errors can be achieved when smart pumps are systematically implemented.[83] There is evidence to suggest, however, that the features of smart pump technology are not being fully utilised by many hospitals that purchase them, limiting the potential for realising safety benefits such as the measurable impact on serious adverse drug events.[84] This highlights the need for promotional and quality improvement activities targeting improved utility of the smart pump features such as increasing nurses' use of the drug libraries.[85]

Although the proportion of ICUs using a clinical information system is not known, there are indications that uptake is on the increase.[86,87] Numerous benefits to healthcare systems that lead to enhanced quality of care have been reported such as improved documentation, legibility, evidence-based decision support, interdisciplinary communication and reduced duplication and medical errors.[88] In intensive care they have reduced documentation time and increased the proportion of time spent on direct care activities.[89] End-user support has been identified as an important factor in the success of clinical information system implementation.[90] Nurses in acute care settings are more accepting of new technologies when implemented well, and dissatisfaction is likely to result from the presence of too many barriers to successful implementation.[88] Barriers that have been identified include issues related to accessibility of staff to computers (e.g. too few in the clinical setting) and the system (e.g. login procedures and time-out rules), accuracy and the speed of operations. Other barriers identified were a lack of: IT support, knowledge and training; experience and confidence in using clinical information systems; time due to increased work demands; and consultation with end-users.[88]

Accuracy of data (correctness and completeness of the data set) from both manual and automated inputs to the information system requires further evaluation. While automated entry eliminates transcription errors from other data sources,[91] the use of 'carry-over' data to fields that require updating by clinicians, finding the right sampling frequency (i.e. the rate at which a clinical information system can record and display patient data) and human interaction such as clinician acceptance of monitor-generated data can all affect data accuracy. For example, if the pulmonary artery waveform is measured at a high frequency rate and displays large variability because of 'noise' and is not checked, erroneously high systolic blood pressure readings will be recorded.[75] Improvements to systems, however, have reportedly led to increased accuracy of data collections,[88,89] suggesting that perhaps developments in technology and the implementation strategies used have mitigated these problems. Errors can also arise, however, if systems are not designed to enhance communication between healthcare workers and facilitate coordination of work processes.[92,93]

Clinical alert functions are designed to improve delivery of care; however they can sometimes lack the specificity required to detect clinically important events[94] and may compromise patient safety when used excessively in clinical settings. For example, one study demonstrated 49–96% of drug safety alerts were overridden by clinicians.[95] A systematic review revealed improvements in prescribing behaviours and reductions in error rates as a result of computerised alerts and prompts; some studies reported a positive impact on clinical and organisational outcomes such as decreased prescribing-related renal impairment, fewer falls in elderly patients and reduced length of hospital stay.[96] In intensive care computerised alerts have been used to improve glucose control in patients without the need for increased blood sampling[97] and increase mean elevations of the head of the bed for patients without contraindications for this aspect of care.[98] The features that might make alerts and prompts more effective, however, are generally unknown and require further research.

Computerised order entry and decision support

Computerised provider order entry (CPOE) is a system that allows orders for medications, intravenous fluids, diagnostic tests and procedures to be entered then rapidly communicated to pharmacies. It can also be used for results management, treatment orders and clinical decision support.[99,100] CPOE is viewed as an important innovation in reducing medical errors, through minimising transcribing errors,[101] triggering alerts for adverse drug interactions and facilitating the adoption of evidence-based clinical guidelines.[99,102]

Implementation of CPOE and related clinical decision support systems have demonstrated significant reductions in medication errors and adverse drug events,[100] redundant or unnecessary order requests[103–105] and improved compliance with practice guidelines.[106,107] Decision support systems interface with hospital databases to retrieve patient-specific and other relevant clinical data and to generate recommended actions at the time and location of decision making.[108] Importantly, clinical decision making at the bedside can be enhanced by providing clinicians with a readily available tool that incorporates relevant clinical information and evidence-based medicine.[109] Clinician alerts (e.g. allergies or interaction effects) or prompts (e.g. to check coagulation when prescribing warfarin) can be generated. A number of studies have demonstrated improved delivery of patient care after the introduction of such reminders.[110,111] As with clinical information system implementation, detailed planning including examination of clinician workflow and care delivery patterns is required for successful implementation of a CPOE process.[112,113] A number of potentially important features of clinical decision support systems have been identified that cover communication content (e.g. provide recommendations with justifications in addition to assessment), clinician–system interaction (e.g. incorporate into clinical workflow, provide at the time and location it is required and request reason for not following recommendations) and other general (e.g. integrate with electronic charting or CPOE) and auxiliary (e.g. provide decision support results and feedback reports) features.[108,114]

Additional developments involving wireless communication, handheld technologies and closed-loop delivery systems may improve the efficiency, effectiveness and adoption of this innovation in clinical practice. Closed-loop delivery offers fully automated treatment without the need for human intervention;[108] it adjusts drug or fluid delivery based on active feedback from the target parameter (e.g. inotropic dosages adjusted to a range for mean arterial pressure). An example of a successfully implemented system includes administering protocols for weaning patients from mechanical ventilation to ventilator machines.[115]

Handheld technologies

Wireless applications enable clinical information access, portability and mobility within a critical care environment at the point of care. Clinical uses for a personal digital assistant (PDA), tablet computer and smartphone technologies continue to evolve at a rapid pace.[116] These handheld computers use operating systems and pen-like styluses that enable touchscreen functionality, handwriting recognition and synchronisation with other hospital-based computer systems. An increasing array of clinical applications and content is available for downloading to these devices, including drug reference information (e.g. Monthly Index of Medical Specialties [MIMS]), clinical guidelines, medical calculators and internet-based literature searches.[117,118]

A systematic review of healthcare applications for smartphones revealed a total of 57 applications for healthcare professionals with the majority focused on disease diagnosis,[21] medical calculators,[8] drug reference information,[6] literature search[6] and health information system client applications.[4] There were eleven applications related to medical or nursing student education. Both healthcare professionals and students reported disease diagnosis, drug reference and medical calculator applications as the most useful.[119]

Personal digital assistant and smartphone use has been reported as a helpful nursing education tool,[120–122] with nursing students reporting specific benefits of using handheld devices such as having access to readily available data, validation of thinking processes and facilitation of care plan re-evaluation.[121] In critical care, handheld devices have been used to document clinical activities, such as logging critical care procedures, which was demonstrated as feasible and useful.[123] They have also been used to deliver point-of-care decision support to improve antibiotic selection[124] and prescribing[105] and an interactive weaning protocol that assisted care providers wean patients from mechanical ventilation more efficiently when compared with the use of a paper-based weaning protocol.[125]

The benefits of this mobile computing also create concerns, particularly regarding confidentiality of patient information. Health services therefore need policies for managing handheld devices, including password protection, data encryption, authenticated synchronisation and physical security.[126] In particular, wireless applications require appropriate standards for data security.[127] As these issues are addressed, these technologies will form an integral component of routine clinical practice in critical care.

Practice tip

While handheld devices can assist nurses in their practice, with a range of helpful clinical applications now available, ensure patient confidentiality is not breached and the devices are secure.

Telehealth initiatives

Remote critical care management (tele-ICU) using telemedicine/telehealth technologies is expanding as the necessary high bandwidths for transmitting large amounts of data and digital imagery become available between partner units or hospitals. Videoconferencing functions enable direct visualisation and communication of patients and on-site staff with the 'virtual' critical care clinician or team. Review of real-time physiological data, patient flowcharts and other documents (e.g. electrocardiograms, laboratory results) or images (e.g. radiographs) provides a comprehensive data set for patient assessment and management.[116]

This technology-enabled remote care initiative is of particular value for critical care units where no or limited on-site intensivist resources are available. Despite various methodological limitations,[128] several studies using 'before and after' comparisons have indicated improved outcomes such as decreases in severity-adjusted hospital mortality, incidence of ICU complications, ICU length of stay and ICU costs.[129–131] Other studies, however, have not found improvement in patient outcomes as a result of telemedicine technology,[132–134] highlighting the complex nature of these initiatives and the difficulties evaluating them. More recently, a systematic review and meta-analysis of the literature found that tele-ICU coverage was associated with reduced ICU mortality and length of stay but not hospital mortality or length of stay.[117] The constantly evolving nature of technology and innovative ideas from healthcare workers can bring about novel approaches to healthcare delivery. One study, for example, demonstrated improved outcomes for neurological ICU patients through the use of a robotic tele-ICU system that made rounds in response to nurse paging.[131]

There are also characteristics of tele-ICU that are likely to impact on both the process and outcomes of care. Benefits are likely to be generated from the availability of extra resources and the ability of the tele-ICU to serve as a quality improvement trigger (e.g. checking compliance with evidence-based medicine) and to provide medication management support, software alerts and real-time patient monitoring by camera.[116] For these benefits to be realised, however, the technology needs to be accepted and used appropriately by ICU staff. Further studies that include detailed descriptions of system implementation are required to determine the most effective elements of this technology in critical care settings as well as their impact on care processes and outcomes.[128,135]

In addition to remote patient assessment and management, telecommunications have been used to deliver continuing education to rural healthcare professionals for many years via audio, video and computer.[136] Distance education delivered via web-based courses accessed over the internet is now commonplace.[137] One example of a web-based educational tool was used to provide information about the classification of pressure ulcers and the differentiation between pressure ulcers and moisture lesions to both student and qualified nurses.[138] The potential use of web logs or 'blogs',[139] online communities and virtual preceptorships[137] in nursing education and intensive care practice has also been discussed.[119] Professional development opportunities are also provided online; for example, AusmedOnline contains a range of resources and learning activities that count towards continuing professional development for registration requirements. However, more work is required to determine how successful these technological advances are in terms of educational outcomes.[139]

Patient safety

The signing of the Declaration of Vienna in 2009[140] committed critical care organisations around the world, including the World Federation of Critical Care Nurses, to patient safety. Patient safety is viewed as a crucial component of quality.[141-144] Over the years, numerous definitions of patient safety have emerged in the literature. The Institute Of Medicine described it as the absence of preventable harm to a patient during the process of health care,[141] whereas the World Health Organization describes it as the reduction of risk of unnecessary harm to an acceptable level.[143]

Three techniques used to understand patient risk are: 1) analysing reports of adverse events, 2) root cause analyses and 3) failure mode and effect analysis. Research on adverse events in critical care has helped to better understand patient risks and target improvement activities. For example, medications, indwelling lines and equipment failure were the three most frequent types of adverse events in a study of 205 intensive care units worldwide.[1] Focusing on analysing the narratives written about adverse events is viewed as an important way to learn from errors. Root cause analysis is a structured process generally used to analyse catastrophic or sentinel events.[145,146] In root cause analysis, the various situations that led to the event are documented and analysed in order to identify contributing factors to the event and make recommendations for system changes to prevent the event from occurring again. Learning from both incident reporting and root cause analyses is based on the premise that the information they contain is of sufficient quality to allow accurate analysis, interpretation and detection of the root causes of problems and, even more importantly, the formulation and implementation of corrective actions. Failure mode and effect analysis identifies potential failures and their effects, calculating their risk and prioritising potential failure modes based on risk.[147] In addition to examining patient risk, another strategy has focused on understanding the safety culture of a unit or organisation, with subsequent activities aimed at improving components of this culture.

Practice tip

By undertaking a root cause analysis, the contributing factors to the event can be identified and strategies to mitigate future adverse events can be implemented.

Safety culture

Measurement of the baseline safety culture facilitates an action plan for improvement. Safety culture has been defined as 'the product of individual and group values, attitudes, perceptions, competencies, and patterns of behaviour that determine the commitment to, and the style and proficiency of, an organisation's health and safety management.'[148] It is commonly referred to as 'the way we do things around here.'[149] A systematic review found evidence for a relationship between safety culture and patient outcomes at both the hospital and unit level.[150] A widely used instrument to measure safety culture, the Safety Attitudes Questionnaire (SAQ), focuses on six domains: teamwork climate, safety climate, job satisfaction, perceptions of management, working conditions and stress recognition.[151] Interestingly, two studies in the USA[152,153] and one Australian study conducted in 10 ICUs[154] showed that nurses and doctors differed in their perceptions of safety culture. The Australian study also identified some differences between bedside nurses and nursing leaders.[154] Using the SAQ, a Palestinian neonatal intensive care unit study found wide variation in the perceptions of the safety culture held by 164 nurses and 40 physicians in 16 hospitals.[155] Another recent European study of 378 patients in 57 ICUs showed a relationship between safety culture and fewer errors.[156]

Practice tip

A positive safety culture is associated with better patient outcomes.

One strategy to improve the safety culture has involved identifying factors that make organisations safe, which in turn allows initiatives to be developed that target areas of specific need. For example, five characteristics of organisations that have been able to achieve high reliability include:[157]

1 safety viewed as a priority by leaders
2 flattened hierarchy that promotes speaking up about concerns
3 regular team training
4 use of effective methods of communicating
5 standardisation.

There are a number of other resources available to those interested in improving patient safety. For example,

WHO has published a patient safety curriculum guide to assist organisations in this endeavor.[158] Leadership, teamwork and behaviour change strategies provide a foundation for improvements in safety culture.[159] In the USA, the Comprehensive Unit-Based Safety Program has emerged as one specific safety intervention.[160] Three others shown to be beneficial in systematic reviews were executive or multidisciplinary wards and multi-faceted interventions, which included a comprehensive unit-based safety program, and team training, which included tools to improve communication. Another American critical care quality improvement program found that a nurse-led safety program that included executive walkrounds and a multidisciplinary team tasked with identifying and resolving safety issues were effective.[161] The three top safety issues identified related to nursing, supplies and daily unit operations with 36–70% of the issues being resolved. In summary, understanding the various dimensions of safety culture in a unit can be used as a foundation for the development and implementation of programs targeted at specific aspects that may benefit from improvements. To be successful, safety programs have to be supported by the leaders as well as other members of the unit.

Rapid response systems

Rapid response systems (RRS) are systems that have developed to recognise and provide emergency response to patients who experience acute deterioration.[162–165] One 2013 systematic review of RRS found moderate evidence for the claim that RRS were associated with reduced rates of cardiopulmonary arrest and mortality.[164] A second 2013 systematic review concluded that much of the available evidence on the effects of RRS was of poor quality.[165] The Australian Commission on Safety and Quality in Health Care have identified eight essential elements in a RRS (Table 3.6).[162]

RRS have three components.[166] First, there are some criteria and a system for identifying and activating the rapid response team, often referred to as the afferent limb.[166,167] Second, there is the response, also termed the efferent limb.[166] Finally, there is an administrative and quality improvement component.[166] Each of these components is briefly described.

Afferent limb

Recognising the deteriorating patient, the afferent limb has focused on measuring clinical signs including vital signs, level of consciousness and oxygenation as well as acting on abnormalities in these measurements.[166] They may also include concerns expressed by clinicians and families.[168,169] Various scoring systems to identify ward patients with clinical deterioration have evolved as part of the development of critical care outreach,[170] including the Medical Emergency Team (MET),[169] early warning scoring[170] and patient-at-risk criteria[171] (see Table 3.7). All systems identify abnormalities in commonly measured parameters (e.g. respiratory rate, heart rate, blood pressure,

TABLE 3.6

Essential elements of a rapid response system (RRS)

DOMAIN	ELEMENT	DESCRIPTION
Clinical processes	Measurement and documentation	Vital signs, oxygen saturation and level of consciousness should be undertaken regularly on all acute care patients
	Escalation of care	A protocol for the organisation's response in dealing with abnormal physiological measures and observations including appropriate modifications to nursing care, increased monitoring, medical review and calling for assistance
	Rapid response systems	When severe deterioration occurs, medical emergency teams, outreach teams or liaison nurses are available to respond
	Clinical communication	Structured communication protocols are used to hand over information about the patient
Organisational prerequisites	Organisational supports	Executive and clinical leadership support and a formal policy framework for recognition and response systems should exist
	Education	Education should cover clinical observation, identification of deterioration, escalation protocols, communication strategies and skills in initiating early interventions
	Evaluation, audit and feedback	Ongoing monitoring and evaluation are required to track changes in outcomes over time and to check that the RRS is operating as planned
	Technological systems and solutions	As relevant technologies are developed, they should be incorporated into service delivery, after considering evidence of their efficacy and cost as well as potential unintended consequences

Adapted from Australian Commission on Safety and Quality in Health Care: National Consensus Statement: Essential Elements for Recognising and Responding to Clinical Deterioration. Sydney: ACSQHC; 2010, with permission.

TABLE 3.7

Commonly used risk assessment scores

CLINICAL PARAMETER	MEDICAL EMERGENCY TEAM CALLING CRITERIA[216]	PATIENT-AT-RISK SCORE[173]	MODIFIED EARLY WARNING SCORE[172]
	CALL FOR ALL CONDITIONS LISTED BELOW	ANY 3 OR MORE OF THE FOLLOWING PRESENT	SCORE OF ≥3 REQUIRES REFERRAL
Airway	Threatened	–	–
Breathing	Respiratory arrest rate <5/min or >36/min	Respiratory rate 1 = 20–29 breaths/min 2 = <10 or 30–39 breaths/min 3 = ≥40 breaths/min Oxygen saturation: 1 = 90–94% 2 = 85–89% 3 = <85%	Respiratory rate: 1 point = 15–20/min 2 points = <8 or 21–29/min 3 points = ≥30/min
Cardiac	Cardiac arrest pulse <40/min or >140/min	Heart rate: 1 = 40–49 or 100–114/min 2 = 115–129/min 3 = >130/min	Heart rate: 1 = 40–50/min or 101–110/min 2 = <40/min or 111–129/min 3 = ≥130/min
	Systolic blood pressure (SBP) <90 mmHg	SBP: 1 = 80–99 mmHg 2 = 70–79 or ≥180 mmHg 3 = <70 mmHg	SBP: 1 = 81–100 mmHg 2 = 71–80 or >200 mmHg 3 = <70 mmHg
Disability (neurological)	Decrease in Glasgow Coma Score >2 repeated/prolonged seizures	1 = confused 2 = responds to voice 3 = responds to pain/unresponsive	1 = responds to voice 2 = responds to pain 3 = unconscious
Other parameters	Any patient who does not fit the criteria above is causing clinical concern	Temperature: 1 = 35.0–35.9° or 37.5–38.4°C 2 = <35° or >38.5°C Urine output: 1 = >3 mL/kg/h 2 = <0.5 mL/kg/h 3 = nil	

neurological status). Other parameters used in patient assessment are oxygen saturation, temperature and urine output in patient-at-risk and early warning scores. The early warning scoring/patient-at-risk systems include an ordinal scoring approach used as calling criteria for contacting the admitting medical team, ICU staff, the critical care outreach team or the MET, depending on the severity of the patient's clinical deterioration and the resources available in the local clinical environment. Yet, observation charts are not always being completed and, when they are, sometimes the RRT is not called even when the calling criteria are met. However, an Australian study showed that a new observation chart incorporating the modified early warning score along with training significantly improved the documentation of vital signs in the first 24 hours after patients had been discharged from the ICU.[172]

Efferent limb

The efferent limb involves the team responding to clinical deterioration.[166] Some teams will include physicians and nurses, known as MET or RRT, whereas others such as critical care outreach teams[166] and ICU liaison nurses are nurse-led.[173] Irrespective of the title of the model used, the RRT generally assess deteriorating patients and then initiate emergency treatments. A 2014 systematic review of critical care transitions programs in general found they were associated with a reduced risk of ICU readmission.[174] This positive association was also found when the only service considered was an ICU liaison nurse.[174]

Administrative and quality improvement

The third component of an RRS focuses on administration and quality improvement.[166] Generally, this involves the collection and analysis of RRS data including the reason for the call, the treatments administered and patient outcomes. Analysing RRS data provides managers, clinicians and policy makers with guidance for future improvements. A single site evaluation of a two-tiered RRS provides one example of how local RRS data can be collected and analysed.[175] In summary, RRS have evolved to provide emergency care to patients whose condition is deteriorating, and who are not already in the critical care unit. RRS involve a mechanism to identify these patients and call for help, as well as a response team. They also generally involve some administrative and quality improvement components to improve the service. RRT rely on team members working together, which leads to the next section on non-technical skills.

Non-technical skills

Nurses need to have current knowledge and skills in critical care to ensure safe, high quality care, but these technical skills are not sufficient. They also need to possess other, non-technical skills (NTS) to ensure patient safety. This section provides an overview of four inter-related[176,177] non-technical skills: situational awareness, decision making, communication and teamwork. Another important non-technical skill, leadership, is described in Chapters 1 and 2. Understanding the importance of non-technical skills in providing safe, high quality care, has led to the development of a number of training programs, which are briefly described in this section.

Situational awareness

Situational awareness has been described as the cognitive, social and personal skills that complement technical skills and contribute to safe and efficient task performance.[178] It describes the awareness and understanding of a situation and its possible outcomes.[179] Situations may be categorised on a continuum from routine and easily managed to confusing and dangerous, requiring specific skills and expertise.[180] Endsley,[181] whose work has been particularly influential, describes three levels of situational awareness. Level 1, *perception*, involves gathering data about the current situation. Level 2, *comprehension*, reflects interpretation and understanding the data. Level 3, *projection*, is concerned with predicting what can happen in the future. Figure 3.3 demonstrates application of these three levels of situational awareness using the scenario of a postoperative patient whose blood pressure has dropped. Importantly, situational awareness is viewed as a necessary precursor for good quality decision making.[179]

Team situational awareness is a term applied to teams and reflects the notion that team members possess the situational awareness needed to perform their tasks in the team.[179] This team situational awareness has also been termed shared situational awareness.[181] In the critical care environment, nurses and physicians will have some unique but related tasks to undertake including during procedures such as central line insertions, intubations

---

FIGURE 3.3 Situational awareness example.

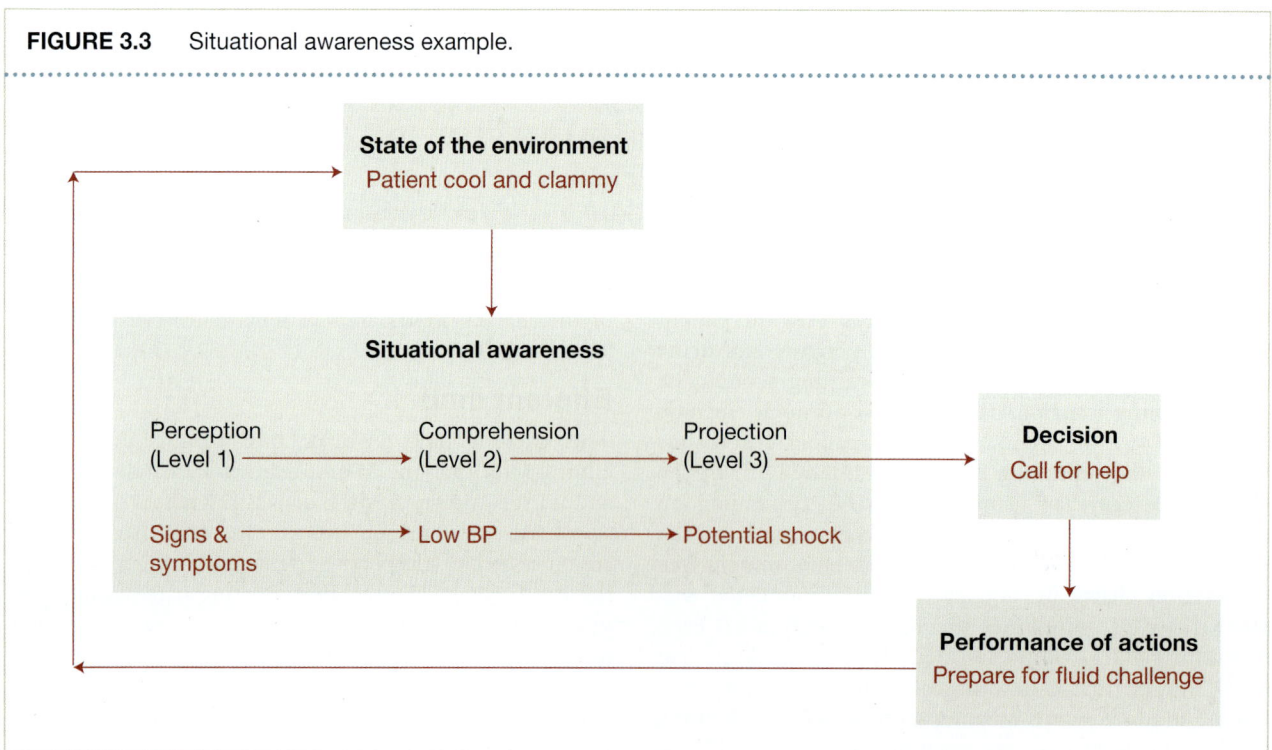

and bronchoscopies, and these tasks will require both complementary and shared situational awareness. The extent of team or shared situational awareness will influence the quality of decisions and subsequent team performance.[179]

Practice tip

Team briefings before undertaking a complex procedure can help to develop team situational awareness.

One review identified that both individual factors and interpersonal behaviours influenced situational awareness.[177] Lapses in situational awareness can occur because of issues such as distractions, fatigue, time pressures and team dynamics such as assertive authority figures. A number of strategies are recommended to overcome these lapses. They include thorough briefings about the nature and risk of a given activity, minimising distractions and interruptions during critical tasks, receiving regular updates, good time management, being physically and mentally fit for work and speaking up when not sure of a goal, procedure or next step.[181,182,183]

Decision making

Decision making involves a judgement or choosing an option (i.e. a course of action) to meet the needs of a given situation.[181] In critical care, multiple, complex decisions are made in rapid succession.[184] Decision making entails defining a problem, generating and considering one or more alternatives, selecting and implementing an option and reviewing the outcome. Clinical decision making is a complex process and is influenced by a number of factors. For example, environmental factors such as the team, the patient and resources can influence decision making as can situational awareness. Individual factors such as fatigue, affective state interruption in work and distractions can also influence decision making.[185,186]

Critical care nursing practice has been the focus of many studies on decision making. One study demonstrated that critical care nurses generate one or more hypotheses about a situation prior to decision making.[184] Other studies indicated that experienced and inexperienced nurses differ in their decision-making skills,[185–187] and that role models or mentors are important in assisting to develop decision-making skills.[188] A Greek study classified ICU nurses' decisions as urgent or non-urgent and as independent or dependent.[189] The researchers observed that 75% (962/1281) of decisions were non-urgent and 60% (220/368) were independent.[189] It is intuitive that good quality clinical decisions, irrespective of what they are about, will likely improve patient care and outcomes.

Recommendations for developing clinical decision-making skills

Several strategies that can be used to help critical care nurses to develop their clinical decision-making abilities

---

TABLE 3.8

Strategies to develop clinical decision making

STRATEGY	DESCRIPTION
Iterative hypothesis testing[190] (Narayan and Corcoran-Perry, 2008)	Description of a clinical situation for which the clinician has to generate questions and develop hypotheses; with additional questioning the clinician will develop further hypotheses. Three phases: 1 asking questions to gather data about a patient 2 justifying the data sought 3 interpreting the data to describe the influence of new information on decisions
Interactive model[190] (Narayan and Corcoran-Perry, 2008)	Schema (mental structures) used to teach new knowledge by building on previous learning. Three components: 1 advanced organisers – blueprint that previews the material to be learned and connects it to previous materials 2 progressive differentiation – a general concept presented first is broken down into smaller ideas 3 integrative reconciliation – similarities and differences and relationships between concepts explored
Case study[191] (Rivett and Jones, 2008)	Description of a clinical situation with a number of cues followed by a series of questions. Three types: 1 stable – presents information, then asks clinicians about it 2 dynamic – presents information, asks the clinicians about it, presents more information, asks more questions 3 dynamic with expert feedback – combines the dynamic method with immediate expert feedback
Reflection on action[190] (Narayan and Corcoran-Perry, 2008)	Clinicians are asked to reflect on their actions after a particular event. This pondering focuses on clinical judgements made, feelings surrounding the actions and the actions themselves. Reflection on action can be undertaken as an individual or group activity and is often facilitated by an expert
Thinking aloud[190] (Narayan and Corcoran-Perry, 2008)	A clinical situation is provided and the clinician is asked to 'think aloud' or verbalise their decisions. Thinking aloud is generally facilitated by an expert and can be undertaken individually or in groups

are identified in Table 3.8.[190,191] These strategies can be used by nurses at any level to develop their own decision-making skills or by educators in planning educational sessions. It is important to note, however, that a review of interventions to improve decision making concluded that most studies in this area were of relatively poor quality.[192]

Communication

Communication has been described as 'the exchange of information, feedback or response, ideas and feelings'.[176,p 69] Good quality communication is viewed as a two-way sharing of information, whereby the sender encodes some idea into a message and transmits it to a receiver. The receiver then decodes the message to gain an understanding of it. Next, the receiver becomes the sender, encoding and transmitting a subsequent message.[176] There are various types of communication including verbal and non-verbal. Non-verbal communication includes written communication and body cues or gestures.

Reason,[193] a well-known safety researcher, suggests that there are three kinds of communication failure that contribute to accidents. The first, system failure, occurs when there are either no channels of communication or the channels that exist are not working or are not used. The second, message failure, happens when necessary information is not communicated. And finally, reception failure occurs when the information is misinterpreted or arrives too late.

P r a c t i c e t i p

Using closed loop communications, where the receiver acknowledges the message was heard, can prevent miscommunication.

Experts recommend that communication be explicit, efficient and closed-loop.[194] By being explicit, a person is being clear in what they are saying. Being efficient means that the message is conveyed using only as many words as necessary. And closed-loop communication is a term used to signify that a receiver acknowledges or responds to the sender of information. This response lets the initiator know that the message was heard. Other strategies to improve communication include ensuring it is timely and assertive.[194] Timely communication means that the sender is cognisant of the other activities that the receiver may be doing and, because of this, provides information at a relevant time. Assertiveness involves standing up for yourself while respecting others.

In the critical care setting two specific communication situations have been the focus of recent research – clinical handover and rounds. Handover is more than the transfer of patient information; it has been described as the transfer of professional responsibility and accountability for some or all aspects of care for a patient, or group of patients, from one care provider to another.[195] Besides sharing patient information, handovers provide

nurses with opportunities for social bonding, coaching and educating and team building.[196,197] A contemporary Australian study focused on the content of ICU nursing handover.[198] The researchers found that while ≥95% of observed handovers included identifying nursing care needs, vital sign observations, changes in patient condition and the medical management of the patient, ≤40% included a discussion of discharge or long-term plans, cross-checking and reporting on resuscitation status.[198] A second study of 157 nursing shift-to-shift handovers conducted in seven ICUs in three countries (Australia, Israel and the United Kingdom)[199] found handovers were more comprehensive when: 1) the oncoming nurse did not know the patient; 2) the patient was expected to die during the shift; or 3) the family were present. Over 70% of nurses in Israel had cared for the patient in the previous 48 hours, whereas only 29% and 20% of UK and Australian nurses had. Over 75% of the handover communication included the goals for care and 73% included pain management, but legal issues such as advance directives and identification of a health proxy were mentioned in less than 10% of the handovers.

A 2013 review identified three important features of good quality handover including: 1) face-to-face, two way communication; 2) standardised templates or checklists that incorporate a minimum dataset; and 3) content that includes the patient's current diagnosis and clinical situation.[200] In order to improve the quality of handovers, a group of Australians has developed an interactive, 3-dimensional computer simulation (virtual world) for training intensive care nurses in shift-to-shift handover.[201]

Multidisciplinary rounds are seen to be one way to promote shared situational awareness, yet seminal research in the 1990s showed that nurses were not participating in medical rounds.[202] In fact, this study revealed communication between doctors and nurses accounted for 2% of all activities but 37% of all errors. In another study published in 2006, nurses did not believe they were allowed to talk during rounds in two of four ICUs studied.[203] A 2013 systematic review of ICU rounds concluded that 'rounds conducted using a standardized structure and a best practice checklist by a multidisciplinary group of providers, with explicitly defined roles and a goal-orientated approach, had the strongest supporting evidence'.[200, p 2025] Table 3.9 provides more specific details of the recommendations from this review.

Teamwork

Teams have been described as two or more individuals with specialised roles and responsibilities who act interdependently to achieve some common goal,[204] although a systematic review noted teamwork is a broad term with varying definitions.[205] High performing teams share an understanding of the activity they are working on; they understand the aim or mission of that activity, and

> **TABLE 3.9**
> Recommendations for ICU rounds
>
> | BEST PRACTICE | STRENGTH OF RECOMMENDATION |
> |---|---|
> | Implement multidisciplinary rounds (including at least a medical doctor, registered nurse and pharmacist) | Strong – definitely do it |
> | Standardise location, time and team composition | Strong – definitely do it |
> | Define explicit roles for each HCP participating on rounds | Strong – definitely do it |
> | Develop and implement structured tool (best practices checklist) | Strong – definitely do it |
> | Reduce nonessential time-wasting activities | Strong – definitely do it |
> | Minimise unnecessary interruptions | Strong – definitely do it |
> | Focus discussions on development of daily goals and document all discussed goals in health record | Strong – definitely do it |
> | Conduct discussions at bedside to promote patient-centeredness | Weak – probably do it |
> | Conduct discussions in conference room to promote efficiency and communication | Weak – probably do it |
> | Establish open collaborative discussion environment | Weak – probably do it |
> | Ensure clear visibility between all HCP | Weak – probably do it |
> | Empower HCP to promote team-based approach to discussions | Weak – probably do it |
> | Produce visual presentation of patient information | No specific recommendation |
>
> HCP = health care professional.
> *Adapted from* Lane D, Ferri M, Lemaire J, McLaughlin K, Stelfox HT. A systematic review of evidence-informed practices for patient care rounds in the ICU. Crit Care Med 2013;41(8):2015–29, with permission.

they know each other's roles and expectations. They are also trained and skilled in leadership, conflict resolution, back-up behaviour and closed-loop communication. Important aspects of leadership include coordinating the team, distributing workloads equitably and monitoring the team's performance. Conflict resolution often requires clarification of roles and responsibilities, fostering useful debate and assertive communication. Back-up behaviour is when one team member can step in to assist another in their role, providing support to other team members. In essence, teamwork is dependent on each member being able to anticipate the needs of others, adjust to others' actions and the changing environment and have a shared understanding of how a task should be performed. In their systematic review, Dietz and colleagues found standardised protocols (such as using checklists), implementing daily rounds and training were the three main solutions used to improve ICU teamwork.[205]

Non-technical skills training

Increasing recognition of the importance of non-technical skills has led to the development of a number of training programs. These programs recognise that, while human error cannot be eliminated, it can be minimised, trapped or mitigated.[176] A systematic review of non-technical skills training to enhance patient safety documented both the content of and training methods used in non-technical skills training.[206]

Figure 3.4 demonstrates the content covered in the team training studies reviewed by Gordon and colleagues.[206] In addition to the core non-technical skills described in this section, the review also identified training programs focused on understanding error and systems such as the human/technology interface. Two well-known teamwork experts noted that factors such as how the team training is implemented, the method of its delivery and leadership all influence the effectiveness of team training on both processes and outcomes.[207]

Figure 3.5 provides an overview of these training methods.[206] Most of the team training studies reviewed took a multidisciplinary approach, reflecting contemporary clinical practice. Simulation has attracted a lot of attention recently as a team training strategy. Simulation allows clinicians to practise skills and reflect on their performance in a simulated environment. That is, it increases both knowledge and performance. In their 2013 systematic review, Schmidt and colleagues[208] asserted that simulation as a patient safety strategy had four purposes: 1) education; 2) assessment; 3) research; and 4) health system integration. It is evident that teamwork and NTS team training are core components of patient safety. In summary, patient safety involves understanding the risks to patients and developing strategies to minimise these risks. Safety culture and non-technical skills are two important aspects of patient safety, with a number of strategies and programs available to enhance both.

FIGURE 3.4   Analysis of non-technical skills training teaching methods.

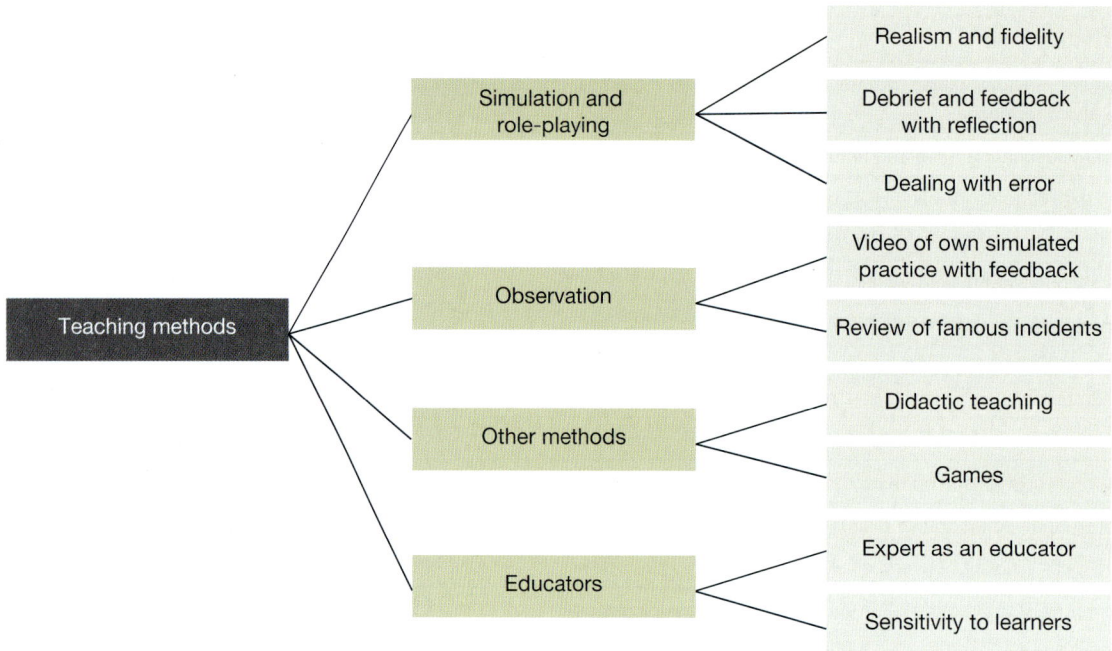

Reproduced from Gordon M, Darbyshire D, Baker P. Non-technical skills training to enhance patient safety: a systematic review. Med Educ 2012;46(11):1042–54, with permission.

FIGURE 3.5   Analysis of non-technical skills training content themes.

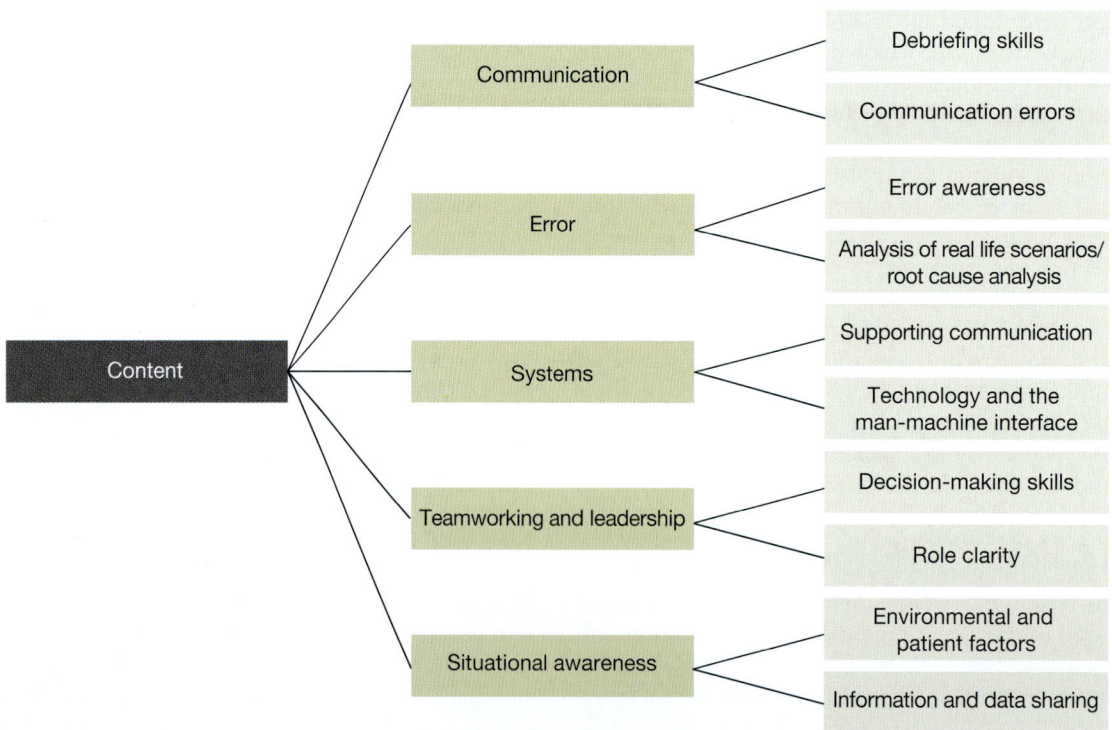

Reproduced from Gordon M, Darbyshire D, Baker P. Non-technical skills training to enhance patient safety: a systematic review. Med Educ 2012;46(11):1042–54, with permission.

Summary

In summary, this chapter has provided an overview of safety and quality in critical care. EBN is viewed as an important foundation to promote quality as is the development and use of good quality clinical practice guidelines. Quality and safety monitoring underpin understanding the risks that patients face in critical care. The use of care bundles, checklists and information and communication technologies may improve quality of care. Improving patient safety is multifaceted, but often includes understanding the safety culture as well as the risks faced by patients in a particular clinical area. Techniques such as the analysis of clinical incidents, root cause analyses and failure mode and effects analysis help in understanding situations that place patients at risk of adverse events. One particular high-risk scenario is the deteriorating patient, with a number of RRS now being implemented to respond to this scenario. Other initiatives to improve patient safety include NTS training. Understanding situations that place patients at risk of harm as well as the safety culture of a unit or organisation provides the foundation to improve safety culture.

Case study

You have just been asked to participate in a working group tasked with identifying and detailing important content for clinical decision support within your unit's new CPOE system. As a member of this group you are required to contribute one key area that requires decision support – glycaemic management. The question below asks you to plan your contribution to this working group.

CASE STUDY QUESTION

1   Use the information contained in this chapter and related learning activities to prepare a brief outline of what needs to be incorporated into the design and functionality of the clinical decision support system. The outline should include the following:

   • aim(s) of the clinical decision support system (e.g. reduce hypoglycaemic events)
   • target patient population and potential users of the system
   • features that will be important to the success of this particular system
   • methods for evaluating its effectiveness.

Recommended reading for this case study:

Mann EA, Salinas J: The use of computer decision support systems for the critical care environment. AACN Adv Crit Care 2009;20(3):216–219.

RESEARCH VIGNETTE

Karra V, Papathanassoglou ED, Lemonidou C, Sourtzi P, Giannakopoulou M. Exploration and classification of intensive care nurses' clinical decisions: a Greek perspective. Nurs Crit Care 2014;19(2):87–97

Abstract

Aim: The recording, identification, coding and classification of clinical decisions by intensive care nurses.

Background: Clinical decision-making is an essential dimension of nursing practice as through this process nurses make choices to meet the goals of patient care. Intensive care nurses' decision-making has received attention because of the complexity and urgency associated with it, however, the types of nurses' clinical decisions have not been described systematically.

Methods: Qualitative content analysis of daily diaries of clinical decisions recorded during nursing work by 23 purposefully selected intensive care nurses from three major hospitals of Greece. The process of data collection and analysis continued until the point of theoretical saturation.

Findings: Eight categories of nursing clinical decisions emerged including decisions related to: (1) evaluation, (2) diagnosis, (3) prevention, (4) intervention, (5) communication with patients, (6) clinical information seeking, (7) setting of clinical priorities and (8) communication with health care professionals. Psychological assessment and support decisions were scarce, whereas patient input in care decisions appeared to be limited. The most frequent types of decisions were regarding intervention (29%), evaluation (25%) and clinical setting of priorities (17%), while clinical information seeking (3%) and communication with patients' decisions (2%) were the least frequent. Additionally, recorded decisions were ranked in order of degree of urgency and of dependency on medical order. Non-urgent decisions were 78% of the total and 60% of nurses' intervention decisions were independent of medical order and were related to basic nursing care.

Conclusions: Intensive care nurses make multiple decisions that seem to be in line with the nursing process, although the latter is not officially implemented in Greek ICUs.

Relevance to clinical practice: The types and frequency of clinical decisions made by intensive care nurses are related to features of ICU work environment, their professional autonomy and accountability, as well as their perceptions of their clinical role.

Critique

This interesting study focused on identifying and classifying the decisions Greek ICU nurses made. It received institutional approval and individual nurses consented to be part of the study. The nurses in this study were drawn from three major hospitals and were all registered nurses. They were purposely sampled to ensure they had a range of education and experience, but all had at least 5 years of clinical experience and 2 years of ICU experience. This sampling technique was appropriate and resulted in a variation in participants and contexts, something that helps ensure 'rich data' are collected. While qualitative research does not aim to identify generalisable findings, using three hospitals may increase the applicability of the findings to other contexts. Nurses recorded the decisions they made during one 8-hour shift on a 'log sheet' that they referred to as a 'diary of decisions'. While the authors explained that they considered other methods to collect the data such as the 'think aloud' technique, the diary of decisions was the method favoured by participants. It is possible that there may have been missing or inaccurate information recorded during times when the nurses were particularly busy, given writing these notes would have taken time away from patient care and other normal work activities. Data collection occurred over eight months in late 2011 and all three shifts (day, evening and night), suggesting good sampling in terms of the times the decisions were made and recorded. The researchers clearly explained how they undertook data analysis using content analysis. They noted that, while they used an inductive approach to analysis, many of their emerging categories reflected the nursing process (assess, plan, implement, evaluate). They were also able to classify the emerging categories as urgent or non-urgent and independent or dependent. Overall, the findings were clearly and logically presented. The tables were clear and complemented the text. The discussion of the findings was insightful and easy to understand. Overall, this was an interesting study that may provide ideas to others for how they could investigate decision making in their own context.

Learning activities

1   Using each domain of quality and safety as headings (i.e. structure, process, culture, outcome), list some of the key considerations for a quality improvement project targeting shift-to-shift nursing handover in your unit.

2   After identifying a CPG that guides nurses in providing care in your unit, assess it against the NHMRC criteria of: 1) its evidence base; 2) consistency of the primary research findings; 3) proposed clinical impact of the evidence; 4) generalisability of the evidence; and 5) applicability of the evidence to your unit's context.

3   Examine the patterns of incidence for a high-frequency adverse event in your unit over the past 12 months. What were the causes of incidents? What targeted strategies could be used to reduce the incidence of these adverse events?

4   Identify and provide a rationale for an aspect of care that might benefit from the use of a checklist in your unit. Develop some specific checklist items that you think should be included.

5   Describe how technology is used in your unit to improve care delivered to patients. Using the information outlined in the section on information and communication technologies, identify where there is potential to use technology to improve care delivery further. Use examples specific to your unit.

Online resources

Agency for Healthcare Research and Quality, www.ahrq.gov

Australian Commission on Safety and Quality in Health Care (ACSQHC), www.safetyandquality.gov.au

Australian Council on Healthcare Standards (ACHS), www.achs.org.au

Institute for Healthcare Improvement (IHI), USA, www.ihi.org/ihi

Intensive Care Coordination and Monitoring Unit (ICCMU), New South Wales Health, http://intensivecare.hsnet.nsw.gov.au

Joint Commission (USA), www.jointcommission.org

National E-Health Transition Authority, www.nehta.gov.au/

National Health and Medical Research Council, www.nhmrc.gov.au

National Quality Forum, www.qualityforum.org

Quality Use of Medicines, www.health.gov.au/internet/main/publishing.nsf/Content/nmp-quality.htm

World Health Organization Patient Safety, www.who.int/patientsafety/en

Further reading

Ausserhofer D, Schubert M, Desmedt M, Blegen MA, De Geest S, Schwendimann R. The association of patient safety climate and nurse-related organizational factors with selected patient outcomes: a cross-sectional survey. Int J Nurs Stud 2013;50(2):240–52.

Australian Commission on Safety and Quality in Health Care. Safety and Quality Improvement Guide Standard 9: Recognising and responding to clinical deterioration in acute health care. Sydney: ACSQHC; 2012.

Browne M, Cook P. Inappropriate trust in technology: implications for critical care nurses. Nurs Crit Care 2011;16(2):92–8.

Craze L, McGeorge P, Holmes D, Bernardi S, Taylor P, Morris-Yates A et al. Recognising and responding to deterioration in mental state: a scoping review. Sydney: ACSQHC; 2014.

Dubois C-A, D'Amour D, Tchouaket E, Clarke S, Rivard M, Blais R. Associations of patient safety outcomes with models of nursing care organization at unit level in hospitals. Int J Qual Health Care 2013;25(2):110–7.

Garrouste-Orgeas M, Soufir L, Tabah A, Schwebel C, Vesin A, Adrie C et al; Outcomerea Study Group. A multifaceted program for improving quality of care in intensive care units: IATROREF study. Crit Care Med 2012;40(2):468–76.

Groves PS. The relationship between safety culture and patient outcomes: results from pilot meta-analyses. West J Nurs Res 2014;36(1):66–83.

Guidet B, Gonzalez-Roma V. Climate and cultural aspects in intensive care units. Crit Care 2011;15(6):312.

Nemeth CP. Improving healthcare team communication: building on lessons from aviation and aerospace. Hampshire, England: Ashgate; 2008.

Odell M. Human factors and patient safety: changing roles in critical care. Aust Crit Care 2011;24(4):215–7.

Reason JT. The human contribution: unsafe acts, accidents and heroic recoveries. Surrey, England: Ashgate; 2008.

Rossi PJ, Edmiston CE, Jr. Patient safety in the critical care environment. Surg Clin North Am 2012;92(6):1369–86.

Runciman B, Merry A, Walton M. Safety and ethics in healthcare. Hampshire, England: Ashgate; 2007.

Thompson DN, Hoffman LA, Sereika SM, Lorenz HL, Wolf GA, Burns HK et al. A relational leadership perspective on unit-level safety climate. J Nurs Adm 2011;41(11):479–87.

References

1 Valentin A, Capuzzo M, Guidet B, Moreno RP, Dolanski L, Bauer P et al. Patient safety in intensive care: results from the multinational Sentinel Events Evaluation (SEE) study. Intensive Care Med 2006;32(10):1591–8.

2 Lohr K, Schroeder S. A strategy for quality assurance in medicine. New Engl J Med 1990;322:1161-71.

3 Henneman EA, Gawlinski A, Giuliano KK. Surveillance: a strategy for improving patient safety in acute and critical care units. Crit Care Nurse 2012;32(2):e9-e18.

4 Cullum N, Cilicska D, Haynes RB, Marks S. Evidence-based nursing: an introduction. Oxford, UK: Blackwell; 2008.

5 Cooke A, Smith D, Booth A. Beyond PICO: the SPIDER tool for qualitative evidence synthesis. Qual Health Res 2012;22(10):1435-43.

6 National Health and Medical Research Council. How to use the evidence: assessment and application of scientific evidence. Canberra: Commonwealth of Australia, <https://www.nhmrc.gov.au/guidelines-publications/cp69>; 2000 [accessed 25.03.14].

7 National Health and Medical Research Council. NHMRC additional levels of evidence and grades for recommendations for developers of guidelines. Canberra: Commonwealth of Australia, <https://www.nhmrc.gov.au/guidelines/archived-public-consultations/nhmrc-additional-levels-evidence-and-grades-recommendations>; 2009 [accessed 25.03.14].

8 Eccles MP, Grimshaw JM, Shekelle P, Schunemann HJ, Woolf S. Developing clinical practice guidelines: target audiences, identifying topics for guidelines, guideline group composition and functioning and conflicts of interest. Implement Sci 2012;7:60.

9 Grol R, Grimshaw J. From best evidence to best practice: effective implementation of change in patients' care. Lancet 2003;362(9391):1225-30.

10 Ilott I, Rick J, Patterson M, Turgoose C, Lacey A. What is protocol-based care? A concept analysis. J Nurs Manag 2006;14(7):544-52.

11 Miller M, Kearney N. Guidelines for clinical practice: development, dissemination and implementation. Int J Nurs Stud 2004;41(7):813-21.

12 Intensive Care Coordination and Monitoring Unit, New South Wales Department of Health, <http://intensivecare/hsnet.nsw.gov.au/>; 2014 [accessed 25.03.14].

13 Merlin T, Weston A, Tooher R. Extending an evidence hierarchy to include topics other than treatment: revising the Australian "levels" of evidence. BMC Med Res Methodol 2009;9:34.

14 Hillier S, Grimmer-Somers K, Merlin T, Middleton P, Salisbury J, Tooher R et al. FORM: an Australian method for formulating and grading recommendations in evidence-based clinical guidelines. BMC Medical Research Methodol 2011;11(1):23.

15 Brouwers MC, Kho ME, Browman GP, Burgers JS, Cluzeau F, Feder G et al. AGREE II: advancing guideline development, reporting and evaluation in health care. CMAJ 2010;182(18):E839-42.

16 Cahill NE, Suurdt J, Ouellette-Kuntz H, Heyland DK. Understanding adherence to guidelines in the intensive care unit: development of a comprehensive framework. J Parenteral Enteral Nutr 2010;34(6):616-24.

17 Iver N, Jamtvedt G, Flottorp S, Young JM, Odgaard-Jensen J, French SD et al. Audit and feedback: effects on professional practice and healthcare outcomes (Review). Cochrane Database Syst Rev 2012;6:CD000259. doi: 10.1002/14651858.pub3. 1-227.

18 Donabedian A. Evaluating the quality of medical care. Milbank Q 2005;44(3):691-729.

19 Pronovost PJ, Sexton JB, Pham JC, Goeschel CA, Winters BD, Miller MR. Measurement of quality and assurance of safety in the critically ill. Clin Chest Med 2009;30(1):169-79, x.

20 Wilson RM, Van Der Weyden MB. The safety of Australian healthcare: 10 years after QAHCS. Med J Aust 2005;182(6):260-1.

21 Curtis JR, Cook DJ, Wall RJ, Angus DC, Bion J, Kacmarek R et al. Intensive care unit quality improvement: a "how-to" guide for the interdisciplinary team. Crit Care Med 2006;34(1):211-8.

22 Scales DC, Dainty K, Hales B, Pinto R, Fowler RA, Adhikari NK et al. A multifaceted intervention for quality improvement in a network of intensive care units: a cluster randomized trial. JAMA 2011;305(4):363-72.

23 Speroff T, O'Connor GT. Study designs for PDSA quality improvement research. Qual Manag Health Care 2004;13(1):17-32.

24 Baker GR, Norton PG, Flintoft V, Blais R, Brown A, Cox J et al. The Canadian Adverse Events Study: the incidence of adverse events among hospital patients in Canada. CMAJ 2004;170(11):1678-86.

25 Brennan TA, Leape LL, Laird NM, Hebert L, Localio AR, Lawthers AG et al. Incidence of adverse events and negligence in hospitalized patients. Results of the Harvard Medical Practice Study I. N Engl J Med 1991;324(6):370-6.

26 Wilson RM, Runciman WB, Gibberd RW, Harrison BT, Newby L, Hamilton JD. The Quality in Australian Health Care Study. Med J Aust 1995;163(9):458-71.

27 Davis P, Lay-Yee R, Briant R, Ali W, Scott A, Schug S. Adverse events in New Zealand public hospitals I: occurrence and impact. N Z Med J 2002;115(1167):U271.

28 Nilsson L, Pihl A, Tagsjo M, Ericsson E. Adverse events are common on the intensive care unit: results from a structured record review. Acta Anaesthesiol Scand 2012;56(8):959-65.

29 de Vries EN, Ramrattan MA, Smorenburg SM, Gouma DJ, Boermeester MA. The incidence and nature of in-hospital adverse events: a systematic review. Qual Safety Health Care 2008;17(3):216-23.

30 Welters ID, Gibson J, Mogk M, Wenstone R. Major sources of critical incidents in intensive care. Crit Care 2011;15(5):R232.

31 Stockwell DC, Kane-Gill SL. Developing a patient safety surveillance system to identify adverse events in the intensive care unit. Crit Care Med 2010;38(6 Suppl):S117-25.

32 Kiekkas P, Karga M, Lemonidou C, Aretha D, Karanikolas M. Medication errors in critically ill adults: a review of direct observation evidence. Am J Crit Care 2011;20(1):36-44.

33 Capuzzo M, Nawfal I, Campi M, Valpondi V, Verri M, Alvisi R. Reporting of unintended events in an intensive care unit: comparison between staff and observer. BMC Emerg Med 2005;5(1):3.

34 Henneman EA. Unreported errors in the intensive care unit: a case study of the way we work. Crit Care Nurse 2007;27(5):27-34; quiz 5.

35 Wolff AM, Bourke J, Campbell IA, Leembruggen DW. Detecting and reducing hospital adverse events: outcomes of the Wimmera clinical risk management program. Med J Aust 2001;174(12):621-5.

36 Wu AW, Holzmueller CG, Lubomski LH, Thompson DA, Fahey M, Dorman T et al. Development of the ICU safety reporting system. J Patient Saf 2005;1(1):23-32.

37 Beckmann U, West LF, Groombridge GJ, Baldwin I, Hart GK, Clayton DG et al. The Australian Incident Monitoring Study in Intensive Care: AIMS-ICU. The development and evaluation of an incident reporting system in intensive care. Anaesth Intensive Care 1996;24(3):314-9.

38 Ohta Y, Sakuma M, Koike K, Bates DW, Morimoto T. Influence of adverse drug events on morbidity and mortality in intensive care units: the JADE study. Int J Qual Health Care 2014;26(6):573-8.

39 Moyen E, Camire E, Stelfox HT. Clinical review: medication errors in critical care. Crit Care 2008;12(2):208.

40 Latif A, Rawat N, Pustavoitau A, Pronovost PJ, Pham JC. National study on the distribution, causes, and consequences of voluntarily reported medication errors between the ICU and non-ICU settings. Crit Care Med 2013;41(2):389-98.

41 Bucknall TK. Medical error and decision making: learning from the past and present in intensive care. Aust Crit Care 2010;23(3):150-6.

42 Runciman WB, Roughead EE, Semple SJ, Adams RJ. Adverse drug events and medication errors in Australia. Int J Qual Health Care 2003;15 Suppl 1:i49-59.

43 Taxis K, Barber N. Ethnographic study of incidence and severity of intravenous drug errors. Br Med J 2003;326(7391):684.

44 Classen DC, Metzger J. Improving medication safety: the measurement conundrum and where to start. Int J Qual Health Care 2003;15 Suppl 1: i41-7.

45 Roughead EE, Semple SJ. Medication safety in acute care in Australia: where are we now? Part 1: a review of the extent and causes of medication problems 2002–2008. 2009 [cited 30 Sept 2014]. Available from http://www.anzhealthpolicy.com/content/6/1/18.

46 Malashock CM, Shull SS, Gould DA. Effect of smart infusion pumps on medication errors related to infusion device programming. Hosp Pharm 2004;39:460-9.

47 Rothschild JM, Landrigan CP, Cronin JW, Kaushal R, Lockley SW, Burdick E et al. The Critical Care Safety Study: the incidence and nature of adverse events and serious medical errors in intensive care. Crit Care Med 2005;33(8):1694-700.

48 Apkon M, Leonard J, Probst L, DeLizio L, Vitale R. Design of a safer approach to intravenous drug infusions: failure mode effects analysis. Qual Saf Health Care 2004;13(4):265-71.

49 Westbrook JI, Woods A, Rob MI, Dunsmuir WT, Day RO. Association of interruptions with an increased risk and severity of medication administration errors. Arch Intern Med 2010;170(8):683-90.

50 Kliger J. Giving medication administration the respect it is due: comment on: "association of interruptions with an increased risk and severity of medication administration errors". Arch Intern Med 2010;170(8):690-2.

51 Sherman H, Castro G, Fletcher M, Hatlie M, Hibbert P, Jakob R et al. Towards an International Classification for Patient Safety: the conceptual framework. Int J Qual Health Care 2009;21(1):2-8.

52 Australian Council on Healthcare Standards (ACHS). Intensive care indicators. Sydney: ACHS; 2013.

53 Ilan R, Fowler R. Brief history of patient safety culture and science. J Crit Care 2005;20(1):2-5.

54 Esmail R, Kirby A, Inkson T, Boiteau P. Quality improvement in the ICU. A Canadian perspective. J Crit Care 2005;20(1):74-6; discussion 6-8.

55 Pinto A, Burnett S, Benn J, Brett S, Parand A, Iskander S et al. Improving reliability of clinical care practices for ventilated patients in the context of a patient safety improvement initiative. J Eval Clin Pract 2011;17(1):180-7.

56 Pronovost P, Needham D, Berenholtz S, Sinopoli D, Chu H, Cosgrove S et al. An intervention to decrease catheter-related bloodstream infections in the ICU. N Engl J Med 2006;355(26):2725-32.

57 Bion J, Richardson A, Hibbert P, Beer J, Abrusci T, McCutcheon M et al. 'Matching Michigan': a 2-year stepped interventional programme to minimise central venous catheter-blood stream infections in intensive care units in England. BMJ Qual Saf 2013;22(2):110-23.

58 Pronovost P, Berenholtz S, Dorman T, Lipsett PA, Simmonds T, Haraden C. Improving communication in the ICU using daily goals. J Crit Care 2003;18(2):71-5.

59 Narasimhan M, Eisen LA, Mahoney CD, Acerra FL, Rosen MJ. Improving nurse–physician communication and satisfaction in the intensive care unit with a daily goals worksheet. Am J Crit Care 2006;15(2):217-22.

60 Vincent JL. Give your patient a fast hug (at least) once a day. Crit Care Med 2005;33(6):1225-9.

61 Pronovost PJ, Goeschel CA, Marsteller JA, Sexton JB, Pham JC, Berenholtz SM. Framework for patient safety research and improvement. Circulation 2009;119(2):330-7.

62 Crunden E, Boyce C, Woodman H, Bray B. An evaluation of the impact of the ventilator care bundle. Nurs Crit Care 2005;10(5):242-6.

63 Bloos F, Muller S, Harz A, Gugel M, Geil D, Egerland K et al. Effects of staff training on the care of mechanically ventilated patients: a prospective cohort study. Br J Anaesth 2009;103(2):232-7.

64 Morris AC, Hay AW, Swann DG, Everingham K, McCulloch C, McNulty J et al. Reducing ventilator-associated pneumonia in intensive care: impact of implementing a care bundle. Crit Care Med 2011;39(10):2218-24.

65 Alsadat R, Al-Bardan H, Mazloum MN, Shamah AA, Eltayeb MF, Marie A et al. Use of ventilator associated pneumonia bundle and statistical process control chart to decrease VAP rate in Syria. Avicenna J Med 2012;2(4):79-83.

66 Rello J, Afonso E, Lisboa T, Ricart M, Balsera B, Rovira A et al. A care bundle approach for prevention of ventilator-associated pneumonia. Clin Microbiol Infect 2013;19(4):363-9.

67 Hales B, Terblanche M, Fowler R, Sibbald W. Development of medical checklists for improved quality of patient care. Int J Qual Health Care 2008;20(1):22-30.

68 Halm MA. Daily goals worksheets and other checklists: are our critical care units safer? Am J Crit Care 2008;17(6):577-80.

69 Hewson-Conroy KM, Elliott D, Burrell AR. Quality and safety in intensive care – a means to an end is critical. Aust Crit Care 2010;23(3):109-29.

70 Dobkin E. Checkoffs play key role in SICU improvement. Healthcare Benchmarks and Quality Improvement 2003;10(10):113-5.

71 Wall RJ, Ely EW, Elasy TA, Dittus RS, Foss J, Wilkerson KS et al. Using real time process measurements to reduce catheter related bloodstream infections in the intensive care unit. Qual Saf Health Care 2005;14(4):295-302.

72 DuBose JJ, Inaba K, Shiflett A, Trankiem C, Teixeira PG, Salim A et al. Measurable outcomes of quality improvement in the trauma intensive care unit: the impact of a daily quality rounding checklist. J Trauma 2008;64(1):22-7; discussion 7-9.

73 Chua C, Wisniewski T, Ramos A, Schlepp M, Fildes JJ, Kuhls DA. Multidisciplinary trauma intensive care unit checklist: impact on infection rates. J Trauma Nurs 2010;17(3):163-6.

74 Weiss CH, Moazed F, McEvoy CA, Singer BD, Szleifer I, Amaral LA et al. Prompting physicians to address a daily checklist and process of care and clinical outcomes: a single-site study. Am J Respir Crit Care Med 2011;184(6):680-6.

75 Ward NS. The accuracy of clinical information systems. J Crit Care 2004;19(4):221-5.

76 Clemmer TP. Computers in the ICU: where we started and where we are now. J Crit Care 2004;19(4):201-7.

77 Seiver A. Critical care computing. Past, present, and future. Crit Care Clin 2000;16(4):601-21.

78 Levy MM. Computers in the intensive care unit. J Crit Care 2004;19(4):199-200.

79 Clemmer TP. Monitoring outcomes with relational databases: does it improve quality of care? J Crit Care 2004;19(4):243-7.

80 Rubenfeld GD. Using computerized medical databases to measure and to improve the quality of intensive care. J Crit Care 2004;19(4):248-56.

81 Kirkbride G, Vermace B. Smart pumps: implications for nurse leaders. Nurs Adm Q 2011;35(2):110-8.

82 Wilson K, Sullivan M. Preventing medication errors with smart infusion technology. Am J Health Syst Pharm 2004;61(2):177-83.

83 Pang RKY, Kong DCM, deClifford J-M, Lam SS, Leung BK. Smart infusion pumps reduce intravenous medication administration errors at an Australian teaching hospital. J Pharm Pract Res 2011;41:192-5.

84 Trbovich PL, Cafazzo JA, Easty AC. Implementation and optimization of smart infusion systems: are we reaping the safety benefits? J Health Qual 2013;35(2):33-40.

85 Harding AD. Increasing the use of 'smart' pump drug libraries by nurses: a continuous quality improvement project. Am J Nurs 2012;112(1): 26-35; quiz 6-7.

86 Colpaert K, Vanbelleghem S, Danneels C, Benoit D, Steurbaut K, Van Hoecke S et al. Has information technology finally been adopted in Flemish intensive care units? BMC Med Inform Decis Mak 2010;10:62.

87 Ryan A, Abbenbroek B. Intensive Care Clinical Information System (ICCIS) Program Overview: NSW HealthShare, <http://www.hss.health.nsw.gov.au/__documents/programs/iccis/iccis_hs12-07a_iccis-project-overview.pdf>; 2013 [accessed 05.09.14].

88 Mills J, Chamberlain-Salaum J, Henry R, Sando J, Summers G. Nurses in Australian acute care settings: experiences with and outcomes of e-health: an integrative review. IJMIT 2013;3(1):1-8.

89 Bosman RJ. Impact of computerized information systems on workload in operating room and intensive care unit. Best Pract Res Clin Anaesthesiol 2009;23(1):15-26.

90 Gruber D, Cummings GG, LeBlanc L, Smith DL. Factors influencing outcomes of clinical information systems implementation: a systematic review. Comput Inform Nurs 2009;27(3):151-63; quiz 64-5.

91 Ward NS, Snyder JE, Ross S, Haze D, Levy MM. Comparison of a commercially available clinical information system with other methods of measuring critical care outcomes data. J Crit Care 2004;19(1):10-5.

92 Morrison C, Jones M, Blackwell A, Vuylsteke A. Electronic patient record use during ward rounds: a qualitative study of interaction between medical staff. Crit Care 2008;12(6):R148.

93 Ballermann M, Shaw NT, Mayes DC, Gibney RT. Critical care providers refer to information tools less during communication tasks after a critical care clinical information system introduction. Stud Health Technol Inform 2011;164:37-41.

94 Manjoney R. Clinical information systems market – an insider's view. J Crit Care 2004;19(4):215-20.

95 van der Sijs H, Aarts J, Vulto A, Berg M. Overriding of drug safety alerts in computerized physician order entry. J Am Med Inform Assoc 2006;13(2):138-47.

96 Schedlbauer A, Prasad V, Mulvaney C, Phansalkar S, Stanton W, Bates DW et al. What evidence supports the use of computerized alerts and prompts to improve clinicians' prescribing behavior? J Am Med Inform Assoc 2009;16(4):531-8.

97 Meyfroidt G, Wouters P, De Becker W, Cottem D, Van den Berghe G. Impact of a computer-generated alert system on the quality of tight glycemic control. Intensive Care Med 2011;37(7):1151-7.

98 Lyerla F, LeRouge C, Cooke DA, Turpin D, Wilson L. A nursing clinical decision support system and potential predictors of head-of-bed position for patients receiving mechanical ventilation. Am J Crit Care 2010;19(1):39-47.

99 Rothschild J. Computerized physician order entry in the critical care and general inpatient setting: a narrative review. J Crit Care 2004;19(4): 271-8.

100 Maslove DM, Rizk N, Lowe HJ. Computerized physician order entry in the critical care environment: a review of current literature. J Intensive Care Med 2011;26(3):165-71.

101 Koppel R. What do we know about medication errors made via a CPOE system versus those made via handwritten orders? Crit Care 2005;9(5):427-8.

102 Christian S, Gyves H, Manji M. Electronic prescribing. Care Crit Ill 2004;20(3):68-71.

103 Fernandez Perez ER, Winters JL, Gajic O. The addition of decision support into computerized physician order entry reduces red blood cell transfusion resource utilization in the intensive care unit. Am J Hematol 2007;82(7):631-3.

104 Thursky KA, Buising KL, Bak N, Macgregor L, Street AC, Macintyre CR et al. Reduction of broad-spectrum antibiotic use with computerized decision support in an intensive care unit. Int J Qual Health Care 2006;18(3):224-31.

105 Sintchenko V, Iredell JR, Gilbert GL, Coiera E. Handheld computer-based decision support reduces patient length of stay and antibiotic prescribing in critical care. J Am Med Inform Assoc 2005;12(4):398-402.

106 Eslami S, de Keizer NF, Abu-Hanna A, de Jonge E, Schultz MJ. Effect of a clinical decision support system on adherence to a lower tidal volume mechanical ventilation strategy. J Crit Care 2009;24(4):523-9.

107 Sucher JF, Moore FA, Todd SR, Sailors RM, McKinley BA. Computerized clinical decision support: a technology to implement and validate evidence based guidelines. J Trauma 2008;64(2):520-37.

108 van Wyk JT, van Wijk MA, Sturkenboom MC, Mosseveld M, Moorman PW, van der Lei J. Electronic alerts versus on-demand decision support to improve dyslipidemia treatment: a cluster randomized controlled trial. Circulation 2008;117(3):371-8.

109 Kucher N, Koo S, Quiroz R, Cooper JM, Paterno MD, Soukonnikov B et al. Electronic alerts to prevent venous thromboembolism among hospitalized patients. N Engl J Med 2005;352(10):969-77.

110 Ali NA, Mekhjian HS, Kuehn PL, Bentley TD, Kumar R, Ferketich AK et al. Specificity of computerized physician order entry has a significant effect on the efficiency of workflow for critically ill patients. Crit Care Med 2005;33(1):110-4.

111 Coleman RW. Translation and interpretation: the hidden processes and problems revealed by computerized physician order entry systems. J Crit Care 2004;19(4):279-82.

112 Kawamoto K, Houlihan CA, Balas EA, Lobach DF. Improving clinical practice using clinical decision support systems: a systematic review of trials to identify features critical to success. Br Med J 2005;330(7494):765.

113 Jouvet P, Farges C, Hatzakis G, Monir A, Lesage F, Dupic L et al. Weaning children from mechanical ventilation with a computer-driven system (closed-loop protocol): a pilot study. Pediatr Crit Care Med 2007;8(5):425-32.

114 Mitchell MB. How mobile is your technology? Nurs Manage 2012;43(9):26-30.

115 Duffy M. Tablet technology for nurses. Am J Nurs 2012;112(9):59-64.

116 Craig AE. PDAs and smartphones: clinical tools for nurses, <http://www.medscape.com>; 2009 [accessed 01.09.14].

117 Mosa AS, Yoo I, Sheets L. A systematic review of healthcare applications for smartphones. BMC Med Inform Decis Mak 2012;12:67.

118 George LE, Davidson LJ, Serapiglia CP, Barla S, Thotakura A. Technology in nursing education: a study of PDA use by students. J Prof Nurs 2010;26(6):371-6.

119 Kuiper R. Metacognitive factors that impact student nurse use of point of care technology in clinical settings. Int J Nurs Educ Scholarsh 2010;7:Article5.

120 Phillippi JC, Wyatt TH. Smartphones in nursing education. Comput Inform Nurs 2011;29(8):449-54.

121 Martinez-Motta JC, Walker RG, Stewart TE, Granton J, Abrahamson S, Lapinsky SE. Critical care procedure logging using handheld computers. Crit Care 2004;8(5):R336-R42.

122 Bochicchio GV, Smit PA, Moore R, Bochicchio K, Auwaerter P, Johnson SB et al. Pilot study of a web-based antibiotic decision management guide. J Am Coll Surg 2006;202(3):459-67.

123 Iregui M, Ward S, Clinikscale D, Clayton D, Kollef MH. Use of a handheld computer by respiratory care practitioners to improve the efficiency of weaning patients from mechanical ventilation. Crit Care Med 2002;30(9):2038-43.

124 Lapinsky SE, Wax R, Showalter R, Martinez-Motta JC, Hallett D, Mehta S et al. Prospective evaluation of an internet-linked handheld computer critical care knowledge access system. Crit Care 2004;8(6):R414-21.

125 Frassica JJ. CIS: where are we going and what should we demand from industry? J Crit Care 2004;19(4):226-33.

126 Afessa B. Tele-intensive care unit: the horse out of the barn. Crit Care Med 2010;38(1):292-3.

127 Rosenfeld BA, Dorman T, Breslow MJ, Pronovost P, Jenckes M, Zhang N et al. Intensive care unit telemedicine: alternate paradigm for providing continuous intensivist care. Crit Care Med 2000;28(12):3925-31.

128 Breslow MJ, Rosenfeld BA, Doerfler M, Burke G, Yates G, Stone DJ et al. Effect of a multiple-site intensive care unit telemedicine program on clinical and economic outcomes: an alternative paradigm for intensivist staffing. Crit Care Med 2004;32(1):31-8.

129 Vespa PM, Miller C, Hu X, Nenov V, Buxey F, Martin NA. Intensive care unit robotic telepresence facilitates rapid physician response to unstable patients and decreased cost in neurointensive care. Surg Neurol 2007;67(4):331-7.

130 Westbrook JI, Coiera EW, Brear M, Stapleton S, Rob MI, Murphy M et al. Impact of an ultrabroadband emergency department telemedicine system on the care of acutely ill patients and clinicians' work. Med J Aust 2008;188(12):704-8.

131 Thomas EJ, Lucke JF, Wueste L, Weavind L, Patel B. Association of telemedicine for remote monitoring of intensive care patients with mortality, complications, and length of stay. JAMA 2009;302(24):2671-8.

132 Morrison JL, Cai Q, Davis N, Yan Y, Berbaum ML, Ries M et al. Clinical and economic outcomes of the electronic intensive care unit: results from two community hospitals. Crit Care Med 2010;38(1):2-8.

133 Yoo EJ, Dudley RA. Evaluating telemedicine in the ICU. JAMA 2009;302(24):2705-6.

134 Curran VR. Tele-education. J Telemed Telecare 2006;12(2):57-63.

135 Skiba DJ. MOOCs and the future of nursing. Nurs Educ Perspect 2013;34(3):202-4.

136 Kreideweis J. Indicators of success in distance education. Comput Inform Nurs 2005;23(2):68-72.

137 Simpson RL. See the future of distance education. Nurs Manage 2006;37(2):42, 4, 6-51.

138 Beeckman D, Schoonhoven L, Boucque H, Van Maele G, Defloor T. Pressure ulcers: e-learning to improve classification by nurses and nursing students. J Clin Nurs 2008;17(13):1697-707.

139 Maag M. The potential use of "blogs" in nursing education. Comput Inform Nurs 2005;23(1):16-24; quiz 5-6.

140 Moreno RP, Rhodes A, Donchin Y. Patient safety in intensive care medicine: the Declaration of Vienna. Intensive Care Med 2009;35(10):1667-72.

141 Institute of Medicine. Crossing the quality chasm: A new health system for the 21st century. Washington, DC: National Academy Press; 2001.

142 Institute of Medicine. Patient safety: Achieving a new standard of care. Washington DC: National Academy Press; 2003.

143 World Health Organization. What is patient safety?, <http://www.who.int/patientsafety/about/en/>; [accessed 5.03.14].

144 World Health Organization. Conceptual Framework for the International Classification for Patient Safety, Version 1.1: World Health Organization, <http://www.who.int/patientsafety/taxonomy/icps_full_report.pdf>; 2009 [accessed 05.09.14].

145 Bagian JP, Gosbee J, Lee CZ, Williams L, McKnight SD, Mannos DM. The Veterans Affairs root cause analysis system in action. Jt Comm J Qual Improv 2002;28(10):531-45.

146 Middleton S, Walker C, Chester R. Implementing root cause analysis in an area health service: views of the participants. Aust Health Rev 2005;29(4):422-8.

147 McDonough JE. Proactive hazard analysis and health care policy. New York: Milbank Memorial Fund; 2002.

148 Sorro JS, Nieva VF. Hospital survey on patient safety culture. Rockville, MD: Agency for Healthcare Research and Quality; 2004.

149 Davies HT, Nutley SM, Mannion R. Organisational culture and quality of health care. Qual Health Care 2000;9(2):111-9.

150 Dicuccio MH. The relationship between patient safety culture and patient outcomes: a systematic review. J Patient Saf 2014.

151 Sexton JB, Helmreich RL, Neilands TB, Rowan K, Vella K, Boyden J et al. The Safety Attitudes Questionnaire: psychometric properties, benchmarking data, and emerging research. BMC Health Serv Res 2006;6:44.

152 Thomas EJ, Sexton JB, Helmreich RL. Discrepant attitudes about teamwork among critical care nurses and physicians. Crit Care Med 2003;31(3):956-9.

153 Huang DT, Clermont G, Sexton JB, Karlo CA, Miller RG, Weissfeld LA et al. Perceptions of safety culture vary across the intensive care units of a single institution. Crit Care Med 2007;35(1):165-76.

154 Chaboyer W, Chamberlain D, Hewson-Conroy K, Grealy B, Elderkin T, Brittin M et al. CNE article: safety culture in Australian intensive care units: establishing a baseline for quality improvement. Am J Crit Care 2013;22(2):93-102.

155 Hamdan M. Measuring safety culture in Palestinian neonatal intensive care units using the Safety Attitudes Questionnaire. J Crit Care 2013;28(5):886 e7-14.

156 Steyrer J, Schiffinger M, Huber C, Valentin A, Strunk G. Attitude is everything? The impact of workload, safety climate, and safety tools on medical errors: a study of intensive care units. Health Care Manage Rev 2013;38(4):306-16.

157 Clarke JR, Lerner JC, Marella W. The role for leaders of health care organizations in patient safety. Am J Med Qual 2007;22(5):311-8.

158 World Health Organization. WHO patient safety curriculum guide: multi-professional edition. Geneva, <http://www.who.int/patientsafety/education/curriculum/en/>; 2011 [accessed 25.03.14].

159 Weaver SJP, Lubomksi LH, Wilson RF, Pfoh ER, Martinez KA, Dy SM. Promoting a culture of safety as a patient safety strategy: a systematic review. Ann Intern Med 2013;158(5):369.

160 Morello RT, Lowthian JA, Barker AL, McGinnes R, Dunt D, Brand C. Strategies for improving patient safety culture in hospitals: a systematic review. BMJ Qual Saf 2013;22(1):11-8.

161 Saladino L, Pickett LC, Frush K, Mall A, Champagne MT. Evaluation of a nurse-led safety program in a critical care unit. J Nurs Care Qual 2013;28(2):139-46.

162 Australian Commission on Safety and Quality in Health Care. National Consensus Statement: Essential Elements for Recognising and Responding to Clinical Deterioration. Sydney: ACSQHC; 2010.

163 Centre for Clinical Practice at NICE (UK). Acutely Ill Patients in Hospital: Recognition of and Response to Acute Illness in Adults in Hospital. (NICE Clinical Guideline 50) London: National Institute for Health and Clinical Excellence (UK), <http://www.ncbi.nlm.nih.gov/books/NBK45947/pdf/TOC.pdf>; 2007 [accessed 01.09.14].

164 Winters BD, Weaver SJ, Pfoh ER, Yang T, Pham JC, Dy SM. Rapid-response systems as a patient safety strategy: a systematic review. Ann Intern Med 2013;158(5 Pt 2):417-25.

165 McNeill G, Bryden D. Do either early warning systems or emergency response teams improve hospital patient survival? A systematic review. Resuscitation 2013;84(12):1652-67.

166 DeVita MA, Braithwaite RS, Mahidhara R, Stuart S, Foraida M, Simmons RL. Use of medical emergency team responses to reduce hospital cardiopulmonary arrests. Qual Saf Health Care 2004;13(4):251-4.

167 Hueckel RM, Mericle JM, Frush K, Martin PL, Champagne MT. Implementation of condition help: family teaching and evaluation of family understanding. J Nurs Care Qual 2012;27(2):176-81.

168 McArthur-Rouse F. Critical care outreach services and early warning scoring systems: a review of the literature. J Adv Nurs 2001;36(5):696-704.

169 Lee A, Bishop G, Hillman KM, Daffurn K. The medical emergency team. Anaesth Intensive Care 1995;23(2):183-6.

170 Morgan RJM, Williams F, Wright MM. An early warning scoring system for detecting developing critical illness. Clin Intens Care 1997;8:100.

171 Goldhill DR, McNarry AF, Mandersloot G, McGinley A. A physiologically-based early warning score for ward patients: the association between score and outcome. Anaesthesia 2005;60(6):547-53.

172 Hammond NE, Spooner AJ, Barnett AG, Corley A, Brown P, Fraser JF. The effect of implementing a modified early warning scoring (MEWS) system on the adequacy of vital sign documentation. Aust Crit Care 2013;26(1):18-22.

173 Eliott S, Chaboyer W, Ernest D, Doric A, Endacott R. A national survey of Australian Intensive Care Unit (ICU) Liaison Nurse (LN) services. Aust Crit Care 2012;25(4):253-62.

174 Niven DJ, Bastos JF, Stelfox HT. Critical care transition programs and the risk of readmission or death after discharge from an ICU: a systematic review and meta-analysis. Crit Care Med 2014;42(1):179-87.

175 Aitken LM, Chaboyer W, Vaux A, Crouch S, Burmeister E, Daly M et al. Effect of a 2-tier rapid response system on patient outcome and staff satisfaction. Aust Crit Care 2014; doi: 10.1016/j.aucc.2014.10.044.

176 Flin RH, O'Connor P, Crichton MD. Safety at the sharp end: a guide to non-technical skills. Burlington, VT: Ashgate; 2008.

177 Stubbings L, Chaboyer W, McMurray A. Nurses' use of situation awareness in decision-making: an integrative review. J Adv Nurs 2012;68(7):1443-53.

178 Tenney YJ, Pew RW. Situation awareness catches on: what? so what? now what? Reviews of Human Factors and Ergonomics 2006;2(1):1-34.

179 Wright MC, Endsley MR. Building shared situation awareness in healthcare settings. In: Nemeth CP, ed. Improving healthcare team communication: building on lessons from aviation and aerospace. Burlington, VT: Ashgate; 2008. pp 97-116.

180 Bucknall TK. Critical care nurses' decision-making activities in the natural clinical setting. J Clin Nurs 2000;9(1):25-35.

181 Endsley MR. Toward a theory of situation awareness in dynamic systems. Hum Factors 1995;37(1):32-64.

182 Croskerry P, Singhal G, Mamede S. Cognitive debiasing 1: origins of bias and theory of debiasing. BMJ Qual Saf 2013;22 Suppl 2:ii58-ii64.

183 Sendelbach S, Funk M. Alarm fatigue: a patient safety concern. AACN Adv Crit Care 2013;24(4):378-86; quiz 87-8.

184 Aitken LM. Critical care nurses' use of decision-making strategies. J Clin Nurs 2003;12(4):476-83.

185 Currey J, Botti M. The influence of patient complexity and nurses' experience on haemodynamic decision-making following cardiac surgery. Intensive Crit Care Nurs 2006;22(4):194-205.

186 Thompson C, Dalgleish L, Bucknall T, Estabrooks C, Hutchinson AM, Fraser K et al. The effects of time pressure and experience on nurses' risk assessment decisions: a signal detection analysis. Nurs Res 2008;57(5):302-11.

187 Hoffman KA, Aitken LM, Duffield C. A comparison of novice and expert nurses' cue collection during clinical decision-making: verbal protocol analysis. Int J Nurs Stud 2009;46(10):1335-44.

188 Hough MC. Learning, decisions and transformation in critical care nursing practice. Nurs Ethics 2008;15(3):322-31.

189 Karra V, Papathanassoglou ED, Lemonidou C, Sourtzi P, Giannakopoulou M. Exploration and classification of intensive care nurses' clinical decisions: a Greek perspective. Nurs Crit Care 2014;19(2):87-97.

190 Narayan S, Corcoran-Perry S. Teaching clinical reasoning in nursing education. In: Higgs J, Jones MA, Loftus S, Christensen M, eds. Clinical reasoning in the health professions. 3rd ed. Philadelphia: Butterworth-Heinemann; 2008: pp 405-30.

191 Rivett DA, Jones MA. Using case reports to teach clinical reasoning. In: Higgs J, Jones M, eds. Clinical reasoning in the health professions. Philadelphia: Butterworth-Heinemann; 2008: pp 477-84.

192 Thompson C, Stapley S. Do educational interventions improve nurses' clinical decision making and judgement? A systematic review. Int J Nurs Stud 2011;48(7):881-93.

193 Reason JT. Managing the risks of organizational accidents. Aldershot, England: Ashgate; 1997.

194 Orasanu J, Fischer U. Improving healthcare communication: lessons from the flightdeck. In: Nemeth CP, ed. Improving healthcare team communication: building on lessons from aviation and aerospace. Burlington, VT: Ashgate; 2008: pp 23-46.

195 Australian Commission on Safety and Quality in Health Care (ACSQHC). OSSIE guide to clinical handover improvement. Sydney, NSW: ACSQHC; 2010.

196 Chaboyer W, McMurray A, Wallis M. Bedside nursing handover: a case study. Int J Nurs Pract 2010;16(1):27-34.

197 Halm MA. Nursing handoffs: ensuring safe passage for patients. Am J Crit Care 2013;22(2):158-62.

198 Spooner AJ, Chaboyer W, Corley A, Hammond N, Fraser JF. Understanding current intensive care unit nursing handover practices. Int J Nurs Pract 2013;19(2):214-20.

199 Ganz FD, Endacott R, Chaboyer W, Benbinishty J, Ben Nun M, Ryan H et al. The quality of intensive care unit nurse handover related to end of life: a descriptive comparative international study. Int J Nurs Stud 2015;52(1):49-56.

200 Lane D, Ferri M, Lemaire J, McLaughlin K, Stelfox HT. A systematic review of evidence-informed practices for patient care rounds in the ICU*. Crit Care Med 2013;41(8):2015-29.

201 Brown R, Rasmussen R, Baldwin I, Wyeth P. Design and implementation of a virtual world training simulation of ICU first hour handover processes. Aust Crit Care 2012;25(3):178-87.

202 Donchin Y, Gopher D, Olin M, Badihi Y, Biesky MR, Sprung CL et al. A look into the nature and causes of human errors in the intensive care unit. Crit Care Med 1995;23(2):294-300.

203 Patterson ES, Hofer T, Brungs S, Saint S, Render ML. Structured interdisciplinary communication strategies in four ICUs: an observational study. Proc Hum Fact Ergon Soc Annu Meet 2006;50(10):929-33.

204 Brannick MT, Prince C. An overview of team performance measurement. In: Brannick MT, Salas E, Prince C, eds. Team performance assessment and measurement: theory, methods, and applications. Mahwah, N.J: Lawrence Erlbaum Associates; 1997: pp 3-16.

205 Dietz AS, Pronovost PJ, Mendez-Tellez PA, Wyskiel R, Marsteller JA, Thompson DA et al. A systematic review of teamwork in the intensive care unit: what do we know about teamwork, team tasks, and improvement strategies? J Crit Care 2014;29(6):908-14.

206 Gordon M, Darbyshire D, Baker P. Non-technical skills training to enhance patient safety: a systematic review. Med Educ 2012;46(11):1042-54.

207 Salas E, Rosen MA. Building high reliability teams: progress and some reflections on teamwork training. BMJ Qual Saf 2013;22(5):369-73.

208 Schmidt E, Goldhaber-Fiebert SN, Ho LA, McDonald KM. Simulation exercises as a patient safety strategy: a systematic review. Ann Intern Med 2013;158(5 Pt 2):426-32.

Chapter 4

Recovery and rehabilitation

Janice Rattray, Leanne Aitken

Learning objectives

After reading this chapter, you should be able to:

- discuss the physical, psychological and cognitive sequelae present for some survivors of a critical illness

- outline the common functional, psychological, cognitive and health-related quality of life (HRQOL) instruments used to assess patient outcomes after a critical illness

- describe the benefits and challenges for implementing rehabilitation interventions in ICU, in hospital after ICU discharge and after hospital discharge.

Introduction

Millions of people each year experience a critical illness requiring admission to an intensive care unit (ICU). Although overall survival rates approximate 90% at hospital discharge,[1] recovery for individuals is delayed often beyond 6 months postdischarge.[2] Physical de-conditioning and neuromuscular dysfunction[3] as well as psychological[4,5] and cognitive sequelae[6] are common, adding to the burden of illness for survivors, carers, the healthcare system and broader society.

Although ICU clinicians have traditionally focused on survival as the principal indicator of patient outcome and unit performance,[7] physical and psychological functioning and health-related quality of life (HRQOL) have now emerged as legitimate patient outcomes from both practice and research perspectives.[2] With this shifting focus towards long-term health and wellbeing has also come a reconsideration and re-conceptualisation of critical care as only one component in the continuum of care for a critically ill patient. An episode of critical illness is now viewed as a continuum that begins with the onset of acute clinical deterioration, includes the ICU admission and continues until the patient's risk of late sequelae has returned to the baseline risk of a similar individual who has not incurred a critical illness[7] (see Figure 4.1). Timing of this recovery trajectory is variable, and related to a number of individual, illness and treatment factors.

FIGURE 4.1 The continuum of critical illness.[7]

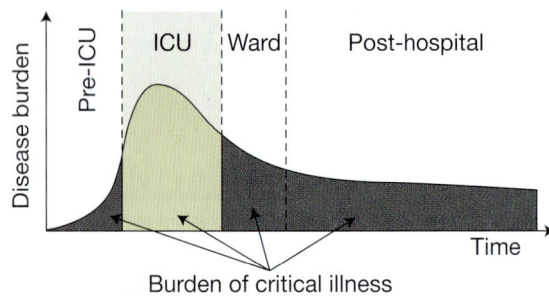

Adapted with permission from Angus DC, Carlet J. Surviving intensive care: a report from the 2002 Brussels Roundtable. Intensive Care Med 2003;29(3):368–77.

Reviews of numerous observational studies confirm delayed recovery in HRQOL,[8] with physical, psychological and cognitive symptoms prevalent:

- weakness: approximately 40%[3,9]
- delirium: up to 74%[10,11]
- anxiety: up to 45%[12,13]
- depression: approximately 30%[5]
- post-traumatic stress symptoms: approximately 20%[4]
- cognitive dysfunction: 36–62%.[14]

Recognition of the frequency, and co-occurrence, of these elements of compromise has led to the development of the term 'post-intensive care syndrome' (PICS) to 'describe new or worsening impairments in physical, cognitive, or mental health status arising after critical illness and persisting beyond acute care hospitalisation' (p. 505).[2] While significant sequelae therefore exist for a substantial proportion of critical illness survivors, little evidence is currently available to support specific interventions for improving their recovery.[2,15]

In further chapters of this book psychological issues including sedation management and delirium monitoring while in ICU (Chapter 7) and breathing trials and weaning from mechanical ventilation (Chapter 15) are discussed. Common physical and psychological sequelae associated with a critical illness, and how this impacts on a survivor's HRQOL, are discussed in this chapter. Common instruments measuring physical, psychological and HRQOL are described. Physical rehabilitation strategies, commencing with exercise and early mobility in-ICU, post-ICU and post-hospital services are also discussed.

Compromise following a critical illness

Examination of patient outcomes beyond survival is an important contemporary topic for critical care practice and research.[4,5,8,16] Patient outcomes after a critical illness or injury were traditionally measured using a number of objective parameters (e.g. number of organ failure-free days, 28-day status, or 1-year mortality). Other measures that examined patient-centred concepts such as functional status, HRQOL, psychological health and cognitive function have become more prevalent in the past 10 years.[2,15] As the recovery trajectory from a critical illness may be long and incomplete, mapping this path is a complex process.

Health-related quality of life

Survivors of critical illness experience compromised health-related quality of life for varying periods of time after leaving ICU. Health-related quality of life covers a number of physical, psychological, emotional and social domains of life and is now generally accepted as an important outcome measure. Within this chapter, we guide the reader to the commonly used measures but present the physical and psychological issues separately. Ongoing physical and psychological problems tend to impact negatively on social, environmental and economic elements in life,[17] and many patients and families experience a significant economic challenge during the recovery process. Although some patients recover quickly and do not report ongoing issues, others report significant and protracted compromise in their quality of life.[16] It is clear that survivors of critical illness have markedly lower health-related quality of life than other members in the community when matched for age and gender. Although there is convincing evidence of this widespread compromise, we also know that recovery patterns vary for individual patients, with some recovering rapidly. Factors that have been shown to influence components of quality of life include age, lower socioeconomic status, gender, severity of illness, primary diagnosis and length of ICU stay, although few of these factors appear to affect people in a consistent manner.[4,5,16]

ICU-acquired weakness

Critical illness myopathy (CIM), polyneuropathy (CIP) and neuromyopathy (CINM) syndromes occur in 50–100% of ICU survivors.[18–20] ICU-acquired weakness (ICU-AW) has come into use as a term that encompasses these syndromes of muscle wasting and functional weakness in patients with a critical illness who have no other plausible aetiology.[20] The three syndromes above form the sub-categories of ICU-AW, with CINM used when both myopathy and axonal polyneuropathy are evident. Development of ICU-AW is associated with a number of risk factors that occur during intensive care treatment:[18,21]

- critical illness: sepsis, systemic inflammatory response syndrome (SIRS), multi-organ system failure, catabolic state
- treatments: mechanical ventilation, hyperglycaemia, glucocorticoids, sedatives, neuromuscular blocking agents, immobility.

Local and systemic inflammation acts synergistically with bed rest and immobility to alter metabolic and structural function of muscles,[22] resulting in muscle atrophy and contractile dysfunction, loss of flexibility, CIP, heterotopic ossification and entrapment neuropathy.[20] Muscle strength can reduce by 1–1.5% per day with a total loss of 25–50% of body strength possible following immobilisation.[23] Patients can lose up to 2% of muscle mass per day,[24] which contributes to weakness and disability and a prolonged recovery period. These neuromuscular dysfunctions are diagnosed by clinical assessment, diagnostic studies (electrophysiology, ultrasound) or histology of muscle or nerve tissue.

The syndrome of ICU-AW manifests as prolonged weaning time, inability to mobilise and reduced functional capacity. Patients with ICU-AW also experience increased mortality.[25] Some groups of ICU survivors report relatively poor HRQOL due to prolonged weakness that may persist for months and years after discharge, particularly for those recovering from acute lung injury/adult respiratory distress syndrome (ARDS).[9]

Clinical assessment

Clinical assessment includes identification of generalised weakness following the onset of a critical illness, exclusion of other diagnoses (e.g. Guillain–Barré syndrome) and measurement of muscle strength. Instruments are available to assess both volitional and non-volitional muscle strength.[26]

Manual muscle testing is commonly assessed using the Medical Research Council (MRC) Scale,[27] a 0–5 point ordinal scale:

0 = no contraction

1 = flicker or trace of muscle contraction

2 = full range of active movement with gravity eliminated

3 = reduced power but active movement against gravity

4 = reduced power but active movement against gravity and resistance

5 = normal power against gravity and full resistance.

For patients who are awake and cooperative, each muscle group is assessed sequentially for strength and symmetry:

- upper limb: deltoid, biceps, wrist extensors
- lower limb: quadriceps, gluteus maximus, ankle dorsiflexion.

Ordinal data are obtained in response to a subjective evaluation of muscle strength.[26] In 1991 an MRC sum-score, ranging from 0–60, was first introduced.[28] Weakness is evident with an MRC sum score of <48 (<4 in all testable muscle groups), and re-tested after 24 hours. Weakness (<4 MRC Scale) was associated with an increased hospital mortality.[29] Inter-rater reliability following appropriate training using the MRC has been demonstrated.[30]

Hand-held dynamometry and handgrip dynamometry can also be used to measure volitional muscle strength using a calibrated device for patients who are conscious and cooperative. The benefit of these measures is increased objectivity to obtain continuous data.[26]

All volitional strength measurements may be affected by the level of awareness and cooperation of patients, as well as their motivation, although inter-rater reliability of the MRC sum score as well as hand-held dynamometry and handgrip dynamometry has been shown to be good to very good.[26] Further, dynamometry was demonstrated to be a reliable, rapid and simple alternative to comprehensive manual muscle testing assessment,[29] and may be a surrogate measure for global strength.[20]

Diagnostic testing

Electrophysiological testing (nerve conduction studies, needle electromyography) may be useful to differentiate between CIM and CIP, although this distinction is difficult and often not required in the clinical setting.[18,20] Histology for CIP is primarily noted as distal axonal degeneration in both sensory and motor fibres, while the characteristic findings in CIM are patchy loss of myosin (thick filaments), necrosis and fast twitch fibre atrophy.[20]

> ### Practice tip
>
> Current clinical recommendations to limit muscle wasting include:
>
> - minimising patient exposure to corticosteroids and neuromuscular blocking agents
> - limiting excessive analgesia and sedation
> - moderate glycaemic control
> - early mobilisation.

Psychological health

Psychological responses to a critical illness and patients' memories of experiences during an ICU admission have been explored using quantitative[31-35] and/or qualitative approaches.[36,37] Some survivors reported increased anxiety, including transfer anxiety (discharge from ICU);[38] depression;[5] post-traumatic stress;[4,39-41] hallucinations;[42-44] and continuing cognitive dysfunction.[6,11,45]

For some patients, recovery from a critical illness results in short- and long-term psychological dysfunction (e.g. anxiety, depression and post-traumatic stress symptoms), which potentially result in additional health problems, reduced HRQOL,[46,47] reduction in social activities and functioning and failure to engage with rehabilitation programs.[48] Our understanding of these sequelae has improved over the past decade in part due to increased research activity and evaluations of intensive care follow-up clinics in the UK (discussed in a later section). However, despite testing a variety of interventions, it is still unclear how best to identify at-risk patients and initiate an effective intervention in a timely way.

Anxiety and depression

Reported prevalence of anxiety and depression after ICU discharge varies depending upon the questionnaire and 'cut-off' scores used, and the research design, and ranges from 7% 3 months after discharge[49] to 18% 1 year after discharge.[50] Both studies used the Hospital Anxiety and Depression Scale (HADS) with scores of ≥11 to indicate an anxiety or depressive problem.

Prevalence of depression tends to be high in the immediate weeks after ICU discharge and Davydow and colleagues[48] report significant depressive symptoms in 36% of medical-surgical patients 3 months after hospital discharge. This figure reduced to 18% at 12 months.[48] A summary of studies reporting the prevalence of anxiety and depression is provided in Table 4.1. These differences may be explained by differences in case mix or timing of assessment.

TABLE 4.1
Summary of studies examining anxiety and depression in survivors of a critical illness

FIRST AUTHOR/ COUNTRY	DESIGN	N/% MALES	COHORT	ACUITY[a]/ICU LOS DAYS	AGE	INSTRUMENT/ CUT-OFF SCORE	MAIN FINDINGS
Eddleston (2000)[49]/UK	Cross-sectional	143/52%	Follow-up clinic 3 months postdischarge	15/3.7	51	HADS[b] ≥11	7% met the criteria for anxiety, and 3% depression / Females more likely to have higher anxiety scores
Nelson (2000)[51] UK	Cross-sectional, postal survey	24/58%	19 months (mean) after acute lung injury	58[d]/27	40	GDS[c]/16	Positive correlation ($r = 0.30$) between depression scores and days of sedation; 69% of patients not depressed prior to ICU scored >16
Scragg (2001)[52] UK	Cross-sectional postal survey	80/52%	Survival from ICU over 2 years	–/–	57	HADS >8	43% scored above 8 for anxiety and 30% for depression
Jones (2001)[53] UK	Cohort	30/67%	2 and 8 weeks after ICU discharge	17/8	57	HADS ≥11	Patients with no factual but some delusional memories were more likely to be anxious and depressed at 2 weeks
Jones (2003)[54] UK	RCT	116/61%	General ICU patients – 3 hospitals; 8 weeks and 6 months after discharge	17/14	58	HADS >11	No statistically significant differences between the two groups; there was a trend to reduced depression scores for those with scores >11 at 8 weeks
Jackson (2003)[55] USA	Prospective cohort	34/53%	Medical and coronary ICU; 6 month follow-up	24.9/–	53.2	GDS-SF ≥6	Patients with neuropsychological impairment were more likely to score above the threshold at 6 months (36% v 17%)
Hopkins (2004)[56]/USA	Prospective longitudinal	66/50%	ARDS; 12 month follow-up	18.1/34	46	BDI >30 BAI >30	9% severe levels of anxiety and 6% severe levels of depression at 12 months
Hopkins (2005)[57]/USA			2 year follow-up				Anxiety and depression persisted up to 2 years with 23% reporting moderate-to-severe levels
Rattray (2005)[50] UK	Prospective longitudinal	80/64%	General ICU; Hosp discharge, 6 and 12 months	17.7/4.9	54.7	HADS ≥11	Anxiety and depression significantly reduced between 6 and 12 months; 18% demonstrated probable anxiety, 11% probable depression

FIRST AUTHOR/ COUNTRY	DESIGN	N/% MALES	COHORT	ACUITY[a]/ICU LOS DAYS	AGE	INSTRUMENT/ CUT-OFF SCORE	MAIN FINDINGS
Sukantarat (2007)[58]/UK	Prospective	51/43%	ICU patients ≥3 days; 3 and 9 months	15.3/16.9	57.4	HADS: anxiety ≥10 HADS: depression ≥8	24% had anxiety scores ≥10 at both 3 and 9 months; 35% had depression scores ≥8 at 3 months and 45% at 6 months
Dowdy (2009)[59]/ USA	Prospective cohort	161/55%	Acute lung injury; 6 months	≤20 = 80%/≤10 = 51%	49	HADS ≥11	11% scored above threshold at 6 months
Myhren (2009)[61]/ Norway	Cross-sectional	255/63%	4–6 weeks post-ICU discharge	SAPS[e] 37/12	48	HADS ≥11	Mean anxiety (5.6 vs 4.2) and depression (4.8 vs 3.5) scores higher than general population norms
Myhren (2010)[60]/ Norway	Longitudinal		As above and 3 and 12 months				Unemployment and optimism were predictors of anxiety scores; surgery and optimism predicted depression
Peris (2011)[62]/ Italy	Cross-sectional using historical controls	Control: 86/72.1% Intervention: 123/83.7%	Major trauma 12 months	Control[e]: 38.5/20.1 Intervention[e]: 44.1/17.8	Control: 44.9 Intervention: 43.7	HADS ≥11	Intervention group had lower rate of anxiety 8.9% vs 17.4% and depression 6.5% vs 12.8%
Wade (2012)[63]/UK	Prospective	100/52%	Level 3 patients 3 months	22/8[f]	57	CES-D ≥19 STAI ≥44	Probable depression 46.3% Probable anxiety 44.4%
Schandl (2013)[64]/ Sweden	Prospective	150/41.5%	General ICU 2 months	55[e]/1.5/6	Adverse psychological outcome group = 54 No adverse psychological outcome group = 60	HADS ≥8	Overall 31% had adverse psychological outcomes 35 (23%) high anxiety scores 19 (12.6%) high depression scores
Kowalczyk (2013)[65]/ Poland	Retrospective, cross-sectional	195/57.5%	General ICU Variable length of time after ICU	14.9/not reported	48.1	HADS >10	64 (34.4%) scored above anxiety threshold 51 (27.4%) above depression threshold

a APACHE II score.
b Hospital Anxiety and Depression Scale.
c Geriatric Depression Scale – Short Form.
d APACHE III score.
e Simplified Acute Physiology Score.
f Median value.
BAI = Beck Anxiety Instrument; BDI = Beck Depression Instrument; CES-D = Center for Epidemiologic Studies – Depression Scale; GDS = Geriatric Depression Scale – Short Form; ICU LOS = intensive care unit length of stay.

Patients often exhibit high levels of distress at the time of hospital discharge and these tend to reduce during the first year after discharge.[50,51] However, the episodic timing of assessments may not fully capture patterns of anxiety and depression, and establish whether full resolution is achieved, or identify a later onset problem. For example, in patients with ARDS, levels of depression increased from 16% at 1 year after discharge to 23% at 2 years.[57] This may reflect prolonged recovery in general for this subgroup of patients, who tend to be among the most critically ill patients, with a mean ICU stay of 34 days noted. A rise in depression scores may therefore be a reflection of that prolonged physical recovery.

Depression is also associated with other aspects of recovery and, in particular, HRQOL. Depressed patients tend to rate their HRQOL as poorer than those who are not.[50,57] However, what is less clear is the direction of this relationship; it could be that patients with a poorer HRQOL tend to be depressed rather than depression leading to perceptions of poorer HRQOL. Patients who have psychological problems prior to intensive care are likely to develop these after discharge. Although assessment of pre-ICU status is difficult, in some cases this information can be obtained from relatives or caregivers.

It is becoming increasingly clear that depression is closely associated with post-traumatic stress symptomatology,[66] and while these may be related they have distinct differences and treatments. Patients who are depressed are likely to exhibit post-traumatic stress symptoms and vice versa. Diagnosis, however, can be difficult.[67]

Post-traumatic stress

In recent years there has been increasing interest in the development of post-traumatic stress reactions such as post-traumatic stress disorder (PTSD) as a response to critical illness,[68,69] and there is increasing recognition of these symptoms as a problem for some intensive care survivors.[4,70] Individuals are required to meet a number of criteria before a diagnosis of PTSD is considered, and in 2013 the American Psychiatric Association presented the DSM-V criteria for PTSD (see Box 4.1 for these criteria).

Many symptoms of post-traumatic stress that patients experience in the initial days after intensive care discharge may be considered a normal reaction, and it is important that practitioners clearly separate the normal from the abnormal response. This is achieved by assessing the severity and duration of symptoms, and their effect on an individual's life. PTSD should not be diagnosed until at least 1 month after the event, and until the symptoms have been present for 1 month. Symptoms commonly cause problems in relation to work, social or other important activities;[72] this is important to consider when developing critical care follow-up services. Importantly, PTSD symptoms may be reactivated after some time, and being in ICU may serve as a catalyst for some patients, e.g. reliving a war event.[44]

Signs of post-traumatic symptomatology include four main symptom areas (this is a change from *Diagnostic and Statistical Manual of Mental Disorders* (DSM-IV) criteria where three symptom groups were recognised): intrusive thoughts, avoidance behaviours, negative alterations in cognitions and mood and hyper-arousal symptoms.[72] Individuals can re-experience a traumatic event through involuntary unwanted thoughts, often in the form of 'flashbacks' and/or 'nightmares'. Individuals experiencing these thoughts often develop avoidant behaviours in the belief this action will reduce the intrusive thoughts. Avoidant behaviours for intensive care patients can range from simply avoiding television programs about hospitals, not talking about their ICU experience or, more seriously, non-attendance at a follow-up clinic or other hospital out-patient appointments. The latter also compounds the issue of accurate prevalence. Negative alterations in cognitions and mood may include continuing self-blame or blaming others about the cause or consequences of the critical illness.[72] Hyper-arousal behaviours include difficulties in concentrating or falling asleep. Future assessment of post-traumatic stress in survivors of a critical illness should examine all four symptom areas.

As with other psychological symptoms such as anxiety and depression, it has been difficult to establish the prevalence of PTSD after intensive care because of the use of self-report measures, different research designs, varied patient case-mix and international variations in the delivery of intensive care. These variations have resulted in overestimation of the prevalence of PTSD and post-traumatic stress symptoms (PTSS),[73] although note that patients with significant PTSS, particularly avoidant behaviours, may be less likely to participate in research studies. Patients may have significant PTSS without developing PTSD and it is mainly these symptoms that are assessed using the self-report measures. Reported prevalence of a significant post-traumatic stress reaction or PTSD ranges from 5% to 64%.[63,70]

What is emerging from the literature is that there are certain non-modifiable and modifiable risk factors that predict subsequent anxiety, depression and post-traumatic stress symptoms, although not consistently. The non-modifiable factors are those associated with individuals and include: previous psychiatric history,[48] previous stressful events,[66] admission as a result of trauma,[67] women rather than men[49,50,74] and younger patients more anxious than older patients.[50] Interestingly, individual characteristics such as employment and level of education also appear to predict those most at risk.[5,61,64] The modifiable factors tend to be those associated with the critical illness experience. Patients with a longer ICU stay,[50,51] longer duration, type and dose of sedation and/or neuromuscular blockade,[63] mechanical ventilation,[41,59] use of restraints and in-ICU stress or agitation[63,75] are more likely to report post-traumatic stress symptoms. Early signs of acute stress or depression are a strong predictor of ongoing problems.[50] Other consequences of being in intensive care such as neuropsychological impairment can also predict significantly higher depression scores.[55]

What is also evident in the emerging literature is the effect of patients' subjective intensive care experiences. These experiences tend to be reported as unpleasant memories of being in ICU[31,44,61,76,77] and are discussed later in this chapter.

BOX 4.1

Post-traumatic stress disorder diagnostic criteria[71]

Criterion A: Stressor – The person was exposed to: death, threatened death, actual or threatened serious injury or actual or threatened sexual violence, as follows (one required):

1 Direct exposure
2 Witnessing, in person
3 Indirectly, by learning that a close relative or close friend was exposed to trauma. If the event involved actual or threatened death, it must have been violent or accidental
4 Repeated or extreme indirect exposure to aversive details of the event(s) usually in the course of professional duties. This does not include indirect non-professional exposure through electronic media, television, movies or pictures

Criterion B: Intrusion symptoms – The traumatic event is persistently re-experienced in the following way (one required):

1 Recurrent, involuntary and intrusive memories
2 Traumatic nightmares
3 Dissociative reactions (e.g. flashbacks), which may occur on a continuum from brief episodes to complete loss of consciousness
4 Intensive or prolonged distress after exposure to traumatic reminders
5 Marked physiological reactivity after exposure to trauma-related stimuli

Criterion C: Avoidance – Persistent effortful avoidance of distressing trauma-related stimuli after the event (one required):

1 Trauma-related thoughts or feelings
2 Trauma-related external reminders

Criterion D: Negative alterations in cognitions and mood – Negative alterations in cognitions and mood that began or worsened after the traumatic event (two required):

1 Inability to recall key features of the traumatic event (usually dissociative amnesia: not due to head injury, alcohol or drugs)
2 Persistent (and often distorted) negative beliefs and expectations about oneself or the world (e.g. I am bad, the world is completely dangerous)
3 Persistent distorted blame of self or others for causing the traumatic event or for resulting consequences
4 Persistent negative trauma-related emotions (e.g. fear, horror, anger, guilt or shame)
5 Markedly diminished interest in (pre-traumatic) significant activities
6 Feeling alienated from others (e.g. detachment or estrangement)
7 Constricted affect: persistent inability to experience positive emotions

Criterion E: Alterations in arousal and reactivity – Trauma-related alterations in arousal and reactivity that began or worsened after the traumatic event (two required):

1 Irritable or aggressive behaviour
2 Self-destructive or reckless behaviour
3 Hypervigilance
4 Exaggerated startle response
5 Problems in concentration
6 Sleep disturbance

Criterion F: Duration
Persistence of symptoms (in Criteria B, C, D and E) for more than 1 month

Criterion G: Functional significance
Significant symptom-related distress or functional impairment (e.g. social, occupational)

Criterion H: Exclusion
Disturbance is not due to medication, substance use, or other illness

Memories and perceptions

Interestingly, illness severity does not consistently predict a PTSS reaction,[40,50] but such a reaction is more likely to be influenced by patients' perceptions of their intensive care experience. This is one of the unique features of being in intensive care: patients have limited recall for factual events and often report large gaps where they remember very little about their critical illness. Some patients will report upsetting or unpleasant factual memories such as pain, oxygen masks on a patient's face and difficulty breathing.[78] However, frequently, patients' accounts include disturbing recollections with memories of 'odd perceptual experiences',[79,80] 'nightmares' or 'hallucinations'.[31,44,78] While not all patients experience these, those who do so tend to report memories that are persecutory in nature,[78] are often associated with feelings of being elsewhere,[80] reliving a previous life event[81] or fighting for survival.[80]

These memories often seemed 'real' and were distressing to patients at the time, and may be recalled in detail some months afterwards.[44] Having delusional rather than factual memories is more likely to result in distress;[31,50,82] and lack of memory for factual events may result in longer term psychological problems,[53] with the important element being the content of the ICU memories rather than the number of memories. Studies exploring post-traumatic stress after ICU are summarised in Table 4.2.

Cognitive dysfunction

Cognitive impairment in survivors of critical illness has only been recognised and measured in the past decade. Although there is some variation in prevalence and severity, in general more than 50% of survivors report cognitive impairment at the time of hospital discharge and approximately one-quarter continue to have problems 12 months later (Table 4.3).[6,11] Cognitive problems include memory,

TABLE 4.2

Summary of studies examining post-traumatic stress symptoms (PTSS) in survivors of critical care

FIRST AUTHOR/ COUNTRY	DESIGN	N/% MALES	COHORT	ACUITY[a]/ ICU LOS	AGE	INSTRUMENT/ CUT-OFF SCORE	MAIN FINDINGS
Perrins (1998)[83]/ UK	Prospective	38/–	General ICU; 6 weeks, 6 and 12 months post-ICU discharge	–/6	49	IES/–	Avoidance and intrusion scores reduced at 12 months; scores associated with patients' recollection of ICU – those with no recall had higher scores
Schelling (1998)[49]/Germany	Retrospective cross-sectional	80/51%	ARDS; patients discharged over 10-year period	22/31	36	PTSS >35	25% scored above cut-off score; symptoms associated with the number of traumatic memories of ICU
Nelson (2000)[51]/ UK	Cross-sectional	24/58%	19 months (mean) after acute lung injury	58/27	40	7-item questionnaire	Significant correlation with days of sedation and days of neuromuscular blockade and PTSS scores
Scragg (2001)[52]/ UK	Cross-sectional	80/52%	Admitted to ICU over previous 2 years	–/–	57	IES ≥20	12% high levels of avoidance, 8% high levels of intrusive thoughts. Younger patients had higher IES scores
Jones (2001)[53]/ UK	Cohort study	30/66%	General ICU; 2 and 8 weeks	17/8	57	IES	Patients with no factual but who reported delusional memories had higher IES scores at 8 weeks
Jones (2003)[54]/ UK	RCT	116/61%	General ICU patients – 3 hospitals; 8 weeks and 6 months after discharge	17/14	58	IES >19	Patients who received 6-week rehabilitation program had lower IES scores at 8 weeks but not 6 months; 51% scored >19 at 6 months
Kress (2003)[85]/ USA	RCT	32/58%	Medical ICU; 11–14 months after hospital discharge	Control 18.4/12.8; Intervention 16.2/6.9	48	IES; structured clinical interview	Evaluated the effect of daily sedation withdrawal; patients in the intervention group reported lower IES scores (not statistically significant); 6 patients in the control group were diagnosed with PTSD compared with no patients in the intervention group
Cuthbertson (2004)[41]/UK	Prospective cohort	78/72%	General ICU 3 months after discharge	18/5.6	58	DTS ≥27 – high level ≥40 PTSD	22% demonstrated high level of PTS symptoms and 12% confirmed PTSD
Kapfhammer (2004)[47]/Germany	Cross-sectional	46/52%	ARDS; median 8 years after treatment	22.5/–	36	PTSS-10 >35	24% of patients diagnosed with PTSD; a further 17% had sub-threshold PTSD; those with PTSD reported a poorer HRQOL
Rattray (2005)[50]/ UK	Prospective longitudinal	80/64%	General ICU; hospital discharge, 6 and 12 months	17.7/4.9	55	IES ≥20	12% reported severe avoidant behaviour, 18% severe intrusive thoughts at 12 months; scores did not reduce over 12 months and were associated with reported ICU memories and age
Sukantarat (2007)[58]/UK	Prospective	51/43%	In ICU ≥3 days; 3 and 9 months after ICU discharge	15.3/16.9	57.4	IES: intrusion ≥21; avoidance ≥18	Intrusion in 24% at 3 months and 20% at 9 months; avoidance in 36% at 3 months and 38% at 9 months

FIRST AUTHOR/ COUNTRY	DESIGN	N/% MALES	COHORT	ACUITY[a]/ ICU LOS	AGE	INSTRUMENT/ CUT-OFF SCORE	MAIN FINDINGS
Wallen (2008)[86]/ Australia	Predictive cohort	100/68%	≥24 hours ICU LOS; medical/surgical ICU; 1 month after discharge	13.0/2.4	63	IES-R ≥33	Mean IES-R=17.8; 13% scored higher than cut-off score; those ≤65 years were 5.6 times more likely to report PTSS
Weinert (2008)[82]/ USA	Prospective	149/52%	Medical and surgical ICUs; 2 and 6 months	–/–	54	PTSD 6 positive responses across 3 domains	PTSD prevalence at 2 months was 17% and this had reduced to 15% by 6 months; patients who reported delirious memories had higher PTSD scores
Myhren (2009)[61] Norway	Cross-sectional	255/63%	Medical/surgical ICUs and CCU; 4–6 weeks postdischarge	SAPS 37/12 days	48	IES ≥35	25% above threshold
Myhren (2010)[60] Norway	Longitudinal		3 and 12 months				27% above threshold at 12 months; no differences in scores across time; high education level, optimism trait, factual recall, memory of pain were independent predictors of PTSD
Peris (2011)[62]/ Italy	Cross-sectional using historical controls	Control: 86/72.1% Intervention: 123/83.7%	Major trauma 12 months	Control[e]: 38.5/20.1 Intervention[e]: 44.1/17.8	Control: 44.9 Intervention[e]: 43.7	IES-R	Intervention group had lower risk of PTSD (21.1% vs 57%)
Wade (2012)[63]/UK	Prospective	100/52%	Level 3 patients 3 months	22/8[f]	57	PDS ≥18	Probably PTSD 27.1% Strongest predictors were in-ICU mood, intrusive memories, perceived illness and psychological history
Bienvenu (2013)[87]/USA	Prospective	186/55%	Acute lung injury 3, 6, 12, and 24 months	23/13		IES-R item mean score ≥1.6	35% had PTSD symptoms during the 2-year follow-up Symptoms enduring
Schandl (2013)[64]/ Sweden	Prospective	150/415%	General ICU 2 months	55[e]/1.5/6	Adverse psychological outcome group = 54 No adverse psychological outcome group = 60	PTSS-10 >35	Overall 31% had adverse psychological outcomes 21 (14%) high PTSS scores

[a]APACHE II score.
[b]Hospital Anxiety and Depression Scale.
[c]Geriatric Depression Scale – Short Form.
[d]APACHE III score.
[e]Simplified Acute Physiology Score.
[f]Median value. ARDS = adult respiratory distress syndrome; DTS = Davidson Trauma Scale; HRQOL = health-related quality of life; ICU LOS = intensive care unit length of stay; IES = Impact of Event Scale; PTSD = post-traumatic stress disorder; PTSS = post-traumatic stress symptoms; SAPS = Simplified Acute Physiology Score.

TABLE 4.3

Summary of recent studies examining cognitive function after critical illness

AUTHOR/COUNTRY	DESIGN	N/% MALES	COHORT	ACUITY/ICU LOS	AGE	INSTRUMENT	MAIN FINDINGS
Adhikari 2009[89]/ Canada	Prospective cohort; variable follow-up including 6 months and 1, 2, 3 and 4 years	109 (71 completed cognitive assessment)/–	ARDS patients	APACHE II (median) – 23 (IQR 15–27); ICU LOS (median) – 27 (IQR 16–51) days	Median = 42 (IQR 35–56)	Memory Assessment Clinics Self-Rating Scale (MAC-S)	MAC-S scores were 76 (IQR 61–93) for Ability and 91 (IQR 77–102) for Frequency of Occurrence; 8% and 16% of respondents were >2 and 1.5 SD, respectively, below USA norms
Duning 2010[90]/ Germany	Case-control study of patients who experienced ≥1 episode of hypoglycaemia or not	74/44 (59%)	Surgical ICU patients	SAPS – mean 39 ± 2.3; ICU LOS – mean 15.2 ± 1.6 days	Mean 66.3 ± 1.3 years	MMSE; Boston Naming Test; Nuernberg Gerontopsychological Inventory; WMS-R; Trailmaking Tests A and B; Color word interference task (interference condition); Regensburg Word Fluency Test; Rey-Osterrieth Complex Figure Test; Auditory verbal learning test; Recognition	Impaired neurocognitive function (compared to age-matched healthy controls) was identified in most tests; patients who experienced hypoglycaemia experienced significant impairment of visuospatial skills compared to those who did not experience hypoglycaemia; other domains were similar between the groups
Ehlenbach 2010[91]/ USA	Prospective cohort	Total study population 2,929; n=41 experienced critical illness/ 23 (56%)	Older individuals (> 65 years) with critical illness	Not described	Mean = 75.4 (SD 6.6)	Cognitive Abilities Screening Instrument (CASI) = continuous score 0 to 100 'Cases of dementia'	Critical illness hospitalisation resulted in a change in reduction in CASI by –1.5 (-3.0–1.0) for the interval that included a critical illness hospitalisation (not significant). 31.1 cases of dementia per 1,000 person-years (95% CI 12.9–74.6) for critically ill 14.6 cases per 1,000 per years (95% CI 12.6–17.0) for never hospitalised
Girard 2010[14]/ USA	Prospective cohort	126 (77 completed cognitive assessment/ 40 (52%)	Medical ICU patients	APACHE II – median 29 (23–34)	Median 61 (IQR 47–71) years	Digit Span; Trailmaking Tests A and B; Digit Symbol Coding; RAVLT; Rey-Osterreith Complex Figure (copy test and 30-minute delay); Verbal Fluency Text, MMSE	Cognitive function at 3 mths: no impairment – 16/76 (21%); mild/moderate impairment – 13/76 (17%); severe impairment – 47/76 (62%); cognitive function at 12 months: no impairment – 15/52 (29%); 18/52 (35%); 19/52 (36%); Duration of delirium was an independent predictor of cognitive impairment 3 and 12 months after ICU
Jackson 2010[93]/ USA	Sub-study of Awakening and Breathing Controlled (ABC) trial (RCT) with 3- and 12-month follow-up	180/89 (49%)	Medical ICU patients	APACHE II – 28; SOFA – 9		Digit Span; Digit Symbol Coding; MMSE; RAVLT Rey-Osterreith Complex Figure – Copy; Rey-Osterreith Complex Figure – Delayed Recall; Trailmaking Tests A and B; Verbal Fluency Test	Cognitive impairment identified in 79% of all patients at 3 months and 71% at 12 months Fewer patients in the intervention group (70% versus 91%) impaired at 3 months, similar number of patients in both groups impaired at 12 months Composite cognitive scores similar in both groups at 3 and 12 months

AUTHOR/COUNTRY	DESIGN	N/% MALES	COHORT	ACUITY / ICU LOS	AGE	INSTRUMENT	MAIN FINDINGS
Sacanella 2011[94]/Spain	Prospective cohort	230 (112 assessed at 1 year)/57%	Medical ICU patients aged ≥ 65 years	APACHE II – mean 19 ± 6.0; ICU LOS – mean 9.4 ± 10.2	Mean 73 ± 5.5 years	MMSE	10% of patients had an MMSE score <24 at 12 months
Torgersen 2011[95]/ Norway	Prospective cohort with 3- and 12-month follow-up	55/ –	Mixed, primarily surgical ICU patients	SAPS II – mean 35 ± 14.0; ICU LOS – mean 10 ± 9.5 days	Mean 51 ± 16.2 years	Cambridge Neuropsychological Test Automated Battery (CANTAB)	At hospital discharge 18/28 (64%) patients had cognitive impairment; at 3 months 4/35 (11%) and 3/30 (10%) at 12 months continued to have cognitive impairment; cognitive impairment was not associated with any pre-ICU or in-ICU factors tested
Jackson 2012[92]/USA	Pilot RCT: in-home rehabilitation over 3 months	21/11 (52%)	Medical/surgical ICU patients	APACHE II Control – 25.5 (19.5–33.0); Intervention – 23 (19–27); ICU LOS (d) Control – 5.8 (4.3–7.0); Intervention – 3 (2.1–7.9)		TOWER: Delis-Kaplan Tower Test: 'normal' 7 to 13 Mini-Mental State Examination The Dysexecutive questionnaire	3 month scores: TOWER: higher in intervention than controls (median and IQR: 13.0 (11.5-14.0) vs 7.5 (4.0–8.5) p<0.01 Mini-Mental State Exam: Control 26.5 (24.8–28.5); Intervention 30.0 (29.0-30.0) Dysexecutive: Control 16.0 (7.8–19.2); Intervention 8.0 (6.0–13.5)
Mikkelsen 2012[96]/USA	Cohort study (sub-study of FACTT by ARDSNet)	213 (122 tested in ≥1 domain; 75 tested at 12 months in all domains)/43%	ARDS patients	APACHE III – mean 85 (63–102)	Median 49 (40–58)	WAIS-III: Vocabulary; WAIS-III: Similarities; WMS-III: Logical Memory I; Controlled Oral Word Association Test; Hayling Sentence Completion Test	Cognitive impairment present in 41/75 (55%) participants at 12 months. When considering all participants tested in ≥ 1 domain: Vocabulary – 3/98 (3%) Reasoning – 3/98 (3%) Memory – 12/92 (13%) Verbal fluency – 15/96 (16%) Executive function – 57/100 (57%) Lower PaO₂, conservative fluid-management strategy and lower CVP were associated with cognitive impairment at 12 months
Panhariparde 2013[11]/USA	Cohort study with 3- and 12-month follow-up	821/420 (51%)	Medical/surgical ICU patients	APACHE II median 25 (19–31)	Median 61 (51–71) years	RBANS Trailmaking Test B	Median RBANS cognition scores at 3 and 12 months were 79 (IQR 70–86) and 80 (IQR 71–87) respectively; these scores were 1.5 SD below age adjusted population mean and were similar to scores for patients with mild cognitive impairment 40% of patients at 3 months and 34% of patients at 12 months had scores similar to those for patients with moderate traumatic brain injury

APACHE = Acute Physiology and Chronic Health Evaluation; ARDSNet = Acute Respiratory Distress Syndrome Clinical Trials Network; FACTT = Fluid and Catheter Treatment Trial; MMSE = Mini-Mental State Examination; RAVLT = Rey Auditory Verbal Learning Test; Rey-O = Rey-Osterrieth Complex Figure; SAPS = Simplified Acute Physiology Score; WAIS-R = 'Wechsler Adult Intelligence Scale = Revised; WMS-R = Wechsler Memory Scale – Revised.

attention and executive function, which in turn includes reasoning and decision making.[45] These can have significant impact upon the daily life of not just patients but families, and have been linked to longer term dementia. Patients who have been admitted to ICU for treatment of acute respiratory distress appear to be more likely to experience cognitive impairment than other critical illness survivors.[6]

Various factors have been linked to cognitive impairment including delirium, hypoxaemia, hypotension, glucose dysregulation, use of sedatives, sepsis and inflammation and sleep efficiency.[6,11,88] Although many of these relationships appear inconsistent, and may be more problematic in specific sub-groups of the critical care population, delirium has repeatedly been shown to be highly predictive of cognitive impairment.

Measuring patient outcomes following a critical illness

The measurement of health outcomes after critical illness is vital – both to determine patient recovery and inform decisions about ongoing care. Measures related to HRQOL and physical, psychological and cognitive function are discussed.

It is unclear how long patient outcomes following critical illness should be measured, but given ongoing compromise exists for months to years post hospital discharge, such measurement should continue for a similar time, for example 6–12 months. In the research setting there is a need to extend follow-up of patients beyond 2 years to determine the long-term morbidities associated with critical illness and care.[2]

Measures of health-related quality of life after a critical illness

The range of HRQOL instruments available is large, but can be divided into two groups: generic to all illnesses or specific to a particular disease state. One limitation of generic instruments is that, while they can be applied to a broad spectrum of populations, they may not be responsive to specific disease characteristics,[97] and this is problematic in the usually heterogeneous critical care population. A generic instrument that measures baseline HRQOL and exhibits responsiveness in a recovering critically ill patient with demonstrated reliability and validity has been elusive, although recent review papers have identified some useful instruments[7,16] (see Table 4.4). SF-36 is the most commonly used and validated instrument in the literature, including with a variety of critically ill patient groups (e.g. general ICU, ARDS, trauma and septic shock). In a comparison of two related instruments the 15D was considered to be more sensitive to clinically important differences in health status than Euro-Qol – 5 dimensions (EQ-5D) in a critical care cohort.[98]

TABLE 4.4
Health-related quality of life (HRQOL) instruments used for patients following a critical illness

INSTRUMENT	ITEMS	CONCEPTS/DOMAINS
Medical outcomes study (SF-36)[100,101]	36	Physical: functioning, role limitations, pain, general health; mental: vitality, social, role limitations, mental health; health transition; variable response levels (2–5)
Euro–Qol-5 dimensions (EQ-5D)[98,102]	5	Mobility, self-care, usual activities, pain/discomfort, anxiety/depression; 3 response levels; cost-utility index
15D[98,103]	15	Mobility, vision, hearing, breathing, sleeping, eating, speech, elimination, usual activities, mental function, discomfort, distress, depression, vitality and sexual activity; 5-point ordinal scale (1 = full function; 5 = minimal/no function)
Quality of life–Italian (QOL–IT)[104]	5	Physical activity; social life; perceived quality of life; oral communication; functional limitation; varied response levels (4–7)
Assessment of Quality of Life (AQOL)[105]	15	Illness (3 items); independent living (3 items); physical senses (3 items); social relationships (3 items); psychological wellbeing (3 items); 4 response levels; enables cost-utility analysis
Quality of life–Spanish (QOL–SP)[106]	15	Basic physiological activities (4 items); normal daily activities (8 items); emotional state (3 items)
Sickness impact profile (SIP)[107]	68	Physical: somatic autonomy; mobility control; mobility range psychosocial: psychic autonomy and communication; social behaviour; emotional stability; developed from original 136-item[170]
Nottingham Health Profile (NHP)[108]	45	Experience: energy, pain, emotional reactions, sleep, social isolation, physical mobility; daily life: employment, household work, relationships, home life, sex, hobbies, holidays
Perceived quality of life (PQOL)[99]	11	Satisfaction with: bodily health; ability to think/remember; happiness; contact with family and friends; contribution to the community; activities outside work; whether income meets needs; respect from others; meaning and purpose of life; working/not working/retirement; each scored on 0–100 scale

Measures of physical function following a critical illness

Numerous instruments have been developed to examine the physical capacity of individuals, usually focusing on functional status ranging from independent to dependent.[109,110] Common instruments used with individuals after an acute or critical illness are summarised in Table 4.5. Many other instruments exist for specific clinical cohorts, including Katz's ADL index[111] and the instrumental activities of daily living,[112] but these have not been used commonly with survivors of a critical illness.

Physical activity associated with cardiac or pulmonary dysfunction may be assessed using perceived breathlessness (dyspnoea) during exercise by the modified Borg scale,[113] ranging from 0 (no dyspnoea) to 10+ (maximal). The Borg scale is commonly used with other physical activity instruments, e.g. the 6-minute walk test (6MWT).[114]

Measures of psychological function after a critical illness

The psychological recovery process and trajectory for survivors of a critical illness remains an important but relatively under-researched area.[88] Exploration of the impact of the intensive care experience, including ongoing stress and distress[13,79,122,123] and memories for the patient,[76,77] has now emerged in the literature as an important area of research and practice. Instruments that assess mood and mental wellbeing after a critical illness focus on psychological constructs, including anxiety, depression, fear and post-traumatic stress symptoms[124] (see Table 4.6). Constructs that relate to an individual

during a critical illness episode also include agitation and confusion/delirium[39] (discussed further in Chapter 7).

Assessment of psychological outcomes has relied mainly on self-report questionnaires administered via either a postal survey or a structured interview format. Few studies have included clinical assessments such as the Clinical Administered PTSD Scale, the 'gold standard' for diagnosing PTSD.[125] This means, therefore, that such questionnaires are screening tools that can be used to identify individuals at risk of developing a significant clinical problem. They are not diagnostic and this is an important point when considering designing, implementing and evaluating any intervention. A number of standardised questionnaires have demonstrated reliability and validity in this patient group, but the use of different questionnaires makes it difficult to generalise findings. Studies that assessed anxiety and depression used the HADS,[31,49,50,59–61] Beck Anxiety Inventory,[56] State Trait Anxiety Inventory (STAI)[85] and the Beck Depression Inventory.[56,85] Post-traumatic stress has been assessed using the Impact of Event Scale (IES),[50,53,61,85] Post-traumatic Stress Syndrome 10-Questions Inventory (PTSS-10),[40] Davidson Trauma Scale,[41] the Experience after Treatment in Intensive Care 7 (ETIC-7) item scale,[52] Kessler-10,[126] Post-traumatic Stress Symptom Checklist – civilian version 5 (PCL-5)[127] and Post-traumatic Stress Diagnostic Scale (PDS).[128]

These instruments often include 'cut-off' or 'threshold' scores that enable screening for the presence or severity of a disorder. For example, a score of 8–10 on either subscale of the HADS indicates the possible presence of a disorder, while a score of 11 or above

---

TABLE 4.5

Common measures of physical function following a critical illness

INSTRUMENT	MEASUREMENT	SCORE RANGE/COMMENTS
St George's Respiratory Questionnaire (SGRQ),[121] (SGRQ-C)[120]	COPD-specific items assessing three domains: symptoms (7 items), activity (2 multi-part items), impacts (5 multi-part items)	Item responses have empirical weights; higher scores indicate poorer health; used with patients with chronic lung disease, including ARDS
Six-minute walk test (6MWT)[114]	Walk distance, reflects functional capacity in respiratory or cardiac diseases	Assesses walk function in patients with moderate heart failure, ARDS
Barthel Index (BI)[118,119]	10 items of functional status (activities of daily living [ADLs])	Dependence: total = 0–4; severe = 5–12; moderate = 13–18; slight = 19; independent = 20
Functional Independence Measure (FIM)[117]	Severity of disability in inpatient rehabilitation settings	18 activities of daily living in two themes: motor (13 items), cognitive (5 items); 7-point ordinal scales; score range 18–126 (fully dependent–functional independence)
Timed Up and Go (TUG)[116]	Functional ability to stand from sitting in a chair, walk 3 m at regular pace and return to sit in the chair	≤10 seconds = normal; ≤20 seconds = good mobility, independent, can go out alone; 21–30 seconds = requires supervision/walk aid
Shuttle walk test (SWT)[115]	10-m shuttle walk with pre-recorded audio prompts to complete a shuttle turn	Participant keeps pace with audio sounds; 12 levels of speed (0.5–2.37 m/second)

ARDS = adult respiratory distress syndrome.

TABLE 4.6

Examples of common measures of psychological function after critical illness

INSTRUMENT	MEASUREMENT	SCORE RANGE
Impact of Event Scale (IES);[130] IES-R[131]	15-item; assesses levels of post-traumatic distress; two subscales: intrusive thoughts, avoidance behaviours; revised form (IES-R) adds hyper-arousal subscale (7 items)[131]	Frequency of thoughts over past 7 days; 0 = no thoughts; 5 = often; higher scores indicate greater distress: scores ≥26 (combined intrusion and avoidance) are significant
Hospital Anxiety and Depression Scale (HADS)[129]	14-item (4-point scale); measures mood disorders in non-psychiatric patients; focuses on psychological rather than physical symptoms of anxiety and depression	Combined score ≥11 indicates a clinical disorder
Center for Epidemiologic Studies – Depression Scale (CES–D)[132]	20-item self-report scale assesses frequency and severity of depressive symptoms experienced in the previous week	Score range 0–60; higher scores reflect increased symptoms and severity
Kessler 10 (K-10)[133]	10-item (5-point scale) self-report measure of non-specific psychological distress over the past 4 weeks	Score range 10–50; higher scores reflect greater distress
Post-traumatic stress disorder (PTSD) checklist (PCL)[134]	20-item (5-point scale) self-report assessment of symptoms of PTSD corresponding to DSM-V criteria	Score range 20–100; higher scores reflect increased symptoms of PTSD
Post-traumatic Stress Symptoms 14 (PTSS 14)[135]	14-item extended version of the PTSS 10 to cover all aspects of PTSD consistent with *Diagnostic and Statistical Manual of Mental Disorders* (DSM-IV) symptom categories	2 parts: Part A – Assessment of traumatic memories from ICU; Part B – Post-traumatic stress disorder symptoms; score range 14–98

indicates probable presence of such a condition.[129] One limitation of these self-report measures is that while sensitivity (ability to correctly identify all patients with the condition) can be high, specificity (ability to correctly identify all patients without the condition) is less easy to determine, and therefore the incidence of psychological distress may be overstated. This makes estimation difficult and is one of the challenges in establishing the actual magnitude of psychological distress after a critical illness. Other challenges include the recruitment of different cohorts or subgroups of patients (e.g. patients with adult respiratory distress syndrome[56] or acute lung injury[51]). Variations in the international provision of ICU services also mean that differences may exist in case-mix in the areas of illness severity, planned or unplanned admissions, ages and reasons for admission.

Measures of cognitive function after a critical illness

Cognitive or neuropsychological assessment of critical illness survivors has only become more common in the past 10 years. Comprehensive and lengthy testing batteries exist, although those used in studies examining recovery after critical illness have tended to favour the slightly shorter testing (Table 4.7). More than 30 minutes is generally still required for this assessment, which may tire some people, particularly early in their recovery phase after critical illness. Neuropsychological instruments are non-invasive; however, many of them need to be used

in an in-person format, so testing over the phone or via mailed questionnaires is limited. Repeated testing with the same instrument on multiple occasions may lead to practice effects, in other words the critical illness survivor learning how to perform better on the test; hence instruments with multiple versions prove beneficial in some circumstances. Further, some of the tests need to be administered by qualified psychology or psychiatry personnel. Where neuropsychological testing can be carried out, it enables assessment of the nature, severity, prevalence and incidence of cognitive impairment.[136] Cross-cultural differences do exist in some of the domains measured in neuropsychological assessment so where comparison to normative data is required for analysis and interpretation, for example in the Repeatable Battery for the Assessment of Neuropsychological Status (RBANS), country-specific data are required.[137]

The most commonly used brief measure is the Mini Mental Status Examination MMSE);[138] however, criticisms of insensitivity, susceptibility to ceiling effects and limited capacity to differentiate between cognitive domains are often levelled at brief measures.[137] In contrast, more lengthy measures such as the RBANS,[139] Trail Making Test,[140] the Wechsler Memory Scale – revised[141] and the Wechsler Adult Intelligence Scale – revised[142] provide more detail and better differentiation of memory problems but often tire those being tested, particularly older people. Scales such as the Memory Assessment Clinics Self-rating Scale (MAC-S)[143] and Cognistat[144] offer an option in between these two extremes.

TABLE 4.7
Neuropsychological instruments to assess cognitive function in patients following a critical illness

INSTRUMENT	MEASUREMENT	SCORE RANGE / COMMENTS
Mini-Mental State Examination (MMSE)[138]	11 items in 5 domains including orientation, memory, attention and concentration, delayed recall, language	Score of ≤23, or 2 points below maximum in any domain, indicates the presence of moderate-to-severe cognitive impairment; 5–10 minutes to administer
Repeatable Battery for the Assessment of Neuropsychological Status (RBANS)[139]	Measurement of multiple areas of cognitive functioning across 5 indices covering the domains of immediate memory, visuospatial/constructional, language, attention, delayed memory	RBANS must be administered by a qualified psychologist; designed as a paper-and-pencil screening battery; has multiple versions to allow for multiple testing without problems of practice effect
Trail Making Test[140]	Part A requires the rapid connection of 25 sequential numbers; Part B measures visual scanning, visuospacial sequencing and cognitive set shifting by requiring connection of 25 alternate numbers and letters in ascending sequence	Score is obtained as the number of seconds required to complete each part (the examiner points out errors as they occur so correction time is included); this is then converted to a 10-point scale with 10 as the best possible score in each part; Total score ≤12 indicates impairment
Memory Assessment Clinics Self-Rating Scale (MAC-S)[143]	42 items grouped into 2 scales including 21 ability items, 24 frequency of occurrence items and 4 global rating items; assessment on a 5-point Likert scale from *very poor* to *very good*	Ability domains include remote personal memory; numeric recall; everyday task-oriented memory; word recall/semantic memory; spatial/topographic memory. Frequency of occurrence domains include word and fact recall or semantic memory; attention/concentration; everyday task-oriented memory; general forgetfulness; facial recognition
Neurobehavioural Cognitive Status Examination (NCSE)[144] (now known as Cognistat)	Screening test to assess 5 domains including language, construction, memory, calculations and reasoning	Available in web-based format and has been translated into multiple languages, normative data exist for adolescents and adults aged 60–64, 65–74 and 75–84 years (http://www.cognistat.com)
Wechsler Memory Scale – Revised (WMS-R)[141]	Measures different memory functions in adults; 7 sub-tests including spatial addition, symbol span, design memory, general cognitive screener, logical memory, verbal paired associates, visual reproducing	Performance reported as 5 index scores including auditory memory, visual memory, visual working memory, immediate memory and delayed memory
Wechsler Adult Intelligence Scale – Revised (WAIS-R)[142]	Measures intelligence in adults and older adolescents; although it is used to measure intelligence rather than cognition, it is often used in combination with WMS-R	10 core sub-tests and 5 supplemental sub-tests; 4 index scores (verbal comprehension and working memory that combine to provide Verbal IQ Index; perceptual organisation and processing speed that combine to provide Performance IQ Index) as well as the overall full scale IQ

Improving recovery following a critical illness

Survivors of critical illness experience multidimensional and protracted compromise over weeks to months and often extending to years. Interventions to improve recovery following critical illness can be delivered at multiple time points in the critical illness continuum. Some of these interventions are the primary responsibility of the multidisciplinary critical care team, are delivered while the patient remains in ICU and are directed towards limiting the detrimental effects of intensive care or promoting recovery as early as possible. Other interventions to improve recovery may be delivered after the patient has left the ICU but remains in the hospital or after discharge from hospital. These later strategies are often delivered in collaboration with other members of the healthcare team. Although there is limited evidence of specific strategies that are effective in improving recovery, there is building evidence of the principles that should underpin these strategies.[15]

Interventions delivered in ICU

Interventions to improve long-term recovery that are delivered in the ICU focus on strategies to minimise the detrimental effects of critical illness and the associated care. These interventions might focus on one aspect of care, for example sedation minimisation or early mobilization, or might be multidimensional, for example targeting sedation minimisation, optimisation of sleep and limitation of the use of restraints as a combined intervention. The majority of interventions delivered within the ICU are targeted at improving physical function.

Interventions to minimise ICU-AW, particularly in relation to muscle de-conditioning from disuse (e.g. sedation; bed-rest) have recently focused on active exercises and mobility, including while patients are intubated and ventilated.[145] Multiple studies have demonstrated the safety and feasibility of ICU-based early mobilisation interventions,[146–149] although few interventions have had sufficient testing yet to show improvement in patient outcomes. Interventions that have shown initial benefit in small studies include in-bed cycling using an ergometer,[150] a combination of functional electrical stimulation and cycling[151] or early exercise and mobilsation[152] (see Table 4.8).

In addition, strategies primarily directed towards minimising sedation, and therefore facilitating more patient movement, have demonstrated effectiveness. In a Danish setting the use of a 'no sedation' strategy resulted in less mechanical ventilation time and a shorter stay in ICU, although it should be noted that patients in the 'no sedation' group did receive morphine for analgesia and sedative agents such as propofol and haloperidol when needed.[155] On a similar theme, patients who received a combined spontaneous awakening trial and spontaneous breathing trial also spent less time ventilated and in ICU.[156]

An early multidimensional intervention that combined many of the above elements and was referred to by the acronym ABCDE has been proposed to minimise physical, psychological and cognitive sequelae in ICU survivors.[157] This bundle of care incorporates:

A awakening the patient daily

B breathing trials (to minimise mechanical ventilation duration)

C coordination (of daily awakening and spontaneous breathing trials)

D delirium monitoring

E exercise/early mobility (requires a patient to be awake, alert and cooperative).

Effective implementation of any of these interventions requires a change in how critical care clinicians care for their patients and this requires a cultural shift with a multidisciplinary team approach and changes in care processes.[158,159] Strong leadership in the process and a culture of safety and improvement within the ICU are perceived as important factors to aid implementation of interventions such as early mobilisation.[158] Involving the family in interventions to support recovery, including early mobilisation, has also been proposed,[160] and although this has not yet been confirmed in research as an effective strategy, it has great potential and few disadvantages if appropriate preparation is provided.

Implementation of 'early' activity for ICU patients relates to after clinical stabilisation is evident, and includes those still intubated. Factors to ensure patient safety during mobilisation have been identified, including confirming that a patient has sufficient cardiovascular and respiratory reserve and cognitive function.[161] Potential barriers to mobilisation during mechanical ventilation (e.g. acute lung injury, vasoactive infusions) have also been examined and include clinical instability, excessive staff turnover, morale issues and a lack of respect among disciplines.[148,158]

Physiotherapy recommendations for physical de-conditioning include development of 'exercise prescriptions' and 'mobilising plans'.[161] Activities range from passive stretching and range of motion exercises for limbs and joints to positioning, resistive muscle training to electrical stimulation, aerobic training and muscle strengthening and ambulation.[150,162] Specific mobility activities include:

- in-bed (range of motion, roll, bridge, sitting on the edge of the bed)
- standing at the side of the bed
- standing on the tilt-table
- transfer to and from bed to chair
- marching on the spot
- walking
- neuromuscular electrical stimulation
- bedside cycle ergometry.

Patient support for each activity ranges from assistance with 1–2 staff through to independence under supervision. Inspiratory muscle training has been used for weakness associated with prolonged mechanical ventilation, using resistance and threshold-training devices. While there is beginning evidence that inspiratory muscle training is effective,[163] this evidence is not consistent.[164]

A survey of practices in Australian ICUs noted that 94% of physiotherapists prescribed exercise frequently for both ventilated and non-ventilated patients, but practices did vary widely and no validated functional outcome measures were used.[165] When mobilisation practices were explored in point prevalence assessments in both Australia and Germany, almost no mechanically ventilated patient was mobilised[166,167] with activity of the mechanically ventilated limited to in-bed exercise or sitting on the edge of the bed.

As noted earlier, a culture of patient wakefulness and early in-ICU activity and mobility is advocated but challenged by the status quo of work practices and health professional role delineations.[158,159,168] A re-engineering of work processes and practices to promote patient activity is therefore required to ensure optimal outcomes for survivors of a critical illness. Few reports of achieving this change are available, but initial evidence suggests it is possible to change practice in the local environment so that more patients are mobilised.[169]

TABLE 4.8

Recent studies of in-ICU mobility

FIRST AUTHOR/ COUNTRY	DESIGN	N/AGE	COHORT	INTERVENTION	MAIN FINDINGS
Morris 2008[147]/ USA	Cohort	330/55	Acute respiratory failure < 48 hours MV	'Mobility team'[a] > 20 min 3×/day	Out of bed: 5 vs 11 days (p < 0.001) ICU LOS: 5.5 vs 6.9 days (p = 0.025) Hospital LOS: 11.2 vs 14.5 days (p = 0.006)
Burtin 2009[150]/ Belgium	Randomised controlled trial	90/57	Prolonged ICU (expected 12 day LOS)	Daily exercise; 20 mins with bedside cycle ergometer[b] from day 5, 5 days/week	6MWD (hospital discharge): 196 vs 143 m (<0.05) Isometric quadriceps: 2.37 vs 2.03 Newton (n.s.) SF-36 PF: 21 vs 15 (p < 0.01) ICU LOS: 25 vs 24 days (n.s.) Hospital LOS: 36 vs 40 days (n.s.)
Schweickert 2009[152]/USA	2-site randomised controlled trial	104/56	ICU patients with <72 hours MV	Exercise and mobilisation (PT and OT)[c] for stable and awake patients; activity based on patient stability and tolerance	Independent function (hospital discharge): 59% vs 35% (p = 0.02) Ventilator free days: 23.5 vs 21.1 (n.s.) ICU LOS: 5.9 vs 7.9 days (n.s.) Hospital LOS: 13.5 vs 12.9 days (n.s.) Barthel Index (hospital discharge): 75 vs 55 (n.s.) 1 serious adverse event in 498 therapy sessions (desaturation <80%) and 4% sessions discontinued due to patient instability
Bourdin 2010[153]/ France	Cohort	20/68	≥7 days ICU ≥2 days MV	Protocol of chair sitting, tilt-table, walking activities; 33% during MV	Contraindication to mobility intervention on 230/524 (43%) patient days 425 mobility interventions performed, complete data on 275 (65%) 91 (33%) interventions during MV Common interventions were sitting in chair (55%), tilt-up ± arm support (33%), walking 11% Adverse event occurred in 3% interventions (no harm)
Needham 2010[154]/USA	Before/ after Quality Improvement (QI) project	57/52	≥2 days MV	Structured QI model, multi-disciplinary team, new PT and OT referral and sedation reduction guidelines	Reduced benzodiazepine dose (pre: 50%, post: 25%, p = 0.02) Increased number of functional mobility treatments (pre: 56%, post: 78%, p = 0.03)
Pohlman 2010[148]/USA	Intervention arm of randomised controlled trial	49/58	<3 days MV with expected further MV	Sedation interruption, PT/OT rehabilitation protocol,[d] sessions 25–30 minutes	Intubated participants sat at edge of bed in 60%, stood in 33% and ambulated in 15% of sessions
Denehy 2013[149]/ Australia	Randomised controlled trial	150/61	>5 days in ICU	Exercise rehabilitation in ICU, ward and outpatients	No major adverse events No significant differences at hospital discharge, 3, 6 or 12 months in 6MWD, TUG, AQoL, SF-36
Parry 2014[151]/ Australia	Observational	16/63	Septic ICU patients, >48 hours MV, in ICU >4 days	FES-cycling intervention[e] 20–60 minutes daily, 5 times/week	Number of cycling sessions – 8/patient Total cycling sessions provided 69 (73%) out of possible 95 1 minor adverse event (S_pO_2 86% requiring F_iO_2 increase)

6MWD = 6-minute walk distance; AQOL = Assessment of Quality of Life instrument; FES = Functional Electrical Stimulation; MV = mechanical ventilation; n.s. = not significant; OT = occupational therapy; PT = physiotherapy; SF-36 = Short Form 36 Health Survey; TUG = Timed Up and Go test.

[a]Registered nurse, nursing assistant, physical therapist team; passive range of motion (ROM), turning, active resistance, sitting, transfer.
[b]Passive or active cycling, 6 levels of increasing resistance; sedated patients received passive cycling at 20 cycles/minute.
[c]Daily passive ROM for unresponsive; after daily interruption of sedation, assisted and independent active ROM supine, bed mobility (transferring to upright sitting and balance) and activities of daily living (ADLs), transfer training (sit-to-stand from bed to chair), pre-gait exercises, walking.
[d]Passive ROM for unresponsive; assisted and independent active ROM supping, bed mobility (lateral rolling, transferring to upright sitting), balance, ADLs, transfer training, walking.
[e]Supine motorised cycle ergometer attached to a current-controlled stimulator, muscles were stimulated at specific stages throughout cycling phase based on normal muscular activation patterns regulated by the bicycle software.

Further development and testing of potential interventions also remain to be undertaken, particularly in terms of patient selection, when to commence and the duration, intensity and frequency of the rehabilitation interventions. Activities may also be adopted and adapted from other established rehabilitation programs such as those for stroke and chronic respiratory disease patients. Technological devices, such as virtual reality rehabilitation,[170] may also prove to be beneficial in this cohort with further development and testing.

Interventions to improve psychological recovery

Although there is now strong empirical evidence that some patients experience significant psychological dysfunctions after a critical illness, it is less clear how and when to treat these symptoms.[171] There is some evidence to support the minimisation of sedation, particularly with benzodiazepines, while the patient is in ICU, and strategies to achieve this that are relevant to each ICU context should be implemented.[67,172]

Evidence is emerging of the benefits of in-ICU psychological care as a way of reducing anxiety, depression and post-traumatic stress symptoms.[173] These results are promising but this was a single centre study in a subgroup of trauma patients; therefore, further work is necessary before considering wider implementation.

Early detection and identification of patients at risk of psychological problems are important and there have been recent developments of at-risk screening tools specifically for this patient population.[64] From an initial 21 potential predictors, univariate analysis identified 6 key variables (pre-existing disease, parent to children < 18 years, previous psychological problems, in-ICU agitation, unemployed/sick leave at ICU admission and appeared depressed in ICU).[64] This is an interesting development and one that requires further testing. For example, depression was not measured using a standardised tool, and the study was unable to capture patients' memories of being in ICU.

Systematic follow-up services may offer appropriate assessment support during recovery for individuals identified with psychological disturbances. Intensive care follow-up clinics where patients have the opportunity to discuss their intensive care experiences and receive information about what had happened to them could be a useful intervention, although there are currently no empirical data to support this,[13] and further research work is required.

Diaries for patients are also thought to be important in providing missing pieces of information that might help a patient make sense of their critical illness experience. A diary approach has been adopted in a number of European ICUs;[174,175] however, there has been a great deal of variation in how the diaries were compiled and viewed by a patient, as well as how much support was offered to them to explain diary content.[176] To this point in time the use of such diaries tends to be atheoretical,[176] with limited long-term exploration of the effect of the diary intervention on patient outcomes. While there is a small amount of evidence that supports their use,[177] further empirical work is necessary to ensure the patient experiences no harm on receipt of a diary. Note, however, that not all patients may wish to be reminded of their ICU experience; this is especially the case for patients who demonstrate avoidant behaviours. Two studies have reported that approximately 50% of patients do not wish to know what has happened to them during intensive care.[50,178] Others may wish not to be reminded of being critically ill but wish to concentrate on recovery.[13] Further research that incorporates these issues during assessment of post-traumatic stress symptoms will establish the effectiveness of diary use.

The UK NICE guidelines[179] emphasised regular assessment of patient recovery including psychological recovery. Assessment periods include during intensive care, ward-based care, before discharge home or community care and 2–3 months after ICU discharge, with the use of existing referral pathways and stepped care models to treat identified psychological dysfunctions. These services are usually well established and allow patients to be treated by appropriately qualified practitioners. The role of critical care practitioners may therefore be to establish the causes of psychological disturbances associated with critical illness, identifying at-risk patients through systematic and standardised screening activities, closely monitoring identified patients and referring to appropriate specialties where appropriate, to optimise their recovery trajectory while not introducing any further harm. Once a patient has a diagnosis of anxiety, depression or post-traumatic stress, treatment should follow national guidelines, for example NICE guidelines for the management of adult patients with depression (see the NICE website, http://www.nice.org.uk/Guidance/CG90).

Ward-based post-ICU recovery

Follow-up services for survivors of a critical illness in Australia and New Zealand have occurred sporadically in individual units with interested clinician teams,[180] but there is currently no widespread systematic approach to recovery and rehabilitation and the management of physical, psychological or cognitive dysfunctions beyond clinical stability and deterioration with ICU liaison services[181,182] or medical emergency teams (MET).[183]

Commencement or continuation of rehabilitation activities in the general wards after discharge from ICU highlights a potentially different set of challenges, particularly in terms of physiotherapy resources, involvement of other medical teams and compliance to a prescribed plan. Although some cohorts of critically ill patients (e.g. pulmonary, cardiac, stroke, brain injury) have defined rehabilitation pathways,[184] patients with other clinical presentations may not be routinely prescribed a rehabilitation plan or be referred to a rehabilitation specialist.

For patients who survive to ICU discharge, approximately 3–5% will die prior to hospital discharge.[185] Some work in Europe on prognosis post-ICU discharge using the 4-point Sabadell Score (0 = good prognosis; 1 = long-term poor prognosis; 2 = short-term poor prognosis; 3 = expected hospital death)[186] demonstrated that subjective intensivist assessment was able to predict the risk of patient mortality,[187] and conversely those patients potentially suitable for rehabilitation.

Specific ward-based rehabilitation interventions following ICU discharge are beginning to be investigated. Designing and implementing such an intervention is challenging because of the heterogeneous nature of intensive care patients who have increasing complexity and ill-defined recovery trajectories. Furthermore, these patients tend to be 'scattered' throughout the hospital making coordination of care post-ICU difficult. Some exploratory work in the UK implemented a generic rehabilitation assistant to support enhanced physiotherapy and nutritional rehabilitation in collaboration with ward-based staff.[188,189] Following the MRC framework for complex interventions, the intervention focused primarily on physical recovery from ICU discharge to 3 months. The generic rehabilitation assistant was able to provide information and explanation of the patient's time in intensive care, facilitate discussions with the multidisciplinary team, assist in goal setting and provide enhanced ward-based rehabilitation.[190] Results from this study will be published shortly.

The benefits of physical exercise training for patients with COPD was affirmed in a recent review, with recommendations focused on maintenance of health behaviour change,[191] and these guidelines could be applied to some cohorts of critically ill survivors. Identification of the most effective level of intervention, however, remains elusive. One Australian study of acute medical patients (not after critical illness) noted that individually tailored physical exercise (20–30 minutes twice daily, 5 days per week) in hospital was not sufficient to influence functional activity at discharge.[192] Further research is therefore required to test specific interventions during the post-ICU hospital period aimed at improving the recovery trajectory and health outcomes for patients with limited physical function. As noted with in-ICU rehabilitation, the optimal duration, intensity and frequency of interventions is not yet clear.

Recovery after hospital discharge

Of patients who survive their critical illness to hospital discharge, 5% will die within 12 months, and their risk of death is 2.9 times higher than for the general population.[1] Functional recovery can be delayed in some individuals for 6–12 months[8,16,193,194] or longer.[195] In a Norwegian study, only half of 194 patients had returned to work or study 1 year after surviving their critical illness.[194]

There is, however, only limited research and mixed study findings identifying specific interventions during the post-hospital period that may improve a patient's recovery trajectory and health outcomes. Most work has involved practice evaluations or studies of outpatient 'ICU follow-up' clinics,[54,196,197] while there is some work exploring home-based programs.[198]

ICU follow-up clinics

Systematic follow-up for survivors of a critical illness after hospital discharge emerged in the UK in the early 1990s, after a number of government reviews on the cost and effectiveness of critical care services highlighted the need to evaluate longer term patient outcomes, in particular quality of life,[199] and recognised that patients had sequelae that were best understood and managed by ICU clinicians. In 2000, the UK Department of Health published a comprehensive review of critical care services. With emerging albeit limited evidence of the benefits of an ICU follow-up clinic, the review recommended the provision of follow-up services for those patients expected to benefit.[200] Importantly, this review also recommended collection of patient recovery and outcome data; this has been facilitated through follow-up clinics. The review did not, however, indicate how these services should be delivered or funded. Although this review is now quite dated, strategies have not changed significantly over time and the emerging pattern in the UK has continued to be inviting patients to a follow-up clinic.

The first intensive care follow-up clinics were established in the UK in the early 1990s,[201] driven by a few interested and committed intensive care clinicians. A recent UK survey indicated that approximately 27% of UK ICUs offered a follow-up service.[202] Although there are few reports of clinics operating outside the UK, occasional clinics do exist.[203] Different clinic models have evolved as nurse-led, doctor-led or a combination of multidisciplinary team members with more than half in the UK nurse-led. Many clinics restrict patients invited to return to those with an ICU length of stay of at least 3 or 4 days. This decision is often based upon resources rather than evidence, as patients who have a shorter stay may also have subsequent physical and psychological problems.[196]

Common practice is to invite patients to attend a first clinic appointment approximately 2–3 months after discharge from intensive care or hospital, although timing has to be flexible given the length of hospital stay for some patients. For many, one appointment is sufficient,[204] but others have continuing problems and may need to return on a number of occasions. Some clinics routinely offer return appointments up to 1 year after discharge, determined on an individual patient basis. Attendance can be problematic; only 70–90% in some studies.[180,196] Non-attendance can occur because a patient has no identified problems (shorter ICU length of stay, less ill) or, more importantly, because of individual limitations (limited mobility, living a distance away from the clinic or significant post-traumatic stress symptoms including avoidant behaviours).[205]

While these services developed in a relatively ad hoc manner, tended to be underfunded and used a variety of models in their delivery, the purposes for such a service are similar (see Box 4.2).

BOX 4.2

Purpose of an intensive care follow-up service

- Review and assess patient progress
- Facilitate early identification of problems and refer to appropriate specialties where necessary
- Coordinate care
- Support a rehabilitation program
- Discuss the intensive care experience and offer patient the opportunity to comment on care
- Offer patient the opportunity to visit the ICU
- Provide a forum for relatives to ask questions
- Use information to inform delivery of intensive care

Clinic activities

Patient progress is reviewed for identification of subsequent problems and timely referral to appropriate services for further treatment. A major advantage of follow-up clinics is the increased understanding of patient recovery, as a range of physical and psychological assessments can be conducted (see an example in Table 4.9). Content of assessment is informed by the understanding and knowledge of the problems patients commonly face during their recovery period. Critical care and rehabilitation staff, however, need to ensure that issues are not 'problematising' for aspects of recovery that are not of concern to the patient.

Content of an assessment tool structures the clinic visit and identifies any patient problems. These assessments can include the use of standardised questionnaires of HRQOL, physical function, psychological status and cognitive function and other free-text responses that incorporate patient comments and other issues. Use of standardised questionnaires is, however, inconsistent,[201,202] which limits evaluation and comparisons of clinic outcomes. Common examples of questionnaires were previously listed in Tables 4.4, 4.5, 4.6 and 4.7. The issue of respondent burden must be considered and questionnaire fatigue recognised. This can be managed in part by asking patients to bring completed questionnaires with them to the clinic appointment. Administration, scoring and interpretation of questionnaires must also be managed in accordance with instrument guidelines.

Referral to appropriate specialists using a systematic approach and timely response times are necessary, as other healthcare professionals will not usually be present when patients attend the clinic. Delays in treatment following identification of significant post-traumatic symptomatology can result in PTSD that is enduring and lasts for several years.[47] Implementing defined referral criteria and

TABLE 4.9

Sample clinic assessment tool

SUBJECT AREA	RATIONALE
General health	Assessed on a linear analogue or forced choice response to elicit a patient's subjective account of how they view their general health and how it has changed since critical illness
Medications	Review of medications commenced during the critical illness and continued postdischarge, with advice provided to the patient's general practitioner[196]
Movement and mobility, household management and joints	Assess mobility problems, often due to continuing fatigue and weakness, but also perhaps joint problems;[207] identify impact on daily activities[179]
Breathing and tracheostomy	Breathlessness is common after critical illness and there are a number of potential difficulties post-tracheostomy; these can be identified and the patient referred to the appropriate specialist
Sleep and eating	Sleep and concentration disturbances are common, and muscle loss and weakness are important contributors to delayed recovery[179]
Urology/reproduction, skin and senses	Patients may have sexual problems[206] and skin and nail problems
Recreation, work and lifestyle change	Patients may experience difficulties reintegrating into society and in particular returning to work
Memory, concentration, decision making	This will provide an indication of ongoing cognitive problems that may influence ongoing recovery[6]
Intensive care experience	Patients rarely remember factual events of their time in ICU, but their memories are often of unpleasant and disturbing events;[78] offering an opportunity to discuss actual events and sometimes distressing memories can be beneficial[204]
Quality of life	The ultimate aim of treatment and care is to return a patient to an acceptable and optimal quality of life; it is important to gauge how patients perceive their life quality, and may identify areas for practice improvement

pathways can, however, be challenging particularly when a clinic is nurse-led.[196] While identification of referrals during a follow-up clinic reflects a potential unmet need for these patients, one survey reported that 51% of clinics had no formal referral mechanisms.[201] This referral activity also reflects an additional function of the clinic in coordinating patient care after hospital discharge.

Coordination of care for these patients with complex needs often includes multiple outpatient appointments and investigations at a time when they are least able to cope with this complexity. An additional patient benefit of returning to a follow-up clinic is in supporting them to negotiate their way through this complex care, coordinate outpatient appointments and to have someone whom they know help them understand and interpret the entire critical illness and recovery experience.[196] The follow-up clinic can also be a vehicle for supporting and evaluating a rehabilitation program.[54] Rehabilitation in the form of a 6-week supported self-help manual with weekly telephone calls and completion of a diary demonstrated an improvement in physical recovery at 8 weeks and 6 months after intensive care discharge.

As noted earlier, a unique element of a patient's intensive care experience is their limited recall of factual events but a common experience of 'nightmares' and 'hallucinations' that can be distressing both at the time and during recovery. The benefits of having an opportunity to discuss their experiences with intensive care staff should not be underestimated, and as such effective communication skills are vital for those delivering ICU clinic services.[208] Patients value being able to speak to 'experts' about their experience, being given information about what happened to them in ICU and also receiving reassurances about the length of time that recovery will take and that their distressing memories are common. Clinics also offer patients the opportunity to comment on their care both during and after intensive care.[180,204] This is important not just for the patient but to inform care delivery. For ICUs that complete patient diaries, the follow-up clinic is often the place where these are introduced and discussed with the patient.[177,209,210]

Offering the patient an opportunity to visit the ICU is possible during the follow-up clinic appointment. As noted earlier, the lack of factual memory of intensive care often leaves patients with gaps that may be distressing. Visiting the ICU may therefore be beneficial for some patients, particularly when they report odd perceptual experiences, and enable them to make sense of some of these experiences. However, care should be taken, as some patients may find this experience distressing and appropriate explanation and support is essential.

A follow-up clinic also provides an important forum for relatives. Relatives may have different needs to a patient, and it is common to encourage relatives to attend with the patient. Relatives may not only have short- and long-term consequences for their emotional wellbeing and physical health,[211] but also be faced with supporting a patient who has unrealistic expectations about their recovery.

Clinic attendance by relatives varies[196] and may be related to them having no identified problems or unanswered questions about the patient's recovery, or being unable to attend because of work commitments. Some relatives, however, may not attend because of also adopting avoidant strategies if they are experiencing post-traumatic stress symptomatology,[212] depression[213] or other health problems.

Clinic evaluation

Given the development of follow-up clinics and the nature of implementation, formal evaluation is difficult and this is reflected in the paucity of empirical evidence. Anecdotally, nurses who deliver these clinics consider them beneficial and patients seem to value them. Intuitively, it is a good idea for intensive care practitioners who have unique insights into patient experiences to follow their patients after discharge. Three approaches to follow-up clinic evaluation are evident: a service evaluation,[180] a qualitative study[204] and a pragmatic, randomised controlled trial;[196] each provides different insights.

Twenty-five interviews were performed to evaluate one service, with a number of important themes evident: patients valued easy access to the clinic, being well-treated by staff and not having to wait long to be seen. Some patients attended because they simply received the appointment, while others identified the need to have questions answered, and wanted to discuss their distressing dreams and hallucinations.[180] While there was an insightful account of the development and initial evaluation, no demonstrable patient benefits were evident.

Four main themes emerged from another study of 34 patients: continuity of care; receiving information; importance of expert reassurance; and giving feedback to intensive care staff.[204] Continuity of care enabled reassurance to patients that their progress was being monitored and any problems dealt with if referral to other specialties was needed. Opinions varied about the number of clinic appointments and this reflects individual perceptions and needs. Receiving information was invaluable because of the poor memory for factual events. General information about what had happened to them in ICU was also important for gauging the length of time needed for recovery. Patients also found specific information about tracheostomy scars and other specific areas beneficial. While much of this information could be delivered by non-ICU staff, it was noted patients and relatives were specifically reassured by experts familiar with their ICU experiences.[204] Being informed that other patients had similar experiences, particularly with problems sleeping or the nightmares and hallucinations, was also comforting to patients. Clinics also offered the patient the opportunity to give feedback to ICU staff, and allowed patients and relatives to thank staff for the care received.

The PRaCTICaL study randomised eligible patients to a control group of usual care (in-hospital review by a liaison nurse) or intervention group (a physical rehabilitation handbook and a nurse-led intensive care follow-up clinic 2–3 months after discharge and 6 months later).[196]

Referral pathways were developed with 'fast-track' access to psychiatric or psychological services. There were no demonstrated differences between groups for the primary (HRQOL: SF-36) or secondary outcome measures (anxiety and depression: HADS; post-traumatic stress: Davidson Trauma Scale). There were also no differences between patients who had a short intensive care stay and those with longer stays.[196]

Despite the lack of evidence to support any improvement in outcome, there is little doubt that patients value intensive care follow-up.[214] There are a number of reasons for the lack of empirical evidence. Our contemporary understanding of patient recovery is evolving constantly. The clinics tend to see all patients at the same time in the recovery process and this may not be appropriate, and perhaps the timing of the clinic is either too late or too early for some patients. It may be that studies have been based on an outdated intervention that did not recognise other challenges such as the effects of delirium or cognitive compromise. Sample sizes tend to be relatively small and often fail to identify what can be small subgroups of patients who might benefit from a specific intervention.

Other models that incorporate a more person-centred approach and allow more flexibility should therefore be considered. Telephone contact in the initial weeks after discharge can offer some reassurance to patients and also identify early problems. Patients could then be referred to other specialties, have their outpatient appointments coordinated or be invited to return to a follow-up clinic if they experience identified difficulties. Home visits could also be an option for those who are physically or practically unable to return to a clinic or for those with avoidant behaviours.

Other considerations

It is important to consider that while interventions may not always benefit patients, it also has to be demonstrated that they cause no harm and, therefore, initiating a new service has governance issues. There are also knowledge and skill-set development issues. Intensive care nurses tend not to have training in managing patients on an outpatient basis and new skills have to be learned. They may also not have knowledge and experience in managing many of the patient problems evident at follow-up, in particular the psychological and cognitive issues. Other considerations include accommodation, documentation, communication with other healthcare professionals and evaluation processes. Table 4.10 provides an example of how these

TABLE 4.10

Examples of considerations in setting up a nurse-led follow-up service

CONSIDERATION	ACTION
Staff preparation and training	• Attend at least one established clinic • Arrange to access educational preparation in relation to psychiatric problems • Discussion and frequent contact with relevant healthcare practitioner, e.g. consultant psychiatrist, psychologist • Observe or 'shadow' a community psychiatric nurse
Accommodation	• Arrange outpatient accommodation with an area close to but separate from the ICU
In-hospital follow-up	• Introduce patients to the presence of the follow-up clinic prior to hospital discharge • Identify how best to communicate with the patient after discharge, i.e. telephone consultation, home visit or clinic appointment
Timing of clinic and number of appointments	• Initial appointment 2–3 months after ICU discharge • Further appointments determined by patient need or request • All patients can contact the follow-up nurse without formal appointments
Structure of clinic	• Patient's case notes reviewed prior to the clinic appointment and discussed between nurse and intensivist • General assessment questionnaire forms the basis of the discussion between the nurse and patient • Standardised measures include for example Short-Form 36, Hospital Anxiety and Depression Scale and Intensive Care Experience Questionnaire and the Mini-Mental State Examination • Consider offering patients a visit to the ICU but ensure they are ready for this, e.g. if they do not 'trigger' referral on the Hospital Anxiety and Depression Scale
Documentation	• General assessment questionnaire will form the basis of the record of appointment; the nurse records any additional information on this form
Referral criteria	• Develop and negotiate clear referral criteria for the relevant specialties, in collaboration with intensivists, other medical specialties and allied health professionals
Letter to general practitioner	• A letter summarising the appointment and any recommendations is sent to the patient's GP

issues were addressed when setting up a follow-up service in a Scottish teaching hospital, an evolving service that developed from the PRaCTICaL study.[196] A more flexible approach is used with different options discussed with the patient regarding delivery, with a telephone consultation, home visit and/or clinic appointment.

Home-based care

Although there are home-based programs to manage ongoing care for some clinical cohorts (e.g. patients with heart failure), no specific follow-up programs currently exist to support survivors of a critical illness. Initial studies in this setting are also yet to identify an optimal intervention to improve recovery. A small number of studies have been undertaken where various interventions lasting from 6 to 12 weeks after hospital discharge have been examined; inconsistent results have been identified.

Two studies have been conducted in the UK. In the first patients were provided with a self-help manual that included instructions for exercise; they also received two phone calls in the 6-week period.[215] In this group of 126 patients improvement in physical function as measured on the SF-36 instrument was reported. In contrast, a self-help manual was used by Cuthbertson and colleagues over a 3-month period after hospital discharge and no difference in either physical function or mental health on the SF-36 was reported by the 192 participants.[196] In Australia two studies have also been undertaken. In the first, 195 patients

received a graded, individualised endurance and strength training intervention at home that incorporated a printed manual, three home visits and four follow-up phone calls over 8 weeks post hospital discharge.[198] No difference in physical function on the SF-36 or 6-minute walk test was reported. More recently, Denehy and colleagues provided 150 patients with an exercise program that commenced in ICU and continued through their ward stay and first 8 weeks post hospital discharge; patients attended outpatients clinics for exercise twice a week for 60 minutes in this post-hospital phase.[149] No difference in physical function was identified. One home-based study has been conducted in the USA where 21 patients received a multi-component intervention incorporating physical, functional and cognitive training.[92] Despite the small patient numbers, improved physical and cognitive functions were identified in patients who received the intervention.

Further research is therefore required to determine what elements of interventions are effective, and at what time-points these interventions should be delivered; a number of these are currently underway.[216,217] With further study, future continuity of care and follow-up services after hospital discharge should enable the development of a series of seamless services that start recovery and rehabilitation activities for a patient while in ICU, are carried through to hospital discharge and continue into the community setting.

Summary

In summary we now have increasing evidence of the significant burden of health issues faced by critical illness survivors. We know many face a prolonged and difficult recovery period that will include physical and psychological problems and that these affect not just the patient themselves but family members and other carers. Patients' lives may be significantly altered after critical illness, placing a social and economic burden on the patient and family but also on the healthcare system. Quality of life is often viewed as diminished and we now need to look to focusing on two main areas by identifying a) effective interventions that will reduce these burdens and improve overall life quality and b) the patients most likely to benefit from these interventions. Currently health systems are not organised in such a way as to recognise these problems and, therefore, care after ICU discharge tends to be ad hoc and does not follow a recognised rehabilitation pathway. We perhaps need to look at and learn from other long-term conditions and to adopt approaches that recognise the concept of survivorship after critical illness[218] and develop the appropriate systems and processes that will improve life after critical care.

Case study

Mr Smith was a 70-year-old man admitted to ICU with community-acquired pneumonia. He required 14 days of mechanical ventilation and was sedated through much of this time. Mr Smith's wife and extended family visited him each day while he was in the ICU; on some days he didn't appear to recognise his family members immediately, although as they spoke to him he would become more oriented and recognise them. Mr Smith was then discharged to the high dependency unit for 3 days and then to a medical ward for a further 10 days. An ICU liaison nurse saw him three times prior to discharge from the ward where he initially had some confusion, could not remember what had happened to him and was suffering from hallucinations. He was sent an out-patient appointment to attend the nurse-led ICU follow-up clinic around 3 months after hospital discharge.

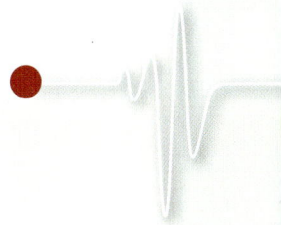

Mr Smith and his wife both attended the clinic. He seemed to be progressing well physically although he struggled a bit at times, but had returned to his usual activities of walking to the corner shop each day as well as starting to do a little weeding in his garden, which he cherished. Despite this aspect of recovery, Mr Smith found it was really upsetting him that he had continuing memory loss. He complained he had to write everything down or he would forget appointments. His wife also commented he still had vivid dreams about being in intensive care and these seemed to upset him. He almost did not attend the clinic appointment. He was a bit irritable with his family and at times was short-tempered. Mr Smith had visited his general physician and described these problems, but was told it was quite common to experience these problems after a lengthy hospitalisation and time in the ICU.

CASE STUDY QUESTION

1   How and when should Mr Smith have been screened or assessed specifically for psychological symptoms?

RESEARCH VIGNETTE

Corner EJ, Soni N, Handy JM, Brett SJ. Construct validity of the Chelsea critical care physical assessment tool: an observational study of recovery from critical illness. Crit Care 2014;18(2):R55

Abstract

Introduction: Intensive care unit-acquired weakness (ICU-AW) is common in survivors of critical illness, resulting in global weakness and functional deficit. Although ICU-AW is well described subjectively in the literature, the value of objective measures has yet to be established. This project aimed to evaluate the construct validity of the Chelsea Critical Care Physical Assessment tool (CPAx) by analyzing the association between CPAx scores and hospital-discharge location, as a measure of functional outcome.

Methods: The CPAx was integrated into practice as a service-improvement initiative in an 11-bed intensive care unit (ICU). For patients admitted for more than 48 hours, between 10 May 2010 and 13 November 2013, the last CPAx score within 24 hours of step down from the ICU or death was recorded (n=499). At hospital discharge, patients were separated into seven categories, based on continued rehabilitation and care needs. Descriptive statistics were used to explore the association between ICU discharge CPAx score and hospital-discharge location.

Results: Of the 499 patients, 171 (34.3%) returned home with no ongoing rehabilitation or care input; 131 (26.2%) required community support; 28 (5.6%) went to inpatient rehabilitation for <6 weeks; and 25 (5.0%) went to inpatient rehabilitation for >6 weeks; 27 (5.4%) required nursing home level of care; 80 (16.0%) died in the ICU, and 37 (7.4%) died in hospital. A significant difference was found in the median CPAx score between groups (P<0.0001). Four patients (0.8%) scored full marks (50) on the CPAx, all of whom went home with no ongoing needs; 16 patients (3.2%) scored 0 on the CPAx, all of whom died within 24 hours. A 0.8% ceiling effect and a 3.2% floor effect of the CPAx is found in the ICU. Compliance with completion of the CPAx stabilised at 78% of all ICU admissions.

Conclusion: The CPAx score at ICU discharge has displayed construct validity by crudely discriminating between groups with different functional needs at hospital discharge. The CPAx has a limited floor and ceiling effect in survivors of critical illness. A significant proportion of patients had a requirement for post-discharge care and rehabilitation.

Critique

This study is the second by this group of authors examining the development of a physical assessment instrument – the Chelsea Critical Care Physical Assessment tool (CPAx). Content and construct validity, internal consistency and inter-rater reliability were demonstrated initially in a small pilot study.[219] In this second study the authors have explored construct validity in a larger cohort by examining the association between CPAx scores on ICU discharge and hospital discharge location and support. In addition, they have examined usability of the CPAx and floor and ceiling effects as well as future care needs for survivors of critical illness.

Ten components of physical function are assessed using the CPAx, including respiratory function, cough, moving within the bed, dynamic sitting, standing balance, sit to stand, transferring bed to chair, stepping and grip strength. Each of these components is assessed on a 6-point scale from 0 (complete dependence) to 5 (independence). The instrument is designed to be used by physiotherapists during their routine treatment of critically ill patients, with only the grip strength assessment representing assessment that is not routinely undertaken. Hospital discharge location/support incorporated five survival categories including home with no rehabilitation needs, home with community support, short inpatient rehabilitation (<6 weeks), long inpatient rehabilitation (>6 weeks) or nursing home care. In addition, two non-survival categories were incorporated: non-survival in ICU and non-survival in hospital.

Good separation of CPAx scores was identified between most of the seven discharge groups, with gradual reduction of scores from the category requiring no rehabilitation support to those who died in ICU. The only discharge location that was not distinct in terms of CPAx scores was the non-survival in hospital group, possibly reflecting the many different reasons patients die while they are in hospital wards.

Further, few patients scored the extreme scores of 0/50 (complete dependence) or 50/50 (complete independence) suggesting few problems with floor or ceiling effects, in other words a large grouping of patients at the minimum or maximum score due to insufficient spectrum of the function being measured. All 16 (3%) of the patients who scored 0 died within 24 hours of this score, and all four (1%) of the patients who scored 50 were discharged home without requiring support.

A number of limitations of this study should be considered. The CPAx is designed, and has only been tested, when used by physiotherapists. It is not known if the reliability and validity would remain consistent when used by other members of the healthcare team, particularly nurses; therefore this limits generalisability to ICUs that have limited or no physiotherapy service. Despite this, the fact that scoring using the CPAx requires only 2 minutes in addition to routine assessment should be seen as a strength as this improves feasibility of completion.

The average length of stay for patients included in this study was 6 days (median). In addition, patients had a relatively low APACHE II score[16] for this length of stay and no information has been provided regarding the proportion of patients who received mechanical ventilation. These characteristics should be taken into account when considering if the cohort examined in this study reflects the usual cohort in each individual ICU. In the study centre (Chelsea and Westminster Hospital, London, UK) only 1524 patients were admitted to ICU over 3.5 years, representing approximately 435 patients per year – this is low throughput for an 11-bed ICU and raises the question of whether there is something unique about the population that is not reflected in the general demographic description. Some post hoc analysis had limited power, but this was clearly noted by the authors.

Despite these limitations, good construct validity has been demonstrated suggesting that, with further testing, final CPAx scores before discharge from ICU might be appropriate to use to plan discharge support both prior to leaving ICU and throughout the patient's ward stay.

When considering the applicability of these results to each individual setting, generalisability is further affected by individual patient characteristics, for example age, desire for rehabilitation and level of family support as well as local facilities such as rehabilitation services. In this particular cohort 34% of patients required no further support after hospital discharge, 26% required ongoing community healthcare support, 11% required inpatient rehabilitation and 5% were discharged to a nursing home. Recognising that more than 40% of critical illness survivors require ongoing support is important to inform planning for future services.

The CPAx is consistent with the Function Status Score for the ICU (FSS-ICU) first described by Zanni and colleagues,[220] which incorporates multiple different components such as rolling, sitting, standing and walking that are each scored on a multi-level scale. In contrast, the ICU Mobility Scale[221] considers these components in one continuous domain, with patients receiving a score that represents their maximum ability; this instrument has undergone initial reliability testing only at this stage. Although all of these scales are in an early phase of their development, the potential to measure progress and identify patients who require assistance with physical function is an important step forward in our planning to provide appropriate support across the critical care continuum.

Learning activities

1 Patients transferred from ICU to the ward may have complex care needs. In your hospital, if a follow-up service was planned, how do you think this should be developed?

2 Review the evidence for psychological assessment and management of patients after a critical illness and intensive care admission.

3 What are the educational implications for staff in relation to supporting the physical and psychological problems patients experience after ICU?

Online resources

I-CAN UK (Intensive Care After Care Network), www.i-canuk.co.uk/default.aspx

ICU Steps, www.icusteps.com

Patient-reported Outcome and Quality of Life Instruments Database (PROQOLID), www.proqolid.org

Patient-Centered Outcomes Research Institute, www.pcori.org

PTSD NICE Guidelines, www.nice.org.uk/CG26

Further reading

National Institute for Health and Clinical Excellence. Rehabilitation after critical illness. NICE clinical guideline 83. 2009 March: 1–91, <http://www.nice.org.uk/CG83>; 2009 [accessed 03.02.15].

References

1 Williams TA, Dobb GJ, Finn JC, Knuiman MW, Geelhoed E, Lee KY, et al. Determinants of long-term survival after intensive care. Crit Care Med 2008;36(5):1523-30.

2 Needham DM, Davidson J, Cohen H, Hopkins RO, Weinert C, Wunsch H, et al. Improving long-term outcomes after discharge from intensive care unit: report from a stakeholders' conference. Crit Care Med 2012;40(2):502-9.

3 Stevens RD, Dowdy DW, Michaels RK, Mendez-Tellez PA, Pronovost PJ, Needham DM. Neuromuscular dysfunction acquired in critical illness: a systematic review. Intensive Care Med 2007;33(11):1876-91.

4 Davydow D, Gifford J, Desai S, Needham D, Bienvenu O. Posttraumatic stress disorder in general intensive care unit survivors: a systematic review. Gen Hosp Psychiatry 2008;30(5):421.

5 Davydow DS, Gifford JM, Desai SV, Bienvenu OJ, Needham DM. Depression in general intensive care unit survivors: a systematic review. Intensive Care Med 2009;35(5):796-809.

6 Wilcox ME, Brummel NE, Archer K, Ely EW, Jackson JC, Hopkins RO. Cognitive dysfunction in ICU patients: risk factors, predictors, and rehabilitation interventions. Crit Care Med 2013;41(9 Suppl 1):S81-98.

7 Angus DC, Carlet J. Surviving intensive care: a report from the 2002 Brussels Roundtable. Intensive Care Med 2003;29(3):368-77.

8 Oeyen SG, Vandijck DM, Benoit DD, Annemans L, Decruyenaere JM. Quality of life after intensive care: a systematic review of the literature. Crit Care Med 2010;38(12):2386-400.

9 Fan E, Dowdy DW, Colantuoni E, Mendez-Tellez PA, Sevransky JE, Shanholtz C et al. Physical complications in acute lung injury survivors: a two-year longitudinal prospective study. Crit Care Med 2014;42(4):849-59.

10 van den Boogaard M, Schoonhoven L, Maseda E, Plowright C, Jones C, Luetz A et al. Recalibration of the delirium prediction model for ICU patients (PRE-DELIRIC): a multinational observational study. Intensive Care Med 2014;40(3):361-9.

11 Pandharipande PP, Girard TD, Jackson JC, Morandi A, Thompson JL, Pun BT, et al. Long-term cognitive impairment after critical illness. N Engl J Med 2013;369(14):1306-16.

12 Rattray J, Johnston M, Wlldsmith JW. Predictors of emotional outcomes of intensive care. Anaesthesia 2005;60:1085-92.

13 Rattray J, Hull A. Emotional outcome after intensive care: literature review. J Adv Nurs 2008;64(1):2-13.

14 Girard TD, Jackson JC, Pandharipande PP, Pun BT, Thompson JL, Shintani AK, et al. Delirium as a predictor of long-term cognitive impairment in survivors of critical illness. Crit Care Med 2010;38(7):1513-20.

15 Rubenfeld GD. Interventions to improve long-term outcomes after critical illness. Curr Opin Crit Care 2007;13(5):476-81.

16 Dowdy DW, Eid MP, Sedrakyan A, Mendez-Tellez PA, Pronovost PJ, Herridge MS, et al. Quality of life in adult survivors of critical illness: a systematic review of the literature. Intensive Care Med 2005;31:611-20.

17 Griffiths J, Hatch RA, Bishop J, Morgan K, Jenkinson C, Cuthbertson BH, et al. An exploration of social and economic outcome and associated health-related quality of life after critical illness in general intensive care unit survivors: a 12-month follow-up study. Crit Care 2013;17(3):R100.

18 Kress JP, Hall JB. ICU-acquired weakness and recovery from critical illness. N Engl J Med 2014;371(3):287-8.

19 Batt J, dos Santos CC, Cameron JI, Herridge MS. Intensive care unit-acquired weakness: clinical phenotypes and molecular mechanisms. Am J Respir Crit Care Med 2013;187(3):238-46.

20 Stevens RD, Marshall SA, Cornblath DR, Hoke A, Needham DM, de Jonghe B, et al. A framework for diagnosing and classifying intensive care unit-acquired weakness. Crit Care Med 2009;37(10 Suppl):S299-308.

21 de Jonghe B, Lacherade JC, Sharshar T, Outin H. Intensive care unit-acquired weakness: risk factors and prevention. Crit Care Med 2009;37 (10 Suppl):S309-15.

22 Winkelman C. Mechanisms for muscle health in the critically ill patient. Crit Care Nurs Q 2013;36(1):5-16.

23 Sliwa JA. Acute weakness syndromes in the critically ill patient. Archives of Physical Medicine & Rehabilitation 2000;81(3 Suppl 1):S45-54.

24 Puthucheary ZA, Rawal J, McPhail M, Connolly B, Ratnayake G, Chan P, et al. Acute skeletal muscle wasting in critical illness. JAMA 2013;310(15):1591-600.

25 Hermans G, Van Mechelen H, Clerckx B, Vanhullebusch T, Mesotten D, Wilmer A, et al. Acute outcomes and 1-year mortality of intensive care unit-acquired weakness. A cohort study and propensity-matched analysis. Am J Respir Crit Care Med 2014;190(4):410-20.

26 Vanpee G, Hermans G, Segers J, Gosselink R. Assessment of limb muscle strength in critically ill patients: a systematic review. Crit Care Med 2014;42(3):701-11.

27 O'Brien M for the Guarantors of Brain. Aids to the examination of the peripheral nervous system. 5th Ed. Edinburgh: Saunders Elsevier; 2010.

28 Kleyweg RP, van der Meche FG, Schmitz PI. Interobserver agreement in the assessment of muscle strength and functional abilities in Guillain–Barré syndrome. Muscle Nerve 1991;14(11):1103-9.

29 Ali NA, O'Brien JM, Jr, Hoffmann SP, Phillips G, Garland A, Finley JC, et al. Acquired weakness, handgrip strength, and mortality in critically ill patients. Am J Respir Crit Care Med 2008;178(3):261-8.

30 Fan E, Ciesla ND, Truong AD, Bhoopathi V, Zeger SL, Needham DM. Inter-rater reliability of manual muscle strength testing in ICU survivors and simulated patients. Intensive Care Med 2010;36(6):1038-43.

31 Jones C, Griffiths R, Humphris G, Skirrow P. Memory, delusions and the development of acute post-traumatic stress disorder-related symptoms after intensive care. Crit Care Med 2001;29:573-80.

32 Granja C, Gomes E, Amaro A, Ribeiro O, Jones C, Carneiro A, et al. Understanding posttraumatic stress disorder-related symptoms after critical care: the early illness amnesia hypothesis. Crit Care Med 2008;36(10):2801-9.

33 Granja C, Lopes A, Moreira S, Dias C, Costa-Pereira A, Carneiro A, et al. Patients' recollections of experiences in the intensive care unit may affect their quality of life. Crit Care 2005;9:R96-R109.

34 Jones C, Humphris G, Griffiths RD. Preliminary validation of the ICUM tool: a tool for assessing memory of the intensive care unit experience. Clin Intensive Care 2000;11:251-5.

35 Boyle M, Murgo M, Adamson H, Gill J, Elliott D, Crawford M. The effect of chronic pain on health related quality of life amongst intensive care survivors. Aust Crit Care 2004;17:104-13.

36 Stein-Parbury J, McKinley S. Patients' experiences of being in an intensive care unit: a select literature review. Am J Crit Care 2000;9(1):20-7.

37 Lof L, Berggren L, Ahlstrom G. ICU patients' recall of emotional reactions in the trajectory from falling critically ill to hospital discharge: follow-ups after 3 and 12 months. Intensive Crit Care Nurs 2008;24(2):108-21.

38 Strahan EH, Brown RJ. A qualitative study of the experiences of patients following transfer from intensive care. Intensive Crit Care Nurs 2005;21(3):160-71.

39 Griffiths J, Fortune G, Barber V, Young JD. The prevalence of post traumatic stress disorder in survivors of ICU treatment: a systematic review. Intensive Care Med 2007;33(9):1506-18.

40 Schelling G, Stoll C, Haller M, Briegel J, Manert W, Hummel T, et al. Health-related quality of life and posttraumatic stress disorder in survivors of the acute respiratory distress syndrome. Crit Care Med 1998;26(4):651-9.

41 Cuthbertson BH, Hull A, Strachan M, Scott J. Post-traumatic stress disorder after critical illness requiring general intensive care. Intensive Care Med 2004;30:450-5.

42 Rundshagen I, Schnabel K, Wegner C, am Esch S. Incidence of recall, nightmares, and hallucinations during analgosedation in intensive care. Intensive Care Med 2002;28(1):38-43.

43 Magarey JM, McCutcheon HH. 'Fishing with the dead' – recall of memories from the ICU. Intensive Crit Care Nurs 2005;21(6):344-54.

44 Adamson H, Murgo M, Boyle M, Kerr S, Crawford M, Elliott D. Memories of intensive care and experiences of survivors of a critical illness: an interview study. Intensive Crit Care Nurs 2004;20(5):257-63.

45 Sukantarat KT, Burgess PW, Williamson RCN, Brett SJ. Prolonged cognitive dysfunction in survivors of critical illness. Anaesthesia 2005;60:847-53.

46 de Miranda S, Pochard F, Chaize M, Megarbane B, Cuvelier A, Bele N, et al. Postintensive care unit psychological burden in patients with chronic obstructive pulmonary disease and informal caregivers: a multicenter study. Crit Care Med 2011;39(1):112-8.

47 Kapfhammer HP, Rothenhausler HB, Krauseneck T, Stoll C, Schelling G. Posttraumatic stress disorder and health-related quality of life in long-term survivors of acute respiratory distress syndrome. Am J Psychiatry 2004;161(1):45-52.

48 Davydow DS, Zatzick D, Hough CL, Katon WJ. A longitudinal investigation of posttraumatic stress and depressive symptoms over the course of the year following medical-surgical intensive care unit admission. Gen Hosp Psychiatry 2013;35(3):226-32.

49 Eddleston JM, White P, Guthrie E. Survival, morbidity, and quality of life after discharge from intensive care. Crit Care Med 2000;28(7):2293-9.

50 Rattray JE, Johnston M, Wildsmith JA. Predictors of emotional outcomes of intensive care. Anaesthesia 2005;60(11):1085-92.

51 Nelson BJ, Weinert CR, Bury CL, Marinelli WA, Gross CR. Intensive care unit drug use and subsequent quality of life in acute lung injury patients. Crit Care Med 2000;28(11):3626-30.

52 Scragg P, Jones A, Fauvel N. Psychological problems following ICU treatment. Anaesthesia 2001;56(1):9-14.

53 Jones C, Griffiths RD, Humphris G, Skirrow PM. Memory, delusions, and the development of acute posttraumatic stress disorder-related symptoms after intensive care. Crit Care Med 2001;29(3):573-80.

54 Jones C, Skirrow P, Griffiths RD, Humphris GH, Ingleby S, Eddleston J, et al. Rehabilitation after critical illness: a randomized, controlled trial. Crit Care Med 2003;31(10):2456-61.

55 Jackson JC, Hart RP, Gordon SM, Shintani A, Truman B, May L, et al. Six-month neuropsychological outcome of medical intensive care unit patients. Crit Care Med 2003;31(4):1226-34.

56 Hopkins RO, Weaver LK, Chan KJ, Orme JF, Jr. Quality of life, emotional, and cognitive function following acute respiratory distress syndrome. J Int Neuropsychol Soc 2004;10(7):1005-17.

57 Hopkins RO, Weaver LK, Collingridge D, Parkinson RB, Chan KJ, Orme JF, Jr. Two-year cognitive, emotional, and quality-of-life outcomes in acute respiratory distress syndrome. Am J Respir Crit Care Med 2005;171(4):340-7.

58 Sukantarat K, Greer S, Brett S, Williamson R. Physical and psychological sequelae of critical illness. Br J Health Psychol 2007;12:65-74.

59 Dowdy D, Bienvenu O, Dinglas V, Mendez-Tellez P, Sevransky J, Shanholtz C, et al. Are intensive care factors associated with depressive symptoms 6 months after acute lung injury? Crit Care Med 2009;37(5):1702.

60 Myhren H, Ekeberg O, Toien K, Karlsson S, Stokland O. Posttraumatic stress, anxiety and depression symptoms in patients during the first year post intensive care unit discharge. Crit Care 2010;14(1):R14.

61 Myhren H, Toien L, Ekeberg A, Karlsson S, Sandvik L, Stokland O. Patients' memory and psychological distress after ICU stay compared with expectations of the relatives. Intensive Care Med 2009;35(12):2078.

62 Peris A, Bonizzoli M, Iozzelli D, Migliaccio ML, Zagli G, Bacchereti A, et al. Early intra-intensive care unit psychological intervention promotes recovery from post traumatic stress disorders, anxiety and depression symptoms in critically ill patients. Crit Care 2011;15(1):R41.

63 Wade DM, Howell DC, Weinman JA, Hardy RJ, Mythen MG, Brewin CR, et al. Investigating risk factors for psychological morbidity three months after intensive care: a prospective cohort study. Crit Care 2012;16(5):R192.

64 Schandl A, Bottai M, Hellgren E, Sundin O, Sackey PV. Developing an early screening instrument for predicting psychological morbidity after critical illness. Crit Care 2013;17(5):R210.

65 Kowalczyk M, Nestorowicz A, Fijalkowska A, Kwiatosz-Muc M. Emotional sequelae among survivors of critical illness: a long-term retrospective study. Eur J Anaesthesiol 2013;30(3):111-8.

66 Paparrigopoulos T, Melissaki A, Tzavellas E, Karaiskos D, Ilias I, Kokras N. Increased co-morbidity of depression and post-traumatic stress disorder symptoms and common risk factors in intensive care unit survivors: a two-year follow-up study. Int J Psychiatry Clin Prac 2014;18(1):25-31.

67 Long AC, Kross EK, Davydow DS, Curtis JR. Posttraumatic stress disorder among survivors of critical illness: creation of a conceptual model addressing identification, prevention, and management. Intensive Care Med 2014;40(6):820-9.

68 Tedstone JE, Tarrier N. Posttraumatic stress disorder following medical illness and treatment. Clin Psychol Rev 2003;23(3):409-48.

69 Capuzzo M, Valpondi V, Cingolani E, Gianstefani G, De Luca S, Grassi L, et al. Post-traumatic stress disorder-related symptoms after intensive care. Minerva Anestesiol 2005;71(4):167-79.

70 Jones C, Bäckman C, Capuzzo M, Flaatten H, Rylander C, Griffiths R. Precipitants of post-traumatic stress disorder following intensive care: a hypothesis generating study of diversity in care. Intensive Care Med 2007;33(6):978-85.

71 US Department of Veterans Affairs. PTSD: National Center for PTSD Washington, DC: US Department of Veterans Affairs, <http://www.ptsd.va.gov>: 2014 [accessed 29.08.14].

72 American Psychiatric Association. Diagnostic and statistical manual of mental disorders. 5th ed. Arlington, VA: American Psychiatric Association; 2013.

73 Jackson JC, Hart RP, Gordon SM, Hopkins RO, Girard TD, Wesley E. Post-traumatic stress disorder and post-traumatic stress symptoms following critical illness in medical intensive care unit patients: assessing the magnitude of the problem. Crit Care 2007;11:1-11.

74 Schandl A, Bottai M, Hellgren E, Sundin O, Sackey P. Gender differences in psychological morbidity and treatment in intensive care survivors – a cohort study. Crit Care 2012;16(3):R80.

75 Samuelson KAM, Lundberg D, Fridlund B. Stressful memories and psychological distress in adult mechanically ventilated intensive care patients – a 2-month follow-up study. Acta Anaesthesiol Scand 2007;51:671-8.

76 Hopkins RO. Haunted by delusions: trauma, delusional memories, and intensive care unit morbidity. Crit Care Med 2010;38(1):300-1.

77 Ringdal M, Plos K, Ortenwall P, Bergbom I. Memories and health-related quality of life after intensive care: a follow-up study. Crit Care Med 2010;38(1):38-44.

78 Wade DM, Brewin CR, Howell DC, White E, Mythen MG, Weinman JA. Intrusive memories of hallucinations and delusions in traumatized intensive care patients: an interview study. Br J Health Psychol 2014.

79 Rattray J, Johnston M, Wildsmith JA. The intensive care experience: development of the ICE questionnaire. J Adv Nurs 2004;47(1):64-73.

80 Granberg A, Engberg IB, Lundberg D. Acute confusion and unreal experiences in intensive care patients in relation to the ICU syndrome. Part II. Intensive Crit Care Nurs 1999;15(1):19-33.

81 Russell S. An exploratory study of patients' perceptions, memories and experiences of an intensive care unit. J Adv Nurs 1999;29(4):783-91.

82 Weinert C, Sprenkle M. Post-ICU consequences of patient wakefulness and sedative exposure during mechanical ventilation. Intensive Care Med 2008;34(1):82-90.

83 Perrins J, King N, Collings J. Assessment of long-term psychological well-being following intensive care. Intensive Crit Care Nurs 18(6):320-31 1998; 14(3):108-16.

84 Schelling G, Stoll C, Vogelmeier C, Hummel T, Behr J, Kapfhammer HP, et al. Pulmonary function and health-related quality of life in a sample of long-term survivors of the acute respiratory distress syndrome. Intensive Care Med 2000;26(9):1304-11.

85 Kress JP, Gehlbach B, Lacy M, Pliskin N, Pohlman AS, Hall JB. The long-term psychological effects of daily sedative interruption on critically ill patients. Am J Respir Crit Care Med 2003;168(12):1457-61.

86 Wallen K, Chaboyer W, Thalib L, Creedy DK. Symptoms of acute posttraumatic stress disorder after intensive care. Am J Crit Care 2008;17(6):534-43; quiz 44.

87 Bienvenu OJ, Gellar J, Althouse BM, Colantuoni E, Sricharoenchai T, Mendez-Tellez PA, et al. Post-traumatic stress disorder symptoms after acute lung injury: a 2-year prospective longitudinal study. Psychol Med 2013;43(12):2657-71.

88 Jackson JC, Mitchell N, Hopkins RO. Cognitive functioning, mental health, and quality of life in ICU survivors: an overview. Crit Care Clin 2009;25(3):615-28, x.

89 Adhikari NK, McAndrews MP, Tansey CM, Matte A, Pinto R, Cheung AM, et al. Self-reported symptoms of depression and memory dysfunction in survivors of ARDS. Chest 2009;135(3):678-87.

90 Duning T, van den Heuvel I, Dickmann A, Volkert T, Wempe C, Reinholz J, et al. Hypoglycemia aggravates critical illness-induced neurocognitive dysfunction. Diabetes Care 2010;33(3):639-44.

91 Ehlenbach WJ, Hough CL, Crane PK, Haneuse SJ, Carson SS, Curtis JR, et al. Association between acute care and critical illness hospitalization and cognitive function in older adults. JAMA 2010;303(8):763-70.

92 Jackson JC, Ely EW, Morey MC, Anderson VM, Denne LB, Clune J, et al. Cognitive and physical rehabilitation of intensive care unit survivors: results of the RETURN randomized controlled pilot investigation. Crit Care Med 2012;40(4):1088-97.

93 Jackson JC, Girard TD, Gordon SM, Thompson JL, Shintani AK, Thomason JW, et al. Long-term cognitive and psychological outcomes in the awakening and breathing controlled trial. Am J Respir Crit Care Med 2010;182(2):183-91.

94 Sacanella E, Perez-Castejon JM, Nicolas JM, Masanes F, Navarro M, Castro P, et al. Functional status and quality of life 12 months after discharge from a medical ICU in healthy elderly patients: a prospective observational study. Crit Care 2011;15(2):R105.

95 Torgersen J, Hole JF, Kvale R, Wentzel-Larsen T, Flaatten H. Cognitive impairments after critical illness. Acta Anaesthesiol Scand 2011;55(9):1044-51.

96 Mikkelsen ME, Christie JD, Lanken PN, Biester RC, Thompson BT, Bellamy SL, et al. The adult respiratory distress syndrome cognitive outcomes study: long-term neuropsychological function in survivors of acute lung injury. Am J Respir Crit Care Med 2012;185(12):1307-15.

97 Buckley TA, Cheng AY, Gomersall CD. Quality of life in long-term survivors of intensive care. Ann Acad Med, Singapore 2001;30(3):287-92.

98 Vainiola T, Pettila V, Roine RP, Rasanen P, Rissanen AM, Sintonen H. Comparison of two utility instruments, the EQ-5D and the 15D, in the critical care setting. Intensive Care Med 2010;36(12):2090-3.

99 Patrick DL, Danis M, Southerland LI, Hong G. Quality of life following intensive care. J Gen Intern Med 1988;3:218-23.

100 Ware JE, Jr. SF-36 health survey update. Spine 2000;25(24):3130-9.

101 Ware JE, Snow KK, Kosinski M. SF-36 Health Survey: Manual and Interpretation Guide. Lincoln: Quality Metric Incorporated; 2000.

102 Brooks R. EuroQol: the current state of play. Health Policy 1996;37(1):53-72.

103 Sintonen H. The 15D instrument of health-related quality of life: properties and applications. Ann Med 2001;33:328-36.

104 Capuzzo M, Grasselli C, Carrer S, Gritti G, Alvisi R. Validation of two quality of life questionnaires suitable for intensive care patients. Intensive Care Med 2000;26(9):1296-303.

105 Hawthorne G, Richardson J, Osborne R. The Assessment of Quality of Life (AQoL) instrument: a psychometric measure of health-related quality of life. Qual Life Res 1999;8(3):209-24.

106 Fernandez RR, Cruz JJ, Mata GV. Validation of a quality of life questionnaire for critically ill patients. Intensive Care Med 1996;22:1034-42.

107 de Bruin AF, Diederiks JP, de Witte LP, Stevens FC, Philipsen H. The development of a short generic version of the Sickness Impact Profile. J Clin Epidemiol 1994;47(4):407-18.

108 Hunt S, McKenna S, McEwan J, Backett E, Williams J, Papp E. Measuring health status: a new tool for clinicians and epidemiologists. J R Coll Gen Pract 1985;35:185-8.

109 Elliott D, Denehy L, Berney S, Alison JA. Assessing physical function and activity for survivors of a critical illness: a review of instruments. Aust Crit Care 2011;24(3):155-66.

110 Tipping CJ, Young PJ, Romero L, Saxena MK, Dulhunty J, Hodgson CL. A systematic review of measurements of physical function in critically ill adults. Crit Care Resusc 2012;14(4):302-11.

111 Katz S, Ford A, Moskowitz R. Studies of illness in the aged: the index of ADL: a standardized measure of biological and psychosocial function. JAMA 1963;185:914-9.

112 Karnofsky D, Abelmann W, Craver L, Burchenal J. The use of nitrogen mustards in the palliative treatment of cancer. Cancer 1948;1:634-56.

113 Borg GA. Psychophysical bases of perceived exertion. Med Sci Sports Exerc 1982;14:377-81.

114 American Thoracic Society. Guidelines for the six-minute walk test. Am J Respir Crit Care Med 2002;166:111-7.

115 Singh SJ, Morgan MD, Scott S, Walters D, Hardman AE. Development of a shuttle walking test of disability in patients with chronic airways obstruction. Thorax 1992;47(12):1019-24.

116 Podsiadlo D, Richardson S. The timed "Up & Go": a test of basic functional mobility for frail elderly persons. J Am Geriatr Soc 1991;39(2):142-8.

117 Dodds TA, Martin DP, Stolov WC, Deyo RA. A validation of the functional independence measurement and its performance among rehabilitation inpatients. Arch Phys Med Rehabil 1993;74(5):531-6.

118 Wade DT, Collin C. The Barthel ADL Index: a standard measure of physical disability? Int Disabil Stud 1988;10(2):64-7.

119 Mahoney F, Barthek D. Functional evaluation: the Barthel Index. Md State Med J 1965;14:61-5.

120 Meguro M, Barley EA, Spencer S, Jones PW. Development and validation of an improved, COPD-specific version of the St. George Respiratory Questionnaire. Chest 2007;132(2):456-63.

121 Jones PW, Quirk FH, Baveystock CM. The St George's Respiratory Questionnaire. Respir Med 1991;85(Suppl B):25-31; discussion 3-7.

122 Jones C. Aftermath of intensive care: the scale of the problem. Br J Hosp Med (London, England: 2005) 2007;68(9):464-6.

123 Jones C, Twigg E, Lurie A, McDougall M, Heslett R, Hewitt-Symonds M, et al. The challenge of diagnosis of stress reactions following intensive care and early intervention: a review. Clin Intensive Care 2003;14:83-9.

124 Brewin CR. Systematic review of screening instruments for adults at risk of PTSD. J Trauma Stress 2005;18(1):53-62.

125 Hull AM, Rattray J. Competing interests declared: early interventions and long-term psychological outcomes. Crit Care 2013;17(1):111.

126 Kessler RC, Andrews G, Colpe LJ, Hiripi E, Mroczek DK, Normand SL, et al. Short screening scales to monitor population prevalences and trends in non-specific psychological distress. Psychol Med 2002;32(6):959-76.

127 Weathers FW, Litz BT, Herman DS, Huska JA, Keane TM, editors. The PTSD Checklist (PCL): reliability, validity and diagnostic utility. Annual Meeting of International Society for Traumatic Stress Studies; 1993; San Antonio, TX.

128 Foa EB, Cashman L, Jaycox L, Perry K. The validation of a self-report measure of posttraumatic stress disorder: The Posttraumatic Diagnostic Scale. Psychological Assessment 1997;9(4):445-51.

129 Zigmond A, Snaith R. The Hospital Anxiety and Depression Scale. Acta Psychiatr Scand 1983;67(6):361-70.

130 Horowitz MJ, Wilner N, Alvarez W. Impact of Event Scale: a measure of subjective stress. Psychosom Med 1979;41(3):209-18.

131 Weiss DS. The Impact of Event Scale – Revised. In: Wilson JP, Keane TM, editors. Assessing psychollogical trauma and PTSD. 2nd ed. New York: The Guilford Press; 2004.

132 Radloff LS. The CES-D Scale: a self-report depression scale for research in the general population. ApplPsychol Measurement 1977;1(3):385-401.

133 Kessler RC, Barker PR, Colpe LJ, Epstein JF, Gfroerer JC, Hiripi E, et al. Screening for serious mental illness in the general population. Arch Gen Psychiatry 2003;60(2):184-9.

134 Weathers FW, Litz BT, Keane TM, Palmieri PA, Marx BP, Schnurr PP. The PTSD Checklist for DSM-5 (PCL-5). National Center for PTSD at www.ptsd.va.gov, 2013.

135 Stoll C, Kapfhammer HP, Rothenhausler HB, Haller M, Briegel J, Schmidt M, et al. Sensitivity and specificity of a screening test to document traumatic experiences and to diagnose post-traumatic stress disorder in ARDS patients after intensive care treatment. Intensive Care Med 1999;25(7):697-704.

136 Jackson JC, Gordon MW, Ely EW, Burger C, Hopkins RO. Research issues in the evaluation of cognitive impairment in intensive care unit survivors. Intensive Care Med 2004;30:2009-16.

137 Green A, Garrick T, Sheedy D, Blake H, Shores A, Harper C. Repeatable Battery for the Assessment of Neuropsychological Status (RBANS): preliminary Australian normative data. Aust J Psychol 2008;60(2):72-9.

138 Folstein MF, Folstein SE, McHugh PR. Mini-mental state. A practical method for grading the cognitive state of patients for the clinician. J Psychiatr Res 1975;12(3):189-98.

139 Randolph C, Tierney MC, Mohr E, Chase TN. The Repeatable Battery for the Assessment of Neuropsychological Status (RBANS): preliminary clinical validity. J Clin Exp Neuropsychol 1998;20(3):310-9.

140 Reitan RM. The relation of the trail making test to organic brain damage. J Consult Psychol 1955;19(5):393-4.

141 Wechsler D. Wechsler Memory Scale – Revised. San Antonio, TX: Psychological Corporation; 1997.

142 Wechsler D. Wechsler Adult Intelligence Scale – Revised. San Antonio, TX: Psychological Corporation; 1997.

143 Crook TH, Larrabee GJ. A self-rating scale fo revaluating memory in everyday life. Psychol Aging 1990;5(1):48-57.

144 Kiernan RJ, Mueller J, Langston JW, Van Dyke C. The Neurobehavioral Cognitive Status Examination: a brief but quantitative approach to cognitive assessment. Ann Intern Med 1987;107(4):481-5.

145 Calvo-Ayala E, Khan BA, Farber MO, Ely EW, Boustani MA. Interventions to improve the physical function of ICU survivors: a systematic review. Chest 2013;144(5):1469-80.

146 Bailey P, Thomsen GE, Spuhler VJ, Blair R, James J, Bezdjian L, et al. Early activity is feasible and safe in respiratory failure patients. Crit Care Med 2007;35(1):139-45.

147 Morris PE, Goad A, Thompson C, Taylor K, Harry B, Passmore L, et al. Early intensive care unit mobility therapy in the treatment of acute respiratory failure. Crit Care Med 2008;36(8):2238-43.

148 Pohlman MC, Schweickert WD, Pohlman AS, Nigos C, Pawlik AJ, Esbrook CL, et al. Feasibility of physical and occupational therapy beginning from initiation of mechanical ventilation. Crit Care Med 2010;38(11):2089-94.

149 Denehy L, Skinner EH, Edbrooke L, Haines K, Warrillow S, Hawthorne G, et al. Exercise rehabilitation for patients with critical illness: a randomized controlled trial with 12 months of follow-up. Crit Care 2013;17(4):R156.

150 Burtin C, Clerckx B, Robbeets C, Ferdinande P, Langer D, Troosters T, et al. Early exercise in critically ill patients enhances short-term functional recovery. Crit Care Med 2009;37(9):2499-505.

151 Parry SM, Berney S, Warrillow S, El-Ansary D, Bryant AL, Hart N, et al. Functional electrical stimulation with cycling in the critically ill: a pilot case-matched control study. J Crit Care 2014;29(4):695 e1-7.

152 Schweickert WD, Pohlman MC, Pohlman AS, Nigos C, Pawlik AJ, Esbrook CL, et al. Early physical and occupational therapy in mechanically ventilated, critically ill patients: a randomised controlled trial. Lancet 2009;373(9678):1874-82.

153 Bourdin G, Barbier J, Burle JF, Durante G, Passant S, Vincent B, et al. The feasibility of early physical activity in intensive care unit patients: a prospective observational one-center study. Respir Care 2010;55(4):400-7.

154 Needham DM, Korupolu R, Zanni JM, Pradhan P, Colantuoni E, Palmer JB, et al. Early physical medicine and rehabilitation for patients with acute respiratory failure: a quality improvement project. Arch Phys Med Rehabil 2010;91(4):536-42.

155 Strom T, Martinussen T, Toft P. A protocol of no sedation for critically ill patients receiving mechanical ventilation: a randomised trial. Lancet 2010;375(9713):475-80.

156 Girard TD, Kress JP, Fuchs BD, Thomason JW, Schweickert WD, Pun BT, et al. Efficacy and safety of a paired sedation and ventilator weaning protocol for mechanically ventilated patients in intensive care (Awakening and Breathing Controlled trial): a randomised controlled trial. Lancet 2008;371(9607):126-34.

157 Pandharipande P, Banerjee A, McGrane S, Ely EW. Liberation and animation for ventilated ICU patients: the ABCDE bundle for the back-end of critical care. Crit Care 2010;14(3):157.

158 Carrothers KM, Barr J, Spurlock B, Ridgely MS, Damberg CL, Ely EW. Contextual issues influencing implementation and outcomes associated with an integrated approach to managing pain, agitation, and delirium in adult ICUs. Crit Care Med 2013;41(9 Suppl 1):S128-35.

159 Fan E. What is stopping us from early mobility in the intensive care unit? Crit Care Med 2010;38(11):2254-5.

160 Rukstele CD, Gagnon MM. Making strides in preventing ICU-acquired weakness: involving family in early progressive mobility. Crit Care Nurs Q 2013;36(1):141-7.

161 Gosselink R, Bott J, Johnson M, Dean E, Nava S, Norrenberg M, et al. Physiotherapy for adult patients with critical illness: recommendations of the European Respiratory Society and European Society of Intensive Care Medicine Task Force on Physiotherapy for Critically Ill Patients. Intensive Care Med 2008;34(7):1188-99.

162 Kayambu G, Boots R, Paratz J. Physical therapy for the critically ill in the ICU: a systematic review and meta-analysis. Crit Care Med 2013;41(6):1543-54.

163 Moodie L, Reeve J, Elkins M. Inspiratory muscle training increases inspiratory muscle strength in patients weaning from mechanical ventilation: a systematic review. J Physiotherapy 2011;57(4):213-21.

164 Condessa RL, Brauner JS, Saul AL, Baptista M, Silva AC, Vieira SR. Inspiratory muscle training did not accelerate weaning from mechanical ventilation but did improve tidal volume and maximal respiratory pressures: a randomised trial. J Physiotherapy 2013;59(2):101-7.

165 Skinner EH, Berney S, Warrillow S, Denehy L. Rehabilitation and excercise prescription in Australian intensive care units. Physiotherapy 2008;94(3):220-9.

166 Nydahl P, Ruhl AP, Bartoszek G, Dubb R, Filipovic S, Flohr HJ, et al. Early mobilization of mechanically ventilated patients: a 1-day point-prevalence study in Germany. Crit Care Med 2014;42(5):1178-86.

167 Berney SC, Harrold M, Webb SA, Seppelt I, Patman S, Thomas PJ, et al. Intensive care unit mobility practices in Australia and New Zealand: a point prevalence study. Crit Care Resusc 2013;15(4):260-5.

168 Bailey PP, Miller RR, 3rd, Clemmer TP. Culture of early mobility in mechanically ventilated patients. Crit Care Med 2009;37(10 Suppl):S429-35.

169 Drolet A, DeJuilio P, Harkless S, Henricks S, Kamin E, Leddy EA, et al. Move to improve: the feasibility of using an early mobility protocol to increase ambulation in the intensive and intermediate care settings. Phys Ther 2013;93(2):197-207.

170 Van de Meent H, Baken BC, Van Opstal S, Hogendoorn P. Critical illness VR rehabilitation device (X-VR-D): evaluation of the potential use for early clinical rehabilitation. J Electromyogr Kinesiol 2008;18(3):480-6.

171 Mehlhorn J, Freytag A, Schmidt K, Brunkhorst FM, Graf J, Troitzsch U, et al. Rehabilitation interventions for postintensive care syndrome: a systematic review. Crit Care Med 2014;42(5):1263-71.

172 Wade D, Hardy R, Howell D, Mythen M. Identifying clinical and acute psychological risk factors for PTSD after critical care: a systematic review. Minerva Anestesiol 2013;79(8):944-63.

173 Perris A, Bonizzoli M, Iozzelli D, Migliaccio M, Zagli G, Bacchereti A, et al. Early intra-intensive care unit psychological intervention promotes recovery from post traumatic stress disorders, anxiety and depression symptoms in critically ill patients. Crit Care 2011;15:R41.

174 Backman CG, Walther SM. Use of a personal diary written on the ICU during critical illness. Intensive Care Med 2001;27(2):426-9.

175 Bergbom I, Svensson C, Berggren E, Kamsula M. Patients' and relatives' opinions and feelings about diaries kept by nurses in an intensive care unit: pilot study. Intensive Crit Care Nurs 1999;15(4):185-91.

176 Aitken LM, Rattray J, Hull A, Kenardy JA, Le Brocque R, Ullman AJ. The use of diaries in psychological recovery from intensive care. Crit Care 2013;17(6):253.

177 Jones C, Backman CG, Capuzzo M, Egerod I, Flaatten H, Granja C, et al. Intensive care diaries reduce new onset post traumatic stress disorder following critical illness: a randomised, controlled trial. Crit Care 2010;14(5):168-78.

178 Rattray J, Crocker C, Jones M, Connaghan J. Patients' perception of and emotional outcome after intensive care: results from a multicentre study. Nurs Crit Care 2010;15(2):86-93.

179 National Institute for Health and Clinical Excellence. Rehabilitation after critical illness. NICE clinical guideline 83, <http://www.nice.org.uk/CG83>; 2009 [accessed 03.02.15].

180 Cutler L, Brightmore K, Colqhoun V, Dunstan J, Gay M. Developing and evaluating critical care follow-up. Nurs Crit Care 2003;8:116-25.

181 Eliott SJ, Ernest D, Doric AG, Page KN, Worrall-Carter LJ, Thalib L, et al. The impact of an ICU liaison nurse service on patient outcomes. Crit Care Resusc 2008;10(4):296-300.

182 Williams TA, Leslie G, Finn J, Brearley L, Asthifa M, Hay B, et al. Clinical effectiveness of a critical care nursing outreach service in facilitating discharge from the intensive care unit. Am J Crit Care 2010;19(5):e63-72.

183 Hillman K, Chen J, Cretikos M, Bellomo R, Brown D, Doig G, et al. Introduction of the medical emergency team (MET) system: a cluster-randomised controlled trial. Lancet 2005;365(9477):2091-7.

184 Morris PE, Herridge MS. Early intensive care unit mobility: future directions. Crit Care Clin 2007;23(1):97-110.

185 Moran JL, Bristow P, Solomon PJ, George C, Hart GK. Mortality and length-of-stay outcomes, 1993–2003, in the binational Australian and New Zealand intensive care adult patient database. Crit Care Med 2008;36(1):46-61.

186 Fernandez R, Baigorri F, Navarro G, Artigas A. A modified McCabe score for stratification of patients after intensive care unit discharge: the Sabadell score. Crit Care 2006;10(6):R179.

187 Fernandez R, Serrano JM, Umaran I, Abizanda R, Carrillo A, Lopez-Pueyo MJ, et al. Ward mortality after ICU discharge: a multicenter validation of the Sabadell score. Intensive Care Med 2010;36(7):1196-201.

188 Salisbury LG, Merriweather JL, Walsh TS. Rehabilitation after critical illness: could a ward-based generic rehabilitation assistant promote recovery? Nurs Crit Care 2010;15(2):57-65.

189 Salisbury LG, Merriweather JL, Walsh TS. The development and feasibility of a ward-based physiotherapy and nutritional rehabilitation package for people experiencing critical illness. Clin Rehabil 2010;24(6):489-500.

190 Ramsay P, Salisbury LG, Merriweather JL, Huby G, Rattray JE, Hull AM, et al. A rehabilitation intervention to promote physical recovery following intensive care: a detailed description of construct development, rationale and content together with proposed taxonomy to capture processes in a randomised controlled trial. Trials 2014;15:38.

191 Langer D, Hendriks E, Burtin C, Probst V, van der Schans C, Paterson W, et al. A clinical practice guideline for physiotherapists treating patients with chronic obstructive pulmonary disease based on a systematic review of available evidence. Clin Rehabil 2009;23(5):445-62.

192 de Morton NA, Keating JL, Berlowitz DJ, Jackson B, Lim WK. Additional exercise does not change hospital or patient outcomes in older medical patients: a controlled clinical trial. Aust J Physiotherapy 2007;53(2):105-11.

193 Adamson H, Elliott D. Quality of life after a critical illness: a review of general ICU studies 1998-2005. Aust Crit Care 2005;18:50-60.

194 Myhren H, Ekeberg O, Stokland O. Health-related quality of life and return to work after critical illness in general intensive care unit patients: a 1-year follow-up study. Crit Care Med 2010;38(7):1554-61.

195 Cuthbertson BH, Roughton S, Jenkinson D, Maclennan G, Vale L. Quality of life in the five years after intensive care: a cohort study. Crit Care 2010;14(1):R6.

196 Cuthbertson BH, Rattray J, Campbell MK, Gager M, Roughton S, Smith A, et al. The PRaCTICaL study of nurse led, intensive care follow-up programmes for improving long term outcomes from critical illness: a pragmatic randomised controlled trial. BMJ 2009;339:b3723.

197 McWilliams DJ, Atkinson D, Carter A, Foex BA, Benington S, Conway DH. Feasibility and impact of a structured, exercise-based rehabilitation programme for intensive care survivors. Physiotherapy Theory and Practice 2009;25(8):566-71.

198 Elliott D, McKinley S, Alison J, Aitken LM, King M, Leslie GD, et al. Health-related quality of life and physical recovery after a critical illness: a multi-centre randomised controlled trial of a home-based physical rehabilitation program. Crit Care 2011;15(3):R142.

199 UK NHS Audit Commission. Critical to Success. The place of efficient and effective critical care services within the acute hospital. London: Audit Commission; 1999.

200 UK Department of Health. Comprehensive critical care: a review of adult critical care services. London: HMSO, 2000.

201 Griffiths JA, Barber VS, Cuthbertson BH, Young JD. A national survey of intensive care follow-up clinics. Anaesthesia 2006;61(10):950-5.

202 Connolly B, Douiri A, Steier J, Moxham J, Denehy L, Hart N. A UK survey of rehabilitation following critical illness: implementation of NICE Clinical Guidance 83 (CG83) following hospital discharge. BMJ Open 2014;4(5):e004963.

203 Modrykamien AM. The ICU follow-up clinic: a new paradigm for intensivists. Respir Care 2012;57(5):764-72.

204 Prinjha S, Field K, Rowan K. What patients think about ICU follow-up services: a qualitative study. Crit Care 2009;13(2):R46.

205 Cutler L. From ward-based critical care to educational curriculum 1: a literature review. Intensive Crit Care Nurs 2002;18:162-70.

206 Griffiths J, Gager M, Alder N, Fawcett D, Waldmann C, Quinlan J. A self-report-based study of the incidence and associations of sexual dysfunction in survivors of intensive care treatment. Intensive Care Med 2006;32(3):445-51.

207 Griffiths RD, Jones C. Seven lessons from 20 years of follow-up of intensive care unit survivors. Curr Opin Crit Care 2007;13(5):508-13.

208 Hazzard A, Harris W, Howell D. Taking care: practice and philosophy of communication in a critical care follow-up clinic. Intensive Crit Care Nurs 2013;29(3):158-65.

209 Akerman E, Granberg-Axell A, Ersson A, Fridlund B, Bergbom I. Use and practice of patient diaries in Swedish intensive care units: a national survey. Nurs Crit Care 2010;15(1):26-33.

210 Egerod I, Storli SL, Akerman E. Intensive care patient diaries in Scandinavia: a comparative study of emergence and evolution. Nurs Inq 2011;18(3):235-46.

211 Paul F, Rattray J. Short- and long-term impact of critical illness on relatives: literature review. J Adv Nurs 2008;62(3):276-92.

212 Paul F, Hendry C, Cabrelli L. Meeting patient and relatives' information needs upon transfer from an intensive care unit: the development and evaluation of an information booklet. J Clin Nurs 2004;13(3):396-405.

213 Choi J, Sherwood PR, Schulz R, Ren D, Donahoe MP, Given B, et al. Patterns of depressive symptoms in caregivers of mechanically ventilated critically ill adults from intensive care unit admission to 2 months postintensive care unit discharge: a pilot study. Crit Care Med 2012;40(5):1546-53.

214 Williams TA, Leslie GD. Beyond the walls: a review of ICU clinics and their impact on patient outcomes after leaving hospital. Aust Crit Care 2008;21(1):6-17.

215 Jones C, Skirrow P, Griffiths RD, Humphris GH, Ingleby S, Eddleston J, et al. Rehabilitation after critical illness: a randomized, controlled trial. Crit Care Med 2003;31(10):2456-61.

216 Batterham AM, Bonner S, Wright J, Howell SJ, Hugill K, Danjoux G. Effect of supervised aerobic exercise rehabilitation on physical fitness and quality-of-life in survivors of critical illness: an exploratory minimized controlled trial (PIX study). Br J Anaesth 2014;113(1):130-7.

217 O'Neill B, McDowell K, Bradley J, Blackwood B, Mullan B, Lavery G, et al. Effectiveness of a programme of exercise on physical function in survivors of critical illness following discharge from the ICU: study protocol for a randomised controlled trial (REVIVE). Trials 2014;15(1):146.

218 Iwashyna TJ. Survivorship will be the defining challenge of critical care in the 21st century. Ann Intern Med 2010;153(3):204-5.

219 Corner EJ, Wood H, Englebretsen C, Thomas A, Grant RL, Nikoletou D, et al. The Chelsea critical care physical assessment tool (CPAx): validation of an innovative new tool to measure physical morbidity in the general adult critical care population; an observational proof-of-concept pilot study. Physiotherapy 2013;99(1):33-41.

220 Zanni JM, Korupolu R, Fan E, Pradhan P, Janjua K, Palmer JB, et al. Rehabilitation therapy and outcomes in acute respiratory failure: an observational pilot project. J Crit Care 2010;25(2):254-62.

221 Hodgson C, Needham D, Haines K, Bailey M, Ward A, Harrold M, et al. Feasibility and inter-rater reliability of the ICU Mobility Scale. Heart Lung 2014;43(1):19-24.

Chapter 5

Ethical issues in critical care

Maureen Coombs, Carol Grech

Learning objectives

After reading this chapter, you should be able to:

- appreciate the diversity and complexities of ethical issues involved in critical care practice
- understand key ethical and legal principles in health care and how to apply them in everyday practice as a critical care nurse
- identify and access additional resource material that may inform and support ethical professional conduct in critical care
- discuss ethical decision making involved in withdrawing and withholding of treatment, brain death and the organ donation decision-making process
- describe the ethical conduct of human research, in particular issues of patient risk, protection and privacy, and how to apply ethical principles within research practice.

KEY WORDS

autonomy
beneficence
confidentiality
consent
euthanasia
futility
Human Research
  Ethics Committee
justice
non-maleficence
patient rights
privacy
quality of life

Introduction

Nursing work, regardless of the context, will always involve an ethical dimension: it is therefore essential that nurses are guided by ethical principles. This is well-recognised by the International Council of Nurses (ICN) who in 1953 adopted a Code of Ethics for Nurses,[1] which ICN continue to refine. This code informs the ethical standards and guidelines developed by nursing authorities across the world. As a result, nurses are expected to provide compassionate and ethically coherent care, meet professional standards as stated by their regulatory authority and act in accordance with relevant codes of ethics at all times (see Box 5.1).

So why is ethics so important? Critical care nurses regularly encounter clinical situations that require them to employ ethical reasoning. However, the application of such reasoning that informs clinical decision making can be challenging and demanding. The vulnerability of patients in critical care settings, the distress experienced by their families, issues related to the adequacy of informed consent, quandaries that arise from life-sustaining technologies, potential conflict related to withdrawal of life support, equitable allocation of resources and many other challenges encountered in caring require nurses to utilise rational and logical reasoning to determine the right course of action(s) in the face of conflicting choices.

Codes of ethics from selected countries

Australia: Nursing and Midwifery Board of Australia Code of Ethics for Nurses (2008), http://www.nursingmidwiferyboard.gov.au/Codes-Guidelines-Statements/Codes-Guidelines.aspx

and

Nursing and Midwifery Board of Australia Code of Professional Conduct for Nurses (2008), http://www.nursingmidwiferyboard.gov.au/Codes-Guidelines-Statements/Codes-Guidelines.aspx

Canada: Canadian Nurses Association – Code of Ethics for Registered Nurses (2008), http://www.cna-aiic.ca/en/on-the-issues/best-nursing/nursing-ethics

European Union: European Federation of Nursing Regulators – The Code of Ethics and Conduct for European Nursing (2007), http://nej.sagepub.com/content/15/6/821.full.pdf

Hong Kong: The Nursing Council of Hong Kong Code of Professional Conduct and Code of Ethics for Nurses in Hong Kong (2002), http://www.nchk.org.hk/en/code_of_conduct_and_practice/code_of_professional_conduct_and_code_of_ethics_for_nurses_in_hong_kong/index.html

India: Indian Nursing Council Code of Ethics & Professional Conduct, http://www.indiannursingcouncil.org

International Council of Nurses (ICN): Code of Ethics for Nurses (revised 2012), http://www.icn.ch/images/stories/documents/about/icncode_english.pdf

Ireland: Irish Nursing Board Draft Code of Professional Conduct and Ethics for Registered Nurses and Registered Midwives for consultation (2013), http://www.nursingboard.ie/en/professional_practice.aspx

Japan: Japanese Nursing Association The Code of Ethics for Nurses (2003), http://www.nurse.or.jp/jna/english/activities/pdf/ethics2003.pdf

Malaysia: Nursing Board Malaysia Code of Professional Conduct for Nurses (1998), http://nursing.moh.gov.my/uploads/PDdownloads/nursing_board_malaysia-code_of_professional_conduct_1998.pdf

New Zealand: Nursing Council of New Zealand Code of Conduct for Nurses (2013), http://www.nzno.org.nz/Portals/0/publications/Code%20of%20Ethics,%20(2010,%202013).pdf

United Kingdom: Nursing and Midwifery Council (NMC) The Code: Standards of conduct, performance and ethics for nurses and midwives (2008), http://www.nmc-uk.org/Publications/Standards/The-code/Introduction

United States of America: American Nurses Association Code of Ethics for Nurses with Interpretive Statements (2001) [Note: Code was updated June 2014], http://www.nursingworld.org/MainMenuCategories/EthicsStandards/CodeofEthicsforNurses

Working in contemporary health care, where health technology is constantly evolving and life expectancy is increasing, requires increasingly complex decisions to be made about patient and health resource management. Difficult situations now arise where no consensus has developed about the ethical decision making or where all the alternatives in a given situation have specific short-comings. These types of situations are referred to as 'ethical dilemmas'. Dilemmas are different from problems, because problems have potential solutions.[2] It is in this world that critical care nurses often find themselves. This chapter therefore seeks to provide a resource to understand some of the current ethical issues across the continuum of critical care services. The chapter has three sections. The first section outlines the broad principles that underpin ethical decision making. There is exploration about the distinction between ethics, morality and values and of key ethical concepts. In linking ethics with the law, legal positions that inform health care are also described. The second part of the chapter explores the application of ethical principles in critical care, with particular emphasis on withholding and withdrawing of treatment and the decision-making principles that inform this. The third section of the chapter explores key ethical issues that arise from clinical research in the context of critical care.

Ethics and the law

When debates about clinical situations occur in critical care, these inevitably involve focused consideration on what the legal and ethical issues are. Although ethics are often made evident through the laws of society, the principles and frameworks of ethics, as they are used in society, can be very different. Understanding the distinction between ethics and the law becomes increasingly important as clinical situations encountered become more complicated.

Distinction between ethics, morality and values

Ethics is concerned with the many clinical situations that invite reflection and raise questions about health professionals' inherent values informing decision making, as distinct from specific diagnostic or technical questions. Ethics involves the study of rational processes to inform a course of action in response to a particular situation where conflicting options exist.[3] Morality, however, can be understood as the norms widely shared by a community or among a professional group about what is 'right' or 'wrong' about human conduct, the widely held views then forming stable social consensus.[4] Values are the beliefs and attitudes that individuals hold about what is important and therefore influence individual actions and decision making.[5] It is important that critical care nurses be aware of, and reflect on, their personal and professional ethical, moral and value positioning to understand how they will approach ethical decision making in clinical practice.

Where personal ethics can be described as a personal set of moral values that an individual chooses to live by, professional ethics refer to agreed standards and behaviours expected of members of a particular professional group.[6] The value statements developed to underpin nursing and medical practice were originally informed by the moral traditions of Western civilisations with the resultant standards intended to guide and justify professional conduct. Interest in ethical practice in the healthcare area has now developed to such an extent that bioethics has emerged as a subject area concerned with moral issues raised by biological science developments and health care.

Although this section has clearly delineated the differences in definitions of ethics and morality, these concepts are sometimes used interchangeably when professional organisations articulate codes of professional conduct, for example in the Australian *Code of professional conduct for nurses*.[7]

Ethical principles

Key ethical principles often used to explore healthcare ethics include autonomy, beneficence, non-maleficence, justice, veracity and fidelity.[4] While these are important in understanding the ethical dimensions of care, there are other ethical concepts important to understanding health care including integrity, best interests, informed consent and advance directives. All are applicable to critical care practice. These are explored individually in the following paragraphs or incorporated as part of the discussion of clinical issues, such as treatment withdrawal.

Autonomy

An autonomous person is an individual who is capable of deliberation, self-determination and action without the influence of external coercion. To respect autonomy is to give weight to, and respect, the autonomous person's considered opinions and choices and to not obstruct their actions unless these are detrimental to themselves or others. To show lack of respect for an autonomous agent or to withhold information necessary for that person to make a considered judgement when there are no reasons to do so, is to reject that person's judgement. To deny a competent individual their autonomy is to treat that person paternalistically. All individuals, including critical care patients, should be treated as autonomous agents and be able to self-determine, unless otherwise indicated. However, individuals with diminished autonomy, for example an unconscious person, are entitled to protection and, depending on the risk of harm and likely benefit of protecting them, paternalism may be considered justifiable.[4,8] In such cases, healthcare professionals should act to respect the autonomy of the individual as much as

possible, for example by attempting to discover what the patient's preferences and decisions would have been in the circumstances.

> **Practice tip**
>
> A competent person has a right to make an informed choice about his or her treatment. When giving information about care options to a patient, keep the discussion accurate and factual. Do not direct or influence the patient's decision making. Respect the right of the person to make self-determining decisions.

Beneficence and non-maleficence

The principle of beneficence (i.e. to do good) requires that actions are undertaken to promote the wellbeing of another person. This incorporates the actions of doing no harm and maximising possible benefits while minimising possible harm (non-maleficence).[9] In healthcare practice, treatment is focused on 'doing no harm'. However, there may be times where, to 'maximise benefits' for health outcomes, it may be ethically justifiable to expose the patient to a 'higher risk of harm'. For example, consider a clinical situation in the coronary care unit (CCU). A patient requires a central venous catheter (CVC) to optimise fluid and drug therapy, but this intervention is not without its own inherent risks (e.g. infection, pneumothorax on insertion). To minimise possible harm to the patient, evidence-based protocols are therefore developed to ensure safe insertion of a CVC and subsequent care.

Justice

Justice may be defined as fair, equitable and appropriate treatment in light of what is due or owed to an individual. The fair, equitable and appropriate distribution of health care, as determined by justified rules or 'norms', is termed distributive justice.[4] There are well-regarded theories of justice in health care including egalitarian theories that propose people be provided with an equal distribution of particular goods or services. However, it is recognised that justice does not always require equal sharing of all possible social benefits. In situations where there is insufficient resource to be equally distributed, guidelines (e.g. intensive care unit [ICU] admission policies) may be developed in order to ensure treatment is as fair and equitable as possible.

Conditions of scarcity and competition for resources lead to the main problems associated with fair and equitable allocation of resources (distributive justice). For example, a shortage of intensive care beds may result in critically ill patients having to 'compete' for access to the ICU. There is considerable debate about ICU admission criteria that varies across institutions, jurisdictional boundaries and countries with differing health funding structures. Such resource limitations can impact on distributive justice if decisions about access are influenced by economic factors as distinct from clinical need.[10]

Veracity and fidelity

The principle of veracity is concerned with telling the truth and is based on respect for persons and the concept of autonomy. To provide the opportunity for patients, or those authorised by law to act on their behalf, to make informed decisions about treatment options they must be provided with full and honest disclosure so that they can weigh up the risks and benefits of treatments.[3] It is also important to note that the principle of veracity can be violated through omission of important information – deliberately withholding information or using medical jargon or language that may camouflage or mislead the patient or their legal guardian. Critical care environments are highly complex, as are the technologies and procedures patients are exposed to. Patients and their families can easily feel overwhelmed by the critical care environment and by the choices that they may be faced with during critical illness.[11] Ensuring patients and families are informed and fully involved in the decision making is pivotal. Nurses and medical staff need to be vigilant in ensuring they convey information to patients and their families using language that can be readily understood and ensuring support services are drawn on (e.g. social workers, religious and spiritual advisors) to provide additional help to augment understanding so that patients or their legal guardian can make informed choices about care.

Practice tip

If you know a person's treatment is not working for them, you must help get their voice heard. This means having the courage to raise the matter with a more senior nurse or the doctor in a way that will be heard and considered in a timely way.

Fidelity refers to the concepts of keeping promises and honouring contracts and commitments[12] and is based upon the fundamental nursing virtue of caring. This principle encompasses qualities including loyalty, fairness, providing compassionate care to patients, advocacy and being responsible and accountable for the standard of nursing practice provided.

The principles of veracity and fidelity underpin the practice of every nurse. These values relate to professional ethics and the expectation that nurses are honest in all professional interactions, and demonstrate compliance with the professional codes of conduct, practice standards and regulatory reporting requirements.

Practice tip

Communicate with patients honestly and respectfully. If you tell a patient that you will be back in 10 minutes, mean it. However, if you know that you are busy and unlikely to meet that timeline, explain this to the patient instead of making false assurances.

Ethics and the law

Although distinct, ethics and the law overlap in many important ways. Moral rightness or wrongness may be quite distinct from legal rightness or wrongness and, while ethical decision making will always require consideration of the law, there may be conflict about the morality of the law. Ethically based nursing practice, such as confidentiality, respect for human rights and consent, are also legal requirements for health practice.[6,13]

The law enforces rules that are desirable for social good in every country. The terms 'legislation' and 'law' are used to refer generically to statutes, regulation and other legal instruments that may be the forms of law used in a particular country. A general distinction can be made between civil law jurisdictions (e.g. in counties like France, Germany, Spain), which codify laws and in which the law is almost entirely based on legislative enactments and considered binding for all, and common law systems (e.g. in England, the USA, Australia and New Zealand (NZ)), where the law continually evolves in addition to being amended by laws passed by parliament.[3] In some countries, religion informs law such as Sharia or Islamic law that specifically influences the legal code in some Muslim countries.

Laws related to health care are often created on the basis of what is considered morally right and of benefit to members of society. Statute law, i.e. written law set down by a legislature (e.g. parliament), has particular relevance to ethics in the critical care context. An example of how a statute law in one jurisdiction might be applied in practice pertaining to, for example, consent for life-sustaining measures is the *Consent to Medical Treatment and Palliative Care Act 1995* (SA).[14] This Act at s17 (2) states that: 'in the absence of an express direction by the patient or the patient's representative to the contrary, [the doctor is] under no duty to use, or to continue to use, life sustaining measures'.[14]

In some countries such as Australia, each state and territory has many different Acts pertaining to healthcare practices, and this can be confusing when practitioners work across jurisdictional borders. This is less problematic in some countries, such as New Zealand, where health Acts are applicable across the whole country. Therefore, when sourcing laws relevant to health care in specific countries, it is important to use validated sources such as government websites.

Privacy and confidentiality

Although not an ethical principle as such, privacy and confidentiality are fundamental human entitlements recognised in all major international treaties and agreements on human rights. Nearly every country in the world acknowledges privacy as a fundamental human right in their constitution, either explicitly or implicitly. The right to privacy has been involved in new areas of debate given technology's increasing erosion of privacy, for example via video surveillance cameras, the internet and use of social media. Recently drafted constitutions now include specific rights to access and control one's personal information, with a growing trend towards comprehensive privacy and data protection legislation around the world. Currently, over 40 countries and jurisdictions have, or are in the process of enacting, such laws.[15] Countries are adopting these laws to ensure compatibility with international standards developed by the European Union, the Council of Europe and the Organization for Economic Cooperation and Development.

In New Zealand, privacy legislation is described in the *Privacy Act 1993*[16] and in Australia in the *Commonwealth Privacy Act 1988*.[17] In addition, each state and territory in Australia has additional jurisdictional regulatory guidelines that apply to privacy matters and disclosure of health information.[18] Increasingly, government departments and hospitals also have dedicated policies on the use of social media.

Practice tip

Details about a patient's personal circumstance, condition and medical treatment must always be kept private and confidential. Do not discuss patients in inappropriate environments (e.g. in corridors and elevators where others could overhear). Do not take handover sheets or papers that have recorded patient details outside the unit where they could be found by unauthorised personnel or members of the public; and never discuss patients, colleagues or work-related matters on social media.

Patients' rights

Patients' rights arise from human rights law that universally recognises that everyone is born free and with equal rights irrespective of nationality, place of residence, gender, ethnic origin, race or religion.[19] Statements with a focus on patients' rights relate to the particular moral interests that a person might have in a healthcare context and any particular protection required when a person assumes the role of a patient.[6] Institutional-based charters (position statements), such as those in hospitals, are helpful in developing a shared understanding amongst patients/consumers, families and carers of the rights of people receiving health care and of the entitlements and special interests to be respected. Such charters also emphasise to healthcare professionals that relationships with patients are constrained ethically and bound by certain associated duties.[6] The World Federation of Critical Care Nurses has recognised the importance of this and developed a Position Statement on the rights of the critically ill patient (see the World Federation of Critical Care Nurses website, http://wfccn.org).

To further protect patients' rights, attention should be paid to cultural differences in the provision of health care and to ensure cultural safety of both patients and the healthcare team. Clinical situations are culturally safe when patients and their families feel that cultural and spiritual needs are acknowledged and that those needs are met without prejudice.[20,21] Cultural competency, as a health

concept, has received little exploration in the literature to date[22] although some resources exist[23] to inform practice. Professional codes of conduct should incorporate an understanding of patients' rights and acknowledge that nurses accept the rights of individuals to make informed choices about their treatment and care. Box 5.2 provides some useful tips to ensure that the needs of diverse populations in critical care may be met.

BOX 5.2

Needs of diverse population groups in critical care

To cater for the needs of diverse population groups in critical care it is important to:

- organise and use qualified interpreters and cultural advisors when required
- create care environments that facilitate optimal patient and family control of decisions
- work collaboratively with other healthcare workers in a culturally sensitive and competent manner to ensure optimal outcomes
- identify and address bias, prejudice and discrimination in healthcare service delivery
- integrate measures of patient satisfaction into improvement programs.

Consent

Any procedure that involves intentional contact by a healthcare practitioner with the body of a patient is considered an invasion of the patient's bodily integrity and requires patient consent. A healthcare practitioner must not assume that a patient provides a valid consent purely on the basis that the individual has been admitted to a hospital.[24] All healthcare staff (nurses, doctors, allied health professionals) are expected to give information on management, care and alternative options to the patient to enable informed consent and decision making to occur.[25] The responsibility for obtaining consent for medical treatment rests with the medical practitioner and generally may not be delegated to a nurse.[24]

Patients have the right, as autonomous individuals, to discuss any concerns or raise questions at any time with staff. Hospitals should provide detailed patient admission information, including information regarding 'patients' rights and responsibilities' and a broad explanation of the consent process within that institution. In many countries there is no distinction between the obligation to obtain valid consent from the patient and the overall duty of care that a practitioner has in providing treatment to a patient. Obtaining consent is part of the overall duty of care.[14]

In order to provide safe care where patients are able to make choices with informed consent, clear systems and processes are required. Critical care nurses need to be aware of relevant professional, organisational and unit-based policies and understand their individual obligations and responsibilities in this area. While the treating medical officer is legally regarded as the person who informs the patient about associated risks,[26] it is incumbent on all critical care nurses to be aware of the potential risks in critical care and ensure that informed consent is gained cognisant of these. Due to the nature of critical illness, direct informed consent is often difficult in critical care and surrogate consent may be the only option in emergency situations. Consent issues in critical care may be concerned with healthcare treatment or, as discussed later, participation in human research and the use and disclosure of personal health information.[27]

Practice tip

Make sure that informed consent is consistently applied in every healthcare encounter. As such, consent is required for turning a patient and making them comfortable, for making sure that the patient understands the procedure that they are undergoing or that they understand what is involved in the research study that they have recently enrolled in. If a patient does not understand, stop and ensure appropriate information is given by the person whose responsibility it is before continuing your intervention further.

Consent to treatment

A competent individual has the right to decline or accept healthcare treatment. This right is enshrined in common law in Australia (with some variation across state or territory jurisdictions) and in the *Code of Health and Disability Consumers' Rights in New Zealand (1996)*.[28] With the introduction of human rights Acts (for example in the United Kingdom [UK])[29] there is global awareness of the individual rights of patients in health care and of patients being actively encouraged to participate in treatment decisions.

Informed consent provides assurance that patients and others are neither deceived nor coerced in decision making; this recognises the person's autonomy. Consent procedures should minimise the potential for deception and coercion and should be designed to give patients control over the amount of information received and the opportunity to rescind consent already given.[30] However, clinical information can be complex and confusing for patients and obtaining informed consent can be problematic. Improved communication skills for doctors and nurses go some way toward resolving this problem. Shared decision making in clinical care can best be achieved by framing the relevant information in a comprehensible way to the patient, while understanding that some patients may not wish to make such choices themselves, preferring to have decisions made by clinicians.[31] Box 5.3 lists key criteria that describe valid consent.

Patients must have the mental capacity and be competent in order to give informed consent in healthcare decisions. To be competent, an individual must be able to comprehend and retain information, must not be impervious to reason or incapable of judgement after reflection and must be

> **BOX 5.3**
>
> ### Criteria for consent
>
> Consent is considered VALID if:
>
> * informed (the patient must understand the broad nature and effects of the proposed intervention and the material risks it entails)
> * voluntarily given
> * it encompasses the act to be performed
> * given by a person legally competent to do so.

able to weigh that information up (i.e. consider the effects of having or not having the treatment). Many jurisdictions around the world have legislation that addresses situations where adults lack the capacity to give consent. In emergencies, healthcare treatment may be provided without the consent of a person. However, consent should be obtained for all procedures that involve 'doing' to a patient (e.g. administering an injection). Consent should never be implied irrespective of the situation of the person or the place of care, e.g. critically ill in ICU.[25] In many countries, if patients perceive that informed consent was not obtained, a civil court case can be actioned on the grounds of battery (deliberate touching without their consent) or negligence (receiving insufficient information about risk). Doctors and nurses therefore need to make clear what they are proposing to do to a patient and why they need to do it, with a 'reasonable' amount of information about any risks involved.[32]

If a person is assessed as not having capacity, consent must be sought from someone who has lawful authority to consent on his or her behalf. If the courts have appointed a person to be guardian for an individual, then the guardian can provide consent on behalf of that individual. However, even for legally appointed guardians, consent cannot be given for certain procedures and the consent of a guardianship statutory authority may be required. Some states have legislated to allow this authority to be delegated to a 'person responsible' or 'statutory health authority' without prior formal appointment. This person would usually be a spouse, next-of-kin or unpaid carer of the individual. As with formally appointed guardians, the powers of a 'person responsible' are limited by statute.[27]

Application of ethical principles in the care of the critically ill

Any health professional working with critically ill patients knows that critical care is complex and the number of decisions about clinical interventions that should, or should not, be offered to those who are critically ill are ever increasing. Given this, it becomes even more important that clinical questions raised about medical and nursing care be underpinned by consideration of the ethical dimensions of that care.[33]

Alongside the increasing number of technological developments in critical care, critical care nursing has also evolved in scope and practice. Critical care nurses are more autonomous in their role, using more developed assessment and diagnostic skills and more advanced respiratory, cardiac and renal patient interventions. With such increased autonomy comes increased responsibility,[34] and this increases the potential for ambiguity in the role and conflict with others in the interdisciplinary team. To minimise such risks it is important that critical care nurses understand the fundamental ethical principles that apply to, and underpin, their clinical practice. This is not always an easy task. As demonstrated in findings from a Portuguese study,[35] ethical issues pervade many aspects of day-to-day care including: patient privacy issues (confidentiality); patient and family interaction (right to self-determination); teamwork relationships and role responsibilities (equity, paternalism); end-of-life decision making (respecting autonomy); and healthcare access (equality, distributive justice).

When faced with operating in such a difficult environment, nurses in clinical practice feel vulnerable when managing such a range of ethical responsibilities.[36] The ongoing challenge of navigating practice while upholding professional values, responsibilities and duties can lead nurses to experience moral distress resulting in increased levels of emotional distress, withdrawal from patient care, decreased job satisfaction and, ultimately, increased attrition in nursing.[37] However, proactively addressing ethical issues at a clinical team level through dedicated case reviews, support systems and processes, including clinical supervision, debriefing, case conferences and mortality and morbidity meetings, can help in maintaining ethical awareness in healthcare organisations.

End-of-life decision making

With technological advances in health care, it is now more possible than ever before to restore, sustain and prolong life with the use of technology and associated therapies including mechanical ventilation, extracorporeal oxygenation, intra-aortic balloon counter pulsation and haemodialysis. Each new medication or treatment on the market seems to promise added benefits to patients with improved outcomes and fewer side effects. However, in many cases managing the critically ill patient is more concerned with provision of supportive therapies, rather than curative ones.[38]

A common ethical dilemma experienced by doctors and nurses in critical care concerns the opposing decision-making positions of 'maintaining life at all costs' and 'relieving suffering associated with the prolongation of life'. However, there are critically ill patients who receive life-sustaining therapies for prolonged periods with a limited evidence-base about survival rates or longer term quality of life indicators. These are complex, emotive and much debated areas requiring decision making around the withdrawal and withholding of life support treatments and substantial deliberation with the patient, their family and all clinical teams involved.[39]

Withdrawing and withholding treatment

The incidence of withholding and withdrawal of life support from critically ill patients has increased to the extent that these practices now precede the majority of deaths in intensive care[40] with evidence that the majority of clinicians in the USA[41–43] and Europe[44,45] have been involved in the withholding or withdrawal of treatments for critically ill patients. Although there is a legal and moral presumption in favour of preserving life, avoiding death should not always be the pre-eminent goal.[46] The withholding or withdrawal of life support is considered ethically acceptable and clinically desirable if it reduces unnecessary patient suffering in those whose prognosis is considered hopeless (i.e. 'futile'). Patients' preferences, as evidenced through advanced care planning conversations, documented current advance directives or accounts from proxy decision makers, should be used to inform decision making in this area. Treatments that may be withdrawn (removed) or withheld (not commenced) in critical care may include the provision of ventilator support, inotropic support, haemodialysis, blood transfusions and antibiotics. The assumption is that, after the withholding or withdrawal of such treatments, the patient will most probably die from their underlying disease.[47] This is an area of health care receiving increased attention of late. In Australia, work is underway to develop a consensus statement with the aim of setting out expected standards of care and agreed practice for recognising and responding to people in need of end-of-life care in acute hospitals,[48] including in situations where treatments are withheld or withdrawn for the critically ill. In the United Kingdom, care pathways have been used with some success,[49] although this remains a contentious area.

There are marked differences in the foregoing of life-sustaining treatments between countries and even within states. What may be adopted legally and ethically in one country may not be acceptable in another. For example, a recent publication highlights current challenges experienced by clinicians in Japan where, despite clear support from end-of-life guidelines, the practice of treatment withdrawal is limited.[50] Further, complexities in care arise due to the differing views held internationally on whether withdrawal and withholding treatment is ethically the same.[51] In Australasia, when active treatment is withdrawn or withheld, the same legal and ethical principles apply. The Australian and New Zealand Intensive Care Society (ANZICS) and College of Intensive Care Medicine of Australia and New Zealand (CICM) recommend that, when treatment withdrawal or withholding has been discussed and agreed with the family, an 'alternative care plan' with a focus on dignity and patient comfort be implemented. It is suggested that such discussions be recorded in the patient notes including the basis for the decision, those involved in the discussions and the specifics of treatment(s) being withheld or withdrawn.[52]

Although doctors and nurses appear clear in their support for treatment withdrawal in cases of futility, the public at large hold different perceptions about this aspect of care. This is demonstrated in results from the Ethicatt study[53] where questionnaires on end-of-life decision making were administered to 1899 doctors, nurses, patients and family members across intensive care units in six European countries. The results demonstrated that less than 10% of doctors and nurses wanted their life prolonged by all available means, compared to 40% of patients and 32% of families. When asked where they would prefer to be cared for if they had a terminal illness with a short time to live, more doctors and nurses preferred care at home or in a hospice and more patients and families preferred care in intensive care. Differences in responses were based on the respondent's country.[53] A similar spread of views across healthcare staff and the general public was demonstrated when consulted about physician-assisted suicide in the USA.[54] It is therefore interesting that North American observational studies demonstrate healthcare staff consult families more often than European healthcare staff[53,55] with some seriously ill patients indicating a willingness to participate in end-of-life decisions, while others did not.[56]

It is clear that having in-depth knowledge of the critical care environment and of futile treatments influences clinicians' views on the practice of treatment withdrawal or limitation. Cultural, religious, philosophical and professional attitudes also influence views held in this area. In a UK study[57] reviewing the use of treatment withdrawal guidelines, staff reported concern over the legal, moral, ethical and professional accountability issues involved in this area. The study demonstrated that medical decisions to withdraw treatment were inconsistent within medical teams and in similar patients. With such a range of factors influencing decision making about withdrawal and withholding of treatment, it is not surprising that gaining consensus on complex clinical situations, such as withdrawal of treatment, can be difficult. In cases where there is uncertainty about the efficacy or appropriateness of a life-sustaining treatment, it may be considered preferable to commence treatment, with an option to withdraw treatment after broad consultation has occurred. However, managing such situations can be challenging as conflicts can occur about when and how to withdraw life-sustaining treatment;[10] this is an area that critical care nurses can actively contribute to in supporting the processes of decision making at end of life.[45]

Although it is essential that all members of the critical care team contribute to such discussions, legal responsibility and accountability for the decision lies with the senior treating doctor. Where conflict arises with family members, especially if a family member has medical power of attorney (or equivalent), the doctor must take this into consideration and respect the rights of any patient legal representative. It is unlikely that withdrawal of treatment will occur until a consensus decision is reached. This is a different situation to that of a person who is legally declared brain dead[52] where different ethical challenges are posed[58] (see *Brain death* section).

Once a decision to limit or withdraw treatment has been agreed, a plan is made as to how this will occur, which treatments will be withdrawn/withheld, when and by whom. It is at this stage that critical care nurses play an important role in managing end-of-life care.[59] Concepts of caring for the dying patient in a critical care unit are no different to those in a hospital ward or hospice. The principles of care encompass privacy, dignity, relief of pain, provision of comfort and support for patient and relatives. Recognising and being respectful of the religious, spiritual and cultural needs of the patient and family are also important. Care given at this time continues beyond the moment of the patient's death with particular attention placed on how the death of the person is pronounced, how the family is notified of this death and the immediate bereavement support offered to the family, including discussions about possible autopsy. Compassionate care to the family at this time is essential.

Decision-making principles

Despite significant advances in critical care medicine, approximately 20% of patients admitted to intensive care units do not survive.[60] The majority of patients who die in critical care do so after planned withdrawal of life-prolonging therapies, as opposed to dying after unexpected and unsuccessful cardiopulmonary resuscitation.[61] In order for care and treatment to be oriented away from active intervention to palliation requires communication to occur with the patient (if able), with the patient's family and with the health team. Communication can be a complicated process especially when difficult and challenging information is required to be exchanged within a short timeframe, as sometimes happens at end of life in critical care.

Lack of communication or misunderstood communication about end-of-life issues can lead to decisions being made that do not respect patient autonomy and that are not made in the patient's best interests. This can result in patients receiving burdensome and expensive treatments that they may not want. Such communication issues may result from the lack of professional guidance for end-of-life practices or from fear of litigation.[62] With the profiled role that family members hold as key decision makers in critical care, complex family dynamics cause a further challenge when working with relatives as surrogate decision makers or patient advocates. Collectively, these factors can lead to misunderstandings and confusion about what the patient wants, what the family wish for and what critical care staff feel is achievable.

End-of-life decision making can be difficult leading to inconsistencies in the initiation of end-of-life care and the withdrawal of life-supporting treatment.[39] A further area that contributes to conflict between medical and nursing staff during end-of-life decisions is the impact of different professional ethical decision-making frameworks. While the values of patients' rights, justice and quality of life are central to medicine's ethical framework, empirical work demonstrates that nursing staff focus on patient dignity, comfort and respect for patients' wishes that are central

FIGURE 5.1   Factors influencing decision-making processes in healthcare ethics.

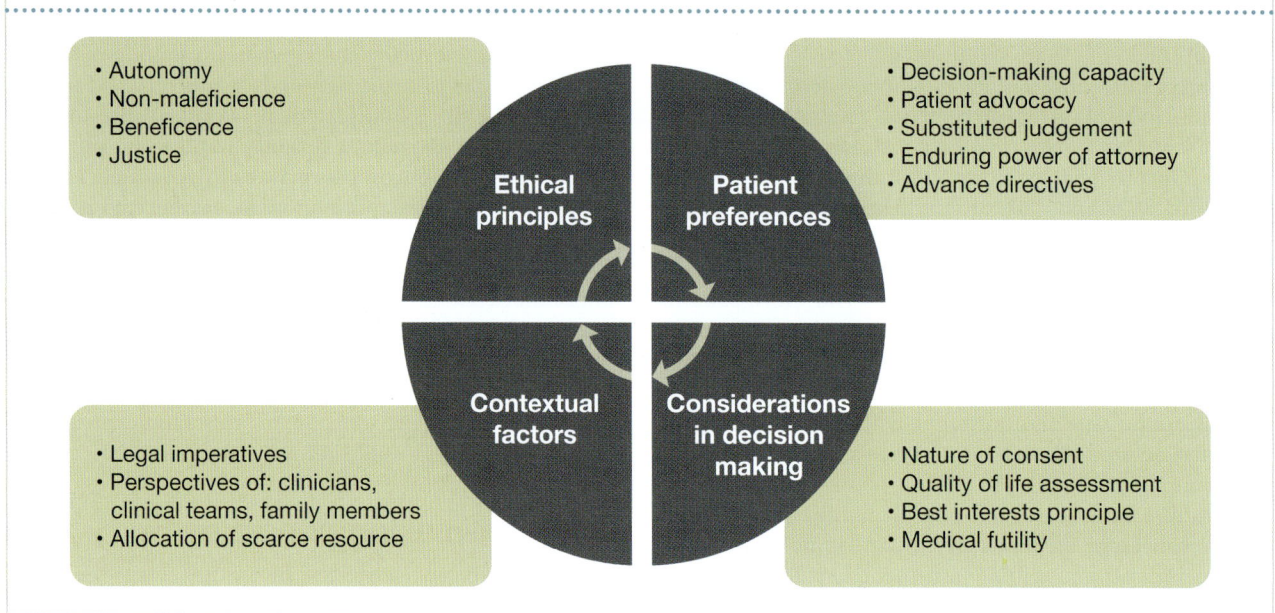

- Autonomy
- Non-maleficience
- Beneficence
- Justice

Ethical principles

Patient preferences

- Decision-making capacity
- Patient advocacy
- Substituted judgement
- Enduring power of attorney
- Advance directives

Contextual factors

Considerations in decision making

- Legal imperatives
- Perspectives of: clinicians, clinical teams, family members
- Allocation of scarce resource

- Nature of consent
- Quality of life assessment
- Best interests principle
- Medical futility

to nurses' ethical framework.[63] In enacting these values, nurses provide important support to patients and families enabling them to become involved in end-of-life decisions ensuring that decisions match with stated care preferences, expectations, values and circumstances[64] (see Figure 5.1).

Quality of life

Despite the importance placed on quality of life in influencing clinical decision making in critical care, there is no single agreed definition of what quality of life is. Debate about quality of life is often engaged with when justifying the continuation or discontinuation of life-sustaining treatment in critical care.[6] Definitions of quality of life focus on subjective components related to the notions of desires and wellbeing (e.g. personal satisfaction or happiness) and objective components related to the meeting of personal needs (work, income, housing, leisure factors) with both aspects needing consideration when making quality-of-life assessments.[10] When making decisions about medical treatments based on quality-of-life arguments, it is important therefore that consideration is given to the personal preferences and wellbeing of the individual together with review of the person's independent health and welfare status.

Best interests

Best interest is a guiding principle for making decisions in, and about, health care. It is defined as acting in a way that optimally promotes good for the individual and is referred to when one person makes a decision on behalf of another, as when a doctor makes a decision to cease life-sustaining treatment for a particular patient. The best interest principle is often invoked in situations where the patient may be assessed as incompetent and therefore unable to participate in the decision-making process.

The best interest principle relies on decision makers holding an understanding of, and knowing the views held by, the person in question (e.g. critically ill patient) and of articulating those views relevant to decisions being made. The best interest principle poses particular challenges including how assumptions are made about what quality of life means for individuals and how a person's views can change over time and not be communicated to significant others. As a case example, Mary witnessed her mother's death several years ago on a ventilator after an acute exacerbation of chronic obstructive respiratory disease. After this, Mary said to her family that she would never want to be ventilated. However, after a sudden collapse following a perforated duodenal ulcer, Mary required emergency surgery and, due to unexpected intraoperative bleeding, required postoperative ventilation until she was stabilised. Although Mary's doctors and family were aware of her views, they made the decision for short-term ventilation as it was seen to be in her best interests. Ethical justification of medical decisions using the best interest principle therefore requires a relevant and current understanding of what quality of life means to that particular person.[65]

Patient advocacy

Patient advocacy has, at its heart, a focus on patient rights, values and interests and seeks to promote autonomy when patients are unable or incapable of participating in making decisions about their health care. Internationally, there are many recognised titles for individuals acting in the role of patient advocate. 'Medical or healthcare agent', 'medical power of attorney' and 'enduring guardian' are terms and roles related to the concept of patient advocacy. With regards to health care, a patient advocate is usually someone chosen by an individual (e.g. a partner, child, good friend over 18 years of age) to make medical decisions on behalf of that person, should a situation arise where that person lacks decisional capacity. Most patient advocates are known to, and appointed by, the person or are representatives of recognised bodies (e.g. guardianship boards, Office of the Public Advocate) appointed into the role to safeguard vulnerable persons who lack capacity to make decisions. Each country has legislation in place to protect the patient, patient advocate and healthcare team and such legal provision should be consulted to fully understand the conditions and safeguards in place.

Substituted judgement

If a person does not have the mental capacity to make medical decisions, a surrogate decision maker should be identified. Substituted judgement is where an appropriate surrogate attempts to determine what the patient would have wanted in his/her present circumstances[66] by utilising the values and preferences of the patient. In order to do this, the proxy decision maker needs an in-depth knowledge of the patient's values. Making a substituted judgement is a relatively informal process, in the sense that the patient has not formally appointed the proxy decision maker. Rather, the role of proxy tends to be assumed on the basis of an existing relationship between proxy and patient, for example, next of kin or family member. However, this informal arrangement means that making an accurate substituted judgement can be difficult and that the proxy might not be the most appropriate person for this role.[67]

Medical futility

Treatment with no apparent benefit to the patient is generally considered futile. In this it is acknowledged that the physiological decay of the body due to old age and/or illness exceeds the body's response to medical treatments.[68] Futility is a concept in widespread use in healthcare ethics and poses clinical challenges and debate at an international level.[69] Futility is often used by critical care doctors and nurses as a rationale for why medical treatments, including life-saving or sustaining treatments, are considered not to be in the patient's best interest. At times, the concept of futility may be used inappropriately and unethically, for example if the argument of 'futility' is used to coerce relatives into agreeing to stop treatment of a patient.[70] It is therefore important that a clear working understanding of 'futility' is held by healthcare practitioners.

Treatment is considered futile if the medical therapy will never enable the person to achieve a state beyond permanent unconsciousness or if, even with the treatment, it is unlikely that the person will ever be discharged alive from intensive care.[66] Futility can be used to describe situations where the predicted success of the treatment is unlikely (physiological futility) or where the benefit of recovery is outweighed by the burden of survival (e.g. the person survives but with potential of physical or mental incapacity).[4]

Physiological futility is being referred to when practitioners discuss 'useless treatments' in patient management. In such situations, clinicians usually reflect on their past

clinical experiences, experiential knowledge gained from colleagues and reported empirical data to conclude that treatments are futile.[71] There is no international definition of futility although some country-specific and profession-specific guidance exists to inform care.[14] It is generally agreed that healthcare practitioners should help the sick and that treatments should be offered, if of benefit to the patient. Futile interventions are seen to cause pain and discomfort at end of life, give false hope to patients and family, delay palliative care and expend limited medical resources. However, determining which interventions are beneficial to patients can be difficult, especially as the views of patients, families and clinicians may differ. While the ethical requirement to respect patient autonomy entitles a patient to choose or reject the medically acceptable treatment options, it does not entitle patients to receive whatever treatments they would want. Clinicians are only required to offer treatments consistent with professional standards and that give benefit to the patient. With respect to the law governing withholding and withdrawing treatment in such circumstances, although there have been few cases in Australia and New Zealand where these decisions have been litigated, the courts have been consistent in concluding that there is no duty to provide life-sustaining treatment that is futile.[72]

Advance directives

For individuals wanting to document preferences about their future health care should situations arise where they are no longer competent to make decisions, anticipatory direction or advance directive forms are able to be completed. With the increasing availability of medical technology, use of advance directives has improved.[73,74] Advance directives inform health professionals how medical decisions are to be made and who is to make them, should the person be no longer able to make those decisions for themselves. An advance directive, also known as a living will, a personal directive or an advance care directive, sets out instructions from a competent individual specifying what actions should be taken for their health in the event that they are no longer able to make decisions due to illness or incapacity. The five wishes advance directive created by 'Aging with Dignity', a non-profit organisation in the USA, is one example of an advance directive.[75] There are also national frameworks for advanced care directives[76] and specialty specific exemplars, e.g. the Western Australian Cancer and Palliative Care Network Advance Health Directive.[77]

Some people are hesitant to document their end-of-life care plan so there is legal provision for the appointment of a person holding enduring power of attorney for matters of health.[55] The enduring power of attorney can make healthcare decisions on their behalf should the person loose capacity (for example, become unconscious).

Do not resuscitate considerations

Cardiopulmonary resuscitation (CPR) remains the only intervention that patients explicitly state that they do or do not want.[78] If patients have acute, reversible illness conditions, they should have the right to CPR. However, discussions may occur regarding the withholding of CPR in patients with irreversible or terminal illnesses. This is an important point to consider as every patient will have CPR, unless documented otherwise. The decision to withhold CPR may be termed a 'do not resuscitate' (DNR), 'do not attempt resuscitation' (DNAR) or 'not for resuscitation' (NFR) order. While such 'orders' reflect a decision against any resuscitation treatment, there are other types of resuscitation orders seen written in patient notes that use limited treatment, including 'for defibrillation only' or 'for one round of ALS only'. These can be confusing for staff and families who may perceive such orders to be half-hearted attempts at resuscitation or, indeed, that no care is meant to be given.[78] As each patient case is considered on its own merit, it is important that any medical orders or directives are clearly documented in the patient's notes or on the appropriate forms so that misinterpretations do not occur. It is important that clear discussion and broad consultation across the clinical team(s) and patient/family occurs. A management plan that incorporates assessment of patient and family understanding, disclosure of the patient's situation, discussion and consensus gaining with the patient and family may be particularly useful.[79]

Euthanasia

Euthanasia continues to be the subject of ongoing international debate. Generally understood as the termination of a person's life in order to relieve suffering, in most cases euthanasia is carried out because it is requested by the person. Although the concept of euthanasia is supported in some areas, it remains illegal in Australia and New Zealand. With confusion occurring about the difference between treatment withdrawal and euthanasia, the primary distinction between the two relates to the issue of 'intent'. If the primary intention of the intervention (e.g. a lethal injection) is to cause death, this is regarded as euthanasia. If the primary intention of the intervention is to reduce pain and suffering, this may not be regarded as euthanasia but this may still be tested legally in a court of law. It is this complexity that causes the vigorous 'for' and 'against' debates about euthanasia. Those opposing euthanasia do so in the belief of the sanctity of life and that life is God-given and that effective symptom control should be able to keep individuals comfortable. Other opponents raise the concern that, if euthanasia were made legal, the laws regulating it could be abused and this would lead to euthanasia being used with people not expressing a wish to die. Those in support of euthanasia argue that a civilised society should support a person's autonomy and self-determinism and that people should die in dignity and without pain. If people are not able to terminate their own life, others should be allowed to help them to do so.

Several countries have considered the physician's role in euthanasia (termed physician-assisted suicide) including the USA and the Netherlands. Many other countries, including the UK, New Zealand and Australia, have ongoing public,

professional and legal debate on this matter. Oregon was the first state in the USA to legalise physician-assisted suicide when it passed the *Death with Dignity Act* in 1997.[80] The *Death with Dignity Act* outlines a rigorous process for assisted dying with strict criteria requiring details pertaining to: the patient's request; the patient's suffering; information provided to the patient; the presence of reasonable alternatives; consultation with another physician; and the applied method of ending life. Under the *Death with Dignity Act*, physicians may not administer the medication; patients must ingest it independently.

Since 2002 euthanasia and physician-assisted suicide in the Netherlands are not punishable if the attending physician acts in accordance with criteria of due care. These criteria are similar to the Oregon areas outlined above. In reporting on a review of 158 reported euthanasia and physician-assisted suicide cases from the Netherlands, Buiting et al[81] identified that medical care including medication (89%), radio- or chemotherapy (21%) and palliative care options (46%) had been administered with continued unbearable suffering leading to the request for physician-assisted suicide. This is clearly a contentious area and so, to guide current practice in Australasia, when requests for euthanasia are made, it would be appropriate to explore alternative treatment options to support symptom relief and develop an agreed future treatment plan. Assistance from other specialist teams and professionals, for example palliative care, a counsellor or other qualified professional, may also be useful.[79]

Brain death

Death can occur in the critical care setting due to unexpected cardiac arrest, expected death after a planned treatment withdrawal or treatment withholding, and as a result of the diagnosis of brain death. Brain death occurs in the setting of a severe brain injury associated with marked elevation of intracranial pressure. To ascertain that brain death has occurred requires that the patient be in an unresponsive coma and demonstrate no brainstem reflexes or respiratory centre functioning. Clear clinical or neuroimaging evidence of acute brain pathology (e.g. traumatic brain injury, intracranial haemorrhage, hypoxic encephalopathy) consistent with the irreversible loss of neurological function is also required.[82] However, cases have been reported where brainstem death has occurred without injury or death of the cerebral hemispheres, for example in patients with severe Guillain–Barré syndrome or isolated brainstem injury.[83]

Defining brain death is a complex area with different international interpretations of death in this context. In Australia and New Zealand, the standard definition of brain death is cell death within the brain stem and cerebral hemispheres. This contrasts with the UK where brainstem death (even in the presence of cerebral blood flow) is the standard. In the USA, according to the *Uniform Determination of Death Act*, brain death occurs when a person permanently stops breathing, the heart stops beating and 'all functions of the entire brain, including the brain stem' cease. Yet determining brain death is a complex process that requires a series of tests to ensure the correct diagnosis is made. With that in mind, the American Academy of Neurology issued guidelines in 2010[84] to remove some of the uncertainty and variability amongst doctors in their procedures. Periodically, there are news reports about patients in long-term coma who regain consciousness, or reports of conflict about the management of people in a persistent vegetative state. However, brain death should not be confused with persistent vegetative state, where limited brain activity remains.

The international variation in brain death definition and procedures was highlighted in a survey of 89 countries undertaken a decade ago.[85] Results from this study demonstrated that practice guidelines for brain death in adults were present in 88% of countries surveyed with legal standards on organ transplantation present in 69% of countries. All guidelines agreed on the presence of irreversible coma, absent motor response and absent brainstem reflexes to determine brain death. Although there was broad agreement on the role of apnoea testing (59% of the surveyed countries), differences across the guidelines were noted with regard to the length of time of observation and the professional credentials for the physicians examining for brain death. ANZICS recommends that testing for brain death be undertaken independently by two medical practitioners with specific experience and qualifications pertinent to this area. It is recommended that the two sets of tests be performed separately, using the same procedures and assessments. Although it is recognised that brain death will have occurred sometime before the brain stem testing, the time of death of that patient is recorded as the time of completion of the second set of tests.[82]

Certification of brain death, while a distinct diagnosis with an associated set of diagnostic testing procedures, is often associated in clinical practice with organ donation as this allows for retrieval of well-perfused organs from patients who have already been certified dead ('beating-heart donors'). There is also increasing international recognition of the role of donation after cardiac death (DCD) where organs are retrieved after the circulation has ceased and the person has died.[86] DCD has not gained the level of support within the healthcare community as brain death donation,[87] and this may be because of ethical concerns that are different to those encountered in brain death organ donation. Key issues reported in DCD include concerns about whether appropriate efforts are undertaken to save patients, whether irreversibility exists and difficulties associated with the decision to remove mechanical or organ-perfusion support.[88]

While the diagnosis of brain death and cardiac death for any patient must be unequivocal, it is particularly important when organs are being retrieved that the diagnosis of death is a systematic, comprehensive and transparent process so that it is fully understood by the family and the healthcare team as the absolute diagnosis.[89]

Organ donation

The retrieval of organs and tissues after death has important legal and ethical perspectives that need to be considered. As a result, there is legislative guidance in Australia and New Zealand for the removal of organs and tissues after death for the purpose of transplantation. Human tissue Acts in both counties prohibit trading in human organs or tissue and there are guidelines to support practice in this area,[89] together with specific resources that are useful for critical care clinicians (see Table 5.1). Although organ and tissue donation are spoken about together in clinical practice, it is often organ donation that provokes the greatest ethical debate and discussion, and this is now explored in more depth here.

Nurses' attitudes to, and knowledge of, organ donation

Even where there are dedicated nurses who coordinate tissue and organ donation, nurses who work in critical care areas should still be able to raise and discuss donation matters with patients, families and the wider clinical team. In order to competently manage this, nurses need to have well-developed communication and interpersonal skills[75] and an understanding of the ethical and legal frameworks within which donation occurs. Organ donation can challenge the personal ethical and belief systems for some nurses. This situation can be further

Table 5.1
Organ donation resources

RESOURCE	DESCRIPTION
Organ and Tissue Donation by Living Donors: Guidelines for Ethical Practice for Health Professionals 2007[78]	These guidelines outline ethical practice for health professionals involved in living organ and tissue donation and provide guidance on how these principles can be put into practice
Organ and Tissue Donation After Death, for Transplantation: Guidelines for Ethical Practice for Health Professionals[51]	These guidelines outline ethical principles for health professionals involved in donation after death and provide guidance on how these principles can be put into practice
Making a Decision about Organ and Tissue Donation after Death; this booklet is derived from *Organ and Tissue Donation after Death, for Transplantation: Guidelines for Ethical Practice for Health Professionals*[78]	This booklet aims to help people think through some ethical issues and make informed decisions about organ and tissue donation after death.

complicated by the general public misunderstanding the concept of brain death and easily confusing brain death with profound coma or massive brain damage.[90] More worryingly, this confusion can even reside within families of deceased patients involved in organ donation. An Australian study reported that 20% of bereaved families of brain dead patients remained concerned about whether their family member had actually been dead at the time of withdrawal of the ventilator.[91] It is understandable why this confusion can occur as researchers have described the contradictions associated with caring for brain dead patients, in particular the ambiguity of caring for a pink and warm brain dead body, a body that is exhibiting traditionally accepted signs of life.[92,93] In another study of experienced intensive care nurses, almost half the participants did not regard brain death as a state of death.[94] Participants who were non-accepting or ambivalent towards brain death did not perceive that the medico-legal construct of brain death was congruent with their 'personal foundational death notions'.[94] It is therefore important that critical care nurses possess a thorough understanding of brain death and are supported to reflect on their personal understanding of death, including the concept of brain death.

Such ambiguity for staff and families surrounding brain death can be illustrated by nursing and medical staff continuing to talk to a patient who is brain dead while providing direct care. This can cause confusion for relatives who have already been informed that the patient is brain dead with no possibility of recovery or being able to comprehend/hear. Alternatively, staff and family members may be comforted by staff talking to their family member: they may perhaps be demonstrating a respectful attitude towards that person and who that person was. It is clear that there is no right and wrong here, rather that such situations reinforce the need for all staff to be sensitive to how their actions may be perceived and be clear with families as to what is informing such actions. Another area to consider is the language used by healthcare staff with families. Depersonalising terms such as 'cadaver' and 'harvesting' may be inadvertently used during organ donation and, although these may serve to psychologically protect staff, they can also act as a barrier to effective communication and understanding with grieving families.[95] What is important here is that doctors and nurses have a heightened awareness as to the emotional distress that families may be under at this time, and to ensure that communication with families is timely, clear and compassionate.

Critical care nurses are therefore in a strong position to foster a positive attitude and understanding of organ donation through provision of education and support to families of such patients. It is important that families have time to consider organ and tissue donation only after the subject of the patient's death has been discussed. If organ donation is to be raised, it may be useful to note that the majority of donor families would make the decision to donate, if in that situation again.[96] See Chapter 29 for further details.

Supporting the family of the person who is brain dead is stressful.[97] There is often concern from critical care nurses that discussing organ donation may further increase the distress of the grieving family. However, consenting to organ donation has been shown to neither hinder nor prolong the grief process of bereaved families.[98] Empirical work demonstrates that nurses possessing higher knowledge about organ donation hold more positive attitudes towards organ donation[99] and are more likely to discuss organ donation with families.[89] The role of healthcare staff in raising awareness and education about organ donation is important as donation rates continue to be low,[100] with only half of those who support organ donation actually consenting to donate.[96] In 2009, the Australian Organ and Tissue Authority (AOTA)[101] was established with the mandate to significantly improve organ and tissue donation and transplantation. This national reform program was based on the world's best practice approach using learning from leading country performers, e.g. Spain, France, Belgium, Austria and the USA. Awareness and engagement with the general public, healthcare sector, non-government sectors and donor families was seen as paramount to improve donor rates.[89,101] This raises a debate about the mechanism of consent, with many European countries using 'opt-out' consent processes, as opposed to 'opt-in' processes. Equally important is adequate training of health professionals to sympathetically and sensitively approach the grieving family with full knowledge of the donation process.[89]

The role of the critical care nurse in ethical decision making

With the most frequently occurring and most stressful ethical issues for nurses being protecting patients, autonomy and informed consent to treatment, staffing patterns, advanced care planning and surrogate decision making,[102] ethical issues challenge nurses on a daily basis. As the bedside role allows nurses to have an intimate understanding of the patient/family and their views on direction of care and treatments being delivered, nurses are well-placed to support patient autonomy and help the patient/family make choices congruent with their values and wishes.[103] This view is reflected in the Australian Code of Ethics for Nurses: specifically, that nurses should ensure patients are appropriately informed to make choices about their treatment and to maintain optimal self-determination (Value statement 2.3).[7] Practice is made more challenging when further ethical conflicts for doctors and nurses result from organisational ethical issues, e.g. allocation of funding and resources, and administration support – or lack of it.[104] In such times, it is important that person-centred care becomes the focus of care delivery with patients and their families being the lead advocates in care and, where this is not possible, advocacy being collaborative rather than any one professional taking a paternalistic role. In situations where complex ethical dilemmas are faced, access to a clinical ethicist or a clinical ethics committee[105] may help in bringing together those involved and offer an ethical review to mediate the problem.

Many aspects of critical care nursing hold moral and ethical challenges. Ethical issues in practice range from the 'big' subjects, such as assisted dying or treatment (or non-treatment) based on religious beliefs, through to the 'everyday' ethical challenges of nursing practice,[106] such as the use of chemical versus physical restraints for patients. It is important that critical care nurses understand such dimensions of their work and have considered the personal and professional positions from which they operate.

Ethics in research

When it comes to conducting research, ethical codes of conduct and ensuring all criteria for valid consent are met are requirements for all those conducting human research. There are various ethical guidelines for the conduct of research, for example the Declaration of Helsinki is regarded as an authoritative source.[107] In the UK, the General Medical Council provides clear overall modern guidance in the form of its Good Medical Practice Statement.[108] Other organisations, such as the Medical Protection Society in the UK, are often consulted by British doctors regarding issues relating to ethics. With this guidance developed at a national level to inform research ethics, there is also guidance for local research and ethics boards to ensure that research ethics are attended to at the institutional level. There is usually country-specific guidance to inform the expected composition of these local research and ethics bodies.[9,109]

Healthcare research in Australia is performed in accordance with guidelines issued by the National Health and Medical Research Council (NHMRC), while in New Zealand the guidelines are issued by the Health Research Council (HRC). Both councils have statutory authority, and health service and university human research ethics committees (HRECs) (Australia) and both health and disability ethics committees (HDECs) and institutional ethics committees (IECs) (NZ) are required to consider research proposals in accordance with the relevant recommended processes and procedures outlined by these Research Councils (see *Online resources* at the end of the Chapter for a list of relevant resources provided by the NHMRC and HRC).

Application of ethical principles

When considering human clinical research in the context of critical care, the concept of *respect for persons* is linked to the ethical principle of autonomy.[9] In human research, respect for persons demands that participants receive adequate information and choose to participate voluntarily in the research without coercion. Similar criteria as for consent to treatment should be applied by researchers seeking to recruit participants into their study. Although there may be some variation between organisations and jurisdictions, Box 5.4 provides the type of information that potential participants should be provided with to meet

---

BOX 5.4

Information requirements for participant consent in medical research

Consent to medical research documentation should include the following:[23]

- A statement that the study involves research
- An explanation of the purposes of the research
- The expected duration of the subject's participation
- A description of the procedures to be followed
- Identification of any procedures that are experimental
- A description of any reasonably foreseeable risks or discomforts to the subject
- A description of any benefits to the subject or to others that may reasonably be expected from the research
- A disclosure of appropriate alternative procedures or courses of treatment, if any, that might be advantageous to the subject
- A statement describing the extent, if any, to which confidentiality of records identifying the subject will be maintained
- For research involving more than minimal risk, an explanation as to whether any compensation, and an explanation as to whether any medical treatments are available, if injury occurs and, if so, what they consist of, or where further information may be obtained
- An explanation of whom to contact for answers to pertinent questions about the research and research subjects' rights, and whom to contact in the event of a research-related injury to the subject
- A statement that participation is voluntary, refusal to participate will involve no penalty or loss of benefits to which the subject is otherwise entitled, and the subject may discontinue participation at any time without penalty or loss of benefits, to which the subject is otherwise entitled

---

ethical requirements for consent in medical research.[27] When research studies are being considered in critical care areas, surrogate consent may be applicable.[110]

Other important and relevant ethical principles for consideration in human research are beneficence and non-maleficence. *Beneficence* in the research context is expressed by the researcher's responsibility to minimise the risk of harm or discomfort to research participants.[9] Research protocols should be designed to ensure that respect for dignity and wellbeing takes precedence over any expected knowledge benefits from the research. With regard to *justice* in research, this requires that within a population there is a fair distribution of 'benefits and burdens' for research participation. In using this concept it is the scientific objective, as opposed to membership of either a privileged or vulnerable population, that should determine the participants for a study, and the sample population should be selected to most equitably share the risks and benefits of the research.

When recruiting research participants it is important to ensure that any initial approach is made appropriately. When the study involves recruitment of hospital inpatients, this approach should be made by someone directly involved in their care, with the aim of seeking permission to then be approached by the investigators specifically about the research. If the study involves recruitment of individuals from the community, this can be done by public display (e.g. flyers, published advertisements) that provides the contact details of the researcher. Control for involvement in the research is then with the participant to make contact with the researcher. While these processes may be interpreted as putting an extra barrier to recruitment, the principles of respect and autonomy for persons are upheld as the potential for coercive recruitment is reduced. Another guiding value in ethical research is that of *integrity*. This requires that the researcher be committed to the search for knowledge and to the principles of ethical research, conduct and results dissemination.[9]

Human research ethics committees

HRECs play a central role in the ethical supervision of research involving humans. Individual research institutes/centres, universities, regional/local health authorities and hospitals will have an HREC (or equivalent body) and articulate requirements for research to be conducted in their institution. The HREC will review proposals for research involving humans to ensure that the research is soundly designed, and conducted according to high ethical standards such as those articulated in Australia in the *National Statement on Ethical Conduct in Human Research 2007* (known as the National Statement).[9] Individual HRECs have protocols for submission of ethics applications, compliance, monitoring and complaints handling processes. Importantly, no research study involving humans can be commenced until ethical clearance has been formally given by the relevant HREC(s).

The role of an HREC should not be confused with another form of clinical ethics committee that has been established in some hospitals and health services to provide closed forums for clinicians to raise ethical and legal concerns associated with particular clinical treatments or decisions. These are advisory committees that can also take into account patients' and or their families' wishes when this raises complex decision making with clinicians. In addition to providing clinicians with advice on particular cases these committees may also assist with the development of organisational policies on patient care and facilitate staff and patient education about ethical issues.

Research involving unconscious persons

The question of whether it is justifiable to include an unconscious patient in a research project without his or

her consent is a problematic issue that most critical care researchers and HRECs have to attend to.[9,111] Paramount in these considerations is the careful weighing of potential risks and benefits by a competent individual. However, analysis of these risks and benefits by a surrogate on behalf of an incompetent individual poses a range of ethical difficulties. Most national and international guidelines concur that such research is justified as long as safeguards are in place. Both the National Statement[9] and the Operational Standards[112] outline categories of vulnerable persons and the relevant ethical considerations that apply to these groups. The governing bodies recommend careful consideration of these highly vulnerable groups. Of note, the New Zealand Operational Standards[112] recognise that research on unconscious patients is appropriate, but emphasise the need for communication with the family or other legal representatives wherever possible. These Standards do note that in emergency situations consultation with the family/legal representatives may not be possible, but that the 'health care practitioner must always act in the best interests of the consumer.'[112]

Clinical trials

Clinical trials are a specific type of research study that explores whether a medical treatment or device is safe and effective for humans. As these trials use people/patients as subjects in the study, these studies must follow strict scientific standards that are set within each country. The Therapeutic Goods Administration (TGA) in Australia has adopted the *Note for Guidance on Good Clinical Practice* to replace the *Guidelines for Good Clinical Research Practice*,[113] but at the same time note there is some overlap with The National Statement, which prevails. The TGA has published an annotated version for the Australian regulatory context. The *Note for Guidance on Good Clinical Practice*[113] is an internationally accepted standard for the designing, conducting, recording and reporting of clinical trials.

The Australian government, through the NHMRC, has funded and established the Australian Clinical Trial Registry (ACTR) at the NHMRC Trials Centre in Sydney, which complies with these requirements. Clinical trials can be registered online. For trials commencing recruitment after 1 July 2005, registration must occur prior to subject recruitment, as there are important implications for future research publication in journals. In parallel, as more national trial registries emerge, the World Health Organization (WHO) is developing an approval process to assess trial register compliance. The WHO International Clinical Trial Registry Platform (ICTRP)[114] is a global project to facilitate access to information about controlled trials and their results. The Clinical Trials Search Portal provides access to a central database containing the trial registration data sets provided by the registries listed. It also provides links to the full original records. To facilitate the unique identification of trials, the Search Portal bridges (groups together) multiple records about the same trial.[114]

Ethics in publication

One of the key ways in which research findings are disseminated is through publication in peer-reviewed journals. Many international high quality journals, including *Australian Critical Care*, support the implementation of the *Committee of Publication Ethics (COPE) Code of Conduct and Best Practice Guidelines*[115] for journal editors and publishers. These guidelines recognise the important roles of editors, editorial boards and publishers in promoting and supporting ethical practices in reporting research. Therefore, journal editors are increasingly requiring that researchers demonstrate evidence of their ethics review process before a manuscript/study is considered for publication.

In Australia the NHMRC *Australian Code for the Responsible Conduct of Research (2007)*[116] provides guidance on the minimum requirements for authorship of research. Authorship is defined as substantial participation, where all the following conditions are met:

- conception and design, or data collection or analysis/interpretation of data
- drafting the article, or revising it critically for important intellectual content
- final approval of the version to be published.[116]

Authors must also ensure that all those who have contributed to the work are recognised and acknowledged. Acquisition of research funding or general supervision of a research group is not considered sufficient for authorship. Intellectual honesty should be paramount and used to inform publication ethics and to prevent misconduct.[116] Furthermore, under best practice guidelines, journals should ensure processes whereby researchers are obliged to disclose any potential competing interests before a manuscript is published and ensure all published reports and reviews of research papers have been peer reviewed by suitably qualified persons and, where needed, publish corrections, clarifications, retractions and apologies.[115]

Summary

Effectively dealing with ethical issues in any healthcare setting is complex and at times contentious. This is even more so in the critical care environment, where the patient cohort is predominantly vulnerable and lacking capacity and competence regarding autonomous decision making. Hence, critical care nurses need to be familiar with guiding ethical principles in the care of the critically ill and with the ethical considerations relating to the conduct of clinical human research. While a broad knowledge of these principles is a requirement for all health professionals as critical care nurses are often involved in these discussions and debates, they need to be particularly well informed in order to actively participate in ethical decision making. They must also be cognisant of the dynamic nature of the world we inhabit where rapidly changing communication media (e.g. the use of social media) and digital health technologies will create new and emerging ethical conundrums and legal challenges associated with privacy and confidentiality.

Critical care nurses have a unique position, being with the patient around the clock, often side-by-side with their relatives. Responsibilities include acting as patient advocate, frequently with a counselling and listening role at the bedside with patients and relatives. With medical officers having specific legal responsibilities surrounding consent and end-of-life decision making, a multidisciplinary approach is therefore important and indeed prudent to ensure all pertinent ethical matters are considered appropriately and according to guiding ethical principles.

Case study

This study reports on a high profile case from the UK. The case was a noteworthy ethico-legal dilemma and vividly illustrates key ethical principles that inform clinical reasoning in the face of a challenging event. Firstly, the case is presented and then the ethical issues arising from this case are explored. Finally, learning activities are included in the form of questions to stimulate thinking and help reflection on ethical areas of practice.

On 17 September 2007 Kerrie Wooltorton, a 26-year-old woman, drank 350 mL of ethylene glycol (antifreeze) and called an ambulance. She took with her a letter written by her and dated 14 September 2007, stating that she knew the consequences of her actions and wanted no life-saving treatment but had come to hospital so that she could be made comfortable as she did not want to die alone. The letter stated:

To whom this may concern, if I come into hospital regarding taking an overdose or any attempt of my life, I would like for NO lifesaving treatment to be given. I would appreciate if you could continue to give medicines to help relieve my discomfort, painkillers, oxygen etc. I would hope these wishes will be carried out without loads of questioning.

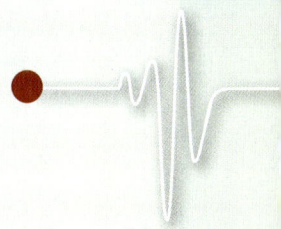

Please be assured that I am 100% aware of the consequences of this and the probable outcome of drinking anti-freeze, e.g. death in 95–99% of cases and if I survive then kidney failure, I understand and accept them and will take 100% responsibility for this decision.

I am aware that you may think that because I call the ambulance I therefore want treatment. THIS IS NOT THE CASE! I do however want to be comfortable as nobody wants to die alone and scared and without going into details there are loads of reasons I do not want to die at home which I realise that you will not understand and I apologise for this.

Please understand that I definitely don't want any form of Ventilation, resuscitation or dialysis, these are my wishes, please respect and carry them out.

Yours sincerely

Kerrie Wooltorton[117]

After admission, Kerrie Wooltorton was questioned by doctors on several occasions and over that period of time she continued to refuse medical treatment. Kerrie was known to hospital services and had taken overdoses on previous occasions and received treatment. Consultation was carried out with the full clinical team and the medical director and legal advice was taken. Kerrie Wooltorton was assessed as having mental capacity and therefore had the right to refuse treatment.

Kerrie Wooltorton died on 19 September 2007, from ethylene glycol toxicity.

CASE STUDY QUESTIONS

1 What legal and ethical issues were raised by this case?

2 How can capacity be assessed?

3 Does a person's autonomy have limits?

4 Ethically, is there a difference between a competent person making a well-thought-through request as opposed to an irrational one?

RESEARCH VIGNETTE

Bloomer MJ, Morphet J, O'Connor M, Lee S, Griffiths D. Nursing care of the family before and after a death in the ICU – an exploratory pilot study. Aust Crit Care 2013;26(1):23–8

Abstract

This qualitative descriptive study was undertaken in two metropolitan ICUs utilising focus groups to describe the ways in which ICU nurses care for the families of dying patients during and after the death. Participants shared their perspectives on how they care for families and their concerns about care, and detailed the strategies they use to provide timely and person-centred family care. Participants identified that their ICU training was inadequate in equipping them to address the complex care needs of families leading up to and following patient deaths, and they relied on peer mentoring and role-modelling to improve their care. Organisational constraints, practices and pressures impacting on the nurse made 'ideal' family care difficult. They also identified that a lack of access to pastoral care and social work after hours contributed to their concerns about family care. Participants reported that they valued the time nurses spent with families, and the importance of ensuring families spent time with the patient, before and after death.

Critique

Introduction and aims: This qualitative descriptive study explores how nurses facilitate 'a good death' for families of dying patients in intensive care. The paper reports on the preparedness of nurses to provide this care and on the organisational factors that impact on care delivered. At the beginning of the paper, the context of the study is well presented. Reference is made to the body of international work exploring how decisions are made with families during end-of-life care in the ICU and identifies that our understanding is less developed about nursing challenges when caring for dying patients. This then sets the scene for the aims of this work, one of which provides the focus for the title of this exploratory pilot study. The study reads as if the original intention of the research team was to undertake a small study. The intention may have been that this would lead to a larger study (hence pilot) in an area considered poorly explored in the research literature, hence the need for 'exploration'. An alternative title for this paper could have been: 'a qualitative exploratory study'.

Methods: As a qualitative study, no hypotheses are put forward for testing and no research question is used. However, several study aims are used that align with the preceding literature and subsequent study design and findings. The particular qualitative approach employed (e.g. phenomenology) is not acknowledged; this may be due to the applied nature of this clinical research. Ethical approval and funding support particulars are supplied, details of the sample and setting are provided and the recruitment strategy is well detailed. Specifics about the open questions used in the focus groups (for example, was a template used?) and the use of 'body language and participation' field notes would have been useful. Although there is good detail about the inductive method of data analysis, the rationale for content analysis is not clear. However, such lack of detail can easily result from choices made by authors to meet word limits set for published papers.

Results and discussion: In describing findings of the study, details are provided about the number and duration of focus groups but the overall sample size is not given. It may be that the authors considered this and chose not to report on specific data in what is, potentially, a sensitive area. Four themes develop from the data incorporating aspects of the nursing role (e.g. presence), constraints on the nursing role (e.g. time and place) and preparedness of nurses (e.g. culture). The themes are well-supported by data extracts. The discussion section of the paper explores all salient points raised by the data, using recent references to support assertions made. However, there is less evidence of data saturation to support discussion about poor educational preparation and lack of organisational support.

Conclusion: The paper concludes with a clear exploration of study limitations together with recommendations for future work in the area. This study, undertaken by an interdisciplinary team and published in a peer-reviewed, clinical journal, contributes to our knowledge about the role of nurses during end of life in intensive care.

Learning activities

1   Consider the issues of mental capacity raised by the Case study. How are assessments about someone's mental capacity made in your clinical area? What legal, professional and organisational processes and guidance are in place to assist this? What actions would you take if your assessment of a patient's mental capacity were not reflective of others in your team?

2   If a similar case to Kerrie Wooltorton's presented to your hospital, how would it be managed – similarly or differently? Why? What were the key issues from a legal perspective that might have prevented the medical team in this case being seen as aiding and abetting her suicide?

3   In your practice, are there decisions made by adult patients with capacity that challenge you in thinking there are limits to someone's autonomy? What are those circumstances and how are these managed in practice?

4   What would you do if a competent patient made a request about their treatment that you considered irrational?

Online resources

AUSTRALIA

Australian Organ and Tissue Authority (AOTA), www.donatelife.gov.au

Australian state and territory privacy law, www.oaic.gov.au/privacy/other-privacy-jurisdictions/state-and-territory-privacy-law

Human research ethics committees and the therapeutic goods legislation, Department of Health and Aged Care, Canberra, 2001, www.tga.gov.au/pdf/access-hrec.pdf

National Health and Medical Research Council (NHMRC), An ethical framework for integrating palliative care principles into the management of advanced chronic or terminal conditions, www.nhmrc.gov.au/_files_nhmrc/publications/attachments/rec31_ethical_framework_palliative_care_terminal_110908.pdf

National Health and Medical Research Council (NHMRC), Challenging ethical issues in contemporary research on human beings, 2007, current, www.nhmrc.gov.au/_files_nhmrc/publications/attachments/e73.pdf

National Health and Medical Research Council (NHMRC), Ethical considerations relating to healthcare resources allocation decisions, 1993, current, www.nhmrc.gov.au/_files_nhmrc/publications/attachments/e24.pdf

National Health and Medical Research Council (NHMRC), Health ethics, research integrity, www.nhmrc.gov.au/health-ethics/research-integrity

National Health and Medical Research Council (NHMRC), National Statement on Ethical Conduct in Human Research 2007, updated 2014, www.nhmrc.gov.au/guidelines/publications/e72

National Health and Medical Research Council (NHMRC), Revision of the Joint NHMRC/AVCC Statement and Guidelines on Research Practice 2007, www.nhmrc.gov.au/_files_nhmrc/publications/attachments/r39.pdf

National Health and Medical Research Council (NHMRC), Values and ethics: Guidelines for ethical conduct in Aboriginal and Torres Strait Islander health research, 2003 and current, www.nhmrc.gov.au/_files_nhmrc/publications/attachments/e52.pdf

NEW ZEALAND

Health Act 1956 (NZ), www.legislation.govt.nz/act/public/1956/0065/latest/DLM305840.html

Health Research Council of New Zealand (HRCNZ), Ethics overview, www.hrc.govt.nz/ethics-and-regulatory/nz-ethics-overview and www.hrc.govt.nz/ethics-and-regulatory

Health Research Council of New Zealand (HRCNZ), Guidelines for researchers on health research involving Maori, revised 2010, www.hrc.govt.nz/news-and-publications/publications/guidelines-researchers-health-research-involving-m%C4%81ori

National Ethics Advisory Committee NZ, http://neac.health.govt.nz/home

New Zealand multi-region ethics committees, http://ethics.health.govt.nz/about-committees/archived-minutes-and-reports-pre-2012/multi-region-committee

New Zealand Privacy Commissioner website, www.privacy.org.nz

Public Health and Disability Act 2000 (NZ), Amended as NZ Public Health and Disability Amendment Bill 2010, www.parliament.nz/en-nz/pb/legislation/bills/digests/49PLLawBD17731/new-zealand-public-health-and-disability-amendment-bill

OTHERS

Council for International Organisations of Medical Sciences (CIOMS), International guidelines for biomedical research involving human subjects, 1993, revised in August 2002; International guidelines for epidemiological research, 1991, www.cioms.ch

International Committee of Medical Journal Editors (ICMJE) Recommendations (The Uniform Requirements), www.icmje.org

Medical Research Council of Canada (MRC), National Science and Engineering Research Council of Canada (NSERC) and the Social Science and Humanities Research Council of Canada (SSHRC), Tri-Council Policy Statement: Ethical conduct for research involving humans, Ottawa, MRC, NSERC & SSHRC, 1998, www.ncehr-cnerh.org/english/code_2

NHS Organ Donation Register Wall of Life, www.walloflife.org.uk

US Department of Health and Human Services and Other Federal Agencies Common Rule, www.hhs.gov/ohrp/human subjects/commonrule

World Health Organization, Operational guidelines for ethics committees that review biomedical research, 2000, www.who.int/tdr/publications/training-guideline-publications/operational-guidelines-ethics-biomedical-research/en

World Medical Association, Declaration of Helsinki, updated 2013, www.wma.net/en/30publications/10policies/b3

Further reading

Benatar S. Reflections and recommendations on research ethics in developing countries. Soc Sci Med 2002;54(7):1131–41.

DeAngelis CD, Drazen JM, Frizelle FA, Haug C, Hoey J, Horton R et al. Clinical trial registration: a statement from the International Committee of Medical Journal Editors. JAMA 2004;292:1363–4.

Emmanuel EJ, Wendler D, Killen J, Grady C. What makes clinical research in developing countries ethical? The benchmarks of ethical research. J Infect Dis 2004;189:930–7.

Hurley C. A model to support the ethical elements of decisions made by advanced level practitioners. Nurs Crit Care 2011;16:53–4.

Kim Y-S, Kang SW, Ahn JA. Moral sensitivity relating to the application of the code of ethics. Nurs Ethics 2013;20(4):470–8.

Laabs CA. (2012). Confidence and knowledge regarding ethics among advanced practice nurses. Nurs Educ Perspectives 2012;33(1):10–4.

Lavery JV, Grady C, Wahl ER, Emanuel EJ. Ethical issues in international biomedical research: a casebook. Oxford: Oxford University Press; 2007.

McGowan CM. Legal issues. Legal aspects of end-of-life care. Crit Care Nurs 2011;31(5):64–9.

Organ Donation Taskforce Implementation Programme. Working together to save lives: The Organ Donation Taskforce Implementation Programme's Final Report, 2011. London: Department of Health. Available from http://www.nhsbt.nhs.uk/to2020/resources/TheOrganDonationTaskforcImplementationProgrammesFinalReport2011.pdf.

Settle PD. Nurse activism in the newborn intensive care unit: actions in response to an ethical dilemma. Nurs Ethics 2014;21(2):198–209.

Woods M. Beyond moral distress: preserving the ethical integrity of nurses. Nurs Ethics 2014;21:127–8.

References

1 International Council of Nurses (ICN). Code of Ethics, <http://www.icn.ch/publications/position-statements/>; 2014 [accessed 05.14].
2 Tschudin V. The words private and costly certainly figure large in nurses work. Nurs Ethics 2002;9(2):119.
3 McIlwraith J, Madden B. Health care and the law. 6th ed. Sydney, NSW: Thomson Reuters (Professional) Australia; 2014.
4 Beauchamp TL, Childress JF. Principles of biomedical ethics. 5th ed. New York: Oxford University Press; 2001.
5 McPherson P, Stakenberg S. Values, ethics and advocacy. In: Berman A, Snyder S, Levett-Jones T, Dwyer T, Hales M, Harvey N et al., eds. Kozier and Erb's Fundamentals of Nursing, volume 1. 2nd Australian ed. Frenchs Forest, NSW: Pearson; 2010.
6 Johnstone M-J. Bioethics : A nursing perspective. 5th ed. Chatswood, NSW: Churchill Livingstone Elsevier; 2009.
7 Nursing and Midwifery Board of Australia (NMBA). Code of Ethics for Nurses and Midwives in Australia 2013; May 2014. Available from: http://www.nursingmidwiferyboard.gov.au/Codes-Guidelines-Statements/Codes-Guidelines.aspx.
8 The National Commission for the Protection of Human Subjects of Biomedical & Behavioral Research. The Belmont Report: Ethical principles and guidelines for the protection of human subjects of research. 1979; (78-0014), <http://videocast.nih.gov/pdf/ohrp_appendix_ belmont_report_vol_2.pdf>.
9 National Health and Medical Research Council (NHMRC). National Statement on Ethical Conduct in Human Research 2007, updated March 2014, <http://www.nhmrc.gov.au/guidelines/publications/e72>; 2014 [accessed 05.14].
10 Bailey S. Ethically defensible decision-making in health care: challenges to traditional practice. Aust Health Rev 2002;25(2):27–31.
11 Nelson JE, Puntillo KA, Pronovost PJ, Walker AS, McAdam JL, Ilaoa D et al. In their own words: patients and families define high-quality palliative care in the intensive care unit. Crit Care Med 2010;38(3):808–18.
12 Angelucci P, Carefoot S. Working through moral anguish. Nurs Manage. 2007;38(9):10, 12.
13 Staunton P, Chiarella M. Nursing and the law. 6th ed. Chatswood, NSW: Churchill Livingston Elsevier; 2008.
14 South Australian Government. Consent to Medical Treatment and Palliative Care Act 1995, <http://www.legislation.sa.gov. au/lz/c/a/consent%20to%20medical%20treatment%20and%20palliative%20care%20act%201995/current/1995.26.un.pdf>; 2010.
15 Global Internet Liberty Campaign. Privacy and human rights: An international survey of privacy laws and practice, <http://gilc.org/privacy/survey>; 2014.
16 New Zealand Government. Privacy Act 1993: Reprint 2014, <http://www.legislation.govt.nz/act/public/1993/0028/latest/viewpdf.aspx>; 2014.
17 Commonwealth of Australia. Privacy Act 1988 – C2014C00669, <http://www.comlaw.gov.au/Details/C2014C00669>; 2014.
18 Australian state and territory privacy law, <http://www.oaic.gov.au/privacy/other-privacy-jurisdictions/state-and-territory-privacy-law>.
19 United Nations. The Universal Declaration of Human Rights 1948, <http://www.un.org/en/documents/udhr/hr_law.shtml>; 2014.
20 Grech C. Factors affecting the provision of culturally congruent care to Arab Muslims by critical care nurses. Aust Crit Care 2008;21(3):167–71.
21 Bloomer MJ, Al-Mutair A. Ensuring cultural sensitivity for Muslim patients in the Australian ICU: considerations for care. Aust Crit Care 2013;26(4):193–6.
22 Høye S, Severinsson E. Professional and cultural conflicts for intensive care nurses. J Adv Nurs 2010;66(4):858–67.
23 National Health and Medical Research Council (NHMRC). Cultural competency in health: A guide for policy, partnerships and participation. Canberra: Australian Government, <https://www.nhmrc.gov.au/guidelines/publications/hp19-hp26>; 2006 [accessed 10.14].
24 Gulam H. Consent: tips for healthcare professionals. Aust Nurs J 2004;12(2):17–9.
25 Aveyard H. Implied consent prior to nursing care procedures. J Adv Nurs 2002;39(2):201–7.
26 Rogers vs Whitaker (1992). 175 CLR 479. In: McIlwraith J, Madden B, eds. Health care and the law. Sydney: Thomson Reuters; 2014.
27 Rischbieth A, Blythe D. Ethics handbook for researchers, Australian and New Zealand Intensive Care Society (ANZICS) Clinical Trials Group (CTG). Melbourne: Wakefield Press; 2005.
28 Health and Disability Commissioner. Annual report of the Health and Disability Commissioner for the year ended 30 June 2002. Auckland: New Zealand Government; 2002.

29 Government of the United Kingdom. *Human Rights Act, 1998*. London, <http://www.legislation.gov.uk/ukpga/1998/42>.

30 O'Neill O. Some limits of informed consent. J Med Ethics 2003;29(1):4–7.

31 Doyal L. Informed consent: moral necessity or illusion? Qual Health Care 2001;10(suppl 1):i29–i33.

32 McConnell T. Inalienable rights: the limits to informed consent in medicine and the law. New York: Oxford University Press; 2000.

33 Hurley C. A model to support the ethical elements of decisions made by advanced level practitioners. Nurs Crit Care [Editorial]. 2011;16:53–4.

34 Weng L, Joynt G, Lee A, Du B, Leung P, Peng J et al. Attitudes towards ethical problems in critical care medicine: the Chinese perspective. Intensive Care Med 2011;37(4):655–64.

35 Fernandes MIIM. Ethical issues experienced by intensive care unit nurses in everyday practice. Nurs Ethics 2013;20(1):72–82.

36 Langeland K, Sørlie V. Ethical challenges in nursing emergency practice. J Clin Nurs 2011;20(13–14):2064–70.

37 Pauly BM, Varcoe C, Storch J. Framing the issues: Moral distress in healthcare. HEC Forum 2012;24:1–11.

38 Hall K. Intensive care ethics in evolution. Bioethics 1997;11(3–4):241–5.

39 Oberle K, Hughes D. Doctors' and nurses' perceptions of ethical problems in end-of-life decisions. J Adv Nurs 2001;33(6):707.

40 Luce JM. Making decisions about the forgoing of life-sustaining therapy. Am J Respir Crit Care Med 1997;156(6):1715–8.

41 Prendergast TJ, Claessens MT, Luce JM. A national survey of end-of-life care for critically ill patients. Am J Respir Crit Care Med 1998;158:1163–67.

42 Society of Critical Care Medicine Ethics Committee. Attitudes of critical care professionals concerning forgoing life-sustaining treatments. Crit Care Med 1992;20:320–6.

43 Asch DA, Hansen-Flaschen J, Lanken PN. Decisions to limit or continue life-sustaining treatment by critical care physicians in the United States: conflicts between physicians' practices and patients' wishes. Am J Respir Crit Care Med 1995;151(2):288–92.

44 Sprung CL, Cohen SL, Sjokvist P, Baras M, Bulow HH, Hovilehto S et al. End-of-life practices in European intensive care units: the Ethicus Study. JAMA 2003;290(6):790–7.

45 Latour JM, Fulbrook P, Albarran JW. EfCCNa survey: European intensive care nurses' attitudes and beliefs towards end-of-life care. Nurs Crit Care 2009;14(3):110–21.

46 Orlowski J. Ethics in critical care medicine. Baltimore Md: University Publishing Group; 1999.

47 Rocker G, Dunbar S. Withholding or withdrawal of life support: the Canadian critical care society position paper. J Palliat Care 2000;16:S53–62.

48 Australian Commission on Safety and Quality in Health Care (ACSQHC). National consensus statement: Essential elements for safe and high-quality end-of-life care in acute hospitals: Consultation draft, <http://www.safetyandquality.gov.au/ wp-content/uploads/2014/01/ Draft-National-Consensus-Statement-Essential-Elements-for-Safe-and-High-Quality-End-of-Life-Care-in- Acute-Hospitals.pdf>; 2014.

49 Walker R, Read S. The Liverpool care pathway in intensive care: an exploratory study of doctor and nurse perceptions. Int J Palliat Nurs 2010;16(6):267–73.

50 Makino J, Fujitani S, Twohig B, Krasnica S, Oropello J. End-of-life considerations in the ICU in Japan: ethical and legal perspectives. J Intensive Care 2014;2(1):9.

51 Wilkinson D, Savulescu J. A costly separation between withdrawing and withholding treatment in intensive care. Bioethics 2014;28(3):127–37.

52 Australian and New Zealand Intensive Care Society (ANZICS), College of Intensive Care Medicine of Australia and New Zealand. The ANZICS Statement on Withholding and Withdrawing Treatment, <http://www.cicm.org.au/cms_files/IC-14%20Statement%20on%20 Withholding%20 and%20Withdrawing%20Treatment.pdf>; 2010.

53 Sprung CL, Carmel S, Sjokvist P, Baras M, Cohen SL, Maia P et al. Attitudes of European physicians, nurses, patients, and families regarding end-of-life decisions: the ETHICATT study. Intensive Care Med 2007;33(1):104–10.

54 Bachman JG, Alcser KH, Doukas DJ, Lichtenstein RL, Corning AD, Brody H. Attitudes of Michigan physicians and the public toward legalizing physician-assisted suicide and voluntary euthanasia. New Engl J Med 1996;334(5):303–9.

55 Sjokvist P, Cook D, Berggren L, Guyatt G. A cross-cultural comparison of attitudes towards life support limitation in Sweden and Canada. Clin Intensive Care 1998;9(2):81–5.

56 Uhlmann RF, Pearlman RA, Cain KC. Physician' and spouses' predictions of elderly patients' resuscitation preferences. J Gerontol 1988;43(5):M115–21.

57 Ravenscroft AJ, Bell M. 'End-of-life' decision making within intensive care – objective, consistent, defensible? J Med Ethics 2000;26(6):435.

58 National Health and Medical Research Council (NHMRC). Organ and Tissue Donation after Death, for Transplantation: Guidelines for Ethical Practice for Health Professionals, <http://www.nhmrc.gov.au/files_nhmrc/publications/attachments/e75.pdf>; 2007.

59 Long-Sutehall T, Willis H, Palmer R, Ugboma D, Addington-Hall J, Coombs M. Negotiated dying: a grounded theory of how nurses shape withdrawal of treatment in hospital critical care units. Int J Nurs Stud 2011;48(12):1466–74.

60 Barber K, Falvey S, Hamilton C, Collett D, Rudge C. Potential for organ donation in the United Kingdom: audit of intensive care records, <http://www.bmj.com/bmj/early/2005/12/31/bmj.38804.658183.55.full.pdf>; 2006.

61 Wunsch H, Harrison DA, Harvey S, Rowan K. End-of-life decisions: a cohort study of the withdrawal of all active treatment in intensive care units in the United Kingdom. Intensive Care Med 2005;31(6):823–31.

62 The A-M, Hak T, Koëter G, van der Wal G. Collusion in doctor–patient communication about imminent death: an ethnographic study, <http://www.bmj.com/content/321/7273/1376.full.pdf+html>; 2000.

63 Çobanoglu N, Alger L. A qualitative analysis of ethical problems experienced by physicians and nurses in intensive care units in Turkey. Nurs Ethics 2004;11(5):444–58.

64 Murray MA, Miller T, Fiset V, O'Connor A, Jacobsen MJ. Decision support: helping patients and families to find a balance at the end of life. Int J Palliat Nurs 2004;10(6):270–7.

65 Bailey S. In whose interests? The best interests principle under ethical scrutiny. Aust Crit Care 2001;14(4):161–4.

66 Degrazia D. Value theory and the best interests standard. Bioethics 1995;9(1):50–61.

67 Bailey S. Decision making in health care: limitations of the substituted judgement principle. Nurs Ethics 2002;9(5):483–93.

68 Morgan J. End-of-life care in UK critical care units – a literature review. Nurs Crit Care 2008;13(3):152–61.

69 Coombs M, Long-Sutehall T, Shannon S. International dialogue on end of life: challenges in the UK and USA. Nurs Crit Care 2010;15(5):234–40.

70 Bailey S. The concept of futility in health care decision making. Nurs Ethics 2004;11(1):77–83.

71 Schneiderman LJ, Jecker NS, Jonsen AR. Medical futility: response to critiques. Ann Intern Med. 1996;125(8):669–74.

72 Willmott L, White B, Downie J. Withholding and withdrawal of 'futile' life-sustaining treatment: unilateral medical decision-making in Australia and New Zealand. J Law Med 2013;20(4):907–24.

73 Childress JF. Dying patients: who's in control? J Law Med Ethics 1989;17(3):227–31.

74 Caring Connections. Planning ahead, <http://www.caringinfo.org/i4a/pages/index.cfm?pageid=3289>; 2014 [accessed May 2014].

75 Wynn F. Reflecting on the ongoing aftermath of heart transplantation: Jean-Luc Nancy's L'intrus. Nurs Inquiry 2009;16(1):3–9.

76 Australian Health Ministers Advisory Council (AHMAC). A National Framework for Advanced Care Directives, <http://www.ahmac.gov.au/cms_documents/AdvanceCareDirectives2011.pdf>; 2011 [accessed 2014].

77 Government of Western Australia. WA Cancer and Palliative Care Network Advance Health Directive, My Advance Care Plan 2013, <http://www.health.wa.gov.au/advancehealthdirective/docs/ACP_form.pdf>; 2014.

78 Lachman V. Do-not-resuscitate orders: nurse's role requires moral courage. Med Surg Nurs 2010;19(4):249–52.

79 New South Wales Government. Advanced Care Directives (NSW) – Using. Sydney: NSW Government, <http://www0.health.nsw.gov.au/policies/gl/2005/pdf/GL2005_056.pdf>; 2005.

80 Prokopetz JJZ, Lehmann LS. Redefining physicians' role in assisted dying. New Engl J Med 2012;367(2):97–9.

81 Buiting H, van Delden J, Onwuteaka-Philpsen B, Rietjens J, Rurup M, van Tol D et al. Reporting of euthanasia and physician-assisted suicide in the Netherlands: descriptive study. BMC Med Ethics 2009;10.

82 Australia and New Zealand Intensive Care Society (ANZICS). The ANZICS statement on death and organ donation. Melbourne: ANZICS, <http://www.google.com.au/url?sa=t&rct=j&q=&esrc=s&frm=1&source=web&cd=1&ved=0CBwQFjAA&url=http%3A%2F%2Fwww.anzics.com.au%2Fdownloads%2Fdoc_download%2F867-the-anzics-statement-on-death-and-organ-donation-edition-3-2&ei=JM-XU6HsLIn3kAWTrIFo&usg=AFQjCNH_mSYzfAyhP70YauI0o31CdBrkYw>; 2013.

83 Ogata J, Imakita M, Yutani C, Miyamoto S, Kikuchi H. Primary brainstem death: a clinico-pathological study. J Neurol Neurosurg Psychiatry 1988;51:646–50.

84 Greer DM, Varelas PN, Haque S, Wijdicks EFM. Variability of brain death determination guidelines in leading US neurologic institutions. Neurology 2008;70(4):284–9.

85 Wijdicks EFM. Brain death worldwide: accepted fact but no global consensus in diagnostic criteria. Neurology 2002;58(1):20–5.

86 Jay CL, Skaro AI, Ladner DP, Wang E, Lyuksemburg V, Chang Y et al. Comparative effectiveness of donation after cardiac death versus donation after brain death liver transplantation: recognizing who can benefit. Liver Transpl. 2012;18(6):630–40.

87 Mandell MS, Zamudio S, Seem D, McGaw LJ, Wood G, Liehr P et al. National evaluation of healthcare provider attitudes toward organ donation after cardiac death. Crit Care Med 2006;34(12):2952–8.

88 DeVeaux TE. Non–heart-beating organ donation: issues and ethics for the critical care nurse. J Vasc Nurs 2006;24(1):17–21.

89 National Health and Medical Research Council (NHMRC). Australian Organ and Tissue Donation and Transplant Authority: National Protocol for Donation after Cardiac Death, <http://www.donatelife.gov.au/sites/default/files/files/DCD%20protocol%20 020311-0e4e2c3d-2ef5-4dff-b7ef-af63d0bf6a8a-1.PDF>; 2010.

90 Sundin-Huard D, Fahy K. The problems with the validity of the diagnosis of brain death. Nurs Crit Care 2004;9(2):64–71.

91 Pearson Y, Bazeley P, Spencer-Plane T, Chapman JR, Robertson P. A survey of families of brain dead patients: their experiences, attitudes to organ donation and transplantation. Anaesth Intens Care 1995;23:88–95.

92 Pearson A, Robertson-Malt S, Walsh K, Fitzgerald M. Intensive care nurses' experiences of caring for brain dead organ donor patients. J Clin Nurs 2001;10(1):132–9.

93 Sadala MLA, Mendes HWB. Caring for organ donors: the intensive care unit nurses' view. Qual Health Res 2000;10(6):788–805.

94 White G. Intensive care nurses' perceptions of brain death. Aust Crit Care 2003;16(1):7–14.

95 Kirklin D. The altruistic act of asking. J Med Ethics 2003;29(3):193–5.

96 DeJong W, Franz H, Wolfe S, Nathan H, Payne D, Reitsma W et al. Requesting organ donation: an interview study of donor and nondonor families. Am J Crit Care 1998;7(1):13–23.

97 Smith J. Organ donation: what can we learn from North America? Nurs Crit Care 2003;8(4):172–8.

98 Cleiren M, Zoelen A. Post-mortem organ donation and grief: a study of consent, refusal and well-being in bereavement. Death Stud 2002; 26(10):837–49.

99 Ingram JE, Buckner EB, Rayburn AB. Critical care nurses' attitudes and knowledge related to organ donation. Dimens Crit Care Nurs 2002;21(6):249–55.

100 Kerridge IH, Saul P, Lowe M, McPhee J, Williams D. Death, dying and donation: organ transplantation and the diagnosis of death. J Med Ethics 2002;28(2):89–94.

101 Australian Government. Australian Organ and Tissue Authority. Canberra: Australian Government department of Health, <http://australia.gov. au/directories/australia/aodtta>; 2014 [accessed 2014].

102 Ulrich CM, Taylor C, Soeken K, O'Donnell P, Farrar A, Danis M et al. Everyday ethics: ethical issues and stress in nursing practice. J Adv Nurs 2010;66(11):2510–9.

103 Wlody G. Critical care nurses: moral agents in the ICU. In: Orlowski JP, ed. Ethics in critical care medicine. Hagerstown, Md: University Publishing Group; 1999.

104 Gaudine A, LeFort SM, Lamb M, Thorne L. Ethical conflicts with hospitals: the perspective of nurses and physicians. Nurs Ethics 2011;18(6):756–66.

105 Hall RM. Ethical consultations in the ICU: by whom and when? Crit Care Med 2014;42(4):983–4.

106 Holt J, Convey H. Ethical practice in nursing care. Nurs Stand 2012;27(13):51–6.

107 World Medical Association (WMA). The WMA Declaration of Helsinki – Ethical Principles for Medical Research Involving Human Subjects, 2013, <http://www.wma.net/en/30publications/10policies/b3/>; 2013.

108 General Medical Council. Consent guidance: patients and doctors making decisions together. London: GMC, <http://www.gmcuk.org/ guidance/ethical_guidance/consent_guidance_index.asp>; 2014 [accessed 2014].

109 Research and Ethical Boards USA. Policy and procedures manual: Research ethics board, <http://www.psi.org/sites/ default/files/REB-Policy-Procedures-Manual.pdf>; 2013.

110 The SAFE Study Investigators. A comparison of albumin and saline for fluid resuscitation in the intensive care unit. New Engl J Med 2004;350(22):2247.

111 Council for International Organizations of Medical Sciences (CIOMS). International Ethical Guidelines for Biomedical Research Involving Human Subjects, <http://www.cioms.ch/publications/guidelines/guidelines_nov_2002_blurb.htm>; 2002 [accessed 2014].

112 New Zealand Ministry of Health. Operational Standard for Ethics Committees: Updated edition. Wellington: Ministry of Health, <http://wwwparliamentnz/resource/0000162273>; 2006.

113 Australian Therapeutic Goods Administration (TGA). Note for Guidance on Good Clinical Practice (CPMP/ICH/135/95) Annotated with TGA comments, <http://www.tga.gov.au/pdf/euguide/ich13595an.pdf>; 2000.

114 World Health Organization (WHO). International Clinical Trials Registry Platform (ICTRP), <http://apps.who.int/trialsearch/>; 2014.

115 Committee on Publication Ethics (COPE). Code of Conduct and Best Practice Guidelines, <http://publicationethics.org/resources/code-conduct>; 2011.

116 National Health and Medical Research Council (NHMRC). Australian Code for the Responsible Conduct of Research, <https://www.nhmrc.gov. au/guidelines/publications/r39>; 2007.

117 Armstrong W. Notes of extracts from summing up by Coroner in Kerrie Wooltorton Inquest. Great Norfolk District: British Coronial System; 2009.

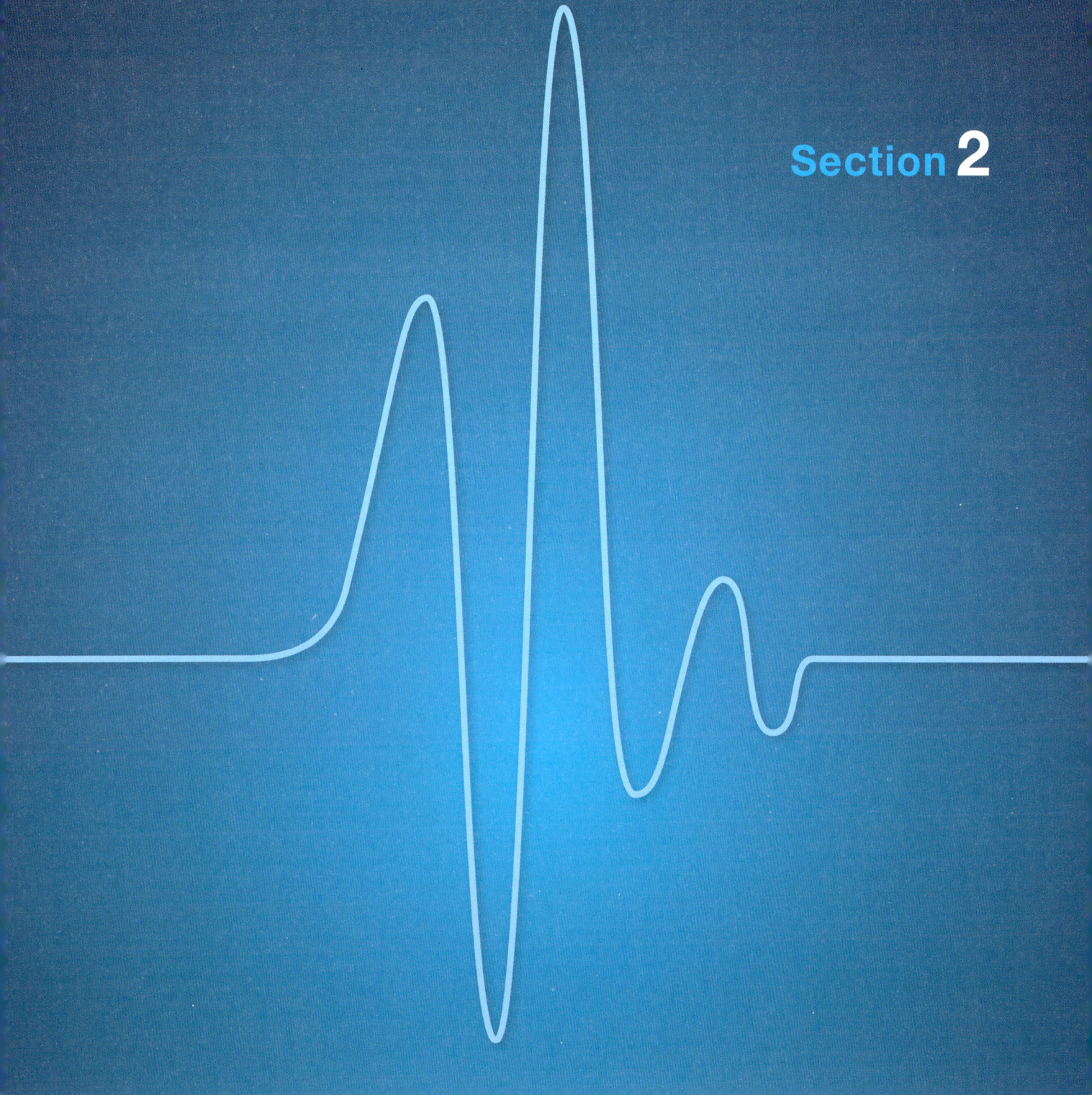

Principles and practice
of critical care

Chapter 6

Essential nursing care of the critically ill patient

Bernadette Grealy, Fiona Coyer

Learning objectives

After reading this chapter, you should be able to:

- identify risks posed to critically ill patients relating to inadequate physical care and hygiene
- describe best practice in the provision of physical care and hygiene
- understand the key elements of safe transfer of critically ill patients within the hospital setting
- understand the principles of infection-control risk identification and management for critically ill patients.

Introduction

This chapter is about essential nursing care. Because it is often referred to as basic nursing, nurses may not always perceive it as deserving of priority. Yet, how well patients are cared for has a direct effect on their sense of wellbeing and their recovery. 'Interventional patient hygiene' is a systematic, evidence-based approach to nursing actions designed to improve patient outcomes using a framework of hygiene, catheter care, skin care, mobility and oral care.[1] This chapter focuses on the physical care, infection control, preventative therapies and transport of critically ill patients. The first two areas are closely linked: poor-quality physical care increases the risk of infection. The final areas are essential features of critical care nursing.

Comfort is a paramount concern in intensive care. The two key areas of care – reducing risk and providing quality care – are closely related and served by a series of principles (see Table 6.1). The implementation of evidence-based essential nursing care is a key strategy to reduce avoidable errors and improve patient outcomes.[1,2] Thus, good risk management is an important component of quality care; if patients are assessed thoroughly and on a continuing basis, problems may be detected and treated early, preventing the development of unnecessary complications. These principles underpin this chapter. Additionally, it is important always to treat the patient as a person. Although this chapter focuses on the physical dimension of nursing care, patients' psychosocial care should not be ignored (see Chapters 7 and 8). Further, while this chapter describes essential nursing care, care bundles, which encompass a number of these activities, are described in Chapter 3.

TABLE 6.1
Principles of practice

REDUCING RISKS TO PATIENTS	PROVISION OF QUALITY CARE
• Recognition of the specific needs of critically ill patients, particularly those who are unconscious, sedated or immobile • Recognition of specific complications that may require special observation or treatment • Vigilant monitoring and early recognition of signs of deterioration • Selection, implementation and evaluation of specific preventive measures • Management of potentially detrimental environmental factors that may affect the patient	• Development of knowledge and skills for practice • Evidence-based practice • Optimal use of protocol-driven therapy • Competent, efficient and safe practice • Selection and application of appropriate nursing interventions • Monitoring the consequences of nursing interventions • Review and evaluation of nursing practices • Continuity of care • Effective critical care team functioning

Practice tip

Make sure patients know your name when you are caring for them; introducing yourself is professionally appropriate and reassuring to patients.

Personal hygiene

It is important to provide the critically ill patient with effective personal hygiene as poor hygiene may increase the risk of bacterial colonisation and subsequent infection.[3] Daily bed-baths are usually provided for most critically ill patients, although their effectiveness at reducing bacterial colonisation is questionable.[3] However, bed-baths provide an opportunity to achieve other clinical goals such as skin examination, comfort and stimulating circulation. Personal hygiene is closely related to an individual's esteem and sense of wellbeing. It may also influence family members' perception of the quality of care the patient is receiving and the confidence they have in the staff's ability to care for their loved one.

Consideration of the patient's specific condition may influence when and how personal hygiene is performed. For example, the patient may have to be moved slowly when changing bed linen because of their cardiovascular instability, or they may require a blanket while bathing if they are hypothermic. Finally, providing essential care should be timed to promote optimal rest.

Assessment of personal hygiene

Assessment of critical care patients' personal hygiene should be undertaken on two levels: first, determining what patients are able and want to do for themselves and, second, the nurse's assessment of what is required. As with all aspects of care, the patient has the right to refuse personal hygiene measures. Many critical care patients are unable to participate in decision making, and in these cases it falls to the nurse at the bedside to determine what level of care is necessary.[4] Washing patients provides opportunities for the nurse to assess the patient's skin and tissue. Often this enables the nurse to: pick up vital clues about the patient's health status; identify tissue damage that requires treatment; and identify dressings or wounds that require attention.[4] There are a number of areas to consider when assessing the skin (see Table 6.2). Excessive moisture on the patient's skin from sweat can be problematic, particularly in skinfolds. Perspiration is a normal insensible loss, and is invisible. Body sweat is usually related to temperature and is observed on all skin surfaces, especially the forehead, axillae and groins. Emotional sweating is stress-related and is observed on the palms of the hands, soles of the feet, forehead and axillae.

Essential hygiene care

A daily bed-bath with intermittent washes of the face and hands is standard care; however, patients who are sweating, incontinent, bleeding or with leaking wounds should be washed and their linen changed as often as necessary. Wet, creased sheets may contribute to changes in the support surface microclimate and cause pressure on dependent areas, increasing the risk of pressure injury development.[5] For many critically ill patients, being moved is painful and it may be appropriate to give prophylactic pain relief before commencing a bed-bath.

Personal hygiene including bed-baths should be timed to avoid disruption to patients' sleep.[4] When several nurses are required to move the patient, it makes sense to consult with colleagues to coordinate their availability. Planning ahead with respect to events such as medical rounds, chest X-ray requirements and family visits helps avoid unnecessary delays in completing personal hygiene and interruptions that affect the dignity of the patient. Privacy for the patient during personal hygiene should be of paramount concern.

The length of time taken to wash a patient and the environmental temperature are factors that affect cooling. Water on exposed skin causes rapid heat loss through conduction, convection and radiation, and for many years tepid sponging was used in critical care as a method of cooling pyrexic patients. Vasoconstriction increases the patient's perception of cold and the possibility of shivering,[6] which can affect the patient's cardiovascular stability. When shivering occurs, vulnerable patients, with low energy reserves, can rapidly use energy to keep warm. The higher oxygen consumption associated with shivering may be particularly significant in elderly patients.[6]

A range of cleansing solutions is available for washing. Although soap is effective in facilitating the removal of

TABLE 6.2
Skin and tissue assessment

FACTOR	OBSERVATIONS
Colour of the skin	• Jaundice, erythema, pallor, cyanosis
Condition of the skin	• Skin turgor (elasticity): evidence of oedema (taut skin), dehydration (dryness, tenting of the skin), age-related or steroid-related damage (thin, papery, easily torn skin), skin tears • Presence of: rash, cellulitis, irritation, bruising, swelling
Tissue perfusion	• Hypoperfusion: capillary refill time, cool extremities, pulse strength and volume, blanching of the skin • Hyperaemia: very warm, red areas of skin • Thrombus formation: warm, red, swollen areas (especially calves)
Moisture	• Excessive sweating • Skin damage caused by moisture, especially in skinfolds: under the breasts, in the groin, between the buttocks
Wounds, drains, cannulae, catheters	• Evidence of inflammation, infection, pressure damage, skin excoriation caused by leaking exudates, correct positioning of drains, need to redress wounds

bacteria, it can cause dryness of the skin. Use of a pH appropriate skin cleanser is recommended.[5] The patient's skin should be dried thoroughly to protect the skin from excess moisture and water-based emollients applied to maintain skin hydration.[5] Baby care products are often used, although these may be the least effective due to their low oil content.[7] Specific topical treatments may be required for patients with skin diseases such as dermatitis. Disposable cloths should be used for washing, as linen flannels have been shown to harbour bacteria. Complete disposable wash kits are available with potential advantages of being effective for patients' skin cleaning without requiring rinsing and therefore drying the skin, and being disposable may reduce potential for infection and certainly reduces linen costs.[3]

Personal hygiene involves washing the patient's hair as necessary, shaving the patient, management of cerumen in ears and care of finger and toe nails. While normal shampoo can be used, hair caps and washing products are available that are easier to use for bedridden patients. Male facial hair should be managed as per the patient's normal routine, such as maintaining a beard or shaving. Ears should be gently inspected for debris or injury. If assessed as appropriate, wax softening drops may be needed for 3–5 days if cerumen is present and causing the patient difficulties with their hearing.[8] Maintaining clean nails is another aspect of personal hygiene. Care should be taken if nails require trimming, especially if the patient has brittle nails or is diabetic.

Practice tip

Although personal grooming is not vital from a health perspective, it is a factor in how we see ourselves and how others identify with us. With the many changes that come with illness and therapies applied in critical care, it is important to keep the patient's 'look' as normal as possible – simple things such as styling hair or trimming beards – if not for the patients themselves, who might be unaware, then for their families.

Skin tears

Dependent patients who require total care are at greatest risk of skin tears. Injuries result from routine activities such as dressing, positioning and transferring.[9] The elderly, those with fragile skin (particularly those with a history of previous skin tears), those who require the use of devices to assist lifting, those who are cognitively or sensorially impaired and those who have skin problems such as oedema, purpura or ecchymosis are at greatest risk. Most skin tears occur on the arms and the back of the hands. The International Skin Tear Advisory Panel (ISTAP) classification system[9] uses three categories to describe skin tears: skin tears without tissue loss; skin tears with partial tissue (flap) loss; and skin tears with complete tissue (flap) loss.

Skin tears can be prevented by careful handling of patients to reduce skin friction and shear during repositioning and transfers. Padded bed rails, pillows and blankets can be used to protect and support arms and legs. Paper-type or non-adherent dressings should be used on frail skin, and should be removed gently and slowly. Wraps or nets can be used instead of surgical tape to secure dressings and drains in place. Application of a moisturising lotion to dry skin helps to keep it adequately hydrated. Treatment of skin tears[9] is outlined in Table 6.3. The focus of nursing care should be on careful cleansing and protection of the skin tear to prevent further damage and documentation of interventions and healing progress.

Practice tip

Monitor any bruising regularly, as these areas may be at risk of developing skin tears.

TABLE 6.3

Treatment of skin tears

FACTOR	INTERVENTIONS
Cleansing	• Gently clean skin with saline or non-toxic wound cleaner • Allow to dry or pat dry carefully
Skin flap	• Approximate the skin tear flap/tissue, if present, as closely as possible
Dressing	• Provide appropriate topical wound care, such as a moist wound dressing • Remove any product with an adhesive backing with utmost care to avoid further trauma • Secure non-adherent dressing with a gauze or tubular non-adhesive wrap • Change dressings according to the manufacturer's recommendations
Documentation	• Record details of skin tear, describe or photograph wound, record details of dressings and implementation of measures to reduce the risk of further occurrences

Eye care

The eyes are one of the most sensitive parts of the human body. If their eyes are not properly cared for, critical care patients may experience unnecessary discomfort. Simple bedside procedures such as turning on lights at night or assessing pupil reactions can be uncomfortable. There are a number of physiological processes that protect the eye. For example, the eye is protected from dryness by frequent lubrication facilitated by blinking. Antimicrobial substances in tears help prevent infection, and the tear ducts provide drainage. When the eye is unable to close properly, the tear film evaporates more quickly.[10] If any of these defense mechanisms are compromised the eyes are at greater risk.

There is considerable risk to patients' eyes while they are in the ICU.[11] The blink response may be slowed or absent in some patients, such as individuals receiving sedatives and muscle relaxants, or those with Guillain–Barré syndrome.[12] A number of complications can result, such as keratopathy, corneal ulceration and viral or bacterial conjunctivitis.[11] Corneal abrasions may occur within 48 hours of ICU admission[13] and in up to 40–60% of critically ill patients.[11] When the eyes are exposed they are at greater risk of injury and infection, and conjunctival oedema can lead to sub-conjunctival haemorrhage.[11] For the intensive care patient, who often has multiple intravenous lines, nasogastric tubes, ventilation tubes and their various connections, there is potential to unintentionally damage one of the eyes with one of these devices during position changes.[13]

Eye assessment

Eye assessment should be undertaken at least every 12 hours, even for conscious patients who are able to blink spontaneously. The risk of corneal abrasion or iatrogenic trauma is greatest when patients are unable to close their eyes spontaneously,[14] so these patients are at greatest risk of injury. The second at-risk group is those patients receiving positive pressure ventilation, who may develop conjunctival oedema (chemosis), sometimes referred to as 'ventilator eye'.[11] Third, patients who are exposed to high flows of air/oxygen, such as that with continuous positive airway pressure (CPAP) systems, may be vulnerable to its drying effects. Finally, all patients are at risk of eye inflammation and infection. Serious infections with bacteria such as pseudomonas can progress rapidly, resulting in blindness if not treated promptly.

The general principles of eye assessment are shown in Table 6.4, including a full examination of the eye's external structure, colour and response. Various assessment tools have been developed for this purpose.[11] Thorough eye assessment should assess appearance (which may provide indications of disease or trauma) and physical and neurological functions. If there is concern about any aspect of a patient's eyes, a referral for assessment should be made to an ophthalmologist.

TABLE 6.4

Assessment of the eyes

EXTERNAL STRUCTURE	COLOUR	REACTION
• Is it bulging or misshapen? • Is the pupil circular? • What size are the pupils? • Are both pupils the same size? • Is the pupil clear? • Is there any visible trauma? • Is it weeping? • Does it look dry or moist?	• Is the sclera its normal off-white colour or is there evidence of jaundice or haemorrhage? • Does it look red and inflamed?	• Is the blink reflex present? • Do both pupils react to light with equal speed? • Is there a composite reaction to light in the opposite eye?

Essential eye care

The goals of eye care are to provide comfort and protect the eyes from injury and infection. Eye care and the administration of artificial tears should be provided as required, if the patient complains of sore or dry eyes or if there is visible evidence of encrustation. If a patient is receiving high-flow oxygen therapy via a mask, they may benefit from regular 4-hourly administration of artificial tears to lubricate the eyes,[11,14] although this may be unnecessary while they are sleeping.

The Intensive Care Collaborative project team offer an evidence-based eye care guideline for critically ill patients, which makes a number of practice recommendations relating to the assessment and management of ophthalmologic complications in the critically ill.[15] These recommendations are outlined in Table 6.5. Further recommendations relate to regular monitoring, reporting and timely referral of ophthalmologic complications.

For at-risk patients, the general consensus is that eye care should be performed using a sterile technique, cleansing the eye from the inside to the outside usually with saline and gauze; however, eye care regimens have not been rigorously researched.[11] Cotton wool is not recommended because of the presence of particulates that may cause corneal abrasions. Eye-drops should be administered gently, inserting the drop in the uppermost part of the opened eye and as close to the eye as possible without touching it. Sometimes eye-drops can sting, so it is advisable to warn the patient of this possibility. Regular scheduled eye care with an ocular lubricant plus eye closure with tape or wrap is used to reduce the potential for corneal abrasions or subsequent corneal ulceration or infection in patients who are either paralysed or heavily sedated.[16,17]

Practice tip

Another source of irritant to the eyes can be the constant air flow from air-conditioning vents or fans, so check that your patient at risk is not positioned directly in line with these vents or poorly-positioned fans.

Conjunctival oedema (chemosis)

Conjunctival oedema (chemosis) is a common problem associated with positive pressure ventilation, positive end-expiratory pressure (PEEP) above 5 cmH_2O and prone positioning.[11] Although the oedema itself usually resolves without treatment when ventilation is discontinued, it may be advisable to seek an ophthalmic opinion if there is concern. The literature is inconclusive concerning the best method of treatment for conjunctival oedema, but evidence supports the use of artificial tear ointment and maintaining eye closure as effective measures to reduce corneal abrasions.[11]

Severe oedema often results in the patient's inability to maintain eye closure. Under such circumstances, the majority opinion is that eye closure may be maintained by applying a wide piece of adhesive tape horizontally to the upper part of the eyelid.[10,11] This usually anchors the lid in the closed position, while allowing the eyelid to be opened for pupil assessment and access for eye care. It is not necessary to change the tape at each pupil assessment using this method. However, the use of tape may be inappropriate for patients whose skin is very friable. Furthermore, if the eyelid becomes sore and inflamed, taping should be discontinued and an alternative method employed to close the eyes, e.g. gel eye pads.[10,11] When it is not possible to close the eyes, artificial tear ointment has been shown to reduce the incidence of corneal abrasion.[15]

If it is difficult to maintain eye closure by taping the upper part of the eyelid, the entire eye can also be covered with polyethylene film, which has been shown to reduce the incidence of corneal abrasion.[17] This should be changed 4-hourly with eye care and assessment. Commercially available eye-closing tape products are also available along with gel eye dressings, which may be used instead of polyethylene film.[18,19] Current evidence indicates that polyethylene film is the superior and most cost-effective product for maintaining the ocular surface.[11,19]

Oral hygiene

Poor oral hygiene is unpleasant, causing halitosis and discomfort. Although mouth care is one of the most

---

TABLE 6.5

Eyecare in the critically ill

Assessment	Patients must be assessed for risk factors for iatrogenic eye complications
	Daily assessment of the ability of the patient to maintain eyelid closure
	Weekly assessment of iatrogenic eye complication (at the microepithelial level) using instillation or fluorescein or a cobalt blue pen torch
Management	Eyelid closure should be maintained either passively or mechanically
	All patients who cannot achieve eyelid closure should receive 2-hourly eye care
	Eye care should be cleaning with saline-soaked gauze and administration of an eye-specific lubricant

Adapted from Marshall A, Elliott R, Rolls K, Schacht S, Boyle M. Eye care in the critically ill: clinical practice guideline. Aust Crit Care 2008;21(2);97–109, with permission.

basic nursing activities, in some cases lack of oral hygiene can lead to serious complications or increase their risk, such as ventilator-associated pneumonia in the ventilated patient.[20] Attendance to oral hygiene including the removal of dental plaque that harbours pathogens is an important component of nursing care.[21] Using a well-developed oral protocol can improve the oral health of ICU patients. However, the practice of mouth care is not always evidence based,[22,23] although evidence supports having a standardised oral care protocol to improve oral hygiene.[24] Factors associated with poor quality of oral care include lack of education, insufficient time, non-prioritising of oral care and the perception that it is unpleasant.[25]

Saliva produces protective enzymes, but absence of mastication, for example due to the presence of an endo-tracheal tube (ETT) or deep sedation, leads to a reduction in saliva production. An ETT can cause pressure areas in the mouth (which may be exacerbated if the patient is oedematous) and may thus need to be relocated regularly to a different position in the patient's mouth.

Oral assessment

Mouth care should be reviewed regularly based on a thorough assessment of the oral cavity.[24] Oral assessment tools have been designed specifically for intubated patients.[26] Essentially, a healthy mouth is characterised by several factors,[27] as identified in Box 6.1, and all of these areas should be assessed as a basis for good oral care.

BOX 6.1

Characteristics of a healthy mouth

- Pink, moist oral mucosa and gums. Absence of coating, redness, ulceration or bleeding
- Pink, moist tongue. No coating, cracking, blisters or areas of redness
- Clean teeth/dentures; free of debris, plaque and dental caries
- Well-fitting dentures
- Adequate salivation
- Smooth and moist lips. No cracking, bleeding or ulceration
- No difficulties eating or swallowing (uncommon in ICU)

Essential oral care

Oral care aims to ensure healthy oral mucosa, prevent halitosis, maintain a clean and moist oral cavity, prevent pressure sores from devices such as ETTs, prevent trauma caused by grinding of teeth or biting of the tongue and reduce bacterial activity that leads to local and systemic infection.[20] Oral care for an un-intubated conscious patient with a healthy mouth generally involves daily observation of the mucosa and twice-daily tooth brushing with a non-irritant fluoride toothpaste.[22] In general, for unconscious patients oral care should be performed 2-hourly, although the evidence is inconclusive and frequency ranges from

2- to 12-hourly.[22] If the mouth is unhealthy, it may be necessary to provide oral hygiene as often as hourly.

The basic method for oral care is to use a soft toothbrush and toothpaste (even for intubated patients), as this will assist with gum care as well as cleaning teeth.[23] Toothpaste loosens debris[24] and fluoride helps to prevent dental caries.[28] However, if it is not rinsed away properly, toothpaste dries the oral mucosa. Using mouth swabs only for oral hygiene is ineffective, and toothbrushes perform substantially better than foam swabs in removing plaque.[28,29] Mouth rinses have not conclusively shown benefit;[29] however, they may be comfortable for the patient to use. Tooth brushing every 8 hours was recommended in a study as being an adjunct to other ventilator-associated pneumonia prevention practices[30] while use of chlorhexidine tooth brushing was found to be of benefit in another study.[31]

Although it is an effective saliva stimulant, practices such as the use of lemon and glycerine are outdated, as glycerine causes reflex exhaustion of the saliva process, resulting in a dryer mouth.[29] Lemon juice is to be avoided, as it can decalcify enamel.[29] Commercial mouthwashes moisten and soften the mucosa and help to loosen debris, which can be washed away.[21] They must be used with caution in patients with oral problems, due to their potential to cause irritation and hypersensitivity.[26] In addition to tooth brushing, regular sips of fluid or mouth washing with water is recommended. A recent report identified thirst as one of the three most prevalent, intensive and distressing symptoms critically ill patients suffer.[32] If the patient is able to suck and swallow, small pieces of ice are very refreshing. Patients with clean mouths, who are febrile and/or receiving antibiotics, should also have their mouths moistened often with water to prevent drying, coating and subsequent discomfort. Immunosuppressed patients or those on high-dose antibiotics may also require antifungal treatment to treat oral thrush.

There are many oral hygiene products and solutions available to suit the needs of all patients.[21] Commercial mouthwashes should be used as a comfort measure to supplement toothbrushing.[33] A range of other products is available to treat oral problems, for example benzydamine hydrochloride (anti-inflammatory), aqueous lignocaine (anaesthetic) and nystatin (antifungal). For patients intubated for more than 24 hours, rates of nosocomial pneumonia may be reduced by using twice-daily chlorhexidine gluconate mouthwashes,[31,34] which also prevent plaque accumulation. This has the disadvantage of an unpleasant taste and can discolour teeth.[27] For patients with crusty build-up on their teeth, a single application of warm dilute solution of sodium bicarbonate powder with a toothbrush is effective in removing debris and causes mucus to become less sticky, although its use has not been definitively tested.[33] However, it can cause superficial burns and its use should be followed immediately by a thorough water rinse of the mouth to return the oral pH to normal. Hydrogen peroxide has an antiplaque effect but, if incorrectly diluted, it can cause pain and burns to the oral mucosa and a predisposition to candida colonisation.[35] It is not pleasant tasting and is sometimes rejected by patients although it is the substance that impregnates some of the foam sticks available for oral care.[28] As a preventive measure, to reduce the incidence of fungal colonisation, natural yoghurt may be used. Normal oral hygiene is followed by coating the mouth and tongue with yoghurt. While evidence suggests that probiotics are safe complete consideration of the risk–benefit ratio before administration to the critically ill patient is recommended.[36]

Plastic water ampoules (10 mL) can be used to drip water into the mouth for convenient administration to patients unable to easily open their mouths or swallow. A Yankauer suction catheter facilitates rinsing of toothpaste from the mouth, and a bite-guard device may be used temporarily to prevent patients from inadvertently biting on the toothbrush or their tongue. They should not be used long term due to the risk of pressure sores. Lanolin may be applied to help maintain integrity of the lips.

Practice tip

If the patient objects to the taste of the chlorhexidine gluconate mouthwash, consider a follow-up rinse of water.

Practice tip

Performing oral hygiene with toothbrush and toothpaste in an intubated patient and ensuring the mouth is rinsed well may be assisted by the use of a dental sucker, which is flexible. This disposable device attached to a continuous suction system can be positioned in the mouth to aid in the continual removal of fluids while brushing and rinsing is performed. The dental sucker can also be used for continuous oral suction in patients with excessive saliva.

Patient positioning and mobilisation

Positioning patients correctly is important for their comfort and the reduction of complications associated with pressure areas[5,37] and joint immobility. Lying in bed for long periods can be a painful experience.[38] Researchers[39–41] describe neuromyopathy from critical illness and disuse atrophy from prolonged immobility contributing to intensive care acquired weakness. This weakness may contribute to prolonged ventilation and intensive care length of stay as well as delayed return to physical normality.[42–45] Cardiovascular stability, respiratory function and cerebral or spinal function are all factors that influence the positioning of patients in critical care areas. Modern beds and pressure-relieving devices have helped considerably to enhance the care of critically ill patients.

The primary goals of essential nursing care for patient positioning are:

- to position the patient comfortably
- to enhance therapeutic benefits

- to prevent pressure injuries, also known as pressure ulcers
- to ensure the limbs are supported appropriately and to maintain flexible joints
- to facilitate patient activity to minimise muscle atrophy
- to implement early mobilisation as the patient's condition allows.

There is growing evidence that early mobilisation is an important aim for critically ill patients[42–45] and an essential goal of nursing care is to support the patient in maintaining or attaining a normal level of physical function for mobility. As with many other aspects of care for the critically ill, this is best achieved through multidisciplinary team members working together. Here, physiotherapists and occupational therapists have a lead role in assessing patients and planning programs of care and activity to facilitate attaining the goals of normal physical function, while nurses contribute by ensuring the programs of care are delivered when other personnel are not available.

Practice tip

Movement of the lower legs, ankles and feet can be achieved in conjunction with a gentle massage or application of moisturiser. Family members may wish to undertake this, giving them an opportunity to provide the patient with care and touch.

Assessment of body positioning

A risk assessment should be undertaken and those patients at highest risk of complications related to their position are those who are unable to move for long periods, for whatever reason.[46] For example, unstable patients whose status is compromised when they are moved, patients who are in critical care for a long time, elderly and frail or malnourished patients and patients who are unable to move themselves (e.g. due to sedation, trauma, surgery or obesity) are all at risk. Numerous significant risk factors exist, for example age, length of intensive care stay, use of adrenaline and/or noradrenaline infusions; patients with restricted movement; patients with comorbidities such as cardiovascular disease and diabetes and unstable patients.[47] However, even previously fit patients who experience a critical illness can develop severe limitations in their mobility. The common short- and long-term complications of immobility are pressure injuries, venous thromboembolism and pulmonary dysfunction, each of which carries a significant comorbidity.[46] Regular musculoskeletal assessment should be made, focusing on the patient's major muscles and joints and the degree of mobility. Table 6.6 offers a simple guide to assessment, which includes visual and physical assessment of all limbs and joints. Provided there are no contraindications, function should be stimulated by regular passive then active movements of all limbs and joints to maintain both flexibility and comfort.

TABLE 6.6
Musculoskeletal assessment

MUSCLES AND JOINTS	MOBILITY
• Power/strength	• Degree of independence
• Range of movement	• Need for assistance
• Symmetry	• Adherence/compliance
• Tenderness and pain	with physiotherapy/
• Inflammation, swelling,	mobility regimen
wasting	• Need for planned rest
	periods
	• Use of splints or collar

Positioning and mobilising patients

Positioning the patient to achieve maximum comfort, therapeutic benefit and pressure area relief and employing active and passive exercises to maintain muscle and joint integrity and progress to regaining mobility are important nursing activities. Provided there are no specific contraindications, the immobile patient should be positioned with the head raised by 30° or more, as research has demonstrated that it improves mortality[48] and helps reduce ventilator-associated pneumonia.[49] When combined with thromboembolic prophylaxis, gastric ulcer prophylaxis and daily sedation assessment, ventilator-associated pneumonia may be reduced by around 45%.[49] Good body positioning and alignment helps prevent muscle contracture, pressure injuries and unnecessary pain or discomfort for the patient.[50,51]

Mobilisation for the critically ill patient can be described as a graduated increase in range of activity from positioning, passive movement, sitting upright in bed, sitting in a chair to actually ambulating.[50,52] Stiller[52] describes a range of safety factors that need to be considered prior to mobilising the critically ill patient, which fall into two groups: those specific to the patient and their physical and physiological condition and those extrinsic to the patient such as the environment, staffing and patient devices attached. Creating an individualised mobility plan that can be adapted according to patient assessment and general health progress will optimise early movement and mobilisation.[52,53]

Practice tip

From the perspective of patient comfort, even small readjustments in positioning may be advantageous, and often can be made without much effort by the nurse or disturbance to the resting patient. Most electric beds provide for adjustments to the backrest angle, knee bend and bed tilt, and adjustments can be easily made. In addition to comfort, these adjustments will aid in pressure changes between re-positioning of the patient.

Practice tip

When planning to reposition the patient, ensure that there are enough staff to give the patient a feeling of security during the procedure and that all the patient's devices (e.g. IV lines) are managed. Check that all devices are placed to accommodate the repositioning before you begin to move the patient.

Active and passive exercises

Spontaneous physical activity decreases by as much as 50% in hospitalised patients[54] and physical activity is essential to healthy functioning and beneficial for the cardiovascular system.[44] Inactivity, age and the inflammatory process that occurs during critical illness combine to progress muscle breakdown and loss of physical function in older hospitalised patients with muscle mass reduction, which occurs as early as several hours from the onset of immobility.[54] Active exercises are those that can be performed by the patient with no, or minimal, assistance. Passive exercises are performed when patients are either too weak or incapable of active exercise. Exercises can be employed to help the recovering patient develop power and regain function, to assist in venous return and maintain the normal sensation of movement.[54] They should be performed at least daily. Passive exercises put the main joints through their range of movement, which helps reduce joint stiffness and maintain muscle integrity, preventing contractures. Shoulders, hands, hips and ankles are particularly at risk of stiffness and muscle contracture.[54] It is important, however, to ensure that joints and muscles are not overstretched, as this is painful for patients and can cause permanent injury. Splints may be used when the patient is resting, to maintain joints in a neutral position.[54] The physiotherapist's advice should be sought regarding the correct range of movement and the frequency of passive exercises. This is particularly important for burn-injured patients. Concern has been expressed about the effects of limb movements on head-injured patients; however, two dated yet seminal studies detected no significant cardiovascular or neurological changes during passive exercises in neurosurgical patients,[55] and found no detrimental effects on cerebral perfusion or intracranial pressure (ICP), whether ICP was raised or not.[56]

Changing body position

Mobility is defined as the ability to change and control body position.[57] The complications of immobilisation in critically ill patients are well documented, and include pressure injury, venous thromboembolism and pulmonary dysfunction such as atelectasis, retained secretions, pneumonia and aspiration.[45] The routine standard for immobilised patients in ICU is 2-hourly body repositioning, although this does not always happen,[46] and the optimal interval for turning critically ill patients is unknown.[58] In addition to providing pressure relief, it is recommended that the patient's position be changed often to ensure comfort, relaxation and rest; to inflate both lungs, improve oxygenation[58] and help mobilise airway secretions; to orient the patient to the surroundings and for a change of view; and to improve circulation to limbs through movement.[42] The frequency of body repositioning should be determined according to the patient's pressure injury risk (preferably using one of the assessment tools described below), clinical stability and comfort.

Good body alignment helps prevent pressure points, contractures and unnecessary pain or discomfort for the patient.[50] Here, careful consideration should be given to factors (outlined in Table 6.7) such as haemodynamic and cardiopulmonary responses of the patient,[59] the timing and method of positioning patients and whether there are any restrictions on movement. It is important to fully consider the individual needs of patients: they may have a history of back or neck problems, and the selective use of soft or firm pillows and mattresses may be relevant. Pillows can optimise the patient's position so that the shoulders and chest are squared, and may reduce the work of breathing for patients with chronic airways disease.[42] Some pressure-relieving mattresses have an adjustable pressure control, which can be changed according to pressure relief assessment and patient comfort.[5] When patients are positioned lying on one side, consideration should be given to their feeling of security; for example, ensuring that they are well supported by pillows and the bed rails are raised. Provided cerebral perfusion pressure is maintained above 50 mmHg, even severely head-injured patients can be moved safely;[56] however, it is important to maintain the neck in alignment to promote venous drainage (see Chapter 17) and, for those with spinal injuries, log-rolling may be required (see Chapter 17).

Pressure area care

The term 'pressure injury' rather than 'pressure ulcer' is now used in Australasia. Terms that have been used to describe pressure injuries are numerous and include bed sore and decubitus ulcer. This new term recognises the general consensus that the majority of pressure injuries are preventable adverse events.[5] The prevalence of pressure injuries in an ICU ranges from 5% to 50%[47] and the risk of developing a pressure injury is cumulative: 5% risk after 5 days; 30% risk after 10 days; and 50% risk after 20 days in the ICU.[60] Pressure injury risk for critically ill patients can be attributed to their immobility, lack of sensory protective mechanisms, suboptimal tissue perfusion and environmental factors that cause pressure and friction.[5,47] The commonest locations for pressure injuries are the sacrum, the heels and the head.[5] Significant risk factors include the age of the patient, the number of days since admission, malnutrition[47] and delays in the use of pressure-relieving mattresses.[60]

Pressure risk assessment tools can help nurses identify at-risk patients.[5,37] However, it is unusual for a patient in critical care to be assessed as low-risk. There are several pressure injury risk assessment tools available such as the Braden score[57] and the revised Jackson/Cubbin pressure risk calculator[61] (Table 6.8) that was designed specifically for use in ICU and provides an awareness of the many factors that need to be considered and monitored prior to and during procedures for pressure injury prevention. Risk assessment should be undertaken as soon as possible after the patient's admission and within 8 hours of admission.[5] A comprehensive head-to-toe skin assessment for pressure should be scheduled at least daily and include a review of pressure-relieving devices for effectiveness or requirement for change. Skin should be inspected at each episode of patient repositioning. Skin assessment should include

---

TABLE 6.7

Factors to consider when positioning patients

FACTORS	COMMENTS
Haemodynamic and cardiopulmonary responses	• Placing patients in the left lateral position can cause a (usually harmless) fall in oxygenation for a few minutes
Timing	• Position the patient to avoid clashes with treatment/investigations such as chest physiotherapy or chest X-ray • Consider the need for the patient to rest
Method	• The need to use lifting devices • The availability of staff to perform a safe manoeuvre • The placement of pillows to support limbs, to facilitate both comfort and respiratory efficiency • Use of bed adjustments to create 'chair' positions to prepare patients to sit out of bed
Restrictions on positioning	• The need for spinal alignment • Cerebral injury • Haemodynamic instability • Respiratory compromise • Access to devices for therapies • Body size

TABLE 6.8

Components of the revised Jackson/Cubbin pressure area risk calculator[61]

RISK ASSESSMENT CATEGORIES	SCORING

• Age
• Weight/tissue viability
• Past medical history affecting condition
• General skin condition
• Mental status
• Mobility
• Haemodynamics
• Respiration
• Oxygen requirements
• Nutrition
• Incontinence
• Hygiene
	• Score range = 12–48
	• One point is deducted for each of the following:
	  ○ The patient has spent time in surgery/scan in the past 48 hours
	  ○ The patient has received blood products
	  ○ The patient is hypothermic
	• A lower score indicates higher risk
	• A score of <29 indicates high risk

testing for blanching response and checking for areas of oedema, induration, redness or localised heat.[37]

Pressure injury prevention practices include alternating the use of pressure-relief mattresses, low-pressure mattresses and air-flow mattresses.[37,60] For bariatric patients (usually those heavier than 150 kg), specialist beds and mattresses are required.

Intensive care patients are at risk of pressure injuries and injury from a number of devices in everyday use, such as endotracheal tubes and blood pressure cuffs (see Table 6.9). Close attention to detail with frequent observation of the patient, the patient's position and the presence and location of equipment is required to prevent skin damage.[62] It is important to remove aids such as compression stockings and cervical collars to assess the skin. Vulnerable patients, such as those with poor tissue perfusion, anaemia, oedema, diaphoresis and poor sensory perception,[37] can develop pressure injuries relatively quickly, and pressure injuries caused by equipment are entirely avoidable.

All pressure points and any pressure injuries should be monitored closely. The key areas of monitoring are identified in Table 6.10, and it is important to use standardised methods to objectively assess pressure injuries and their response to therapy. If a patient develops one pressure injury, there is a good chance he/she could develop another. Nursing intervention includes the placing of patients in positions that avoid pressure on the affected area(s), employing measures such as good fluid management to improve tissue perfusion, reducing the risk of infection and promoting tissue granulation with the use of appropriate dressings.

The International NPUAP–EPUAP Pressure Ulcer Classification System[37] grades pressure injuries as follows:

• Stage I: Non-blanchable redness of intact skin
• Stage II: Partial thickness skin loss or blister

TABLE 6.9

Risk of pressure injuries from commonly used equipment

RISK FACTOR	COMMENTS
Endotracheal tubes (ETTs)	The ETT should be repositioned from one corner of the mouth to the other on a daily basis to prevent pressure on the same area of oral mucosa and lips. Care should also be taken when positioning and tying ETT tapes: friction burns may be caused if they are not secure; pressure sores may be caused if they are too tight (particularly above the ears and in the nape of the neck). Moist tapes exacerbate problems and harbour bacteria
Oxygen saturation probes	Repositioning of oxygen saturation probes 1–2-hourly prevents pressure on potentially poorly perfused skin. If using ear probes, these must be positioned on the lobe of the ear and not on the cartilage, as this area is very vulnerable to pressure and heat injury
Blood pressure cuffs	Non-invasive blood pressure cuffs should be regularly reattached and repositioned. If left in position without reattachment for long periods of time they can cause friction and pressure damage to skin. Care should be taken to ensure that tubing is not caught under the patient, especially after repositioning
Urinary catheters, central lines and wound drainage	The patient should be checked often to ensure that invasive lines are not trapped under the patient. In addition to causing skin injury, they may function ineffectively
Bed rails	Limbs should not press against bed rails; pillows should be used if the patient's position or size makes this likely
Oxygen masks	Use correct-size mask and hydrocolloid protective dressing on the bridge of the nose to assist with prevention of pressure from non-invasive or continuous positive airway pressure masks, especially when these are in constant or frequent use
Splints, traction and cervical collars	Devices such as leg/foot splints, traction and cervical collars can all cause direct pressure when in constant use and friction injury if they are not fitted properly. ICU patients often have rapid body mass loss (especially muscle) following admission, so daily assessment is required

- Stage III: Full thickness skin loss (fat visible)
- Stage IV: Full thickness tissue loss (muscle/bone visible)
- Unstageable pressure injury: depth unknown
- Suspected deep tissue injury: depth unknown

Further, the NPUAP differentiates skin injuries from mucosal injuries. Mucosal pressure injuries are defined as injuries found on mucous membranes with a history of a medical device in use at the location of the injury. These injuries cannot be staged.[63]

The use of standardised tools to both assess pressure risk and stage pressure injuries is vital to effective continuity of care. Treatment of pressure injuries is complex and based on individual patient factors; however, the main issues include:

- protecting tissue from further damage with pressure re-distribution techniques
- preventing infection either localised or systemic by closely observing the injury for signs of infection such as friable, oedematous, pale or dusky tissue
- aiding wound healing such as use of negative pressure wound therapy for deep injuries or foam and alginate dressings to control heavy exudate.[5,37]

Practice tip

It is worthwhile knowing the key features of the beds and mattresses commonly used in your area so that you can use them effectively to match patient requirements for bed functions, bed type (e.g. bariatric suitability) and pressure prevention (e.g. high-, medium- or low-risk mattress systems).

Rotational therapy

Continuous lateral rotation therapy or kinetic bed therapy is an intervention in which the patient is rotated continually, on a specialised bed, through a set number of degrees; it helps to relieve pressure areas and can significantly improve oxygenation.[64,65] Continuous lateral rotation therapy may reduce the prevalence of ventilator-associated pneumonia in patients requiring long-term ventilation.[66] Appropriate evaluation of the benefits and suitability of the patient for Continuous lateral rotation therapy should be undertaken by the team and the therapy implemented according to local protocols.[64] In implementing this therapy, the goal is to achieve continuous rotation through the maximum angle that the patient tolerates for 18 hours per day.[67]

Venous thromboembolism (VTE) prophylaxis

Deep vein thrombosis (DVT) and pulmonary embolism (PE) are separate conditions collectively referred to as venous thromboembolism (VTE).[68,69] DVT is a blood clot in a major vein of the lower body, i.e. leg, thigh or pelvis, which causes disruption to venous blood flow and is often first noticed by pain and swelling of the leg. The blood clot forms due to poor venous flow, endothelial injury to the vein or increased blood clotting that may be caused by trauma, venous stasis or coagulation disorders.[70] Pulmonary emboli occur when a part of a thrombosis moves through the circulation and lodges in the pulmonary circulation. VTE is a major risk factor for hospitalised patients in general and critically ill patients in particular, due to blood vessel damage, coagulation disorders and limited mobility leading to venous stasis.[69] Further, around 50% of patients with DVT will also suffer a pulmonary embolism, which can be fatal causing around 10% of hospital deaths in Australia.[69,71] Patients with VTE may also develop post-thrombotic syndrome where tissue injury occurs leading to pain, paraesthesia, pruritus, oedema, venous dilatation and venous ulcers.[68,70]

It is important to consider the individual patient (age, body mass index) and their history (previous VTE, coagulation disorders) along with their current condition whether it be surgical or medical and features of their treatment (immobilisation) when determining risks

---

TABLE 6.10

Monitoring pressure injuries (PIs)

FACTOR	ACTIONS
Size	• Objectively assess length, width and depth
Stage/grading	• Use a standardised measure to grade the injury (e.g. International NPUAP & EPUAP Pressure Ulcer Classification System)
Documentation	• Note the absence/presence/location of PIs on admission and discharge • Keep a record of nursing interventions and treatments used to treat PIs
Treatment	• Monitor response to therapy by assessing the size and stage/grade of the PI on a daily basis
Observing other sites	• Dependent areas of the body are susceptible: sacrum, heels, back of the head, hips, shoulders, elbows, knees • Areas of the body where equipment is causing pressure are susceptible: nose, ears, corners of the mouth, fingertips • Areas of the body where tissue perfusion is poor are susceptible: extremities

for VTE.[72–74] Both the risk assessment and the patient's current condition will determine the most appropriate VTE prophylaxis strategy.[73] Prophylaxis consists of a combination of pharmacological and mechanical interventions that may be used together or separately according to the degree of risk for VTE and/or contraindications to particular therapies. The use of combined therapies is supported by recent reviews and guidelines.[70,73] The National Health and Medical Research Council *Clinical practice guideline for the prevention of venous thromboembolism (deep vein thrombosis and pulmonary embolism) in patients admitted to Australian hospitals*[69] provides a comprehensive guide to risks and management relating to VTE for critical care in Australia.

Low-molecular-weight heparin or unfractionated heparin is the most common pharmacological therapy prescribed, while other medications will be prescribed for patients according to individual factors.[69,74] Special consideration of an appropriate regimen for pharmacological prophylaxis will need to be given to patients with renal and hepatic impairment.[74] Heparin-induced thrombocytopenia (HIT) may develop in some patients[75] so, as with all heparin therapy, close monitoring of the patient's platelet count and assessing for signs of bleeding such as bruising or haematuria will form part of the nurse's role in managing VTE prophylaxis.

In principle, it is advised that graduated compression stockings are used for all general, cardiac, thoracic and vascular surgical patients until full mobility is achieved irrespective of pharmacological prophylaxis.[69,73] Mechanical prophylaxis is provided through a range of graduated compression stockings and various pneumatic venous pump or sequential compression devices.[76,77] It is important to make sure that the relevant devices are fitted correctly and monitored closely. Comparisons between a number of pneumatic pumps have been published[75–77] with all displaying relative effectiveness. The availability of battery-operated sequential compression devices can assist with the continuous application of the therapy during patient transports away from their bedside, such as to the imaging department for radiological procedures.[77]

Along with pharmacological and mechanical venous thromboembolism prophylaxis, maintaining patients' hydration and implementing early mobilisation are key components of care in preventing VTE.[69,72] Rauen et al[68] describe the most common reasons cited for lack of proper VTE prophylaxis as being lack of knowledge among healthcare providers and underestimation of the risk of VTE along with overestimation of the potential risk of bleeding from prophylaxis. Given the risks of VTE for critically ill patients, it is clearly important that nurses contribute to lowering risks for their patients by knowing the range of risk factors for their patients, along with the appropriate pharmacological prophylaxis that may be prescribed. It is also important to know how to appropriately implement and manage the mechanical prophylactic devices and, most importantly, facilitate the early mobilisation of the patient.

Bowel management

Although bowel care is an essential aspect of critical care nursing care, there is limited research on the topic specific to this cohort of patients. Good bowel care promotes patient comfort and reduces the risks of further associated problems such as nausea, vomiting and abdominal/pelvic discomfort. Maintaining good bowel care in the critically ill patient can have changing foci from promoting defecation to containing diarrhoea, as throughout the critical illness gut function is influenced by changing therapies, medications, nutrition, hydration and mobility of the patient. Enteral feeding is often cited in the literature as a cause of diarrhoea,[78] but poor gastric fluid intake causes constipation, and improved gut motility decreases the risk of aspiration and subsequent pneumonia. Additional to the need to manage faecal incontinence, the two spectrums of constipation and diarrhoea are particular challenges for nurses to provide patient-specific, effective management in a sensitive and dignified way for their critically ill patient.

Causes of constipation in critically ill patients range from shock and reduced gut motility to changes in nutrition and lack of mobility. The consequences of constipation are not well defined but can include increased abdominal distension and resulting impedance of lung function, inability to establish adequate enteral nutrition and increased acquired bacterial infections.[79] The prevention of constipation is particularly important for patients with high cervical spinal injuries, as if left untreated it may cause potentially fatal autonomic dysreflexia.[79] de Azevedo et al[80] discussed the need to determine whether constipation is a marker of severity and poor prognosis in critically ill patients or if it is a dysfunction contributing to a worsening clinical condition. However, the need for effective prevention and management of constipation in critically ill patients is clear.

Bowel care can be one of the most distressing aspects of nursing care, from a patient's perspective. Often patients find bowel care to be awkward and embarrassing, and the routines that individuals may have developed, especially the elderly, to sustain effective bowel function in their daily lives are then interrupted by their illness, and their loss of control over their body for this function can be particularly distressing. Sensitive nursing care that respects the dignity of the patient is paramount.

Bowel assessment

Initial bowel assessment should be undertaken to determine the patient's usual bowel habits, as a daily bowel action is not common for most of the population. In general, older patients are more susceptible to constipation.

Gut function should be assessed at the start of each nursing shift[78] (see Box 6.2). Several authors have developed bowel care protocols for intensive care patients and studies suggest that use of a protocol improves bowel care in critically ill patients.[81,82] Rectal examination should be undertaken if the patient has not had their bowels open for 3 consecutive days.[81] If the bowels have not been

---

BOX 6.2

Assessment of gut function

- Observation of nasogastric aspirate volume
- Visual inspection and palpation of abdomen, noting any tenderness, pain or distension
- Recording the frequency, nature and quantity of bowel actions
- The presence or absence of bowels sounds

---

opened during this period, action should be taken.[81] For some patients in whom defecation is problematic, it may be appropriate to objectively assess the quality of faecal stools using a tool such as the Bristol stool form scale, which uses a 7-point grading system to assess stool consistency (see Table 6.11).[83] Establishing the cause of faecal incontinence is important as this will direct the treatment and management plan. Faecal incontinence may occur in conditions such as neurological and spinal conditions, intestinal diseases such as Crohn's, cognitive impairment such as dementia or be the result of anal sphincter or rectal injury or dysfunction, medications or intestinal impaction and overflow.[84]

Practice tip

When undertaking bowel assessment you should also consider the patient's normal diet and any laxatives routinely taken, as this information may influence any bowel regimen developed for the patient.

Essential bowel care

Nursing care is based on managing privacy and embarrassment, increasing exercise where possible, ensuring adequate fibre and fluid in the diet, reducing unnecessary use of drugs that cause constipation and appropriate use

TABLE 6.11
Bristol stool form scale

GRADE	DESCRIPTION
0	No bowel movement
1	Separate hard lumps; like nuts; hard to pass
2	Sausage-shaped but lumpy
3	Like a sausage but with cracks on the surface
4	Like a sausage or snake but smooth and soft
5	Soft blobs with clear-cut edges; easily passed
6	Fluffy pieces with ragged edges; a mushy stool
7	Watery; no solid pieces; entirely liquid

Adapted from Riegler G, Esposito I. Bristol scale stool form. A still valid help in medical practice and clinical research. Tech Coloproctol 2001;5(3):163–4, with permission.

of laxative agents. Where bowel care is concerned, it is always appropriate to first explain to patients what is to be done, and to gain their consent if they are conscious. Constant reassurance is important so that patients feel safe and secure in the knowledge that their privacy will be maintained to the greatest degree possible.

Peristaltic movement of the gut is stimulated by exercise. Although difficult in the intensive care setting, many patients are awake, and even those who require sedation should be sedated with the minimal amount necessary for their safety, as this will enable some degree of movement. Promoting patient mobility, especially voluntary movement, is helpful as it will improve gut motility.

Diet and fluids

Diet and fluids are two important considerations in maintaining normal bowel function. Ensuring the appropriate administration of fluid and an adequate dietary fibre intake[81] helps to prevent constipation. Although enteral feeding increases faecal bulk and provides gastric fluid, which helps to maintain gut motility, Bishop et al[85] found a higher rate of enteral nutrition was strongly associated with a looser type of stool. Chapter 19 contains an in-depth discussion on the principles of enteral feeding.

Drugs

The use of sedatives is often an ascribed cause of constipation in critically ill patients. This is not due to their direct effect, but due to the subsequent immobility of patients when sedatives are used. Opiates, which are often used to control pain, slow propulsive gut contraction. In a small cohort study, Sawh et al[86] reported the successful resumption of target enteral feeding after treating opioid-induced constipation with subcutaneous methylnaltrexone. The main drugs that cause constipation in critical care settings are analgesics, anaesthetic agents, anticonvulsants, diuretics and calcium channel blockers. Although it is difficult to avoid giving these drugs, their judicious use in tandem with other preventive measures will help avoid constipation. Anti-emetic and pro-kinetic agents can also be used in critical care patients and Bishop et al[85] found the administration of ondansetron was a significant predictor of defecation on that day in their critical care patient cohort.

Constipation

From practice we know that constipation is a common issue for critically ill patients, but reported incidence varies enormously from 5–83%.[87] Variations in incidence may be attributed to the lack of a consistent definition for constipation. Constipation is described as fewer than three bowel movements per week, incomplete evacuation, hard or difficult to pass stools or the requirement of manual faecal removal, according to the American Gastroenterological Association.[88]

Non-pharmacological methods to reduce constipation include exercise or moving, increasing fluid intake and adding dietary fibre.[78] These means should be implemented routinely before the need to use laxatives arises. There are many types of laxatives available, which can be given to prevent or treat constipation. Bulk-forming agents work by increasing faecal size; stimulants, such as senna, increase peristalsis; and osmotic agents draw fluid into the gut. Faecal impaction should be treated with enemas, not stimulant laxatives. In general, existing protocols advise that treatment of constipation should commence with senna administration and, if ineffective after 2–3 days, lactulose should be commenced.[81]

Diarrhoea

Diarrhoea can be a major problem for intensive care patients, and in severe cases may lead to electrolyte imbalances, dehydration, malnutrition (see also Chapter 19) and skin breakdown. Furthermore, it can be very distressing for the patient, who may also suffer from abdominal distension, nausea and cramp-like pain. Investigations should be implemented to determine the cause of the diarrhoea and the patient should be managed with appropriate precautions to prevent cross-contamination if the cause is infectious. If laxatives are being given they should be stopped, and a stool specimen should be obtained for microbiological examination. Anti-motility drugs may be used, except with bloody diarrhoea or proven infection with *E. coli*.[81] Appropriate re-hydration should be implemented. If patients are being fed enterally there may be a reduction in episodes of diarrhoea if fibre-enriched feed is used.[78]

Faecal containment devices should be used in severe cases of diarrhoea in conjunction with all other measures to support the patient's comfort.[89] The patient should be assessed for suitability for using the incontinence system as per the manufacturer's guidelines as there are significant contraindications for use of some systems. Broadly, indications for use of a faecal containment device are persistent diarrhoea, diagnosis of *C. difficile* infection, peri-anal wound or skin breakdown in the presence of incontinence, plus the patient must have anal sphincter tone to enable securement of the device balloon.[90,91] There are many conditions and factors that may prevent a patient being suitable for these devices such as allergy to the materials in the product and including the risk of autonomic dysreflexia in spinal cord injury patients, but mostly they relate to rectal and anal conditions.[90,91] It is imperative that both medical and nursing consultation occurs, along with patient consent before use of such devices as the potential for complications ranges from discomfort and failure of the device through to infection and rectal and bowel injuries. Significant rectal haemorrhage associated with the use of faecal management devices has been described in case reports[92–95] as well as the development of recto-urethral and ano-vaginal fistulas.[93,95] An appropriate bowel therapy regimen and close monitoring of these systems should be implemented to optimise functioning and reduce risk.

> ### Practice tip
>
> Monitoring the security and position of a faecal management system is necessary for effective functioning of the system as well as the prevention of pressure-related injury and potential rectal bleeding.

Urinary catheter care

Urinary catheters are inserted into many critically ill patients. Catheter-associated urinary tract infections (CAUTI) are a common cause of infection in this group, and are associated with increased mortality and length of stay in the ICU.[96] Monitoring the incidence of CAUTI is a requirement in many jurisdictions. In principle, urinary catheters should be inserted only when deemed clinically necessary, and they should be removed as soon as they are no longer required clinically. Alternatives to urinary catheterisation should be considered; however, most critically ill patients require accurate monitoring of their urinary output and fluid balance, and a catheter is required for this reason.[97] CAUTI are primarily caused by contamination from the healthcare worker or from the patient's own flora during catheter insertion or management of the urinary drainage system or via reflux of contaminated urine.[98,99] While routine screening for urinary tract infection is not required,[98] critical care nurses should be mindful of the risk factors for CAUTI such as prolonged catheterisation, older patients, impaired immunity and any breaches in good practices related to the insertion and maintenance of urinary catheters and drainage.[98] The consequences of poor urinary catheter care and management are not only distressing to the patient but detrimental to their health.

Urinary catheterisation assessment

The rationale for urinary catheter insertion outlined in Table 6.12 should be carefully considered. Once it is established that a urinary catheter is necessary, the type of catheter should be determined. While the primary purpose of urinary catheters is management of urine drainage, the choice of catheter type may be influenced by the concurrent need for urinary temperature monitoring. The smallest size catheter possible is used to reduce urethral damage[98] although narrow-bore tubes flex easily, which can be problematic in male catheterisation where the urethra rounds the prostate gland. Larger-diameter catheters may be required to drain haematuria and clots. The routine use of antibiotic-impregnated catheters or silver alloy catheters is not currently recommended.[98]

Urinary catheterisation essential care

Catheter insertion and maintenance should be according to facility policies and undertaken by people appropriately trained in the procedures.[98,99] Aseptic techniques should be adhered to during catheter insertion, and hand hygiene should be performed before and after and gloves used during any manipulation of the catheter or drainage system.[98]

TABLE 6.12
Urinary catheter quick reference

COMPONENT OF CARE	CONSIDERATIONS
Rationale for insertion and/or continuing use *Re-evaluate continuing use daily against rationale and remove catheter as soon as possible when no longer required*	Acute urinary retention or bladder obstruction Need for accurate measurement of urinary output in critically ill patients Perioperative use for selected surgical procedures Assist in healing of open sacral or perineal wounds in incontinent patients Patient requiring prolonged immobilisation, e.g. spinal injury Patient admitted with chronic indwelling catheter Exceptional circumstances such as to improve end-of-life care
Insertion *Use principles of aseptic non-touch technique*	Follow documented facility policy on urinary catheter insertion Staff performing procedure follow policy and are trained in technique Use sterile equipment, including sterile drape Use aseptic technique when inserting catheter and connecting to sterile drainage system Clean meatus with sterile normal saline before catheter insertion Use appropriate sterile, single use lubricant or anaesthetic gel Secure catheter after insertion to prevent movement and urethral traction Document insertion information in patient record
Maintenance *Consider each shift:* • *How long has the catheter been in situ?* • *Is the catheter still required?* • *Are there any indications of infection or complications?* • *Is the drainage system being managed appropriately?*	Maintain aseptic continuously closed system drainage Perform hand hygiene and use non-sterile gloves prior to any manipulation of the drainage system Position drainage bag to prevent backflow or contact with floor Empty drainage bag frequently to maintain urine flow and prevent reflux and empty before patient transport Use separate urine collection container for each patient, avoiding contact between drainage bag and container. This collection container should be discarded if single use or cleaned and sterilised if reusable Change drainage bags only according to manufacturers' guidelines or patients clinical need, without clamping as it is unnecessary Daily meatal hygiene via routine hygiene Avoid use of bladder irrigation, instillation or washouts as routine measures to prevent catheter-associated infections Document all related assessment and procedures for the catheter and drainage system

Adapted from NHMRC Australian guidelines for the prevention and control of infection in healthcare, <http://www.nhmrc.gov.au>; 2010 [accessed 06.14].

The urine drainage system should be sterile and continuously closed with an outlet designed to avoid contamination. It should have a sample port for taking urine samples. Where appropriate, patients should be given a choice of system suited to their needs: for example, a shorter drainage tube with a leg-bag may be more comfortable for a patient who is mobile. All procedures involving the catheter and drainage system should be documented in the clinical notes, including size and type of catheter, balloon size and the date of insertion. If an anticipated date of removal is also documented at the time of insertion and subsequent assessments, it may trigger staff to remove the catheter as soon as possible.

Catheter maintenance

The ongoing need for a urinary catheter should be assessed on a daily basis. The introduction of criteria that enable registered nurses to remove catheters without a medical review may result in a reduction in catheter-related infections. Routine hygiene at appropriate intervals for patient comfort is adequate for urethral meatal care.[98]

Cleansing with antiseptic solution is not recommended and can lead to multi-resistant organism infection.

Urinary catheters should be changed according to clinical need and with regard to the manufacturer's guidelines, and the closed drainage system should be broken only for limited, clearly defined clinical reasons. Bladder washout or irrigation should be avoided and only performed for a specific clinical reason, such as intermittent irrigation for clots or debris. If obstruction is likely, a closed continuous irrigation system may be utilised.

Critically ill patients should be provided with appropriate information about their catheters and drainage system, according to their needs and ability to understand. The drainage system should be simple to operate with one hand and easy to position, and the tap should have an open–close device. Contamination of the outlet must be avoided during emptying. An aseptic technique and sterile equipment must be used when taking a urine sample via the sample port. The sample port should be cleaned with an alcohol wipe for 30 seconds before and after sampling. Urine samples should be taken on clinical need and must be refrigerated if more than 1 hour is expected to elapse before the specimen reaches the laboratory.

The whole drainage system should be maintained with patient comfort in mind, and care should be taken to ensure that the patient is not lying on the drainage tube, which can cause pressure sores and blockage. Furthermore, the catheter itself should be positioned and then secured so that it is not pulling on the urethra or kinked. The drainage bag should be kept below the level of the bladder at all times to maintain an unobstructed flow of urine,[98] and it should be emptied into a disinfected or single-use container. The drainage bag should be changed according to the manufacturer's instructions, which is usually in the range of 5–7 days. In addition, it should be replaced if it is leaking, if there has been a break in the closed system or whenever the catheter is changed.

> **Practice tip**
>
> Using a catheter support device or bandage on the leg to secure the urinary catheter is recommended. This lessens tension and irritation from catheter movement, patient comfort is improved, and it also promotes effective drainage and, in restless patients, may prevent accidental catheter removal as well.

Care of the elderly

Older and elderly patients are being admitted to the intensive care unit in greater numbers as this section of the population continues to grow.[100] There are no absolute definitions of elderly, but the United Nations describes 60 plus years as older, while many developed countries use 65 plus years as older. Some groupings of chronological age may have an older person between 65 and 75, elderly person between 75 and 85 and very elderly over 85 years. However, ageing is more than chronological age, especially related to health, where biological and psychological ageing may be more of a factor. In an Australian and New Zealand cohort, those over 80 years were more often admitted to the ICU with cardiac and gastrointestinal conditions than patients in younger age groups, although rates of admissions for sepsis were comparable between the elderly and young groups.[100]

There are a multitude of physiological changes that result from ageing and critical care nurses should be aware of these differences so that therapies and care can be titrated and adjusted accordingly.[101]

Common causes of anemia in the elderly are iron deficiency and the presence of chronic disease or inflammation followed by chronic kidney dysfunction. The presence of anemia not only adversely affects outcomes from illness, but adds to the elderly patient's difficulties with mobility and managing daily activities. When critically ill, this may contribute to the elderly patient's fatigue, so careful consideration should always be given to planning activities such as hygiene and mobilisation. Some elderly patients are quite fragile, this being the

result of anorexia of ageing,[102,103] and, after 65 years of age, a person may have less body fat and lower weight as a consequence of reduced food intake. Other consequences include impaired muscle function and decreased bone mass, which will impair mobility and lead to increased falls. The decrease in bone mass is also age-related and the decline begins in the 40s, so in the elderly this is quite significant.[101] Mobility problems are exacerbated by both loss of muscle mass and function and degenerative joint disease.[101] Loss of muscle mass and then muscle activity reduces metabolic function and subsequently causes loss of body heat, so care should be taken to ensure the older patient is well covered at all times with additional lightweight warming devices available to be used as required.

Skin, the biggest organ, is often the most visible sign of age in the older patient. The epidermis atrophies especially in exposed areas of the body, and once over 65 years, blistered skin takes longer to repair than in a young adult. From fragile to easily bruised skin or moist skin folds in those who are overweight, careful hygiene care is required and consideration should be given to the use of specific products for these patients.

> **Practice tip**
>
> Pay extra attention to the positioning of devices when used in elderly patients and check them more frequently than normal, as the patient may not have full sensation in the affected area or the physical ability to adjust the device themselves, or the confidence to tell you that the device is causing pressure or discomfort. Examples may be non-invasive blood pressure cuffs that are left on too long or sequential compression device leggings that have slipped.

Persistent abdominal discomfort and pain should be triggers for considering bowel obstruction in the elderly, as with age the colon is hypotonic resulting in slower stool transit and subsequent increased hardening of the stool from dehydration.[101] Faecal incontinence in the elderly can be as a result of loss of anal sphincter tone and, therefore, planning for toileting is a practical way of managing continence and eliminating the distress caused by this problem. Symptoms of urinary tract infection such as dysuria and frequency are less likely to be as obvious in the elderly as the young, as the capacity of the bladder decreases with age and especially if the patient suffers from stress incontinence already.[101] As with other functions, ageing blunts the immune system response, which results in increased susceptibility of the elderly to infection. This, along with the additional deterioration in skin integrity and likely increased exposure to antibiotics over time, means that this group of patients may be at greater risk of hospital-acquired infections and multi-resistant organisms.

Consideration should be given to a suitable environment for the elderly, such as increased sound proofing, more comfortable and supportive chairs and cutlery and utensils that are easy to grip to enable more comfortable meals.

Above all, nurses should adjust some of their behaviours with the older person, such as speaking clearly, listening carefully without interruption, anticipating frequent personal care needs and allowing time to enable mobilisation without haste, all of which may help to facilitate feelings of independence and control of their circumstances for these patients.

Bariatric considerations

Obesity continues to be a major health issue around the world. While many bariatric patients will present to hospital with various health issues, obesity has its own physiological impact to be considered, such as impaired chest expansion and respiration from a large abdomen or insulin resistance related to altered glucose metabolism.[104,105] Close glucose monitoring regimens should be implemented and appropriately calculated dosages for medications prescribed. Adapted techniques to enhance patient assessment may be required, such as auscultating over the left lateral chest wall to hear heart sounds while the patient is positioned towards their left side or using a thigh or regular blood pressure cuff on the patient's forearm.[104]

Studies have found that persons who are obese contend with a negative bias within a social context,[106] but this same negative bias from health professionals including nurses may then interfere with their ability to obtain quality health care.[107,108] According to Susan Bejciy-Spring, the key to providing quality, patient-centred, sensitive care to the bariatric patient is R-E-S-P-E-C-T: **r**apport, **e**nvironment/**e**quipment, **s**afety, **p**rivacy, **e**ncouragement, **c**aring/**c**ompassion and **t**act.[108] Simple things such as an appropriately sized gown and suitable bed linen that provide the patient with adequate covering are often not well-organised for this patient group, unless the nurse takes the time to arrange specific supplies if they are not routinely available.

Sedation in the bariatric patient needs to be carefully managed to avoid the resultant risk of respiratory failure and need for ventilation. Reducing narcotic usage through use of combinations of other analgesia along with sedatives will also reduce the risk of respiratory failure.[109] Bispectral index monitoring can be used to assist in the titration of sedations during procedures where levels of sedation that eliminate awareness and recall are necessary.[109]

The use of arterial monitoring rather than non-invasive blood pressure measurements for patients receiving titrated vasoactive infusions should be considered, because of the difficulty in obtaining accurate readings if the cuff is not sized or positioned correctly. Use specific bariatric equipment and techniques to move patients safely for both the patient and the staff involved. It is important to be aware of the weight capacities of various facilities, such as lifts and equipment, which may be required in the care of the bariatric patient.

Overweight patients can be challenging in any setting, and it is important to consider the health and safety of the staff involved in lifting and moving patients. Equally important is maintaining the patients' dignity and feelings of safety and minimising their self-consciousness during repositioning, irrespective of the method required. Lifts and hoists and other equipment that are designed for heavier people should be used.[110,111] A well-thought-out strategy by an interdisciplinary group can work through the local issues within a hospital or unit and produce a bariatric kit, containing a range of equipment appropriate to the needs of the bariatric patients in various settings including the ICU.[111]

A major concern in the ICU is the positioning of the morbidly obese patient with respect to airway management and oxygenation. Boyce et al found no differences in the difficulty of airway management when patients were in the 30° reverse Trendelenburg (head up, feet down), supine-horizontal or 30° back-up position.[112] However, when patients were positioned in the reverse Trendelenburg position, their oxygen saturation dropped the least and took the shortest time to recover. While the reverse Trendelenberg position should decrease pressure on the diaphragm and therefore decrease intrathoracic pressure, a likely outcome of using this position is the patient slipping down the bed and then having to be re-positioned, so frequent tilt adjustments may assist with limiting this consequence. Ask patients about techniques that work for them at home when re-positioning and mobilising. As with all patients, bariatric patients are vulnerable to fears and anxieties resulting from their illness; however, additional concerns for their physical safety may be experienced, such as during re-positioning, if the activity is not arranged competently and with sensitivity. Care should be given to monitoring the obese patient, especially those post bariatric surgery with prolonged immobility, for pressure-induced rhabdomyolysis.[113]

As obese persons often have venous stasis disease, VTE prophylaxis in bariatric patients is vital especially for those patients having bariatric surgery. Routine prophylaxis is recommended with weight-adjusted dosing of medications.[70,105] Combining pharmacological and mechanical prophylaxis is recommended for this high-risk group. The application of leggings or sleeves for sequential compression devices or pneumatic venous pumps can often be easier than applying graduated compression stockings in any patient when they are supine in bed. Care must be taken with measuring the limb to obtain the correct size legging or stocking. Careful monitoring of the limb for signs of skin deterioration from moisture or of pressure from an ill-fitting legging, sleeve or stocking must be undertaken diligently in the bariatric patient.[70] The insertion of a removable inferior vena cava (IVC) filter as a component of pulmonary embolism prophylaxis for patients undergoing bariatric surgery may occur in some institutions,[105] especially patients with BMI >50 kg/m², or with prior history of thromboembolism. The post-operative management of the bariatric patient will include nutrition to support tissue repair. The use of post pyloric enteral nutrition may be of benefit in reducing the risk of aspiration in the bariatric patient, as these patients often experience postoperative vomiting and nausea.[109] For critically ill patients who are obese, nutritional goals are similar to those of other patients but may include weight reduction while preserving lean muscle.[114] Unless there is a particular rationale for the use of a urinary catheter for the patient, plans should be in place for assisting the bariatric patient with toileting, as many obese patients have stress incontinence.

General principles of infection control in critical care

Effective infection control is vital in the critical care setting to prevent further health risks to critically ill patients already compromised by their disease or trauma (Box 6.3). And a vital factor of infection control is effective hand hygiene. Critically ill patients often require multiple invasive devices and therapies to manage their illness and these increase the potential risk to the patient of infection. While using therapeutic medical devices is often vital to the management of the patient, they are not without risk. Ventilator-associated pneumonia (VAP), catheter-associated urinary tract infections (CAUTIs) and central line-associated bacteraemia (CLAB) are all aligned with invasive device use and form a significant source of healthcare-acquired infections (HAIs) within critical care.[99] Critical care staff themselves need to protect against contracting infections while providing care for their patients.

When patients are admitted to critical care it is impossible to identify whether or not they are newly colonised with bacteria, or are carrying an infection, without further investigation. Standard Precautions are applied in the management of all patients regardless of the reason for their admission. Standard Precautions include: hand hygiene, respiratory hygiene and cough etiquette; the use of appropriate personal protective equipment; safe handling of sharps, waste and used linen; appropriate cleaning and environmental controls; appropriate re-processing of reusable equipment; and the use of aseptic non-touch techniques during procedures.[99]

With the advent of influenza outbreaks, there has been an emphasis on respiratory hygiene and cough etiquette, which effectively means covering the mouth with a tissue when coughing or sneezing and then immediately disposing of the tissue into waste bins, followed by effective hand hygiene.[99] Further Transmission-based Precautions are implemented as required in response to suspicion (while awaiting confirmation from tests) or diagnosis of a condition in which Standard Precautions may not be sufficient to control the transmission of microorganisms.[99] Transmission-based Precautions appropriately applied to specific microorganisms disrupt their method of transmission to other patients, visitors and healthcare workers. Transmission-based Precautions include continuation of Standard Precautions, the use of personal protective equipment specific to the risk of transmission, individual patient equipment where possible and specific cleaning

---

BOX 6.3

Infection-control guidelines for the prevention of transmission of infectious diseases in the healthcare setting[99]

- Healthcare-associated infections are those acquired in care establishments ('nosocomial' infections) and infections that occur as a result of healthcare interventions ('iatrogenic' infections). The infection may manifest after people leave the healthcare establishment.

- A healthcare establishment is any facility that delivers healthcare services.

- Healthcare workers (HCWs) are all people delivering healthcare services, including students, trainees and mortuary attendants, who have contact with patients or with blood and body substances.

- Standard precautions are standard operating procedures that apply to the care and treatment of all patients, regardless of their perceived infection risk. They are work practices required to achieve a basic level of infection control and are recommended for the treatment and care of all patients.

- Transmission-based precautions are required when standard precautions may not be sufficient to prevent the transmission of infectious agents (e.g. in tuberculosis, measles, Creutzfeldt–Jakob disease). These precautions are tailored to the specific infectious agent concerned and may include measures to prevent airborne, droplet or contact transmission, and healthcare-associated transmission agents (see Table 6.13).

- Transmission-based precautions are recommended for patients known or suspected to be infected or colonised with disease agents that cause infections in healthcare settings and that may not be contained by standard precautions alone.

Adapted from NHMRC Australian guidelines for the prevention and control of infection in healthcare, <http://www.nhmrc.gov.au>; 2010 [accessed 06.14].

---

protocols for shared equipment, placement of patients in single rooms (or cohorted if appropriate) and specific air filtration or circulation and environmental cleaning protocols.[99]

There are three types of Transmission-based Precautions recommended to counteract the various infectious agents: Contact Precautions, Droplet Precautions and Airborne Precautions[99] (see Table 6.13). These types of precautions are applied with refinement to the use of personal protective equipment, room requirements and recommendations for visitors specific to the mode of transmission of the organism. Critical care nurses should be knowledgeable about both local and national guidelines and protocols for infection control in order to provide safe

TABLE 6.13

Transmission-based precautions and infectious conditions

TRANSMISSION-BASED PRECAUTIONS	EXAMPLES OF INFECTIOUS CONDITIONS
Contact	MROs : MRSA, MRGN, VRE, ESBL, CRE Gastrointestinal pathogens: *C. difficile*, norovirus Highly contagious skin infections
Droplet	Influenza RSV Meningococcal
Airborne	Pulmonary TB Chickenpox (varicella), measles (rubella) SARS, MERS

CRE = carbapenem resistant Enterobacteriaceae; ESBL = extended-spectrum beta-lactamase-producing (Enterobacteriaceae); MERS = Middle East respiratory syndrome coronovirus; MRGN = ; MRO = multi-resistant organism; MRSA = methicillin-resistant Staphylococcus aureus; RSV = pertussis; SARS = severe acute respiratory syndrome; TB = tuberculosis; VRE = vancomycin-resistant enterococcus.

Adapted from NHMRC Australian guidelines for the prevention and control of infection in healthcare, <http://www.nhmrc.gov.au>; 2010 [accessed 06.14], with permission.

care to all their patients. Breaks to the consistent application of Standard Precautions and, when implemented, Transmission-based Precautions put patients at risk, especially those who are critically ill.

Although good hand hygiene is the single most effective tool in infection control,[115,116] the key components of effective infection control are surveillance, prevention and control, which are described in more detail.

Surveillance

ICU patients may be colonised or infected with a multi-resistant organism (MRO) prior to admission,[117] so routine screening should be undertaken to detect the presence of bacteria. Ideally, all critically ill patients will be screened for multi-resistant *Staphylococcus aureus* (MRSA) and vancomycin-resistant *Enterococcus* (VRE) on admission.[117] Regular surveillance to identify rates of nosocomial infection, with feedback to critical care staff, helps to improve compliance with infection control guidelines.[99] In the 1980s, a landmark study established that hospital-acquired infection may be reduced by around a third if surveillance and prevention programs are implemented.[118]

Prevention

The Australian Government Department of Health and Ageing provides guidelines for infection control within the healthcare setting (see Box 6.3).[99] All health services should apply designated guidelines and operate within clearly defined infection-control procedures, which are based on Standard Precautions. Although formerly referred to as 'Universal Precautions' and 'Additional Precautions', the recent guidelines on infection control from the National Health and Medical Research Council uses the terms 'Standard Precautions' and 'Transmissions-based Precautions', respectively, to clearly describe these levels of precautions.[99] Critical care nurses should refer to their specific hospital infection-control policies regarding details of procedures that must be followed.

Control

Once an organism has been identified, the goal is to limit its spread. Although patients may be colonised with bacteria, they may not be infected. Colonisation refers to the presence of microorganisms in any amount, whereas infection means that pathological tissue injury or disease has occurred due to the invasion and multiplication of the microorganism.[119] Typically, surveillance measures identify many patients who are colonised with MRSA or VRE and, although they themselves are not infected, it is important to stop the spread of bacteria to patients more vulnerable and thus more susceptible to opportunistic infection, by implementing Transmission-based Precautions.[120] Several measures demonstrated to be effective in managing multi-resistant bacterial infections in ICUs are summarised in Box 6.4. Due to the vulnerable nature of critically ill patients, specific issues are described in more detail including: hand hygiene, personal protective equipment (PPE), MROs, HAIs, VAP and CLAB.

BOX 6.4

Preventative measures to reduce the spread of MRO infection

- Identifying the infected patient – infection control notification in patient's record
- Hand washing with antiseptic solution before and after contact with the patient
- Contact precautions using gloves and gowns during direct patient contact
- Separation of stethoscopes, sphygmomanometers and thermometers for individual use
- Separation of other articles and equipment for exclusive use of the patient
- Daily surface cleaning and disinfection

Adapted from:
NHMRC. Australian guidelines for the prevention and control of infection in healthcare, <http://www.nhmrc.gov.au>; 2010 [accessed 06.14], with permission.
Haley RW, Culver DH, White JW, Morgan WM, Emori TG, Munn VP et al. The efficacy of infection surveillance and control programs in preventing nosocomial infections in US hospitals. Am J Epidemiol 1985;121(2):182–205, with permission.

Hand hygiene

At the core of Standard Precautions is effective hand hygiene. Good hand hygiene is a simple yet effective technique that reduces the spread of bacteria. It is the most effective and least expensive method of preventing healthcare-associated or nosocomial infection.[115] However, hand hygiene compliance is poor,[99,115] but can be improved significantly if regular education programs, feedback and reminders are employed.[99,116] For example, the five moments for hand hygiene (see Box 6.5) created by the World Health Organization (WHO) in 2009[115] can be adopted for local implementation, such as by Hand Hygiene Australia.[116] Evidence has led to the current recommendation of using an alcohol-based hand rub for hand hygiene unless the hands are soiled.[115,116,121] The use of alcohol hand rubs is associated with higher rates of hand hygiene compliance and effectiveness although effectiveness is dependent on technique.[115,116,121]

BOX 6.5

WHO '5 moments' of hand hygiene

Hand hygiene is performed:

- before touching a patient
- before commencing a procedure
- after a procedure or exposure to body fluids
- after touching a patient
- after touching a patient's environment

plus

- after the removal of gloves.

Adapted from Grayson L, Russo P, Ryan K. Hand hygiene. Australia manual. Australian Commission for Safety and Quality in Healthcare 2009, <http://www.hha.org.au/>; [accessed 11.10], with permission.

Personal protective equipment (PPE)

PPE may include any and all of the following: plastic aprons, gowns (single use or sterile), gloves (single use or sterile), masks ranging from surgical to particulate filter N95 mask or P2 respirators and eye protection such as goggles or face shields that also protect mucous membranes of the mouth and nose.[99] Specific sequences have been outlined for putting on and taking off PPE that minimise the risk of contamination.[99]

Epidemic outbreaks of severe acute respiratory syndrome (SARS) coronavirus occurred in Canada, China, Hong Kong, Singapore and Vietnam[122] in 2003 and cases were reported in over 25 countries.[123] SARS was transmitted between patients, healthcare workers and hospital visitors, and large within-hospital outbreaks were associated with aerosol-generating procedures such as bronchoscopy, endotracheal intubation and the use of aerosol therapy,[123] which are commonplace in critical care areas. In Hong Kong, more than 20% of cases were healthcare workers.[124] Because of the high level of morbidity and mortality associated with SARS,[125] the risk to healthcare staff is considerable and, during the Hong Kong SARS outbreak, healthcare workers wore full head covers with a visor.[126]

Previous research has demonstrated relatively low rates of compliance with standard precautions, ranging from 16% to 44%.[127] The SARS outbreaks emphasised the need for effective infection-control procedures, especially for airborne pathogens. With airborne pathogens such as pulmonary TB or the Middle East respiratory syndrome coronavirus (MERS-CoV),[128,129] Airborne Precautions[129] using properly fitted N95 masks (face mask with 95% or greater filter efficiency), gowns and gloves are implemented to reduce the spread of the organism, plus the use of airborne infection isolation rooms or negative air pressure rooms with room exhaust via high-efficiency particulate air (HEPA) filtration and strict control of family visiting.[129] Additional measures may include the use of high-efficiency bacterial filters to filter patients' expired air, closed suction systems and ventilator scavenging systems.[126]

MERS-CoV was first reported in 2012 in Saudi Arabia and, up to 2014, there were nearly 700 cases in countries near to the KSA and from travelers returning home from the area.[129] The severity of respiratory infection symptoms varies, but as of 2014 the mortality is around 30% for confirmed MERS-CoV infections.[129]

The influenza H1N1 pandemic alerted everyone to the need for vigilance in infection control. The use of Droplet

Precautions is the main feature of infection control for influenza, along with early testing.[130] The influenza outbreak also drew attention to the need for vaccinations. Influenza vaccines are developed as the influenza A virus changes. All healthcare workers and especially those in critical care should be knowledgeable of the vaccinations that may be available to them through their employers and those that are recommended by local jurisdictions. A variation of the avian influenza A (H7N9) virus was first reported in China in 2013.[131]

> ### Practice tip
>
> Reminder: hand hygiene is performed before putting on PPE and after removing PPE. Hand hygiene is also performed after removal of gloves.

Multi-resistant organisms

MROs, or multi-drug-resistant organisms, is a collective term for a number of infections from multi-resistant organisms. While the early diagnosis of an MRO and immediate implementation of organism-specific Transmission-based Precautions is key to management, it is true that MRSA and extended-spectrum beta-lactamase-producing *Enterobacteriaceae* (ESBL-E) have reached epidemic proportions. Multiple strains of MRSA have been identified, and in many studies ICUs have the highest incidence.[120] In the past decade VRE has become a serious health issue and, more recently, carbapenem-resistant *Enterobacteriaceae* (CRE).[132] Other multi-resistant organisms include multi-drug resistant *Pseudomonas aeruginosa* and *Acinetobacter* spp.[119] As with MRSA, transmission of these other MROs is associated with contact.

There are a number of methods for reducing the spread of MROs (see Box 6.4), although not all methods may be effective and, if the organism is not identified, its spread will continue unseen. Another key component of management of MROs is surveillance, such as the routine screening for MRSA and VRE of all patients on admission to critical care areas and on a regular basis thereafter. Once diagnosed, it is common practice to use single rooms for patients with MROs to reduce cross-infection. Growing antimicrobial resistance can be reduced with effective infection prevention and control and prescribing antibiotics only when needed.

Healthcare-acquired infections (HAI)

Nosocomial, or hospital- or healthcare-acquired, infection (HAI) is a major problem in critical care that may affect up to 20% of patients, with a mortality of around 30%.[117] Critically ill patients are 5–10 times more likely to become infected than hospital ward patients.[119] Multi-drug-resistant bacteria are a worldwide problem; their acquisition by patients can lead to infection with the same bacteria, and multiple antibiotic therapy encourages the proliferation of resistant organisms.[119] The introduction of antibiotic stewardship assists in focusing on the optimal use of antibiotics.[99]

Medical devices or therapies may expose patients to the potential risk of acquiring an HAI. This risk may occur during the insertion procedure or subsequent maintenance care of the medical device, unless appropriate techniques are used. The use of an aseptic technique during insertion of a device is a feature of infection control, asepsis being the elimination of pathogens. Aseptic non-touch technique is a format for guiding practice in the application.[133,134] Standard aseptic non-touch technique involves standard hand hygiene, a general aseptic field and non-sterile or sterile gloves and is used for minor procedures that are simple and of short duration, that is, less than 20 minutes. Examples of procedures include simple wound dressings and intravenous cannulation or urinary catheterisation by proficient practitioners. Surgical aseptic non-touch technique is used for complex or lengthy procedures such as insertion of a central venous catheter and involves the use of full barrier precautions (sterile gown and gloves, face mask), extensive drapes and critical aseptic field.[99] Box 6.6 provides some basic points to guide management of the use of medical devices in critical care.

The commonest HAIs occur at surgical sites, the urinary tract, lower respiratory tract and bloodstream. For the critically ill patient intravascular cannulas including central venous catheters, urinary catheters, enteral or nasogastric tubes and artificial airways and ventilation are some of the healthcare devices associated with risk. See the section on urinary catheters for information regarding catheter-associated urinary tract infections.

Ventilator-associated pneumonia

Ventilator-associated pneumonia (VAP) is common in intensive care and usually occurs within 48 hours of initiating ventilation.[135] Changing entire team practices

> ### BOX 6.6
>
> #### Invasive device management
>
> - Does the patient need the invasive device for effective management of their condition?
> - Is the chosen device the most suitable for the individual patient, e.g. size and type of device?
> - Are the healthcare professional/s trained to safely insert and manage the device?
> - Use the appropriate aseptic procedure for device insertion.
> - Follow management protocols to minimise the risk of infection while the device is in situ.
> - Monitor the patient for signs and symptoms of infection.
> - Review the need for the device in the management of the patient daily and remove as early as possible.
>
> *Adapted from:* NHMRC. Australian guidelines for the prevention and control of infection in healthcare, <http://www.nhmrc.gov.au>; 2010 [accessed 06.14], with permission.

and behaviours is critical to successful reduction of VAP within an intensive care unit.[136,137] A number of strategies that are effective in helping to prevent infection[135] are identified in Table 6.14, and two of the simplest and most effective are raising the head of the bed and frequent oral hygiene.[31] Effective analgesia and minimising sedation plus avoidance of muscle-relaxant medications along with early mobilisation are some of the other strategies that may contribute to the reduction of VAP. Using a heat and moisture exchanger (HME) limits the need to change ventilator circuits, while maintaining a closed ventilator circuit and the use of closed suction systems for endotracheal suction assist with prevention strategies.

Selective digestive decontamination has been studied extensively. In theory, the use of antimicrobial agents to reduce gut flora in intubated intensive care patients reduces the risk of pneumonia due to micro aspiration (see Chapter 19). Although most studies have demonstrated a reduction in the incidence of VAP, there has been an inconsistent reduction in ICU mortality, and there remains concern about the promotion of antimicrobial resistance with its prolonged use.[138] Related information on respiratory failure, VAP and ventilation can be found in Chapters 14 and 15.

Central line-associated bacteraemia (CLAB)

The use of central lines is common in critical care areas. Catheter-related sepsis is defined by the International Sepsis Forum as at least one peripheral positive blood culture plus at least one of the following: a positive catheter tip culture, a positive hub or exit-site culture or a positive paired central and peripheral blood culture where the central culture is positive ≥2 hours earlier than the peripheral culture or has 5 times the growth.[139] CLAB is one of the most important and severe infections that can occur in ICU. Renal failure may significantly increase the risk of infection.[140] Berenholtz et al demonstrated that implementing quality improvement measures to ensure adherence to evidence-based infection control guidelines results in a significant reduction of catheter-related bloodstream infection.[141]

Southworth et al[142] noted that, after implementing strategies to reduce CLAB, staff engagement in constant vigilance is required to maintain success. The use of antibiotic-impregnated catheters has been shown to reduce bacteraemia[143] and, although it is common practice in many critical care units to routinely change intravenous administration sets, with antiseptic-coated catheters they can be used safely for up to 7 days.[144] Currently available evidence supports the use of maximal barriers (head cap, face mask, sterile body gown, sterile gloves and full-size body drape) during routine insertion of central venous catheters along with antiseptic solutions to prepare the skin, and catheter insertion by appropriately trained personnel.[99] Chapter 3 contains information on central line care bundles and checklists. Although chlorhexidine solutions are recommended, their effectiveness depends upon the strength of the solution. In Australia decontamination of the insertion site is with 0.5% chlorhexidine gluconate in 70% isopropyl alcohol.[99] Nurses are responsible for the maintenance of central venous catheters once inserted, including care of the insertion site dressing and infusion line management. The types of dressing commonly used are transparent semi-permeable and, more recently, chlorhexidine gluconate gel dressings.[99,145] Transparent dressings are advantageous because they allow direct observation of the entry site of the catheter. Dressings should be replaced whenever their seal is broken or every 7 days.[99] Catheter hubs are another site of colonisation for microorganisms such as *Staphylococcus epidermidis*, and effective hand hygiene combined with non-touch aseptic techniques when accessing the catheter hub should be implemented. Intravenous administration sets containing blood products or lipids or parenteral nutrition infusions are changed when the infusion completes or daily, while others are changed according to local protocols. Infusions such as

---

TABLE 6.14
Strategies to prevent VAP

MEASURE	INTERVENTIONS
Infection control measures	• Hand hygiene • Active surveillance • Appropriate PPE when managing ventilation-related devices, e.g. ETT, ventilator circuits, tracheal suctioning
Gastrointestinal tract	• 2-hourly oral hygiene • Stress ulcer prophylaxis • Avoid gastric over-distention • Enteral nutrition
Patient position	• Semi-recumbent with head raised to >30° • Rotational bed therapy
Artificial airway	• Respiratory airway care • Avoid unplanned extubations • Secure tracheal airway cuff • Inline or intermittent subglottic secretion removal
Mechanical ventilation	• Maintenance of ventilation equipment, heat and moisture exchangers, safe removal of condensate from circuits • Minimisation of ventilation time • Daily interruption to sedation and/or assessment for readiness to wean therapy and/or extubate • Non-invasive mechanical ventilation

ETT = endotracheal tube; PPE = personal protective equipment; VAP = ventilator associated pneumonia.

Adapted from NHMRC. Australian guidelines for the prevention and control of infection in healthcare, <http://www.nhmrc.gov.au>; 2010 [accessed 06.14], with permission.

propofol or nitroglycerine may have additional manufacturer guidelines regarding administration set changes.[99]

After removal of the catheter, and once homeostasis has been established, the site should be covered with an occlusive dressing, which should be left in place for 48 hours to minimise the risk of infection. The catheter should be examined after removal and any damage reported. It may be hospital or unit policy to send the catheter tip for culture and sensitivity; however, a recent single-centre study has shown that colonisation is heaviest at the intravascular proximal segment compared to the distal tip of the catheter.[146]

Practice tip

Unless contraindicated in a specific patient, a central venous catheter dressing should be changed whenever there is evidence of fluid accumulation or loss of the dressing's occlusive seal.

Transport of critically ill patients: General principles

The transport of a critically ill patient may occur for several reasons, such as from an accident site, categorised as pre-hospital transport, or to move a patient to another facility for treatment, which is known as inter-hospital transport, or within a hospital from one department to another, this being intra-hospital transport.[147] This section will focus on intra-hospital transport, while inter-hospital transport is described in Chapter 23. A large proportion of intra-hospital transports occur from the emergency department[148] to the critical care unit. Another significant group is the deteriorating patient within a hospital ward who requires emergency transfer to the ICU. Patients within the ICU may require transport to imaging departments for scans or operating theatres for procedures or cardiac cathlab for angiography.

Guidelines for the transport of critically ill patients are available in many countries including Australia and New Zealand[147,149] with the principles applying to intra-hospital and other transport.[147,150] Specific guidelines may need to be observed for certain groups of patients, for example those with head injury. A careful assessment of risk versus benefit should be undertaken before making a decision to transport a patient.[150,151] To reduce the risk of adverse events during transport, various diagnostic tests or surgical procedures should be evaluated in terms of their potential to be undertaken in the critical care unit.[149]

Considerations

Fanara et al[152] outlined a diversity of adverse events during intra-hospital transport. In one study 16.8% of intra-hospital transport adverse events were considered serious.[153] Recognition of the risk of adverse events during intra-hospital transports has long been a concern in critical care and remains so today.[154,155]

The primary focus of assessment should be on patient safety and the prevention of adverse events. A transport 'event' can be any event that has an adverse impact and can be patient-, staff- or equipment-related.[152,155] The patient may be adversely affected during transport, ranging from anxiety or pain to respiratory or cardiovascular compromise.[152] Staff may have difficulty with managing the patient's needs during transport and equipment-related problems during transport of critically ill patients are a major consideration along with device dislodgement.[154,155] Risk–benefit assessment is helpful to identify patients with a high risk of complications.[151] For example, the potential risk of moving a severely head-injured patient with unstable intracranial pressure may outweigh the potential benefit of a CT scan. Parmentier-Decrucq et al[153] 'found sedation of the patient before transport, PEEP >6 cmH$_2$O and the need for fluid infusion for transport, to be risk factors for any adverse event during intra-hospital transport'. Meticulous planning for all aspects of the transport, based on a thorough assessment of the patient's anticipated needs, is the key to safe intra-hospital transport.[147,151] Consideration of specific patient needs such as the availability of lifting devices for transferring bariatric patients from bed to CT table or appropriate warming devices for the use of elderly patients during lengthy interventional radiological procedures need to be communicated to the procedural areas prior to transport commencing so that no delays occur. A comprehensive outline of information addressing key components of intra-hospital transport of critically ill patients should be available to personnel at every hospital.[147,149]

Safe transport requires accurate assessment and stabilisation of the patient before transport.[147] Key elements[150] are identified in Box 6.7. Securing vascular accesses should be a primary concern, while some consideration may be given to having two intravenous accesses in situ. All equipment should be checked for functionality prior to transport and, while it is vital to ensure that sufficient

BOX 6.7

Key elements of safe transfer

- Experienced staff
- Appropriate equipment
- Full assessment and investigation
- Extensive monitoring
- Careful stabilisation of patient
- Reassessment
- Continuing care during transfer
- Direct handover
- Documentation and audit

Adapted from Wallace PGM, Ridley SA. ABC of intensive care: transport of critically ill patients. Br Med J 1999;319(7206): 368–71, with permission.

equipment is taken to maintain the patient, unnecessary equipment complicates the logistics of managing the transport smoothly. Specifically constructed transport beds or attachments such as equipment tables designed to support equipment safely during transfer are useful.[147,151] The period of transport should ideally be as short as possible, although safety should not be sacrificed for speed. Pre-planning the route of transport and good dialogue between department staff can help to maximise the efficiency of transport and reduce unnecessary delays.[149] At all times, the team must be confident that all safety considerations have been made. Flabouris et al[156] noted both 'haste' and 'pressure to proceed' with transport as contributing factors in adverse events.

> **Practice tip**
>
> Transport preparation should include: 1) establishing the need and purpose of transport; 2) time duration relating to the route to be taken, length of procedure and return journey; 3) necessary equipment; 4) patient preparation; 5) appropriately skilled and numbers of staff; 6) supplies required to continue therapies during transport event; and 7) consideration of emergency and contingency plans.

Essential nursing care during transport

Essential care during transport involves three components: the patient, the personnel and the equipment and monitoring. Importantly, the patient and their family should be given an explanation of why the transport is necessary, how long the procedure is expected to take and that the transport process includes a team accompanying the patient to continue monitoring and provide any required treatment.

Nursing responsibilities during transport of the patient include all aspects of patient and therapy monitoring, comfort and maintaining appropriate documentation. Continuous or frequent monitoring of the patient's vital signs and physiological parameters and equipment alarms and parameters should be undertaken throughout the transport event, and all equipment should be checked regularly to ensure correct functioning. Gas reserves of oxygen cylinders and battery time of all devices require pre-transport calculation before being used and vigilant attention during transport. Patient safety is paramount and close attention to detail is required. Throughout the transport, patients should be reassured regarding their condition and the progress of the purpose of the transport.

The level of experience and specialty of personnel involved in the transport of critically ill patients are factors influencing safe transport.[147,149] Staff should be trained in the various aspects of patient transport,[147,154] including competent management and troubleshooting of all equipment required for particular patient needs,

e.g. intra-aortic balloon pump. Team members should be aware of their specific roles and ensure excellent communication throughout the transport procedure.

> **Practice tip**
>
> Staff involved in patient transports should be knowledgeable of the most efficient route to take as well as the facilities at their destination such as power and gas supplies.

Equipment used during patient transport must be robust, lightweight and battery-powered,[151] and must adhere to relevant national manufacturing and safety standards. Equipment-related complications occur in around a third of transports.[154] All equipment must be adequately secured during transport, and must be available continuously to the operator.[147] Oxygen requirements should be calculated in advance (or it should be established that piped oxygen is available at the destination department) to ensure an adequate supply, both for the journey and for the duration of the investigation/procedure. Standard equipment for inter-hospital transport is identified in Table 6.15[147] and, while some items may be unnecessary for all intra-hospital transport, this table provides a useful checklist so that all necessary equipment is taken. Additional specialist equipment may be required for certain patients, such as spare tracheostomy tubes in case of accidental extubation.

> **Practice tip**
>
> To ensure safe equipment preparation, especially during emergency transport events, have two nurses perform independent checks against a transport checklist that includes battery life and gas cylinder data for equipment in your unit as a standard transport preparation practice.

Before transport, all equipment should be prepared and checked, including the function of visible and audible alarms. All non-essential therapy should be discontinued temporarily during the transport, such as enteral nutrition. Where possible, therapies should be simplified, such as exchanging chest drainage systems for one-way valves, or disconnecting completed infusion administration sets from intravenous lines. The patient's physical safety should be maintained and care should be taken to ensure that bed rails are used and the patient's limbs are secure and not likely to be injured by equipment. All vital monitoring and therapy equipment should be transferred to portable equipment, and the patient should be stabilised before being moved. Some transport equipment ventilators may not provide identical parameters or functioning to a ventilator the patient is already using, so time must be taken to adjust the transport ventilator to effective ventilation for the patient. If the patient is being transported for magnetic resonance imaging (MRI), it is important to ensure that all equipment is compatible.

TABLE 6.15
Standard equipment for intra-hospital transport

RESPIRATORY SUPPORT EQUIPMENT	CIRCULATORY SUPPORT EQUIPMENT	OTHER EQUIPMENT	PHARMACOLOGICAL AGENTS
• Airway management equipment, including intubation set, range of endotracheal tubes and laryngeal mask airways, hand ventilation set with PEEP valve and emergency surgical airway set • Oxygen, masks, nebuliser • Pulse oximeter and capnography • Sufficient oxygen supply • Suction equipment • Portable ventilator with disconnect and high-pressure alarms • Pleural drainage equipment	• Monitor/defibrillator/external pacer combined unit • Non-invasive blood pressure device • IV cannula, IV fluids, pressure infusion set, infusion pumps • Arterial cannulae and arterial monitoring device • Syringes and needles, sharps disposal container • Pericardiocentesis equipment	• Nasogastric tube and bag • Dressings, antiseptic lotions, bandages, tape, • Torch • Thermal insulation and temperature monitor • PPE for transport team	• Checked and clearly labelled drugs: standard resuscitation drugs and those specific to the patient's condition

IV = intravenous; PPE = personal protective equipment.

Adapted from College of Intensive Care Medicine Australia and New Zealand (CICM). Guidelines for transport of critically ill patients, <http://www.cicm.org.au>; 2013 [accessed 06.14], with permission.

Practice tip

If ceasing nutrition during patient transport, make sure that the patient is not at risk of hypoglycaemia from concurrent insulin therapy.

The need for monitoring relates to both the patient and equipment, and is identified in Table 6.16.[147] Some monitoring should be continuous, such as cardiac, oxygen saturation, capnography if the patient is intubated and arterial, pulmonary artery and intracranial monitoring if the respective devices are in situ. Intermittent monitoring of central venous pressure (CVP), non-invasive blood pressure and respiratory rate should be undertaken as indicated by the patient's condition.[147]

A complete record should be kept of all details of the patient's condition, personnel involved, clinical events, observations and therapy given during transport. The transporting team should hand over directly to the receiving team providing continuing care for the patient[151,154] or should remain during the intervention/procedure to manage the patient's care.

TABLE 6.16
Monitoring during transport

CLINICAL PATIENT MONITORING	EQUIPMENT MONITORING
• Circulation • Respiration • Oxygenation • Neurological • Pain score • Patient comfort	• Pulse oximeter, and capnography • Breathing system alarms • Electrocardiograph • Physiological pressures • Other clinically indicated equipment • Audible and visual equipment alarms

Adapted from College of Intensive Care Medicine Australia and New Zealand (CICM). Guidelines for transport of critically ill patients, <http://www.cicm.org.au>; 2013 [accessed 06.14], with permission.

Summary

In the management of critically ill patients there is always an initial focus on assessing and treating the patient's most life-threatening and immediate problems. Early attention should then be given to the implementation of preventative therapies such as VTE prophylaxis and pressure injury prevention, along with a thorough assessment of physical care needs and a subsequent plan of management. Recovery for patients to normal functioning after a critical illness is dependent upon a multitude of factors and is a dynamic process over time; however, much of the essential nursing care given to critically ill patients assists in both reducing deficits associated with their episode of illness and reducing the time taken to achieve normal functioning.

Good personal hygiene is at the heart of essential nursing care, and many other aspects of essential care (e.g. eye care and oral care) are closely related. Personal hygiene is often attended to when patients are repositioned, and whenever they are moved the nurse has an opportunity to assess patients, particularly their dependent pressure areas. Bowel and urinary catheter care are vital but often neglected areas of care. When patients are critically ill, the development of preventable complications such as constipation and urinary tract infection may have significant consequences for them. All critically ill patients are at risk of infection, and essential nursing care requires effective application of surveillance, prevention and control measures that should be applied equally to all patients. This principle is embedded in the recommended use of standard precautions.

Critically ill patients are often transferred to other departments for further investigation or specific interventions. All transports pose a potential risk to patients, particularly if they are unstable. Essential nursing care of patients during transfer is based on thorough assessment and preparation in an attempt to anticipate their every need so that adverse events do not occur. This chapter has provided a comprehensive overview of the general but essential nursing care of critically ill patients. It offers a guideline for nurses that is relevant for most patients, most of the time. As with all other aspects of nursing practice, nursing care and intervention should be based on a thorough assessment of each individual patient and tailored to their needs and preferences.

Case study

Mrs C is a 70-year-old female living in a supported residential care home. She presented to the emergency department with abdominal pain, fevers and general malaise. Mrs C was febrile with mild tachycardia and her blood pressure was slightly lower than her normal reading. Initial investigations revealed a urinary tract infection and pyelonephritis. Her white cell count was 47 and IV antibiotics were initiated and she was admitted to a medical ward. Mrs C has diabetes controlled with oral hypoglycaemics and hypertension managed with medication.

Mrs C is a widow with one daughter who lives interstate. Mrs C moved to the residential home 5 years ago because of her increasing inability to cope with daily living in her own home, exacerbated by long-term depression and increasing obesity. Mrs C lives a relatively solitary life, having become increasingly withdrawn from interactions with other residents, and has almost become bed bound due to limited mobility. She presented to hospital with a stage 2 pressure injury on her sacrum and oedema of her lower limbs.

The day after being admitted to the medical ward, Mrs C was in increasing abdominal discomfort and was found to have midline suprapubic abdominal wall distension. An ultrasound showed a suprapubic abdominal wall collection. Reviewed by a surgeon, and on suspicion of necrotising fasciitis, it was determined that debridement needed to be undertaken urgently. A CVC and arterial catheter had been inserted in preparation for theatre to provide vascular access for an aramine infusion and to monitor Mrs C's decreasing blood pressure.

After a 7-hour operation involving plastic, urology and general surgeons performing a laparotomy, pelvic exploration and extensive surgical debridement through to abdominal rectus, Mrs C was transferred to the intensive care unit. Preparatory handover from the anaesthetic team prior to Mrs C's transfer from the operating theatre enabled her to be placed directly onto a suitable pressure relief mattress system bed in the ICU. She arrived in the ICU intubated and ventilated, still under the effects of the anaesthetic and with a noradrenaline infusion sustaining a mean arterial pressure of 70 mmHg. She had an indwelling catheter with temperature sensor in situ displaying a temperature of 39°C but, despite intraoperative fluids of 7 units of packed red cells and 2 units of fresh frozen plasma, had minimal urine output. Her limbs were oedematous with knee-high leggings in situ for sequential compression therapy and a bolus of intravenous albumin was administered. Mrs C's abdominal wound extended down to the perineum and was packed but not closed.

Over the following days Mrs C's management was focused on the treatment of sepsis, management of an extensive open wound and prevention of further infection and prevention of other complications related to invasive devices, ventilation, reduced mobility and poor skin condition. Ideally, wound management would have included the use of negative pressure wound management systems; however, the extent of Mrs C's wound and the inability to seal the wound negated this as an option. Use of prostan-soaked dressings with 4-hourly irrigation kept the wound clean and moist between returns to the operating theatre for debridement. Because of the involvement of the perineum in the wound area, the wound was compartmentalised and dressed in sections. Undertaking frequent wound care in a manner that was safe and effective for both Mrs C and the nursing team meant good preparation of wound care supplies and planning of various nursing roles for participation in the dressing and re-positioning of Mrs C a number of times during the dressing procedure. As well as pain management, comfort and reassurance were provided for Mrs C during this time-consuming and intrusive procedure. A faecal containment system was inserted to manage faecal incontinence but, due to lack of rectal tone, leakage occurred and it was removed. As with any transport of a critically ill patient outside the ICU, returns to theatre for wound debridement required patient preparation, appropriate equipment and liaison with the theatre personnel for timing, so that other activities related to Mrs C's care could continue.

Positioning Mrs C for pressure injury prevention, wound care and comfort required good planning and appropriate equipment and sufficient personnel.

After six daily returns to the operating theatre for wound debridement, Mrs C's clinical condition had improved sufficiently and she was extubated. And 3 days afterward, she was stable enough for transfer to the surgical ward with ongoing infectious diseases review regarding the duration of antibiotic therapy.

CASE STUDY QUESTIONS

1 What is necrotising fasciitis and what are the most common bacteria involved?
2 Outline the extrinsic and intrinsic factors of tissue tolerance that may have had significance for Mrs C during her stay in ICU.

RESEARCH VIGNETTE

Duncan CN, Riley TV, Carson KC, Budgeon CA, Siffleet J. The effect of acidic cleanser versus soap on the skin pH and micro-flora of adult patients: a non-randomised two group crossover study in an intensive care unit. Int Crit Care Nurs 2013;29:291–296

Abstract

Objective: To test the effects of two different cleansing regimens on skin surface pH and micro-flora, in adult patients in the intensive care unit (ICU).

Methods: Forty-three patients were recruited from a 23-bed tertiary medical/surgical ICU. The 19 patients in group one were washed using soap for daily hygiene care over a 4-week period. In group two, 24 patients were washed daily using an acidic liquid cleanser (pH 5.5) over a second 4-week period. Skin pH measurements and bacterial swabs were sampled daily from each patient for a maximum of 10 days or until discharged from the ICU.

Results: Skin surface pH measurements were lower in patients washed with a pH 5.5 cleanser than those washed with soap. This was statistically significant for both the forearm ($p = 0.0068$) and leg ($p = 0.0015$). The bacterial count was not statistically significantly different between the two groups. Both groups demonstrated that bacterial counts were significantly affected by the length of stay in ICU ($p = 0.0032$).

Conclusions: This study demonstrated that the product used in routine skin care significantly affects the skin pH of ICU patients, but not the bacterial colonisation. Bacterial colonisation of the skin increases with length of stay.

Critique

This small study was a single site non-randomised and unblinded study. The study was labelled a prospective descriptive crossover design. The design was used to prevent product substitution with the intervention (soap or a pH 5.5 liquid cleanser). However, this study appears to be an A-B intervention design, where a group of participants received treatment A over a 4-week period and the next group of participants received treatment B over a 4-week period. In a crossover design participants serve as their own controls (i.e. they receive the intervention and crossover to receive the placebo), but this did not occur in this study; therefore, the term 'crossover' appears misleading. Comparing the same participants also provides less statistical variance in the results; however, this would be difficult to manage in the critically ill patient population.

All patients admitted to the ICU during the study period (n = 344) were screened. Those with an anticipated length of stay of greater than 48 hours were recruited. Patients were excluded if they had pre-existing skin conditions or known allergies to the skin cleanser. Forty-three patients were recruited to the study over an 8-week period, with 19 patients in group one and 24 patients in group two. It would have been helpful if participant progress through the phases of the two groups (that is, enrolment, intervention allocation, follow-up and data analysis) was provided diagrammatically. Transparent reporting of trials is an important issue. Given only 12.5% (43/344) of potential patients were enrolled in the study it would have been interesting to note the reasons for exclusion.

A clear description of the study procedures was provided. Details about the study procedures, processes and interventions allow others to replicate them in future research. However, the researchers did not mention collecting data on intervention fidelity, or the extent to which the bed-bathing protocol was performed as was planned. Further, it is not clear what 'usual care' for bed-bathing was at the study site.

The study results were presented clearly. Importantly, this study did not use methods of randomisation. Randomisation is a method to try to ensure the groups are similar in all known and unknown characteristics, which is important in that this will control for the effect of potential confounders. The researchers noted the characteristics between the two groups were similar but these specific characteristics were not reported. Only the potential confounder of length of stay was acknowledged and found to be associated with increased bacterial colonisation. In other words, the longer the patient remained in ICU, the greater the chance of the skin becoming colonised with bacteria.

The researchers acknowledged and explained study findings, identifying the importance of the relationship between skin pH and potential disruption of the skin integrity, the stratum corneum, through critical illness. Overall, the researchers should be commended on undertaking this important small descriptive study. Finally, and very importantly, other researchers interested in this work could use the results of this study to inform a larger three-arm randomised controlled trial.

Learning activities

1 List the benefits and risks of faecal containment devices.
2 Outline ICU patient preparation for transfer to the operating theatre.
3 What criteria do you use to evaluate the positioning in bed of your patients?
4 Name some of the significant infection risks for patients in ICU.

Online resources

Australian Department of Health, www.health.gov.au

Australian Wound Management Association, www.awma.com.au

Cochrane Collaboration, www.cochrane.org

College of Intensive Care Medicine of Australia and New Zealand (CICM), www.cicm.org.au

Communicable Diseases Network Australia (CDNA), www.health.gov.au/cdna

European Pressure Ulcer Advisory Panel, www.epuap.org

Hand Hygiene Australia, www.hha.org.au

National Health and Medical Research Council, www.nhmrc.gov.au

National Institute of Clinical Studies (NICS), www.nhmrc.gov.au/nics/index.htm

Skin Tear Advisory Panel, www.skintears.org/pdf/Skin-Tear-Resource-Kit.pdf

Therapeutic Goods Australia, www.tga.gov.au/index.htm

US Centers for Disease Control and Prevention, www.cdc.gov

World Health Organization, www.who.int/en

Further reading

College of Intensive Care Medicine Australia and New Zealand (CICM). Guidelines for transport of critically ill patients, <http://www.cicm.org.au>; 2013 [accessed 06.14].

Khoury J, Jones M, Grim A, Dunne WM Jr, Fraser V. Eradication of methicillin-resistant *Staphylococcus aureus* from a neonatal intensive care unit by active surveillance and aggressive infection control measures. Infect Control Hosp Epidemiol 2005;26(7):616–21.

Wright MO, Hebden JN, Harris AD, Shanholtz CB, Standiford HC, Furuno JP et al. Concise communications: aggressive control measures for resistant *Acinetobacter baumannii* and the impact on acquisition of methicillin-resistant *Staphylococcus aureus* and vancomycin-resistant *Enterococcus* in a medical intensive care unit. Infect Control Hosp Epidemiol 2004;25(2):167–8.

References

1 Vollman KM. Interventional patient hygiene: discussion of the issues and a proposed model for implementation of nursing care basics. Intensive Crit Care Nurs 2013;29:250–255.

2 Burns SM, Day T. A return to the basics: 'Interventional patient hygiene'. Intensive Crit Care Nurs 2013;29:247–249.

3 Larson EL, Ciliberti T, Chantler C, Abraham J, Lazaro EM, Venturanza M et al. Comparison of traditional and disposable bed baths in critically ill patients. Am J Crit Care 2004;13(3):235–41.

4 Coyer F, O'Sullivan J, Cadman N. The provision of patient personal hygiene in the intensive care unit: a descriptive exploratory study of bed-bathing practice. Aust Crit Care 2011;24(3):198–209.

5 Australian Wound Management Association. Pan Pacific Clinical Practice Guideline for the Prevention and Management of Pressure Injury. AWMA; March 2012. Osborne Park, WA: Cambridge Publishing.

6 Holtzclaw BJ. Shivering in acutely ill vulnerable populations. AACN Clin Issues 2004;15(2):267–79.

7 Burr S, Penzer R. Promoting skin health. Nurs Stand 2005;19(36):57–65.

8 NHS Quality Improvement Scotland. Ear Care Best Practice Statement, <http://www.nhshealthquality.org/nhsqi/files/EARCARE_BPS_MAY06.pdf>; 2006 [accessed 11.10].

9 LeBlanc K, Baranoski S, the International Skin Tear Advisory Panel 2013. Skin tears: the state of the science: consensus statements for the prevention, prediction, assessment and treatment of skin tears. Adv Skin Wound Care 2011;24(9 Suppl):2–15.

10 Nair PN, White E. Care of the eye during anaesthesia and intensive care. Anaesthesia Intensive Care Med 2014;15(1):40-43.

11 Joyce N. Eye care for the intensive care patient. Adelaide: Joanna Briggs Institute for Evidence Based Nursing and Midwifery; 2002.

12 Newswanger DL, Warren CR. Guillain–Barré syndrome. Am Fam Physician 2004;69(10):2405–10.

13 Rosenberg JB. Eye care in the intensive care unit: narrative review and meta-analysis. Crit Care Med 2008;36(12);3151-3155.

14 Dawson D. Development of a new eye care guideline for critically ill patients. Intensive Crit Care 2005;21(2):119–22.

15 Marshall A, Elliott R, Rolls K, Schacht S, Boyle M. Eye care in the critically ill: clinical practice guideline. Aust Crit Care 2008;21(2);97-109.

16 Bates J, Dwyer R, O'Toole L, Kevin L, O'Hegarty N, Logan P. Corneal protection in critically ill patients: a randomized controlled trial of three methods. Clin Intensive Care 2004;15(1):23–6.

17 Koroloff N, Boots R, Lipman J, Thomas P, Rickard C, Coyer F. A randomised controlled study of the efficacy of hypromellose and Lacri-Lube combination versus polyethylene/cling wrap to prevent corneal epithelial breakdown in the semiconscious intensive care patient. Intensive Care Med 2004;30(6):112–16.

18 Ezra DG, Chan MP, Solebo L, Malik AP, Crane E, Coombes A et al. Randomised trial comparing ocular lubricants and polyarylamide hydrogel dressings in the prevention of exposure keratopathy in the critically ill. Intensive Care Med 2009;35(3):455–61.

19 So HM, Lee CC, Leung AK, Lim JM, Chan CS, Yan WW. Comparing the effectiveness of polyethylene covers (Gladwrap) with lanolin (Duratears) eye ointment to prevent corneal abrasions in critically ill patients: a randomized controlled study. Int J Nurs Stud 2008;45(11):1565–71.

20 Micik S, Besic N, Johnson N, Han M, Hamyln S, Ball H. Reducing risk for ventilator associated pneumonia through nurse sensitive interventions. Intensive Crit Care Nurs 2013;29:261-265.

21 Berry AM, Davidson PM. Beyond comfort: oral hygiene as a critical nursing activity in the intensive care unit. Intens Crit Care Nurse 2006;22(6):318–28.

22 Binkley C, Furr LA, Carrico R, McCurren C. Survey of oral care practices in US intensive care units. Am J Infect Control 2004;32(3):161–9.

23 Dale C, Angus JE, Sinuff T, Mykhalovskiy E. Mouth care for orally intubated patients: a critical ethnographic review of the nursing literature. Intensive Crit Care Nurs 2013;29:266-274.

24 O'Reilly M. Oral care of the critically ill: a review of the literature and guidelines for practice. Aust Crit Care 2003;16(3):101–10.

25 Furr LA, Binkley C, McCurren C, Carrico R. Factors affecting quality of oral care in intensive care units. J Adv Nurs 2004;48(5):454–62.

26 Prendergast V, Kleiman C, King M. The Bedside Oral Exam and the Barrow Oral Care Protocol: translating evidence-based oral care into practice. Intensive Crit Care Nurs 2013;29:282-90.

27 Evans G. A rationale for oral care. Nurs Stand 2001;15(43):33–6.

28 Pearson LS, Hutton JL. A controlled trial to compare the ability of foam swabs and toothbrushes to remove dental plaque. J Adv Nurs 2002;39(5):480–89.

29 Berry AM, Davidson PM, Masters J, Rolls K. Systematic literature review of oral hygiene practices for intensive care patients receiving mechanical ventilation. Am J Crit Care 2007;16(6):552–62.

30 Fields LB. Oral care intervention to reduce the incidence of ventilator-associated pneumonia in the neurologic intensive care unit. J Neurosci Nurs 2008;40(5):291–8.

31 Munro CJ, Grap MJ, Jones DJ, McClish DK, Sessler CN. Chlorhexidine, toothbrushing, and preventing ventilator-associated penumonia in critically ill adults. Am J Crit Care 2009; 18(5):428–37.

32 Puntillo KA, Nelson JE, Weissman D, Curtis R, Weiss S, Frontera J et al. Palliative care in the ICU: relief of pain, dyspnea and thirst – a report from the IPAL ICU Advisory Board. Int Care Med 2014;40(2):235-48.

33 Berry AM. A comparison of Listerine® and sodium bicarbonate oral cleansing solutions on dental plaque colonization and incidence of ventilator associated pneumonia in mechanically ventilated patients: a randomized control trial. Intensive Crit Care Nurs 2013;29:275-81.

34 Houston S, Hougland P, Anderson JJ, LaRocco M, Kennedy V, Gentry LO. Effectiveness of 0.12% chlorhexidine gluconate oral rinse in reducing prevalence of nosocomial pneumonia in patients undergoing heart surgery. Am J Crit Care 2002;11(6):567–70.

35 Tombes MB, Gallucci B. The effects of hydrogen peroxide rinses on the normal oral mucosa. Nurs Res 1993;42(6):332–7.

36 Didari T, Solki S, Mozaffari S, Nikfar S, Abdollahi M. A systematic review of the safety of probiotics. Expert Opin Drug Saf 2014;13(2):227-39.

37 National Pressure Ulcer Advisory Panel, European Pressure Ulcer Advisory Panel. Pressure ulcer prevention and treatment clinical practice guideline. Washington DC: National Ulcer Advisory Panel; 2009.

38 Fan E, Zanni JM, Dennison CR, Lepre SJ. Critical illness neuromyopathy and muscle weakness in patients in the intensive care unit. AACN Advanced Crit Care 2009;20(3):243–53.

39 de Jonghe B, Lacherade JC, Sharshar T, Outin H. Intensive care unit-acquired weakness: risk factors and prevention. Crit Care Med 2009;37(10):S309–15.

40 Griffiths RD, Hall JB. Intensive care unit-acquired weakness. Crit Care Med 2010;38(3):779–87.

41 Needham DM. Mobilizing patients in the intensive care unit: improving neuromuscular weakness and physical function. J Med Assoc 2008;300(14):1685–90.

42 Needham DM, Korupolu R, Zanni JM, Pradhan P, Colantuoni E, Palmer JB et al. Early physical medicine and rehabilitation for patients with acute respiratory failure: a quality improvement project. Arch Phys Med Rehabil 2010;91(4):536–42.

43 Vollman KM. Introduction to progressive mobility. Crit Care Nurse 2010;30(2):S3–5.

44 Schweickert WD, Pohlman MC, Pohlman AS, Nigos C, Pawlik AJ, Esbrook CL et al. Early physical and occupational therapy in mechanically ventilated, critically ill patients: a randomised controlled trial. Lancet 2009;373(9678):1874–82.

45 Truong AD, Fan E, Brower RG, Needham DM. Bench-to-bedside review: mobilizing patients in the intensive care unit – from pathophysiology to clinical trials. Crit Care 2009;13(4):167.

46 Krishnagopalan S, Johnson EW, Low LL, Kaufman LJ. Body positioning of intensive care patients: clinical practice versus standards. Crit Care Med 2002;30(11):2588–92.

47 Tayyib N, Coyer F, Lewis P. Pressure injuries in the adult intensive care unit: a literature review of patient risk factors and risk assessment scales. J Nurs Educ Prac 2013;3(11):28-42.

48 Berenholtz SM, Dorman T, Ngo K, Pronovost PJ. Qualitative review of intensive care unit quality indicators. J Crit Care 2002;17(1):1–12.

49 Resar R, Pronovost P, Haraden C, Simmonds T, Rainey T, Nolan T. Using a bundle approach to improve ventilator care processes and reduce ventilator-associated pneumonia. Joint Commiss J Qual & Patient Safety 2005;31(5):243–8.

50 Clavet H, Hebert PC, Fergusson D, Doucette S, Trudel G. Joint contracture following prolonged stay in the intensive care unit. Can Med Assoc J 2008;178(6):691–7.

51 Jankowski IM. Tips for protecting critically ill patients from pressure ulcers. Crit Care Nurse 2010;30(2):S7–9.

52 Stiller K. Safety issues that should be considered when mobilizing critically ill patients. Crit Care Clin 2007;23(1):35–53.

53 Timmermann RA. A mobility protocol for critically ill adults. Dimens Crit Care Nurs 2007;26(5):175–9.

54 Casey CM. The study of activity: an integrative review. J Gerontol Nurs 2013;39(8):12-25.

55 Koch SM, Fogarty S, Signorino C, Parmley L, Mehlhorn U. Effect of passive range of motion on intracranial pressure in neurosurgical patients. J Crit Care 1996;11(4):176–9.

56 Brimioulle S, Moraine JJ, Norrenberg D, Kahn RJ. Effects of positioning and exercise on intracranial pressure in a neurosurgical intensive care unit. Phys Ther 1997;77(12):1682–9.

57 Powers GC, Zentner T, Nelson F, Bergstrom N. Validation of the mobility subscale of the Braden Scale for predicting pressure sore risk. Nurs Res 2004;53(5):340–46.

58 Jastremski C. Back to basics: can body positioning really make a difference in the intensive care unit? Crit Care Med 2002;30(11):2607–8.

59 Jones A, Dean E. Body position change and its effect on hemodynamic and metabolic status. J Acute Crit Care 2004;33(5):281–90.

60 Weststrate J, Heule F. Prevalence of pressure ulcers, risk factors and use of pressure-relieving mattresses in ICU patients. Connect 2001;1(3):77-82.

61 Jackson C. The revised Jackson/Cubbin Pressure Area Risk Calculator. Intens Crit Care 1999;15(3):169–75.

62 Coyer F, Stotts NA, Blackman VS. A prospective window into medical device-related pressure ulcers in intensive care. Int Wound J 2013. doi: 10.1111/iwj.12026.

63 National Pressure Ulcer Advisory Panel. Mucosal pressure ulcers: An NPUAP position statement. Washington DC: National Ulcer Advisory Panel; 2009.

64 Swaderner-Culpepper L. Continuous lateral rotation therapy. Crit Care Nurse 2010;30(2):S5–7.

65 Goddard R. Use of rotational therapy in the treatment of early acute respiratory distress syndrome (ARDS): a retrospective case report. Connect 2004;3(3):82–5.

66 Kirschenbaum L, Azzi E, Sfeir T, Tietjen P, Astiz M. Effect of continuous lateral rotational therapy on the prevalence of ventilator-associated pneumonia in patients requiring long-term ventilatory care. Crit Care Med 2002;30(9):1983–6.

67 Goldhill DR, Imhoff M, McLean B, Waldman C. Rotational bed therapy to prevent and treat respiratory complications: a review and meta-analysis. Am J Crit Care 2007;16(1):50–62.

68 Rauen CA, Flynn-Makic MB, Bridges E. Evidence-based practice habits: transforming research into bedside practice. Crit Care Nurse 2009;29(2):46–59.

69 NHMRC. Clinical practice guideline for the prevention of venous thromboembolism (deep vein thrombosis and pulmonary embolism) in patients admitted to Australian hospitals. Melbourne: National Health and Medical Research Council; 2009.

70 Kakkos SK, Caprini JA, Geroulakos G, Nicolaides AN, Stansby GP, Reddy DJ. Combined intermittent pneumatic leg compression and medication for prevention of deep vein thrombosis and pulmonary embolism in high-risk patients. Coch Database Syst Rev 2011; 4 (CD005258. pub2). doi: 10.1002/14651858.

71 Access Economics. The burden of venous thromboembolism in Australia. 2008. Report for the Australian and New Zealand working party on the management and prevention of venous thromboembolism, <http//www.accesseconomics.com.au/ publicationsreports/showreport.php>; [accessed 11.10].

72 Geerts WH, Bergqvist D, Pineo GF, Heit JA, Samama CM, Lassen MR et al. Prevention of venous thromboembolism: American College of Chest Physicians evidence-based clinical practice guidelines (8th edition). Chest 2008; 133: S381–453.

73 Sachdeva A, Dalton M, Amaragiri SV, Lees T. Elastic compression stockings for prevention of deep vein thrombosis. Coch Database Syst Rev 2010;7(CD001484). doi: 10.1002/14651858).

74 Douketis J, Cook D, Meade M, Guyatt G, Geerts W, Skrobik Y et al. Prophylaxis against deep vein thrombosis in critically ill patients with severe renal insufficiency with the low-molecular-weight heparin dalteparin: an assessment of safety and pharmacodynamics: the DIRECT study. Arch Intern Med 2008;168:1805–12.

75 Griffen M, Kakkos SK, Geroulakos G, Nicolaides AN. Comparison of three intermittent pneumatic compression systems in patients with varicose veins: a hemodynamic study. Int Angiol 2007;26(2):158–64.

76 Lachiewicz PF, Kelley SS, Haden LR. Two mechanical devices for prophylaxis of thromoboembolism after total knee arthroplasty. A prospective, randomised study. J Bone Joint Surg 2004;86(8):1137–41.

77 Kakkos SK, Griffin M, Geroulakos G, Nicolaides AN. The efficacy of a new portable sequential compression device (SCD Express) in preventing venous statis. J Vasc Surg 2005;42(2):296–303.

78 Rushdi TA, Pichard C, Khater YH. Control of diarrhea by fiber-enriched diet in ICU patients on enteral nutrition: a prospective randomized controlled trial. Clin Nutr 2004;23(6):1344-52.

79 Gacouin A, Camus C, Gros A, Isslame S, Marque S, Lavoue S et al. Constipation in long-term ventilated patients; associated factors and impact on intensive care outcomes. Crit Care Med 2010;38(10):1933-1938.

80 de Azevedo RP, Machado FR. Constipation in critically ill patients: much more than we imagine. Rev Bra Ter Intensiva 2013;25(2):73-4.

81 Dorman BP, Hill C, McGrath M, Mansour A, Dobson D, Pearse T et al. Bowel management in the intensive care unit. Intensive Crit Care Nurs 2004;20(6):320–29.

82 McPeake J, Gilmore H, MacIntosh G. The implementation of a bowel management protocol in an adult intensive care unit. Nurs Crit Care 2011;16(5):235-42.

83 Riegler G, Esposito I. Bristol scale stool form. A still valid help in medical practice and clinical research. Tech Coloproctol 2001;5(3):163–4.

84 Bianchi J, Segovia-Gomez T. The dangers of faecal incontinence in the at-risk patient. Wound Int 2012;3(3):15-21 [cited June 2014]. Available from http://www.woundsinternational.com.

85 Bishop S, Young H, Goldsmith D, Buldock D, Chin M, Bellomo R. Bowel motions in critically ill patients: a pilot observational study. Crit Care Resusc 2010;12(3):182-5.

86 Sawh SB, Selvaraj IP, Danga A, Cotton AL, Moss J, Patel PB. Use of methylnaltrexone for the treatment of opioid-induced constipation in critical care patients. Mayo Clin Proc 2012;87(3):255-9.

87 Mostafa SM, Bhandari S, Ritchie G, Gratton N, Wenstone R. Constipation and its implications in the critically ill patient. Br J Anaesth 2003;91(6):815-9.

88 Locke GR, Pemberton JH, Phillips SF. American Gastroenterological Association Medical Position Statement: guidelines on constipation. Gastroenterology 2000;119(6):1761-6.

89 Padmanabhan A, Stern M, Wishin J, Mangino M, Richey K, DeSane M. Clinical evaluation of a flexible fecal incontinence management system. Am J Crit Care 2007;16(4):384–93.

90 All Wales Guidelines for Faecal Management Systems, <http://welshwoundnetwork.org/dmdocuments/all_wales_faecal_systems.pdf>; 2010 [accessed 06.14].

91 Yates A. Faecal incontinence: a joint approach to guideline development. Nursing Times 2011;107(12):12, <http://www.nursingtimes.net/continence>; [accessed 06.14].

92 Bright E. Fishwick G, Berry D, Thomas M. Indwelling bowel management system as a cause of life-threatening rectal bleeding. Case Rep Gastroenterol 2008;2(3):341-55.

93 Massey J, Gatt M, Tolan DJ, Finan PJ. An ano-vaginal fistula associated with the use of a faecal management system: a case report. Colorectal Dis 2010;12(July (7)):e173-4.

94 Reynolds M, van Haren F. A case of pressure ulceration and associated haemorrhage in a patient using a faecal managment system. Aust Crit Care 2012;25(3):188.

95 A'Court J, Yiannoullou P, Pearce L, Hill J, Donnelly D, Murray D. Rectourethral fistula secondary to a bowel management system. Intensive Crit Care Nurs 2014;30:226-30.

96 Chant C, Smith OM, Marshall JC, Friedrich, JO. Relationship of catheter associated urinary tract infection to mortality and length of stay in critically ill patients: a systematic review and meta-analysis of observational studies. Crit Care Med 2011;39(5):1167-73.

97 Marklew A. Urinary catheter care in the intensive care unit. Nurs Crit Care 2004;9(1):21–7.

98 Mitchell B, Ware C, McGregor A, Brown D, Wells A, Stuart RL et al. ASID (HICSIG)/AICA Position Statement: preventing catheter-associated urinary tract infections in patients. Healthcare Infection 2011;16:45-52, <http://www.publish.csiro.au/journals/hi>; [accessed 06.14].

99 NHMRC. Australian guidelines for the prevention and control of infection in healthcare, <http://www.nhmrc.gov.au>; 2010 [accessed June 2014].

100 Bagshaw SM, Webb SAR, Delaney A, George C, Pilcher D, Hart GK et al. Very old patients admitted to intensive care in Australia and New Zealand: a multi-centre cohort analysis. Crit Care 2009;13:R45 (doi:10.1186/cc7768), <http://ccforum.com/ content/13/2/R45de>; [accessed 06.14].

101 Pisani MA. Considerations in caring for the critically ill older patient. J Intensive Care Med 2009;24(2):83-95.

102 Boer A, Ter Horst GJ, Lorist MM. Physiological and psychosocial age-related changes associated with reduced food intake in older persons. Ageing Res Rev 2013;12(1):316-28.

103 Atalayer D, Astbury NM. Anorexia of aging and gut hormones. Aging Dis 2013;4(5):264-75.

104 Hurst S, Blanco K, Boyle D, Douglass L, Wikas A. Bariatric implications care nursing. Dimens Crit Care Nurs 2004;23(2):76–83.

105 Pieracci FM, Barie PS, Pomp A. Critical care of the bariatric patient. Crit Care Med 2006;34(6):1796–804.

106 Puhl R, Brownell KD. Confronting and coping with weight stigma: an investigation of overweight and obese adults. Obesity 2006;14:1802–15.

107 Brown I. Nurses' attitudes towards adult patients who are obese: literature review. J Adv Nurs 2006;53:221–32.

108 Bejciy-Spring SM. Respect: a model for the sensitive treatment of the bariatric patient. Bariatric Nurs Surg Patient Care 2008;3(1):47-56.

109 King DR, Velmahos GC. Difficulties in managing the surgical patient who is morbidly obese. Crit Care Med 2010;38(9):S478–82.

110 Hignett S, Griffiths P. Risk factors for moving and handling bariatric patients. Nurs Stand 2009;24(11):40–48.

111 Nowicki T, Burns C, Fulbrook P, Jones J. Changing the mindset: an inter-disciplinary approach to management of the bariatric patient. Collegian 2009;16:171–5.

112 Boyce JR, Ness T, Castroman P, Gleysteen JJ. A preliminary study of the optimal anesthesia positioning for the morbidly obese patient. Obes Surg 2003;13(1):4–9.

113 Reed MJ, Gabrielsen J. Bariatric surgery patients in the ICU. Crit Care Clin 2010;26:695-98. doi:10.1016/j.ccc.2010.09.001.

114 McClave SA, Martindale RG, Vanek VW, McCarthy M, Roberts P, Taylor B et al. Guidelines for the provision and assessment of nutritional support therapy in the adult critically ill patient: Society of Critical Care Medicine (SCCM) and American Society for Parenteral and Enteral Nutrition (ASPEN). J Parenteral Enteral Nutr 2009;33(3):277-316.

115 WHO. Guidelines on hand hygiene in healthcare, <http://www.who.int/gpsc/5may/tools>; 2009 [accessed 06.14].

116 Grayson L, Russo P, Ryan K. Hand hygiene. Australia manual. Australian Commission for Safety and Quality in Healthcare, <http://www.hha.org.au/>; 2009 [accessed 11.10].

117 Orsi GB, Raponi M, Franchi C, Rocco M, Mancini C, Venditti M. Surveillance and infection control in an intensive care unit. Infect Control Hosp Epidemiol 2005;26(3):321–5.

118 Haley RW, Culver DH, White JW, Morgan WM, Emori TG, Munn VP et al. The efficacy of infection surveillance and control programs in preventing nosocomial infections in US hospitals. Am J Epidemiol 1985;121(2):182–205.

119 Lim S-M, Webb SAR. Nosocomial bacterial infections in intensive care units. Organisms and mechanisms of antibiotic resistance. Anaesthesiology 2005;60(9):887–902.

120 Hardy KJ, Hawkey PM, Gao F, Oppenheim BA. Methicillin resistant *Staphylococcus aureus* in the critically ill. Br J Anaesth 2004;92(1):121–30.

121 Johnson PDR, Martin R, Burrell LJ, Grabsch EA, Kirsa SW, O'Keeffe J et al. Efficacy of an alcohol/chlorhexidine hand hygiene program in a hospital with high rates of nosocomial methicillin-resistant staphylococcus aureus (MRSA) infection. Med J Aust 2005;183(10):509–14.

122 Gamage B, Moore D, Copes R, Yassi A, Bryce E. Protecting health care workers from SARS and other respiratory pathogens: a review of the infection control literature. Am J Infect Control 2005;33(2):114–21.

123 Lee NE, Siriarayapon P, Tappero J, Chen K, Shuey D. SARS Mobile Response Team Investigators. Infection control practices for SARS in Lao People's Democratic Republic, Taiwan and Thailand: experience from mobile SARS containment teams. Am J Infect Control 2004;32(7):377–83.

124 Lau PY, Chan CWH. SARS (severe acute respiratory syndrome): reflective practice of a nurse manager. J Clin Nurs 2005;14(1):28–34.

125 Ho W, Hong Kong Hospital Authority Working Group on SARS Central Committee of Infection Control. Guideline on management of severe acute respiratory syndrome (SARS). Lancet 2003;361(9366):1313–15.

126 Chan D. Clinical management of SARS patients in ICU. Connect 2003;2(3):76–9.

127 Moore D, Gamage B, Bryce E, Copes R, Yassi A, other members of The BC Interdisciplinary Respiratory Protection Study Group. Protecting health care workers from SARS and other respiratory pathogens: organizational and individual factors that affect adherence to infection control guidelines. Am J Infect Control 2005;33(2):88–96.

128 WHO. Middle East respiratory syndrome coronavirus [MERS-CoV] summary and literature update – as of 11 June 2014, <http://www.who.int/crs/disease/coronavirus_infections/archive_updates/en/>; [accessed 11.14].

129 CDC. Middle East Respiratory Syndrome (MERS), <http://www.cdc.gov/coronavirus/MERS/index.html>; [accessed 07.14].

130 Webb SA, Seppelt IM, ANZIC Influenza Investigators. Pandemic (H1N1) 2009 influenza ("swine flu") in Australia and New Zealand intensive care. Crit Care Resus 2009;11(3):170–2.

131 CDC. Avian influenza A (H7N9) virus, <http://www.cdc.gov/avianflu/h7n9-virus.html>; [accessed 07.14].

132 Australian Commission on Safety and Quality in Health Care (ACSQHC). Recommendations for the control of multi-drug resistant Gram-negatives: carbapenem resistant *Enterobacteriaceae*, <http://www.safetyandquality.gov.au/>; 2013 [accessed 07.14].

133 Pratt RJ, Pellowe CM, Wilson JA, Loveday HP, Harper PJ, Jones SR et al. National evidence-based guidelines for preventing healthcare associated infections in NHS hospitals in England. J Hosp Infect 2007;65:S1–64.

134 Rowley S, Clare S. Improving standards of aseptic practice through an ANTT trust-wide implementation process: a matter of prioritisation and care. Br J Infect Prevention 2009;10(1):S18–23.

135 Coffin S, Klompas M, Classen D, Arias K, Podgorny K, Anderson DJ et al. Strategies to prevent ventilator-associated pneumonia in acute care hospitals. Infect Control Hosp Epidemiol 2008;29(1):S31–40.

136 Sole ML. Overcoming the barriers: a concerted effort to prevent ventilator-associated pneumonia. Aust Crit Care 2005;18(3):92–4.

137 Sedwick MB, Lance-Smith M, Reeder SJ, Nardi J. Using evidence-based practice to prevent ventilator-associated pneumonia. Crit Care Nurs 2012;32(4):41-50.

138 Safdar N, Crnich CJ, Maki DG. The pathogenesis of ventilator-associated pneumonia: its relevance to developing effective strategies for prevention. Respir Care 2005;50(6):725–39.

139 Calandra T, Cohen J. The international sepsis forum consensus conference on definitions of infection in the intensive care unit. Crit Care Med 2005;33(7):1538–48.

140 Hosoglu S, Akalin S, Kidir V, Suner A, Kayabas H, Geyik MF. Prospective surveillance study for risk factors of central venous catheter-related bloodstream infections. Am J Infect Control 2004;32(3):131–4.

141 Berenholtz S, Pronovost P, Lipsett P, Hobson D, Earsing K, Farley JE et al. Eliminating catheter-related bloodstream infections in the intensive care unit. Crit Care Med 2004;32(10):2014–20.

142 Southworth SL, Henman LJ, Kinder LA, Sell JL. The journey to zero central catheter-associated bloodstream infections: culture change in an intensive care unit. Crit Care Nurs 2012;32(2):49-54.

143 Hanna HA, Raad II, Hackett B, Wallace SK, Price KJ, Coyle DE et al. Antibiotic-impregnated catheters associated with significant decrease in nosocomial and multidrug-resistant bacteremias in critically ill patients. Chest 2003;124(3):1030–8.

144 Rickard C, Lipman J, Courtney M, Siversen R, Daley P. Routine changing of intravenous administration sets does not reduce colonization or infection in central venous catheters. Infect Control Hosp Epidemiol 2004;25(8):650–5.

145 Moureau NL, Deschneau M, Pyrek J. Evaluation of the clinical performance of a chlorhexidine gluconate antimicrobial transparent dressing. J Infect Prevention 2009;10:S13–7.

146 Koh DBC, Robertson IK, Watts M, Davies AN. Density of microbial colonization on external and internal surfaces of concurrently placed intravascular devices. Am J Crit Care 2012;21(3):162-71.

147 College of Intensive Care Medicine Australia and New Zealand (CICM). Guidelines for transport of critically ill patients, <http://www.cicm.org.au/>; 2013 [accessed 06.14].

148 Gray A, Gill S, Airey M, Williams R. Descriptive epidemiology of adult critical care transfers from the emergency department. Emergency Med J 2003;20(3):242–6.

149 Warren J, Fromm RE, Orr RA, Rotello LC, Horst M; ACoCCM. Guidelines for the inter- and intrahospital transport of critically ill patients. Crit Care Med 2004;32(1):256–62.

150 Gray A, Bush S, Whiteley S. Secondary transport of the critically ill and injured adult. Emergency Med J 2004;21(3):281–5.

151 Wallace PGM, Ridley SA. ABC of intensive care: transport of critically ill patients. Br Med J 1999;319(7206):368–71.

152 Fanara B, Mazon C, Barbot O, Desmettre T, Capellier G. Recommendations for the intra-hospital transport of critically ill patients. Crit Care 2010;14:R87.

153 Parmentier-Decrucq E, Poissy J, Favory R, Nseir S, Onimus T, Guerry M et al. Adverse events during intrahospital transport of critically ill patients: incidence and risk factors. Ann Intensive Care 2013;3:10.

154 Chang YN, Lin LH, Chen WH, Liao HY, Hu PH, Chen SE et al. Quality control work group focusing on practical guidelines for improving safety of critically ill patient transportation in the emergency department. J Emerg Nurs 2010;36(2):140–5.

155 Venkategowda PM, Rao SM, Mutkule DP, Taggu AN. Unexpected events occurring during the intra-hospital transport of critically ill patients. Indian J Crit Care Med 2014;18(6):354-7.

156 Flabouris A, Runciman WB, Levings B. Incidents during out of hospital patient transportations. Anaesth Intensive Care 2006;34(2):228-36.

Chapter 7

Psychological care

Leanne Aitken, Rosalind Elliott

Learning objectives

After reading this chapter, you should be able to:

- implement appropriate evidence-based strategies to reduce patient anxiety
- describe the different instruments available to assess sedation needs in critically ill patients and discuss the benefits and limitations of each
- describe the subtypes of delirium
- recognise risk factors for the development of delirium in the critically ill
- implement and evaluate delirium assessment screening instruments for the critically ill
- implement appropriate evidence-based strategies to manage patients' sedative needs
- integrate best practice into pain assessment and management
- determine methods to promote rest and sleep for critically ill patients.

Introduction

Care of the psychological health and wellbeing of patients is essential in the complex and multifactorial care of critically ill patients. Patients experience ongoing compromise of their psychological health well beyond hospitalisation, with this psychological compromise also affecting their physical health. Aspects of psychological health most relevant in the care of the critically ill include the recognition and management of anxiety, delirium, sedation needs, pain and sleep and inclusion of the patient's family in promoting psychological health. Although each of these concepts is reviewed sequentially through this chapter, in reality it is often difficult to separate the issues as their effects are often additive or synergistic. While it is important to ensure that assessment incorporates each of the individual concepts, management may often target multiple aspects concurrently.

KEY WORDS

anxiety

delirium

pain assessment and pain management

sedation assessment and management

sedation protocols

sleep promotion

Anxiety

Anxiety can occur both during and following a period of critical illness. Anxiety has been defined as an unpleasant emotional state or condition.[1] Within that broad definition Spielberger recognises two related, but conceptually different constructs, specifically state and trait anxiety. Trait anxiety, a personality characteristic, refers to the relatively stable tendency of people to perceive stressful situations as stressful or anxiety-provoking.[1] In contrast, and of more immediate concern during the care of critically ill patients, is state anxiety, an emotional state that exists at a given moment in time and is characterised by 'subjective feelings of tension, apprehension, nervousness, and worry'.[1] In addition, activation of the autonomic nervous system is present during state anxiety.

Factors that have been identified as precipitating anxiety include:[2,3]

- concern about current illness as well as any underlying chronic disease
- current experiences and feelings such as pain, sleeplessness, thirst, discomfort, immobility
- current care interventions including mechanical ventilation, indwelling tubes and catheters, repositioning and suctioning
- medication side effects
- environmental considerations such as noise and light
- concern about the ongoing impact of illness on recovery.

Anxiety has been identified in approximately half of critically ill patients, with the majority of patients reporting moderate-to-severe anxiety in most cohorts.[4–6] Patients have reported varying patterns of anxiety over their ICU stay, with some patients reporting high anxiety early in their stay and others reporting high anxiety later in their ICU stay.[5] The presence of anxiety appears to be an international issue, with the presence of anxiety in acute myocardial patients being reported as similar across multiple cultures.[4]

There are both physiological and psychological responses to anxiety, associated with feelings of apprehension, uneasiness and dread from a perceived threat. These responses reflect a stress response and incorporate avoidance behaviour, increased vigilance and arousal, activation of the sympathetic nervous system and release of cortisol from the adrenal glands.[7] The humoral response, mediated by the hypothalamic–pituitary–adrenal (HPA) axis, regulates this activity. Physiological changes occur to multiple body systems, with the most relevant including inhibition of salivation and tearing, constriction of blood vessels, increased heart rate, relaxation of airways, increased secretion of epinephrine and norepinephrine as well as increased glucose production,[7] all of which contribute to the range of clinical indicators outlined in Table 7.1. These physiological manifestations illustrate the importance of early identification, active reduction and minimisation of anxiety in critically ill patients.

Clinical indicators of anxiety are broad and relate to four major categories including physiological, behavioural, psychological/cognitive and social (Table 7.1).[8–10] Appropriate recognition of anxiety is important as there is beginning evidence that the physiological effects of anxiety can have important effects on outcomes for critical care patients. Many of the clinical signs listed in Table 7.1, for example increased blood pressure and respiratory rate, are likely to lead to poorer outcomes for the critically ill patient. In addition, in acute myocardial infarction patients, anxiety has been identified as a significant predictor of in-hospital complications such as recurrent ischaemia, infarction and significant arrhythmias.[11,12]

TABLE 7.1

Clinical indicators of anxiety

PHYSIOLOGICAL	BEHAVIOURAL	PSYCHOLOGICAL/ COGNITIVE	SOCIAL
• Heart rate	• Restlessness	• Confusion	• Seeking reassurance
• Blood pressure	• Agitation	• Anger	• Need for attention/ companionship
• Chest pain	• Sleeplessness	• Negative thinking	• Limiting interaction
• Respiratory rate	• Hypervigilance	• Verbalisation of anxiety	
• Shortness of breath	• Fighting ventilator	• Crying	
• Altered O_2 saturation	• Facial grimacing/tension	• Inability to retain and process information	
• Coughing/choking feeling	• Uncooperative		
• Diaphoresis	• Rapid speech		
• Pallor	• Difficulty verbalising		
• Cold and clammy	• Distrustful/suspicious		
• Dry mouth	• Desire to leave stressful area		
• Pain			
• Headache			
• Nausea and vomiting			
• Swallowing difficulty			

Anxiety assessment

The importance of anxiety assessment, with the aim of reducing or preventing the adverse effects it produces, is supported by the literature. However, recognition and interpretation of anxiety is complex, particularly when signs and symptoms are masked by critical illness, the effects of medications and/or mechanical ventilation. Further, alterations in levels of biochemical markers such as cortisol and catecholamines that are frequently associated with anxiety may also be attributed to physiological stress.[13] Thus, anxiety rating scales are advocated and may offer benefits not found with unstructured clinical assessment.

The relationship between a patient's self-report of anxiety and clinician assessment of anxiety has been inconsistent. When chart reviews were undertaken to determine the relationship between clinicians' routinely documented anxiety and patient self-report of anxiety, no relationship was found.[14] In contrast, when clinicians were prompted to assess anxiety in intensive care patients their rating of the severity of anxiety did have moderate correlation with patients' self-report of anxiety.[6]

A number of self-reporting scales exist for measuring anxiety (Table 7.2). These scales require cognitive interpretation and an ability to communicate responses, which presents challenges to many critically ill patients. In addition, some of these scales have up to 21 items, making them both time-consuming and unmanageable for regular use in the critical care setting. Patients with visual and auditory impairments will require additional assistance, such as larger print, hearing aids or glasses in order to complete the forms.

The visual analogue scale (VAS) – anxiety is fast and simple to complete as it is a single-item measure. It has been evaluated against a recognised anxiety scale (the State Anxiety Inventory) with 200 mechanically ventilated patients.[15] The VAS – anxiety comprises a 100-millimetre vertical line, with the bottom marker labelled 'not anxious at all' and the top marker labelled 'the most anxious I have ever been'. Patients were able to successfully mark, or indicate, their present level of anxiety.

The Faces Anxiety Scale, another single-item scale that has been developed by a group of Australian researchers, has five possible responses to assess anxiety (see Figure 7.1).[16] Testing in critically ill patients indicates that the self-reporting single-item scale appears to accurately detect a patient's anxiety.[17,18]

Anxiety management

Critical care nurses recognise that anxiety is detrimental to patients and that anxiety management is important.[26] Although pharmacological interventions such as anxiolytic and pain-relieving medication are well-recognised and are frequently used to reduce anxiety, non-pharmacological treatments are also useful, and can be divided into environmental and nurse-initiated interventions.

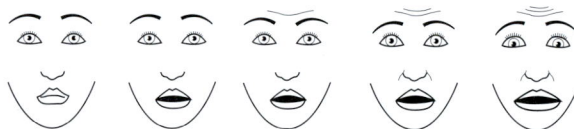

FIGURE 7.1   Faces anxiety scale.

Adapted from McKinley S, Coote K, Stein-Parbury J. Development and testing of a Faces Scale for the assessment of anxiety in critically ill patients. J Adv Nurs 2003;41(1):73–9, with permission.

TABLE 7.2
Anxiety self-report scales

SCALE	NUMBER OF ITEMS	COMMENTS
Hospital Anxiety and Depression Scale (HADS)[19]	14 (including 7 anxiety items)	Easy and fast to complete Extensively used and therefore international comparisons are available Demonstrated validity[20]
Depression Anxiety and Stress Scale 21 (DASS 21)[21,22]	21 (including 7 anxiety items)	Items measured on scale of 0 (did not apply to me at all) to 3 (applied to me very much or most of the time) Demonstrated validity in clinical populations[17]
Spielberger State Anxiety Inventory (SAI)[1]	20 items	Items measured on a scale of 1 (not at all) to 4 (very much so) Validity demonstrated in various populations[1] Too long for routine clinical use, but may be useful in associated research; attempts to shorten the SAI have provided inconsistent results[24,25]
Visual Analogue Scale – Anxiety (VAS–A)	1 item	10 cm/100 mm line from 'not at all anxious' to 'very anxious' Demonstrated validity[23]
Faces Anxiety Scale[16]	1 item	5 possible responses or 'faces' to reflect anxiety Fast and easy to use Validity has been demonstrated in a small number of ICU cohorts[17,18]

Non-pharmacological treatments

An advantage of the non-pharmacological treatments is that they can be nurse-initiated or implemented when units are designed or refurbished (see Table 7.3). Although the benefits of some non-pharmacological treatments may be widely accepted in the community, incorporation of complementary therapies into critical care is dependent on their acceptance within the clinical context and appropriate patient consent. Beneficial effects that have been reported include lowered blood pressure, heart rate and respiratory rate; improved sleep; and reduced stress, anxiety and pain,[27] although the benefits of some therapies have only been demonstrated in hospitalised, rather than critical care, patients. As with any therapy, each non-pharmacological treatment may have different effects on individual patients; consequently, ongoing assessment is essential. In addition, the safety of these therapies within the critical care environment has not been well demonstrated, necessitating a high level of monitoring throughout administration.

> ### Practice tip
>
> Ask your patient or their family if they like music to help relax. Have the family bring in a music player with some favourite music and headphones. Prepare the patient for a rest period. Ensure that pain relief is sufficient, all interventions are complete, and the patient is comfortable. Assess the anxiety or level of sedation beforehand and then commence at least 30 minutes of uninterrupted music. Reassess after the session, and record and report results.

> ### Practice tip
>
> Prioritise the assessment and treatment of discomfort, pain and anxiety. This will greatly reduce sedative medication requirements.

Other strategies to reduce anxiety include interpersonal interventions such as communication and information sharing by the healthcare team and inclusion of family members in care processes. The presence of a family member can provide additional reassurance and can facilitate communication between the health team and patients (see Chapter 8 for additional information).

TABLE 7.3

Non-pharmacological measures to reduce anxiety

NURSE-INITIATED TREATMENTS	ENVIRONMENTAL FACTORS
Patient massage[28,29]	Provision of natural light[30]
Aromatherapy[31,32]	Calming wall colours such as blue, green and violet
Music therapy[27,33]	Noise reduction with consideration of alarms, paging systems, talking etc[34]

Pharmacological treatment for anxiety

Treatment for pain and other reversible physiological causes of anxiety and agitation should be a priority. Should anxiety and agitation continue, despite the incorporation of non-pharmacological interventions, pharmacological treatment with relevant agents may be initiated. A brief overview of these medications in the treatment of unrelieved anxiety is provided in Table 7.4. In general, non-benzodiazepine sedative medications such as propofol are recommended over benzodiazepines.[35]

Delirium

Delirium is a significant concern for critically ill patients and the clinicians who care for them. It is a category of central nervous dysfunction where behaviours and physiological responses are not conducive to healing and recovery. Early detection and treatment of delirium is vital, as it is associated with adverse clinical outcomes such as prolonged duration of ventilation and length of ICU and hospital stay and higher rates of morbidity and mortality.[37–40] Furthermore, increased duration of delirium has been associated with long-term cognitive impairment[41,42] and an increase in delusional memories.[43] Arguably, the condition has been under-recognised and under-treated[44] and has only recently received the attention it deserves. Under-recognition is probably related to a number of factors including the high incidence of the hypoactive subtype as well as lack of use of formal screening instruments – without which there exists a high degree of subjectivity when assessing delirium.

There are three subtypes of delirium: hypoactive, hyperactive and combined (a combination of both).[45,46] Disturbances in attention (e.g. reduced ability to direct, focus, sustain and shift attention) and awareness (e.g. reduced orientation to the environment) that develop over a short period of time (e.g. hours to a few days) are characteristic of all subtypes of delirium.[47] This is in contrast to dementia in which cognitive decline occurs over months and years. Cognitive and perceptive ability often fluctuates through the day worsening at night. A change in an additional cognitive domain such as memory deficit, disorientation or language disturbance that is not better accounted for by a pre-existing, established or evolving other neurocognitive disorder and does not occur in the context of a severely reduced level of arousal such as coma is diagnostic of delirium. There should also be evidence from the patient's history, physical examination or laboratory findings that the disturbance is a direct physiological consequence of another medical condition or substance intoxication or withdrawal.[47]

Lethargy, slow quiet speech and reduced alertness are typical behaviours of hypoactive delirium.[46] It is hypothesised that clinicians may not recognise the 'quietly' confused patient so the condition may be untreated or misdiagnosed as depression.[46] Behaviours evident in hyperactive delirium such as hyperactivity and agitation cannot go unnoticed by clinicians and present overt risks of self harm such as unintentional extubation/decannulation and

TABLE 7.4

Anxiety drug therapy[35,36]

DRUG GROUP	DRUG/DOSE RANGE	ACTION	SIDE EFFECTS	COMMENT
Sedative hypnotic agent	Propofol 10–100 mcg/kg/min (infusion)	General anaesthetic agent	• Hypotension • Respiratory depression • Myocardial depression when given as bolus • Reported to affect memory • May cause dreams	• Dedicated intravenous line • Infusions recommended • High metabolic clearance • Patients wake quickly once drug is ceased • Expensive
Non-benzodiazepine sedative	Dexmedetomidine 0.2–0.7 mcg/kg/h (infusion)[36]	Highly selective alpha-2-adrenoceptor agonist	• Initial hypertension may be experienced • Hypotension • Bradycardia may persist • Hyperglycaemia	• Minimal respiratory depression • No amnesic effect • Rapid onset • Infusions preferred • Role as first line agent not yet demonstrated
Benzodiazepine sedative	Diazepam 5–10 mg bolus	Block encoding on GABA receptors	• Long-acting metabolites • Hypotension • Respiratory depression	• No analgesia properties
	Midazolam 0.5–10 mg/h (infusion) 1–2 mg (bolus)		• Less likely to have above side effects, but they may still occur	• Useful as continuous infusion • Rapid onset • No analgesia properties • Amnesic effect
	Lorazepam 0.01–0.1 mg/kg/h (≤10 mg/h)		• Less likely to have above side effects, but they may still occur	• Not licensed for use in some countries • Strong anxiolytic

intravenous/arterial device removal. Combined delirium is characterised by fluctuations in activity and attention levels including the behaviours of both hyperactive and hypoactive subtypes.

Reports in the healthcare literature about the prevalence of delirium in ICU vary widely from 10% to 80%,[48–51] an unsurprising finding given that it is notoriously difficult to diagnose in patients who are unable to communicate verbally. The prevalence in other critical care areas such as emergency departments is generally documented to be lower, likely because of the varying illness severity of patients.[39,52]

The exact pathophysiology of delirium is not yet fully understood; however, imbalances in brain cholinergic and dopaminergic neurotransmitter systems are thought to be responsible.[46] Many predisposing and precipitating risk factors have been identified (Table 7.5) and current opinion suggests that there is an additive effect: patients with more than one predisposing factor will require less noxious precipitating factors to develop delirium than patients who have none. Predisposing risk factors are those that exist prior to the occurrence of critical illness, while precipitating risk factors occur during the course of critical illness and may be disease-related or iatrogenic. Prevention and therapeutic management of risk factors is the mainstay of treatment for delirium.

TABLE 7.5

Risk factors for delirium

PREDISPOSING RISK FACTORS[38,51,53,54]	PRECIPITATING RISK FACTORS[51,53,55–58]
• Advanced age	Increased severity of illness
• Dementia	Metabolic, fluid and electrolyte disturbance
• Illicit substance use	Infection
• Excessive intake of alcohol	Hypoxia
• Smoking	Acute injury affecting the CNS
• Sensory deficits	Medications that affect acetylcholine transmission, e.g. atropine, fentanyl
• Renal insufficiency	Psychoactive medications, e.g. benzodiazepines, opioids
• Previous cerebral damage	Prolonged pain
• Hypertension	Excessive noise
• Congestive heart failure	Sleep deprivation
• History of depression	Immobility
• Genetic propensity	

> **Practice tip**
>
> Interview the patient or their family to identify predisposing risk factors for delirium. Document your findings and incorporate these into the plan of care.

Assessment of delirium

The higher morbidity and mortality associated with delirium and the relative ease of assessing its occurrence make it imperative to incorporate relevant assessment in routine care. Delirium is diagnosed when both the features of acute onset of mental status changes or fluctuating course and inattention are present, together with either disorganised thinking or altered level of consciousness. A practical delirium assessment screening instrument for the critically ill cannot be reliant on patient–assessor verbal communication. Both the Intensive Care Delirium Screening Checklist (ICDSC)[59] (Figure 7.2) and the Confusion Assessment Method for the Intensive Care Unit (CAM–ICU)[60] (Figure 7.3) have been shown to fulfil these requirements, although clinical

FIGURE 7.2 Intensive care delirium screening checklist (ICDSC).

PATIENT EVALUATION	DAY 1	DAY 2	DAY 3	DAY 4	DAY 5
Altered level of consciousness* (A-E)					
If A or B do not complete patient evaluation for the period					
Inattention					
Disorientation					
Hallucination – delusion – psychosis					
Psychomotor agitation or retardation					
Inappropriate speech or mood					
Sleep/wake cycle disturbance					
Symptom fluctuation					
TOTAL SCORE (0-8)					

Level of consciousness*:		Score
	A: no response	none
	B: response to intense and repeated stimulation (loud voice and pain)	none
	C: response to mild or moderate stimulation	1
	D: normal wakefulness	0
	E: exaggerated response to normal stimulation	1

SCORING SYSTEM:
The scale is completed based on information collected from each entire 8-hour shift or from the previous 24 hours.
Obvious manifestation of an item = 1 point. No manifestation of an item or no assessment possible = 0 point.
The score of each item is entered in the corresponding empty box and is 0 or 1.

1. Altered level of consciousness:
A) No response or B) the need for vigorous stimulation in order to obtain any response signified a severe alteration in the level of consciousness precluding evaluation. If there is coma (A) or stupor (B) most of the time period then a dash (-) is entered and there is no further evaluation during that period.
C) Drowsiness or requirement of a mild to moderate stimulation for a response implies an altered level of consciousness and scores 1 point.
D) Wakefulness or sleeping state that could easily be aroused is considered normal and scores no point.
E) Hypervigilance is rated as an abnormal level of consciousness and scores 1 point.

2. Inattention: Difficulty in following a conversation or instructions. Easily distracted by external stimuli Difficulty in shifting focuses. Any of these scores 1 point.

3. Disorientation: Any obvious mistake in time, place or person scores 1 point.

4. Hallucination, delusion or psychosis: The unequivocal clinical manifestation of hallucination or of behaviour probably due to hallucination (e.g, trying to catch a non-existent object) or delusion. Gross impairment in reality testing. Any of these scores 1 point.

5. Psychomotor agitation or retardation: Hyperactivity requiring the use of additional sedative drugs or restraints in order to control potential dangerousness (e.g, pulling out IV lines, hitting staff), hyperactivity or clinically noticeable psychomotor slowing. Any of these scores 1 point.

6. Inappropriate speech or mood: Inappropriate, disorganised or incoherent speech. Inappropriate display of emotion related to events or situation. Any of these scores 1 point.

7. Sleep/wake cycle disturbance: Sleeping less than 4 hours or waking frequently at night (do not consider wakefulness initiated by medical staff or loud environment). Sleeping during most of the day. Any of these scores 1 point.

8. Symptom fluctuation: Fluctuation of the manifestation of any item or symptom over 24 hours (e.g, from one shift to another) scores 1 point.

Adapted from Bergeron N, Dubois MJ, Dumont M, Dial S, Skrobik Y. Intensive Care Delirium Screening Checklist: evaluation of a new screening tool. Intensive Care Med 2001;27(5):859–64, with permission.

FIGURE 7.3   Confusion Assessment Method – Intensive Care Unit (CAM-ICU).

CAM-ICU Worksheet

Feature 1: Acute Onset or Fluctuating Course Positive if you answer 'yes' to either 1A or 1B.	Positive	Negative
1A: Is the patient different than his/her baseline mental status? Or 1B: Has the patient had any fluctuation in mental status in the past 24 hours as evidenced by fluctuation on a sedation scale (e.g. RASS), GCS, or previous delirium assessment?	Yes	No
Feature 2: Inattention Positive if either score for 2A or 2B is less than 8. Attempt the ASE letters first. If patient is able to perform this test and the score is clear, record this score and move to Feature 3. If patient is unable to perform this test or the score is unclear, then perform the ASE Pictures. If you perform both tests, use the ASE Pictures' results to score the Feature.	Positive	Negative
2A: ASE Letters: record score (enter NT for not tested) Directions: Say to the patient, "*I am going to read you a series of 10 letters. Whenever you hear the letter 'A', indicate by squeezing my hand.*" Read letters from the following letter list in a normal tone. SAVEAHAART Scoring: Errors are counted when patient fails to squeeze on the letter "A" and when the patient squeezes on any letter other than "A".	Score (out of 10):_____	
2B: ASE Pictures: record score (enter NT for not tested) Directions are included on the picture packets.	Score (out of 10):_____	
Feature 3: Disorganised Thinking Positive if the combined score is less than 4	Positive	Negative
3A: Yes/No Questions (Use either Set A or Set B, alternate on consecutive days if necessary): Set A / Set B 1. Will a stone float on water? / 1. Will a leaf float on water? 2. Are there fish in the sea? / 2. Are there elephants in the sea? 3. Does one pound weigh more than two pounds? / 3. Do two pounds weigh more than one pound? 4. Can you use a hammer to pound a nail? / 4. Can you use a hammer to cut wood? Score___(Patient earns 1 point for each correct answer out of 4) 3B: Command Say to patient: "Hold up this many fingers" (Examiner holds two fingers in front of patient) "Now do the same thing with the other hand" (Not repeating the number of fingers). (If pt is unable to move both arms, for the second part of the command ask patient "Add one more finger") Score___(Patient earns 1 point if able to successfully complete the entire command)	Combined Score (3A + 3B): _____ (out of 5)	
Feature 4: Altered Level of Consciousness Positive if the Actual RASS score is anything other than "0" (zero)	Positive	Negative
Overall CAM-ICU (Features 1 and 2 and either Feature 3 or 4):	Positive	Negative

Adapted from Ely EW, Margolin R, Francis J, May L, Truman B, Dittus R et al. Evaluation of delirium in critically ill patients: validation of the Confusion Assessment Method for the Intensive Care Unit (CAM-ICU). Crit Care Med 2001;29:1370–9, with permission.

judgement should also be retained in the diagnostic process.[61,62]

The ICDSC contains eight items based on the *Diagnostic and Statistical Manual of Mental Disorders* (DSM-IV) criteria for delirium and was validated in a study conducted within ICU.[59] It is also simple to use and easily integrated into existing patient documentation. All features of delirium are incorporated such as sleep pattern disturbances and hypo- or hyperactivity. The first step in using the ICDSC is an assessment of conscious level using

a five point scale (A–E). Only patients who are adequately conscious, that is, responsive to moderate physical stimuli (C–E on the scale), are able to be assessed. The eight items of the ICDSC are rated present (1) or absent (0). A score of four or higher is considered to be indicative of delirium.[59]

The CAM–ICU has also been shown to be valid for diagnosing delirium in the ICU population (see *Further reading* for more information).[60] Acute onset of mental status changes or fluctuating course is assessed using neurological observations conducted over the previous

24 hours. Inattention is tested in patients who are unable to communicate verbally by using either picture recognition or a random letter test. Disorganised thinking is assessed by listening to the patient's speech and, for patients who are unable to verbally communicate, a simple instruction is administered such as asking the patient to hold up some fingers. Any conscious level other than 'alert' is considered 'altered'. Scores are not derived from the CAM–ICU; delirium is either present or absent.[60]

Prevention and treatment of delirium

As previously stated, prevention and management of risk factors is the mainstay of delirium treatment; therefore patients' risk factors should be identified and where possible modified (even in the absence of delirium). Potential preventative measures include:

- adequate pain relief
- reassurance to reduce anxiety
- judicious use of sedative medications, particularly benzodiazepine medications
- correction of the physiological effects of critical illness (for example hypoxia, hypotension and fluid and electrolyte imbalance)
- optimisation of the sleep cycle
- early mobilisation
- treatment of the underlying illness.

Research into preventative interventions that target delirium on its own has not been conducted in ICU; however, trials conducted in acute care with the elderly show that many risk factors are potentially modifiable. In one trial a multifaceted intervention that included reorientation strategies, a non-pharmacological sleep regimen, frequent mobilisation, provision of hearing devices and glasses and early treatment of dehydration led to a significant reduction in the incidence of delirium.[63] There is also beginning evidence that bundles of interventions directed towards prevention of delirium among other aspects of care in ICU patients can be beneficial,[34,64] although both of these studies were before and after cohort studies that do not represent high level evidence. Despite these methodological concerns, the creation of environmental conditions that are conducive to rest and sleep, in particular noise reduction and adjusting light levels appropriate for the time of day, as well as sedation minimisation, delirium monitoring and early mobilisation, have not been shown to cause harm and therefore represent good practice for any critically ill patients.

In cases where non-pharmacological strategies have not succeeded atypical antipsychotic medications (e.g. olanzapine) may reduce the duration of delirium in adult ICU patients.[35] Although frequently used, it should be noted that there is no evidence indicating the benefit of haloperidol in reducing the duration of delirium in adult ICU patients.[35] It should also be noted that any medication designed to enhance cognition has the potential to make it worse and there are many unwanted

side effects (e.g. Q-T interval prolongation); therefore any psychoactive medication should be used judiciously in the critically ill.

Sedation

Maintaining adequate levels of sedation is a core component of care in critical care environments, where patients are treated with invasive and difficult-to-tolerate procedures and treatments. A primary aim of nursing critically ill patients is to provide comfort, and adequate sedation is fundamental to this. Individualising sedation management is crucial to the effective management of each patient, with accurate assessment a core nursing skill. An appropriate level of sedation is essential for all patients – this may be no sedation for some patients while other patients may require a significant level. The provision of adequate sedation is paramount for those patients receiving muscle relaxants. In association with sedation management, it is essential that adequate pain relief and anxiolysis are provided to all critically ill patients.

There has been growing evidence of the detrimental effects of sedation on outcomes in critically ill patients. A light, rather than deep, level of sedation in critically ill patients is associated with shorter duration of mechanical ventilation and shorter length of ICU stay.[35] There is also beginning, although sometimes conflicting, evidence to suggest that lighter levels of sedation are beneficial for improved psychological recovery.[35] Strategies to achieve light sedation are now the mainstay of sedation assessment and management for critically ill patients.

Assessment of sedation

Assessment of the effect of all sedative treatments is essential. When pharmacological agents are used there is always a risk of over- or under-sedation, and both can have significant negative effects on patients.[65] Over-sedation may lead to detrimental physiological effects including cardiac, renal and respiratory depression and can result in longer duration of mechanical ventilation, associated complications and recovery. Under-sedation has the opposite effect on the cardiac system, with hypertension, tachycardia, arrhythmias, ventilator dyssynchrony, agitation and distress, with the potential for incidents concerning patient safety. There is beginning evidence to suggest that heavy sedation is associated with psychological recovery, particularly in relation to delusional memories.[66,67]

Objective sedation scales provide an effective method of assessing and monitoring a patient's level of consciousness or arousal, as well as evaluating parameters such as cognition, agitation and patient–ventilator synchrony (Figures 7.4 and 7.5). A number of different sedation scales have been developed for use in the intensive care environment (Table 7.6), with variable strengths and weaknesses of each.[68] Essential requirements of an effective sedation scale include that it measures what is intended, is reliable and is easy to use.[69]

TABLE 7.6
Sedation scales

SCALE	DESCRIPTION	COMMENT
Ramsay sedation scale[73]	• Scores from 1 (agitated/restless) to 6 (no response) • 4 levels of sedation, 1 level of 'cooperative, oriented and tranquil' and 1 level of 'anxious, agitated or restless'	• Easy to administer • No differentiation between different levels of anxiety, restlessness and agitation • Unable to distinguish between a light plane of unconsciousness and a deep coma • Lack of clarity between each score • Limited testing of psychometric properties
Richmond Agitation–Sedation Scale (RASS)[74]	• Scores from −5 (unarousable) to +4 (combative) • 4 levels of agitation, 1 level for 'calm and alert', 5 levels of sedation	• Assesses patient's responses in relation to the type of stimulus given (i.e. verbal or physical), plus consideration of cognition and sustainability • Thorough testing of psychometric properties with positive results including good inter-rater reliability
Sedation–Agitation Scale (SAS)[75]	• Scored from 1 (unarousable) to 7 (dangerous agitation) • 3 levels of agitation, 1 level of 'calm and cooperative', 3 levels of sedation	• Multiple criteria for each level which, although increase complexity, result in better discrimination between scores • Thorough testing of psychometric properties with positive results including good inter-rater reliability
Motor Activity Assessment Scale (MAAS)[76]	• Scored from 0 (unresponsive) to 6 (dangerously agitated) • 3 levels of agitation, 1 level of 'calm and cooperative', 3 levels of sedation	• Very similar to SAS • Multiple criteria for each level which, although increase complexity, result in better discrimination between scores • Limited psychometric testing
Vancouver Interactive and Calmness Scale (VICS)[77]	• Two domains (interaction and calmness) each containing 5 questions • Each question is scored on a 6-point scale from 'strongly agree' to 'strongly disagree', resulting in a potential total score of 30 for each domain	• Thorough assessment of calmness (in contrast to agitation) with multiple levels of scoring available • Differentiation between each of the points on the 6-point scale difficult • Moderate psychometric testing completed, with positive results
Adaptation to the Intensive Care Environment (ATICE)[72]	• Designed to measure the level of adaptation of mechanically ventilated patients to the ICU environment • Two domains – consciousness (awakeness and comprehension items) and tolerances (calmness, ventilator synchrony and face relaxation items)	• Different scales for assessment of each item • Moderate psychometric testing completed, with positive results
Minnesota Sedation Assessment Tool (MSAT)[78]	• Two domains – motor activity (assessed on 4-point scale) and arousal (assessed on 6-point scale) • Assessed over previous 10 min	• Good descriptive differentiation of points on scales • Moderate psychometric testing completed, with positive results

Bispectral index monitoring is an assessment tool that provides an objective measure of sedation. It uses a self-adhesive pad secured to the patient's forehead to continuously record cortical activity that is scored on a scale from 0 (absence of brain activity) to 100 (completely awake). There is not yet consensus on the most appropriate level of activity for intensive care patients or what role bispectral index might offer in their care.[70,71] Continued studies to evaluate the efficacy of bispectral index are required.

Sedation protocols

The sedation needs of patients are complex, with various reports of patients receiving sub-optimal care and inconsistent practice in this area.[79,80] One of the responses to this gap in nursing practice has been the development of protocols.

Sedation protocols offer a framework, or algorithm, within which health professionals can manage specific

FIGURE 7.4 Richmond Agitation–Sedation Scale (RASS).

Richmond Agitation Sedation Scale (RASS)

Sore	Term	Description	
+4	Combative	Overtly combative, violent, immediate danger to staff	
+3	Very agitated	Pulls or removes tube(s) or catheter(s); aggressive	
+2	Agitated	Frequent non-purposeful movement, fights ventilator	
+1	Restless	Anxious but movements not aggressive vigorous	
0	Alert and calm		
−1	Drowsy	Not fully alert, but has sustained awakening (eye-opening/eye contact) to *voice* (≥10 seconds)	Verbal Stimulation
−2	Light sedation	Briefly awakens with eye contact to *voice* (<10 seconds)	
−3	Moderate sedation	Movement or eye opening to *voice* (but not eye contact)	
−4	Deep sedation	No response to voice, but movement or eye opening to *physical* stimulation	Physical Stimulation
−5	Unarousable	No response to *voice* or *physical* stimulation	

Procedure for RASS Assessment

1. Observe patient
   a. Patient is alert, restless, or agitated. (score 0 to +4)
2. If not alert, state patient's name and *say* to open eyes and look at speaker.
   b. Patient awakens with sustained eye opening and eye contact. (score −1)
   c. Patient awakens with eye opening and eye contact, but not sustained. (score −2)
   d. Patient has any movement in response to voice but no eye contact. (score −3)
3. When no response to verbal stimulation, physically stimulate patient by shaking shoulder and/or rubbing sternum.
   e. Patient has any movement to physical stimulation. (score −4)
   f. Patient has no response to any stimulation. (score −5)

Adapted from Sessler CN, Gosnell M, Grap MJ, et al. The Richmond Agitation–Sedation Scale: validity and reliability in adult intensive care patients. Am J Respir Crit Care Med 2002;166:1338–44, with permission.

FIGURE 7.5 Sedation–Agitation Scale (SAS).

Riker Sedation-Agitation Scale (SAS)

Score	Term	Description
7	Dangerous agitation	Pulling at ET tube, trying to remove catheters, climbing over bedrail, striking at staff, thrashing side-to-side
6	Very agitated	Requiring restraint and frequent verbal reminding of limits, biting ETT
5	Agitated	Anxious or physically agitated, calms to verbal instructions
4	Calm and cooperative	Calm, easily arousable, follows commands
3	Sedated	Difficult to arouse but awakens to verbal stimuli or gentle shaking, follows simple commands but drifts off again
2	Very sedated	Arouses to physical stimuli but does not communicate or follow commands, may move spontaneously
1	Unarousable	Minimal or no response to noxious stimuli, does not communicate or follow commands

Guidelines for SAS Assessment

1. Agitated patients are scored by their most severe degree of agitation as described.
2. If patient is awake or awakens easily to voice ('awaken' means responds with voice or head shaking to a question or follows commands), that's a SAS 4 (same as calm and appropriate – might even be napping).
3. If more stimuli such as shaking is required but patient eventually does awaken, that's SAS 3.
4. If patient arouses to stronger physical stimuli (may be noxious) but never awakens to the point of responding yes/no or following commands, that's a SAS 2.
5. Little or no response to noxious physical stimuli represents a SAS1.

Adapted from Riker RR, Picard JT, Fraser GL. Prospective evaluation of the Sedation–Agitation Scale for adult critically ill patients. Crit Care Med 1999;27(7):1325–9, with permission.

patient care with prearranged outcomes. Protocol-directed sedation is ordered by a doctor or advanced practice nurse with prescribing rights, contains guidance regarding sedation management and is usually implemented by nurses although it may have input from pharmacists or other members of the healthcare team. Aspects of sedation management that are incorporated into sedation protocols include:

- the sedation scale to be used, as well as frequency of assessment
- an algorithm-based process for selecting the most appropriate sedative agent
- the range of sedative agents that might be considered and associated administration guidelines
- when to commence, increase, decrease or cease use of sedative agents
- when to seek review by a medical officer.

Many sedation protocols will also incorporate an analgesia component.

The aim of sedation protocols is to improve sedation management by encouraging regular discussion of sedation goals among the healthcare team, while enabling nurses to manage the ongoing sedative needs of the patient. Not all patients' sedative needs will be met within the sedation protocol; in these instances specific care should be planned and implemented by the multidisciplinary healthcare team.

Although sedation protocols have widespread support, there is mixed evidence regarding the benefits of implementation of such protocols. A number of studies have demonstrated the benefits associated with nurse-led sedation protocols, yet other studies do not demonstrate a benefit.[81] Until further research is undertaken, sedation protocols should be considered on a local basis where current practice conditions indicate potential benefit from standardisation of care. Appropriate evaluation of the impact of protocol implementation should be undertaken.

Daily interruption of sedation

A specific form of sedation protocol is the daily interruption of sedation. This intervention has been used in practice in some settings for more than 10 years based on the original study by Kress and colleagues of 128 patients in a single centre in the USA.[82] In this study improved patient outcomes were seen in the form of reduced duration of mechanical ventilation and ICU length of stay. In a sub-study of 18 patients from this cohort and a further 14 patients from a similar time period no adverse psychological outcomes were noted.[83] These initial benefits have not been demonstrated in subsequent work. In both a meta-analysis of data from studies including 699 patients and a multicentre study of 423 patients in 16 centres across Canada and the USA, no improvement in duration of mechanical ventilation, ICU or hospital length of stay or rates of delirium was seen.[84,85] Further, in the multicentre study patients who received daily interruption of sedation required higher daily doses of some sedative and analgesic

agents and greater nurse workload was required for patients in this group.[85] Given this evidence, daily interruption of sedation cannot be recommended. Instead, the mainstay of achieving good practice in this area is setting and maintaining appropriate targets for sedation levels based on the individual needs of the patient.

Pain

Pain is an unobservable, inherently subjective, experience. The nebulous multifaceted nature of pain has led to significant difficulties in not only understanding the mechanisms underlying the experience for individuals but also assessing and managing the phenomenon.

Pain is almost certainly a sensation widely experienced by critical care patients as it is one of the stressors most commonly reported by former and current ICU patients.[86,87] In particular, procedures such as chest drain removal and the insertion of arterial catheters are reported to be painful (median 5/10 and 4/10 respectively).[88] Arguably, pain management is not always afforded the same emphasis as more 'life-threatening' conditions such as haemodynamic instability in critical care. However, its alleviation is an essential element of critical care nursing. Myths such as the possibility that patients may become addicted to analgesics and that the very young and elderly have higher tolerance for pain, and our cultural tendency to reward high pain tolerance may lead to inadequate pain management. In critical care, nurses assume a fairly autonomous role in titrating pain-relieving medication. With this increased autonomy comes a responsibility to be knowledgeable and aware of effective pain management and assessment of the 'fifth vital sign'.

Pathophysiology of pain

Pain is defined as 'an unpleasant sensory and emotional experience associated with actual or potential tissue damage'.[89,p.250] Although unpleasant it has a role in protecting against further injury.[90] There are three categories of pain receptors or nociceptors: mechanical nociceptors, which respond to damage such as cutting and crushing; thermal nociceptors, which respond to temperature; and polymodal nociceptors, which respond to all types of stimuli including chemicals released from injured tissue. Prostaglandins released from fatty acids in response to tissue damage reduce the threshold for activation of the nociceptors.[90]

Pain is transmitted to the central nervous system via one of two pathways. The fast pain pathway occurs when the stimuli are carried by small myelinated A-delta fibres, producing a sharp, prickling sensation that is easily localised. The slow pathway acts in response to polymodal nociceptors, is carried by small unmyelinated C fibres and produces a dull, aching or burning sensation. It is difficult to locate, acts after fast pain, and is considered to be more unpleasant than fast pain.[90]

Perceptions of pain are thought to occur in the thalamus, whereas behavioural and emotional responses occur in the hypothalamus and limbic system.[90] Perceptions of pain are influenced by prior experience, and by cultural and normative practices, which helps to explain individual reactions to pain.[90]

There are negative physiological effects of pain that include a sympathetic response with increased cardiac work, thus potentially compromising cardiac stability.[91] Respiratory function may be impaired in the critically ill undergoing surgical procedures when deep-breathing and coughing is limited by increased pain, thus reducing airway movement and increasing the retention of secretions and possibility of nosocomial pneumonia. Other known effects of unrelieved pain are nausea and vomiting.

Adverse psychological sequelae of poorly-treated pain include diminished feelings of control and self-efficacy and increased fear and anxiety. Inattention with an inability to engage in rehabilitation and health-promoting activities is not uncommon. Pain is commonly cited by patients as a significant negative memory of their ICU experience.[86,87,92,93] The long-term effects of pain are not clearly understood but they almost certainly impact on recovery and may even lead to worsening chronic pain.[94] When these unwanted outcomes are considered alongside the physiological effects of poorly treated pain, the vital importance of pain management is evident.

Pain assessment

'Pain is whatever the experiencing person says it is, existing whenever he says it does.'[95,p.26] The nebulous quality and subjective nature of the pain experience lead to considerable problems in assessing it. Compounding this is the challenge of assessment in the critically ill who often have insufficient cognitive acumen to articulate their needs and an inability to communicate verbally. A common language and process in which to assess pain is essential in ameliorating some of these challenges. Furthermore, accurate assessment and consistent recording are fundamental aspects of pain management. Without these vital components, it is impossible to evaluate interventions designed to reduce pain.[96] Despite the importance of assessing pain there is evidence to suggest that formal assessment (or at least documentation of that assessment) only occurs about 50% of the time.[50]

Since the pain experience is subjective, all attempts should be made to facilitate communication by the patient of the nature, intensity, body part affected and characteristics of their pain. For example, the patient's usual communication aids such as glasses and hearing aid should be used. Whenever patients cannot verbally communicate other strategies must be established and used consistently. For example, strategies involving nodding, hand movements, facial expressions, eye blinks, mouthing answers and writing can be highly effective, not only for the self-assessment of pain but also to express other feelings and concerns. In extremely challenging cases when there is very limited motor function but the patient is cognitively able, the speech pathologist may be able to advise on alternative communication strategies.

If at all possible, a history of the patient's health status, including any existing painful conditions, should be taken. A family member or close friend may be willing to assist if the patient is unable to provide one. Quite apart from the presenting condition, which may be painful, many critical care patients have significant comorbidities such as rheumatoid/osteoarthritis and chronic back pain. It is imperative that the patient's usual pain management strategies are identified and implemented if possible. For example, factors that relieve the pain or increase its intensity should be recorded, along with its relationship to daily activities such as sleep, appetite and physical ability.

Regardless of the patient's communication capability, strategies to ensure consistent objective assessment and management should be implemented. Laminated cards displaying body diagrams, words to describe pain and pain intensity measures (including visual analogues and numerical scales) are useful instruments in meeting these requirements. Verbal numerical scales and visual analogue scales (VAS) are commonly used. These are outlined in Table 7.7. VAS can be difficult to administer to critically ill patients; however, a combined VAS and numerical scale includes the benefit of a visual cue with the ability to quantify pain intensity.

Other physiological and behavioural pain indicators may be used to assess pain in less responsive or unconscious patients.[97] Research indicates that consistent assessment of a number of indicators together provides an adequate substitute for self-assessments.[97,98] Several instruments have been developed and validated for use in the critically ill adult patient including the Behavioural Pain Scale (BPS) (Figure 7.6),[99] Checklist of Nonverbal Pain Indicators (CNPI)[100] and the Critical Care Pain Observation Tool (CPOT)[101] (Figure 7.7). Briefly, scores are assigned to categories such as altered body movements, restlessness and synchronisation with the ventilator, providing a global score for comparison after pain relief interventions. The BPS and the CPOT are considered to be the most valid and reliable behavioural pain assessment instruments,[102] and the BPS is one of the most widely used scales for patients unable to communicate verbally.[99,103,104]

Nurses are urged not to solely rely on changes in physiological parameters, including cardiovascular (elevated blood pressure and heart rate) and respiratory recordings, as other pathophysiological or treatment-related factors may be responsible.[97] Classic reactions to stressors (e.g. pain), such as increased heart rate and blood pressure, do not always occur in critically ill patients and are therefore unreliable methods of assessing pain in this patient group.[105] A potential explanation is that autonomic tone may be dysfunctional in a large proportion of ICU patients.[106] In haemodynamically-stable long-term critical patients, vital signs may be useful if used in conjunction with other forms of assessment.[97]

In addition, it is particularly important to regularly consider and search for potential sources of pain in

TABLE 7.7
Pain scales

SCALE	DESCRIPTION	COMMENTS
Verbal numeric scale	• Self-rating scale • Single-item scale • Scale from 0 (no pain) to 10 (worst pain ever)	• Patient has to be able to communicate verbally • Needs to understand concept of rating pain • Dependent on prior pain experiences • Simple, easy to use
Visual Analogue Scale (VAS)	• Self-rating scale • Single-item • A horizontal line with equal divisions is used for the patient to rate current pain level (no pain is on far left and worst pain is far right)	• Patient can communicate by pointing • Needs to understand concept of rating pain • Dependent on patient's prior pain experiences • Simple, easy to use
McGill short pain questionnaire[167]	• Measures quality of pain • Uses 15 descriptor words to measure sensory effect of pain • Can be used in conjunction with a pain intensity scale	• Gives more information about the patient's pain[107] • Takes longer to administer
Behavioural Pain Scale (BPS) (Figure 7.6)[99]	• Based on pain-related behaviours: the sum of three items • Higher scores indicate higher pain intensity (range: 3–12)	• Patient does not have to communicate • Simple, easy to use • Includes 'ventilator compliance' (may no longer be relevant for pain assessment when using modern ventilators)
Checklist of Nonverbal Pain Indicators (CNPI)[100]	• Developed for cognitively impaired adults • Based on the presence/absence of 5 non-verbal pain behaviours (one is non-verbal vocalisation, e.g. groaning) and verbal complaints • Score 0 to 6 (score of 1 allocated for the presence of a pain behaviour/verbal complaint), higher scores indicate more pain	• Patient does not have to communicate • Simple, easy to use • No patient report at all • Not as reliable for immobile patients[100]
Critical Care Pain Observation Tool (CPOT)[101] (Figure 7.7)	• Based on previously developed instruments using pain-related behaviour to assess pain, e.g. BPS • 4 items: facial expression, body movements, muscle tension and compliance with ventilator or vocalisation • Higher scores indicate more pain (range: 0–8)	• Patient does not have to communicate • Simple, easy to use • Includes 'ventilator compliance' (may no longer be relevant for pain assessment when using modern ventilators) or vocalisation in extubated patients

unresponsive patients and those who are unable to communicate. Nurses are implored to assume pain is present if there is a reason to suspect pain. If pain is suspected an analgesic trial may assist in diagnosing sources of pain. As a general rule, analgesia medication should be administered to patients who are heavily sedated or receiving muscle relaxants as a precaution.

Pain management

Although pain management is discussed here independently, in practice pain management is often combined with sedative administration to reduce anxiety. However, pain management should always be the first goal for achieving overall patient comfort. Efforts to improve patient comfort for intubated patients often favour the concurrent use of both sedative and analgesic forms of medication.[96] This practice therefore makes it difficult to assess the single effect of each medication on the patient's pain, and highlights its multidimensional properties. In addition to pharmacological treatment of pain, non-pharmacological strategies can prove effective as an adjunct to drug therapy or as an alternative.

Pain relief may be required for pre-existing injuries or prior to specific procedures to prevent the occurrence of pain. Being turned is often cited as the most painful procedure; however, wounds, drain removal, tracheal suction, femoral catheter removal, placement of a central-line catheter and non-burn wound dressings and coughing may also cause considerable discomfort.[91,107] Guidelines and written protocols for procedures such as

FIGURE 7.6   Behavioural Pain Scale.

Item	Description	Score
Facial expression	Relaxed	1
	Partially tightened (e.g. brow lowering)	2
	Fully tightened (e.g. eyelid closing)	3
	Grimacing	4
Upper limbs	No movement	1
	Partially bent	2
	Fully bent with finger flexion	3
	Permanently retracted	4
Compliance with ventilation	Tolerating movement	1
	Coughing but tolerating ventilation for most of the time	2
	Fighting ventilator	3
	Unable to control ventilation	4

Adapted from Payen JF, Bru O, Bosson JL, Lagrasta A, Novel E, Deschaux I et al. Assessing pain in critically ill sedated patients by using a behavioral pain scale. Crit Care Med 2001;29(12):2258–63, with permission.

FIGURE 7.7   Critical Care Pain Observation Tool.

Indicator	Description	Score	
Facial expression	No muscular tension observed	Relaxed, neutral	0
	Presence of frowning, brow lowering, orbit tightening, and levator contraction	Tense	1
	All of the above facial movements plus eyelid tightly closed	Grimacing	2
Body movements	Does not move at all (does not necessarily mean absence of pain)	Absence of movements	0
	Slow, cautious movements, touching or rubbing the pain site, seeking attention through movements	Protection	1
	Pulling tube, attempting to sit up, moving limbs/thrashing, not following commands, striking at staff, trying to climb out of bed	Restlessness	2
Muscle tension Evaluation by passive flexion and extension of upper extremities	No resistance to passive movements	Relaxed	0
	Resistance to passive movements	Tense, rigid	1
	Strong resistance to passive movements, inability to complete them	Very tense or rigid	2
Compliance with the ventilator (intubated patients)	Alarms not activated, easy ventilation	Tolerating ventilation movement	0
	Alarms stop spontaneously	Coughing but tolerating	1
	Asynchrony: blocking ventilation, alarms frequently activated	Fighting ventilator	2
OR Vocalization (extubated patients)	Talking in normal tone or no sound	Talking in normal tone or no sound	0
	Sighing, moaning	Sighing, moaning	1
	Crying out, sobbing	Crying out, sobbing	2
Total, range			0–8

Adapted from Gélinas C, Fillion L, Puntillo KA, Viens C, Fortier M. Validation of the critical-care pain observation tool in adult patients. Am J Crit Care 2006;15(4):420–7, with permission.

femoral sheath removal and insertion of a central-line catheter can significantly reduce pain intensity as they often contain reminders to provide analgesia.[108] Some procedures, such as insertion of a central-line catheter, require additional pain management and considerations such as administration of local anaesthetic. This highlights the potential need for additional pain protocols linked to key standard procedures (e.g. patient turning) to reduce patients' pain experience.

Pain-relieving medication can be given via a number of routes, including oral, enteral feeding tube, intravenous, rectal, topical, subcutaneous, intramuscular, epidural and intrathecal. For all routes of administration, assessment of the patient's suitability and contraindications for use are an essential part of the decision-making process. Patient-controlled analgesia for intravenous and, more recently, epidural analgesia is commonly part of critical care nursing.

Epidural pain management requires additional evaluation, including sensory and functional assessment, due to the use of local anaesthetic agents in addition to opioid drugs. Sensory function should be regularly checked using a dermatome chart to gauge segments that are blocked by the local anaesthetic agent. In addition to sensory blockade, regular assessment for lower limb motor deficit is required to detect changes in motor response, which may impair the ability to mobilise safely. Sudden or subtle changes may also indicate a complication such as epidural haematoma. The Bromage Assessment Scale is often used for assessing motor response. Regular checks of the catheter site are essential to identify complications such as bleeding, haematoma and infection early but also to ensure catheter patency. Intrathecal administration of analgesic medications has similar contraindications and complications to epidural analgesia and requires similar precautions. It is important to note that intrathecal (as compared to intravenous) administration does not eliminate all of the side effects of opioids (see *Further reading*).

Practice tip

Epidural administration of medication does not preclude mobilisation. However, certain safety measures should be taken. Ensure that the epidural catheter is well secured: view the site before mobilising and apply extra tape. Monitor blood pressure and heart rate before and during the initial stages of mobilising. Two healthcare personnel should assist during the first attempt to mobilise.

Non-pharmacological treatment for pain

Non-pharmacological strategies to reduce pain are linked to some key strategies to reduce stress. Excessive pain may lead to stress as the body attempts to maintain homeostasis and stress can exacerbate pain. Strategies to reduce stress and pain include both comfort measures and diversional interventions, which require the critical care nurse to individualise and adapt strategies to match the patient's needs and preferences. Diversional methods may include strategies to distract the patient, and aim to refocus the patient's thinking away from the pain and on to other more pleasant thoughts or activities. Research has highlighted the importance patients place on the presence of family members in the facilitation of emotional and physical strategies of pain management.[109,110] Some interventions that may be effective are listed in Table 7.8.

Non-pharmacological interventions have the benefit of being nurse-initiated, non-invasive and able to be personalised for each patient. These strategies alone may not achieve a pain-free experience but they have the capacity to enhance the effects of analgesic medication and humanise the critically ill patient's experience, particularly when family members are included.[110,111]

TABLE 7.8
Non-pharmacological treatment for pain

COMFORT MEASURES	DIVERSIONAL MEASURES
• Repositioning[35]	• Relaxation
• Oral and endotracheal suctioning	• Breathing exercises
• Mouth, oral and/or wound care	• Visual imagery
• Reassurance and information	• Music therapy[168]
• Massage	• Family presence[109]

Pharmacological treatment for pain

Pharmacological treatment for pain in critically ill patients centres on opioid medications, which act as opioid agonists binding to the μ-receptors in the brain, central nervous system and other tissues.[35] Opioid medications have a rapid action and are readily titrated, and their metabolites, if present, are less likely to accumulate. Morphine sulfate and fentanyl are routinely used in critical care, and their properties, side effects and nursing implications are outlined in Table 7.9. For ischaemic chest pain, nitrates will be used together with morphine sulfate as first-line pain measures (see Chapter 10).

Other medications such as non-steroidal anti-inflammatory drugs (NSAIDs) act by inhibition of an enzyme within the inflammatory cascade, and may produce analgesia (especially when combined with opioids) for bone and soft tissue injuries. As with all medication, side effects and contraindications for use can be serious and, in the case of NSAIDs, include gastrointestinal bleeding, renal insufficiency and exacerbation of asthma. Paracetamol is another medication that may be highly effective for mild pain and, when combined with opioid medications, provides analgesia for bone and soft tissue injuries.

An alternative to opioid medication for procedural pain is ketamine.[112,113] Single doses of the medication are effective in achieving analgesia during severely painful interventions such as deep wound care (for example, a burn injury). Ketamine is usually administered in conjunction with midazolam to reduce any potential emergent effects.

Pain relief is a primary goal for critical care nursing and requires regular assessment of pain intensity using reliable, objective, patient friendly instruments. No single medication is ideal for all patients, and clinicians need to carefully select, monitor and titrate the doses of any agent selected. In the case of, for example, cardiac surgery patients, patient-controlled analgesia may provide the most effective pain management strategy (see Chapter 12). Non-pharmacological strategies add to the relief of pain and come under the domain of nursing care. Without adequate pain management, patients will be unable to achieve adequate rest and sleep, both essential to healing processes and wellbeing.

TABLE 7.9

Analgesics

DRUG/DRUG DOSE	PROPERTIES	SIDE EFFECTS	NURSING IMPLICATIONS
Morphine sulfate 1–10 mg/h (IV infusion), 1–4 mg (IV bolus)	• Water-soluble • Peak effect 30 min • Half-life: 3–7 h • Sedative effect and release of histamines[35]	• Vasodilatory effect • Decreased gastric motility • Respiratory depression • Nausea and vomiting[88]	• Intermittent doses, rather the need for continuous infusions[35]
Fentanyl 25–200 mcg/h (IV infusion), 25–100 mcg/h (IV bolus)	• Lipid-soluble • Synthetic opioid • 80–100 times more potent than morphine • Peak effect in 4 min • Half-life: 1.5–6 h[35]	• Respiratory depression • Bradycardia • Muscular rigidity	Useful where: • Hypotension or tachycardia needs to be avoided • Gastric and/or histamine side effects occur with morphine
Tramadol hydrochloride 100 mg (IV bolus), then 50–100 mg 4–6/24 h	• Soluble in water and ethanol • Synthetic • Centrally acting opioid-like analgesic	• Nausea, vomiting • Dizziness, dry mouth • Headache • Sweating	• Intermittent doses only
NSAIDs	• Analgesia and antipyretic	• Gastrointestinal • Some have anticoagulant side effects	• Oral or rectal • Renal clearance
Ketamine 20 mg (IV bolus), then 10–20 mg every 5–10 min[90]	• Analgesic and dissociative anaesthetic for painful procedures • Onset of action 1–2 min • Analgesic/anaesthetic effects last 5–15 min • Half-life 3 h	• Hypertension and respiratory depression (administer slowly) • Increased intracranial pressure • Hallucinations	• Use for painful procedures e.g. wound dressings • Administer 2 mg of midazolam at the start of the procedure or continue midazolam infusion to minimise the dysphoric and hallucinogenic side effects

NSAIDs = non-steroidal anti-inflammatory drugs.

Sleep

The function of sleep is not yet fully understood; however, it is considered to be required for many bodily functions.[114] It is vital for wellbeing and sleep disruption or deprivation leads to psychological and physical ill health.[115–117] Sleep is considered to be physically and psychologically restorative and essential for healing and recovery from illness. Arguably, critically ill people are in greater need of undisrupted sleep but are more likely to experience poor quality sleep.[118]

Evidence suggests that, although critically ill patients may experience normal quantities of sleep, the quality is poor with very few experiencing deep or rapid eye movement sleep.[119–121] Sleep is highly disrupted and distributed across 24 hours with roughly equal amounts occurring in the day and at night.[122,123] These findings, obtained using polysomnography (PSG), have been corroborated by patients' self-reports of their sleep in critical care.[124,125] Patients consistently rate the overall quality of their sleep as poor and, more specifically, they report light sleep with frequent awakenings and considerable difficulty falling asleep and returning to sleep.[126–128]

Many factors are thought to affect the patient's ability to sleep, including discomfort, treatment, medications, environmental noise and illness.[123]

Sleep in the healthy adult comprises one consolidated period of 6–8 hours (mean 7.5 hours) in each 24-hour period occurring at night according to natural circadian rhythms.[129] There are two main sleep states: rapid eye movement sleep (REM) (approximately 25% of total sleep time [TST]) and non-rapid eye movement sleep (non-REM) (approximately 75% of TST). Non-REM sleep is composed of four stages: stages 1 and 2 or light sleep and stages 3 and 4 or slow wave sleep (SWS) or deep sleep, which must be completed in sequence in order to enter REM sleep. The consolidated sleep period consists of four to six sleep cycles: stages 1–4 followed by REM sleep, which lasts 60–90 minutes. (More recent sleep staging guidelines have combined stages 3 and 4 so that there are now only 3 stages of non-REM sleep;[130] however, the foremost textbook on sleep medicine uses the conventional 1–4 staging nomenclature.[129]) Time spent awake during the sleep period is less than 5% of TST.[129] All sleep stages are important to health and, unfortunately, critically ill patients commonly experience very little deep or REM sleep.

There are changes in sleep architecture over the adult lifespan that require consideration in the context of critical care nursing. TST and the percentage of SWS decline (TST by 10 minutes and SWS by 2% per decade) and light sleep increases slightly (only by 5% between 20 and 70 years) with age.[131] REM sleep remains fairly constant with an approximate 0.6% decline per decade until age 70 when REM increases with a simultaneous decrease in TST.[132] Time spent awake after sleep onset increases with age by 10 minutes per decade after age 30.[131]

Sleep assessment/monitoring

An assessment of the patient's sleep history should be performed as soon as possible after admission. The person closest to the patient (ideally living in the same home) may be willing to provide a sleep history if the patient is unable to communicate verbally. The requirement for nocturnal non-invasive ventilation or sleep medication should be conveyed to the medical team for consideration. Particular attention should be paid to reports of daytime sleepiness, dissatisfaction with sleep and bed partner reports of excessive snoring as these may indicate an undiagnosed sleep disorder. Usual sleep habits such as 'going to bed', 'getting up' and shower times should be accommodated while the patient is treated in critical care whenever possible.

Unfortunately, few objective methods of assessing sleep reliably in the critically ill are available. PSG, a method of recording electroencephalography, electrooculography and electromyography, is the 'gold standard' for assessing sleep. PSG data are analysed according to Rechtschaffen and Kales' (R & K)[133] criteria and provide TST and sleep stage times. However, a trained operator is required to ensure satisfactory signal quality, continuous recording and interpretation.[129] In addition, recently sleep researchers have highlighted the difficulties applying standard R & K sleep criteria to critically ill patients' sleep data: for example, EEG waveforms may be abnormal as a result of sedative medications, mediators of systemic inflammatory response and the disease process.[134] These drawbacks preclude its routine use in clinical practice in critical care. Actigraphy is another method of recording sleep that has been attempted in the critically ill. Modern actigraphs are small wristwatch devices (they may also be located on the trunk or leg) containing accelerometers that detect motion in a single axis or multiple axes.[135,136] Data obtained from actigraphy provides an overestimation of sleep time (critically patients are typically immobile for long periods regardless of sleep state). The other objective method that has been attempted in critical care is bispectral index monitoring.[137,138] At present, considerable algorithm development using comparisons with PSG data are required before it is a viable option to measure sleep accurately in any setting.

The most reliable option for the critical care clinician to assess sleep is a patient self-report (in any case, the patient is best placed to judge the quantity and quality of their sleep if they are able). Two instruments have been specifically developed for use in critical care: the Richards-Campbell Sleep Questionnaire (RCSQ)[139] and the Sleep in Intensive Care Questionnaire (SICQ).[125] The RCSQ comprises five 100-mm visual analogue scales (VAS): sleep depth, latency, awakenings, time awake and quality of sleep. It was pilot-tested in medical ICU patients (n = 9, 100% male)[140] and validated in a more extensive investigation involving 70 male patients.[139] There was a moderate correlation between total RCSQ score and PSG sleep efficiency index, r = 0.58, ($p < 0.001$).[139] The SICQ is better suited for use when assessing a unit/organisation-wide change in practice rather than for individual patient's sleep (see Table 7.10).

TABLE 7.10

Sleep assessment instruments

INSTRUMENT	DESCRIPTION	COMMENTS
Richards Campbell Sleep Questionnaire[139]	• Five visual analogue scales (0–100 mm) • Total score derived from average of the 5 scales (high scores indicate good sleep)	• Patient does not need to be able to write (nurse can mark the line as instructed by patient) • Patient requires sufficient level of cognitive function to use it
Sleep in Intensive Care Questionnaire[125]	• Seven questions (some have more than one item) • Likert scales 1–10 • No global score • Good for organisational changes in practice	• Patient does not need to be able to write (nurse can circle the response as instructed by patient) • Patient requires sufficient level of cognitive function to use it • Not yet validated
Nurses' observation checklist[141]	• Tick box table • Assignment of a category: 'awake', 'asleep', 'could not tell' and 'no time to observe' every 15 min	• No training required • Typically, nurses tend to overestimate sleep • Better for trend over several nights

Up to 50% of all patients treated in critical care may be unable to complete a self-assessment of their sleep, in which case the only remaining option is nurse assessment.[126,136] The Nurses' Observation Checklist (NOC)[141] can be used to obtain the bedside nurses' assessments of the quantity of the patient's sleep. It is a relatively simple instrument to use. However, evidence from many studies suggests that nurses tend to overestimate sleep time, so sleep time derived from the NOC may be better used as a trend rather than a definitive report for an individual night's sleep.[136,142–144]

Sleep promotion and maintenance

In the absence of conclusive evidence to support sleep-promoting interventions in ICU, recommendations are based on practices that would be likely to improve sleep and health, e.g. noise reduction, limiting the number of interruptions to which patients are subjected and maintenance of an environment that is generally conducive to normal night-time sleep. Individualised approaches to all aspects of care are best and this is particularly important when promoting and maintaining sleep in the critically ill. The following information, based on research and expert opinion, provides some general advice that may promote and maintain sleep and, at the very least, create conditions conducive to rest.

Comfort measures

- Ensure pain relief is offered and administered if pain is suspected.
- Reduce anxiety by providing information and the opportunity to have questions answered. Anxiolytics such as benzodiazepines may also be required.
- Provide night-time sedation as required (remember sedation is not natural sleep and patients may only appear to be asleep; however, it is possible to be sedated and asleep).
- Provide a light massage unless contraindicated.[140]
- Offer guided relaxation and imagery (audio–guided relaxation and imagery sessions may be purchased).[145]
- Provide an extra cover for warmth (metabolic rate typically drops during sleep).
- Request the patient's family to provide some of the patient's own personal belongings such as pillows and toiletries.
- Ear plugs and eye covers may assist some patients; however, it should be highlighted that studies have shown that neither provides protection from excessive noise and light levels.[146] Patients provided with ear plugs and eye covers should have the ability to remove them without assistance if they wish.

Care activities

- Attend to nursing care at the beginning of the night to reduce the likelihood of disturbing sleep during the night, for example:
  - redress wounds and empty drainage bags
  - wash, clean teeth and change gown and sheets

  - reposition with suitable pressure support measures
  - level the transducer at the phlebostatic axis to ensure accurate haemodynamic monitoring so you do not need to disturb the patient again later
  - ensure intravenous lines and drains are accessible.
- Plan care activities to allow the patient 1.5–2-hour periods of undisturbed time during the night. (Negotiate with other healthcare personnel to allow these uninterrupted periods at night and during daytime rest times). 'Cluster care', for example, time medication administration and blood samples to coincide with pressure area care.
- Provide the daily bath to suit patient needs rather than organisational needs (either before settling for the night or during normal waking hours).

> **Practice tip**
>
> The importance of sleep to critically ill patients cannot be overstated. Enabling the patient to experience good quality and quantities of sleep should be a major priority for critical care nursing. Demonstrate your commitment to improving rest and sleep for intensive care patients by incorporating sleep into the treatment reminder system used in the unit you work in (e.g. FASTHUG becomes FASSTHUG).

Environmental

- Reduce noise levels especially during rest times and at night (this may require a unit-wide change in practice) as several studies conducted in critical care have highlighted the association between noise levels and sleep disruption.[34,119,147–149] Continuous noise levels in adult critical care areas consistently exceed hospital noise standards, for example, the Environmental Protection Agency 35 dB(A) at night and 45 dB(A) during the day[150] and the Australian Standard AS/NZS 2107/2000 minimum 40 dB(A) and maximum 45 dB(A).[151–153]
- Ensure lights are sufficiently dimmed and window blinds drawn during rest times and at night and that lighting is bright and blinds opened at all other times. It is known that critically ill patients' melatonin metabolism is non-circadian so it is particularly important to attempt to use lighting that encourages normal circadian rhythm.[154,155] Generally, critical care areas contain fluorescent lights that may emit up to 600 lux.[156] Light levels between 50 and 100 lux at night, even for relatively brief periods, are known to suppress melatonin production, a vital hormone in the promotion of sleep and maintenance of circadian rhythm.[129] It is well known that artificial lights emit light with sufficient short wave content to affect melatonin secretion.

Treatments

- Discuss the need for alternative mechanical ventilation settings at night with the medical team. Hyperventilation caused by inappropriately high inspiratory pressure can cause hypocapnia, which may lead to central apnoeas and sleep disturbance.[157]

- Many medications administered in critical care affect sleep architecture. Even vasoactive medications such as adrenaline have the capacity to affect the quality of sleep. Sedatives, especially benzodiazepines and opioids, reduce time in stages 3 and 4 and REM, thus reducing the amount and quality of sleep.[158,159] However, pain relief and anxiolysis may be essential for sleep to occur, but an awareness of potential adverse medication reactions is important in the prevention of escalating sleep disturbances.

- Specific sleep-promoting medications may be administered once non-pharmacological interventions have been attempted. Table 7.11 contains a summary of the commonly used medications for the general management of insomnia. It should be noted that investigations of the effectiveness of these medications have not been undertaken in the critically ill.

TABLE 7.11

Summary of commonly used sleep-promoting medications

MEDICATION	MEDICATION CLASS	TYPICAL HYPNOTIC DOSE RANGE (ADULT)	CAUTIONS
Temazepam	Benzodiazepine	Oral/enteral: 10–20 mg once per night (30 min before settling)	Reduce dose in liver failure Check liver function
Propofol	Intravenous sedative/ anaesthetic agent	Intravenous: Mechanical ventilation: 1.0–3.0 mg/kg/h Self-ventilating: no greater than 0.5 mg/kg/h	Short-term use only Continuous respiratory monitoring Check liver function
Zolpidem	Non-benzodiazepine hypnotic	Oral/enteral: 5–10 mg once per night (immediately before settling)	Short-term use only (2–4 weeks) Associated with hallucinations Extended half-life in liver impairment
Zopiclone	Nonbenzodiazepine hypnotic	Oral/enteral: 3.75–7.5 mg once per night (immediately before settling)	Short-term use only (2–4 weeks) Associated with hallucinations Extended half-life in liver impairment
Haloperidol	Typical antipsychotic	Provide maintenance doses used for treatment of delirium for night-time settling Intravenous (slow): 2–10 mg which can be repeated Oral/enteral: 5–15 mg per day	Monitor QT interval and liver function Observe for extrapyramidal symptoms No more than 100 mg/day
Olanzapine	Atypical antipsychotic	Oral/enteral: 2.5–20 mg once per night several hours before settling	Short-term use only May cause hypotension
Quetiapine	Atypical antipsychotic	Oral/enteral: 25–200 mg once per night 1 h before settling	Short-term use only May cause hypotension Monitor QT interval
Amitriptyline	Tricyclic antidepressant	Oral/enteral: 25–150 mg once per night 1–2 h before settling	Monitor QT interval and for anticholinergic effects Increased seizure risk
Doxepin	Tricyclic antidepressant	Oral/enteral: 25–150 mg once per night 1–2 h before settling	Monitor QT interval and for anticholinergic effects Increased seizure risk
Mirtazapine	Noradrenergic and specific serotonergic antidepressant	Oral/enteral: 15–60 mg once per night 1–2 h before settling	Higher doses may have a stimulatory effect
Dexmedetomidine	Alpha agonist	Intravenous: Loading dose 1 mcg/kg over 10–20 min followed by maintenance infusion 0.2–1 mcg/kg/h titrated to effect	Not to be used as a continuous infusion for more than 24 h Continuous respiratory monitoring

A note on melatonin

Melatonin is used for the short-term alleviation of insomnia. This naturally-occurring hormone is both sleep-promoting and -maintaining. Despite its use as a treatment for primary insomnia, e.g. jet lag and shift work, the effectiveness of exogenous melatonin as a treatment for most sleep disorders has not been established.[160,161] Investigations performed in ICU did not use polysomnography and were largely inconclusive.[162–164] Difficulties occur in emulating the typical endogenous pulsatile secretion of the hormone[165] and, together with its short half-life, these probably explain why many study results are inconclusive. The high doses required to achieve an adequate plasma level overnight when administered once at the beginning of the night are likely to persist in the body and may upset normal circadian rhythm. Some studies investigating the effect of melatonin on insomnia suggest that it may be more effective when administered to adults older than 55 years as there is an age-related decrease in endogenous melatonin.[166] The typical dose is 2 mg once a day (1–2 hours before settling).

The current advice of the authors is that it is better to provide conditions that encourage the normal circadian secretion of endogenous melatonin (i.e. provide lighting and activity levels appropriate for the time of day) than to administer exogenous melatonin.

Summary

Meeting the psychological needs of patients is essential in the care of critically ill patients. This chapter outlines various methods that are available to assess and then effectively manage aspects of patient care related to anxiety, delirium, pain, sedation and sleep. Assessment of these aspects of patient condition requires thorough clinical assessment, with a range of instruments available to help improve consistency over time and between clinicians, as well as to inform decisions regarding the most appropriate interventions. Although these aspects of care have been reviewed sequentially in this chapter, in reality they are closely interrelated and should be considered concurrently.

Case study

A 49-year-old woman, Violet Jones, was admitted to the intensive care unit (ICU) with community-acquired pneumonia. Her twin sister visited her at home after Violet's employers expressed their concern that she had not attended work for 2 consecutive days and had not called them. Violet's sister found her unconscious at her home in bed and called an ambulance.

On arrival in the emergency department Violet was unresponsive to voice but groaned to sustained tactile stimulation, and was profoundly hypotensive and pyrexial. She was intubated and initially stabilised in the emergency department before being transferred to the ICU. There were widespread infiltrates on her chest X-ray.

Despite initial stabilisation in the emergency department her blood pressure on arrival in ICU remained low; therefore, several litres of intravenous saline were administered and a vasopressor was started. Her peak airway pressures were high and arterial blood gases poor so pressure control ventilation was instigated with a high fraction of inspired oxygen and machine-delivered respiratory rate. Whenever the rate of sedative medication infusion was reduced she became agitated and reached for her endotracheal tube. Over the next day Violet's lungs were increasingly difficult to ventilate and she experienced several hypoxic episodes. On day 3 in ICU she was diagnosed with acute respiratory distress syndrome (ARDS). In an attempt to improve gaseous exchange she was placed in a prone position for long periods of the day. Throughout

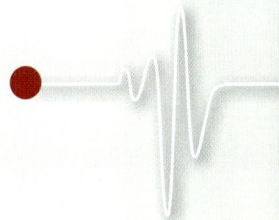

this time high-dose benzodiazepine medication with low-dose opioid medication was administered along with vasopressors. On day 4 her family was informed that she had a high risk of dying. By day 6 Violet had improved so she was returned to a supine position. However, the sedative medication infusion rate could not be reduced appreciably without her becoming tachypnoeic and agitated. A head CT scan was performed but showed no abnormalities.

On day 8 Violet's respiratory condition had improved sufficiently for her to undergo a tracheostomy, which enabled the sedative medication to be reduced. It took several days for the ventilator support to be reduced; she remained on pressure control with pressure support until day 16 when she was placed on pressure support exclusively. By day 18 Violet was breathing spontaneously without ventilator support for several hours of the day.

Once she received her tracheostomy Violet was no longer agitated but was withdrawn and tearful; she was rarely seen to close her eyes and was hypervigiliant and non-communicative, even with her family. Her family, in particular her sister, was very distressed. She said, 'She is not herself. This is not like her'. Serial delirium assessments (using the CAM-ICU) revealed that Violet was not likely to be experiencing delirium. The tracheostomy was still in situ and, although Violet could tolerate the cuff being deflated for short periods, she struggled to speak loudly enough to be heard and did not have enough 'huff' to complete long sentences. In addition, she was too weak to write and was frustrated and easily tired using alphabet boards. Therefore, in order to facilitate a more meaningful assessment of Violet's psychological wellbeing the speech pathologist was consulted to explore alternative communication strategies. A specialised swallowing and speaking (Passy-Muir®) valve was provided to allow Violet to speak.

After careful questioning it transpired that Violet was feeling acutely anxious and frightened (Faces Anxiety Scale =5/5). She described memories of 'voices of concern' (ICU healthcare personnel talking at her bedside) and times when she was 'gasping for breath' when she was acutely unwell earlier during her ICU stay. She was fearful and pessimistic about her future.

TREATMENT

Violet was provided with information about the likely recovery trajectory after critical illness. The physiotherapist reassured her that her current level of physical weakness was not permanent. Violet's primary nurse validated her feelings and provided additional information about the emotional and psychological recovery process. In addition, Violet's primary nurse developed a care plan in consultation with Violet to address her acute anxiety:

- Violet was moved to a quieter area of the intensive care unit.
- Violet was provided with regular opportunities to express her feelings verbally and describe her memories: the tracheostomy cuff was deflated and the Passy-Muir valve used for as long as she could tolerate it.
- A daily routine was negotiated in which several periods of the day were dedicated to sleep/rest and listening to music.
- A masseur was employed by the family to provide a head and neck massage each evening.
- A small dose of diazepam (2 mg) was provided prior to chest physiotherapy as Violet found this particularly frightening.
- Her dog was brought in to visit by her sister twice a week (this arrangement was negotiated with the hospital infection control department and hospital governance).

Violet's mood and emotional wellbeing improved and she became more engaged in her rehabilitation in ICU. She was transferred to the hospital ward after 30 days in ICU. Approximately 2 weeks after this she was discharged home.

RECOVERY

Violet's recovery was complicated by a pulmonary embolism 2 months after her return home but this did not necessitate treatment in hospital. However, she fully recovered psychologically. She visited the ICU and expressed her gratitude for the assistance she had been given to overcome her anxiety.

DISCUSSION

Violet's illness and recovery trajectory are not uncommon. She was severely unwell and the respiratory nature of her illness placed her at risk of becoming acutely anxious. She was provided with the means to communicate verbally and several strategies both pharmacological (benzodiazepine medication is anxiolytic) and non-pharmacological were implemented to reduce her anxiety. Her mood improved dramatically and, subsequently, her ability to engage in rehabilitation increased. This may have been a result of the ability to fully express herself, the other interventions or, most likely, a combination of both. The multifaceted multidisciplinary healthcare team approach to addressing her obvious psychological distress while she was a patient in ICU was highly likely to have contributed to her full psychological long-term recovery.

CASE STUDY QUESTIONS

1 When Violet was able to communicate verbally she expressed her fear and anxiety related to memories of 'voices of concern' (ICU healthcare personnel talking at her bedside) and times when she was 'gasping for breath' when she was acutely unwell earlier during her ICU stay. Outline some nursing interventions that could have been implemented when she was acutely unwell that may have ameliorated her fear and reduced the likelihood of her having unpleasant memories of that time.

2 One of the non-pharmacological interventions used to treat Violet's anxiety was massage. Describe the proposed underlying physiological mechanism(s) for the relaxing effect of massage.

RESEARCH VIGNETTE

Rose L, Fitzgerald E, Cook D, Kim S, Steinberg M, Devlin JW, et al. Clinician perspectives on protocols designed to minimize sedation. J Crit Care 2015;30:348–52

Abstract

Purpose: Within a multicenter randomized trial comparing protocolized sedation with protocolized sedation plus daily interruption (DI), we sought perspectives of intensive care unit (ICU) clinicians regarding each strategy.

Methods: At 5 ICUs, we administered a questionnaire daily to nurses and physicians, asking whether they liked using the assigned strategy, reasons for their responses, and concerns regarding DI.

Results: A total of 301 questionnaires were completed, for 31 patients (15 protocol only and 16 DI); 117 (59 physicians and 58 nurses) were the first questionnaire completed by that healthcare provider for that patient and were included in analyses. Most respondents liked using the assigned strategy (81% protocol only and 81% DI); more physicians than nurses liked DI (100% vs 61%; $P < 0.001$). Most common reasons for liking the assigned sedation strategy were better neurologic assessment (70% DI), ease of use (58% protocol only), and improved patient outcomes (51% protocol only and 44% DI). Only 19% of clinicians disliked the assigned sedation strategy (equal numbers for protocol only and DI). Respondents' concerns during DI were respiratory compromise (61%), pain (48%), agitation (45%), and device removal (26%). More questionnaires from nurses than physicians expressed concerns about DI.

Conclusions: Most respondents liked both sedation strategies. Nurses and physicians had different preferences and rationales for liking or disliking each strategy.

Critique

ICU clinicians' (nursing and medical) perspectives regarding the use of protocolised sedation with and without daily interruption (DI) of sedation were sought in this survey-based study. This study was conducted within the framework of the SLEAP trial (randomized controlled trial of protocolised sedation alone versus protocolised sedation with DI). Clinicians in 5 of the 16 hospitals participating in the SLEAP trial were provided with questionnaires at the time they were caring for study participants. In the SLEAP trial, where no differences in patient outcomes were identified between the two sedation strategies, perceived workload was assessed as significantly higher for nurses in the protocol only group compared to the protocolised sedation plus DI group.[84]

Clinicians participating in this sub-study generally liked both the protocol only and protocol with DI strategies, although clinicians from different professions had differing views in relation to the strategy that incorporated DI with fewer nurses (only 61%) indicating support compared to 100% of medical clinicians. In addition, more nurses raised concerns with the strategy incorporating DI in relation to aspects such as patient discomfort and the potential for respiratory compromise, pain and cardiac instability. The most common reason for liking the strategy that incorporated DI was the improved neurological assessment that was possible.

Strengths of this study include that clinicians from 5 centres across Canada participated, although no participants from the SLEAP trial centres in the USA participated. Further, as identified by the investigators, asking participants to answer questions in regard to a specific patient being managed by one of the strategies helps provide real-time perspectives rather than general opinions. This is the first examination of how clinicians view protocolisation of sedation, particularly with the addition of DI, and is essential information to inform effective implementation of such a strategy in practice. Given the evidence and associated guidelines[35] it is essential that we identify effective methods to minimise sedation levels in critically ill patients; understanding clinicians' views of the benefits and challenges of procolised sedation as one method to achieve this is vital.

The investigators of both this survey and the parent SLEAP trial have made the assertion that nurse led sedation protocols provide one method to minimise sedation and have therefore designed both this and the parent SLEAP study with protocolised sedation as the standard care. This is unfortunate given the lack of evidence of effectiveness of nurse led sedation protocols.[82] Despite this, the responses to the survey provide differentiation between the two alternatives of the protocolisation that were offered in this setting and therefore give some general guidance on clinicians' views of protocolisation, as well as the incorporation of DI.

In summary, this study represents an important element of the larger issue of how best to achieve sedation minimization when caring for critically ill patients. Results demonstrate that, although both nursing and medical clinicians were generally supportive of using protocolised sedation with or without DI, nursing clinicians in particular raised a number of concerns. In the context of the overall results of the SLEAP trial, where protocolised sedation with DI provided no additional benefits over procolised sedation alone, daily sedation interruption should not be used as a routine component of caring for critically ill patients.

Learning activities

1   The assessment of anxiety, sedation and pain intensity is integral to critical care nursing.
    - Discuss the assessment strategies you would use to differentiate between anxiety and pain. List any special considerations associated with your choices.
    - Suggest a non-pharmacological strategy you could employ to reduce pain.
    - Consider how family could help with the management of the patient's anxiety.

2   Critically ill patients who experience delirium require highly skilled and informed nursing. The following exercises may enhance your ability to manage delirium:
    - Identify nursing interventions that may reduce the potential for delirium, including some interventions that involve the family in care.
    - Describe the rationale for your selection of nursing interventions using current research.
    - Outline the differences between delirium and dementia.
    - Develop a nursing plan for a patient you cared for previously with delirium. Identify interventions you did not use but would use in the future.

3   Compare and contrast the various sedation assessment instruments, and discuss the relative merits and disadvantages of using each of these instruments. Now repeat the exercise for each of the pain assessment instruments and the delirium assessment instruments.

4   Using the references provided in this chapter:
    - highlight the importance of good quality sleep in health and illness
    - identify theories that explain the function of sleep.

5 Think about the last time you experienced fragmented sleep or insufficient sleep and describe how you felt in terms of your:
- mood
- cognitive function
- physical function
- appetite
- motivation.

Online resources

Australasian Sleep Association, www.sleep.org.au

ICU Delirium and Cognitive Impairment Study Group, www.icudelirium.org

Further reading

Ballantyne J, Bonica JJ, Fishman S. Bonica's management of pain. Philadelphia: Lippincott Williams & Wilkins; 2009.

Barr J, Fraser GL, Puntillo K, Ely EW, Gelinas C, Dasta JF et al. Clinical practice guidelines for the management of pain, agitation, and delirium in adult patients in the intensive care unit. Crit Care Med 2013,41:263–306.

Bergeron N, Dubois MJ, Dumont M, Dial S, Skrobik Y. Intensive Care Delirium Screening Checklist: evaluation of a new screening tool. Intensive Care Med 2001;27:859–64.

Ely EW, Inouye SK, Bernard GR, Gordon S, Francis J, May L et al. Delirium in mechanically ventilated patients: validity and reliability of the confusion assessment method for the intensive care unit (CAM-ICU). JAMA 2001;286:2703–10.

Hardin KA. Sleep in the ICU: potential mechanisms and clinical implications. Chest 2009;136:284–94.

Kyranou M, Puntillo K. The transition from acute to chronic pain: might intensive care unit patients be at risk? Ann Intensive Care 2012;2:36.

References

1 Spielberger C, Gorsuch R, Lushene R. Manual for the state-trait anxiety inventory. Palo Alto, CA: Consulting Psychologist Press; 1983.
2 Chlan L. A review of the evidence for music intervention to manage anxiety in critically ill patients receiving mechanical ventilatory support. Arch Psychiatr Nurs 2009;23(2):177–9.
3 Sessler CN, Varney K. Patient-focused sedation and analgesia in the ICU. Chest 2008;133(February):552–65.
4 De Jong MJ, Chung ML, Roser LP, Jensen LA, Kelso LA, Dracup K et al. A five-country comparison of anxiety early after acute myocardial infarction. Eur J Cardiovasc Nurs 2004;3(2):129–34.
5 Chlan L, Savik K. Patterns of anxiety in critically ill patients receiving mechanical ventilatory support. Nurs Res 2011;60(3 Suppl):S50–7.
6 McKinley S, Stein-Parbury J, Chehelnabi A, Lovas J. Assessment of anxiety in intensive care patients by using the Faces Anxiety Scale. Am J Crit Care 2004;13(2):146–52.
7 Bear M, Connors B, Paradiso M. Neuroscience, exploring the brain. 2nd ed. Baltimore, MD: Lippincott Williams & Wilkins; 2001.
8 Tate JA, Devito Dabbs A, Hoffman LA, Milbrandt E, Happ MB. Anxiety and agitation in mechanically ventilated patients. Qual Health Res 2012;22(2):157–73.
9 Porth C, Matfin G. Pathophysiology: Concepts of altered health states. 8th ed. Philadelphia, PA: Lippincott, Williams & Wilkins; 2009.
10 Moser DK, Chung ML, McKinley S, Riegel B, An K, Cherrington CC et al. Critical care nursing practice regarding patient anxiety assessment and management. Intensive Crit Care Nurs 2003;19(5):276–88.
11 Moser DK, Riegel B, McKinley S, Doering LV, An K, Sheahan S. Impact of anxiety and perceived control on in-hospital complications after acute myocardial infarction. Psychosom Med 2007;69(1):10–6.
12 Huffman JC, Smith FA, Blais MA, Januzzi JL, Fricchione GL. Anxiety, independent of depressive symptoms, is associated with in-hospital cardiac complications after acute myocardial infarction. J Psychosom Res 2008;65(6):557–63.
13 Schelling G. Effects of stress hormones on traumatic memory formation and the development of posttraumatic stress disorder in critically ill patients. Neurobiol Learn Mem 2002;78(3):596–609.
14 Frazier SK, Moser DK, O'Brien JL, Garvin BJ, An K, Macko M. Management of anxiety after acute myocardial infarction. Heart Lung 2002;31(6):411–20.

15 Chlan LL. Relationship between two anxiety instruments in patients receiving mechanical ventilatory support. J Adv Nurs 2004;48(5):493–9.

16 McKinley S, Coote K, Stein-Parbury J. Development and testing of a Faces Scale for the assessment of anxiety in critically ill patients. J Adv Nurs 2003;41(1):73–9.

17 Gustad LT, Chaboyer W, Wallis M. Performance of the Faces Anxiety Scale in patients transferred from the ICU. Intensive Crit Care Nurs 2005;21(6):355–60.

18 McKinley S, Madronio C. Validity of the Faces Anxiety Scale for the assessment of state anxiety in intensive care patients not receiving mechanical ventilation. J Psychosom Res 2008;64(5):503–7.

19 Zigmond AS, Snaith RP. The hospital anxiety and depression scale. Acta Psychiatr Scand 1983;67(6):361–70.

20 Snaith RP, Taylor CM. Rating scales for depression and anxiety: a current perspective. Br J Clin Pharmacol 1985;19 Suppl 1:17S–20S.

21 Lovibond S, Lovibond P. Manual for the Depression Anxiety Stress Scales. 2nd ed. Sydney Psychology Foundation; 1995.

22 Ng F, Trauer T, Dodd S, Callaly T, Campbell S, Berk M. The validity of the 21-item version of the Depression Anxiety Stress Scales as a routine clinical outcome measure. Acta Neuropsychiatrica 2007;19:304–10.

23 Hornblow AR, Kidson MA. The visual analogue scale for anxiety: a validation study. Aust N Z J Psychiatry 1976;10(4):339–41.

24 Abed MA, Hall LA, Moser DK. Spielberger's state anxiety inventory: development of a shortened version for critically ill patients. Issues Ment Health Nurs 2011;32(4):220–7.

25 Chlan L, Savik K, Weinert C. Development of a shortened state anxiety scale from the Spielberger State-Trait Anxiety Inventory (STAI) for patients receiving mechanical ventilatory support. J Nurs Meas 2003;11(3):283–93.

26 Frazier SK, Moser DK, Daley LK, McKinley S, Riegel B, Garvin BJ et al. Critical care nurses' beliefs about and reported management of anxiety. Am J Crit Care 2003;12(1):19–27.

27 Davis T, Jones P. Music therapy: decreasing anxiety in the ventilated patient: a review of the literature. Dimens Crit Care Nurs 2012;31(3):159–66.

28 Tracy MF, Chlan L. Nonpharmacological interventions to manage common symptoms in patients receiving mechanical ventilation. Crit Care Nurse 2011;31(3):19–28.

29 Papathanassoglou ED, Mpouzika MD. Interpersonal touch: physiological effects in critical care. Biol Res Nurs 2012;14(4):431–43.

30 Rashid M. Two decades (1993–2012) of adult intensive care unit design: a comparative study of the physical design features of the best practice examples. Crit Care Nurs Q 2014;37(1):3–32.

31 Lytle J, Mwatha C, Davis KK. Effect of lavender aromatherapy on vital signs and perceived quality of sleep in the intermediate care unit: a pilot study. Am J Crit Care 2014;23(1):24–9.

32 Halm MA. Essential oils for management of symptoms in critically ill patients. Am J Crit Care 2008;17(2):160–3.

33 Chlan LL, Weinert CR, Heiderscheit A, Tracy MF, Skaar DJ, Guttormson JL et al. Effects of patient-directed music intervention on anxiety and sedative exposure in critically ill patients receiving mechanical ventilatory support: a randomized clinical trial. JAMA 2013;309(22):2335–44.

34 Patel J, Baldwin J, Bunting P, Laha S. The effect of a multicomponent multidisciplinary bundle of interventions on sleep and delirium in medical and surgical intensive care patients. Anaesthesia 2014;69(6):540–9.

35 Barr J, Fraser GL, Puntillo K, Ely EW, Gelinas C, Dasta JF et al. Clinical practice guidelines for the management of pain, agitation, and delirium in adult patients in the intensive care unit. Crit Care Med 2013;41(1):263–306.

36 Reardon DP, Anger KE, Adams CD, Szumita PM. Role of dexmedetomidine in adults in the intensive care unit: an update. Am J Health Syst Pharm 2013;70(9):767–77.

37 Lin SM, Liu CY, Wang CH, Lin HC, Huang CD, Huang PY et al. The impact of delirium on the survival of mechanically ventilated patients. Crit Care Med 2004;32(11):2254–9.

38 Ouimet S, Kavanagh BP, Gottfried SB, Skrobik Y. Incidence, risk factors and consequences of ICU delirium. Intensive Care Med 2007;33(1):66–73.

39 Han JH, Shintani A, Eden S, Morandi A, Solberg LM, Schnelle J et al. Delirium in the emergency department: an independent predictor of death within 6 months. Ann Emerg Med 2010;56(3):244–52 e1.

40 Ely EW, Gautam S, Margolin R, Francis J, May L, Speroff T et al. The impact of delirium in the intensive care unit on hospital length of stay. Intensive Care Med 2001;27(12):1892–900.

41 Girard TD, Jackson JC, Pandharipande PP, Pun BT, Thompson JL, Shintani AK et al. Delirium as a predictor of long-term cognitive impairment in survivors of critical illness. Crit Care Med 2010;38(7):1513–20.

42 van den Boogaard M, Schoonhoven L, Evers AW, van der Hoeven JG, van Achterberg T, Pickkers P. Delirium in critically ill patients: impact on long-term health-related quality of life and cognitive functioning. Crit Care Med 2012;40(1):112–8.

43 Svenningsen H, Tonnesen EK, Videbech P, Frydenberg M, Christensen D, Egerod I. Intensive care delirium – effect on memories and health-related quality of life – a follow-up study. J Clin Nurs 2014;23(5–6):634–44.

44 Spronk PE, Riekerk B, Hofhuis J, Rommes JH. Occurrence of delirium is severely underestimated in the ICU during daily care. Intensive Care Med 2009;35(7):1276–80.

45 Peterson JF, Pun BT, Dittus RS, Thomason JW, Jackson JC, Shintani AK et al. Delirium and its motoric subtypes: a study of 614 critically ill patients. J Am Geriatr Soc 2006;54(3):479–84.

46 Meagher D. Motor subtypes of delirium: past, present and future. Intl Rev Psychiatry (Abingdon, England) 2009;21(1):59–73.

47 American Psychiatric Association. Diagnostic and statistical manual of mental disorders. 5th ed. Arlington, VA: American Psychiatric Association; 2013.

48 Ely EW, Shintani A, Truman B, Speroff T, Gordon S, Harrell F, Jr et al. Delirium as a predictor of mortality in mechanically ventilated patients in the intensive care unit. JAMA 2004;291:1753–62.

49 Shehabi Y, Botha JA, Boyle MS, Ernest D, Freebairn RC, Jenkins IR et al. Sedation and delirium in the intensive care unit: an Australian and New Zealand perspective. Anaesth Intensive Care 2008;36(4):570–8.

50 Elliott D, Aitken LM, Bucknall TK, Seppelt IM, Webb SA, Weisbrodt L et al. Patient comfort in the intensive care unit: a multicentre, binational point prevalence study of analgesia, sedation and delirium management. Crit Care Resusc 2013;15(3):213–9.

51 van den Boogaard M, Schoonhoven L, Maseda E, Plowright C, Jones C, Luetz A et al. Recalibration of the delirium prediction model for ICU patients (PRE-DELIRIC): a multinational observational study. Intensive Care Med 2014;40(3):361–9.

52 Kennedy M, Enander RA, Tadiri SP, Wolfe RE, Shapiro NI, Marcantonio ER. Delirium risk prediction, healthcare use and mortality of elderly adults in the emergency department. J Am Geriatr Soc 2014;62(3):462–9.

53 Dubois M-J, Bergeron N, Dumont M, Dial S, Skrobik Y. Delirium in an intensive care unit: a study of risk factors. Intensive Care Med 2001;27:1297–304.

54 Ely EW, Girard TD, Shintani AK, Jackson JC, Gordon SM, Thomason JW et al. Apolipoprotein E4 polymorphism as a genetic predisposition to delirium in critically ill patients. Crit Care Med 2007;35(1):112–7.

55 Girard TD, Pandharipande PP, Ely EW. Delirium in the intensive care unit. Crit Care 2008;12 Suppl 3:S3.

56 Aldemir M, Ozen S, Kara IH, Sir A, Bac B. Predisposing factors for delirium in the surgical intensive care unit. Crit Care 2001;5(5):265–70.

57 Pandharipande P, Shintani A, Peterson J, Pun BT, Wilkinson GR, Dittus RS et al. Lorazepam is an independent risk factor for transitioning to delirium in intensive care unit patients. Anesthesiology 2006;104(1):21–6.

58 McPherson JA, Wagner CE, Boehm LM, Hall JD, Johnson DC, Miller LR et al. Delirium in the cardiovascular ICU: exploring modifiable risk factors. Crit Care Med 2013;41(2):405–13.

59 Bergeron N, Dubois MJ, Dumont M, Dial S, Skrobik Y. Intensive Care Delirium Screening Checklist: evaluation of a new screening tool. Intensive Care Med 2001;27(5):859–64.

60 Ely EW, Margolin R, Francis J, May L, Truman B, Dittus R et al. Evaluation of delirium in critically ill patients: validation of the Confusion Assessment Method for the Intensive Care Unit (CAM-ICU). Crit Care Med 2001;29:1370–9.

61 Shi Q, Warren L, Saposnik G, Macdermid JC. Confusion assessment method: a systematic review and meta-analysis of diagnostic accuracy. Neuropsychiatr Dis Treat 2013;9:1359–70.

62 Neto AS, Nassar AP, Jr, Cardoso SO, Manetta JA, Pereira VG, Esposito DC et al. Delirium screening in critically ill patients: a systematic review and meta-analysis. Crit Care Med 2012;40(6):1946–51.

63 Inouye SK, Bogardus ST, Jr., Charpentier PA, Leo-Summers L, Acampora D, Holford TR et al. A multicomponent intervention to prevent delirium in hospitalized older patients. N Engl J Med 1999;340(9):669–76.

64 Balas MC, Burke WJ, Gannon D, Cohen MZ, Colburn L, Bevil C et al. Implementing the awakening and breathing coordination, delirium monitoring/management, and early exercise/mobility bundle into everyday care: opportunities, challenges, and lessons learned for implementing the ICU Pain, Agitation, and Delirium Guidelines. Crit Care Med 2013;41(9 Suppl 1):S116–27.

65 Jackson DL, Proudfoot CW, Cann KF, Walsh T. A systematic review of the impact of sedation practice in the ICU on resource use, costs and patient safety. Crit Care 2010;14(2):R59.

66 Samuelson KA, Lundberg D, Fridlund B. Light vs. heavy sedation during mechanical ventilation after oesophagectomy – a pilot experimental study focusing on memory. Acta Anaesthesiol Scand 2008;52(8):1116–23.

67 Treggiari MM, Romand JA, Yanez ND, Deem SA, Goldberg J, Hudson L et al. Randomized trial of light versus deep sedation on mental health after critical illness. Crit Care Med 2009;37(9):2527–34.

68 Robinson BR, Berube M, Barr J, Riker R, Gelinas C. Psychometric analysis of subjective sedation scales in critically ill adults. Crit Care Med 2013;41(9 Suppl 1):S16–29.

69 Sessler CN, Grap MJ, Ramsay MA. Evaluating and monitoring analgesia and sedation in the intensive care unit. Crit Care 2008;12 Suppl 3(3):S2.

70 Anderson J, Henry L, Hunt S, Ad N. Bispectral index monitoring to facilitate early extubation following cardiovascular surgery. Clin Nurse Spec 2010;24(3):140–8.

71 Weatherburn C, Endacott R, Tynan P, Bailey M. The impact of bispectral index monitoring on sedation administration in mechanically ventilated patients. Anaesth Intensive Care 2007;35(2):204–8.

72 De Jonghe B, Cook D, Griffith L, Appere-de-Vecchi C, Guyatt G, Theron V et al. Adaptation to the Intensive Care Environment (ATICE): development and validation of a new sedation assessment instrument. Crit Care Med 2003;31(9):2344–54.

73 Ramsay MA, Savege TM, Simpson BR, Goodwin R. Controlled sedation with alphaxalone-alphadolone. Br Med J 1974;2(5920):656–9.

74 Sessler CN, Gosnell M, Grap MJ, et al. The Richmond Agitation–Sedation Scale: validity and reliability in adult intensive care patients. Am J Respir Crit Care Med 2002;166:1338–44.

75 Riker RR, Picard JT, Fraser GL. Prospective evaluation of the Sedation–Agitation Scale for adult critically ill patients. Crit Care Med 1999;27(7):1325–9.

76 Devlin JW, Boleski G, Mlynarek M, Nerenz DR, Peterson E, Jankowski M et al. Motor Activity Assessment Scale: a valid and reliable sedation scale for use with mechanically ventilated patients in an adult surgical intensive care unit. Crit Care Med 1999;27(7):1271–5.

77 de Lemos J, Tweeddale M, Chittock D. Measuring quality of sedation in adult mechanically ventilated critically ill patients: the Vancouver Interaction and Calmness Scale. Sedation Focus Group. J Clin Epidemiol 2000;53(9):908–19.

78 Weinert C, McFarland L. The state of intubated ICU patients: development of a two-dimensional sedation rating scale for critically ill adults. Chest 2004;126(6):1883–90.

79 Jackson DL, Proudfoot CW, Cann KF, Walsh TS. The incidence of sub-optimal sedation in the ICU: a systematic review. Crit Care 2009;13(6):R204.

80 Mehta S, McCullagh I, Burry L. Current sedation practices: lessons learned from international surveys. Crit Care Clin 2009;25(3):471–88, vii–viii.

81 Aitken LM, Bucknall T, Kent B, Mitchell M, Burmeister E, Keogh SJ. Protocol directed sedation versus non-protocol directed sedation to reduce duration of mechanical ventilation in mechanically ventilated intensive care patients. Coch Database Syst Rev 2015;Issue 1:Art. No.: CD009771. doi: 10.1002/14651858.CD009771.pub2.

82 Kress JP, Pohlman AS, O'Connor MF, Hall JB. Daily interruption of sedative infusions in critically ill patients undergoing mechanical ventilation. N Engl J Med 2000;342(20):1471–7.

83 Kress JP, Gehlbach B, Lacy M, Pliskin N, Pohlman AS, Hall JB. The long-term psychological effects of daily sedative interruption on critically ill patients. Am J Respir Crit Care Med 2003;168(12):1457–61.

84 Augustes R, Ho KM. Meta-analysis of randomised controlled trials on daily sedation interruption for critically ill adult patients. Anaesth Intensive Care 2011;39(3):401–9.

85 Mehta S, Burry L, Cook D, Fergusson D, Steinberg M, Granton J et al. Daily sedation interruption in mechanically ventilated critically ill patients cared for with a sedation protocol: a randomized controlled trial. JAMA 2012;308(19):1985–92.

86 Roberts BL, Rickard CM, Rajbhandari D, Reynolds P. Factual memories of ICU: recall at two years post-discharge and comparison with delirium status during ICU admission – a multicentre cohort study. J Clin Nurs 2007;16(9):1669–77.

87 Rotondi AJ, Chelluri L, Sirio C, Mendelsohn A, Schulz R, Belle S et al. Patients' recollections of stressful experiences while receiving prolonged mechanical ventilation in an intensive care unit. Crit Care Med 2002;30(4):746–52.

88 Topolovec-Vranic J, Gelinas C, Li Y, Pollman-Mudryj MA, Innis J, McFarlan A et al. Validation and evaluation of two observational pain assessment tools in a trauma and neurosurgical intensive care unit. Pain Res Manag 2013;18(6):e107–14.

89 Bonica JJ. The need of a taxonomy. Pain 1979;6(3):247–8.

90 Fishman SM, Ballantyne JC, Rathmell JP, eds. Bonica's Management of pain. 4th ed. Philadelphia, Pa: Lippincott Williams & Wilkins; 2009.

91 Milgrom LB, Brooks JA, Qi R, Bunnell K, Wuestfeld S, Beckman D. Pain levels experienced with activities after cardiac surgery. Am J Crit Care 2004;13(2):116–25.

92 Adamson H, Murgo M, Boyle M, Kerr S, Crawford M, Elliott D. Memories of intensive care and experiences of survivors of a critical illness: an interview study. Intensive Crit Care Nurs 2004;20(5):257–63.

93 Wade DM, Brewin CR, Howell DC, White E, Mythen MG, Weinman JA. Intrusive memories of hallucinations and delusions in traumatized intensive care patients: an interview study. Br J Health Psychol 2014. doi: 10.1111/bjhp.12109.

94 Boyle M, Murgo M, Adamson H, Gill J, Elliott D, Crawford M. The effect of chronic pain on health related quality of life amongst intensive care survivors. Aust Crit Care 2004;17(3):104–6, 8–13.

95 McCaffery M. Understanding your patient's pain. Nursing (Lond) 1980;10(9):26–31.

96 Gélinas C, Fortier M, Viens C, Fillion L, Puntillo K. Pain assessment and management in critically ill intubated patients: a retrospective study. Am J Crit Care 2004;13(2):126–35.

97 Herr K, Coyne PJ, Key T, Manworren R, McCaffery M, Merkel S et al. Pain assessment in the nonverbal patient: position statement with clinical practice recommendations. Pain Manag Nurs 2006;7(2):44–52.

98 Puntillo KA, Miaskowski C, Kehrle K, Stannard D, Gleeson S, Nye P. Relationship between behavioral and physiological indicators of pain, critical care patients' self-reports of pain, and opioid administration. Crit Care Med 1997;25(7):1159–66.

99 Payen JF, Bru O, Bosson JL, Lagrasta A, Novel E, Deschaux I et al. Assessing pain in critically ill sedated patients by using a behavioral pain scale. Crit Care Med 2001;29(12):2258–63.

100 Feldt KS. The Checklist of Nonverbal Pain Indicators (CNPI). Pain Manag Nurs 2000;1(1):13–21.

101 Gélinas C, Fillion L, Puntillo KA, Viens C, Fortier M. Validation of the critical-care pain observation tool in adult patients. Am J Crit Care 2006;15(4):420–7.

102 Gélinas C, Puntillo KA, Joffe AM, Barr J. A validated approach to evaluating psychometric properties of pain assessment tools for use in nonverbal critically ill adults. Semin Respir Crit Care Med 2013;34(2):153–68.

103 Young J, Siffleet J, Nikoletti S, Shaw T. Use of a Behavioural Pain Scale to assess pain in ventilated, unconscious and/or sedated patients. Intensive Crit Care Nurs 2006;22(1):32–9.

104 Aissaoui Y, Zeggwagh AA, Zekraoui A, Abidi K, Abouqal R. Validation of a behavioral pain scale in critically ill, sedated, and mechanically ventilated patients. Anesth Analg 2005;101(5):1470–6.

105 Arbour C, Gélinas C. Are vital signs valid indicators for the assessment of pain in postoperative cardiac surgery ICU adults? Intensive Crit Care Nurs 2010;26(2):83–90.

106 Frazier SK, Moser DK, Schlanger R, Widener J, Pender L, Stone KS. Autonomic tone in medical intensive care patients receiving mechanical ventilation and during a CPAP weaning trial. Biol Res Nurs 2008;9(4):301–10.

107 Puntillo KA, White C, Morris AB, Perdue ST, Stanik-Hutt J, Thompson CL et al. Patients' perceptions and responses to procedural pain: results from Thunder Project II. Am J Crit Care 2001;10(4):238–51.

108 Puntillo KA, Wild LR, Morris AB, Stanik-Hutt J, Thompson CL, White C. Practices and predictors of analgesic interventions for adults undergoing painful procedures. Am J Crit Care 2002;11(5):415–29; quiz 30–1.

109 Gélinas C, Arbour C, Michaud C, Robar L, Cote J. Patients and ICU nurses' perspectives of non-pharmacological interventions for pain management. Nurs Crit Care 2013;18(6):307–18.

110 Fredriksen ST, Svensson T. The bodily presence of significant others: intensive care patients' experiences in a situation of critical illness. Int J Qual Stud Health Well-being 2010;5(4).

111 Alpers LM, Helseth S, Bergbom I. Experiences of inner strength in critically ill patients – a hermeneutical approach. Intensive Crit Care Nurs 2012;28(3):150–8.

112 MacPherson RD, Woods D, Penfold J. Ketamine and midazolam delivered by patient-controlled analgesia in relieving pain associated with burns dressings. Clin J Pain 2008;24(7):568–71.

113 Zor F, Ozturk S, Bilgin F, Isik S, Cosar A. Pain relief during dressing changes of major adult burns: ideal analgesic combination with ketamine. Burns 2010;36(4):501–5.

114 Siegel JM. Why we sleep. Sci Am 2003;289(5):92–7.

115 Bonnet MH, Berry RB, Arand DL. Metabolism during normal, fragmented, and recovery sleep. J Appl Physiol 1991;71(3):1112–8.

116 Banks S, Dinges DF. Behavioral and physiological consequences of sleep restriction. J Clin Sleep Med 2007;3(5):519–28.

117 Ferrie JE, Shipley MJ, Cappuccio FP, Brunner E, Miller MA, Kumari M et al. A prospective study of change in sleep duration: associations with mortality in the Whitehall II cohort. Sleep 2007;30(12):1659–66.

118 Kamdar BB, Needham DM, Collop NA. Sleep deprivation in critical illness: its role in physical and psychological recovery. J Intensive Care Med 2012;27(2):97–111.

119 Freedman NS, Gazendam J, Levan L, Pack AI, Schwab RJ. Abnormal sleep/wake cycles and the effect of environmental noise on sleep disruption in the intensive care unit. Am J Respir Crit Care Med 2001;163(2):451–7.

120 Friese RS, Diaz-Arrastia R, McBride D, Frankel H, Gentilello LM. Quantity and quality of sleep in the surgical intensive care unit: are our patients sleeping? J Trauma 2007;63(6):1210–4.

121 Hardin KA, Seyal M, Stewart T, Bonekat HW. Sleep in critically ill chemically paralyzed patients requiring mechanical ventilation. Chest 2006;129(6):1468–77.

122 Elliott R, McKinley S, Cistulli P, Fien M. Characterisation of sleep in intensive care using 24-hour polysomnography: an observational study. Crit Care 2013;17(2):R46.

123 Drouot X, Cabello B, d'Ortho M-P, Brochard L. Sleep in the intensive care unit. Sleep Medicine Reviews [Internet]. 2008 070808; doi:10.1016/j.smrv.2007.11.004.

124 McKinley S, Fien M, Elliott R, Elliott D. Sleep and psychological health during early recovery from critical illness: an observational study. J Psychosom Res 2013;75(6):539–45.

125 Freedman NS, Kotzer N, Schwab RJ. Patient perception of sleep quality and etiology of sleep disruption in the intensive care unit. Am J Respir Crit Care Med 1999;159(4 Pt 1):1155–62.

126 Frisk U, Nordström G. Patients' sleep in an intensive care unit – patients' and nurses' perception. Intensive Crit Care Nurs 2003;19(6):342–9.

127 Knapp-Spooner C, Yarcheski A. Sleep patterns and stress in patients having coronary bypass. Heart Lung 1992;21(4):342–9.

128 Nicolás A, Aizpitarte E, Iruarrizaga A, Vázquez M, Margall A, Asiain C. Perception of night-time sleep by surgical patients in an intensive care unit. Nurs Crit Care 2008;13(1):25–33.

129 Kryger MH, Roth T, Dement WC. Principles and practice of sleep medicine. 5th ed. Philadelphia: Elsevier Saunders; 2011.

130 Iber C, Ancoli-Israel S, Chesson A, Quan SF, eds. AASM Manual for the Scoring of Sleep and Associated Events: Rules, Terminology and Technical Specification. 1st ed. Westchester, IL: American Academy of Sleep Medicine; 2007.

131 Ohayon MM, Carskadon MA, Guilleminault C, Vitiello MV. Meta-analysis of quantitative sleep parameters from childhood to old age in healthy individuals: developing normative sleep values across the human lifespan. Sleep 2004;27(7):1255–73.

132 Floyd JA, Janisse JJ, Jenuwine ES, Ager JW. Changes in REM-sleep in percentage over the adult lifespan. Sleep 2007;30(7):829–36.

133 Rechtschaffen A, Kales A. A manual of standardized terminology: Techniques and scoring system for sleep stages of human subjects. Los Angeles: UCLA Brain Information Service/Brain Research Institute; 1968.

134 Watson PL, Pandharipande P, Gehlbach BK, Thompson JL, Shintani AK, Dittus BS et al. Atypical sleep in ventilated patients: empirical electroencephalography findings and the path toward revised ICU sleep scoring criteria. Crit Care Med 2013;41(8):1958–67.

135 Ancoli-Israel S, Cole R, Alessi C, Chambers M, Moorcroft W, Pollak CP. The role of actigraphy in the study of sleep and circadian rhythms. Sleep 2003;26(3):342–92.

136 Bourne RS, Minelli C, Mills GH, Kandler R. Clinical review: sleep measurement in critical care patients: research and clinical implications. Crit Care 2007;11(4):226.

137 Nieuwenhuijs D, Coleman EL, Douglas NJ, Drummond GB, Dahan A. Bispectral index values and spectral edge frequency at different stages of physiologic sleep. Anesth Analg 2002;94(1):125–9, table of contents.

138 Sleigh JW, Andrzejowski J, Steyn-Ross A, Steyn-Ross M. The Bispectral Index: A measure of depth of sleep? Anesth Analg 1999;88:659–61.

139 Richards KC, O'Sullivan PS, Phillips RL. Measurement of sleep in critically ill patients. J Nurs Meas 2000;8(2):131–44.

140 Richards KC. Effect of a back massage and relaxation intervention on sleep in critically ill patients. Am J Crit Care 1998;7(4):288–99.

141 Edwards GB, Schuring LM. Pilot study: validating staff nurses' observations of sleep and wake states among critically ill patients, using polysomnography. Am J Crit Care 1993;2(2):125–31.

142 Beecroft JM, Ward M, Younes M, Crombach S, Smith O, Hanly PJ. Sleep monitoring in the intensive care unit: comparison of nurse assessment, actigraphy and polysomnography. Intensive Care Med 2008;34(11):2076–83.

143 Aurell J, Elmqvist D. Sleep in the surgical intensive care unit: continuous polygraphic recording of sleep in nine patients receiving postoperative care. Br Med J (Clin Res Ed) 1985;290(6474):1029–32.

144 Richardson A, Crow W, Coghill E, Turnock C. A comparison of sleep assessment tools by nurses and patients in critical care. J Clin Nurs 2007;16(9):1660–8.

145 Richardson S. Effects of relaxation and imagery on the sleep of critically ill adults. Dimens Crit Care Nurs 2003;22(4):182–90.

146 Richardson A, Allsop M, Coghill E, Turnock C. Earplugs and eye masks: do they improve critical care patients' sleep? Nurs Crit Care 2007;12(6):278–86.

147 Aaron JN, Carlisle CC, Carskadon MA, Meyer TJ, Hill NS, Millman RP. Environmental noise as a cause of sleep disruption in an intermediate respiratory care unit. Sleep 1996;19(9):707–10.

148 Gabor JY, Cooper AB, Crombach SA, Lee B, Kadikar N, Bettger HE et al. Contribution of the intensive care unit environment to sleep disruption in mechanically ventilated patients and healthy subjects. Am J Respir Crit Care Med 2003;167(5):708–15.

149 Dennis CM, Lee R, Woodard EK, Szalaj JJ, Walker CA. Benefits of quiet time for neuro-intensive care patients. J Neurosci Nurs 2010;42(4):217–24.

150 Environmental Protection Agency US. EPA identifies noise levels affecting health and welfare, <http://www.epa.gov/history/topics/noise/01.htm>; 1974 [accessed 21.11.08].

151 Ryherd EE, Waye KP, Ljungkvist L. Characterizing noise and perceived work environment in a neurological intensive care unit. J Acoust Soc Am 2008;123(2):747–56.

152 Tijunelis MA, Fitzsullivan E, Henderson SO. Noise in the ED. Am J Emerg Med 2005;23(3):332–5.

153 Topf M, Davis JE. Critical care unit noise and rapid eye movement (REM) sleep. Heart Lung 1993;22(3):252–8.

154 Frisk U, Olsson J, Nylén P, Hahn RG. Low melatonin excretion during mechanical ventilation in the intensive care unit. Clin Sci (Lond) 2004;107(1):47–53.

155 Olofsson K, Alling C, Lundberg D, Malmros C. Abolished circadian rhythm of melatonin secretion in sedated and artificially ventilated intensive care patients. Acta Anaesthesiol Scand 2004;48(6):679–84.

156 Perras B, Meier M, Dodt C. Light and darkness fail to regulate melatonin release in critically ill humans. Intensive Care Med 2007;33(11):1954–8.

157 Cabello B, Thille AW, Drouot X, Galia F, Mancebo J, d'Ortho MP et al. Sleep quality in mechanically ventilated patients: comparison of three ventilatory modes. Crit Care Med 2008;36(6):1749–55.

158 Bourne RS, Mills GH. Sleep disruption in critically ill patients – pharmacological considerations. Anaesthesia 2004;59(4):374–84.

159 Hardin KA. Sleep in the ICU: potential mechanisms and clinical implications. Chest 2009;136(1):284–94.

160 Buscemi N, Vandermeer B, Hooton N, Pandya R, Tjosvold L, Hartling L et al. Efficacy and safety of exogenous melatonin for secondary sleep disorders and sleep disorders accompanying sleep restriction: meta-analysis. Br Med J 2006;332(7538):385–93.

161 Buscemi N, Vandermeer B, Hooton N, Pandya R, Tjosvold L, Hartling L et al. The efficacy and safety of exogenous melatonin for primary sleep disorders. A meta-analysis. J Gen Intern Med 2005;20(12):1151–8.

162 Ibrahim MG, Bellomo R, Hart GK, Norman TR, Goldsmith D, Bates S et al. A double-blind placebo-controlled randomised pilot study of nocturnal melatonin in tracheostomised patients. Crit Care Resusc 2006;8(3):187–91.

163 Bourne RS, Mills GH, Minelli C. Melatonin therapy to improve nocturnal sleep in critically ill patients: encouraging results from a small randomised controlled trial. Crit Care 2008;12(2):R52.

164 Shilo L, Dagan Y, Smorjik Y, Weinberg U, Dolev S, Komptel B et al. Effect of melatonin on sleep quality of COPD intensive care patients: a pilot study. Chronobiol Int 2000;17(1):71–6.

165 Claustrat B, Brun J, Chazot G. The basic physiology and pathophysiology of melatonin. Sleep Med Rev 2005;9(1):11–24.

166 Brzezinski A, Vangel MG, Wurtman RJ, Norrie G, Zhdanova I, Ben-Shushan A et al. Effects of exogenous melatonin on sleep: a meta-analysis. Sleep Med Rev 2005;9(1):41–50.

167 Melzack R. The short-form McGill Pain Questionnaire. Pain 1987;30(2):191–7.

168 Nilsson U. The anxiety- and pain-reducing effects of music interventions: a systematic review. AORN J 2008;87(4):780–807.

Family and cultural care of the critically ill patient

Marion Mitchell, Denise Wilson, Robyn Aitken

Learning objectives

After reading this chapter, you should be able to:

- describe models of care and evaluate how they meet patient and family needs
- recognise appropriate resources to enhance communication
- develop an understanding of the needs of families and patients who die in the ICU
- evaluate and implement appropriate strategies for working with families from a diversity of cultures
- recognise and implement the needs of the critically ill and/or dying patient who is either an Aboriginal or Torres Strait Islander person or Māori
- recognise the various religious considerations for patients who are dying or who have died.

Introduction

Care of critically ill patients is complex and multifactorial. Although management of the haemodynamic parameters and healthcare interventions is an essential component of effective care of the critically ill, the psycho-social health and wellbeing of patients are intimately related to their wellness and eventual illness outcome. There is a tendency, due to the technologically complex nature of nursing in critical areas, for novice nurses to focus their attention on the management of medical treatment regimens. This is an important part of their learning trajectory. However, nurses need to be guided to see beyond the waveforms and physical parameters to see the patient in the bed as an individual with unique needs. The previous chapter examined specific aspects of the psychological wellbeing of the critically ill with strategies to improve patient outcomes. This chapter extends the focus to incorporate the family into the caring paradigm and introduces the concept of person-centred, patient-centred and family-centred care. Nursing practices that incorporate the patient's family into the care of the critically ill acknowledge the vital part families play in the illness continuum.

The assessment, understanding and incorporation of the patient's and family's cultural needs are essential elements of nursing the critically ill, and involve the entire multidisciplinary team. These elements are important for both the recipients of the care (the patient and family) and the critical care nurse, as the practice of nursing all aspects of the patient's wellbeing brings humanity into critical care nursing. Cultural factors include social factors and human behaviours associated with emotional and spiritual needs.[1] In this chapter, models of nursing are examined with particular reference to the philosophy of family-centred care, which may be an appropriate nursing model for use within critical care settings. The specific needs of the families of critically ill patients are discussed, also the implications for critical care nursing. The differing world views on health and illness are highlighted for consideration of appropriate care. Many of the populations where we practise exhibit diversity of ethnicity, country of origin and cultural practices. Effective communication is crucial to meet both family members' needs and those of the patient. The complexity of patient communication together with the addition of linguistically diverse patients is outlined and suggestions for clinical practice provided. End-of-life care is discussed in general terms and specific cultural considerations are highlighted with particular reference to Aboriginal and Torres Strait Islander people of Australia and New Zealand Māori patients and families.

Overview of models of care

The ways that nurses manage their daily activities and patient care are affected by both the critical care unit's model of care delivery and the nurse's personal philosophy of what and how nursing is constructed. Alternative models of care are examined in this section and their use in critical care areas discussed. Nursing models define shared values and beliefs that guide practice. Various philosophies and models of nursing care delivery have evolved over the decades and contrast with the 'medical model', which focuses on the diagnosis and treatment of disease.[2] Models such as primary nursing and team nursing include organisational or management properties, whereas patient-centred practice is another model in which a partnership relationship is developed between health professionals and the patient and family.[3–8]

Patient-centred care

Patient-centered care shifts control in health-related decisions from the healthcare professional to the patient – the recipient of care, thus challenging some existing paradigms.[9] This model has patient empowerment as the core element. To facilitate empowerment, patients need to be well informed in such a way that they can understand the information to help with their decisions.[6] It is incumbent upon critical care nurses to ask patients about their illness perceptions, priorities and future plans. Having a clear understanding of patients' concepts of illness, their cultural beliefs and intent is vital.[3,6] Treating patients with respect and providing care that is responsive to individual patient preferences, needs and values is fundamental to acknowledging empowerment.[10]

Implementation of patient-centred care requires a culture change and therefore needs support at an individual professional level and at an organisational level.[11] A study in the USA examined how critical care nurses communicate with patients and families within a patient-centred care framework that was operating within their unit. They found that nurses predominantly communicated information related to the patient's acute biophysical status. Although the nurses in the study supported the importance of shared power and responsibility, they exhibited few examples in practice. They reflected that they felt sharing power fell within the domain of intensivists' discussions with patients and families rather than theirs.[12] Nurses deferring responsibility for communication in such a way highlights the importance of a whole-of-team approach to patient-centred care where healthcare professionals share the responsibility of meaningfully involving patients and their families in decisions and care options.

Person-centred care

More recently, the term person-centred care has gained favour over patient-centred care.[13–15] The *Oxford Dictionary* defines 'patient' in passive terms as the receiver of care whereas a 'person' is acknowledged as being an individual.[16] Those who read about patient-centred care (as outlined above) will understand that the word patient in the context of patient-centred care is far from the passive role in this dictionary definition. However, if consumers are to understand healthcare organisations' working paradigms, semantics and first impressions are important. The term 'person-centred care' emphasises the individual nature of the person with the illness. It promotes the perception (and reality) of equal power and a shared partnership between the person and healthcare provider/s. Here, the person is an acknowledged expert for their own health values and goals. The partnership is both collaborative and respectful and highlights the importance of knowing the person behind the patient and understanding that the patient is more than their illness.[4,13]

No evaluations of person-centred care in critical care areas could be found. However, some evidence is coming out of the Centre for Person-centred Care in the University of Gothenburg in Sweden. In one in-hospital study of chronic heart failure patients, length of stay was reduced by a third with no compromise in their perceived quality of care when person-centred care was compared to usual care. The individualised care plan based on understanding each patient's needs was seen to be a major contributing factor in reducing hospital stay.[14] In another study of patients with chronic heart failure in the USA, person-centred care was explored in five wards in a single hospital that implemented a person-centred care approach.[12] Person-centred care was evaluated in relation to how it reduced patients' uncertainty about their illness. The differing organisational and operational features of the ward were examined. In wards where goal setting, planning, control and stability were evident, patients' uncertainty in illness was reduced, which the authors linked to a person-centred approach to care.[12] Within an ICU environment, however, a truly shared partnership with the patient may be problematic, where critical illness restricts patient involvement in decision making and care planning.[17] In reality, it is generally family members who provide the link between the patient and healthcare team.

During the 1980s, the role of the family was one focus of nursing debate and discussion. Friedman believed families were the greatest social institution influencing individuals' health in our society.[18] A worldwide trend is for health professionals to value the role of family members in providing ongoing, post-acute care,[19] with the reality being that families provide considerable support during rehabilitation phases of critical illnesses.[20–22] The family is strongly incorporated within the three philosophies of patient-centred, person-centred and family-centred care. Whichever model is selected, it must be practical and understood in the clinical setting for which it is intended.[2]

Family-centred care

Family-centred care shares the responsibility of patient care decisions with the family and thus highlights the importance of family in critical care areas. The family-centred model of care, developed during the early 1990s, primarily in North America in the area of children's nursing, considered incorporating the family was fundamental to the care of the patient.[23] Over the past two decades, the scope and extent of family-centred care has broadened and the Institute for Family-Centered Care defines family-centred care as 'an innovative approach to the planning, delivery,[24] and evaluation of healthcare that is governed by mutually beneficial partnerships among healthcare providers, patients and families'.[25] Patient-and-family-centred care applies to patients of all ages, and it may be practised in any healthcare setting.

Family-centred care is founded on mutual respect and partnership among patients, families and healthcare providers. It incorporates all aspects of physical and psychosocial care, from assessment to care delivery and evaluation.[26] Healthcare providers that value the family/patient partnership during a critical illness strive to facilitate relationship building and provide amenities and services that facilitate families being near their hospitalised relative.[19] When a clinical unit's staff embrace a family-centred care philosophy and partner with families to make changes to the physical environment, such as improved privacy and aesthetically pleasing decor, it can have the added advantage of positive culture changes for the staff. Such outcomes indicate there is a benefit beyond the family members for whom the changes were initiated.[27]

In trying to understand family-centred care, neonatal and paediatric ICU studies have focused on parents' perceptions of care in the three key components of family-centred care: respect, collaboration and support.[28–30] In the area of respect, families rated most highly 'feeling welcome when I come to the hospital' and 'I feel like a parent, not a visitor'.[28] Within the area of collaboration, feeling well-prepared for discharge and being given honest

information about care were rated the highest. The familiarity of nurses with the special needs of patients was rated highest in the area of support.[28]

Many nurses also value family involvement in the care of their own sick relative.[31,32] Strategies to improve family-centred care within adult critical care areas include involving family members in partnering with the nursing staff to consider the involvement they would like, which may include providing fundamental care to their sick relative.[33] Family members can decide in consultation and negotiation with the bedside nurse the care that they want, and are able to provide. This care may vary from moisturising their relative's skin to a full sponge and will require negotiation. Such acts of caring allow family members to connect in what they see as a meaningful way with their sick relative. In addition, it can also improve communication with critical care nurses and facilitate close physical and emotional contact with their relative.[34] An independent nursing intervention such as partnering with family to provide care constitutes an example of how to operationalise a family-centred care model in the clinical setting and assists in the evaluation of other future interventions directed to improve an area's family-centred approach. Further research on the benefits of family-centred care is needed in all critical care areas.[33,35,36]

It is acknowledged that taking care of critically ill patients requires considerable knowledge and skill. When family members are incorporated into the caring paradigm, as advocated within family-centred care, health professionals equally need specific knowledge and skills.[28] This information should be initiated in foundation degrees, postgraduate studies and via ongoing professional development opportunities.[12,37]

Beyond the educational needs for nurses there is an international policy drive to include families as a quality and safety measure in patient care.[38–40] The family knows the patient best, has their best interest foremost and is the one constant throughout the critical illness. Family members provide ongoing care and involving them during the critical illness phase supports their ability to provide immediate feedback and prolonged care to their relative. Involving and supporting families is not necessarily time-consuming but, to be able to do this, an understanding of the needs of families is required.[18,41]

Needs of family during critical illness

Family members of critically ill patients contribute a significant and ongoing involvement to patients' wellbeing.[42] Patients need and want their family members with them[43] and healthcare professionals also need family members' input.[44] Family members' satisfaction with the care their relative receives is considered a legitimate quality indicator in many areas that routinely assess family satisfaction.[45,46]

On a very practical level within a critical illness situation, family members are often the decision makers on treatment options due to the impaired cognitive state of the patient. Their contribution to healthcare decisions is sought in both acute and ongoing care situations as they have insight and knowledge of the patient on an entirely different level to health professionals.[47] In addition, family members provide not only support in the critical illness situation, but also continuity of care through rehabilitation. This responsibility together with the often sudden critical illness may create stress, anxiety, depression and/or post-traumatic stress disorder (PTSD) for family members.[48,49] A primary aim of family-centred care is to reduce the risk of stress-related reactions to the ICU experience, which is often traumatic for family members.[50,51]

Practice tip

Suggest to a family member(s) that they might like to remain by the bedside (when you would normally ask them to leave). At first it may feel daunting, as the family member may seem to watch your every move and action, but if you start doing this when you are performing interventions with which you feel confident, you will find that having them there seems natural. There is less fuss with family coming and going and talking about what you are doing, and it promotes information sharing and understanding.

Stress and anxiety associated with having a critically ill relative can hinder a family's coping ability, adaptation, decision making[52] and long-term health with the possibility that post-traumatic stress disorder (PTSD) may develop in family members of ICU patients.[50] Families that experience stress before the critical illness do not cope as well, and may need additional assistance.[53] As many as half of family members report symptoms of anxiety and depression, indicating it is a very real problem.[32] These figures are concerning, particularly when symptoms continue beyond 6 months post ICU.[50,54] In addition, post-traumatic stress symptoms are reported by family members, which is consistent with a moderate-to-major risk of PTSD, resulting in ongoing health-related concerns for the family members.[50] Early identification and prevention strategies are an important area for further research.[50,55] Meeting the needs of families during this stressful and demanding time has the capacity to reduce their stress and promote positive coping strategies.

A combined healthcare team approach is needed to meet the family's needs, as differing perceptions among the healthcare team can result in non-unified approaches[56] that are potentially confusing. The needs of families with critically ill relatives are complex and multifactorial, reinforcing the need for an all-of-team approach.[56] Family members' needs were recognised in Molter's influential study in 1979 in which she researched the specific needs of ICU patients' family members. Although Molter's sample was small ($n = 40$), 45 potential needs of family members were identified and ranked in order of importance.[57] Family needs continue to be researched[48,58–63] and can be generally grouped into the need for: 1) information,

2) reassurance, 3) closeness, 4) support and 5) comfort.[52] More specifically, families' needs include the following:[52]

- to know their relative's progress and prognosis
- to have their questions answered honestly
- to speak to a doctor at least once a day
- to be given consistent information by staff
- to feel their relative is looked after by competent and caring people
- to feel confident that staff will call them at home if changes occur in their relative's condition
- to be given a sense of hope
- to know about transfer plans as they are being made.

Meeting information needs

Families' needs for information and reassurance are paramount during a critical illness, which is often unexpected or unexplained. Seven out of the top ten needs of families are related to information needs.[64] When information is provided, it is important to spend sufficient time with family members.[65] A self-designated family member can act as the primary receiver of information and take the responsibility of relaying the information to others. However, the information has to make sense to them and it is imperative that healthcare professionals check their understanding.[59] It is not sufficient to think, 'But I told them all that yesterday'. Communication is a two-way process and as such needs to be received in a meaningful way as well as given appropriately. Repeated and current information is suggested as it helps to reduce family members' anxiety.[59] In a case study report of a mother and her adult war-injured son, the mother tells how she tried to remember things the staff told her. She said, 'I loved how my questions would be answered when we asked (except for the daily one about his brain damage) and how most people did not take offense at me writing down everything. I know that I was scared to death most of the entire time'.[48, p.18]

Strategies to improve communication with family members include nurse-led education sessions designed to identify and meet the needs of family members. Once the needs have been identified, a specific program can be developed to meet those needs. This strategy was found to be effective when two 1-hour sessions were conducted with family members who reported significantly lower levels of anxiety and higher levels of satisfaction.[60] Other units may choose to have a designated critical care nursing position in their unit that focuses on family advocacy within a family-centred care philosophy.[66]

Multidisciplinary patient rounds that meaningfully include the family show an inclusive and open communication process that values all contributors as they make an individual plan of care for the patient.[48] Alternatively, consider routine family meetings with the healthcare team aimed at improving communication and understanding.[61,62] Frequently, family meetings are called when the family is needed to make critical decisions about the ongoing care of their relative rather than as a proactive and positive strategy that allows for patient and family preferences to be integrated into patient care.[62]

Family conferences with the interdisciplinary team should be organised in a staged and planned manner with the first occurring within the first 48 hours of admission, the second after 3 days and a third when there is a significant change in treatment goals.[24,64] Fundamental topics for the interdisciplinary meetings with the family could include the patient's condition and prognosis together with short- and long-term treatment goals.[24,45,67] Family conferences provide time for discussion among family members with the healthcare team as a resource and also for the team to make an assessment of the family's understanding of the situation. In addition, they provide an opportunity to develop an awareness of specific family needs that the team can endeavour to meet.[45] Unhurried family conferencing allows opportunities for families to pose questions and longer family conferences can result in families feeling greater support and significantly reduced PTSD symptoms.[68] Some authors suggest the family should be given a meeting guide prior to the family conference that outlines the purpose of the meeting and points for discussion relating to current and future patient care. A meeting guide prompts family members to jot down their questions prior to coming to the conference to ensure these are discussed,[69] as it is well recognised that families forget, or are hesitant to ask their questions.

Although family conferencing has been found beneficial, it is advocated that multiple modes of communication and information sharing are required. Individualised or general information via leaflets, brochures and internet-based information and support strategies are also helpful.[45,68,70]

To promote communication, nurses can discuss with the family whether they would like a phone call at night updating them on their relative's condition. Alternatively, nurses can give them a time to phone before change of shift. This will help to allay their anxiety and promotes positive communication and trust. When patients are transferred from critical care, families and patients may become anxious or concerned by the reduced level of care in the new ward area. This can be alleviated by providing families with verbal and individualised written transfer information as a means to help prepare them for transfer.[71] In addition, a structured transferring plan helps critical care nurses feel better equipped to ensure they give families the information they need at this important time of transfer.[72]

Visiting practices

One of the primary needs of families is the need to be physically close to their sick relative. Patient confidentiality and privacy remain central and need to be balanced with family presence.[73] Patients find that family provides a link with their pre-illness self and provides support and comfort.[74]

Family-friendly policies with few restrictions that centre on genuine patient care issues require the support of critical care nurses and medical officers for them to work effectively.[75] This is particularly relevant for patients' families who live large distances from the hospital and have to travel for many hours in order to be with their sick relative. Flexible visiting policies have been found to improve quality indicators with higher patient and family satisfaction levels and fewer formal complaints.[76] Restrictive visiting policies limit families' access to their relatives and restrict their involvement. Family members are different from other visitors in critical care areas because of their intimate relationship, which helps to form crucial components of the patient's identity.[77–79] Remember that there are often different meanings or interpretations of 'family', with family often meaning more than just the immediate nuclear family (e.g. the Māori *whānau* [extended family] and the Aboriginal 'compound' family). Negotiation of visiting processes that take into account these cultural understandings is imperative and is discussed later in this chapter.

There is a genuine concern by some parents or carers that children should not visit family members who are critically ill as they may find the ICU environment and visit traumatic. However, this needs to be balanced against a child who experiences separation anxiety, which can be intense and have a negative impact on their adaptive functioning. In addition, when children are appropriately supported in visiting a critically ill close family member, they are more likely to be not frightened but rather curious about their surroundings.[37] Children may have questions and it is recommended that they be prepared well with adequate information before, during and after their time with their relative in the critical care area.

Patients, however, may want visiting restricted as some patients find them stressful or tiring.[21] Contrary to popular belief, unrestricted visiting hours are not associated with long visits. In two separate European studies where unrestricted visiting hours were introduced, the number of hours family members spent with the patient was low. They stayed for 1 to 2 hours per day and usually came during the day. This suggests that when family members have free access to their sick relative they do not perceive a sense of duty to be there all day and night.[14,80]

Barriers that restrict family presence require attention as family attendance is beneficial to the patient[43] and a primary need for family members.[70] Although some critical care staff indicate they experience performance anxiety with the family present during procedures[43,81] or with extended family visits,[21] many nurses are comfortable providing care with the family present.[82] Staff who do not feel comfortable with this methodology require support and mentoring to facilitate this fundamental aspect of family-centred care.

Participating in patient care is one way for family members to feel closer to their critically ill family member[74,83,84] and at the same time promotes family integrity.[83] Most family members, however, will not ask if they can help with care[32] as this is seen as the nurses'

TABLE 8.1

Family participation in patient care

PRINCIPLE	PROCEDURE
Consent	Gain patient consent beforehand where possible
Building of trust	Introduce the concept of family members' involvement in care after a period during which a rapport is developed
Individualise for patient and family	Offer suitable options from which family members can choose: for example, massaging feet and hands, cleaning teeth and feeding may be appropriate options for short-term patients, whereas additional options may exist for long-term patients
Safety	The registered nurse should remain physically close by at all times
Promote achievement of goals	Provide sufficient information to the family member to support successful completion of the care
Reflect on outcomes	Provide feedback to family members on how they performed the task
Continuity of care	Document the care the family members participated in and any relevant information

domain in adult critical care areas.[85,86] Nurses, therefore, should invite family members to be part of the patient's care, with massaging and providing a sponge being popular activities.[6,33,86] Providing care allows the family members to feel connected emotionally with their relative and provides a means to get to know and communicate with the nurses, which families consider important. Family members appreciate invitations from nurses as this allows them to feel more in control[24] in a situation where family members do not often experience this.[87,88]

For family participation to work effectively and safely, a number of guiding principles should be incorporated, as outlined in Table 8.1. It is useful for critical care nurses to explore their beliefs and practices concerning family participation, as many support family participation but do not always implement these beliefs in their practice.[89]

Communication

The ability to communicate effectively is an underlying tenet of nursing practice and a fundamental need for people. As mentioned previously in the context of caring for family members, for communication to occur, there needs to be a two-way passage of ideas or information. In the patient context the inability to communicate causes, or adds to, anxiety, frustration and stress[90–92] as they lose control over their life and decisions.[93] It is therefore imperative for healthcare professionals to find ways to communicate with patients in simple non-technical language. Critically ill patients commonly have

communication difficulties due to either mechanical devices (e.g. endotracheal tubes),[90] cognitive impairment from the disease and/or pharmacological medications or language difficulties.[94] Therefore, effective communication is challenging, and nurses need additional knowledge and understanding of these complex situations to meet medico-legal obligations and to assist in meeting the key information needs of patients and families.[95] As many critically ill patients are unconscious, it is important to understand the need for verbal communication to continue. Such communication did not occur in one Jordanian setting where in-depth interviews and observations in three critical care areas identified that nurses communicated less with unconscious patients than with conscious patients.[96] It has been known for decades that sedated and unconscious patients can hear and recall some verbal communication once they regain consciousness.[97,98]

Meeting information needs builds trust between the nurse and patient and their family as a relationship develops.[95] The nurse's understanding of the person behind the patient is important to families, and can be achieved by talking to the family about the patient's life before the illness.[99]

Good communication is a prime patient need and inspires patient confidence, making patients feel safe.[100] When nurses reassure patients they provide a sense of hope and a feeling of safety, which is further supported by family members' presence and the patients' religious beliefs, which may include the desire to have their priest or religious leader visit.[93,100] Constructive strategies should be identified to overcome difficulties with patient communication. This is worthwhile pursuing as it reduces both nurse and patient frustration and improves nursing care.[91] The following methods of communication may be used individually or together to enhance communication, and should be readily employed in critical care settings:[90,101]

- body language
- lip reading
- writing
- alphabet boards
- communication boards
- pictures
- gestures, including nodding and blinking of the eyes.

Although electronic voice output communication aids are used with disabled children and adults, they have not been evaluated sufficiently with an ICU population. These aids use prerecorded digitalised voice messages or synthesised speech, with the phrases accessed by the patient via a computer screen or keyboard.[101] This device would be restricted to those patients who are dexterous and able to select an appropriate key, which limits its utility in the ICU setting. However, some patients in a small study found electronic voice output beneficial, particularly when communicating with family.[101]

Practice tip

Routinely, both document and inform the nurse taking over the patient's care of any points of patient and family discussion and any codes that have been developed during the shift to promote communication. This fosters continuity of care and consistency in information sharing and is useful to the entire healthcare team.

An effective strategy to promote good communication is for health professionals to seek and maintain eye contact (if culturally appropriate). This may mean the nurse or doctor sitting down on a chair beside the bed to facilitate face-to-face communication.[95] This act also conveys a sense of the importance the health professional is placing on the interaction by taking time to ensure they understand each other. Associated with this is the need to use commonly understood language. One method of checking patients' responses is to repeat these back to them. A quiet environment reduces extraneous noise and potential interruptions, and may promote communication and concentration. Codes may also be developed by the nurse and patient, with facial expression, head nods and eye blinks used to respond to questions.[91] These codes should be passed on to the next nurse and recorded in the patient's notes to promote continuity of care.

When communication seems unsuccessful, talking loudly will not improve the interaction; one good strategy is for the nurse and patient to agree to try again later.[91] Communication can also occur through physical contact, and touch often communicates empathy and provides spiritual comfort.[1] Spiritual needs may further be met by providing comfort, reassurance and respect for privacy, and by helping patients relate to others.[102]

Practice tip

Communication with the family is essential. When family members describe the patient, Ling-Chi, as the 55-year-old wife of Lee and mother of two adult children, June and Maggie, who works full-time as an enrolled nurse, they help the staff to see the person beyond the patient with an illness. This assists the critical care nurse to individualise care.

Language barriers may necessitate the assistance of an interpreter with knowledge of healthcare terminology to ensure the content is adequately translated. An independent person ensures that the patient receives the message in its entirety from the health professional.[95] Interviews with previously intubated patients after discharge from the ICU capture, from the patients' perspective, issues with communication and highlight the need for further improvement and understanding of the two-way process. An example of this is from an ex-patient, who related her situation: 'They would come into the room in masses to talk to me. One doctor would stand there and read off a

summary: '[Subject's name], we find her this and that', and they'd be saying stuff and I'd think, 'Oh no!' They would ask me, 'Do you understand?', 'Are there any questions?' And I would think … 'I don't even know what you just said; how do I know if I have questions or not?'[93] In this case, both parties were trying to communicate with each other, but it is apparent that the patient was not able to take in and process the information about her current condition and therefore had difficulty comprehending. Basic principles of patient autonomy and respect need to be used cautiously with critically ill patients who may appear competent, when in reality their cognitive ability is impaired.[17] Effective communication with the family is vital in order to determine the cultural beliefs and practices of patients and their family to further enhance communication and understanding.

Cultural care

The challenge for critical care nurses is to establish positive working relationships with the patient (when possible) and the family so their important values, beliefs and practices can be shared and incorporated in plans of intervention and treatment. It is not always possible to 'know' another person's culture in any great depth, or 'know' all cultural beliefs and practices of the patients and families a critical care nurse comes into contact with. Therefore, establishing relationships with the patient and the family during their critical care experience is crucial, and also demonstrates both respect for, and valuing of, patients and their families and the cultural beliefs and practices they hold. This enables critical care teams to better meet their needs.

Although people's ethnicities may provide a clue to their culture, it is not a reliable indicator and ignores the multiple cultural groups people belong to that extend beyond ethnicity, such as age and gender. Furthermore, with increasing migration globally and inter-ethnic marriages, some people identify with more than one ethnic group. Making assumptions about a person's culture and reliance on universal approaches to direct nursing practice engenders risks to nursing practice and potentially compromises the outcomes of interactions and interventions. Even within cultural groups (e.g. indigenous and immigrant groups), variations in beliefs and practices can exist. Such differences result from factors such as colonisation, interactions with the various groups a person belongs to, responses to societal changes and the socialisation of immigrants into a new country. Thus, person-centred care of patients and their families is imperative to incorporating specific cultural needs in the planning and delivery of interventions. This section outlines important strategies critical care nurses can develop for working with patients and their families to identify the essential beliefs and practices they need to have incorporated into treatment and intervention plans during a stressful time in an unfamiliar environment. Such actions can optimise their spiritual wellbeing and lessen some of the stress they feel.

Defining culture

Wepa describes culture: 'Our way of living is our culture. It is our taken-for-grantedness that determines and defines our culture. The way we brush our teeth, the way we bury people, the way we express ourselves through art, religion, eating habits, rituals, humour, science, law and sport; the way we celebrate occasions … is our culture. All these actions we carry out consciously and unconsciously'.[103,p.31] Simply, culture refers to the values, beliefs and practices that patients, family members and nurses undertake on a daily basis. It determines how they view the world, and their orientation to health, illness, life and death.[104,105]

Culture involves a shared set of rules and perspectives acquired through the processes of socialisation and internalisation. These provide a frame of reference to guide how members interpret such phenomena as health and illness and death and dying. This, in turn, influences their actions and interactions.[105] Culture is a more specific way of describing how groups of people function on a daily basis, influenced by their beliefs, relationships and the activities they engage in.

Understanding that culture, ethnicity and race are not the same thing is crucial to meeting the cultural needs of patients and their families. Race is generally determined on the basis of physical characteristics and is often used to socially classify people broadly as Caucasians, Europeans, Polynesians or Asians, for example.[106] However, assigning people to a homogeneous group is problematic, the antithesis of cultural diversity,[103] particularly as globally countries are becoming increasingly ethnically diverse. Furthermore, homogenisation does not account for the diversity that exists within many groups in contemporary society. Ethnicity extends beyond the physical characteristics associated with race to include such factors as common origins, language, history and dress – it is usually associated with nations,[103] although a number of ethnic groups may exist within a nation.

Differing world views

Culture influences how people view the world, what they believe in and how they do things, particularly with regard to practices around health, dying and death. The critical care environment is unfamiliar for patients and families, especially as health professionals' beliefs, practices and world views may not align with their own. What is important for critical care nurses may not be important for the patient or the family, and may lead to tension and dissatisfaction when patients' and families' views are at variance. This does not mean that one world view is necessarily more right or wrong – they are different.

The biomedical model influences the way healthcare services are structured and delivered.[107] As a dominant model it heavily influences the necessary focus on the physical wellbeing of patients within critical care environments. Focusing on the management of disease and illness, and using processes that lead to health issues being fragmented and reduced to presenting signs and symptoms

and diagnoses, risks excluding what is important for the patient and family.[108] This contrasts with indigenous cultures, for example, which tend to have a holistic eco-spiritual world view, with a strong spiritual dimension that extends beyond a disease and illness focus.[109] The world view of critical care nurses is influenced by the cultural beliefs, practices and life circumstances of each nurse, and the 'world view' of the critical care service that drives its service delivery. The result is that, consequently, patients and their families become sandwiched between differing world views.

Research highlights the lack of alignment that can occur between the needs of consumers of health services and the intentions of healthcare providers such as nurses.[110] It is the potential for the non-alignment between patients and families and healthcare providers that critical care nurses need to be aware of, as dissatisfaction with the care being delivered may arise when the patient's and family's needs are not recognised or attended to,[111] leading to unnecessary tensions and conflicts between patients, families and nurses. A nurse's willingness to acknowledge and respect patients' world views and the things that are important to them minimises the occurrence of any dissatisfaction,[108] as it values their specific needs during their critical care experience.

> **Practice tip**
>
> Being able to deliver culturally responsive nursing care requires the nurse to undergo a process of education and self-examination of culture, own cultural beliefs and practices, and the possible influences these may have on practice.

Where the world views of patients and families are considerably different from that of the nurse, nurses should identify the beliefs they hold about the patient and family, the impact of these interactions on the patient and family and the power the nurse can utilise during such interactions.[103] Sometimes the nurse's personal beliefs will be in conflict with professional nursing beliefs, which necessitates choosing between personal and professional beliefs in the practice setting. For example, a nurse's personal beliefs about life, death and body tissues may be compromised by the duty to care for a patient with brain death awaiting the removal of organs for transplant. This may also be compounded by nursing staff shortages, less-than-desirable skill mixes and the acuity and complexity that critical care nurses are faced with on a daily basis. Therefore, it is vital, not only for the individual nurse, but also for the team of critical care nurses to develop strategies, such as processes and procedures, that can optimise the development of working relationships with patients from different cultural backgrounds.[112]

Cultural responsiveness

Cultural responsiveness refers to strategies for responding to a patient's and their family's cultural backgrounds, and depends on the cultural competence of nurses so that they feel cultural safety. Different models exist to assist in the integration of the cultural beliefs and practices of patients and their family in critical care nursing practice. For example, Leninger's cultural care diversity and universality theory[113] requires nurses to deliver culturally congruent nursing care for people of varying or similar cultures. Ramsden's work on cultural safety[114,115] focuses on the delivery of nursing care to patients (whose cultural beliefs and practices differ from that of the nurse) that is determined appropriate and effective by the patients and families who are the recipients of that care. These models have been used to guide nursing practice in Australia, New Zealand and North America. Such models require that critical care nurses recognise patients' and families' views of their health experience[107] and any that subsequently have discordant priorities. Wood and Schwass have described three levels at which a nurse may practise with respect to cultural issues (see Table 8.2).[116] These levels, ranging from cultural awareness to cultural safety, describe the differing characteristics of nurses' cultural care. For example, a nurse practising in an organisation where cultural safety is required would need not only to recognise differences between groups of people, but also to deliver differing cultural care to patients and their families after undergoing appropriate education.

From a transcultural nursing perspective, culturally responsive nursing care requires the nurse to incorporate cultural knowledge, the nurse's own cultural perspective and the patient's cultural perspective into intervention plans.[117] However, it is not possible to collate cultural knowledge specific to various groups owing to the diversity that exists both among and within groups.[118] Therefore, critical care nurses are advised to critically examine theories and models to guide their practice, to ensure they deliver appropriate and effective care for the patients and families they work with.

Competence is an important dimension of nursing practice, as it provides users of nursing services with confidence in nurses' knowledge, skills and attitudes necessary to undertake their practice. Given the importance of culture in the delivery of nursing care, the measurement of cultural competence is also important. There is evidence of numerous variations on the concept of cultural competence.[118–120] The attributes of cultural competence include cultural awareness, cultural knowledge, cultural understanding, cultural sensitivity, cultural interaction and cultural skill.[119–121] However, the inherent need for the acquisition and use of culturally specific information limits the application of these attributes: the collation of culturally specific information is becoming increasingly problematic as our communities become more diverse in their composition.

Practice tip

The ability to deliver culturally competent nursing practice involves self-awareness, the nurse's actions undertaken to improve the patient's and family's health experience and integrating their beliefs and practices into treatment and intervention plans.

Cultural responsiveness is about practising in a sound manner rather than about behaving correctly.[122] Durie encouraged the development of cultural safety (which focuses on the patient's and their family's experience and determination of the appropriateness of care received), to a construct that can measure the capability of the health worker, such as the critical care nurse.[122] Culturally competent nursing practice is about:

- the nurses' knowledge about their own cultural beliefs and practices and the impact these may have on others
- the actions of the nurse to improve the patient's health experience, and the integration of culture in clinical practice
- delivering culturally competent and safe care.[123]

Cultural competence provides a framework to objectively measure the nurse's performance, although there is variation in frameworks.[112] Fundamental for the critical care nurse to deliver culturally responsive care, which is competent and safe, is determining the cultural needs of patients and families, and the provision of patient-centred care that focuses on their individual needs.

Determining the cultural needs of patient and family

The concepts of health and illness are generally constructed within the context of people's sociocultural environment and the groups they belong to; these vary from person to

TABLE 8.2
Levels of cultural practice

LEVEL OF CULTURAL PRACTICE	INDICATORS
1 Awareness	Recognition that differences between groups of people extend beyond socioeconomic differences
2 Sensitivity	Recognition that difference is valid, which initiates a critical exploration of personal cultural beliefs and practices as a 'bearer' of culture that may affect others
3 Safety	Delivery of a safe service as a result of undergoing education about culture and nursing practice, and reflecting on their own and others' practice

Adapted from Wood PJ, Schwass M. Cultural safety: a framework for changing attitudes. Nurs Prax NZ 1993;8(1): 4–15, with permission.

person and group to group. To this end, culture influences how health and illness experiences are constructed and lived. When people become critically ill, their cultural beliefs and practices can be just as important as their physical health status.[124] Yet cultural beliefs and practices are often compromised when healthcare providers' concern about physical health takes precedence – invariably, health services also do things differently than patients and families would do them. While the importance of psychosocial and cultural needs is the focus of this chapter, the presence of life-threatening events or crises experienced by the patient in critical care must rightfully take precedence. However, on stabilisation of the patient, establishing a positive working relationship with the family can facilitate the determination of their perspectives and needs and negotiation about how these can be included in a potentially complex plan of care. Incorporating cultural requirements becomes vital in a delivery of nursing care that is both appropriate and acceptable. Therefore, given the nature of critical care settings, the quality of interactions with the patient's family is just as crucial as interactions with the patient.

Promoting a genuine, welcoming atmosphere and the use of effective communication invite the family to be involved early in the patient's critical care experience, and are essential to determine the cultural needs of the patient and family. While communication has been mentioned earlier, interpreting cultural needs requires the critical care nurse to be attentive to communication. Nurses are advised to talk less, attend to details that may arise and simply listen. The need to intervene and to dominate discussions and 'interviews' with the family[125] from the nurse's perspective needs to be curbed, so time is made available for cultural beliefs and practices to be shared.[27,108,125] Understanding and supporting the patient and family can be improved by the nurse's empowering them through the processes of listening, understanding and validating what they have to say.[124,126] Conning and Rowland's research on the attitudes of mental health professionals towards management practices and the process of assessing patients and decision making found that those who had a greater 'client orientation' (versus management orientation) were more likely to engage in assessment processes that facilitate patient-centred care that focuses on the individual needs of patients and their family.[127,128]

Working in partnership with a family can bridge the cultural 'gap'. However, this is not always easy to achieve in challenging situations, such as when various members of a large family come and go, compounded by changing nurses with shift changes. Receiving clear and consistent information about the patient, including his/her progress, from all members of the healthcare team can reduce cross-cultural confusion and misunderstanding, especially as messages are prone to distortion and change when many are involved. A strategy to manage this may involve discussing the management of information dissemination with the family, and the identification of one or two family members who become the point of contact through which staff discuss and communicate information about the patient.[108] Often, apparent 'cultural conflicts' will arise

as a result of communication problems with the family; communicating information in a clear and understandable manner helps prevent these problems from occurring.

An Indigenous health workforce

Increasing the representation of indigenous people within the health workforce has been recognised internationally as an important mechanism for improving cultural safety within healthcare facilities.[129] Research has demonstrated that indigenous people are more likely to access mainstream health services if there is an indigenous workforce.[130]

In Australia, there have been efforts to increase the number of Aboriginal registered nurses to improve the competency of the Australian nursing workforce in delivering appropriate care to Aboriginal people. This move is supported by the 'getting 'em 'n' keeping 'em' report of the Indigenous Nursing Education Working Group.[131] Similar strategies for improving culturally responsive care by increasing the participation of First Nations people within the healthcare workforce exist in North America (see, for example, the National Aboriginal Health Organization[132] and the First Nations Authority[133]).

Cultural responsiveness and patient-centred, individualised care

'Individualised care requires the patient and nurse to work together to identify a path towards health that maintains the integrity of the patient's sense of self and is compatible with their personal circumstances'.[134,p.46] This means the critical care nurse ideally working in collaboration with the family to identify important cultural needs and the inclusion of beliefs and practices that need to be observed during the patient's critical care experience; in other words, eliciting a patient's view to ensure person-centred care.[135] It is recognised that 'the work' of the nurse involves responding, anticipating, interpreting and enabling, all of which are crucial for individualised care.[136] Indeed, partnership requires the nurse not only to work with the patient and family but also to identify the power that the nurse possesses and the potential for its inadvertent misuse.[108] Patient- and family-centred care requires critical care nurses to observe each of the following:

- respectfully interacting with the patient and their family, and treating them with dignity
- communicating clearly, without jargon
- sharing information fully and honestly
- using the strengths of the family to enhance their sense of control and independence
- working with patients and their family collaboratively.[136]

Facilitating the inclusion of cultural beliefs and practices requires identification and then incorporation in the patient's plan of care. However, given the resource constraints and the culture of some health services, universal approaches to planning care may be adopted for convenience. The critical care nurse is discouraged from adopting a 'one-size-fits-all' approach to nursing practice, as this disregards the cultural systems of the patient and family.[108] Patient-centred care is optimised by nurses having sufficient information about the patient and family in order to identify their needs and plan interventions. Incorporating each family's cultural beliefs and practices provides a 'bigger picture' of the patient[124] than would have been gained by simply focusing on the presenting disease or illness and its management. Such an approach to patient-centred care enables the critical care nurse to become familiar with the context of the patient's life circumstances and how they interpret illness, and also improves the quality of care and interactions they have with patients and families.[137,138]

Sometimes the nurse will want to have a full understanding of a cultural belief or practice before being willing to incorporate it. For example, several years ago a Māori patient was dying and the family wanted to organise the patient's expedient removal from the hospital environment on the patient's death. This was necessary so that the spiritual and cultural grieving processes could be commenced. But the nurse blocked the family's desire to plan and organise a prompt postmortem on death because the patient had not yet died. This created unnecessary tension and conflict between the nurse and the family. Clearly, the nurse's and the family's beliefs about death and dying were different, and the apparent position of 'power' adopted by the nurse did not encourage communication and negotiation about how this situation could be resolved to the satisfaction of both parties. This is an example of where the identification and acceptance of cultural beliefs and practices of the family (to the extent that they will not deliberately harm the patient), and working with the family on how these are incorporated in an intervention plan, can be beneficial to all parties. Once this has occurred, it is crucial this information is documented, thereby making visible the patient's individualised care.[139]

Practice tip

Determining cultural needs means the critical care nurse must:

- identify a spokesperson to communicate information to so the messages the family receives are consistent
- engage in genuine communication and partnership with the patient and family
- be willing to listen, understand and validate information received.

Practice tip

To optimise interactions with people from a culture different from yours as a critical care nurse:

- avoid making assumptions
- avoid culturally offensive practices that are known and learned
- remember that actions speak louder than words.

Working with culturally and linguistically diverse patients and families

Globalisation has resulted in increasing immigration and migration to both Australia and New Zealand, similar to other countries, thus populations are increasing in their cultural and linguistic diversity. Thirty-three percent of Australians,[140] 25% of New Zealanders,[141] 20.6% of Canadians[142] and 13% of Americans[143] were born overseas. Immigrants arrive from various countries globally, but especially the European, Asian and African continents. Labels assigned to groups of 'immigrants', such as Asians, are misleading and far from the homogeneity they infer. Added to the complexity of trying to determine ways of working with culturally and linguistically diverse patients and families is the variation in their degree of acculturation – for example, some may be second- or third-generation Australian- or New Zealand-born and highly acculturated into the respective culture, or they may be new immigrants with traditional cultural beliefs and practices. Therefore, given this diversity it is difficult to provide specific guidelines on working with culturally and linguistically diverse patients and their families, although some common principles exist.

A fundamental starting point for working with culturally and linguistically diverse patients is to establish their capacity to communicate in English. Determining the language a patient uses on a daily basis, and whether they can speak and write in English, will indicate whether an interpreter is needed. Family members or friends can be used as interpreters when care is being undertaken on a daily basis, although a professional or accredited interpreter should be used when important information is to be shared or when decisions need to be made. This avoids the potential for family members or friends 'censoring' the information conveyed during discussions. How the patient prefers to be addressed, cultural values and beliefs related to communication (e.g. eye contact, personal space or social taboos), preferences related to healthcare providers (that is culture, gender or age), the nature of family support and usual food and nutrition are other areas that should be explored with the patient or family, whichever is appropriate.

Given the great diversity that occurs within contemporary cultural groups, it is crucial to develop a relationship so important cultural values, beliefs and practices can be identified and incorporated into the patient's plan of care. Critical care nurses can then better understand a patient's or family's behaviours when the patient is critically unwell. Discovering the values and beliefs a patient and their family have about health, illness, death and dying, and what they believe may make their health worse, is a good starting point, and will provide insight into the type of support and caring behaviours that may be observed. In addition to this, identifying how health and illnesses are managed will provide an indication of whether traditional healers are used, along with healing remedies such as herbs and prayer, for example. Understanding the patient's locus of control can also provide an indication of whether they will play an active role in the outcome of an illness, or whether there is a fundamental belief that illnesses are caused by some external force.

For many cultural groups the presence of family is vital to both the patient's and family's spiritual wellbeing. Therefore, facilitating family presence at the patient's bedside and possibly including them in the care of the patient is important. For some cultures there is a belief that family members should shoulder the burden of information and decision making so the patient can expend their energy and focus on getting better. In some cases to burden the patient with information about their condition, especially its gravity, or having to make decisions, is believed to contribute to a negative outcome. Thus, positively engaging families and, where practical, patients in collaborative relationships, involving them in the care and decision making and ensuring their cultural values, beliefs and practices are protected are ways critical care nurses can respect the cultural traditions of those patients who are from different cultural and linguistic backgrounds.

Campinha-Bacote's[144] mnemonic, ASKED, provides a process for self-reflection to make explicit your knowledge and skills and desires to work with people who are culturally and linguistically diverse. The following questions can be asked:

- **A**wareness: what awareness do you have of the stereotypes, prejudices and racism that you hold about those in cultural groups that are different from your own?
- **S**kill: what skills do you have to undertake a cultural assessment in an appropriate and safe manner?
- **K**nowledge: how knowledgeable are you about the world views of the various cultural and ethnic groups within your community?
- **E**ncounters: what face-to-face interactions have you initiated with people from different cultural groups than yourself?
- **D**esire: what is the extent of your desire to be culturally safe or competent in your nursing practice?

When critical care nurses understand their position on nursing people from other cultures, strategies can be adopted to improve their responsiveness and the quality of care delivered. Working with culturally and linguistically diverse people should be based on the following framework:

1 Partnership: aim to work in partnership with the patient and family. Prior negative experiences may influence the development of a productive relationship. A respectful, genuine, non-judgemental attitude is necessary to develop a productive relationship with the patient and family, and providing time for responses is important.

2 Participation: where possible involve the patient and family in their care, if this is appropriate. This will involve the critical care nurse explaining the treatment and intervention routines.

3 Protection: determine specific cultural and spiritual values, beliefs and practices, and enable these to be practised during the patient's time in the critical care unit. Where possible these should be accommodated, although there may be instances when this is not possible. In such situations, the patient and family should be fully informed of the rationale for this.

Considerations when caring for Aboriginal and Māori peoples are reviewed in the next sections. Closely related to cultural aspects of care is spirituality, which for some is based in religion. Aspects to consider when patients have religious needs are reviewed later in this chapter.

Working with Māori patients and families

Māori are the indigenous people of New Zealand and, like other indigenous people who have survived the processes of colonisation, they experience poorer health status and health outcomes and socioeconomic disadvantage compared to other groups in the New Zealand population.[145] Māori were not a homogeneous group of people before settlement by European people, and contemporary Māori continue to be diverse in their *iwi* (tribal) affiliations, cultural identity, backgrounds, beliefs and practices,[146] and in the colour of their hair, eyes and skin. The critical care nurse ideally needs to recognise the diversity that exists, and have a sociopolitical and historical perspective of contemporary Māori. This positions the critical care nurse to understand the importance of and respect the need to undertake assessments with Māori patients and *whānau* regarding their cultural needs (see Table 8.3).

TABLE 8.3

Considerations for working with Aboriginal or Māori people

ISSUE	ABORIGINAL CONSIDERATION	MĀORI CONSIDERATION
Holistic, spiritual world view	• Health is not just the physical wellbeing of the individual but the social, emotional and cultural wellbeing of the whole community	• Most Māori have a holistic and spiritual world view, this means *whānau* (extended family) and their *wairua* (spiritual wellbeing) are important • *Whānau* members generally have a strong connection and sense of obligation to each another, which means that they want to be present with patient, especially when they are unwell

ISSUE	ABORIGINAL CONSIDERATION	MĀORI CONSIDERATION
Beliefs around hospitalisation and places to die	• Identify any previous encounters with family members dying, or stories from communities that reinforce these views • Provide honest responses to questions about a patient's condition • Avoid communication that expects people to 'read between the lines'	• Many Māori have had negative experiences in hospitals with *whānau* dying. They have also been subjected to judgemental staff and discriminatory attitudes and behaviours. Therefore, Māori *whānau* may be wary and possibly defensive – approaching them in consistent, genuine and non-judgemental ways can instill confidence that the patient will be cared for well • Talk to *whānau* about concerns they may have about the patient and the care they will be receiving, and any specific cultural practices they would like observed • It is important to avoid doing things that may breach *tapu*: by keeping body tissues and fluids, and body parts, away from food and utensils; removing food and drink when undertaking cares, not putting food where hairbrushes are, for instance. Body parts (particularly the head for some Māori), tissues and fluids are considered *tapu* (spiritually restricted)
Traditional healing	• Explore how traditional medicine can complement western medicine • Facilitate access by traditional healers when requested	• Explore how traditional healing and medicines can complement western medicine. Traditional healers (*tohunga*) may play an important role • Discuss with the *whānau* any specific healing modalities that need to be considered, e.g. a *tohunga* to be present or the use of *rongoā* or *karakia* (prayer)
Connections	• Acknowledge Aboriginal people's needs to connect to the land and possible need to return to their land to die • Compound families are common and identifying kinship relationships is important	• Acknowledge that connections with other people and the land may be important • Whakapapa and kinship may be important, so having *whānau* present may be very important • Note that *whānau* is broader than the nuclear concept of family, and *kaupapa whānau* (*whānau* groups formed between those members who do not share genealogical connections) are equally important for some as *whakapapa whānau* • Enquire whether body tissue/fluids/parts need to be returned for burial
Elders	• Respect of community elders • Elders are often spokespersons for the family so the spokesperson needs to be identified	• Elders are respected members of society that hold *mana* and important status. Thus, an unwell elder may have a lot of visitors because of his/her respected status • Elders may be the spokeperons for the *whānau*, or will designate spokesperson(s) for staff to communicate with
Establishing relationships	• Aboriginal health workers and liaison officers provide vital links to Aboriginal communities • Establish relationships with Aboriginal people through sharing community knowledge: family, friends, football, food	• Showing attitudes and actions that are genuine, and a willingness to listen and to share where you have come from and who you are, are helpful in establishing relationships with Māori *whānau* • The principles of the Treaty of Waitangi, partnership, participation, protection, provide a useful framework for working with Māori • Establish and maintain a positive partnership relationship that promotes participation of *whānau* and that protects their values and beliefs • Develop a relationship with the Māori health service within the hospital
Diversity	• Aboriginal communities have different lores • Talk to family, community elders about community lore	• Māori are diverse, so patient-centred assessment and planning is important. This recognises the diverse values, beliefs and practices of Māori
Language	• Facilitate use of interpreters • Cauliously engage family or trained community members • Have culturally appropriate resources developed	• Facilitate use of interpreters for Māori whose main language is te reo Māori • Always check out understanding of the information shared • Avoid using healthcare jargon when explaining things

The Treaty of Waitangi (commonly known as 'the Treaty') is based on an agreement between Māori and the Queen of England, Queen Victoria, which established the rights of Māori as *tangata whenua*, or people of the land. There are two versions of the Treaty – one in English and one in *te reo* Māori (Māori language). Māori understood that, while they gave governorship to the Queen under Article One of the Treaty, they would retain their right to control and self-determination over their lands, villages and *taonga* (which includes health) under Article Two. Under Articles Three and Four Māori are guaranteed protection and the same rights as British citizens, including the protection of beliefs and customs. Nurses working within the New Zealand health setting can be considered agents of the Crown;[147] therefore they have a responsibility and obligation to honour the Treaty when working with Māori. The principles of partnership, participation and protection[148] are used to apply the Treaty in practice within health settings such as critical care.

The commitment that critical care nurses have to establish, and maintain, a positive relationship with Māori patients and their families is as important as being willing to facilitate the inclusion of cultural beliefs and practices in the care of the patient. Such a commitment can influence the outcome of the critical care experience for Māori patients and their *whānau*. It is not the purpose of this section to provide a 'recipe' for working with Māori in the critical care setting. An overview of the fundamental issues to consider, and the importance of critical care nurses establishing working relationships with local Māori health services and/or local *iwi* and Māori community groups, is stressed.

Māori have a collective, rather than an individual, orientation, with *whakapapa* and kinship having an important place.[149] Reilly outlines the variations that occur in the contemporary social organisation of Māori.[149] The *whānau* is the social group that critical care nurses will generally interact with. *Whānau* encompasses more than the common notion of the family.[150] *Whānau* are inclusive and are made up of multiple generations, extending widely to include those who have 'kinship' ties. This contrasts with the 'nuclear' family concept. Elders, especially *kuia* (older respected women) and *kaumatua* (older respected men) possess *mana* (power, authority and prestige) and important status that commands respect. Because of the status of *kuia* and *kaumatua* in Māori society, if they become ill it is especially important for the *whānau* and wider Māori community to support them during this time.

Practice tip

Māori elders may prefer to speak in *te reo* Māori (Māori language). In these instances, a *whānau* member may be able to assist in interpreting explanations about care.

Because of the collective orientation of many Māori, *whānau* support is exceedingly important. Thus, critical care nurses often have to explore how they manage relationships with large numbers of people within confined physical spaces, which may necessitate establishing relationships and identifying one or two people who will be the point of contact through which information can be communicated.[124] Establishing connections and links can be a positive way of engaging with Māori patients and *whānau*; this is often called *whanaungatanga*, and Māori will often do this by sharing their *whakapapa*, or genealogy. This means identifying where you have come from and who you are. It is crucial that the critical care nurse be able to demonstrate a genuine intent and a willingness to listen to what the *whānau* feel is important. Forming effective working relationships with Māori *whānau* can never be underestimated. It is also useful for critical care nurses to establish working relationships with Māori health services within their health service and to get to know the local Māori community.

Practice tip

Often when a *whānau* member is seriously or critically ill, the wider *whānau* members will have a strong sense of obligation to want to visit and to *manaaki* (care for) the immediate *whānau* members. This may mean many *whānau* members will be present at the hospital. In situations such as this it is often important to get the *whānau* to identify a spokesperson with whom to engage in explanations and discussions about the patient, and the needs of the critical care staff to care for the patient and other patients. This assists in meeting the needs of both the *whānau* and the critical care staff.

Many Māori view themselves as spiritual beings,[146,149] and ill health may therefore be seen to have a spiritual as opposed to a physical cause. The way Māori interpret the world is a unique blend of cultural artefacts from the past and present, and also reflects the nature of their interactions within contemporary society.[146] Despite the diversity that exists, many Māori have a world view that is holistic and eco-spiritual in nature.[150] This holistic and spiritual world view interconnects the physical world and the world of others.[149] Māori creation stories are cosmological in nature, and establish the link Māori have to the *atua* (gods) and *tupuna* (ancestors) who created the world and all living things through the separation of Ranginui (the 'sky father' in mythology) and Papatuanuku (the 'earth mother' in mythology).[151] For some Māori, acknowledging *atua* and *tupuna* in *karakia* (ritual chants or prayer) is spiritually important, as well as maintaining their strong links to others and the land. Some Māori also have religious faiths originating from the processes of colonisation, and may include Christianity or the Māori-based Ratana and Ringatu faiths.[149]

The activities of individuals and groups of Māori that serve to control human activities and life, and maintain health and wellness, are restricted spiritually and practically (through rituals) by the concept of *tapu* (sacred or restricted).[122,149] Breaches of *tapu*, while spiritual in nature, often manifest in physical forms such as illness. Often illness is seen as a failure to observe *tikanga* (custom) and *tapu*,[149] and is known as *makatu* (a spell or curse) or *mate* Māori (sickness or death). Traditional healers and healing practices (such as the use of *rongoa* [medicine] and *karakia* [ritual chant or prayer]) play an important role in healing someone who is ill. Accessing traditional healers, such as a *tohunga* (expert), may be an important part of the critically ill person's recovery or dying process. However, cultural expressions of spirituality differ among Māori and, for some, traditional cultural approaches may not be acceptable. The critical care nurse needs to identify the beliefs and practices related to wellbeing and illness.

There are some things that are done in one culture that are perceived to be offensive in another, and thus disrupt the formation of relationships. The concept of *tapu* (sacred or restricted), mentioned above, is also associated with the concept of *noa* (common), or to make ordinary. Thus, a person's body, body fluids and body parts are considered *tapu*, whereas food is often used to make something ordinary. In practical terms this means that food should be kept separate from the person's body and body fluids. For example, do not put urine in urinals or collecting chambers for faeces in pans on surfaces where food will be put. Body tissues and body parts and their placement and disposal are a major consideration in the care of Māori. For some Māori, having their body parts and any tissues removed returned to them so they can bury them is spiritually important: they are returning these to Papatu-anuku (the Earth Mother). However, again it is important to identify what is important for each patient and their *whānau*, as some Māori may not want their body tissues or parts returned to them.

Practice tip

Before proceeding with care that involves touching the head or disposal of body fluids, for instance, ask the patient or family member if there are any considerations that need to be observed.

Working with people of Australia

Aboriginal and Torres Strait Islander peoples are the traditional owners of Australia but currently represent only 3% of the entire population. Of this population 90% identify as Aboriginal, 6% identify as Torres Strait Islander people and 4% identify as both Aboriginal and Torres Strait Islander people.[152] In line with culturally acceptable practices, excepting for when distinctions between Aboriginal and Torres Strait Islander people are required, the term Aboriginal will be used for the remainder of this section to refer to both population groups.

Practice tip

Acknowledging identity is an important contributor to establishing respectful cross-cultural relationships. Be mindful of Australia's history of colonisation of Aboriginal and Torres Strait Islander people and take the time to ask Aboriginal people what community/traditional name they identify with, e.g. Koori, Yolngu, Kaurna, Barundji, Gurindji etc.

The contribution of Aboriginal people as a small component of the overall Australian population means that critical care nurses will have varying levels of interaction with them. For example, Aboriginal people represent 30% of the population of the Northern Territory and between 45% and 65% of intensive care admissions.[153,154] Therefore, working with Aboriginal people is core business for critical care nurses in the Northern Territory. In contrast, 6.4% of patients admitted to a tertiary intensive care unit in Western Australia identify as Aboriginal,[155] which is slightly higher than the national figures where Aboriginal people represent on average 5.6% of intensive care admissions.[156] This section therefore aims to provide information that will assist critical care nurses to understand some of the complexities of care unique to Aboriginal people no matter where they work and to improve the experience for both nurses and patients regardless of whether this is a familiar or unfamiliar situation for all concerned.

The information presented is broadly applicable to the diverse cultural and language groups of Aboriginal people and their communities in Australia. However, it is essential that each episode of nursing care provided for an Aboriginal person and his/her family is individualised to the person, their distinct cultural heritage, local Aboriginal law, identified family relationships and unique connection with particular land and country.

Health status of Aboriginal people

Critically ill Aboriginal people vary from their non-indigenous counterparts. Aboriginal persons admitted to Australian ICUs are on the whole younger (mean age 40 compared to 48 years) and sicker than non-indigenous people. Emergency admissions for sepsis, septic shock, pneumonia, cardiopulmonary arrest and trauma are most common for Aboriginal people. The high rates of infection are reflective of the high burden of chronic disease within the Aboriginal population and the challenging socioeconomic setting in which Aboriginal people live.[153] Injury, poisoning, motor vehicle accidents, assaults, self-inflicted harm and falls are the second most common causes of hospitalisation for Aboriginal people.[157] Hospitalisation for assault is 34 times higher for Aboriginal women than other women. Aboriginal men aged 15–24 years have the highest rate of trauma of any age group and experience violence twice as frequently as non-indigenous men.[158] Aboriginal people also have disproportionately higher rates of presentation to ICU following suicide attempts compared to their proportion of the overall population.[159] Aboriginal males are also more likely to choose hanging as a method of suicide, survive and require a subsequent admission to ICU following hanging than non-indigenous people.

Although mortality rates for Aboriginal people admitted to intensive care units are comparable to outcomes for non-indigenous people, the reality is that they have a higher severity of illness (APACHE II score), which is related to their high levels of chronic disease.[153,154] Rates of diabetes are three times higher for Aboriginal people than for non-indigenous people, and they are also 3.9 and 5.7 times more likely to be hospitalised for diabetes than non-indigenous males and females, respectively. In 2012, Aboriginal people died from diabetes at almost seven times the rate of non-indigenous people. Between 2008 and 2012 the rate of end stage renal disease was 7.3 times higher for Aboriginal people than for non-indigenous people. The most common reason for hospitalisation of Aboriginal persons was care involving dialysis. Chronic liver disease is also high amongst Aboriginal people, with the hospitalisation rate for alcoholic liver disease six times the rate for non-indigenous people. Rheumatic heart disease, which is rare among non-indigenous Australians, is prevalent amongst Aboriginal people aged 45–54 years.[157,160]

Each of these chronic diseases is preventable. The high incidences reflect the socioeconomic disadvantage experienced by Aboriginal people and the decreasing access to primary health care the further people live from major cities.[158] In broad terms, the 'social determinants of health' reflect the disadvantage Aboriginal people suffer in terms of employment, physical infrastructure (including running water and housing), education, connection to land, racism and incarceration.[161] Together, these factors result in Aboriginal people presenting to hospital further along the trajectory of their disease process than non-indigenous people. In the critical care setting many chronic health conditions, including severe cardiovascular disease, may not have been diagnosed until the person presents with life-threatening complications. Similarly, life-threatening complications of acute illness exacerbate underlying chronic disease and result in more complicated and often longer lengths of stay in critical care.[155] With even this very brief overview of the status of Aboriginal health, it should be clear that understanding both the physiological and social determinants of health is essential for optimal nursing care of the critically ill Aboriginal person.

A long way from home and family in an unfamiliar environment

The geographical distribution of the Aboriginal population not only impacts on how much contact the critical care nurse might have with them, but also impacts on people's experiences of an admission to critical care. Only 32% of Aboriginal people live in major cities. An estimated 43% of Aboriginal people live in regional areas and 25% in remote areas.[157] Therefore, most Aboriginal people admitted to critical care units have come from somewhere else, and are often a long way from home. This demographic has a

particularly important impact on the patient themselves and their accompanying family members.

The concept of 'culture shock' provides an explanation for the tension and anxiety, feelings of isolation and sensations of loss, confusion and powerlessness that people encounter when entering an environment characterised by an unfamiliar culture.[162,163] The critical care environment is unfamiliar to most people. However, in the case of Aboriginal people an admission to critical care may be the first time the patient and their family has encountered this level of invasive healthcare treatment and/or city life. The conditions in remote communities where one-quarter of Aboriginal people live are very different to the circumstances encountered in a major city or even regional hospital. For example, most Australian hospitals are multistorey. Travelling in a lift may be a significant challenge[164] for family members. Being 'up in the air' away from direct contact with the earth and enclosed in an air-conditioned environment can be unsettling so that frequent visits outside are often necessary to renew contact with the natural and more familiar external environment. The highly technical environment of the critical care unit adds another layer of unfamiliarity and contributes further to a sense of anxiety. There are specific hospital routines, corridors and spaces, unfamiliar smells, technology, restraints on movement, protocols for safety, limitations to visiting, biomedical customs and practices, professional and personal relationships to negotiate and language and jargon to interpret, along with expectations of compliance to systems and procedures that reinforce the dominance of western medicine.

Critical care nurses have a significant role in determining how well Aboriginal patients and their families manage such culture shock. A first step is being aware of the contributing factors and the feelings these may invoke for Aboriginal people. The authors of *Binan Goonj*[165] have identified factors characteristic of six cross-cultural stressors within institutions such as hospitals. Figure 8.1 depicts these stressors and some of the concerns and reactions experienced by Aboriginal people. Acknowledging these stressors and reactions is a first step in assisting the patient and their family to adapt to the unfamiliar culture of the critical care unit.

Establishing trust to promote adaptation[165] should be a priority of the critical care nurse. Understanding the conditions that underpin culture shock for Aboriginal patients and their families is a particularly good starting point for developing trust. Understanding the importance of family within Aboriginal culture and how the culture influences beliefs about health and illness is also essential for developing a therapeutic relationship and minimising the impact of culture shock during the critical care experience. Elements of family relationships and health beliefs that are particularly relevant to the critical care setting are discussed in the next section.

Family

'Family' is cited as one of the most enabling and enduring pillars of Aboriginal culture, and the fundamental unit of

FIGURE 8.1 Bridging cultures in Aboriginal health.

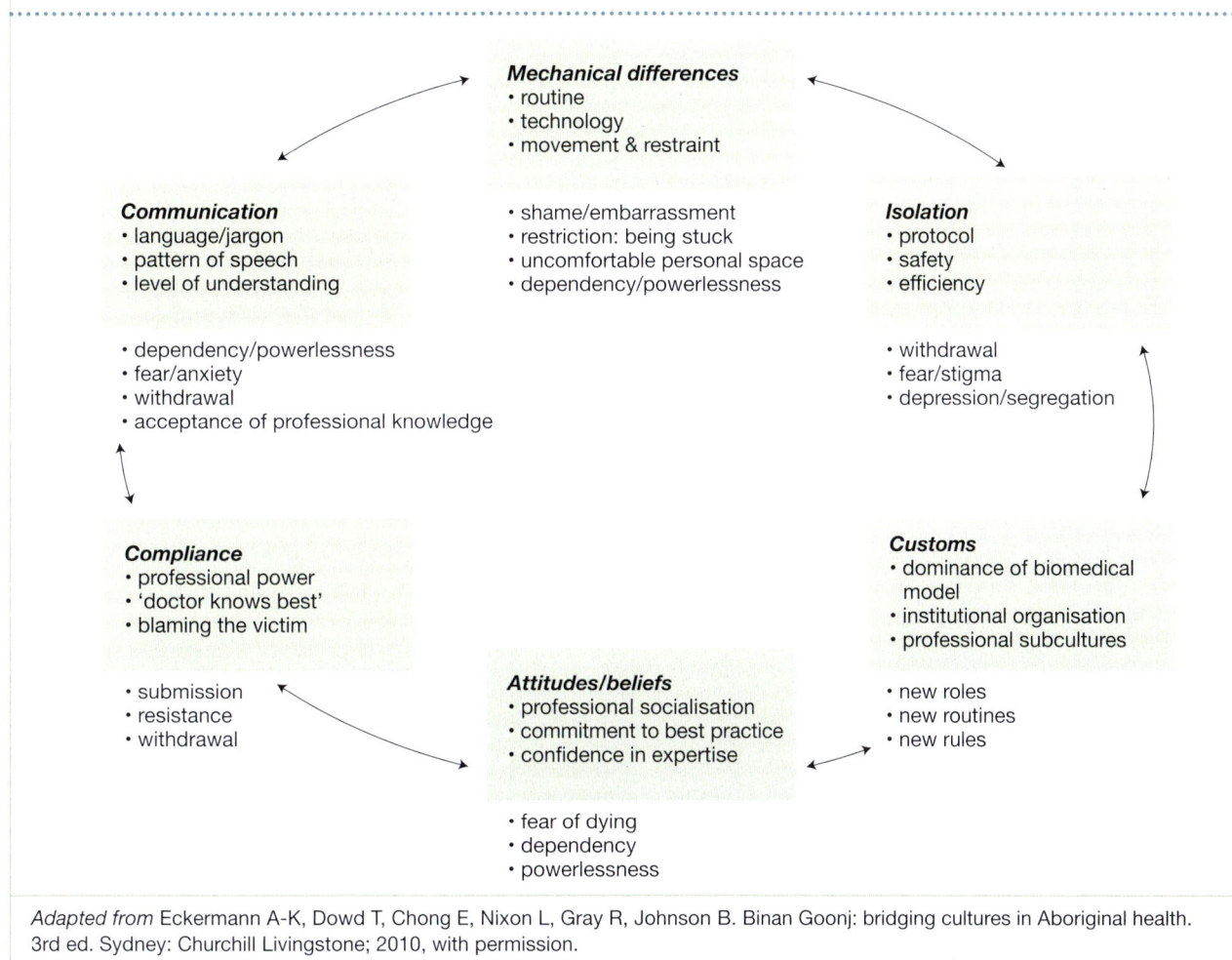

Adapted from Eckermann A-K, Dowd T, Chong E, Nixon L, Gray R, Johnson B. Binan Goonj: bridging cultures in Aboriginal health. 3rd ed. Sydney: Churchill Livingstone; 2010, with permission.

contemporary Indigenous society.[166] Concepts of family are, however, a potential point of cultural tension between Aboriginal people and health professionals educated in dominant models of health that emphasise a strong ethical and legal commitment to individual rights, confidentiality and autonomy. In contrast, health may not be an individual issue within Aboriginal family constructs. The construct of an extended family with a complex set of kinship rules and different levels of sharing and support is often cited as distinguishing Aboriginal from western culture.[165]

Within the Aboriginal extended family, relationships are defined through the traditions of culture so that the biological mother's sisters are also called mother, while her brothers are uncles. The sisters' children become brothers and sisters rather than cousins. The children of the father's brothers are also considered brothers and sisters rather than cousins and the father's brothers are called uncle. This system carries over to grandparents and grandchildren.

In the critical care environment, the kinship system has significance in terms of the western concept of 'next of kin'. Spokespeople such as 'aunties' or 'uncles' are often nominated to speak on behalf of the Aboriginal family,

but would not usually fulfill this role for non-indigenous people.

Another feature of traditional Aboriginal kinship systems is avoidance relationships. Kinship laws determine who can and cannot speak to each other, associate with each other or have physical contact with each other. This might mean that certain visitors are not able to be present in the room at the same time – an important consideration for the critical care nurse when convening a family conference. Some Aboriginal communities also have lores that dictate that only women speak about 'women's business' or only men speak about 'men's business'.

Practice tip

It is important to identify who is the spokesperson of the patient from the outset and who is the right person to talk to about all aspects of the patient's care. Identifying the right person is of additional importance when the patient is a long way from home. Early notification of family when an important decision is to be made is essential if they are required to travel long distances to join their critically ill family member.

Kinship systems also mean that Aboriginal people may have a number of names. A person may have a European first name and surname, a bush name, a skin name and maybe a nickname. A person's name may also change over the period of their life. If a person shares a name with a person who dies, they may be given a new name at that time.

Practice tip

Retrieving past results/records may be essential to inform current care, so knowing if the patient has multiple names or medical histories is important, particularly if these need to be retrieved from regional hospitals or remote health clinics.

Respecting kinship structures may assist in relieving some culture shock experienced by Aboriginal patients and their families. However, it is also important to acknowledge that the traditional 'extended' family has been somewhat eroded through forcible removal of Aboriginal children from their families (the 'stolen generation'); policies of assimilation; disconnection from traditional lands, community, family and cultural values; and socioeconomic disadvantage. The latter has particularly led to disruption of Aboriginal family structures, gravitation of youth to regional centres and capital cities and family structures being disrupted by incarceration, domestic violence and drug and alcohol abuse.[167] 'Compound families' are the urban and contemporary equivalent to the traditional extended family. A compound family is a group of people who share a dwelling and where the household head agrees to accept cohabitation with a diversity of relatives and other persons not related biologically, but who are considered 'kin'. Another new form of family structure is the grandparent family where grandmothers, in particular, take responsibility for child-rearing. This occurs due to parents being unable to look after their children because of the need to relocate for work, parents who misuse drugs, family violence or parents who are too young to cope. Regardless, individual decision making continues to be influenced by communal relationships and family groupings that may go beyond a specific locality, and shared health beliefs.

Aboriginal view of health and health beliefs

Aboriginal people have a view of health that incorporates notions of body, spirit, family and community. The National Aboriginal Health Strategy (1989)[168] identifies that: 'Health to Aboriginal peoples is a matter of determining all aspects of their life, including control over their physical environment, of dignity, of community self-esteem, and of justice. It is not merely a matter of …. the absence of disease and incapacity'. In the context of these beliefs, understanding how Aboriginal people conceptualise disease and illness is particularly important in the critical care environment. Despite 200 years of colonisation, significant changes to the traditional lifestyles of Aboriginal people and the cultural diversity among Aboriginal groups and communities themselves, 'traditional' beliefs regarding the cause of illness appear to have persisted in a consistent way.[169] The interconnected aspects of connection to country and kinship obligations place an emphasis on social and spiritual dysfunction causing illness. Mobbs[170] proposes that there are five categories of illness causation. Natural causes (diet, physical assault, injury and emotions such as homesickness, anger and jealousy) and environmental causes (including the wind, the moon and excessive heat or cold) may be considered responsible for temporary states of weakness such as loss of appetite, weight loss, diarrhoea, coughs, lung complaints and headaches. Suicide and attempted suicide are also considered to be the result of such emotional factors.

Alternatively, these ailments may be associated with more serious 'direct supernatural' causes that result from transgressing Aboriginal law. Such transgressions include breaching taboos relating to place (sacred sites), ceremony, relationships (parenthood, childhood, avoidance, incest and mortuary), women's business (pregnancy and menstruation) or spirits of the dead. Persistent sickness, mental illness and death may also result from transgressing these lores/laws.

'Indirect supernatural' causes of illness result from more serious offences involving transgressions of social or spiritual law or intergroup or intragroup conflict and are believed to have multiple effects including death, serious illness and injury, sterility, congenital abnormalities and physical deformities. Illnesses in this category may have been precipitated by 'pointing the bone', 'singing' and 'painting'.[171] The concept of supernatural intervention provides a culturally embedded explanation for why one person and not another becomes sick or dies.[172] It links illness and death to personal and social conflict and the breach of cultural and spiritual lores.[173]

The final category of illness causation is 'western influences', deemed responsible for alcohol-related illnesses, substance abuse, infectious diseases, heart disease, cancer and sexually transmitted diseases, which fall into this category.

On the other hand, for Aboriginal people preventative measures to ensure wellbeing include actions that avoid repercussions such as observing kinship obligations to others; containing anger, violence or jealousy; respecting and honouring elders and the dead; and leading a moral life.

Traditional treatment includes the use of bush medicines, involvement of a traditional healer, singing/chanting or employing counter spells and charms to remove evil influences. Traditional healers provide strong spiritual support and can identify the underlying causes of a serious injury or illness. In contrast to the western biomedical model, upon which most western health care is based, the Aboriginal world view does not see the primary function of the western healthcare provider as being able to remove the cause of the illness, except for illnesses relating to colonisation. Instead, the role of western medicine is often that of relieving symptoms and hastening the cure, provided it does not conflict with traditional beliefs.[174] For the critical care nurse, this means that making an effort to understand and assist patients and families to link into Aboriginal health beliefs (such as facilitating the presence of a healer), while at the same time explaining western interventions, can ensure maximum effect of critical care therapies.

'Payback' is a traditional physical or psychological punishment for transgressing Aboriginal laws. Whereas a person sustaining an injury as a result of payback may never engage with western medicine, the fear of being blamed for failure of a medical intervention and suffering payback as a result may influence decision making by families in relation to consenting to treatment of a critically ill patient. For this reason, it is important that the correct family members are consulted. For example, Western Australian desert people divide themselves into two separate groups for important cultural occasions, including when someone dies or is critically ill. The *tilitja* belong to the same generation as the ill/dying person and are the activists and the *yirrkapirri*, the partners and children, are the mourners. In the case of an unconscious or dying relative, when serious healthcare interventions or procedures are being considered, the *tilitja* are the ones that should be consulted first and it is their duty to then consult with family members before final decisions can be made. Being aware of, and respecting, this process encourages the right people to come forward, allows those who wait and mourn to be able to do so and ensures decisions become shared according to cultural laws and not the decision of one person who may be at risk of recriminations.[175]

Communication

Aboriginal culture is based on a deep sense of spirituality and oral history. Traditionally, knowledge has been passed down from generation to generation through storytelling and yarning. In some communities traditional languages are still being used, and English may be a second or third language for many Aboriginal people. Critical care nurses should therefore identify interpreters to optimise communication with patient and family. Family members are frequently the first choice and there are advantages and disadvantages of this practice.[176] On the positive side, family may be the most expedient choice for interpreting because they are immediately available, and can translate culture and context as well as language. If the family member has the appropriate cultural authority there may also be significant trust, which an interpreter would not be able to foster. On the negative side, there is the potential for bias, inaccurate information, selective transfer of information, transgressing laws relating to gender and kinship, and for relatives receiving information that the person would prefer they did not know.[177] Utilising the important cultural brokerage abilities of Aboriginal health practitioners, health workers or liaison officers is an important strategy to enhance communication between Aboriginal patients, their families and health professionals.[178] However, health professionals have been known to use health workers to excuse their own deficits in communication,[179] rather than observing some basic verbal and non-verbal communication cues and principles when working with Aboriginal people. Table 8.4 provides some guidance in this respect.

TABLE 8.4

Communication cues and principles

PRINCIPLE	CONSIDERATIONS
Establish a relationship	The first few minutes of your initial interaction with an Aboriginal person are critical for effective communication Avoid perpetuating Aboriginal people's experiences with western systems where language has reinforced dominant and submissive power relationships Obtaining information is regarded as a privilege, not a right This may mean a person has to prove they are worthy and can be trusted with the receipt of knowledge Spend time building rapport and establishing common ground before exploring the 'business at hand' Be prepared to share information about yourself. As family and country are important to Aboriginal people, positioning yourself within your family context and your 'place' is important. For example, sharing where you are from, relationships you are comfortable talking about (children, brothers, sisters, grandparents), the football team you support and food you like is culturally appropriate
Consider kinship relationships	Certain people will have rights to access particular knowledge and make specific decisions within family and community The passing of information often depends on a person's position in the family/community or relationship with the holder of information Find out the relationships between the Aboriginal patient, and his/her attending family and friends and the relationships between family and friends Identify any avoidance relationships Establish spokespersons – remembering that there might be different spokespersons for different elements of the person's life Identify who can make decisions on behalf of the patient (e.g. in the capacity of next of kin) Consider what might constitute 'women's and men's business' in conversations

TABLE 8.4 *continued*

PRINCIPLE	CONSIDERATIONS
Body language	Become familiar with non-verbal forms of communication amongst Aboriginal people, e.g. hand signs and facial gestures Don't assume Aboriginal people do not make direct eye contact. However, if the person is avoiding eye contact this does not mean that they are not listening or are being rude Body language may also extend into close proximity within the client's personal space, this is particularly evident when the opposite sex is conducting the consultation; ask for permission to conduct any physical examinations
Use of silence	Use of silence is a key feature of communication with and between Aboriginal people. Pauses or silence during an interaction may mean that a person is thinking carefully before speaking or divulging information. It may also be a time for translation between languages. Pauses may be quite pronounced and time should be allowed for responses before seeking to fill in the silence by repeating the question Cultural protocols may also mean there are times when it is culturally inappropriate to respond Try reframing the question in a different way, or ask if the person may like someone else to respond
Shame	Shame is a term often used in Aboriginal society. 'Shame' describes a person's feeling of utmost embarrassment about something. It is used in both serious and humorous terms
Providing information and asking questions	'Reading between the lines' is a concept that is difficult to understand if English is not your first language and western culture is unfamiliar Be direct in your communication – carefully consider how to describe clinical progression, while at the same time not diminishing the severity of a situation because family may need to be informed and travel long distances to join the patient Don't assume nodding or saying yes means that a message is understood – it is often easier to say yes – this is known as gratuitous concurrence. Perceived/actual power relationships between the health professional and Aboriginal person may prompt the person not to contradict or disappoint and may lead to the person providing what they think is an agreeable response Improve communication outcomes by: • providing opportunities for more than one person to ask questions • following up on individual messages in different ways to ensure full understanding has been gained • using open rather than closed questions • avoiding compound questions (e.g. 'Is it this way, that way or the other way?') • avoiding asking questions in a way that is framed in expectation of a positive response • asking only one question at a time

---

Practice tip

Developing a relationship with Aboriginal patients and their families is an invaluable start to good communication and establishing trust. Introducing yourself in a conversation based on the four 'F's' may be useful: family, food, football and fun.[180] Not only does this approach open up shared space for conversation, it also positions you as a nurse within a family and community of your own, which is important to Aboriginal people.

A major complaint of Aboriginal people is that communication occurs too late, particularly when a health professional has attempted to deliver bad news gently, oblivious to the recipient not being able to 'read between the lines' within the subtleties of English language.[179] 'People need the full story so they can die with dignity, with their family members fully involved ... it is a good way to let them drive the process' (p 156).

Issues around death and dying and the importance of country

Aboriginal people also have a strong connection to the land they live on. Community is linked to land, a shared history and mutual responsibility and is the basis of physical, social, spiritual and emotional wellbeing.[181] 'People talk about country the same way they would talk about a person: they speak to country, sing to country, visit country, worry about country, feel sorry for country and long for country.'[182,p.7]

The ties Aboriginal people have to their people and land are so strong that, rather than receiving life-saving care, many prefer to refuse the treatment and die on the land that they belong in, with their family and community present. This means that patients often do not present to healthcare settings until their illness is very advanced. When transfer to hospital occurs it is often traumatic for both patients and accompanying family. The following research quote summarises some of the stresses experienced: 'They split the family up, one family in one hostel, one family in another …. So how can you lean on one another in time of grieving and in that time and if it comes the time to turn something off.'[183,p.3] The reality is that Aboriginal people frequently die in hospital. Stress relating to hospital admissions for many Aboriginal people is that their knowledge of city hospitals draws upon previous encounters with family members dying, or of hospitals as places where you go to die.[179,183]

In this situation the most important consideration for Aboriginal families may be the need for the patient to go 'back to country', back to their traditional lands to die or to heal. The critical care nurse should allow time and facilitate discussion with the team around these issues. However, return to country is rarely medically possible. Instead, ensuring the relevant family or community members are present is a priority. However, financial constraints and geographical distance may make family visiting difficult.

For those members of Aboriginal families who do manage to gather around the dying person, having the opportunity to pass on knowledge through stories to family members is important. The critical care nurse can facilitate this by allowing time and space for storytelling to occur and should also be aware of the culture shock described earlier, kinship relationships and the logistical practicalities in the critical care unit. The following quote demonstrates the interrelationship of these issues and the negative impact nurses can have on the family's experience.

It was really hard to sit down and talk … they are all close together, very close and … you haven't got the privacy. You say something and … it might offend the person next to you or whatever … And this does happen you know. I mean when they are in the intensive care part, there are little rooms that can only have about 4 people … because the machines are everywhere hooked up to the ceiling. And you have some in there, some outside the door you know, and then we have nurses say 'We can't have that many in here' …. That's family, that's a son, that's a daughter, that's the other son, you can't chuck them out.[183,p.6]

It is anticipated that the information presented in this chapter will assist in overcoming such dissonance between nurses' and Aboriginal people's expectations in the critical care setting. When an Aboriginal patient dies in the critical care setting there are also certain protocols that need to be considered. Gender-appropriate care may be needed, as often male elders will not allow women into their room, and a male nurse may be required to provide care. Some Aboriginal communities may not allow health professionals to handle the body after death. The critical care nurse needs to discuss with the family issues that relate to handling of the body, whether cremation is acceptable and arrangements for the person to be returned home.

The potential for organ donation may also be raised. Despite anecdotal reports that broaching this subject is inappropriate for Aboriginal people, research has identified that culturally sensitive discussion about organ donation and transplantation may not be met with any negative reactions from Aboriginal people.[154] Currently, there are low rates of both organ donation and organ transplantation amongst Aboriginal people. This situation has been attributed to beliefs relating to the importance of a body being buried whole and issues relating to transference of the spirit of the donor into the body of the recipient. Both concerns are related to transgressing the connection between a person and their own country. Discussing the principles and purpose of organ donation with identified family decision makers well before an expected death occurs, rather than approaching an individual family member with a request for consent when death occurs, is recommended.[150] This discussion should take place within a culturally supportive environment where collective decision making is possible.

When death occurs, it is associated with a period of intense grieving. Although many western nurses associate singing after death with 'wailing' in anguish, death is often accompanied by singing to help the spirit move on to the traditional place of rest.[179] 'Sorry business' is the term commonly used to describe the complex bereavement practices and protocols that occur in Aboriginal communities. There is no set time for *sorry business* to conclude, but to avoid prolonging the grief, the name of the deceased person is not used again once they have passed away. A discussion with the family will establish how critical care personnel can refer to the deceased person in a culturally acceptable way.

Aboriginal people have a distinct history, health profile, culture and health beliefs that affect their experiences of western medicine and health care in the critical care environment. It cannot be stressed enough that the integration of the patient's culture into the critical care setting is important to achieving optimal health outcomes and improved relationships between patients, family and healthcare professionals. Critical care nurses are placed in an ideal situation where the experiences of Aboriginal people and their families who are critically ill or dying can be positive while maintaining their cultural integrity. To achieve these aims critical care nurses need to be culturally safe, become familiar with specific factors influencing Aboriginal patient's and their family's experiences of hospitalisation, pay attention to verbal and non-verbal communication cues and develop therapeutic relationships built on trust.

Religious considerations

Religious beliefs and practices contribute to a person's spiritual wellness, on one hand, while on the other a critical care nurse's religion may influence how care is delivered.[184] Religious beliefs can be closely aligned with a person's culture and vary in how life, dying and death are viewed, and may dictate how life is conducted.[1,185,186] Any breaches can have profound effects on a patient's wellbeing and, in some cases, how a family member may consequently interact with the patient. This has important implications for critical care nurses undertaking everyday practices and common procedures where religious beliefs dictate a different approach. A common example is blood transfusions for those belonging to the Jehovah's Witness religion. Having a standardised list of religions and procedural considerations is flawed due to the variations that exist, and in some instances the variations are great. Thus, as part of the initial assessment the critical care nurse should determine whether the patient has religious beliefs and practices that must be observed or not, and incorporate these into the care plan.

When a family member becomes critically ill, religious beliefs and practices become an important coping mechanism in terms of making sense of the experience, as well as being a source of faith and hope. While it can be helpful to the critical care nurse to have an overview of the main religious beliefs and practices (see Table 8.5), caution must be used, and should not preclude working with the patient's family to ascertain exactly what their beliefs and preferences are. Having said this, a patient may have adopted a religion that is separate from their family's. In such circumstances family cannot be relied upon as informants and, in some situations, there may be a conflict between the religious values and practices of the patient and those of the family. Religious beliefs and practices, like

TABLE 8.5
Overview of key religious beliefs and practices

RELIGION	PRACTICES TO BE AWARE OF	BELIEFS ABOUT ILLNESS, LIFE AND DEATH
Protestantism	Prayer and the Bible are important for support. Minister, vicar or pastor may visit the sick person and the family	Illness is an accepted part of life, although euthanasia is not allowed. There is a belief in the afterlife, with the dead being buried or cremated
Roman Catholicism	Prayer and the Bible are important. Some may have restrictions on eating meat on Fridays of Lent, Ash Wednesday and Good Friday. Priest may undertake communion with and anoint the sick person	Illness is an accepted part of life, although euthanasia is forbidden. There is a belief in the afterlife, with the dead being buried or cremated
Judaism	There are orthodox and non-orthodox forms of Judaism. Procedures should be avoided on the Sabbath (from sundown on Friday to sundown on Saturday). Dietary restrictions around pork, shellfish and the combination of meat and dairy products extend to the use of dishes and utensils. Frequent praying, especially for the sick person who should not be left alone. The Rabbi will attend the sick person	Illness is an accepted part of life, with euthanasia being forbidden, thus prolonging life is important and those on life support stay on it until death. The Sabbath is a time that is considered sacred and when restrictions on activities are observed. There is a belief that the human spirit is immortal. There are special processes for managing the dead person, who should be buried as soon as possible after death. Thus, consultation with the Rabbi is important. Postmortem examination is allowed only if necessary
Buddhism	Prayer and meditation are important, using prayer books and scriptures, supported by teacher and Buddhist monks. The Buddhist is generally vegetarian. Patients may refuse treatments (e.g. narcotic medications) that alter consciousness	Illness originates from a sin in a previous life. There is a belief in afterlife, and the dead are buried or cremated. Living things should not be killed; this belief extends to euthanasia
Hinduism	Prayer and meditation are important, and are supported by a Guru. Some Hindus are vegetarian. The dying patient may have threads tied around the neck or wrist and be sprinkled with water; these threads are sacred and are not removed after death. The body is not washed after death	Illness is usually a punishment and must be endured. Some Hindus have healing practices based on their faith. There is a belief that the dead are reincarnated; they are usually cremated
Islam (Muslims)	Private prayer, facing Mecca several times a day, requires a private space. The patient may like to be positioned towards Mecca. Guided by the Qur'an (Koran), which outlines the will of Allah (the creator of all) as given through Muhammad (the prophet). Muslims fast during Ramadan, and eating pork and drinking alcohol are forbidden. Stopping treatment goes against Allah. Talking about death should be avoided; designated male relatives will decide what information patient and family should receive	Life and death are predetermined by Allah, and any suffering must be endured in order to be rewarded in death. It is believed that dying the death of a martyr will be rewarded in death by going to paradise. Thus, staying true to the Qur'an is crucial. There is a belief in the afterlife, and the dead are buried as soon as possible after death, on the side facing Mecca

Adapted from Blockley C. Meeting patients' religious needs. Kai Tiaki Nurs NZ. 2001/2002;7(11):15–7, with permission.

cultural beliefs and practices, will vary between orthodox or traditional and contemporary interpretations.

Patients generally fall into three groups with regard to their religious practices.[187] There are those who:

1 practise their religious beliefs regularly

2 practise their religious beliefs on an irregular basis, often in times of need and stress

3 have no religious interests.

All patients should have access to religious support where they indicate a need. Therefore, it is beneficial for critical care nurses to have knowledge of how to access the relevant religious resources if needed. The focus of the critical care setting often involves going to extreme lengths to keep patients alive, which may well be in direct opposition to some religious beliefs. Religious beliefs can either facilitate or disrupt the process of living or dying.[185,186] There are a number of useful principles underpinning practice when nursing patients with specific religious needs (see Table 8.6).

In addition to these principles, contact and communication between the patient, family and the critical care nurse are important,[1] and can enable a person's spiritual or religious needs to be determined. The critical care nurse should ascertain whether the patient and family have any spiritual or religious beliefs and practices to be observed during their time in the critical care setting.[1,187] Once the spiritual or religious beliefs and practices have been determined, the critical care nurse can facilitate opportunities for the patient and/or family to carry out their beliefs and practices, and avoid any insensitive actions and pay attention to any spiritual distress evident in the patient and family members.[187]

A person's spirituality, whether informed by religion or some other basis, manifests in a variety of relationships with self, others, nature and 'divine' beings. It is the essence of who a person is, or who groups of people are. While assessing spiritual or religious needs is one aspect, presence and being with, empathetic listening, reality orientation of the family and enabling visiting and contact are all important nursing activities that can support the spiritual and religious needs of patients and their families.[1] When families are confronted with the possibility of death, the documentation of a death plan that outlines the preferred care during the process of dying and death is recommended.[187] Death plans are about empowerment, and differ from advance directives, which outline what is not wanted (e.g. cardiopulmonary resuscitation). Through formal discussion with the patient and/or family, religious and end-of-life needs can be determined and a management plan developed for implementation.

TABLE 8.6
Principles for recognising religious needs

PRINCIPLE	AREAS FOR CONSIDERATION
Diversity exists between and within the various religions	Determine values and beliefs related to health, illness, dying, death and any specific requirements for undertaking everyday nursing cares and procedures
Spirituality is an essential part of care planning and the delivery of quality care	Spiritual and religious needs should be documented in the care plan to ensure continuity and quality of care
Interpersonal skills and therapeutic use of self are essential to engaging and being present with the patient and family	Approach the patient with a genuine, non-judgemental attitude Avoid imposing own religious or spiritual beliefs on the patient and family
Being knowledgeable about a patient's religious values about life, health, illness, death and dying enables the critical care nurse to be respectful and accommodating in their care	Consult family, if they share same religion, and/or consult appropriate representative of the patient's religion. Areas to explore should include the following to determine: • religious values regarding life, health, illness, dying and death • nature of the ideal environment • processes surrounding dying, if appropriate to the patient • beliefs regarding nutrition and hydration • use of touch • gender-specific care • family presence, involvement and support • care after death
Philosophies and policies should be cognisant of the cultural and religious diversity within the critical care patient population	Policies should be cognisant of cultural and religious diversity, and include management of the following: • visiting • modesty • gender-specific care • communication • language and the use of interpreters

End-of-life issues and bereavement

Internationally, mortality rates in ICUs vary considerably and are a feature of the models of care including admission criteria and discharge destinations.[188] Specifically, within Australia and New Zealand the Intensive Care Society Centre for Resource and Evaluation reported on data from 140 Australasian ICUs about discharge of 128,095 patients. The mortality rates across these tertiary, metropolitan, rural, paediatric and private ICUs ranged from 2% to 8%. The impact is that 6000 families in these two countries alone were bereaved during the reporting year of 2010/2011.[189] End-of-life questions and bereavement in critical care areas are therefore important issues involving patients, families and staff. Death can occur as a result of sudden decline in the patient's condition, or as a result of withdrawal of life support in anticipation of demise. Patient death in critical care areas is found to have a significantly different effect on family members from a death in another in-hospital area.[190] This is perhaps due to the heightened anxiety associated with a critical care environment[190] or to the perception of an ability to cure in highly medicalised areas.[191] Where possible, family-centred decision making with patient involvement, together with effective communication and attention to symptom management, is optimal. Practical and emotional support for family and patients is important and scrutiny of the way we manage these important areas provides quality indicators for critical care areas.[45,192]

Patient comfort and palliative care

Maintaining patient comfort and support for families and staff are primary requirements of nursing patients during the end stages of life. Advanced directives and 'not for resuscitation' orders should be in place to prevent mismanagement and misunderstanding of patient care (see Chapter 5).[45] Maintenance of patient comfort through care guidelines to facilitate a 'good death in ICU'[193] is designed to control symptoms such as agitation, pain and breathlessness and is extremely important from the patient, family and nurses' perspective.[194–196] Although this may seem fundamental, there is evidence to suggest this is not always achieved, with 78% of over 900 North American critical care nurses perceiving that patients received inadequate pain medications 'sometimes' or 'frequently' during end-of-life nursing in critical care areas.[197]

Collaboration and early involvement by palliative care teams is one way to integrate end-of-life care for patients who either remain in critical care areas or are transferred from the unit to other areas.[195] Withdrawal of mechanical ventilator support requires adequate provision for management of potential agitation, pain and hypoxia.[196] Opioid and benzodiazepine agents should be considered for administration before and after extubation to prevent agitation and pain. Choices of bolus or infusion administration need to be based on patient comfort issues. Oxygen therapy is continued in the most appropriate form, and an oral airway may improve patient comfort and aid secretion clearance. Atropine and scopolamine have been reported to successfully reduce copious oral secretions and enhance comfort.[198]

The attainment of humane nursing care must include heightened efforts in achieving quality indicators, such as mentioned above – adequate management of pain and nausea, agitation and restlessness. Both critical care staff and families should continue to communicate with the patient by speaking and touching as this can have a calming influence. Comfort measures to enhance holistic care delivery should continue and may include:

- hygiene care
- position changes
- foot and hand massages
- hair washes and other individual preferences
- artificial nutrition and hydration.[195]

Patient dignity should be a priority, with gowns or personal attire essential elements of care. The management of symptoms further allows patients to maintain their dignity. Privacy for patients and their families allows an opportunity for them to communicate without the constraints of observers.[199] As indicated in previous sections of this chapter, patient and family culture, beliefs and spiritual values are important considerations that underpin care.[193]

Family care

Care of the family is supported by proactive palliative care interventions that include empathic, informative communication with interdisciplinary team meetings and family conferences that are not rushed where families are integral to decision making and goal planning.[45,70,200] The desire to participate in decision making varies from family to family, and cannot be assumed. Ascertaining individual families' needs for decision making is therefore recommended[201] as families are best placed to have an understanding of patients' wishes, which can be taken into account when decisions are made.[202] Structured communication between the healthcare team and families can assist with earlier decisions and goal formation about care.[203] Emotional and practical support can be given to families by providing written material about the critical care area, local facilities and specific information on bereavement.[70] Privacy is not always possible in the busy critical care environment, but maximising efforts in this regard for dying patients and their families provides a more conducive environment for strengthening patient–family relationships and communication.[204] Communication is enhanced with family conferences, which provide a structured process where family members and patients' healthcare teams can share goals and understanding of end-of-life care.

Family conferences are a way to meet family needs, and enhance communication and understanding of the patient situation. These become an essential element of care when end-of-life discussions are needed. Privacy, away from the direct clinical environment, is important to allow uninterrupted time for families to meet with their relative's healthcare team.[205] When family conferences have been instituted early in the admission, a family/staff relationship will be established that supports ongoing communicating about end-of-life care.[24,206]

It is important to have the interprofessional team (for example: intensivist, social worker, case manager, direct care nurse, chaplain) meeting with the patient's family at this time to ensure a comprehensive approach to the coordination of patient care and family support.[67,207] This approach enhances understanding and information consistency. Where possible, involving all significant family members in the family conference allows them to hear the same information, ask individual questions and discuss options. These collectively reduce family and/or family/staff conflict[87] and support those families that prefer to make decisions as a collective.

Family members of ICU patients are at a high risk of anxiety and depression. In a large ICU multicenter French study, 73% of family members had anxiety and 35% were diagnosed with depression around the time of discharge or death of their relative.[208] This mental health morbidity is likely related to the burden of the critical illness and potential or imminent demise of a loved one. Family member's depression, grief and anxiety can be manifested by physiological, behavioural, psychological/cognitive and social indicators. The physiological stress response with increased cortisol excretion and poor sleep patterns[51] can affect family interactions with each other and with staff. At times of end-of-life discussions, family members may exhibit confusion, anger and/or threatening behavior, making it difficult for everyone involved. Importantly, these emotions make it difficult for family to grasp and understand the often complex patient situation. Strategies such as family conferences are important as they improve communication channels and promote understanding, thereby reducing conflict situations.[209]

Planning for the family conference around end-of-life issues involves ensuring a common time for significant family members and the critical care team to meet. If a key family member is away or overseas, a conversation over the internet may be the best option as video facilities will allow better communication than with a telephone call. Where there are complex family situations with extended families or previous partners, care must be taken to try to avoid a poorly functioning group. There may also be an estranged partner who wants to be included, which may add to the dynamics of the situation. The critical care team will need to exhibit great diplomacy in such complex situations to keep the group and meeting meaningful and productive. There is no rule as how to manage these situations but the foremost consideration is how to serve the best interests of the patient. Family members unable to attend the family conferences should be relayed information in a timely way by a self-designated family spokesperson. This person is generally one who is more resilient and coping better than others with the end-of-life discussions who can take the responsibility for communicating the situation to other family members. Reassurance that the patient will not be abandoned and care will remain of the highest quality is important to families.[210,211]

A well-organised critical care team will meet prior to the family conference and ensure all relevant information is gathered and that there is a shared understanding. Curtis and colleagues[212] suggest the use of a five-point approach during the family conference, which may be useful around end-of-life meetings. This approach is termed 'VALUE': 1) **v**aluing family statements, 2) **a**cknowledging emotion, 3) **l**istening, 4) **u**nderstanding the patient as a person and 5) **e**liciting questions. The critical care team's ability to listen to the family is a key element and has been found to significantly increase a family's satisfaction with end-of-life care.[200,213,214]

The healthcare team that provides information and discusses palliation and end-of-life care needs to clearly indicate to families that, although they are involved in much of the decision making,[24] the decision to withdraw treatment is a medical one in Australia. This notwithstanding, consensus and shared decision making is the aim as careful consideration of the patient's wishes, the family perspective and the futility or otherwise of further treatment are considered within an ethical framework.[24,205]

While the family grapple with the process of grieving,[215] nurses need to provide physical and psychological care for patients and families.[216] This can be achieved when there is patient- and family-centred decision making, good communication, continuity of care and emotional and practical support; and spiritual support can assist with this.[217] Individualising the care to the family is essential, and support measures should be instituted after a full assessment of their needs. This should be informed by the notion that grief manifests in different ways, and that grieving is a complex process. Bereaved families in intensive care demonstrate complex bereavement processes and, without support, prolonged grief reactions can occur. In a longitudinal study nearly half (46%) of bereaved family members had complicated grief 1 year later when measured by the Inventory of Complicated Grief Scale.[218] Complicated grief patterns decrease the family's ability to cope with everyday needs, increase the need for health services and may progress to unresolved grief.[219,220]

The detrimental effects of long-term unresolved grief after the death of a loved one are well documented.[220] Current terminology favours the term 'prolonged grief disorder' (previously called complicated grief), which has clinically disabling grief symptoms including, amongst others, a preoccupation with thoughts of the loss, avoidance of reminders of the loss, disbelief over the person's death, feeling lonely since the loss, feeling that the future holds no purpose and feeling stunned or shocked by the loss.[221] These symptoms can result in elevated morbidity and mortality levels associated with depression, cardiac events (including a higher risk of sudden cardiac death), hypertension, neoplasms, ulcerative colitis, suicidal tendencies and social dysfunction (including alcohol abuse and violence).[51,220,222] These potentially harmful outcomes provide strong motivation for critical care clinicians to initiate family support mechanisms such as bereavement services.[195] Bereavement programs aim to reduce the immediate physical and emotional distress for those grieving, while improving the long-term morbidity associated with unresolved grief.[223]

Although critical care clinicians in the UK,[224,225] USA,[195] Europe and Canada[201] are conducting dialogue and developing guidelines for bereavement care in critical care, little evidence-based research has been conducted on bereavement care strategies.[195] An exception is a bereavement program developed by a group of nurses from a British ICU, who instituted a booklet on 'coping with bereavement', an after-care form for the clinical nurse to complete with details for follow-up with the family and a sympathy card and letter inviting family to participate in support group meetings.[224] Although initial evaluation of the program through feedback from participating family members was positive, the team acknowledges that this does not constitute rigorous research. Evaluation of bereavement services in Australian adult ICUs was also reported to be inadequate, as no data could be located concerning bereavement services in other areas of critical care. Only 30% of ICUs provided some follow-up care, and only four units had any evaluation other than anecdotal evidence.[226] It is imperative to assess new and existing bereavement interventions and how well they meet the needs of families through rigorous evaluation. Legitimising research on this vulnerable group is required to improve end-of-life care for families and patients.[224]

Care of the critical care nurse

The two previous sections have focused on care for the dying patient and the patient's family. Critical care nurses who care for both patients and families also require care in bereavement situations. Caring for dying patients is emotionally draining and highly demanding of the critical care nurse, who often fails to notice or acknowledge the need to grieve.[227,228] In addition, critical care nurses may not have the knowledge and understanding of palliative

care and death in the critical care environment, and a specific educational program and unit guidelines on palliative care may provide support and reduce burnout and caregiver burden.[193,195,229,230]

Once the patient has died, nurses may not have the opportunity to mourn publicly and may feel they are acting unprofessionally if they show overt signs of grief.[227] Dealing with the death of patients may be exacerbated in some critical care environments, particularly in the rural setting, where the nurse may know the patient outside the work environment. Collaboration with colleagues from oncology areas or palliative care teams will provide guidance and support to critical care nurses as they develop better organisational and emotional support for each other.[231] Effective palliation occurs when the multidisciplinary team, including senior management, collectively develops a philosophy for palliative care and bereavement services.[195,217]

Nurses depend on colleagues and friends for support when patients die, and value debriefing sessions.[224] 'Debriefing' sessions can have a number of interpretations. For example, debriefing in critical care often takes the form of an opportunity to share feelings. Alternatively, it may involve a procedural clinical review of events where the objective is to understand and learn from the situation.[231] Both components of debriefing are important, together with the opportunity to provide mutual support within the multidisciplinary team. The effectiveness of sessions should be evaluated.

A 'grief team' provides more formalised support from colleagues that have been given additional education on grief, dying and death.[227] This enables a program of care, and may include such strategies as assessing the welfare of the staff immediately after the death of the patient, being present for staff members to express their feelings and providing follow-up and information on coping mechanisms during grief.[227] Accessing experts from outside the unit's usual resources may be helpful with debriefing in especially challenging situations.[231] Dealing with death is never easy; however, an awareness of colleagues' needs is the key to providing the support they require.

Summary

The psychosocial, cultural and religious needs of critically ill patients and their families are just as important as their physical needs, and care needs to be taken not to overlook these. This chapter presents a holistic and person-, patient- and family-centred approach to practice, which enables individualised plans of care that include specific psychosocial, cultural and religious needs of critically ill patients and their families. Māori and Aboriginal people generally have a holistic and spiritual world view, and consequently have specific cultural practices that are vital to their spiritual wellbeing. Culturally and linguistically diverse patients and families also have specific cultural values, beliefs and practices that critical care nurses need to determine, which may involve the assistance of an interpreter. These patients require the critical care nurse to interact with them in a manner that facilitates the identification of their needs on an individual basis. The old adage 'actions speak louder than words' is worthy of consideration when working with these patients in the critical care setting. It is important that individual plans of care be developed that include the participation of Māori, Aboriginal and culturally and linguistically diverse patients and *whānau* or family, reflecting the beliefs and practices that need to be included in their critical care experience. In order to meet the needs of the critically ill patient and family, the critical care nurse is advised to identify personal beliefs, practices and expectations that may influence professional decision making and interactions with the patient and family.

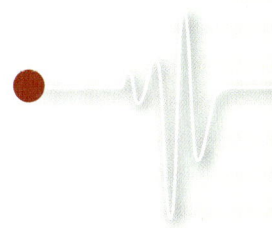

Case study

Mereana is a 40-year-old woman who has just been admitted to the critical care unit post-bariatric surgery. In the past, Mereana has been an active member of her community advocating for the support of young families with limited resources. However, she has been unwell for some time, as a consequence of being morbidly obese and having diabetes, hypertension, sleep apnoea and restricted mobility. During her bariatric surgery (Roux-en-Y), Mereana had significant blood loss and cardiac arrhythmias. At the bedside the critical care nurse is challenged by a number of concerned family members, including Mereana's partner, children, siblings, cousins, aunties and uncles, who all want to be with Mereana. Some of the family members are exhibiting defensive and negative attitudes, and the critical care nurses are somewhat concerned. Aware of the problem with having too many people within the restricted space of the critical care unit, the critical care nurse's immediate thought is to restrict visitors to her partner and children – as per the critical care visitation policy. This action is also reinforced by the need to assess Mereana, and ensure she gets the necessary rest she needs post-surgery. Nevertheless, the critical care nurse is aware that the family has indicated that this is totally unacceptable and that they need to be with the patient. Instead of acting on her immediate thoughts to restrict the family, the critical care nurse instead opts to explain to the family what she needs to do in the interim for Mereana and requests that, while this is occurring, they decide upon someone to be the spokesperson for the family, and who could be the person that staff then communicate with. She also asks them to consider what cultural needs that Mereana and the family have that should be included in Mereana's plan of care.

MAJOR ISSUES

There are a number of issues evident within this situation:

1 The family's request to be present will impact on the critical care environment, given the number of people wanting to be with Mereana.

2 The critical care nurse does not fully appreciate or understand the need for the wider group of family members to be present and support the patient, although she recognises it is important for them.

3 The critical care nurse is concerned about a potentially volatile situation, particularly with some family members.

DISCUSSION

This situation is not uncommon for people belonging to indigenous or other minority groups who culturally have collective world views that contrast with dominant biomedical approaches to health care, which predominately focus on individuals. For these cultural groups, the individual has less prominence; instead, the predominant focus is collectively on ensuring the wellbeing of family members. This means, as in the case of Mereana (and not dissimilar to many Māori and Indigenous Australian families), family members who are both close and distant relatives will come from near and far to be with an unwell person. This creates tension for critical care nurses who have to manage visitation, particularly when their mind is on keeping the patient stable and improving his or her outcome. Critical care nurses may be concerned about the increased traffic caused by large families within the critical care environment, especially when there is restricted space, and the need for the patient to rest is uppermost in their minds. On the other hand, the family may be interested in having unrestricted access to the patient and somewhere to sleep.[232] The critical care nurse in this case study managed an immediate situation prudently – she explained the work that she had to do, and asked the family to decide on a spokesperson. Having a spokesperson is one way that critical care nurses can manage family needs, in particular their cultural needs. Communicating and working with the family through the spokesperson can defuse potentially volatile situations whereby family members feel the critical care nurses are obstructing their need to be with the patient. Foci of communication with families should be on: 1) understanding the family's cultural and general needs, 2) explaining the critical care unit functioning and needs and other patients' needs and the reasons and 3) negotiating the specifics of how the family members can be with the patient. For example, this may mean that the numbers of family members are restricted unless there are important cultural practices, such as *karakia* (prayer), when more people may be able to be present for this short time. Such approaches enable the facilitation and balancing of the family needs to be with the patient with the family's cultural needs, the patient's needs and the nurses' needs.

CASE STUDY QUESTIONS

1   When confronted by large family groups, reflect on 1) how this makes you feel, think and act and 2) how this is similar or different to your own family of origin. Identify how your own personal cultural orientation impacts on working with patients and their families within the critical care setting, particularly when their requests and activities may differ markedly from your own views.

2   When confronted by large family groups, reflect on your thoughts, the actions you undertake and how you evaluate whether your actions are driven by your personal and/or professional values and beliefs, and if you are being culturally responsive in such situations.

3   Having worked with the family, how will you ensure that their needs are integrated into the patient's plan of care, and communicated to other critical care nurses and staff?

RESEARCH VIGNETTE

Henrich NJ, Dodek P, Heyland D, Cook D, Rocker G, Kuitsogiannis D et al. Qualitative analysis of an intensive care unit family satisfaction survey. Crit Care Med 2011;39(5):1000–5

Abstract

Objectives: To describe the qualitative findings from a family satisfaction survey to identify and describe the themes that characterize family members' intensive care unit experiences.

Design: As part of a larger mixed-methods study to determine the relationship between organizational culture and family satisfaction in critical care, family members of eligible patients in intensive care units completed a Family Satisfaction Survey (FS-ICU 24), which included three open-ended questions about strengths and weaknesses of the intensive care unit based on the family members' experiences and perspectives. Responses to these questions were coded and analyzed to identify key themes.

Setting: Surveys were administered in 23 intensive care units from across Canada.

Participants: Surveys were completed by family members of patients who were in the intensive care unit for >48 hours and who had been visited by the family member at least once during their intensive care unit stay.

Interventions: None.

Measurements and main results: A total of 1381 surveys were distributed and 880 responses were received. Intensive care unit experiences were found to be variable within and among intensive care units. Six themes emerged as central to respondents' satisfaction: quality of staff, overall quality of medical care, compassion and respect shown to the patient and family, communication with doctors, waiting room, and patient room. Within three themes, positive comments were more common than negative comments: quality of the staff (66% vs 23%), overall quality of medical care provided (33% vs 2%), and compassion and respect shown to the patient and family (29% vs 12%). Within the other three themes, positive comments were less common than negative comments: communication with doctors (18% vs 20%), waiting room (1% vs 8%), and patient rooms (0.4% vs 5%).

Conclusions: The study provided improved understanding of why family members are satisfied or dissatisfied with particular elements of the intensive care unit and this knowledge can be used to modify intensive care units to better meet the physical and emotional needs of the families of intensive care unit patients.

Critique

Although the research question was not overtly stated, the aim of the study was to gain insight into the ICU experience from the perspective of family members to improve the capacity of ICU staff to meet their emotional needs. The authors note that most evaluations of family satisfaction in the ICU involve quantitative data assessing characteristics of the ICU experience such as satisfaction with overall care, the decision making process and communication. The survey tool used in this study included both closed and open-ended questions. This paper reports on the data analysis of the open-ended questions. The mixed-methods approach is appropriate to both compare the results with previous quantitative surveys and generate new knowledge by exploring known themes in greater depth. For example, a qualitative approach can explore why families are satisfied or dissatisfied with specific aspects of ICU care that they rated on the Likert scale as 'excellent' or 'poor', respectively.

The authors compare and contrast their results with five other quantitative studies and provide references for five qualitative studies to support the inclusion of free-text questions as a way to improve understanding of experiential aspects of ICU. It is unclear from these short précis the depth and breadth of other studies about patient satisfaction in the ICU and what is already known about this topic. The paper would therefore have benefited from including more information about the existing literature and results of previous studies when comparing and contrasting the findings to their own.

In the absence of this more comprehensive information it appears from the introduction that the quantitative element of the survey tool is based on the previously validated 24-item Family Satisfaction Survey (FS-ICU), but that this study included three new, yet to be validated questions seeking suggestions and comments about things that were done well and ways to improve.

Despite the qualitative element of the survey tool appearing not to have been validated or even piloted prior to use, the sample size adds validity and reliability to the tool. Surveys to 40 family members of ICU survivors and 40 family members of ICU non-survivors who had spent a minimum of 48 hours in the ICU and who had a family member visit them at least once during the stay were distributed in participating units. The family members of surviving patients were recruited in person when their relative was ready for discharge. The family members of non-surviving patients were recruited by mail 2–3 weeks after the death of their relative. It would have been beneficial to include a definition of 'family member' given the potential variety of family composition across Canada, which has both a multicultural population and a First Nations population.

Almost half (48%) of respondents identified as the patient's spouse, with the other relationships being husband, partner, sibling or parent. Interestingly, there were no respondents who identified as the children of the ICU patient, although there are missing data in relation to this variable for 250 respondents. Of the reported relationships, 69% were female with the highest number (34% of all respondents) identifying as the patient's wife, then mother (8%) and sister (4%). It is unclear from the paper how many family members of each patient were represented, i.e. did a wife, mother and sister of some patients all respond to the survey, or just one member of each family? Although the size of the ICU where the respondent's family member stayed is reported (1–10 beds, 11–20 beds or >20 beds), it would also have been pertinent to identify the types of ICUs and their distribution across the country. Given the aim of the study is to improve families' experiences, these characteristics may have important ramifications in terms of recommendations for improving care.

The qualitative components of the surveys were analysed using the qualitative software *NVIVO*, which is an appropriate tool for thematic analysis. Twenty-two themes were identified, each of which were coded according to the positive or negative nature of the responses. Six themes were mentioned by at least 5% of all respondents across all sites and are those themes discussed in this paper. The six themes included: 1) staff quality and quantity; 2) overall care: competency and quality; 3) compassion/respect for family and patient: kindness meeting individual patient/family needs; 4) communication: quality, frequency, directness, timing; 5) waiting rooms: characteristics; 6) patient rooms: characteristics. These themes are set out in tables that make it easy to gain a sense of the results at a quick glance. The narrative provides more detail.

The most common theme identified by 66% of respondents was the high quality of staff, their competency, professionalism, concern and positive attitudes. Negative comments related to lack of interpersonal skills including rudeness, abruptness, insensitivity and 'dodging' interaction with family members as well as 'unprofessional' conversations between each other. Respondents also worried about shortages of nurses compared to patient demands. Competency ranked as the second most common positive theme, with only 2% of respondents making negative comments. Staff treating patients/family with kindness contributed to the third most common theme of compassion and respect for family/patient, with only 12% of respondents reporting negative experiences such as not being provided adequate space or time to grieve their family member's death.

Slightly more respondents were not happy with communication from ICU staff (20%) compared to those who were (18%). Negative communication experiences included infrequent communication/invisibility of doctors, excluding family from decision making and not being informed how long they may have to wait for a procedure to take or how long they would be excluded from the room when asked to leave. They also wanted to know logistical information to reduce the 'scariness' of ICU as a place. Family members wanted communication to be honest, particularly when it comes to discussing death. Positive comments appreciated clinicians who made communication with family a priority, made themselves available, were honest and direct and answered questions thoroughly. Waiting room conditions such as phones, couches, television, décor and a generally unwelcoming environment were ranked negatively. Lack of privacy and not catering for large numbers of people were the primary complaints relating to the patient room.

The authors identified that themes and subthemes were interconnected but that, when attempting to address overall dissatisfaction or improve satisfaction, breaking themes into their individual parts is useful for achieving change. Recommended changes included: establishing regular clinician/family meetings; improving doctors' interpersonal skills and decreasing inappropriate communication through education; providing more chairs in patient rooms; providing more informational pamphlets about the ICU environment; and making waiting rooms more welcoming. The authors identified that most of these recommendations are consistent with the American College of Critical Care Medicine/Fellow of the American College of Critical Care Medicine Guidelines.[233]

The authors also noted the insight qualitative responses gave to quantitative assessment of family satisfaction, and that these findings confirmed results from previous quantitative studies. Having said this, it was disappointing that the authors did not relate the two elements of their survey in this paper.

Strengths of this study are identified by the authors as providing an opportunity for respondents to articulate their opinions and the large size of the sample, which means that these comments most likely are representative of the diversity of families across Canadian ICUs. Limitations of the research were poorly identified. The authors identified that there were different recruitment techniques between survivor and non-survivor families. They also identified that the perspectives of families who opted not to respond may have been different to those who did. Additional limitations include the absence of information related to whether there were versions of the survey in both French and English, as would be expected in bi-lingual Canada, and the potential shortcoming of failure to identify responses from specific cultural groups in the multicultural Canadian environment. The degree of illness of the patient was not analysed, which has previously been identified as impacting on satisfaction rates. Similarly, it would have been good to know if there were differences in satisfaction based on length of stay and survival.

Overall, this paper provides an interesting perspective on family satisfaction. The quotations drawn from the data powerfully illustrate the family's perspective. The six identified themes are significant because, as the authors note, they reveal that, for each element that can be handled poorly, elements that contribute to family satisfaction can also be handled well with some awareness and effort informed by research such as this paper.

Learning activities

1   Delivering patient- and person- or family-centred nursing care can be assisted by working through your own philosophy for nursing practice. To develop and articulate your own nursing philosophy, or way of doing things, complete the following activities:

   • List any organisational practices you can identify in the clinical practice setting in which you most recently worked that might influence the model of nursing.

   • Write out a list of characteristics of a clinician you admire and indicate how these complement good nursing care.

   • If you were a patient in the critical care unit in which you recently worked, what would be important to you about the nursing care you received?

- If you had a family member in a critical care unit, write down the top eight things you consider most important about the care that you and your family member receive. Compare this with the list provided earlier in the chapter in the section *Needs of family during critical illness*.

- Having completed the above four activities, write three sentences that reflect your desired way of nursing that can constitute your philosophy of nursing.

2 Ascertain the personal and professional beliefs you hold as a critical care nurse about 1) health and illness and 2) life, death and dying, by identifying situations when your personal and professional beliefs are in conflict. Once these beliefs have been identified, the critical care nurse may ask:

- 'How do these personal and professional beliefs influence my practice?'

- 'What strategies do I need to implement to minimise negative impacts?'

- 'When faced with a conflict between personal and professional beliefs and practices, which one is more likely to direct practice decisions, and why?'

3 Using the information established in Learning activity 2, identify:

- your personal cultural beliefs and practices, and the impact these have on the patients and families that use the services of critical care

- what actions you take to meet the patient's and family's needs during their critical care experience

- how you can integrate culture into nursing practice and the critical care setting that you work in. This information can serve as a baseline for the development of strategies to improve practice.

4 The patient you are caring for today is to be the focus of a family conference that you will attend. Consider the following:

- What would you do if this was your first ever family conference?

- What information would you prepare in readiness for the family conference?

- If you have not cared for the patient before, how and from whom would you seek additional information?

- How would you vary your approach if children were to be present?

- What would you record in the patient's notes following the family conference?

Online resources

Australian Indigenous Health InfoNet, www.healthinfonet.ecu.edu.au

Cooperative Research Centre for Aboriginal Health, www.crcah.org.au/index.cfm

eMedical Journal of Australia articles on Aboriginal health, www.mja.com.au/Topics/Aboriginal%20health.htm

Hauora: Māori standards of health IV: A study of the years 2000–2005, www.Maori.org.nz/tikanga/?d=page&pid=sp44&parent=42

Information about Māori protocol and beliefs, www.Maori.org.nz/tikanga/?d=page&pid=sp44&parent=42)

New Zealand Ministry of Health website (access to Māori health-related publications and resources), www.moh.govt.nz

Office of Aboriginal Health–WA, http://www.aboriginal.health.wa.gov.au/home

Patient-centred care: Improving quality and safety by focusing care on patients and consumers, www.safetyandquality.gov.au/wp-content/uploads/2012/01/PCCC-DiscussPaper.pdf

Further reading

Carson B, Dunbar T, Chenhall RD, Bailie R, eds. Social determinants of Indigenous health. Crows Nest, NSW: Allen and Unwin; 2007.

Durie M. Whaiora. Auckland, NZ: Oxford University Press; 1998.

Eckermann A-K, Dowd T, Chong E, Nixon L, Gray R, Johnson SM. Binan Goonj: Bridging cultures in Aboriginal health. 3rd ed. Sydney: Churchill Livingstone; 2010.

Wepa D. Cultural safety in Aotearoa New Zealand. Auckland, NZ: Pearson Education; 2004.

Wright LM, Leahey M. Nurses and families: A guide to family assessment and intervention. 5th ed. Philadelphia: FA Davis; 2009.

References

1 Nussbaum GB. Spirituality in critical care: patient comfort and satisfaction. Crit Care Nurs 2003;26(3):214–20.

2 Alsop-Shields L. The parent-staff interaction model of pediatric care. J Pediatr Nurs 2002;17(6):442–9.

3 Gallant MH, Beaulieu MC, Carnevale FA. Partnership: an analysis of the concept within the nurse–client relationship. J Adv Nurs 2002;40:149–57.

4 Franck LS, Callery P. Re-thinking family-centred care across the continuum of children's healthcare. Child: Care Health Dev 2004;30:265–77.

5 Briggs LA, Kirchhoff KT, Hammes BJ, Song M-K, Colvin ER. Patient-centered advance care planning in special patient populations: a pilot study. J Prof Nurs 2004;20(1):47–58.

6 Davidson JE, Powers K, Hedayat KM, Tieszen M, Kon AA, Shepard E et al. Clinical practice guidelines for support of the family in the patient-centred intensive care unit: American College of Critical Care Medicine Task Force 2004–2005. Crit Care Med 2007;35:605–22.

7 Wilkins S, Pollock N, Rochon S, Law M. Implementing client-centred practice: why is it so difficult to do? Can J Occ Health 2001;68(2):70–9.

8 Berry LL, Seiders K, Wilder SS. Innovations in access to care: a patient-centered approach. Ann Intern Med 2003;139(7):568–74.

9 Berwick DM. What "patient-centered" should mean: confessions of an extremist. Health Affairs 2009;28(4):w555–w65.

10 Institute of Medicine. Crossing the quality chasm: a new health system for the 21st century. Washington DC: IOM; 2001. Available from http://www.iom.edu/Reports/2001/Crossing-the-Quality-Chasm-A-New-Health-System-for-the-21st-Century.aspx.

11 Epstein RM, Fiscella K, Lesser CS, Stange KC. Why the nation needs a policy push on patient-centered health care. Health Affairs 2010;29(8):1489–95.

12 Slatore CG, Hansen L, Ganzini L, Press N, Osborne ML, Chestnutt MS et al. Communication by nurses in the intensive care unit: qualitative analysis of domains of patient-centered care. Am J Crit Care 2012;21:410–8.

13 Ekman I, Swedberg K, Taft C, Lindseth A, Norberg A, Brink E et al. Person-centered care – ready for prime time. Euro J Cardio Nurs 2011;10:248–51.

14 Fumagalli S, Boncinelli L, Lo Nostro A, Valoti P, Baldereschi G, Di Bari M et al. Reduced cardiocirculatory complications with unrestrictive visiting policy in an intensive care unit: results from a pilot, randomized trial. Circ 2006;113(7):946–52.

15 University of Gothenburg Centre for Person-Centred Care, <http://gpcc.gu.se/english/>; 2012 [accesed 01.09.14].

16 Oxford Dictionary, <www.oxforddictionaries.com/definitions/english/>; 2014.

17 Misak CJ. The critical care experience: a patient's view. Am J Resp Crit Care Med 2004;170(4):357–9.

18 Friedman M. Family nursing: research, theory and practice. 5th ed. Stamford: Appleton & Lange; 2003.

19 Wright LM, Leahey M. Nurses and families: a guide to family assessment and intervention. 5th ed. Philadelphia: F A Davis & Company; 2009.

20 Hook ML. Partnering with patients – a concept ready for action. J Adv Nurs 2006;56:133–43.

21 Olsen KD, Dysvik E, Hansen BS. The meaning of family members' presence during intensive care stay: a qualitative study. Intens Crit Care Nurs 2009;25(4):190–8.

22 Shields L, Pratt J, Davis L, Hunter J. Family-centred care for children in hospital. Cochrane Database Syst Rev 2007;CD004811.

23 Espezel HJE, Canam CJ. Parent–nurse interactions: care of hospitalized children. J Adv Nurs 2003;44(1):34–41.

24 Cyprus BS. Family conference in the intensive care unit: a systematic review. Dimensions Crit Care Nurs 2011;30(5):246–55.

25 Institute of Patient- and Family-Centered Care. What is patient- and family-centered care?, <http://www.ipfcc.org/faq.html>; 2010.

26 Webster P, Johnson B. Developing family-centered vision, mission, and philosophy of care statements. Bethesda, MD: Institute of Family Centered Care; 1999.

27 Frost M, Green A, Gance-Cleveland B, Kersten R, Irby C. Improving family-centered care through research. J Pediat Nurs 2010;25(2):144–7.

28 Galvin E, Boyers L, Schwartz PK, Jones MW, Mooney P, Warwick J et al. Challenging the precepts of family-centered care: testing a philosophy. Pediat Nurs 2000;26:625–32.

29 Shields L, Tanner A. Pilot study of a tool to investigate perceptions of family-centered care in different care settings. Pediat Nurs 2004;30:189–97.

30 Bruce B, Letourneau N, Ritchie J, Larocque S, Dennis C, Elliott MR. A multisite study of health professionals' perceptions and practices of family-centered care. J Fam Nurs 2002;8(4):408–29.

31 Engström B, Uusitalo A, Engströmemail Å. Relatives' involvement in nursing care: a qualitative study describing critical care nurses' experiences. Intensive Crit Care Nurs 2011;27(1):1–9.

32 Garrouste-Orgeas M, Willems V, Timsit J-F, Diaw F, Brochon S, Vesin A et al. Opinions of families, staff, and patients about family participation in care in intensive care units. J Crit Care 2010;25:634–40.

33 Mitchell M, Chaboyer W, Burmeister E, Foster M. Positive effects of a nursing intervention on family-centered care in adult critical care. Am J Crit Care 2009;18(6):543–52.

34 Mitchell M. Family-centred care – are we ready for it? An Australian perspective. Nurs Crit Care 2005;10(2):54–5.

35 Courtney M. Evidence for nursing practice. Sydney: Churchill Livingstone; 2005.

36 Shields L. Questioning family-centred care. J Clin Nurs 2010;19:2629–38.

37 Knutsson SE, Bergbom IL. Custodians' viewpoints and experiences from their child's visit to an ill or injured nearest being cared for at an adult intensive care unit. J Clin Nurs 2007;16(2):362–71.

38 Australian Commission on Safety and Quality in Health Care. Patient centred care: improving quality and safety by focusing care on patients and consumers, <http://www.safetyandquality.gov.au/wp-content/uploads/2012/01/PCCC-DiscussPaper.pdf>; 2010 [accessed 01.09.14].

39 Scottish Government. The healthcare quality strategy for NHS Scotland. Edinburgh: The Scottish Government; 2010.

40 de Silva D. Helping measure person-centred care. London: The Health Foundation; 2014.

41 Kean S, Mitchell ML. How do ICU nurses perceive families in intensive care? Insights from the United Kingdom and Australia. J Clin Nurs 2014;23(5-6):663–72.

42 McKiernan M, McCarthy G. Family members' lived experience in the intensive care unit: a phenomenological study. Intens Crit Care Nurs 2010;26(5):254–61.

43 Duran CR, Oman KS, Abel JJ, Koziel VM, Szymanski D. Attitudes toward and beliefs about family presence: a survey of healthcare providers, patients' families, and patients. Am J Crit Care 2007;16:270–9.

44 Johnson BH, Abraham MR, Shelton TL. Patient- and family-centered care: partnerships for quality and safety. N C Med J 2009;70(2):125–30.

45 Nelson JE, Mulkerin CM, Adams LL, Pronovost PJ. Improving comfort and communication in the ICU: a practical new tool for palliative care performance measurement and feedback. Qual Safe Health Care 2006;15:264–71.

46 Ekwall A, Gerdtz M, Manias E. The influence of patient acuity on satisfaction with emergency care: perspectives of family, friends and carers. J Clin Nurs 2008;17:800–9.

47 Szalados JE. Legal issues in the practice of critical care medicine: a practical approach. Crit Care Med 2007;35(2 Suppl):S44–58.

48 Aiken LJ, Bibeau PD, Cilento BJ, Boutin R. A personal reflection: a case study in family-centered care at the National Naval Medical Center in Bethesda, Maryland. DCCN 2010;29(1):13–9.

49 Hwang DY, Yagoda D, Perrey HM, Currier PF, Tehan TM, Guanci M et al. Anxiety and depression symptoms among families of adult intensive care unit survivors immediately following brief length of stay. J Crit Care 2014;29:278–82.

50 Azoulay E, Pochard F, Kentish-Barnes N, Chevret S, Aboab J, Adrie C et al. Risk of post-traumatic stress symptoms in family members of intensive care unit patients. Am J Resp Crit Care Med 2005;171:987–94.

51 Buckley T, Sunari D, Marshall A, Bartrop R, McKinley S, Tofler G. Physiological correlates of bereavement and the impact of bereavement interventions. Dialogues Clin Neurosci 2012;14:129–39.

52 Lee LY, Lau YL. Immediate needs of adult family members of adult intensive care patients in Hong Kong. J Clin Nurs 2003;12(4):490–500.

53 Leske JS. Protocols for practice: applying research at the bedside, interventions to decrease family anxiety. Crit Care Nurs 2002;22(6):61–5.

54 Jones C, Skirrow P, Griffiths R, Humphris G, Ingleby S, Eddleston J et al. Post-traumatic stress disorder-related symptoms in relatives of patients following intensive care. Intensive Care Med 2004;30(3):456–60.

55 Paparrigopoulos T, Melissaki A, Efthymiou A, Tsekou H, Vadala C, Kribeni G et al. Short-term psychological impact on family members of intensive care unit patients. J Psychosom Res 2006;61:719–22.

56 Kinrade T, Jackson AC, Tomnay JE. The psychosocial needs of families during critical illess comparison of nurses' and family members' perspectives. Aust J Adv Nurs 2009;27(1):82–8.

57 Molter NC. Needs of relatives of critically ill patients: a descriptive study. Heart Lung 1979;8(2):332–9.

58 Ågård AS, Harder I. Relatives' experiences in intensive care – finding a place in a world of uncertainty. Intensive Criti Care Nurs 2007;23(3):170–7.

59 Alvarez GF, Kirby AS. The perspective of families of the critically ill patient: their needs. Curr Opin Crit Care 2006;12(6):614–8.

60 Chien W-T, Chiu YL, Lam L-W, Ip W-Y. Effects of a needs-based education programme for family carers with a relative in an intensive care unit: a quasi-experimental study. Int J Nurs Stud 2006;43(1):39–50.

61 Davidson JE, Daly BJ, Agan D, Brady NR, Higgins PA. Facilitated sensemaking: a feasibility study for the provision of a family support program in the intensive care unit. Crit Care Nurs Q 2010;33(2):177–89.

62 Hickman RLJ, Douglas SL. Impact of chronic critical illness on the psychological outcomes of family members. AACN Adv Crit Care 2010;21(1):80–91.

63 Kentish-Barnes N, Lemiale V, Chaize M, Pochard F, Azoulay E. Assessing burden in families of critical care patients. Crit Care Med 2009;37(10 Suppl):S448–56.

64 Mitchell ML, Courtney M, Coyer F. Understanding uncertainty and minimizing families' anxiety at the time of transfer from intensive care. Nurs Health Sci 2003;5(3):207–17.

65 Azoulay E, Pochard F, Chevret S, Lemaire F, Mokhtari M, Le Gall JR et al. Meeting the needs of intensive care unit patient families: a multicenter study. Am J Resp Crit Care Med 2001 (163):1.

66 Nelson DP, Polst G. An interdisciplinary team approach to evidence-based improvement in family-centered care. Crit Care Nurs Q 2008;31(2):110–8.

67 Moore C, Bernardini GL, Hinerman R, Sigond K, Dowling J, Wang DB et al. The effect of a family support intervention on physician, nurse and family perceptions of care in the surgical, neurological and medical intensive care units. Crit Care Nurs 2012;35(4):378–87.

68 Soltner C, Lassalle V, Galienne-Bouygues S, Pottecher J, Floccard B, Delapierre L et al. Written information that relatives of adult intensive care unit patients would like to receive – a comparison to published recommendations and opinion of staff members. Crit Care Med 2009;37:2197–202.

69 Nelson JE, Walker AS, Luhrs CA, Cortez TB, Pronovost PJ. Family meetings made simpler: a toolkit for the intensive care unit. J Crit Care 2009;24(626):e7–e14.

70 Lautrette A, Darmon M, Megarbane B, Joly LM, Chevret S, Adrie C et al. A communication strategy and brochure for relatives of patients dying in the ICU. N Engl J Med 2007;356(5):469–78. PubMed PMID: 17267907.

71 Mitchell M, Courtney M. An intervention study to improve the transfer of ICU patients to the ward – evaluation by ICU nurses. Aust Crit Care 2005;18(3):123–8.

72 Mitchell ML, Courtney M. An intervention study to improve the transfer of ICU patients to the ward – evaluation by family members. Aust Crit Care 2005;18(2):61–9.

73 Kirchhoff KT, Faas AI. Family support at end of life. AACN Adv Crit Care 2007;18(4):426–35.

74 Gonzalez CE, Carroll DL, Elliott JS, Fitzgerald PA, Vallent HJ. Visiting preferences of patients in the intensive care unit and in a complex care medical unit. Am J Crit Care 2004;13(3):194–8.

75 Gavaghan SR, Carroll DL. Families of critically ill patients and the effect of nursing interventions. DCCN 2002;21(2):64–71.

76 Roland P, Russell J, Richards KC, Sullivan SC. Visitation in critical care: processes and outcomes of a performance improvement initiative. J Nurs Care Q 2001;15(2):18–26.

77 Carnevale FA. Avoiding family induced stress: effective strategies for working with families. 29th Australian and New Zealand Annual Scientific Meeting on Intensive Care; 7-10 October. Melbourne, Australia; 2004.

78 Molter NC. Families are not visitors in the critical care unit. DCCN 1994;13(1):2–3.

79 Mitchell ML, Chaboyer W. Family centred care – a way to connect patients, families and nurses in critical care: a qualitative study using telephone interviews. Intensive Crit Care Nurs 2010;26(3):154–60.

80 Garrouste-Orgeas M, Philippart F, Timsit JF, Diaw F, Willems V, Tabah A et al. Perceptions of a 24-hour visiting policy in the intensive care unit. Crit Care Med 2008;36(1):30–5.

81 Lee MD, Friedenberg AS, Mukpo DH, Conray K, Palmisciano A, Levy MM. Visiting hours policies in New England intensive care units: strategies for improvement. Crit Care Med 2007;35(2):497–501.

82 Whitcomb JJ, Roy D, Blackman VS. Evidence-based practice in a military intensive care unit family visitation. Nurs Res 2010;59(1 Suppl): S32–9.

83 Van Horn ER, Kautz D. Promotion of family integrity in the acute care setting: a review of the literature. DCCN 2007;26(3):101–7.

84 Maxwell KE, Stuenkel D, Saylor C. Needs of family members of critically ill patients: a comparison of nurse and family perceptions. Heart Lung 2007;36(5):367–76.

85 Davidson JE, Powers K, Hedayat KM, Tieszen M, Kon AA, Shepard E et al. Clinical practice guidelines for support of the family in the patient-centered intensive care unit: American College of Critical Care Medicine Task Force 2004–2005. Crit Care Med 2007;35:605–22.

86 Williams CMA. The identification of family members' contribution to patients' care in the intensive care unit: a naturalistic inquiry. Nurs Crit Care 2005;10(1):6–14.

87 Davidson JE. Meeting the needs of patients' families and helping families to adapt to critical illness. Crit Care Med 2009;29(3):28–34.

88 Arockiasamy V, Holsti L, Albersheim S. Fathers' experiences in the neonatal intensive care unit: a search for control. Pediatrics 2008; 121(2):e215–e22.

89 Azoulay É, Pochard F, Chevret S, Arich C, Brivet F, Brun F et al. Family participation in care to the critically ill: opinions of families and staff. Intensive Care Med 2003;29(9):1498–504.

90 Patak L, Gawlinski A, Fung NI, Doering L, Berg J, Henneman EA. Communication boards in critical care: patients' views. Appl Nurs Res 2006;19:182–90.

91 Hemsley B, Sigafoos J, Balandin S, Forbes R, Taylor C, Green VA et al. Nursing the patient with severe communication impairment. J Adv Nurs 2001;35:827–35.

92 Casbolt S. Communicating with the ventilated patient – a literature review. Nurs Crit Care 2002;7(4):198–202.

93 Hupcey JE, Zimmerman HE. The need to know: experiences of critically ill patients. Am J Crit Care 2000;9:192–8.

94 Happ MB, Tuite P, Dobbin K, DiVirgilio-Thomas D, Kitutu J. Communication ability, method, and content among nonspeaking nonsurviving patients treated with mechanical ventilation in the intensive care unit. Am J Crit Care 2004;13:210–8.

95 Travaline JM. Communication in the ICU: an essential component of patient care. J Crit Illn 2002;17:451–6.

96 Alasad J, Ahmad M. Communication with critically ill patients. J Adv Nurs 2005;50(4):356–62.

97 Lawrence M. The unconscious experience. Am J Crit Care 1995;4(3):227–32.

98 Green A. An exploratory study of patients' memory recall of their stay in an adult intensive therapy unit. Intens Crit Care Nurs 1996;12(3): 131–7.

99 Benner P. Seeing the person beyond the disease. Am J Crit Care 2004;13(1):75–8.

100 Hupcey JE. Feeling safe: the psychosocial needs of ICU patients. J Nurs Schol 2000;32:361–7.

101 Happ MB, Roesch TK, Garrett K. Electronic voice-output communication aids for temporarily nonspeaking patients in a medical intensive care unit: a feasibility study. Heart Lung 2004;33(2):92–101.

102 Narayanasamy A, Clissett P, Parumal L, Thompson D, Annasamy S, Edge R. Responses to the spiritual needs of older people. J Adv Nurs 2004;48(1):6–16.

103 Wepa D. Cultural safety in Aotearoa New Zealand. Auckland, NZ: Pearson Education New Zealand; 2005.

104 Dempsey J, Hillage S, Hill R, eds. Fundamentals of nursing and midwifery: a person-centred approach to care. 2nd Australian and New Zealand ed. Sydney: Lippincott, Williams and Wilkins; 2013.

105 Charon JM. Symbolic interactionism: an introduction, an interpretation, an integration. 10th ed. Upper Saddle River, NJ: Prentice-Hall; 2009.

106 Gushue GV, Mejia-Smith BX, Fisher LD, Cogger A, Gonzalez-Matthews M, Lee Y-J et al. Differentiation of self and racial identity. Couns Psych Q 2013;26:343–61.

107 Ryan A, Carryer J, Patterson L. Healthy concerns: Sociology for New Zealand nursing and midwifery students. Auckland: Pearson Education; 2003.

108 Wilson D. The nurse's role in improving indigenous health. Contemp Nurs 2003;15(3):232–40.

109 Mosley S. Ki te whaiao: an introduction to Māori culture and society. Auckland: Pearson Education; 2004.

110 Jackson D, Brady W, Stein I. Towards (re)conciliation: (re)constructing relationships between indigenous health workers and nurses. J Adv Nurs 1999;29(1):97–103.

111 McKinnon J. The case for concordance: value and application in nursing practice. Brit J Nurs 2013;22(13):766–71. PubMed PMID: 24261092.

112 Gill GK, Babacan H. Developing a culturally responsive framework in healthcare systems: an Australian example. Divers Equal Health Care 2012;9:45–4.

113 Leininger MM. Cultural care diversity and universality: a theory of nursing. New York: National League for Nursing Press; 2001.

114 Ramsden I. Kawa whakaruruhau: cultural safety in nursing education. Wellington: Ministry of Health; 1990.

115 Ramsden I. Cultural safety and nursing education in Aotearoa and Te Waipounamu. Wellington, New Zealand: Victoria University of Wellington; 2002.

116 Wood PJ, Schwass M. Cultural safety: a framework for changing attitudes. Nurs Prax NZ 1993;8(1):4–15.

117 Giger JN. Transcultural nursing: assessment and intervention. St Louis: Elsevier Mosby; 2012.

118 McDonough S, Chopra P, Tuncer C, Schumacher B, Bhat R. Enhancing cultural responsiveness: the development of a pilot transcultural secondary consultation program. Aust Psych 2013;21(5):494–8.

119 Dudas KI. Cultural competence: an evolutionary concept analysis. Nurs Educ Perspect 2012;33:317–21.

120 Perng S-J, Watson R. Construct validation of the nurse cultural competence scale: a hierarchy of abilities. J Clin Nurs 2012;21:1678–84.

121 Ingram RR. Using Campinha-Bacote's process of cultural competence model to examine the relationship between health literacy and cultural competence. J Adv Nurs 2012;68:695–704.

122 Durie M. Cultural competence and medical practice in New Zealand. Australian and New Zealand Boards and Council Conference; November 21; Wellington, New Zealand; 2001.

123 Wilson D. The significance of a culturally appropriate health service for indigenous Maori women. Contemp Nurs 2008;28(1–2):173–88.

124 Wilson D, Roberts M. Māori health initiatives. In: Wepa D, ed. Cultural safety in Aotearoa/New Zealand. Auckland: Pearson Education; 2004.

125 Funnell MM, Anderson RM. Empowerment and self-management of diabetes. Clin Diabetes 2004;22(3):123–7.

126 Chambers-Evans J, Stelling J, Godin M. Learning to listen: serendipitous outcomes of a research training experience. J Adv Nurs 1999; 29(6):1421–6.

127 Conning AM, Rowland LA. Staff attitudes and the provision of individualised care: what determines what we do for people with long-term psychiatric disabilities? J Mental Health 1992;1(1):71–80.

128 Ciufo D, Hader R, Holly C. A comprehensive systematic review of visitation models in adult critical care units within the context of patient- and family-centered care. Int J Evidence-Based Healthcare 2011;9(4):362–87.

129 Usher K, Cook J, Miller M, Turale S, Goold S. Meeting the challenges of recruitment and retention of Indigenous people into nursing: outcomes of the Indigenous Nurse Education Working Group. Collegian 2005;12(3):27–31.

130 Ring I, Brown N. The health status of indigenous peoples and others: the gap is narrowing in the United States, Canada, and New Zealand, but a lot more is needed. Br Med J 2003;327(7412):404–5.

131 Commonwealth Department of Health and Ageing and Office of Aboriginal and Torres Strait Islander Health. Getting em n keeping em: report of the Indgenous Nursing Education Working Group. 2002.

132 National Aboriginal Health Organization. Strategic framework to increase the participation of First Nations, Inuit and Metis in health, <http://www.naho.ca/documents/naho/english/pdf/hhr_StrategicFramework.pdf>; 2006 [accessed 01.09.14].

133 First Nations Health Authority. First Nations health human resources tripartite strategic approach, http://www.fnha.ca/ Documents/First_Nations_Health_Human_Resources_Tripartite_Strategic_Approach.pdf>; 2012.

134 Procter S. Whose evidence? Agenda setting in multi-professional research: observations from a case study. Health Risk Society 2002;4(1):45–59.

135 Petroz U, Kennedy D, Webster F, Nowak A. Patients' perceptions of individualized care: evaluating psychometric properties and results of the individualized care scale. CJNR 2011;43:80–100.

136 Shaw JSCL. Shadowing: a central component of patient and family-centred care. Nurs Manage – UK 2014;21(3):20–3.

137 Bredemeyer S, Reid S, Polverino J, Wocadlo C. Implementation and evaluation of an individualized developmental care program in a neonatal intensive care unit. J Spec Pediatr Nurs 2008;13(4):281–91.

138 Suhonen R, Välimäki M, Leino-Kilpi H. Individualized care, quality of life and satisfaction with nursing care. J Adv Nurs 2005;50:283–92.

139 Kärkkäinen O, Bondas T, Eriksson K. Documentation of individualized patient care: a qualitative metasynthesis. Nurs Ethics 2005;12(2):123–32.

140 (ABS) ABoS. Cultural diversity in Australia: Reflecting a nation: Stories from 2011 Census, <http://www.abs.gov.au/ausstats/abs@.nsf/Lookup/2071.0main+features902012-2013>; 2012 [accessed 01.09.14].

141 Statistics New Zealand. 2013 Census QuickStats about national highlights, <http://www.stats.govt.nz>; 2013.

142 Statistics Canada. Immigration and ethnocultural diversity in Canada, <http://www12.statcan.gc.ca/nhs-enm/2011/as-sa/99-010-x/99-010-x2011001-eng.cfm>; 2011 [accessed 01.09.14].

143 United States Census Bureau. State and country quick facts, <http://quickfacts.census.gov/qfd/states/00000.html>; 2014 [accessed 01.09.14].

144 Campinha-Bacote J. The process of cultural competence in the delivery of health services, <http://www.transculturalcare.net>; 2002 [accessed 01.09.14].

145 Health Mo. Tatau kahukura: Maori health chart book. Wellington, New Zealand: Author; 2010.

146 Ka'ai T, Higgins R. Te ao Māori: Māori worldview. In: Ka'ai TM, Moorfield JC, Reilly MPJ, Mosley S, eds. Ki te whaiao: an introduction to Māori culture and society. Auckland: Pearson Education; 2004: p 13–25.

147 Wilson D. The Treaty of Waitangi, nurses and their practice. N Z Nurs Rev 2002;3(4):18.

148 Reilly MPJ. Whanaungatanga – kinship. In: Ka'ai TM, Moorfiled JC, Reilly MPJ, Mosley S, eds. Te ao Māori: Māori worldview. Auckland: Pearson Education; 2004: pp 61–72.

149 Reilly MPJ. Te timatanga mai o ngā atua. In: Ka'ai T, Moorfield JC, Reilly MPJ, Mosley S, eds. Te ao Māori: Māori worldview. Auckland: Pearson Education; 2004.

150 Ministry of Health. He Korowai Oranga: Māori health strategy 2014. Wellington, New Zealand: Author. <http://www.health.govt.nz/publication/guide-he-korowai-oranga-maori-health-strategy>; 2014.

151 Stenhouse J, Paterson L. Ngā poropiti me ngā Hatu – prophets and the churches. In: Ka'ai TM, Moorfield JC, Reilly MPJ, Mosley S, eds. Ki te whaiao: an introduction to Māori culture and society. Auckland: Pearson; 2004: pp 163–70.

152 Australan Bureau of Statistics (ABS). Australian Aboriginal and Torres Strait Islander health survey: updated results, 2012–2013, <http://www.abs.gov.au/ausstats/abs@.nsf/Lookup/4727.0.55.006main+features12012-12>; 2014 accessed 01.09.14].

153 Secombe PJ, Stewart PC, Brown A. Functional outcomes in high risk ICU patients in central Australia: a prospective case series. Rural Remote Health 2013;13(1):2128.

154 Stephens DP. Exploring pathways to improve indigenous organ donation. Intern Med J 2003;37:713–6.

155 Ho KM, Finn J, Dobb GJ, Webb SAR. The outcome of critically ill Indigenous patients. Med J Aust 2006;184:496–9.

156 Drennan K, Hart G, Hicks P. Intensive care resources and activity: Australia and New Zealand 2006/2007. Melbourne, VIC: ANZICS; 2008.

157 Australian Institute of Health and Welfare. Indigenous identification in hospital separation data: quality report (AIHW Catalogue No IHW 90). Canberra: Australian Institute of Health and Welfare. <http://www.aihw.gov.au/publication-detail/?id=60129543215>; 2013.

158 Australian Indigenous Health *InfoNet*. Overview of Australian Indigenous health status, 2014, <http://www.healthinfonet.ecu.edu.au/health-facts/overviews>; 2014 [accessed 01.09.14].

159 Walker X, Lee J, Koval L, Kirkwood A, Taylor JK, Gibbs J et al. Predicting ICU admissions from attempted suicide presentations at an Emergency Department in Central Queensland. Aust Med J 2013;6:536–41.

160 Australan Bureau of Statistics (ABS). Australian and Torres Strait Islander health survey: updated results 2012–13, <http://www.abs.gov.au/ausstats/abs@.nsf/Lookup/4727.0.55.006main+features12012-13>; 2013 [accessed 01.09.14].

161 Carson B, Dunbar T, Chenhall RD, Bailie R, eds. Social determinants of Indigenous health. Crows Nest: Allen and Unwin; 2007.

162 Oberg K. Culture shock. Indianapolis: Bobb-Merrill Series in Social Science A-329; 1954.

163 Oberg K. Culture shock and the problem of adjustment to new cultural environments, <http://www.worldwide.edu/travel_planner/culture_shock.html>; 2006 [accessed 01.09.14].

164 Kildea S. And the women said . . . reporting on birthing services for Aboriginal women from remote Top End communities. Government Printer of the Northern Territory: Women's Health Strategy Unit, Territory Health Services; 1999.

165 Eckermann A-K, Dowd T, Chong E, Nixon L, Gray R, Johnson B. Binan Goonj: bridging cultures in Aboriginal health. 3rd ed. Sydney: Churchill Livingstone; 2010.

166 McEwan A, Tsey K. The role of spirituality in social and emotional wellbeing initiatives: the family wellbeing program of Yarrabah. Discussion paper series No. 7. Northern Territory: Cooperative Centre for Aboriginal Health, James Cook University, <https://www.lowitja.org.au/sites/default/files/docs/DP7_FINAL.pdf>; 2009.

167 Burgess P, Morrison M. Country. In: Carson B, Dunbar T, Chenhall RD, Bailie R, eds. Social determinants of Indigenous health. Crows Nest: Allen and Unwin; 2007: pp 177–202.

168 National Aboriginal Health Strategy Working Party. National strategic framework for Aboriginal and Torres Strait Islander health: context. Canberra: NATSIHC; 1983.

169 Natham P, Japanangka DL. Health business. Melbourne: Heinemann Educational Australia; 1983.

170 Mobbs R. In sickness and health: the sociocultural context of Aboriginal well-being, illness and healing. In: Reid J, Trompf P, eds. The health of Aboriginal Australia. Sydney: Harcourt Brace Javanovich; 1991.

171 Maher P. A review of 'traditional' Aboriginal health beliefs. Aust J Rural Health 1999;7:229–36.

172 Reid J, Mununggurr D. We are losing our brothers: sorcery and alcohol in an Aboriginal community. Med J Aust 1977;2Suppl:1-5.

173 Reid J, Williams N. 'Voodoo death' in Arnhem land: whose reality? Am Anthro 1984;86:121–33.

174 Morgan DL, Slade MD, Morgan CM. Aboriginal philosophy and its impact on health care outcomes. Aust N Z J Pub Health 1997;21:597–601.

175 Ngangala TB, Nangala GM, McCoy B. Who makes decisions for the unconscious Aboriginal patient? Aboriginal and Torres Strait Island Health Worker J 2008;32(1):6–9.

176 Ho A. Using family members as interpreters in the clinical setting. J Clin Ethics 2008;19:223–33.

177 Gray B, Hilder J, Donaldson H. Why do we use trained interpreters for all patients with limited English proficiency? Is there a place for using family members? Aust J Prim Health 2011;17:240–9.

178 Shahid S, Finn LD, Thompson SC. Barriers to participation of Aboriginal people in cancer care: communication in the hospital setting. Med J Aust 2009;190(10):574–9.

179 Trudgeon R. Why warriors lie down and die. Adelaide: Openbook Print; 2000.

180 Lenthal S, Gordon V, Knight S, Aitken R, Ivanhoe T. Do not move the furniture and other advice for new remote area nurses. Aust J Rural Health 2012;20:44–5.

181 Pearson N. Our right to take responsibility. Cairns: Noel Pearson; 2000.

182 Rose D. Nourishing terrains: Australian Aboriginal views of landscape and wilderness. Canberra: Australian Heritage Commission; 1996.

183 Stamp G, Miller D, Coleman H, Milera A, Taylor J. Transfer issues for rural and remote Australia. Anaesth Intens Care 2006;31:294–9.

184 Latour J, Fulbrook P, Albarran J. EfCCna survey: European intensive care nurses' attitudes and beliefs towards end-of-life care. Nurs Crit Care 2009;14(3):110–21.

185 Halligan P. Caring for patients of Islamic denomination: critical care nurses' experiences in Saudi Arabia. J Clin Nurs 2006;15:1565–73.

186 Kongsuwan W, Locsin RC. Promoting peaceful death in the intensive care unit in Thailand. Int Nurs Rev 2009;56(1):116–22.

187 Blockley C. Meeting patients' religious needs. Kai Tiaki Nurs NZ. 2001/2002;7(11):15–7.

188 Murthy S, Wunsch H. Clinical review: international comparisons in critical care – lessons learned. Crit Care 2012;16(2):1–7.

189 Australia and New Zealand Intensive Care Society. Intensive care: Centre for Outcome and Resource evaluation. Resource and activity report 2010–2011. Carlton: ANZICS Centre for Outcome and Resource Evaluation (CORE); 2013.

190 Warren NA. Critical care family members' satisfaction with bereavement experiences. Crit Care Nurs Q 2002;25(2):54–60.

191 Puri VK. Death in the ICU: feelings of those left behind. Chest 1003;124(1):11–3.

192 Gries CJ, Randall Curtis J, Wall RJ, Engelberg RA. Family member satisfaction with end-of-life decision making in the ICU. Chest 2008; 133(3):704–12.

193 Gaeta S, Price KJ. End-of-life issues in critically ill cancer patients. Crit Care Clin 2010;26:219–27.

194 Rocker G, Heyland D, Cook D, Dodek P, Kutsogiannis D, O'Callaghan C. Most critically ill patients are perceived to die in comfort during withdrawal of life support: a Canadian multicentre study. Can J Anesth 2004;51:623–30.

195 Kuschner WG, Gruenewald DA, Clum N, Beal A, Ezeji-Okoye SC. Implementation of ICU palliative care guidelines and procedures: a quality improvement initiative following an investigation of alleged euthanasia. Chest 2009;135(1):26–32.

196 Mularski RA, Puntillo K, Varkey B, Erstad BL, Grap MJ, Gilbert HC et al. Pain management within the palliative and end-of-life experience in the ICU. Chest 2009;135:1360–9.

197 Puntillo K, Benner P, Drought T, Drew B, Stotts N, Stannard D et al. End-of-life issues in intensive care units: a national random survey of nurses' knowledge and beliefs. Am J Crit Care 2001;10:216–29.

198 O'Mahony S, McHugh M, Zallman L, Selwyn P. Ventilator withdrawal: procedures and outcomes. Report of a collaboration between a critical care division and a palliative care service. J Pain Symptom Manage 2003;26:954–61.

199 Enes SP. An exploration of dignity in palliative care. Palliat Med 2003;17:263–9.

200 Schaefer KG, Block SD. Physician communication with families in the ICU: evidence-based strategies for improvement. Curr Opin Crit Care 2009;15:569–77.

201 Cook D, Rocker G, Heyland D. Dying in the ICU: strategies that may improve end-of-life care. Can J Anesth 2004;51(3):266–72.

202 Johnson N, Cook D, Giacomini M, Willms D. Towards a "good" death: end-of-life narratives constructed in an intensive care unit. Cult Med Psychiatry 2000;24(3):275–95.

203 Mosenthal AC, Murphy PA, Barker LK, Lavery R, Retano A, Livingston DH. Changing the culture around end-of-life care in the trauma intensive care unit. J Trauma 2008;64:1587–93.

204 Clarke EB, Curtis R, Luce JM, Levy M, Danis M et al. Quality indicators for end-of-life care in the intensive are unit. Crit Care Med 2003; 31(9):2255–62.

205 Siegal MD. End-of-life decision making in the ICU. Clin Chest Med 2009;30:181–94.

206 Seaman JB. Improving care at end of life in the ICU. J Gerontol Nurs 2013;39(8):52–8.

207 Kaufer M, Murphy PA, Barker KK, Mosenthal AC. Family satisfaction following the death of a loved one in an inner city MICU. Am J Hosp Palliat Med 2008;25(4):318–25.

208 Pochard F, Darmon M, Fassier T, Bollaert PE, Cheval C, Coloigner M et al. Symptoms of anxiety and depression in family members of intensive care unit patients before discharge or death: a prospective multicenter study. J Crit Care 2005;20:90–6.

209 Studdert C, Burns JP, Mello MM, Puopolo AL, Truog RD, Brennan TA. Nature of conflict in the care of pediatric intensive care patients with prolonged stay. Pediat 2003;112:553–8.

210 Stapleton RD, Engelberg RA, Wenrich MD, Goss CH, Curtis JR. Clinician statements and family satisfaction with family conferences in the intensive care unit. Crit Care Med 2006;43:1679–85.

211 West HF, Engelberg RA, Wenrich MD, Curtis JR. Expressions of nonabandonment during the intensive care unit family conference. J Palliat Med 2005;8:797–807.

212 Curtis JR, Ciechanowski PS, Downey L, Gold J, Nielson EL, Shannon SE et al. Development and evaluation of an interprofessional communication intervention to improve family outcomes in the ICU. Contemporary Clinical Trials 2012;33:1245–54.

213 Lautrette A, Ciroldi M, Ksibi H, Azoulay E. End-of-life family conference: rooted in the evidence. Crit Care Med 2006;34(Suppl 11):S346–72.

214 McDonagh JR, Elliott TB, Engelberg RA, Treece PD, Shannon SE, Rubenfeld GD et al. Family satisfaction with family conferences about end-of-life care in the ICU: increased proportion of family speech is associated with increased satisfaction. Crit Care Med 2004;32:1484–8.

215 Krueger G. Meaning-making in the aftermath of sudden infant death syndrome. Nurs Inq 2006;13:3163–71.

216 Campbell M, Thill M. Bereavement follow up to families after death in the intensive care unit. Crit Care Med 2000;28(4):1252–3.

217 Nelson JE, Angus DC, Weissfeld LA, Puntillo K, Danis M et al. End-of-life care for the critically ill: a national intensive care unit survey. Crit Care Med 2006;31:2547–53.

218 Anderson WG, Arnold RM, Angus DC, Bryce CL. Post-traumatic stress and complicated grief in family members of patients in the intensive care unit. J Gen Intern Med 2008;23(11):1871–6.

219 Fauri D, Ettner B, Kovacs P. Bereavement services in acute care settings. Death Studies 2000;24:51–64.

220 Stroebe S, Schut H, Stroebe W. Health outcomes of bereavement. Lancet 2007;370:1960–73.

221 Golden A-MJ, Dalgleish T. Is prolonged grief distinct from bereavement-related posttraumatice stress? Psych Res 2010;178:208–15.

222 Casarett D, Kutner J, Abraham J. Life and death: a practical approach to grief and bereavement. Ann Intern Med 2001;134(3):208–15.

223 Fauri D, Oliver R, Sturtevant J, Scheetz J, Fallat M. Beneficial effects of a hospital bereavement intervention program after traumatic childhood death. J Trauma 2001;50:440–8.

224 Williams R, Harris S, Randall L, Nichols R, Brown S. A bereavement after-care service for intensive care relatives and staff: the story so far. Nurs Crit Care 2003;8(3):109–15.

225 Department of Health. Bereavement care services: a synthesis of the literature. London: Department of Health; 2011.

226 Valks K, Mitchell ML, Inglis-Simmons C, Limpus A. Dealing wth death: an audit of family bereavement programs in Australian intensive care units. Aust Crit Care 2005;18:257–68.

227 Brosche TA. Death, dying and the IC nurse. DCCN 2003;22(4):173–9.

228 Main J. Management of relatives of patients who are dying. J Clin Nurs 2002;11:794–801.

229 Shaw DJ, Davidson JE, Smilde RI, Sondoozi T, Agan D. Multidisciplinary team training to enhance family communication in the ICU. Crit Care Med 2014;42:265–71.

230 Quenot JP, Rigaud JP, Prin S, Barbar S, Pavon A, Hamet M et al. Suffering among carers working in critical care can be reduced by an intensive communication strategy on end-of-life practices. Intens Care Med 2012;38(1):55–61.

231 Rogers S, Babgi A, Gomez C. Educational interventions in end-of-life care: part 1. Adv Neonatal Care 2008;8(1):56–65.

232 Wallace M, Sarles S. EB49 Changing culture to cultivate patient- and family-centered care. Crit Care Med 2012;32(2):e30-e.

233 Henrich NJ, Dodek P, Heyland D, Cook D, Rocker G, Kutsogiannis D et al. Qualitative analysis of an intensive care unit family satisfaction survey. Crit Care Med 2011;39:1000–5.

Chapter 9

Cardiovascular assessment and monitoring

Thomas Buckley, Frances Lin

Learning objectives

After reading this chapter, you should be able to:

- describe the normal blood flow through the cardiovascular system
- define each stage of the cardiac action potential and its application to electrocardiography
- describe the determinants of cardiac output and their interpretation in cardiovascular assessment and monitoring
- describe the reasons for the assessment and monitoring of critically ill patients
- summarise the key principles underpinning cardiac assessment and monitoring
- identify the recommended anatomical landmarks for cardiac auscultation and identify normal and common abnormal heart sounds
- describe the physiological bases and reasons for different types of haemodynamic monitoring
- critique and evaluate current clinical practice on haemodynamic monitoring and integrate best evidence in clinical practice.

Introduction

This chapter reviews the support of cardiovascular function in the face of many compromises to the system. It is essential for the reader to have a thorough knowledge of both electrical and mechanical functions of the cardiac system. Methodology for assessment of cardiovascular elements is discussed, along with best practice ideas and diagnostic techniques.

Related anatomy and physiology

The cardiovascular system is essentially a transport system for distributing metabolic requirements to, and collecting byproducts from, cells throughout the body. The heart pumps blood continuously through two separate circulatory systems: to the lungs and to all other parts of the body (see Figure 9.1). Structures on the right side of the heart pump blood through the lungs (the pulmonary circulation) to be oxygenated. The left side of the heart pumps oxygenated blood throughout the remainder of the body (the systemic circulation).[1,2] The two systems are connected, so the output of one becomes the input of the other.

Cardiac macrostructure

The heart is cone-shaped and lies diagonally in the mediastinum towards the left side of the chest. The point of the cone is called the apex and rests just above the diaphragm; the base of the cone lies just behind the mediastinum. The adult heart is about the size of that individual's fist, weighs around 300 g and is composed of chambers and valves that

form the two separate pumps. The upper chambers, the atria, collect blood and act as a primer to the main pumping chambers, the ventricles. As the atria are low-pressure chambers, they have relatively thin walls and are relatively compliant. As the ventricles propel blood against either pulmonary or systemic pressure, they have much thicker and more muscular walls than the atria. As pressure is higher in the systemic circulation, the left ventricle is much thicker than the right ventricle. Dense fibrous connective tissue rings provide a firm anchorage for attachments of atrial and ventricular muscle and valvular tissue.[1,4]

FIGURE 9.1 The systemic and pulmonic circulations.[3]

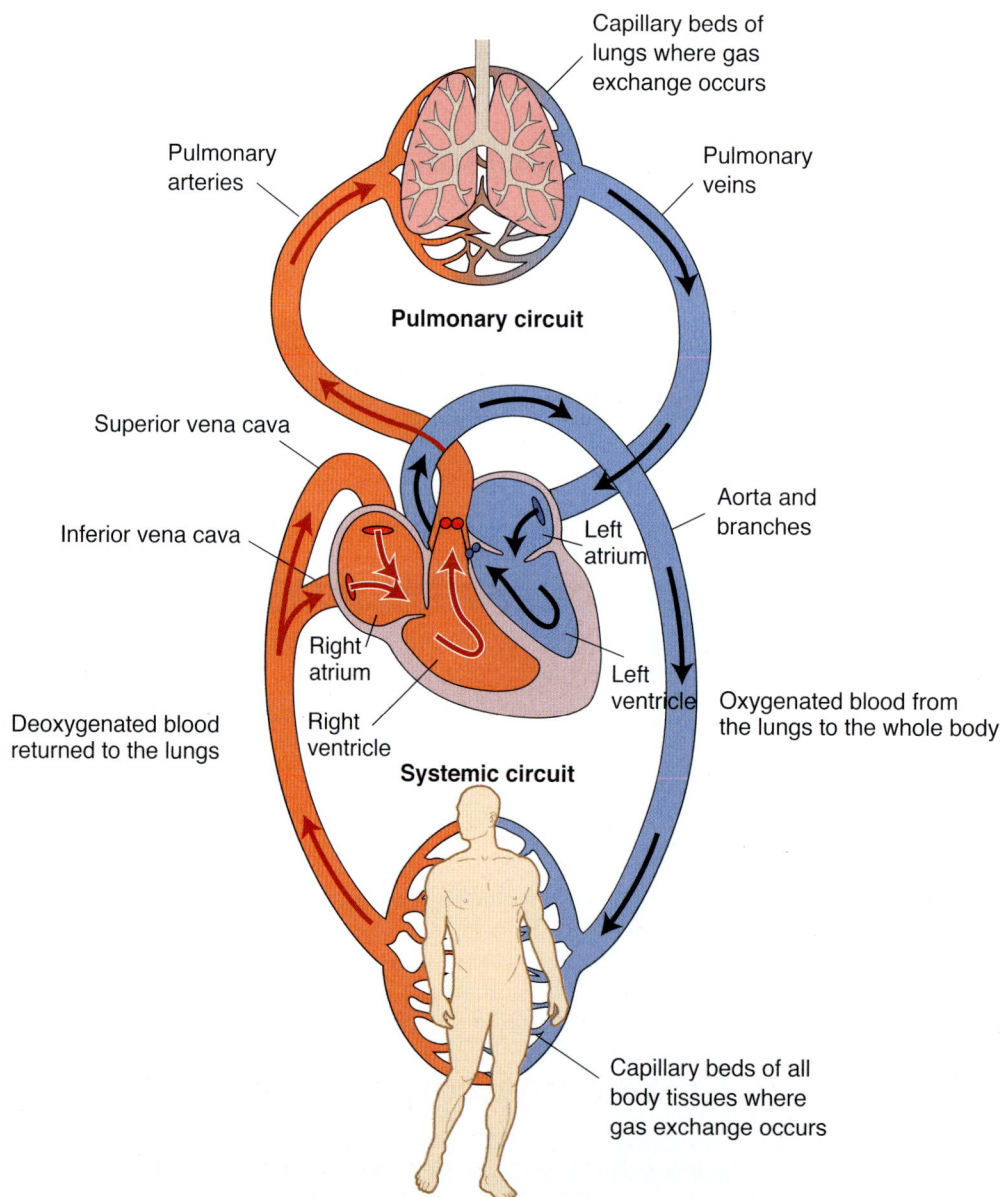

Adapted from Novak B, Filer L, Latchett R. The applied anatomy and physiology of the cardiovascular system. In: Hatchett R, Thompson D, eds. Cardiac nursing: a comprehensive guide. Philadelphia: Churchill Livingstone Elsevier; 2002, with permission.

One-way blood flow in the system is facilitated by valves. Valves between the atria and ventricles are composed of cusps or leaflets sitting in a ring of fibrous tissue and collagen. The cusps are anchored to the papillary muscles by chordae tendinae so that the cusps are pulled together and downwards at the onset of ventricular contraction. The atrioventricular valves are termed the tricuspid valve in the right side of the heart and the mitral or bicuspid valve in the left side of the heart. Semilunar valves prevent backflow from the pulmonary artery (pulmonic valve) and aorta (aortic valve) into the corresponding right and left ventricles. The muscles in the ventricles follow a distinct spiral path so that, during contraction, blood is propelled into the respective outflow tracts of the pulmonary artery and aorta. The aortic valve sits in a tubular area of mostly non-contractile collagenous tissue, which contains the opening of the coronary arteries. The coronary arteries run through deep grooves that separate the atria and ventricles. The two sides of the heart are divided by a septum, which ensures that two separate but integrated circulations are maintained.[1,4]

The heart wall has three distinct layers: the outer protective pericardium, a medial muscular layer or myocardium and an inner layer or endocardium that lines the heart. The pericardium is a double-walled, firm fibrous sac that encloses the heart. The two layers of the pericardium are separated by a fluid-filled cavity, enabling the layers to slide over each other smoothly as the heart beats. The pericardium provides physical protection for the heart against mechanical force and forms a barrier to infection and inflammation from the lungs and pleural space. Branches of the vagus nerve, the phrenic nerves and the sympathetic trunk enervate the pericardium.

The myocardium forms the bulk of the heart and is composed primarily of myocytes.[5] Myocytes are the contractile cells, and autorhythmic cells, which create a conduction pathway for electrical impulses. Myocytes (see Figure 9.2) are cylindrical in shape and able to branch to interconnect with each other. The junctions between myocytes are termed intercalated discs and contain desmosomes and gap junctions.[6] Desmosomes act as anchors to prevent the myocytes from separating during contraction. Gap junctions

FIGURE 9.2 Diagram of an electron micrograph of cardiac muscle showing mitochondria, intercalculated discs, tubules and sarcoplasmic reticulum.

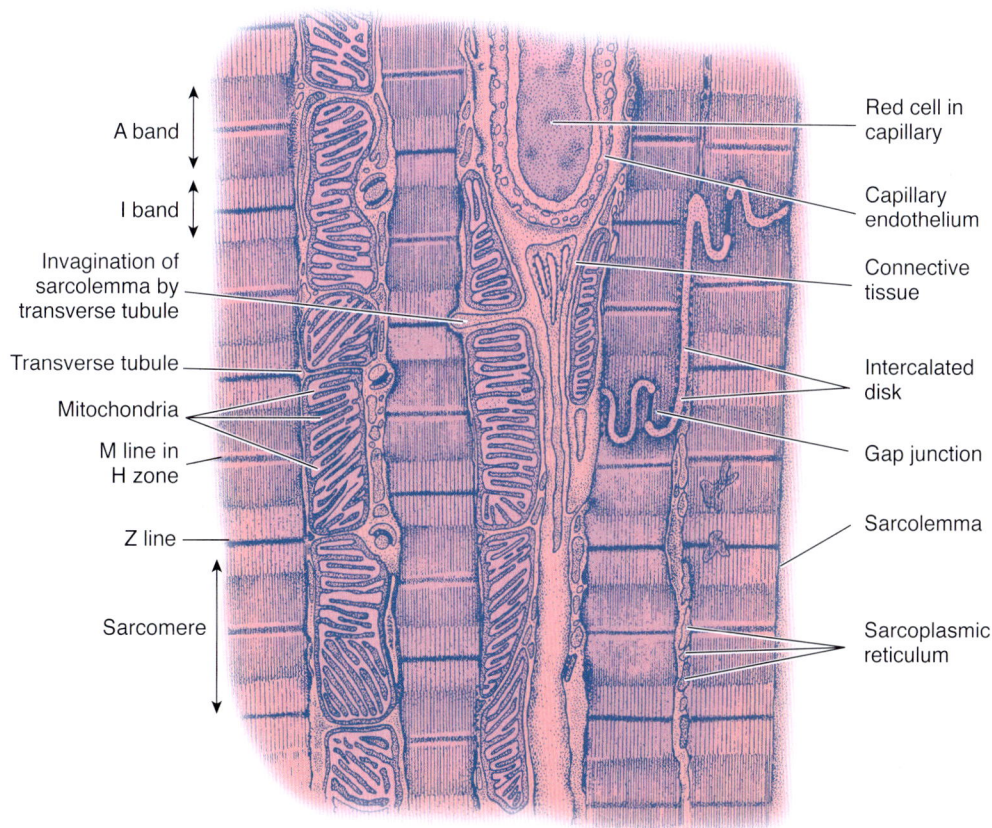

A band

I band

Invagination of sarcolemma by transverse tubule

Transverse tubule

Mitochondria

M line in H zone

Z line

Sarcomere

Red cell in capillary

Capillary endothelium

Connective tissue

Intercalated disk

Gap junction

Sarcolemma

Sarcoplasmic reticulum

Adapted from Urden L, Stacy KL, Lough ME, eds. Thelan's critical care nursing: Diagnosis and management. 6th ed. St Louis: Mosby/Elsevier; 2010, with permission.

contain connexons, which allow ions to move from one myocyte to the next. The movement of ions from cell to cell ensures that the whole myocardium acts as one unit, termed a functional syncytium. When ischaemia occurs, the gap junctions may uncouple, so ions do not move as freely. Uncoupling may also contribute to the poor conduction evidenced on ECG during ischaemia.

The endocardium is composed primarily of squamous epithelium, which forms a continuous sheet with the endothelium that lines all arteries, veins and capillaries. The vascular endothelium is the source of many chemical mediators, including nitric oxide and the endothelin involved in vessel regulation. It has been theorised that the endocardium may also have this function.[1,4]

Coronary perfusion

The heart is perfused by the right and left coronary arteries that arise from openings in the aorta called the coronary ostia (see Figure 9.3). The right coronary artery (RCA) branches supply the atrioventricular node, right atrium and right ventricle, and the posterior descending branch supplies the lower aspect of the left ventricle. The left coronary artery divides into the left anterior descending artery (LAD) and the circumflex artery (CX) shortly after its origin. The LAD supplies the interventricular septum and anterior surface of the left ventricle. The CX supplies the lateral and posterior aspects of the left ventricle. This is the most common distribution of the coronary arteries, but it is not uncommon for the right coronary artery to be small and the CX to supply the inferior wall of the left ventricle. The coronary arteries ultimately branch into a dense network of capillaries to support cardiac myocytes. Anastomoses between branches of the coronary arteries often occur in mature individuals when myocardial hypoxia has been present. These anastomoses are termed collateral arteries, but the contribution to normal cardiac perfusion during occlusion of coronary arteries is unclear.[1]

The cardiac veins collect venous blood from the heart. Cardiac venous flow is collected into the great coronary vein and coronary sinus and ultimately flows into the right atrium. Lymph drainage of the heart follows the conduction tissue and flows into nodes and into the superior vena cava.

Physiological principles

An understanding of the principles of cardiac physiology is essential for safe management of the critically ill patient. While the primary role of the circulatory system is to provide sufficient blood flow to meet metabolic demands, this requires adequate myocardial contraction, coordinated electrical conduction and adequate intravascular volume.

Mechanical events of contraction

Energy is produced in the myocytes by a large number of mitochondria contained within the cell. The mitochondria produce adenosine triphosphate (ATP), a molecule that is able to store and release chemical energy. Other organelles in the myocyte, called sarcoplasmic reticulum, are used to store calcium ions. The myocyte cell membrane (sarcolemma) extends down into the cell to form a set of transverse tubules (T tubules), which rapidly transmit external electrical stimuli into the cell. Cross-striated

---

FIGURE 9.3 Location of the coronary arteries.

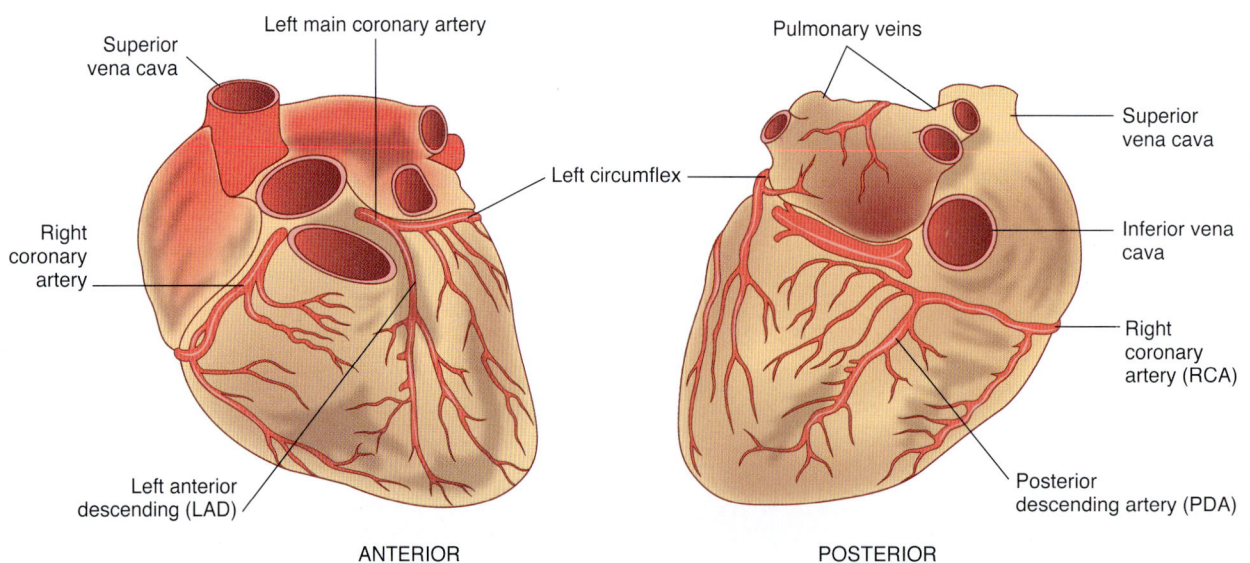

ANTERIOR   POSTERIOR

Adapted from Urden L, Stacy KL, Lough ME, eds. Thelan's critical care nursing: Diagnosis and management. 6th ed. St Louis: Mosby/Elsevier; 2010, with permission.

FIGURE 9.4 Actin and myosin filaments and other cross-bridges responsible for cell contraction.

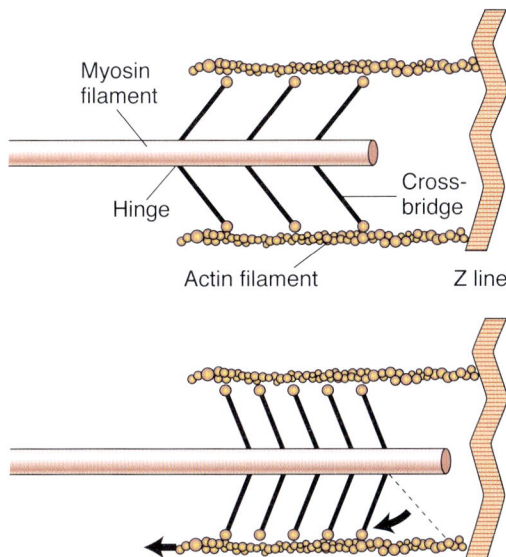

Adapted from Urden L, Stacy KL, Lough ME, eds. Thelan's critical care nursing: Diagnosis and management. 6th ed. St Louis: Mosby/Elsevier; 2010, with permission.

FIGURE 9.5 **A** Action potential in a 'fast response', non-pacemaker myocyte: phases 0–4, resting membrane potential –80 mV, absolute refractory period (ARP) and relative refractory period (RRP). **B** Action potential in a 'slow response', pacemaker myocyte. The upward slope of phase 4, on reaching threshold potential, results in an action potential.[7]

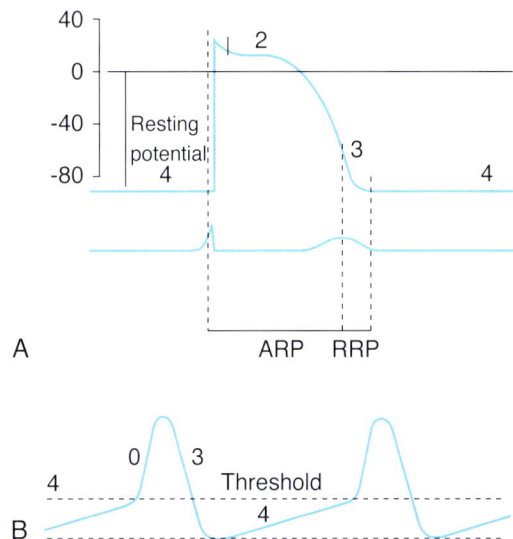

Adapted from Bersten AD, Soni N, Oh TE. Oh's intensive care manual. 7th ed. Oxford: Butterworth-Heinemann; 2013, with permission.

muscle fibrils, which contain contractile units, fill up the myocyte. These fibrils are termed sarcomeres.

The sarcomere contains two types of protein myofilaments, one thick (myosin) and one thin (actin, tropomyosin and troponin) (see Figure 9.4). The myosin molecules of the thick filaments contain active sites that form bridges with sites of the actin molecules on the thin filaments. These filaments are arranged so that during contraction, bridges form and the thin filaments are pulled into the lattice of the thick filaments. As the filaments are pulled towards the centre of the sarcomere, the degree of contraction is limited by the length of the sarcomere. Starling's law states that, within physiological limits, the greater the degree of stretch, the greater the force of contraction. The length of the sarcomere is the physiological limit because too great a stretch will disconnect the myosin–actin bridges.

Electrical events of depolarisation, resting potential and action potential

Automaticity and rhythmicity are intrinsic properties of all myocardial cells. However, specialised autorhythmic cells in the myocardium generate and conduct impulses in a specific order to create a conduction pathway. This pathway ensures that contraction is coordinated and rhythmical, so that the heart pumps efficiently and continuously. Electrical impulses termed action potentials are transmitted along this pathway and trigger contraction in myocytes. Action potentials represent the inward and outward flow of negative and positive charged ions across the cell membrane (see Figure 9.5).

Cell membrane pumps create concentration gradients across the cell membrane during diastole to create a resting electrical potential of −80 mV. Individual fibres are separated by membranes but depolarisation spreads rapidly because of the presence of gap junctions. There are five key phases to the cardiac action potential:

0 depolarisation
1 early rapid repolarisation
2 plateau phase
3 final rapid repolarisation
4 resting membrane phase.[8]

The contractile response begins just after the start of depolarisation and lasts about 1.5 times as long as the depolarisation and repolarisation (see Figure 9.6).

The action potential is created by ion exchange triggered by an intracellular and extracellular fluid trans-membrane imbalance. There are three ions involved: sodium, potassium and calcium. Normally, extracellular fluid contains approximately 140 mmol/L sodium and 4 mmol/L potassium. In intracellular fluid these concentrations are reversed. The following is a summary of physiological events during a normal action potential:

• At rest cell membranes are more permeable to potassium and, consequently, potassium moves slowly and passively from intracellular to extracellular fluid.

FIGURE 9.6 Action potential.

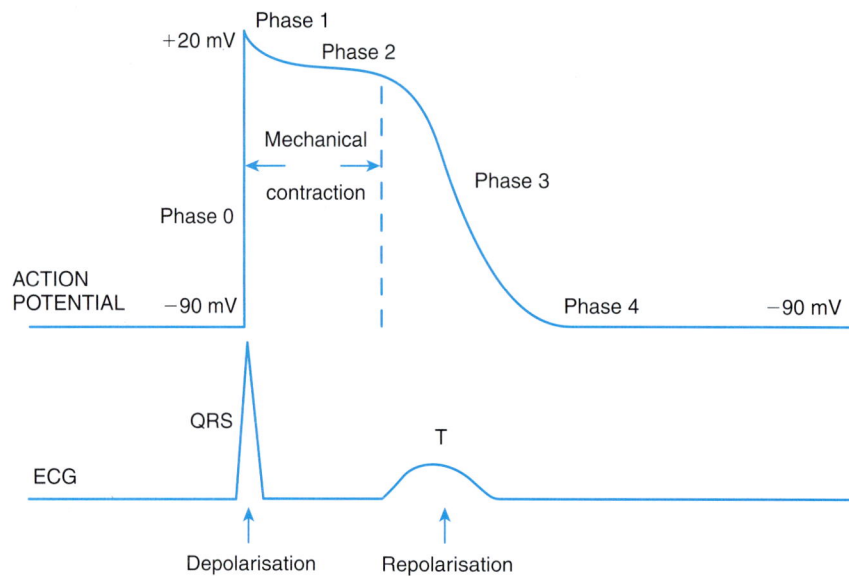

Adapted from Urden L, Stacy KL, Lough ME, eds. Thelan's critical care nursing: Diagnosis and management. 6th ed. St Louis: Mosby/Elsevier; 2010, with permission.

At this time fast sodium and slow calcium channels are closed and the resting membrane potential is very negative (-90 mV).

- During depolarisation (phase 0), rapid ion movement caused by sodium flowing into the cell alters the electrical potential from -90 mV to +30 mV. At this time potassium channels close.

- In phase 1 the sodium channels close and potassium begins to leave the cell. This is followed by a brief influx of calcium via the fast channel and then more via the slower channel to create a plateau (phase 2), the duration of which determines stroke volume due to its influence on the contractile strength of the muscle fibres.

- The third phase occurs when the calcium channels are inactivated allowing potassium to leave the cell more rapidly, restoring the negative charge and causing rapid depolarisation.

- The final resting phase occurs when slow potassium leakage allows the cell to increase its negative potential or charge (phase 4) to ensure that it is more negative than surrounding fluid, before the next depolarisation occurs and the cycle repeats.[6]

Cardiac muscle is generally slow to respond to stimuli and has relatively low ATPase activity. Its fibres are dependent on oxidative metabolism and require a continuous supply of oxygen. The lengths of fibres and the strength of contraction are determined by the degree of diastolic filling in the heart. The force of contraction is enhanced by catecholamines.[2]

Depolarisation is initiated in the sinoatrial (SA) node and spreads rapidly through the atria, then converges on the atrioventricular (AV) node; atrial depolarisation normally takes 0.1 second. There is a short delay at the AV node (0.1 s) before excitation spreads to the ventricles. This delay is shortened by sympathetic activity and lengthened by vagal stimulation. Ventricular depolarisation takes 0.08–0.1 sec, and the last parts of the heart to be depolarised are the posteriobasal portion of the left ventricle, the pulmonary conus and the upper septum.[8]

The electrical activity of the heart can be detected on the body surface because body fluids are good conductors; the fluctuations in potential that represent the algebraic sum of the action potentials of myocardial fibres can be recorded on an electrocardiogram (see later in this chapter).

Cardiac macrostructure and conduction

The electrical and mechanical processes of the heart differ but are connected. The autorhythmic cells of the cardiac conduction pathway ensure that large portions of the heart receive an action potential rapidly and simultaneously. This ensures that the pumping action of the heart is maximised. The conduction pathway is composed of the sinoatrial (SA) node, the atrioventricular (AV) node, the bundle of His, right and left bundle branches and Purkinje fibres (see Figure 9.7). The cells contained in the pathway conduct action potentials extremely rapidly, 3–7 times faster than general myocardial tissue. Pacemaker cells of the sinus and atrioventricular nodes differ, in that they are more permeable to potassium, so that potassium easily 'leaks' back out of the cells triggering influx of sodium and calcium back into cells. This permits the spontaneous automaticity of pacemaker cells.

FIGURE 9.7 Cardiac conduction system. AV = atrioventricular; LBB = left bundle branch; RBB = right bundle branch.

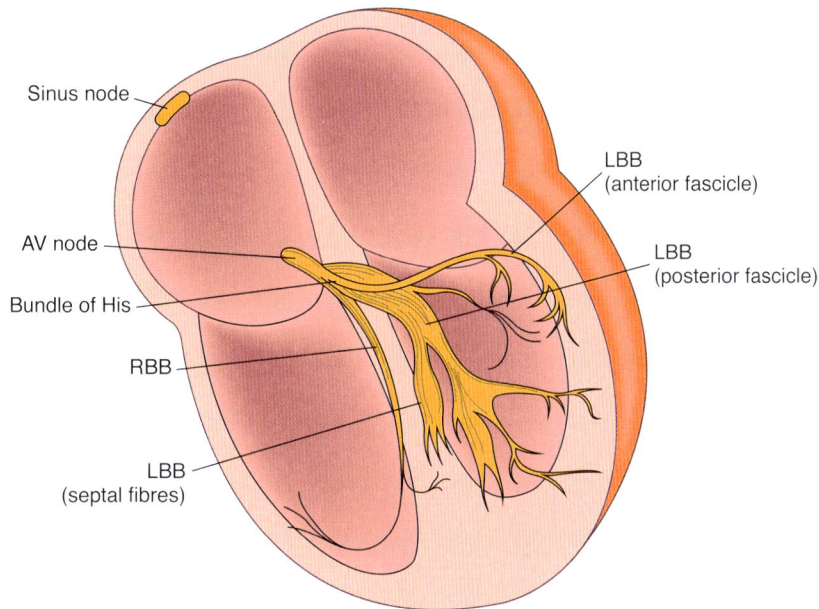

Adapted from Urden L, Stacy KL, Lough ME, eds. Thelan's critical care nursing: Diagnosis and management. 6th ed. St Louis: Mosby/Elsevier; 2010, with permission.

At the myocyte, the action potential is transmitted to the myofibrils by calcium from the interstitial fluid via channels. During repolarisation (after contraction), the calcium ions are pumped out of the cell into the interstitial space and into the sarcoplasmic reticulum and stored. Troponin releases its bound calcium, enabling the tropomyosin complex to block the active sites on actin, and the muscle relaxes.

The cardiac conduction system and the mechanical efficiency of the heart as a pump are directly connected. Disruption to conduction may not prevent myocardial contraction but may result in poor coordination and lower pump efficiency. Interruption to flow through the coronary arteries may alter depolarisation. Disrupted conduction from the SA to the AV node may allow another area in the conduction system to become the new dominant pacemaker and alter cardiac output. Although the autonomic nervous system influences cardiac function, the heart is able to function without neural control. Rhythmical myocardial contraction will continue because automaticity and rhythmicity are intrinsic to the myocardium.

Cardiac output

Cardiac performance is altered by numerous homeostatic mechanisms. Cardiac output is regulated in response to stress or disease, and changes in any of the factors that determine cardiac output will result in changes to cardiac output (see Figure 9.8). Cardiac output is the product of heart rate and stroke volume; alteration in either of these will increase or decrease cardiac output, as will alteration in preload, afterload or contractility.

Determinants of cardiac output

In the healthy individual, the most immediate change in cardiac output is seen when heart rate rises. However, in the critically ill, the ability to raise the heart rate in response to changing circumstances is limited, and a rising heart rate may have negative effects on homeostasis, due to decreased diastolic filling and increased myocardial oxygen demand.

Preload is the load imposed by the initial fibre length of the cardiac muscle before contraction (i.e. at the end of diastole). The primary determinant of preload is the amount of blood filling the ventricle during diastole and, as indicated in Figure 9.8, it is important in determining stroke volume. Preload influences the contractility of the ventricles (the strength of contraction) because of the relationship between myocardial fibre length and stretch. However, a threshold is reached when fibres become overstretched, and force of contraction and resultant stroke volume will fall.

Preload reduces as a result of large-volume loss (e.g. haemorrhage), venous dilation (e.g. due to hyperthermia or drugs), tachycardias (e.g. rapid atrial fibrillation or supraventricular tachycardias), raised intrathoracic pressures (a complication of intermittent positive pressure ventilation [IPPV]), and raised intracardiac pressures (e.g. cardiac tamponade). Some drugs such as vasodilators can cause a decrease in venous tone and a resulting decrease in preload. Preload increases with fluid overload, hypothermia or other causes of venous constriction, and ventricular failure. Body position will also affect preload, through its effect on venous return.

FIGURE 9.8 Determinants of cardiac function and oxygen delivery.[9]

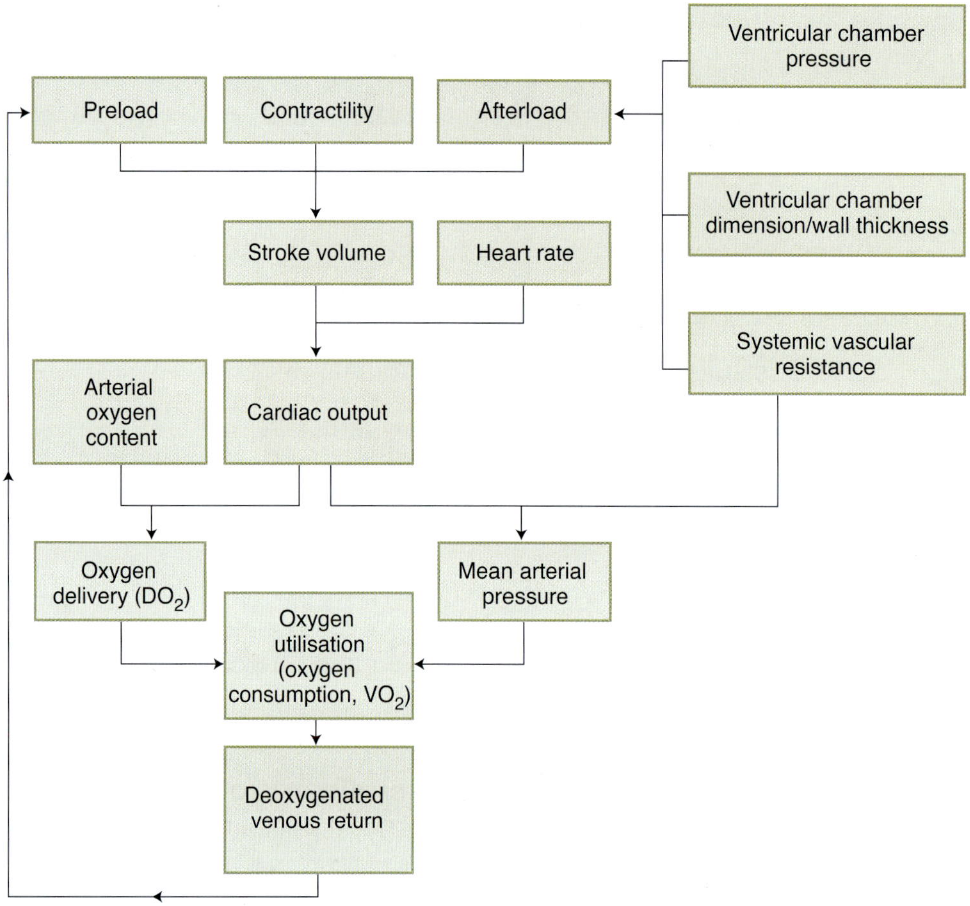

Adapted from Elliott D. Shock. In: Romanini J, Daly J, eds. Critical care nursing: Australian perspectives. Sydney: Harcourt Brace; 1994, with permission.

The volume of blood filling the ventricles is also affected by atrial contraction: a reduction in atrial contraction ability, as can occur during atrial fibrillation, will result in a reduction in ventricular volume, and a corresponding fall in stroke volume and cardiac output.

Preload of the left side of the heart, assessed at the end of filling of the left ventricle from the left atrium using the pulmonary capillary wedge pressure (PCWP), is assumed for clinical purposes to reflect left ventricular end–diastolic volume (LVEDV). Due to the non–linear relationship between volume and pressure,[10] caution must, however, be taken when interpreting these values, as rises in LVEDP may indicate pathology other than increased preload. Preload of the right side of the heart is indirectly assessed at the end of filling of the right ventricle from the right atrium through central venous pressure (CVP) monitoring.

Afterload is the load imposed on the muscle during contraction, and translates to systolic myocardial wall tension. It is measured during systole, and is inversely related to stroke volume and therefore cardiac output, but it is not synonymous with systemic vascular resistance

(SVR), as this is just one factor determining left ventricular afterload. Factors that increase afterload include:

- increased ventricular radius
- raised intracavity pressure
- increased aortic impedance
- negative intrathoracic pressure
- increased SVR.

As afterload rises, the speed of muscle fibre shortening and external work performed falls, which can cause a decrease in cardiac output in critically ill patients. Afterload of the right side of the heart is assessed during the ejection of blood from the right ventricle into the pulmonary artery. This volume is indirectly assessed by calculating pulmonary vascular resistance. Ventricular afterload can be altered to clinically affect cardiac performance. Reducing afterload will increase the stroke volume and cardiac output, while also reducing myocardial oxygen demand. However, reductions in afterload are associated with lower blood pressure, and this limits the extent to which afterload can be manipulated.

Contractility is the force of ventricular ejection, or the inherent ability of the ventricle to perform external work, independent of afterload or preload. It is difficult to measure clinically. It is increased by catecholamines, calcium, relief of ischaemia and digoxin. It is decreased by hypoxia, ischaemia and certain drugs such as thiopentone, beta-adrenergic blockers, calcium channel blockers or sedatives. Such changes affect cardiac performance, with increases in contractility causing increased stroke volume and cardiac output. Increasing contractility will increase myocardial oxygen demand, which could have a detrimental effect on patients with limited perfusion. Stroke volume is the amount of blood ejected from each ventricle with each heartbeat. For an adult, the volume is normally 50–100 mL/beat, and equal amounts are ejected from the right and left ventricle.

Cardiac output is dependent on a series of mechanical events in the cardiac cycle (see Figure 9.9). As normal

FIGURE 9.9 The cardiac cycle.

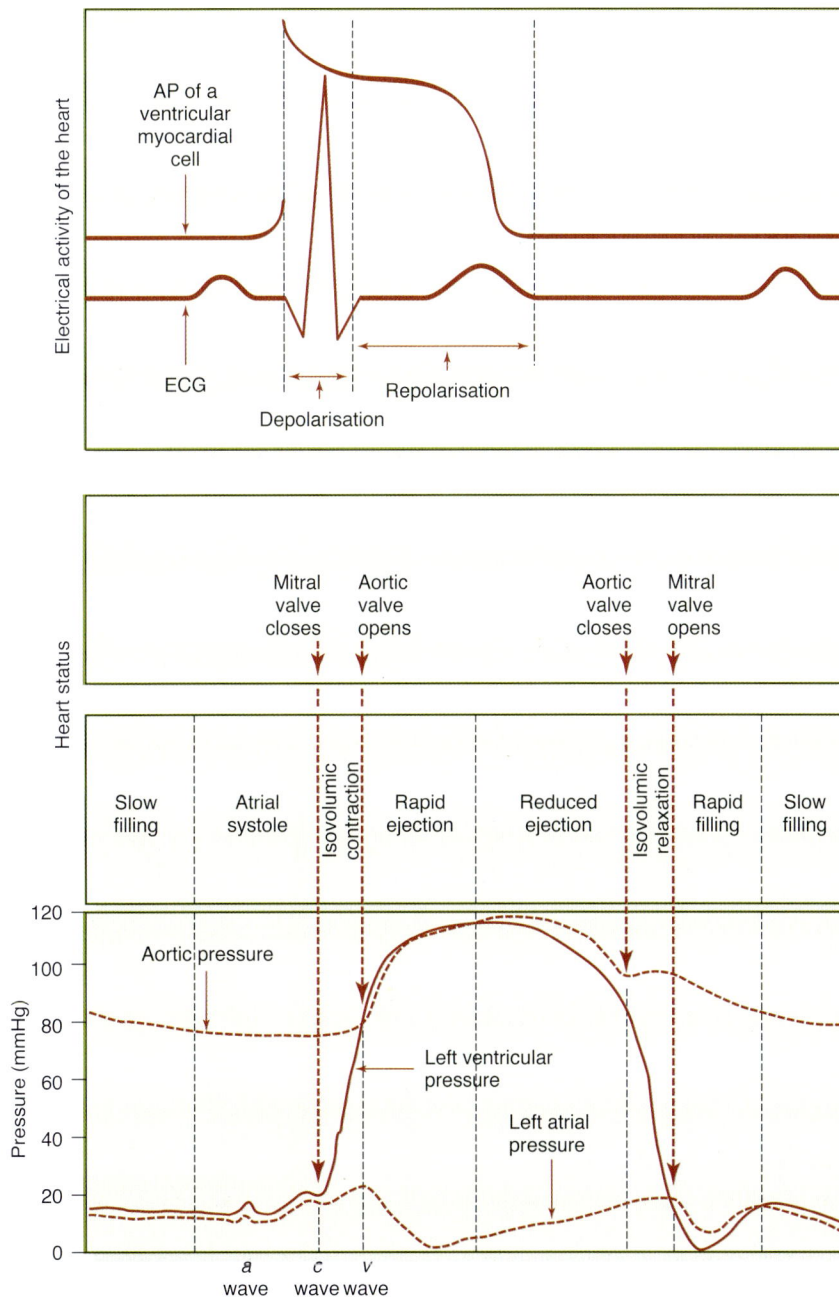

Adapted from Urden L, Stacy KL, Lough ME, eds. Thelan's critical care nursing: Diagnosis and management. 6th ed. St Louis: Mosby/Elsevier; 2010, with permission.

average heart rate is maintained at approximately 70 beats/min the average phases of the cardiac cycle are completed in less than a second (0.8 s). Electrical stimulation of myocardial contraction ensures that the four chambers of the heart contract in sequence. This allows the atria to act as primer pumps for the ventricles, while the ventricles are the major pumps that provide the impetus for blood to flow through the pulmonary and systemic vascular systems. The phases of the cardiac cycle are characterised by pressure changes within each of the heart chambers, resulting in blood flow from areas of high pressure to areas of lower pressure.

During late ventricular diastole (rest), pressures are lowest in the heart and blood returns passively to fill the atria. This flow also moves into the ventricle through the open AV valves, producing 70–80% of ventricular filling. The pulmonic and aortic valves are closed, preventing backflow from the pulmonary and systemic systems into the ventricles. Depolarisation of the atria then occurs, sometimes referred to as atrial kick, stimulating atrial contraction and completing the remaining 20–30% of ventricular filling.

During ventricular systole (contraction), the atria relax while the ventricles depolarise, resulting in ventricular contraction. Pressure rises in the ventricles, resulting in the AV valves closing. When this occurs, all four cardiac valves are closed, blood volume is constant and contraction occurs (isovolumetric contraction). When the pressure in the ventricles exceeds the pressure in the major vessels the semilunar valves open. This occurs when pressure in the left ventricle reaches approximately 80 mmHg and in the right ventricle approximately 27–30 mmHg. During the peak ejection phase, pressure in the left ventricle and aorta reaches approximately 120 mmHg and in the right ventricle and pulmonary artery approximately 25–28 mmHg.

During early ventricular diastole, the ventricles repolarise and ventricular relaxation occurs. The pressure in the ventricles falls until the pressures in the aorta and pulmonary artery are higher and blood pushes back against the semilunar valves. Shutting of these valves prevents backflow into the ventricles, and pressure in the ventricles declines further. During ventricular contraction, the atria have been filling passively, so the pressure in the atria rises to higher than that in the ventricles and the AV valves open, allowing blood flow to the ventricles. Any rise in heart rate will shorten the resting period, which may impair filling time and coronary artery flow as these arteries fill during diastole.[1]

Regulation of cardiac output

The heart is a very effective pump and is able to adapt to meet the metabolic needs of the body. The activities of the heart are regulated by two responsive systems: intrinsic regulation of contraction and the autonomic nervous system.

Intrinsic regulation of contraction responds to the rate of blood flow into the chambers. Blood flow into the heart depends on venous return from systemic and pulmonic veins and varies according to tissue metabolism, total blood volume and vasodilation. Venous return contributes to end-diastolic volume (preload) and pressure, which are both directly related to the force of contraction in the next ventricular systole. The intrinsic capacity of the heart to respond to changes in end-diastolic pressure can be represented by a number of length–tension curves and the Frank-Starling mechanism (see Figure 9.10). According to this mechanism, within limits, the greater the stretch of the cardiac muscle fibre before contraction, the greater the strength of contraction. The ability to increase strength of contraction in response to increased stretch exists because there is an optimal range of cross-bridges that can be created between actin and myosin in the myocyte. Under this range, when venous return is poor, fewer cross-bridges can be created. Above this range, when heart failure is present, the cross-bridges can become partially disengaged, contraction is poor and higher filling pressures are needed to achieve adequate contractile force.

Ventricular contraction is also intrinsically influenced by the size of the ventricle and the thickness of the ventricle wall. This mechanism is described by Laplace's law, which states that the amount of tension generated in the wall of the ventricle required to produce intraventricular pressure depends on the size (radius and wall thickness) of the ventricle.[1] As a result, in heart failure, when ventricular thinning and dilation are present, more tension or contractile force is required to create intraventricular pressure and therefore cardiac output.

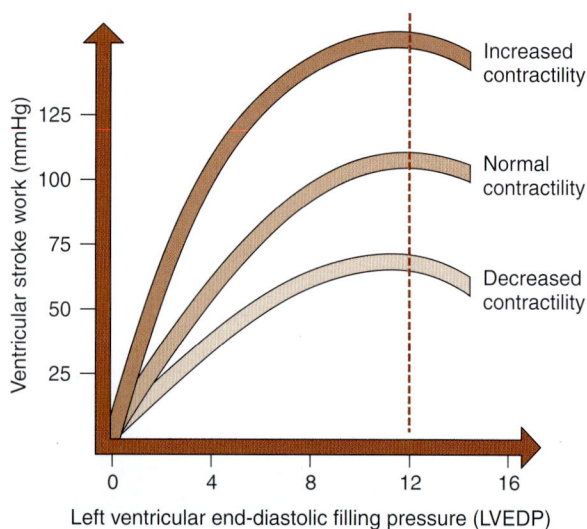

FIGURE 9.10 The Frank-Starling curve. As left ventricular end-diastolic pressure increases, so does ventricular stroke work.

Adapted from Urden L, Stacy KL, Lough ME, eds. Thelan's critical care nursing: Diagnosis and management. 6th ed. St Louis: Mosby/Elsevier; 2010, with permission.

The heart's ability to pump effectively is also influenced by the pressure that it is required to generate above end-diastolic pressure to eject blood during systole. This additional pressure is usually determined by how much resistance is present in the pulmonary artery and aorta, and is in turn influenced by the peripheral vasculature. This systemic vascular resistance, known and measured as afterload, causes resistance to flow in relation to the left ventricle and is influenced by vascular tone and disease.

Autonomic nervous system control and regulation of heart rate

Although the pacemaker cells of the heart are capable of intrinsic rhythm generation (automaticity), inputs from the autonomic nervous system regulate heart rate changes in accordance with body needs by stimulating or depressing these pacemaker cells. Cardiac innervation includes sympathetic fibres from branches of T1–T5 and parasympathetic input via the vagus nerve.[11] The heart rate at any moment is a product of the respective inputs of sympathetic stimuli (which accelerate) and parasympathetic stimuli (which depress) on heart rate. Rises in heart rate can thus be achieved by an increase in sympathetic tone or by a reduction in parasympathetic tone (vagal inhibition). Conversely, slowing of the heart rate can be achieved by decreasing sympathetic or increasing parasympathetic activity.[4]

Hormonal, biochemical and pharmacological inputs also exert heart rate influences by their effects on autonomic neural receptors or directly on pacemaker cells. In mimicking the effects of direct nervous inputs, these influences may be described as sympathomimetic or parasympathomimetic. Sympathomimetic stimulation (e.g. through the use of isoprenaline) achieves the same cardiac end points as direct sympathetic activity, increasing the heart rate, while sympathetic antagonism (e.g. beta-blockade therapy) slows the heart through receptor inhibition. By contrast, parasympathomimetic agonist activity slows the heart rate, while parasympathetic antagonism (e.g. via administration of atropine sulfate) raises the heart rate by causing parasympathetic receptor blockade.[4]

The vascular system

The vascular system is specialised according to the different tissues it supplies, but the general functions and characteristics are similar. All vessels in the circulatory system are lined by endothelium, including the heart. The endothelium creates a smooth surface, which reduces friction and also secretes substances that promote contraction and relaxation of the vascular smooth muscle. Arteries function to transport blood under high pressure and are characterised by strong elastic walls that allow stretch during systole and high flow. During diastole, the artery walls recoil so that an adequate perfusion pressure is maintained. Arterioles are the final small branches of the arterial system prior to capillaries, and have strong muscular walls that can contract (vasoconstrict) to the point of closure and relax (vasodilate) to change the artery lumen rapidly in response to tissue needs. The lumen created by the arterioles is the most important source of resistance to blood flow in the systemic circulation (just under 50%).

Capillaries function to allow exchange of fluid, nutrients, electrolytes, hormones and other substances through highly permeable walls between the blood plasma and interstitial fluid (see Figure 9.11). Just before the capillary beds are precapillary sphincters, bands of smooth muscle that adjust flow in the capillaries. Venules collect blood from the capillaries to veins. Excess tissue fluid is collected by the lymphatic system. Lymphatic veins have a similar structure to the cardiovascular system veins described below, with lymph returning to this system at the right side of the heart.

Veins collect and transport blood back to the heart at low pressure and serve as a reservoir for blood. Therefore, veins are numerous and have thinner, less muscular walls, which can dilate to store extra blood (up to 64% of total blood volume at any time). Some veins, particularly in the lower limbs, contain valves to prevent backflow and ensure one-way flow to the heart. Venous return is promoted during standing and moving by the muscles of the legs compressing the deep veins, promoting blood flow towards the heart.[1,4]

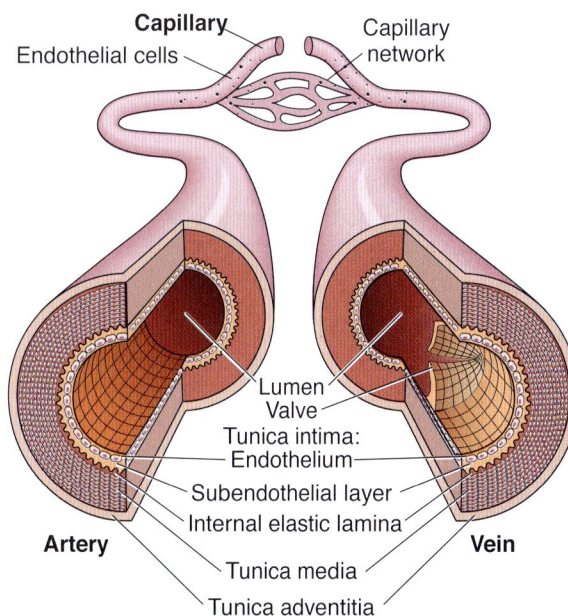

FIGURE 9.11 The structure of arteries, veins and capillaries.

Adapted from Novak B, Filer L, Latchett R. The applied anatomy and physiology of the cardiovascular system. In: Hatchett R, Thompson D, eds. Cardiac nursing: a comprehensive guide. Philadelphia: Churchill Livingstone Elsevier; 2002, with permission.

Blood pressure

Blood flow is maintained by pulsatile ejection of blood from the heart and pressure differences between the blood vessels. Traditionally, blood pressure is measured from the arteries in the general circulation at the maximum value during systole and the minimum value occurring during diastole. The cardiovascular system must supply blood according to varying demands and in a range of circumstances, with at least a minimal blood flow to be maintained to all organs. At a local level this is achieved by autoregulation of individual arteries, such as the coronary arteries, in response to the metabolic needs of the specific tissue or organ. The exact mechanism is unknown, but it has been proposed that increased vascular muscle stretch and/or metabolites and decreased oxygen levels are detected and cells release substances such as adenosine.[4] These substances result in rapid vasodilation and increased perfusion. The vascular endothelium actively secretes prostacyclin and endothelial-derived relaxing factor (nitric oxide), both vasoactive agents.

There are three main regulatory mechanisms of blood pressure control: (a) short-term autonomic control, (b) medium-term hormonal control and (c) long-term renal system control.

Autonomic control

The cardiovascular control centre connects with the hypothalamus to control temperature, the cerebral cortex and the autonomic system to control cardiac activity and peripheral vascular tone. Information about blood pressure and resistance is sensed by neural receptors (baroreceptors) in the aortic arch and the carotid sinuses, which detect changes in blood supply to the body and the brain. Impulses from these receptors initiate a blood-pressure regulating reflex in the cardiovascular centre, which activates the parasympathetic system and sympathetic system to alter cardiac activity and dilation or constriction of arterioles and veins to lower or raise blood pressure. The cardiovascular system also maintains a constant resting tone of intermediate tension in the arteries.

Hormonal control

Changes in blood pressure are also detected by the adrenal medulla, which secretes catecholamines as cardiac output declines. The two main catecholamines, adrenaline (epinephrine) and noradrenaline (norepinephrine), mimic the action of the sympathetic system by binding to and stimulating adrenergic receptors. Adrenergic receptors are located in smooth muscle cells of vascular beds including the peripheral veins and arterioles supplying the skin, kidneys, skeletal muscles and mucosa.

The main action of adrenaline occurs by binding to the beta-1 adrenoreceptors (located mainly in the heart but also found in platelets and the non-sphincter part of the gastrointestinal tract), causing an increase in the rate and contraction of the heart, aggregation of platelets and relaxation of the non-sphincter part of the gastrointestinal tract. Adrenaline also binds to beta-2 receptors, located on blood vessels, the bronchi, gastrointestinal tract, skeletal muscle, liver and mast cells (inflammatory cells). Activation results in vasodilatation of small coronary arteries, bronchodilation, relaxation of the gastrointestinal tract, glycogenolysis (breakdown of glycogen to glucose) in the liver, tremor in skeletal muscle and inhibition of histamine (an inflammatory amine responsible for increased permeability of capillaries).

Noradrenaline binds to both beta and alpha receptors. Alpha-1 and alpha-2 adrenoreceptors are found in the central and peripheral nervous system and are located on vascular and non-vascular smooth muscle. Alpha-1 adrenergic stimulation causes vasoconstriction and is the main mechanism of the vasopressor action of noradrenaline. Presynaptic alpha-2 receptors inhibit the release of noradrenaline and thus serve as an important receptor in the negative feedback control of noradrenaline release. Postsynaptic alpha-2 receptors are located on liver cells, platelets and the smooth muscle of blood vessels and, when activated, cause platelet aggregation and blood vessel constriction. Noradrenaline results in very little beta-2 activity. Clinically, the positive inotropic and chronotropic effects of noradrenaline, from beta-1 simulation, are counterbalanced by the increased afterload from elevated systemic vascular resistance (alpha-1 adrenergic agonist effect).

Renal control

Renal control of blood pressure in the long term occurs via control of blood volume. Generally, as blood pressure or volume rises, the kidneys produce more urine; conversely, as blood pressure or volume falls, the kidneys produce less urine.

In addition to longer term fluid regulation, during acute illness or time of acute hypotension, the renin–angiotensin–aldosterone system (RAAS) plays an important role in maintaining blood pressure. This negative feedback system both reabsorbs intravascular fluid and increases peripheral resistance, in an effort to increase blood pressure. Further details on the RAAS system can be found in Chapter 18.

Assessment

It is essential that the critical care nurse conducts a comprehensive cardiac assessment on a critically ill patient. The nursing assessment aims to define patient cardiovascular status as well as inform implementation of an appropriate clinical management plan. The focus of the cardiovascular assessment varies according to the setting, clinical presentation and treatments commenced, if any. However, the main priority should be to determine whether the patient is haemodynamically stable or requiring initiation or adjustment of supportive treatments.

A thorough cardiac assessment requires the critical care nurse to be competent in a wide range of interpersonal, observational and technical skills. A cardiac assessment should be performed as part of a comprehensive patient assessment and should consider the following elements.

It is important to create a health history, if not already obtained. This history should aim to elicit a description of the present illness and chief complaint. A useful guide in taking a specific cardiac history is to use direct questions to seek information regarding symptom onset, course, duration, location and precipitating and alleviating factors. Some common cardiovascular disease-related symptoms to be observed for include: chest discomfort or pain, palpitations, syncope, generalised fatigue, dyspnoea, cough, weight gain or dependent oedema. Chest pain, discomfort or tightness should be initially considered indicative of cardiac ischaemia until proven otherwise by further examination and diagnostic assessment. Additionally, a health history should be inclusive of known cardiovascular risk factors, such as hyperlipidaemia or hypertension, and any medications the patient may be taking including over-the-counter medications.

Prior to inspecting or palpating the patient, the nurse should observe the patient's general appearance noting whether the patient is restless, able to lie flat, in pain or distress, is pale or has decreased level of consciousness. Patients with compromised cardiac output will likely have decreased cerebral perfusion and may have mental confusion, memory loss or slowed verbal responses. Additionally, assessment of any pain should be noted.

Specific physical assessment in relation to cardiovascular function should be inclusive of:

- vital signs
- respiratory assessment for signs of pulmonary oedema (shortness of breath or basal crepitations)
- assessment of neck vein distension for signs of right-sided venous congestion
- assessment for signs of peripheral oedema
- capillary refill time with >3 s return indicative of sluggish capillary return
- 12-lead ECG for signs of ischaemia or cardiac pathology
- appearance and temperature of the skin for signs of peripheral constriction or dehydration
- core body temperature measurement
- urine output with <0.5 mL/kg/h a potential indicator of decreased renal perfusion.[12]

Assessment of pulse

In the critical care environment, the heart rate can be observed from a cardiac monitor; however, this does not give qualitative information about the arterial pulse. Routinely performed as part of most patient assessments, information gathered from pulse assessment can give useful cues and direct further assessments. Although the radial pulse is distant from the central arteries, it is useful for gathering information on rate, rhythm and strength. Heart rate below 60 beats per minute is defined as 'bradycardia' (*brady* is Greek for slow, and *kardia* means heart). A heart rate greater than 100 beats per minute is called 'tachycardia' (*tachy* is Greek meaning swift). An important aspect of pulse assessment involves assessment for regularity. Detection of an irregular pulse should trigger further investigation and prompt ECG assessment for atrial fibrillation, a condition in which atrial contraction becomes lost due to chaotic electrical activity with variable ventricular response. In addition to rate and rhythm, assessment of pulse, especially if palpated in the carotid or femoral artery, can reveal a bounding pulse that may be indicative of hyperdynamic state or aortic regurgitation. An alternating strong and weak pulse, known as *pulsus alternans*, may be observed in advanced heart failure.

Auscultation of heart sounds

Auscultation of the heart involves listening to heart sounds over the pericardial area using a stethoscope. While challenging to achieve competence in, cardiac auscultation is an important part of cardiac physical examination and relies on a sound understanding of cardiac anatomy, cardiac cycle and physiologically associated sounds. For accurate auscultation, experience in assessment of normal sounds is critical and can only be obtained through constant practice. When auscultating heart sounds, normally two sounds are readily audible and they are known as the first (S1) and second (S2) sounds. A useful technique when listening to heart sounds is to feel the carotid pulse at the same time as auscultation, which will help identify the heart sound that corresponds with ventricular systole.

> **Practice tip**
>
> When learning to interpret heart sounds, feel the carotid pulse at the same time as auscultation of the heart, which will help identify the heart sound that corresponds with ventricular systole (S1 will be heard simultaneously with the pulse).

The first heart sound (S1) occurs at the beginning of ventricular systole, following closure of the intracardiac valves (mitral and tricuspid valves). This heart sound is best heard with the diaphragm of the stethoscope and loudest directly over the corresponding valves (4th intercostal space [ICS] left of the sternum for the tricuspid and 5th ICS left of the mid-clavicular line for the mitral valve). Following closure of these two valves, ventricular contraction and ejection occurs and a carotid pulse may be palpated at the same time that S1 is audible.

The second heart sound (S2) occurs at the beginning of diastole, following closure of the aortic and pulmonary valves and can be best heard over these valves (2nd ICS to the right and left of the sternum, respectively). It is important to remember that both S1 and S2 result from events occurring in *both* left and right sides of the heart. As left-sided heart sounds are normally loudest and occur slightly before right-sided events, careful listening during inspiration and expiration may result in left and right events being heard separately. This is known as physiological splitting of heart sounds, a normal physiological event.

TABLE 9.1

Guide to placement of the stethoscope when listening to heart sounds

STETHOSCOPE PLACEMENT		AUDITABLE REGION OF HEART
2nd intercostal space	right of sternum	Aortic valve
2nd intercostal space	left of sternum	Pulmonary valve
4th intercostal space	left side of sternum	Tricuspid valve
5th intercostal space	Mid-clavicular line	Mitral valve

A guide to placement of the stethoscope when listening to heart sounds is presented in Table 9.1.

In assessment of the critically ill patient extra heart sounds, labelled S3 and S4, may be heard during times of extra ventricular filling or fluid overload. Often referred to as 'gallops', these extra heart sounds are accentuated during episodes of tachycardia. S3, ventricular gallop, occurs during diastole in the presence of fluid overload. Considered physiological in children or young people, due to rapid diastolic filling, S3 may be considered pathological when due to reduced ventricular compliance and associated increased atrial pressures. As S3 occurs early in diastole, it will be heard and associated more closely with S2.

S4 is a late diastolic sound and may be heard shortly before S1. S4 occurs when ventricular compliance is reduced secondary to aortic or pulmonary stenosis, mitral regurgitation, systemic hypertension, advanced age or ischaemic heart disease. In patients with severe ventricular dysfunction, both S3 and S4 may be audible although, when coupled with tachycardia, these may be difficult to differentiate and will require specialist assessment.

The critical care nurse auscultating the heart should also listen for a potential pericardial rub. This 'rubbing' or 'scratching' sound is secondary to pericardial inflammation and/or fluid accumulation in the pericardial space. To differentiate pericardial rub from pulmonary rub, if possible the patient should be instructed to hold their breath for a short duration as pericardial rub will continue to be audible in the absence of breathing, heard over the 3rd ICS to the left of the mid sternum. Detection of pericardial rub warrants further investigation by ultrasound.

Practice tip 2

To differentiate pericardial rub from pulmonary rub, ask the patient to hold their breath for a short duration, as pericardial rub will continue to be audible in the absence of breathing and pleural rub will not be audible while the patient is not breathing.

In addition to pericardial rub, murmurs may also be audible. Murmurs are generally classified and characterised by location with the most common murmurs associated with the mitral or aortic valves, due to either stenosis or regurgitation at these locations. Murmurs are best thought of as turbulent flow or vibrations associated with the corresponding valve and can be of variable pitch. Specialist cardiac referral is indicated upon detection of cardiac murmurs to differentiate pathological murmurs, as seen during valvular dysfunction or myocardial infarction, from innocent systolic 'high flow' murmurs detected in children or adolescents as a result of vigorous ventricular contraction. Murmurs may be classified using the Levine scale,[12] shown in Table 9.2.

Continuous cardiac monitoring

In the case of the critically ill patient, there are two main forms of cardiac monitoring, both of which are used to generate essential data: continuous cardiac monitoring and the 12-lead ECG. Internationally, a minimum standard for an ICU requires availability of facilities for cardiovascular monitoring.[13,14] Continuous cardiac monitoring allows for rapid assessment and constant evaluation with, when required, the instantaneous production of paper recordings for more detailed assessment or documentation into patient records. In addition, practice standards for electrocardiographic monitoring in hospital settings have been established.[15]

It is now common practice for five leads to be used for continuous cardiac monitoring, as this allows

TABLE 9.2

Classification of heart murmurs using the Levine scale

Grade 1	Low intensity and difficult to hear
Grade 2	Low intensity, but audible with a stethoscope but no palpable thrill
Grade 3	Medium intensity and easily heard with a stethoscope
Grade 4	Loud and audible and with palpable thrill
Grade 5	Very loud but cannot be heard outside the praecordium and with palpable thrill
Grade 6	Audible with the stethoscope away from the chest

Adapted from Johnson K, Rawlings-Anderson K. Oxford handbook of cardiac nursing. 2nd ed. New York: Oxford University Press; 2014, with permission.

a choice of seven views. The five electrodes are placed as follows:

- right and left arm electrodes: placed on each shoulder
- right and left leg electrodes: placed on the hips or level with the lowest ribs on the chest
- V-lead views can be monitored: for V1 place the electrode at the 4th ICS, right of the sternum; for V6 place the electrode at the 5th ICS, left mid-axillary line.

The monitoring lead of choice is determined by the patient's clinical situation. Generally, two views are better than one. V1 lead is best to view ventricular activity and differentiate right and left bundle branch blocks; therefore, one of the channels on the bedside monitor should display a V lead, preferably V1, and the other display lead II or III for optimal detection of arrhythmias. When the primary purpose of monitoring is to detect ischaemic changes, leads III and V3 usually present the optimal combination.[15]

The skin must be carefully prepared before electrodes are attached, as contact is required with the body surface and poor contact will lead to inaccurate or unreadable recordings, causing interference or noise. Patients who are sweaty need particular attention, and it may be necessary to shave the areas where the electrodes are to be placed in very hairy people.

12-lead ECG

The Dutch physiologist Einthoven was one of the first to represent heart electrical conduction as two charged electrodes, one positive and one negative.[16] The body can be likened to a triangle, with the heart at its centre, and this has been called Einthoven's triangle. Cardiac electrical activity can be captured by placing electrodes on both arms and on the left leg. When these electrodes are connected to a common terminal with an indifferent electrode that remains near zero, an electrical potential is obtained. Depolarisation moving towards an active electrode produces positive deflection.

The 12-lead ECG consists of six limb leads and six chest leads. The limb leads examine electrical activity along a vertical plane. The standard bipolar limb leads (I, II, III) record differences in potential between the two limbs by using two limb electrodes as positive and negative poles (see Figure 9.12):[17] leads I, II, and III all produce positive deflections on the ECG because the electrical current flows from left to the right and from upwards to downwards. Placement should be:

- I = negative electrode in right arm and positive electrode in left arm
- II = negative electrode in right arm and positive electrode in left leg
- III = negative electrode in left arm and positive electrodes in left leg.

The three unipolar limb leads (aVR, aVL, aVF) record activity of the heart's frontal plane. Each of these unipolar leads has only one positive electrode (the limb electrode

FIGURE 9.12 Einthoven's triangle formed by standard limb leads.

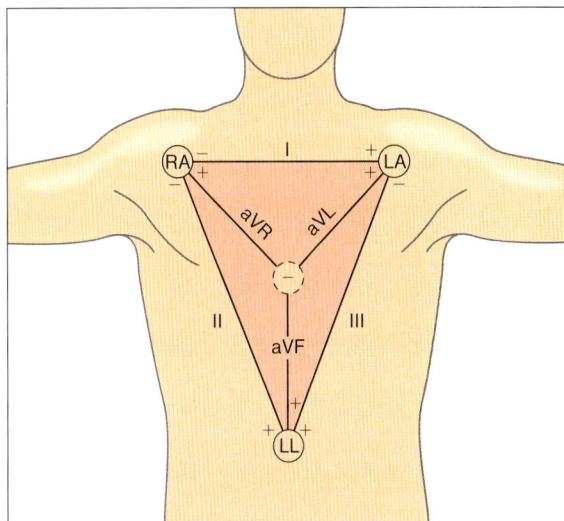

Adapted from Urden L, Stacy KL, Lough ME, eds. Thelan's critical care nursing: Diagnosis and management. 6th ed. St Louis: Mosby/Elsevier; 2010, with permission.

such as left arm, right arm or left leg), with the centre of Einthoven's triangle acting as the negative electrode. The waveforms of these leads are usually very small; therefore, they are augmented by the ECG machine to increase the size of the potentials on the ECG strip.[17] These three leads view the heart at different angles:

- Lead aVR produces a negative reflection because the electrical activity moves away from the lead. Lead aVR does not provide a specific view of the heart.
- Lead aVL produces a positive deflection because the electrical activity moves towards the lead. Lead aVL views the electrical activity from the lateral wall.
- Lead aVF also produces a positive deflection on the ECG because the electrical activity flows toward this lead. It views the electrical activity from the inferior wall.

The six unipolar chest leads (precordial leads) are designated V1–6 and examine electrical activity along a horizontal plane from the right ventricle, septum, left ventricle and the left atrium. They are positioned in the following way (see Figure 9.13):

- V1 = 4th ICS, to the right of the patient's sternum
- V2 = 4th ICS, to the left of the patient's sternum
- V3 = equidistant between V2 and V4
- V4 = 5th ICS on the mid-clavicular line
- V5 = 5th ICS, anterior axillary line
- V6 = 5th ICS on the mid-axilla line

Amplitude (voltage) in the ECG is measured by a series of horizontal lines on the ECG trace (see Figure 9.14).

Lines are 1 mm apart and represent increments of 0.1 mV. Amplitude reflects the wave's electrical force and has no relation to the muscle strength of ventricular contraction.[8]

FIGURE 9.13   Position of chest leads.

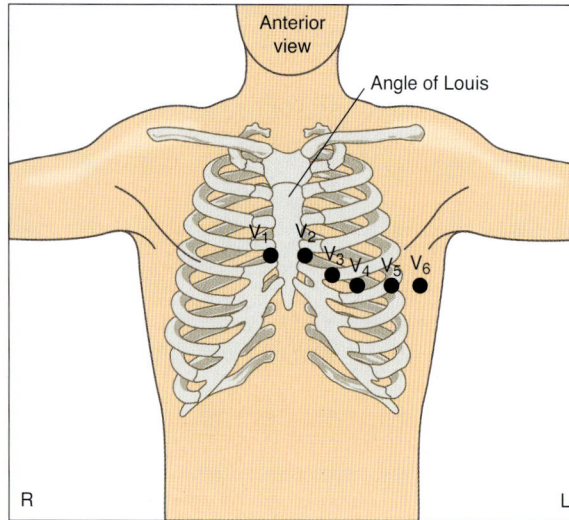

Anterior view

Angle of Louis

V₁ V₂ V₃ V₄ V₅ V₆

R   L

Adapted from Urden L, Stacy KL, Lough ME, eds. Thelan's critical care nursing: Diagnosis and management. 6th ed. St Louis: Mosby/Elsevier; 2010, with permission.

Duration of activity within the ECG is measured by a series of vertical lines also 1 mm apart (see Figure 9.14). The time interval between each line is 0.04 s. Every 5th line is printed in bold, producing large squares. Each represents 0.5 mV (vertically) and 0.2 s (horizontally).

Key components of the ECG

Key components of the cardiac electrical activity are termed PQRST (see Figure 9.15):

- The P wave represents electrical activity caused by spread of impulses from the SA node across the atria and appears upright in lead II. Inverted P waves indicate atrial depolarisation from a site other than the SA node. Normal P wave duration is considered to be less than 0.12 s.

- The P–R interval reflects the total time taken for the atrial impulse to travel through the atria and AV node. It is measured from the start of the P wave to the beginning of the QRS complex, but is lengthened by AV block or some drugs. Normal P–R interval is 0.12–0.2 s.

- The QRS complex is measured from the start of the Q wave to the end of the S wave and represents the time taken for ventricular depolarisation. Normal QRS duration is 0.08–0.12 s. Anything longer than 0.12 s is abnormal and may indicate conduction disorders such as bundle branch block. The deflections

FIGURE 9.14   ECG graph paper.

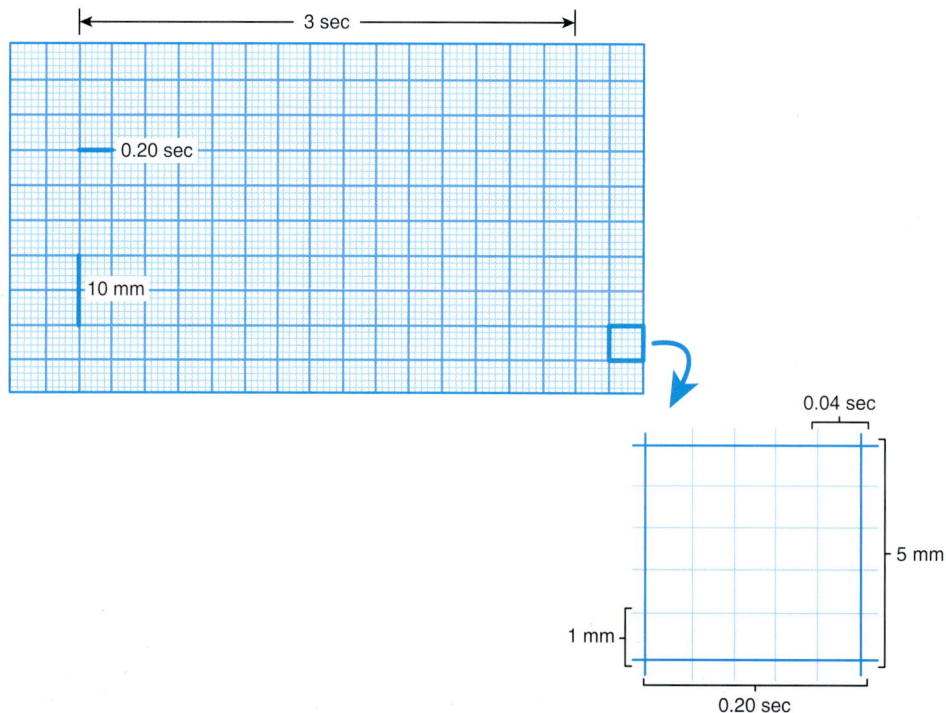

3 sec

0.20 sec

10 mm

0.04 sec

5 mm

1 mm

0.20 sec

Adapted from Urden L, Stacy KL, Lough ME, eds. Thelan's critical care nursing: Diagnosis and management. 6th ed. St Louis: Mosby/Elsevier; 2010, with permission.

seen in relation to this complex will vary in size, depending on the lead being viewed. However, small QRS complexes occur when the heart is insulated, as in the presence of pericardial effusion. Conversely, an exaggerated QRS complex is suggestive of ventricular hypertrophy. Normal, non-pathological Q waves are often seen in leads I, aVL, V5, V6 from septal depolarisation, which are less than 25% of the R height and 0.04 s. A 'pathological' Q wave (>0.04 s plus >25% of R wave height) may indicate a previous myocardial infarction; however, not every myocardial infarction will result in a pathological Q wave[18] and some abnormal Q waves, in combination with other ECG changes and patient symptoms, may indicate a current myocardial infarction.[19] Pathological Q waves could also be seen in non-ischaemic conditions such as Wolff–Parkinson–White syndrome (WPW).[20]

- The Q–T interval is the time taken from ventricular stimulation to recovery. It is measured from the beginning of the QRS to the end of the T wave. Normally, this ranges from 0.35 to 0.45 s, but shortens as heart rate increases. It should be less than 50% of the preceding cycle length.

- The T wave reflects repolarisation of the ventricles. A peaked T wave indicates hyperkalaemia, myocardial infarction (MI) or ischaemia,[21] while a flattened T wave usually indicates hypokalaemia. An inverted T wave occurs following an MI, or ventricular hypertrophy. A normal T wave is 0.16 s. The height of the T wave should be less than 5 mm in all limb leads, and less than 10 mm in the precordial leads.[17]

- The ST segment is measured from the J point (junction of the S wave and ST segment) to the start of the T wave. It is usually isoelectric in nature, and elevation or depression indicates some abnormality in the onset of recovery of the ventricular muscle, usually due to myocardial injury.

- The U wave is a small positive wave sometimes seen following the T wave. Its cause is still unknown but it is exaggerated in hypokalaemia. Inverted U waves may be seen and are often associated with coronary heart disease (CHD), and these may appear transiently during exercise testing.[18]

Practice tip

The 6-second measurement for heart rate calculation is particularly useful when the patient's heart rate is irregular. Count the R waves on a 6-s strip and multiply by 10 to calculate the rate for 1 minute.

ECG interpretation

Interpretation of a 12-lead ECG is an experiential skill, requiring consistent exposure and practice. Some steps to aid interpretation are noted below.

- Calculate heart rate
  - There are many ways to calculate the heart rate. One way is to count the R waves on a 6-s strip and multiply by 10 to calculate the rate (the top of the ECG paper is usually marked at 3-s intervals).
  - Use an ECG ruler if one is available.

FIGURE 9.15 Normal ECG.

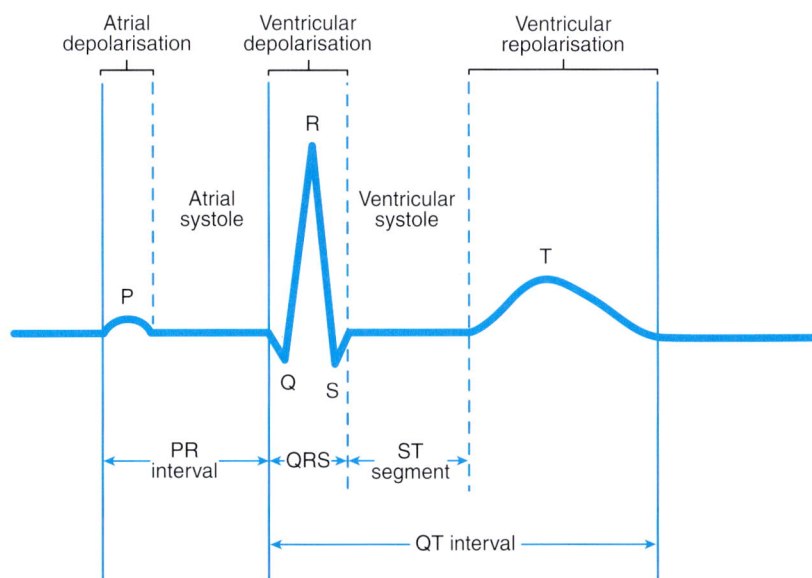

Adapted from Urden L, Stacy KL, Lough ME, eds. Thelan's critical care nursing: Diagnosis and management. 6th ed. St Louis: Mosby/Elsevier; 2010, with permission.

- Check R–R intervals (rhythm)
  - Are the rhythms regular?
  - To assess regularity, mark the duration of two neighbouring R waves (R–R interval) on a plain piece of paper and move this paper to check other R–R intervals on the ECG strip. R–R intervals should be uniform in a normal ECG, which means the patient has a regular ECG rhythm.
- Locate P waves (check atrial activity)
  - Observe for the presence or absence of P waves.
  - Check regularity and shape.
  - Is the P wave positive?
  - The relationship between P waves and QRS complexes: is there a P wave preceding every QRS complex?
  - What is the duration of the P wave?
- Measure P–R interval (check AV node activity)
  - What is the duration of the P–R interval?
- Measure QRS duration (check ventricular activity)
  - Is the ventricular electrical activity normal?
  - Is the QRS complex too wide or narrow?
  - Check the presence of a Q wave. If present, is it normal or pathological?
- Note other clues
  - Observe whether the isoelectric line is present between the S and T waves.
  - Examine the T wave to see whether it is positive, negative or flat: is it less than 0.16 s?
  - Examine the duration of the Q–T interval: is it too long?
  - Observe for any extra complexes and note their rate and shape, and whether they have the same or different morphology.

Practice tip

The presence of Q waves does not always indicate past myocardial infarction. Q waves may be secondary to:

- physiological and positional effects
- myocardial injury or replacement
- ventricular enlargement
- altered ventricular conduction.

Other patient clinical information is needed to interpret the significance of Q waves. ECG interpretation should always take a patient's clinical information (patient symptoms, complaints, other haemodynamic information) into account.

Practice tip

Think of the leads I, II, III, aVR, aVL, aVF, V1–V6 as the 'eyes' that are looking at the heart's electrical activity from different angles and view the heart's different areas.

Haemodynamic monitoring

The dynamic movement of the blood in the cardiovascular system is referred to as haemodynamics. Haemodynamic monitoring is performed to provide the clinician with a greater understanding of the pathophysiology of the problem being treated than would be possible with clinical assessment alone. Knowledge of the evidence that underpins the technology and the processes for interpretation is therefore essential to facilitate optimal usage and evidence-based decisions.[22]

This section explores the principles related to haemodynamic monitoring and the different types of monitoring available, and introduces the most recent and appropriate evidence related to haemodynamic monitoring. The reasons for haemodynamic monitoring are generally threefold:

1 to establish a precise health-related diagnosis
2 to determine appropriate therapy
3 to monitor the response to that therapy.

Haemodynamic monitoring can be non-invasive or invasive, and may be required on a continuous or intermittent basis depending on the needs of the patient.[23] In both cases, signals are processed from a variety of physiological variables, and these are then clinically interpreted within the individual patient's context.[22]

Non-invasive monitoring does not require any device to be inserted into the body and therefore does not breach the skin. Directly measured non-invasive variables include body temperature, heart rate, blood pressure, respiratory rate and urine output, while other processed forms can be generated by the ECG, arterial and venous Dopplers, transcutaneous pulse oximetry (using an external probe on a digit such as the finger or on the ear) and expired carbon monoxide monitors.

Invasive monitoring requires the vascular system to be cannulated and pressure or flow within the circulation interpreted. Invasive haemodynamic monitoring technology includes:

- systemic arterial pressure monitoring
- central venous pressure
- pulmonary artery pressure
- cardiac output.

Invasive monitoring has also facilitated greater use of blood component analyses, such as arterial and venous blood gases.

The invasive nature of this monitoring allows the pressures that are sensed at the distal ends of the catheters to be transduced, and to continuously display and monitor the corresponding waveforms. The extent of monitoring should reflect how much information is required to optimise the patient's condition, and how precisely the data are to be recorded. As Muller argues, a great deal of information is generated by this form of monitoring, and the clinical value of this is questionable.[23] It is important to note that these invasive monitoring strategies are not substitutes for careful examination and do not replace the clinicians' clinical decision making. The accuracy of the values obtained and the critical care professionals' ability to interpret the data and choose an appropriate intervention directly affect the patient's condition and outcome.[23]

Principles of haemodynamic monitoring

A number of key principles need to be understood in relation to invasive haemodynamic monitoring of critically ill patients. These include haemodynamic accuracy, the ability to trend data and the maintenance of minimum standards. These are reviewed below.

Haemodynamic accuracy

Accuracy of the value obtained from haemodynamic monitoring is essential as this information is used to guide patient care.[23] Electronic equipment for this purpose has four components (see Figure 9.16):

1 an invasive catheter attached to high-pressure tubing
2 a transducer to detect physiological activity
3 a flush system
4 a recording device, incorporating an amplifier to increase the size of the signal, to display information.

FIGURE 9.16 Haemodynamic monitoring system.

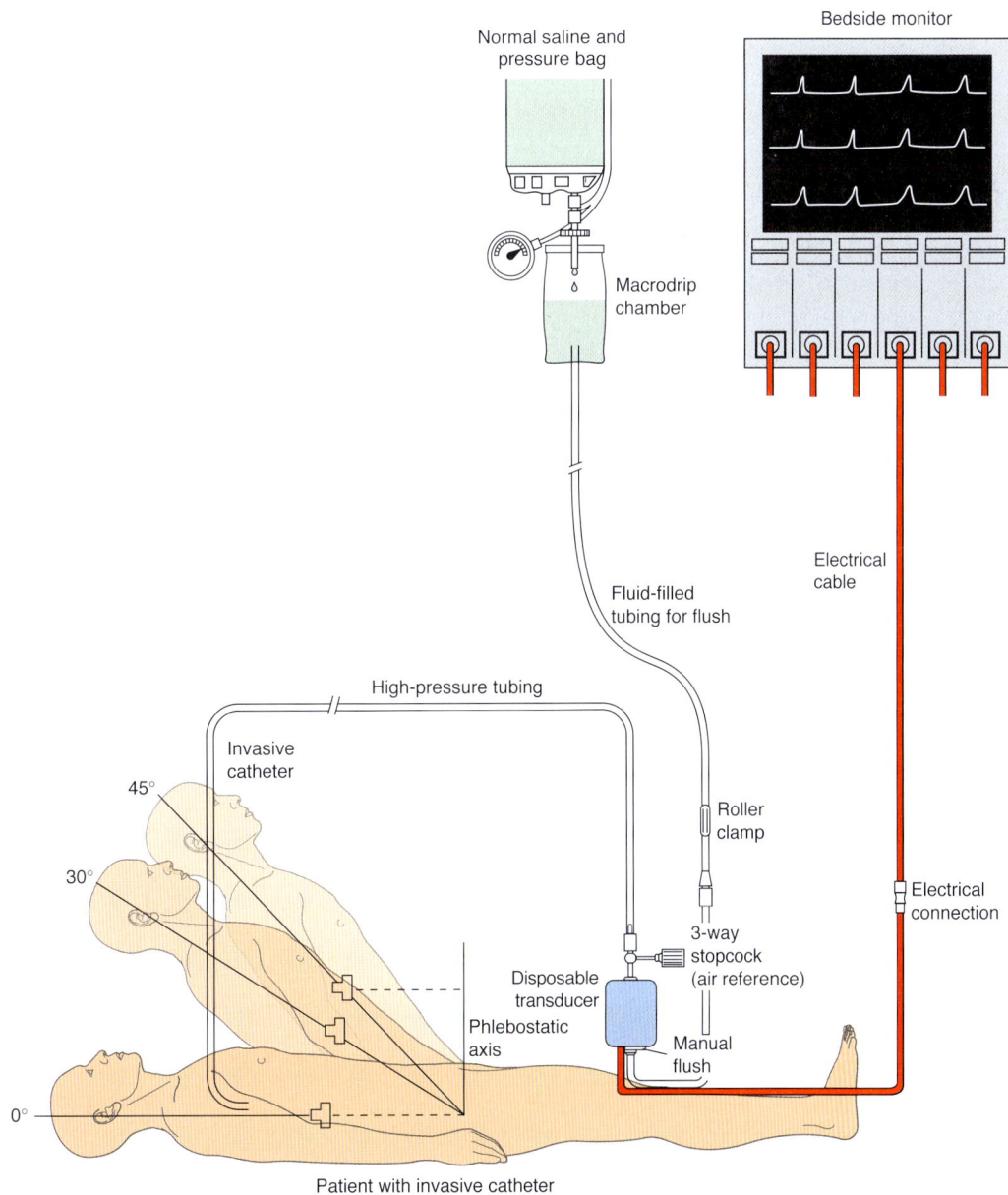

Adapted from Urden L, Stacy KL, Lough ME, eds. Thelan's critical care nursing: Diagnosis and management. 6th ed. St Louis: Mosby/Elsevier; 2010, with permission.

High-pressure (non-distensible) tubing reduces distortion of the signal produced between the intravascular device and the transducer; the pressure is then converted into electrical energy (a waveform). Fluid (0.9% sodium chloride) is routinely used to maintain line patency using a continuous pressure system; the pressure of the flush system fluid bag should be maintained at 300 mmHg, which normally delivers a continual flow of 3 mL/h.

Accuracy is dependent on levelling the transducer to the appropriate level (and altering this level with changes in patient position as appropriate), then zeroing the transducer in the pressure monitoring system to atmospheric pressure (called calibration) as well as evaluating the response of the system by fast-flush wave testing. The transducer must be levelled to the reference point of the phlebostatic axis, at the intersection of the 4th intercostal space and the mid-thoracic anterior–posterior diameter (not the mid-axillary line). Error in measurement can occur if the transducer is placed above or below the phlebostatic axis. Measurements taken when the patient is in the lateral position are not considered as accurate as those taken when the patient is lying supine or semi-recumbent up to an angle of approximately 60°.[24]

Zeroing the transducer system to atmospheric pressure (calibration of the system) is achieved by turning the three-way stopcock nearest to the transducer open to the air, and closing it to the patient and the flush system. The monitor should display zero (0 mmHg), as this equates to current atmospheric pressure (760 mmHg at sea level). With the improved quality of transducers, repeated zeroing is not necessary as, once zeroed, the drift from the baseline is minimal.[25] Some critical care units, however, continue to recalibrate transducer(s) at the beginning of each clinical shift.

Fast-flush square wave testing, or dynamic response measurement, is a way of checking the dynamic response of the monitor to signals from the blood vessel.[25] It is also a check on the accuracy of the subsequent haemodynamic pressure values. The fast-flush device within the system, when triggered and released, exposes the transducer to the amount of pressure in the flush solution bag (usually 300 mmHg). The pressure waveform on the monitor will show a rapid rise in pressure, which then squares off before the pressure drops back to the baseline (see Figure 9.17).

Interpretation of the square wave testing is essential; the clinician must observe the speed with which the wave returns to the baseline as well as the pattern produced. One to three rapid oscillations should occur immediately after the square wave, before the monitored waveform resumes. The distance between these rapid oscillations should not exceed 1 mm or 0.04 s.[25] Absence, or a reduction, of these rapid oscillations, or a 'square wave' with rounded corners, indicates that the pressure monitoring system is overdamped; in other words, its responsiveness to monitored pressures and waveforms is reduced (see Figure 9.18). An underdamped monitoring system will produce more rapid oscillations after the square wave than usual.

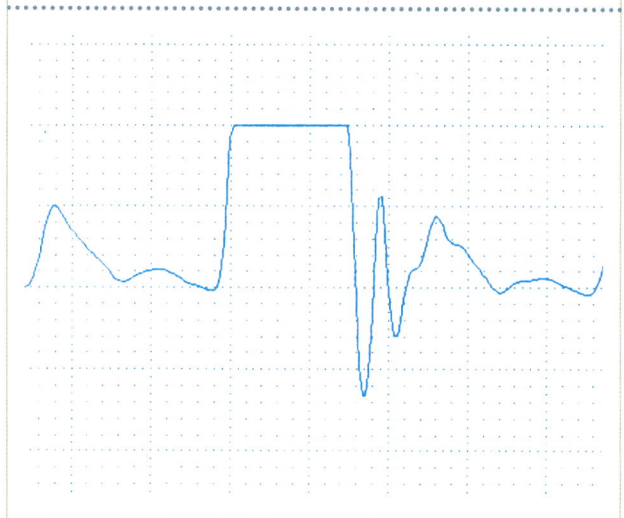

FIGURE 9.17   Normal dynamic response test.

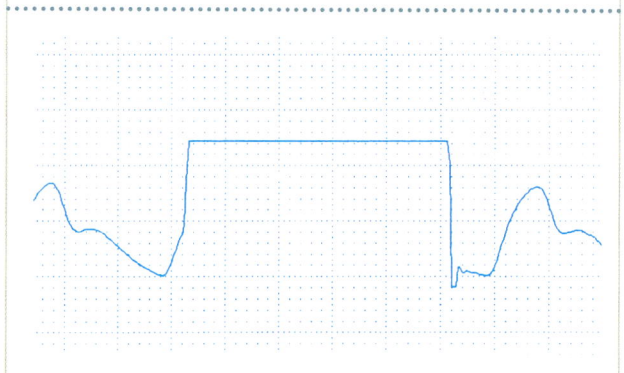

FIGURE 9.18   Over-damped dynamic response test.

Data trends

The ability to trend data via a monitor or a clinical information system is essential for critical care practice. Current monitoring systems can retain data for a period of time, produce trend graphs and link to other devices to allow review of data from locations other than the immediate bedside. The data trends can be used to assess the progression of a patient's clinical condition and monitor the patient's response to treatment.

Haemodynamic monitoring standards

There are stated minimum standards for critical care units worldwide. The standards require that patient monitoring include circulation, respiration and oxygenation, with the following essential equipment available for every patient: an ECG that facilitates continual cardiac monitoring; a mechanical ventilator, pulse oximeter; and other equipment available where necessary to measure intra-arterial and pulmonary pressures, cardiac output, inspiratory pressure and airway flow, intracranial pressures and expired carbon dioxide.[26]

Blood pressure monitoring

Indirect and direct means of monitoring blood pressure are widely used in critical care units. These are outlined in more detail below.

Non-invasive blood pressure monitoring

Non-invasive blood pressure monitoring requires the use of a manual or electronic sphygmomanometer. Oscillation in the pressure generated by alterations in arterial flow is captured either through auscultation or automatic sensing. On auscultation, a number of Korotkoff sounds can be heard as the cuff pressure is released:[27]

- a sharp thud that is heard when the patient's systolic pressure is reached
- a soft tapping, intermittent in nature
- a loud tapping, intermittent in nature
- a low, muffled noise that is continuous in nature and is heard when the diastolic pressure is reached; as the cuff pressure diminishes further, the sound disappears.

For critically ill patients, this method of blood pressure monitoring has limitations and is often used when invasive methods cannot be utilised.[22] It is a less accurate alternative, as results vary with the size of cuff used, equipment malfunction and incorrect placement of the sphygmomanometer (this must be placed at heart level). In addition, the pressures generated by the inflating cuff, particularly those generated by automatic machines, can be high, and frequent measurements of blood pressure by this method may become uncomfortable for the patient. It is therefore important that skin integrity be checked regularly to prevent ischaemia and that the frequency of automated inflations be minimised.[22]

Invasive intra-arterial pressure monitoring

Arterial pressure recording is indicated when precise and continuous monitoring is required, especially in periods of fluid volume, cardiac output and blood pressure instability.[22] An arterial catheter is commonly placed in the radial artery, although other sites can be accessed, including the brachial, femoral, dorsalis pedis and axillary arteries. Arterial catheter insertion is performed aseptically, and it is important that collateral circulation, patient comfort and risk of infection be assessed before insertion is attempted. The radial artery is the most common site, as the ulnar artery provides additional supply to extremities if the radial artery becomes compromised.

Complications of arterial pressure monitoring include:

- infection
- arterial thrombosis
- distal ischaemia
- air embolism
- accidental disconnection (the insertion sites should be always visible)

- accidental drug administration through the arterial catheter; all arterial lines and connections should be clearly identified as such (e.g. marked with red stickers or have red bungs).

Blood pressure is the same at all sites along a vertical level but when the vertical level is varied, pressure will change. Consequently, referencing is required to correct for changes in hydrostatic pressure in vessels above and below the heart; if not, the blood pressure will appear to rise when this is not really the case. It is important to zero the monitoring system at the left atrial level.[24]

Arterial waveform

A steep upstroke (corresponding to ventricular systole) is followed by brief, sustained pressure (anacrotic shoulder). At the end of systole pressure falls in the aorta and left ventricle, causing a downward deflection (see Figure 9.19). A dicrotic notch can be seen in the downward deflection which represents the closure of the aortic valve. The systolic pressure corresponds to the peak of the waveform. The arterial pressure waveform changes its contours when recorded at different sites. It can become sharper in distal locations.

Disease process has an effect on waveforms: for example, atherosclerosis causes an increase in systolic waveform, as well as a decrease in the size of the diastolic wave and dicrotic notch due to changes in elasticity. Cardiomyopathy causes reduced stroke volume and mean arterial pressure, and there is a late secondary systolic peak seen on the waveform.

Invasive arterial pressure versus cuff pressure

At times, the accuracy of the invasive arterial pressure reading may be checked by comparing the reading against that generated by a non-invasive device using an inflating cuff. However, there is no basis for comparing these values. Invasive blood pressure values are a measure of the actual pressure within the artery whereas those from the cuff depend on flow-induced oscillations in the arterial wall. Pressure does not equal flow, as resistance does not

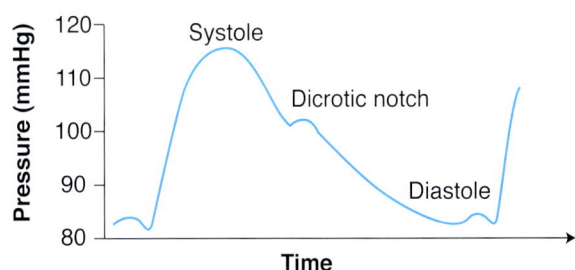

FIGURE 9.19 Arterial pressure waveform.

Adapted from Urden L, Stacy KL, Lough ME, eds. Thelan's critical care nursing: Diagnosis and management. 6th ed. St Louis: Mosby/Elsevier; 2010, with permission.

remain constant. Studies found that the non-invasive cuff blood pressure method can be unreliable in measuring systolic blood pressure when the blood pressure is low, for example, when a patient is in shock.[22] In addition, radial arterial pressure is normally higher than that obtained by brachial non-invasive pressure monitoring because the smaller vessel size exerts greater resistance to flow, and therefore generates a higher pressure reading.[24]

Invasive cardiovascular monitoring

For many critically ill patients, haemodynamic instability is a potentially life-threatening condition that necessitates urgent action. Accurate assessment of the patient's intra-cardiac status is therefore essential. A number of values can be calculated; the measurements commonly made are listed in Tables 9.3 and 9.4 .

Preload

As noted earlier, preload is the filling pressure in the ventricles at the end of diastole. Preload in the right ventricle is generally measured as CVP, although this may be an unreliable predictor because CVP is affected by intrathoracic pressure, vascular tone and obstruction.[28] Left ventricular preload can be measured as the pulmonary capillary wedge pressure (PCWP), but again, due to unreliability, this parameter provides an estimate rather than a true reflection of volume.[29,30] In view of this, other modalities are now being explored, including right ventricular end-diastolic volume evaluation via fast-response pulmonary artery catheters, left ventricular end-diastolic area measured by echocardiography and intrathoracic blood volume measured by transpulmonary thermodilution.[22]

Central venous pressure monitoring

CVP is defined as the pressure of the blood within the systemic venous return.[23] Central venous catheters are inserted to facilitate the monitoring of CVP; facilitate the administration of large amounts of IV fluid or blood; provide long-term access for fluids, drugs, specimen collection and/or parenteral feeding. CVP monitoring has been used for many years to evaluate circulating blood volume, despite discussion as to its validity to do so.[22] However, it is a common monitoring practice and

continues to be used. Therefore, clinicians need to be aware of possible limitations to this form of measurement and interpret the data accordingly. CVP monitoring can produce erroneous results: a low CVP does not always mean low volume and it may reflect other pathology, including peripheral dilation due to sepsis. Hypovolaemic patients may have normal CVP due to sympathetic nervous system activity increasing vascular tone. An increase in CVP can also be seen in patients on mechanical ventilation with application of PEEP.[31]

Central venous catheters used for haemo-dynamic monitoring are classed as short-term percutaneous (non-tunnelled) devices. Short-term percu-taneous catheters are inserted through the skin, directly into a central vein, and usually remain in situ for only a few days or for a maximum of 2–3 weeks.[28] They are easily removed and changed, and are manufactured as single- or multi-lumen types. However, they can be easily dislodged, are thrombogenic due to their material and are associated with a high risk of infection.[28,32]

A number of locations can be used for central venous catheter insertion. The two commonly used sites in critically ill patients are the subclavian and the internal jugular veins. Other less common sites are the antecubital fossa (generally avoided but may be used when the patient cannot be positioned supine), the femoral vein (associated with high infection risk and the external jugular vein (although the high incidence of anomalous anatomy and the severe angle with the subclavian vein make this an unpopular choice).[32]

Internal jugular cannulation has a high success rate for insertion; however, complications related to insertion via this route include carotid artery puncture and laceration of local neck structures arising from needle probing.[32,33] There are a number of key structures adjacent to the vein, including the vagus nerve (located posteriorly to the internal jugular vein), the sympathetic trunk (located behind the vagus nerve) and the phrenic nerve (located laterally to the internal jugular).[34] Damage can also occur to the sympathetic chain, which leads to Horner's syndrome (constricted pupil, ptosis and absence of sweat gland activity on that side of the face). Central venous catheters inserted in the internal jugular vein pose a number of nursing challenges that can cause fixation

TABLE 9.3
Haemodynamic pressures

PARAMETER	RESTING VALUES
Central venous pressure	0 to +8 mmHg (mean)
Right ventricular pressure	+15 to +30 mmHg systolic; 0 to +8 mmHg diastolic
Pulmonary artery wedge pressure	+5 to +15 mmHg (mean)
Left atrial pressure	+4 to +12 mmHg (mean)
Left ventricular pressure	90 to 140 mmHg systolic; +4 to +12 mmHg diastolic
Aortic pressure	90 to 140 mmHg systolic; 60 to 90 mmHg diastolic; 70 to 105 mmHg (mean)

TABLE 9.4

Normal haemodynamic values

PARAMETER	DESCRIPTION	NORMAL VALUES
Stroke volume (SV)	Volume of blood ejected from left ventricle/beat SV = CO/HR	50–100 mL/beat
Stroke volume index (SVI)	Volume of blood ejected/beat indexed to BSA	25–45 mL/beat
Cardiac output (CO)	Volume of blood ejected from left ventricle/min CO = HR $\times$ SV	4–8 L/min
Cardiac index (CI)	A derived value reflecting the volume of blood ejected from left ventricle/min indexed to BSA CI = CO/BSA	2.5–4.2 L/min/m² (normal assumes an average weight of 70 kg)
Mean arterial pressure (MAP)	[(2 $\times$ diastolic) + systolic] /3	70–105 mmHg
Flow time corrected (FTc)	Systolic flow time corrected for heart rate	330–360 ms
Systemic vascular resistance (SVR)	Resistance left heart pumps against SVR = [(MAP – RAP) $\times$ 79.9]/CO	900–1300 dyn•s/cm⁵
Systemic vascular resistance index (SVRI)	Resistance left heart pumps against indexed to body surface area SVRI = [(MAP – RAP) $\times$ 79.9]/CI	1700–2400 dyn•s/cm⁵/m²
Pulmonary vascular resistance (PVR)	Resistance right heart pumps against PVR = [(mPAP – LVEDP) $\times$ 79.9]/CO	20–120 dyn•s/cm⁵
Pulmonary vascular resistance index (PVRI)	Resistance right heart pumps against indexed to body surface area PVRI = [(mPAP – LVEDP) $\times$ 79.9]/CI	255–285 dyn•s/cm⁵/m²
Mixed venous saturation (SvO₂)	Shows the balance between arterial O_2 supply and oxygen demand at the tissue level	70%
Left ventricular stroke work index (LVSWI)	Amount of work performed by LV with each heartbeat (MAP – LVEDP) $\times$ SVI $\times$ 0.0136	50–62 g-m/m²
Right ventricular stroke work index (RVSWI)	Amount of work performed by RV with each heartbeat (mPAP – RAP) $\times$ SVI $\times$ 0.0136	7.9–9.7 g-m/m²
Right ventricular end-systolic volume (RVESV)	The volume of blood remaining in the ventricle at the end of the ejection phase of the heartbeat	50–100 mL/beat
Right ventricular end-systolic volume index (RVESVI)		30–60 mL/m²
Right ventricular end-diastolic volume (RVEDV)	The amount of blood in the ventricle immediately before a cardiac contraction begins	100–160 mL/beat
Right ventricular end-diastolic volume index (RVEDVI)		60–100 mL/m²

BSA = body surface area; HR = heart rate; RAP = right atrial pressure.

Adapted from:
Leeper B. Monitoring right ventricular volumes: a paradigm shift. AACN Clinical Issues 2003;14(2):201–19, with permission.
Schummer W. Central venous pressure. Validity, informative value and correct measurement. Anaesthetist 2009;58(5):499–505, with permission.

problems and the need for repeated dressing changes. These include beard growth, diaphoresis and poor control of oral secretions.

The subclavian approach is used often, perhaps because of a reported lower risk of catheter-related bloodstream infection.[34,35] Coagulopathy is a significant contraindication for this approach, as puncture of the subclavian artery is a known complication. There is also a risk of pneumothorax, which rises if the patient is receiving intermittent positive pressure ventilation (IPPV).[35] Complications of any central venous access catheter include air embolism, pneumothorax, hydrothorax and haemorrhage.[22,23,32]

Pulmonary artery pressure monitoring

Pulmonary artery pressure (PAP) monitoring began in the 1970s, led by Drs Swan, Ganz and colleagues,[36] and was subsequently adopted in ICUs worldwide. Pulmonary artery catheterisation facilitates assessment of filling

FIGURE 9.20 Pulmonary artery catheter.

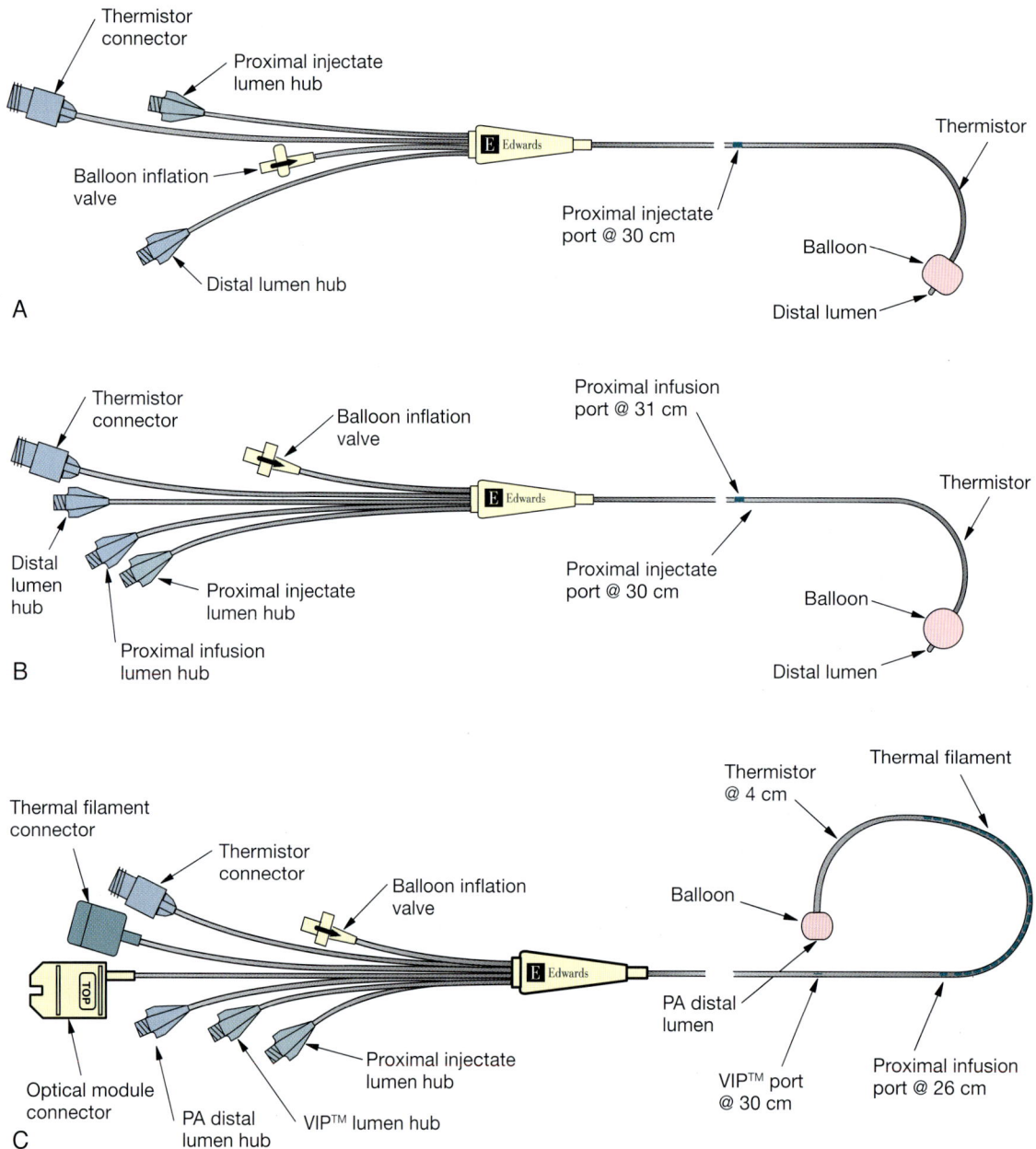

A

B

C

Adapted from Urden L, Stacy KL, Lough ME, eds. Thelan's critical care nursing: Diagnosis and management. 6th ed. St Louis: Mosby/Elsevier; 2010, with permission.

pressure of the left ventricle through the pulmonary artery wedge (occlusion) pressure (see Figure 9.20).[22,33,37] By using a thermodilution pulmonary artery catheter (PAC), cardiac output and other haemodynamic measurements can also be calculated. PAP monitoring is a diagnostic tool that can assist in determination of the nature of a haemodynamic problem and improve diagnostic accuracy. In addition to measuring PA pressures, PAC may also be used for accessing blood for assessment of mixed-venous oxygenation levels (see Chapter 13).

The benefits of PAP monitoring have been scrutinised in recent years. A Cochrane systematic review on PAC use by Rajaram et al[38] suggests that there was no difference in mortality rates, hospital length of stay and ICU length of stay in patients with or without PACs, and there was no difference in clinical benefit or harm in either group of patients. The PAC insertion is invasive, and increases the cost of patients' hospitalisation.[38] Consequently, the use of PAC in clinical practice has dropped 50–65% in recent years,[38] although the PAC is still considered a useful monitoring tool that helps with diagnosis in clinical practice.

Thus, the indications of PAP monitoring are largely based on health professionals' clinical experience and expertise. It has been suggested that PAP monitoring may be indicated for adults in severe hypovolaemic or cardiogenic shock, where there may be diagnostic uncertainty, or where the patient is unresponsive to initial therapy. The PAP is used to guide administration of fluids, inotropes and vasopressors. PAP monitoring may also be utilised in other cases of haemodynamic instability when the diagnosis is unclear. It may be helpful when clinicians want to differentiate hypovolaemia from cardiogenic shock or, in cases of pulmonary oedema, to differentiate cardiogenic from non-cardiogenic origins.[39] However, in their Cochrane review, Rajaram et al[38] concluded that more studies are needed to investigate the benefit of PAC use in subgroup patients including reversing shock states and improving organ function. Complications do arise from PACs, as these catheters share all the complications of central lines and are additionally associated with a higher incidence of arrhythmia, valve damage, pulmonary vascular occlusion, emboli/infarction (reported incidence of 0.1–5.6%) and, very rarely, knotting of the catheter.[32]

A number of measurements can be taken via the PAC, either by direct measurement, for example using pulmonary capillary wedge pressure (PCWP), which is an estimate of left ventricular preload (LVEDV), or through calculation of derived parameters such as cardiac output (CO) and cardiac index (CI) (see Table 9.4 for descriptors and normal values).

Pulmonary capillary wedge pressure (PCWP) monitoring

PCWP, or pulmonary artery occlusion pressure (PAOP), is measured when the pulmonary artery catheter balloon is inflated with no more than 1–1.5 mL air. The inflated balloon isolates the distal measuring lumen from the pulmonary arterial pressures, and measures pressures in the capillaries of the pulmonary venous system, and indirectly the left atrial pressure. The PAP waveform looks similar to that of the arterial waveform, with the tracing showing a systolic peak, dicrotic notch and a diastolic dip (see Figure 9.21). When the balloon is inflated, the waveform changes shape and becomes much flatter in appearance, providing a similar waveform to the CVP. There are two positive waves on the tracing: the first reflects atrial contraction and the second reflects pressure changes from blood flow when the mitral valve closes and the ventricles contract.[40] The PCWP should be read once the 'wedge' trace stops falling at the end-expiratory phase of the respiratory cycle (see Figure 9.21).

FIGURE 9.21 Pulmonary artery pressure and wedge waveforms.

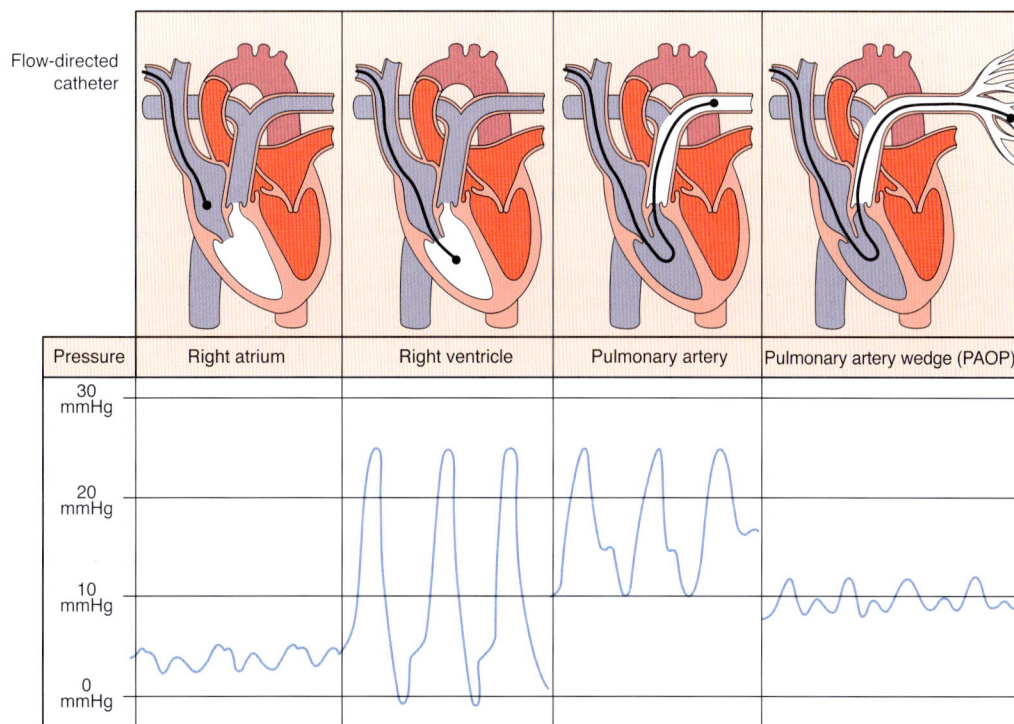

Adapted from Urden L, Stacy KL, Lough ME, eds. Thelan's critical care nursing: Diagnosis and management. 6th ed. St Louis: Mosby/Elsevier; 2010, with permission.

If balloon occlusion occurs with <1 mL of air, the balloon is wedged in a small capillary and consequently will not accurately reflect LA pressure. Conversely, if 1.5 mL air does not cause occlusion, the balloon may have burst (which can result in an air embolus) or it may be floating in a larger vessel. If balloon rupture is suspected, no further attempts to inflate the balloon should be made, and interventions to minimise the risk of air embolism should be initiated.[7]

Note: it is essential that the balloon be deflated as soon as the wedge has been recorded, as continued occlusion will cause distal pulmonary vasculature ischaemia and infarction.[40]

Left atrial pressure monitoring

Left atrial pressure (LAP) monitoring directly estimates left heart preload. It used to require an open thorax to enable direct cannulation of the atrium. It was used only in the postoperative cardiac surgical setting, although such use has been infrequent since the widespread use of PAC. Recent advancement in cardiac implantable devices development enables the patients to self-monitor LAP under their doctors' guidance, which was found to be a valuable tool to improve the management of patients with advanced heart failure.[41] Other modes of monitoring can also be used to achieve comprehensive left atrial assessment, such as Doppler echocardiography.[42]

Afterload

As previously noted, afterload is the pressure that the ventricle produces to overcome the resistance to ejection generated in the systemic or pulmonary circulation by the arteries and arterioles. It is calculated by cardiac output studies: left heart afterload is reflected as systemic vascular resistance (SVR), and right heart afterload is reflected as pulmonary vascular resistance (PVR) (see Table 9.4).

Systemic and pulmonary vascular resistance

Systemic vascular resistance (SVR) is a measure of resistance or impediment of the systemic vascular bed to blood flow. An elevated SVR can be caused by vasoconstrictors, hypovolaemia or late septic shock. A lowered SVR can be caused by early septic shock, vasodilators, morphine, nitrates or hypercarbia. Afterload is a major determinant of blood pressure, and gross vasodilation causes peripheral pooling and hypotension, reducing SVR. The precise estimation of SVR enables safer use of therapies such as vasodilators (e.g. sodium nitroprusside) and vasoconstrictors (e.g. noradrenaline).[43]

Pulmonary vascular resistance (PVR) is a measure of resistance or the impediment of the pulmonary vascular bed to blood flow. An elevated PVR ('pulmonary hypertension') is caused by pulmonary vascular disease, pulmonary embolism, pulmonary vasculitis or hypoxia. A lowered PVR is caused by medications such as calcium channel blockers, aminophylline or isoproterenol, or by the delivery of O_2.[43]

Contractility

Contractility reflects the force of myocardial contraction, and is related to the extent of myocardial fibre stretch (preload, see above) and wall tension (afterload, see above). It is important because it influences myocardial oxygen consumption. Contractility of the left side of the heart is measured by calculating the left ventricular stroke work index (LVSWI), although the clinical use of this value is not widespread.

Right ventricular stroke work index (RVSWI) can be similarly calculated. Contractility can decrease as a result of excessive preload or afterload, drugs such as negative inotropes, myocardial damage such as that occurring after MI and changes in the cellular environment arising from acidosis, hypoxia or electrolyte imbalances. Increases in contractility arise from drugs such as positive inotropes.[44]

Cardiac output

As discussed earlier in the chapter, the cardiac output (CO) refers to the blood volume ejected by the heart in one minute. Stroke volume (SV) is the blood ejected by the heart in one beat. Therefore cardiac output can be calculated as the heart rate multiplied by stroke volume. Stroke volume is determined by the heart's preload, afterload and the contractility.

The variety of cardiac output measurement techniques has grown over the past decade since the development of thermodilution pulmonary artery catheters, pulse-induced contour devices, less invasive techniques such as Doppler and non-invasive continuous haemodynamic monitoring methods. As many critically ill patients require mechanical ventilation support, the associated rises in intrathoracic pressure, as well as changing ventricular compliance, make accurate haemodynamic assessment difficult with the older technologies. Therefore, volumetric measurements of preload, such as right ventricular end-systolic volume (RVESV), right ventricular end-diastolic volume (RVEDV) and index (RVESVI/RVEDVI) as well as measurements of right ventricular ejection fraction (RVEF) are now being used to more accurately determine cardiac output. The parameters RVEF, CO and/or CI and SV are generated using thermodilution technology, and from these the parameters of RVEDV/RVEDVI and RVESV/RVESVI can be calculated (see Table 9.4 for normal values).[10] The availability of continuous modes of assessment has further improved a clinician's ability to accurately assess, and then effectively treat, these patients.[10]

The Fick principle

Several cardiac output measurement methods use the Fick principle. In 1870, Fick proposed that 'in an organ, the uptake or release of an indicator substance is the product of the arterial–venous concentration of this substance and the blood flow to the organ'.[45] Using oxygen as the indicator substance, the calculation of cardiac output is as follows:

$$CO = VO_2/(CaO_2 - CvO_2)$$

whereVO_2 is oxygen consumption, CaO_2 is arterial oxygen concentration, and CvO_2 is venous oxygen concentration.

Thermodilution methods

Thermodilution methods calculate cardiac output by using temperature change as the indicator in Fick's method. Cardiac output and associated pressures such as global end-diastolic volume can be calculated using a thermodilution PA catheter. Cardiac output can be monitored intermittently or continuously using the PA catheter. Intermittent measurements obtained every few hours produce a snapshot of the cardiovascular state over that time. By injecting a bolus of 5–10 mL of crystalloid solution, and measuring the resulting temperature changes, an estimation of stroke volume is calculated. Cold injectate (run through ice) was initially recommended, but studies now support the use of room temperature injectate, providing there is a difference of 12° Celsius between injectate and blood temperature.[46] Three readings are taken at the same part of the respiratory cycle (normally end expiration), and any measurements that differ by more than 10% should be disregarded (see Table 9.4 for normal values). Since the 1990s, the value of having continuous measurement of cardiac output has been recognised[37] and this has led to the development of devices that permit the transference of pulses of thermal energy to pulmonary artery blood – the pulse-induced contour method.[23]

Pulse-induced contour cardiac output

Pulse-induced contour cardiac output (PiCCO) provides continuous assessment of CO, and requires a central venous line and an arterial line with a thermistor (not a PAC).[47] A known volume of thermal indicator (usually room temperature saline) is injected into the central vein. The injectate disperses both volumetrically and thermally within the cardiac and pulmonary blood. When the thermal signal is detected by the arterial thermistor, the temperature difference is calculated and a dissipation curve generated. From these data, the cardiac output can be calculated. These continuous cardiac output measurements have been well researched and appear to be equal in accuracy to those produced by intermittent injections required for the earlier catheters.[48] The parameters measured by PiCCO[47] include the following:

- Pulse-induced contour cardiac output (PiCCO): derived normal value for cardiac index, 2.5–4.2 L/min/m^2.

- Global end-diastolic volume (GEDV): the volume of blood contained in the four chambers of the heart; assists in the calculation of intrathoracic blood volume. Derived normal value for global end-diastolic blood volume index, 680–800 mL/m^2.

- Intrathoracic blood volume (ITBV): the volume of the four chambers of the heart plus the blood volume in the pulmonary vessels; more accurately reflects circulating blood volumes, particularly when a patient is artificially ventilated. Derived normal value for intrathoracic blood volume index, 850–1000 mL/m^2.

- Extravascular lung water (EVLW): the amount of water content in the lungs; allows quantification of the degree of pulmonary oedema (not evident with X-ray or blood gases). Derived normal value for extravascular lung water index is 3–7 mL/kg. EVLW has been shown to be useful as a guide for fluid management in critically ill patients.[46] An elevated EVLW may be an effective indicator of severity of illness, particularly after acute lung injury or in ARDS, when EVLW is elevated due to alterations in hydrostatic pressures.[49] Other patients at risk of high EVLW are those with left heart failure, severe pneumonia and burns. There may be an association between high EVLW and increased mortality, the need for mechanical ventilation and a higher risk of nosocomial infection.[49] A decision tree outlining processes of care guided by information provided by PiCCO is provided in Figure 9.22.

PiCCO removes the impact of factors that can cause variability in the standard approach of cardiac output measurement, such as injectate volume and temperature, and timing of the injection within the respiratory cycle.[48] The additional fluid volume injected with the standard technique is significant in some patients; with the continuous technology, this is eliminated. A further advantage is that virtually real-time responses to treatment can be obtained, removing the time delay that was a potential problem with standard thermodilution techniques.[48]

An arterial catheter is widely used in critical care to enable frequent blood sampling and blood pressure monitoring, and is used to measure beat-by-beat cardiac output, obtained from the shape of the arterial pressure wave. The area under the systolic portion of the arterial pulse wave from the end of diastole to the end of the ejection phase is measured and combined with an individual calibration factor. The algorithm is capable of computing each single stroke volume after being calibrated by an initial transpulmonary thermodilution.

PiCCO preload indicators of intrathoracic blood volume (ITBV) and global end-diastolic volume (GEDV) are more sensitive and specific to cardiac preload than the standard cardiac filling pressures of CVP and PCWP, as well as right ventricular end-diastolic volume. One advantage of ITBV and GEDV is that they are not affected by mechanical ventilation and therefore give correct information on the preload status under almost any condition. Extravascular lung water (EVLW) correlates moderately well with severity of ARDS, length of ventilation days, ICU stay and mortality,[50] and appears to be of greater accuracy than the traditional assessment of lung oedema by chest X-ray. Disadvantages of PiCCO include its potential unreliability when heart rate, blood pressure and total vascular resistance change substantially.[10,47]

FIGURE 9.22 PiCCO decision tree.

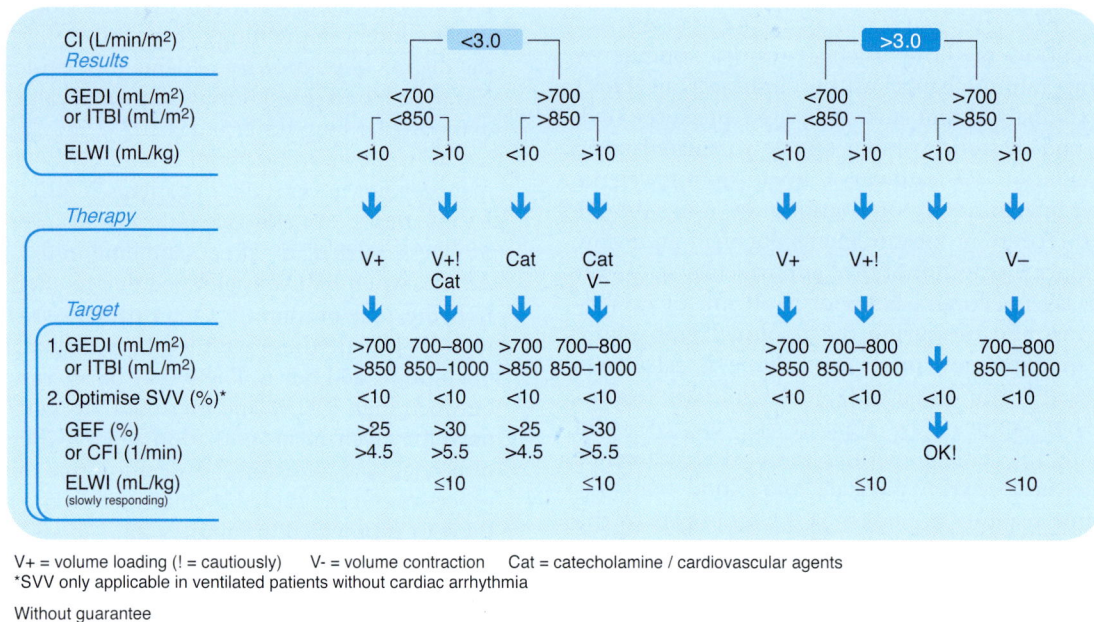

CI (L/min/m²) Results	<3.0				>3.0			
GEDI (mL/m²) or ITBI (mL/m²)	<700		>700		<700		>700	
	<850		>850		<850		>850	
ELWI (mL/kg)	<10	>10	<10	>10	<10	>10	<10	>10
Therapy	↓	↓	↓	↓	↓	↓	↓	↓
	V+	V+! Cat	Cat	Cat V−	V+	V+!		V−
Target	↓	↓	↓	↓	↓	↓	↓	↓
1. GEDI (mL/m²) or ITBI (mL/m²)	>700 >850	700–800 850–1000	>700 >850	700–800 850–1000	>700 >850	700–800 850–1000	↓	700–800 850–1000
2. Optimise SVV (%)*	<10	<10	<10	<10	<10	<10	<10	<10
GEF (%) or CFI (1/min)	>25 >4.5	>30 >5.5	>25 >4.5	>30 >5.5			↓ OK!	
ELWI (mL/kg) (slowly responding)		≤10		≤10			≤10	≤10

V+ = volume loading (! = cautiously)   V− = volume contraction   Cat = catecholamine / cardiovascular agents
*SVV only applicable in ventilated patients without cardiac arrhythmia

Without guarantee

Courtesy Pulsion Medical Systems.

Doppler ultrasound methods

Oesophageal Doppler monitoring enables calculation of cardiac output from assessment of stroke volume and heart rate, but uses a less invasive technique than those outlined previously.[51] Stroke volume is assessed by measuring the flow velocity and the area through which the forward flow travels. Flow velocity is the distance one red blood cell travels forward in one cardiac cycle, and the measurement provides a time velocity interval. The area of flow is calculated by measuring the cross-sectional area of the blood vessel or heart chamber at the site of the flow velocity measurement.[42] Oesophageal Doppler monitoring can be performed at the level of the pulmonary artery, mitral valve or aortic valve.

According to Doppler principles, the movement of blood produces a waveform that reflects blood flow velocity, in this case in the descending thoracic aorta (see Figure 9.23), that is captured by the change in frequency of an ultrasound beam as it reflects off a moving object.[23] This measurement is combined with an estimate of the cross-sectional area of the aorta so that the stroke volume, cardiac output and cardiac index can be calculated, using the patient's age, height and weight.[42]

Oesophageal Doppler monitoring provides an alternative for patients who would not benefit from PAC insertion,[42,52] and can be used to provide continuous measurements under certain conditions: the estimate of cross-sectional area must be accurate; the ultrasound beam must be directed parallel to the flow of blood; and there should be minimal variation in movement of the beam between measurements. There is some debate at present among clinicians about the accuracy of oesophageal Doppler monitoring for calculating cardiac

output.[53] This form of monitoring can be used perioperatively and in the critical care unit, on a wide variety of patients.[52] It should not, however, be used in patients with aortic coarctation or dissection, oesophageal malignancy or perforation, severe bleeding problems or with patients on an intra-aortic balloon pump.[54]

The Doppler probe that sits in the oesophagus is approximately the size of a nasogastric tube, is semi-rigid and is inserted using a similar technique. The patient is usually sedated but the method has been used in awake patients. In such cases, however, the limitation is that the probe is more likely to require more frequent repositioning.[54]

The waveform that is displayed on the monitor is triangular in shape (see Figure 9.23) and captures the systolic portion of the cardiac cycle – an upstroke at the beginning of systole, the peak reflecting maximum systole and the downward slope of the ending of systole. The waveform captures real-time changes in blood flow and can therefore be seen as an indirect reflection of left ventricular function. Changes to haemodynamic status will be reflected in alterations in the triangular shape (see Figure 9.23).

Ultrasonic cardiac output monitor

The ultrasonic cardiac output monitor (USCOM) monitors CO non-invasively using continuous Doppler ultrasound waves by placing an ultrasound transducer probe supra- or parasternally. The principles of CO calculation in this method are the same as for oesophageal Doppler monitoring. Empirical study suggests that the use of non-invasive ultrasonic cardiac output monitor (USCOM) provided adequate clinical data in patients in different shock categories, and it was safe and cost effective.[55]

FIGURE 9.23   Oesophageal Doppler waveforms.

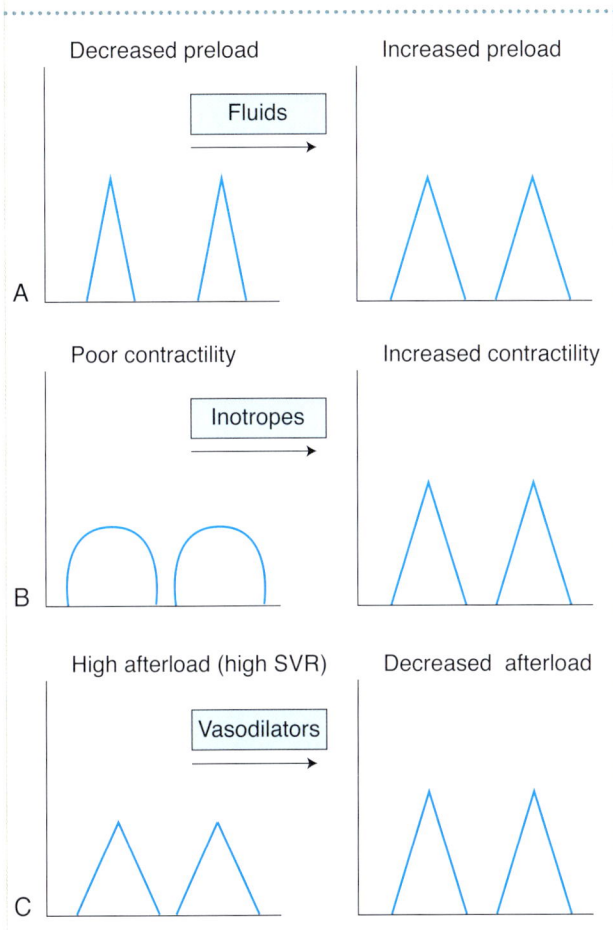

Decreased preload   Increased preload

Fluids

A

Poor contractility   Increased contractility

Inotropes

B

High afterload (high SVR)   Decreased afterload

Vasodilators

C

Impedance cardiography

Transthoracic bioimpedance (impedance cardiography) is another form of non-invasive monitoring used to estimate cardiac output, and was first introduced by Kubicek in 1966.[56] It measures the amount of electrical resistance generated by the thorax to high-frequency, very-low-magnitude currents. This measure is inversely proportional to the content of fluid in the thorax: if the amount of thoracic fluid increases, then transthoracic bioimpedance falls.[23] Changes in cardiac output can be reflected as a change in overall bioimpedance. The technique requires six electrodes to be positioned on the patient: two in the upper thorax/neck area and four in the lower thorax. These electrodes also monitor electrical signals from the heart.

Overall, transthoracic bioimpedance is determined by: 1) changes in tissue fluid volume, 2) volumetric changes in pulmonary and venous blood caused by respiration and 3) volumetric changes in aortic blood flow produced by myocardial contractility.[57] Accurate measurements of changes in aortic blood flow are dependent on the ability to measure the third determinant, while filtering out any interference produced by the first two determinants. Any changes to position or to electrode contact will cause alterations to the measurements obtained, and recordings

should therefore be undertaken with the electrodes positioned in the same location as previous readings. Caution is required for patients with high levels of perspiration (which reduces electrode contact), atrial fibrillation (irregular R–R intervals make estimation of the ventricular ejection time difficult) or pulmonary oedema, pleural effusions or chest wall oedema (which alter bioimpedance readings irrespective of any changes in cardiac output). The use of transthoracic bioimpedance in critically ill patients is variable, due in part to limitations of its usefulness in patients who have pulmonary oedema.[58,59]

> **Practice tip**
>
> Current evidence-based literature suggests that haemo-dynamic measurements such as CVP, PAWP and PAP can be accurately measured with a patient position of supine to head – up to 60°.

Diagnostics

Apart from the haemodynamic monitoring methods to facilitate cardiac assessment of a patient's clinical condition, various diagnostic tests are often used. Echocardiography and blood tests are the most commonly used in critical care. Other tests such as computerised tomography (CT) and nuclear medicine cardiac examination are also used when indicated. Exercise stress tests and cardiac angiography are also used and are reviewed in Chapter 10.

Echocardiography

Echocardiography (frequently shortened to ECHO) is often used in critical care to assess cardiovascular conditions such as heart failure, hypertensive heart disease, valve disease and pericardial disease in critically ill patients. It adopts a technique of detecting the echoes produced by a heart from a beam of very high frequency sound – ultrasound. Two-dimensional, three-dimensional and contrast ECHO images can be obtained using the non-invasive transthoracic technique or the invasive transoesophageal technique (TOE). The transthoracic ECHO uses a transducer probe externally to the heart to obtain images (same as a normal ultrasound technique). This method is painless and does not require sedation. The TOE technique involves placing a transducer probe into the oesophageal cavity to assess the function and structure of the heart. This method produces better images of the heart than the normal transthoracic ECHO.[45] However, this method requires sedation during the procedure and the patient needs to fast for a few hours prior to the examination.

Two-dimensional ECHO images are valuable resources for assessment of the function and structure of the heart. Three-dimensional images offer more realistic visualisation of its structure and function. Contrast ECHO provides enhanced images of left and right ventricular definition to facilitate the diagnosis of complex cardiac conditions such as congenital heart defects, valve stenosis and regurgitation.[60,61] The contrast ECHO technique uses gas air microbubbles, produced by hand-agitating a syringe containing 10 mL of normal saline with a small amount of air, injected into the peripheral vein to produce images of the heart functions.[45]

In the critical care setting, the preparation of critically ill patients for this examination is important. The nurse needs to help the sonographer to position the patient to achieve the best results. For TOE preparation, fasting time must be followed to avoid complications such as respiratory aspiration. The nurse will also need to assist the anaesthetist and the TOE operator, and continue to monitor the patient's clinical conditions during the procedure.

Blood tests

A number of blood tests are often conducted to assist the clinical assessment of critically ill patients in the critical care setting.

Full blood count

The full blood count (FBC) assesses the status of three major cells that are formed in the bone marrow: red blood cells (RBC), white blood cells (WBC) and platelets. Although normal values have been given (see *Appendix A*), for critically ill patients changes will occur under certain conditions. For example, haemoglobin (Hb) is reduced in the presence of haemorrhage and also in acute fluid overload causing haemodilution.

Haemoconcentration can occur during acute dehydration, which would show up as a high Hb. Similar conditions will also affect the haematocrit. WBC levels will be elevated during episodes of infection, tissue damage and inflammation. When infections are severe, the full blood count will show a dramatic rise in the number of immature neutrophils. Platelets are easily lost during haemorrhage, and spontaneous bleeding is a danger when the count falls to below 20×10^9/L.[62,63]

Electrolytes

The assessment of electrolyte levels in critically ill patients is important in diagnosing the patient's condition. Electrolyte imbalances, such as potassium and calcium level changes, can cause cardiovascular abnormalities such as arrhythmias. Electrolyte levels are often checked regularly in critically ill patients.

The functions of electrolytes and their cardiac implications are listed in Table 9.5.

Cardiac enzymes

Cardiac biochemical markers, such as troponin, are proteins that are released from damaged myocardial cells that are detectable by performing blood tests. Troponin elevation is considered a significant biomarker for patients with MI; however, it can also be elevated in non-MI patients.[64] Thus, diagnosis for critically ill patients with elevated cardiac troponin levels should be made with support from other data.[64] See Table 9.6 for cardiac enzyme parameters and normal values. For abnormal cardiac enzymes in MI, please refer to Chapter 10.

TABLE 9.5

Electrolyte functions and pathophysiology

ELECTROLYTE	FUNCTIONS	COMMON IMBALANCES AND CAUSES	SIGNS AND SYMPTOMS
Potassium	Maintains normal functions of nerve and muscle cells Acid–base balance	*Hyperkalaemia* Renal failure, dehydration, diabetes, diuretic medications	Muscle weakness, ECG changes in cardiac toxicity, severe hyperkalaemia (serum K between 6 and 6.5 mEq/L) needs prompt attention because it can cause life-threatening arrhythmia
		Hypokalaemia Kidney disease, diarrhoea, vomiting, diuretic medications	Muscle weakness, respiratory failure, ECG changes
Sodium	Regulates body fluid movement Maintains cell functions Acid–base balance	*Hypernatraemia* Renal failure, dehydration, diarrhoea, vomiting	Thirst, confusion, hyperreflexia, seizures
		Hyponatraemia Acute renal failure, heart failure, pancreatitis, peritonitis, burns	Altered personality, confusion, seizures, coma, death
Calcium	Bone metabolism Blood coagulation Muscle contraction Nerve conduction	*Hypercalcaemia* Hyperparathyroidism, vitamin D toxicity, cancer	Polyuria, constipation, nausea, vomiting, muscle weakness, confusion, coma, ECG changes (shortened QT intervals)
		Hypocalcaemia Hypoparathyroidism, vitamin D deficiency, renal disease	Paraesthesias, tetany. In severe cases, seizures, encephalopathy, ECG changes (prolonged ST and QT intervals), heart failure

ELECTROLYTE	FUNCTIONS	COMMON IMBALANCES AND CAUSES	SIGNS AND SYMPTOMS
Magnesium	Activates sodium–potassium pumps Inactivates calcium channels Neuromuscular transmission	*Hypermagnesaemia* Renal failure	Hypotension, respiratory depression, AV conduction disturbances, which can lead to cardiac arrest (often in renal failure patients)
		Hypomagnesaemia Inadequate intake and absorption, or increased excretion, due to hypercalcaemia or diuretics	Anorexia, nausea, vomiting, lethargy. It may contribute to hypokalaemia development therefore cardiac arrhythmias may be present *Note*: associated hypocalcaemia is common in hypomagnesaemia
Phosphorus	Intracellular energy production (ATP) and enzyme regulation Tissue oxygen delivery Bone metabolism	*Hyperphosphataemia* Kidney failure, metabolic and respiratory acidosis	Usually asymptomatic. However, when concurrent hypocalcaemia, symptoms of hypocalcaemia may be present
		Hypophosphataemia Burns, diuretic medications, respiratory alkalosis, acute alcoholism	Usually asymptomatic. Severe cases may have muscle weakness, heart failure, coma

For cardiac implications of electrolytes imbalances, see Chapter 10 and Chapter 11.

Adapted from:
Urden LD, Stacey KM, Lough ME, eds. Critical care nursing: diagnosis and management. St Louis, Mo: Elsevier; 2014, with permission.
Moser DK, Reigel B. Cardiac nursing: a companion to Brauwald's heart disease. St Louis: Elsevier; 2008, with permission.

TABLE 9.6
Cardiac biochemical markers – description and normal values

ENZYME	DESCRIPTION	NORMAL VALUE
Troponin T (cTnT)	Detected within 2–3 h after infarction, and may remain elevated for 7–10 d	<0.1 ng/mL
Troponin I (cTnI)	Detected within 2–3 h of infarction, and may remain elevated for up to 14 d	<0.03 ng/mL
Creatine kinase (CK)	Serum CK are elevated following muscle or neurological injury. Creatine kinase myocardial bound (CK–MB) is useful in quantifying the degree of infarction and timing of onset. Levels rise 3–6 h and peak 12–24 h after infarction	Adult female: 30–135 units U/L; Adult male: 55–170 units U/L CK-MB: 0–5% of total CK
Aspartate aminotransferase (AST)	Detection and monitoring of liver cell damage. No cardiac-specific isoenzymes; today rarely used because it is released after renal, cerebral and hepatic damage	<40 U/L
Lactate dehydrogenase (LDH)	Of no value in the diagnosis of myocardial infarction. Occasionally useful in the assessment of patients with liver disease or malignancy (especially lymphoma, seminoma, hepatic metastases); anaemia when haemolysis or ineffective erythropoiesis suspected. Although it may be elevated in patients with skeletal muscle damage, it is not useful in this situation. Post-AMI, cardiac-specific isoenzyme LDH[1] peaks between 48 and 72 h	110–230 U/L
D-Dimer	Presence indicates deep vein thrombosis, myocardial infarction, DIC	<0.25 ng/L

DIC = disseminated intravascular coagulation.
Adapted from Pragana KD, Pragana TJ. Mosby's diagnostic and laboratory test reference. 12th ed. St Louis: Elsevier; 2015.

Chest X-ray

Chest X-ray is the oldest non-invasive way to visualise the heart and blood vessels, and is one of the most commonly taken diagnostic procedures in critical care. To interpret a chest X-ray for cardiac diagnosis, basic knowledge of the normal anatomical cardiac structure is important to identify abnormality, and a basic understanding of the chest X-ray is essential. Please review the basic concepts, such as what water, air and bone show on X-ray, and the concepts of anteroposterior (AP) and posteroanterior (PA) films, in Chapter 13 before you move on to the next section.

Cardiac chest X-ray interpretation

To interpret the chest X-ray for cardiac assessment, the following steps should be followed to ensure a thorough diagnosis:

1   The heart size needs to be checked first to see if the size of the heart is appropriate. The cardiac silhouette should be no more than 50% of the diameter of the thorax; this is called the cardiothoracic ratio.[65] The position of the heart should be ⅓ of the heart shadow to the right of the vertebrae and ⅔ of the shadow to the left of the vertebrae.[65] The size of the heart can be determined in a matter of seconds, even by the novice clinician, since this can be simply determined by visualising the cardiothoracic ratio.

2   The shape of the heart should be inspected next. The border of the heart on the X-ray film is determined by the heart anatomy. The border is formed by: the right atrial shadow as the right convex cardiac border, the superior vena cava as the superior border and the left ventricle as the left heart border and cardiac apex. In the frontal chest X-ray, the right ventricle is not a border-forming structure because it is directly superimposed on the cardiac silhouette. Similarly, the normal left atrium should not be visible on a posteroanterior (PA) film. The border of the heart should be sharp. If the left atrium is enlarged, a convex superior left heart border is seen.[65]

3   On the superior border the aortic arch and the pulmonary arteries should be identified next. The aortic arch is called the knob. The pulmonary arteries and their branches radiate outward from the hila (see Figure 9.24). The hilum in the mediasternal region is formed by the pulmonary arteries and the main stem bronchi shadows on the film. The focus of this step is to check for prominence of vessels in this region, as this suggests vascular abnormalities.[66]

Chest X-ray in diagnosing cardiac conditions

For coronary heart disease assessment, an initial chest X-ray film is useful to exclude other causes of chest pain, such as pneumonia, pneumothorax and aortic aneurysm, and to assess whether heart failure and/or pulmonary congestion are present. Patients with chronic heart failure show cardiomegaly, Kerley B lines or pulmonary oedema. Cardiomegaly is seen as an enlarged heart on the X-ray film. Kerley B lines on the X-ray film are the result of pulmonary congestion and fluid accumulation in the interstitium. Although cardiomegaly and pulmonary oedema indicate heart failure, the chest X-ray alone cannot diagnose the condition. Other tests are needed to thoroughly assess patients for accurate diagnosis.[67]

FIGURE 9.24   Chest PA radiograph. The convex right cardiac border is formed by the right atrium (thin arrows), and the heavy arrows indicate the location of the superior vena cava.

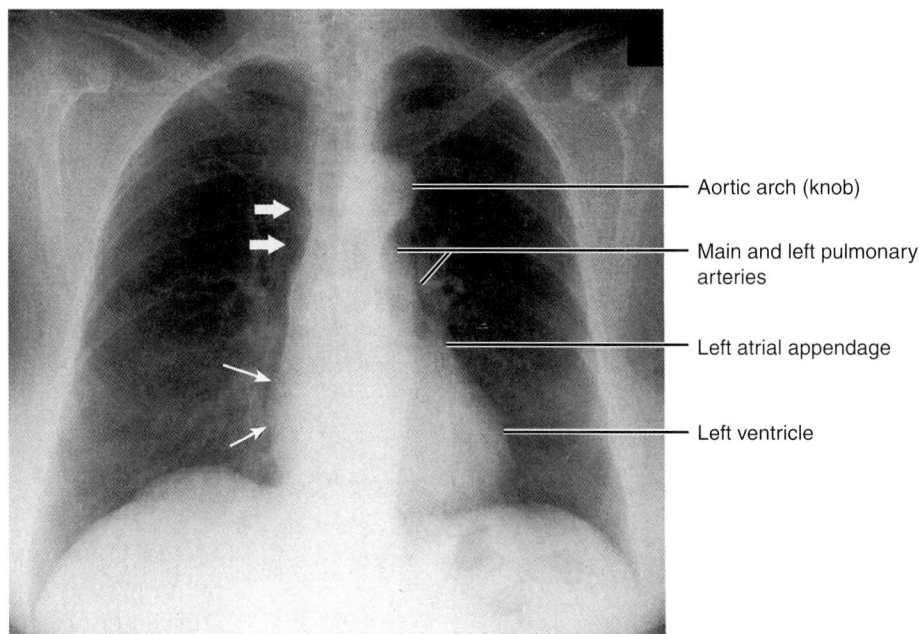

- Aortic arch (knob)
- Main and left pulmonary arteries
- Left atrial appendage
- Left ventricle

Adapted from Erkonen WE, Wilbur LS. Radiology 101: The basics and fundamentals of imaging. 3rd ed. Philadelphia, PA: Lippincott Williams & Wilkins; 2009, with permission.

A widened mediastinum and abnormal aortic contour may indicate aortic dissection. Similar to heart failure, further tests such as TOE, magnetic resonance imaging (MRI) or angiography are needed to confirm the diagnosis. Subtle abnormalities in the hilar region may indicate pulmonary hypertension (PAH). A decrease in pulmonary vascular markings and prominent main and hilar pulmonary arterial shadows in the lung fields on the chest film are classic signs of pulmonary hypertension. However, the sensitivity of this for excluding PAH is lacking.[68] In pericardial disease, the chest X-ray often appears normal unless the accumulated fluid in the pericardial space is over 250 mL. Note that accumulation of fluid is indicated in many cardiac conditions; therefore, other tests need to be carried out to confirm the diagnosis.[69]

The positions of a pulmonary artery catheter, a central venous catheter and pacing wires can be identified on the chest X-ray. The positions of these catheters need to be checked regularly to ensure the catheters and wires are in appropriate places. More details on how to identify the catheters and pacing wires are given in Chapter 13.

Due to individual variations in shape, size and rotation of the heart, and the complexity of cardiac signs, chest X-rays often play a minor role in cardiac diagnosis. A patient's clinical condition and other diagnostic test results must be taken into account when diagnosing a cardiac condition.[68]

Other diagnostic tests of cardiac function

Since 2000, more non-invasive diagnostic imaging techniques are used to aid cardiac assessment. Some of these techniques have shown significant advantages, such as lowered cost, but they also have their limitations.[45]

Cardiac computed tomography

Cardiac computed tomography (cardiac CT) is a recent development in diagnosing cardiac conditions such as suspected coronary heart disease and in the evaluation of coronary artery bypass grafts. It provides a method for visualising the anatomical structures of the heart and coronary arteries reliably and accurately in patients.[70] However, limitations remain with this method including the inability to assess the haemodynamic relevance of a coronary artery lesion. In addition, the most appropriate radiation and contrast doses have not been determined.[71]

Magnetic resonance imaging

Magnetic resonance imaging (MRI) is a non-invasive method that can provide cardiac-specific biochemical information about factors such as tissue integrity, cardiac aneurysms, ejection fraction and cardiac output. These techniques are sometimes considered superior to radiography and ultrasound examination methods because the MRI is not affected by bone structure. The techniques include perfusion imaging, atherosclerosis imaging and coronary artery imaging.[72] MRI is considered an accurate method for predicting the presence of significant coronary artery disease.[73] However, MRI use in critically ill patients has its limitations. Because of the magnetic field required for this method, the patient cannot be fitted with any pumps or machines that have metal parts in them. Organising appropriate equipment for critically ill patients who are undergoing this test can be a challenge.

Nuclear medicine cardiac studies

There are several types of radionuclide imaging methods available to assess a patient's cardiac status, including radionuclide isotopes, thallium scan and stress test radionuclide scan.[17] The purpose of radionuclide imaging is to assess the perfusion status of cardiac muscle. When lowered perfusion in cardiac muscle is identified this may indicate heart muscle damage. Radionuclide imaging is often used in patients who have been diagnosed with a myocardial infarction when further investigation is required to determine if interventions such as cardiac stent or coronary artery bypass surgery are likely to benefit the patient.

Nursing care of patients undergoing diagnostic tests

All of the above methods have advantages and benefits in assessing the cardiac condition of a patient. For the critical care nurse, preparation of patients for these examinations is important because patients often need to be transported to the radiology or nuclear medicine departments. Important considerations include:

- Patient's allergy profile in relation to imaging contrast needs to be evaluated before the requests are made.
- These tests all require the patient to lie still for certain periods of time; therefore, explanation is essential and sedation may be required during the procedure.
- Appropriate equipment, such as non-metal equipment, needs to be organised beforehand if the patient is having an MRI study.

Summary

The cardiovascular system is essentially a transport system for distributing metabolic requirements to, and collecting byproducts from, cells throughout the body. A thorough understanding of anatomical structures and physiological events is critical to inform a comprehensive assessment of the critically ill patient. Findings from assessment should define patient cardiovascular status as well as inform the implementation of a timely clinical management plan. A thorough cardiac assessment requires the critical care nurse to be competent in a wide range of interpersonal, observational and technical skills.

Current minimum standards for critical care units in Australia and New Zealand require that patient monitoring include circulation, respiration and oxygenation. For many critically ill patients, haemodynamic instability is a potentially life-threatening condition that necessitates urgent action. In the critical care environment two main forms of cardiac monitoring are commonly employed: continuous cardiac monitoring and the 12-lead ECG. Accurate assessment of the patient's intracardiac status is frequently employed and often considered essential to guide management. Strong research evidence has shown that there is no increased harm or benefit in using pulmonary artery monitoring in critically ill patients; therefore the decision to use pulmonary artery monitoring as a diagnostic tool depends on the clinical need and clinician expertise. In day-to-day management of critically ill patients, critical care nurses must ensure they are skilled and educated in the techniques of non-invasive and invasive cardiovascular monitoring techniques and technologies, and be able to synthesise all data gathered and base their practice on the best available evidence to date.

Case study

Mr Andrew is a 40-year-old man who was admitted to the intensive care unit 14 days ago via the emergency department. He weighs 82 kg and is 173 cm tall. The following is a summary of the key events to date and his haemodynamic status currently.

Past medical history:

1 Long history of thrombocythaemia
2 Portal vein thrombosis

Regular medications on admission to hospital:

- Warfarin (titrated to INR range 2.0–3.0)
- Propranolol (80 mg sustained-release once a day)

Drug, alcohol and smoking habits:

- Nil

Allergies:

- None known

Presenting symptoms:

Admitted to emergency department with a 2-day history of PR bleeding and haematemesis. Commenced on Hartmann's solution (active ingredients sodium lactate, sodium chloride, potassium chloride, calcium) IV shortly after admission.

Sequence of events:

- Admitted to ICU 14 days ago from emergency with Sengstaken–Blakemore (SB) tube in situ and gastric balloon inflated.
- Patient was sedated and ventilated (see settings below).
- Recurrent PR bleeding on day 2 and became haemodynamically unstable.
- Transferred to theatre: SB tube removed and surgical banding of oesophageal varices attempted and failed. Gastrotomy performed and large clot removed from stomach. Actively bleeding varix over-sewn.
- Returned to ICU.
- Difficulties with ventilation 1 day postoperatively.
- Patient became haemodynamically unstable and pulmonary artery catheter inserted.
- Chest X-ray: bilateral pulmonary infiltrates.

- Cultures taken and commenced on IV antibiotics.
- Spiking high temperatures despite negative cultures.
- Sedated on morphine and midazolam infusion and commenced on synchronised intermittent mandatory volume (SIMV) control ventilation.

Patient observations and status currently:

Respiratory:

Size 8 ET tube,   ET cuff pressure 17 mmHg

Ventilated SIMV + pressure support (PS)

Ventilator settings: rate 12, TV 500 mL, FiO_2 0.6, PEEP 6 cmH_2O, PS 10 cmH_2O, flow 35 Lpm

Upper alarm (peak inspiratory pressure) set at 25 cmH_2O

I:E = 1:2.3

Minimal secretions on suction

Last arterial blood gas:

pH	7.30
PCO_2	49.0 mmHg
PO_2	78 mmHg
HCO_3	16 mmol/L
BE	−6.5
SaO_2	95%
Na	148 mmol/L
K	3.1 mmol/L

Cardiovascular:

BP   102/63 mmHg

ECG as follows (lead II)

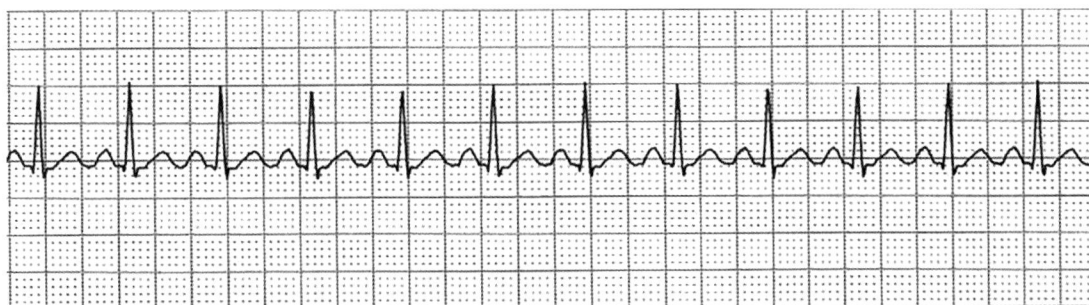

Haemodynamic parameters from pulmonary artery catheter:

CI	4.4 L/min/m^2
CVP	18 mmHg
PCWP	21 mmHg
SVRI	2311 dynes/s/cm^5/m^2

Neurological:

Opens eyes to command

Withdraws to painful stimuli

Pupils equal size 2–3 mm and reacting

Renal:

Urine output for last hour: 15 mL

Average urine output for past 6 hours 10–15 mL/h

Hydration:

N/saline @ 120 mL/h

Heparin infusion (25,000 IU in 500 mL) @ 20 mL/h

Midazolam (50 mg in 50 mL) @ 2 mL/h

Morphine (60 mg in 60 L) @ 2 mL/h

Noradrenaline (8 mg in 100 mL) @ 18 mL/h

20% Albumex @ 10 mL/h

Mannitol @ 10 mL/h

Previous days' balance + 3868

GIT/nutrition:

No nasogastric (NG) tube in situ

Blood sugar level (BSL) 6.1 mmol

Bowels: no record in patient notes

Integumentary/hygiene:

Temperature 38.4°C

Pressure areas intact

Currently supine

Dry dressing intact to abdominal wound

+2 pitting oedema in dependent areas

Sociopsychological:

Patient's wife and 3 children visit daily

DISCUSSION

This case study illustrates the complexities of critical illness in the presence of several risk factors and comorbidities. Initial non-invasive assessments following admission focused on assessment and management of intravascular volume depletion secondary to blood loss. When the patient's bleeding was controlled during surgery, he was transferred to the intensive care unit and invasive monitoring was required to guide patient management. As the patient's haemodynamic status became unstable, continuous invasive arterial monitoring aided titration of vasoconstrictor therapy and insertion of a central venous line aided with directing fluid therapy. At this stage, it would have been easy to have continued focusing on treating the patient's hypovolaemia but, in this case, the value of invasive pulmonary artery monitoring readings guided management direction with evidence of septic shock (hyperdynamic status, low intravascular filling pressures and peripheral vasodilation), prompting the commencement of a noradrenaline infusion.

For the critical care nurse at the bedside, this case demonstrates the need to be able to synthesise all assessment findings, invasive and non-invasive, and titrate prescribed therapies to achieve optimal tissue perfusion while providing holistic nursing care in a complex and changing environment. Without invasive monitoring, management of this patient would have been technically challenging and required a trial-and-error approach, especially with fluid and drug therapy, until a successful treatment plan was accomplished. This patient did ultimately get discharged from ICU to the medical ward several weeks later and was eventually discharged back home after 12 weeks hospitalisation.

CASE STUDY QUESTIONS

1 What is the patient's MAP from the BP reading above and how is it calculated?

2 What is the patient's rhythm on the rhythm strip above?

3 Calculate the patient's heart rate from the rhythm strip above.

4 The patient in this case study required invasive arterial monitoring. Discuss some of the potential complications of such monitoring and measures to prevent them.

5 In the case study above, the patient's SVRI is 2311 dynes/s/cm^5/m^2. Discuss SVRI: how it is derived and what high or low values indicate clinically.

RESEARCH VIGNETTE

Sotomi Y, Sato N, Kajimoto K, Sakata Y, Mizuno M, Minami Y et al. Impact of pulmonary artery catheter on outcome in patients with acute heart failure syndromes with hypotension or receiving inotropes: From the ATTEND Registry. Int J Cardiol 2014;172(1):165–172

Abstract

Background: Randomized controlled trials concerning pulmonary artery catheters (PACs) use have yielded little evidence of their beneficial effects on survival. This study aimed to evaluate the association between PACs and in-hospital mortality in patients with acute heart failure syndromes (AHFS).

Methods: The Acute Decompensated Heart Failure Syndromes (ATTEND) Registry is a prospective, observational, multicenter cohort study performed in Japan, since April 2007. We analyzed data from the ATTEND Registry and evaluated the effectiveness of PAC in AHFS treatment using propensity score-matching and the Cox proportional hazards model.

Results: Final follow-up examinations of the 4842 patients were conducted in December 2012. During the study period, 813 patients (16.8%) were managed with PACs, of which 502 patients (PAC group) were propensity score-matched with 502 controls (Control group). Of the 1004 score-matched patients, 22 (4.4%) patients from the Control group and 7 (1.4%) from the PAC group died. The risk of all-cause death was lower in the PAC group than that in the Control group [hazard ratio (HR), 0.3; 95% confidence interval (CI), 0.13–0.70; p = 0.006]. PAC-guided therapy decreased all-cause mortality in patients with lower systolic blood pressure (SBP $\leq$ 100 mmHg; HR, 0.09; 95% CI, 0.01–0.70; p = 0.021) or inotropic therapy (HR, 0.22; 95% CI, 0.08–0.57; p = 0.002).

Conclusions: This study revealed that appropriate PAC use effectively decreases in-hospital mortality in AHFS patients, particularly those with lower SBP or receiving inotropic therapy, suggesting that real-world PAC use could improve AHFS management.

Critique

In this paper the results of a multicentre, prospective observational study on the use of a pulmonary artery catheter (PAC) in acute heart failure syndromes (AHFS) are reported. The aim of the study was to evaluate the impact of PAC use in AHFS patients. The outcome measure was in-hospital mortality.

Data were collected using the Acute Decompensated Heart Failure Syndromes (ATTEND) Registry in Japanese hospitals from April 2007 to December 2011. Patients were assigned to two groups: the study group (with PAC inserted) and the control group (no PAC use). Please note, that the hospital follows the Japanese guidelines for treatment of AHFS, which recommend PAC use in AHFS patients. The allocation of the two groups was not randomised. To overcome the randomisation issue, the researchers used a propensity score-matching technique to eliminate the potential confounding factors in both groups. In simpler terms, the groups were comparable in terms of diagnosis, severity of illness and comorbidities. They score-matched a total of 502 patients in each group for final analysis.

The authors found that appropriate PAC use in AHFS patients effectively decreased in-hospital mortality, especially for those patients who had lower systolic blood pressure or who received inotropic therapy. Recent strong evidence suggests that PAC use does not alter mortality and hospital/ICU length of stay and that further study is needed to study the usefulness of PAC use in subgroup patients, such as patients in shock states, and in improving organ functions.[38] This study adds to the literature on PAC use in heart failure patients.

In their Cochrane review, Rajaram and colleagues[38] recommended that the PAC is a useful diagnostic tool to assist with patient management. Insertion and management of a PAC requires the operator to have a high level of clinical expertise to ensure patient safety. For the critical care nurse, competence in caring for patients with PACs is important. Being able to understand and manage the PAC, and recognise potential PAC-associated complications, is imperative. In recent years, the decreased use of PAC in clinical practice may be attributed to the available research evidence that suggests a PAC does not improve patient survival. Some argued that this reduced PAC use may have consequently contributed to the decrease in PAC clinical expertise.[22] Subsequently, critical care nurses may not have adequate exposure to PAC use in clinical practice, which adds challenge to managing staff training in PAC use.

Learning activities

1 Briefly discuss the main ion movement at each of the following phases of the cardiac action potential:
   - depolarisation
   - early rapid repolarisation
   - plateau phase
   - final rapid repolarisation
   - resting membrane phase.

2 Describe the correct placement of the precordial leads when doing a 12-lead ECG.

3 Describe what PQRST represents on an ECG and identify what is the normal duration for each segment.

4 Describe what systematic vascular resistance (SVR) is and what clinical condition can cause an elevated or lowered SVR.

5 Describe what are the limitations of central venous pressure (CVP) monitoring and why.

Online resources

American Heart Association, www.americanheart.org

Australian and New Zealand Intensive Care Society, www.anzics.com.au

Australian College of Critical Care Nurses, www.acccn.com.au

Australian Institute of Health and Welfare, www.aihw.gov.au

British Association of Critical Care Nurses, www.baccn.org.uk

Critical Care Forum, www.ccforum.com/home

Intensive Care, www.intensivecare.com

National Heart Foundation of Australia, www.heartfoundation.org.au

World Federation of Critical Care Nurses, www.wfccn.org

Further reading

Chung F-T, Lin S-M, Lin S-Y, Lin H-C. Impact of extravascular lung water index on outcomes of severe sepsis patients in a medical intensive care unit. Resp Med 2008;102(7):956–61.

Erkonen WE, Wilbur LS. Radiology 101: the basics and fundamentals of imaging. 3rd ed. Philadelphia, PA: Lippincott Williams & Wilkins; 2009.

Patil H, Vaidya O, Bogart D. A review of causes and systemic approach to cardiac troponin elevation. Clin Cardiol 2011;34(12):723–728.

Rajaram SS, Desai NK, Kalra A, Gajera M, Cavanaugh SK, Brampton W et al. Pulmonary artery catheters for adult patients in intensive care. Cochrane Database Syst Rev 2013;2:CD003408.

References

1 McCance K, Brashers VL. Structure and function of the cardiovascular and lymphatic systems. In: Huether SE, McCance K, eds. Understanding pathophysiology. 5th ed. St. Louis, Mo: Mosby; 2012.

2 Copstead L, Banasik J. Pathophysiology. 5th ed. St Louis, Mo: Elsevier Saunders; 2013.

3 Novak B, Filer L, Hatchett R. The applied anatomy and physiology of the cardiovascular system. In: Hatchett R, Thompson D, eds. Cardiac nursing: a comprehensive guide. Philadelphia: Churchill Livingstone Elsevier; 2002.

4 Guyton AC. Textbook of medical physiology. 12th ed. Philadelphia: Elsiever Saunders; 2010.

5 Boron WF, Boulpaep EL. Medical physiology. 2nd ed. Philadelphia: Saunders; 2008.

6 Craft J, Gordon C, Huether SE, Brashers VL. Understanding pathophysiology. Sydney: Mosby/Elsevier; 2011.

7 Bersten AD, Soni N, Oh TE. Oh's intensive care manual. 7th ed. Oxford: Butterworth-Heinemann; 2013.

8 Bucher L, Gallagher R. Nursing management: ECG monitoring and arrhythmias. 3rd ed. In: Brown D, Edwards H, eds. Lewis' medical and surgical nursing. Sydney: Mosby/Elsevier; 2012.

9 Elliott D. Shock. In: Romanini J, Daly J, eds. Critical care nursing: Australian perspectives. Sydney: Harcourt Brace; 1994. p 687.

10 Leeper B. Monitoring right ventricular volumes: a paradigm shift. AACN Clinical Issues 2003;14(2):208–19.

11 Sugerman RA. Structure and function of the neurological system. In: McClance KL, Huether SE, Brasher VL, Rote NS, eds. Pathophysiology: the biological basis for disease in adults and children. 6th ed. Maryland Heights: Mosby Elsevier; 2010.

12 Johnson K, Rawlings-Anderson K. Oxford handbook of cardiac nursing. 2nd ed. New York: Oxford University Press; 2014.

13 Australian and New Zealand College of Intensive Care Medicine (CICM). Minimum standards for intensive care units, <http://www.cicm.org.au/cms_files/IC-01MinimumStandardsForIntensiveCareUnits-Current September2011.pdf>; [accessed 05.14].

14 Andreas V, F. Patrick. Recommendations on basic requirements for intensive care units: structural and organizational aspects. Intensive Care Med 2011;37(10):1575-87.

15 Drew BJ, Califf RM, Funk M, Kaufman ES, Krucoff MW et al. Practice standards for electrocardiographic monitoring in hospital settings: an American Heart Association scientific statement from the Councils on Cardiovascular Nursing, Clinical Cardiology, and Cardiovascular Disease in the Young: Endorsed by the International Society of Computerized Electrocardiology and the American Association of Critical-Care Nurses. Circulation 2004;110(17):2721–6.

16 Shoemaker WC. Routine clinical monitoring in acute illness. In: Shoemaker WC, Vehmohos GC, Demetridas D, eds. Procedure and monitoring for the critically ill. Philadelphia: W.B. Saunders; 2002. pp 155–66.

17 Urden L, Stacy KL, Lough ME, eds. Critical care nursing: diagnosis and management. 6th ed. St Louis: Mosby/Elsevier; 2010.

18 Conover MB. Understanding electrocardiography. 8th ed. St Louis: Mosby; 2003.

19 Bayes de Luna. Clinical electrocardiography: A textbook. 4th ed. Chicester: Wiley; 2012.

20 Thygesen, K, Alpert JS, Jaffe AS, Simoons ML, Chaitman BR, White HD. Third universal definition of myocardial infarction. Am Coll Cardiol 2012;60(16):1581-1598.

21 Sims DB, Sperling LS. ST-segment elevation resulting from hyperkaelemia. Circulation 2005;111:295-296.

22 Tsang R. Hemodynamic monitoring in the cardiac intensive care unit. Congenital Heart Dis 2013;8(6):568-575.

23 Muller JC, Kennard JW, Browne JS, Fecher AM, Hayward TZ. Hemodynamic monitoring in the intensive care unit. Nutr Clin Pract 2012;27(3):340-51.

24 McGhee BH, Bridges MEJ. Monitoring arterial blood pressure: what you may not know. Crit Care Nurse 2002;22(2):60–79.

25 Quaal SJ. Improving the accuracy of pulmonary artery catheter measurements. J Cardiovas Nurs 2001 15(2):71–82.

26 Australian Council on Health Standards. Clinical indicator user manual 2012: intensive care version 4. Melbourne, Australia; ACHS; 2012. p 68.

27 O'Sullivan J, Allen J, Murray A. The forgotten Korotkoff phases: how often are phases II and III present and how often do they relate to the other Korotkoff phases? Am J Hypertension 2002;15(3):264–8.

28 Woodrow P. Central venous catheters and central venous pressure. Nurs Stand 2002;16(26):45–51.

29 Bellomo R, Uchino S. Cardiovascular monitoring tools: use and misuse. Curr Opin Crit Care 2003;9(3):225–9.

30 Kumar A, Anel R, Bunnell E, Habet K, Zanotti S, Marshall S et al. Pulmonary artery occlusion pressure and central venous pressure fail to predict ventricular filling volume, cardiac performance, or the response to volume infusion in normal subjects. Crit Care Med 2004;32(3):691–9.

31 Schummer W. Central venous pressure. Validity, informative value and correct measurement. Anaesthetist 2009;58(5):499–505.

32 McGee DC, Gould MK. Current concepts: preventing complications of central venous catheterization. N Engl J Med 2003;348(12):1123–33.

33 Truwit JD. Technique and measurements: getting a line on the hemodynamic undercurrent. J Crit Illness 2003;18(1):9–20.

34 Ruesch S, Walder B, Tramèr MR. Complications of central venous catheters: internal jugular versus subclavian access – a systematic review. Crit Care Med 2003;30(2):454–60.

35 Rubinson L, Diette GB. Best practices for insertion of central venous catheters in intensive care units to prevent catheter-related bloodstream infections. J Lab Clin Med 2004;143(1):5–13.

36 Swanz HJ, Ganz W, Forrester J, Marcus H, Diamond G, Chonette D. Catheterisation of the heart in man with use of flow-directed balloon-tipped catheter. N Engl J Med 1970;283(9):447–51.

37 Truwit JD. The pulmonary artery catheter in the ICU, part 2: clinical applications; how to interpret the hemodynamic picture. J Crit Illness 2003;18(2):63–71.

38 Rajaram SS, Desai NK, Kalra A, Gajera M, Cavanaugh SK, Brampton W et al. Pulmonary artery catheters for adult patients in intensive care. Cochrane Database Syst Rev 2013;2:CD003408.

39 Cruz K, Franklin C. The pulmonary artery catheter: uses and controversies. Crit Care Clinics 2001;17(2):271–91.

40 Bridges EJ. Pulmonary artery pressure monitoring: when, how, and what else to use. AACN Adv Crit Care 2006;7(3):286–303.

41 Ritzema J, Troughton R, Melton I, Crozier I, Doughty R, Krum H et al. Physician-directed patient self-management of left atrial pressure in advanced chronic heart failure. Circulation 2010;121(9):1086–95.

42 Roşca M, Lancellotti P, Popescu BA, Piérard LA. Left atrial function: pathophysiology, echocardiographic assessment, and clinical applications. Heart 2011;97(23):1982-89.

43 Carelock J, Clark AP. Heart failure: pathophysiologic mechanisms. Am J Nurs 2001;101(12):26–33.

44 Lough ME, Thompson CL. Cardiovascular diagnostic procedures. In: Urden LD, Stacey KM, Lough ME, eds. Critical care nursing: diagnosis and management. St Louis, Mo: Elsevier; 2014. pp 502-13.

45 Moser DK, Reigel B. Cardiac nursing: a companion to Brauwald's heart disease. St Louis: Elsevier; 2008.

46 Faybik P, Hetz H, Baker A, Yankovskaya E, Krenn CG, Steltzer H. Iced versus room temperature injectate for assessment of cardiac output, intrathoracic blood volume and extravascular lung water by single transpulmonary thermodilution. J Crit Care 2004;19(2):103–7.

47 Cottis R, Magee N, Higgins DJ. Haemodynamic monitoring with pulse-induced contour cardiac output (PiCCO) in critical care. Intens Crit Care Nurs 2003;19(5):301–7.

48 Litton E, Morgan M. The PiCCO monitor: a review. Anaesthesia Intensive Care 2012;40:393-409.

49 Chung F-T, Lin S-M, Lin S-Y, Lin H-C. Impact of extravascular lung water index on outcomes of severe sepsis patients in a medical intensive care unit. Resp Med 2008;102(7):956–61.

50 Martin GS, Eaton S, Mealer M, Moss M. Extravascular lung water in patients with severe sepsis: a prospective cohort study. Crit Care 2005;9(2):74–82.

51 King S, Lim T. The use of the oesophageal Doppler monitor in the intensive care unit. Crit Care Resusc 2004;6(2):113–22.

52 Singer M. Oesophageal Doppler. Curr Opin Crit Care 2009;15:244-8.

53 Wilson RJT. Oesophageal Doppler monitoring – the emperor's new clothes? Anaesthesia 2013;68:1072-85.

54 Turner MA. Doppler-based haemodynamic monitoring. AACN Clin Issues 2003;14(2):220-31.

55 Haas LEM, Tjan DHT, van Wees J, van Zanten ARH, eds. Validation of the USCOM-1A cardiac output monitor in hemodynamic unstable intensive care patients. Conference Paper: Annual Intensive Care Society Congress, Netherlands; 2006.

56 Lasater M, VonRueden KT. Outpatient cardiovascular management utilizing impedance cardiography. AACN Clin Issues 2003;14(2):240–50.

57 Kamath SA, Drazner MH, Tasissa G, Rogers JG, Stevenson LW, Yancy CW. Correlation of impedance cardiography with invasive hemodynamic measurements in patients with advanced heart failure: the BioImpedance CardioGraphy (BIG) substudy of the Evaluation Study of Congestive Heart Failure and Pulmonary Artery Catheterization Effectiveness (ESCAPE) Trial. Am Heart J 2009;158(2):217-33.

58 Sageman WS, Riffenburgh RH, Spiess BD. Equivalence of bioimpedance and thermodilution in measuring cardiac index after cardiac surgery. J Cardiothoracic Vasc Anesthesia 2002;16(1):8–14.

59 Raaijmakers E, Faes TJ, Scholten RJ, Goovaerts HG, Heethaar RM. A meta-analysis of three decades of validating thoracic impedance cardiography. Crit Care Med 1999;27(6):1203–13.

60 Almeida AG, Sargento L, Gabriel HM, da Costa JM, Morais J, Madeira F et al. Evaluation of aortic stenosis severity: role of contrast echocardiography in comparison with conventional echocardiography and cardiac catheterization. Portuguese J Cardiol 2002;21(5):555–72.

61 Baumgartner H, Hung J, Bermejo J, Chambers JB, Evangelista A, Griffin BP et al. Echocardiographic assessment of valve stenosis: EAE/ASE Recommendations for clinical practice. Morrisville, NC: American Society of Echocardiography; 2010.

62 Royal College of Pathologists Australasia. RCPA manual. Version 46, <http://www.rcpa.edu.au/ Publications/RCPAManual.htm>; 2011 [accessed 03.11].

63 Pagana KD. Mosby's diagnostic and laboratory test reference. 8th ed. St Louis: Mosby/Elsevier; 2007.

64 Patil H, Vaidya O, Bogart D. A review of causes and systemic approach to cardiac troponin elevation. Clin Cardiol 2011;34(12):723-28.

65 Erkonen WE, Wilbur LS. Radiology 101: the basics and fundamentals of imaging. 3rd ed. Philadelphia, PA: Lippincott Williams & Wilkins; 2009.

66 Lareau C, Wootton J. The 'frequently' normal chest x-ray. Canadian J Rural Med 2004;9(3):183–6.

67 Malcolm J, Arnold O. Heart failure. The MERCK manual for healthcare professionals, <http://www.merckmanuals.com/ professional/sec07/ch074/ch074a.html>; 2009.

68 McGoon M, Gutterman D, Steen V, Barst R, McCrory DC, Fortin TA et al. Screening, early detection, and diagnosis of pulmonary arterial hypertension: ACCP evidence-based clinical practice guidelines. Chest 2004;126(1 Suppl):S14–34.

69 Parmet S, Lynm C, Glass RM. Pericarditis. JAMA 2003;289(9):1194.

70 Wijesekera NT, Duncan MK, Padley SPG. X-ray computed tomography of the heart. Brit Med Bull 2010;93:49–67.

71 Ropers D. Multislice computer tomography for detection of coronary artery disease. J Interventional Cardiol 2006;19:574–82.

72 Lima J, Desai M. Cardiovascular magnetic resonance imaging: current and emerging applications. J Am College Cardiol 2004;44:1164–71.

73 Paetsch I, Gebker R, Fleck E, Nagel E. Cardiac magnetic resonance imaging: a noninvasive tool for functional and morphological assessment of coronary artery diease: current clinical applications and potential future concepts. J Interventional Cardiol 2003;16:457–63.

Chapter 10

Cardiovascular alterations and management

Robyn Gallagher, Andrea Driscoll

Robyn Gallagher, Andrea Driscoll

KEY WORDS

acute coronary
   syndrome

acute heart failure

aortic aneurysm

arrhythmia

cardiomyopathy

endocarditis

hypertensive
   emergencies

left ventricular failure

myocardial
   infarction

percutaneous
   coronary
   intervention

right ventricular
   failure

ventricular
   aneurysm

Learning objectives

After reading this chapter, you should be able to:

- explain the pathophysiology of coronary artery disease, clinical manifestations of acute coronary syndromes and management of events
- discuss the collaborative care for a patient with chest pain
- list the diagnostic tests used to assess myocardial ischaemia
- outline the actions and contraindications of thrombolytic drugs
- outline the clinical manifestations of right and left ventricular failure
- discuss the goals of heart failure treatment
- discuss the pathophysiologies of the four different types of cardiomyopathy and how they affect cardiac function
- outline the actions of angiotensin-converting enzyme inhibitors, beta-blockers, loop diuretics and spironolactone and how they relate to the pathophysiology of heart failure.

Introduction

This chapter reviews the support of cardiovascular function in the face of many compromises to the system. It focuses on two of the most prevalent and fatal diseases affecting the heart: coronary heart disease and heart failure. These diseases are also a common comorbidity in elderly patients admitted to critical care units. The first section on coronary heart disease reviews the pathophysiological concepts of myocardial ischaemia and associated complications, with detailed consideration of the clinical implications, assessment and associated management. Heart failure is discussed in terms of the body's compensatory mechanisms and the clinical sequelae and associated clinical features of heart failure. Nursing and medical management is outlined including the management of acute exacerbations of heart failure. Finally, other cardiovascular disorders commonly managed in critical care units are reviewed, ranging from other forms of heart failure to hypertensive emergencies and aortic aneurysms. The case study presented at the end of the chapter highlights the key aspects of the management of coronary heart disease and heart failure in patients admitted to critical care units.

Coronary heart disease

Coronary heart disease (CHD) is the term used to describe the effects of a reduction or complete obstruction of blood flow through the coronary arteries due to narrowing from atherosclerosis and/or thrombus. Although some patients may be asymptomatic, the most common manifestations of CHD are chest pain due to angina, acute coronary syndrome (ACS, a term used to collectively describe acute myocardial infarction [AMI] and unstable angina) and sudden death. CHD may also cause arrhythmias and heart failure.[1]

CHD is now the leading single cause of death, premature death and disability both globally[2] and in Australia and New Zealand.[3–5] In 2011, more than 21,500 people died of CHD in Australia, more than 5000 in New Zealand in 2006 and in 2010 more than 7 million worldwide.[2–5] Death rates have fallen by about 76% since the 1960s, primarily due to improvements in risk factors and health care for those at risk. However, the burden of CHD remains high, with 11% of males and 9% of females impacted by the disease in Australia.[3] Furthermore, the impact of this disease worldwide is forecast to be substantial, with an increase of 28% in deaths between 1990 and 2010.[2]

Myocardial ischaemia

When coronary blood flow is insufficient to meet myocardial tissue demand for oxygen, myocardial ischaemia occurs. Critical restriction to blood flow occurs when the diameter of the lumen of the blood vessel is reduced by more than half. Coronary blood flow is also determined by perfusion pressure, which can be adversely affected by abnormalities in blood flow (valvular disease), vessel wall (coronary spasm) and the blood (anaemia, polycythaemia).[6] Myocardial oxygen demand is influenced by heart rate, strength of myocardial contraction and left ventricular wall tension. The myocardium receives most of its blood supply during diastole; hence a rise in heart rate that decreases the duration of diastole will also decrease coronary perfusion. Sympathetic stimulation increases the force of contraction and therefore oxygen demand. Left ventricular wall tension increases with the changes in preload associated with filling and afterload associated with systemic vascular resistance. During activity, pyrexia and arrhythmias, these effects may compound due to sympathetic stimulation, causing increased oxygen demand and reduced coronary perfusion.

Angina

Angina (angina pectoris) is the most common manifestation of CHD and is the term used to describe the symptoms of discomfort that occur during myocardial ischaemia. The classic angina pattern consists of retrosternal constricting pain/discomfort, which may radiate to the arms, throat, jaw, teeth, back or epigastrium. Associated symptoms often include shortness of breath, nausea, vomiting, sweating, palpitations and weakness.

A fixed coronary artery lesion, causing limitation of oxygen supply at times of increased demand, results in stable angina. Therefore, symptoms arise during periods of physical and emotional stress and resolve within 2–10 minutes of rest. Symptoms tend to be worse in the morning (coinciding with a peak in blood pressure), after heavy meals and in cold weather. The severity of symptoms has little correlation with the progress of the disease. However, a patient with a typical history of angina has a high probability of CHD and a higher risk of AMI and coronary death during the next 5 years.[7]

Unstable angina and acute myocardial infarction

Unstable angina and AMI form a continuum on the basis of reduction in coronary blood flow and subsequent damage to myocardial cells. Unstable angina may indicate transient ischaemia, whereas AMI indicates myocardial tissue death. The term 'acute coronary syndrome' (ACS) is now used to represent this continuum.[8,9] ACS results from the rupture or erosion of an atherosclerotic plaque, leading to release of vasoconstrictor substances and potentially triggering coagulation activity (see Figure 10.1). Formation of thrombi results in intermittent and/or prolonged obstruction of the coronary artery. Therefore, ACS typically presents as a recent history of angina (within the past 4–6 weeks); a change in symptoms including increased frequency, more easily provoked or occurring in the absence of physical or emotional stress, more severe or prolonged and/or less responsive to nitrate therapy. ACS is a medical emergency, with up to a third of ACS patients at risk of AMI and death within 3 months.[9] There is a high risk of death if the patient experiences more than 20 minutes of pain at rest (pain at rest is associated with changes in ST segment of 1 mm or more on a 12-lead ECG), if there was myocardial infarction within the previous 2 weeks or if pulmonary oedema or mitral regurgitation is present.[8]

Myocardial infarction (MI) occurs when blood flow to the myocardium is severely impaired for more than 20 minutes as myocardial cell necrosis begins. A coronary artery thrombus arising from an atherosclerotic plaque is found in the majority of patients dying of AMI.[10] Cellular death begins in the subendocardial layer and progresses through the full muscle thickness, so that by 2 hours with total occlusion a full 'transmural' infarction will result. However, the full extent of tissue death may occur as a single incident or evolve over several days, depending on the degree of obstruction to blood flow.

The size and location of the infarction will influence the clinical manifestations and risk of death and determine treatment. The size of the infarction is determined by the extent, severity and duration of the ischaemic event, the amount of collateral circulation and the metabolic demands placed on the myocardium. Usually the ventricle wall is affected, with a small infarction often resulting in a dyskinetic wall (altered movement), whereas a large infarction may result in akinesis (no movement).

FIGURE 10.1 **(A)** Plaque rupture exposes thrombogenic lipid. A white thrombus is formed by activated platelets adhering. This lesion is unstable and may lead to thrombin activation. **(B)** Thrombin activation leads to a mesh of fibrin and red blood cells, leading to a 'red thrombus'.

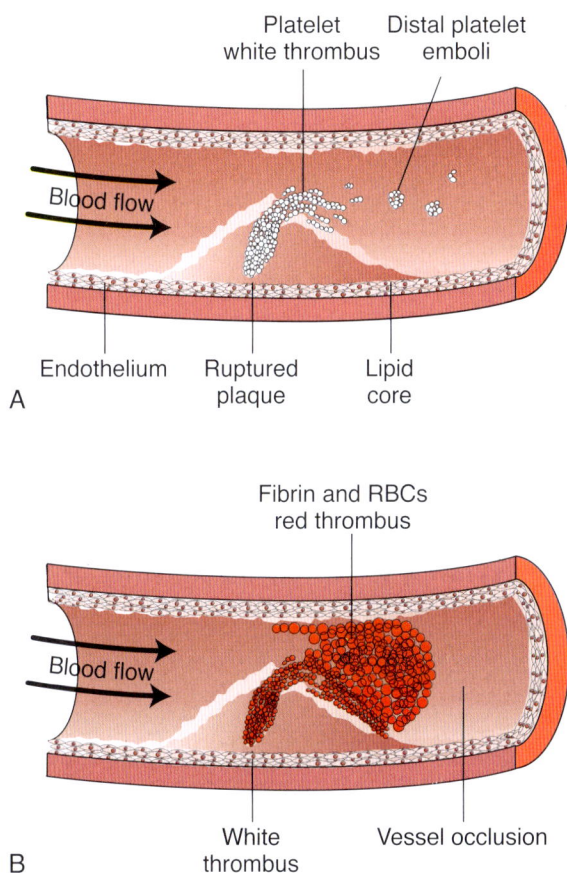

Platelet white thrombus   Distal platelet emboli

Blood flow

Endothelium   Ruptured plaque   Lipid core

A

Fibrin and RBCs red thrombus

Blood flow

White thrombus   Vessel occlusion

B

Adapted from Bersten AD, Soni N, Oh TE. Oh's intensive care manual. 5th ed. Oxford: Butterworth-Heineman; 2003, with permission.

The location and impact of the infarction will depend on which coronary artery has been obstructed:

- Left anterior descending (LAD) affects the function of the left ventricle and interventricular septum, including ventricular conduction tissue. Patients with anteroseptal MI are at high risk of heart failure, cardiogenic shock and mortality due to pump deficits.

- Circumflex (CX) affects the left ventricle lateral and posterior walls and the SA node in 50% of people.[6] The impact on pump efficiency of lateral and posterior wall necrosis is not as severe as anteroseptal infarctions, although patients are at more risk of arrhythmias.

- Right coronary artery (RCA) affects the inferior wall of the left ventricle and the right ventricle, as

well as the AV node in most patients and the SA node in 50% of people. There is potentially severe impact on ventricular function if both the inferior wall and the right ventricle are affected, as well as a high risk of arrhythmias due to SA and AV node involvement.

Clinical features

Patients with AMI most often present with chest pain. This pain is described as central crushing retrosternal pain, which lasts longer than 20 minutes and is not relieved by nitrate therapy. The pain may radiate to the neck, jaw, back and shoulders and is often accompanied by 'feelings of impending doom', sweating and pallor. Nausea is often associated with the pain, due to vagal nerve stimulation. Depending on the size and location of the AMI, patients may also present as sudden death and with varying degrees of syncope and heart failure. Women may present with different symptoms.

Patient assessment and diagnostic features

A key feature of assessment of the patient with chest pain is the use of protocols and guidelines to promote rapid assessment so that revascularisation procedures such as thrombolysis and percutaneous coronary intervention (PCI) can be implemented as soon as possible. This means that assessment may begin as early as in the ambulance, with ECG transmission to the hospital emergency department where rapid, early triage models of care are in place.[11] Additionally, assessment needs to determine whether there are any contraindications for thrombolysis.

The assessment method used depends on the condition of the patient but should occur within 10 minutes of arrival.[10] This initial history will focus on the nature of symptoms such as pain. Pain assessment is complex, and the use of an acronym such as PQRST (see Table 10.1) is useful to incorporate precipitating and palliative factors, qualitative descriptors, location, radiation, severity and length of time. A pain scale is included to help rate the intensity of pain. Asking patients for descriptive words is useful in assessment as many patients will deny pain and instead use words such as pressure, tightness or constriction. It is essential not to ignore other presentations, as patients with atypical symptoms, such as women, often have a delayed diagnosis and treatment and a higher mortality (50%) than those with typical symptoms (18%).[8] Differentiating this pain from any previous pain is also useful. The brief history should include a short cardiovascular risk profile: 1) previous cardiac history such as angina, MI, revascularisation and 2) family history, smoking, hypertension, diabetes.

A more complete history, which includes detailed information about risk factors, can be acquired when the patient is stabilised. This information will be essential to guide patient education and rehabilitation and to plan discharge. Recurrent chest discomfort requires urgent reassessment, including immediate ECG.

TABLE 10.1

The PQRST criteria for assessing chest pain[12]

P	Precipitating	Exercise and activity
		Stress and anxiety
		Cold weather
	Palliating	Stop activity
		Rest
		Nitroglycerin
Q	Quality	Heavy, tight, choking, vice-like, constricting
R	Region, Radiation	Left side of chest, shoulder, arm and jaw
		Retrosternal and radiating to the neck
S	Severity	Rate pain on scale of 1 (no pain) to 10 (worst pain possible)
T	Time	Pain lasts longer than 10 min despite nitroglycerin
		Pain comes and goes but lasts longer than 20 min

Adapted from Hudak CM, Gallo BM, Morton PG. Critical care nursing, A holistic approach. 7th ed. Philadelphia: Lippincott; 1998, with permission.

Practice tip

Because of changes in neuroreceptors, older patients and diabetic patients may not describe the typical anginal pain. Women also may not describe classic angina symptoms and may use different descriptors from men.[8] Be alert for prodromal symptoms, such as increased shortness of breath, weakness and fainting.

Physical examination

Physical manifestations vary and depend on the impact of pain, size and location of the infarction in the individual. Heart rate and blood pressure may be raised due to anxiety. Impaired left ventricular function may result in dyspnoea, tachycardia, hypotension, pallor, sweating, nausea and vomiting. Impaired right ventricular function may be indicated by jugular vein distension and peripheral oedema. Abnormalities in heart sounds may be present, including a muffled and diminished first heart sound due to decreased contractility. A fourth heart sound is common, whereas a third heart sound is uncommon. Many patients develop a pericardial rub after about 48–72 hours due to an inflammatory response to the damaged myocardium. Additional findings occur with complications, and these are discussed in the related specific sections below.

Electrocardiographic examination

Patients with chest discomfort should be assessed by an appropriately qualified person and have a 12-lead ECG recorded within 5 minutes of arrival at a healthcare facility to determine the presence and extent of myocardial

ischaemia, the risk of adverse events and to provide a baseline for subsequent changes.[8] Most importantly, the ECG is essential to determine whether emergency reperfusion is required, and is recommended as the sole test for selecting patients for PCI or thrombolysis. Where ST-segment monitoring is available, this should be continuous. Alternatively, if chest discomfort persists, ECGs should be repeated every 15 minutes. Even when chest pain resolves it is important to record a series of 12-lead ECGs during admission to determine changes over time. (The normal ECG is covered in Chapter 9, whereas this section addresses ischaemic changes in the ECG.)

Myocardial ischaemia, injury or infarction causes cellular alterations and affects depolarisation and repolarisation.[13] Myocardial ischaemia may be a transient finding on the ECG. Ischaemia results in T-wave inversion or ST-segment depression in the leads facing the ischaemic area.[14] Ischaemic T waves are usually symmetrical, narrower and more pointed. ST-segment depression of 1 mm for 0.08 seconds is indicative of ischaemia, especially when forming a sharp angle with an upright T wave.[15] These changes are reversible with reduction in demand (e.g. by rest, nitrates).

On acute presentation, myocardial injury (infarction) is most commonly associated with ST-segment elevation on the ECG, although this is not universal. In addition, a typical pattern of ECG changes over time (evolution of the ST segments, Q-wave development and T-wave inversion) is often seen (described below), but these changes too are not universal. The distinction between the various acute coronary syndromes, including ST-elevation acute coronary syndrome (STEACS), ST-elevation myocardial infarction (STEMI) and non-ST-elevation myocardial infarction (non-STEMI), is important for ensuring appropriate assessment and protocol-based treatment[16] for the various presentations.

The location and extent of ischaemia or infarction may be evident on the ECG leads overlying the affected area, as follows:

- anteroseptal wall of left ventricle, V1–V4
- anterior wall of the left ventricle, V1–V6, I and aVL
- lateral wall of left ventricle, I, aVL, V5 and V6
- inferior wall of left ventricle, II, III and aVF.

Additional leads are needed to view the right ventricle and posterior wall. Chest electrodes can be placed on the right chest wall using the same landmarks as the left chest to view the right ventricle (see Chapter 9). Further electrodes, V7–V9, may be placed over the posterior of the left chest to view the posterior wall. Other indicative signs of posterior wall damage are a small r wave in V1 and/or ST depression in V3 and V4, as these may be reciprocal changes. The endocardial surface of the posterior wall faces the precordial leads of the ECG so the signs of ischaemia and infarction, such as ST depression or a small r wave, are reversed or reciprocal. If these signs are present a left-sided

ECG, V7–V9, should be done to confirm or rule out a posterior infarction.

Continuous ECG monitoring is essential to detect arrhythmias, which often accompany AMI and are a common cause of death. The arrhythmia may be due to poor perfusion of the conduction tissue. More often, arrhythmias occur because ischaemic tissue has a lower fibrillatory threshold and ischaemia is not being managed. Arrhythmias also result from left ventricular failure.

Typical ECG evolution pattern

The initial ECG features of myocardial infarction are ST-segment elevation with tall T waves recorded in leads overlying the area of damaged myocardium. These changes gradually change, or evolve, over time, with ST segments returning to baseline (within hours), while Q waves develop (hours to days) and T waves become inverted (days to weeks). The time course for the evolutionary changes is accelerated by reperfusion, e.g. PCI, thrombolysis or surgery. Thus, an almost fully-evolved pattern may be seen within hours if successful reperfusion has been undertaken (see Figures 10.2–10.4 for examples). Given the expected time course for evolution, it is possible to approximate how recently infarction has occurred, which is essential in determining management:

- Acute (or hyperacute): there is ST elevation but Q waves or T inversion has not yet developed (see Figure 10.5).

- Recent: Q waves have developed. ST-segment elevation may still be present. Evolution is underway. The infarction is more than 24 hours old.

- Old (fully evolved): Q waves and T inversion are present. ST segments are no longer elevated. Infarction occurred anything from a few days to years ago.

Biochemical markers

Intracellular cardiac enzymes enter the blood as ischaemic cells die, and elevated levels are used to confirm myocardial infarction and estimate the extent of cell death. The cardiac troponins T and I (cTnT and cTnI) have been found to be both sensitive and specific measures of cardiac muscle damage.[17] Troponin I is rapidly released into the bloodstream, so it is especially useful for the diagnosis and subsequent risk stratification of patients presenting with chest pain in the early stages. High sensitivity troponin T assays are being used increasingly, but lack specificity, especially when trauma and renal disease are present. Troponin I is also a more appropriate marker to use in postoperative and trauma patients than creatine kinase-MB (CK-MB), as CK-MB levels will be affected by muscle damage. However, CK-MB is less costly and more readily available, and so is still often used, particularly in the presence of a non-diagnostic ECG. C-reactive protein assays may prove to be useful, as baseline and discharge levels are predictive of subsequent cardiac events. However, the laboratory facilities are not readily available.

FIGURE 10.2 Acute inferoposterior infarction: ST elevation in indicative leads II, III and aVF. The ST-segment depression in I and aVL is reciprocal to the inferior infarction. As well, ST depression in anterior leads (V1–V3) is reciprocal to posterior wall infarction. Posterior leads (not shown here) were recorded and revealed ST elevation in V7, V8 and V9. This patient had acute (100%) obstruction at the ostium of the right coronary artery.

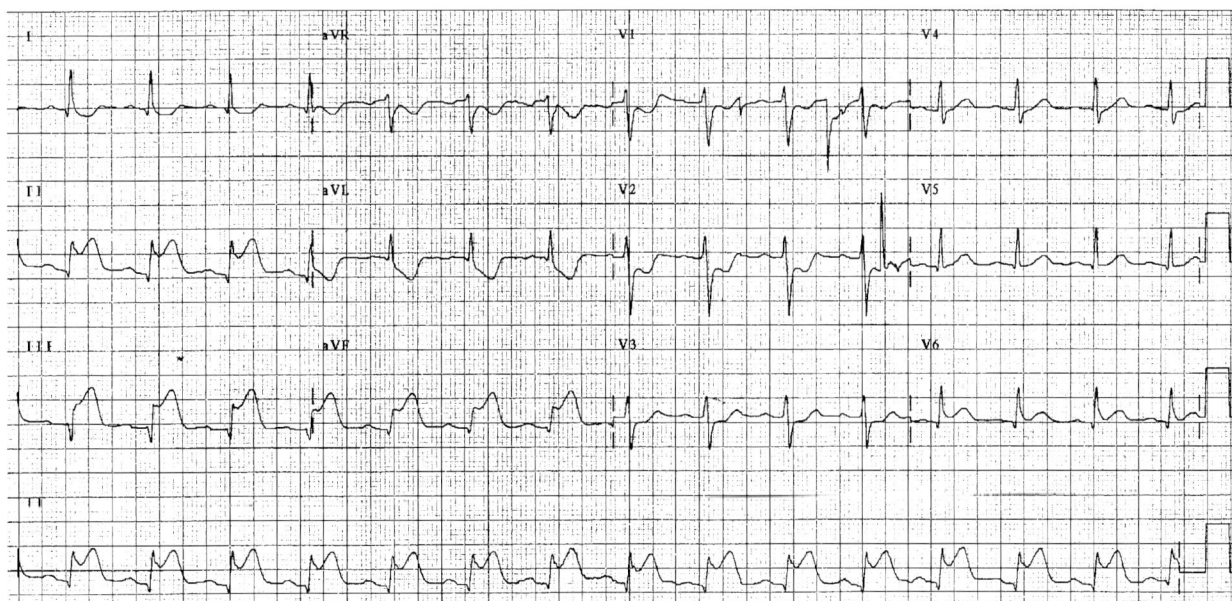

FIGURE 10.3   The same patient as above, recorded only 1 hour later, after stenting of the right coronary artery with an evolving inferoposterior infarction. Note the ST segments in II, III and aVF are still elevated but returning to baseline. The reciprocal ST depression is likewise diminishing and can now be seen only in aVL, V1 and V2. Q waves have already developed in inferior leads.

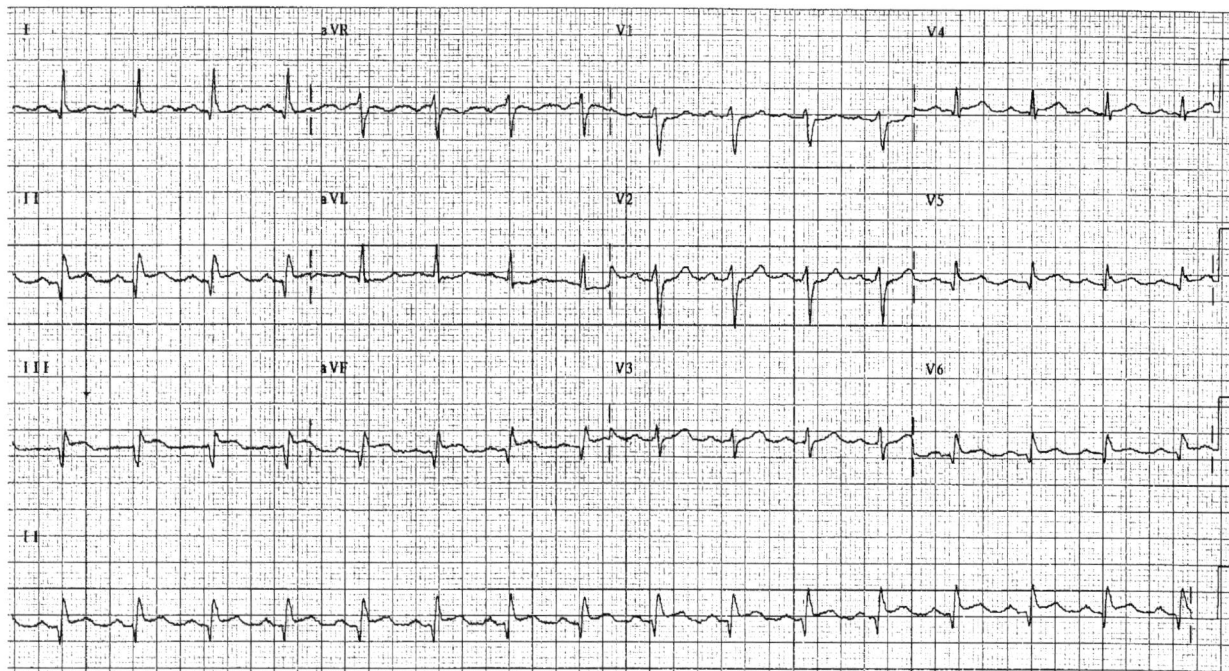

FIGURE 10.4   The same patient again, recorded a further 21 hours later. An almost fully evolved pattern is now present. Note the ST segments inferiorly have almost completely returned to baseline (as have the reciprocal changes). The Q waves remain, and T waves have now inverted inferiorly.

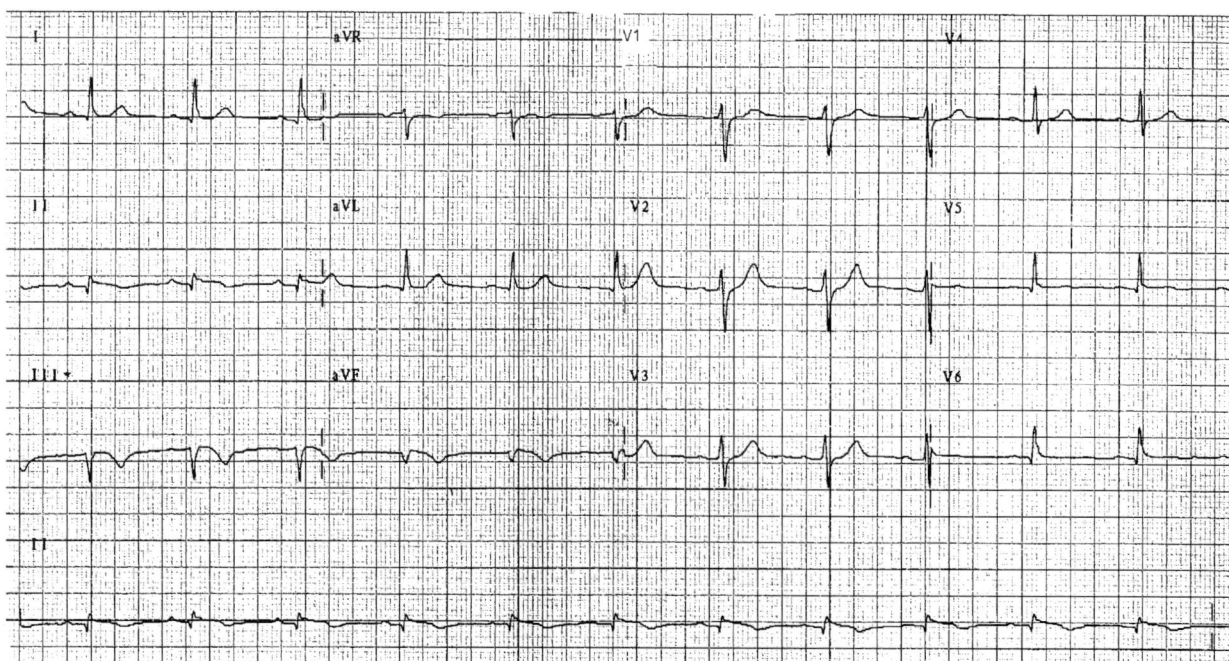

FIGURE 10.5 Acute anterolateral infarction in a patient with left anterior descending coronary artery obstruction. Note the ST elevation and tall (hyperacute) T waves across the chest leads V1–V6. ECG recorded on admission.

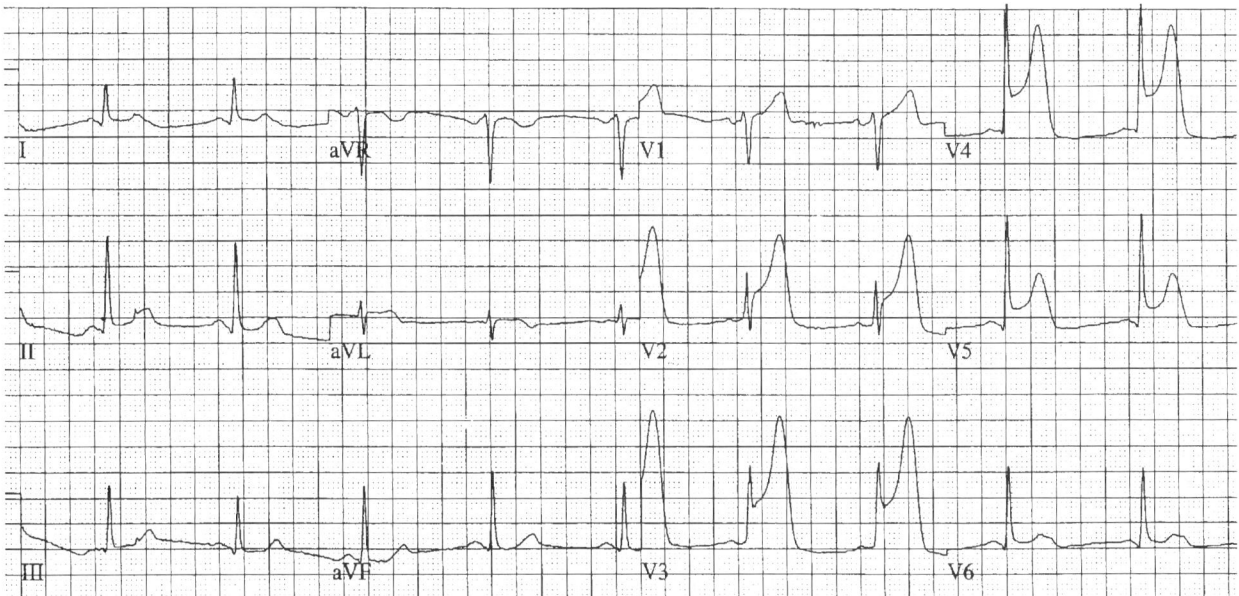

Coronary angiography and left heart catheterisation

Coronary angiography gives a detailed record of coronary artery anatomy and pathophysiology. Specially designed catheters are advanced with the assistance of a guidewire into the ascending aorta via the femoral or brachial arteries and manoeuvred into the ostium of each coronary artery. Contrast media is then injected and images are taken from several views to provide detailed information on the extent, site and severity of coronary artery lesions and the blood flow into each artery. This flow is graded using the Thrombolysis in Myocardial Infarction (TIMI) studies system (see Table 10.2).[1] Typically, a left ventricular angiogram is performed during the same procedure to assess the appearance and function of the left ventricle, mitral and aortic valves. If CHD is present, treatment is determined as appropriate according to the severity

(percutaneous coronary intervention [PCI], coronary artery bypass grafting or medical therapy). The nursing care for coronary angiography is similar to PCI, and is covered under that section.

Exercise test

Exercise testing with ECG monitoring forms part of the diagnostic screen for patients suspected of stable angina. The Bruce protocol is used most often and considered positive for CHD if there is 1 mm or more of reversible ST-segment depression.[19] False-positive tests are more common in populations with a lower incidence of CHD, including women.[20]

Chest radiography

An initial chest X-ray film is useful to exclude other causes of chest pain, such as pneumonia, pneumothorax

TABLE 10.2

Thrombolysis in myocardial infarction (TIMI) flow grades in coronary arteries[18]

TIMI 0	No perfusion and no antegrade flow beyond the occlusion
TIMI 1	Penetration with minimal perfusion, and contrast does not opacify the entire bed distal to the stenosis during the picture run
TIMI 2	Partial perfusion and contrast opacifies the entire coronary bed distal to the stenosis, although entry to this area is slower than with unaffected coronary beds
TIMI 3	Complete perfusion and filling and clearance of contrast is rapid and comparable to other coronary beds

Adapted from Belenkie I, Knudtson ML, Roth DL, Hansen JL, Traboulsi M, Hall CA et al. Relation between flow grade after thrombolytic therapy and the effect of angioplasty on left ventricular function: a prospective randomized trial. Am Heart J 1991; 121(2 Pt 1):407–16, with permission.

and aortic aneurysm, and to assess whether heart failure and/or pulmonary congestion are present. If the diagnosis is clearly ACS or AMI, this step can wait until after thrombolysis or PCI.

Patient management

The management of stable angina patients is aimed at: 1) secondary prevention of cardiac events, 2) symptom control with medication, 3) revascularisation and 4) rehabilitation (see Figure 10.6). (Revascularisation by coronary artery bypass graft is reviewed in Chapter 12; revascularisation by percutaneous coronary angioplasty is reviewed in the next section.)

Treatment of acute coronary syndrome aims at rapid diagnosis and prompt re-establishment of flow through the occluded artery to ensure myocardial perfusion and reduce the size of infarction. In addition, treatment aims to:[21]

- minimise the area of myocardial ischaemia by increasing coronary perfusion and decreasing myocardial workload
- maximise oxygen delivery to tissues
- control pain and sympathetic stimulation
- counter detrimental effects of reperfusion
- preserve ventricular function
- reduce morbidity and mortality.

The ideal place to manage ACS or MI patients is in the coronary care unit, where continuous, specialised nursing care is available and there is rapid access to treatments.[22] Secondary prevention of cardiac events includes the provision of medications, such as antiplatelet therapy and lipid-lowering therapy.[23]

Reperfusion therapy

Reperfusion therapy includes coronary angioplasty, ideally with stent and thrombolytic therapy (also termed fibrinolysis). Patients fast-tracked for reperfusion therapy have one or more of the following indications: 1) ischaemic or infarction symptoms for longer than 20 minutes; 2) onset of symptoms within 12 hours; 3) ECG changes (ST elevation of 1 mm in contiguous limb leads, ST elevation of 2 mm in contiguous chest leads; left bundle branch block).

Thrombolytic therapy

Thrombolytic therapy has been demonstrated to produce a significant reduction in mortality in the high-risk group described above.[24] The greatest reduction in mortality occurs if the reperfusion occurs within the first 'golden' hour of presentation.[25] Thrombolysis can be delivered effectively in many settings where other methods of reperfusion are not available.

Clots formed in response to injury normally dissolve using the body's fibrinolytic processes as tissue repair takes place. This requires the presence of the proenzyme plasminogen, which is converted into the enzyme plasmin when activated by macrophages and degrades the clot. Thrombolytic agents, including streptokinase and tissue-type

plasminogen activator (tPA), have been developed that trigger conversion of plasminogen to plasmin and therefore break down clots. It is essential to screen patients for contraindications to thrombolysis quickly but thoroughly so that therapy can be commenced as soon as possible. Contraindications are given in the National Health Foundation of Australia (NHFA) Guidelines.[8]

Tenecteplase is the most commonly prescribed thrombolytic agent and is a drug tissue-type plasminogen activator (tPA) that is available as alteplase, tenecteplase and reteplase. These agents are of human origin, made by recombinant DNA techniques.[26] The drug activates only plasminogen present in blood clots, so the risk of haemorrhage is decreased. Unlike streptokinase, tPA can be given repeatedly without risk of anaphylactic reaction. Often patients with anterior ischaemic changes are treated with tPA (alteplase) based on the GUSTO-1 trial that showed improved outcomes in terms of reduction of ischaemia.[27] Alteplase is usually given by infusion, whereas reteplase, which has a longer half-life, can be given in two bolus injections.

Nursing management of patients post-thrombolysis focuses on monitoring and detection of bleeding complications and/or return of ischaemia. Care is as follows:

- Observations: assess neurological state including orientation, any IV sites and urinalysis for the presence of bleeding. Along with vital signs, these are attended every 15 minutes for the first hour, half-hourly for an hour and then hourly according to the patient's condition; however, patients are advised to report any bleeding post-discharge as well.
- ECG monitoring: includes 12-lead ECG on return and ongoing ECG monitoring and chest pain assessment to detect reocclusion. Patients need to be requested to inform nursing staff of any chest pain or discomfort.
- IV anticoagulants such as heparin and/or oral antiplatelet drugs, such as clopidogrel or ticlopidine: may be given following thrombolysis to prevent reocclusion in the stent. Assess International Normalised Ratio (INR), prothrombin (PT) and partial thromboplastin time (PTT), as bleeding is more likely to occur if anticoagulants are above the therapeutic range.

Coronary angioplasty

Percutaneous transluminal coronary angioplasty (PTCA) procedures are being used about twice as frequently as coronary artery bypass graft surgery, with 155 PTCA procedures performed for every 100,000 population in Australia in 2008–09.[3] PTCA rates have grown dramatically in patients aged over 75 years. In this procedure, a catheter is introduced by the brachial or femoral artery into the coronary arteries and advanced into the area of occlusion or stenosis under the guidance of imagery and specifically designed catheters. A balloon attached to the end of the catheter is then inflated to widen the lumen

FIGURE 10.6 Management of acute coronary syndromes.

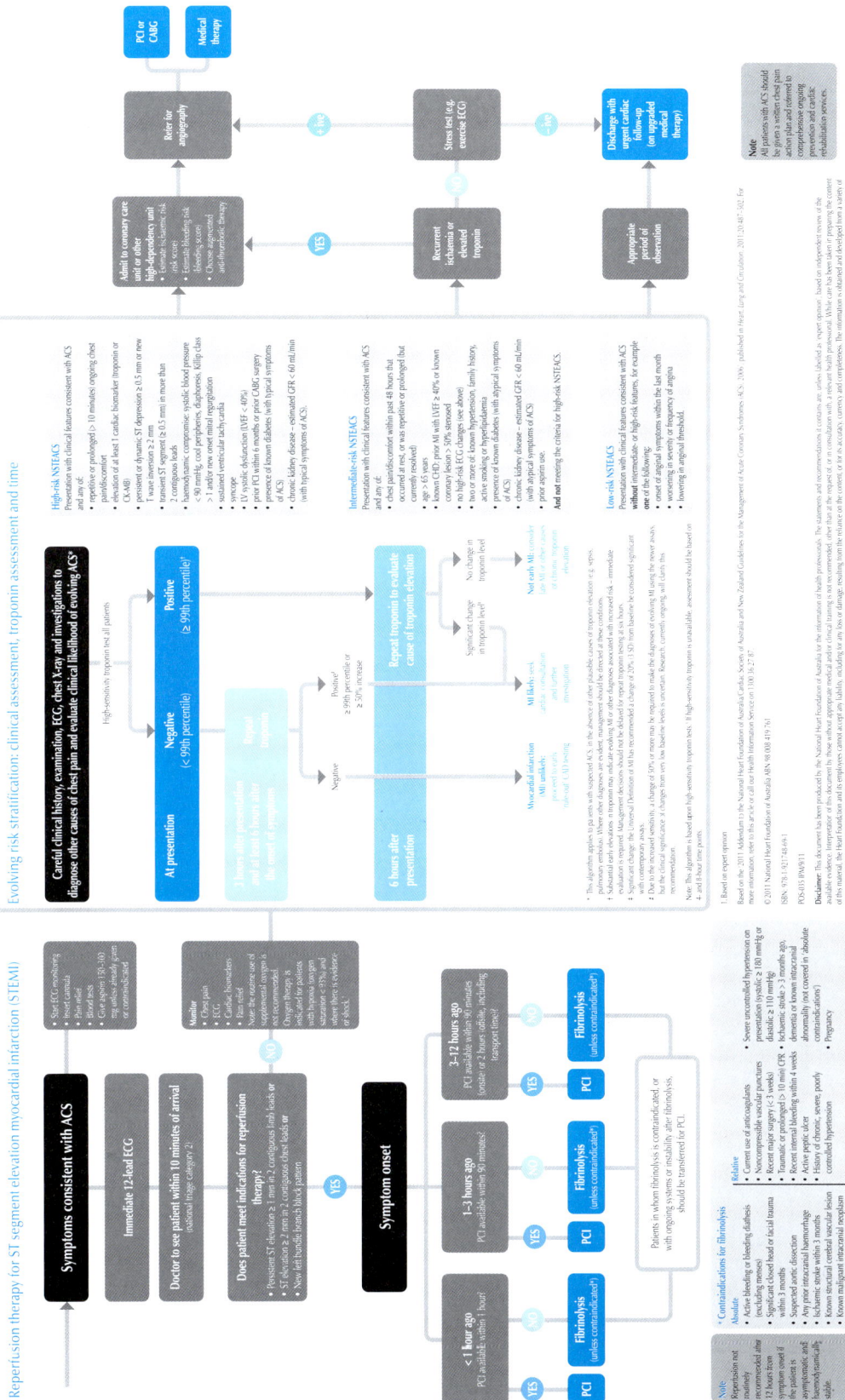

Acute coronary syndromes treatment algorithm   Updated September 2011

2011 National Heart Foundation of Australia, http://www.heartfoundation.org.au/acute-coronary-syndrome.

FIGURE 10.7 PTCA procedure.[28]

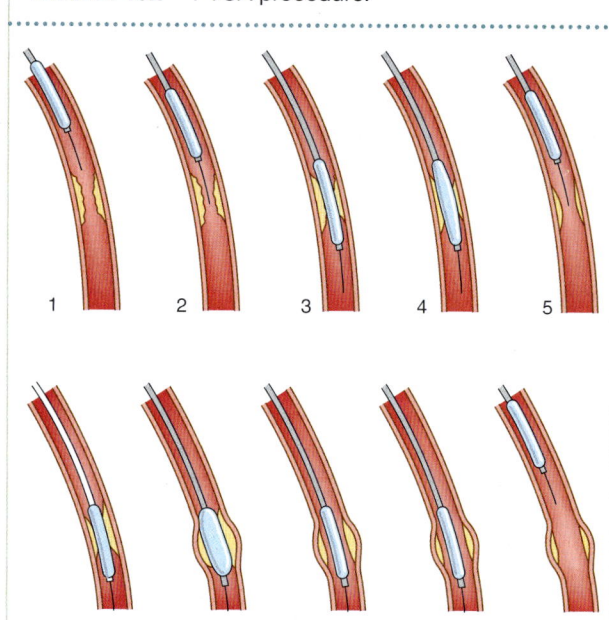

of the artery by stretching the vessel wall, rupturing the atheromatous plaque and cracking the intima and media of the artery (see Figure 10.7).

PTCA tends to be reserved for patients with single- or double-vessel disease as assessed on coronary artery angiograms. Angioplasty provides better symptom relief than medication alone, but there is no evidence of survival benefits.[29] Primary angioplasty results in a higher rate of patency of the affected artery in AMI (>90%), lower rates of cerebrovascular accident (CVA) and reinfarction and higher short-term survival than thrombolysis in ACS.[30] PTCA is recommended in all patients presenting with chest pain who meet the indications for reperfusion when: 1) facilities are available and it can be achieved within 60 minutes; 2) there are contraindications to fibrinolytic therapy described above; 3) ischaemia would result in large anterior AMI within 4 hours; or 4) haemodynamic instability or cardiogenic shock is present.

A stent is usually inserted to prevent abrupt closure and maintain patency for longer.[30] The structure of the stent within the vessel enlarges the lumen and prevents vessel stricture. Restenosis due to intimal hyperplasia is a relatively common complication, occurring 10–12 weeks post-implantation. In response to this problem, drug-eluting stents have been developed. The drug coatings include sirolimus, a macrolide antibiotic that has been demonstrated to effectively decrease hyperplasia and prevent reduction of flow.[31] Paclitaxel has also shown promise in a series of studies.[32] In addition to dactinomycin, these drugs are undergoing approval processes and, while short-term benefits are clear, long-term benefits are not.[33,34]

Nursing management of patients post-PTCA includes care of the puncture site to prevent bleeding and detect arterial changes (including clot and aneurysm).[35] The process used to create and maintain access for insertion of the catheters can damage the blood vessel(s) and alter perfusion to the limb. The sheath used to aid insertion and maintain access is usually maintained for 1–2 hours postprocedure for emergency access. Care is as follows:

- Observations: observe access site for haemorrhage and haematoma; assess perfusion to the lower limb, including colour, warmth and pulses. This monitoring needs to be done often in the first few hours, when complications are most likely to occur.

- ECG monitoring: includes 12-lead ECG on return and ongoing ECG monitoring and chest pain assessment to detect reocclusion. Patients need to be requested to inform nursing staff of any chest pain or discomfort.

- Vital signs: are recorded every 15 minutes for the first hour, half-hourly for one hour and then hourly according to the patient's condition.

- Removal of sheath: is usually performed by medical or specially trained nursing staff.

- Achievement of haemostasis: use either application of pressure for at least 5 minutes or vascular sealing.[35]
  ○ Pressure application can be by a manual compression device (such as Femostop, RADI Medical Systems, Uppsala, Sweden) and less often digital, to maintain a pressure of about 20 mmHg.
  ○ Vascular sealing uses a device such as the Angioseal Vascular Closure Device (St Jude Medical Inc, St Paul, MN). This includes a collagen plug and a small biodegradable plate inside the artery, which is held in place by a small suture, tamping tube and small spring on the exterior. The tension spring is removed and the suture trimmed half an hour after application. This enables the patient to mobilise and reduces nursing time.[36]

- Assess: International Normalised Ratio (INR), prothrombin (PT) and partial thromboplastin time (PTT), as bleeding is more likely to occur if anticoagulants are above the therapeutic range. Weight-adjusted heparin (100 units/kg) is usually used during PTCA to prevent thrombus formation, and glycoprotein IIb/IIIa inhibitors such as abciximab may be used to prevent platelet aggregation and thrombus formation for patients at high risk of occlusion.

- Bedrest (2–6 hours): is used to discourage the patient from moving the joint of the insertion site to prevent clot displacement and haematoma formation. Initially, the patient should lie relatively flat if femoral artery access has been used, then progress to sitting. The period of rest has been demonstrated to be safely reduced to 1 hour in low-risk patients (normotensive and normal platelet count).[35]

- Pain relief: is used primarily to promote comfort for patients who find bedrest causes pain and discomfort.

- Urine output: adequate urine output is essential as radiographic IV contrast is cleared by the kidneys, so it is vital that nurses ensure good hydration and monitor initial urine output.

- Oral antiplatelet drugs, such as clopidogrel or ticlopidine: may be given prior to the procedure to prevent later reocclusion in the stent. Usually patients will be discharged on this medication to continue for up to 3 months while endothelium lines the stent/injured area. Unless contraindicated, all patients will take aspirin for the rest of their lives.[36,37]

Many patients find the PTCA procedure and confirmation of CHD diagnosis stressful.[38] It is an important nursing role to provide patients with preparatory information about the procedure and care required during recovery. As family members provide valuable support and reminders about recovery, these people should be included in any information sessions. The patient and family need to be provided with information about the possibility of restenosis, mobility restrictions at home and the lifestyle changes needed to reduce the risk of worsening CHD.

Practice tip

Increased hydration can aggravate problems with urination when on bedrest, particularly in older men with prostate enlargement. If a femoral access site is used in these patients, it is easier for the patient to urinate while turned on the side, using pillow support to maintain the position.

Practice tip

If a femoral access site has been used, bleeding may track between the patient's legs and pool, and this will be invisible to a cursory inspection, particularly if the patient is obese. Always move the patient's thigh during regular inspections.

Nursing management of ACS and MI patients

The nursing role in patients with ACS and MI includes reducing myocardial workload and maximising cardiac output, provision of treatments, careful monitoring to determine the effects of treatment and detect complications, rapid treatment of complications, comfort and pain control, psychosocial support and teaching and discharge planning.

Reduction of myocardial workload includes ensuring the patient has bedrest, providing support with activities and limiting stress. A calm, caring manner during nursing care is essential to lower patient and family stress levels. Individual evaluation of the patient and the family is necessary to determine the most appropriate management of visiting. ECG monitoring (preferably including ST monitoring) and evaluation of heart rate, shortness of breath, chest discomfort and blood pressure are essential to determine ischaemia, treatment effects, myocardial workload and complications. This monitoring should occur hourly during the acute phase, reducing as the patient recovers. Oxygen saturation levels should be routinely assessed and provision of oxygen by mask or nasal cannulae provided if levels are reduced. Conventional practice was to provide O_2 in the first 6 hours to raise SaO_2 levels in the myocardium; however, there is no evidence of patient benefit if SaO_2 levels are not decreased.[10] Symptom relief should be provided, including analgesia for pain. Analgesia management should be conducted by nurses because of their continued contact and thus more accurate assessment and treatment of pain.[20] It is essential to treat pain, not only for the distress it causes patients but also because pain causes stimulation of the sympathetic nervous system (SNS). SNS responses include elevated heart rate and potential for arrhythmias, peripheral vasoconstriction and increased myocardial contractility and, therefore, an overall increase in myocardial oxygen demand. Effective treatments for pain include IV morphine and nitrates. The IV route is preferable, as absorption is predictable and additional punctures in thrombolysed patients are not required. Morphine has the additional benefit of reducing anxiety in a distressing situation and should be initially provided at a dose of 2.5–5 mg at 1 mg/min, followed by 2.5-mg doses as indicated. While there is little randomised controlled trial evidence to support this particular practice, it is generally accepted to be appropriate. A standardised method of pain evaluation and charting should be used to ensure consistent assessment and treatment. An antiemetic such as metoclopramide should be given concurrently to lessen and prevent nausea. Other drugs, such as beta-blockers and nitrates, decrease myocardial workload, contributing to pain reduction.

Nursing care specific to thrombolysis

Patients receiving thrombolytics require constant observation and regular non-invasive blood pressure measurement for hypotension. Continuous ECG monitoring for arrhythmias and ST-segment changes is essential. Some arrhythmias, particularly idioventricular arrhythmias, are associated with reperfusion and tend to be benign. ST-segment monitoring and assessment of pain help evaluate the effectiveness of the thrombolysis. Thrombolysis is considered to have failed if the patient is still in pain and the ST segment has not resolved within 60–90 minutes.[20] If thrombolysis fails, patients are at high risk for other interventions, so repeat thrombolysis is often the only treatment option. Salvage or rescue angioplasty may be undertaken if available at the site.

Medications

Provision of medications and assessment of the effectiveness of treatment is a major component of the nurse's role in caring for the cardiac patient. Many of the medications are accompanied by side effects and interactions with other drugs, which the nurse must monitor. An array of medications is used to treat AMI patients, including aspirin, lipid-lowering agents, beta-blockers and organic nitrates (see Table 10.3).

TABLE 10.3
Medications used in the treatment of ACS

AGENT	ACTION	SIDE EFFECTS/CAUTION	COMMENTS
ANTIPLATELET AGENTS			
Aspirin	Prevents platelet synthesis of thromboxane A2, a vasoconstrictor and stimulant of platelet aggregation. May provide benefits from anti-inflammatory properties in reducing plaque rupture[34]	Gastrointestinal irritation and bleeding; use enteric-coated tablets to minimise	Noted to reduce the risk of AMI by 50%,[33] although often underutilised.[6] Lifelong use is recommended in angina patients
Clopidogrel	Adenosine diphosphate (ADP) receptor agonist; prevents the binding of ADP to its platelet receptor, thus inhibiting platelet aggregation	Inhibits P450 liver enzyme; care is required when delivering with other drugs and other anticoagulants[25]	Clopidogrel produces fewer GI effects than aspirin and is more effective in patients with recent stroke, MI and peripheral vascular disease[37]
Ticlopidine	As for clopidogrel	Severe side effects including neutropenia	
Tirofiban, eptifibatide, lamifiban, abciximab[37]	Glycoprotein IIb/IIIa receptor antagonists prevent the final step of platelet aggregation; used most commonly to inhibit thrombus formation in acute coronary syndrome angina[37]	Bleeding, thrombocytopenia, nausea, fever and headache;[25] doses need to be reduced in renal failure	Early decreases in mortality in ACS and MI, particularly when given in combination with aspirin and heparin, have been seen
BETA-BLOCKERS			
	Reduce cardiac workload (↓ heart rate and force of contraction) by blocking beta-adrenergic receptors, preventing sympathetic stimulation of the heart	Contraindications include significant AV block, bradycardia, hypotension, history of asthma or uncontrolled heart failure	Recommended for patients during the acute MI phase, reducing risk of further MI
NITRATES			
Glyceryl trinitrate (IV, sublingual and spray), isosorbide mononitrate	Potent peripheral vasodilators, particularly in venous capacitance vessels, thereby reducing preload and to a lesser extent afterload, to reduce myocardial workload. Dilate normal and atherosclerotic coronary blood vessels to increase myocardial oxygen supply. Used to manage unstable angina and reduce blood pressure in the critical care setting, where there is some evidence for symptomatic relief	Reflex tachycardia, hypotension, syncope and migraine-like headache; generally occur in first few days of treatment, then subside. Blood pressure should be monitored	Tolerance to the vasodilator effect occurs, so intermittent treatment is most effective. In the case of transdermal delivery, if treatment is withheld for 8–12 h in every 24 h, therapeutic activity is restored
LIPID-LOWERING STATINS			
Atorvastatin, simvastatin, fluvastatin, pravastatin	Inhibit 3-hydroxy-3-methylglutaryl-coenzyme-A (HMG-CoA) reductase, the enzyme that limits the rate of cholesterol synthesis in the liver, thereby reducing plasma cholesterol	Headache, gastrointestinal upset, inflammation of voluntary muscles and altered liver function; taking statins with food may reduce GI symptoms	To lower and maintain cholesterol at 5 mmol/L, evidence that statin medications can reduce mortality for up to 5 years after AMI.[39] Education needs to include monitoring for muscle soreness and regular GP visits for liver function tests

Adapted from Bryant B, Knights K, Saterno E. Pharmacology for health professionals. Sydney: Mosby Elsevier; 2006.

Symptom control

Control of anginal symptoms with medication usually includes sublingual glyceryl trinitrate (GTN) for immediate symptom control and one or more antianginal medications for sustained symptom management.[21] Beta-blockers are usually commenced unless contraindicated. Calcium channel blockers may be used in patients who do not have cardiac failure or heart block. (These medications are described in the next section.) The choice of medication may depend on how acceptable the patient finds the reduction in symptoms and the presence of side effects. Patients need to take antianginal agents continuously, regardless of symptoms. Patients should also be encouraged to take sublingual GTN prophylactically.

Angina may also be managed by avoiding situations that trigger angina. Education needs to be directed at awareness of symptoms and management of unstable angina and AMI symptoms, and the need for emergency care. Although these patients are at low risk of further cardiovascular events in the short term, in the medium to long term, risk may accumulate. Patients with angina are encouraged to attend cardiac rehabilitation programs to learn how to deal with symptom management.[39]

Angiotensin-converting enzyme (ACE) inhibitors have been recommended for all post-AMI patients while in hospital, with review of prescription at 4–6 weeks post-discharge. Patients with left ventricular failure should be maintained on ACE inhibitors. Similarly, diuretics provide the mainstay of the management of left ventricular failure if it is present (see Chapter 19). Diabetic patients have a higher mortality after AMI in both acute and long-term phases. Provision of an insulin-glucose infusion for BSL >11 mmol/L during the acute phase, followed by subcutaneous injections for at least 3 months, has been demonstrated to significantly reduce mortality up to 3 years post-AMI.[40]

Transfer to a step-down unit or general ward usually occurs when the patient is pain-free and is haemodynamically stable. Stability means that patients are not dependent on IV inotropic or vasoactive support and have no arrhythmias. Discharge home after AMI varies, but usually occurs at day 3 for low-risk patients.[20]

Emotional responses and patient and family support

ACS or AMI is usually accompanied by feelings of acute anxiety and fear, as most patients are aware of the significant threat posed to their health.[18] For many patients it may also be the first experience of acute illness and associated aspects such as ambulance transport, emergency care and hospitalisation, so they may experience shock and disbelief as well. Fast-track processes such as prehospital triage require patients and their families to process a large amount of information and make decisions quickly, and this, added to an alien environment, full of unfamiliar technology and personnel, can be quite distressing. However, the environment can also promote a feeling of security for patients and their families. Patients' perceptions of the CCU environment have been linked to recovery, in a study conducted in 1996, which remains surprisingly relevant today.[41]

Anxiety is a common response to the stress of an acute cardiac event and leads to important physiological and psychological changes.[42] The sympathetic nervous system is stimulated, resulting in increased heart rate, respiration and blood pressure. These responses increase the workload of the heart and therefore myocardial oxygen demand. In an acute cardiac event, these demands occur when perfusion is already poor and may lead to worse outcomes, including ventricular arrhythmias and increased myocardial ischaemia. Therefore, staff working in emergency and coronary care should employ strategies to reduce a patient's anxiety. Chapter 7 provides a more detailed description of psychological care.

Increasing a patient's sense of control, calm and confidence in care reduces the patient's sense of vulnerability, whether it is realistic or not.[42] This can be achieved by:

- providing order and predictability in routines, allowing the patient to make choices, providing information and explanations and including the patient in decision making
- using a calm, confident approach
- communicating with patients and families, while reducing conversation demands, as excessive conversation by patients may unnecessarily raise heart rate[43]
- restricting the number and type of visitors in the acute phase is customary, but many patients feel safer if a family member is present
- provision of comprehensive information to families, with more concise information in understandable language for patients.

Nurses need to monitor patients for signs of excessive anxiety, including facial expressions and behavioural changes. However, overt behaviours may be controlled by the patient, so careful conversation and/or use of specific assessments may be necessary to detect anxiety. The move to the step-down or general ward may also be stressful to the patient and family. This move needs to be planned and discussed, and promoted as a sign of recovery.

Cardiac rehabilitation

Coronary heart disease is a chronic disease process, which often presents with acute events such as ACS or AMI. Like all chronic illnesses, it has implications for patients in terms of lifestyle change, uncertainty of long-term outcomes, functional changes and social and economic alterations. Cardiac rehabilitation aims to address these issues. The World Health Organization describes cardiac rehabilitation as 'the sum of activities required to influence favourably the underlying cause of the disease, as well as to ensure the patients the best possible physical, mental and social conditions so that they may, by their own efforts, preserve, or resume when lost, as normal a place as possible in the life of the community'.[44] Systematic, individualised rehabilitation and secondary prevention need to be offered to all AMI patients and considered for all patients who have coronary heart disease. Participation in well-structured, multidisciplinary programs has been demonstrated to reduce mortality by almost 30% in AMI and by 13% in other coronary heart disease conditions.[45] Additional benefits have been shown for improvements in exercise tolerance, symptoms, serum lipids, psychological wellbeing and cessation of smoking.[46,47]

Cardiac rehabilitation is structured around four phases, beginning with phase I, during admission.[48] The components of phase I include:

- information regarding the disease process, the prognosis, and an optimal approach to recovery, early mobilisation and discharge planning

- assessment of patients' understanding of their diagnosis and treatment as a foundation for self-management

- discharge planning, which incorporates discussions on adaptation to the functional and lifestyle changes needed for secondary prevention – dietary intake of lipids, exercise, smoking cessation, stress management and symptom monitoring, and management of acute symptoms

- early mobilisation as an inpatient to encourage a positive approach to recovery with monitoring of the response to activity in heart rate, shortness of breath and chest pain to determine the rate of progress. (Most hospital units use an activity progress chart for this purpose based on metabolic equivalents [METs].)

The phases that follow, from II to IV, are managed in the outpatient setting and begin with assessment, liaison with multidisciplinary professionals and health education. Phase II occurs in the immediate post-discharge period and includes liaison with community-based carers and services and further assessment. In phase III, tailored, supervised exercise programs are usually conducted and there is a range of psychosocial interventions, such as support sessions and stress management. Finally, in phase IV the focus is on chronic disease management and maintaining risk modification behaviours. All phases require incorporation of the principles of adult learning to maximise learning and behaviour change. These principles include recognition of 'readiness to learn'.[48] Adults are ready to learn most effectively when they are physically and emotionally stable and are aware of the problem or need to learn. Nurses, because of their expertise and continual presence, are best placed to assess and provide education at optimal times.

Complications of myocardial infarction

Despite declines in death rates from myocardial infarction,[3–5] many patients will experience complications, most of which occur within the first 24 hours.

Cardiogenic shock

Cardiogenic shock occurs as a complication of MI in about 5–10% of patients and is the most common cause of death in hospitals.[49] It arises from loss of contractile force, and generally occurs when ventricular damage is more than 40% and ejection fraction less than 35%. Cardiogenic shock and the related management are described in more detail in Chapter 12.

Arrhythmias

Arrhythmias often occur in ACS and AMI and are often the cause of death in the prehospital phase. Management of the prehospital phase focuses on community education and an effective, rapidly responsive ambulance service, as exemplified in Seattle in the USA.[50] Arrhythmias may be generated by poorly perfused tissue and electrolyte alterations, and increased sympathetic tone during infarction, but are more often due to a failing left ventricle. They may also complicate reperfusion after successful revascularisation.[51] It is essential to rapidly and effectively treat arrhythmias in the ACS and AMI context. The goal of treatment is to maintain cardiac output while reducing workload. Arrhythmias and management are described in Chapter 11.

Pericarditis

Pericarditis is an inflammation of the visceral and parietal layers of the pericardium that cover the heart. This inflammation occurs in approximately 20% of AMI patients within the following 2–3 days.[13] The patient experiences chest pain, which may be confused with ischaemic pain. This confusion with an ischaemic event may be compounded by the additional presence of ST-segment elevation on the ECG. However, pericardial pain increases with deep inspiration and a pericardial rub is often present. Electrocardiographically, the elevated ST segments of pericarditis are typically concave upwards (saddle-shaped) and often widespread, contrasting with convex ST-segment elevation limited to the distribution of a single coronary artery in infarction.[52] Pericarditis normally responds to anti-inflammatory treatment by aspirin, indomethacin and/or corticosteroids. Approximately 1–5% of AMI patients develop pericarditis as a late complication, 2 weeks to a few months post-AMI.[21] Usually, this late-onset pericarditis is associated with Dressler's syndrome and may be an autoimmune response to myocardial injury. This is a chronic condition requiring systemic corticosteroid treatment.

Structural defects

Myocardial tissue death may be catastrophic if it is extensive or results in rupture of ventricular or papillary muscle. These conditions are rare and symptoms develop rapidly. Intraventricular septal rupture is usually associated with anterior MI. The patient develops progressive dyspnoea, tachycardia and pulmonary congestion, as well as a loud systolic murmur associated with a thrill felt in the parasternal area. If a pulmonary artery catheter is present, blood samples from the right atrium and right ventricle will reveal a higher than usual oxygen content. Diagnosis must be confirmed by cardiac catheterisation, and urgent surgery is required.

Papillary muscle rupture most often occurs 2–7 days after MI. Patients experience a sudden onset of pulmonary oedema secondary to pulmonary hypertension and cardiogenic shock. Additional heart sounds and a systolic murmur will be heard. Urgent surgery is required, as the mortality rate for papillary muscle rupture is 95%.[53] Cardiac rupture most often occurs within 5 days of MI and is commonest in older women. The patient experiences continuous chest pain, dyspnoea and hypotension as tamponade develops. Symptoms may worsen rapidly and result in pulseless electrical activity (PEA) unless surgery is undertaken immediately.

Heart failure

In normal circumstances, the heart is a very effective, efficient pump with reserve mechanisms available to allow output to meet changing demands. These mechanisms include: 1) increasing heart rate to increase total cardiac output, 2) dilation to create muscle stretch and more effective contraction, 3) hypertrophy of myocytes over time to generate more force and 4) increasing stroke volume by increasing venous return and increased contractility. Heart failure is a complex clinical condition that is characterised by an underlying structural abnormality or dysfunction that results in the inability of the ventricle to fill with or eject blood.[54] The condition is also known as congestive cardiac failure, a term commonly used in the USA but not in Australia. Chronic heart failure (CHF) describes the long-term inability of the heart to meet metabolic demands.

The burden of disease associated with heart failure is on the rise due to our ageing population, the prevalence of coronary heart disease and hypertension, the decrease in fatality from acute coronary syndrome and improved methods of diagnosis.[54] Survival rates and prognosis for heart failure patients are extremely poor. Approximately 50% of patients diagnosed with heart failure will die within 5 years of diagnosis.[55,56] When compared with patients with cancer, heart failure patients have the poorest 5-year survival rate, with the exception of lung cancer.[57] In Australia during 2007–08, 49,307 patients were hospitalised with a primary diagnosis of CHF (0.6% of all hospitalisations).[58] Internationally, heart failure is the most common cause of hospitalisation in patients aged over 70 years.[59] Approximately 40% of patients admitted to hospital with heart failure will be readmitted or die within 1 year.[59] In the USA approximately 5.1 million people have been diagnosed with heart failure.[60] Approximately, 1 million hospital admissions annually have a primary diagnosis of heart failure.[60]

Over 50% of patients newly diagnosed with heart failure have concurrent ischaemic heart disease, hypertension is present in 65% and idiopathic dilated cardiomyopathy in 5–10% of cases.[54] The causes of heart failure can be categorised according to: 1) myocardial disease, 2) arrhythmias, 3) valve disease, 4) pericardial disease and 5) congenital heart disease.[61] Myocardial disease may be caused by myocardial infarction and fibrosis from prolonged ischaemic heart disease, which accounts for approximately two-thirds of systolic heart failure causing systolic dysfunction and a reduced ejection fraction.

Arrhythmias, including both brady- and tachyarrhythmias, may cause heart failure due to changes in filling time affecting preload and resultant cardiac output. Myocardial oxygen demand is increased and, if the heart is poorly perfused, muscle contraction will be affected. Frequent premature contractions and atrial fibrillation disturb mechanical coordination so that the ventricles may not be adequately filled for efficient contraction. Heart failure patients are also at high risk of sudden cardiac death due

to ventricular fibrillation or tachycardia. Valvular disease causing heart failure usually involves valves on the left side of the heart (mitral and/or aortic valves). Aortic stenosis results in an increase in afterload and ventricular hypertrophy develops with reduced diastolic compliance resulting in a reduced ejection fraction. Mitral stenosis is usually due to rheumatic heart disease. Valvular incompetence results in a dilated ventricle to accommodate the regurgitant volume. Stroke volume increases in an attempt to empty its contents and ventricular muscle mass increases. However, over time the ventricle is unable to maintain the increased workload and heart failure develops. Valvular heart disease and treatment are described in more detail in Chapter 12.

There are several terms used to describe the pathology and signs and symptoms of heart failure. These include:

- Backward failure: refers to the systemic and pulmonary congestion that occurs as a result of failure of the ventricle to expel its volume.

- Forward failure: is due to an inadequate cardiac output and leads to decrease in vital organ perfusion.

- Acute heart failure: includes the initial hospitalisation for the diagnosis of heart failure and exacerbations of chronic heart failure.

- Chronic heart failure: develops over time as a result of the inability of compensatory mechanisms to maintain an adequate cardiac output to meet metabolic demands.

- Heart failure with reduced ejection fraction (HF*r*EF) or systolic heart failure: refers to the inability of the ventricle to contract adequately during systole resulting in a reduced ejection fraction and an increased end-diastolic volume. This is the most common form of heart failure.

- Heart failure with preserved ejection fraction (HF*p*EF) or diastolic heart failure: indicates normal systolic function with a normal ejection fraction but impaired relaxation so there is a resistance to filling with increased filling pressures. Diastolic dysfunction usually occurs in conjunction with systolic dysfunction and is more common in the elderly.

- Low cardiac output syndrome: this occurs in response to hypovolaemia and/or hypertension. Severe vasoconstriction further reduces the cardiac output.

- High cardiac output syndrome: is the result of an increase in metabolic demands causing a decrease in systemic venous return leading to an increase in stroke volume and cardiac output. Burns and sepsis are the main causes.

- Left-sided heart failure: occurs when there is a reduced left ventricular stroke volume resulting in accumulation of blood in the pulmonary system.

- Right-sided heart failure: is the congestion of blood in the systemic system due to the inability of the right ventricle to expel its blood volume.

Responses to heart failure

When heart failure occurs, several adaptive responses are initiated by the body in an attempt to maintain normal perfusion (see Figure 10.8). These mechanisms are successful in the normal heart, but contribute to decreased effectiveness in the failing heart. The compensatory mechanisms include:

- sympathetic nervous system response
- renin–angiotensin–aldosterone system (RAAS)
- Frank-Starling response
- neurohormonal response.

The sympathetic nervous system is the first response to be stimulated in heart failure. It occurs within seconds of a reduction in cardiac output and the parasympathetic system becomes inhibited. The baroreceptor reflexes are activated in response to a reduced arterial pressure. The beta-adrenergic receptors located in the heart are activated, resulting in an increase in heart rate and contractility to increase stroke volume and cardiac output. Sympathetic nervous system response in the peripheral vascular system results in vasoconstriction, which increases systemic venous return and mean systemic filling pressures. This results in an increase in venous return, preload and afterload (see Figure 10.8). The consequence of this activation is increased myocardial oxygen demand. Although blood flow to essential organs is maintained, perfusion to the kidneys, gastrointestinal system and skin is reduced and peripheral resistance increased. Chronic activation of vasoconstrictors contributes to the progression of cardiac failure through increased resistance and effects on cardiac structure, causing hypertrophy and fibrosis and downregulation of beta-adrenergic receptors and endothelial dysfunction. Chronic poor perfusion to skeletal muscles may contribute to changes in muscle metabolism, resulting in further reductions in exercise tolerance.

The next compensatory mechanism to be activated is the RAAS. This is stimulated within minutes, in response to a decrease in kidney perfusion resulting in a decrease in glomerular filtration rate. Activation of this response results in an increase in systemic venous return and sodium and water reabsorption, which then increases the circulating blood volume, systemic filling pressures and venous return enhancing preload and afterload (see Chapter 9).

The Frank-Starling response is also activated. As the end-diastolic volume increases (preload) in response to sympathetic nervous system stimulation, ventricular dilation occurs stimulating the Frank-Starling response. As the myocardial fibres are stretched during diastole the

FIGURE 10.8 Flowchart of the pathophysiology of heart failure.[62]

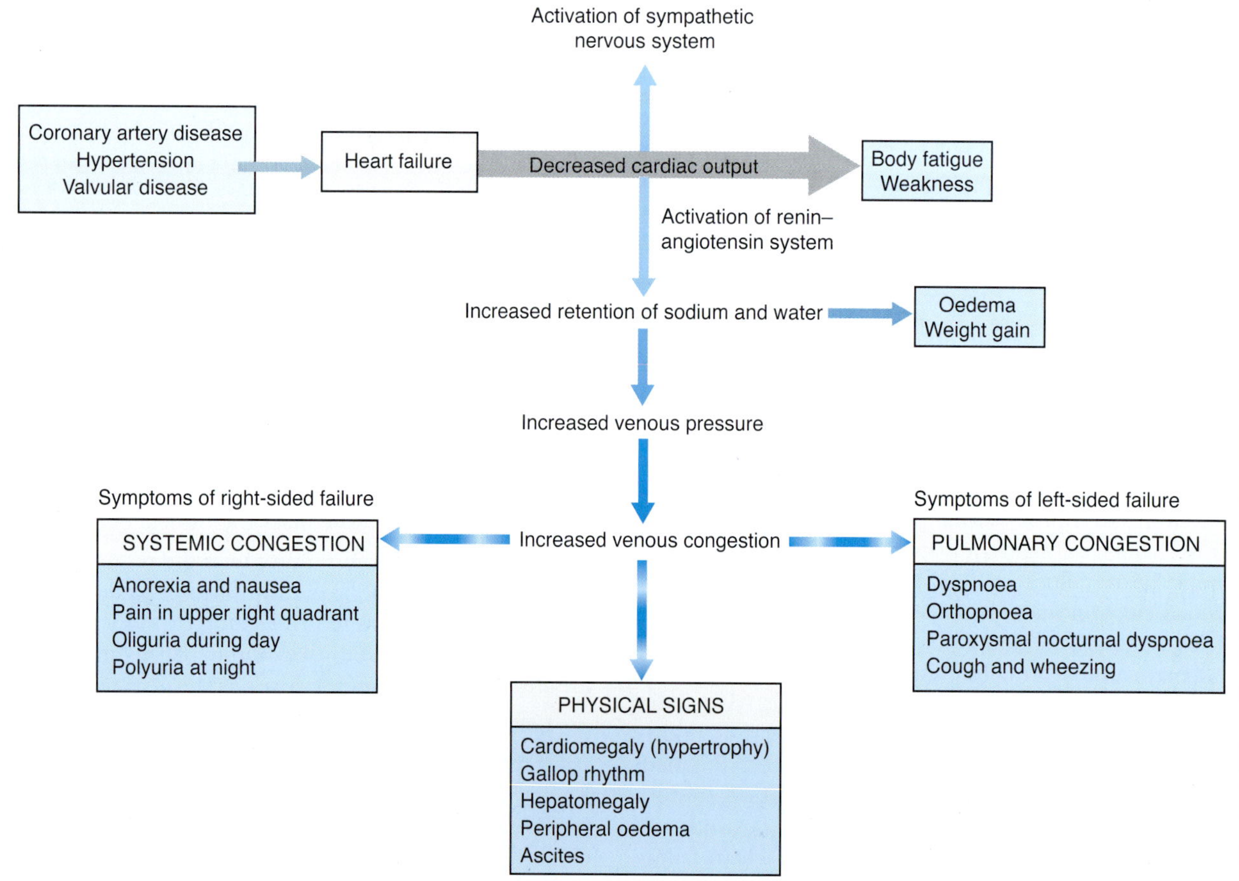

force of contractility also increases to expel the increasing preload. This is a major mechanism of the heart to maintain a normal cardiac output. Optimal contractility occurs when the diastolic volume is 12–18 mmHg.[63] However, when the ventricle is damaged, such as in MI, the sympathetic nervous system increases heart rate and contractility, further increasing cardiac workload and exacerbating myocardial dysfunction, which increases end-diastolic volume (preload) and ventricular dilation further, and heart failure progresses. As ventricular dilation continues, ventricular hypertrophy results. The myocardium also increases its muscle mass in an attempt to increase contractility, called ventricular remodelling. However, over time ventricular hypertrophy results in changes to end-diastolic compliance and contractility due to the thickened ventricular wall, impaired muscle function and growth of collagen. These result in further impairment of ventricular function (see Figure 10.9).[58] Ventricular hypertrophy also has a depressant effect on ventricular compliance, heart rate and contractility resulting in an increase in end-diastolic pressure with no associated increase in contractility. As the pulmonary artery pressures increase, pulmonary oedema and cardiogenic shock develop.

The final compensatory mechanism to be activated is the neurohormonal response, which takes days to be activated. This response involves the activation of vasopressin and atrial natriuretic peptide (ANP). Vasopressin is a potent vasoconstrictor and also an antidiuretic hormone. ANP is important in the regulation of cardiovascular volume homeostasis. It is released from the atria in response to atrial stretching due to an increased circulating blood volume. ANP blocks the effect of the sympathetic nervous system, RAAS and vasopressin. It reduces tachycardia via the baroreceptors and reduces circulating blood

volume by increasing salt and water excretion in the kidneys. Plasma ANP is increased in acute heart failure but depleted in chronic heart failure.

While in the healthy heart these compensatory mechanisms would result in an adequate cardiac output, in heart failure they do not, depending on the aetiology. In ischaemic heart failure the damaged myocardium is unable to respond adequately to the Frank-Starling response and ventricular remodelling develops. Heart failure caused by hypertension or valvular heart disease results in persistent pressure or volume overload, which is exacerbated by the Frank-Starling response and sympathetic nervous system compensatory mechanisms. This causes ventricular remodelling and depletion of norepinephrine and a reduction of inotropic response to the cardiac sympathetic nervous system. These all exacerbate the reduction in circulating blood volume and kidney perfusion. Many patients with heart failure often have a high plasma renin activity due to the continual activation of the RAAS compensatory mechanism.

In heart failure patients the inadequate cardiac output results in signs and symptoms of hypoperfusion (oliguria, cognitive impairment and cold peripheries) and congestion of the venous and pulmonary systems (acute pulmonary oedema, dyspnoea, hypoxaemia, peripheral oedema and liver congestion). Classification of signs and symptoms is usually considered in the context of left or right ventricular failure.

Left ventricular failure

Left ventricular failure (LVF), compared with other forms of heart failure, is characterised by breathlessness, orthopnoea and paroxysmal nocturnal dyspnoea, irritating cough and fatigue (see Table 10.4). Left ventricular failure or HF*p*EF exists when the ventricle has an ejection fraction of less than 40%, resulting in increased end-diastolic volume and increased intraventricular pressure.[61] The left atrium is unable to empty into the left ventricle adequately and pressure in the left atrium rises. This pressure is reflected in the pulmonary veins and causes pulmonary congestion. When pulmonary venous congestion exceeds 20 mmHg, fluid moves into the pulmonary interstitium. Raised pulmonary interstitial pressure reduces pulmonary compliance, increases the work of breathing and is experienced by the patient as shortness of breath. Increased blood volume in the lung also initiates shallow, rapid breathing and the sensation of breathlessness. Patients also experience orthopnoea (dyspnoea while lying flat) and paroxysmal nocturnal dyspnoea because, when lying down, blood is redistributed from gravity-dependent areas of the body to the lung. Sitting upright or standing, and sleeping with additional pillows, relieves breathlessness at night.[63]

Acute pulmonary oedema results when pulmonary capillary pressure exceeds approximately 30 mmHg, and then fluid from the vessels begins to leak into the alveoli (see Figure 10.10).[65] This fluid leak decreases the area available for normal gas exchange and severe shortness of breath

FIGURE 10.9 Function curves of left ventricular pressure during various stages of heart failure.[64]

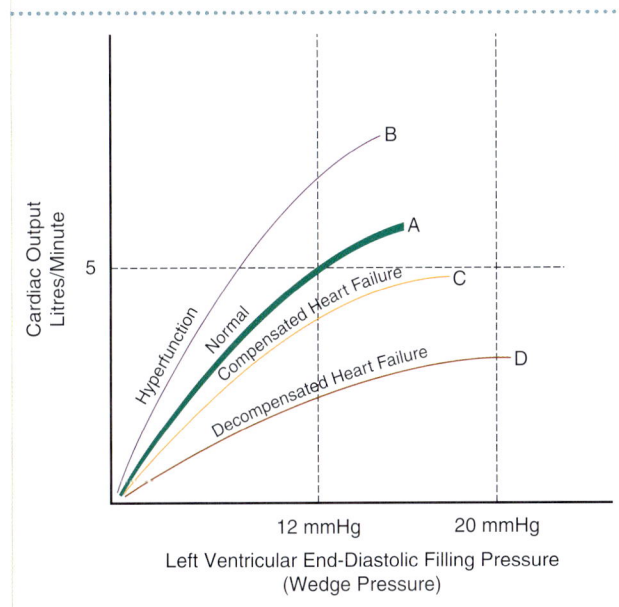

TABLE 10.4

Clinical manifestations of failure of right and left sides of the heart

LEFT VENTRICULAR FAILURE		RIGHT VENTRICULAR FAILURE	
SIGNS	**SYMPTOMS**	**SIGNS**	**SYMPTOMS**
Tachypnoea	Dyspnoea	Peripheral oedema	Fatigue
Tachycardia	Orthopnoea	Raised jugular venous pressure	Weight gain
Bibasal crackles	Paroxysmal nocturnal	Raised central venous pressure	Anorexia
Haemoptysis	dyspnoea	Ascites	
Cough	Fatigue	Hepatomegaly	
Pulmonary oedema	Nocturia		
Raised pulmonary artery pressure			
S3 heart sound			

FIGURE 10.10 Pathophysiology of pulmonary oedema. As pulmonary oedema progresses, it inhibits oxygen and carbon dioxide exchange at the alveolar–capillary interface. **(A)** Normal relationship. **(B)** Increased pulmonary capillary hydrostatic pressure causes fluid to move from the vascular space into the pulmonary interstitial space. **(C)** Lymphatic flow increases and pulls fluid back into the vascular or lymphatic space. **(D)** Failure of lymphatic flow and worsening of left-sided heart failure causes further movement of fluid into the interstitial space and then into the alveoli.[23]

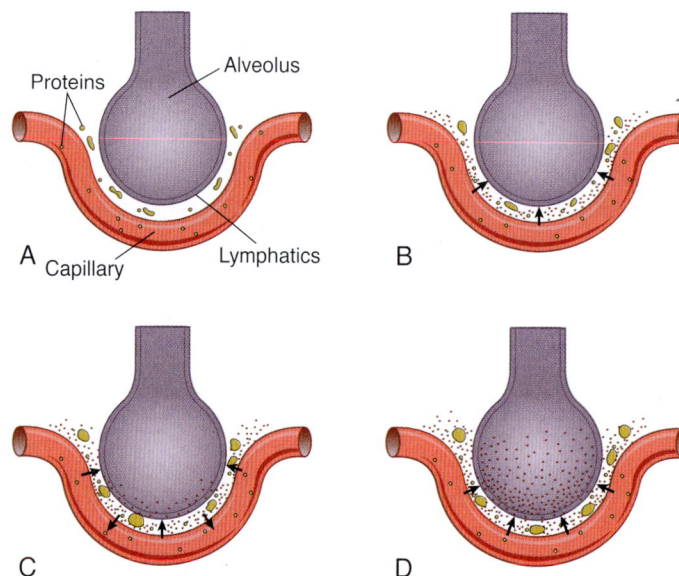

results, often accompanied by pink, frothy sputum and noisy respirations. This causes patients to experience severe anxiety and decreased oxygen levels. Pulmonary oedema is a medical emergency and requires urgent treatment.

In addition to pulmonary symptoms, patients with left ventricular failure experience signs and symptoms related to decreased left ventricular output, including weakness, fatigue, difficulty in concentrating and decreased exercise tolerance. These symptoms may be present for some time before an accurate diagnosis of heart failure is made, because they are non-specific and are consistent with other diagnoses such as depression. Other signs that are useful in diagnosis include the presence of S3 (ventricular gallop), crackles over lung fields that do not clear with

a cough, cardiomegaly and the presence of pulmonary vessels on chest X-ray.

Right ventricular failure

Right ventricular failure (RVF) does not usually occur in isolation, except in the presence of severe lung disease, such as chronic obstructive pulmonary disease, pulmonary hypertension or a massive pulmonary embolus.[63] In this case, right ventricular failure is due to resistance to outflow. The right ventricle can adapt to fairly large changes in volume; however, when cardiac output decreases, end-diastolic volume increases, and the right atrium is unable to empty adequately. Right atrial pressure rises and is reflected into the venous system. Jugular vein distension occurs, and the veins are usually visible above the clavicle. Symptoms of right heart failure are not as specific as left ventricular failure, and are mostly related to low cardiac output and raised venous pressure (see Table 10.4). Ascites and oedema tend to progress insidiously, and dependent oedema in the feet and ankles is often most prominent. Weight gain is an important sign as 1 kilogram of weight gain equals 1 litre of excess fluid. Liver congestion may result in tenderness, ascites and jaundice. Nausea and anorexia may be present and are a result of an increased intra-abdominal pressure. Many signs are not readily distinguishable from left ventricular failure, including extra heart sounds.

Patient assessment, diagnostic procedures and classification

Assessment and diagnosis are summarised in a diagnostic algorithm (see Figure 10.11).[51] A full assessment and history is essential to determine the cause(s) of CHF and to assess the severity of the disease. A careful physical assessment is important for initial diagnosis and to evaluate the effectiveness of treatments and progress of the disease. The depth and time taken to conduct the assessment depend on the severity of symptoms. The physical examination of the patient focuses on cardiovascular and pulmonary assessment.

Cardiovascular assessment includes:

- Pulse rate and rhythm: the pulse rate is generally elevated due to a low cardiac output. However, if the patient is prescribed beta-adrenergic blocking agents and/or angiotensin-converting enzyme inhibitors (ACEIs), the pulse rate may be low.
- Palpation of the precordium and apical impulse: may be displaced laterally and downward to the left due to an increased heart size.
- Auscultation of a third heart sound (S3 gallop): occurs due to a low ejection fraction and diastolic dysfunction. A fourth heart sound may also be present due to a decrease in ventricular compliance.
- Assessment of jugular venous pressure (JVP): is performed to estimate the degree of venous volume. If raised it reflects hypervolaemia, right ventricular failure and reduced right ventricular compliance. It can also be raised in the presence of tricuspid valve disease. The hepatojugular reflex is also assessed by pressing on the liver and observing an increase in JVP. This results in an increase in blood flow to the right atrium.
- Blood pressure: lying and standing blood pressure are measured to assess postural hypotension due to a low cardiac output and also the prescribing of beta-adrenergic blocking agents and ACEIs.
- Peripheries: look for the presence of cyanosis that may be due to vasoconstriction. Assess the fingers for clubbing, which indicates long-term cyanosis usually as a consequence of congenital heart disease. Also assess the patient for ankle oedema. Peripheral oedema up to the midcalves indicates a moderate amount of excess fluid and the patient may require a bolus dose of diuretic medication.

TABLE 10.5

New York Heart Association functional classification of heart failure[69]

CLASS	DEFINITION
I	Normal daily activity does not initiate symptoms. There are no limitations on activity
II	Ordinary activities initiate onset of symptoms, but symptoms subside with rest. Slight limitation of daily activities
III	A small amount of activity initiates symptoms; patients are usually symptom-free at rest. Marked limitation of activity
IV	Any type of activity initiates symptoms, and symptoms are present at rest

---

Pulmonary assessment includes chest auscultation for inspiratory crepitations that do not clear with coughing. They are initially heard in the bases but as congestion increases they become diffuse. General assessment of the patient includes daily weighing and looking for signs of cachexia (usually associated with severe chronic heart failure), anaemia and dizziness.

Heart failure is usually classified according to the severity of symptoms. In chronic heart failure, the New York Heart Association (NYHA) Functional Classification is commonly used to classify patients on the basis of the activity level that initiates symptoms (see Table 10.5).[65]

Diagnostic tests

Tests used to diagnose heart failure include the following:

- Trans-thoracic echocardiography is the most useful investigation to confirm diagnosis. This is the gold standard diagnostic test for heart failure and should always be undertaken when possible.[54,66] This test is vital, as it can distinguish systolic dysfunction (left ventricular ejection fraction [LVEF] <40%) from diastolic dysfunction, and therefore help determine treatment.[54] Information on left and right ventricular sizes, volumes, left ventricular thrombus and ventricular wall thickness and motion can be provided. Assessment of valve structure and function as well as intracardiac and pulmonary pressures can be determined, without the need for invasive techniques. Pulsed-wave Doppler and tissue Doppler studies can be used to determine diastolic dysfunction.
- Assessment of cardiac function can also be done by invasive techniques (e.g. coronary angiography) and nuclear cardiology tests (e.g. gated radionuclide angiocardiography).
- ECG should be done as an initial investigation. Most common abnormalities include ST-T wave changes, left bundle branch block, left anterior hemiblock, left ventricular hypertrophy, atrial fibrillation and sinus tachycardia.

FIGURE 10.11 Diagnostic algorithm for CHF.

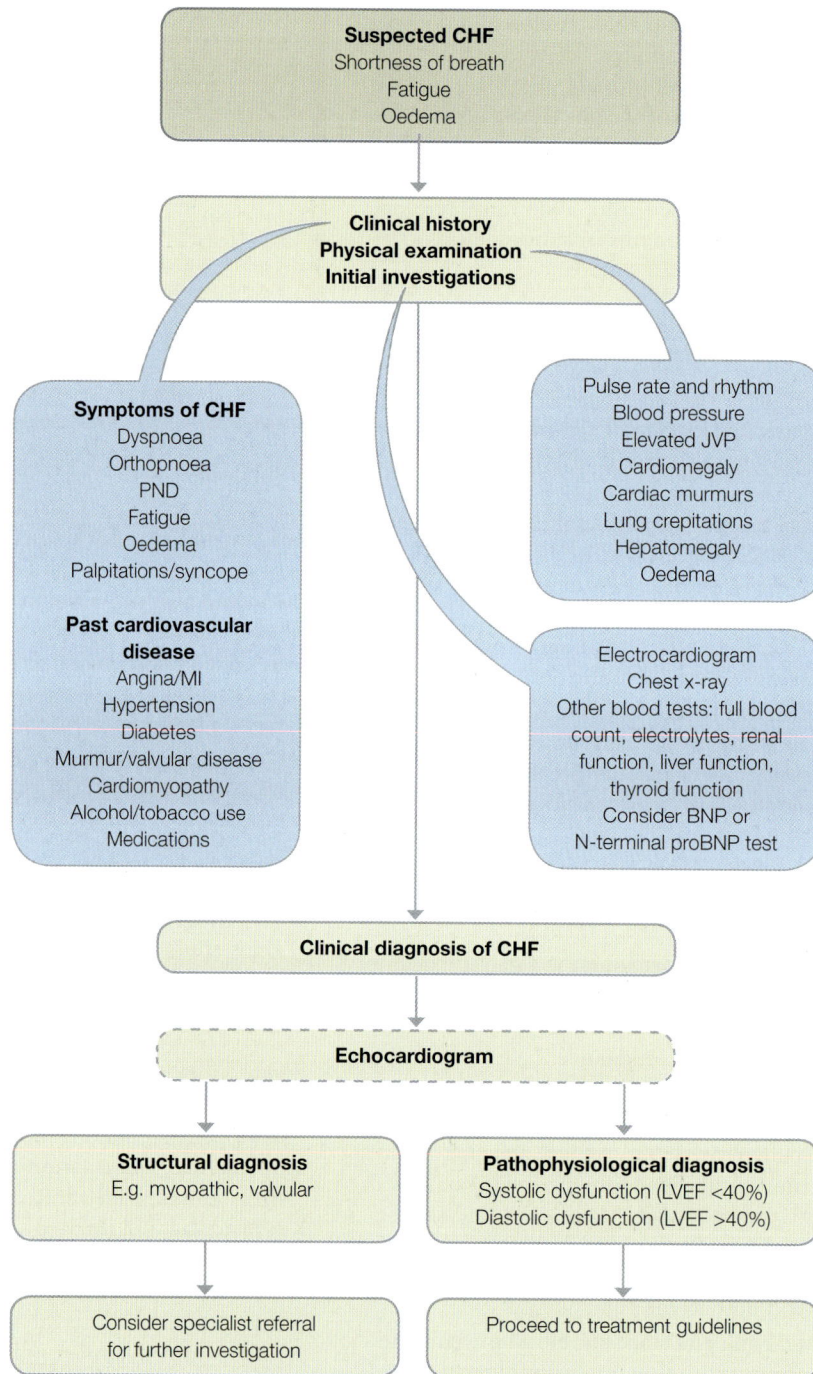

BNP = B-type natriuretic peptide
JVP = jugular venous pressure
LVEF = left-ventricular ejection fraction
MI = myocardial infarction
PND = paroxysmal nocturnal dyspnoea

Courtesy National Heart Foundation of Australia and the Cardiac Society of Australia and New Zealand (Chronic Heart Failure Guidelines Expert Writing Panel). Guidelines for the prevention, detection and management of people with chronic heart failure in Australia. Updated October 2011. Melbourne: National Heart Foundation of Australia; 2011.

- Chest X-ray shows cardiomegaly and pulmonary markings, including evidence of interstitial oedema: perihilar pulmonary vessels, small basal pleural effusions obscuring the costophrenic angles, Kerley B lines (indicating raised left atrial pressure).

- Full blood count checks for anaemia and mild thrombocytopenia. Any signs of anaemia should be further investigated.

- Urea, creatinine and electrolytes tests for dilutional hyponatraemia, hypokalaemia, hyperkalaemia, low magnesium and glomerular filtration rate. These should be closely monitored if there are any changes in clinical status and/or drug therapy such as ACEIs and diuretics.

- Liver function tests check for elevated levels of AST, ALT, lactate dehydrogenase (LDH) and serum bilirubin.

- Thyroid function tests are performed particularly in patients with no history of coronary artery disease and who develop atrial fibrillation.

- Urinalysis is conducted to measure specific gravity and proteinuria.

- Myocardial ischemia and viability need to be assessed in patients with heart failure and coronary artery disease. These can be assessed by a stress ECG, stress echocardiography or a myocardial perfusion study.

  Coronary angiography is useful to determine the contribution of coronary artery disease in these patients.

- Natriuretic peptides include plasma ANP and B-type natriuretic peptide (BNP). BNP or N-terminal proBNP is not recommended to be used as the only test to diagnose chronic heart failure as an elevated BNP may be due to other causes.[54] However, it is useful to use it in conjunction with other diagnostic tests, particularly to differentiate between dyspnoea due to chronic heart failure and dyspnoea due to chronic obstructive pulmonary disease.

- Endomyocardial biopsy should be conducted if there is a suspicion of cardiomyopathy.

Patient management

Treatment of CHF is lifelong and multifactorial, requiring a well-coordinated, multidisciplinary approach. The goals of heart failure treatment are to identify and eliminate the precipitating cause, promote optimal cardiac function, enhance patient comfort by relieving signs and symptoms and help the patient and family cope with any lifestyle changes. Clinical practice guidelines have been developed to guide the treatment of heart failure on the basis of ventricular dysfunction and grade of symptoms (see Figures 10.12–10.14).[54]

Planning for hospital discharge begins early in the admission and aims to promote quality of life for the patient and prevent unnecessary admissions. Several healthcare services have been implemented to support the transition from hospital to home as it is during the first 30 days post-discharge that nearly 35% of heart failure patients are readmitted to hospital.[67] There are currently over 70 outreach heart failure programs throughout Australia that support heart failure patients post-discharge.[68] The main goals of these programs are to reduce symptom burden, improve functional capacity and minimise hospital readmissions. These programs range from in-hospital visits to facilitate discharge planning to nurse-led heart failure outpatient clinics, home visit programs and heart failure-specific exercise programs. Several meta-analyses of home visit programs have shown a reduction in hospital admissions and mortality[69,70] and these programs are now standard care for heart failure patients.[54,59,71] Home visit heart failure programs involve a heart failure nurse visiting the patient at home and providing education to the patient and carer, assessing their symptoms and educating the patients and their carers about self-management strategies. Nurse-led outpatient clinics also reduce hospital admissions and mortality[72,73] and play an important role in the management of heart failure patients post-discharge.

Management of heart failure post the acute phase is based on three principles: self-care management, long-term lifestyle changes and adherence to pharmacotherapy. Management of self-care is the key to non-pharmacological management of heart failure. Self-care refers to the decision-making process of patients concerning their choice of healthy behaviour and response to worsening symptoms when they occur. It involves cognitive decision making, requiring the recognition of signs and symptoms that indicate a change in condition, which is based on knowledge and prior experiences of deterioration.[74,75]

Lifestyle modification and self-care management

Patient education is the key to self-management and must include family members to be effective. Patient education should include information on the following:

- the disease process – this involves discussing what heart failure is, signs and symptoms and why they occur, and strategies to improve their symptoms
- lifestyle changes
- medications and side effects
- self-monitoring and acute symptoms
- importance of adherence to the medications and management plan.

There are numerous resources available for patient and carer education. The Heart Foundation has an excellent resource titled 'Living well with chronic heart failure' (http://www.heartfoundation.org.au/SiteCollectionDocuments/Living well with chronic heart failure.pdf). Also 'heart online' (http://www.heartonline.org.au/Pages/default.aspx) is another excellent resource for health professionals providing information for patients and carers. 'Heartonline' also provides resources for health professionals regarding heart failure management and tools such as surveys.

Restriction of fluid to 1.5–2 L/day is one of the most important strategies that patients can adhere to in order to improve their symptoms. Patients are encouraged to weigh themselves daily and to identify any increase in weight as

FIGURE 10.12 Pharmacological treatment of systolic heart failure.

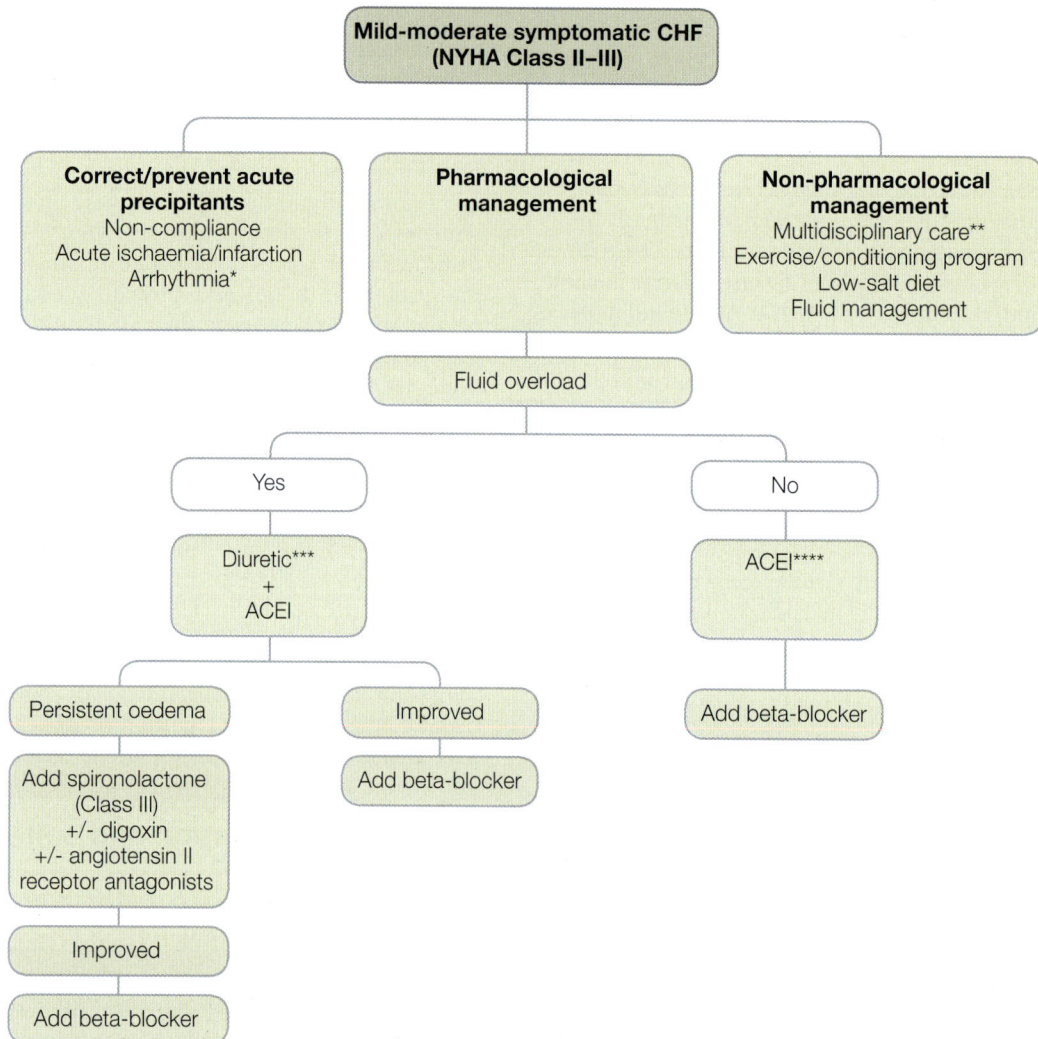

* Patients in atrial fibrillation (AF) should be anticoagulated with a target INR of 2.0–3.0. Amiodarone may be used to control AF rate or attempt cardioversion. Electrical cardioversion may be considered after 4 weeks if still in AF. Digoxin will slow resting AF rate.

** Multidisciplinary care (pre-discharge and home review by a community care nurse, pharmacist and allied health personnel) with education regarding prognosis, compliance, exercise and rehabilitation, lifestyle modification, vaccinations and self-monitoring.

*** The most commonly prescribed first-choice diuretic is a loop diuretic e.g. frusemide; however there is no evidence that loop diuretics are more effective or safer than thiazides.

**** If ACEI intolerant, use angiotensin II receptor antagonists instead.

Courtesy National Heart Foundation of Australia and the Cardiac Society of Australia and New Zealand (Chronic Heart Failure Guidelines Expert Writing Panel). Guidelines for the prevention, detection and management of people with chronic heart failure in Australia. Updated October 2011. Melbourne: National Heart Foundation of Australia; 2011.

an increase of 1 kg equals 1 litre of excess fluid. National guidelines stipulate that, if their weight increases by 2 kg over 2 days, they need to see their local doctor as soon as possible.[54] Patients who adhere to their management plan and closely monitor their daily weight may self-manage their volume status by using a flexible diuretic action plan as developed by their cardiologist. In addition, patients should be advised of early warning signs of excess fluid volume and decompensation, such as increasing dyspnoea, fatigue and peripheral oedema.

Sleep apnoea also occurs commonly in CHF patients. There are two types: obstructive sleep apnoea and central sleep apnoea. Obstructive sleep apnoea occurs due to airway collapse and is associated with obesity. It can be treated

FIGURE 10.13   Pharmacological treatment of refractory systolic heart failure.

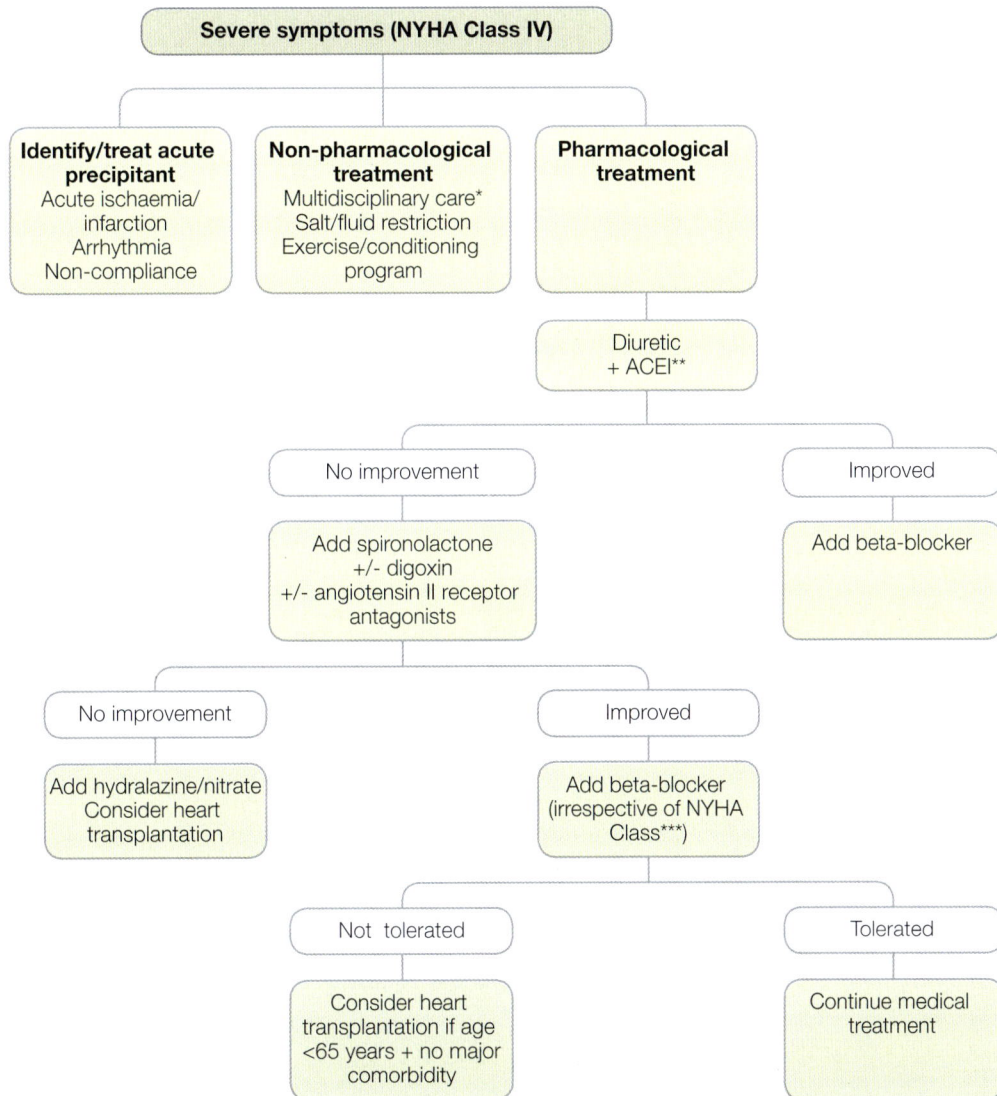

```
                    ┌─────────────────────────────────┐
                    │  Severe symptoms (NYHA Class IV) │
                    └─────────────────────────────────┘
```

Identify/treat acute precipitant
Acute ischaemia/infarction
Arrhythmia
Non-compliance

Non-pharmacological treatment
Multidisciplinary care*
Salt/fluid restriction
Exercise/conditioning program

Pharmacological treatment

Diuretic + ACEI**

No improvement

Improved

Add spironolactone
+/- digoxin
+/- angiotensin II receptor antagonists

Add beta-blocker

No improvement

Improved

Add hydralazine/nitrate
Consider heart transplantation

Add beta-blocker (irrespective of NYHA Class***)

Not tolerated

Tolerated

Consider heart transplantation if age <65 years + no major comorbidity

Continue medical treatment

* Multidisciplinary care (pre-discharge and home review by a community care nurse, pharmacist and allied health personnel) with education regarding prognosis, compliance, exercise and rehabilitation, lifestyle modification, vaccinations and self-monitoring.

** If ACEI intolerant, use angiotensin II receptor antagonists instead.

*** Patients with NYHA Class IV CHF should be challenged with beta-blockers provided they have been rendered euvolaemic and do not have any contraindication to beta-blockers.

Courtesy National Heart Foundation of Australia and the Cardiac Society of Australia and New Zealand (Chronic Heart Failure Guidelines Expert Writing Panel). Guidelines for the prevention, detection and management of people with chronic heart failure in Australia. Updated October 2011. Melbourne: National Heart Foundation of Australia; 2011.

with weight reduction and night-time continuous positive airway pressure (CPAP). The use of CPAP for obstructive sleep apnoea results in an improvement in LVEF due to an increase in left ventricular filling and emptying rates, and a decrease in systolic blood pressure and left ventricular chamber size.[76] Central sleep apnoea (Cheyne–Stokes respiration) occurs due to pulmonary congestion and high sympathetic stimulation in patients with severe heart

failure and may be treated with CPAP. However, the benefits of oxygen therapy have not been proven. Exercise is equally important, to prevent the deconditioning of skeletal muscle that occurs in CHF. Exercise training – including walking, exercise bicycle and light resistance – has been shown to improve functional capacity, symptoms, neurohormonal abnormalities, quality of life and mood in CHF.[65] The Heart Foundation of Australia recommends

FIGURE 10.14 Management of heart failure with preserved ejection fraction (HFpEF).

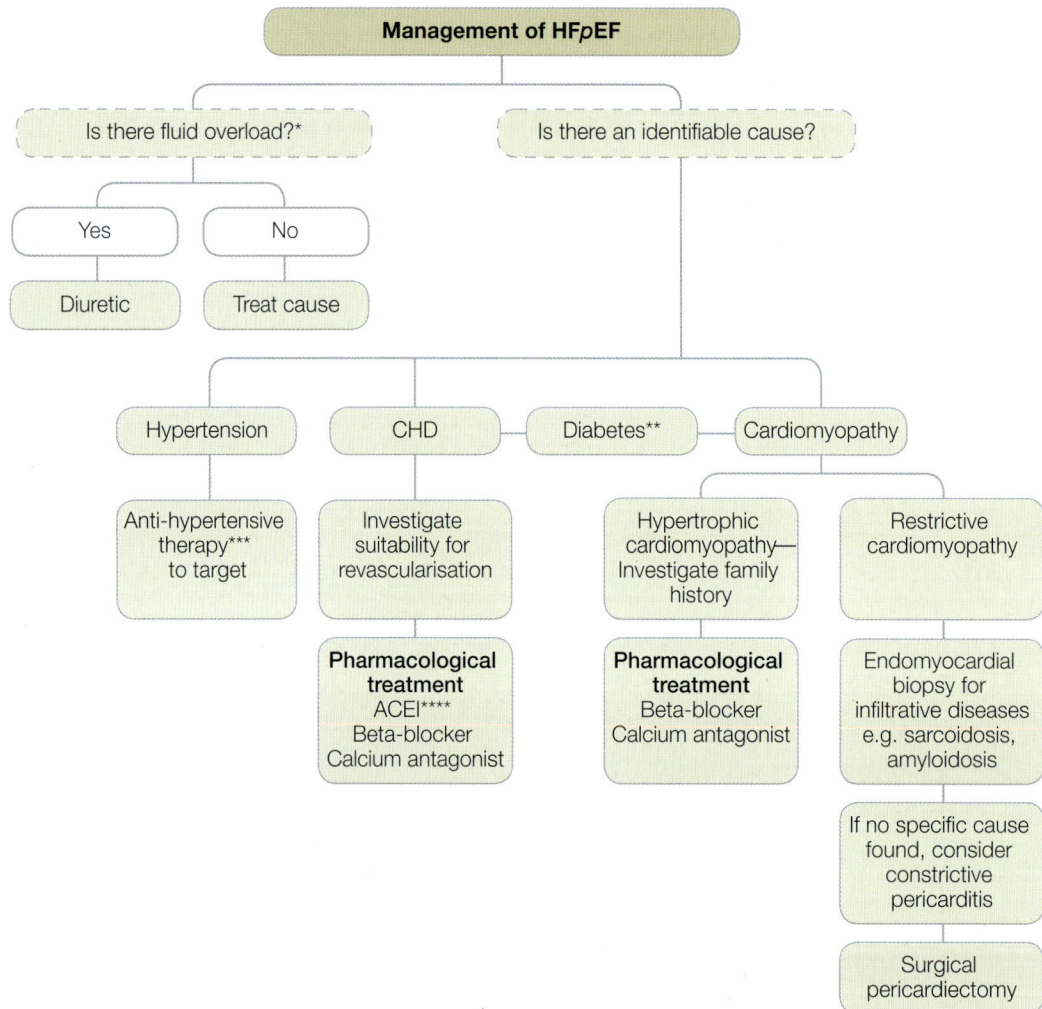

* With rare exception, patients with diastolic heart failure present with symptoms and signs of fluid overload, either pulmonary or systemic congestion or both.

** Better diabetes control.

*** Choice of therapy will vary according to clinical circumstances, e.g. thiazide diuretic — elderly, systolic hypertension; ACEI — LV hypertrophy, diabetes, CHD; beta-blocker — angina.

**** If ACEI intolerant, use angiotensin II receptor antagonist instead.

Courtesy National Heart Foundation of Australia and the Cardiac Society of Australia and New Zealand (Chronic Heart Failure Guidelines Expert Writing Panel). Guidelines for the prevention, detection and management of people with chronic heart failure in Australia. Updated October 2011. Melbourne: National Heart Foundation of Australia; 2011.

that all stable CHF patients, regardless of age, should be considered for referral to a tailored exercise program (preferably a heart failure-specific exercise program) or modified cardiac rehabilitation program.[54] Heart failure exercise programs comprise resistance training and have been shown to improve functional capacity, heart failure symptoms and survival and reduce hospitalisations.[77] In patients with symptomatic heart failure physical activity should be undertaken under the supervision of trained heart failure specialists, e.g. a physiotherapist or exercise physiologist, who can tailor the level of exercise to the

degree of severity of symptoms. Many CHF patients have comorbidities such as arthritis, which make exercise programs difficult, but maintaining general activity should be encouraged.

Dietary sodium intake should be reduced to 2 g/day for patients with moderate-to-severe heart failure and to 3 g/day for mild heart failure.[54] Reduction in sodium intake helps reduce fluid retention, diuretic requirements and potassium excretion. A large proportion of an individual's sodium intake can come from processed foods, so patients are encouraged to read nutrition labels and reduce the intake of these foods. Salt intake can also be reduced by avoiding adding salt in cooking or to meals. As CHF patients who are overweight increase demands on their heart, weight loss by lowering dietary fat intake may improve symptoms and quality of life. These patients may require referral to a dietician for weight loss management. In patients with moderate-to-severe heart failure, cardiac cachexia and anaemia are common, which further exacerbate weakness and fatigue. These patients will require a referral to a dietician for nutritional support. Other lifestyle changes are: cease smoking, ideally cease alcohol intake or otherwise limit alcohol to less than 2 standard drinks/day (alcohol is a myocardial toxin and reduces contractility), limit caffeinated drinks to 1–2 drinks/day (to decrease the risk of arrhythmias), control diabetes and have annual vaccinations for influenza and regular pneumococcal disease vaccinations.[54]

Palliative care may be appropriate for patients with end-stage heart failure who are experiencing significant symptoms, prescribed maximal pharmacotherapy, frequent hospital admissions and poor response to treatment. It is important that all patients have an advanced care plan in place and that this has been discussed with family members. Advanced care plans should be discussed soon after the patient's first hospital admission for treatment of decompensated heart failure.

Pharmacotherapy in patients with heart failure is vital, and includes an array of drugs that require careful management. Nurse practitioners are authorised to titrate some heart failure medications, including diuretics and beta-adrenergic blocking agents. Pharmacists also provide essential patient education, and support the optimisation of medication treatments and management of complex medication schedules. Some major hospitals have a pharmacist outreach program where a pharmacist visits the patient at home.

Practice tip

When considering if a patient is suitable for palliation, discussion also needs to include deactivation of their pacemaker or implantable cardioverter defibrillator (ICD).

Medications

Pharmacological management relies on the following categories of drugs: ACEIs, beta-adrenergic blocking agents, angiotension receptor blocking agents (ARBs), diuretics, digoxin and antiarrhythmic drugs. (Beta-adrenergic blocking agents and antiarrhythmic drugs are reviewed later in this chapter.) The main actions and adverse effects of these drugs in heart failure are summarised in Table 10.6.

TABLE 10.6

Common medications for the treatment of heart failure[58,69]

DRUG/EXAMPLE	ACTION	MAJOR ADVERSE EFFECTS
FIRST-LINE PHARMACOTHERAPY		
ACE inhibitor Captopril Enalapril	Decrease systemic vascular resistance by stopping angiotensin I conversion to II; decreased sodium and water retention	Symptomatic hypotension Hyperkalaemia Unproductive cough Renal failure Rash
Loop diuretics Frusemide	Increase urine volume by decreasing reabsorption of chloride and sodium	Hypokalaemia Ototoxicity Rash
Thiazide diuretics Chlorothiazide Hydrochlorothiazide	Increase urine volume by decreasing reabsorption of sodium	Hypokalaemia Hyperglycaemia Sensitivity: rash
Beta-adrenergic blockers Bisoprolol Carvedilol Metoprolol CR/XL	Reduce systemic vascular resistance and heart rate by blocking adrenoreceptors in arteries and heart	Hypotension Bronchoconstriction
Potassium-sparing diuretics Spironolactone	Increase urine volume by aldosterone blocking and sodium retention	Hyperkalaemia Rash Gynaecomastia
ARB Candesartan Irbesartan	Block the angiotensin II receptor that responds to angiotensin II stimulation; decreased sodium and water retention. Alternative to ACEI	Symptomatic hypotension Hyperkalaemia Renal failure
SECOND-LINE PHARMACOTHERAPY		
Cardiac glycosides Digitalis	Increase myocardial contractility and decrease heart rate by inhibiting sodium pump in myocytes	Tachycardia AV block Nausea and vomiting Disorientation Visual disturbances

Angiotensin-converting enzyme inhibitors

ACEIs are the cornerstone of CHF treatment, as they have been demonstrated to prolong survival, improve patient symptoms and exercise tolerance, prevent hospitalisation and improve ejection fraction in CHF patients.[78,79] All patients with symptomatic systolic LV dysfunction should be prescribed ACEIs.[1,54,59,71] Drugs in this group (captopril, enalapril, lisinopril) act on the renin–angiotensin system by specifically preventing the conversion of angiotensin I to angiotensin II.[80] As a result, systemic vascular resistance (afterload) is decreased. This is particularly important in preventing the progression of CHF, because blockade of the renin–angiotensin system prevents further development of systolic dysfunction. In addition, because angiotensin II also stimulates the release of aldosterone, sodium and water retention are decreased (preload). This may also be beneficial when ACEIs are prescribed with diuretics, as potassium loss is limited. Further, ACEIs inhibit the breakdown of bradykinin (a vasodilator), which also contributes to decreasing vascular resistance. The total reduction of systemic vascular resistance reduces the workload of the heart without affecting heart rate or cardiac output.

Common adverse effects of ACEIs primarily result from hypotension, including dizziness and headache. Other side effects include hyperkalaemia, deterioration of renal function and an unproductive cough, which may respond to asthma prophylactic medications. Initial doses of ACEIs should be low, as severe – though transient – symptomatic hypotension can occur, worsening of renal function and hyperkalaemia. The dose of ACEIs needs to be gradually increased to maximum dose over 2–3 months to optimise the survival and functional capacity benefits. This group of drugs is contraindicated in patients with bilateral renal artery stenosis due to the danger of developing renal failure. One important adverse effect of ACEIs is that they cannot be taken in conjunction with NSAIDs as NSAIDs reduce the action of ACEIs.[81]

Practice tip

A dry, non-productive cough is often associated with the introduction of ACEI medication, but is often mistaken for a symptom of other conditions, so patients may not report the symptom as new. The cough usually begins within 1–2 days of commencing therapy and up-titration of dose.

Practice tip

Heart failure is a disease of the elderly. Many elderly patients have arthritis. However, elderly patients with heart failure must avoid taking NSAID medications, especially when taking ACEIs, as NSAIDs counter the action of ACEIs. In such cases we usually recommend taking long-acting paracetamol or glycosamine for relief from arthritis pain.

Beta-adrenergic blocking agents

All patients with symptomatic systolic left ventricular dysfunction should be prescribed a beta-adrenergic blocking agent. Beta-adrenergic blocking agents (carvedilol, metoprolol, bisoprolol) are used in CHF to inhibit the adverse effects of chronic activation of the sympathetic nervous system and improve ventricular function. In heart failure beta-2 receptors predominate with beta-1 receptors being downregulated. In heart failure beta-adrenergic blocking agents reduce this neurohormonal activity. The addition of a beta-adrenergic blocker has been demonstrated to reduce symptoms, reduce hospitalisations and prolong survival in patients.[82,83] Similar to ACEIs the dose of beta-adrenergic blocking agents needs to be gradually increased. Once the patient is euro-volaemic they should be commenced on low dose and gradually increased to maximal dose over several months.

In patients with COPD, selective beta-1 blockers are prescribed. Patients will require close monitoring for signs of deterioration of their COPD. Other adverse events are: symptomatic hypotension, bradycardia and worsening heart failure. Also, during the up-titration of beta-adrenergic blocking agents many patients complain of feeling vague in the morning; this usually disappears after 2–3 weeks.

Angiotensin receptor blocking agents

The primary use of angiotensin receptor blocking agents (ARBs) is in patients who are intolerant of ACEI symptoms such as ACEI cough. They have a similar action as ACEIs; however, ARBs block the angiotensin II receptor that responds to angiotensin II stimulation. ACEIs, on the other hand, act on the enzyme that produces angiotensin II.[80] They have similar benefits as ACEIs, improving survival, LVEF and heart failure symptoms and reducing hospitalisations.[84,85] Similar to ACEIs, ARBs are commenced on a low dose and gradually up-titrated to optimal dose over 2 months. Adverse effects are: deterioration in renal function, hyperkalaemia and symptomatic hypotension.[80]

Diuretics

Diuretics are one of the mainstays of management of heart failure, primarily to decrease the sodium and water retention response to the low cardiac output state. A combination of diuretics may be used if oedema persists on one diuretic. Most often, diuretics will be used in combination with ACEIs.

- Loop diuretics: (frusemide, ethacrynic acid and bumetanide) act on the ascending limb of the loop of Henle of the nephron. They prevent the reabsorption of chloride and sodium ions from the loop, so that increased concentrations are present in the loop, attracting more water and increasing urine volume. Intravenous administration of frusemide is often used to manage preload in acute exacerbations. In fluid-overloaded patients, the aim is to achieve increased urine output and a weight reduction of 0.5–1 kg daily, until clinical euvolaemia is achieved. Hypokalaemia is a common adverse effect, and patients on long-term diuretics need regular monitoring and may require potassium supplements. Hyponatraemia may also occur at high doses, and needs careful management in heart failure patients. Ototoxicity, presenting as tinnitus, vertigo and deafness, can occur at high doses, so IV delivery of frusemide should be no faster than 4 mg/min.

- Thiazide and thiazide-like diuretics: (chlorothiazide, hydrochlorothiazide, chlorthalidone) act on the ascending loop of the nephron and decrease sodium reabsorption. As a result, the fluid in the collecting ducts is more concentrated and attracts more water. Thiazides also cause peripheral arteriole vasodilation, which may be beneficial in hypertensive patients. Adverse effects are similar to loop diuretics due to potassium and sodium loss, and supplementation may be necessary. When ACEIs are prescribed concurrently, there is less potassium loss (details below). Hyperglycaemia can occur, so diabetics need monitoring. Impotence may also occur, as well as sensitivity due to the presence of sulfonamide in the drug structure.

- Aldosterone antagonists: are potassium-sparing diuretics and include spironolactone.[54] Aldosterone acts on the distal convoluted tubule of the nephron to cause sodium retention and thus water retention, although potassium is lost. Antagonists stop this action, so potassium is not lost and not as much sodium retained, thus there is minor diuresis. Spironolactone is particularly useful in chronic heart failure because there is excessive aldosterone production, causing oedema. There is the potential that spironolactone, by blocking aldosterone systemically, may prevent the negative effects of aldosterone on the heart, such as fibrosis, hypertrophy and arrhythmogenesis. Adverse effects include hyperkalaemia, which may occur more readily in CHF patients because of renal failure, and because of its potentially lethal effects spironolactone requires regular monitoring. Other effects include hyponatraemia and feminisation effects such as gynaecomastia. In patients with HFpEF, spironolactone has been shown to reduce heart failure-related hospitalisations.[86] Spironolactone is recommended for use in patients with severe symptomatic (NYHA class III–IV) systolic heart failure in addition to other pharmacotherapy such as ACEIs. Aldosterone antagonists have additional survival benefits and reduce hospital readmission.[87,88]

Inotropic agents

This category of drugs increases cardiac contractility. The group includes cardiac glycosides (digoxin) and dopamine agonists (dopamine, dobutamine), sympathomimetics (adrenaline, noradrenaline) and calcium sensitising agents (levosimendan). Inotropes are used as IV infusions in severe heart failure, acute exacerbations of chronic heart failure and for palliative care or bridging to transplant in very severe chronic heart failure. These drugs have both inotropic and chronotropic actions, so that cardiac contractility and heart rate are both increased to improve cardiac output. Continuous ambulatory infusions of inotropic agents such as dobutamine are administered to patients with severe heart failure as a bridge to transplantation, which allows these patients to be discharged home with support from a home visit nurse.

Cardiac glycosides

Cardiac glycosides such as digitalis inhibit the sodium pump such that the exchange between sodium and calcium is impaired. This results in calcium stores being released and intracellular calcium levels rising. As more calcium is available for contraction, contractility and cardiac output increase. These changes in ion movement and additional effects, which enhance parasympathetic stimulation, result in decreased impulse generation by the sinoatrial (SA) node. This is known as a negative chronotropic effect. Conduction is also slowed through the atrioventricular (AV) node and ventricles, allowing more filling time, and therefore having a positive effect on cardiac output. The negative chronotropic effects are particularly beneficial in patients with the atrial fibrillation that is so common in CHF. Digitalis may also affect cardiopulmonary baroreceptors to reduce sympathetic tone, which may be a valuable offset to excessive sympathetic stimulation in CHF.

The most important adverse effects of digoxin are caused by changes in conduction: tachycardia, fibrillation and AV block. Digoxin may also cause nausea and vomiting due to direct brain effects and gastrointestinal irritation. Digitalis has a narrow margin of safety, a long half-life and side effects that can be fatal, so assay of plasma drug levels must be conducted regularly and at initiation and change of treatment. Excessive digoxin causes disorientation, hallucinations and visual disturbances. Potassium levels directly alter the effect of digoxin, so that low levels enhance effects and high levels reduce effects.

Arrhythmias are common in heart failure and need to be treated. The agent must be carefully selected, as chronic heart failure patients often have complex medication regimens and interactions may occur. Also, some ventricular antiarrhythmics, such as class 1 agents (e.g. flecainide), are associated with sudden death in CHF. Implantable cardioverter-defibrillator (ICD) therapy may be more effective in treating ventricular arrhythmias. ICDs reduce mortality by 20–30%[89] and are first-line therapy in patients with a history of VF or sustained VT, LVEF ≤30% with NYHA class II–III, at least 40 days post-myocardial infarction, and prescribed optimal pharmacotherapy or NYHA class I with LVEF ≤35% and prescribed optimal pharmacotherapy.[66] Cardiac resynchronisation therapy (CRT) (also known as biventricular pacing) is also indicated in patients with symptomatic heart failure to reduce asynchronous pacing of the left ventricle (QRS duration >150 ms).[71] Systolic function is improved when the left and right ventricles are paced simultaneously. Often patients with a prolonged QRS will have a combination of an ICD with CRT therapy. ICDs and CRT are discussed in more detail in Chapter 11.

In severe heart failure, when patients do not respond to pharmacological treatment, mechanical measures such as cardiopulmonary bypass and left ventricular assist devices may be used. In appropriate candidates, cardiac transplant may also be an option. These procedures are covered under cardiac surgery.

Acute exacerbations of heart failure

Acute exacerbations of CHF usually occur as episodes of decompensation due to progression of the disease or non-adherence to the management plan.[90] Acute episodes usually present as congestive heart failure with associated pulmonary oedema, cardiogenic shock (see Chapter 21) or decompensated CHF.[54] Patients with severe dyspnoea due to pulmonary congestion should be administered oxygen therapy. If their hypoxaemia does not improve, they may benefit from bilevel positive airway pressure (BiPAP) to support ventilation and gas exchange. The use of continuous positive airway pressure ventilation (CPAP) or BiPAP in acute pulmonary oedema will reduce the need for intubation and mechanical ventilation.

The mainstay of treatment of an acute exacerbation is pharmacological, so a combination of the medications is given, usually comprising diuretics, morphine and nitrates. The nitrates and morphine cause vasodilatation. Morphine also reduces the respiratory drive and respiratory workload. Nitrates also cause epicardial artery dilatation and reduce preload, which also helps to relieve symptoms of pulmonary congestion particularly at night when filling pressures are increased due to the recumbent position of sleeping.[54] Diuretics should be administered intravenously to optimise the excretion of intra- and extra-vascular cellular fluid to reduce circulating blood volume to reduce cardiac workload. Fluid restriction, usually to 1–1.5 L in 24 hours, is begun. A urinary catheter may need to be inserted so that accurate, continuous measures of urine output can be gained and an accurate fluid balance calculated. This is necessary, along with consistent daily weighing, to determine the effectiveness of diuretic therapy and renal status. Various positive inotropes may be administered (e.g. IV dobutamine causes vasodilatation; IV dopamine improves renal function) to improve contractility and reduce systemic venous return. Various mechanical devices are also available, e.g. intra-aortic balloon pump, LVAD (discussed in Chapter 12). CRT with or without an ICD may be implanted. CRT is recommended in NYHA class II–III or ambulatory class IV patients on optimal pharmacological therapy, LVEF ≤35%, left bundle branch block with a QRS duration >150 ms, and sinus rhythm.[71] All of these criteria must be fulfilled. Criteria for implantation of an ICD include: symptomatic patients (NYHA class II–IV) and LVEF ≤35%, LVEF <30% at least 40 days post AMI.[71] If a patient is to have an ICD implanted, extensive counselling pre- and post-implantation must be undertaken with the patient and carer to ensure they are aware of the painful and unexpected shocks that may be delivered.[54,71] Figure 10.15 provides an overview of the escalation of treatment for acute heart failure.[54]

FIGURE 10.15 Emergency therapy of acute heart failure.

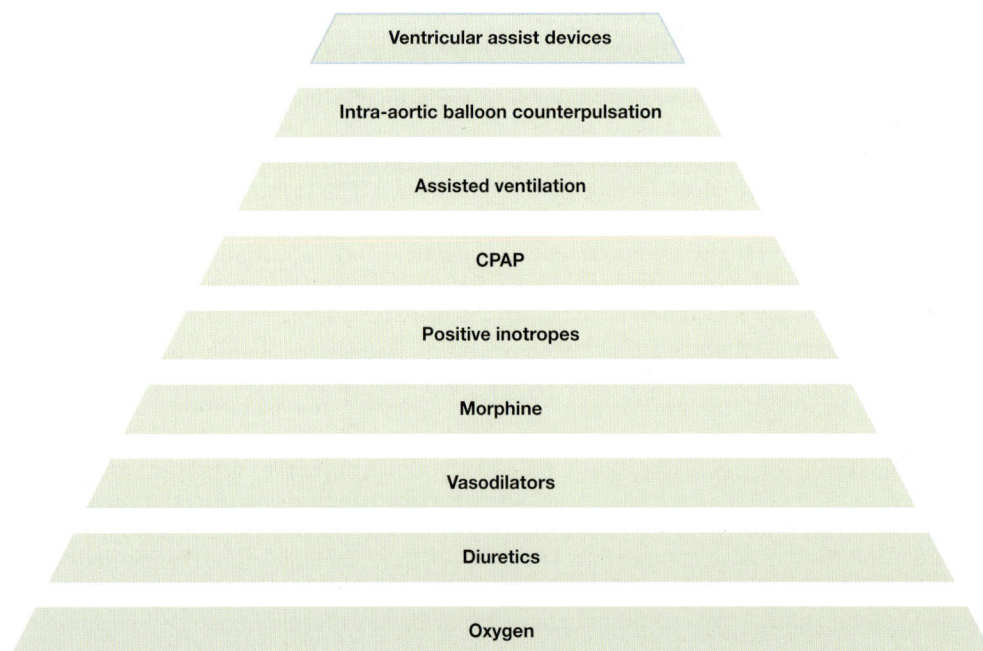

Ventricular assist devices

Intra-aortic balloon counterpulsation

Assisted ventilation

CPAP

Positive inotropes

Morphine

Vasodilators

Diuretics

Oxygen

Courtesy National Heart Foundation of Australia and the Cardiac Society of Australia and New Zealand (Chronic Heart Failure Guidelines Expert Writing Panel). Guidelines for the prevention, detection and management of people with chronic heart failure in Australia. Updated October 2011. Melbourne: National Heart Foundation of Australia; 2011.

Most patients in acute heart failure have poor perfusion of the gastrointestinal system and, combined with dyspnoea, a resultant limited appetite. Small, easily ingested meals are best. While the patient is on bedrest, nursing care to prevent problems related to immobility is important. Skin care is particularly important, as poor skin perfusion and oedema place the CHF patient at higher risk of skin breakdown.

Selected cases

Cardiomyopathy

As the term implies, the cardiomyopathies are primary disorders of the myocardium in which there are systolic, diastolic or combined abnormalities. Classification of the most common forms of cardiomyopathy is made on the basis of the dominant abnormality, which may be dilation, hypertrophy or restricted filling. However, each has different haemodynamic effects and therefore requires different treatment.

Dilated cardiomyopathy

Dilated cardiomyopathy (DCM) is the most common form of cardiomyopathy and is characterised by ventricular and atrial dilation and systolic dysfunction.[91] All four chambers become enlarged, which is not in proportion to the degree of hypertrophy. It presents as heart failure of variable severity, sometimes complicated by thromboembolism, at least partly due to atrial fibrillation, which is common. Conduction abnormalities are common in DCM further exacerbating AV dyssynchrony and left ventricular dysfunction. DCM is the most common cause of sudden cardiac death due to ventricular arrhythmias. Annual mortality from DCM ranges from 10–50%.[91] Idiopathic DCM is the most common cause of heart failure in young people. Aetiology of DCM includes coronary heart disease, myocarditis, cardiotoxins, genetics and alcohol misuse.

Diagnosis

Many of the features of DCM are non-specific. Heart failure, as mentioned, is present with typical symptoms of dyspnoea, fatigue, peripheral oedema and cardiomegaly. S3 and S4 heart sounds may be present on auscultation. Atrial and ventricular arrhythmias are common, particularly atrial fibrillation, ventricular tachycardia, ventricular fibrillation and torsades de pointes. Left bundle branch block (LBBB) is often present, which worsens systolic performance and shortens survival, especially when the QRS interval is markedly prolonged.[91] Echocardiography demonstrates the defining abnormalities and may be useful in revealing atrial thrombus. Occasionally, endocardial biopsy is undertaken to differentiate from myocarditis or rarer causes of cardiomyopathy.

Patient management

Treatment for DCM is similar to that of heart failure and includes beta-adrenergic blocker therapy, ACEIs, diuretics and antiarrhythmic therapy where indicated or, if necessary, an ICD for recurrent haemodynamically significant ventricular arrhythmias.[91] The use of cardiac resynchronisation therapy (CRT) has produced significant clinical improvements and is recommended for DCM patients with NYHA functional class II–III or ambulatory class IV, optimal medical therapy, LVEF ≤35% and sinus rhythm with left bundle branch block with a QRS >150 ms.[71] Cardiac transplantation is considered when standard therapies fail to influence clinical progression and left ventricular assist devices and ICDs may be used as a bridge to transplantation.

Hypertrophic cardiomyopathy

Hypertrophic cardiomyopathy (HCM) is a genetic abnormality that gives rise to inappropriate hypertrophy especially in the intraventricular septum with preserved or hyperdynamic systolic function. The main abnormality with HCM is diastolic rather than systolic as in DCM. The hypertrophy is not a compensatory response to excessive load, such as in aortic stenosis or hypertension. Left ventricular hypertrophy of variable patterns is seen, occasionally with disproportionate septal hypertrophy, which causes left ventricular outflow tract obstruction in which HCM progresses to hypertrophic obstructive cardiomyopathy, or HOCM. In HCM the muscle mass is large and hypercontractile, but the left ventricular cavity is small. The increase in left ventricular systolic pressure and the altered relaxation cause diastolic dysfunction and impaired ventricular filling. Mitral regurgitation is common. These abnormalities combine to produce pulmonary congestion and dyspnoea due to raised end-diastolic pressure. Sudden cardiac death, often after exertion or other increases in contractility, is sometimes seen in HCM and is thought to be partly attributable to outflow obstruction.[71] It is the most common cause of death in athletes.[71]

Diagnosis

Echocardiography will confirm the presence and pattern of hypertrophy and the presence (or absence) of an outflow tract gradient. Examination findings include cardiomegaly and pulmonary congestion. An S4 heart sound is common, and the ECG shows left ventricular hypertrophy and often ventricular arrhythmias. When the obstructive form hypertrophic obstructive cardiomyopathy (HOCM) is present, a systolic murmur, mitral regurgitation murmur and deep narrow Q waves on ECG may be present.[91] The majority of patients are asymptomatic and, when they present to hospital, it will be with severe symptoms of dyspnoea, angina and syncope. Angina is the result of an imbalance between oxygen supply and demand due to the increased myocardial mass and not due to atherosclerosis.

Patient management

Treatment for HCM is aimed at the prevention of sudden cardiac death and pharmacotherapy to increase diastolic filling and to reduce the left ventricular outflow tract obstruction. Pharmacotherapy includes beta-adrenergic blocker or calcium channel blocker therapy, as these decrease contractility and lessen outflow tract obstruction. Care is necessary with medication selection, as vasodilation may worsen obstruction, causing haemodynamics to suffer.[91] The impact of atrial fibrillation, by worsening the ventricular filling defect, can be dramatic in HCM patients and will require antiarrhythmics and anticoagulation. If ventricular arrhythmias are present, or there is a family history of sudden cardiac death, treatment with an ICD should be considered.[92] For severely symptomatic patients or those worsening despite maximal drug treatment, surgical myectomy to reduce the size of the septum and lessen obstruction may be necessary and can result in a marked improvement of symptoms.[92] Septal ablation with alcohol injected into the first septal branch of the left anterior descending artery is a less invasive alternative, a procedure that is usually undertaken with pacemaker insertion as AV block is produced. Although surgical myectomy remains the gold standard, both treatments provide effective symptom relief and improvement in heart failure severity.[92] If the patient with HCM deteriorates and is hospitalised, positive inotropes, chronotropes and nitrates worsen left ventricular outflow tract obstruction and should be avoided. However, beta-adrenergic blockers, amiodarone and calcium antagonists such as verapramil are indicated.[91] Due to the familial nature of HCM, relatives aged 12–18 years also need to be screened for HCM.

Restrictive cardiomyopathy

Restrictive cardiomyopathies (RCMs) limit diastolic distensibility or compliance of the ventricles. The stiff ventricular walls produce diastolic dysfunction and there is impaired ventricular filling. Infiltrates into the interstitium and the replacement of normal myocardium with abnormal tissue hamper this relaxation.[91] Initially, systolic function and wall thickness are normal. However, as the disease progresses systolic dysfunction occurs. RCM is commonly caused by myocardial infiltration, as in amyloidosis, sarcoidosis, fibrosis or cardiac metastases, or may be idiopathic. Endomyocardial disease is more common in tropical countries, but in the Western world, RCMs are the least common form of cardiomyopathy.[91]

Diagnosis

Clinically, there is heart failure (increase in JVP, dyspnoea, S3 and S4 heart sounds and oedema), particularly right ventricular, and infiltration of the conduction system may cause conduction defects and heart block. Low-voltage ECGs are commonly seen. Patients commonly present with decreased exercise tolerance due to the impaired ability to increase heart rate and cardiac output because of reduced ventricular filling. RCM must be distinguished from constrictive pericarditis (which it may closely resemble), as pericarditis may be easily managed.[91] If echocardiography demonstrates a restrictive pattern, a myocardial biopsy may be undertaken to determine its aetiology, especially in the case of systemic infiltrative disease.

Patient management

There is no treatment for RCM so the aim of therapy is to relieve symptoms. This includes diuretics, corticosteroids and pacing. The use of nitrates should be initiated with caution as the filling defect can be worsened by decreased venous return or hypovolaemia. Generally, prognosis is poor with many dying within 1–2 years of diagnosis.[91]

Hypertensive emergencies

Acute, uncontrolled hypertension is often divided into two categories: hypertensive emergencies and hypertensive urgencies. In hypertensive emergencies blood pressure needs to be reduced within 1 hour to prevent end-organ damage, such as hypertensive encephalopathy, papilloedema or aortic dissection.[93] Immediate blood pressure reduction with IV agents under critical care monitoring is needed. By contrast, hypertensive urgencies are those in which end-organ damage is not occurring and, although prompt management is required, this can be approached more gradually with oral antihypertensive agents under close supervision, without necessarily requiring admission to a critical care unit.[93] Previous hypertension is not always present, but because of chronic adaptive vascular changes may provide some level of protection against acute tissue injury. Symptoms may not develop until the blood pressure exceeds 220/110 mmHg, whereas in patients without previous hypertension, hypertensive emergencies may occur at levels of even 160/100 mmHg.[94] When the diastolic pressure is persistently above 130 mmHg, there is risk of vascular damage and it must be treated.

Diagnosis

A thorough history is taken, including any hypertension management, known renal or cerebrovascular disease, eclampsia in previous pregnancies if gravid or use of stimulants or illicit drugs such as cocaine. Patient assessment should include evidence of: end-organ damage, such as back pain (aortic dissection); neurological damage, such as headache, altered consciousness, confusion, visual loss, stupor or seizure activity (encephalopathy); cardiac damage, such as chest pain, ST-segment changes, cardiac enlargement or the development of heart failure or pulmonary oedema; and renal damage, such as oliguria and azotaemia.[93] Serum urea, creatinine, electrolytes, urinalysis, ECG and chest X-ray should be performed.

Patient management

More severe, or malignant, hypertension may cause retinal haemorrhage or papilloedema, and emergency treatment should immediately be instituted. Other contexts in which there is a need for rapid treatment of severe hypertension include intracranial bleeding, acute myocardial infarction, phaeochromocytoma, recovery from cardiac surgery and bleeding from vascular procedure sites. Hypertensive emergencies in pregnancy threaten both the mother and the fetus.[95]

The aim of treatment is to acutely lower the blood pressure, but neither too quickly nor too dramatically.

Recommendations vary, but an initial aim of 150/110–160/100 mmHg within 2–6 hours, or a 25% reduction in mean arterial pressure within 2 hours, has been described.[96,97] Continuous direct arterial pressure monitoring should be in place during treatment. Intravenous sodium nitroprusside, a rapidly acting arterial and venous dilator, is most frequently used, at doses of 0.25–10 mcg/kg/min.[97] Weaning of nitroprusside is undertaken after the later introduction of oral antihypertensives. Care is required to avoid hypotension during treatment, as well as rebound hypertension as nitroprusside is withdrawn. Rapidly acting beta-adrenergic blocking agents with short half-lives, such as IV esmolol, may be used at doses of 50–100 mcg/kg/min (or higher) in patients without standard contraindications to beta-adrenergic blockers (asthma, heart failure).[97] Glyceryl trinitrate infusions at 10–100 mcg/min or higher are used for combined venous and arterial dilation, especially if there is angina.[97] Intravenous frusemide may be introduced during the acute phase. After intravenous therapies have been established and progress towards target pressures is made, oral agents are introduced. These include oral beta-adrenergic blockers, calcium channel blockers, ACEIs and diuretics.

Infective endocarditis

Infective endocarditis remains a potentially life-threatening disorder, with mortality remaining as high as 20–25%[98] even in this era of relative rheumatic fever control. This same era, however, sees other means of developing endocarditis, with factors such as longer life, IV drug use, prosthetic valves, greater rates of cannulation during hospitalisation, cardiac surgery, resistant organisms and increased numbers of immunocompromised patients from immunosuppressant drugs and human immunodeficiency virus/acquired immune deficiency syndrome HIV/AIDS.[99,100]

Infection of the endocardium, often with involvement of the cardiac valves, occurs most commonly due to staphylococcal, streptococcal and enterococcal bacteraemia.[99,100] The definition of infective endocarditis now also includes an infection of any structure within the heart such as prosthetic valves, implanted devices and chordae tendineae.[101] Infective endocarditis can be acute or subacute. Acute infective endocarditis progresses over days to weeks with destruction of valves and metastatic infection. Subacute infective endocarditis occurs over weeks to months and is milder than acute infective endocarditis. Endothelial damage occurs in the endocardium. Platelet-fibrin deposits form and a lesion develops. Bacterial colonisation then occurs and vegetation adheres to the endocardial lesion. Many of the signs and symptoms of infective endocarditis are due to the immune response to the microorganism. The patient presents with fever, and general features of febrile illness, which may include septic shock. Joint pain is common and septic arthritis is sometimes seen. Cardiac symptoms develop when there is valvular involvement, which may manifest as erosion through valve leaflets producing regurgitation, fusing of valve leaflets or vegetations (outgrowths from valve structures), producing valvular stenosis or regurgitation.[100] The mitral valve is more commonly affected, but aortic valve involvement carries a worse prognosis.[98] Conduction system involvement manifests as arrhythmias and conduction defects. Embolic complications are relatively common and multifactorial. Septic emboli, embolisation of atrial thrombi when atrial fibrillation is present and fragmentation of vegetations may all give rise to pulmonary and systemic emboli. These most often present as splenic infarction, stroke, peripheral vascular occlusion and renal failure.[98]

Diagnosis

Diagnosis of infective endocarditis is based on the modified Duke criteria.[100] These are based on the presence of microorganisms (identified in blood cultures), pathological lesions (vegetation or abscess present) and clinical criteria. The clinical criteria are based on two major criteria or one major and three minor criteria or five minor criteria. Major clinical criteria are:

- positive blood culture
- evidence of endocardial involvement (positive echocardiography, abscess, partial dehiscence of a prosthetic valve or new valvular vegetation).

Minor clinical criteria include:

- fever with body temperature ≥38°C
- predisposing heart condition or intravenous drug use
- vascular signs: arterial emboli, intracranial haemorrhage, Janeway lesions (erythematous spots on the palms and feet) or conjunctival haemorrhages
- immunological signs: Osler nodes (painful, reddened nodules on the fingers and the feet) or glomerulonephritis.[98]

Echocardiography may reveal vegetations, abscess and valvular abnormalities, but endocarditis is more a clinical diagnosis based on the appearance of febrile illness, positive blood cultures with organisms known to cause endocarditis, new murmur and vascular features.

Patient management

Prosthetic valve endocarditis must be aggressively managed, as mortality may be as high as 65%.[100] Impaired valvular opening, even obstruction, may occur or the prosthetic valve may become unseated. Reoperation to replace the affected valve should be undertaken when valvular dysfunction is present. Antibiotic therapy is provided empirically until blood culture and sensitivities are established. Cardiac failure, if present, is managed along standard lines (see section on nursing management of acute heart failure). Observations during endocarditis should be directed at detecting embolic complications involving the brain, kidneys, or spleen; development and progress of heart failure; progress of the febrile illness, including hydration and dietary status.

Prophylactic antibiotic coverage should be undertaken for at-risk patients 1 hour before dental procedures are to be performed, in particular for those with previous rheumatic fever or endocarditis, or prosthetic valves.[101] Antibiotic prophylaxis for genitourinary and gastrointestinal procedures is no longer recommended.[101]

Aortic aneurysm

The aorta is the major blood vessel leaving the heart. An aneurysm is a local dilation or outpouching of a vessel wall and comes in several forms (see Figure 10.16).[28] Most aortic aneurysms are fusiform and saccular, and occur in the abdominal aorta. A fusiform aneurysm is uniform in shape with symmetrical dilation that involves the whole circumference of the aorta.[102] A saccular aneurysm has dilation of part of the aortic wall so the dilation is very localised.[102] A dissecting aneurysm occurs when the layers of the wall of the aorta continue to separate and fill with blood, resulting in obstructed blood flow. The aorta is particularly susceptible to aneurysm formation because of constant stress on the vessel wall and the absence of penetrating vasa vasorum that normally provide perfusion to the adventitia. As the blood flows through the aneurysm it becomes turbulent and some blood may stagnate along the walls, allowing a thrombus to form. This thrombus in addition to atherosclerotic debris may embolise into the distal arteries compromising their circulation. Atherosclerosis is the commonest cause of aneurysm, because plaque formation erodes the vessel wall. Other causes include syphilis, infection, inflammatory diseases and trauma. Aneurysms occur most often in men and in people with the risk factors of hypertension or smoking. Approximately 80% of aortic aneurysms rupture into the left retroperitoneum, which may contain the rupture. However, the other 20% rupture into the peritoneal cavity and uncontrolled haemorrhage results.[102]

Patients often experience no symptoms until the aneurysm is extensive or ruptures. Clinical presentation varies and depends on the location and expansion rate. Aneurysms of the ascending aorta tend to affect the aortic root and cause valve regurgitation. Expansion of the aneurysm may also compress the vena cavae, leading to engorged neck and superficial veins, or compress the large airways, causing respiratory distress. The first symptom most patients experience is pain, which may be steady and continuous from local compression or sudden and severe in the case of dissection or rupture, usually in the lower back. In this case, the pain is usually associated with syncope and is an acute emergency. Depending on the site of the aneurysm, there is usually an absence or decrease in the pulses below the site of the aneurysm, most commonly in the limbs. The renal arteries may be affected, resulting in decreased urine output and renal failure. The spinal blood flow may also be affected, resulting in paraplegia and, if the carotid arteries are affected, there may be altered consciousness. Infrarenal aneurysms are the most common form of aortic aneurysm and are located below the renal arteries. Bruits can also be heard over the aneurysm.

Diagnosis

A chest X-ray is usually the first investigation, and may reveal a widened mediastinum or enlarged aortic knob. Some aneurysms will be hidden, so normal chest X-ray does not exclude the diagnosis. If available, a CT scan, using contrast dye, provides accurate information on the location and size of the aneurysm. Transoesophageal echocardiography (TOE) provides an accurate diagnosis and is the preferred investigation in dissecting aneurysms. TOE can clearly identify the tear/flap, to enable classification of the aneurysm. There are some limitations in viewing the ascending aorta, and patients with respiratory dysfunction may have difficulty with lying flat for the procedure and having a light anaesthetic.

Patient management

Management of asymptomatic aneurysms is conservative, unless the size of the aneurysm is >1.5 times the normal

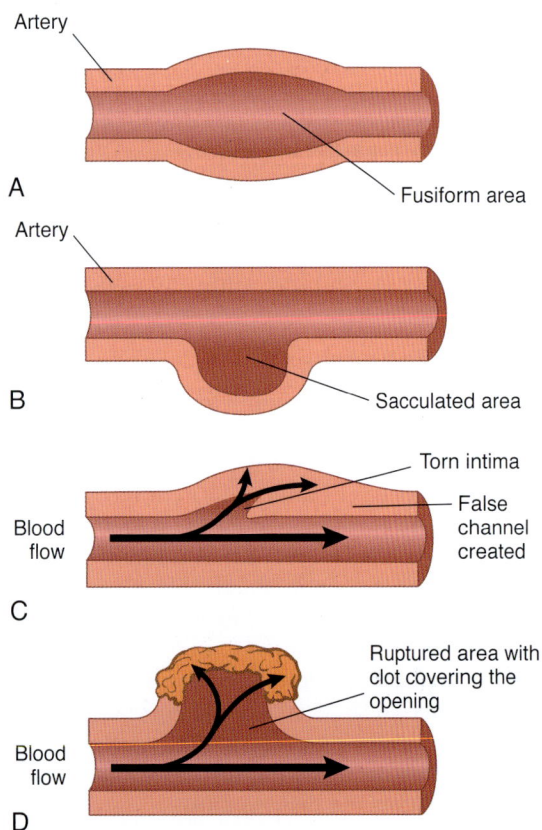

FIGURE 10.16 Aneurysm. Major types of aneurysm: **(A)** fusiform aneurysm has an entire section of an artery dilated, occurring most often in the abdominal aorta due to atherosclerosis; **(B)** sacculated aneurysm affects one side of an artery, usually in the ascending aorta; **(C)** dissecting aneurysm results from a tear in the intima, causing blood to shunt between the intima and media; **(D)** pseudoaneurysm usually results from arterial trauma, such as intra-aortic balloon pump catheter or an arterial introducer; the opening does not heal properly and is covered by a clot that can burst at any time.[28]

Artery

A Fusiform area

Artery

B Sacculated area

Torn intima
False channel created
Blood flow
C

Ruptured area with clot covering the opening
Blood flow
D

size of the aortic segment[102] or the situation is acute. The primary aim is to lower hypertension and prevent increases in thrombus size and emboli through the administration of aspirin. Usually, the patient has regular monitoring to assess the aneurysm and to determine the timing and need for surgical repair.

Acute and dissecting aortic aneurysms are life-threatening emergencies, and surgery is often the only option. The development of new or worsening lower back pain may indicate impending rupture and there may be a palpable pulsatile abdominal mass. The faster treatment is initiated, the higher the chances of survival with optimal recovery. The primary goal is to control blood pressure. If hypertensive, beta-adrenergic blockers or sodium nitroprusside is used to reduce further arterial wall stress. If the patient is hypotensive, IV fluid and inotropes may be necessary.

Nursing management of dissecting aortic aneurysm involves the following:

- support during the diagnostic phase
- assessment of pain and provision of analgesia
- stabilising and monitoring the clinical condition
- providing psychological support to patient and family
- preparation for surgery and long-term care.

Assessment of the patient's symptoms and effects of the aneurysm is essential. This includes careful assessment and recording of symptoms, including pain level and intensity, peripheral pulses, oxygen saturation levels, blood pressure in both arms and neurological symptoms to assist with diagnosis and detect progression. Intravenous analgesia is essential to control the severe pain, and an antiemetic is useful to prevent opiate side effects. Opiates may also contribute to a sedative effect and slight vasodilation, which are both beneficial. Oxygen therapy via mask should be administered as indicated by oxygen saturation levels. Blood pressure control is vital, and usually IV medications are titrated to a narrow MAP range of 60–75 mmHg. Close observation of fluid balance to detect changes in renal perfusion and maintain appropriate blood volume is also essential. Finally, preparation for surgery is necessary, and must include the patient and family.

Ventricular aneurysm

Less than 5% of patients post-STEMI, particularly a transmural anterior infarction, develop a left ventricular aneurysm.[103] Post-STEMI, dyskinetic or akinetic areas of the left ventricle are common and known as regional wall motion abnormalities. It is in these areas that there is a risk of an aneurysm developing. Ventricular aneurysms are more likely to develop post–anterior STEMI with a totally occluded LAD with poor collateral circulation.

Aneurysms form when the intraventricular tension stretches the dyskinetic area and a thin, weak layer of necrotic muscle and fibrous tissue develops and bulges with each contraction of the ventricle resulting in a reduction in stroke volume. Aneurysms range from 1–8 cm in diameter and are four times more likely to occur at the apex and anterior wall rather than the inferoposterior wall.[103] Large ventricular aneurysms may result in a reduction in stroke volume causing an increase in myocardial oxygen demand resulting in angina and heart failure. The mortality rate in people with ventricular aneurysms is four times higher than those with no aneurysm due to a higher risk of tachyarrhythmias and sudden cardiac death. Unlike aortic aneurysms these aneurysms rarely rupture so their management is usually conservative.

Diagnosis

Diagnosis of a ventricular aneurysm is by echocardiography. Ventricular aneurysm should be considered when ST-segment elevation persists beyond 1 week after myocardial infarction.

Patient management

Management of a left ventricular aneurysm consists of aggressive management of STEMI and reperfusion therapy. Long-term anti-coagulation therapy with warfarin is required. A complication of a ventricular aneurysm includes the development of an intraventricular thrombus within the aneurysmal pocket which, if mobilised, becomes arterial emboli. Also due to the high risk of tachyarrhythmias, antiarrhythmic therapy is indicated. An ICD may also be necessary if antiarrhythmic therapy is unsuccessful in suppressing tachyarrhythmias. Surgical aneurysmectomy may also be required, if heart failure and angina become severe, and is usually successful.

Summary

Compromise of the cardiovascular system, as either a primary or secondary condition, is a common problem that necessitates admission of patients to a critical care area. Prompt and appropriate assessment and treatment are required to ensure adequate oxygen supply to the tissues throughout the body. The most common cardiovascular problems experienced by patients include coronary heart disease, arrhythmias and cardiogenic shock; however, heart failure and selected conditions such as cardiomyopathics, hypertensive emergencies, endocarditis and aortic aneurysm also occur. Appropriate assessment and management are essential to prevent secondary complications arising. Important principles covered in this chapter are summarised below.

- Coronary heart disease:
  - Incorporates myocardial ischaemia, angina and acute coronary syndrome.
  - Early patient assessment and diagnosis are essential to facilitate prompt intervention.

- Initial diagnosis is based on history, clinical assessment, electrocardiographic and biochemical examination, with coronary angiography, exercise testing and chest radiography available to provide later detail.
- Early restoration of blood flow – including reperfusion therapy and coronary angioplasty – to reduce myocardial damage is a core component of treatment.
- Other goals of care include reducing plaque and clot formation in coronary arteries, reducing the workload of the heart, controlling symptoms, providing psychosocial support to the patient and family and educating the patient about the disease process, lifestyle and future responses to illness.
- Heart failure:
  - May affect either the left, right or both ventricles, resulting in different symptoms being displayed by the patient.
  - Diagnosis is usually made on the basis of echocardiography, ECG, chest X-ray, full blood count, electrolytes, liver function tests and urinalysis.
  - In acute heart failure, CPAP or BiPAP may be necessary to improve hypoxaemia.
  - Pharmacological therapy of acute heart failure consists of morphine, nitrates and diuretics. Positive inotropes may also be used, such as IV dopamine and dobutamine, to improve renal perfusion and contractility.
  - Many patients with heart failure will also have a pacemaker with cardiac resynchronisation therapy and/or a defibrillator to improve cardiac function and reduce the incidence of sudden death.
  - Patient care must be lifelong and coordinated between all members of the healthcare team. Broad interventions, including medications, diet and lifestyle modification, may be appropriate for some patients, while palliative care might be more appropriate for other patients.

Case study

Ms Patel is a 60-year-old woman who presented to the emergency department with intermittent chest pain. She presented to her general practitioner (GP) 2 days ago complaining of intermittent chest pain over a 2–3 hour period. An ECG was done showing old Q waves anteriorly and ST depression in V5 and V6. A troponin-I was done by her GP that was 0.16 mcg/L.

Her past medical history included: diabetes mellitus type 2, infrarenal abdominal aortic aneurysm, asthma/COPD, peripheral vascular disease, hypercholesterolaemia and hypertension. Her medications consisted of: diamicron 60 mg daily, glargine 26 units nocte, perindopril 5 mg daily, seretide and ventolin puffers and lipitor 20 mg daily.

One day after visiting her GP, she presented to the emergency department with further intermittent chest pain and upper abdominal pain. Initial 12-lead ECG showed ST elevation in leads II, III and aVF. She was also feeling very tired and nauseated at times. She denied any chest pain. She was afebrile, BP 143/96 mmHg, pulse 120 bpm and regular, respiratory rate 33 bpm and O_2 sat 91% on room air. Her respiration was laboured and her skin was cool and clammy. On chest auscultation there were bibasal crackles to mid-zones. Her jugular venous pressure was +5 and she had peripheral oedema to lower calves. She had dual heart sounds (S1, S2) and a third heart sound (S3). U&E blood test results included: Na 134 mmol/L, K 5.1 mmol/L, urea 5.2 mmol/L, creatinine 86 mcmol/L, ctroponin-I 2.0 mcg/L, CK 590 U/L and random glucose 9.2 mmol/L. Her FBE and LFTs were normal. Fast-track treatment was commenced, including administering aspirin 300 mg orally, oxygen via mask 6 L/min, glyceryl trinitrate patch, morphine 2.5 mg IV, metoclopramide 10 mg IV and frusemide 40 mg IV. Chest X-ray showed horizontal linear interstitial opacities at both bases, which were not present on a previous X-ray taken 6 months ago, which was consistent with the clinical impression of pulmonary oedema. There was also a marked increase in the size of the heart, which also had a slightly globular configuration. There was no evidence of a pericardial effusion.

Within a short time her acute pulmonary oedema was stabilised and so she was considered for a primary PTCA. Coagulation profiles and a brief history of, and contraindications to, fibrinolytic treatment were collected. Preparation for PTCA included locating, assessing and marking peripheral pulses in both right leg and right arm. The coronary angiogram report stated: moderate-to-severe reduction in left ventricular function, ejection fraction 30%; intact left circumflex artery, intact left main coronary artery with minor irregularities (30%) in left anterior descending artery; and severe localised 70–80% stenosis within the proximal third of the right coronary artery and collaterals from the left coronary artery. Her right coronary artery was the dominant vessel. The stenosis was dilated by PTCA with resulting TIMI 3 flow, and a paclitaxel drug-eluting stent was placed.

Post-PTCA, Ms Patel was admitted to CCU with oxygen via mask, PTCA access site and sheath in her right groin. Her observations included: BP 100/60 mmHg, HR 80 beats/min, RR 20/min. She was free of pain. Her ECG was normal except for T inversion in lead III with a generalised widened QRS (200 ms). Post-PTCA she experienced short runs of ventricular tachycardia. These were initially thought to be due to reperfusion arrhythmias. However, the short intermittent runs of ventricular tachycardia continued. Her blood test results were: Na 137 mmol/L, K 4.6 mmol/L, urea 8.8 mmol/L, creatinine 99 mcmol/L, calcium 2.37 mmol/L, magnesium 0.96 mmol/L. Fasting cholesterol profile: total cholesterol 4.3 mmol/L, HDL-C 1.91 mmol/L, LDL-C 2.1 mmol/L, triglycerides 0.7 mmol/L, cholesterol/HDL-C 2.3 mmol/L. Her liver function and full blood examination tests were normal. She was commenced on an intravenous amiodarone infusion and considered for an ICD with CRT, in light of her newly diagnosed heart failure (evident on coronary angiogram) and NYHA class III symptoms.

Post-ICD-implantation, her hospital stay was uneventful. Her fluids were restricted to 1.5 L/day, and she was weighed daily, commenced a beta-adrenergic blocking agent and diuretic and was provided with education concerning heart failure and coronary artery disease. Her husband was also included in the education sessions. She was transferred from CCU to the ward and then a few days later discharged home. On discharge her medications were: bisoprolol 5 mg daily, perindopril 5 mg daily, spironolactone 25 mg daily, co-plavix 100/75 mg daily, spirivia 18 mcg daily, seretide 250/25 mg BD, lantus 36 units nocte, amiodarone 200 mg BD, gliclazide MR 60 mg mane, frusemide 80 mg mane and midi and GTN spray. She was also referred to a heart failure management program and a cardiac rehabilitation program.

CASE STUDY QUESTIONS

1   Identify the key indicators of ST-elevation myocardial infarction (STEMI).

2   Discuss the use of oxygen in acute myocardial infarction.

3   Identify the common complications of myocardial infarction in the early recovery period.

4   What is the significance of an S3 heart sound in the clinical setting of heart failure?

5   What criteria might have been considered when deciding to implant an ICD with CRT in Ms Patel?

6   When the patient was discharged from hospital, why was she prescribed perindopril, bisoprolol, spironolactone and frusemide? Include in your answer the reason for prescribing these medications and their actions and major side effects.

RESEARCH VIGNETTE

Dizon JM, Brener SJ, Maehara A, Witzenbichler B, Biviano A, Godlewski J et al. Relationship between ST-segment resolution and anterior infarct size after primary percutaneous coronary intervention: analysis from the INFUSE-AMI trial. Eur H J Acute Cardiovasc Care 2014;3:78–83

Abstract

Objective: ST-segment resolution after reperfusion therapy has been shown to correlate with prognosis in patients with ST-segment elevation myocardial infarction (STEMI). We investigated whether acute ECG measurements also correlate with ultimate infarct size.

Methods: The INFUSE-AMI trial randomized 452 patients with anterior STEMI to intracoronary bolus abciximab vs. no abciximab, and to thrombus aspiration vs. no aspiration. Infarct size as percentage of total LV mass was calculated by cardiac magnetic resonance imaging (MRI) 30 days post intervention. Five ECG methods were analysed for their ability to predict MRI infarct mass: 1) summed ST resolution across all infarct-related ECG leads (ΣSTR); 2) STR in the single lead with maximum baseline ST-segment elevation (maxSTR); 3) summed residual ST segment elevation across all infarct-related leads at 60 min post intervention (ΣST residual); 4) maximum residual ST-segment elevation in the worst single lead at 60 min post intervention (maxSTresidual); 5) number of new significant Q-waves (Qwave) at 60 min.

Results: All ECG methods strongly correlated with 30-day MRI infarct mass (all p<0.003). Simpler ECG measurements such as maxSTresidual and Qwave were as predictive as more complex measurements. A subset analysis of

158 patients who had microvascular obstruction (MVO) determined by MRI 5 days post intervention also showed strong correlations of MVO with the ECG measures.

Conclusions: ST-segment and Q-wave changes after primary PCI in anterior STEMI strongly correlated with 30-day infarct size by MRI. In particular, maxSTresidual and Qwave at 60 min are simple ECG parameters that offer rapid analysis for prognostication.

Critique

This study investigated the relative importance of ECG measures at the end of the angioplasty procedure for determining cardiac tissue viability after STEMI, an important indicator of prognosis including mortality. International guidelines recommend the use of 12-lead ECG to monitor myocardial ischaemia after STEMI and primary angioplasty, but a variety of ECG markers, including ST-segment markers, are available for this purpose and TIMI flow post procedure is often considered before ECG evidence.

The study was a multicentre study and enrolled patients who had proximal or mid-left anterior descending artery occlusion indicated by STEMI. Participants were then entered into a four-arm randomized controlled trial to receive intracoronary abciximab or not and manual aspiration thrombectomy or not. ECG interpretation was blinded and conducted by two staff at independent laboratories. Both the random allocation to group and the blinding of ECG interpretation are important strengths of the study. Five ECG measurements were used to determine residual ischaemia and/or infarction at varying levels of complexity, for instance, determining change from pre to post intervention from all affected leads (ΣSTR) to percentage ST-segment residual elevation in a single maximally affected lead (maxSTR) or number of new significant Q waves (Qwave). MRI was performed at 30 days to measure infarct size and in a subgroup at 5 days to measure microvascular obstruction.

Of the 482 patients enrolled 91% were alive at 30 days and MRI was performed and assessable in 80% of these participants and paired ECGs available for 73%. All ECG measures correlated well with MRI infarct size, with simpler measures (MaxSTR and Qwave) performing as well as complex measures. Only one ECG measure correlated significantly with mortality at 30 days and this was Qwave.

Several limitations are relevant to the study including that the sample was restricted to patients with anterior infarcts due to proximal or LAD occlusion so the results may not apply to other MI. Loss to follow-up and unusable assessments were low; however, the loss of these participants may limit generalisability. Regardless, the results confirm that in STEMI patients straightforward ECG measures following angioplasty, such as new Q waves and level of ST-segment elevation of the most affected lead, are good indicators of myocardial tissue damage, and therefore of the potential for complications in the early recovery phase. Considerations before changing clinical practice include whether nursing staff are skilled at ECG interpretation, particularly determining the presence and size of Q waves. Also, many other clinical factors aside from the size of the infarction are likely to influence mortality, such as pre-existing cardiovascular fitness and/or ejection fraction as well as the presence of comorbid conditions, and need to be taken into account in determining prognosis.

Learning activities

1   Follow two patient journeys, one each for early triage primary PTCA and elective PTCA, and compare the patient experiences from the two pathways.

2   Describe the key nursing care requirements of a patient immediately following stent placement in an abdominal aortic aneurysm.

3   Discuss the compensatory mechanisms that are activated in heart failure and their effects on the cardiovascular system.

4   Observe an echocardiograph and ask the sonographer to explain what is visualised on the screen, particularly in Doppler mode. Ask them to identify areas of hypokinesis or akinesis and any evidence of dyssynchrony between the ventricles.

Online resources

American Heart Association, www.heart.org/HEARTORG/

Australian Institute of Health and Welfare, www.aihw.gov.au

Cardiac Society of Australia and New Zealand, www.csanz.edu.au

Heart Education Assessment and Rehabilitation Toolkit (HEART), www.heartonline.org.au

National Heart Foundation of Australia, www.heartfoundation.com.au

National Heart Foundation of New Zealand, www.heartfoundation.org.nz

Patient information on living with heart failure, www.heartfoundation.org.au/SiteCollectionDocuments/Living well with chronic heart failure.pdf

Further reading

Woods SL, Froelicher ESS, Motzer SU, Bridges EJ, eds. Cardiac nursing. 6th ed. Baltimore: Lippincott, Williams & Wilkins; 2010.

Zipes DP, Libby P, Bonow RO, Braunwald E, eds. Braunwald's heart disease: a textbook of cardiovascular medicine. 7th ed. Philadelphia: Elsevier Saunders; 2008.

References

1 Badellino K. Pathogenesis of atherosclerosis. In: Moser D, Riegel B eds. Cardiac nursing: A companion to Braunwald's heart disease. St Louis: Saunders Elsevier; 2008.

2 Lozano R, Haghavi M, Foreman K, Lim S, Aboyans V, Abraham J et al. Global and regional mortality from 235 causes of death for 20 age groups in 1990 and 2010: a systematic analysis for the Global Burden of Disease Study. Lancet 2012;380;2095–128.

3 Australian Institute of Health and Welfare (AIHW). Australia's health 2010 update. AIHW Cat. No. 12. Canberra: AIHW; 2010.

4 National Heart Foundation of Australia. Heart Disease Fact Sheet. National Heart Foundation of Australia Fact Sheets; 2012.

5 Ministry of Health. Mortality and Demographic Data 2011. Wellington: Ministry of Health; 2014.

6 Guyton A. Textbook of medical physiology. 8th ed. Philadelphia: WB Saunders; 1991.

7 Rapsomaniki E, Shah A, Perel P, Denaxas S, George J, Nicholas O et al. Prognostic models for stable coronary artery disease based on electronic health record cohort of 102,023 patients. Eur Heart J 2014;35:844-52.

8 NHFA and Cardiac Society of Australia and New Zealand. Guidelines for the management of acute coronary syndrome 2006. Med J Aust 2006;184: S1–32.

9 Bersten AD, Soni N, Oh TE. Oh's intensive care manual. 5th ed. Oxford: Butterworth-Heineman, 2003.

10 Chew DA, Aroney C, Aylward P, White H, Tideman P, Kelly A et al. Addendum to the Guidelines for the Management of Acute Coronary Syndromes 2006. Heart Lung Circ 2011;20(Suppl 2):s111-s112.

11 Bagai A, Dangas GD, Stone GW, Granger CB. Reperfusion strategies in acute coronary syndromes. Circ Res 2014;114:1918-28.

12 Hudak CM, Gallo BM, Morton PG. Critical care nursing: A holistic approach. 7th ed. Philadelphia: Lippincott &Williams; 1998.

13 McCance K. Structure and function of the cardiovascular and lymphatic systems. In: Huether S, McCance K, eds. Understanding pathophysiology. ANZ adaptation by Craft J, Gordon C, Tiziani A. St Louis: Mosby; 2010.

14 Nam J, Caners K, Bowen JM, Welsford M, O'Reilly D. Systematic review and meta-analysis of the benefits of out-of-hospital 12-lead ECG and advance notification in ST-segment elevation myocardial infarction patients. Ann Emerg Med 2014;64(2):176-86.

15 Moliterno DJ, Sgarbossa EB, Armstrong PW, Granger CB, Van de Werf F, Califf RM et al. A major dichotomy in unstable angina outcome: ST depression versus T-wave inversion: GUSTO II results. J Am Coll Cardiol 1996;27(2 Suppl 1):181–2

16 Pollack CV Jr, Diercks DB, Roe MT, Peterson ED. American College of Cardiology/American Heart Association guidelines for the management of patients with ST-elevation myocardial infarction: implications for emergency department practice. Ann Emerg Med 2005;45(4):363–76.

17 Reichlin T, Hochholzer W, Bassetti S, Steuer S, Stelzig C, Hartwiger S et al. Early diagnosis of myocardial infarction with sensitive cardiac troponin assays. N Engl J Med 2009;361:858-67.

18 Belenkie I, Knudtson ML, Roth DL, Hansen JL, Traboulsi M, Hall CA et al. Relation between flow grade after thrombolytic therapy and the effect of angioplasty on left ventricular function: a prospective randomized trial. Am Heart J 1991;121(2 Pt 1):407–16.

19 Froelicher VF Jr, Thompson AJ Jr, Davis G, Stewart AJ, Triebwasser JH. Prediction of maximal oxygen consumption: comparison of the Bruce and Balke treadmill protocols. Chest 1975;68(3):331–6.

20 Melin JA, Wijns W, Vanbutsele RJ, Robert A, DeCostes P, Brasseur LA et al. Alternative diagnostic strategies for coronary artery disease in women: demonstration of the usefulness and efficiency of probability analysis. Circulation 1985;71(3):535–42.

21 Moser D, Riegel B. Care of patients with acute coronary syndrome: ST-segment elevation myocardial infarction. In: Moser D, Riegel B, eds. Cardiac nursing: A companion to Braunwald's heart disease. St Louis: Saunders Elsevier; 2008.

22 Lawrence-Mathew PJ, Wilson AT, Woodmansey PA, Channer KS. Unsatisfactory management of patients with myocardial infarction admitted to general medical wards. J R Coll Phys Lond 1994;28(1):49–51.

23 2011 National Heart Foundation of Australia, <http://www.heartfoundation.org.au/SiteCollectionDocuments/ACS%20therapy%20algorithm-WEB-secure.pdf>.

24 Fibrinolytic Therapy Trialists' (FTT) Collaborative Group. Indications for fibrinolytic therapy in suspected acute myocardial infarction: collaborative overview of early mortality and major morbidity results from all randomised trials of more than 1000 patients. Lancet 1994;343:311–22.

25 Boersma E, Maas AC, Deckers JW, Simoons ML. Early thrombolytic treatment in acute myocardial infarction. J Adv Nurs 1996;12:677–82.

26 Bullock S, Manias E. Fundamentals of pharmacology: a text for nurses and allied health professionals. 7th ed. Sydney: Pearson; 2013.

27 The GUSTO authors. GUSTO-1 Global utilisation of streptokinase and t-PA for occluded coronary arteries. An international randomised trial comparing four thrombolytic strategies for acute myocardial infarction. New Engl J Med 1993;329:673–82.

28 Urden L, Stacy K, Logh M. Thelans' critical care nursing: Diagnosis and management. 5th ed. St Louis: Mosby; 2006.

29 Maron DJ, Spertus JA, Mancini GB, Hartigan PM, Sedlis SP, Bates ER et al. COURAGE Trial Research Group. Impact of an initial strategy of medical therapy without percutaneous coronary intervention in high-risk patients from the Clinical Outcomes Utilizing Revascularization and Aggressive DruG Evaluation (COURAGE) trial. Am J Cardiol 2009;104:1055-62.

30 Zijlstra F, Hoorntje JC, de Boer MJ, Reiffers S, Miedema K, Ottervanger JP et al. Long-term benefit of primary angioplasty as compared with thrombolytic therapy for acute myocardial infarction. New Engl J Med 1999;341:1413–19.

31 van Hout BA, Serruys PW, Lemos PA, van den Brand MJ, van Es GA, Lindeboom WK et al. One year cost effectiveness of sirolimus eluting stents compared with bare metal stents in the treatment of single native de novo coronary lesions: an analysis from the RAVEL trial. Heart 2005;91(4):507–12.

32 Halkin A, Stone GW. Polymer-based paclitaxel-eluting stents in percutaneous coronary intervention: a review of the TAXUS trials. J Intervent Cardiol 2004;17(5):271–82.

33 Zheng F, Xing S, Gong Z, Xing Q. Five-year outcomes for first generation drug-eluting stents versus bare-metal stents in patients with ST-segment elevation myocardial infarction: a meta-analysis of randomised controlled trials. Heart Lung Circ 2014;23:542-8.

34 De Luca G, Dirksen MT, Kelbæk H, Thuesen L, Vink MA, Kaiser C et al. Paclitaxel-eluting versus bare metal stents in primary PCI: a pooled patient-level meta-analysis of randomized trials. J Thromb Thrombolysis 2015;39(1):101–12.

35 Schiks IE, Schoonhoven L, Aengevaeren WR, Nogarede-Hoekstra C, van Achterberg T, Verheugt FW. Ambulation after femoral sheath removal in percutaneous coronary intervention: a prospective comparison of early vs. late ambulation. J Clin Nurs 2009;18:1862–70.

36 Bhatt DL, Hulot JS, Moliterno DJ, Harrington RA. Antiplatelet and anticoagulation therapy for acute coronary syndromes. Circ Res 2014;114(12):1929-43.

37 Nascimento BR, de Sousa MR, Demarqui FN, Ribeiro AL. Risks and benefits of thrombolytic, antiplatelet, and anticoagulant therapies for ST segment elevation myocardial infarction: systematic review. ISRN Cardiol 2014;2014:416253.

38 Trotter R, Gallagher R, Donoghue J. Anxiety in patients undergoing percutaneous coronary interventions. Heart Lung 2011;40(3):185–92.

39 Thompson DR, Bowman GS. Evidence for the effectiveness of cardiac rehabilitation. Clin Effect Nurs 1997;1:64–75.

40 Malmberg K, Norhammer A, Wedel H, Ryden L. Glycometabolic state at admission: important risk marker of mortality in conventionally treated patients with diabetes mellitus and acute myocardial infarction: long term results from the Diabetes and Insulin-Glucose Infusion in Acute Myocardial Infarction (DIGAMI) study. Circulation 1999;99:2626–32.

41 Proctor T, Yarcheski A, Oriscello RG. The relationship of hospital process variables to patient outcome post myocardial infarction. Int J Nurs Stud 1996;33(2):121–30.

42 De Jong M. Impact of anxiety on cardiac disease. In: Moser D, Riegel B, eds. Cardiac nursing: A companion to Braunwald's heart disease. St Louis: Saunders Elsevier; 2008.

43 Baker CF, Garvin BJ, Kennedy CW, Polivka BJ. The effect of environmental sound and communication on CCU patients' heart rate and blood pressure. Res Nurs Health 1993;16:415–21.

44 World Health Organization. Needs and action priorities in cardiac rehabilitation and secondary prevention in patients with CHD. Copenhagen: WHO Regional Office for Europe; 1993.

45 Heran BS, Chen JM, Ebrahim S, Moxham T, Oldridge N, Rees K et al. Exercise-based cardiac rehabilitation for coronary heart disease. Cochrane Database Syst Rev 2011;(7):CD001800.

46 Oldridge N, Guyatt G, Jones N, Crowe J, Singer J. Effects on quality of life with comprehensive cardiac rehabilitation after acute myocardial infarction. Am J Cardiol 1991;74:1240–44.

47 Gulanick M, Berra K. Cardiac rehabilitation. In: Moser D, Riegel B, eds. Cardiac nursing: A companion to Braunwald's heart disease. St Louis: Saunders Elsevier; 2008.

48 National Heart Foundation of Australia and Australian Cardiac Rehabilitation Association. Recommended framework for cardiac rehabilitation. 2004. National Heart Foundation of Australia.

49 Kim U, Park JS, Kang SW, Kim YM, Park WJ, Lee SH et al., Korea Acute Myocardial Infarction Registry Investigators. Outcomes according to presentation with versus without cardiogenic shock in patients with left main coronary artery stenosis and acute myocardial infarction. Am J Cardiol 2012;110:36-9.

50 Møller Nielsen A, Lou Isbye D, Knudsen Lippert F, Rasmussen LS. Engaging a whole community in resuscitation. Resuscitation 2012;83(9):1067-71.

51 Bonnemeier H, Ortak J, Wiegand UK, Eberhardt F, Bode F, Schunkert H et al. Accelerated idioventricular rhythm in the post-thrombolytic era: incidence, prognostic implications, and modulating mechanisms after direct percutaneous coronary intervention. Ann Noninvas Electrocardiol 2005;10(2):179–87.

52 Wagner GS, Marriott HJL. Marriott's practical electrocardiography. 10th ed. Baltimore: Lippincott, Williams & Wilkins; 2000.

53 Appel S. Care of patients with complications of acute myocardial infarction. In: Moser D, Riegel B, eds. Cardiac nursing: A companion to Braunwald's heart disease. St Louis: Saunders Elsevier; 2008.

54 National Heart Foundation of Australia and the Cardiac Society of Australia and New Zealand (Chronic Heart Failure Guidelines Expert Writing Panel). Guidelines for the prevention, detection and management of people with chronic heart failure in Australia. Updated October 2011. Melbourne: National Heart Foundation of Australia; 2011.

55 Najafi F, Dobson AJ, Jamrozik K. Recent changes in heart failure hospitalizations in Australia. Eur J Heart Fail 2007;9:228–33.

56 Roger VL, Weston SA, Redfeild MM, Hellermann-Homan JP, Killian J, Yawn BP et al. Trends in heart failure incidence and survival in a community-based population. JAMA 2004;292:344–50.

57 Stewart S, MacIntyre K, Hole DA, Capewell S, McMurray JJV. More malignant than cancer? Five-year survival following a first admission for heart failure in Scotland. Eur J Heart Fail 2001;3:315–22.

58 Australian Institute of Health and Welfare. Cardiovascular disease: Australian facts 2011. Cardiovascular disease series. Cat. no. CVD 53. Canberra: AIHW; 2011.

59 McMurray JJ, Adamopoulos S, Anker SD, Auricchio A, Böhm M, Dickstein K et al. Task force for the diagnosis and treatment of acute and chronic heart failure 2012 of the European Society of Cardiology. ESC Guidelines for the diagnosis and treatment of acute and chronic heart failure. Eur Heart J 2012;33:1787–847. doi:10.1093/eurheartj/ehs104.

60 Go AS, Mozaffarin D, Roger VL, Benjamin EJ, Berry JD, Borden WB et al. Heart disease and stroke statistics: 2014 update a report from the American Heart Association. Circulation 2013;127(1):e6–e245.

61 Abraham WT, Krum H. Heart failure: a practical approach to treatment. New York: McGraw Hill Medical; 2007.

62 Bryant B, Knights K, Saterno E. Pharmacology for health professionals. Sydney: Mosby Elsevier; 2003.

63 Soine L. Heart failure and cardiogenic shock. In: Woods SL, Froelicher ESS, Motzer SU, Bridges EJ, eds. Cardiac nursing. 6th ed. Baltimore: Lippincott, Williams & Wilkins; 2010.

64 Michaelson CR. Congestive heart failure. St Louis: Mosby; 1983.

65 Gould M. Chronic heart failure. In: Hatchett R, Thompson D, eds. Cardiac nursing: a comprehensive guide. Edinburgh: Churchill Livingstone Elsevier; 2002.

66 Krum H, Driscoll A. Management of heart failure. Med J Aust 2013;199(5):174-178.

67 Ezekowitz JA, Bakal JA, Kaul P, Westerhout CM, Armstrong PW. Acute heart failure in the emergency department: short and long-term outcomes of elderly patients with heart failure. Eur J Heart Fail 2008; 10:308-14.

68 Driscoll A, Worrall-Carter L, Hare DL, Davidson PM, Riegel B, Tonkin A et al. Evidence-based chronic heart failure management programs: myth or reality. Qual Safe Health Care 2009;18(6):450–5.

69 McAlister FA, Stewart S, Ferrua S, McMurray JJ. Multidisciplinary strategies for the management of heart failure patients at high risk for readmission: a systematic review of randomised trials. J Am Coll Cardiol 2004; 44(4): 810–9.

70 Whellan DJ, Hasselblad V, Peterson E, O'Connor CM, Schulman KA. Meta-analysis and review of heart failure disease management randomised controlled clinical trials. Am Heart J 2005;149:722–9.

71 Yancy CW, Jessup M, Bozkurt B, Butler J, Casey DE Jr, Drazner MH et al. 2013 ACCF/AHA Guideline for the Management of Heart Failure: A Report of the American College of Cardiology Foundation/American Heart Association Task Force on Practice Guidelines. Circulation 2013. <http://circ.ahajournals.org/content/early/2013/06/03/CIR.0b013e31829e8776.citation>.

72 Phillips CO, Singa RM, Rubin HR, Jaarsma T. Complexity of program and clinical outcomes of heart failure disease management incorporating specialist nurse-led heart failure clinics. A meta-regression analysis. Eur J Heart Fail 2005;7:333–41.

73 Driscoll A, Toia D, Gibcus J, Srivastava PM, Hare DL. Heart failure nurse practitioner clinic: an innovative approach for optimisation of beta-blockers. Heart Lung Circulation 2008;17(1):S13.

74 Driscoll A, Davidson P, Clark R, Huang N, Aho Z on behalf of National Heart Foundation Consumer Resource Working Group. Tailoring consumer resources to enhance self-care in chronic heart failure. ACC 2009;22(3):133–40.

75 Riegel B, Carlson VV. A situation-specific theory of heart failure self-care. J Cardiovasc Nurs 2008;23(3):190–6.

76 Kaneko Y, Floras JS, Usui K, Plante J, Tkacova R, Kubo T et al. Cardiovascular effects of continuous positive airway pressure in patients with chronic heart failure and obstructive sleep apnoea. N Engl J Med 2003;348:1233–41.

77 Piepoli MF, Davos C, Francis DP, Coats AJ for the ExTraMATCH Collaborative. Exercise training meta-analysis of trials in patients with chronic heart failure (ExTraMATCH). Br Med J 2004;328(7443:189–200.

78 CONSENSUS Trial Study Group. Effects of enalapril on mortality in severe congestive cardiac failure. Results of the Cooperative North Scandinavian Enalapril Survival Study (CONSENSUS). N Engl J Med 1987;316:1429–35.

79 SOLVD Investigators. Effect of enalapril on survival in patients with reduced left ventricular ejection fractions and congestive heart failure. N Engl J Med 1991;325:293–302.

80 Opie LH, Pfeffer MA. Inhibitors of angiotensin-converting enzyme, angiotesin II receptor, aldosterone and renin. In: Opie LH, Gersh BJ, eds. Drugs for the heart. 7th ed. Philadelphia: Saunders; 2009.

81 Ailabouni W, Eknoyan G. Nonsteroidal anti-inflammatory drugs and acute renal failure in the elderly. A risk–benefit assessment. Drugs Aging 1996;9(5):341–51.

82 Hjalmarson A, Goldstein S, Fagerberg B, Wedel H, Waagstein F, Kjekshus J et al. Effects of controlled-release metoprolol on total mortality, hospitalizations, and well-being in patients with heart failure: the Metoprolol CR/XL Randomized Intervention Trial in congestive heart failure (MERIT-HF). MERIT-HF Study Group. JAMA 2000;283:1295–302.

83 Packer M, Fowler MB, Roecker EB, Coats AJ, Katus HA, Krum H et al. Effect of carvedilol on the morbidity of patients with severe chronic heart failure: results of the carvedilol prospective randomized cumulative survival (COPERNICUS) study. Circulation 2002;106:2194–9.

84 McMurray JJ, Ostergren J, Swedberg K, Granger CB, Held P, Michelson EL et al. Effects of candesartan in patients with chronic heart failure and reduced left-ventricular systolic function taking angiotensin converting-enzyme inhibitors: the CHARM-Added trial. Lancet 2003;362(9386):767–71.

85 Cohn JN, Tognoni G, for the Valsartan Heart Failure Trial Investigators. A randomized trial of the angiotensin receptor blocker valsartan in chronic heart failure. N Engl J Med 2001;345(23):1667–75.

86 Pitt B, Pfeffer MA, Assmann SF, Boineau R, Anand IS, Claggett B et al. for the TOPCAT Investigators. Spironolactone for heart failure with preserved ejection fraction. N Engl J Med 2014;370:1383–92.

87 Pitt B, Zannad F, Remme WJ, Cody R, Castaigne A, Petez A et al. The effect of spironolactone on morbidity and mortality in patients with severe heart failure. Randomized Aldactone Evaluation Study Investigators. N Engl J Med 1999;341:709–17.

88 Pitt B, Remme W, Zannad F, Neaton J, Martinez F, Roniker B et al. Eplerenone, a selective aldosterone blocker, in patients with left ventricular dysfunction after myocardial infarction. N Engl J Med 2003;348:1309–21.

89 Bokhari F, Newman D, Greene M, Korley V, Mangat I, Dorian P. Long-term comparison of the implantable cardioverter defibrillator versus amiodarone: eleven-year follow-up of a subset of patients in the Canadian Implantable Defibrillator Study (CIDS). Circulation 2004;110:112–6.

90 Moser D, Mann D. Improving outcomes in heart failure: it's not unusual beyond usual care (Editorial). Circulation 2002;105:2810–2.

91 Wynne JA, Braunwald E. The cardiomyopathies and myocarditides. In: Zipes DP, Libby P, Bonow RO, Braunwald E, eds. Braunwald's heart disease: a textbook of cardiovascular medicine. 7th ed. Philadelphia: Elsevier Saunders; 2008. p 1404.

92 Ralph-Edwards A, Woo A, McCrindle BW, Shapero JL, Schwartz L, Rakowski H et al. Hypertrophic obstructive cardiomyopathy: comparison of outcomes after myectomy or alcohol ablation adjusted by propensity score. J Thorac Cardiovasc Surg 2005; 129(2): 351–8.

93 Kaplan NM. Systemic hypertension: mechanisms and diagnosis. In: Zipes DP, Libby P, Bonow RO, Braunwald E, eds. Braunwald's heart disease: a textbook of cardiovascular medicine. 7th ed. Philadelphia: Elsevier Saunders; 2008. p 807.

94 González PH, Morales VN, Núñez Urquiza JP, Altamirano CA, Juárez HU, Arias MA et al. Patients with hypertensive crises who are admitted to a coronary care unit: clinical characteristics and outcomes. J Clin Hypertens 2013;15:210–4.

95 Vidaeff AC, Carroll MA, Ramin SM. Acute hypertensive emergencies in pregnancy. Crit Care Med 2005;33(Suppl 10):S307–12.

96 Shapiro S. Cardiac problems in critical care. In: Bongard FS, Sue DY, eds. Current critical care: Diagnosis and treatment. 2nd ed. New York: Lange Medical Books/McGraw-Hill; 2002.

97 Baas LS. Hypertensive emergencies. In: Baird MS, Keen JH, Swearingen PL, eds. Manual of critical care nursing: Nursing interventions and collaborative management. 5th ed. St Louis: Elsevier Mosby; 2005.

98 Karchmer AW. Infective endocarditis. In: Zipes DP, Libby P, Bonow RO, Braunwald E, eds. Braunwald's heart disease: a textbook of cardiovascular medicine. 7th ed. Philadelphia: Elsevier Saunders; 2008. p 1077.

99 Baas LS. Acute infective endocarditis. In: Baird MS, Keen JH, Swearingen PL, eds. Manual of critical care nursing: Nursing interventions and collaborative management. 5th ed. St Louis: Elsevier Mosby; 2005.

100 Nakagawa T, Wada H, Sakakura K, Yamada Y, Ishida K, Ibe T et al. Clinical features of infective endocarditis: comparison between the 1990s and 2000s. J Cardiol 2014;63:145–8.

101 Bashore T, Cabell CH, Fowler V. Update on infective endocarditis. Current Prob Cardio 2006;31:274–352.

102 Isselbacher EM, Eagle KA, Descanctis RW. Diseases of the aorta. In: Zipes DP, Libby P, Bonow RO, Braunwald E, eds. Braunwald's heart disease: a textbook of cardiovascular medicine. 7th ed. Philadelphia: Elsevier Saunders; 2008. p 1546.

103 Antman EM. ST-Elevation myocardial infarction: management. In: Zipes DP, Libby P, Bonow RO, Braunwald E, eds. Braunwald's heart disease: a textbook of cardiovascular medicine. 7th ed. Philadelphia: Elsevier Saunders; 2008. p 1215.

Chapter 11

Cardiac rhythm assessment and management

Malcolm Dennis, David Glanville

KEY WORDS

ablation

antiarrhythmic

antitachycardia
 pacing

arrhythmia

atrial

atrioventricular

bradycardia

cardiac
 resynchronisation
 therapy

cardioversion

failure to capture

failure to pace

failure to sense

implantable
 cardioverter
 defibrillator

junctional

oversensing

pacemaker

sinoatrial

tachycardia

threshold

ventricular

Learning objectives

After reading this chapter, you should be able to:

- describe the various arrhythmogenic mechanisms implicated in the development and propagation of cardiac arrhythmias
- recognise the features of the various commonly observed arrhythmias and discuss the aetiological factors that predispose to the development of each
- discuss the actual or potential haemodynamic consequences and prognostic implications of each of the commonly observed arrhythmia types
- describe the general and specific assessment and treatment strategies applicable to each of the various arrhythmia types
- discuss the principles and indications for pacemaker therapy
- recognise abnormal pacemaker activity on the ECG and discuss the causes and corrective actions for complications during temporary pacing
- describe the principles and benefits of cardiac resynchronisation therapy (CRT), including the factors that limit the effectiveness of the therapy
- discuss the principles and indications for treatment of arrhythmias including ablation therapies, permanent pacing, cardioverter defibrillators, cardioversion and defibrillation.

Introduction

Cardiac arrhythmias occur as primary diagnoses or as a complication of cardiac, other organ or systemic abnormalities. In broad terms most arrhythmias occur with greater frequency and with greater impact in the critically ill patient. Early detection and interpretation of arrhythmias and their impacts are essential with initiation of appropriate arrhythmia management that takes into account biochemical and metabolic variation and pharmacological interventions in critical illness.

The clinical impact of arrhythmia is highly variable and depends upon the type and rate of the arrhythmia and the presence of any underlying cardiac disease. When occurring in the critically ill patient, the impact is likely worsened due to coexistent circulatory, metabolic or biochemical abnormalities and the high oxygen demand states of many critical illnesses. Symptomatic impact ranges from lethargy, exercise intolerance, dyspnoea, lightheadedness and palpitations, to marked haemodynamic instability and syncope. Arrhythmias may present as, or progress to, cardiac arrest. Physiological effects of tachyarrhythmias include increased myocardial oxygen demand at the same time that reduced oxygen delivery is occurring, with scope for resultant myocardial ischaemia. The metabolic impact of compromising arrhythmias is effectively the same as the outcomes of shock from other aetiologies, with escalating stress responses, along with reduced oxygen delivery and consumption, increased oxygen extraction and lactic acidosis.

Practice tip

Morbid obesity (BMI ≥40 kg/m2) is associated with discrete ECG alterations including low chest lead voltages, leftward QRS, T wave and P wave axis shifts, left atrial abnormalities and T wave flattening in the inferior and lateral leads. However, the mean resting heart rate and incidence of conduction abnormalities do not differ from those with a normal BMI and any alteration in these parameters in obese patients should be considered abnormal. Similarly, a localised T wave inversion pattern should always be considered abnormal in persons with significant obesity.

Arrhythmia incidence in critical care units is far greater than in the general community. The most common compromising arrhythmia is atrial fibrillation (AF). Its community incidence is 8–9% over the age of 80,[1,2] but it occurs in 20% of critically ill patients.[3] Subgroup incidence is even greater with half of septic shock patients[4] and 30–40% of post cardiac surgical patients[3,5] developing atrial fibrillation. Ventricular arrhythmias occur in less than 2% of critically ill patients.[6]

The arrhythmia landscape continues to change for the critical care nurse. The increasing multiculturalism of most populations increases the chances of encountering arrhythmic syndromes previously only encountered in certain countries, such as the Brugada syndrome and arrhythmogenic right ventricular dysplasia. In addition, the increased survival of children to adulthood with congenital structural and arrhythmic diseases (e.g. long QT syndromes) further adds to the complexity of arrhythmias with which critical care nurses must be familiar.

Practice tip

Reduced amplitude of ECG complexes may occur in critical illness (e.g. severe sepsis, renal failure). It is important to adjust the bedside cardiac monitor 'gain' size in response to this phenomenon and to be mindful of the potential 'masking' effect it may have on underlying 12-lead ECG cardiac hypertrophic voltage enlargement criteria and the possible suppression of ST segment changes.

The cardiac conduction system

The normal heartbeat sequence occurs through rhythmic stimulation of the heart via its specialised conduction system. Through inherent automaticity, the sinus node spontaneously generates an activation current that conducts across preferential atrial pathways (producing a P wave on the surface ECG) and then to the atrioventricular node. After a brief physiological slowing, this wavefront conducts to the bundle of His and then to the ventricles via the right and left bundle branches. These terminate distally as branching Purkinje fibres, which activate the ventricles. This ventricular activation (or depolarisation) sequence produces a QRS complex on the surface ECG and subsequent repolarisation gives rise to the T wave.

The ability to spontaneously generate a cardiac rhythm is termed automaticity and, in health, automaticity is tightly controlled by neurohormonal inputs to match heart rate to metabolic rate. Excitatory influences increase automaticity, accelerating the heart rate, while automaticity depressant influences slow the heart rate. Arrhythmias may thus arise from alterations in automaticity (increased or decreased), failure of the conduction pathways described above or via reentry or triggered mechanisms (described below).[7,8]

Arrhythmogenic mechanisms

Arrhythmias result from three primary electrophysiological mechanisms: abnormal automaticity, triggered activity and reentry.

Abnormal automaticity

The action potentials of sinus and atrioventricular (AV) conducting tissues differ from that of the myocardium in that phase 4 of their action potentials undergo spontaneous depolarisation (automaticity). This property allows these tissues to assume the role of electrophysiological pacemaker dominance. However, in some circumstances, such as myocardial ischaemia or under cardiostimulatory influences, regional levels of spontaneous automaticity can be abnormally accelerated, stimulating ectopic locations (foci) within the atria, ventricles or AV node to discharge more rapidly.[9,10] Conversely, depressed automaticity gives rise to bradyarrhythmias and accompanies myocardial and conduction system disease, pharmacological and biochemical influence and often, strikingly, vagal (parasympathetic) stimulation.

Triggered activity

Arrhythmias may occur through the occurrence of abnormal oscillations within the early and late repolarisation stages of the cardiac action potential. Normally, all areas of the myocardium repolarise in a uniform manner. However, when adjacent areas of myocardium show different rates of repolarisation, voltage differences between these areas at the critical 'superexcitable' phase in the relative refractory period can be sufficient to re-excite tissues, generating premature ectopic beats or accelerated ectopic rhythms. Such variations in repolarisation and the consequent 'self-triggering' of depolarisation at least partially explain the arrhythmias accompanying long QT intervals.

Voltage oscillations are classified as either 'early after depolarisations', which occur during phases 2 and 3 of the action potential, or 'late after depolarisations', which occur during phase 4. Digitalis toxicity, ischaemia, hypokalaemia, hypomagnesaemia and elevated catecholamine levels are the more common causes of triggered activity.[11] Excessive prolongation of the action potential duration enhances the risk of triggered activity and, as such, these mechanisms are implicated in the development of certain subtypes of ventricular tachyarrhythmias, in particular torsade de pointes (refer to description later in this chapter).

Reentry

The most common cause of tachyarrhythmias is reentry, in which current can continue to circulate through the heart because of different rates of conduction and repolarisation in different areas of the heart. Slow conduction through a region of the heart may allow enough time for other tissues that have already been depolarised to recover, and then to be re-excited by the arrival of this slowly conducting wavefront. Once this pattern of out-of-phase conduction and repolarisation is established, a current may continue to circulate continuously around a reentry circuit. Each 'lap' of the circuit gives rise to another depolarisation (P wave or QRS complex).[10,12] The ultimate rate of the tachycardia depends on the size of the circuit (micro versus macro reentry) and the conduction velocity around the circuit.

Arrhythmias and arrhythmia management

Arrhythmias may arise from myocardial or conduction system tissue, appearing as inappropriate excitation or depression of automaticity, impaired conduction or altered refractoriness.[9]

The clinical impact of tachyarrhythmias is highly variable and is influenced by the rate and duration of the arrhythmia, the site of origin (ventricular vs supraventricular) and the presence or absence of underlying cardiac disease. As a result, arrhythmias may require no treatment, at least in the short term, or at worst may present as cardiac arrest and require treatment according to advanced life support algorithms (see Chapter 25).

Bradyarrhythmias may be due to failure of sinus node discharge (sinus bradycardia, pause, arrest or exit block) or to failure of AV conduction (AV block). Unless junctional or ventricular escape rhythms emerge asystole or ventricular standstill results.

Arrhythmias of the sinoatrial node and atria

The sinus node controls the heart rate according to metabolic demand, responding to autonomic, adrenal and other inputs, which vary according to exertion or other stressors. In response to needs, the sinus node discharge rate typically varies from as low as 50 beats/min to as high as 160 beats/min. In the conditioned heart (e.g. athletes), this range extends down as low as 40 beats/min and as high as 180 beats/min. Peak activity in the elite athlete may even achieve sinus rates of 200/min, though this represents the extreme end of the sinus rate (see Figure 11.1 for an illustration of sinus rhythm). An individual's maximal sinus rate is approximately 220 beats/min minus their age. The ECG rhythm criteria for arrhythmias of the sinoatrial node and atria are summarised in Table 11.1.

Sinus node disease predominantly manifests as inappropriately slow rather than fast sinus rates. Sinus tachycardia is therefore not generally an expression of sinus node dysfunction but a physiological response to some stressor (see below). A rare exception to this is 'inappropriate sinus tachycardia' that appears most commonly in young women,[13] in whom the resting daytime heart rate chronically exceeds 100/min. Treatment includes beta-blockers, calcium channel blockers or the novel selective sinus node inhibitor agent ivabradine.[14]

Sinus tachycardia

In adults, a sinus rate above 100/min is termed sinus tachycardia and may occur with normal exertion[15,16] (see Figure 11.2). When sinus tachycardia occurs in the patient at rest, reasons other than exertion must be sought and include compensatory responses to mental or physiological stress, hypotension, anaemia, hypoxaemia, hypoglycaemia or pain, in which there is increased neurohormonal drive. Inotropes and sympathomimetics also accelerate the sinus rate. Sinus tachycardia should therefore be

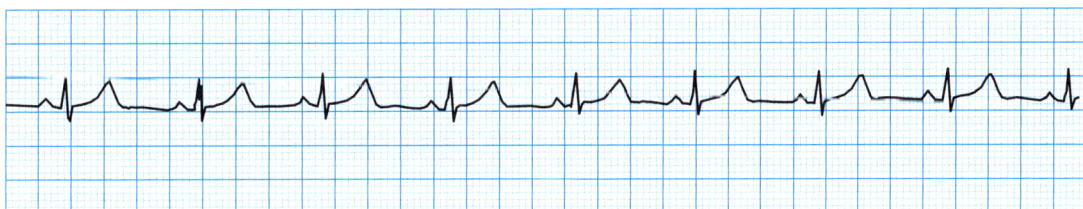

FIGURE 11.1 Sinus rhythm, rate 78/min. All P waves are followed by QRS complexes of normal duration after a P–R interval of around 0.16 s.

TABLE 11.1

ECG rhythm criteria for arrhythmias of the sinoatrial node and atria

RHYTHM	ECG CRITERIA
Sinus rhythm (SR)	Upright P waves in inferior leads. Rate 60–100/min. Regular
Sinus tachycardia (ST)	Upright P waves in inferior leads. Rate 100–180/min. Regular
Sinus bradycardia (SB)	Upright P waves in inferior leads. Rate <60/min. Regular
Sinus arrhythmia	Upright P waves in inferior leads but they are irregular, with gradual increase and decrease in rate. Usually in phase with respiration
Sinus pause	Abrupt drop in P wave rate, absent P waves (usually <3 s duration)
Sinus exit block	Abrupt drop in P wave rate P–P interval spanning the pause is a multiple of the preceding P–P interval
Sinus arrest	Abrupt cessation in P wave rate (>3 s duration)
Atrial ectopic beats (AEs) Also: premature atrial contractions (PACs)	Premature ventricular complexes of normal morphology P' waves of altered morphology precede premature ventricular complexes Compensatory pause may occur after premature ventricular complex
Atrial tachycardia	Atrial rate regular 140–230/min AV conduction may be 1:1, 2:1 or less P waves may be hidden in T waves P wave when visible usually different morphology to sinus P wave Ventricular rate usually regular May show 'warm up' in rate at onset
Atrial flutter (AFl)	Atrial rate 220–430/min, commonly close to 300/min. Regular atrial rhythm Flutter waves appear as sawtooth baseline in II, III, aVF, but more like discrete P waves in V1/MCL1, and as fibrillatory waves in I and aVL 1:1 uncommon in adults, unless flutter rate is slow 2:1, 3:1, 4:1 AV block more common (therefore ventricular rate often close to 150, 100, 75/min)
Atrial fibrillation (AF)	Atrial rate 300–500/min. Ventricular rate rarely >180/min Discrete P waves not seen – irregular fibrillatory baseline Ventricular rhythm markedly irregular (irregularly irregular) Ventricular rate >100/min = 'uncontrolled' AF If ventricular rhythm regular – escape or complete heart block

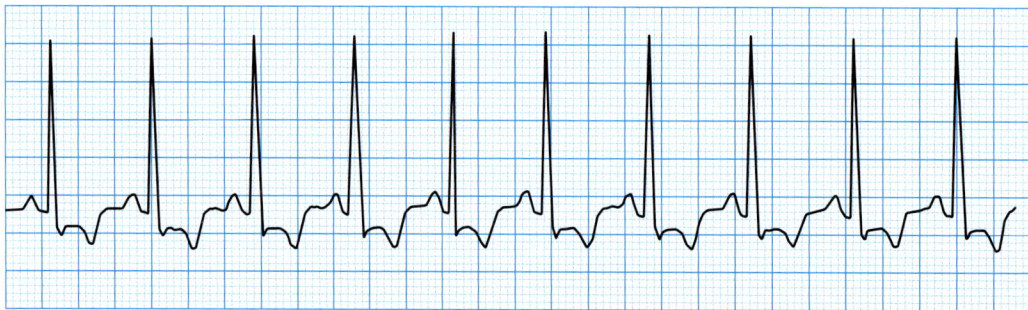

FIGURE 11.2 Sinus tachycardia. The rhythm is slightly irregular and varies between 105/min and 115/min.

regarded as a response to a physiological stimulus rather than an arrhythmia arising from sinus node dysfunction, with treatment directed at the trigger for the tachycardia, not the tachycardia itself. As sinus tachycardia may point to covert events such as internal bleeding or pulmonary embolism, there should be a thorough investigation for unexplained sinus tachycardia.

Sinus bradycardia

A sinus rate of less than 60 beats/min is termed sinus bradycardia[15,16] (see Figure 11.3). In general terms the slower the rate, the more likely it is to produce symptoms related to low cardiac output. Slowing of the rate to less than 50/min is common during sleep, especially in the athletic heart, but is otherwise uncommon. Bradycardia may

FIGURE 11.3 Sinus bradycardia. The rhythm is regular and at a rate of 50/min. Borderline first-degree AV block: the P–R interval is 0.20 s.

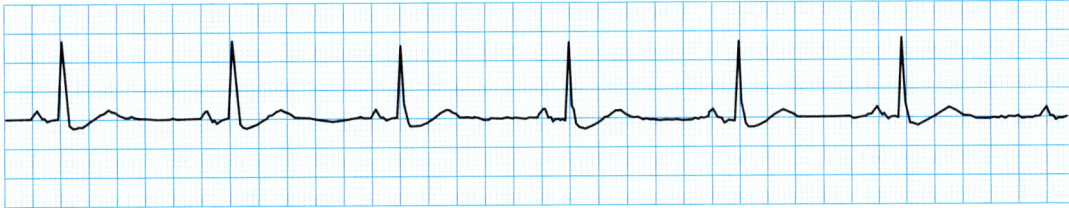

accompany myocardial ischaemia (especially when due to right coronary artery disease), conduction system disease, hypoxaemia and vagal stimulation (e.g. nausea, vomiting or painful procedures). As vagal stimulation may also produce vasodilation, hypotension may be more marked during vagally mediated bradycardia. Bradycardia also accompanies beta-blocker, digitalis, antiarrhythmic or calcium channel blocker treatment.[17] Treatment of sinus bradycardia reflects the treatment of AV block and is covered below under the management of atrioventricular block.

Although sinus bradycardia strictly is defined as less than 60 beats/min, many people have sinus rates that may be normal but that are inappropriately slow for a given level of activity. This behaviour is usually described as chronotropic incompetence[18] and, if it causes activity limitation, can be an indication for pacemaker implantation.

Sinus arrhythmia

When the rhythm is clearly sinus in origin but is irregular, then the term sinus arrhythmia is used (see Figure 11.4). Generally, a gradual rise and fall in rate can be appreciated in synchrony with respiration. The gradual rise and fall in rate is important: it distinguishes sinus arrhythmia from the abrupt prematurity with which atrial ectopic beats make their appearance, or the abrupt slowing of the sinus rate seen in sinus pause and sinus arrest. Sinus arrhythmia may accompany sinus node dysfunction but is seen also in the normal heart. Of itself, sinus arrhythmia does not require treatment.

Sinus pause and sinus arrest

Abrupt interruption to the sinus discharge rate has spawned a variety of descriptive terms, based partly on physiology and partly on severity. Sinus pause is self-descriptive: during a period of sinus rhythm, there is a sudden pause during which the sinus node does not discharge.[17] The heart rate abruptly drops, during which time there may be bradycardic symptoms. Sinus arrest tends to be used as a descriptor when the pause is longer rather than shorter (usually greater than 3 seconds, while less than 3 seconds might be called sinus pause) (see Figure 11.5). The longer the period of sinus arrest, the greater the likelihood of symptoms, and syncope is possible.[17] Sinus pause may be indistinguishable from sinus exit block (in which there are sinus discharges that fail to excite the atria), as both result in missing P waves. The distinction

FIGURE 11.4 Sinus arrhythmia with marked rate variation in synchrony with respiration. The rhythm is clearly sinus but is irregular, accelerating from 75 to 120/min before slowing back to 75/min by the end of the strip.

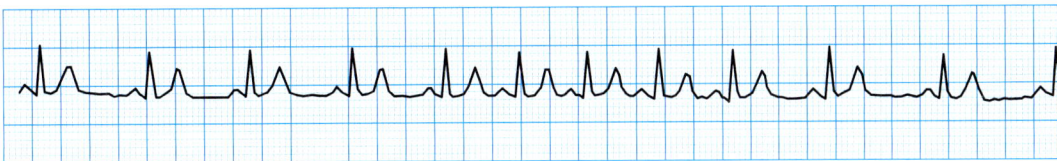

FIGURE 11.5 Sinus pause and sinus arrest. Sinus rhythm at 60/min followed by an abrupt rate drop. Using 3 s as a cut off between sinus pause and sinus arrest, the first long interval of 2.5 s would qualify as sinus pause whereas the next interval (3.2 s) would be classified as sinus arrest.

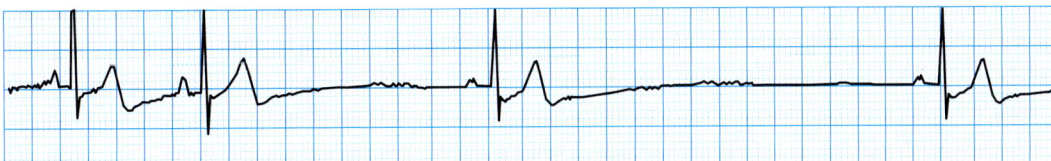

FIGURE 11.6 Sinus exit block. An abrupt rate drop follows the first three sinus beats. As the P–P interval spanning the pause is exactly twice the P–P interval of the preceding beats, the pause here could be due to sinus exit block. It could equally simply be a sinus pause.

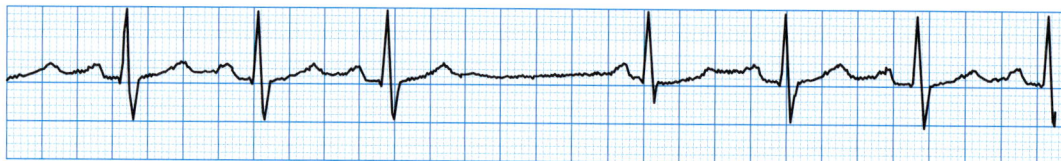

is academic, however, as both arrhythmias arise from the same groups of causes, and are significant only when they cause symptomatic bradycardia. Pauses in which the P–P intervals spanning the pause are multiples of the pre-pause P–P interval favour the diagnosis of exit block (Figure 11.6).[11] Recurrent syncopal pauses may require acute responses for symptomatic bradyarrhythmias. If episodes continue, consideration should be given to permanent pacemaker implantation.

Special contexts for reducing the rate during sinus rhythm

In general, treatment of tachycardia is directed at the cause of the rhythm disturbance and will be considered when physiological instability is experienced. In select situations, however, elevated sinus rates (not necessarily reaching tachycardia) may be counterproductive and heart rate reduction may commence earlier. This is particularly the case in patients with angina or moderate-to-severe heart failure, where sinus rate reduction confers a mortality and morbidity benefit.[19] In the ischaemic population, heart rate reduction reduces myocardial oxygen demand and prolongs diastole, during which coronary perfusion occurs. In the heart failure population, in addition to these effects, heart rate reduction increases diastolic ventricular filling time. In the recent landmark SHIFT study,[20] use of a novel selective sinus node inhibitor (ivabradine) to lower the sinus rate in moderate-to-severe heart failure patients significantly lowered composite end points of cardiovascular death or heart failure-related rehospitalisation compared to placebo (see Chapter 10 for related information).

> ### Practice tip
>
> Sinus tachycardia is usually the compensatory response to raised metabolic needs; however about 1% of the population experience a syndrome known as 'inappropriate sinus tachycardia', which is characterised by the presence of a high resting heart rate (average HR >90 bpm over a 24-hour period) coupled with an excessive heart rate response to minimal physical effort. This exaggerated chronotropic response – which is unrelated to structural heart disease, underlying pathological processes or lack of physical conditioning – is usually asymptomatic and benign but may uncommonly result in palpitations.

Arrhythmias of the atria and atrioventricular node

The term supraventricular tachycardia (SVT) is often used to group the tachyarrhythmias that arise from tissues above the ventricles. In its more common usage, SVT is thus an umbrella term, and includes any of the tachyarrhythmias arising from the sinus node, the atria or the atrioventricular node.[21] However, when a specific arrhythmia can be classified, the specific term is used rather than the more general term SVT. On occasion the electrocardiographic distinction between atrial flutter, atrial tachycardia and atrioventricular nodal reentry tachycardia may be difficult to make, and it may be useful in that context to use the more general term SVT. Supraventricular arrhythmias may occur as single-beat ectopics arising from atrial or junctional tissue or runs of consecutive premature beats, and thus be termed supraventricular tachycardias. SVTs may be self-limiting (paroxysmal) or sustained (until treatment), recurrent or incessant (sustained despite treatment). The ECG rhythm criteria for arrhythmias of the atria and atrioventricular node are summarised in Tables 11.1 and 11.2 (later).

Atrial ectopy

Impulses arising from atrial sites away from the sinus node (atrial foci) conduct through the atria in different patterns to sinus beats, and so generate P waves of different morphologies. These altered P waves define atrial ectopy, and their prematurity, or faster discharge rate, sees them more completely described as premature atrial beats. A characteristic P wave morphology cannot be provided, as ectopy may arise anywhere within the atria, causing upright, inverted or biphasic P waves. However a P wave morphology different to the prevailing sinus P wave is the norm. Ectopic P waves are often so premature that they become hidden within the preceding T wave. At such times evidence of their presence can be concluded only because they deform the T wave, and because premature QRS complexes of normal morphology follow, suggesting a supraventricular origin of those beats. Premature atrial beats may conduct normally, aberrantly or not at all, depending on their degree of prematurity and the state of AV nodal and intraventricular conduction (see Figure 11.7).

FIGURE 11.7   Sinus rhythm with frequent atrial ectopics. The notched P waves at a rate of 75–80/min are the Ps of the dominant sinus rhythm, while the more rapidly firing P waves with peaked configurations are the atrial ectopic beats. Note that the ectopic P waves have some variability in their shapes and firing rate. They should therefore be described as multifocal atrial ectopics.

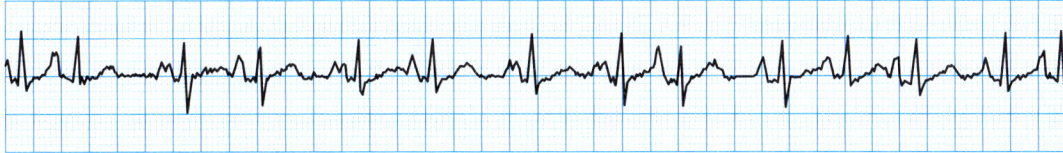

Atrial tachycardia

A rapidly discharging atrial focus or the presence of an atrial reentry circuit may give rise to a rapid rate, which is termed atrial tachycardia. Rates range from 140–230 beats/min and the rhythm is typically very regular once established.[11] Onset is usually abrupt but, when the cause is increased automaticity, a short 'warm up' phase occurs during which the rate gradually accelerates up to the final tachycardia rate. During atrial tachycardia P waves may be difficult to identify, as they become hidden in T waves. At such times, the presence of narrow QRS complexes confirms supraventricular conduction and aids discrimination from ventricular tachycardia. Distinction from other supraventricular arrhythmias may rely on the absence of characteristic features of other SVTs (e.g. the sawtooth baseline of flutter, the irregularity of fibrillation or the pseudo-R waves and onset pattern of atrioventricular nodal reentry tachycardia). When the atrial rate exceeds the conduction capability of the AV node, some degree of AV block occurs. Atrial tachycardia may be paroxysmal, sustained or incessant (see Figure 11.8). Symptoms vary and are partly dependent on the rate of the arrhythmia, and the presence or absence of myocardial dysfunction.

Multifocal atrial tachycardia

When multiple atrial sites participate in generating atrial ectopic beats at a rapid rate, the term multifocal atrial tachycardia is used (see Figure 11.9). The different foci produce P waves of varying morphology, and the strict regularity of normal atrial tachycardia is not seen.[17] Multifocal atrial tachycardia is something of a signature arrhythmia for pulmonary disease as it in particular complicates chronic obstructive pulmonary disease (COPD), as well as other pulmonary diseases as part of the cor pulmonale spectrum.[22]

FIGURE 11.8   Atrial tachycardia. In this narrow complex tachycardia the rhythm is very regular and the rate close to 210/min. It is not possible to clearly identify P waves within the T waves.

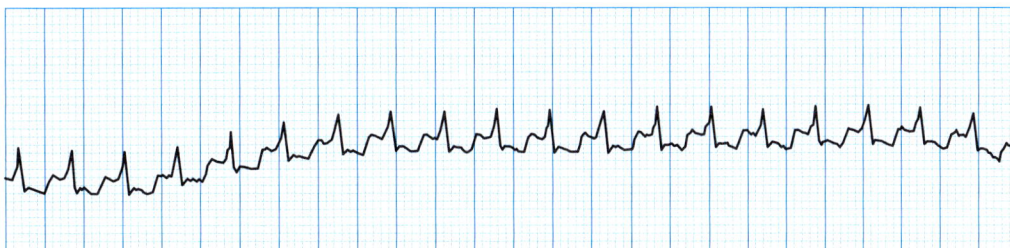

FIGURE 11.9   Multifocal atrial tachycardia. After three beats of sinus rhythm, the rate abruptly rises during a paroxysm of multifocal atrial tachycardia, which spontaneously reverts. The resultant tachycardia is irregular, and P waves of varying shapes can sometimes be clearly seen while others can be gleaned only by the deformity of T waves.

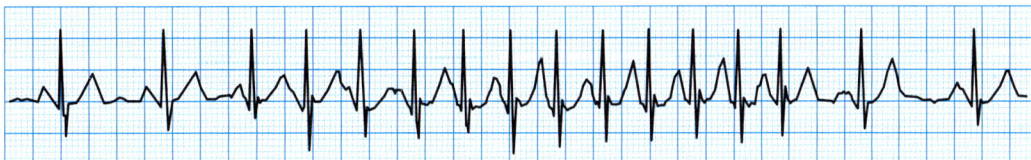

AV conduction during supraventricular tachyarrhythmias

The rapid atrial rates associated with atrial arrhythmias may exceed the conduction capability of the AV node, with the result that not all of the atrial impulses can be conducted (see Figures 11.10 and 11.11). This usually occurs when the atrial rate exceeds 200/min. Thus, during atrial flutter, or rapid atrial tachycardia, it is common to see 2:1 block or greater. During atrial fibrillation the ventricular response rate rarely exceeds 180/min unless there is an accessory pathway of the Wolff-Parkinson-White syndrome linking the atria and ventricles. Using these pathways the ventricular rate may reach 300/min or more.

Atrial flutter

Atrial flutter is a rapid, organised atrial tachyarrhythmia (see Figure 11.11). The atrial rate may be anywhere between 240 and 430/min, but most commonly the rate is close to 300/min.[17] At these rates the atrial depolarisation waves (flutter waves) run together to produce the characteristic ECG feature of this arrhythmia: the so-called 'sawtooth' baseline, because of its resemblance to the teeth of a saw. This sawtooth baseline is generally best shown in the inferior leads. By contrast, in lead V1 the flutter waves usually appear more like discrete P waves, while in leads I and aVL they have more the appearance of fibrillatory waves. The atrial rate of close to 300/min rarely conducts on a 1:1 basis to the ventricles in adults. Rather, 2:1, 3:1, 4:1 or variable levels of AV block intervene to limit the ventricular response rate, often to between 75 and 150/min.[9] When the AV block is variable, beats at 3:1, 4:1 or other ratios are seen together in a single strip. When there is 2:1 block, the flutter waves are often concealed within the QRS and/or T wave, and so definite identification may be difficult (see Figure 11.12). At such times, the presence of a narrow QRS tachycardia at a fixed rate close to 150/min is particularly suggestive of atrial flutter with 2:1 block. The tendency for flutter waves to appear as discrete P waves in lead V1 can be useful in identifying atrial flutter with 2:1 block as the flutter waves are more easily visualised in this lead. Where there is uncertainty about the diagnosis, vagal manoeuvres, or adenosine administration, may increase the degree of block and so reveal the flutter waves (Figure 11.12).[15,16]

Atrial fibrillation

Atrial fibrillation is a chaotic atrial rhythm in which multiple separate foci either discharge rapidly or participate in reentry circuits, resulting in rapid and irregular depolarisations. None of these gain complete control of the atria.[15,17] Discrete P waves (representing the coordinated depolarisation of the atria) are therefore not seen; rather, there is a continuous undulation of the ECG baseline (fibrillatory

FIGURE 11.10 Atrial tachycardia with high-degree block (many consecutive P waves do not conduct). The atrial rate is around 190/min but, because there is variable AV block (3:1 to 4:1), the resultant ventricular rate is between 50 and 60/min. This patient had digitalis toxicity, which should always be considered with atrial tachycardia and high-degree AV block.

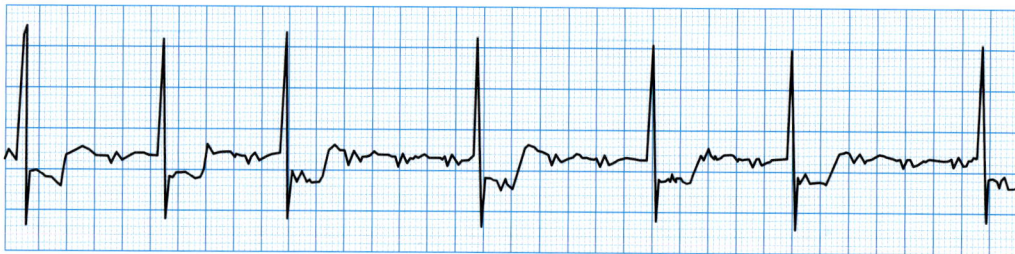

FIGURE 11.11 Atrial flutter with variable block. Note the sawtooth baseline, which characterises atrial flutter. The atrial rate is regular and is a little faster than 300/min, while the ventricular rate is irregular because of the variable block. At times the ventricular rate is close to 150/min (when there is 2:1 block) and at other times close to 100/min (when there is 3:1 block).

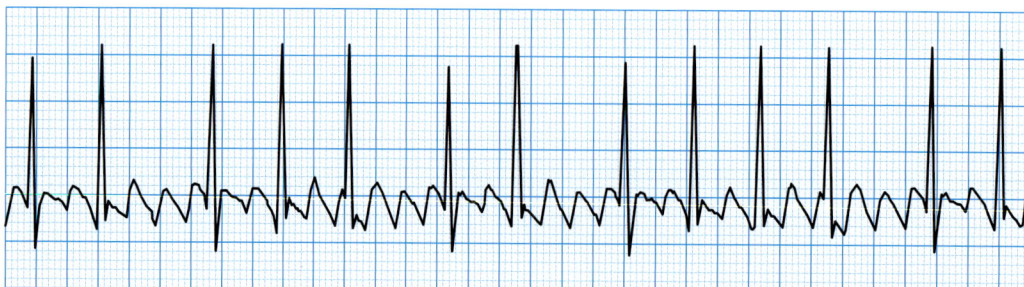

FIGURE 11.12 A regular narrow complex tachycardia at a rate of 165/min could be any number of supraventricular rhythms, among them atrial flutter with 2:1 block. Administration of IV adenosine produces momentary high-degree AV block, during which flutter waves at a rate of 330/min become apparent. Carotid sinus massage or other vagal manoeuvres may produce the same diagnostic impact via transient AV block.

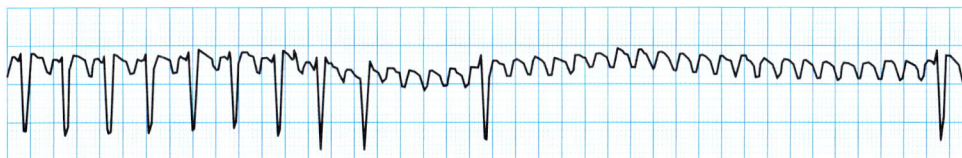

waves at a rate between 300 and 500/min), reflecting the continuous erratic electrical activity within the atria. This erratic, uncoordinated electrical activity results in uncoordinated contraction, and the atria can be seen not so much to contract but to quiver continuously. It is this quivering (fibrillatory) motion that gives atrial fibrillation its name.

The irregularity of the atrial rate results in an irregular arrival of impulses at the AV node and, as a result, conduction to the ventricles at irregular intervals.[15] Thus, a hallmark of atrial fibrillation is the marked irregularity of the ventricular rhythm. The ventricular response rate to the rapid atrial rate is determined by the state of AV nodal conduction and, in patients with normal AV conduction, is often in the range of 140–180/min (rapid, or uncontrolled, atrial fibrillation) (see Figure 11.13). Alternatively, when AV conduction is impaired, or limited by drug effect, slower ventricular rates are seen. When atrial fibrillation is accompanied by a ventricular rate less than 100/min, it may be termed controlled atrial fibrillation. Excessive antiarrhythmic treatment or AV conduction disease may result in more pronounced AV block and genuinely slow (but still irregular) ventricular rates.

Atrial fibrillation is the most common significant arrhythmia[23] and, while not usually immediately life-threatening, it contributes significantly to morbidity, especially in patients with existing cardiac failure. The loss of organised atrial contraction (atrial kick), as well as the rapid rates, deprive the ventricles of adequate filling, and so hypotension and low cardiac output may result. The congestion and altered flow patterns through the atria enhance the risk of thrombus formation and embolic stroke. When atrial fibrillation becomes chronic, lifelong antithrombotic prophylaxis is usually necessary. In addition, the incomplete atrial emptying results in congestion of first the atria and then the pulmonary circulation, and contributes to dyspnoea, increased work of breathing and hypoxaemia. Patients with left ventricular failure rely more heavily on atrial kick, and so symptoms and the severity of their heart failure typically worsen during atrial fibrillation. At times, atrial fibrillation is debilitating in this group, and shock and/or acute pulmonary oedema may develop.

Antiarrhythmic therapy aims at reverting atrial fibrillation, or limiting the ventricular rate (rate control) even if fibrillation persists.[23] For patients with chronic atrial fibrillation in whom adequate rate control cannot be achieved pharmacologically, it is sometimes necessary to perform radiofrequency ablation of the AV node itself, thereby inducing complete heart block. Permanent pacemaker implantation is therefore also necessary.

Common causes of atrial fibrillation are left atrial enlargement (secondary to heart failure), hyperthyroidism, low serum potassium or magnesium and physiological stress.[2] More recently, it has been identified that the pulmonary veins, at sites near their entry to the left atrium, may give rise to electrical impulses that communicate with the atria and give rise to atrial fibrillation.[24] Circumferential ablation of the pulmonary veins, known as pulmonary vein isolation, can isolate these electrical foci and cure atrial fibrillation from this cause.

FIGURE 11.13 Atrial fibrillation with a rapid (uncontrolled) ventricular response. The rate is around 170/min and the rhythm clearly irregular. Because of the rapid rate there is little opportunity to identify the fibrillatory baseline, but enough can be seen for confirmation.

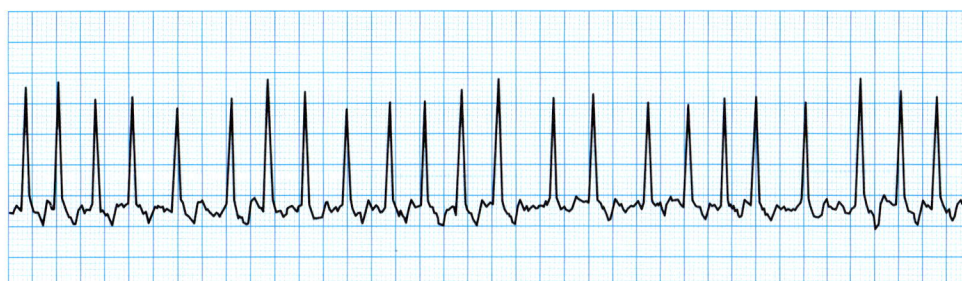

Extremely rapid atrial fibrillation in Wolff-Parkinson-White syndrome

The usual maximal ventricular response rate to atrial fibrillation is around 180/min, representing peak conduction capability of the AV node. However, in patients with Wolff-Parkinson-White (WPW) syndrome, an accessory pathway links the atria to the ventricles. These pathways can conduct more rapidly than the AV node and so it is possible for the ventricular response rate to reach or even exceed 300/min during atrial fibrillation.[16,17] This will present as a wide complex tachycardia that is largely monomorphic but with an irregular rhythm. At such rates syncope may occur and the rhythm may degenerate into ventricular fibrillation. Flecainide is an effective drug in this context, but digoxin should be avoided as it accelerates conduction across accessory pathways.[11]

Atrioventricular nodal reentry tachycardia

Atrioventricular nodal reentry tachycardia (AVNRT) is the most common type of paroxysmal supraventricular tachycardia, accounting for greater than 50% of cases of paraoxysmal SVT.[11] (Note that the term paraoxysmal SVT as used here does not include atrial flutter or fibrillation.) AVNRT is more common in women (75% of cases), more often occurs in younger than older patients, and in some individuals there is an identifiable link to stress, anxiety or stimulants. As the name suggests the arrhythmia arises because of reentry involving the AV node. Normally, atrial impulses reach the AV node via both slow and fast AV nodal pathways that link the atria to the AV node proper. The resultant P–R interval is <0.20 s and represents conduction across the fast AV nodal pathway. In AVNRT, the trigger mechanism is a premature atrial ectopic that is blocked by the fast pathway because it (paradoxically)

has longer refractoriness. Conduction into the AV node and to the ventricles is still possible by the slow AV nodal pathway, but the resultant P–R interval will be quite long (AV delay plus slow conduction into the AV node). Following this atrial ectopic with its long P–R interval is the onset of the tachycardia.[25]

The tachycardia develops because the initiating impulse, the atrial ectopic, is delayed in reaching the AV node. Once it does reach the AV node it conducts to the ventricles, but also now finds the previously refractory fast pathway recovered and able to conduct retrogradely back to the atria. There is now a functional circuit for reentry between the atria and the AV node. Impulses conduct slowly into the AV node, lengthening the P–R interval, but on reaching the AV node conduct just as quickly to atria as to the ventricles. As a result, the P waves appear at much the same time as the QRS.[25] In some instances of AVNRT it is not possible to identify P waves because they are hidden within the QRS. Often, however, the P waves can be seen distorting the final part of the QRS complex, appearing as small R waves in V1 and small S waves in lead II. Because they are P waves rather than part of the QRS, this ECG appearance has been dubbed 'pseudo-R waves' in V1 and 'pseudo-S waves' in lead II[11,25] (Figure 11.14). AVNRT is regular, and most commonly at rates between 170 and 240/min but may be slower. The QRS is narrow unless there is concomitant bundle branch block. AVNRTs sometimes respond well to vagal manoeuvres, including coughing, bearing down and carotid sinus massage. Adenosine may interrupt the arrhythmia, and other AV blocking drugs or antiarrhythmics may be necessary to prevent recurrence. Elective cardioversion is sometimes necessary and, if the arrhythmia is chronically troublesome, slow pathway ablation may be undertaken.[11,13]

TABLE 11.2

ECG rhythm criteria for arrhythmias of the atrioventricular node

RHYTHM	ECG CRITERIA
Junctional ectopic beats	Premature QRS complexes of normal morphology P waves inverted in inferior leads. They may precede QRSs with short P–R intervals or may be (partially) concealed within the QRS or ST segment
Junctional escape beat	Normal QRS following a pause in the rhythm, escape rate 40–60/min P waves may precede the QRS with short P–R intervals or may be (partially) concealed within the QRS or ST segment. P waves inverted in inferior leads
Junctional escape rhythm	Regular rhythm with normal QRS, rate 40–60/min P waves inverted inferiorly and may precede QRS with short P–R interval, or may be (partially) concealed within the QRS or ST segment
Accelerated junctional rhythm	Regular rhythm with normal QRS, rate 60–100/min P wave behaviour as per junctional escape rhythms
Junctional tachycardia	Regular rhythm with normal QRS, rate >100/min P wave behaviour as per junctional rhythms
Atrioventricular nodal reentry tachycardia AVNRT)	Narrow QRS tachycardia. Rate 170–230/min (sometimes slower) P waves may be absent or seen to distort terminal part of QRS ('pseudo R wave' in V1, 'pseudo S wave' in II) Typical onset is via premature atrial ectopic with long P–R (>0.30 s) ahead of onset of tachycardia

FIGURE 11.14   Atrioventricular nodal reentry tachycardia (AVNRT). Lead V1. There is sinus rhythm initially. A premature atrial ectopic conducts with a long P–R interval (0.36 s), initiating onset of AVNRT at a rate of 140/min. Note the P waves during the tachycardia can be seen distorting the end of the QRS (the 'pseudo R wave in V1' of AVNRT), which is not present before the tachycardia.

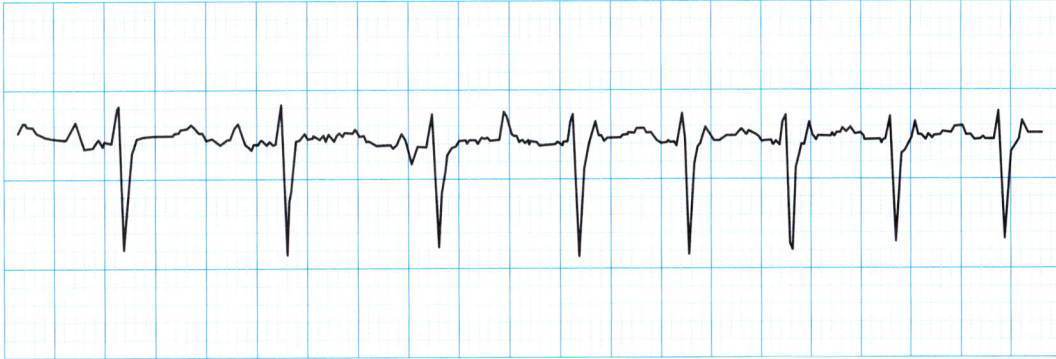

Management of patients with atrial arrhythmias

General symptoms of atrial tachyarrhythmias include: palpitations, dyspnoea/tachypnoea, fullness in the throat/neck, fatigue, lightheadedness, syncope, chest pain and angina symptoms and nausea and/or vomiting. Management of atrial tachyarrhythmias includes: 1) searching for and correction of the cause; 2) rate control limiting the ventricular response, even if the arrhythmias cannot be suppressed;[2,26,27] 3) reversion of the arrhythmias by vagal manoeuvres, medication, cardioversion or overdrive pacing; 4) ablation;[26,28] 5) prophylactic anticoagulation; and 6) prevention of recurrence using cardiac resynchronisation therapies such as biventricular pacing if necessary.[29]

Bradyarrhythmias and atrioventricular block

Bradycardia, a slowing of the ventricular rate to less than 60 beats/min, may occur in the form of slowing of the sinus node rate or failure of conduction at the level of the AV node. As the rate slows, escape rhythms should intervene, limiting the severity of the bradycardia. However, these may also fail, rendering the patient asystolic or with catastrophic bradycardia.[30–32] The ECG rhythm criteria for atrioventricular block are summarised in Table 11.3.

Bradycardic influences

Conduction system depression may occur with abnormal autonomic balance (increased vagal or decreased sympathetic

TABLE 11.3

ECG rhythm criteria for atrioventricular (AV) block

RHYTHM	ECG CRITERIA
First-degree AV block (1° AVB)	1:1 AV conduction. P–R interval >0.20 s
Second-degree AV block Mobitz type I (Wenckebach)	Intermittent non-conducted P waves P–R intervals show progressive P–R interval prolongation until 'dropped' beat
Second-degree AV block Mobitz type II	Intermittent non-conducted P waves P–R intervals of conducted beats show constant P–R interval (i.e., not the progressive increase in P–R interval in advance of dropped beats)
Third-degree AV block (3° AVB) Also: complete heart block (CHB)	No P waves conduct. No uniform P–R intervals or P–R relationships Bradycardia, appearing as: Junctional escape rhythm – normal QRS, regular, rate 40–60/min Ventricular escape rhythm – wide QRS, regular, rate 20–40/min
High-degree AV block	Intermittent non-conducted P waves Some P waves conduct but unlike 2° block there are consecutive non-conducted P waves (2 or more at a time)
Ventricular standstill	Absence of QRS complexes. The term is perhaps more often applied when there are P waves but no QRSs

tone), decreased endocrine stimulation (reduced catecholamine or thyroid hormone secretion) or from pathological influences such as conduction system disease or congestive, ischaemic, valvular or cardiomyopathic heart diseases. Many biochemical and pharmacological factors cause conduction system depression with resultant bradycardia.[18] The causes of bradycardia and AV block include:[30]

- drugs – virtually all antiarrhythmics, calcium channel or beta-blockers and digitalis preparations may contribute to bradycardia and AV conduction disturbance to a greater or lesser extent

- decreased sympathetic activity or blockade of neural transmission (e.g. spinal injury, anaesthetic or receptor blockade)

- increased parasympathetic activity – vagal stimulation such as nausea, vomiting, carotid sinus pressure, increased abdominal pressure, femoral manipulation or instrumentation

- hypoxaemia – the respiratory or ventilated patient with acute disturbance of oxygenation may develop sudden and marked bradycardia; in this situation increased oxygen administration is first-line and often definitive treatment.

In the absence of stimulation by the SA node, other tissues within the conduction system and myocardium can generate cardiac rhythms at rates slower than the normal sinus rate. Thus, sinus node failure need not severely compromise the patient, as the inherent automaticity of the AV node can generate a (junctional or nodal) rhythm at a rate of 40–60 beats/min. Similarly, should the AV node fail and the ventricles receive no stimuli, there is an additional layer of protection, as the ventricles themselves can generate (ventricular) rhythms at rates of 20–40 beats/min.[15]

Junctional escape rhythms

When sinus bradycardia falls to a rate slower than the inherent automatic rate of the AV node, then the junctional tissues discharge.[15,17] Typical rates are 40–60/min but may be slower, as the cause of the primary bradycardia may also suppress the firing of escape foci. Intraventricular conduction may be normal or aberrant. P waves may or may not be evident and are inverted because of retrograde conduction, as atrial activation spreads from the AV node and upwards through the atria. These P waves may at times be seen in advance of the QRS (at shorter than normal P–R intervals), within the ST segment, or may be hidden within the QRS complexes (see Figure 11.15).

Ventricular escape rhythms

When either the sinus or AV node fails and stimulation of the ventricles does not occur, the ventricles can autoexcite themselves, usually at a rate of 20–40 beats/min (Figure 11.16). Symptoms of bradycardia commonly accompany these idioventricular rates, and acute rate restoration may be necessary. However, true cardiac arrest requiring cardiopulmonary resuscitation is less common, with the escape rhythm providing sufficient cardiac output to sustain vital functions in the short term. ECG features of idioventricular escape beats include:

- single ventricular ectopic beats occurring after a pause in the dominant rhythm, or as groups of beats at the slow escape rate

- QRS >0.12 s, often notched, larger in amplitude and bizarre

- ST segment and T wave displacement in the opposite direction to the major QRS direction.

When these beats occur at a rate of 20–40/min the rhythm is termed ventricular escape, or idioventricular rhythm. Under excitatory influences the ventricular pacemaker cells may increase their firing rate to between 60 and 100/min (accelerated idioventricular rhythm) or to faster than 100/min (ventricular tachycardia).[33]

Accelerated idioventricular rhythm

Accelerated idioventricular rhythm (AIVR) has assumed a special place in cardiology because of its relatively common appearance during postinfarction reperfusion, thus often indicating successful revascularisation following percutaneous coronary intervention or thrombolytic therapy.[33,34] It may therefore imply therapeutic success rather than mishap, and usually needs no treatment. The arrhythmia is commonly due to increased automaticity and, as with other automaticity, arrhythmias may show a 'warm-up' in rate, i.e.

FIGURE 11.15 Sinus bradycardia followed by onset of junctional escape rhythm. Note that the sinus rate is initially around 37/min. It then slows into the escape rate range of the AV node, which then discharges at 35/min. The junctional beats are not preceded by P waves: the more slowly discharging sinus node probably has its P waves hidden first in the QRS of the second-last beat and then distorts the ST segment of the last beat.

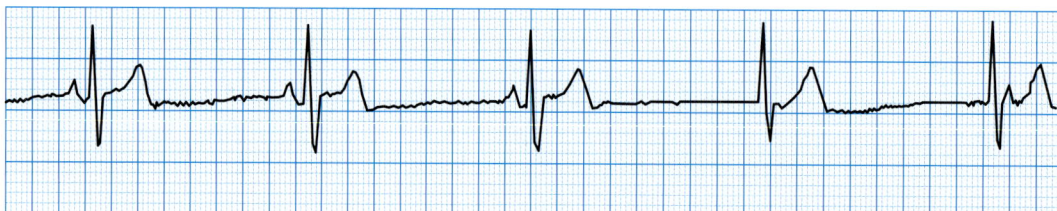

FIGURE 11.16 Ventricular escape rhythm (idioventricular rhythm). Note that after the first sinus beat, the slow rate allows the ventricular escape rhythm to emerge. The resultant rhythm is at a rate of 35/min, with wide QRS complexes and absent P waves.

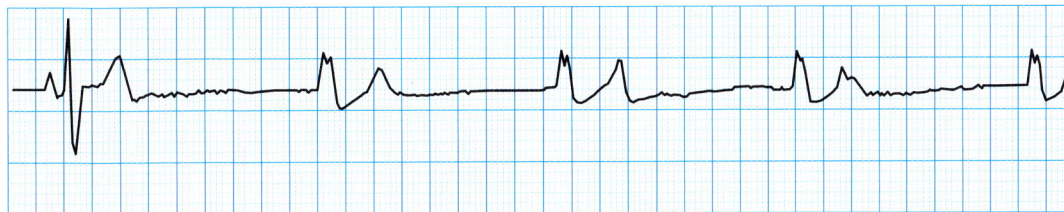

it may commence and then gradually accelerate and settle at a faster rate. This behaviour can be useful in differentiating arrhythmias from reentry, which typically display an abrupt change in rate at onset. When it occurs outside of the context of reperfusion, AIVR should be regarded as inappropriate ventricular excitation (Figure 11.17).

Atrioventricular conduction disturbances

Atrioventricular conduction disturbances make their appearance as delayed or blocked conduction from atria to ventricles, and thus appear as altered P–QRS (or P–R) relationships. The conventional classifications for AV block are based purely on the patterns of conduction. The classification as first-, second- and third-degree partially represents the severity of AV node or His-bundle dysfunction.[15,17] AV block may complicate heart disease and is also seen commonly with drug therapy (e.g. digitalis, calcium channel blockers, beta-blockers and other

antiarrhythmics).[33] It may occur abruptly following vagal stimulation. When accompanying myocardial infarction, it is more likely to be transient following inferior infarction, whereas its appearance following anterior infarction is more likely to be permanent.

Degrees of atrioventricular block

First-degree AV block

All atrial impulses are conducted to the ventricles but conduction occurs slowly, with a P–R interval >0.20 s. 1:1 AV conduction is maintained (see Figure 11.18). First-degree AV block by itself may be a benign occurrence. It is more concerning when the P–R interval lengthens over time as this may precede the development of higher degrees of AV block. If this occurs with the introduction of digoxin or antiarrhythmic therapy, drug cessation or dose modification should be considered. If the P–R is so long that P waves coincide with the T wave of the previous beat, effective loss of atrial kick develops due

FIGURE 11.17 Accelerated idioventricular rhythm (AIVR) following reperfusion in myocardial infarction. An accelerated ventricular focus emerges at 65/min, taking over from the slower sinus rate of 60/min. It then accelerates gradually until settling at a rate of 85/min by the end of the second strip. This display of rate 'warm-up' at onset is a characteristic of arrhythmias due to increased automaticity. The distortion of the ST segment from the third beat of AIVR onwards is due to retrograde conduction to the atria, and explains the absence of the sinus P waves.

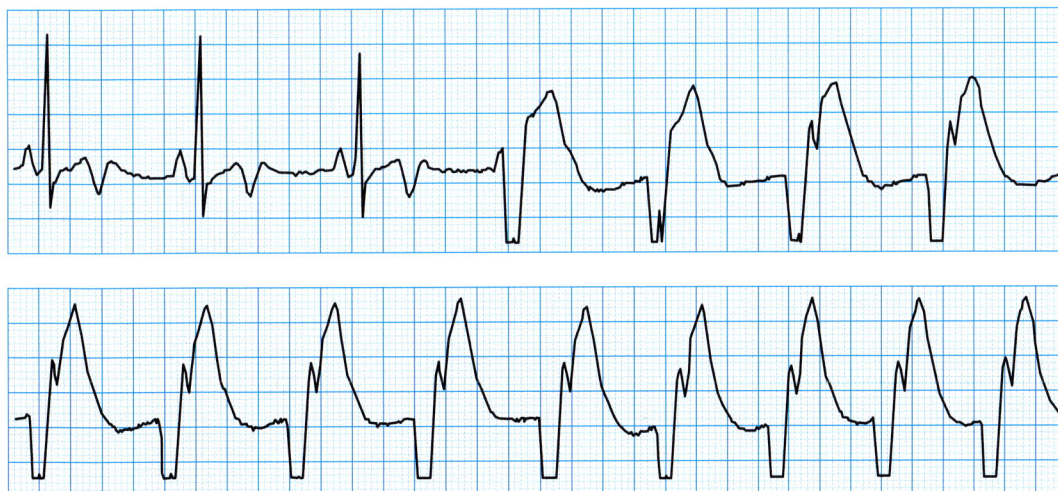

FIGURE 11.18 Sinus rhythm with first-degree AV block. Rhythm is regular, rate 100/min, 1 : 1 AV conduction, with a P–R interval of 0.24 s.

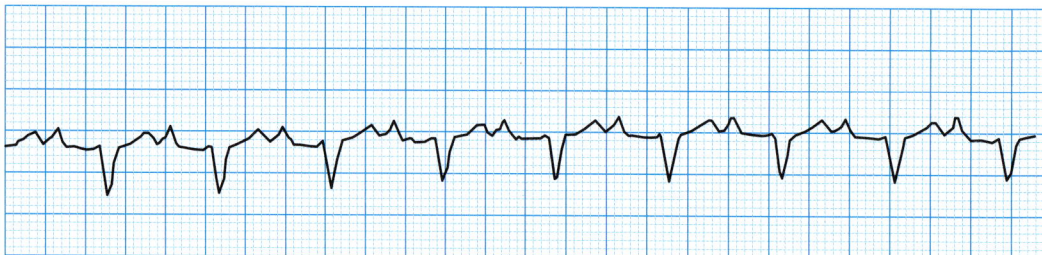

to the atria contracting while the mitral and tricuspid valves are closed. Remember that ventricular systole lasts roughly until the latter part of the T wave. Hypotension or reduced cardiac output and cannon *a* waves, caused by contraction of the atria against closed AV valves, become visible in the jugular veins and CVP waveforms.

Second-degree AV block

This is an intermediate level of block in which some P waves conduct to the ventricles while others do not. Thus there are periodic non-conducted P waves, or 'dropped' beats. A further distinction is made into either type I or type II second-degree AV block:

- Second-degree AV block Mobitz type I (Wenckebach): a cyclical pattern of AV conduction is seen in which the conducted P waves show a progressive lengthening of the P–R interval until one fails altogether to be conducted (blocked, or dropped, P wave). Cycles begin with a normal or prolonged P–R interval, which then extends over succeeding beats until there is a dropped beat. After the dropped beat the cycle recurs, commencing with a P–R interval equivalent to that commencing previous cycles[17] (Figure 11.19). The frequency of dropped beats partially represents the severity of AV block. When, for example, every fifth P wave is not conducted, 5:4 conduction is said to be present. If AV conduction deteriorates further, more frequent P waves fail to be conducted (4:3, 3:2 conduction).

- Second-degree AV block Mobitz type II: dropped beats (non-conducted P waves) are also present, but the conducted beats show a uniform P–R interval rather than any progressive lengthening[17] (Figure 11.20). The dropping of beats may be regular, e.g. every fourth P wave (termed 4:1 block), progressing to 3:1, or even 2:1 block as AV nodal, or His bundle conduction, worsens. Alternatively, the dropping of beats may be more irregular (variable block), with combinations of 2:1, 3:1, 4:1 or other levels of block evident in a given strip. The more frequent the dropped beats, the slower the ventricular rate and the greater the likelihood of symptoms. Second-degree type II AV block is often associated with intraventricular conduction delay, with corresponding widening of QRS complexes. When this is seen it represents conduction impairment not just of the AV node but of intraventricular conduction as well. Progression to complete AV block is more common.[17]

A final form of second-degree block is 'high-degree' AV block, in which some conducted P waves can be seen, and these conducted P waves show a uniform P–R interval. However, rather than single periodic dropped beats, multiple consecutive non-conducted P waves can be seen (Figure 11.21). The impact on ventricular rate and therefore haemodynamic status is typically more severe.

FIGURE 11.19 Sinus rhythm with second-degree AV block type I. Every third P wave is not conducted (3 : 2 conduction). The P–R interval can be seen to lengthen before the dropped beats(*). After the dropped beats the cycle starts with a P–R interval of 0.18 s. It then extends to 0.25 s before again dropping a beat.

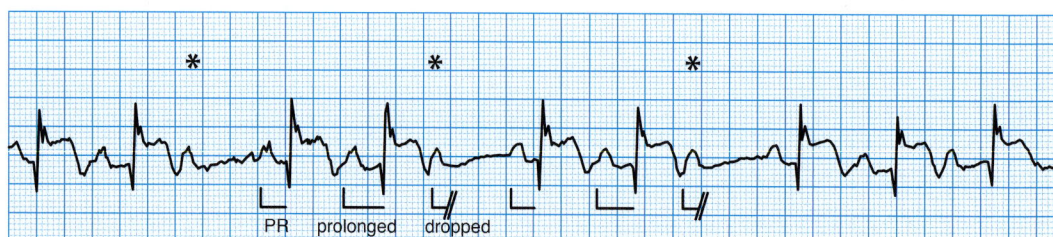

FIGURE 11.20 Second-degree AV block type II. A non-conducted beat confirms the second-degree block. There is no progressive prolongation of the P–R interval before the dropped beat (*), rather, the uniformity of all P–R intervals distinguishes this as type II.

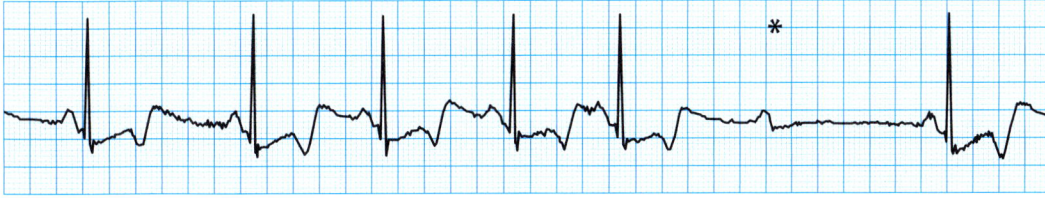

FIGURE 11.21 Sinus rhythm with high-degree AV block. At the beginning and end of the strip there is second-degree block (2:1). Alternate P waves fail to conduct, qualifying as at least second-degree AV block. The appearance of consecutive non-conducted P waves in the middle of the strip (5 in a row), however, escalates the classification to 'high-degree' block.

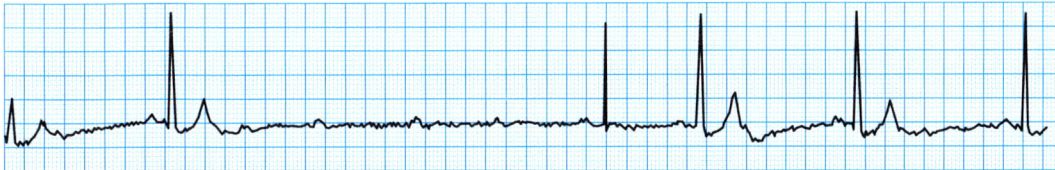

Third-degree (complete) AV block

None of the atrial impulses are conducted to the ventricles, resulting in a loss of any relationship between P waves and QRS complexes (AV dissociation). Usually, a slower pacemaker assumes control of the ventricular rate, and this focus may be either junctional (narrow QRS, at a rate of 40–60/min) or ventricular (wide QRS, at a rate of 20–40/min). These escape rhythms will typically be regular (Figure 11.22).[17] Symptom severity depends on the rate of the escape rhythm and the presence of underlying ventricular dysfunction.

Patient management during AV block

AV block may be progressive in nature, worsening with advancing heart disease or after introduction, or dose modification, of drugs that depress AV conduction.[35–37] Thus, monitoring should include P–R interval measurement and, where the P–R interval becomes prolonged, there should be an increase in vigilance directed towards further prolongation or the development of dropped beats, to identify advancing AV block. Treatment of AV block and bradycardia includes assessment of cardiovascular status or other symptoms, including chest pain, dyspnoea, conscious state and nausea. The cause should be identified and treated where possible. Patients need to rest in bed, provided with reassurance and oxygen by mask or nasal prongs. If the patient is hypotensive, IV fluids should be administered and the patient laid flat. Standardised protocols for bradycardia should be applied if the patient is symptomatic, and these usually include:[30]

- atropine sulfate 0.5–1.0 mg IV[37]
- isoprenaline hydrochloride in 20–40 mcg increments,[38] with an infusion at 1–10 mcg/min

FIGURE 11.22 Sinus rhythm with third-degree AV block. Note the P waves (*) at a rate of 90–100/min and the ventricular rate of 40/min. The P waves bear no relationship to the QRS complexes – they are dissociated. (The seventh asterisked P wave is premature and different in morphology from the others, and is therefore possibly an atrial ectopic P wave.)

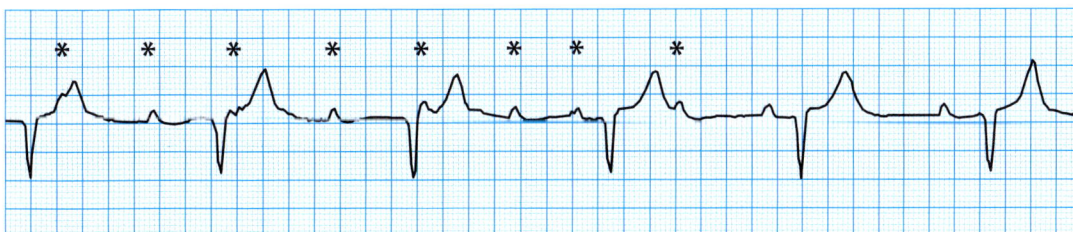

- transthoracic pacing (usually with sedation)
- possibly low-dose adrenaline infusion.

If the patient is pulseless or unconscious, standard advanced life support should be administered (see Chapter 25). Persistent or recurrent symptomatic bradycardia or AV block may require permanent pacemaker implantation.[30,31]

Ventricular arrhythmias

Ventricular ectopic rhythms may either occur as a response to slowing of the dominant cardiac rhythm (escape beats or escape rhythms) or emerge at faster rates than the dominant rhythm (as premature ectopic beats, couplets or 'runs' of ventricular tachycardia).[17] Escape rhythms (occurring after a pause) should be regarded as physiological, as they protect against otherwise severe bradycardia (see Figure 11.16), whereas premature beats (occurring in advance of the dominant rhythm) and rapid ventricular ectopic rhythms occur when pathology gives rise to increased automaticity, or reentrant or triggered behaviours (Figure 11.23).[15,17] Single ectopic beats may be benign occurrences, often seen in the absence of heart disease. However, their new appearance accompanying cardiac or systemic disease may precede the development of more serious arrhythmias, such as ventricular tachycardia or fibrillation, and thus warrant close monitoring. Ectopic beats, whether premature or late (escape), show characteristic features as follows:

- wide QRS complexes (>0.12 s) that are of different morphology (large and bizarre in shape)[39]
- commonly, notching of the QRS
- ST segments and T waves in the opposite direction to the major QRS deflection.

Ectopic beats may occur as single or coupled beats, or in runs of consecutive beats. Ventricular tachycardia is defined as more than 3 consecutive ventricular beats occurring at a rate greater than 100/min.[11,39]

Causes of ventricular tachyarrhythmias include:[9,16]

- myocardial disease
- myocardial ischaemia, infarction
- cardiomyopathies/cardiac failure
- hypertrophy
- myocarditis

- excess sympathetic stimulation
- biochemistry: hypokalaemia, hypomagnesaemia, pH derangements
- hypoxaemia, hypoglycaemia
- shock, hypotension
- excitatory pharmacology (positive chronotropes or inotropes)
- adrenaline, isoprenaline, dobutamine, dopamine, levosimendan, atropine
- arrhythmic syndromes, Brugada syndrome, long QT syndromes, arrhythmogenic right ventricular dysplasia.

Patterns of ectopy

Some patterns of ectopic frequency and morphology may warn of increasing risk for the development of serious arrhythmias such as ventricular tachycardia or fibrillation, and therefore earn a particular mention in monitoring. Historically, ectopic patterns have been graded according to their pre-emptive risk of serious arrhythmia development or 2-year mortality.[40] Studies undertaken in 2003 and 2005 did, however, call into question the predictive status of certain 'high-risk' ectopic patterns (such as 'R on T' ectopy), instead postulating that other factors such as a patient's underlying left ventricular function and level of autonomic responsiveness may play a more significant role in the generation of life-threatening ventricular tachyarrhythmias, independent of the prior presence or pattern of ectopy present.[41,42] However, in the critical care context it is reasonable to respond to certain patterns (as shown in Box 11.1) by investigating and managing potential contributing causes. If the patient can be seen to be advancing through stages of increased arrhythmic complexity, consideration for antiarrhythmic therapy should be given. The ECG rhythm criteria for ventricular arrhythmias are summarised in Table 11.4.

Ventricular tachycardia

Ventricular tachycardia (VT) is described as a 'run' of three or more consecutive ventricular ectopic beats, at a rate greater than 100/min (Figure 11.24).[23] The arrhythmia varies in its clinical impact, but when sustained is typically symptomatic with some degree of haemodynamic compromise. Ventricular tachycardia often presents

---

FIGURE 11.23   Sinus rhythm with premature ventricular ectopic beats occurring bigeminally. The second, fourth and sixth beats arise prematurely, appearing in advance of the dominant rhythm, and are clearly wider than the intervening supraventricular beats.

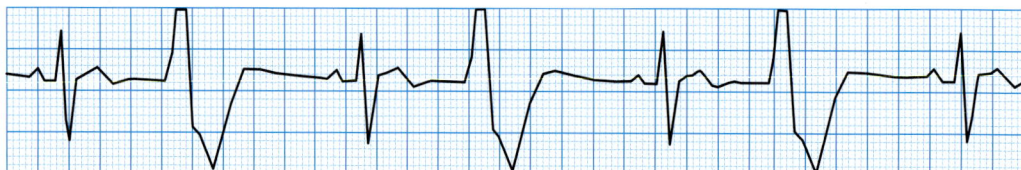

TABLE 11.4

ECG rhythm criteria for ventricular arrhythmias

RHYTHM	ECG CRITERIA
Ventricular ectopic beats (VEs) Also: premature ventricular contractions (PVCs)	Broad complex QRS (>0.12 s duration), often notched ST-T waves in opposite direction to major QRS deflection Occur prematurely – earlier than the prevailing rhythm Compensatory pause post ectopic usually seen
Ventricular escape rhythm (idioventricular rhythm)	Broad complex QRS (as above) rhythm during slowing of sinus rate or AV block Rate 20–40/min. Regular
Accelerated idioventricular rhythm (AIVR)	Broad complex QRS rhythm (as above) but at rates of 40–100/min. P waves may be absent, retrogradely conducted, or dissociated from ventricular rhythm
Ventricular tachycardia (VT)	3 or more consecutive wide QRS beats (>0.12 s), at rate >100/min Rate range 100–240/min P waves may be absent, dissociated or retrogradely conducted after each QRS Usually regular, sometimes irregular at onset of rhythm and prior to reversion
Ventricular fibrillation (VF)	No recognisable/organised QRS. Irregular baseline deflections of variable amplitude at 300–500/min. P waves not discernible
Ventricular flutter (VFl)	Very regular. Ventricular rate 270–330/min. 'Zig-zag' deflections where it is difficult to identify which is QRS and which is T wave
Torsades de pointes (TdP)	Broad complex tachycardia. Some irregularity. Rate 220–330/min Obvious polymorphism of QRS with 'sinusoidal twisting' around the baseline and transitions between polarity of QRS complexes – first positive then negative. Baseline ECG shows QT prolongation May appear monomorphic in some leads
Asystole	Absence of QRS complexes. ECG baseline may show some slow undulation
Agonal rhythm	Extremely slow ventricular rate (<20/min). Usually with markedly wide QRS complexes. The wide QRS and T wave amalgam often referred to as a 'sine wave' rhythm. Commonly a terminal rhythm

BOX 11.1

Patterns suggesting higher risk of arrhythmia

- Increasing frequency of ectopy
- Trigeminy, bigeminy
- Polymorphic ectopics (multiple QRS shapes), regarded as more important than monomorphic ectopics (single QRS shape)
- Two ectopic beats in a row (couplets)
- Three or more beats in a row (defined as ventricular tachycardia)
- R-on-T ectopics
- Bradycardia-dependent ectopics when the Q-T interval is long

as cardiac arrest, with the patient pulseless and unconscious, and is one of the major mechanisms of sudden cardiac death. The severity of symptoms depends partly on the rate (which may be 100–250/min), the duration of the arrhythmia, the presence of cardiac disease and the presence of comorbidities.[17,33] When it develops, VT may be categorised as self-limiting (terminating without treatment), sustained for some period of time (minutes or

longer), incessant (persisting until or despite treatment) or intermittent. Additional defining terminology includes monomorphic (all beats of the same morphology) or polymorphic (in which the rhythm conforms to the other features of VT but there is variability in the QRS shapes). ECG features of ventricular tachycardia include:[11,39,43]

- Three or more ventricular beats occur at a rate >100/min, uncommonly >240/min.
- Rhythm typically regular; there may be minor irregularity, especially on commencement and sometimes preceding self-termination.
- P waves may be absent. Atrial activity, whether dissociated or retrograde, is usually difficult to identify electrocardiographically.
- Morphology: QRS is wide (>0.12 s). QRS often notched or bizarre in shape.
- Any axis is possible (normal axis, left or right axis deviation). An axis in the range of −90 to −180° ('no man's land') provides strong support for the diagnosis of ventricular tachycardia, as it implies the QRS originates at the left ventricular apex and spreads through the ventricles upwards and to the right.
- ST-segment and T-wave displacement is in the opposite direction to the major QRS direction.

FIGURE 11.24 Sinus rhythm at 65/min before the onset of ventricular tachycardia. Note a ventricular ectopic emerges from the T wave of the third sinus beat (R-on-T ventricular ectopic), precipitating ventricular tachycardia (VT). The VT is then sustained at a regular rate of 220/min, with the characteristic wide QRS and ST/T in the opposite direction to the QRS.

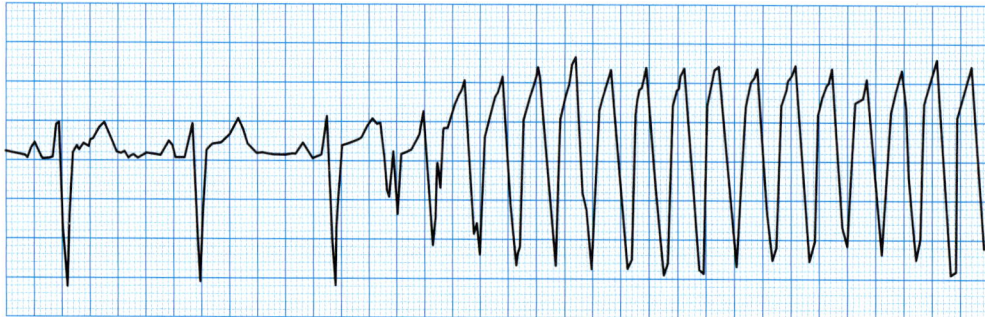

If VT is not self-limiting, treatment depends on the severity of the symptoms. If the patient becomes pulseless and unconscious, advanced life support is initiated (see Chapter 25). If the patient is conscious and has a pulse, therapy can be undertaken less aggressively. Occasionally, robust coughing may revert VT in the cooperative patient. Antiarrhythmic therapy (at slower administration rates than during cardiac arrest) is usually undertaken first, along with biochemical normalisation. If unsuccessful, sedation and elective cardioversion may be necessary. Consideration for internal cardioverter defibrillator (ICD) implantation should be given to patients surviving ventricular tachycardia or fibrillation.[31,44,45]

Practice tip

Initial tolerance of VT may be evident, only to be followed by abrupt deterioration when reserves or compensatory mechanisms are exhausted. Emergency responses should always be activated on initial identification.

Ventricular flutter

This uncommon arrhythmia is most likely just a subset of ventricular tachycardia, but because of its rapid rate (at times up to 300/min or more) and the appearance of QRS complexes that are largely indistinguishable from the T waves, ventricular flutter has earned its own classification.[17,43] It is typically very regular and monomorphic. An example is shown in Figure 11.25 in which it is difficult to say which deflection is the QRS and which is the T wave. The diagnostic separation from other types of VT is clinically unimportant, and treatment should follow normal guidelines for VT.

Ventricular fibrillation

During ventricular fibrillation (VF) there are no recognisable QRS complexes. Instead, there is an irregular and wholly disorganised undulation or erratic deflections about the baseline.[11,17] There are deflections, which at times approach rates of 300–500/min, but these are typically of low amplitude and none convincingly

FIGURE 11.25 Probable ventricular flutter. The complexes are broad, regular and monomorphic (one shape), but it is difficult to know which is the QRS deflection and which is the T wave. This feature plus the very fast rate of 300/min or more are the typical defining characteristics of this uncommon but serious arrhythmia, recorded during recovery from tricyclic antidepressant overdose in a 16-year-old female.

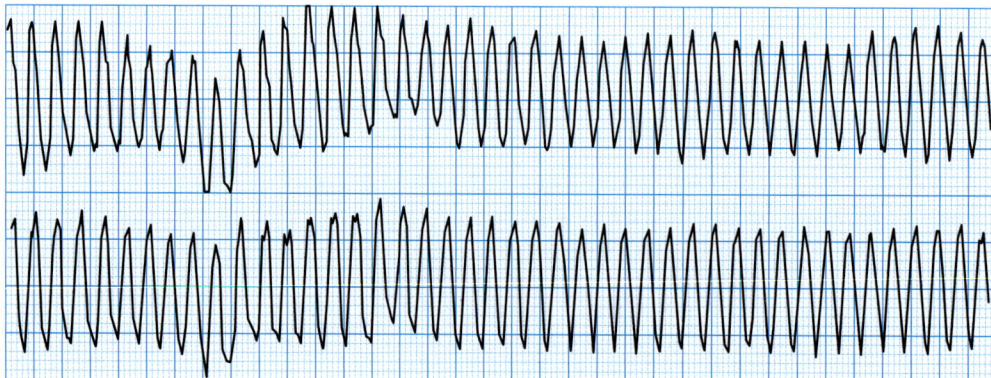

FIGURE 11.26 Ventricular fibrillation. Rapid, irregular and wholly disorganised deflections from the baseline are present, and produce nothing resembling QRS complexes.

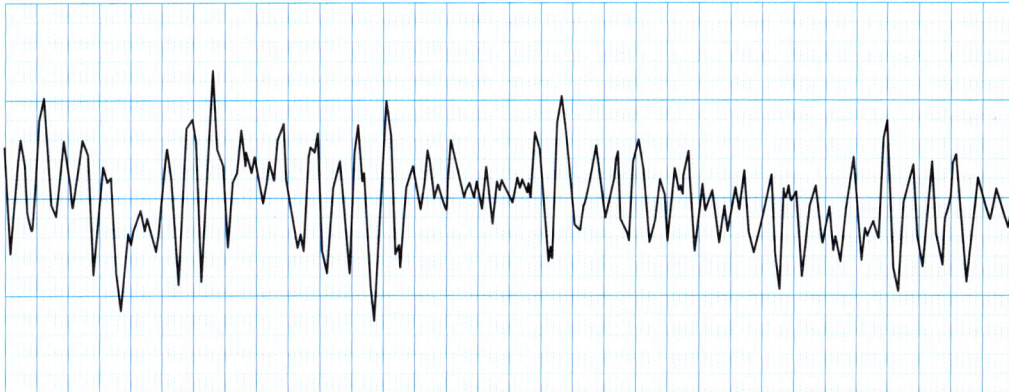

resemble QRS complexes (Figure 11.26). In the absence of organised QRS complexes the patient becomes immediately pulseless, and unconsciousness follows within seconds. Immediate defibrillation is required. If VF persists treatment occurs according to standing basic and advanced life support guidelines. Ventricular fibrillation is the leading cause of sudden cardiac death worldwide. For survivors of sudden cardiac death an implantable cardioverter defibrillator (ICD) is generally indicated unless there are reversible or transient causes, e.g. primary VF in the acute phase of myocardial infarction.[46]

Polymorphic ventricular tachycardias

These forms of VT do not have a single QRS morphology. Rather, the QRS complexes during the rhythm vary from one shape to another, either alternating between two discrete morphologies on a beat-to-beat basis (seen most commonly in digitalis intoxication) or switching between groups of beats, with first one morphology and then another (bidirectional VT).[17] The more common form of polymorphic VT is torsades de pointes (TdP), in which the QRS undergoes a gradual transition from one QRS pattern to another. The descriptive French term, literally 'twisting of the points', refers to the appearance of the 'points' (QRS

direction), which is first positive and then negative, usually with an ill-defined transition between the two. In addition to the changing directions there is a gradual rise and fall in amplitude, giving an overall appearance sometimes described as a 'sinusoidal twisting' (Figure 11.27).[47,48]

ECG features of torsades de pointes are:[47,48]

- broad complex rhythm
- QRS polymorphic, with the transitions between polarity as described above
- in some leads the QRS complexes may appear monomorphic
- rate often very rapid, in the range of 300/min
- regularity: the evident complexes are often regular but, particularly within the transition between QRS directions, there may be irregularity
- often self-limiting but recurrent
- Q–T prolongation evident during normal rhythm
- commonly pause-dependent, with bradycardia or single beat pauses precipitating onset
- ventricular bigeminy common in advance of onset of torsades de pointes
- onset commonly via R-on-T ectopic beats.

FIGURE 11.27 Torsades de pointes polymorphic ventricular tachycardia. After three beats of sinus rhythm a ventricular ectopic beat emerges from the T wave and precipitates onset of a rapid and sustained polymorphic ventricular rhythm. The characteristic sinusoidal twisting around the baseline and changing direction of the QRS are clearly apparent and, along with the rate of 300/min, define this as torsades de pointes.

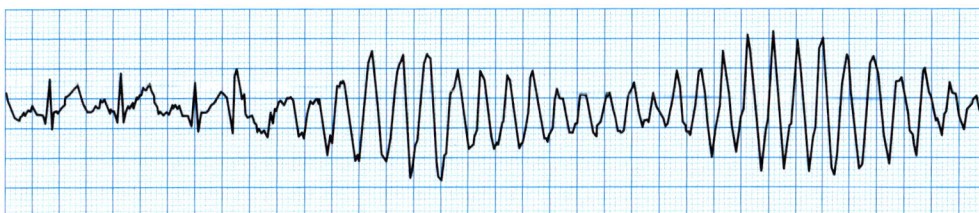

Because of the very rapid rate, syncope and cardiac arrest are common, and advanced life support is required. A thorough search for possible causes of Q–T prolongation should be undertaken. Causes include: class IA (procainamide, quinidine, disopyramide) or class III (amiodarone, sotalol) antiarrhythmics,[11,17] erythromycin, antidepressants, hypocalcaemia, hypokalaemia and hypomagnesaemia.[49] Congenital long Q–T syndromes also exist.[47,49] Apart from the general ventricular arrhythmia management principles listed below, the treatment of torsades de pointes includes cessation of Q–T prolonging agents, a greater emphasis on IV magnesium and the use of isoprenaline and/or pacing to shorten the Q–T interval and prevent bradycardia.[50]

Bradycardia in patients with long Q–T requires special mention as torsades de pointes is so often bradycardia or pause dependent. Bradycardia and pauses prolong the Q–T interval further and favour ectopy, which more easily finds the T wave, triggering torsades de pointes. The roles of pacing and isoprenaline are to both prevent pauses and shorten the Q–T interval[47,51] Pacing rates of 90 to 120 may be necessary to prevent torsades de pointes recurrence. Overdrive pacing (pacing at a rate greater than the tachycardia) is an effective treatment to terminate monomorphic forms of ventricular tachycardia, but is not effective in terminating torsades de pointes episodes.

Rapid differential diagnosis of extremely fast ventricular rates

For broad complex tachycardias approaching rates of 300/min in an adult, differential diagnosis becomes relatively straightforward using the following approach:

- if perfectly regular and with one morphology – likely ventricular flutter
- if largely regular but with obvious polymorphism – likely torsades de pointes
- if irregular, and with largely one morphology – likely atrial fibrillation with WPW.

Management of patients with ventricular arrhythmias

The emergency management algorithm for life-threatening ventricular arrhythmias is described in the chapter on resuscitation. In general terms, the management of ventricular arrhythmias should include the following:[50]

- a search for and correction of causes, including
  - ischaemia: ECG, cardiac enzymes
  - biochemical: potassium derangement, hypomagnesaemia
  - metabolic: shock, hypoxaemia, pH derangement, hypoglycaemia
  - drug effect: inotrope, chronotrope, recreational drugs
  - pulmonary artery or intracardiac catheters[52]
  - cardiomyopathy, hypertrophy, myocarditis
  - long Q–T interval and Q–T prolonging influences
  - proarrhythmia from antiarrhythmic drugs

- immediate CPR and cardioversion/defibrillation for pulseless, unconscious ventricular arrhythmias (cardiac arrest).[50] In conscious patients, initial treatment is usually pharmacological and, if necessary, cardioversion is applied under the influence of short-acting anaesthetics (e.g. propofol)
- antiarrhythmic therapy
  - immediately: IV amiodarone, lignocaine, sotalol[50]
  - ongoing: oral amiodarone, sotalol, procainamide, flecainide, beta-blockers[53]
- heart failure management, which needs to be aggressive if contributory
- electrophysiological testing, which should be performed for serious arrhythmias to identify foci or pathways and confirm effectiveness of treatment[53]
- pacing strategies
  - cardiac resynchronisation therapy using biventricular pacemaker, providing benefit for the heart failure patient at greater risk for ventricular arrhythmias[54]
  - overdrive pacing therapy: antitachycardia pacing strategies via implantable cardioverter defibrillator[44,45]
- implantable cardioverter defibrillator therapy, which should be considered for all survivors of sudden cardiac death not due to transient or reversible factors,[44,45] especially those with low ejection fraction and recurrent sustained ventricular arrhythmias[55]
- where a myocardial scar can be confirmed as the arrhythmic focus, surgical resection may sometimes be undertaken.

Arrhythmia identification and analysis

Arrhythmia differentiation requires knowledge of ECG criteria and a systematic approach to interpretation. The flow diagram in Figure 11.28 aids identification of the site of origin of rhythms or location of conduction disturbances.

Antiarrhythmic medications

Antiarrhythmic drugs are classified partly on the basis of beta-receptor or membrane channel activity, and partly by their physiological effects on the cardiac action potential. This is represented by the Vaughan Williams classification system (see Table 11.5).[51] However, as action potential abnormalities cannot be expediently identified at the bedside, matching antiarrhythmic agents to cellular physiology cannot realistically be undertaken. Instead, antiarrhythmics are chosen partly on the basis of their known efficacy, by their effectiveness on atrial or ventricular arrhythmias and after consideration of the side effects and contraindications to known comorbidities in a given patient.[53,56]

The classification of the major acute antiarrhythmics in use, along with doses, arrhythmic indications, precautions and side effects, are depicted in Table 11.6. Class I agents all slow phase 1 (depolarisation) and so may slow conduction and prolong the QRS. The subgroups of class I agents denote strength (A = weakest, C = strongest) and affect repolarisation, with class IA (prolonging), IB (shortening) and IC (not affecting) repolarisation duration. Class II

FIGURE 11.28 Stepwise approach to arrhythmia identification.

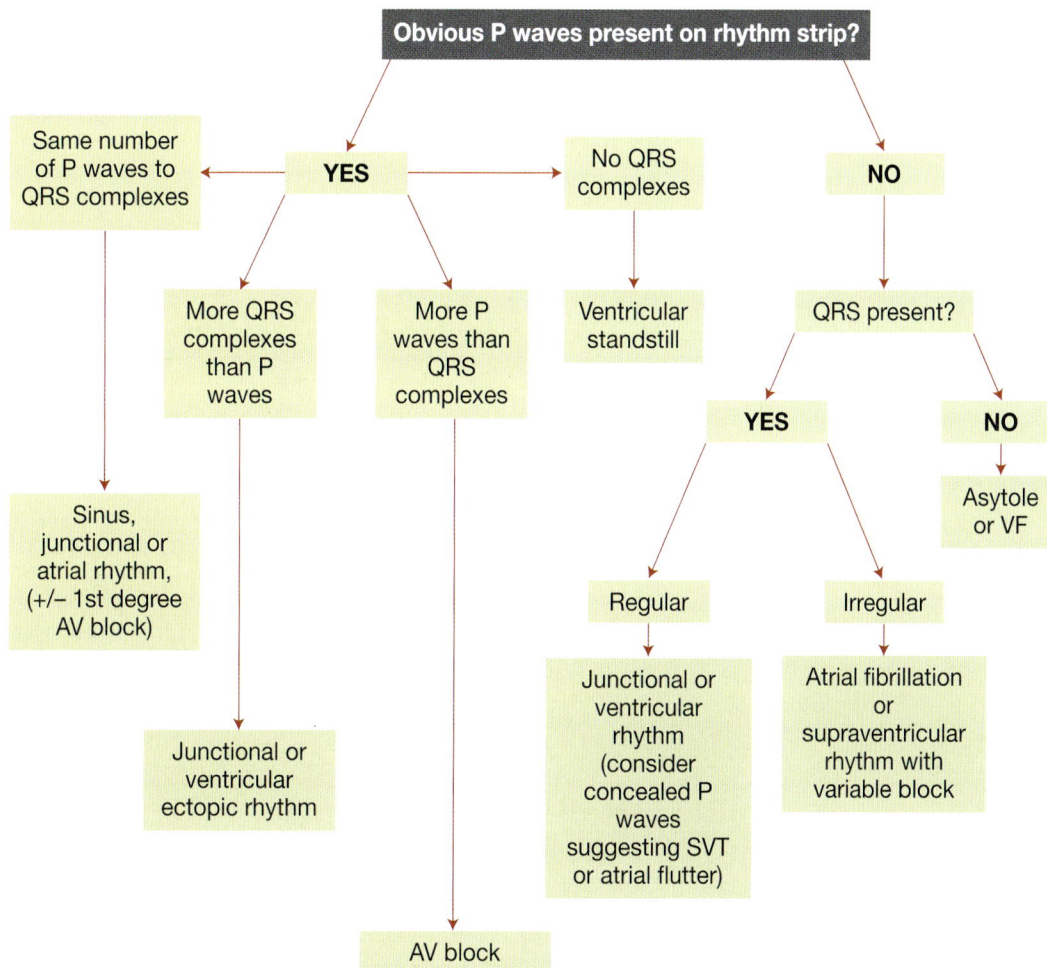

TABLE 11.5

Antiarrhythmic classifications[43]

CLASS	ACTION	DRUGS
IA	Sodium channel blockers: action potential prolongation	quinidine procainamide disopyramide
IB	Sodium channel blockers: accelerate repolarisation; shorten action potential duration	lignocaine mexiletine
IC	Potent sodium channel blockers: little effect on repolarisation	flecainide
II	Beta-blockers: depress automaticity (prolong phase 4); indirect prolongation phase 2	metoprolol propanolol esmolol
III	Potassium (outward) channel blockers: prolong duration of action potential (prolonged repolarisation)	amiodarone sotalol (beta-blocker with class II actions)
IV	Calcium channel blockers	verapamil diltiazem

TABLE 11.6
Acute antiarrhythmic characteristics[41,44,45]

AGENT	DOSE	ARRHYTHMIC INDICATION	CONSIDERATIONS	SIDE EFFECTS
quinidine (class IA)	Oral treatment only	Supraventricular WPW	Avoid hypokalaemia Increased risk torsades following elective cardioversion	QRS prolongation Q-T prolongation Hypotension GI intolerance
procainamide (class IA)	50 mg increments per minute IV (up to 10 mg/kg)	Supraventricular Ventricular WPW	Potentiates class IA and class III	QRS prolongation Hypotension Q-T prolongation AVB
lignocaine (class IB)	1 mg/kg over 2 min; 1–4 mg/min infusion 24 h	Ventricular	If hepatic/renal dysfunction: dose modification necessary to avert toxicity Avoid hypokalaemia	Hypotension, bradycardia, AVB CNS disturbance
flecainide (class IC)	IV 1–2 mg/kg over 10 min; infusion 0.150–0.025 mg/kg/min	Supraventricular Ventricular WPW	Proarrhythmia more marked in structural heart disease	Hypotension Bradycardia, AVB Proarrhythmia QRS prolongation
esmolol (class II)	0.5 mg/kg/min over 1 min, followed by decremental infusion protocol	Supraventricular		Hypotension Bradycardia, AVB Symptom provocation in asthma, COAD, diabetes, peripheral vascular disease Q-T prolongation ++ (sotalol)
metoprolol (class II)		Supraventricular		
sotalol (class III + beta-blocker, class II)	5 mg increments per min up to 80 mg total; maintenance 160–280 mg/day	Supraventricular Ventricular	Potentiation of class IA and III agents	
amiodarone (class III, also strong class I, with some class II and IV activity)	150–300 mg (over 2 min in cardiac arrest, otherwise over 20 min); maintenance 400–800 mg/day	Supraventricular Ventricular	Slow GI absorption Long half-life 25–110 days Potentiation of digoxin, warfarin, class IA, class III effects	Hypotension Bradycardia, AVB Q-T prolongation Thyroid, hepatic dysfunction Pulmonary fibrosis Photosensitivity
verapamil (class IV)	5–10 mg IVI	Supraventricular Selected use in ventricular	Potentiates digoxin	Hypotension Bradycardia AVB
adenosine (class IV-like)	6–12 mg rapid IVI bolus followed by flush (repeatable)	Supraventricular	Experience may be disturbing. Consider pre-sedation. Half-life 10 s	Transient AVB/ ventricular standstill
ivabradine (If channel inhibitor)	Oral 5–7.5 mg twice daily	Modest selective slowing of sinus rate Heart failure or ischaemic heart disease where rate reduction required	Selective sinus node inhibitor	Bradycardia Hypotension Visual disturbances

AVB = atrioventricular block; CNS = central nervous system; COAD = chronic obstructive airway disease; GI = gastrointestinal; If = sinoatrial funny channel; WPW = Wolff-Parkinson-White syndrome.

agents (beta-blockers) depress automaticity, slowing the heart rate and prolonging the action potential. The class III agents notably prolong repolarisation, action potential duration and the Q–T interval. Class IV drugs are calcium channel blockers, decreasing automaticity and prolonging the action potential.[48]

Amiodarone ranks as the most effective agent in converting tachyarrhythmias, but its use must be weighed against its considerable side effects.[57,58] As with other class III drugs (e.g. sotalol) and class IA agents, there is a risk of Q–T interval prolongation and the development of torsades de pointes.[47,49,59,60] Although sotalol carries the greatest risk of this arrhythmia, it may be selected when amiodarone side effects need to be avoided, or when combined antiarrhythmic–beta-blocker therapy is desired, (e.g. arrhythmias postinfarction or in the setting of heart failure). Lignocaine, the front-line ventricular antiarrhythmic for many years, lacks the efficacy of amiodarone, but is well tolerated and effective in the setting of ischaemic myocardium.[61] Whatever the choice of antiarrhythmic, attention should also be directed to biochemical correction, in particular serum magnesium, potassium and pH.[50]

Cardiac pacing

Artificial cardiac pacing is most commonly used to provide protection against bradycardia and/or AV block. Slow heart rates can be sustained at more physiological rates by repetitive electrical stimulation, delivered by a pacemaker at a programmed rate. Temporary pacing may be provided in an emergency, providing rhythm protection while reversible factors are overcome (biochemical or drug influence, myocardial ischaemia) or as a bridge to permanent pacemaker implantation.[62] Separate from such bradycardia protection, pacing may be undertaken to improve haemodynamic status, or to treat or suppress tachyarrhythmias.

Principles of pacing

A paced rhythm can be achieved by delivering electrical stimuli through pacing leads connected to the myocardium. Electrical impulses are delivered to the heart via the negative electrode of the circuit, while the positive electrode completes the electrical circuit and enables sensing (detection) of the patient's intrinsic cardiac rhythm.[63,64] Electrical impulses of sufficient strength stimulate the myocardium to depolarise (and then to contract) at a selected rate.

Pacing leads (electrodes) may be positioned in contact with the endocardium via transvenous access, or attached to the epicardium at the time of cardiac surgery.[65] For epicardial pacing, two separate leads or 'wires' are usually attached to each chamber paced, with one wire connected to each of the negative and positive terminals of the pulse generator (pacemaker). For transvenous pacing, a single lead is advanced to the apex of the right ventricle. These leads have a pacing electrode at their tip and a circumferential (or 'ring') sensing electrode slightly proximal to this. In an emergency, these transvenous ventricular pacing wires can be inserted promptly and establish a supportive

ventricular rate.[66] Temporary transvenous pacing is almost always undertaken as ventricular pacing only. While there are transvenous leads available for temporary atrial pacing, they are more difficult to position, and their use is very infrequent. By contrast, in the cardiac surgical patient, where direct lead attachment is straightforward, pacing may be undertaken as single chamber (atrial or ventricular) or dual chamber (atrial and ventricular).

Temporary transvenous wires are particularly vulnerable to movement.[65] Unlike permanent pacing leads, which are 'fixed' in some manner to the myocardium,[55,67] temporary leads are simply blunt-ended leads that rely on lodging in muscular folds (trabeculae) near the apex of the right ventricle to hold the lead in position. Activity limitation and strict rest in bed are therefore recommended for the patient with temporary transvenous pacing who is pacemaker-dependent.

The details and descriptions of pacing in this section apply equally to temporary and permanent pacing. However, the strategies for the correction of problems are oriented more towards temporary pacing. Additional features and issues related to permanent pacing are provided at the end of this section.

Major pacemaker controls

All temporary pacemakers give the operator control over pacing rate, pacemaker output (strength of the applied electrical stimulus), sensitivity (to intrinsic rhythm) and (in dual-chamber modes) the AV interval. Additional controls such as mode selection, output pulse width, upper tracking rate and the post ventricular atrial refractory period (for DDD mode) are available on some temporary and all permanent devices. Table 11.7 describes the major parameters that can be directly controlled on most temporary devices.

Pacing terminology

To aid in communication when discussing pacing functions, international agreement on terminology has been reached (see Table 11.8). A 5-letter code[68] describes the pacing (and/or defibrillation) capabilities of any given device in terms of chambers involved in pacing, sensing or other functions such as rate responsive pacing capabilities. A pacemaker designated as **VVIR**, for example, is capable of **V**entricular pacing, sensing of **V**entricular activity, **I**nhibiting pacing in response to sensing of ventricular activity, as well as possessing **R**ate responsiveness. While the first three positions in the terminology relate to all types of pacing, the fourth and fifth letters relate only to permanent pacing and have not been used in this chapter.

Capture

A pacing stimulus that successfully generates a P wave or QRS complex is said to have 'captured' the atria or ventricles, respectively. If pacing stimuli are not followed by a P wave or a QRS complex, 'failure to capture' is said to be occurring and requires immediate corrective action (Figure 11.29).

TABLE 11.7

Pacemaker controls and settings

CONTROL	FUNCTION
Base rate	Sets the rate at which the pacemaker will discharge: pacing occurs at this rate unless the patient's own rate is faster and is sensed by the pacemaker. Typically set at 60–100/min
Ventricular output	The size, or strength, of the stimulus delivered to the ventricles. In temporary devices this is an adjustable current (measured in milliamperes [mA]). Output is increased until capture (successful stimulation) is achieved. The minimum current required to achieve capture is termed the output threshold. Impulses delivered below the threshold value will not capture the myocardium. Temporary pacemakers have an adjustable output range of 0.1–25 mA
Atrial output	The size or strength of the stimulus delivered to the atria. Range 0.1–20 mA
Atrial and ventricular pulse width	Only adjustable on some devices. Allows adjustment of the duration for which the pacemaker output is applied to the myocardium. Selectable range typically 1.0–2.0 milliseconds (ms) in 0.25-ms increments. Increasing the pulse width enhances ability to gain capture
Atrioventricular delay	The interval between the delivery of the atrial and ventricular pacing stimuli. Normally this is set in the same range as normal P–R intervals (between 0.12 and 0.20 s)
Sensitivity	Affects the ability of the pacemaker to detect the presence of spontaneous cardiac activity. Sensitivity settings can be adjusted between 1.0 and 20 millivolts (mV). Set at 1.0 mV the device is very sensitive (able to sense small electrical signals from the heart). Set at higher values, the device becomes less sensitive (higher voltage signals required to be detected), with the risk that QRS complexes or P waves will not be sensed

TABLE 11.8

Pacemaker terminology[56]

CHAMBER PACED	CHAMBER SENSED	RESPONSE TO SENSING	PROGRAMMABLE FUNCTIONS	ANTITACHYARRHYTHMIA FUNCTIONS
O, none	O, none	O, none	O, none	O, none
A, atrium	A, atrium	T, triggered	P, simple programmable	P, pacing
V, ventricle	V, ventricle	I, inhibited	M, multi-programmable	S, shock
D, dual (A & V)	D, dual (A & V)	D, dual (T & I)	C, communicating	D, dual (P & S)
			R, rate modulation	

FIGURE 11.29 Ventricular pacing at 86/min. There is capture on the first five beats but none of the remaining pacing spikes are followed by the expected wide QRS of capture. Note that, while there is capture, the patient's own rhythm is suppressed. When capture is lost, the patient's slower rate emerges. Consistent capture needs to be re-established, by either increasing the pacemaker output or correcting factors that depress myocardial responsiveness.

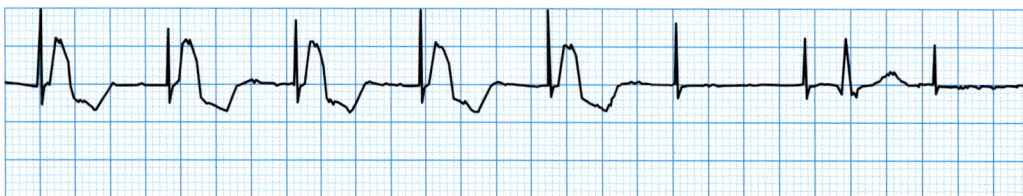

Output and threshold

The strength of the pacing stimulus applied is termed the pacing 'output', and is adjustable by the operator. For temporary pacing this is more often an adjustable current, and with permanent pacing is an adjustable voltage. When first establishing pacing, the output is typically increased gradually until 100% capture is achieved. The minimum output required to achieve capture is termed the output threshold. This pacing threshold may vary significantly with changes in biochemistry, arterial pH, myocardial perfusion, drugs and other factors.[65,69–71] To accommo-date potential threshold changes, output settings on the pulse generator are set with a 'safety margin', i.e. the pulse generator is set to deliver outputs that are at least double the threshold value.[70]

Practice tip

Thresholds for stimulation are more volatile in the temporary pacemaker patient in whom ischaemia or postoperative biochemical, pH and haemodynamic changes are common. Monitoring should be focused on confirming capture and low heart rate limits should be set to 5 or 10 beats below the base pacing rate.

Demand versus asynchronous pacing

Pacing can be configured in either demand (sensing) or asynchronous (non-sensing) modes.

Demand pacing

The most common approaches to pacing are the so-called 'demand' modes. In these modes, pacing is provided only on demand: that is, when the heart rate falls below a nominated level (demand rate) (Figure 11.30). Demand pacing requires pacemaker detection of the patient's intrinsic cardiac rhythm. If an intrinsic rhythm is sensed, it 'inhibits' the pacemaker from delivering a pacing stimulus. The demand modes ensure that pacing is provided only when needed, and also protect against pacing during arrhythmically vulnerable moments in the cardiac cycle.

Ventricular pacing delivered at the time of the T wave may induce ventricular tachyarrhythmias[72] (Figure 11.31), while atrial pacing during atrial repolarisation (shortly after the P wave) may precipitate atrial tachyarrhythmias.[60]

Asynchronous pacing

Pacing may be delivered in an asynchronous mode, that is, without the capability of sensing the heart's inherent rhythm. When in an asynchronous mode, the pulse generator will pace perpetually at the set rate, irrespective of whether the patient is generating his/her own rhythm. The main applications of non-sensing (asynchronous) modes are: 1) when there is oversensing, or risk of oversensing, such as in environments with strong electromagnetic fields and 2) when patients would otherwise be asystolic or critically bradycardic if pacing were interrupted (pacemaker-dependent).[63,73,74] In demand modes of pacing, false sensing of electromagnetic interference is able to inappropriately inhibit pacing, returning patients to their own unreliable rhythm.[73] Temporary reprogramming to non-sensing modes (AOO, VOO, DOO) is commonly undertaken during surgery to prevent false pacemaker inhibition by electrocautery. For permanent pacing this is achieved by reprogramming, or by magnet application over the device causing asynchronous pacing at elevated rates (90–100/min) while the magnet is in place. The appropriateness of continuing in an asynchronous mode should always be reconsidered if the patient's rate re-emerges in competition with the pacing due to the risk of precipitating arrhythmias.

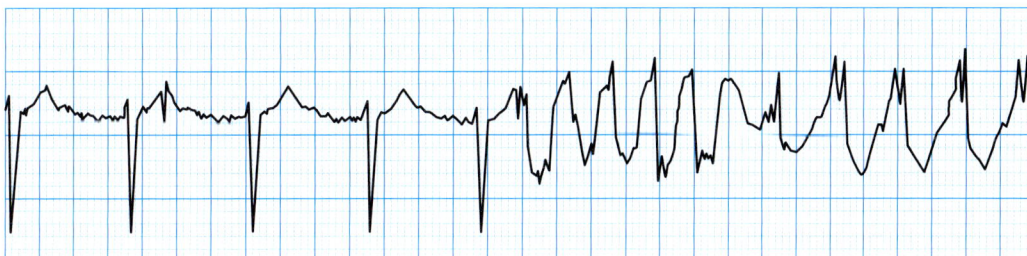

FIGURE 11.30   Demand ventricular pacing at a rate of 60/min. The patient's rate increases after the first two paced beats and inhibits the pacemaker. It then slows to below 60/min and the pacemaker recommences 'on demand'.

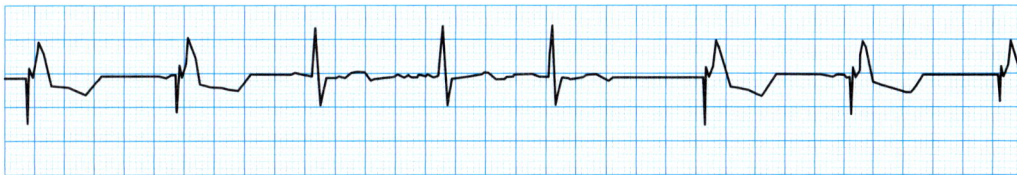

FIGURE 11.31   Intermittent asynchronous pacing due to incomplete sensing. Set pacing rate 66/min. The 1st, 3rd and fourth beats are sensed and appropriately inhibit pacing. However, a pacing spike can be seen at the apex of the T wave of the second beat, which does not cause arrhythmia. The next pacing spike, just after the apex of the T wave of the fifth beat, arrives during the period of increased excitability in the action potential and precipitates ventricular tachycardia.

Ventricular pacing

Stimulation of just the ventricles results in the generation of a ventricular ectopic rhythm. Functionally this will be no different from an intrinsic ventricular rhythm. There will be loss of atrioventricular synchrony, and the loss of atrial kick may cause low cardiac output and hypotension. To offset the loss of atrial kick, ventricular pacing is sometimes undertaken at slightly higher rates than normally seen in the resting patient (e.g. 70–80/min, rather than 50–60/min).

The delivered pacing stimulus should be followed immediately by a QRS complex that is wide (>0.12 s) and often notched, resembling a ventricular ectopic rhythm. Pacing from near the apex will produce an ECG that closely resembles left bundle branch block morphology, with left axis deviation. ST segments and T waves will appear in the opposite direction to the major QRS direction in all leads.[69]

Ventricular pacing provides protection against bradycardia or AV block by stimulating the ventricles at a set rate (Figure 11.32). Temporary ventricular pacing may also be undertaken to prevent bradycardia-dependent tachyarrhythmias such as torsades de pointes.[75] In this context, pacing at faster rates provides protection by reducing the QT interval, as well as preventing pauses that give rise to ectopy and onset of torsades de pointes.[75]

> ### Practice tip
>
> If haemodynamic status is suboptimal during ventricular pacing (low blood pressure and/or cardiac output), consider changing the pacing rate. A faster pacing rate may offset the loss of atrial kick and so restore cardiac output despite low stroke volume. Alternatively, turning down the pacing rate may reveal an underlying (slower) sinus rhythm that produces improved cardiac output due to the inclusion of atrial kick.

Atrial pacing

Atrial pacing alone is indicated when there is sinus node dysfunction in the presence of reliable AV conduction.[62,74]

The characteristic arrhythmias of such patients are symptomatic sinus bradycardia and/or sinus pause/arrest that may be syncopal. For atrial-only pacing to be undertaken, there needs to be confidence that AV conduction is intact, and that it will remain intact in the future[76] as the annual incidence of progression to AV block is 1% in these patients.[77] If there is AV block, atrial pacing alone is unsuitable, and dual-chamber pacing should be considered.[62,74,76] In permanent pacing the reliability of AV conduction is sometimes assessed by pacing the atria rapidly (e.g. at rates of up to 120 to 150/min). If AV block does not develop at these faster rates there can be confidence that AV conduction is reliable. The advantage of atrial pacing over ventricular pacing is the provision of atrial kick, which may contribute substantially to cardiac output and blood pressure. In this respect atrial pacing is superior to ventricular-only pacing.

Atrial pacing tends to produce low-amplitude P waves, which vary from the typical P waves seen during sinus rhythm (Figure 11.33). They may at times be difficult to identify on the ECG. Appropriate lead selection is important to reveal the atrial depolarisation and confirm atrial capture. It is common for the AV interval (P–R interval) to extend slightly (e.g. to 0.20–0.22 s) during atrial pacing compared with sinus rhythm, as the time taken for atrial impulses to traverse the atria from the pacing focus is longer than the sinus-to-AV node conduction interval.

Atrial pacing and AV block

Any degree of AV block is possible during atrial pacing and it must be remembered that AV block is rate dependent.[76,77] Thus, the severity of AV block may be worsened not only by AV node dysfunction but also by changes in the atrial pacing rate. A patient with first-degree block may develop second-degree block if the atrial pacing rate is increased, without this implying worsening AV node function. Conversely, AV block developing during atrial pacing may be lessened or overcome by reducing the atrial pacing rate. An example of such rate-dependent AV block behaviour is demonstrated in Figures 11.34 to 11.36, which are sequential strips from the same patient.

FIGURE 11.32 Onset of ventricular pacing. At the start of the strip the patient's heart rate is around 70/min. The pacemaker is then turned on with the rate set at 80/min. Capture is achieved immediately and, because the pacing rate is faster, there is suppression of the patient's own rhythm. Note the wide QRS and ST elevation during pacing. This is the expected appearance.

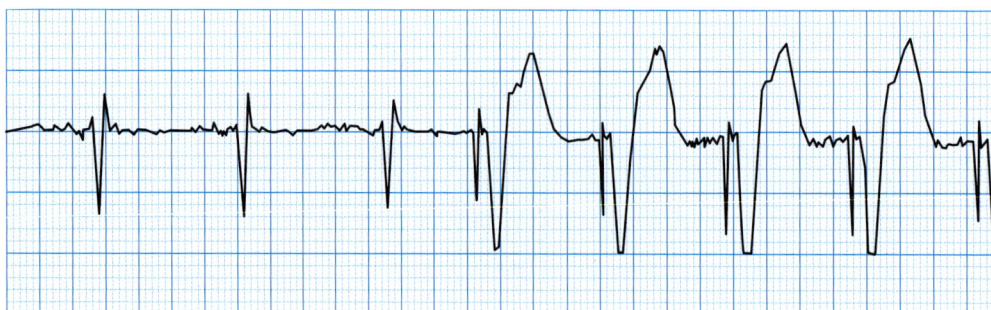

FIGURE 11.33 Commencement of atrial pacing. The patient's own sinus rhythm is around 65/min at the start of the strip. Pacing is turned on at a rate of around 70/min, and causes suppression of the slower sinus rhythm. Note that the commonly seen changes during pacing compared with sinus rhythm are present here – paced P waves are lower in amplitude than the sinus beats, and the P–R interval prolongs slightly during pacing.

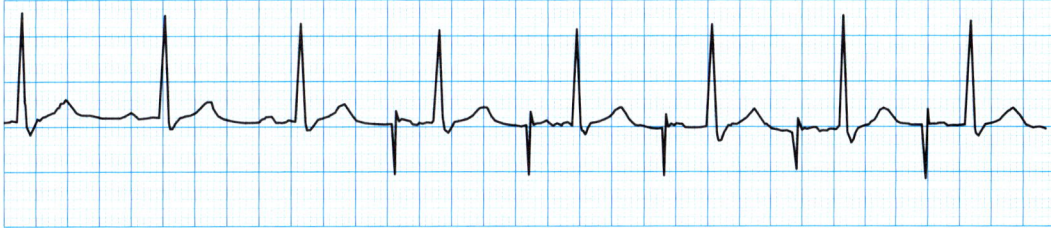

FIGURE 11.34 Atrial pacing at 70/min with first-degree AV block. Note the long P–R interval, at almost 0.4 s; particular caution is warranted in increasing the rate as, although AV conduction is 1:1, it is already very slow. See Figures 11.35 and 11.36 for worsening of AV block as the atrial rate is increased.

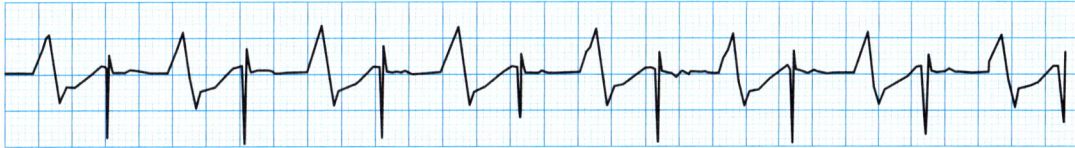

FIGURE 11.35 Second-degree AV block type I with 3:2 conduction. The same patient as above, with worsening AV block after increasing the atrial pacing rate to 80/min. Note the 1:1 conduction has been lost and there are dropped beats. After each of the dropped beats the P–R is 0.30 s, which extends to 0.46 s on the next beat, before dropping of the third beat of each cycle.

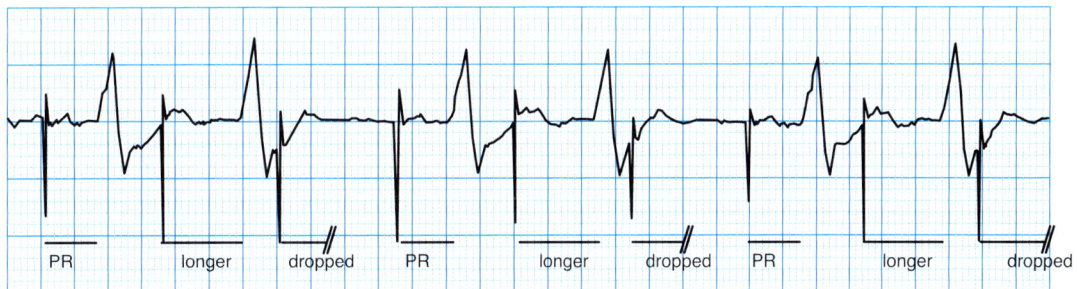

FIGURE 11.36 The same patient again, now with the atrial pacing at 86/min. At the faster atrial rate, AV conduction has worsened further. There is now a 2:1 block yielding a ventricular rate of 43/min.

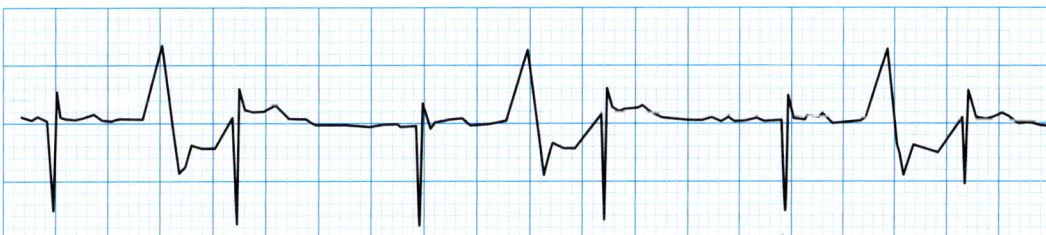

Dual-chamber pacing

Pacing of both the atria and ventricles offers the benefit of atrial kick as well as a guarantee of a ventricular response. Thus, it provides protection against bradycardia and AV block. As with either atrial or ventricular pacing, demand modes have been preferred in dual-chamber pacing, unless oversensing and pacemaker dependence warrant asynchronous pacing. Particular features of the DDD pacing mode have made it the predominant mode in both permanent and postsurgical temporary pacing.

Pacing stimuli are delivered to the atria and ventricles at a selected rate. After delivery of the atrial stimulus there is a delay of usually 0.16–0.24 seconds (equivalent to a P–R interval) before delivery of the ventricular pacing stimulus (Figure 11.37). If the patient is able to conduct the atrial depolarisation to the ventricles themselves before the ventricular pacing is due, then the pacemaker senses the resultant QRS and inhibits ventricular pacing.

A dual-chamber pacemaker may demonstrate atrial and ventricular pacing at the set rate and at the set AV delay as described above, or may operate as simply atrial pacing if normal AV node conduction occurs before the programmed AV delay has elapsed. Deliberately prolonging the programmed AV delay provides greater opportunity for patients to conduct to the ventricles by themselves. In some patients intrinsic ventricular conduction produces a contractile pattern that is superior to the contraction from ventricular pacing; however the difference will be minor. There has been increasing interest in permitting native AV conduction because of the above reasons, and also on the basis of recent data from the DAVID trial, which revealed that chronic ventricular pacing induces negative ventricular remodelling and worsening of heart failure.[78] Prolonging AV delays to permit native conduction has become commonplace in permanent pacemakers, but carries some slight arrhythmic risk[79] (Figure 11.38).

DDD pacing: the 'universal' pacing mode

The introduction of the DDD mode of pacing (**D**ual chamber pacing, **D**ual chamber sensing and **D**ual responses [inhibition and triggered ventricular pacing]) added an important new dimension to dual-chamber pacing: the ability to synchronise ventricular pacing to spontaneous atrial activity in patients with AV block.[74] In addition to the normal bradycardia and AV block protection, the DDD mode features a 'triggered' function. If the pacemaker detects a P wave but a QRS does not follow within the preset AV interval (AV block), the pacemaker

FIGURE 11.37   Dual-chamber pacing at a rate of 72/min. Note the atrial spikes are followed by P waves (atrial capture), then after an AV interval of 0.20 s there is a ventricular spike, followed by a QRS complex (ventricular capture).

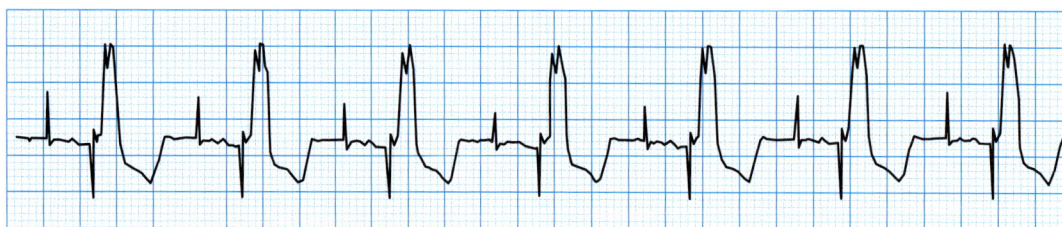

FIGURE 11.38   AV pacing with prolongation of the AV delay to permit native conduction. There is initially AV pacing at a rate of 75/min, with an AV delay of 0.16 s. The AV delay is then increased to 0.30 s, during which the patient can be seen to conduct spontaneously through to the ventricles to produce spontaneous narrow QRS. These are sensed by the pacemaker and inhibit the ventricular pacing.

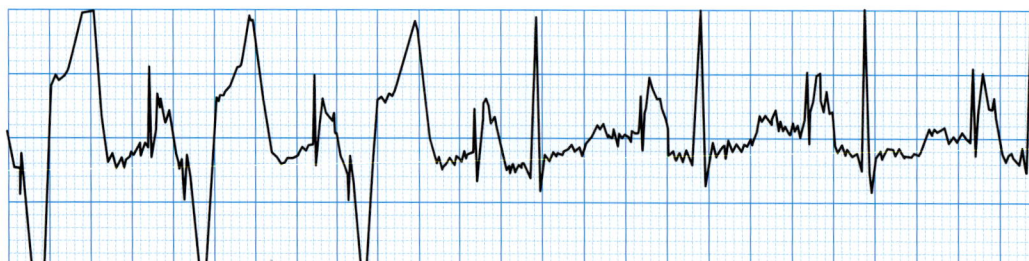

will be triggered to provide ventricular pacing at the end of the programmed AV interval. In short, the pacemaker paces the ventricles after any P wave. This means that the ventricular rate can be brought back under control of the sinus node, even though there is AV block. Consequently, in a DDD pacemaker it is common to see ventricular pacing at a range of different rates as it responds to sinus activity. This triggered behaviour of the DDD device is sometimes called 'P-synchronous ventricular pacing', although 'atrial tracking' is a more practical term as the ventricular pacing 'tracks' the atrial rate.

Atrial tracking allows the pacemaker to pace the ventricles in response to the atrial rate sensed by the pacemaker. This is desirable when the atrial rate is controlled by the sinus node, but is inappropriate during atrial arrhythmias. For example, in the patient with AV block it is beneficial to pace the ventricles after each sinus P wave. In contrast, atrial tracking at a 1:1 rate during atrial flutter would produce an intolerable ventricular rate, and during atrial fibrillation the tracking rate could be even higher. For this reason, an 'upper rate' for atrial tracking is programmed in the DDD pacemaker. The upper rate controls the maximal rate at which ventricular pacing can be provided (how fast it may track the atria at a 1:1 ratio). This is typically set to around 120–130 per minute. In younger patients it may be set higher, e.g. 140–170/min.

This triggering of ventricular pacing in response to sensed P waves is intended to mimic the behaviour of the AV node. It ensures that a QRS follows each P wave and brings the ventricular rate back under the control of the sinus node (see Figures 11.39 and 11.40). Ventricular pacing will thus be seen at a wide range of rates, as the ventricular pacing follows the normal speeding and slowing of the sinus rate in response to activity or illness. If the atrial rate exceeds the upper rate for tracking, then it is no longer possible for all of the atrial beats to be tracked. DDD pacemakers will start 'dropping' beats when the atrial rate exceeds the upper tracking rate in a manner analogous to the behaviour of the AV node.

External ('transcutaneous') pacing

Emergency pacing may be undertaken noninvasively via external pacing electrodes, and is termed 'external' or 'transthoracic' pacing. Adhesive defibrillation pads are applied in either the anteroposterior (preferred) or standard apicobasal positions as per defibrillation. These are connected to a defibrillator with additional pacing capability. Pacing stimuli of large current (10–200 mA) are necessary to achieve myocardial capture, and frequently also cause uncomfortable or painful skeletal muscle stimulation. Its use is therefore usually reserved for highly symptomatic/life-threatening bradyarrhythmias, and only as a short-term bridge to invasive pacing. Sedation is typically required in the conscious patient.

FIGURE 11.39   ECG excerpt from a patient with sinus rhythm and 2:1 AV block. The non-conducted P waves are partially concealed but can be seen distorting the T waves (arrows). Although the sinus node can generate a rate of 75/min, the patient is rendered bradycardic by the AV block.

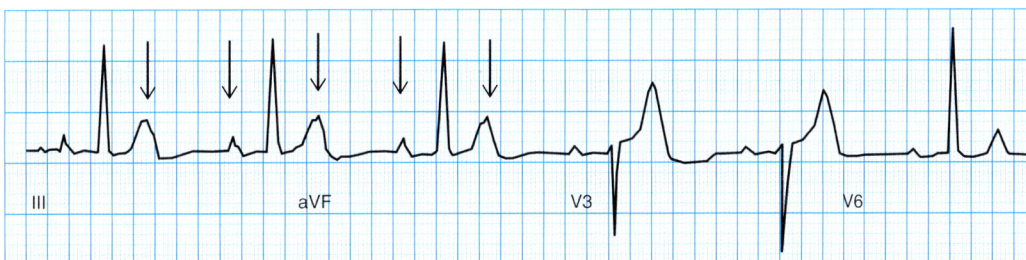

FIGURE 11.40   The same patient as above, 2 hours later. A DDD pacemaker has been inserted and, although some of the pacing spikes are difficult to see, all QRSs are paced beats. The sinus rate is again close to 75/min, and atrial tracking ensures that a paced QRS follows each P wave. The ventricular rate has been brought back under control of the sinus node. Note that, although set to a backup rate of 60/min, the pacemaker is pacing much faster than this because of the triggered behaviour of DDD.

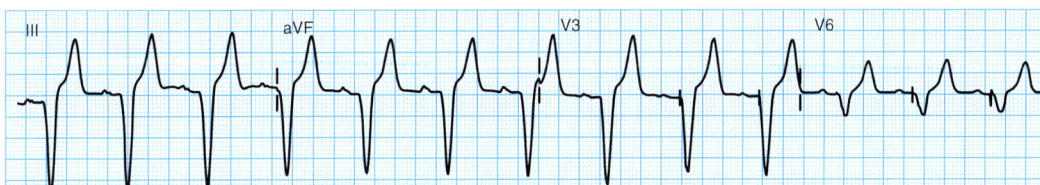

External/transthoracic cardiac pacing provides ventricular pacing only, and the patient should be assessed not only for reliable capture, but also for an adequate pulse and blood pressure during pacing. Pacing may be in either demand or asynchronous mode, usually at rates of 40–80 beats per minute.

Complications of pacing

Effective pacing may be disturbed by problems related to pacing leads, myocardial responsiveness, programmed values, the pulse generator itself (including power sources), and interactions between these factors.[68–72] Four major disturbances to pacing are described below. These provide the bulk of pacing problems encountered and, because they may either interrupt pacing or precipitate serious arrhythmias, critical care nurses need to be competent in their recognition and management.

Failure to capture

When pacing spikes do not successfully stimulate the heart this is termed 'failure to capture'. Pacing spikes are evident on the ECG but are not followed by either QRS complexes (in ventricular pacing) or P waves (in atrial pacing) (see Figures 11.41 and 11.42). Failure to capture may occur when the myocardial responsiveness (threshold) worsens, or when impulses do not reach responsive myocardium. Note that dislodgement of a lead from the myocardium will still show pacing spikes on the ECG as long as the lead is in contact with body fluids or tissue. Repositioning of leads must therefore be included in considerations during management.

Failure to capture may present as a clinical emergency and requires immediate attention. With failure to capture, patients are left to generate their own rhythm, which may

be unacceptably slow. Failure to capture may be complete (all spikes not capturing) or intermittent (with only some spikes achieving capture). Even if there are only occasional spikes that fail to capture, immediate attention is required, as complete failure to capture may ensue. Causes and management of failure to capture[63,70,71,80,81] are listed in Table 11.9.

TABLE 11.9
Failure to capture: causes and management

CAUSES	MANAGEMENT
• Output too low	• Increase output • Increase pulse width if feature is available
• Changing capture threshold	• Check for and treat ischaemia, hyperkalaemia, acidosis or alkalosis • Lead maturation
• Antiarrhythmic drugs	• Consider cessation or dose reduction
• Lead migration/ dislodgement	• Reposition lead if able • Reverse polarity of leads (for epicardial wires) • Position patient on left side (if transvenous lead) • Consider unipolar pacing via application of a skin suture • Treat the resultant rhythm (e.g. atropine, isoprenaline) • Place another lead • Consider external pacing

FIGURE 11.41   Intermittent failure to capture. The 1st, 2nd, 6th and 7th spikes gain ventricular capture but the rest do not. Note the significant pause during failure to capture, in which there is atrial but not ventricular activity. Symptoms during failure to capture depend on the rate of any underlying rhythm.

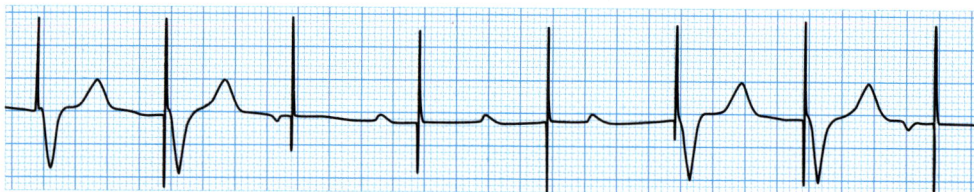

FIGURE 11.42   Atrial pacing with intermittent failure to capture (output set at 14 mA). Note that capture is evident following the 1st, 3rd, 5th, 7th and 8th pacing spikes, but not the others. Fortunately, here the patient has an underlying sinus rhythm, so that the impact of failure to capture is of no great consequence.

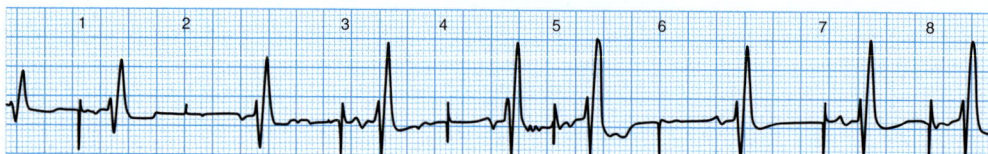

Failure to sense

Sensing of the intrinsic cardiac rhythm is necessary to achieve demand pacing. If rhythms are not sensed, pacing will proceed at a fixed rate and in competition with the native rhythm (Figures 11.43 and 11.44). Pacing spikes may thus be delivered during the excitable period of the action potential and trigger tachyarrhythmias (see Figure 11.31). The risk of arrhythmias is greatest when ventricular pacing spikes are delivered just after the peak of the T wave, especially when there is myocardial ischaemia or infarction, or hypokalaemia. Immediate restoration of appropriate sensing needs to be undertaken. Causes and management of failure to sense[72,80,82] are detailed in Box 11.2. Remember, however, that sensing controls are inverse: lowering numerical settings (e.g. from 5 to 2 mV) *increases* the sensitivity while increasing the value (from 1 to 4 mV) makes the pacemaker *less* sensitive.

Failure to pace

Failure to pace is an imperfect term that is used to describe the event when the pacemaker does discharge but the impulse fails to reach the patient. In this sense it may be useful to regard failure to pace as resulting from an incomplete electrical circuit. The flashing pace indicators on temporary pacemakers confirm that pacing has

BOX 11.2

Failure to sense: causes and management

Causes:
- Sensitivity set too low (too high a number)
- Set in asynchronous mode (AOO, VOO or DOO)
- Altered sensing threshold (lead maturation)
- Decreased myocardial voltages
- Lead movement/dislodgement

Management:
- Increase sensitivity (to a lower number)
- Check/tighten connections
- If epicardial leads, reverse the polarity of the electrodes (reverse connections of positive and negative electrodes)
- Increase the pacing rate to overdrive the competing rhythm
- If underlying rhythm satisfactory, consider turning pacemaker off
- Consider placement of an alternative sensing electrode (skin suture) to create unipolar pacing

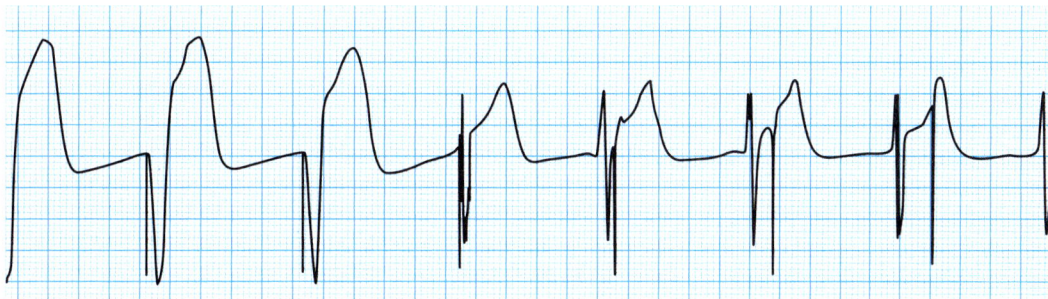

FIGURE 11.43 Ventricular pacing with failure to sense. At the start of the strip there is ventricular pacing. A junctional rhythm appears at a slightly faster rate than the ventricular pacing, but despite this the pacemaker continues to fire, delivering the spikes into the ST segment and T wave. Appropriate sensing of the last three beats of the strip would have caused inhibition of these pacing spikes.

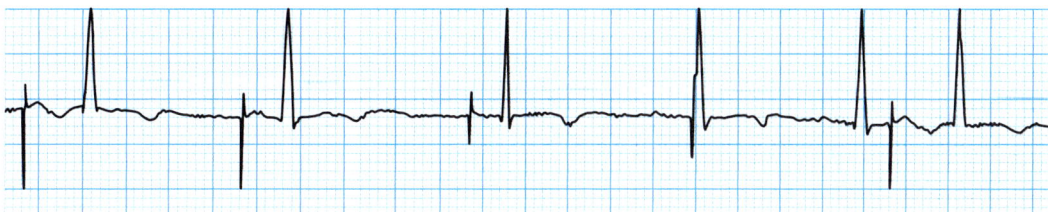

FIGURE 11.44 Atrial failure to sense. The first three beats show atrial pacing. Then there are two spontaneous P waves (fourth and fifth beats). These P waves should have inhibited the atrial pacing, but pacing spikes can be seen at the start of the QRS of the fourth beat and in the ST segment of the fifth beat.

FIGURE 11.45   At the start of the strip there is ventricular pacing at a rate of around 85/min. However, the pacing spikes abruptly cease and the patient is left to generate his/her own slower rate. Spikes do reappear but these are at a slower than the programmed rate. This could be either failure to pace or oversensing during ventricular pacing, and differentiation cannot be made absolutely from this strip. Rather, pacing indicators need to be examined to aid this differentiation. This was a case of ventricular failure to pace due to a poor connection of the pacing leads to the bridging cable.

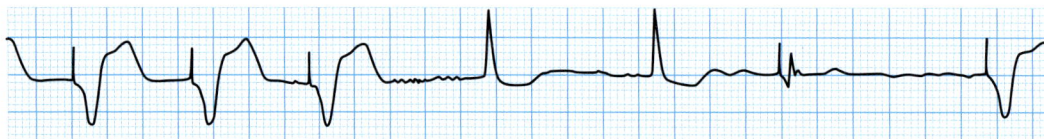

FIGURE 11.46   Atrial pacing with failure to pace. There is sudden disappearance of the pacing spikes after the first three beats. From this strip alone, failure to pace or oversensing cannot be separated as possibilities. However, the pacing indicator was flashing through such pauses, rather than the sensitivity indicator, confirming failure to pace. The connection between the pacing wires and the bridging cable needed tightening and immediately corrected the problem.

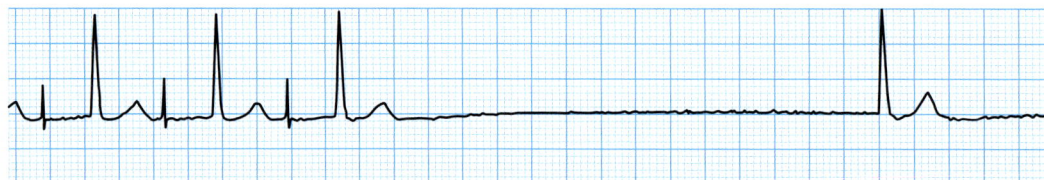

occurred but the spikes fail to appear on the ECG. Most commonly, failure to pace is due to a loose connection in the lead system or a fractured lead or bridging cable, and may involve either the negative or positive limb of the circuit. Electrocardiographically, failure to pace appears as failure of the pacing spikes to appear when expected. As with failure to capture, this leaves patients with whatever rhythm they can generate themselves, which may or may not be adequate. Failure to pace (also termed 'failure to output' in some literature) may present as complete loss of pacing, or just pacing at a slower rate than set (see Figures 11.45 and 11.46). If the patient's rhythm is very slow, failure to pace can be a clinical emergency. Even if there is an adequate rhythm, the situation requires immediate attention. Causes and management of failure to pace[36,63,80,81] are detailed in Box 11.3.

Practice tip

The ECG usually does not help to distinguish between oversensing and failure to pace, and instead – at least with temporary pacing – the distinction is made from inspection of the flashing pacing indicators. If the *pacing* indicator continues to flash during periods where the spikes do not appear, then the problem is failure to pace (an interrupted electrical circuit). Alternatively, if the *sense* indicator is flashing during a period where the spikes do not appear, then the problem is oversensing.

BOX 11.3

Failure to pace: causes and management

Causes:

- Disconnected lead/loose connections – commonest cause
- Pacemaker turned off or dysfunctional
- Output turned off
- Battery depleted
- Fractured lead (may be internally fractured but outwardly intact)

Management:

- Check that pacemaker is turned on
- Check all connections and leads, and tighten/replace if necessary
- Change battery
- Replace the bridging cable between the pacemaker and the pacing leads
- Ensure output is turned on
- Complete circuit with skin suture to positive terminal of the pacemaker, and try each of the existing wires in the negative terminal
- Differentiate from oversensing
- Assess and support rhythm and haemodynamics

Oversensing

As in failure to pace, pacing spikes fail to appear when oversensing occurs. Rather than sensing intrinsic cardiac activity, the pacemaker may sense electrical signals (electromagnetic interference) from other sources. The device will respond as if these are genuine signals and inhibit pacing. Oversensing is a common event during temporary pacing and electrocardiographically may be indistinguishable from failure to pace, as both appear as missing pacing spikes.

Oversensing may result in momentary interruptions to pacing (pauses) or complete cessation of pacing. The clinical impact depends on the duration of oversensing, and on the patient's ability to generate an underlying rhythm. Electromagnetic interference resulting in oversensing may arise from a variety of causes, originating from the patient (muscle movement) or external sources (devices). The sources of oversensing[36,63,82] may be difficult to establish clinically but should be sought and corrected where possible. Causes and management of oversensing are detailed in Box 11.4.

An important distinction must be made between failure to pace and oversensing as both appear electrocardiographically as missing spikes. Examination of the pacemaker indicator lights is most useful: during failure to pace, the *pace* indicator will flash during the periods of missing spikes whereas in oversensing the *sense* indicator will flash.

BOX 11.4

Oversensing: causes and management

Causes:

- Muscle potentials other than QRS complexes:
  - Cardiac: T waves, U waves, P waves
  - Non-cardiac: shivering, fasciculations, seizure activity, any skeletal muscle movement
- External electrical interference:
  - Electrocautery, TENS machines
  - Electrical devices (rare)
- Movement of the connecting pins at the connection to the pulse generator (common)

Management:

- Reduce sensitivity (turn sensitivity to higher number)
- Consider disabling the sensitivity altogether (i.e. asynchronous, VOO, AOO, DOO mode)
- Consider reversing the polarity of the wires (positive to negative)
- Remove the source of interference where it can be identified

---

Practice tip

A ring magnet placed over a permanent pacemaker causes a permanent pacemaker to revert to an asynchronous mode (VOO or DOO). It is thus a management strategy for symptomatic oversensing or for contexts where there is risk of oversensing (e.g. the pacemaker-dependent patient receiving diathermy). The magnet may need to be taped in place while the oversensing risk persists. To avoid possible undersensing of an emerging cardiac rhythm, asynchronous pacing under magnet influence is applied at an elevated rate (e.g. 90–100 beats per minute).

Patient nursing practice

Monitoring and management of the patient and pacing largely fall to the nursing staff of critical care units. Nurses monitor pacing performance and the detection of pacing abnormalities, the integrity of the pacing system, the avoidance of clinical situations or physical changes that may alter pacing effectiveness, patient safety and the prevention of complications.

Nursing responsibilities in the care of the patient with a pacemaker include:

- pacemaker site inspection for inflammation/swelling/haematoma
- avoidance of hip flexion and rest in bed if femoral insertion
- vital signs, circulatory observations etc, at intervals appropriate to the overall patient context
- confirmation of capture and sensing
- identification of return of spontaneous rhythm
- assessment of haemodynamic adequacy during both paced and spontaneous rhythms (BP, CO, perfusion, symptoms)
- strip documentation of rhythm 6-hourly and daily 12-lead ECG
- chest X-ray to confirm the position of the wire/absence of complications
- checking and tightening of all connections (leads to bridging cable, bridging cable to pulse generator) at commencement of the shift and during all pacing adverse events
- confirmation of battery status each shift
- performance of pacemaker threshold assessment each shift or daily.

Protection against microshock

Normally, small electrical stimuli (even static electricity applied to the body) dissipate through body tissues and never reach sufficient current density at the heart to produce arrhythmias. However, pacing wires provide a direct route to the heart, so that even minor electrical sources may achieve sufficient current density at the heart to precipitate arrhythmias. Protection strategies include nursing patients in body- and cardiac-protected areas, insulating lead connector pins when pacing is not in use and using rubber gloves at all times when handling pacing wires.[82]

Battery depletion in a temporary pacemaker

A standard 9V battery powers a temporary pacemaker for up to a week, although this is variable depending on the device and settings. It is prudent to commence treatment with a new battery to avoid unexpected power failure during use.

Indicators of declining battery status are usually displayed when less than 24 hours of battery life remains: flashing battery icons appear on the digital screens of newer generation devices while, on both new and older non-digital screen devices, pacemakers will stop supplying power to the flashing sense/pace LEDs while pacing continues. Battery replacement should be undertaken as soon as reasonably possible as these indicators are not obvious until looked for, so some time may have elapsed before detection by staff.

Changing the battery on a temporary device carries the risk of interrupting pacing, which may be disastrous in the pacemaker-dependent patient. Although the time taken to change a battery may be brief, additional significant time may be lost if the device 'powers down' during the battery change. It is worth noting, however, that temporary pacemakers carry a small stored charge that is enough to sustain pacing for about 10 seconds. If a well-rehearsed procedure is undertaken, battery change can be performed without interrupting pacing for even a single beat. An understanding of the behaviour of the device in use should be established before undertaking battery replacement.

Pacemaker function testing

Routine pacemaker performance checks should be undertaken regularly in the patient with a temporary pacemaker. Temporary pacing leads and wires are prone to movement and other causes of sensing and capture threshold variation. Variations may also be marked when there is myocardial, biochemical and haemodynamic volatility as often seen in the critically ill patient. Pacemaker tests are performed to reveal the return of underlying rhythm, which may be being concealed by pacing, and to measure thresholds for both capture and sensing as these values typically change with time and in response to changing myocardial responsiveness.[66,70,74,80] Regular checking allows detection of threshold changes, and setting of sensing and output safety margins, in order to minimise the development of acute failure to capture or failure to sense.

The practices employed to test temporary pacemakers vary widely, as do attitudes to whether this may or may not be undertaken by nurses. The sample protocol shown in Figure 11.47 provides an organised approach to testing

FIGURE 11.47 Routine temporary pacemaker testing protocol: underlying rhythm, output and sensitivity threshold test.

Pacemaker testing

1. Store current values in memory (for devices with memory). If rhythm difficulty is encountered during testing, these original settings can be immediately re-established by depressing the stored values mode selector.
2. Test for underlying rhythm. Gradually decrease rate in 10 beat/min steps until evidence of underlying rhythm (ULR) emerges:
   (a) If ULR present, observe whether sensing is now occurring.
   (b) If still pacing at 50/min (no emergence of ULR), return to initial settings; do not continue to test sensitivity or output thresholds.
   (c) Document attempt and ULR less than 50/min.
   If underlying rhythm is haemodynamically acceptable, continue.
3. Test sensitivity threshold. Having confirmed haemodynamically adequate underlying rhythm:
   (a) Turn pacing rate to half the patient's rate.
   (b) Turn output to minimum (not off).
   (NB: Sensitivity testing requires that failure to sense is created for a brief period, so steps 3a and 3b are designed to minimise danger of arrhythmias.)
   While observing the sense indicator on the pacemaker:
   • decrease sensitivity (increasing the number) until failure to sense (the sense indicator stops flashing — pacing indicator will now be flashing);
   • increase sensitivity (decreasing the number) until sensing resumes;
   • note the value at which sensing returns — this is the threshold value for sensing; and
   • set sensitivity to half this value minus 1 mV.
4. Test output threshold (continuing from step 3 above the pacing will now be set at a low rate, and at minimum output):
   • Increase the pacing rate to 10 greater than underlying rhythm.
   While watching the monitor:
   • gradually increase the output until capture is achieved;
   • note the value at which capture occurs — this is the threshold value; and
   • set output to double this value plus 1 mA.
5. Store new values in memory and document settings.

during which safety has been emphasised. Because of the varying attitudes to nursing responsibilities, the use of this approach should be ratified at individual institutions before use.

Testing pacemaker thresholds is performed daily or on each shift, but not if the patient is unstable, using the steps described in Figure 11.47. The test should be carried out promptly, with attention to avoiding undue bradycardia or periods of asynchronous pacing. The patient should be advised that pacemaker assessment is being undertaken and to report any sensations of lightheadedness, dyspnoea or other discomfort.

Pacemaker testing in the unstable pacemaker-dependent patient

Greater caution must be applied in the testing of pacemaker functions if the patient has marked haemodynamic instability or has little or no underlying rhythm. It is common for pacemaker testing to be avoided altogether in such circumstances although this may be misguided. Routine testing of pacemaker function as described in Figure 11.47 may not be suitable, but testing for underlying rhythm and some level of testing of capture threshold so as to be confident of safety margins are beneficial. For the patient with haemodynamic instability and/or inotrope use, testing for underlying rhythm becomes of even greater importance as pacing may either prevent or conceal the return of sinus rhythm capability, and cardiac output may be as much as 50% greater with the atrial kick of sinus rhythm than during pacing (see Figure 11.48). It may take several seconds for the sinus node to 'warm up' and express itself,

so decrease the rate gradually and only to reasonable levels (sinus rates of less than 50 are unlikely to be beneficial). Be sure to gain participation of the multidisciplinary team before undertaking testing in this context.

Threshold testing in the pacemaker-dependent patient is also contentious as loss of capture during testing may be poorly tolerated. If the capture threshold is not measured, however, a rising threshold and loss of safety margins cannot be identified, and may only become apparent upon development of acute failure to capture, possibly with outputs already set to maximum and, therefore, no scope for recovering capture. An alternative approach to testing thresholds in this context is useful. Rather than formally measuring threshold by creating loss of capture, the output may be decreased to a value that confirms safety margins are still possible, but without having lost capture at any point, e.g. decreasing output to 10 mA on a device with an output capability of 20 mA. If there is still capture at 10 mA, further reductions can be avoided because a 10 mA safety margin has been demonstrated.

Permanent pacing

For bradyarrhythmias that are not due to temporary, reversible factors or that are likely to be sustained or recurrent, permanent pacemaker implantation may be undertaken. Indications vary, but syncopal events, symptomatic bradycardia, pauses greater than 3 seconds and bradycardia-dependent tachyarrhythmias are general indications for permanent pacing.[75] Dual chamber pacing is usually provided[83] unless the patient has chronic atrial fibrillation as it is not possible to capture the atria during

FIGURE 11.48 Unveiling haemodynamically superior underlying rhythm (strips are continuous). Initially there is ventricular pacing at a rate of 68/min. No atrial activity can be seen and the blood pressure is 85/50 mmHg with noradrenaline support at 8 mcg/min. Across the top strip the paced rate is reduced, allowing P waves to emerge at a rate of 60/min (arrow) and then accelerate to around 70/min across the lower strip. Note the impressive BP increase to 125/65 mmHg allowing discontinuation of noradrenaline infusion. (Note also: cardiac index recorded during V pace 1.7 L/min/m², during sinus rhythm 2.3 L/min/m².) Importantly, there was no suggestion of sinus capability until the pacing rate was reduced.

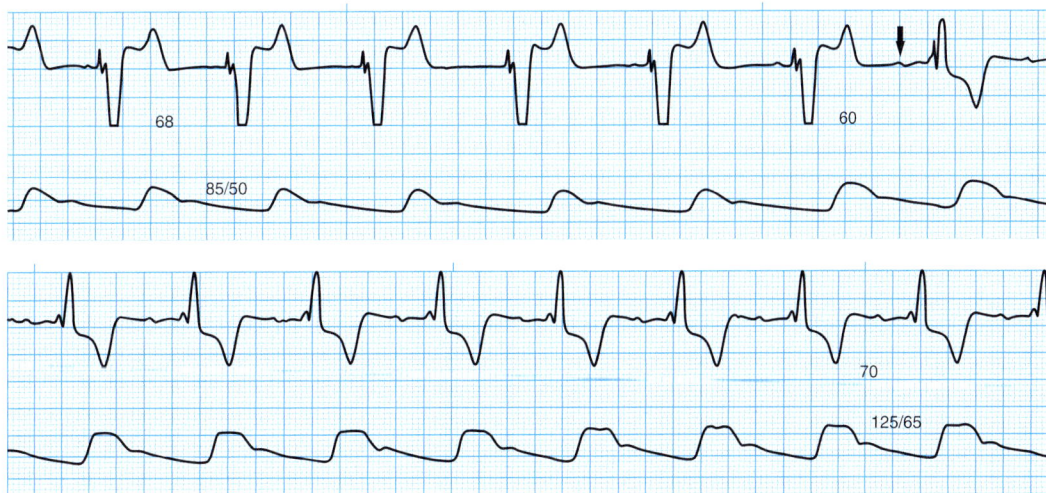

fibrillation. For such patients rate responsive ventricular pacing (VVIR) is the most common mode.[83,84] A dual chamber pacemaker may still sometimes be implanted if there is anticipation of possible future reversion of atrial fibrillation, and the device programmed to DDI or VVI in the interim. Alternatively, the device may be implanted in DDD mode, which allows the device to automatically mode switch to DDI or VVI while the patient is in atrial fibrillation and then automatically switch back to DDD if atrial fibrillation reverts.

The most common mode of pacing with dual chamber devices is DDD, unless the patient has recurrent atrial tachyarrhythmias in which case a non-tracking mode (e.g. DDI) may be selected.[83,84] Patients with sinus node dysfunction are more likely to have rate responsive pacing enabled so that the pacemaker can adjust pacing rates to activity and exercise.

A pulse generator is positioned in a pre-pectoral pocket and leads advanced into the heart either through subclavian vein puncture (from within the pocket) or via cephalic vein cut-down. The cephalic approach avoids intrathoracic complications such as pneumothorax or haemothorax, which may accompany subclavian puncture. Typical pacemaker longevity is 8–12 years.

Permanent pacing leads differ from temporary pacing wires in that, for chronic stability over a lifetime of activity, the leads must be 'fixed' in some manner to the myocardium. 'Active fixation' leads have an extendable helix that is screwed into the myocardium at the time of implantation, much like a corkscrew. 'Passive fixation' leads in contrast are not directly secured to myocardium but have soft tines similar to the barbs of a spear, near the lead tip.[67] The lead is positioned where these tines can embed within muscle infoldings (trabeculae) at the ventricular apex or in the right atrial appendage. Both types of leads have good chronic performance in terms of sensing and stimulation thresholds.[67] However, an inflammatory response does develop at the lead–tissue interface and contributes to an increase in capture thresholds. This is most marked in the first month (acute threshold phase) during which the threshold may double or triple, before settling at a lower chronic threshold.[67] Steroid-tipped leads are now universal and limit the local inflammatory response, reducing the magnitude of the acute threshold increase.[67] Because of the expected threshold change during the first month or so, output safety margins need to be set more generously and patients are typically sent home with outputs set high (e.g. 3.5–5 V) even when thresholds at implantation may have been only 0.5–1 V. Chronic output settings will then be established at the first postoperative visit to the doctor in 6–8 weeks.[48]

Implantation activities

Devices are inserted under light conscious sedation and local anaesthesia. Analgesia may also be administered at the outset of the case, and antibiotics are commenced before skin incision. An anaesthetist is usually only present if judged necessary by the implanting doctor.

Passage of leads into the heart during insertion may result in endocardial contact, causing AV block or bundle branch block. Therefore, a femoral temporary pacing wire may be inserted before progressing to placement of the permanent pacing leads, particularly to ensure reliable ventricular rhythm during the insertion procedure. Ventricular lead placement is most commonly in the right ventricular outflow tract (RVOT) or against the ventricular septum,[78,85] to produce a more normal contractile pattern than from the previously used apex and to prevent the ventricular remodelling seen in chronic RV apical pacing.[78,85] Atrial lead insertion is most commonly at the right atrial appendage, i.e. in the roof of the right atrium. Both ventricular and atrial leads are tested for performance following placement. Leads are then secured within the pacemaker pocket and the pulse generator is attached to the leads and secured in the pocket. The pocket is closed and testing is repeated to confirm secure connections of the leads to the pacemaker. Device and lead testing is repeated on day 1, weeks 6–8 and then every 12 months to confirm operation and to fine tune programming to patient status.[50]

Pacemaker parameters: programming and status reports

Knowing how a patient's pacemaker is programmed is crucial to interpreting pacemaker behaviour in the clinical setting. This has become increasingly important to enable determination of whether a change in behaviour represents a pacing problem or is simply an automated behaviour. Device printouts are available whenever a device is interrogated or reprogrammed. The following section is a guide to how to interpret device printouts to access key information about pacemaker programming, highlighting some of the features of the modern permanent pacemaker, as well as some of the clinical and diagnostic value of the information provided. Device printouts contain an enormous amount of information, but of immediate importance are the summary pages that outline all of the operating parameters, active automated features, results from recent tests and battery status (see Figure 11.49 for an example). Important elements include the following:

- Patient/device details: patient name, type of device, date and time of the printout.

- Battery information: a bar graph displays the progress of the battery towards the elective replacement indicator (ERI); the magnet rate (i.e. the rate that asynchronous pacing will occur at if a magnet is placed over the device); the longevity (indicating the minimum remaining longevity of the device if the patient were to be paced 100% of the time at the current settings).

- Current parameters: basic pacemaker set-up including base rate, maximum rate at which the atrial rhythm will be tracked, AV delay, output settings and pulse widths for both chambers.

- Episodes: summary of any arrhythmia episodes that have been recorded since the last interrogation and any automatic mode switching events that have occurred.

- Events: an event in pacing terms is a beat, rather than a clinical event; every atrial beat (sensed or paced) and every ventricular beat (sensed or paced) is recorded allowing the calculation of the percentage of atrial and ventricular pacing since the last interrogation; this can be compared to previous reports to assess whether pacemaker dependence is increasing or decreasing.

- Test results: the results of device and lead testing performed during the current interrogation as well as testing from the last session performed, including graphic trends of all test results over time shown in a separate section of the report.

- Sense results: the results of the sensing tests carried out in the current interrogation, the last session's values are also shown, and graphic trends of sensing over time can be viewed in a separate section of the report.

- Lead impedance: the results of impedance measurements from the current interrogation and the last session; this provides information about the integrity of the pacing leads, connections and their interface with the myocardium. Impedance is the resistance to current provided by the electrical circuit. Variations in impedance may be seen if the pacing lead insulation is being degraded, the pacing circuit is interrupted or not properly connected or the pacing lead becomes dislodged. Generally, measured impedances do not vary by more than 100 ohms between sessions.

Cardiac resynchronisation therapy

Cardiac resynchronisation therapy (CRT) involves the use of pacing to improve the performance of the left ventricle in heart failure patients. Initially, CRT was undertaken only in patients with severe heart failure (New York Heart Association Class III–IV with ejection fraction <30%) due to dilated cardiomyopathy and with left bundle branch block (LBBB),[86,87] but its proven efficacy in all major randomised controlled studies[88–92] has seen the range of indications expand to include patients with less severe

FIGURE 11.49 FastPath Summary from a St Jude Medical Accent™ dual chamber pacemaker (St Jude Medical Sylmar CA), highlighting basic parameters, events and test results recorded during pacemaker interrogation. Any test results or settings followed by an 'A' in a circle denote automated features. Thus, this device will automatically test capture thresholds and set outputs according to these tests every 8 hours or if ever there is non-capture. Similarly, sensing is automatically tested and automatic sensitivity algorithms allow for changing myocardial voltages. Lead impedance measurements are automatically tested daily, and the pacemaker can automatically switch from bipolar to unipolar to maintain normal capture and sensing if impedance measurements violate alarm limits. See text for additional details.

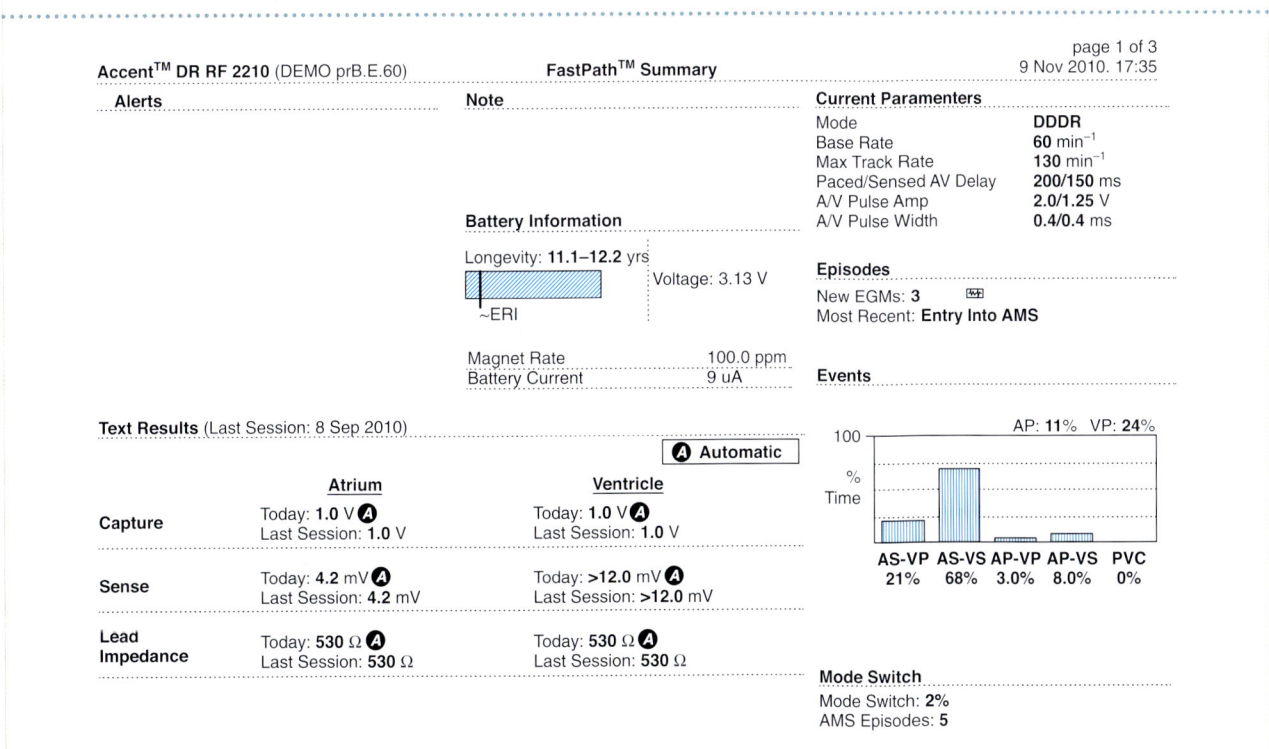

heart failure (New York Heart Association Class I and II).[93] CRT is typically only undertaken after demonstrating failure to respond to optimal pharmacological therapy.

Optimum systolic performance requires all segments of the ventricles to contract more or less synchronously. However, in LBBB septal depolarisation occurs well in advance of the delayed conduction to the posterolateral left ventricular wall. The impact on contraction is to create ventricular dyssynchrony, with the septum contracting before the lateral wall.[94] Similarly, ventricular relaxation becomes dyssynchronous, which may lessen myocardial perfusion and limit ventricular filling, both of which contribute to the severity of heart failure.[94] The majority of patients with LBBB have dyssnchrony and systolic dysfunction, and the impact of this becomes more pronounced when there is existing myocardial disease and/or heart failure.[26,81] With very wide LBBB (e.g. >0.14 s) the impact is greater, as the dyssynchrony between the septal and free wall contraction is exaggerated.[87, 94–96]

In CRT, pacing leads on both the right ventricular (RV) septum and the left ventricular (LV) posterolateral wall are used to stimulate both muscle masses at the same time, with the aim of improving heart failure in patients with significant dyssynchrony.[97] LV and RV pacing stimuli may be delivered simultaneously, although programming of LV stimulation prior to RV pacing by 10–60 milliseconds is more common with the aim to reduce QRS duration to normal duration (<0.12 s).[97] Expected outcomes of CRT include:[88–98]

- improvement in New York Heart Association functional class
- improvement in quality of life
- improvement in physical function
- improvement in ejection fraction and reduction in ventricular size
- reduced hospitalisations for heart failure
- cardiovascular mortality reduction.

The right ventricular lead is implanted in standard fashion, positioned either at the RV apex or outflow tract. Most commonly, the left ventricular lead is also positioned transvenously, with the lead advanced through the coronary sinus into a coronary vein on the lateral or posterolateral LV wall. In a minority of cases a separate mini-thoracotomy may be necessary for secure positioning of an epicardial LV lead when access to the coronary sinus cannot be achieved or where the patient lacks suitable coronary veins.

Two types of devices currently exist: CRT-P (pacemaker), which is a pacemaker achieving resynchronisation, and CRT-D (defibrillator), which adds resynchronisation to an implantable cardioverter defibrillator. The latter devices are more commonly implanted as the combination of severe heart failure and ventricular tachyarrhythmias is frequently present.[99,100]

> **Practice tip**
>
> For the patient with a CRT device whose heart failure is worsening, investigate whether there are device-related factors that may be correctable:
>
> - Is the patient being ventricularly paced >90% of the time? If not, they will be losing the potential benefit of resynchronisation.
> - Can you determine whether there is capture from both the LV and RV leads? Compare with old ECGs where available.

Non-responders to CRT

Disappointingly, up to 25 % of patients who receive CRT devices fail to gain the expected benefits of improved heart function and are termed non-responders.[90,92,101] Failure to respond may be due to device- or lead-related factors, or because of cardiac factors that contribute to worsening heart failure, especially myocardial ischaemia, atrial fibrillation[98] and diminishing responses to adjunctive pharmacological therapy. It should be noted that the preference in CRT is to see *paced* ventricular rhythms rather than the patient's own QRS complexes as pacing produces a synchronised contraction of the LV compared to the patient's native, dyssynchronous contraction. The aim is for >90% of ventricular beats to be paced to achieve the desired benefit from CRT. Amongst device/lead-related factors is loss of capture by either the LV or RV lead, resulting in loss of resynchronisation. Recognition of this can be difficult because loss of capture by only one of the ventricular leads will still appear as capture from the remaining ventricular lead (see below). Atrial fibrillation is a particularly problematic event for CRT patients as they are generally more dependent on atrial kick and the faster rates reduce ventricular filling times. Additionally, because they conduct with their own LBBB rather than receiving biventricular pacing they lose the benefit of resynchronisation.

Optimisation of device programming

Optimum device programming can have a significant impact on the benefit conferred by CRT.[101] It is not practical for all patients to undergo regular echocardiography for programming optimisation and so alternative approaches to optimisation have been developed. The critical timing factors that should be optimised are the atrioventricular (AV) delay and the delay between stimulation of the left and right ventricles (V–V delay). Recent developments allow 'electronic optimisation' whereby CRT devices themselves can calculate optimum settings based on automated measurements of intracardiac conduction,[102,103] but these are not available on all devices. The impact of effective optimisation may be sufficient to convert non-responders to responders.

Recognising failure to capture in a CRT device

Recognising failure to capture in CRT is made difficult by the fact that both ventricles are paced. Failure of pacing to produce QRS complexes will only occur if there is failure to capture from *both* LV and RV leads.[103] The ECG, during failure to capture by just the LV lead, will still show capture from the RV lead, and vice versa. Instead of loss of the QRS, to identify loss of capture it is necessary to look more closely at QRS morphology and vectors to confirm capture or loss of capture from either the left or right ventricular lead.[103] A 12-lead ECG is helpful but, if not available, lead V1 (or MCL1) and lead I are the most helpful in confirming RV, LV or bi-ventricular (Bi-V) capture. Specific changes include:

- RV capture only (loss of LV capture): the QRS will be wide (>0.12 s) with left-axis deviation; lead V1 (or MCL1) will be a negative complex, most commonly as a QS complex. QRS in lead I will be upright, as an R wave or sometimes rSR[104] (see Figure 11.50).

- LV capture only (loss of RV capture): the QRS will be wide (>0.12 s) with right-axis deviation; lead V1 (or MCL1) will be an upright complex, either as an R wave, or less commonly as an rSR. QRS in lead I will be a negative complex, either as a QS or rS complex[104] (see Figure 11.50).

- Bi-ventricular capture: the ECG is less predictable depending upon the timing of the left and right ventricular stimuli. If LV stimulation occurs well ahead of RV, the ECG will look more like LV capture only whereas, if RV stimulation occurs well ahead of LV, the ECG will look more like RV capture only. Nevertheless, the expectation is that, when both leads are capturing, the QRS will become narrower (usually <0.12 s)[98,104] with the axis deviated most commonly to the right. Morphologies are usually somewhere between those seen with RV-only or LV-only pacing. A uniform ECG pattern cannot be described, but in a given patient there should be consistency between serial ECGs (see Figure 11.50).

Phrenic nerve stimulation in CRT patients

The phrenic nerve courses inferiorly behind the left ventricle and it is possible for left ventricular pacing to directly stimulate the phrenic nerve producing repetitive diaphragmatic contraction of varying intensities. These may be continuous and uncomfortable or painful.

FIGURE 11.50 The appearance of lead V1 during alternation of pacing sites with a CRT system. In the top strip there is Bi-V pacing with a narrow QRS, which is negative in V1. In the same strip, loss of LV capture results in RV-only pacing. The QRS widens to beyond 0.12 s and becomes more deeply negative in V1. In the second strip RV-only becomes Bi-V pacing after re-establishing LV capture. The QRS returns to its initial morphology as in strip 1. In the 3rd strip Bi-V pacing is present initially followed by loss of RV capture, resulting in LV-only pacing. Note that the QRS becomes upright in V1 and again widens to well beyond 0.12 s. In the lower strip LV-only pacing precedes the return to the previous Bi-V morphology as RV capture is restored.

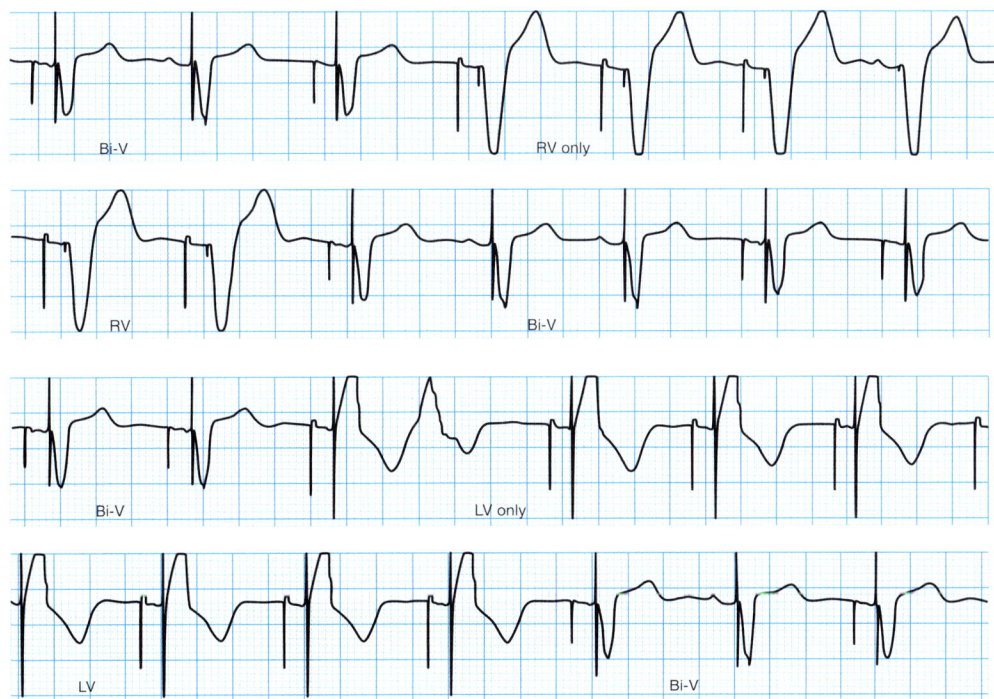

Programming may overcome the problem but, if unsuccessful, reoperation to reposition the left ventricular lead may be necessary, or resynchronisation therapy may need to be abandoned altogether. More recent developments with 'quadripolar' left ventricular leads, featuring four separate pacing electrodes, permit programming to use an alternative electrode rather than the one causing phrenic stimulation and have been successful. Quadripolar leads also provide the ability to program to an electrode (or vector) that has the lowest capture threshold, improving battery longevity.

Multipoint biventricular pacing

The new quadripolar leads mentioned above have also led to newer generation devices that now permit pacing from two separate electrodes on the quadripolar lead.[101] So-called multi-point pacing further improves left ventricular resynchronisation beyond single site pacing and has been shown to improve haemodynamics and patient response rates over conventional CRT configurations.[101,105,106]

Cardioversion

Electrical cardioversion can be applied as an alternative or adjunct to pharmacological therapy in the management of tachyarrhythmias. By far the most common cause of tachyarrhythmias is reentry, in which current can continue to circulate through the heart because of different rates of conduction and recovery in different areas of the heart (temporal dispersion). Conduction through reentry circuits can continue as long as the circulating stimulus encounters non-refractory tissue. The aim of cardioversion is to excite all myocardial cells at the same time with the result that all of the heart will also be refractory at the same time. If this is achieved, the circulating stimulus dies out for lack of non-refractory tissue to conduct through. If the applied shock does not depolarise the greater bulk of myocardium, then non-depolarised cells are still available for conduction and the arrhythmia may persist. External shocks of 100–200 joules (biphasic) are required for sufficient current density to reach the myocardium and depolarise the greater bulk of cells, thus extinguishing available pathways.[107] Drugs or biochemical correction may be necessary to prevent recurrence. Success rates from cardioversion range from 70–95%, depending on the rhythm.[107] Arrhythmias due to increased automaticity are less amenable to cardioversion, as there is a higher chance of early arrhythmia recurrence; and for arrhythmias occurring as a complication of digitalis toxicity, cardioversion (but not defibrillation) is contraindicated.[107]

Early defibrillation increases survival from ventricular fibrillation. The success of public-access defibrillator schemes has warranted their increased availability.[108] Automatic external defibrillators (AEDs) in the home or community simplify the task of applying defibrillation by non-healthcare responders and increase access to definitive electrical management for patients suffering ventricular arrhythmias. For patients who have survived previous arrhythmic cardiac arrest, an implantable cardioverter defibrillator may be necessary. Emergency defibrillation, electrical principles and equipment management are discussed more completely in Chapter 24.

Elective cardioversion

Elective direct current reversion (DCR, or cardioversion) applied under short-acting sedation or anaesthesia is undertaken for non-cardiac arrest arrhythmias.[108] These include atrial fibrillation, tachycardia or flutter, conscious ventricular tachycardia, AV nodal reentry tachycardia and conscious tachyarrhythmias complicating Wolff-Parkinson-White syndrome. The time available for preparation is variable and depends on the haemodynamic impact of the arrhythmia. Patients admitted for reversion of atrial fibrillation or flutter may be stable throughout their hospitalisation, whereas patients with conscious VT may initially demonstrate stability, only to decompensate later without warning.

Unlike emergency defibrillation, cardioversion shocks are synchronised to the cardiac cycle so that they are delivered into the QRS complex. Unsynchronised shocks, if delivered into the T wave, can cause immediate degeneration into ventricular fibrillation. When synchronisation is selected ('ON') on the defibrillator control panel, a marker is inscribed on each detected QRS complex on the monitor screen to confirm successful synchronisation.

When time permits the patient should be thoroughly investigated, including physical examination, neurological assessment, palpation of peripheral pulses, electrocardiograph, biochemistry and serum drug levels where necessary. Fasting should be ensured.[108,109] If atrial fibrillation is present transthoracic echocardiography is undertaken to rule out atrial thrombus, as restoration of atrial contraction may cause pulmonary or systemic arterial embolisation. The patient should be fully informed of the rationale for and nature of the procedure and have all necessary preparatory tasks explained to them.

The cardioversion team should include a minimum of one medical officer, skilled in emergency rhythm management and airway management including intubation, and two critical care nurses, who usually prepare the patient and equipment, assist in sedation, perform the cardioversion, document events and manage aftercare. Usually, there is a cardiologist and anaesthetist present for the separate roles. All team members should confirm readiness and confirm synchronisation selection and correct defibrillator energy settings (in joules). The patient is sedated (e.g. midazolam) or anaesthetised (e.g. propofol), preoxygenated on 100% oxygen delivered by bag and mask and cardioverted under ECG and oximetry monitoring. Electrical safety, and ensuring that all personnel are clear of the bed, is the primary responsibility of the nurse delivering cardioversion, whether via paddles or hands-free electrodes.

After the procedure the patient should be closely monitored for return to wakefulness, airway protection capability, effective respiration and gas exchange, rhythm stability, blood pressure and for any changes in neurological status or peripheral pulses. Pain and inflammation at cardioversion discharge sites may be lessened by application of topical ibuprofen 5% cream 2 hours before elective DCR, where this is feasible.[110] Energy requirements for reversion of atrial tachycardia or flutter may be as little as 50 J.[110,111] The 2010 recommendations of the European Resuscitation Council are for initial shocks at 70–120 J (biphasic) for atrial flutter, and 120–150 J for cardioversion of atrial fibrillation and ventricular tachycardia.[58] If initial shocks are unsuccessful, repeat attempts at higher energy settings (up to 360 J) may be undertaken. Prior to discharge, patients and their families should be informed of the potential for post-procedural chest wall discomfort and topical and oral analgesic advice provided.

Implantable cardioverter defibrillators

Implantable cardioverter defibrillators (ICDs) may be implanted for survivors of sudden cardiac death (SCD) or haemodynamically significant, potentially lethal, ventricular arrhythmias.[112] They have been repeatedly demonstrated in large clinical trials to provide significantly improved survival compared with pharmacological treatment.[113–115] This 'secondary prevention' application of ICDs dominated the early indications for devices, with trial meta-analysis demonstrating a mean 27% mortality reduction compared to antiarrhythmics.[55] However, more recently indications have expanded to 'primary prevention' in patients without prior cardiac arrest, as it has become clear that heart failure patients with ejection fractions <30% (including both ischaemic and non-ischaemic cardiomyopathies) have a high risk of sudden cardiac death due to ventricular arrhythmias, including patients with and without documented non-sustained VT.[116,117] In these contexts patients may receive pure ICDs, or ICDs coupled with cardiac resynchronisation therapy capabilities to also combat their heart failure (CRT-D devices).

The modern ICD features both antibradycardia and antitachycardia capabilities. As antibradycardia devices they possess all the characteristics of standard pacemakers, increasingly in the DDD mode. However, if there is no history of bradycardia, they may be programmed at low base pacing rates (e.g. 40/min). If there is significant heart failure the antibradycardia arm may be provided as biventricular pacing (to achieve cardiac resynchronisation). Antitachycardia features are those therapies provided to treat ventricular tachyarrhythmias and include antitachycardia pacing (ATP), also termed overdrive pacing, as well as cardioversion (for VT) and defibrillation (for very fast VT or VF). Refer to Figure 11.51 for examples of these therapeutic modes.

Devices are inserted in a similar fashion to the pacemaker (see the above section *Permanent pacing*). However, ICDs are most commonly positioned in the left subclavian/pectoral location, leaving the right side of the chest available for conventional placement of external defibrillator paddles should they ever become necessary. Atrial and ventricular leads are placed transvenously via the left subclavian vein. Atrial leads are normal atrial pacing leads, but the ventricular ICD leads are slightly larger than pacing leads and carry the normal ventricular pacing circuitry, as well as coils encircling the lead that emit the high energy shock discharges. Single coil systems have one coil positioned on the lead at the level of the right ventricular cavity, and shocks travel from this coil to the metal casing of the ICD. Dual coil leads feature this same right ventricular coil as well as a second coil in the superior vena cava. In these systems, shocks can be configured to travel from the RV coil to the superior vena cava coil, from the RV coil to the ICD, or from the RV coil to both the superior vena cava coil and the ICD. Configurations can impact significantly on the defibrillation threshold, and changes to the shock vector may be undertaken for patients with high defibrillation thresholds.

All modern ICDs provide biphasic shock waveforms only. Arrhythmia detection and classification usually require only a few seconds, and charging to maximum joules in a new device takes up to 10 seconds. As the battery declines charge time may increase to 15–20 seconds or longer. Maximum energy delivery capabilities vary between manufacturers but are all in the range of 30–40 J. Typically, shocks for ventricular fibrillation are provided at the maximum available capability of the device, but for ventricular tachycardia, lower 'cardioversion' shocks may

FIGURE 11.51 Successful antitachycardia pacing delivered by an implantable cardioverter defibrillator. Three simultaneous strips show the presence of sustained ventricular tachycardia (VT). After the first eight beats, pacing is applied at a rate slightly faster than the tachycardia. Entrainment, or capture, by the pacemaker is best seen in lead II, where the QRS morphology clearly changes. After 11 paced beats, ATP is ceased, revealing interruption of the VT.

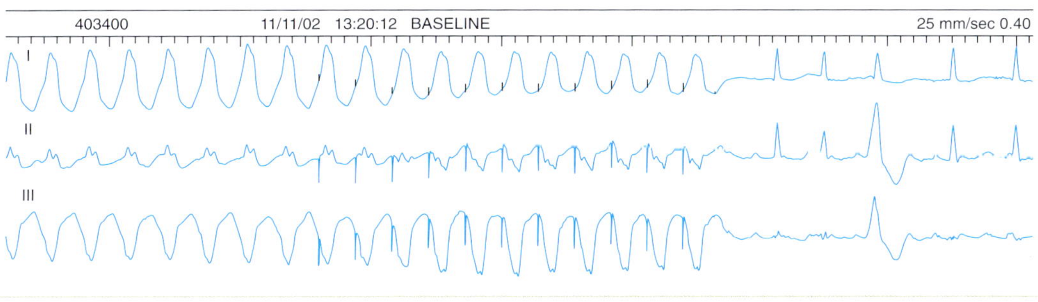

be attempted first (e.g. 15–25 joules). If initial shocks are unsuccessful, devices are usually programmed to increase to maximum joules for subsequent shocks.[112]

Defibrillation thresholds may be measured at the time of implantation of the ICD. It is desirable that a 10-J safety margin exists, i.e. for a device that can deliver 30 J, it is preferred that successful defibrillation can be demonstrated at 20 J or less so that there can be confidence that the device will revert clinical arrhythmias, and to cover any defibrillation threshold increases in the future.[118] Intraoperative defibrillation testing, in which ventricular fibrillation is induced and then defibrillated, has become less common with time, partly because of the risks associated with inducing ventricular fibrillation, and partly because of evidence that spontaneous ventricular fibrillation has different characteristics to induced fibrillation.[119] However, VF induction and defibrillation testing remains the only way to demonstrate whether a device has successfully interrupted VF. If testing is to be performed the patient is prepared for external defibrillation with all safety precautions and subsequent care as outlined above in the section on cardioversion.

ICDs are usually programmed to deliver up to six 'therapies' during a tachyarrhythmia episode. For VF, this usually means six attempts at defibrillation at maximum joules after which further antitachycardia therapies are aborted. No more shocks will be delivered. Antibradycardia pacing operation will continue. If the tachyarrhythmia is interrupted at any point and then recurs, the six-therapy counter will recommence. For ventricular tachycardia, attempts may first be made to overdrive pace. So-called antitachycardia pacing (ATP) aims to interrupt VT by pacing the ventricles slightly faster than the VT rate so as to interrupt reentry, the major cause of VT (see Figure 11.50 for example of reversion). A number of attempts at ATP may be programmed, often with slightly faster rates at each successive attempt. This is especially true if the patient is known to tolerate their VT reasonably well. Persistence of VT after ATP attempts will see the device first attempt low energy cardioversion (15–25 J) and then progress to 30–40 J if unsuccessful. The same limit of six therapies usually applies for an episode.

Tachyarrhythmia detection and classification

ICDs are configured to classify and treat arrhythmias first on the basis of rate. Defibrillation algorithms using high-energy settings (30–40 J) are followed when the rate is very fast (e.g. >200/min), as syncope is likely even if the rhythm is not ventricular fibrillation (e.g. very fast VT). At slower rates, other antitachycardia options may first be attempted as described above. Additionally, at slower rates of tachycardia, attempts are made to discriminate between ventricular and supraventricular (including sinus) tachycardias (SVTs) using a variety of criteria. SVT discrimination by a device uses similar criteria to those by which a clinician would differentiate between VT and SVT and includes regularity or irregularity of the rhythm,

sudden or gradual onset, similar or different morphology to the previous sinus rhythm and atrioventricular relationships. If these discriminators indicate that a tachyarrhythmia is supraventricular, therapy can be withheld, avoiding inappropriate therapy. The major device capabilities and programming options of an ICD are shown in Figure 11.52.

Patients receiving ICDs require particular education and support, as the experience of shocks can be painful and disturbing. Anticipation of shocks can cause anxiety and/or depression,[120] especially in patients who have experienced shocks while conscious. Inappropriate therapy delivery remains a significant problem, and as many as 25% of ICD therapies have been reported as inappropriate, delivered due either to supraventricular arrhythmias or oversensing of electromagnetic interference.[120,121] Refinement of rhythm discrimination behaviours has seen the incidence of inappropriate shocks reduced in recent years. The avoidance of strong electrical fields (welding, magnetic resonance imaging, generators) should be stressed, as well as direct contact with devices such as transcutaneous electrical nerve stimulation (TENS) machines or electrocautery devices.[73] If surgery requiring diathermy becomes necessary, antitachycardia therapies are usually programmed to 'OFF' to avoid inappropriate detection and treatment.

Patients should be encouraged to rest after any therapy delivery and, where multiple discharges occur, they should report to a healthcare facility for assessment.[122] Most doctors advise contact with their rooms if any shocks are received by the patient. If repeated inappropriate therapy continues (shocks delivered despite the patient not being in VT or VF), further shocks may be suspended by the placement of a ring magnet over the device.[123] This suspends the antitachycardia features of the device while the magnet is in place – no therapy will be delivered by the device. Cardiac monitoring is imperative while a magnet is in place to detect any development of genuine ventricular arrhythmias as these would not be treated by the device. Removal of the magnet will immediately reactivate antitachycardia therapies. Back-up (antibradycardia) pacing functions remain active and unaffected during magnet application.

In the event of unsuccessful reversion of a ventricular arrhythmia by ICD therapy, standard advanced life support protocols should be applied. External defibrillation can be undertaken with paddles in normal apicobasal or anteroposterior positions, taking care to avoid positioning paddles over the ICD.[122] External chest compressions can safely be undertaken by rescuers, including during device therapy.[124]

Practice tip

If cardiac arrest occurs in a patient with an ICD in place, all standard therapies should be undertaken, including CPR, drug administration, and immediate preparation for external defibrillation. If device shocks are unsuccessful, proceed to external defibrillation.

FIGURE 11.52 Implantable cardioverter defibrillator (ICD) programmed parameter summary report from St Jude Medical ICD Ellipse™ dual chamber ICD model 2277-36 (St Jude Medical, Sylmar CA). Similar to the report shown earlier for a pacemaker, the report includes battery status and test results for lead impedances, sensing and capture thresholds for the atrial and ventricular lead. The battery status section also displays the most recent time (in seconds) taken for the device to charge to a maximum joule shock and the date. In the parameters section are the programmed settings for pacing and defibrillation behaviours. The tachyarrhythmia treatments are shown at the right of the parameters section and show the device behaviour for tachycardias occurring at different rates. In the so-called 'VF zone', the ICD will respond to any arrhythmia faster than 214 beats per minute (whether it is VF or fast VT). As rhythms at this rate are likely to be syncopal ICDs are usually programmed to proceed directly to delivering shocks rather than spending time delivering antitachycardia pacing (ATP) unless, as here, a single attempt at ATP is selected to be delivered while the device is charging (and therefore not delaying the time to first shock delivery). Shocks in the VF zone are more commonly at maximum joules although 1st shocks may be of lesser strength with subsequent escalation. In the VT-2 zone, a different strategy has been programmed for VT between 181 and 214/min. Three attempts at delivering ATP have been programmed and, if unsuccessful, the ICD will progress to increasing energy levels (20, 30, 36 joules) if reversion is not achieved. An additional strategy has been included for slower forms of VT (150–181/min) (VT-1 zone). As VT at these rates is more likely to be tolerated greater use of ATP is often programmed so as to avoid shocks if possible. Two different ATP regimes have been set, with the second set of 6 pacing attempts more aggressive than the first set of 6. If ATP is unsuccessful, the device progresses to escalating shocks. Details of how the device is set to discriminate between VT and SVT, as well as the set-up of the pacing strategies, are given in separate sections of these reports. Also shown on the summary are any VT/VF episodes since the last device check. In this case there had been two episodes of VT and two of VF. Recordings of these arrhythmias and treatments are recorded elsewhere in the report.

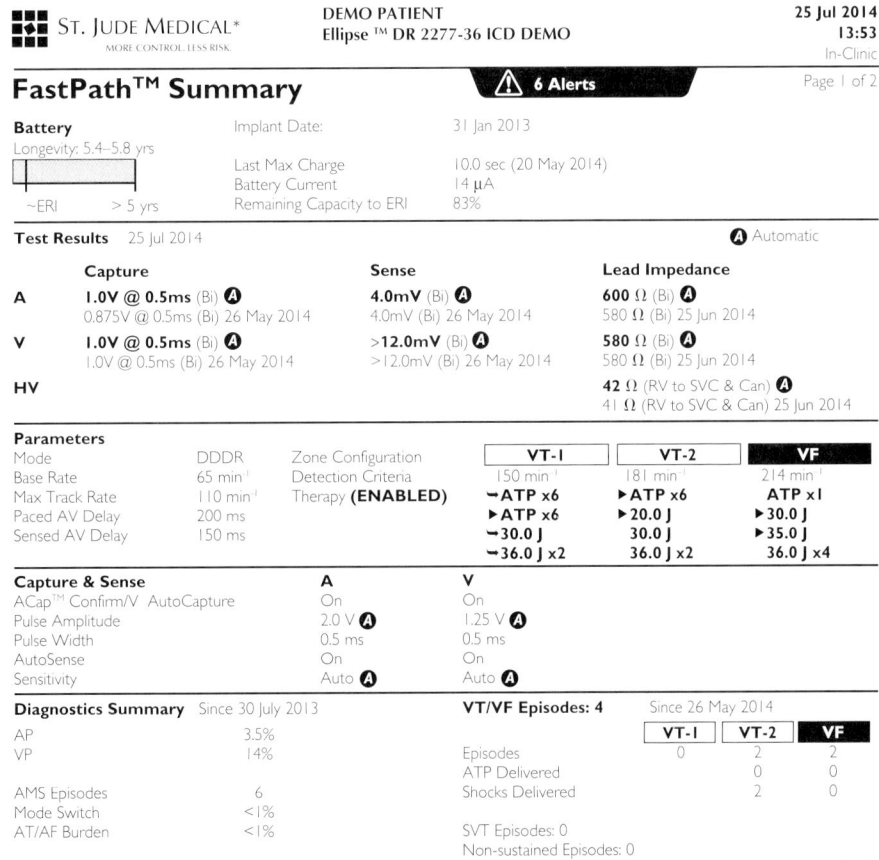

End-of-life care in the patient with an ICD

ICDs often create uncertainty amongst healthcare workers as to how death may occur. In the palliative patient, where active resuscitation for cardiac death is not to be pursued, the decision to disable antitachycardia therapies is often taken. This can be achieved by reprogramming the ICD, and there is often sufficient time to incorporate this step into palliative planning. Alternatively, when active treatment is being withdrawn as a patient progresses more rapidly towards an unexpected (acute) death, there may be a need to disable therapy before the availability of personnel to reprogram the device. In this context, securing a ring magnet over the ICD (tape it in place) will disable tachycardia therapies so that, if the terminal rhythm is VT or VF, therapies will not be delivered.

Other than by disabling therapy, cardiac death may occur by normal mechanisms. However, cardiac depressive factors will not cause bradycardia or asystole because of the pacemaker function. What would otherwise be a brady-arrhythmic death will instead become eventual failure to capture by the pacemaker. Similarly, if the cardiac impact of acute or terminal illness produces tachyarrhythmias, these same influences will increase the defibrillation threshold and antitachycardia therapies will become unsuccessful. Devices offer no protection against pulseless electrical activity.

Ablation

Ablation therapies are aimed at destroying tissues that 1) generate or sustain haemodynamically significant or potentially lethal arrhythmias (arrhythmic foci or reentry pathways) or 2) permit uncontrollable atrial arrhythmias to conduct at rapid rates to the ventricles (the accessory pathways of the Wolff-Parkinson-White syndrome, or at times the AV node itself).[125] Tissue destruction is achieved by the application of radiofrequency energy or cold (cryoablation) to very localised areas of the endocardium, which results in tissue damage and eventual tissue death.[125] Unlike preventive or episode-terminating pharmacological or electrical arrhythmia therapies, successful ablation is curative and can therefore spare patients a lifetime of careful medication compliance, self-monitoring for complications and living under the uncertainty of arrhythmic threat and/or the delivery of therapy from an implantable cardioverter defibrillator.

The use of percutaneous catheter ablation therapies has expanded rapidly as technology and familiarity have developed, and they have been used to treat atrial, ventricular and AV nodal reentry tachyarrhythmias, as well as the abnormal atrioventricular connections of Wolff-Parkinson-White syndrome. For incessant atrial fibrillation, it is sometimes necessary to ablate the AV node to control the ventricular rate. Since this causes complete heart block, a pacemaker must first be implanted. Identification of the pulmonary veins as the culprit arrhythmic foci for many patients with atrial fibrillation has seen the development of ablation techniques to prevent conduction from the pulmonary veins to the atria (pulmonary vein isolation).

For arrhythmia ablation, electrophysiological studies are undertaken to closely map the location of abnormal foci, reentry circuits or accessory pathways, and radiofrequency catheters are then guided to these sites to deliver therapy. Studies are well tolerated as long as patients can remain supine for the sometimes extended periods. The application of radiofrequency and the consequent tissue injury is painless in most cases.[124,125]

Success rates for ablation therapies have been reported as 82–92% for accessory pathway ablation (depending on pathway location), 90–96% for AV nodal reentry tachycardia and 75% for atrial tachycardia and flutter.[126] Complication rates, mostly AV block, have been reported as 2.1–4.4%, with procedure-related mortality below 0.2%.[125,126] When applied to patients with idiopathic ventricular tachycardia, procedural success has been reported as 85–100%.[127] Complications, including death from ventricular wall perforation,[126] have occurred, but major complication rates of less than 1% are generally seen.[127]

Summary

Alteration to the electrophysiological function of the heart is very common in patients admitted to critical care settings. Arrhythmia detection is largely the responsibility of the critical care nurse, who must maintain accurate monitoring, constantly observe for the development of arrhythmias, assess their clinical impact and assist in identifying causative factors. The critical care nurse must also deliver the care and management of arrhythmias, including pharmacological and electrical therapies, being aware of complications and management of complications of these treatments.

Case study

In 1997 Mr Thomas suffered an anterolateral AMI at the age of 37. He subsequently had a prolonged cardiac arrest and was resuscitated from ventricular fibrillation. Prior to this Mr Thomas was a very active windsurfer and competitive solo yachtsman, as well as running his own business as a yacht restorer, and he maintained all these activities after his AMI.

A single chamber implantable cardioverter defibrillator (ICD) was implanted in 1997, with a dual coil ICD lead placed at the apex of the right ventricle. He has subsequently undergone three ICD replacements with each device lasting approximately 4 years before battery depletion. It would normally be anticipated that ICD batteries provide 6 or more years of service; however, frequent shocks diminish battery longevity. In addition to the ICD, Mr Thomas was discharged on oral sotalol 40 mg bd for antiarrhythmic cover.

Between 1997 and 2008 Mr Thomas received repeated shocks for VT at rates of 185 per minute (further details not available due to a change in doctor). In 2008 and 2009 Mr Thomas experienced 10–50 episodes of VT per month, at rates of 185–200/min. While antitachycardia pacing (ATP) reverted many episodes without major symptoms, he regularly received shocks. Sotalol was increased incrementally to 80 mg tds and then 160 mg, although at these doses it began to cause chronic fatigue. In 1999 Mr Thomas suffered a pulmonary embolism and remains on life-long warfarin.

In June of 2009 a new, slower form of sustained VT emerged (175/min) that was recurrent and produced dizziness (systolic blood pressure: 70 mmHg). Mr Thomas' ICD was previously programmed to treat VT above 180/min; therefore this VT did not qualify for ICD treatment – reprogramming of the ICD to treat VT above 160/min was consequently undertaken. A similar scenario, although with VT of 125/min, occurred 3 months later and the ICD was again reprogrammed, this time to treat VT above 120/min.

Mr Thomas continued to receive multiple shocks, often while undertaking his normal activities. One shock was delivered while completing an acrobatic loop on his wind surfer, another while 10 meters under water after having been dumped by a wave while surfing and a third while competing in a solo yacht race. On each occasion he paddled or sailed slowly back to shore and attended ED. Throughout this period Mr Thomas was also experiencing intolerable fatigue from his sotalol treatment. Agreement was reached to undergo VT ablation.

In December 2009 electrophysiological (EP) study revealed Mr Thomas had three separate VT patterns with rates of 150, 180 and 250/min (ventricular flutter), all emerging from different borders of his anteroapical AMI scar. Pace-mapping identified three target sites and radiofrequency ablation was applied to these. After his ablation Mr Thomas' sotalol dose was reduced to 80 mg bd.

Mr Thomas had a review in February 2010 when it was identified that his VT had not decreased significantly with 61 episodes in 2 months that were all terminatd by ATP.

As Mr Thomas' ICD was set to treat VT >120/min, the risk of inappropriate shocks was high and this became reality in October 2010 when Mr Thomas presented to ED after sinus tachycardia and atrial fibrillation accounted for 50 episodes diagnosed as VT with multiple inappropriate shocks. The ICD was reprogrammed with tighter parameters for discriminating between SVT and VT and this proved effective in preventing further inappropriate shocks. Sotalol was also increased back to 160 mg bd.

Six months later Mr Thomas had a routine review that revealed 17 episodes of VT and 5 shocks throughout that period. The argument for amiodarone had become compelling, though not without reservation as warfarin had been commenced some years earlier. Amiodarone inhibits enzymes that degrade warfarin and so International Normalised Ratio (INR) volatility accompanies amiodarone addition. The long half-life of amiodarone and variable rise to peak plasma levels make the management of warfarin more complex. In addition, photosensitivity had weighed against amiodarone use previously given Mr Thomas' outdoor work and leisure activities. Although a beta-blocker was still required because of the original AMI, sotalol was replaced by metoprolol to avoid lengthening the QT interval due to the combined effects of amiodarone and sotalol. The combination of metoprolol and digoxin was used to limit further atrial arrhythmias and for rate control.

After amiodarone (200 mg bd) was commenced there was only one episode of VT in the next 3 years. Digoxin levels were intermittently high (remember amiodarone and digoxin compete for excretion) and digoxin was ultimately withdrawn. Annual thyroid function testing and chest X-ray revealed no complications of amiodarone therapy. After 12 arrhythmia-free months amiodarone was reduced to 200 mg mane, 100 mg nocte.

In 2014 Mr Thomas attended ED after receiving a vibratory notification from his ICD. The ICD was vibrating in his chest as an instruction to seek attention. Device interrogation revealed an out-of-range automatic daily impedance measurement. His ICD lead was now 17 years old and the alert suggested one of the conductors to the shock coils was wearing out. With reprogramming to shock via a different vector the device was able to continue operating normally.

Living with an ICD and the associated threat of unexpected shocks, as well as the side effects of medications and arrhythmias, can be challenging. Both anxiety and depression are experienced by some ICD recipients. Mr Thomas has proven remarkably resilient and demonstrates that it is possible to live life relatively normally. As critical care nurses it is important to recognise the pharmacological and technical challenges in caring for patients with lifelong arrhythmic conditions and ongoing vigilance is required.

CASE STUDY QUESTIONS

1   Sotalol rather than amiodarone was chosen as the first antiarrhythmic agent used for Mr Thomas. What reasons might have prompted this decision?

2   Mr Thomas' ICD was eventually programmed to treat ventricular tachycardia at a rate of 120/min when slower VTs (125/min) developed. What particular risk does this programming change now bring into play?

RESEARCH VIGNETTE

Graham K, Cvach M. Monitor alarm fatigue: standardising the use of physiological monitors and decreasing nuisance alarms. Am J Crit Care 2010;19:28–34

Abstract

Background and purpose: Reliance on physiological monitors to continuously 'watch' patients and to alert the nurse when a serious rhythm problem occurs is standard practice on monitored units. Alarms are intended to alert clinicians to deviations from a predetermined 'normal' status. However, alarm fatigue may occur when the sheer number of monitor alarms overwhelms clinicians, possibly leading to alarms being disabled, silenced, or ignored.

Excessive numbers of monitor alarms and fear that nurses have become desensitized to these alarms was the impetus for a unit-based quality improvement project.

Methods: Small tests of change to improve alarm management were conducted on a medical progressive care unit. The types and frequency of monitor alarms in the unit were assessed. Nurses were trained to individualize patients' alarm parameter limits and levels. Monitor software was modified to promote audibility of critical alarms.

Results: Critical monitor alarms were reduced 43% from baseline data. The reduction of alarms could be attributed to adjustment of monitor alarm defaults, careful assessment and customization of monitor alarm parameter limits and levels, and implementation of an interdisciplinary monitor policy.

Discussion: Although alarms are important and sometimes life-saving, they can compromise patients' safety if ignored. This unit-based quality improvement initiative was beneficial as a starting point for revamping alarm management throughout the institution.

Critique

This study evaluated the pre- and post-intervention effects of a series of alarm management quality improvement measures in a 16-bed mixed medical progressive care unit in Baltimore, USA over a 12-month period. The study's pre-evaluation process included measurement of the quantity and type of alarms occurring in the unit over a consecutive 18-day period, along with a survey that explored the existing alarm setting practices of 30 of the unit's nursing staff. The investigation team then implemented a series of interventions designed to improve staff alarm setting practices including education on troubleshooting practices, the need to individualise patient alarm assignment and revision of the unit's default 'patient' and monitor 'crisis level' settings. These included reduction in lower heart rate level and elevation of upper rate limit, premature ventricular contraction upper limit rise and re-setting of allocated default alarm warning levels within the unit's monitoring system (for example, the re-assignment of heart rate high and low alarms to a 'message' level alert while changing bradycardia and tachycardia from 'advisory' to 'warning' level).

Postintervention evaluation revealed a 43% overall reduction in unit alarm frequency (with heart rate low and high alerts being decreased the most) and improved bedside alarm evaluation and adjustment compliance by staff. Environmental noise levels were also perceived by staff to be lower following the initiatives.

As the authors state, modern physiological monitors are 'set for high sensitivity at the expense of specificity' and the results of this quality improvement initiative demonstrate the potential reduction in 'false positive' alarm events that can be achieved through a program that specifically reviews staff and alarm knowledge and default setting practices.

The issue of excessive 'inappropriate' or 'nuisance' bedside alarms in acute healthcare settings has become a topic of raised emphasis over recent years. Of particular concern is the development of alarm 'fatigue' by staff, with resulting auditory alert desensitisation and reactive alarm silencing and even disablement enhancing the risk of missed critical physiological events, including cardiac arrhythmias. In addition, excessive nuisance alarms disrupt patient care and rest and add significantly to the ambient noise of high acuity care settings. As some previous studies have shown that fewer than 1% of clinical alarms actually result in a change to patient management, it's therefore necessary to explore strategies that reduce the incidence of inappropriate clinical alarm events in order to optimise the clinical relevance and safety of patient bedside monitoring.

The authors have not stated whether the actual or missed 'true positive' critical alarm incidence was monitored during the evaluation periods and this would be vital to ensuring the clinical safety of a clinical monitoring change initiative. The study was also confined to a single clinical setting and staff training and experience levels were not detailed, therefore making it difficult to ascertain whether low technical knowledge or limited clinical exposure significantly influenced the baseline findings.

However, the study's outcomes highlight the significant 'inappropriate' alarm reductions that can be achieved through a focused alarm education and system configuration review and, as such, provide renewed awareness of the important need for individual clinicians and critical care departments to give more detailed attention to the management of bedside and system based alarm settings.

Learning activities

1   Utilise the flowchart in Figure 11.28 to assist in refining your final interpretation of a selection of the ECG rhythm strips presented in pages 314–329 of this chapter.

2   Draw a series of simple diagrams of the heart's conducting system, then sketch and label the differing sequences of sinoatrial, AV junctional and ventricular conduction events that occur with second degree AV block types I and II and third degree AV block. Compare and contrast the relative conduction events occurring with each AV block type and their relationship to the surface ECG rhythm patterns that are typically observed in each.

3   When next at the bedside, take the time to review the number of higher level 'warning' and 'crisis' level alarms that have been stored over the previous 24 hours of monitoring on your allocated patient. Determine the incidence and types of 'false positive' ECG alarm events that have occurred and, with consideration of the patient's current clinical state, readjust the monitor settings to more individually appropriate (yet clinically safe) settings. Which particular ECG monitoring settings would most likely require adjusting?

4   You are caring for a 68-year-old patient with chronic atrial fibrillation who develops intermittent non-sustained runs of ventricular tachycardia. The patient has been admitted to critical care for the management of acute renal failure and has a history of coronary artery disease and chronic obstructive pulmonary disease. With reference to antiarrhythmic classifications (Table 11.5) and with further reading, consider the relative benefits and risks of administering flecainide, sotolol or amiodarone for the treatment of this man's ventricular tachycardia.

Online resources

Arrhythmia and cardiac device presentations, manuals, and learning resources, www.hrsonline.org

ECG quizzes and teaching materials: http://library.med.utah.edu/kw/ecg/, http://ekgreview.com/, http://biotel.ws/quizzes/ekgs/ekgs.htm, www.ecglibrary.com/ecghome.html, http://en.ecgpedia.org, www.learntheheart.com/ecg-review/ecg-quiz

ECRI Institute Alarm Safety Resource site, www.ecri.org/forms/pages/Alarm_Safety_Resource.aspx

European Heart Rhythm Association (EHRA), www.escardio.org/communities/EHRA/Pages/welcome.aspx

European Resuscitation Council, www.erc.edu/index.php/mainpage/en/ECG

Pacing resources, www.sjmprofessional.com, www.medtronic.com/for-healthcare-professionals/education-training

Further reading

Brignole M, Auricchio A, Baron-Esquivias G, Bordachar P, Boriani G, Breithardt OA et al. 2013 ESC Guidelines on cardiac pacing and cardiac resynchronization therapy: the Task Force on cardiac pacing and resynchronization therapy of the European Society of Cardiology (ESC). Developed in collaboration with the European HeartRhythm Association (EHRA). Eur Heart J 2013; 34(29):2281–329. doi:10.1093/eurheartj/eht150. Epub 2013 Jun 24. PubMed PMID: 23801822.

Drew B, Ackerman M, Funk M, Gibler B, Kligfield P, Menon V et al. Prevention of torsades de pointes in hospital settings: a scientific statement from The American Heart Association and The American College of Cardiology Foundation. J Am Coll Cardiol 2010;55(9):934–47.

Epstein A, DiMarco J, Ellenbogen K, Estes NA 3rd, Freedman R, Gettes LS et al. American College of Cardiology Foundation; American Heart Association Task Force on Practice Guidelines; Heart Rhythm Society. 2012 ACCF/AHA/HRS focused update incorporated into the ACCF/AHA/HRS 2008 guidelines for device-based therapy of cardiac rhythm abnormalities: a report of the American College of Cardiology Foundation/American Heart Association Task Force on Practice Guidelines and the Heart Rhythm Society. J Am Coll Cardiol 2013;22:61(3):e6–75. doi: 10.1016/j.jacc.2012.11.007.

References

1 Go AS, Hylek EM, Phillips KA, Chang Y, Henault LE, Selby JV et al. Prevalence of diagnosed atrial fibrillation in adults. JAMA 2001;285(18):2370–5.

2 Medi C, Hankey GJ, Freedman SB. Atrial fibrillation. Med J Aust 2007;186(4):197-203.

3 Arrigo M, Bettex D, Rudiger A. Management of atrial fibrillation in critically ill patients. Crit Care Res Pract [Internet]. 2014;2014:840615, 10 pages. doi: 10.1155/2014/840615.

4 Walkley AJ, Wiener JM, Ghorbrial LH, Curtis LH, Benjamin EJ. Incident stroke and mortality associated with new-onset atrial fibrillation in patients with severe sepsis. JAMA 2011;306(20):2248-55.

5 Auer J, Weber R, Berent R. Risk factors of postoperative atrial fibrillation after cardiac surgery. J Cardiac Surg 2005;20(5):425-31.

6 Annane D, Sebille V, Duboc D, Le Heuzey JY, Sadoul N, Bouvier E et al. Incidence and prognosis of sustained arrhythmias in critically ill patients. Am J Resp Crit Care Med 2008;178(1):20-5.

7 Novak B, Filer L, Hatchett R. The applied anatomy and physiology of the cardiovascular system. In: Hatchett R, Thompson D, eds. Cardiac nursing: A comprehensive guide. Philadelphia: Churchill Livingstone Elsevier; 2002.

8 Hall JE. Guyton and Hall textbook of medical physiology. 12th ed. Philadelphia: WB Saunders; 2010.

9 Issa Z, Miller JM, Zipes DP. Clinical arrhythmology and electrophysiology. 2nd ed. Philadelphia: WB Saunders; 2012.

10 Waldo AL, Wit AL. Mechanisms of cardiac arrhythmias and conduction disturbances. In: Alexander RW, Schlant RC, Fuster V. eds. Hurst's the heart arteries and veins. 9th ed. New York: McGraw-Hill; 1998.

11 Conover MB. Understanding electrocardiography. 8th ed. St Louis: Mosby; 2002.

12 Mines GR. On dynamic equilibrium in the heart. J Physiol 1913;46:349.

13 Olshansky B, Sullivan RM. Inappropriate sinus tachycardia. J Am Coll Cardiol 2013;61(8):793-801.

14 Scheinman M, Vedantham V. Ivabradine. A ray of hope for inappropriate sinus tachycardia. J Am Coll Cardiol 2012;60(15):1330-2.

15 Dunn MI, Lipman BS. Lipmann-Massie clinical electrocardiography. 8th ed. Chicago: Year Book Medical; 1989.

16 Josephson ME. Clinical cardiac electrophysiology. 4th ed. Philadelphia: Lippincott, Williams & Wilkins; 2008.

17 Wagner GS, Strauss DG. Marriott's practical electrocardiography. 12th ed. Baltimore: Lippincott, Williams & Wilkins; 2013.

18 Brubaker PH, Kitzman DW. Chronotropic incompetence: causes, consequences and management. Circulation 2011;123:1010-20.

19 Komajda M. Heart rate and heart failure. In: Fox K, editor. Slow the heart, beat the disease. London: Wiley-Blackwell; 2011.

20 Bohm M, Swedberg K, Komajda M, Borer JS, Ford I, Dubost-Brama A et al. Heart rate as a risk factor in chronic heart failure (SHIFT): the association between heart rate and outcomes in a randomized placebo-controlled trial. Lancet 2010;376(9744):886-894.

21 Chen-Scarabelli C. Supraventricular arrhythmias: an electrophysiology primer. Prog Cardiovasc Nurs 2005;20(1):24–31.

22 McCord J, Borzak S. Multifocal atrial tachycardia. Chest 1998;113(1):203–9.

23 Heeringa J, van der Kuip D, Hofman A, Kors JA, van Herpen, Stricker BH et al. Prevalence, incidence and lifetime risk of atrial fibrillation: the Rotterdam study. Euro Heart J 2006;27(8):949–53.

24 Haissaguerre M, Jais P, Shah DC, Takahashi A, Hocini M, Quiniou G et al. Spontaneous initiation of atrial fibrillation by ectopic beats originating in the pulmonary veins. N Engl J Med 1998;339(10):659–66.

25 Maglana MP, Kam RM, Teo WS. The differential diagnosis of supraventricular tachycardia using clinical and electrocardiographic features. Ann Acad Med Singapore 2000;29(5):653–7.

26 Fuster V, Ryden LE, Cannom DS, Crijns HJ, Curtis AB, Ellenbogen KA et al. ACC/AHA/ESC Guidelines for the management of patients with atrial fibrillation. Circulation 2006;113(7):e257-354.

27 Naccarelli GV, Wolbrette DL, Khan M, Batta L, Hynes J, Samii S et al. Old and new antiarrhythmic drugs for converting and maintaining sinus rhythm in atrial fibrillation: comparative efficacy and results of trials. Am J Cardiol 2003;20(91,6A):15D–26D.

28 Shah D. Catheter ablation for atrial fibrillation: mechanism-based curative treatment. Exp Rev Cardiovasc Ther 2004;2(6):925–33.

29 Schuchert A. Contributions of permanent cardiac pacing in the treatment of atrial fibrillation. Europace 2004;5(Suppl1):S36–41.

30 Kaushik V, Leon AR, Forrester JS Jr, Trohman RG. Bradyarrhythmias, temporary and permanent pacing. Crit Care Med 2000;28(10Suppl):N121–8.

31 Brignole M, Auricchio A, Baron-Esquivias G, Bordachar P, Boriani G, Breithardt OA et al. Cardiac pacing and cardiac resynchronization therapy. ESC clinical practice guidelines. Eur Heart J 2013;34(29):2281-2329.

32 Da Costa D, Brady WJ, Edhouse J. ABC of clinical electrocardiography: bradycardias and atrioventricular conduction block. Br Med J 2002; 324:535-538.

33 Ilia R, Amit G, Cafri C, Gilutz H, Abu-Ful A, Weinstein JM et al. Reperfusion arrhythmias during coronary angioplasty for acute myocardial infarction predict ST-segment resolution. Coron Artery Dis 2003;14(6):439–41.

34 Bonnemeier H, Ortak J, Wiegand UK, Eberhardt F, Bode F, Schunkert H et al. Accelerated idioventricular rhythm in the post-thrombolytic era: incidence, prognostic implications, and modulating mechanisms after direct percutaneous coronary intervention. Ann Noninvas Electrocardiol 2005;10(2):179–87.

35 Deal N. Evaluation and management of bradydysrhythmias in the emergency department. Emerg Med Pract 2013;15(9):1-15.

36 Hales M. Keep up the pace: the prevention, identification and management of common temporary epicardial pacing pitfalls following cardiac surgery. World Crit Care Nurs 2005;4(1):11–19.

37 Brady WJ, Swart G, DeBehnke DJ, Ma OJ, Aufderheide TP. The efficacy of atropine in the treatment of hemodynamically unstable bradycardia and atrioventricular block: prehospital and emergency department considerations. Resuscitation 1999;41(1):47–55.

38 Brady WJ Jr, Harrigan RA. Evaluation and management of bradyarrhythmias in the emergency department. Emerg Med Clin North Am 1998;16(2):361–88.

39 Alzand BSN, Clijns HJG. Diagnostic criteria of broad QRS complex tachycardia: decades of evolution. Europace 2010;13(4):465-472.

40 Lown B, Calvert AF, Armington R, Ryan M. Monitoring for serious arrhythmias and high risk of sudden death. Circulation 1975;52(6Suppl): 189–98.

41 Francis J, Watanabe M, Schmidt G. Heart rate turbulence: a new predictor for risk of sudden cardiac death. Ann Noninvas Electrocardiol 2005;10(1):102–9.

42 Fries R, Steuer M, Schafers H, Böhm M. The R-on-T phenomenon in patients with implantable cardioverter defibrillators. Am J of Cardiol 2003;91(6):752–5.

43 Olgin JE, Zipes DP. Specific arrhythmias: diagnosis and treatment. In: Libby P, Bonow RO, Mann DL, Zipes DP, eds. Braunwald's heart disease: A textbook of cardiovascular medicine. 8th ed. Philadelphia: Saunders Elsevier; 2007: Chap 35.

44 Sweeney MO. Antitachycardia pacing for ventricular tachycardia using implantable cardioverter defibrillators. Pacing Clin Electrophysiol 2004;27(9):1292–305.

45 Finch NJ, Leman RB. Clinical trials update: sudden cardiac death prevention by implantable device therapy. Crit Care Nurs Clin North Am 2005;17(1): 33–8.

46 Epstein AE, DiMarco JP, Ellenbogen KA, Estes NA 3rd, Freedman RA, Gettes LS, et al. ACC/AHA/HRS 2008 guidelines for device-based therapy of cardiac rhythm abnormalities. J Am Coll Cardiol 2008;51(21):e1-62.

47 Goldenberg I, Moss AJ. Long QT syndrome. J Am Coll Cardiol 2008;51(24):2291–300.

48 Wellens HJ, Conover MB. The ECG in emergency decision making. 2nd ed. St Louis: Saunders Elsevier; 2006.

49 Jayasinghe R, Kovoor P. Drugs and the QTc inteval. Aust Prescriber 2002;25(3):63-5.

50 Nolan, JP, Soar J, Zideman DA, Biarent D, Bossaert LL, Deakin C et al. on behalf of the ERC Guidelines Writing Group. European Resuscitation Council Guidelines for Resuscitation 2010. Section 1. Resuscitation 2010;81:1219–76.

51 Spearritt D. Torsades de pointes following cardioversion: case history and literature review. Aust Crit Care 2003;16(4):144–9.

52 Dennis MJ. ECG criteria to differentiate pulmonary artery catheter irritation from other proarrhythmic influences as the cause of ventricular arrhythmias. [abstract]. Am Coll Cardiol 2002; 39(9)[SupplB]:2B.

53 Opie LH, Gersh BJ. Drugs for the heart. 7th ed. Philhadelphia: Elsevier Saunders; 2005.

54 Bristow MR, Saxon LA, Boehmer J, Krueger S, Kass DA, De Marco T et al. Cardiac resynchronization therapy with or without an implantable defibrillator in advanced chronic heart failure. N Engl J Med 2004;350(21):2140–50.

55 Connolly SJ, Hallstrom AP, Cappato R, Schron EB, Kuck KH, Zipes DP et al. Meta-analysis of the implantable cardioverter defibrillator secondary prevention trials. AVID, CASH and CIDS studies. Antiarrhythmics vs Implantable Defibrillator Study, Cardiac Arrest Study Hamburg, Canadian Implantable Defibrillator Study. Eur Heart J 2000;21(24):2071–8.

56 Australian Resuscitation Council. Medications in adult cardiac arrest: Revised Policy Statement PS 11.5. Melbourne: Australian Resuscitation Council; 2010.

57 Piccini P, Berger J, O'Connor C. Amiodarone for the prevention of sudden cardiac death: a meta-analysis of randomized controlled trials. Europ Heart J 2009;30(10):1245–53.

58 Connolly S, Dorian P, Roberts R, Gent M, Bailin S, Fain E et al. Comparison of beta-blockers, amiodarone plus beta-blockers, or sotalol for prevention of shocks from implantable cardioverter defibrillators: the OPTIC Study: a randomized trial. JAMA 2006;295:165–71.

59 Kuhlkamp V, Mermi J, Mewis C, Seipel L. Efficacy and proarrhythmia with the use of d,l-sotalol for sustained ventricular tachyarrhythmias. J Cardiovasc Pharmacol 1997;29(3):373–81.

60 Ahmad K, Dorian P. Drug induced QT prolongation and proarrhythmia: an inevitable link? Europace 2007:iv16–iv22.

61 Sadowski ZP, Alexander JH, Skrabucha B, Dyduszynski A, Kuch, J, Narlowicz E et al. Multicentre randomized trial and systematic overview of lidocaine in acute myocardial infarction. Am Heart J 1999;137(5): 792–8.

62 Ryan TJ, Anderson JL, Antman EM, Braniff BA, Brooks NH, Califf RM et al. ACC/AHA guidelines for the management of patients with acute myocardial infarction. A report of the American College of Cardiology/American Heart Association Task Force on Practice Guidelines (Committee on Management of Acute Myocardial Infarction). J Am Coll Cardiol 1996;28(5):1328-428.

63 Mattingly E. AANA Journal course: update for nurse anesthetists – arrhythmia management devices and electromagnetic interference. AANA J 2005;73(2):129–36.

64 Swerdlow CD, Gillberg JM, Olson WH. Sensing and detection. In: Ellenbogen KA, Kay GN, Lau CP, Wilkoff BL, eds. Clinical cardiac pacing, defibrillation, and resynchronization therapy. 3rd ed. Philadelphia: Elsevier Saunders; 2007.

65 Hayes DL, Friedman PA. Cardiac pacing, defibrillation and resynchronization. 2nd ed. Singapore: Wiley-Blackwell; 2008.

66 Laczika K, Thalhammer F, Locker G, Apsner R, Losert H, Kofler J et al. Safe and efficient emergency transvenous ventricular pacing via the right supraclavicular route. Anesth Analg 2000;90(4):784–9.

67 Kay GN, Shepard RB. Cardiac electrical stimulation. In: Ellenbogen KA, Kay GN, Lau CP, Wilkoff BL, eds. Clinical cardiac pacing, defibrillation, and resynchronization therapy. 3rd ed. Philadelphia; Elsevier Saunders; 2007.

68 Bernstein AD, Camm AJ, Fletcher RD, Gold RD, Rickards AF, Smyth NP et al. The NASPE/BPEG generic pacemaker code for antibradyarrhythmic and adaptive rate pacing and antitachyarrhythmic devices. PACE 1987;10:794–99.

69 Sgarbossa EB, Pinski SL, Gates KB, Wagner GS. Early diagnosis of acute myocardial infarction in the presence of ventricular paced rhythm. Am J Cardiol 1996;77(5):423–44.

70 Schuchert A, Frese J, Stammwitz E, Novák M, Schleich A, Wagner SM et al. Low settings of the ventricular pacing output in patients dependent on a pacemaker: are they really safe? Am Heart J 2002;143(6):1009–11.

71 Ellenbogen KA, Wood MA. Cardiac pacing and ICDs. 4th ed. Oxford: Blackwell Publishing; 2005.

72 Tommaso C, Belic N, Brandfonbrener M. Asynchronous ventricular pacing: a rare cause of ventricular tachycardia. PACE 1982;5(4):561–3.

73 Ahmed FZ, Morris GM, Allen S, Khattar R, Mamas M, Zaidi A. Not all pacemakers are created equal: MRI conditional pacemaker and lead technology. J Cardiovasc Electrophysiol 2013;24(9):1059-65.

74 Hayes DL, Zipes DP. Cardiac pacemakers and cardioverter-defibrillators. In: Braunwald E, Dipes DP, Libby P, eds. Heart disease: a textbook of cardiovascular medicine. 6th ed. Philadelphia: WB Saunders; 2001.

75 Vardas PE, Auricchio A, Blanc JJ, Daubert J-C, Drexler H, Ector H et al. Guidelines for cardiac pacing and cardiac resynchronization therapy. The Task Force for Cardiac Pacing and Cardiac Resynchronization Therapy of the European Society of Cardiology. Europace 2007;9:959–98.

76 Kristensen L, Nielsen JC, Pedersen AK, Mortensen PT, Andersen HR. AV block and changes in pacing mode during long-term follow-up of 399 consecutive patients with sick sinus syndrome treated with an AAI/AAIR pacemaker. Pacing Clin Electrophysiol 2001;24(3):358–65.

77 Brandt J, Anderson H, Fahraeus T, Schüller H. Natural history of sinus node disease treated with atrial pacing in 213 patients: implications for selection of stimulation mode. J Am Coll Cardiol 1992;20(3):633–9.

78 Wilkoff BL, Cook JR, Epstein AE, Greene HL, Hallstrom AP, Hsia H et al. Dual chamber pacing or ventricular backup pacing in patients with an implantable defibrillator: The Dual Chamber and VVI Implantable Defibrillator (DAVID) trial. JAMA 2002;288:3115–23.

79 Dennis MJ, Sparks PB. Pacemaker mediated tachycardia as a complication of the autointrinsic conduction search function. PACE 2004;27(6Pt1):824–6.

80 Finkelmeier BA. Cardiothoracic surgical nursing. 2nd ed. Philadelphia: Lippincott, Williams & Wilkins; 2000.

81 Elmi F, Tullo N, Khalighi K. Natural history and predictors of temporary epicardial pacemaker wire function in patients after open heart surgery. Cardiol 2002: 98(4):175–80.

82 Chen LK, Teerlink JR, Goldschlager N. Pacing emergencies. In: Brown DL, ed. Cardiac intensive care. Philadelphia: WB Saunders; 1998.

83 Connolly SJ, Kerr CR, Gent M. Roberts RS, Yusuf S, Gillis AM et al. Effects of physiologic pacing versus ventricular pacing on the risk of stroke and death due to cardiovascular causes. N Engl J Med 2000;342(19):1385–91.

84 Lamas GA, Lee KL, Sweeney MO, Silverman R, Leon A, Yee R et al. For the Mode Selection Trial in Sinus-Node Dysfunction. Ventricular pacing or dual-chamber pacing for sinus node dysfunction. N Engl J Med 2002;346(2):1854–62.

85 Mond HG, Hikkock RJ, Stevenson IH, McGavigan, AD. The right ventricular outflow tract: the road to septal pacing. Pacing Clin Electrophysiol 2007;30:482–91.

86 Bakker P, Meijburg H, De Vries JW, Mower MM, Thomas AC, Hull ML et al. Biventricular pacing in end-stage heart failure improves functional capacity and left ventricular function. J Interv Card Electrophysiol 2000;4(2):395–404.

87 Hawkins NM, Petrie MC, MacDonald MR, Hogg KJ, McMurray JJ. Selecting patients for cardiac resynchronization therapy: electrical or mechanical dyssynchrony? Eur Heart J 2006;27:1270–81.

88 Linde C, Leclerq C, Rex S, Garrigue S, Lavergne T, Cazeau S et al. Long-term benefits of biventricular pacing in congestive heart failure: results from the MUSTIC study. J Am Coll Cardiol 2002;40:433–40.

89 Cleland JGF, Subert JC, Erdmann E, Freemantle N, Gras D, Kappenberger L et al. Longer-term effects of cardiac resynchronization therapy on mortality in heart failure [The Cardiac Resynchronisation-Heart Failure (CARE-HF) trial extension phase]. Eur Heart J 2006;27:1928–32.

90 Auricchio A, Stellbrink C, Sack S, Block M, Vogt J, Bakker P et al. Pacing Therapies in Congestive Heart Failure (PATH-CHF) Study Group. Long-term clinical effect of hamodynamically optimized cardiac resynchronisation therapy in patients with heart failure and ventricular conduction delay. J Am Coll Cardiol 2002;39:2026–33.

91 Young JB, Abraham WT, Smithe AL, Leon AR, Lieberman R, Wilkoff B et al. Combined cardiac resynchronization and implantable cardioverter defibrillation in advanced chronic heart failure: the MIRACLE ICD trial. JAMA 2003;289:2685–94.

92 Bristow MR, Saxon LA, Boehmer J, Krueger S, Kass, DA, De Marco T et al. Comparison of Medical Therapy, Pacing, Defibrillation in Heart Failure (COMPANION) Investigators. Cardiac resynchronization therapy with or without an implantable defibrillator in advanced chronic heart failure. N Engl J Med 2004;350:2140–50.

93 Ghi S, Constantin C, Klersy C, Serio A, Fontana A, Campana C et al. Interventricular and intraventricular dyssynchrony are common in heart failure patients, regardless of QRS duration. Eur Heart J 2004;25:571–8.

94 Littmann L, Symanski JD. Hemodynamic implications of left bundle branch block. J Electrocardiol 2000;33(Suppl1):115–21.

95 Verrnooy K, Verbeek XA, Peschar M, Crijns HJ, Arts T, Cornelussen RN et al. Left bundle branch block induces ventricular remodelling and functional septal hypoperfusion. Eur Heart J 2005;26:91–8.

96 Sundell J, Engblom E, Koistinen J, Ylitalo A, Naum A, Stolen KQ et al. The effects of cardiac resynchronization therapy on left ventricular function, myocardial energetics and metabolic reserve in patients with dilated cardiomyopathy and heart failure. J Am Coll Cardiol 2004;43:1027–33.

97 Peichl P, Kautzner J, Cihak R, Bytesník J. The spectrum of inter- and intraventricular conduction abnormalities in patients eligible for cardiac resynchronization therapy. Pacing Clin Electrophysiol 2004;27(8):1105–12.

98 Alonso C, Leclercq C, Victor F, Mansour H, de Place C, Pavin D et al. Electrocardiographic predictive factors of long-term clinical improvement with multisite biventricular pacing in advanced heart failure. Am J Cardiol 1998;84:1417–21.

99 Abraham WT, Fisher WG, Smith AL, Delurgio DB, Leon AR, Loh E et al. MIRACLE Study Group. Multicenter InSync Randomized Clinical Evaluation: cardiac resynchronization in chronic heart failure. N Engl J Med 2002;13(346):1845–53.

100 Daubert JC. Atrial fibrillation and heart failure: a mutually noxious association. Europace 2004;5:S1–S4.

101 Pappone C, Ćalović Ž, Vicedomini G, Cuko A, McSpadden LC, Ryu K et al. Multipoint left ventricular pacing improves acute hemodynamic response assessed with pressure-volume loops in cardiac resynchronization therapy patients. Heart Rhythm 2013;11(3)394-401.

102 Meine TJ. An intracardiac EGM method for VV optimization during cardiac resynchronization therapy. Heart Rhythm J 2006;3:AB30–35.

103 Kenny T. The nuts and bolts of cardiac resynchronization therapy. Massachusetts: Blackwell Futura; 2007.

104 Barold SS, Herweg B. Usefulness of the 12-lead electrocardiogram in the follow-up of patients with cardiac resynchronizaiton devices. Part I. Cardiol J 2011;18(5):476-86.

105 Thibault B, Dubuc M, Khairy P, Guerra PG, Macle L, Rivard L et al. Acute haemodynamic comparison of multisite and biventricular pacing with a quadripolar left ventricular lead. Europace 2013;15(7):984-991.

106 Rinaldi CA, Kranig W, Leclercq C, Kacet S, Betts T, Bordachar P et al. Acute hemodynamic benefits of multisite left ventricular pacing in CRT recipients. J Am Coll Cardiol 2012;59(13s1):E972

107 Miller JM, Zipes DP. Management of the patient with cardiac arrhythmias. In: Braunwald E, Zipes DP, Libby P, eds. Heart disease: a textbook of cardiovascular medicine. 6th ed. Philadelphia: WB Saunders; 2001.

108 Deakin C, Nolan J, Sunde, K, Koster R. European Resuscitation Council Guidelines for Resuscitation 2010 Section 3. Electrical therapies: automated external defibrillators, defibrillation, cardioversion and pacing. Resuscitation 2010; 81:1293–304.

109 Valenzuela TD, Bjerke HS, Clark LL, Hardman R, Spaite DW, Nichol G. Rapid defibrillation by nontraditional responders: the Casino Project. Acad Emerg Med 1998;5:414–15.

110 Ambler JJ, Zideman DA, Deakin CD. The effect of topical non-steroidal anti-inflammatory cream on the incidence and severity of cutaneous burns following external DC cardioversion. Resuscitation 2005;65(2):173–8.

111 Pinski SL, Sgarbossa EB, Ching E, Trohman RG. A comparison of 50-J versus 100-J shock for direct current cardioversion of atrial flutter. Am Heart J 1999;137:439–42.

112 Pinski KL, Fahy GJ. Implantable cardioverter defibrillators. Am J Med 1999;106:446–58.

113 The Antiarrhythmics versus Implantable Defibrillators (AVID) Investigators. A comparison of antiarrhythmic-drug therapy with implantable defibrillators in patients resuscitated from near-fatal ventricular arrhythmias. N Engl J Med 1997;337:1576–83.

114 Conolly SJ, Gent M, Roberts RS, Dorian P, Roy D, Sheldon RS et al. Canadian Implantable Defibrillator Study (CIDS): a randomized trial of the implantable cardioverter defibrillator against amiodarone. Circulation 2000;101:1297–302.

115 Kuck KH, Cappato R, Siebels J, Rüppel, R. Randomized comparison of antiarrhythmic drug therapy with implantable defibrillators in patients resuscitated from cardiac arrest. The Cardiac Arrest Study Hamburg (CASH). Circulation 2000;102:748–54.

116 Moss AJ, Hall WJ, Cannom D, Daubert JP, Higgins SL, Klein H et al. Multicentre Automatic Defibrillator Implantation Trial Investigators. Improved survival with an implanted defibrillator in patients with coronary artery disease at high risk for ventricular arrhythmias. N Engl J Med 1996;335(26):1933–40.

117 Mark DB, Nelson CL, Anstrom KJ, Al-Khatib SM, Tsiatis AA, Cowper PA et al. Cost-effectiveness of ICD therapy in the sudden cardiac death in heart failure trial (SCD-HeFT). Circulation 2006;114(2):135-42.

118 Swerdlow MD, Kalyanam Shivkumar MD, Jianxin Zhang MS. Determination of the upper limit of vulnerability using implantable cardioverter defibrillator electrograms. Circulation 2003;107:3028–33.

119 Viskin S, Rosso R. The top 10 reasons to avoid defibrillation threshold testing during ICD implantation. Heart Rhythm 2008;5(3):391–3.

120 Sola CL, Bostwick JM. Implantable cardioverter-defibrillators, induced anxiety, and quality of life. Mayo Clinic Proc 2005;80(2):232–7.

121 Brugada J. Is inappropriate therapy a resolved issue with current implantable cardioverter defibrillators? Am J Cardiol 1993;83:40D–44D.

122 Kruse J, Finkelmeier B. Permanent pacemakers and implantable cardioverter-defibrillators. In: Finkelmeier BA, ed. Cardiothoracic surgical nursing. 2nd ed. Philadelphia: Lippincott, Williams & Wilkins; 2000.

123 Jacob S, Panaich SS, Maheshwari R, Haddad JW, Padanilam BJ, John SK. Clinical application of magnets on cardiac rhythm management devices. Europace 2011;13(9):1222-30.

124 Jacobson C, Gerity D. Pacemakers and implantable defibrillators. In: Woods S, Froelicher E, Underhill Motzer S, eds. Cardiac nursing. 5th ed. Philadelphia: Lippincott, Williams & Wilkins; 2005.

125 Morady F. Radio-frequency ablation as treatment for cardiac arrhythmias. N Engl J Med 1999;340(7):534–44.

126 Scheinman MM. Patterns of catheter ablation practice in the United States: results of the 1992 NASPE survey. North American Society of Pacing and Electrophysiology. PACE 1994;17:873–5.

127 Joshi S, Wilber DJ. Ablation of idiopathic right ventricular outflow tract tachycardia: current perspectives. J Cardiovasc Electrophysiol 2005; 16(Suppl1):S52–8.

Chapter 12

Cardiac surgery and transplantation

Judy Currey, Sher Michael Graan

Learning objectives

After reading this chapter, you should be able to:

- outline cardiac surgical procedures including coronary artery bypass graft surgery and valve repair and replacement

- describe the indications, advantages and disadvantages of using cardiopulmonary bypass

- outline methods of myocardial preservation during cardiac surgery

- outline immediate postoperative management of cardiac surgical patients including haemodynamic, rhythm monitoring, ventilatory support, postoperative bleeding including pericardial tamponade, postoperative pain, fluid and electrolyte and emotional and family support

- outline the principles of counterpulsation in intra-aortic balloon pumping (IABP)

- outline the benefits and timing of balloon inflation and deflation, including conventional and real timing, management and assessment of timing and timing errors

- describe the nursing management of IABP complications, including limb perfusion, bleeding and immobility-related complications

- discuss methods of weaning IABP and management of intra-aortic balloon catheter removal

- discuss the immediate postoperative care of heart transplant recipients

- describe the clinical manifestations of postoperative complications in heart transplant recipients

- identify signs and symptoms of rejection in heart transplant recipients

- evaluate the effectiveness of nursing interventions in the postoperative management of heart transplant recipients.

Introduction

Many critically ill patients experience compromised cardiac function, as either a primary or secondary condition. This chapter follows on from those situations examined in Chapter 10, and reviews patients with conditions that tend to be cared for in specialised critical care units. The burden of cardiovascular disease estimated by the World Health Organization of years of life lost has increased from 14.9% in 2000 to 18.5% in 2012, and ischaemic heart diseases have become

KEY WORDS

arrhythmia

cardiac surgery

cardiopulmonary bypass

denervation

heart transplant

intra-aortic balloon pump

ischaemic reperfusion injury

valve replacement, repair

the leading cause of years of life lost in 2012.[1] In Europe, cardiovascular diseases account for 47% of all deaths; just less than half of mortality is due to coronary heart diseases.[2] Cardiovascular diseases in Australia affect one in six Australians and accounted for 31% of all deaths in 2011,[3] with acute coronary syndrome affecting 69,500 Australians and contributing to 15% of all deaths in 2011.[4] Currently, cardiovascular diseases are the second most common health issue, with the level of burden in Australia slightly lower than other developed nations (25.8% versus 33.7%).[3]

In this chapter three topics will be discussed. First, the management of a patient who requires cardiac surgery for coronary artery disease or valvular disease will be discussed, including the use of cardiopulmonary bypass. Second, the use and management of intra-aortic balloon counterpulsation in cardiac surgical and medical patients will be outlined. Finally, the management of patients following heart transplantation will be described including the prevention and management of immediate postoperative complications.

Cardiac surgery

The focus of this section is on cardiac surgery, for repair of structural abnormalities and repair or replacement of stenotic or regurgitant valves, and bypass grafting of coronary artery lesions. The structural abnormalities resulting from myocardial infarction have been described in Chapter 10. In this chapter, structural and functional abnormalities that are causing valvular disease (mitral, aortic, tricuspid or pulmonic valves) and ventricular defects will be discussed.

Valvular disease

The incidence and types of valvular disease have changed over the past 50 years.[3] Valvular disorders, such as mitral stenosis and aortic regurgitation, often arise from infectious diseases such as rheumatic fever (β-haemolytic streptococcal pharyngitis) and syphilis, which are much less common today. Conversely, there has been a rise in the rate of valvular diseases due to degenerative changes including leaflet degeneration and/or annulus calcification, which are common in ageing. In contrast to these trends, the prevalence of rheumatic fever and rheumatic valvular disorders among Aboriginal people (one of the highest in the world) and Pacific Islanders living in New Zealand is six times higher than the general population.[3] Other causes of valvular diseases are congenital valve diseases (common in the younger population, with respect to e.g. bicuspid valves) and endocarditis.

Two valvular abnormalities that alter the blood flow across the valve are common. Stenotic valves have a tightened, restricted orifice causing the valve to not fully open. There is a restriction to forward flow of blood, which must be forced through the valve at higher pressure (Figure 12.1). The high pressure combined with incomplete emptying of the chamber may increase the end-systolic volume, which will result in hypertrophy and dilation of the affected chamber(s) as a compensatory mechanism. The second valvular abnormality is valve regurgitation, which is also called incompetence or insufficiency. In this condition the incomplete closure of the valve leaflets results in backflow of blood into the chamber increasing its end-diastolic volume, which may cause chamber hypertrophy and dilation.

In both of these conditions heart failure may result as the pressure in the ventricles and atria grows and this pressure is reflected back into the pulmonary or venous system. Although the heart contains four valves, the majority of disorders affect the mitral and aortic valves in the left side of the heart.

Aortic valve disease

The aortic valve is located between the left ventricle and the aorta with a normal surface area of 2–3 cm². Mild aortic stenosis is a narrowing of the opening of the valve area to less than 1.5 cm² and a pressure gradient between the left ventricle and aorta of more than 25 mmHg; severe aortic stenosis is defined as a valve area of less than 1.0 cm² and a pressure gradient of more than 55 mmHg (Figure 12.1). Aortic stenosis often results from degenerative changes or congenital abnormalities such as a bicuspid aortic valve (with a prevalence of 0.5% in the general population), which may also cause regurgitation. Aortic stenosis increases left ventricle afterload, causing impedance to left ventricle ejection. This increases left ventricle end-systolic volume and left ventricle systolic pressure, resulting in left ventricle hypertrophy and dilation. Increased myocardial oxygen demands from the hypertrophied muscle also mean that angina is common.

Clinical manifestations of aortic stenosis include low cardiac output, increased left ventricle workload, angina, dyspnoea, syncope and fatigue. On auscultation, additional heart sounds are heard as a systolic ejection murmur and a loud S4. Left heart failure with pulmonary congestion is usually a late sign. The ECG may show left ventricular hypertrophy with strain patterns.

Aortic regurgitation may occur acutely when the aortic valve is damaged by endocarditis, trauma or aortic dissection, and presents as a life-threatening emergency. Chronic aortic regurgitation usually results from rheumatic heart disease, syphilis or congenital conditions. In aortic regurgitation reflux of blood to the left ventricle during diastole, due to incomplete closure of the valve, increases left ventricle end diastolic pressure and volume. This results in left ventricle dilation and hypertrophy and left heart failure. When left heart failure occurs, left atrial pressure rises and may cause pulmonary congestion and pulmonary hypertension.

In acute aortic regurgitation, the patient presents with signs and symptoms of acute left ventricle failure, cardiogenic shock and acute pulmonary oedema.[6] Patients with chronic aortic regurgitation may remain asymptomatic for years, finally presenting with signs of left heart failure including fatigue, palpitation, syncope, angina and dyspnoea. On auscultation, a diastolic murmur can be

FIGURE 12.1 Valvular stenosis and regurgitation: (**A**) normal position of valve leaflets (cusps) when the valve is open and closed; (**B**) open position of a stenosed valve (left) and closed position of a regurgitant valve (right); (**C**) haemodynamic effect of mitral stenosis shows the mitral valve is unable to open completely during left atrial systole, limiting left ventricular filling; (**D**) haemodynamic effect of mitral regurgitation shows the mitral valve does not close completely during left ventricular systole, allowing blood to re-enter the left atrium.[5]

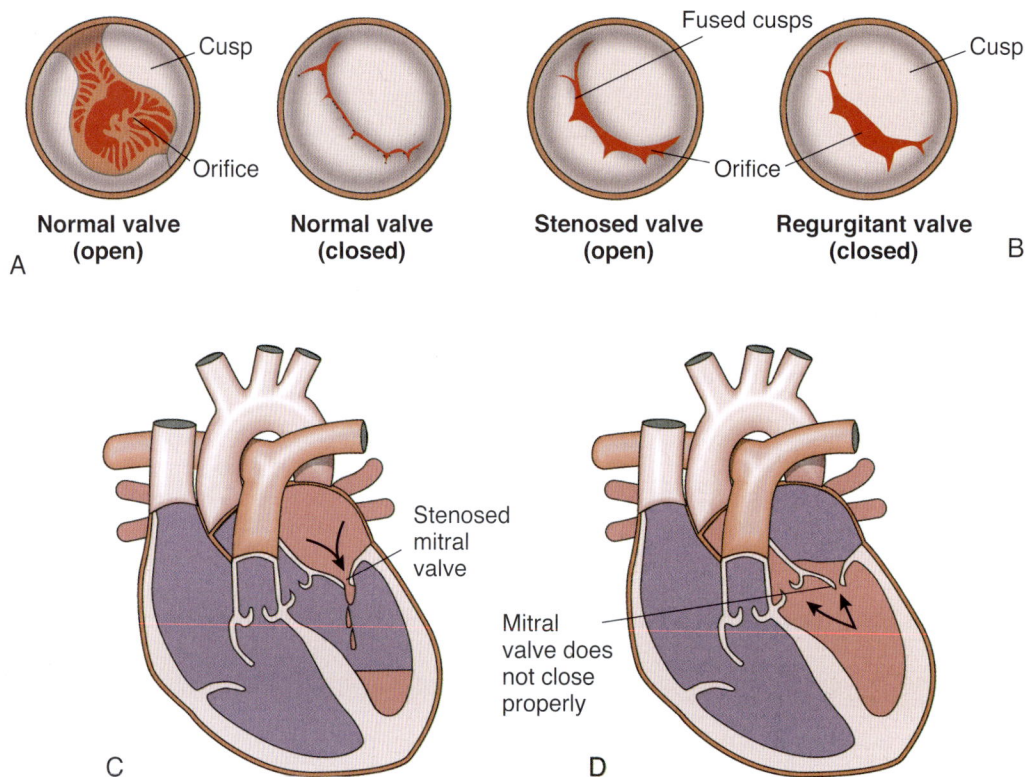

Adapted from Badhwar V, Esper S, Brooks M, Mulukutla S, Hardison R, Mallios D et al. Extubating in the operating room following adult cardiac surgery safely improves outcomes and lowers costs. J Thorac Cardiovasc Surg 2014;148(6):3101-9.e1, with permission.

heard. The ECG may show left ventricular hypertrophy due to volume overload and a chest X-ray may reveal cardiomegaly and features of acute pulmonary oedema.

Mitral valve disease

Mitral stenosis is a chronic and progressive narrowing of the mitral valve orifice (normally 4–6 cm^2), restricting blood flow from the left atrium to the left ventricle. Patients may exhibit symptoms when the valve area is <2 cm^2 and they will have symptoms at rest when the valve area is <1 cm^2.

Mitral valve stenosis often occurs as a result of rheumatic heart disease, degenerative valve diseases and, less often, from systemic lupus erythematosus. These diseases cause damage to the leaflets and chordae tendineae, so that during healing the scars contract and seal, restricting the aperture. The incomplete emptying of the left atrium causes increased left atrial pressure and left atrial enlargement, and results in pulmonary congestion and pulmonary hypertension. In chronic conditions, this pressure may also affect the right ventricle, causing right ventricular

failure, but left ventricular function is usually intact.[5] Lung compliance is reduced, causing dyspnoea, orthopnoea and nocturnal paroxysmal dyspnoea. Patients may complain of fatigue, low exercise tolerance, cough and haemoptysis. On auscultation a low-pitched diastolic murmur and an opening snap can be heard. The ECG may show left atrial enlargement and possibly atrial fibrillation (AF), and a chest X-ray may reveal right ventricular hypertrophy, left atrium enlargement and features of pulmonary oedema.

In mitral valve regurgitation, the mitral valve is not closing during left ventricular systole, causing backflow of blood into the left atrium, which creates elevated atrial and pulmonary pressures, and possibly pulmonary oedema.[5]Acute mitral regurgitation is often caused by acute myocardial infarction (AMI) resulting in papillary muscle rupture, trauma or infectious endocarditis, and patients may present with signs and symptoms of acute left ventricular failure, acute pulmonary oedema and cardiogenic shock. The causes of chronic mitral regurgitation are rheumatic diseases, congenital mitral valve prolapse or degenerative changes. The patient may complain of weakness, fatigue, exertional dyspnoea, palpitation and symptoms of pulmonary congestion and right ventricular failure such as cough, dyspnoea, orthopnoea and lower extremity oedema. On auscultation, a third heart sound and a pansystolic murmur can be heard. ECG may show left atrial enlargement, left ventricular hypertrophy, P mitrale and possibly AF, and a chest X-ray may reveal left ventricular hypertrophy, left atrium enlargement and features of pulmonary oedema.

Tricuspid valve disease

Tricuspid stenosis (normal area is 7 cm^2) is often seen with aortic or mitral valve diseases, and rarely in isolation. The restriction of blood flow from the right atrium to the right ventricle causes systemic venous congestion. On auscultation, a diastolic murmur can be heard. Tricuspid regurgitation is most commonly a functional disorder due to annulus dilation as a result of increased right ventricle pressure and hypertrophy, mitral stenosis, pulmonary embolism, cor pulmonale or right ventricle AMI. The backflow of blood from the right ventricle to the right atrium causes systemic venous congestion. On auscultation, a pansystolic murmur can be heard. In both stenosis and regurgitation of the tricuspid valve patients present with a high central venous pressure (CVP) and jugular venous pressure (JVP), hepatomegaly, ascites and peripheral oedema, and their ECG may show P pulmonale and possibly AF, and a chest X-ray may reveal prominent right heart border.

Pulmonic valve disease

Pulmonic valve stenosis is rare in isolation and is often due to a congenital defect. The restriction to blood flow from the right ventricle to the pulmonary arteries causes right ventricular hypertrophy and dilation, and the patient presents with exertional dyspnoea, syncope, cyanosis and a systolic murmur, and a split S2 heart sound. The ECG may show right ventricular hypertrophy.

Pulmonic valve regurgitation is also a rare condition that is usually caused by a congenital defect or pulmonary hypertension or is iatrogenic (e.g. post balloon valvuloplasty). Patients might be asymptomatic, but in severe cases they present with signs and symptoms of right ventricular failure.

Surgical procedures

The most common cardiac surgical procedures include coronary artery bypass graft (CABG) surgery, to bypass lesions within the coronary arteries, and repair or replacement of stenotic or regurgitant valves. During these procedures preservation of systemic circulation, ventilation and perfusion of the myocardium is required and is often achieved with the aid of cardiopulmonary bypass (CPB).

Coronary artery bypass graft surgery

The pathophysiology and implications of ischaemic heart disease are explained in detail in Chapter 10. Single lesions can be treated by angioplasty and stent; however,

patients with a left main coronary artery lesion, multiple (double- or triple-vessel) disease, longer lesions and failed angioplasty may need CABG surgery.[6]

In CABG a section of vein or artery is used to bypass a blockage in the patient's coronary artery. The vessels used for grafting arise from arteries (internal mammary artery or radial artery and, less commonly, gastroepiploic artery) or veins (saphenous vein). Saphenous veins are harvested from the legs, and the radial artery from the forearm, and each is used as a free graft with anastomoses at the ascending aorta and distal to lesions to one or more coronary arteries. When saphenous veins are used as grafts (SVG), they often develop diffuse intimal hyperplasia, which ultimately contributes to re-stenosis. Patency rates are lowest in saphenous vein grafts attached to small coronary arteries or coronary arteries supplying myocardial scars. Consequently, arterial grafts are used more often, as they are more resistant to intimal hyperplasia. Internal mammary arteries (IMAs) and radial artery grafts may be used.[7] The IMA remains attached to the subclavian artery and is mobilised from the chest wall and anastomosed to the coronary artery distal to the occlusion (Figure 12.2). If the radial artery is being harvested for grafting, the collateral circulation in the forearm is

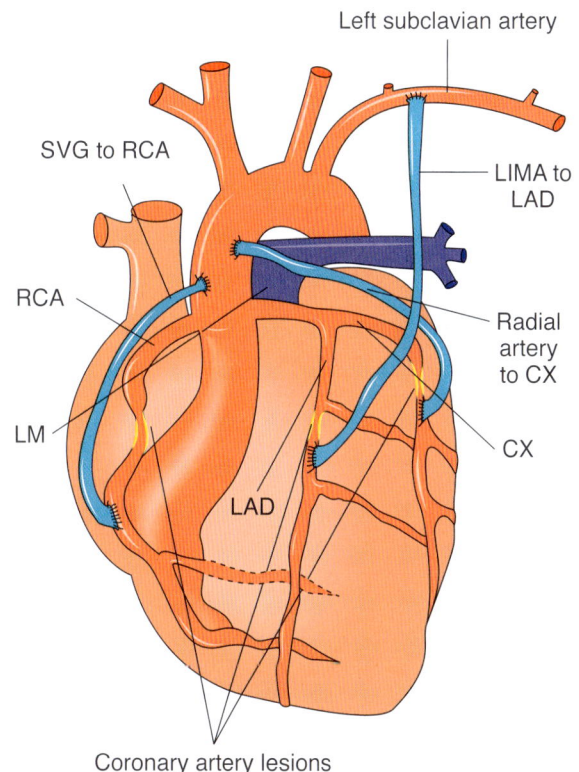

FIGURE 12.2 Coronary artery bypass grafts.
CX = circumflex artery; LAD = left anterior descending; LIMA = left internal mammary artery; LM = left main; RCA = right coronary artery; SVG = saphenous vein graft.

assessed. Echo colour Doppler provides the best accuracy in assessing forearm circulation, although the clinical Allen test is quite commonly used. The disadvantage of the Allen test is that it gives false patency results around 5% of the time.[8] A selection of IMA, SVG and radial artery grafts may be necessary over time as repeat procedures are needed or in patients with extensive disease requiring multiple grafts.

For single-vessel disease, particularly of the left anterior descending (LAD) artery, a new approach to CABG – minimally invasive direct coronary artery bypass grafting (MIDCABG) – has been used. This procedure uses intercostal incisions and a thorascope instead of a sternotomy to access the heart and coronary arteries. MIDCABG is also often performed without cardiopulmonary bypass (off-pump coronary artery bypass, OPCAB); instead, the heart is slowed with beta-blockers to allow the surgery to be performed on a beating heart.[9] OPCAB procedures may also be performed using full or partial sternotomy to provide access for multiple vessel grafting. Both procedures have been successful responses to the drive to reduce the need for transfusion, recovery times, patient stays in hospital and costs.[9,10]

In the last decade robotically assisted cardiac surgery has evolved in America and Europe and has been introduced at a small number of Australian hospitals for CABG and mitral valve surgery. This technique has further reduced the invasiveness of cardiac surgery, as little more than stab wounds are required in the right chest for thoracoscopy and the robotic instruments. Avoiding true thoracotomy or sternotomy improves postoperative pain experience, is associated with quicker recovery and shortens length of stay.[11,12]

Although CABG is the most common cardiac surgical procedure undertaken in Australia, the incidence has declined since 2000/01 from 87 to 61 procedures/100,000 population in 2007–08.[3,13] The decline in surgery rates is due to changes in the treatment of CHD, including the advent of percutaneous coronary intervention (PCI). More procedures are now being performed in older patients, with 73% of current patients aged over 60 years.[3] CABG is used to relieve the symptoms of angina by increasing coronary blood flow distal to occlusive coronary lesions. It is a palliative, not curative, treatment as the underlying disease process continues. CABG is more effective than percutaneous transluminal coronary angioplasty (PTCA) in patients with extensive, multivessel disease with improved survival over a 3–5-year period by 5%, and a 4–7-fold reduction in the need for reintervention.[14] CABG is also used in left main vessel lesions due to the high risk of extensive infarction associated with PTCA in this area. CABG surgery is commonplace, and many cardiothoracic centres have highly efficient, effective systems in place with mortality rates as low as 2%.

Valve repair and replacement

Valve surgery is usually undertaken to repair the patient's valve or, more often, to replace the valve with a mechanical or tissue prosthesis. The clinical decision for valve surgery is primarily based on the clinical state of the patient using the New York Heart Association (NYHA) classification system and echocardiographic findings.[6] The type of surgery used will depend on the valves involved, the valvular pathology, the severity of the condition and the patient's clinical condition. Often valve surgery is not a single procedure, and it may involve multiple valves, CABG and an implantable cardioverter defibrillator (ICD). Valve surgery is palliative, not curative, and patients will require lifelong health care.

Valve repair may involve resecting and/or suturing prolapsed or torn leaflets (valvuloplasty) and repairing the ring of collagen the valve sits in (annuloplasty), and is commonly used for mitral and tricuspid regurgitation. Commissurotomy (incising valve leaflets and debriding calcification) is the treatment of choice for mitral stenosis. Both repair processes have demonstrated lower operative mortality than replacement, although complete valve competence may not be achievable. Open procedures are preferred because thrombi and calcification can thereby be removed.

Valve replacement may be necessary, but could be associated with higher risks due to the long-term disease process and poor underlying left ventricular function. The most common indication for valve replacement is aortic stenosis, which accounts for around 60% of valve surgery.[15] Prosthetic valves may be mechanical or biological. Mechanical valves are made of metal alloys, pyrolite carbon and Dacron (Figure 12.3). Biological valves are constructed from porcine, bovine or human cardiac tissue. Mechanical valves are more durable but have an increased risk of thromboembolism, so lifelong anticoagulation is required. Biological valves suffer from the same problems as the patient's valve (i.e. calcification and degeneration). The choice of valve depends on the age of the patient and potential difficulties with taking anticoagulants.

For elderly patients with high risk of open heart surgery and higher comorbidity, trans-catheter aortic valve implantation (TAVI) of commercial artificial valves (for example Medtronic CORE Valve or Edwards Sapein) has been used. This procedure is usually performed in a catheter laboratory, via femoral artery approach, similar to angiography procedure and light anaesthesia. This procedure carries higher risks of all-cause 1-year mortality of 13.9–16.3%, major vascular complications of 9.3–12.3% and 2.6% incidence of stroke.[16,17]

Mortality is higher for valvular surgery than for CABG, reflecting the underlying loss of ventricular function and additional procedures that are common. Risk stratification models have been developed to help determine the patients that are most likely to have poor recovery and outcomes.[18] The major factors that contribute to poor outcomes are worse left ventricular function and age over 70 years.[15]

Cardiopulmonary bypass

CPB was developed to enable surgery to be performed on a still, relatively bloodless heart, while preserving

FIGURE 12.3 Prosthetic valves: (**A**) the Bjork-Shiley valve, with a pyrolyte-carbon disc that opens to 60°; (**B**) the Starr-Edwards caged-ball valve model 6320, with satellite ball; (**C**) the St Jude Medical mechanical heart valve, with a mechano-central flow disc; (**D**) the Hancock II porcine aortic valve, with stent and sewing ring covered in Dacron cloth 5 (published with permission).

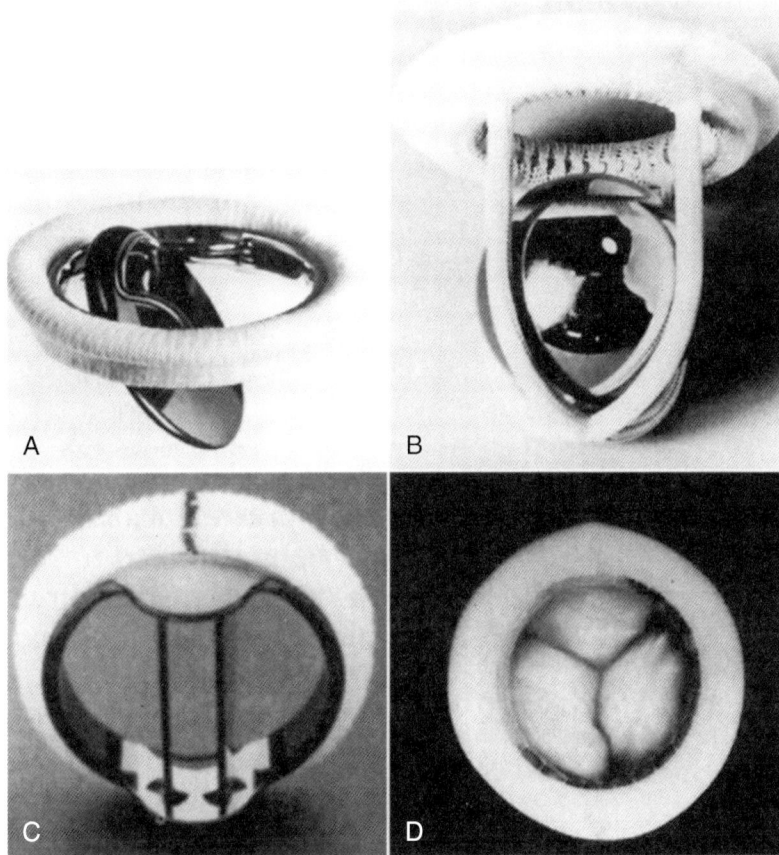

the patient's circulation. CPB temporarily performs the functions of the heart in circulating blood and of the lungs by enabling gas exchange with the blood. Silicone cannulae are inserted into the venae cavae or right atrium, and venous blood is circulated through a circuit outside the body. In this circuit the blood is oxygenated, carbon dioxide removed and blood temperature controlled. Drugs and anaesthetics may be added. A roller pump is generally used to provide the pressure to create blood flow in the circuit and back to the patient's aorta.

Adverse effects of CPB are diverse, and include the following (Table 12.1):[19]

- haematological effects due to exposure of the blood to tubing and gas exchange surfaces, which initiates surface activation of the clotting cycle; also blood component damage due to shear stress from the roller action of the pump, which reduces haematocrit, leucocyte and platelet count.

- pulmonary effects due to activation of systemic inflammatory response syndrome (SIRS), which increases capillary leakage, and lung deflation during surgery leading to postoperative atelectasis

- cardiovascular effects due to volume changes, fluid shifts and decreased myocardial contractility, which decreases cardiac output; this is most severe during the first 6 hours, but usually resolves within 48–72 hours

- neurological effects due to poor cerebral perfusion and generation of thromboemboli from aortic cannulation, which can lead to cerebrovascular accidents

- renal effects due to decreases in cardiac output during initiation of CPB, which decreases renal perfusion

- post-pump delirium or psychosis, which occurs in 32% of CPB patients although the cause has not been identified; symptoms include short-term memory deficit, decreased attention and inability to respond to and integrate sensory information

- activation of a systemic inflammatory response, which may cause vasodilation and increased cardiac output.

TABLE 12.1

Summary of the impact and side effects of CPB

BODY SYSTEM	CPB IMPACT	SIDE EFFECTS
Haematology	Surface activation of clotting cascade	↓ WBC, ↓ HcT, ↓ platelets Thromboembolism formation
Pulmonary	SIRS activation (CPB circuit)	↑ Capillary permeability and leakage Pulmonary congestion ↓ Surfactant production
	Lung deflation (during surgery)	Atelectasis Impaired gas exchange
Cardiovascular	Volume changes SIRS activation	Fluid shift ↓ Myocardial contractility and CO Vasodilation and ↓ SVR
Neurological	Poor cerebral perfusion Thromboembolism	↑ Risk of CVA
	Post pump delirium or psychosis	Short-term memory deficit ↓ Attention Sensory deficit
Renal	↓ CO and renal perfusion	↓ Urine output, and ↑ risk of ARF

ARF = acute renal failure; CO = cardiac output; CPB = cardiopulmonary bypass; CVA = cardiovascular accident; HcT = haematocrit; SIRS = systemic inflammatory response syndrome; SVR = systemic vascular resistance; WBC = white blood cells.

These effects are well documented, and routine CPB management and postoperative care are designed to minimise and treat the complications. Heparin is added at the commencement of CPB and is reversed with protamine (1 mg of protamine for every 100 U of heparin) when CPB ceases; activated clotting times are monitored throughout and after CPB. Blood returning to the circulation is filtered, and surgical procedures proceed carefully to reduce microemboli. Monitoring and maintenance of adequate arterial flow rates are used to prevent low perfusion. Temperature gradients and a rewarming process are instituted slowly so that cardiac output can meet metabolic demands.

Myocardial preservation

One of the processes involved in CPB is that the aorta is clamped where a cannula is inserted to return blood to the circulation. This clamp prevents blood flow into the coronary arteries; therefore, the myocardium must be protected from ischaemia during the cardiac surgical procedure. This protection is achieved through several mechanisms directed towards reducing oxygen demand: first, oxygen demand is reduced by mild-to-moderate hypothermia (28–32°C); second, myocardial temperature is reduced (0–4°C) by infusing cold fluids directly into the coronary arteries; and third, normal conduction is prevented by arresting the heart during diastole, by infusing a concentrated potassium solution into the coronary arteries. Return to normal rhythm is usually achieved by circulation of warm blood, though defibrillation may be necessary.

Patient management

The often-rapid turnaround from complete dependence in intensive care to discharge in post-cardiothoracic surgery patients can provide particularly rewarding nursing experiences. However, this rapid progression is also often marked by haemodynamic instability, arrhythmias and biochemical and haematological changes. The increased emphasis on rapid weaning and extubation, often occurring during turbulent anaesthetic recovery, presents one of the more volatile periods in ventilatory support, requiring knowledgeable and skilled nursing and medical management. In addition to the management of ventilation, temporary pacemaker therapies and mechanical circulatory assist (intra-aortic balloon pumping and ventricular assist) devices provide opportunity for the development of broad and detailed expertise.

Patients are usually admitted to the intensive care unit for 1–2 days although, when early extubation is undertaken, they may spend only hours in a recovery unit before progressing to a cardiothoracic high-dependency area, where nurse-to-patient ratios may be 1:2 to 1:3.

The immediate postoperative period

Patients should be transported to intensive care accompanied by at least an anaesthetist, an appropriately qualified nurse and transport personnel under continuous cardiac monitoring and assisted ventilation. It is a requirement to include capnography during patient transport to detect ventilator disconnection, dysfunction or endotracheal tube migration. Intensive care or theatre nursing staff may be a component of the transport team. The admission to intensive care requires a team approach, with the participation of intensive care nursing and medical staff and/or technician input. The immediate postoperative decision making on patient management is influenced by handover from anaesthetists, settling in procedures and collegial assistance.[20,21] Admission activities are commonly divided between nurses, with one nurse taking responsibility for establishing monitoring and haemodynamic assessment and management, and a second nurse managing ventilation and endotracheal tube security, as well as managing chest drains, gastric tube and urinary catheter. If staffing permits, additional nurses may take responsibility for documentation, performing arterial blood gases, 12-lead ECG and providing assistance as required.

The objectives of immediate postoperative management of cardiac surgical patients may include:

- optimisation of cardiovascular performance
- reestablishment and/or maintenance of normothermia
- promotion of haemostasis
- ventilatory support and management
- prevention and management of arrhythmias
- optimisation of organ perfusion.

Haemodynamic monitoring and support

Typical haemodynamic monitoring includes an intra-arterial catheter for continuous blood pressure monitoring and arterial blood sampling. Cardiac output and preload measurement are achieved most commonly with either a pulmonary artery or central venous catheter configured for pulse contour cardiac output (PiCCO) monitoring (see Chapter 9).

Preload measures provided by the pulmonary artery catheter include right atrial pressure (RAP) to approximate right ventricular filling and pulmonary artery pressure (PAP) to approximate right ventricular systole and provide insight into pulmonary vascular resistance and left heart function. The pulmonary capillary wedge pressure (PCWP) is available to approximate left ventricular filling and left heart function. Alternatively, the PiCCO monitoring system represents preload by intrathoracic blood volume index (ITBVI) and global end-diastolic volume index (GEDVI). In addition, the extravascular lung water index (EVLWI) can demonstrate the accumulation of interstitial lung water.[22]

Cardiac output is measured by either intermittent or continuous thermodilution via pulmonary artery catheters, or measured intermittently and then approximated continuously on a beat-to-beat interpretation of pulse contour by the PiCCO monitoring system. Cardiac output measurement can be combined with other pressure variables to calculate systemic and pulmonary vascular resistance, stroke volume and measures of ventricular work.

Certain common haemodynamic patterns are seen in the early postoperative phase. These must be detected through thorough monitoring and interpretation of variables, and managed according to specific needs. During the initial 2 hours of recovery period, 95% of patients will experience haemodynamic instability.[19,23]

Practice tip

The choice of inotropes and vasoactive drugs should be based on the haemodynamic findings, for example: a patient with low SVR and low contractility (low CO and BP) will need an ino-constrictor such as adrenaline or dopamine; a patient with high SVR and low contractility will need an ino-dilator such as milrinone or dobutamine.

Hypertension

Hypertension is present in up to 30% of patients initially,[24] as hypothermia, stress responses, pain and hypovolaemia contribute to vasoconstriction.[21,24] When the systemic vascular resistance is excessive, the high afterload may contribute to low cardiac output.[24] Rewarming to normothermia with space blankets or heated air blankets, fluid administration, administration of sedation or analgesics and infusion of IV vasodilators (glyceryl trinitrate or sodium nitroprusside) are all commonly used to overcome vasoconstriction when contributing to hypertension.[21,24] Occasionally, beta-blockers are used. Hypertension increases myocardial workload and contributes to bleeding.

Hypotension

Transient hypotension requiring treatment is common at some stage during the postoperative period. Contributing factors to hypotension include hypovolaemia and decreased venous return (from polyuria, bleeding, ventilation and positive end-expiratory pressure and excess vasodilation), contractile impairment (from ischaemia or infarction, hypothermia and negative inotropic influences), pericardial tamponade and vasodilation (from excess vasodilator therapy, or as part of an inflammatory response to cardiopulmonary bypass).[21,25]

Hypotension may present with reduced or elevated preload, reduced or elevated cardiac output and reduced or elevated systemic vascular resistance (SVR). When hypovolaemia is present, cardiac output will be low and SVR usually high. Hypovolaemia is diagnosed by measuring preload indicators, as pressure (RAP, PAP, PCWP) or volume (ITBVI, GEDVI).[22,26] Choice of colloids or crystalloid fluids for volume restoration in the postoperative period has no effect on mortality,[27] but colloids affect clot formation and strength and also produce greater haemodilution, which is associated with more blood product transfusion.[23,28] Blood returned from the cardiopulmonary bypass circuit ('pump blood') usually accompanies the patient to ICU, and this should be readministered at a rate suitable to filling indices and blood pressure.

Hypotension accompanied by elevated preload and low cardiac output usually represents cardiac dysfunction or pericardial tamponade, and the distinction should be quickly sought.[29,30] When such left ventricular dysfunction is present, there is usually compensatory vasoconstriction and tachycardia, although heart rate responses may be unreliable due to cardioplegia, cold, conduction disease[21] and preoperative beta-blocking agents. Inotropic agents, including milrinone hydrochloride, adrenaline, dopamine or dobutamine, may become necessary (these are covered more completely in Table 21.7 and its accompanying text). When the profile of severe left ventricular dysfunction is persistent (either at the time of coming off bypass or later in intensive care), intra-aortic balloon pumping may be instituted. ECG assessment for new ischaemia or infarction should be made, which if of significant size, may warrant surgical re-exploration or angiographic investigation.

Pericardial tamponade is also a cause of hypotension (covered later in this chapter).

A fourth common postoperative profile is hypotension with normal or elevated cardiac output in the presence of low SVR. This may occur with excess vasodilator administration, the use of postoperative epidural infusions and vasodilation from a systemic inflammatory response to cardiopulmonary bypass and other factors such as reinfusion of collected operative site blood.[31] The inotrope milrinone hydrochloride is popular in the postoperative phase because of its dilating effect on radial artery grafts,[32] but often contributes to hypotension through its systemic vasodilator properties. When hypotension is attributable to vasodilation, metaraminol or noradrenaline may be used.[26] Arginine vasopressin, by infusion, could be used as an effective alternative vasoconstrictor for cardiac surgical patients, but early introduction of vasopressin demonstrated improved haemodynamic response.[33,34]

A mean arterial pressure of 70–80 mmHg is generally targeted in the postoperative period.[21] This can sometimes be reduced if there has been ventriculotomy or if there is concern about the status of the aorta. The cardiac index should be maintained above 2.2 L/min/m², as hypoperfusion develops below these values. When at these levels, additional assessments are often undertaken, such as mixed venous oxygen saturation measurement (to assess oxygen delivery deficits) and arterial pH and lactate measurements (to detect metabolic acidosis from anaerobic metabolism).

In addition to assessment of preload, contractility and afterload, heart rate and rhythm should be assessed for their input to cardiac output and blood pressure. Extremes of rate and arrhythmias alter ventricular filling and may need correction. If temporary pacing wires are present, pacing strategies for haemodynamic improvement include rate rises (even if already in the normal range)[21] and the provision of dual-chamber or atrial pacing as alternatives to ventricular pacing only in order to maximise atrioventricular synchrony and the contribution of atrial kick to blood pressure. Alternatively, if ventricular pacing is present, reducing the rate to permit expression of a slower sinus rhythm may, with the provision of atrial kick, improve cardiac output and blood pressure (refer to Chapter 11 for more information on pacing).

Practice tip

Be aware of an apparent paradox: hypertension may occur even if there is hypovolaemia. The intense vasoconstriction often seen postoperatively not only raises blood pressure but aids venous return so that right atrial pressure is normal. It may not be until the patient has warmed and dilated that the true filling status is revealed. When the patient is cold and has normal filling pressures, be prepared for possible hypotension, and the need for significant fluid resuscitation, on rewarming.

Rhythm monitoring and postoperative arrhythmias

Continuous rhythm monitoring is necessary while the patient is in intensive care, and telemetry monitoring is usually continued until discharge from hospital. Lead selection is often haphazard, but a chest lead in the V1 position (or lead MCL1) generally provides the best information on atrial and ventricular activity.[35] Unlike many leads, these two leads reliably demonstrate normal rhythms, bundle branch block and ventricular rhythms,[35] and may be useful in confirming pulmonary artery catheter irritation as the cause of ventricular arrhythmias.[36]

A 12-lead ECG is performed on admission to the ICU and should be compared with the preoperative ECG. It should be assessed for signs of new ischaemia or infarction, new bundle branch block and arrhythmias or conduction disturbances. Pericarditis, a frequent complication of surgery, appears as ST-segment elevation (often, but not always, in many leads), and may mask or mimic myocardial infarction. The nurse should look for the classic concave upward, or 'saddle-shaped' ST segment, to distinguish pericardial changes from the more convex upward ST segment of infarction. Worsening of pain on inspiration and a pericardial rub help to confirm pericarditis.[35]

Atrial fibrillation is the most common postoperative arrhythmia and contributes significantly to postoperative morbidity and hospital length of stay.[37] It occurs in up to 30–50% of patients, most often on days 2–3 postoperatively.[30,37] Many patients revert without treatment, but when treatment becomes necessary beta-blockers and amiodarone appear to be the most successful agents for correction.[37,38] Digitalis is effective for rate control and IV magnesium is often used, although further evidence for its use is needed. Atrial pacing to prevent atrial fibrillation is being increasingly explored but a clear recommendation on pacing sites and protocols has yet to emerge. In contrast, atrial overdrive pacing can be an effective means to immediately and safely interrupt atrial flutter.[37,38]

Ventricular ectopic beats are common and by themselves do not require treatment unless they accompany ischaemia or biochemical disturbance,[39] in which case they may progress to more complex arrhythmias. Consideration should always be given to the pulmonary artery catheter as the cause (including both correctly and incorrectly positioned catheters),[36] as this is an easily corrected influence. Ventricular tachycardia and fibrillation are uncommon and usually denote myocardial disturbance such as ischaemia or infarction, shock, electrolyte disturbance, hypoxia or increased excitation due to high circulating catecholamine levels.[39] Standard approaches to resuscitation according to protocols in Chapter 24 apply, including standard CPR over the recent sternotomy. When ventricular fibrillation cannot be corrected, consideration is often given to re-exploration of the chest to examine graft patency and/or provide internal cardiac massage. The cardiac surgical intensive care unit should be equipped to enable emergency re-exploration for such purposes.

Ventilatory support

Ventilation should be approached according to the general principles described in Chapter 15. As anaesthesia is not typically reversed at the end of the operation, patients are generally admitted apnoeic, and within 1–3 hours return to wakefulness and spontaneous breathing.

Ensuring a secure airway is an initial priority; the following should be undertaken:

- Confirmation of endotracheal tube (ETT) position and its security immediately on admission:
  o auscultation for equal bilateral air entry to rule out right main bronchus intubation
  o recording of the ETT insertion length to detect ETT migration
  o postoperative chest X-ray, taken within 30 minutes, should also be examined for ETT positioning
- Initial ETT care:
  o assessment for air leak around the cuff (via performance of minimal occlusive volume or pressure tests) and auscultation of the neck
  o ensure ETT is adequately secured and positioned so as not to apply undue pressure against soft tissues of the mouth and lips.

There has been a general trend to more rapid ventilatory weaning in recent years, and in some centres 'fast-track' cardiac surgical recovery includes extubation at the end of the operation before transfer to a recovery unit for suitable patients. Indices of respiration show no improvement when intubation is maintained for longer compared with early extubation,[40] and pooled results from randomised early extubation trials show earlier ICU discharge and shorter lengths of stay (by 1 day) when early extubation is undertaken.[40,41]

Apart from these fast-track approaches, ventilation is commonly employed for 2–6 hours in the uncomplicated patient. Reasons for continuing ventilation beyond this time frame may include:

- intraoperative neurological event
- gas exchange deficit with unresolved hypoxaemia
- ventilatory inadequacy
- significant haemodynamic insufficiency
- patients returning from theatre late in the evening may sometimes continue ventilation overnight to optimise postextubation breathing ability.

For many patients, ventilation is provided purely for initial airway and apnoea protection rather than for treatment of pulmonary deficits. In the absence of pulmonary disease, many centres provide fairly uniform approaches to parameter settings that aim at sustaining ventilation and oxygenation, while limiting traumatic risk to the lungs (see Table 12.2). However, approaches to ventilation will need to be tailored in the presence of operative complications or coexisting lung disease.

Ventilation challenges specific to the postoperative cardiac setting include:

- atelectasis due to operative access
- pneumothorax (pleural opening for grafts, or ventilation-induced trauma)
- pulmonary hypertension from cardiac failure or valve disease
- cardiogenic shock/post-pump failure
- systemic inflammatory response syndrome due to cardiopulmonary bypass
- early or rapid weaning that is undertaken before complete readiness, leading to failure at weaning attempt
- surgical pain limiting spontaneous effort and potentially leading to atelectasis or sputum retention.

Approaches to weaning

As patients often have no underlying pulmonary pathology, and have been ventilated for brief periods only, rapid weaning phases have become the norm in most centres. In many instances, as soon as the patient wakes and begins spontaneous breathing activity, he/she may be suitable for at least a trial of spontaneous breathing in CPAP mode, usually with some modest level of pressure support (e.g. 5–10 cmH$_2$O). If tolerated and the patient maintains an adequate minute volume, SpO$_2$ and PaCO$_2$, extubation may be considered within as little as another 30 minutes. Normal demonstrations of airway protection capability (e.g. neuromuscular control, gag, swallow, cough and patient strength) should be sought before extubation (see Chapter 15 for details).

These short ventilation times and rapid weaning carry a greater risk of weaning failure. Patients may initially wake and appear to sustain spontaneous ventilation well for some time, only to lapse back under anaesthetic influence. A return to greater ventilatory support may be necessary. Failure to wean carries greater significance in the cardiac surgical patient with existing pulmonary hypertension, as respiratory acidosis causes pulmonary vasoconstriction, abruptly worsening pulmonary hypertension and the risk of pulmonary oedema and/or right ventricular failure.

When ventilation has been more prolonged due to postoperative pulmonary problems, weaning may be approached more cautiously, as might be applied to the general longer term ventilated patient. Gradual mandatory rate reduction or increasing periods of spontaneous ventilation interspersed with periods of greater assistance have been employed.[40,42]

TABLE 12.2

Postoperative ventilation settings

NOMINAL OR GENERALLY ACCEPTABLE SETTINGS	ALTERNATIVES TO NOMINAL SETTINGS AND REASONS FOR VARIATION
SIMV with volume control ventilation	Pressure control suitable. Generally used only if there is significant hypoxaemia or the need to exert greater control on pulmonary pressure. Hybrid modes such as Autoflow, pressure-regulated volume control or volume control plus (VC+) are also suitable, generally for the same indications as pressure control
Tidal volume 8–10 mL/kg	Lower tidal volumes (6–8 mL/kg) when there is known compliance disorder (atelectasis, pulmonary oedema, fibrosis) or unexplained high plateau pressures
Mandatory rate 10 L/min	Faster rates may be necessary if low tidal volume strategies become necessary. Lower rates if gas trapping risk due to airways disease Adjust according to $PaCO_2$ level
Inspiratory flow 30–50 L/min to provide I:E ratio of 1:2 to 1:4 acceptable	Slower flows to prolong the inspiratory time may be necessary if there is atelectasis and hypoxaemia, or if there is a desire to lessen inspiratory pressures. Faster flows to enhance expiratory time necessary only if gas-trapping risk
PEEP minimum levels of 5 cmH$_2$O	Higher levels of PEEP according to severity of hypoxaemia
Pressure support 5–10 cmH$_2$O	Automated pressure support modes such as automatic tube compensation (autoadjusted pressure support to overcome flow resistance of tracheal tubes) or volume support (autoadjusted pressure support to achieve target tidal volume on spontaneous breaths) exist. There is no pressing indication for their use in uncomplicated cardiac surgical patients
Permissive hypercapnoea rarely necessary	Particularly important to avoid if existing pulmonary hypertension, as may worsen acutely with respiratory acidosis
FiO$_2$ initially 0.8–1.0 then wean down according to PaO$_2$/SaO$_2$	According to PaO$_2$/SaO$_2$

FiO$_2$ = fraction of inspired oxygen; PEEP = positive end expiratory pressure; SIMV = synchronised intermittent mandatory ventilation mode.

Postoperative bleeding

The harvest sites for radial arteries or saphenous veins are uncommon sources of significant blood loss and are generally easily managed with dressings or compression. Intrathoracic bleeding, however, may be torrential and threaten life. Occasionally, surgical bleeding from the aorta, arterial grafts or myomectomy sites may exceed replacement capabilities, and at times patients succumb to overwhelming haemorrhage. Maintenance of drain patency and strict recording of losses and total fluid balance are paramount, and fluid balance assessments over shorter intervals, even every 5–10 minutes, become necessary during active bleeding. Because of the potential rates of bleeding, the cardiac surgical unit must be equipped to institute rapid volume replacement, and have access to adequate blood and blood product stores, blood warmers and all necessary procoagulant therapies. In addition, dedicated equipment should be available to facilitate emergency resternotomy to control haemorrhage.

One or more chest drains are inserted to remove and monitor blood loss, but the positioning of drains is variable, depending in part on the procedure performed, the surgical route taken and surgeon preference. Regardless of these considerations there will always be a retrosternal/anterior mediastinal drain, as the sternum is generally the major source of bleeding in the absence of complications. Additional drains may be inserted in the pericardial or pleural spaces. Pericardial drains are more likely to be inserted following aortic valve surgery, whereas pleural drains become necessary following mammary artery harvesting or when the pleura is opened for any other reason. Pleural drains may be anterior, posterior or 'wrap-around' configurations in which they project over the anterior lung, following the pleural space first from midline to lateral and then, finally, the posterior pleural space.

Reportable postoperative blood losses vary, but greater than 100 mL/h, or greater than 400 mL in the first 4 hours, would generally be regarded as excessive and worthy of surgeon notification. Importantly, excessive bleeding does not always represent a surgical defect that reoperation might correct, as there are many contributors to impaired haemostatic capability in the cardiac surgical patient (see below).

Chest drainage should be monitored closely and, while bleeding is active, volumes should be assessed every 5 minutes and patency of drains ensured to avert tamponade. Sudden cessation of drainage should always raise the possibility of the loss of tube patency and risk of tamponade, but tamponade may also occur while drainage continues, as collections and compressions may occur at sites isolated from drains, or losses may simply be occurring faster than that able to be removed by patent drains.

Chest drains should also be observed for bubbling, to assess for air leaks originating from either system faults or patient leaks. When bubbling can be attributed to the patient, the patency of tubes becomes additionally important to avert tension pneumothorax, which may accumulate rapidly, even over the course of a few breaths in the ventilated patient.

Blood transfusions are not aimed at restoring haemoglobin to normal levels and, despite variations in acceptable levels, relative anaemia is almost universally tolerated. Haemoglobin levels are thus not routinely treated unless below 80 g/L, except in the elderly or when there are significant comorbidities.[43,44] From these levels patients return to normal haemoglobin status within 1 month postoperatively.[43,44]

Contributors to impaired haemostatic capability

Many factors may contribute to postoperative bleeding by their influence on coagulation and haemostatic ability. CPB is used in the majority of cardiac surgical cases and exerts many influences on coagulation, as do additional factors such as preoperative medications, anaemia or coagulopathies. Contributing factors include:

- cardiopulmonary bypass influences:
  - heparinisation, haemodilution, platelet damage and altered function
  - disseminated intravascular coagulation (DIC) following activation of the systemic inflammatory response syndrome post-CPB
- preoperative anticoagulant/antiplatelet medications commonly encountered
- aspirin, warfarin, clopidogrel
- preoperative anaemia due to aortic valve disease, autologous blood donation or the various chronic anaemias
- clotting factor deficiency
- hypothermia
- coexisting coagulopathies
- increased fibrinolytic activity
- surgical defects such as failure of access site closure, or vascular anastomosis defects.

Bedside assessment of bleeding

The activated clotting time (ACT) is the most commonly used assessment of coagulation and heparin activity during cardiac surgery and subsequently in intensive care. It measures the time to onset of fibrin formation (initial clot development). The ACT has been valuable because it can be inexpensively and efficiently performed at the bedside, providing prompt results and requiring only modest personnel training. Bleeding patients with a prolonged ACT come under consideration for administration of

protamine or other agents.[45,46] Treatable levels vary from greater than 120 s to greater than 150 s among different centres.

A limitation of ACT measurements is that they provide no information about clotting processes beyond initial fibrin formation, so clotting deficits such as impaired clot strength or the presence of significant fibrinolysis as contributors to bleeding are not revealed by this test.[47] By contrast, the thromboelastograph (TEG) measures the clotting process as it proceeds over time.[47] TEG monitoring not only reveals abnormalities early in the clot process (time to fibrin formation, as would be demonstrated by the ACT) but also the subsequent development of clot strength, clot retraction and, finally, fibrinolytic activity for each of their contributions in the bleeding patient.[47] TEG monitoring, although considerably more expensive than the ACT, is now available as a bedside or operating room technology and offers better insight into bleeding causes. In addition, because TEG monitoring identifies deficiencies at the various stages of clot formation, development of clot strength and the presence of undue fibrinolytic activity, it may permit better matching of procoagulant, blood product or antifibrinolytic therapy to needs.[47]

No matter which of the above technologies is used at the bedside, the patient with significant bleeding should be evaluated more fully as soon as bleeding develops. Blood should be drawn and sent for laboratory assessment, including full blood examination, clotting profile and measures of fibrinolytic activity.

Heparin reversal

Cardiopulmonary bypass requires full heparinisation (initially 300 IU/kg), which is reversed at end-operation.[45,47] The specific antidote, protamine sulfate, is administered as bypass is ceased, at a dose of 1 mg per 100 IU heparin used (i.e. 3 mg/kg).[45] If reversal is less than complete, as evidenced by a prolonged ACT, further protamine sulfate (at doses of 25–50 mg over 5–10 minutes) may be necessary.

Management of bleeding

Treatment approaches to bleeding once the patient is in intensive care include further protamine administration if the ACT remains prolonged, blood and blood product administration (platelets, clotting factors, fresh frozen plasma), procoagulants (desmopressin acetate [DDAVP]) and antifibrinolytic agents (see Table 12.3 for more details). Other general measures such as rewarming the patient and preventing or treating hypertension should be undertaken.

Autotransfusion

Chest drain systems used in cardiothoracic surgery can be configured for retransfusion of collected blood during rapid blood loss. If losses are fresh, and are collected with reliable sterility, they can be transfused back into the patient. Blood that has been collected and left standing in the drain receptacle rapidly becomes unsuitable for retransfusion, and so autotransfusion is generally limited

TABLE 12.3

Management of the bleeding patient post cardiac surgery[21,33,43,44,48]

THERAPY	DOSE	COMMENTS / ISSUES
Protamine sulfate	25–50 mg slow IV (<10 mg/min); may be repeated if ACT prolonged	Specific antidote to heparin. May cause hypotension. Contraindicated in patient with seafood allergy
Aprotinin (Trasylol)	Continuous infusion of 2 million units over 30 min, then 500,000 units per hour	Antifibrinolytic. Proteinaceous. Anaphylaxis risk on re-exposure. Alert should be posted on history
Desmopressin acetate (DDAVP)	0.4 mcg/kg IV	Promotes factor VIII release; limited evidence for use
'Pump blood' (blood retrieved from bypass circuit at end-operation)	Often 400–800 mL	This is the remaining blood in bypass circuit; usually centrifuged before returning to patient *Note*: this blood contains heparin from CPB
Whole blood/packed cells	As necessary to achieve Hb >80 g/L or more, according to needs	Autologous blood sometimes available when patients have donated blood preoperatively
Fresh frozen plasma	As necessary	'Broad-spectrum' factor replacement; contains most factors. Useful adjunct to massive blood transfusion
Platelet concentrates	As necessary	Generally ABO and Rh compatible preferred
Epsilon-aminocaproic acid (Amicar)	100 mg/kg IV followed by 1–2 g/h	Antifibrinolytic. Inhibits plasminogen activation
Cryoprecipitate	10 units IV	Contains factor VIII and fibrinogen (factor I)
Calcium chloride or gluconate	10 mL 10% solution	Used to offset citrate binding of calcium in stored blood
Prothrombinex	20–50 IU/kg IV	Contains factors II, IX and X

ACT = activated clotting time; CPB = cardiopulmonary bypass.

Adapted from (with permission):
St Andre AC, DelRossi A. Hemodynamic management of patients in the first 24 hours after cardiac surgery. Crit Care Med 2005;33(9):2082–93.
Albright TN, Zimmerman MA, Selzman CH. Vasopressin in the cardiac surgery intensive care unit. Am J Crit Care 2002;11(4):326–30.
Galas F, Almeida JP, Fukushima JT, Osawa EA, Nakamura RE, Silva C et al. Blood transfusion in cardiac surgery is a risk factor for increased hospital length of stay in adult patients. J Cardiothorac Surg 2013;8(54):1–7.
Hajjar LA, Vincent J, Galas FRBG, Nakamura RE, Silva CMP, Santos MH et al. TRACS randomized controlled trial transfusion requirements after cardiac surgery. JAMA 2010;304(14):1559–67.
Bryant B, Knights K, Salerno E. Pharmacology for health professionals. Sydney: Mosby; 2003.

to blood that has collected over 1–2 hours, rarely longer. Blood filters should always be used for protection against clots that may have developed in the drain receptacle.

Pericardial tamponade

Postoperative pericardial tamponade results from the accumulation of blood or effusion fluid within the pericardium. An increasing volume within the pericardial space eventually compresses cardiac chambers, impeding venous return and therefore causing low cardiac output and hypotension. Pericardial tamponade is an emergency, and varies in severity from shock to pulseless electrical activity.[29,49]

Described as one of the extra-cardiac obstructive shocks, pericardial tamponade often resembles cardiogenic shock. The low cardiac output and hypotension result in oliguria, altered mentation, peripheral hypoperfusion and development of lactic acidosis. Compensation includes tachycardia and marked vasoconstriction, elevating the systemic vascular resistance. As in cardiogenic shock, there is usually elevation of the filling pressures (right atrial, pulmonary artery and pulmonary capillary wedge pressures), sometimes with a particularly suggestive merging of the pulmonary artery diastolic, right atrial and pulmonary artery wedge pressures.[29,49] Additional features that may be present include muffled heart sounds, decreased QRS voltage, electrical alternans, narrowing pulse pressure and pulsus paradoxus, along with features of increasing anxiety and/or dyspnoea in the awake patient.

Echocardiography is the definitive assessment tool to reveal the presence of pericardial collections as well as identifying the impact on relaxation, filling and contraction of each cardiac chamber. The chest X-ray is of limited use and may show little, even with significant pericardial collections.

Importantly, the 'classic' or typical haemodynamic profile described above is not uniformly seen in tamponade, and tamponade should never be excluded because the haemodynamic status does not match this profile. This may be because classic tamponade implies uniform compression of the entire heart, which may not be the case with haemorrhagic tamponade. A clot may develop over just one chamber rather than occupying the entire pericardium, and so there may be compromise to only a single chamber rather than the whole heart.[29,49]

Management of pericardial tamponade

The management of pericardial tamponade includes limiting further losses into the pericardium, relief of pericardial pressure through evacuation of blood or clots and management of the haemodynamic impact of tamponade.

Steps to control bleeding and blood pressure as described above may limit further losses into the pericardium. All steps should be taken to maintain or re-establish chest tube patency (crushing clots within tubing, 'milking' when it is truly necessary) and to ensure free flow of blood from the chest by avoiding dependent tubing loops or by instigating side-to-side rolling of the patient to possibly bring collections into proximity of drain tubes. When tube patency is in doubt, the surgeon may even pass a suction catheter through the chest drain under aseptic conditions in an attempt to remove clots at the drain tip.[29,49] If the above measures do not relieve tamponade, consideration is given to re-exploring the pericardium, either by returning to the operating theatre or, in an emergency, to the intensive care unit, although this is less preferable.

Emergency opening of the sternotomy and mediastinal re-exploration requires a coordinated team response and, where possible, operating room staff should be included to manage the sterile field and assist the surgeon. Equipment and disposable materials should be counted and documented in the manner normally applied in theatre. When the situation has been stabilised, consideration should be given to returning to theatre for final assessment and chest closure.[29,49]

> **Practice tip**
>
> Given the variability of presentation of cardiogenic shock, and the importance of accurate identification, clinicians should search for tamponade whenever there is haemodynamic instability postoperatively, especially when the haemodynamic status does not match classic patterns for the major shock states. The management of postoperative cardiac arrest accompanying any arrhythmia, as well as pulseless electrical activity, should include consideration of tamponade.

Assessment and management of postoperative pain

As much an art as a science, pain control in the cardiac surgical patient remains a major challenge and continues to provide uncertainty and opportunities for nursing clinicians and researchers. Principles are similar to those outlined in Chapter 7. Surgical pain is often complicated by pericardial inflammation and pain management must be balanced against the promotion of spontaneous breathing, chest physiotherapy, mobilisation and participation in education and lifestyle modification programs.

Analgesic options for pain control include intravenous, oral or rectal analgesics, non-steroidal anti-inflammatory medications and, less commonly, epidural therapies and nerve blocks. Intravenous opiates and codeine/paracetamol preparations provide the mainstay of postoperative analgesia. When insufficient, or when clinical and electrocardiographic features suggest pericarditis, non-steroidal anti-inflammatory drugs such as rectal indomethacin are appropriate, except in patients with renal impairment due to their renal side effects of reducing glomerular filtration rate and acute deterioration of renal function.[50] The place of IV COX-2 inhibitors such as parecoxib appears uncertain, as analgesic efficacy now must be weighed against emerging data suggesting increased thrombotic complications.[51]

Fluid and electrolyte management

Fluid therapy in the postoperative period is aimed at maintaining blood volume, replacing recorded and insensible losses and providing adequate preload to sustain haemodynamic status. Isotonic dextrose solutions (5%) or dextrose 4% + saline 0.18% are commonly used at approximately 1.5 L/day as maintenance fluids.[21,23]

Potassium replenishment is generally necessary according to measured serum potassium. Polyuria is usually evident in the early postoperative period due to deliberate haemodilution while on cardiopulmonary bypass. With polyuria comes potassium loss, which must be treated to avert atrial or ventricular ectopy and tachyarrhythmias. Because of these predictable potassium losses, protocols for potassium replacement may be instituted, with standing orders for potassium replacement (e.g. 10 mmol over 1 hour if the serum potassium is <4.5 mmol/L, or 20 mmol over 2 hours if <4.0 mmol/L). Main line hydration infusions may also have added potassium to avoid hypokalaemia. Hypomagnesaemia may also develop due to polyuria, and is likewise proarrhythmic. Supplementation (magnesium chloride) is often used for arrhythmia management postoperatively, but its effectiveness has been questioned in many trials.[52]

Hyperkalaemia occurs less often but is seen particularly when there is impaired renal function. Additional contributors to a rising potassium level include acidosis, administration of stored blood, haemolysis, inotrope use and any postoperative use of depolarising muscle relaxants such as suxamethonium.

Emotional responses and family support

The experience of being diagnosed with a cardiac disorder, waiting for surgery, the surgical experience and recovery is an emotional journey for patients and their families. Regardless of low mortality rates, the possibility of death and painful wounds can concern patients. Consequently, patients undergoing cardiac surgery often experience anxiety and depression,[53,54] and women appear to be more vulnerable to these emotions in relation to cardiac surgery than men.[55] In addition, the same levels of anxiety, depression and stress have been experienced by patients' spouses but significantly reduce over time in both patients and their families. It has been suggested that providing appropriate information about the procedures to both patients and their spouses will assist them to deal better with their psychological state in the recovery period.[56]

Similarly, adequate preparation of the patient and their family in the preoperative period will assist them with their stress and anxiety coping strategies as well as reduce their work stress after their return to work.[57] The preoperative preparation is usually provided by nurses and should incorporate information and support about the procedures and recovery period, so that patients and their families are better equipped during their recovery. Emphasis should be on identifying the intrapersonal stressors, such as pain and discomfort, invasive lines and surgical procedures, for individual patients to assist them coping with their perioperative and rehabilitation period.[58] However, patients who have had their surgery postponed or who have been operated on in an emergency setting may need additional support. Also, critical pathways for cardiac surgery do not include assessing the patient's psychological state, so nurses must take care to consider this aspect. Printed information regarding the surgery, recovery and emotions will be useful for the patient and family (for further information refer to Chapter 7, *Psychological care*, and Chapter 8, *Family and cultural care of the critically ill patient*).

Intra-aortic balloon pumping

Intra-aortic balloon pumping (IABP) is a widely-used circulatory assist therapy that has become straightforward in application and relatively free of complications.[59–61] The primary aim of IABP is to assist repairing an existing imbalance between myocardial oxygen supply and demand. The main indications are for cardiogenic shock, myocardial infarction or ischaemia, haemodynamic support for PCI and weaning from cardiopulmonary bypass. The combined effects of increasing cardiac output and mean arterial pressure (increasing oxygen supply) and decreasing myocardial workload (reducing oxygen demand) make IABP therapy ideal for the management of infarct-related cardiogenic shock,[62,63] for which it should be regarded as standard management.

IABP therapy involves placement of a balloon catheter in the descending thoracic aorta. This catheter is most commonly advanced from a percutaneous femoral artery access until the tip of the catheter is situated just below the left subclavian artery (Figure 12.4). A chest X-ray or fluoroscopy should reveal the catheter tip just below the

FIGURE 12.4 Intra-aortic balloon catheter. On the left the inflated catheter can be seen behind the heart, with its tip below the arch of the aorta and the left subclavian artery. The balloon cycles between inflated (during diastole), and deflated (during systole) as on the right. Blood fills the aorta while the balloon is deflated, and with inflation the balloon almost fills the descending aorta, displacing 40 mL blood from the aorta to the coronary and systemic circulation.

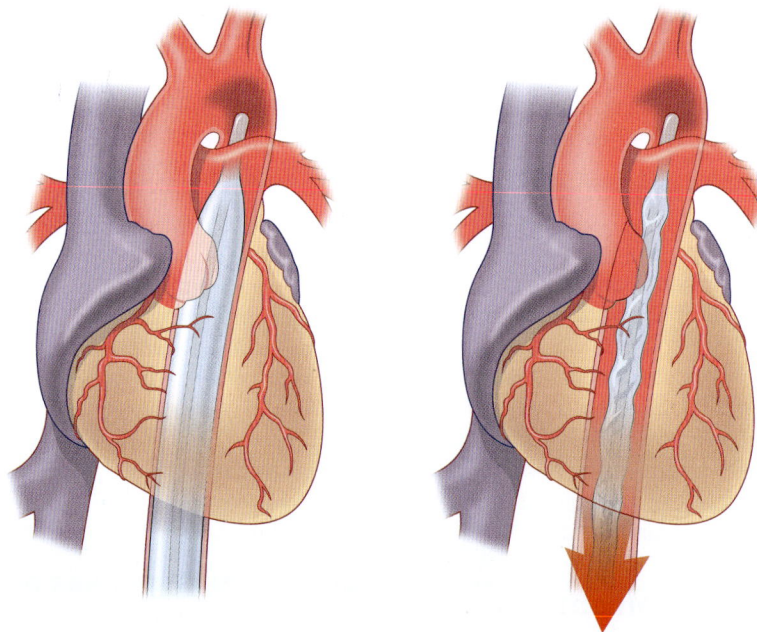

Published with permission from Datascope Corporation, Fairfield, NJ, USA.

FIGURE 12.5 IABP catheter position in CXR; the tip is located in the 2nd intercostal space anterior ribs or 5th intercostal space posterior ribs.

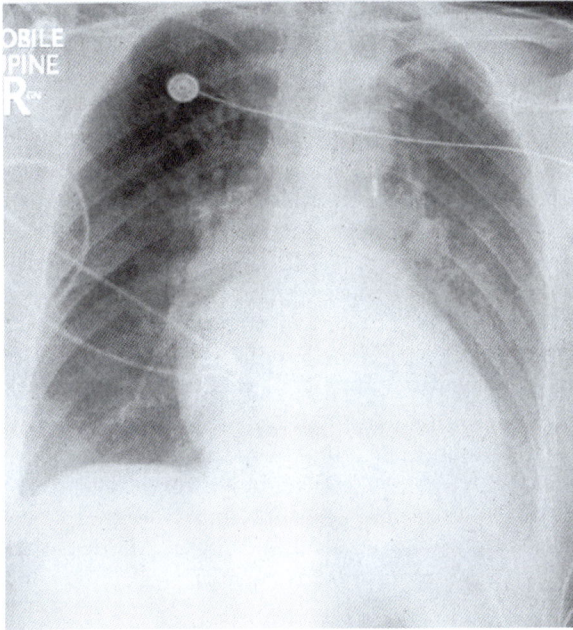

aortic arch, or at the level of the second anterior intercostal space or fifth posterior intercostal space (Figure 12.5). The catheter has two lumens: a monitoring lumen, which opens at the catheter tip from which the aortic pressure waveform is monitored; and a helium drive lumen, through which the helium is shuttled from the pumping console to the catheter balloon. Balloon volumes range from 25 mL (paediatric use) to 34–50 mL in adults (most commonly used is a 40-mL balloon) and are selected according to patient height (e.g. a 40-mL balloon is used for a patient height of 162–183 cm).

Principles of counterpulsation

When intra-aortic balloon pumping is initiated, the balloon will be inflated rapidly at the onset of diastole of each cardiac cycle and then deflated immediately just before the onset of the next systole; this sequence is referred to as counterpulsation.

Balloon inflation

At the onset of diastole, the balloon is rapidly inflated with (most commonly) 40 mL of helium. This inflation causes a sudden rise in pressure in the aortic root during diastole, raising mean arterial pressure and, importantly, coronary perfusion pressure. The blood displaced by the balloon expansion improves blood flow into the coronary circulation (which fills largely during diastole), as well as to the brain and systemic circulation. Thus there is improved myocardial oxygen supply and increased mean arterial pressure, as well as improved systemic perfusion.[6,64] The balloon remains inflated for the duration of diastole. The arterial pressure wave should reveal a sharp rise in pressure at the dicrotic notch, with a second pressure peak now appearing on the waveform, described as the 'augmented diastolic' or 'balloon-assisted peak diastolic' pressure. This peak is usually at least 10 mmHg higher than the systolic pressure (Figure 12.6).

Balloon deflation

As the inflated balloon largely obstructs the aorta, it must be deflated to permit systolic emptying of the left ventricle. Two separate approaches to the timing of balloon deflation have emerged: 'conventional timing' and 'real timing'.

Conventional timing

In conventional timing, the balloon is deflated immediately prior to systole. Rapid deflation induces a precipitous drop in aortic pressure at the end of diastole (a reduced aortic end-diastolic pressure). This reduces the duration of the left ventricle isovolumetric contraction phase of

FIGURE 12.6 IABP during 1:1 assist (counterpulsation on every beat). Balloon inflation at the start of diastole and deflation just before the next systole. IABP during 1:2 assist (counterpulsation on every second beat). Inflation of the balloon rapidly at the inflation point (IP) raises diastolic pressure, producing a peak diastolic pressure (PDP) that exceeds the peak systolic pressure (PSP). The balloon remains inflated during diastole. With balloon deflation just prior to the next systole there is a rapid decline in pressure to the balloon assisted end-diastolic pressure (BAEDP), which is lower than normal non-assisted end-diastolic pressure (EDP), reducing afterload. The ensuing systole is achieved with a reduced systolic pressure (the assisted peak systolic pressure, APSP).

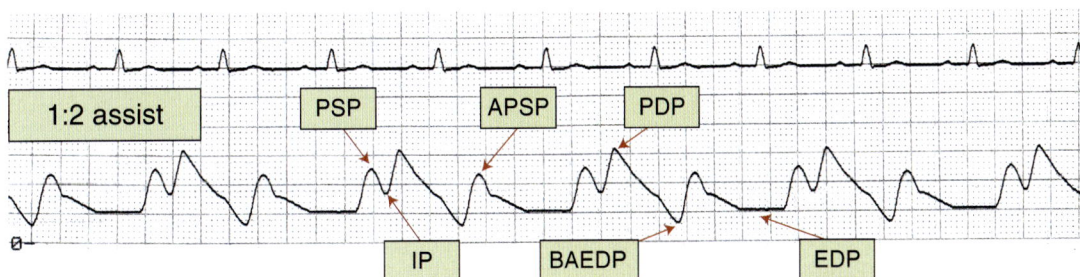

the cardiac cycle (most oxygen-consuming phase of the cardiac cycle), reduces the left ventricular afterload and improves left ventricular emptying, improving stroke volume and cardiac output.[6,64] In addition, less pressure is required for left ventricular emptying, so systolic work and oxygen demands on the myocardium are reduced.[6] Thus, deflation during conventional timing should see the aortic pressure drop to below normal at end-diastole, just in advance of the subsequent systole. Systolic pressure should also be lower than during a non-assisted beat.

Real timing

In contrast to conventional timing, during real timing (also referred to as R wave deflate) the balloon remains inflated for slightly longer, and is deflated not before but at the same time as systole. The reduction in aortic end-diastolic pressure is therefore not seen, but deflating simultaneously with left ventricular contraction still favourably affects left ventricular emptying.[65] Thus, there is improved stroke volume, systolic pressure reduction and decreased ventricular work and oxygen demand as seen during conventional timing.[6,65] Box 12.1 summarises the impact of balloon inflation and deflation on haemodynamic status and the oxygen supply/demand balance.

The arterial pressure wave reveals the impact of IABP therapy on haemodynamic status. Placing the pump into 1:2 assist (balloon pumping on only every second beat) is useful to highlight balloon pump impact and how assisted beats vary from the normal pressure cycle during systole and diastole. Figure 12.6 depicts the impact of IABP on haemodynamic status and the arterial pressure waveform.

BOX 12.1

Effects of intra-aortic balloon counterpulsation

- Balloon inflation:
  - increased aortic diastolic pressure (augmented, or balloon-assisted peak diastolic pressure, balloon aortic end diastolic pressure [BAEDP])
  - increased mean arterial pressure
  - increased myocardial perfusion and oxygen supply
  - increased cerebral and systemic perfusion
- Balloon deflation:
  - decreased afterload
  - increased stroke volume and cardiac output
  - decreased LV congestion, decreased PCWP, decreased pulmonary congestion
  - decreased left ventricular workload
  - decreased systolic pressure
  - decreased myocardial oxygen demand
  - decreased duration of isovolumetric contraction

Complications of intra-aortic balloon pumping

Serious complications are uncommon during IABP treatment and continued to decrease in frequency during the past decade with advances in pump technology and the advent of smaller catheter sizes.[66] Limb ischaemia remains the most common serious complication, especially in patients with existing vasculopathy,[67] providing impetus to the development of smaller catheters, which have now reached 7.5 French gauge. Additional complications, such as bleeding, catheter migration, thromboembolism, insertion-site vascular damage, thrombocytopenia and device-related problems such as timing inaccuracy, device failure and gas leaks, also occur but are less common. These are described below.

Patient management

Prevention of complications, as well as optimisation of the impact of counterpulsation, form the major components of nursing care of a patient being treated with IABP. Thorough understanding of the impact of the presence of the balloon, as well as the beneficial and detrimental effects of counterpulsation, is essential.

Maintenance of limb perfusion

The use of smaller-gauge catheters has reduced the potential for obstruction of arterial flow past the catheter to the lower limbs, as has the trend to sheathless insertion. Nevertheless, the threat of limb ischaemia remains an important issue in patient care, as IABP is most commonly undertaken in patients with atherosclerosis, potentially involving the lower limbs, even in the absence of overt peripheral vascular deficits. Identification of patients at risk (known claudication, chronically cold feet and peripheral vascular diseases) may be useful to ensure appropriate vigilance and prompt intervention where necessary. Peripheral perfusion may also be compromised by arterial embolisation should thrombi develop on the catheter. Although catheter materials are non-thrombogenic, the risk of thrombi formation remains and is heightened if periods of catheter stasis (interrupted pumping) are encountered. Systemic heparinisation is not recommended routinely for thromboembolic prevention as it increases the risk of bleeding except for specific indications.[68]

Hourly assessments of peripheral perfusion (colour, warmth, movement, sensation) should be performed to identify potential deficits. Dorsalis pedis and posterior tibialis pulses should be palpated and may sometimes require examination with a Doppler probe. Deficits should be promptly reported and consideration given to catheter removal or reinsertion on the contralateral limb. When pulses cannot be demonstrated, the limb should be assessed for the development of compartment syndrome. At times, the viability of a limb must be weighed against the potential survival benefit of IABP to the patient.

Prevention and treatment of bleeding

Significant bleeding is uncommon,[51] but blood loss may occur from the femoral arterial access site. In addition to physical factors at the insertion site, contributors to bleeding include heparinisation, thrombocytopenia from the physical effect of the pump on platelets and/or other anticoagulants or antiplatelet agents used for the primary disease. Regular observation should be made of the insertion site for bruising or external bleeding, as well as other possible sites of bleeding due to heparinisation. Treatment includes manual pressure at the insertion site or use of compression devices such as FemoStop, reinforcement of dressings and/or topical procoagulant agents. Monitoring of coagulation status and haemoglobin should be undertaken and blood or blood products may (uncommonly) be required.

Prevention of immobility-related complications

The need for immobilisation of the patient, and in particular the leg, is often overemphasised, and may heighten the risk of atelectasis, pressure area development and venous stasis and thrombosis. Sensible limitation of leg movement is advised, but patients can generally still move in bed, and should still be turned 2-hourly for pressure relief as long as the insertion site is adequately protected and supported. The femoral access limits flexion at the hip beyond 30°, which may also hamper effective chest physiotherapy and increase the risk of atelectasis and pneumonia.

Migration of the balloon catheter towards the aortic arch or towards the abdominal aorta may cause compromised perfusion to the left arm (occlusion of left subclavian artery), kidneys (renal arteries) or abdominal viscera (superior mesenteric artery). Therefore, neurovascular observation of the upper limbs, urine output and bowel sounds are part of nursing management of the patient with IABP in situ.

Weaning of IABP

Weaning of intra-aortic balloon pumping therapy is generally undertaken once the patient has stabilised, is free of ischaemic signs and symptoms and is on minimum or no inotropic support. Algorithms have been offered for approaches to weaning therapy, with no haemodynamic or mortality benefit.[69] Weaning is carried out by either gradual reductions in balloon inflation volume (volume weaning) or gradual reductions in assist frequency from 1:1 through 1:2 and 1:4 (ratio weaning). Hybrids of the two approaches are sometimes used. Support is reduced at intervals while the patient is observed for haemodynamic deterioration, pulmonary congestion and the return of ischaemic signs and symptoms.

Assessment of timing and timing errors

Accurate timing of inflation and deflation in relation to the cardiac cycle is required to maximise IABP benefit. Errors in timing may lessen the potential benefit, or in some cases may worsen cardiac performance and increase demands on the myocardium. Nurses are required to continually assess the haemodynamic impact of balloon pumping and the accuracy of timing via inspection of the arterial pressure waveform, and to adjust timing to optimise the impact of balloon pumping. The development of automated IABP counterpulsation has reduced timing errors by automatic trigger signal recognition and selection, accuracy of automatic setting for optimal inflation and deflation timing and automatic adjustment to changing patient conditions. Therefore the automated mode of counterpulsation is recommended.[70,71]

Early inflation

Early inflation will at times be difficult to differentiate from correct inflation timing but is recognised by the onset of inflation soon after the peak systolic pressure, before the pressure has declined to the level of the dicrotic notch (Figure 12.7). Early inflation may limit the stroke volume and cardiac output, as terminal systole is impeded, and may result in increased myocardial oxygen demands, increased left ventricle workload and premature valve closure. The inflation point should be adjusted (to later) until the inflation upstroke emerges smoothly out of the dicrotic notch.

Late inflation

The arterial pressure waveform reveals the onset of diastole (the dicrotic notch) before balloon inflation commences (Figure 12.8). This generally results in a lower augmented diastolic pressure than could otherwise be achieved. As the duration of balloon inflation is lessened, the desired rise in mean arterial pressure and coronary perfusion will not

FIGURE 12.7 IABP during 1:2 assist. Early inflation. The inflation point (IP) can be seen high in the downstroke of systole, in this case well before the dicrotic notch (DN).

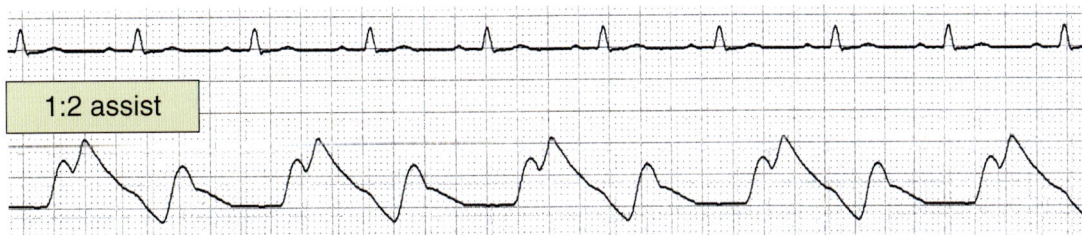

1:2 assist

FIGURE 12.8 IABP during 1:2 assist. Late inflation. Note that the inflation point (IP) occurs well after the dicrotic notch (DN). Late inflation is also obvious in 1:1 assist with balloon inflation well after the dicrotic notch.

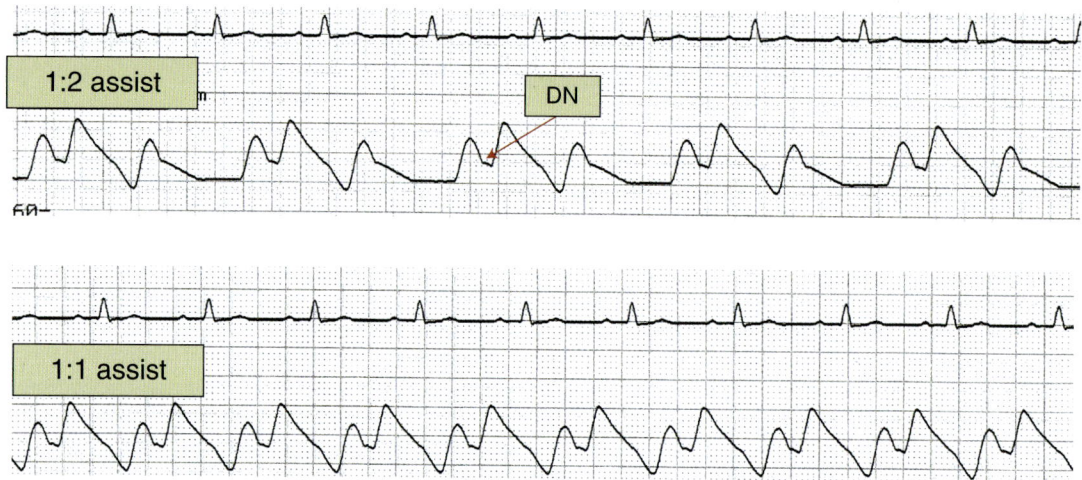

be achieved. The inflation marker should be set to 'earlier' until the inflation upstroke emerges smoothly out of the dicrotic notch.

Early deflation

Deflating the balloon earlier than necessary shortens the duration for which the balloon remains inflated and therefore limits the benefit of IABP. When deflation is very early, it may cause harm. Deflation sees the aortic pressure drop markedly but there is now time for blood to fill the space left by the balloon before systole commences. Aortic end-diastolic pressure increases and may even

exceed the normal end-diastolic pressure, increasing the duration of the isovolumetric phase, worsening left ventricular afterload and increasing myocardial oxygen demand (Figure 12.9). Correction is achieved by setting deflation to later until the pressure drop of deflation occurs just in advance of the succeeding systole.

Late deflation

When deflation begins too late, systole commences before complete emptying of the intra-aortic balloon. The typical reduction of aortic end-diastolic pressure is not seen. When significantly late, the end-diastolic pressure may even be

FIGURE 12.9 IABP during 1:2 assist. Early deflation. The balloon has been deflated well in advance of the subsequent systole. The aortic pressure does drop off (not much from non-assisted diastole) but then begins to rise again before the next systole gets underway, and may even exceed the normal end-diastolic pressure. Early deflation is also obvious in 1:1 assist.

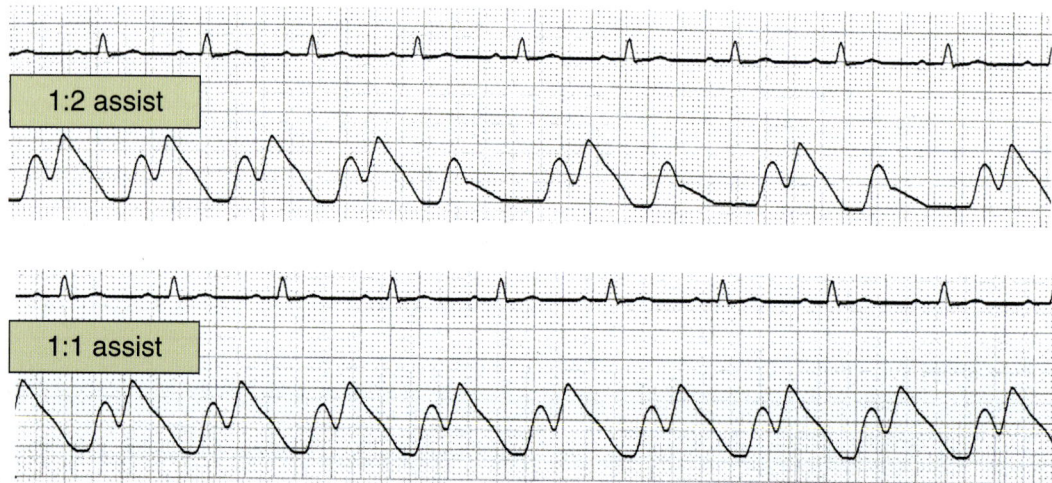

increased, prolonging the duration of the isovolumetric contraction phase and worsening afterload. As systole occurs against an incompletely deflated balloon, the stroke volume and cardiac output suffer and ventricular work and oxygen demand increase (Figure 12.10). Deflation should be set to earlier until the systolic upstroke emerges out of the reduced end–diastolic pressure dip.

Alarm states

Alarm functions vary according to manufacturer and model. The main alarm states common to most devices, and their causes and significance, are shown in Table 12.4. Importantly, in most alarm states the pump consoles will revert to standby, suspending pumping. The balloon is at risk of developing thrombi within the folds of

FIGURE 12.10   IABP during 1:2 assist. Late deflation. The late deflation is seen here as the sharp drop-off before systole and a balloon assisted end-diastole that does not fall to below the normal patient end-diastolic pressure.

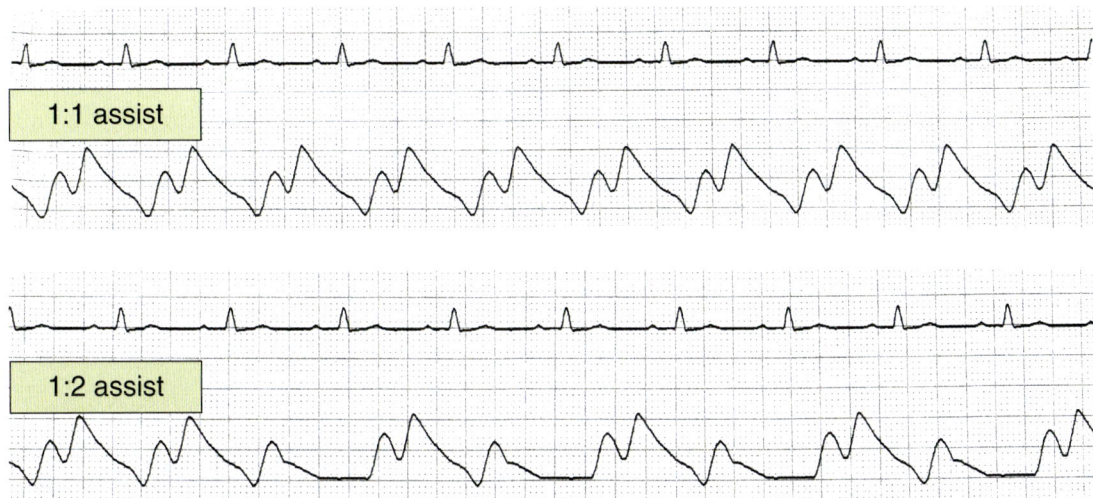

TABLE 12.4

Intra-aortic balloon pump alarm states

ALARM STATE	CAUSES / SIGNIFICANCE
Catheter alarm	Obstruction (complete or subtotal) of the catheter, drive line or balloon Device reverts to standby (non-assist); commonly due to catheter flexion at insertion site due to limb position or excessive surface-to-vessel depth
Loss of trigger	ECG trigger: signal disrupted or low in amplitude, or asystole Pressure trigger: pulse pressure below threshold for detection Pacer trigger: pacing spikes not detected or absent (including demand pacing) Device reverts to standby until restoration of trigger; alternative trigger selection may be necessary
Gas loss alarms	Leak in circuit/drive line or balloon; gas leak may be to the environment or into the patient as a helium embolus Pump reverts to standby; refilling of circuit may be necessary
Low augmentation	Augmented diastolic pressure is lower than operator-selected alarm level; pumping is not interrupted
Pneumatic drive	Functional problem with the pump inflation/deflation pneumatic system Device reverts to standby; alarm may sometimes be activated during tachycardia; 1:2 assist or assist at reduced augmentation may be possible until a replacement device is accessed
Autofill failure	Routine 2-hourly refilling of the system with helium may fail if gas tank is incompletely open or if circuit leaks cause volume loss during the filling attempt Device reverts to standby
System failure	Console self-testing has identified component malfunction Device reverts to standby; restarting may be possible but a replacement device should be accessed
Low helium supply	Helium tank empty or incompletely opened
Low battery	Reconnect to power and recharge

the balloon while deflated, and these can be liberated as arterial emboli on recommencement of pumping. Therefore, it is important to treat alarm states promptly, to limit the duration of balloon stasis. If interruption to pumping is prolonged, intermittent manual inflation of the balloon with a syringe is recommended (e.g. once every 5–10 minutes).

Gas loss alarms

Most devices will determine the severity of gas losses and classify them as slow, rapid or disconnect. In all gas loss states it is imperative that assessments be made to exclude balloon rupture and helium leak into the arterial circulation. Small gas losses of helium may or may not be of clinical significance, but the delivery of sizeable helium volumes may behave as gas emboli and, if delivered into the coronary circulation, may result in lethal arrhythmias or neurological complications if delivered into the cerebral circulation.[59] In all gas loss alarm states, the helium drive line should be inspected for the presence of blood to indicate loss of integrity of the balloon. If blood is present in the drive line (Figure 12.11), pumping should be suspended and no attempts at recommencing balloon pumping should be made. Prompt removal and/ or replacement, along with thorough patient assessment, is essential.

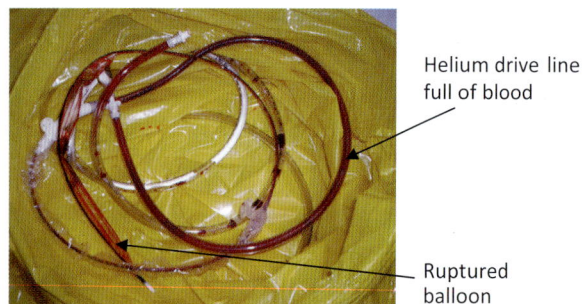

FIGURE 12.11 Intra-aortic balloon rupture and presence of blood in the helium drive line.

Helium drive line full of blood

Ruptured balloon

Heart transplantation

The ultimate goal of organ transplantation is to provide an improved quality of life and long-term survival for patients with end-stage heart disease. To optimise patient outcomes, the early postoperative management of these patients requires critical care clinicians with specific expertise to collaborate with a multidisciplinary team of health professionals. In the following sections, the important management issues in the early postoperative period for heart transplant recipients are discussed. The major long-term complications of heart transplantation are also discussed briefly as survivors may be readmitted to critical care with life-threatening complications years after their transplant.

Patients with certain chronic heart, respiratory and lung diseases may be referred for organ transplantation assessment when their disease state is such that their life expectancy is less than 2 years and quality of life intolerable. Patients who receive organ transplants are commonly debilitated and may have an acute on chronic presentation at the time of surgery. The surgical procedure is lengthy, up to 12 hours, and involves cardiopulmonary bypass. The duration and nature of the surgery in patients with severely compromised health status serve to compound the often critical condition of such patients in the early postoperative period.

The immediate period following surgery is commonly the first contact that critical care clinicians have with transplant recipients and their families. The exception may be patients awaiting heart transplantation who are supported by an intra-aortic balloon pump or mechanical circulatory support, also known as a ventricular assist device (VAD), as a 'bridge to transplantation' (see Figure 12.12). Ideally, patients with mechanical circulatory support are returned to a sound physical, mental and nutritional state prior to receiving a transplant and, as part of their recovery, await transplantation in the ward or home setting. For specific management of patients on mechanical circulatory support, readers are referred to specific resources (e.g. websites and operating manuals for individual mechanical circulatory support devices: HeartWare, Thoratec and SynCardia).

Heart transplantation is a life-saving and cost-effective form of treatment that enhances the quality of life for many people with chronic heart failure. Legislation that defined brain death and enabled beating-heart retrieval was enacted in Australia from 1982. This legislation heralded the establishment of formal transplant programs. In Australia, the first heart program commenced in 1983.[72,73] The success of transplantation in the current era as a viable option for end-stage organ failure is primarily due to the discovery of the immunosuppressive agent cyclosporin A.[74] In this section, heart transplantation as a component of critical care nursing is discussed, with reference to evidence-based practices.

History

Heart transplant surgery for refractory heart failure was first performed in Australia in 1968, only months after the first heart transplant was performed in South Africa in December 1967.[75] However, high mortality rates associated with severe acute rejection and infection within months of surgery led to a reduction in the number of heart transplants performed worldwide, and in effect a moratorium occurred with the procedure. Heart transplantation was finally established in the modern era as a viable treatment option for end-stage heart failure during the early 1980s when cyclosporin A, a then-novel immunosuppressive agent, dramatically improved patients' survival rates by reducing episodes of acute rejection and lowering attendant infectious complications.[76]

FIGURE 12.12 Pump, monitor and controller. (**A**) HeartWareImplanted HVAD® Pump. (**B**) HeartWare® Monitor with HeartWare® Controller and HeartWare® Batteries. (**C**) ThoratecHeartMate II (**A**) and (**B**) Published with permission from HeartWare Inc. (**C**) Published with permission from Thoratec Corporation.

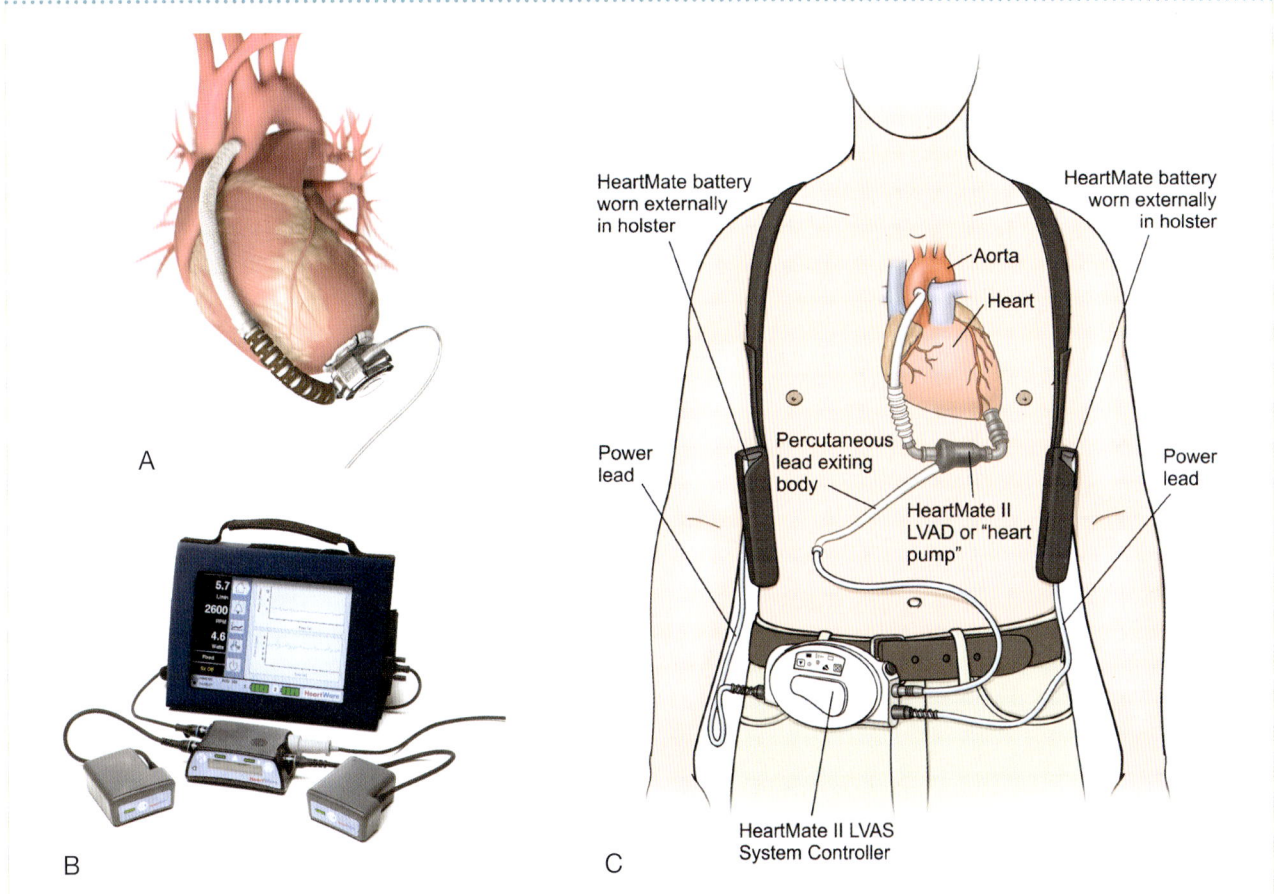

Incidence

Heart transplants in the modern era have been performed in Australia since 1986 and in New Zealand since 1987. In 2013, 86 heart transplants were performed in Australia and New Zealand.[77] In Europe, 589 heart transplants were performed, an annual figure that has been relatively static for the past 5 years.[78] As the annual number of transplants globally is likely to remain relatively stable because of limited organ availability, future management of end-stage heart failure may involve the insertion of a left ventricular assist device (LVAD) designed for long-term permanent mechanical circulatory support, so-called 'destination therapy'. In the early years, the VADs available were primarily used as 'bridge to transplantation' therapy (i.e. support for a failing native heart until a suitable heart became available), not 'destination therapy', although both purposes were shown to be viable options in the REMATCH study.[79] While this is still the case in Australia and New Zealand, recent global reports show about 40% of VADs are now used as 'destination therapy'.[80] This change has been facilitated by improvements in device technologies and the experiences of clinicians in managing this unique cohort. Survival with continuous flow VADs is now

at 81% to the first year and 70% at 2 years.[80] The notion of patients with VADs permanently due to advances in device design and capability (e.g. fully implantable with internal batteries) may not be as futuristic as once thought.

Outcomes from heart transplantation

Currently, the centres around the world that submit data to an international registry achieve survival rates for heart transplant patients of 81% at 1 year, and 69% at 5 years, with a median survival of 11 years.[81] In Australia and New Zealand, approximately 87% of heart transplant patients survive to 1 year, and 82% survive to 5 years.[82]

Indications

The vast majority of patients referred for heart transplantation have persistent NYHA functional class IV symptoms (see Chapter 10), secondary to ischaemic heart disease or some form of dilated cardiomyopathy.[81,83] In ICUs and cardiac units, patients with cardiogenic shock requiring either continuous intravenous inotropic support or cardiovascular support with an intra-aortic balloon pump or VAD are referred for transplant consideration.[83] Commonly, patients listed for transplantation have a life expectancy of less than 2 years without transplantation. Accepted contraindications for heart transplantation include active malignancy,[84] complicated diabetes,[85] morbid obesity,[86] uncontrolled infection, active substance abuse and an inability to comply with complex medical regimens.[87,88] Currently, 50% of transplanted patients globally are between 50 and 64 years of age.[83] Age has become a relative contraindication, with 16 days old being the youngest and 71 years of age being the oldest to have received a transplant to date.[82] However, the presence of multiple comorbidities in patients over 70 years of age would be expected to exclude the majority of such patients from consideration.[84,89] Other relative contraindications include renal failure and an irreversible high transpulmonary gradient (mean pulmonary artery pressure minus pulmonary artery wedge pressure) of greater than 15 mmHg[83,90] (see section on *Early allograft dysfunction and failure* later in this chapter). In the context of a rigorous postoperative regimen of polypharmacy, frequent follow-up medical appointments and routine cardiac biopsies, a strong social support network, absence of psychiatric illnesses and a willingness to participate actively in the recovery process are highly desirable characteristics of prospective recipients.[90]

Patients referred for heart transplant assessment must have exhausted all other accepted pharmacological and surgical treatment options for end-stage heart failure, such as optimal therapeutic doses of common heart failure medications; revascularisation via coronary artery bypass graft surgery or percutaneous transluminal coronary angioplasty; continuous IV infusions of dobutamine in the community/home setting; IV levosimendan (a calcium sensitiser); antiarrhythmic drugs to suppress, or an internal cardiac defibrillator to treat, potentially lethal arrhythmias; and insertion of a biventricular pacemaker (i.e. chronic resynchronisation therapy) to re-establish atrioventricular synchrony (see Chapter 11).

The average costs associated with heart transplantation are high, at approximately A\$35,000 for the first year and approximately A\$15,000 for each ongoing year, depending on the drug regimen and episodes of rejection or infection.[77] As some immunosuppressant drugs have come off patent, these costs have been reduced. However, the high incidence of chronic heart failure and associated hospitalisation costs are also considerable. During 2000, it was estimated that over half a million Australians had chronic heart failure (CHF), with 325,000 patients per annum experiencing symptoms.[91] In Australia during 2007–2008, 49,307 patients were hospitalised with a primary diagnosis of CHF (0.6% of all hospitalisations).[3] Approximately 40% of patients admitted to hospital with heart failure will be readmitted or die within one year.[92] The cost of a single hospital admission for CHF in Australia is currently approximately A\$6000.[93] In New Zealand, hospital admissions for heart failure consume approximately 1% of the healthcare budget.[94] In the context of a 50% mortality rate within 4 years of being diagnosed with chronic heart failure, a 50% mortality rate within 1 year for patients with severe heart failure[95] and the burden of care associated with heart failure exceeding that of all types of cancer,[96] transplantation for end-stage heart failure is actually a viable and economical treatment option for individuals and society; it is, however, a limited resource, available to only a few recipients.

FIGURE 12.13 **Left**: Completion of bicaval transplant technique, showing the inferior vena caval, superior vena caval, aortic and pulmonary artery anastomoses. **Right**: Commencement of the left atrial anastomosis.

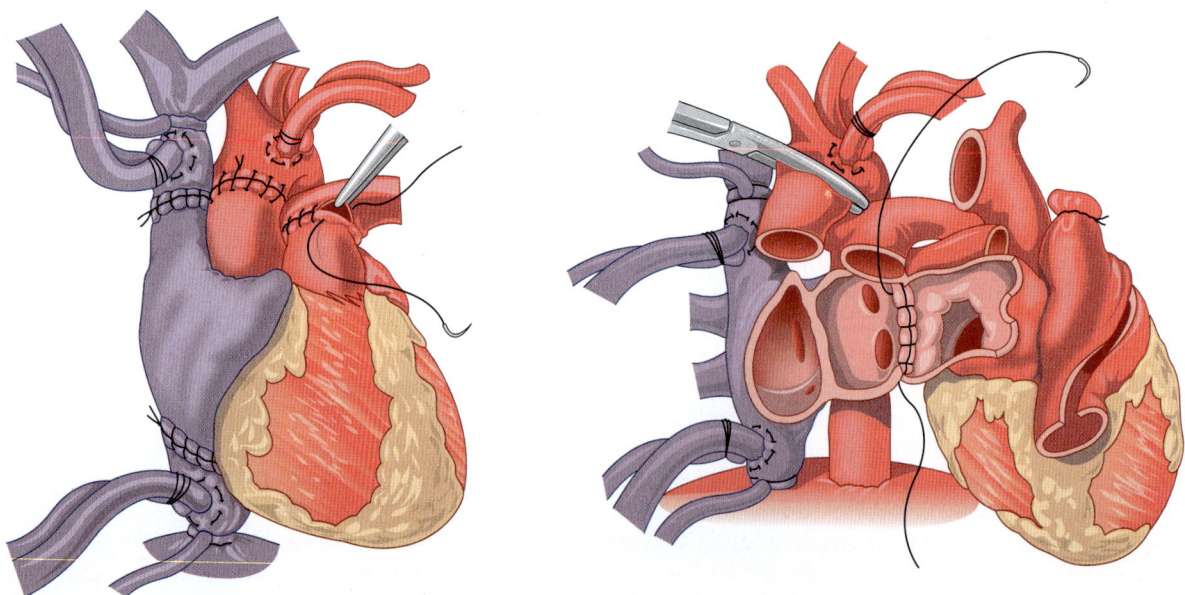

Adapted from Kirklin JK, Young JB, McGiffin DC. Heart transplantation. Philadelphia: Churchill Livingstone; 2002, with permission.

Forms of heart transplant surgery

The most common heart transplant surgery is orthotopic transplantation, with two surgical techniques used: the standard or bicaval approaches. The standard technique has been used since the 1960s and involves anastomoses of the donor and native atria.[97] Complications associated with the standard technique can include abnormal atrial contribution to ventricular filling and tricuspid and mitral valve insufficiency.[98,99] Since the mid-1990s, the bicaval technique as described by Dreyfus et al[100] has gained favour. The main advantage of the bicaval approach is the maintenance of atrial conducting pathways and the likelihood of promoting sinus rhythm and its associated superior atrial haemodynamics[100] (see Figure 12.13). Reported potential disadvantages include stenoses in the inferior and superior vena cava at the anastomosis sites.[100]

The second form of heart transplant surgery is heterotopic transplantation, although these account for only a handful of heart transplants globally.[101] In this procedure, the donor heart is implanted in the right side of the chest next to the native heart[102] to augment native systolic function. Figure 12.14 illustrates a chest X-ray of the donor heart next to the native heart.

FIGURE 12.14   Chest X-ray showing heterotopic heart transplant.

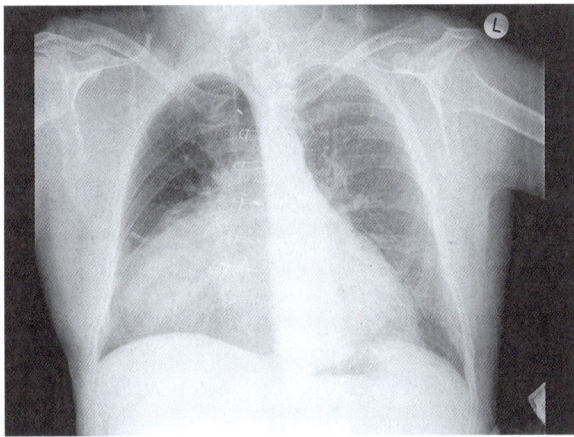

Heterotopic heart transplantation is primarily indicated in patients with pulmonary hypertension refractory to pulmonary vasodilator therapies. It may also be considered in patients with a large body surface area who are unlikely to receive a suitably large-sized donor heart to enable an orthotopic procedure to take place,[97,103] or when the donated organ is unsuitable as an orthotopic graft.[103] Heterotopic transplantation is usually performed to support the left ventricle (LVAD configuration), but can be configured to support biventricular function (Biventricular ventricular assisted device configuration). The LVAD configuration for heterotopic heart transplantation is illustrated in Figure 12.15.

FIGURE 12.15   Heterotopic heart transplant (LVAD configuration).

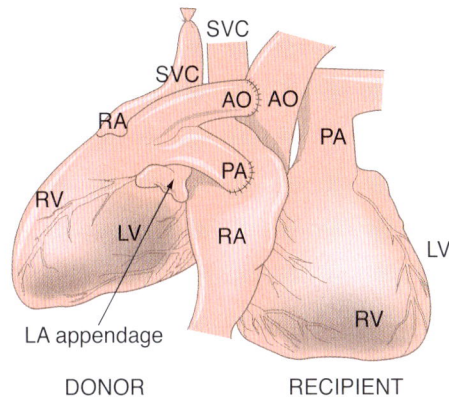

DONOR   RECIPIENT

Adapted from Newcomb AE, Esmore DS, Rosenfeldt FL, Richardson M, Marasco SF. Heterotopic heart transplantation: an expanding role in the twenty-first century? Ann Thorac Surg 2004;78(4):1345–50, with permission.

Patient management

Postoperative nursing and collaborative management of orthotopic heart transplant recipients involve full haemodynamic monitoring with a pulmonary artery catheter (PAC), a triple- or quad-lumen central venous catheter (CVC), arterial line, indwelling urinary catheter and 5-lead cardiac monitoring to assist in arrhythmia discrimination. A 12-lead ECG is also recorded. If the orthotopic transplant is performed with the standard technique, a remnant P wave from the native heart may be visible on the ECG or cardiac monitor (see Figure 12.16). As the native sinus node cannot conduct across the right atrial suture line, the recipient's heart rate is determined by the conduction system of the donor heart, not the native heart. Of interest, it is possible for the native heart to generate a P wave while the donor heart is in atrial fibrillation or other arrhythmia. (More detailed discussion of cardiac monitoring and haemodynamic management of patients with a heterotopic heart transplant is available.[96,104]) Monitoring data are combined with physical assessment information from all body systems to determine nursing and collaborative interventions. Intensive continuous monitoring and assessment of haemodynamic parameters according to

FIGURE 12.16   Rhythm strip post orthotopic transplant (standard technique).

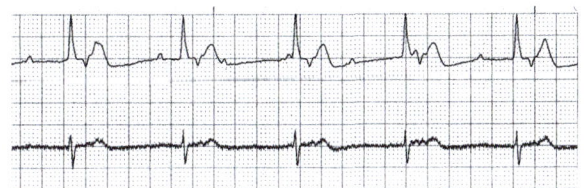

evidence-based practices[87-89] and overall clinical status allow nurses to detect and subsequently respond to emergent postoperative complications. Comprehensive guidelines for the care of heart transplant recipients, supported by the level of evidence for relevant practices, are detailed in a paper published by the International Society for Heart and Lung Transplantation (ISHLT).[105]

Full ventilatory support is required until the patient's haemodynamic status is stable. Respiratory status is monitored via clinical, radiological and laboratory-derived data (see Chapter 13). Enteral feeding is usually commenced on the day of admission. Renal and neurological function are closely monitored, as cyclosporin has a deleterious effect on renal function and can lead to failure[106] as well as neurotoxicity.[107] For the small number of patients who develop allograft dysfunction requiring mechanical circulatory support (i.e. IABP, ECMO or Thoratec LVAD), or acute renal failure requiring haemofiltration, hospitalisation in the critical care unit tends to last weeks rather than days.

The immediate period after transplantation can be a time of great hope and joy for recipients and their family and friends; however, complications and setbacks can make the path to recovery prolonged, unpredictable and difficult. The provision of psychosocial support by all members of the transplant/critical care team to family members and friends is an important part of patients' recovery from organ transplantation. Meetings with family that convey honest and open information about patient progress need to be conducted regularly. Supporting and managing patients and families following transplant is consistent with support provided to other critically ill patients (see Chapter 8). In addition, there is the issue of dealing with lost hope if the transplant fails, a very distressing time for all involved. In the immediate postoperative period, transplant recipients are at risk of developing complications that include hyperacute rejection, acute rejection, infection, haemorrhage and renal failure. In the immediate postoperative period, heart transplant recipients may experience morbidity specific to the heart transplant procedure, such as early allograft dysfunction (i.e. organ failure due to preservation injury), bleeding, right ventricular failure and acute rejection. Long-term complications include chronic renal failure, hypertension, malignancy and cardiac allograft vasculopathy. The common immediate potential complications and associated clinical management for heart recipients are discussed below.

Hyperacute rejection

Hyperacute rejection is now a rare form of humoral rejection that occurs minutes to hours after transplantation and results from ABO blood group incompatibility or the recipient having preformed, donor-specific antibodies.[108] ABO blood group and panel reactive screening of anti-human lymphocyte antigen (anti-HLA) antibodies preoperatively minimises the possibility of hyperacute rejection, particularly in healthcare systems where blood that has been prospectively cross-matched is routinely used. If it occurs, hyperacute rejection leads to organ failure and rapid activation of the complement cascade, producing severe damage to endothelial cells, platelet activation, initiation of the clotting cascade and extensive microvascular thrombosis.[109] There is no effective treatment for hyperacute rejection apart from mechanical circulatory support or interim retransplantation.

Acute rejection

Acute rejection can be classified as either cellular or humoral.[110,111] Cellular rejection involves T-cell infiltration of the allograft. Cellular rejection occurs much more commonly than humoral rejection, but both may occur simultaneously.[112] Humoral or microvascular rejection is thought to be primarily mediated by antibodies. A recent review by key stakeholders has resulted in the publication of standardised nomenclature for antibody-mediated rejection.[110] Humoral rejection may occur due to the presence of a positive donor-specific cross-match or in a sensitised recipient with preformed anti-HLA antibodies.[109]

Percutaneous transvenous endomyocardial biopsy is considered the gold standard for detecting cardiac rejection.[113] Grading of cardiac rejection has a standardised nomenclature globally.[114,115] In humoral rejection, endomyocardial biopsy reveals increased vascular permeability, microvascular thrombosis, interstitial oedema and haemorrhage, and endothelial cell swelling and necrosis.[110,113] An echocardiogram is also performed to evaluate systolic cardiac function.

Therapeutic interventions for rejection vary between centres and are based on the grade of rejection, degree of haemodynamic compromise, clinical findings and time elapsed since transplantation. Asymptomatic mild rejection (grade 1R) is rarely treated, the exception being if there is associated haemodynamic compromise; and only 20–40% of mild cases progress to moderate rejection (grade 2R), usually requiring treatment.[109,116] Grade 3R rejection is always treated, as it represents myocyte necrosis. Cellular rejection is usually treated with higher doses of corticosteroids, such as 'pulse' doses of methylprednisolone (1–3 g IV over 3 days), and antilymphocyte antibody agents (ATG, ATGAM or OKT3). Humoral rejection is treated with plasmapheresis, high-dose corticosteroids, cyclophosphamide therapy and antilymphocyte antibody therapy.[117,118] For both forms of rejection, other immunosuppressant agents such as the calcineurin inhibitor (cyclosporine, tacrolimus) and an antiproliferative cytotoxic agent (azathioprine, mycophenolate mofetil, sirolimus/rapamycin) are continued at the usual doses assuming levels were therapeutic. It may be judicious to review the patient's medications during periods of rejection to ensure that drugs capable of reducing cyclosporin or tacrolimus serum levels, such as certain anticonvulsants and antibiotics, have not been taken. In addition to augmentation of immunosuppression therapy, fluid, pharmacological and mechanical therapeutic interventions are instituted to support cardiac function, depending on the degree of ventricular dysfunction.

Nurses have an important role in detecting acute rejection, as it is diagnosed by clinical signs and supported by histological findings from an endomyocardial biopsy. Low-grade rejection can be suspected when non-specific signs such as malaise, lethargy, low-grade fever and mood changes are present. Acute rejection causing cardiac irritation is revealed by a sinus tachycardia greater than 120 beats/min; a pericardial friction rub; or new-onset atrial arrhythmias such as premature atrial contractions, atrial flutter or fibrillation.[116,119] More severe forms of acute rejection are suspected when signs and symptoms of varying degrees of heart failure emerge. If patients are awake and alert, they may complain of severe fatigue, sudden onset of dyspnoea during minimal physical effort, syncope or orthopnoea. Physical assessment and haemo-dynamic monitoring will reveal clinical signs of left and right cardiac failure (see Chapter 9).

Immunosuppression therapy

In this section, a brief discussion of immunosuppression therapies and associated nursing implications is provided. To prevent rejection of the transplanted organ, recipients receive a triple-therapy regimen of immunosuppression agents for the remainder of their life. Triple-therapy usually consists of corticosteroids (prednisolone or prednisone), a calcineurin antagonist (cyclosporine or tacrolimus [FK506]) and an antiproliferative cytotoxic agent (mycophenolate mofetil, azathioprine or sirolimus/rapamycin).[120,121] For some heart patients sirolimus, also known as rapamycin, may be the cytotoxic drug of choice because of a lower incidence of cardiac allograft vasculopathy at 6 and 24 months, and lower rejection rates with sirolimus compared with azathioprine.[122] A later study also showed mycophenolate mofetil reduced mortality for up to 36 months post-transplantation when compared to azathioprine.[123]

Immunosuppression therapy is commenced pre-operatively or in the operating theatre. A maintenance immunosuppression regimen is usually instituted within hours of admission to ICU, with each patient's immunosuppressive needs individually assessed. For instance, the administration time for introduction of the selected immunosuppressive agent(s) may be delayed in patients with preexisting renal dysfunction. When the administration of the usual regimen of immunosuppression is delayed, induction therapy with anti-lymphocyte agents (anti-thymocyte globulin (ATG), ATGAM or OKT3) or interleukin-2 receptor antagonists (basiliximab, daclizumab) may be used in the immediate postoperative period.[81,124,125] Induction therapy may also be used in circumstances of primary allograft failure perioperatively, e.g. HLA mismatch (rare) or early humoral rejection, or to allow for a delay in initiating cyclosporine in patients at risk of renal failure.[119,126] A recent systematic review has found no support for the routine use of IL-2Ra therapy as routine induction therapy to achieve a survival benefit or reduction in cardiac allograft rejection.[127] The common drugs used to suppress the immune system and the nursing implications are illustrated in Table 12.5. As

highlighted in the table, some immunosuppressive agents are cytotoxic (e.g. mycophenolate mofetil), requiring safety measures during preparation, delivery and disposal. Likewise, some immunosuppressive agents will be given IV (e.g. azathioprine) until patients can eat and drink as they cannot be crushed for nasogastric administration. In addition, as blood levels of some immunosuppression agents (e.g. cyclosporine, sirolimus) are taken regularly to assess efficacy, nurses need to be aware of timing blood sampling to dosage times in order to obtain accurate data to inform doses.

Infection

Infection is a major risk factor for transplant recipients due to their immunosuppressed state. The periods of greatest risk for patients are the first 3 months after transplantation, and after episodes of acute rejection when immunosuppression agents are increased.[128,129] In addition to the nosocomial bacterial infections that all surgical patients are exposed to in critical care (see Chapter 6), immunosuppressed transplant recipients are at risk of acquiring opportunistic bacterial, viral or fungal infections; latent infections acquired from the donor organ such as cytomegalovirus (CMV); or reactivation of their own latent infections (e.g. CMV or *Pneumocystis carinii*). To combat *Pneumocystis carinii*, patients receive trimethoprim with sulfamethoxazole twice weekly.[130] Despite preoperative screening for CMV, the shortage of donor organs often necessitates CMV mismatching. Effective prophylaxis for CMV infection is provided by administering CMV hyperimmune globulin to CMV-positive and CMV-negative recipients who receive a heart from a seropositive donor.[131] This commences within 24–48 hours of surgery.[124] For CMV-negative recipients of organs from seropositive donors, ganciclovir for 1–2 weeks followed by oral therapy for 3 months is required in addition to CMV hyperimmune globulin.[105,131,132]

To prevent infection, standard precautions and meticulous hand washing (see Chapter 6) are performed, rather than isolation procedures.[133] Mandatory measures to prevent overwhelming sepsis are a high level of vigilance by clinicians for signs of infection; obtaining empirical evidence from blood, sputum, urine, wound and catheter-tip cultures; and aggressive and prompt treatment for specific organisms. Although typical signs and symptoms of infection are blunted in transplant recipients, clinicians should suspect infections when patients have a low-grade fever, hypotension, tachycardia, a high cardiac output/index, a decrease in systemic vascular resistance (SVR), changes in mentation, a new cough or dyspnoea.[121,134] Elevated white cell count, the presence of dysuria, purulent discharge from wounds, infiltrates on chest X-ray, sputum production or pain also indicate infection.

Prior to administering blood products, nurses must ascertain the CMV status of the patient and donor. Recipients who are seronegative for CMV and who receive a heart from a seronegative donor must receive

TABLE 12.5

Immunosuppression table[124]

DRUG NAMES	TYPICAL DOSE	IMPORTANT SIDE EFFECTS	NURSING CONSIDERATIONS
Calcineurin antagonists	Maintenance		
cyclosporin	5–10 mg/kg/day (target blood levels)	Renal impairment Hypertension Hypercholesterolaemia Abnormal liver function Headaches Gingival hypertrophy (cyclosporin only) Hirsutism (cyclosporin only) Diabetes (tacrolimus only)	Monitor renal and liver function Mix oral liquid cyclosporin with orange juice or milk in glass Do not crush tablets Time sampling of serum drug levels with dosage times
tacrolimus	0.2–0.5 mg/kg/day (target blood levels)		
Corticosteroids	Maintenance		
prednisolone/prednisone	0.2–0.5 mg/kg/day Augmentation for rejection 'Pulse' of 2 g over 3 days for acute rejection	Mood change Weight gain Glucose intolerance Osteopenia Muscle weakness	Monitor blood glucose levels
Antiproliferative cytotoxic agents	Maintenance		
azathioprine	1–2 mg/kg/day	Bone marrow suppression Gastrointestinal tract irritation (especially mycophenolate mofetil)	Cytotoxic: take full precautions when preparing, administering and disposing of drugs
mycophenolate mofetil	2–3 g/day (adult)		
rapamycin	Starting at 0.03 mg/kg/day (target blood levels)	Bone marrow suppression Hypercholesterolaemia Hypokalaemia	Minimise dietary cholesterol Monitor platelets and serum potassium
interleukin-2 receptor antagonist	Induction of immunosuppression		
basiliximab	20 mg/kg preoperatively and day 4	Few and infrequent	These drugs are often used in patients with pre-existing renal dysfunction Other immunosuppression agents may be delayed with the use of these agents Little information about compatibilities: avoid concurrent administration
daclizumab	1 mg/kg preoperatively and days 14, 28, 42, 56		
Antilymphocyte preparations	Induction or augmentation for rejection		
ATGAM/OKT3	Various, may target T lymphocyte levels	Anaphylaxis Sterile meningitis Pulmonary oedema Serum sickness	Premed of paracetamol, promethazine and hydrocortisone 30 min prior to slow infusion

Adapted from: Farmer DG, McDiarmid SV, Edelstein S, Renz JF, Hisatake G, Cortina G et al. Induction therapy with interleukin-2 receptor antagonist after intestinal transplantation is associated with reduced acute cellular rejection and improved renal function. Transplant Proc 2004;36(2):331–2.

whole blood, packed/red cells or platelets that are CMV-negative, leuco-depleted or both in order to avoid development of a primary CMV infection.[97,105,135]

Haemorrhage/cardiac tamponade

The risk of haemorrhage or cardiac tamponade is greater for heart transplant recipients than for patients undergoing coronary artery bypass graft or valvular surgery. Preoperative anticoagulation for end-stage heart failure or atrial fibrillation, impairment of hepatic function secondary to right heart failure, redo surgery, surgical suture lines connecting major vessels and atria and a larger than usual pericardium are all contributing factors. Good surgical technique is mandatory in preventing postoperative bleeding. As the promotion of haemostasis is a major therapeutic goal postoperatively, blood products, procoagulants and antifibrinolytics are commonly administered according to laboratory and clinical data. Postoperative mortality from bleeding has been reported to occur in up to 6.7% of cases.[136]

Early detection of haemorrhage is achieved by close monitoring of the following: haematological status; chest tube patency, drainage volume and drainage consistency; and trends in haemodynamic data that suggest cardiac tamponade (see earlier in this chapter). Our clinical experience suggests that, if patients are hypotensive sporadically for no readily apparent reason, efforts should be made to eliminate the existence of cardiac tamponade. Suspicion of cardiac tamponade may be confirmed by chest X-ray or echocardiogram if the patient's haemodynamic status is stable. Sudden cardiac arrest or haemodynamic collapse secondary to cardiac tamponade warrants an immediate return to theatre or a sternotomy in critical care.

Acute kidney injury

Acute kidney injury or varying degrees of renal dysfunction can occur in the initial postoperative period due to preexisting renal dysfunction, cyclosporin, nephrotoxic antibiotics or sustained periods of hypotension secondary to cardiopulmonary bypass or allograft dysfunction. Diuretic therapy is invariably needed in the initial postoperative period due to these factors, as well as the fluid retention effects of corticosteroids and raised filling pressures secondary to a transient loss of right and/or left ventricular compliance.[137] High doses or continuous infusions of diuretics may be required in patients who were on diuretic therapy preoperatively. Close monitoring of serum electrolyte levels will indicate the need for any supplements.

In addition to all the usual nursing and collaborative measures that are taken to prevent, detect and support renal dysfunction/failure in patients following cardiac surgery on cardiopulmonary bypass (see earlier in this chapter and Chapter 18), the type and dose of immunosuppressive agents in the postoperative period are carefully selected and initiated according to individual risk factors and clinical status. Experience suggests that early intervention with haemofiltration to support renal function is preferable to continued use of high-dose diuretics and deferred haemofiltration. This is because there is little scope to maintain low doses of renal toxic immunosuppressants for weeks given the imminent risk of rejection and resultant allograft failure.

Early allograft dysfunction and failure

Primary allograft failure is the leading cause of death in the first month and year after surgery.[120,138] In the immediate postoperative period, myocardial performance is depressed due to the clinical sequelae of cardiopulmonary bypass and ischaemic injury associated with surgical retrieval, hypothermic storage, prolonged ischaemic times and reperfusion. Despite a preferred time period between organ retrieval and reimplantation of 2–6 hours, the vast distances between capital cities (up to 3000 km) over which donor hearts may be transported, and a decision to accept marginal, suboptimal organs, led Australian researchers and transplant teams to pioneer prolonged ischaemic times of up to 8 hours (New Zealand, 7 hours).[139]

Heart transplants that encompass long distances with ischaemic periods beyond 6 hours have been, and are likely to continue to be, performed in Australia and New Zealand and other countries, as excellent short-term (30-day mortality) and long-term (ejection fraction at 1 year) outcomes have been reported.[139] These outcomes were achieved by using innovative preservation techniques and postoperative mechanical assistance in the form of intra-aortic balloon counterpulsation and/or a right ventricular assist device.[139,140] Adrenaline is invariably commenced intraoperatively, irrespective of ischaemic time, to provide inotropic support to the transplanted heart.

Early allograft dysfunction can present as left, right or biventricular dysfunction. Management of cardiac dysfunction is dependent on clinical signs and underlying aetiologies that include pulmonary hypertension, acute rejection and ischaemic injury. Right ventricular dysfunction is usually secondary to pulmonary hypertension, whereas left ventricular or biventricular dysfunction results from acute rejection and ischaemic injury.

To prevent right ventricular dysfunction and failure secondary to raised pulmonary pressures, prospective heart transplant recipients are screened preoperatively for the degree and reversibility of pulmonary hypertension. Reversible pulmonary hypertension is a transpulmonary gradient less than 15 mmHg that responds to pulmonary vasodilator therapies, such as prostaglandin E1, prostacyclin or inhaled NO.[141] Right ventricular dysfunction or failure can also occur in the postoperative context due to ischaemic injury, an undersized heart (greater than 20% difference in body surface area between donor and recipient) or hypoxic pulmonary vasoconstriction.[97] Isoprenaline or milronine, dobutamine and adrenaline are administered in this situation.[105]

Left ventricular dysfunction cannot be anticipated preoperatively, so when signs first emerge peri- or postoperatively, fluid management strategies (filling or diuresis as deemed appropriate) and inotropic agents are commenced immediately.[105] In patients with prolonged ischaemic times, mechanical assistance in the form of an IABP is invariably instituted perioperatively.

In the initial postoperative period, cardiac dysfunction can also occur as a result of a low SVR syndrome, characterised by a calculated SVR of less than 750 dynes/sec/cm^{-5} in the presence of an unsustainable high cardiac output.[142,143] The cause of low SVR syndrome is not fully understood, although it has been linked with systemic inflammatory response syndrome (SIRS) associated with cardiopulmonary bypass (see Chapter 21), the chronic use of angiotensin-converting enzyme inhibitors for end-stage heart failure (see Chapter 10) and a deficiency of vasopressin.[142,144] Noradrenaline is titrated to achieve a calculated SVR within normal parameters and to lower the unsustainably high cardiac index. In severe cases, vasopressin may be infused at doses of 0.04–0.1 units/min concurrently with noradrenaline.[145] Experience suggests that the dose of adrenaline should be minimised in the presence of metabolic acidosis, and the noradrenaline infusion increased to achieve normotension, a calculated SVR higher than 900 dynes/sec/cm^{-5} and a sustainable cardiac index.

Patients with depressed left ventricular compliance and contractility due to cardiac dysfunction present clinically with reduced cardiac index, bradycardia, reduced tissue and end-organ perfusion (decreased mental status, oliguria, poor peripheral perfusion, slow capillary refill and raised serum lactate), low systemic venous oxygenation and dyspnoea. Bradycardia may not be evident due to chronotropic support of the denervated heart with atrial pacing and/or isoprenaline. The following discussion focuses on management of right heart dysfunction/failure and left heart dysfunction/failure (see also Chapter 10).

Right heart dysfunction/failure is suspected in patients with preexisting pulmonary hypertension or a haemodynamic profile in the intra- or postoperative context that includes a rising CVP, low-to-normal pulmonary artery diastolic/pulmonary artery wedge pressure (PAWP), high calculated pulmonary vascular resistance, raised pulmonary artery pressures, systemic hypotension and oliguria. The haemodynamic management of patients with right ventricular dysfunction/failure involves optimising right ventricular preload and afterload by titrating fluid and pharmacological therapies to achieve adequate tissue and end-organ perfusion. Fluid resuscitation to a CVP between 14 and 20 mmHg and inotropic therapy are necessary to ensure that the failing right ventricle continues to act as a conduit for the left ventricle. Nitric oxide by inhalation is the therapy of choice, as it provides selective pulmonary vasodilation at doses of 20–40 ppm, thereby reducing right ventricular afterload without producing systemic hypotension.[141,146] A secondary benefit of inhaled NO is improved oxygenation due to reduced mismatching of ventilation/perfusion.[147] If inhaled NO is not available, IV prostaglandin E1 or prostacyclin may be used to reduce right ventricular afterload when pulmonary pressures exceed 50 mmHg.[148]

Mild right ventricular dysfunction may be treated with milrinone at doses of 0.375–0.750 mcg/kg/min or drug combinations that provide afterload reduction and inotropic support (e.g. sodium nitroprusside and adrenaline). Appropriate respiratory management is essential, as hypoxaemia and metabolic or respiratory acidosis can exacerbate right ventricular failure. If pharmacological, fluid and inhaled NO therapies do not produce sustained improvement in right ventricular performance, a right VAD (e.g. Biomedicus centrifugal pump or Abiomed BVS 5000) is indicated to provide temporary support for the failing right ventricle.

The immediate haemodynamic management of left ventricular dysfunction/failure secondary to acute rejection or ischaemic injury often involves fluid resuscitation to a pulmonary artery diastolic of 16–20 mmHg, high-dose inotropes, vasodilator agents and insertion of an IABP to achieve a cardiac index greater than 2.2 L/min/m^2 and adequate end-organ perfusion. The insertion of an LVAD (e.g. Biomedicus centrifugal pump) or full mechanical

circulatory support with extracorporeal membrane oxygenation (ECMO) is indicated when aggressive therapeutic regimens fail to produce a cardiac output that provides adequate end-organ perfusion.[105,149,150] As noted earlier, augmentation of the immunosuppression regimen may also be necessary to manage the acute rejection.

Denervation

Donor heart implantation severs both afferent and efferent nervous system connections to the heart. Hence, the transplanted heart has no direct autonomic nervous system innervation but is responsive to circulating catecholamines. Denervation impairs circulatory system homeostasis, as evidenced by: a volume-expanded state; a tendency to hypertension; no sensation of angina pectoris; a high resting heart rate; a slow or absent baroreceptor reflex (to increase heart rate/cardiac output in response to hypotension); and no rises in heart rate and contractility due to hypovolaemia or vasodilation.[97] As the cardiac allograft is dependent on an adequate preload, the effects of postural changes in recipients are important. (A detailed discussion of physiology of the transplanted heart is provided elsewhere.[97])

There are four important clinical manifestations of denervation in the early postoperative period. First, drugs that act directly on the autonomic nervous system to modify heart rate (e.g. atropine, digoxin) and vagal manoeuvres (carotid sinus massage) are ineffective. Amiodarone and adenosine are effective antiarrhythmic agents. Neither amiodarone nor sotalol interact with immunosuppressive agents.[105] However, as the denervated donor sinus node is more sensitive to exogenous adenosine than a sinus node innervated in the normal way,[151] it has been suggested that adenosine be avoided.[97] That is, a usual adenosine dose may produce toxic-like effects in the context of a denervated heart. Overdrive atrial pacing is a viable alternative to drug therapy to treat a tachyarrhythmia such as atrial flutter.[152]

Second, although a high resting heart rate is possible from efferent cardiac denervation, sinus or junctional bradycardias may occur in the early postoperative period due to transient sinus node dysfunction or preoperative amiodarone. Studies suggest that sinus node dysfunction occurs in about 20% of cases,[153] although anecdotal experience suggests a higher percentage. To prevent low cardiac output secondary to bradycardias, atrial and ventricular epicardial pacing wires are inserted and atrial pacing of >90 beats/min,[105] and often at 110 beats/min, is commenced. Atrial pacing at 110 beats/min appears to 'train' the sinus node to conduct at rates of 70–100 beats/min in the long term. A resting sinus or junctional heart rate below 70 beats/min prior to hospital discharge is predictive of long-term sinus node dysfunction.[97] Insertion of a permanent pacemaker for long-term heart rate control is rarely required. Isoprenaline infusions at doses of 0.5–2 mcg/min may be used for chronotropy in combination with atrial pacing. As noted earlier, atrial arrhythmias such as atrial flutter may be an early indication of acute rejection. Ventricular arrhythmias are rare and often lethal in spite of aggressive resuscitation attempts. Persistent arrhythmias should always prompt investigation of the patient's rejection level.[105]

Third, as patients rely on circulating catecholamines, orthostatic hypotension is common. Patients are educated to sit up slowly from a lying position. Fourth, patients rarely feel anginal pain after surgery; however, there are some reports of patients regaining feelings of angina pectoris.[154]

The inability of patients to feel angina pectoris is important, because all heart transplant recipients are at risk of developing accelerated allograft coronary artery disease.[155] As part of discharge education, patients are taught to identify clinical signs of angina other than chest pain, such as shortness of breath and sweating. A summary of the main clinical manifestations and nursing practice issues for patients following heart transplantation is included in Table 12.6.

TABLE 12.6

Nursing care of patients after heart transplantation

CLINICAL MANIFESTATION	NURSING PRACTICE CONSIDERATIONS
Acute rejection	Detect acute rejection by clinical signs and endomyocardial biopsy Suspect low-grade rejection when malaise, lethargy, low-grade fever and mood changes are present Acute rejection is manifested by a sinus tachycardia >120 beats/min, a pericardial friction rub or new-onset atrial arrhythmias Suspect severe acute rejection with manifestations of left and right heart failure; awake patients may complain of severe fatigue, sudden onset of dyspnoea during minimal physical effort, syncope or orthopnoea
Infection	Standard infection control precautions and meticulous hand washing is required Observe for signs of infection: low-grade fever, hypotension, tachycardia, a high cardiac output/index, a decrease in systemic vascular resistance, changes in mentation, a new cough, dyspnoea, dysuria, sputum production or pain Monitor blood, sputum, urine, wound and catheter-tip cultures, infiltrates on chest X-ray and institute aggressive and prompt treatment for specific infective organisms Check CMV status before administering blood products
Haemorrhage/cardiac tamponade	Monitor haematological status; chest tube patency, drainage volume and drainage consistency; and trends in haemodynamic data that suggest cardiac tamponade Patients who are hypotensive sporadically should be assessed to eliminate cardiac tamponade as a cause
Acute renal failure	Support renal function, including titration of immunosuppressive agents to individual risk factors and clinical status, and early haemofiltration
Early allograft dysfunction	Augment the immunosuppression regimen to manage the acute rejection
Left heart failure	Observe for depressed left ventricular compliance and contractility: reduced cardiac index, possible bradycardia (may not be evident due to atrial pacing and/or isoprenaline), decreased mental status, oliguria, poor peripheral perfusion, slow capillary refill and raised serum lactate, low systemic venous oxygenation and dyspnoea Fluid resuscitate to a PAWP of 14–18 mmHg, high-dose inotropes, vasodilator agents, IABP to achieve a cardiac index >2.2 L/min/m^2 with adequate end-organ perfusion Insertion of full mechanical circulatory support (ECMO or LVAD) is indicated when other interventions do not provide adequate end-organ perfusion
Right heart failure	Observe for right heart dysfunction/failure: rising CVP, low-to-normal PAD/PAWP, high calculated pulmonary vascular resistance, raised pulmonary artery pressures, systemic hypotension and oliguria Optimise right ventricular preload and afterload: titrate fluid and medications to achieve adequate end-organ perfusion; fluid resuscitate to a CVP of 14–20 mmHg; consider inhaled NO (selective pulmonary vasodilation and improved oxygenation from reduced ventilation/perfusion mismatch), prostaglandin E1 or prostacyclin, milrinone or drug combinations with afterload reduction and inotropic support (e.g. sodium nitroprusside and adrenaline) Institute appropriate respiratory management to minimise hypoxaemia and metabolic or respiratory acidosis If no sustained improvement in right ventricular performance, a right VAD is indicated for temporary support
Denervation	Drugs with direct autonomic nervous system actions on heart rate (e.g. atropine, digoxin) and vagal manoeuvres (carotid sinus massage) are ineffective Use overdrive atrial pacing to treat tachyarrhythmias Sinus or junctional bradycardias may occur, and atrial/ventricular epicardial pacing is used to 'train' the sinus node Orthostatic hypotension is common: patients should sit up slowly from a lying position Patients rarely feel anginal pain after surgery: they need to identify other clinical signs of angina, such as shortness of breath and sweating

CMV = cytomegalovirus; CVP = central venous pressure; ECMO = extracorporeal membrane oxygenation; IABP = intra-aortic balloon pump; LVAD = left ventricular assist device; PAD = pulmonary artery diastolic; PAWP = pulmonary artery wedge pressure.

Medium- to long-term complications

There are four long-term complications associated with heart transplantation: 1) cardiac allograft vasculopathy; 2) malignancy; 3) renal dysfunction; and 4) hypertension.[156] Cardiac allograft vasculopathy (CAV) is a diffuse, proliferative form of obliterative coronary arteriosclerosis that affects 30–60% of heart transplant recipients in the first 5 years after surgery.[157] Sudden death, ventricular arrhythmias and symptoms of congestive heart failure may be the first signs of significant CAV. The aetiology of CAV is multifactorial, including immunological factors (e.g. episodes of acute rejection and anti-HLA antibodies), non-immunological cardiovascular risk factors (e.g. hypertension, hyperlipidaemia, preexisting diabetes and new-onset diabetes), the surgical procedure (e.g. donor age, ischaemic time and reperfusion injury) and side effects of immunosuppression drugs such as cyclosporin and corticosteroids (e.g. CMV infection and nephrotoxicity).[105,157–159] Statins at doses less than that prescribed for hyperlipidaemia are commenced within 2 weeks of surgery irrespective of cholesterol levels to reduce episodes of rejection and CAV.[105] Standard use of cyclosporine may be augmented by mycophenolate mofetil, everolimus or sirolimus as they have been shown to reduce the onset and progression of CAV.[105] Diagnosis of CAV is difficult, due to allograft denervation, and because coronary angiogram underestimates the extent of the disease and is insensitive to early lesions.[160] Currently, intravascular ultrasound provides the most reliable quantitative information about the degree of CAV.[160] As the definitive treatment for CAV is retransplantation, ongoing research into the prevention of CAV[161] will be the most important factor in reducing the incidence and associated mortality.

All heart transplant recipients are at a greater risk of developing malignancies than the general population,[162] particularly carcinoma of the skin[162–165]

and lymphoproliferative disorders,[166,167] as a consequence of long-term immunosuppression therapy.[81,168,169] Nurses play an important role in educating patients about how to avoid and reduce the risks of sun exposure. Treatment options in transplant recipients are the same as for the general population (e.g. chemotherapy, radiation therapy and surgical excision), in addition to a reduction in immunosuppression therapy; however, outcomes remain poor.[165]

Long-term renal dysfunction occurs primarily post-transplantation due to cyclosporin nephrotoxicity. Careful monitoring of cyclosporin levels and avoidance of hypovolaemia and other nephrotoxic drugs are important measures in reducing progression to renal failure. Importantly, findings from recent research indicate that chronic cyclosporin nephrotoxicity can be reversed by eliminating cyclosporin from immunosuppression regimens.[108] End-stage renal failure requiring dialysis or renal transplantation has been reported in 3–10% of patients.[170]

Systemic hypertension following transplantation has been linked with cyclosporin-induced tubular nephrotoxicity, peripheral vasoconstriction and fluid retention.[171] Lifestyle modifications such as weight loss, low sodium diet and exercise are recommended along with optimal therapeutic doses of cyclosporin, and combinations of calcium channel blockers and angiotensin-converting enzyme inhibitors and blockers.[105] Such approaches have been reported to achieve blood pressure control in up to 65% of patients.[172]

Lifestyle issues

Following such momentous surgery, patients require sound advice regarding returning to driving, work, exercise and sexual activity. Cardiac rehabilitation with aerobic and resistance exercise is recommended to prevent short-term weight gain and glucose intolerance, as well as adverse effects of immunosuppressive therapy on skeletal muscle.[105] Return to work or education is expected and encouraged after surgery. Driving a vehicle can be considered once the patient's gait, tremor and other neurological issues are normalised, and any bradycardia managed by pacemaker implantation.[105] Pregnancy is possible after 1 year following transplantation; but only under the management of the multidisciplinary team who will explain the considerable risks involved.[105]

Summary

Primary compromise of the cardiovascular system causes patients to require admission to a critical care area and the need for specialised care including intra-aortic balloon pumping and post cardiac surgery management. Appropriate assessment and management are essential to prevent secondary complications arising. Important principles of care are summarised below.

Surgical procedures may be performed as treatment for structural abnormalities, ischaemic lesions within coronary arteries and repair or replacement of cardiac valves. Haemodynamic stability constitutes the most common challenge in the postoperative period and may be managed with fluids, cardiovascular medications, cardiac pacing and intra-aortic balloon pumping. Bleeding in the postoperative period may be due to inadequate reversal or heparin, coagulopathy or surgical bleeding; therefore, appropriate diagnosis must occur before relevant treatment is instigated.

Intra–aortic balloon pumping is one therapy that is used to provide support in the period after cardiac surgery. Major benefits of IABP include increasing cardiac output, increasing myocardial oxygen supply and decreasing myocardial oxygen demand. Appropriate timing is essential to obtain maximum benefits, so correction of timing errors forms a central component of care. In addition, assessment of limb perfusion, with timely intervention when perfusion is inadequate, is essential to prevent limb ischaemia.

Cardiac transplantation may also be used to provide support to the failing heart. Indications for heart transplantation include end-stage heart failure secondary to ischaemic heart disease and cardiomyopathy. Possible complications in the early postoperative period include acute rejection, infection, haemorrhage, renal failure, right ventricular failure and allograft dysfunction (left ventricular dysfunction/failure). A triple-therapy regimen consisting of corticosteroids, a calcineurin antagonist and an antiproliferative cytotoxic agent is used to suppress the immune system after organ transplantation. All cytotoxic agents necessitate specific administration and disposal procedures. Although early signs of low-grade rejection can be non-specific, signs of moderate rejection usually present as organ dysfunction/failure. Nursing practices for managing patients with heart transplantation focus on prevention and management of complications, maintenance of comfort and promotion of long-term recovery.

Case study

Mrs Murphy is a 78-year-old patient admitted for elective CABG surgery. Her past history includes ischaemic heart diseases, hypertension, high cholesterol, type II diabetes and gout. She has had acute myocardial infarction (AMI) 5 years ago, which was treated with percutaneous transluminal coronary angioplasty (PTCA) and a drug-eluting stent to mid LAD lesion. She has had angina pain for the last 6 months and her coronary angiography showed triple vessel diseases in circumflex artery, LAD above the old stent and posterior descending artery (PDA) lesions. Her left ventriculogram revealed apical hypokenesis with moderate left ventricle systolic dysfunction. Preoperative transthoracic echocardiography report revealed normal valves and grade II left ventricle with moderate systolic dysfunction.

Surgery was reported as uncomplicated. Three bypass grafts were performed using left IMA to LAD, left radial artery to mid circumflex artery and SVG to the PDA. Cardiopulmonary bypass was used for 79 minutes and aortic cross-clamp time was 58 minutes. Continuous infusion of glyceryl trinitrate (GTN) at 10 mcg/min and noradrenaline at 2 mcg/min were in progress.

On admission to the ICU the patient was intubated and ventilated. She had a right radial arterial line and a right internal jugular PAC in situ. Two mediastinal and one pericardial drain tube had been placed and had drained 50 mL of blood to the time of admission. There was a small air leak in under water seal drainage system. A urinary catheter was also present. Early chest X-rays confirmed ETT, PAC and chest tube placement. Left lower lobe collapse was noted.

The main dimensions of Mrs Murphy's progress, care and management follow.

NEUROLOGICAL STATUS

She was kept sedated with propofol for 3 hours and then began to wake up, and was obeying commands, able to move all limbs with equal strength. Pupils were normal size and reactive to light. Pain was managed with regular intravenous tramadol, morphine (boluses) and paracetamol suppositories in the initial phase and continued with tramadol for 48 hours and oral paracetamol for 4 days postoperatively.

VENTILATION

Initial parameters: ETT secured at lip level 22 cm, equal air entry bilaterally, but decreased in left lower base. SIMV mode, tidal volume (VT) 500 mL (75 kg), rate 10/min, inspiratory flow 40 L/min, PEEP 5 cmH_2O, FiO_2 1.00, pressure support 10 cmH_2O, producing acceptable peak inspiratory pressures of 22–24 cmH_2O.

Admission ABG (after 20 minutes) revealed the following:

- PaO_2 422 mmHg
- $PaCO_2$ 55 mmHg
- pH 7.30
- HCO_3^- 24 mmol/L
- SaO_2 99.0%.

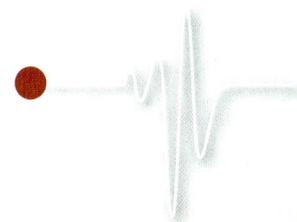

On the basis of the $PaCO_2$ the SIMV rate was increased to 13 breaths per minute, which corrected the $PaCO_2$ and pH. FiO_2 was progressively decreased to 0.40 over the next hour while pulse oximetry revealed a SpO_2 greater than 98%.

Sedation was reduced 3 hours after admission to ICU, and Mrs Murphy started to initiate spontaneous breaths; therefore the ventilation mode switched to CPAP/PS. However, she required further sedation due to events explained next.

CARDIOVASCULAR

Epicardial dual-chamber pacing wires were in place, but pacing was provided in the AAI mode at a rate of 90 beats/min, with no evidence of AV block. Initially, Mrs Murphy's blood pressure was maintained with assistance of noradrenaline infusion at 2 mcg/min to keep MAP above 70 and systolic blood pressure of 110–120 mmHg. Filling pressure (CVP) was kept in the range 10–12 mmHg with colloid administration. She was vasodilated, with an SVR of 676 dynes/sec/cm^{-5}. Her core temperature on admission was 35.3°C, requiring active warming. Chest drainage remained high, with total blood loss of 150 mL in the first hour, and continued to drain 120–150 mL/h for the next 3 hours. Multiple units of red blood cells, fresh frozen plasma, platelets and cryoprecipitate were transfused. Mrs Murphy clinically deteriorated with consistent low blood pressure that escalated the noradrenaline rate to 20 mcg/min and her filling pressures were low, CVP of 5 mmHg and pulmonary artery diastolic pressure of 8 mmHg despite fluid and blood products administration. Her initial cardiac index (CI) was 2.6 L/min/m^2, which dropped to 1.7 L/min/m^2 once she had deteriorated haemodynamically. Her heart rate remained the same at AAI paced rate of 90 beats/min. The surgical team decided to take the patient back to theatre for exploration and to achieve haemostasis.

On return to ICU, Mrs Murphy was sedated with propofol, on noradrenaline at 5 mcg/min and milrinone at 0.250 mcg/kg/min infusions and IABP was inserted in theatre to assist with left ventricle function and recovery (augmented diastolic pressure of 120, systolic pressure of 110, diastolic pressure of 55 and mean arterial pressure of 80 mmHg). One litre of haemoserous collection from the left pleural space and 350 mL from the pericardial sac were drained. The surgical team reported that a small pericardial artery was bleeding, which was clipped. Haemostasis was achieved in theatre before closing the sternum.

Despite returning to theatre, and escalation of care, Mrs Murphy was stable but remained intubated during the night and sedation was turned off at 0600 in view of extubation. IABP was kept at a 1:1 ratio, noradrenaline reduced to 2 mcg/min and milrinone to 0.125 mcg/kg/min, with a CI of 2.4 L/min/m^2. Mrs Murphy was extubated mid-morning and IABP was weaned (ratio wean) on postoperative day 2 over a period of 4 hours without any compromise, and the IABP catheter was removed on day 2 post ICU admission.

FLUID BALANCE

Chest drainage for the first admission was around 750 mL over 3 hours but, after return to ICU for the second time, the total drainage for 48 hours before the drains were removed was 440 mL. Mrs Murphy's urine output remained within the range 0.5–1 mL/kg/h with a small increase in serum urea and creatinine, which returned to normal on day 7. Hourly fluid assessment was maintained for the duration of ICU stay and a positive fluid balance was recorded, a total of 3.2 L positive before discharge from ICU on day 3. Oral fluids were commenced 3 hours post extubation and within 24 hours a light diet was being tolerated. Mrs Murphy remained in the ICU until the third postoperative morning and was then discharged to the step-down unit after removal of all lines and tubes. Mrs Murphy was discharged from hospital to a cardiac rehabilitation centre on day 9.

CASE STUDY QUESTIONS

1 Discuss the steps taken for the management of Mrs Murphy's deterioration with increased drainage from the drain tube post cardiac surgery.
2 Discuss the advantages and disadvantages of IABP counterpulsation use for Mrs Murphy.

RESEARCH VIGNETTE

Sethares KA, Chin E, Costa I. Pain intensity, interference and patient pain management strategies the first 12 weeks after coronary artery bypass graft surgery. Appl Nurs Res 2013;26:174–9

Abstract

Pain is a distressing and often undertreated symptom of cardiac surgery. Little is known about pain levels, interference and treatment strategies beyond the 9 week period. The purpose of this study was to describe pain intensity, interference and strategies used to manage pain in post-operative CABG patients. Baseline data were collected by interview in the hospital after CABG surgery using the Modified Brief Pain Inventory. One to 12 weeks after discharge, weekly telephone interviews were conducted to collect data. Pain levels and interference with activities of daily living were greatest during hospitalization and decreased over 12 weeks. Pain interfered the most with coughing and sleep. Once opioid medications ran out, activity modification was primarily used to manage pain. Activity modification below recommended levels was reported as a pain management strategy. Patients reported pain lasting longer than they expected and the need for more education about activity and pain management strategies.

Critique

The management of postoperative pain is vital for a complete and timely recovery, and to prevent undesirable complications. Few studies have tracked the intensity of pain and its interference with activities of daily living (ADLs) due to cardiac surgical pain beyond the initial period. In this study, a convenience sample of 80 patients participated weekly in telephone interviews for 12 weeks to report their pain intensity scores, sites of pain, how pain interfered with ADLs and coping strategies used to minimise the impact of pain. The sample of patients in this study, 85% of whom completed the study, was a stable, fairly uncomplicated cardiac surgical cohort; only two patients had a history of chronic pain requiring opioid use.

The median pain scores reported from weeks 2 to 12 was below 3 (out of 10); however, the ranges were revealing in that individual scores showed pain intensity up to 5.75 still at week 8. Pain scores for women were consistently higher than men over the entire 12-week period, with statistical significance reached at weeks 4, 6, 10 and 11. The introduction of arm exercises in week 7 during cardiac rehabilitation increased pain scores in the entire cohort. Less than 15% of the cohort fulfilled their opioid prescriptions after the first month, instead choosing to minimise activities as a strategy to minimise pain. At week 8, 10% of the cohort reported a coping strategy of 'bearing it' rather than using analgesic. Based on these results, telephone follow-up is an ideal method of setting and clarifying patients' expectations about pain and related activities, and managing individuals' recoveries. Clearly, the reasons for higher pain scores reported by women need to be considered and addressed. The study was conducted in a single centre that had a number of ethic Portuguese patients who are known to be stoic; however, many patients in Australia and New Zealand have ethnicities (e.g. Anglo-Celtic-Saxon) that have similar stoic attitudes that nurses need to be mindful of while managing pain and recovery. Due to the single site nature of the study and convenience sample, the results may not be generalisable to all cardiac surgical populations.

This article gives an insight into the recovery of patients beyond the early postoperative phase and the important role nurses can play in managing patients' recovery after discharge. Critical care nurses should always be mindful of the education they provide to patients and give written information about expected complications due to incisional pain and appropriate pain management and analgesic advice, including the use of alternatives such as complementary therapies and activity restrictions that are reasonable and not reasonable. The issue of pain being different due to gender is a consideration for all nurses managing post cardiac surgical patients.

Learning activities

1 Compare and contrast the automated and semi-automated modes of intra-aortic ballon counterpulsation.

2 Discuss with a senior colleague the reasons for reduction of IABP therapy complications rate.

3 Discuss how you would identify an intra-aortic balloon catheter rupture and immediate management.

4 Discuss the optimal ventilator setting before extubation of a cardiac surgical patient according to your unit policy and procedures.

5 What haemodynamic values could assist you in deciding the choice of inotropes? Provide rationales.

6 Discuss the management of a patient with cardiac arrest due to pericardial tamponade when an operating theatre is not available.

Online resources

Australian and New Zealand Intensive Care Society (ANZICS), www.anzics.com.au

Australian Institute of Health and Welfare, www.aihw.gov.au

Australian Organ Donor Register (AODR), www.medicareaustralia.gov.au/public/services/aodr/index.jsp

Cardiac Society of Australia and New Zealand, www.csanz.edu.au

Donate Life, www.donatelife.gov.au

National Heart Foundation of Australia, www.heartfoundation.org.au

National Heart Foundation of New Zealand, www.heartfoundation.org.nz

National Health Priorities and Quality, www.health.gov.au/internet/wcms/publishing.nsf/content/pq-cardio

The International Society for Heart and Lung Transplantation (ISHLT), www.ishlt.org

Transplant Nurses' Association (TNA), www.tna.asn.au

Transplantation Society of Australia and New Zealand (TSANZ), www.tsanz.com.au

Further reading

Kurien S, Gallagher C. Ventricular assist device: saving the failing heart. Prog Transplant 2010;20:134–41.

Laing C. LVAD: left ventricular assist devices for end-stage heart failure. Nurse Pract 2014;39:42-7.

Pellegrino V, Hockings LE, Davies A. Veno-arterial extracorporeal membrane oxygenation for adult cardiovascular failure. Curr Opin Crit Care 2014;20:484-92.

Ramakrishna H, Jaroszewski DE, Arabia FA. Adult cardiac transplantation: a review of perioperative management. Ann Card Anaesth 2009;12:155-65.

References

1 World Health Organization. Global health estimates 2014. Summary tables: Causes by age, sex and region, 2000-2012. Geneva, Switzerland: WHO; 2014.

2 Nichols M, Townsend N, Luengo-Fernandez R, Leal J, Scarborough P, Rayner M. European cardiovascular disease statistics 2012. Brussels: European Heart Network; Sophia Antipolis: European Society of Cardiology; 2012.

3 Australian Institute of Health and Welfare. Cardiovascular disease: Australian facts 2011. Canberra: Australian Institute of Health and Welfare; 2011.

4 Australian Institute of Health and Welfare. Australia's health 2014. Canberra: Australian Institute of Health and Welfare; 2014.

5 Urden LD, Satcy KM, Lough ME. Thelan's critical care nursing diagnosis and management. 5th ed. St Louis: Mosby; 2006.

6 Urden L, Stacy K, Lough M. Critical care nursing: diagnosis and management. 7th ed. St Louis: Mosby; 2014.

7 Modine T, Al-Ruzzeh S, Mazrani W, Azeem F, Bustami M, Ilsley C et al. Use of radial artery graft reduces the morbidity of coronary artery bypass graft surgery in patients aged 65 years and older. Ann Thorac Surg 2002;74(4):1144–7.

8 Agrifoglio M, Dainese L, Pasotti S, Galanti A, Cannata A, Roberto M et al. Preoperative assessment of the radial artery for coronary artery bypass grafting: is the Clinical Allen Test adequate? Ann Thorac Surg 2005;79(2):570-2.

9 Kettering K, Dapunt O, Baer FM. Minimally invasive direct coronary artery bypass grafting: a systematic review. J Cardiovasc Surg 2004;45(3):255-64.

10 Birla R, Patel P, Aresu G, Asimakopoulos G. Minimally invasive direct coronary artery bypass versus off-pump coronary surgery through sternotomy. Ann R Coll Surg Engl 2013;95(7):481-5.

11 Jones BA, Krueger S, Howell D, Meinecke B, Dunn S. Robotic mitral valve repair: a community hospital experience. Tex Heart Inst J 2005; 32(2):143-6.

12 Bush B, Nifong LW, Alwair H, Chitwood WR Jr. Robotic mitral valve surgery – current status and future directions. Ann Cardiothorac Surg 2013;2(6):814-7.

13 Australian Institute of Health and Welfare. Australia's health 2010. Canberra: AIHW; 2010.

14 The Task Force on Myocardial Revascularization of the European Society of Cardiology (ESC) and the European Association for Cardio-Thoracic Surgery (EACTS). Guidelines on myocardial revascularization. Eur Heart J 2010;31:2501-55.

15 Curiel-Balsera E, Mora-Ordoñez JM, Castillo-Lorente E, Benitez-Parejo J, Herruzo-Avilés A, Ravina-Sanz JJ et al. Mortality and complications in elderly patients undergoing cardiac surgery. J Crit Care 2013;28:397-404.

16 Chieffo A, Buchanan GL, Van Mieghem NM, Tchetche D, Dumonteil N, Latib A et al. Transcatheter aortic valve implantation with the Edwards SAPIEN versus the Medtronic CoreValve revalving system devices. A multicenter collaborative study: The PRAGMATIC Plus Initiative (Pooled-RotterdAm-Milano-Toulouse in collaboration). J Am Coll Cardiol 2013;61(8):830-6.

17 Popma JJ, Adams DH, Reardon MJ, Yakubov SJ, Kleiman NS,Heimansohn D et al. Transcatheter aortic valve replacement using a self-expanding bioprosthesis in patients with severe aortic stenosis at extreme risk for surgery. J Am Coll Cardiol 2014;63(19):1972-81.

18 Bhukal I, Solanki SL, Ramaswamy S, Yaddanapudi LN, Jain A, Kumar P. Perioperative predictors of morbidity and mortality following cardiac surgery under cardiopulmonary bypass. Saudi J Anaesth 2012;6(3):242-7.

19 Martin CG, Turkelson SL. Nursing care of the patient undergoing coronary artery bypass grafting. J Cardiovasc Nurs 2006;21(2):109-17.

20 Currey J, Browne J, Botti M. Haemodynamic instability after cardiac surgery: nurses' perceptions of clinical decision-making. J Clin Nurs 2006;15(9):1081-90.

21 St Andre AC, DelRossi A. Hemodynamic management of patients in the first 24 hours after cardiac surgery. Crit Care Med 2005;33(9):2082-93.

22 Reuter DA, Felbinger TW, Moerstedt K, Weis F, Schmidt C, Kilger E et al. Intrathoracic blood volume index measured by thermodilution for preload monitoring after cardiac surgery. J Cardiothorac Vasc Anesth 2002;16(2):191-5.

23 Currey J, Botti M. The haemody namic status of cardiac surgical patients in the initial 2-h recovery period. Eur J Cardiovasc Nurs 2005;4(3):207-14.

24 Soto-Ruiz KM, Peacock WF, Varon J. Perioperative hypertension: diagnosis and treatment. Netherlands J Crit Care 2011;15(3):143-8.

25 Larmann J, Theilmeier G. Inflammatory response to cardiac surgery: cardiopulmonary bypass versus non-cardiopulmonary bypass surgery. Best Pract Res Clin Anaesthesiol 2004;18(3):425-38.

26 Sponholz C, Schelenz C, Reinhart K, Schirmer U, Stehr SN. Catecholamine and volume therapy for cardiac surgery in Germany – results from a postal survey. Anesth Card Surg Germany 2014;9(8):1-8.

27 Perel P, Roberts I, Ker K. Colloids versus crystalloids for fluid resuscitation in critically ill patients. Cochrane Database Syst Rev 2013;2:1-71.

28 Skhirtladze K, Base EM, Lassnigg A, Kaider A, Linke S, Dworschak M et al. Comparison of the effects of albumin 5%, hydroxyethyl starch 130/0.4 6%, and Ringer's lactate on blood loss and coagulation after cardiac surgery. Br J Anaesth 2014;112(2):255-64.

29 Ristic AD, Imazio M, Adler Y, Anastasakis A, Badano LP, Brucato A et al. Triage strategy for urgent management of cardiac tamponade: a position statement of the European Society of Cardiology Working Group on Myocardial and Pericardial Diseases. Eur Heart J 2014;35(34):2279-84.

30 Foroughi M, Conte AH. Cardiovascular complications and management after dardiac surgery. In: Dabbagh A, Esmailian F, Aranki SF, eds. Postoperative critical care for cardiac surgical patients. Berlin: Springer; 2014. p. 197-211.

31 Westerberg M, Bengtsson A, Jeppsson A. Coronary surgery without cardiotomy suction and autotransfusion reduces the postoperative systemic inflammatory response. Ann Thorac Surg 2004;78(1):54-9.

32 Majure DT, Greco T, Greco M, Ponschab M, Biondi-Zoccai G, Zangrillo A et al. Meta-analysis of randomized trials of effect of milrinone on mortality in cardiac surgery: an update. J Cardiothorac Vasc Anesth 2013;27(2):220-9.

33 Albright TN, Zimmerman MA, Selzman CH. Vasopressin in the cardiac surgery intensive care unit. Am J Crit Care 2002;11(4):326-30.

34 Mastropietroa CW, Davalosa MC, Walters HL, Deliusa RE. Clinical response to arginine vasopressin therapy after paediatric cardiac surgery. Cardiol Young 2013;23(3):387-93.

35 Wagner GS, Strauss DG. Marriott's practical electrocardiography. 12th ed. Baltimore: Lippincott, Williams & Wilkins; 2014.

36 Dennis MJ. ECG criteria to differentiate pulmonary artery catheter irritation from other proarrhythmic influences as the cause of ventricular arrhythmias [abstract]. Am Coll Cardiol 2002;39(9 [SupplB]):2B.

37 Nair SG. Atrial fibrillation after cardiac surgery. Ann Card Anaesth 2010;13:196-205.

38 Mitchell LB, Crystal E, Heilbron B, Page P. Atrial fibrillation following cardiac surgery. Can J Cardiol 2005;21(SupplB):45B-50B.

39 Peretto G, Durante A, Limite LR, Cianflone D. Postoperative arrhythmias after cardiac surgery: incidence, risk factors, and therapeutic management. Cardiol Res Pract 2014;2014:1-15.

40 Bansal S, Thai HM, Hsu CH, Sai-Sudhakar CB, Goldman S, Rhenman BE. Fast track extubation post coronary artery bypass graft: a retrospective review of predictors of clinical outcomes. World J Cardiovasc Surg 2013;3:81-6.

41 Fitch ZW, Debesa O, Ohkuma R, Duquaine D, Steppan J, Schneider EB et al. A protocol-driven approach to early extubation after heart surgery. J Thorac Cardiovasc Surg 2014;147(3):1344-50.

42 Badhwar V, Esper S, Brooks M, Mulukutla S, Hardison R, Mallios D et al. Extubating in the operating room following adult cardiac surgery safely improves outcomes and lowers costs. J Thorac Cardiovasc Surg 2014;148(6):3101-9.e1.

43 Galas F, Almeida JP, Fukushima JT, Osawa EA, Nakamura RE, Silva C et al. Blood transfusion in cardiac surgery is a risk factor for increased hospital length of stay in adult patients. J Cardiothorac Surg 2013;8(54):1-7.

44 Hajjar LA, Vincent J, Galas FRBG, Nakamura RE, Silva CMP, Santos MH et al. TRACS randomized controlled trial transfusion requirements after cardiac surgery. JAMA 2010;304(14):1559-67.

45 Suárez CJ, Gayoso DP, Gude SF, Gómez ZJM, Rey AH, Fontanillo FM. Method to calculate the protamine dose necessary for reversal of heparin as a function of activated clotting time in patients undergoing cardiac surgery. JECT 2013;45(4):235-41.

46 Hofmann B, Bushnaq H, Kraus FB, Raspé C, Simm A, Silber RE et al. Immediate effects of individualized heparin and protamine management on hemostatic activation and platelet function in adult patients undergoing cardiac surgery with tranexamic acid antifibrinolytic therapy. Perfusion 2013;28:412-8.

47 Galeone A, Rotunno C, Guida P, Assunta B, Rubino G, Schinosa LLT et al. Monitoring incomplete heparin reversal and heparin rebound after cardiac surgery. J Cardiothorac Vasc Anesth 2013;27(5):853-8.

48 Bryant B, Knights K, Salerno E. Pharmacology for health professionals. Sydney: Mosby; 2003.

49 Marcinkiewicz A. Cardiac tamponade and para-aortic hematoma post elective surgical myocardial revascularization on a beating heart – a possible complication of the Lima-stitch and sequential venous anastomosis. BMC Cardiovascular Disorders 2014;14:72.

50 Harirforoosh S, Asghar W, Jamali F. Adverse effects of nonsteroidal antiinflammatory drugs: an update of gastrointestinal, cardiovascular and renal complications. J Pharm Pharm Sci 2013;16(5):821-47.

51 Nussmeier NA, Whelton AA, Brown MT, Langford RM, Hoeft A, Parlow JL et al. Complications of the COX-2 inhibitors parecoxib and valdecoxib after cardiac surgery. New Engl J Med 2005;352(11):1081-91.

52 Bradley D, Cresswell LL, Hogue CW, Epstein AE, Prystowsky EN, Daoud EG. Pharmacologic prophylaxis: American College of Chest Physicians guidelines for the prevention and management of postoperative atrial fibrillation after cardiac surgery. Chest 2005;128(2Suppl):S39-47.

53 Koivula M, Paunonen-Ilmonen M, Tarkka M, Laippala P. Fear and anxiety in patients awaiting coronary artery bypass grafting. Heart Lung 2001;30(4):302-11.

54 Gallagher R, McKinley S, Dracup K. Evaluation of telephone follow-up to promote psychosocial adjustment and risk factor modification in women with coronary heart disease. Heart Lung 2003;32(2):79-87.

55 King K. Emotional and functional outcomes in women with coronary heart disease. J Cardiovasc Nurs 2001;15(3):54-70.

56 Roohafza H, Sadeghi M, Khani A, Andalib E, Alikhasi H, Rafiei M. Psychological state in patients undergoing coronary artery bypass grafting surgery or percutaneous coronary intervention and their spouses. Int J Nurs Pract 2014 Apr 22. doi: 10.1111/ijn.12234.

57 Fiabane E, Giorgi I, Candura SM, Argentero P. Psychological and work stress assessment of patients following angioplasty or heart surgery: results of 1-year follow-up study. Stress Health 2014 Feb 19. doi: 10.1002/smi.2564.

58 Parvan K, Zamanzadeh V, Lak Dizaji S, Mousavi Shabestari M, Safaie N. Patient's perception of stressors associated with coronary artery bypass surgery. J Cardiovasc Thorac Res 2013;5(3):113-7.

59 Parissis H, Soo A, Al-Alao B. Intraaortic balloon pump: literature review of risk factors related to complications of the intraaortic balloon pump. J Cardiothorac Surg 2011;6:147.

60 Wu X, Liu H, Zhao X, Cao J, ZHU P. Factors influencing outcomes of intra-aortic balloon counterpulsation in elderly patients. Chin Med J 2013; 126(14):2632-5.

61 Kale P, Fang JC. Devices in acute heart failure. Crit Care Med 2008;36(1 (Suppl)):S121-S128.

62 Duvernoy CS, Bates ER. Management of cardiogenic shock attributable to acute myocardial infarction in the reperfusion era. J Intens Care Med 2005;20(4):188-98.

63 Cheng LM, Valk SDA, den Uil CA, Van der Ent M, Lagrand WK, Van de Sand M et al. Usefulness of intraaortic balloon counterpulsation in patients with cardiogenic shock from acute myocardial infarction. Am J Cardiol 2009;104:327-32.

64 Onorati F, Santarpino G, Presta P, Caroleo S, Abdalla K, Santangelo E et al. Pulsatile perfusion with intra-aortic balloon pumping ameliorates whole body response to cardiopulmonary bypass in the elderly. Cri Care Med 2009;37(3):902-11.

65 Hanlon-Pena PM, Quaal SJ. Intra-aortic balloon pump timing review of evidence supporting current practice. Am J Crit Care 2011;20(4):323-33.

66 Elahi MM, Chetty GK, Kirke R, Azeem T, Hartshorne R, Spyt TJ. Complications related to intra-aortic balloon pump in cardiac surgery: a decade later. Eur J Vasc Endovasc Surg 2005;29(6):591-4.

67 Meco M, Gramegna G, Yassini A, Bellisario A, Mazzaro E, Babbini M et al. Mortality and morbidity from intra-aortic balloon pumps: risk analysis. J Cardiovasc Surg 2002;43(1):17-23.

68 Pucher PH, Cummings IG, Shipolini AR, McCormack DJ. Is heparin needed for patients with an intra-aortic balloon pump? Interactive CardioVasc Thorac Surg 2012;15:136-40.

69 Manohar VA, Levin RN, Karadolian SS, Usmani A, Timmis RM Dery ME et al. The impact of intra-aortic balloon pump weaning protocols on in-hospital clinical outcomes. J Interv Cardiol 2012;25(2):140-6.

70 Schreuder J, Castiglioni A, Donelli A, Maisano F, Jansen J, Hanania R et al. Automatic intraaortic balloon pump timing using an intrabeat dicrotic notch prediction algorithm. Ann Thorac Surg 2005;79:1017-22.

71 Schreuder J, Maisano F, Donelli A, Jansen J, Hanlon P, Bovelander J et al. Beat-to-beat effects of intraaortic balloon pump timing on left ventricular performance in patients with low ejection fraction. Ann Thorac Surg 2005;79:872-80.

72 Chapman JR. Transplantation in Australia – 50 years in progress. Med J Aust 1992;157(1):46-50.

73 McBride M, Chapman JR. An overview of transplantation in Australia. Anaesth Intensive Care 1995;23(1):60-4.

74 Borel JF, Feurer C, Gubler HU, Stahelin H. Biological effects of cyclosporin-A: a new antilymphocytic agent. Agents Action 1976;6(4):468-75.

75 Barnard CN. A human cardiac transplant: an interim report of a successful operation performed at Groote Schuur Hospital, Capetown. S Afr Med J 1967;41(48):1271-4.

76 Oyer PE, et al. Cyclosporin A in cardiac allografting: a preliminary experience. Transplant Proc 1983;15:1247-52.

77 Excell L, Wride P, Russ GR. Australia and New Zealand organ donation registry, <http://www.anzdata.org/au/anzod/ANZODReport/2010/2010Contents.pdf>; 2010 [accessed 19.08.10].

78 Eurotransplant International Foundation. Annual Report 2013, <http://www.eurotransplant.org/cms/index.php?page=annual_reports>; 2013 [accessed 18.07.14].

79 Rose EA, Moskowitz AJ, Packer M, Sollano JA, Williams DL, Tierney AR et al. The REMATCH trial: rationale, design, and end points. Randomized Evaluation of Mechanical Assistance for the Treatment of Congestive Heart Failure. Ann Thorac Surg 1999;67(3):723-30.

80 Kirklin JK, Naftel, DC, Pagani, FD, Kormos RL, Stevenson LW, Blume ED et al. Sixth INTERMACS annual report: a 10,000-patient database. J Heart Lung Transplant 2014;33(6):555-64.

81 Lund LH, Edwards LB, Kucheryavaya AY, Dipchand AI, Benden C, Christie JD et al. The Registry of the International Society for Heart and Lung Transplantation: Thirtieth Official Adult Heart Transplant Report – 2013; focus theme: age. J Heart Lung Transplant 2013;32(10):951-64.

82 Australia and New Zealand Organ Donation Registry. The ANZROD Annual Report, <http://www.anzdata.org.au/anzod/v1/AR-2013.html>; 2013 [accessed 07.07.14].

83 Mancini D, Lietz K. Selection of cardiac transplantation candidates in 2010. Circulation 2010;122(2):173-83.

84 Mehra MR, Kobashigawa J, Starling R, Russell S, Uber PA, Parameshwa J et al. Listing criteria for heart transplantation: International Society for Heart and Lung Transplantation guidelines for the care of cardiac transplant candidates – 2006. J Heart Lung Transplant 2006;25(9):1024-42.

85 Russo MJ, Chen JM, Hong KN, Stewart AS, Ascheim DD, Argenziano M et al. Survival after heart transplantation is not diminished among recipients with uncomplicated diabetes mellitus: an analysis of the United Network of Organ Sharing database. Circulation 2006;114(21):2280-7.

86 Grady KL, White-Williams C, Naftel D, Costanzo MR, Pitt D, Rayburn B et al. Are preoperative obesity and cachexia risk factors for post heart transplant morbidity and mortality: a multi-institutional study of preoperative weight-height indices. Cardiac Transplant Research Database (CTRD) Group. J Heart Lung Transplant 1999;18(8):750-63.

87 Chacko RC, Harper RG, Gotto J, Young J. Psychiatric interview and psychometric predictors of cardiac transplant survival. Am J Psychiatry 1996;153(12):1607-12.

88 Shapiro PA, Williams DL, Foray AT, Gelman IS, Wukich N, Sciacca R. Psychosocial evaluation and prediction of compliance problems and morbidity after heart transplantation. Transplantation 1995;60(12):1462-6.

89 Macdonald P. Heart transplantation: who should be considered and when? Intern Med J 2008;38(12):911-7.

90 The Transplantation Society of Australia and New Zealand. Eligibility guidelines and allocation protocols, <http://www.tsanz.com.au/organ allocationprotocols/downloads/TSANZ%20Elibility%20and%20Allocation%202nd%20Draft.pdf>; 2010 [accessed 26.08.14].

91 Clarke R, McLennan S, Dawson A, Wilkinson D, Stewart S. Uncovering a hidden epidemic: a study of the current burden of heart failure in Australia. Heart Lung Circ 2004;13(3):266-73.

92 McMurray JJV, Adamopoulos S, Anker SD, Auricchio A, Bohm M, Dickstein K et al. Task force for the diagnosis and treatment of acute and chronic heart failure 2012 of the European Society of Cardiology. ESC Guidelines for the diagnosis and treatment of acute and chronic heart failure. Eur Heart J 2012;33:1787-847.

93 Chronic Heart Failure Working Party, Hospital admission risk program (HARP): Chronic heart failure working group report. Melbourne: Victorian Government Department of Human Services; 2003.

94 Doughty R, Yee T, Sharpe N, MacMahon S. Hospital admissions and deaths due to congestive heart failure in New Zealand, 1988-91. N Z Med J 1995;108(1012):473-5.

95 Garg R, Packer M, Pitt B, Yusuf S. Heart failure in the 1990s: evolution of a major public health problem in cardiovascular medicine. J Am Coll Cardiol 1993;22(4 Suppl A):3A-5A.

96 Australian Institute of Health and Welfare. Heart, stroke and vascular disease: Australian Facts 2001. Perth: Australian Institute of Health and Welfare, The National Heart Foundation, and National Stroke Foundation of Australia; 2001.

97 Kirklin JK, Young JB, McGiffin DC. Heart transplantation. Philadelphia: Churchill Livingstone; 2002.

98 Angermann CE, Spes CH, Tammen A, Stempfle HU, Schutz A, Kemkes BM et al. Anatomic characteristics and valvular function of the transplanted heart: transthoracic versus transesophageal echocardiographic findings. J Heart Transplant 1990;9(4):331-8.

99 Kendall SWH, Ciulli F, Mullins PA, Biocina B, Dunning JJ, Large SR. Total orthotopic heart transplantation: an alternative to the standard technique. Ann Thorac Surg 1992;54:187-92.

100 Dreyfus G, Jebara V, Mihaileanu S, Carpentier AF. Total orthotopic heart transplantation: an alternative to the standard technique. Ann Thorac Surg 1991;52(5):1181-4.

101 Jahanyar J, Koerne, MM, Ghodsizad A, Loebe M, Noon GP. Heterotopic heart transplantation: the United States experience. Heart Surg Forum 2014;17(3):E132-40.

102 Nakatani T, Frazier OH, Lammermeier DE, Marcis MP, Radovancevic B. Heterotopic heart transplantation: a reliable option for a select group of high-risk patients. J Heart Lung Transplant 1989;8(1):40-7.

103 Newcomb AE, Esmore DS, Rosenfeldt FL, Richardson M, Marasco SF. Heterotopic heart transplantation: an expanding role in the twenty-first century? Ann Thorac Surg 2004;78(4):1345-50; discussion 1350-1.

104 Neerukonda SK, Schoonmaker FW, Nampalli VK, Narrod JA. Ventricular dysrthythmia and heterotopic heart transplantation. J Heart Lung Transplant 1992;11:793-6.

105 Costanzo MR, Dipchand A, Starling R, Anderson A, Chan M, Desai S et al. The International Society of Heart and Lung Transplantation Guidelines for the care of heart transplant recipients. J Heart Lung Transplant 2010;29(8):914-56.

106 Busauschina A, Schnuelle P, van der Woude FJ. Cyclosporine nephrotoxicity. Transplant Proc 2004;36(2 Suppl):229S-233S.

107 Serkova NJ, Christians U, Benet LZ. Biochemical mechanisms of cyclosporine neurotoxicity. Mol Interv 2004;4(2):97-107.

108 Trento A, Hardesty RL, Griffith BP, Zerbe T, Kormos RL, Bahnson HT. Role of the antibody to vascular endothelial cells in hyperacute rejection in patients undergoing cardiac transplantation. J Thorac Cardiovasc Surg 1988;95(1):37-41.

109 Laufer G, Laczkovics A, Wollenek G, Buxbaum P, Seitelberger R, Holzinge C et al. The progression of mild acute cardiac rejection evaluated by risk factor analysis. The impact of maintenance steroids and serum creatinine. Transplantation 1991;51(1):184-9.

110 Berry GJ, Laczkovics A, Wollenek G, Buxbaum P, Seitelberger R, Holzinger C et al. The 2013 International Society for Heart and Lung Transplantation Working Formulation for the standardization of nomenclature in the pathologic diagnosis of antibody-mediated rejection in heart transplantation. J Heart Lung Transplant 2013;32(12):1147-62.

111 Stevenson LW,Miller LW. Cardiac transplantation as therapy for heart failure. Curr Probl Cardiol 1991;16(4):217-305.

112 Hammond EH. Pathology of cardiac allograft rejection. In: Cooper DKC, Miller LW, Patterson GA, eds. The transplantation and replacement of thoracic organs. Boston: Kluwer; 1996, pp 239-52.

113 Caves PK, Stinson EB, Billingham ME, Rider AK, Shumway NE. Diagnosis of human cardiac allograft rejection by serial cardiac biopsy. J Thorac Cardiovasc Surg 1973;66(3):461-6.

114 Billingham ME, Cary NR, Hammond ME, Kemnitz J, Marboe C, McCallister HA et al. A working formulation for the standardization of nomenclature in the diagnosis of heart and lung rejection: Heart Rejection Study Group. The International Society for Heart Transplantation. J Heart Transplant 1990;9(6):587-93.

115 Stewart S, Berry C, McMurray JJ. Revision of the 1990 working formulation for the standardization of nomenclature in the diagnosis of heart rejection. J Heart Lung Transplant 2005;24(11):1710-20.

116 Lloveras JJ, Escourrou G, Delisle MB, Fournial G, Cerene A, Bassanetti I et al. Evolution of untreated mild rejection in heart transplant recipients. J Heart Lung Transplant 1992;11(4 Pt 1):751-6.

117 Olsen SL, Wagoner LE, Hammond EH, Taylor DO, Yowell R, Ensley RD et al. Vascular rejection in heart transplantation: clinical correlation, treatment options, and future considerations. J Heart Lung Transplant 1993;12(2):S135-42.

118 Partanen J, Nieminen MS, Krogerus L, Harjula AL, Mattila S. Heart transplant rejection treated with plasmapheresis. J Heart Lung Transplant 1992;11(2 Pt 1):301-5.

119 Williams TJ, Snell GI. Lung transplantation. In: Albert RK, Spiro SG, Jett JR, eds. Clinical respiratory medicine. Philadelphia: Mosby; 2004, pp 831-45.

120 Taylor DO. Cardiac transplantation: drug regimens for the 21st century. Ann Thorac Surg 2003;75(6 Suppl):S72-8.

121 Wade CR, Reith KK, Sikora JH,Augustine SM. Postoperative nursing care of the cardiac transplant recipient. Crit Care Nurs Q, 2004;27(1):17-28; quiz 29-30.

122 Keogh A. Calcineurin inhibitors in heart transplantation. J Heart Lung Transplant 2004;23(5 Suppl):S202-6.

123 Eisen HJ, Kobashigawa J, Keogh A, Bourge R, Renlund D, Mentzer R et al. Three-year results of a randomized, double-blind, controlled trial of mycophenolate mofetil versus azathioprine in cardiac transplant recipients. J Heart Lung Transplant 2005;24(5):517-25.

124 Farmer DG, McDiarmid SV, Edelstein S, Renz JF, Hisatake G, Cortina G et al. Induction therapy with interleukin-2 receptor antagonist after intestinal transplantation is associated with reduced acute cellular rejection and improved renal function. Transplant Proc 2004;36(2):331-2.

125 Morris PJ, Monaco AP. A meta-analysis from the Cochrane Library reviewing interleukin 2 receptor antagonists in renal transplantation. Transplantation 2004;77(2):165.

126 Carey JA, Frist WH. Use of polyclonal antilymphocytic preparations for prophylaxis in heart transplantation. J Heart Transplant 1990;9(3 Pt 2):297-300.

127 Moller CH, Gustafsson F, Gluud C, Steinbruchel DA. Interleukin-2 receptor antagonists as induction therapy after heart transplantation: systematic review with meta-analysis of randomized trials. J Heart Lung Transplant 2008;27(8):835-42.

128 Mason VF, Konicki AJ. Left ventricular assist devices as destination therapy. AACN Clin Issues 2003;14(4):488-97.

129 Miller LW, Naftel DC, Bourge RC, Kirklin JK, Brozena SC, Jarcho J et al. Infection after heart transplantation: a multiinstitutional study. Cardiac Transplant Research Database Group. J Heart Lung Transplant 1994;13(3):381-92; discussion 393.

130 Hughes WT, Rivera GK, Schell MJ, Thornton D, Lott L. Successful intermittent chemoprophylaxis for Pneumocystis carinii pneumonitis. N Engl J Med 1987;316(26):1627-32.

131 Kocher AA, Bonaros N, Dunkler D, Ehrlich M, Schlechta B, Zweytick B et al. Long-term results of CMV hyperimmune globulin prophylaxis in 377 heart transplant recipients. J Heart Lung Transplant 2003;22(3):250-7.

132 Couchoud C. Cytomegalovirus prophylaxis with antiviral agents for solid organ transplantation. Cochrane Database Syst Rev 2000(2):CD001320.

133 Walsh TR, Guttendorf J, Dummer S, Hardesty RL, Armitage JM, Kormos RL et al. The value of protective isolation procedures in cardiac allograft recipients. Ann Thorac Surg 1989;47(4):539-44; discussion 544-5.

134 Rourke TK, Droogan MT, Ohler L. Heart transplantation: state of the art. AACN Clin Issues 1999;10(2):185-201; quiz 307-9.

135 Bowden RA, Slichter SJ, Sayers M, Weisdorf D, Cays M, Schoch G et al. A comparison of filtered leukocyte-reduced and cytomegalovirus (CMV) seronegative blood products for the prevention of transfusion-associated CMV infection after marrow transplant. Blood 1995;86(9):3598-603.

136 Luckraz H, Goddard M, Charman SC, Wallwork J, Parameshwar J, Large SR. Early mortality after cardiac transplantation: should we do better? J Heart Lung Transplant 2005;24(4):401-5.

137 Cooper DKC, Lidsky NM. Immediate postoperative care and potential complications. In: Cooper DKC, Miller LW, Patterson GA, eds. The transplantation and replacement of thoracic organs. Boston: Kluwer; 1996, pp 221-7.

138 McCrystal GD, Pepe S, Esmore DS, Rosenfeld FL. The challenge of improving donor heart preservation. Heart Lung Circ 2004;13:74-83.

139 Rosenfeldt FL, McCrystal G, Pepe S, Esmore D. Myocyte or heart preservation. In: Large S. Towards optimising donor heart quality. Cambridge: publisher; 2002.

140 Esmore DS, Rosenfeldt FL, Mack JA, Waters KN, Bergin P. Long ischaemic time allografts (>6 hr) further expand the transplant donor pool. Washington: International Society of Heart and Lung Transplantation Conference Abstracts; 2002.

141 Kieler-Jensen N, Lundin S, Ricksten SE. Vasodilator therapy after heart transplantation: effects of inhaled nitric oxide and intravenous prostacyclin, prostaglandin E1, and sodium nitroprusside. J Heart Lung Transplant 1995;14(3):436-43.

142 Kristof AS, Magder S. Low systemic vascular resistance state in patients undergoing cardiopulmonary bypass. Crit Care Med 1999;27(6):1121-7.

143 Myles PS, Leong CK, Currey J. Endogenous nitric oxide and low systemic vascular resistance after cardiopulmonary bypass. J Cardiothorac Vasc Anaesth 1997;11(5):571-4.

144 Landry DW, Levin HR, Gallant EM, Ashton RC Jr, Seo S, D'Alessandro D et al. Vasopressin deficiency contributes to the vasodilation of septic shock. Circulation 1997;95(5):1122-5.

145 Argenziano M, Choudhri AF, Oz MC, Rose EA, Smith CR, Landry DW. A prospective randomized trial of arginine vasopressin in the treatment of vasodilatory shock after left ventricular assist device placement. Circulation 1997;96(9 Suppl):II-286-90.

146 Ardehali A, Hughes K, Sadeghi A, Esmailian F, Marelli D, Moriguchi J et al. Inhaled nitric oxide for pulmonary hypertension after heart transplantation. Transplantation 2001;72(4):638-41.

147 Rossaint R, Falke KJ, Lopez F, Slama K, Pison U, Zapol WM. Inhaled nitric oxide for the adult respiratory distress syndrome. N Engl J Med 1993;328(6):399-405.

148 Armitage JM, Hardesty RL, Griffith BP. Prostaglandin E1: an effective treatment of right heart failure after orthotopic heart transplantation. J Heart Lung Transplant 1987;6:348-51.

149 Wang SS, Ko WJ, Chen YS, Hsu RB, Chou NK, Chu SH. Mechanical bridge with extracorporeal membrane oxygenation and ventricular assist device to heart transplantation. Artif Organs 2001;25(8):599-602.

150 Karamlou T, Gelow J, Diggs BS, Tibayan FA, Mudd JM, Guyton SW et al. Mechanical circulatory support pathways that maximize post-heart transplant survival. Ann Thorac Surg 2013;95(2):480-5; discussion 485.

151 Ellenbogen KA, Thames MD, DiMarco JP, Sheehan H, Lerman BB. Electrophysiological effects of adenosine in the transplanted human heart. Evidence of supersensitivity. Circulation 1990;81(3):821-8.

152 Macdonald P, Hackworthy R Keogh A, Sivathasan C, Chang V, Spratt P. Atrial overdrive pacing for reversion of atrial flutter after heart transplantation. J Heart Lung Transplant 1991;10(5 Pt 1):731-7.

153 Mackintosh AF, Carmichael DJ, Wren C, Cory-Pearce R, English TA. Sinus node function in first three weeks after cardiac transplantation. Br Heart J 1982;48(6):584-8.

154 Stark RP, McGinn AL, Wilson RF. Chest pain in cardiac-transplant recipients. Evidence of sensory reinnervation after cardiac transplantation. N Engl J Med 1991;324(25):1791-4.

155 Parry A, Roberts M, Parameshwar J, Wallwork J, Schofield P, Large S. The management of post-cardiac transplantation coronary artery disease. Eur J Cardiothorac Surg 1996;10(7):528-32; discussion 53.

156 Shiba N, et al. Analysis of survivors more than 10 years after heart transplantation in the cyclosporine era: Stanford experience. J Heart Lung Transplant 2004;23(2):155-64.

157 Valantine H. Cardiac allograft vasculopathy after heart transplantation: risk factors and management. J Heart Lung Transplant 2004;23 (5 Suppl):S187-93.

158 Kobashigawa J. What is the optimal prophylaxis for treatment of cardiac allograft vasculopathy? Curr Control Trials Cardiovasc Med 2000;1:166.

159 Rose EA, Pepino P, Barr ML, Smith CR, Ratner AJ, Ho E et al. Relation of HLA antibodies and graft atherosclerosis in human cardiac allograft recipients. J Heart Lung Transplant 1992;11(3 Pt 2):S120-3.

160 Johnson DE, Alderman EL, Schroeder JS, Gao SZ, Hunt S, DeCampli WM et al. Transplant coronary artery disease: histopathologic correlations with angiographic morphology. J Am Coll Cardiol 1991;17(2):449-57.

161 Keogh A, Richardson M, Ruygrok P, Spratt P, Galbraith A, O'Driscoll G et al. Sirolimus in de novo heart transplant recipients reduces acute rejection and prevents coronary artery disease at 2 years: a randomized clinical trial. Circulation 2004;110(17):2694-700.

162 Na R, Grulich AE, Meagher NS, McCaughan GW, Keogh AM, Vajdic CM. De novo cancer-related death in Australian liver and cardiothoracic transplant recipients. Am J Transplant 2013;13(5):1296-304.

163 Krikorian JG, Anderson JL, Bieber CP, Penn I, Stinson EB. Malignant neoplasms following cardiac transplantation. JAMA 1978;240(7):639-43.

164 Ong CS, Keogh AM, Kossard S, Macdonald PS, Spratt PM. Skin cancer in Australian heart transplant recipients. J Am Acad Dermatol 1999;40(1):27-34.

165 Veness MJ, Quinn DI, Ong CS, Keogh AM, Macdonald PS, Cooper SG et al. Aggressive cutaneous malignancies following cardiothoracic transplantation: the Australian experience. Cancer 1999;85(8):1758-64.

166 Armitage JM, Kormos RL, Stuart RS, Fricker FJ, Griffith BP, Nalesnik M et al. Posttransplant lymphoproliferative disease in thoracic organ transplant patients: ten years of cyclosporine-based immunosuppression. J Heart Lung Transplant 1991;10(6):877-86; discussion 886-7.

167 Cole WH. The increase in immunosuppression and its role in the development of malignant lesions. J Surg Oncol 1985;30(3):139-44.

168 Penn I. Cancers following cyclosporine therapy. Transplantation 1987;43(1): 32-5.

169 Penn I, First MR. Development and incidence of cancer following cyclosporine therapy. Transplant Proc 1986;18(2 Suppl 1):210-5.

170 Greenberg A, Thompson ME, Griffith BJ, Hardesty RL, Kormos RL, el-Shahawy MA et al. Cyclosporine nephrotoxicity in cardiac allograft patients – a seven-year follow-up. Transplantation 1990;50(4):589-93.

171 Eisen HJ. Hypertension in heart transplant recipients: more than just cyclosporine. J Am Coll Cardiol 2003;41(3):433-4.

172 Ventura HO, et al. Mechanisms of hypertension in cardiac transplantation and the role of cyclosporine. Curr Opin Cardiol 1997;12(4):375-81.

Chapter 13

Respiratory assessment and monitoring

Mona Ringdal, Janice Gullick

Learning objectives

After reading this chapter, you should be able to:

- understand respiratory anatomy and normal physiology
- understand mechanisms contributing to altered respiratory function
- identify key principles underpinning assessment and monitoring of respiratory function
- describe nursing assessment and monitoring activities for critically ill patients with respiratory dysfunction
- discuss the importance of patient assessment skills, and the contribution of diagnostic and laboratory findings to ongoing clinical management
- outline the physiological basis for different types of monitoring
- describe common diagnostic procedures used in critical care.

Introduction

The respiratory system ensures adequate tissue and cellular oxygenation for the body. It is responsible for gas exchange through the uptake of oxygen and excretion of carbon dioxide (CO_2); assists in optimal organ function; contributes to acid–base balance; and therefore plays a large role in maintaining homeostasis. As respiratory conditions account for 20–26% of admissions to intensive care units (ICUs) in the USA and UK,[1] and up to 33% in Australian hospitals,[2] a thorough understanding of the anatomy, physiology and pathophysiology of this complex system is required to accurately assess critically ill patients and monitor response to treatment or early signs of deterioration.

This chapter provides a comprehensive description of the principles and practice of respiratory assessment, monitoring and diagnostics. These are foundational concepts underpinning timely and effective interventions for critically ill patients. Management of respiratory alterations, oxygenation and ventilation are discussed in Chapters 14 and 15.

KEY WORDS

arterial blood
gases
capnography
diagnostic imaging
gas exchange
hypoxaemia
oxygen delivery
pulse oximetry
work of breathing

Related anatomy and physiology

The thoracic cavity contains the trachea and bronchial tree, the two lungs, pleura and diaphragm. The mediastinum, located between the lungs, houses and protects the heart, great vessels and the oesophagus. Twelve pairs of ribs cover the lungs. Ten are connected to the spine posteriorly, and to the sternum or to the cartilage of the above rib anteriorly (ribs 8–10). The 11th and 12th ribs have no anterior attachment (see Figure 13.1).[3]

The respiratory system is divided into upper and lower respiratory tracts: the upper airways consist of the nose, nasal conchae, sinus and pharynx; the lower respiratory tract includes the larynx, trachea, bronchi and lungs.[5] Larger airways are lined with stratified epithelial tissue, which has a relatively high cellular turnover rate; these cells protect and clear these large airways. Additional specialised features of this tissue include an extensive distribution of mucus/goblet cells and cilia, which facilitate the airways' mucociliary clearance system.

Upper respiratory tract

The nasal cavities contain an extremely vascular and mucoid environment for warming and humidifying inhaled gases. To maximise exposure to this surface area, the nasal conchae create turbulent gas flow. Mucus is moved by the cilia at the top of the epithelial cells lining the conducting airways. Mucus moves towards the pharynx at a rate of 1–2 cm per minute, providing filtration and cleaning of the inhaled air. One litre of mucus is produced every day with only a small part not reabsorbed by the body.[6,7]

The pharynx is a muscular tube that transports food to the oesophagus and air to the larynx. Inferior to the pharynx, the larynx consists mostly of cartilage attached to other surrounding structures and houses the vestibular (false) vocal folds, which do not produce any sounds but help to close the larynx during swallowing. The lower true vocal cords create the vocal sounds (see Figure 13.2).[8] The pyramid-shaped arytenoids, an important pair of cartilages within the larynx, act as attachment points for the vocal cords. This area is easily damaged by pressure from endotracheal tubes; the most significant independent risk factor for injury to the arytenoids is the length of intubation time.[9] The thyroid cartilage ('Adam's apple') and the cricoid cartilage protect the glottis and entrance to the trachea.[7] Another cartilage in the larynx is the triangular-shaped elastic epiglottis, which protects the lower airways from aspiration of food and fluids into the lungs. The epiglottis usually occludes the inlet to the larynx during swallowing. The primitive cough, swallow and gag reflexes further protect the airway.[7]

FIGURE 13.1 Ventilatory structures of the chest wall and lungs, showing the ribs and lobes of the lungs.[4]

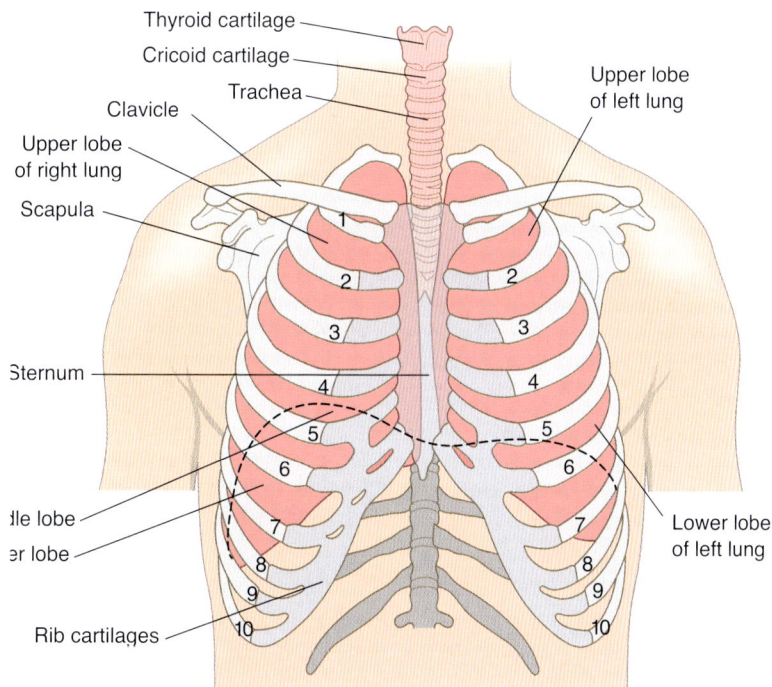

Adapted from Urden L, Stacy K, Lough M. Critical care nursing: Diagnosis and management. 6th ed. St Louis: Mosby; 2010, with permission.

FIGURE 13.2   Larynx. (**A**) Cartilages and ligaments. (**B**) Neck muscles.[10]

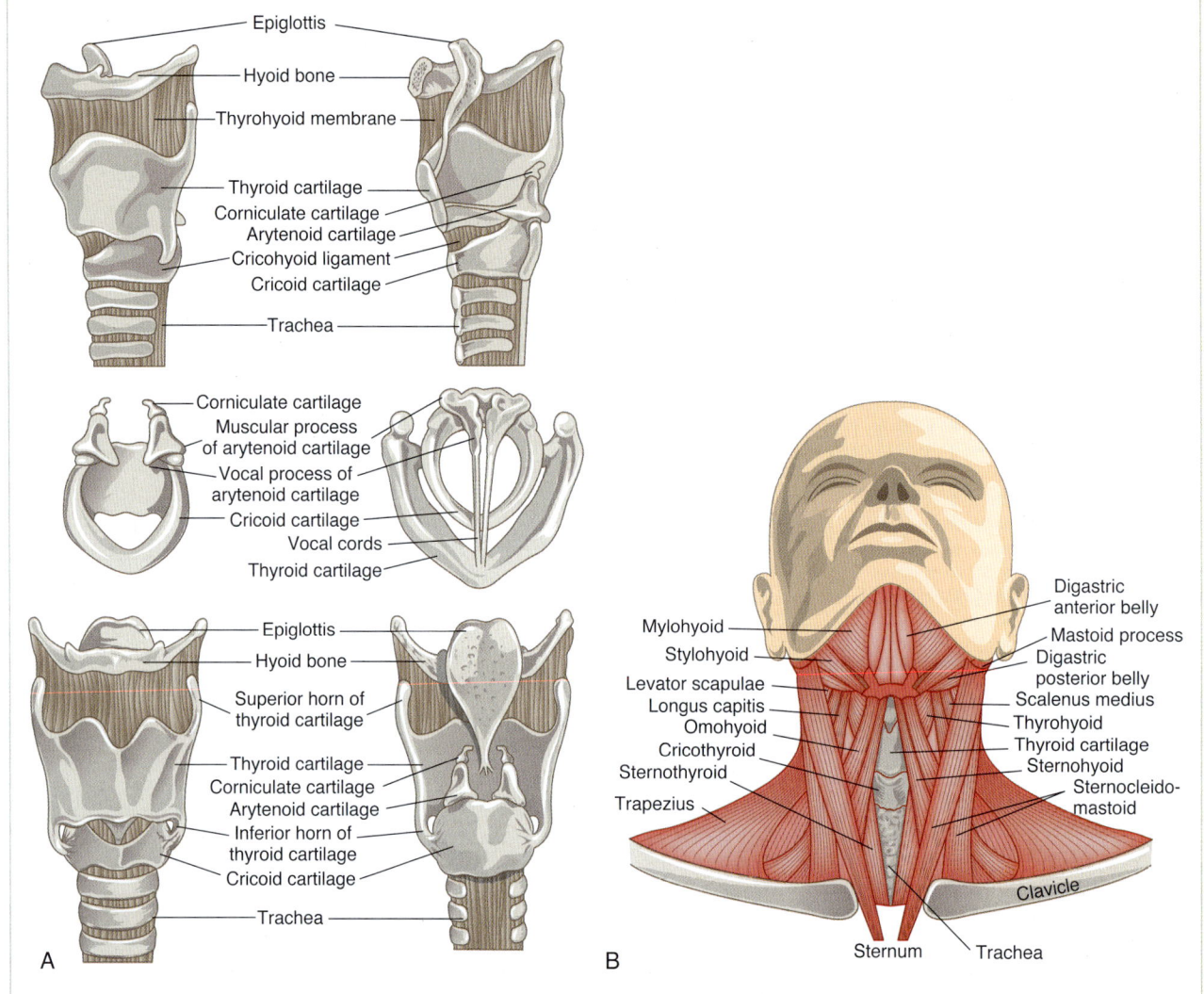

Lower respiratory tract

The trachea is a hollow tube approximately 11 cm long and 2.5 cm in diameter that marks the beginning of the lower respiratory tract. The trachea is supported by 16–20 C-shaped cartilages and is another area at risk of pressure damage from artificial airways. The trachea divides at the carina into the left and right main bronchi. The bronchial tree has two mainstem bronchi that are structurally different. The right bronchus is wider and angles slightly where it divides further into the three lobes of the right lung. The most common site of aspiration of foreign objects is the right bronchus because of its anatomical position. The acutely-angled left main bronchus divides further into the two lobes of the left lung.

The airways within each lung branch further into secondary (or lobar) bronchi then tertiary (or segmental) bronchi. Further divisions within these conducting airways end with the terminal bronchioles, the smallest airways without alveoli. These conducting airways do not participate in gas exchange but form the anatomical dead space (approximately 150 mL).[11]

Larger airways have a greater proportion of supporting cartilage, ciliated epithelium, goblet and serous cells and, hence, a mucous layer. As the airways become smaller, cartilage becomes irregularly dispersed. The number of goblet cells and amount of mucus decrease until, at the alveolar level, there is only a single layer of squamous epithelial cells. Alveolar macrophages present among these epithelial cells phagocytose any small particles that enter the alveoli. Smooth muscle surrounds and supports the bronchioles, enabling airway diameter change and subsequent changes in airway resistance to gas flow.[12]

Thorax/lungs

The lungs and heart are protected within the thoracic cage. When inspiration is triggered, expansion of the thorax creates a negative pressure causing air to flow into the lungs. The thorax then passively compresses to expel air from the lungs during expiration. The diaphragm separates the thorax from the abdomen and is the most important inspiratory muscle, performing approximately 80% of the work of breathing. Inspiration is initiated from the medulla, sending impulses through the phrenic nerve to stimulate the diaphragm to contract and flatten. The phrenic nerve originates in the cervical plexus and involves the third to fifth cervical nerves. It splits into two parts, passing to the left and right side of the heart before it reaches the diaphragm. For this reason, patients can have ventilation difficulties if phrenic nerve damage results from C3–C5 trauma.[12,13]

The conducting airways, ending in the terminal bronchioles, move inspired air towards the respiratory unit. The respiratory unit comprises the respiratory bronchioles, alveolar ducts and alveolar sacs where the diffusion of gas molecules, or gas exchange, occurs. The respiratory unit makes up most of the lung with a volume of 2.5–3 L during rest[11] (see Figure 13.3).

Surfactant

Of particular importance to the structure and function of the respiratory system are the type I and II alveolar epithelial cells. Type I cells provide support of the alveolar unit walls. Type II cells produce an important lipoprotein, surfactant, that lines the inner alveolar surface lowering alveolar surface tension, stabilising the alveoli to optimise lung compliance and facilitating expansion during inspiration.[11] If surfactant synthesis is reduced due to pulmonary disease, lung compliance decreases and the work of breathing increases.[14]

Pleura

Each lung is contained within a continuous thin membrane called the pleura, creating the pleural sac that surrounds each lung. The two pleural sacs, one on each side of the midline, are completely separate from each other. The parietal pleura lines the inner surface of the chest wall and is in close contact with the visceral pleura, which covers the lungs. The pleural space, between these two layers, contains a small amount of serous fluid, which limits friction during lung expansion.

The intrapleural pressure in the pleural space under normal circumstances is always negative with a range of −4 to −10 cmH$_2$O; this negative pressure keeps the lungs inflated. During inhalation the pressure becomes more negative as both the lungs and the chest wall are elastic structures. These elastic fibres of the lung pull the visceral pleura inwards while the chest wall pulls the parietal pleura outward. The pressure difference between the alveolar pressure (0 cmH$_2$O pressure in the lungs) and the intrapleural pressure (−4 cmH$_2$O) across the lung wall is termed the trans-pulmonary pressure (+4 cmH$_2$O [0 − (−4) = +4]), and is the force that holds the lungs open[6,7] (see Figure 13.4).

Pulmonary circulation

The circulatory system of the lung receives the entire cardiac output but operates as a low pressure system; it only directs blood back to the left side of the heart (unlike the systemic circulation, which pumps blood to different regions of the entire body). Within the pulmonary circulation, the right ventricle pumps oxygen-depleted blood

FIGURE 13.3 Lower airway branches.[10]

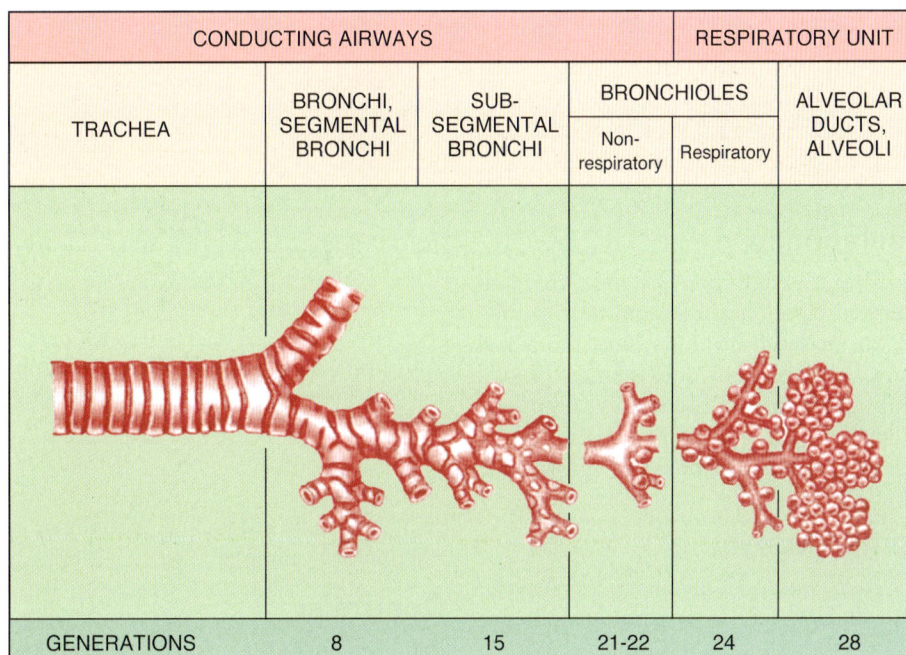

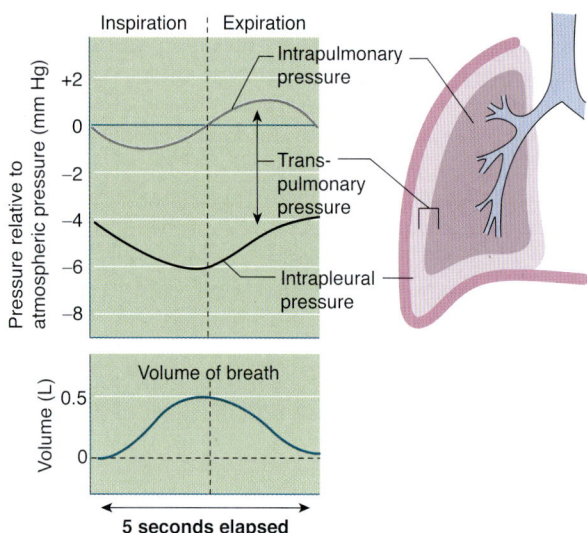

FIGURE 13.4 Changes in intrapleural and intrapulmonary pressure during inspiration and expiration.[7]

Adapted from Marieb E, Hoehn K. Human anatomy and physiology. 4th ed. San Francisco: Pearson Benjamin Cummings; 2010, with permission.

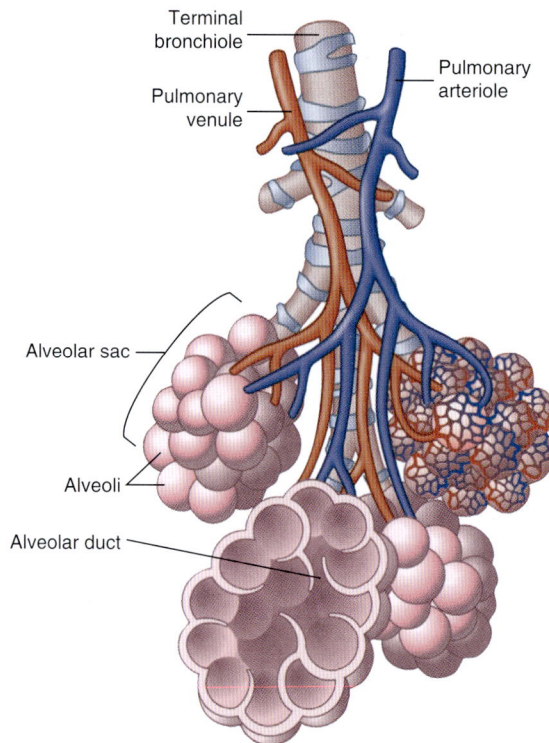

FIGURE 13.5 Terminal ventilation and perfusion units of the lung.[10]

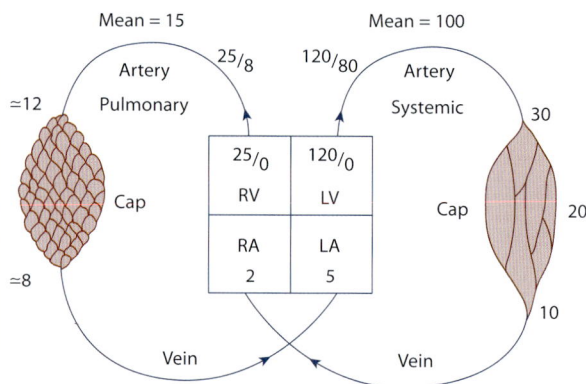

FIGURE 13.6 Comparison of pressure in the pulmonary and systematic circulations (mmHg).[15]

Adapted from West J. Respiratory physiology: the essentials. 8th ed. Philadelphia: Lippincott, Williams & Wilkins; 2008, with permission.

to the lungs via the pulmonary artery, with oxygen-rich blood returning to the left atrium via the pulmonary veins. Pulmonary blood vessels follow the path of the bronchioles, with capillaries forming a dense network in the walls of the alveoli. As illustrated in Figure 13.5,[10] the entire surface area of the alveolar wall is covered by capillaries, just large enough for a red blood cell to pass through, allowing gas exchange.

Pulmonary vessels are short and thin and have relatively little smooth muscle. The pressure inside the vessels is remarkably low (normal pulmonary artery pressure is only 25/8 mmHg; mean 15 mmHg).[11] This low pressure system ensures that right heart workload is minimised, while promoting efficient gas exchange in the lungs[11] (see Figure 13.6).

Bronchial circulation

The bronchial circulation, part of the systemic circulation, supplies oxygenated blood, nutrients and heat to the conducting airways (to the level of the terminal bronchioles) and to the pleura. Drainage of this deoxygenated blood is predominantly through the bronchial network, although some capillaries drain into the pulmonary arterial circulation, contributing to venous admixture or right-to-left shunt[11] (see *Pathophysiology* below for further discussion).

Control of ventilation

Normal breathing occurs automatically and is a complex function not fully understood. It is coordinated by the respiratory centre, regulated by controllers in the brain, effectors in the muscles and sensors including chemoreceptors and mechanoreceptors. There are also protective reflexes such as coughing and sneezing that respond to respiratory tract irritation.

Controller

In the brainstem, the medulla oblongata and the pons regulate automatic ventilation while the cerebral cortex regulates voluntary ventilation (see Figure 13.7). The respiratory rhythmic centre in the medulla can be divided into inspiratory and expiratory centres, with the following functions:[12]

- The inspiratory centre (or dorsal respiratory group) triggers inspiration.
- The expiratory centre (or ventral respiratory group) only functions during forced respiration and active expiration.
- The pneumotaxic and apneustic centre in the pons adjusts the rate and pattern of breathing.
- The cerebral cortex provides conscious voluntary control over the respiratory muscles. This voluntary control cannot be maintained when the partial pressure of carbon dioxide in the arterial blood ($PaCO_2$) and the hydrogen ion (H^+) concentration become markedly elevated; an example is the inability to hold your breath for very long.[12] Emotional and autonomic activities also affect the pace and depth of breathing.

Effectors

The diaphragm is the major muscle of inspiration, although the external intercostal muscles also contribute. The accessory muscles of inspiration (scalenes, sternocleidomastoid muscles and the pectoralis minor) are active only during exercise or strenuous breathing. Expiration is a passive act and only the internal intercostal muscles are involved at rest. During exercise, the abdominal muscles also contribute to expiration. Inspiration is triggered by stimulus from the medulla, causing downward contraction of the diaphragm, and contraction of external intercostal muscles, lifting the thorax up and out. This action lowers pressure within the alveoli (intra-alveolar pressure) relative to atmospheric pressure. Air rushes into the lungs to equalise the pressure gradient. After contraction has ceased, the ribs and diaphragm relax, the pressure gradient reverses, and air is passively expelled from the lungs, which return to their resting state due to elastic recoil.

Sensors

A chemoreceptor is a sensor that responds to a change in the chemical composition of the blood; there are two types: central and peripheral. Central chemoreceptors account for 70% of the feedback controlling ventilation, and respond quickly to changes in the pH of cerebrospinal fluid and increases in $PaCO_2$.[7,13] If the $PaCO_2$ remains high for a prolonged period, as in chronic obstructive pulmonary disease (COPD), a compensatory change in bicarbonate (HCO_3^-) occurs and the pH in cerebrospinal fluid returns to its near normal value.[11]

Central chemoreceptors located in the medulla respond to changes in H^+ concentration in the surrounding cerebrospinal fluid. A change in the $PaCO_2$ causes movement of CO_2 across the blood–brain barrier into the cerebrospinal fluid and alters the H^+ concentration. This increase in H^+ stimulates ventilation. Central chemoreceptors do not, however, respond to changes in the partial pressure of oxygen in arterial blood (PaO_2). Opiates also have a negative influence on these chemoreceptors, reducing sensitivity to changing H^+ concentration.[11] Hyperventilation may reduce $PaCO_2$ to a level that could

---

FIGURE 13.7 Respiratory centres and reflex.[7]

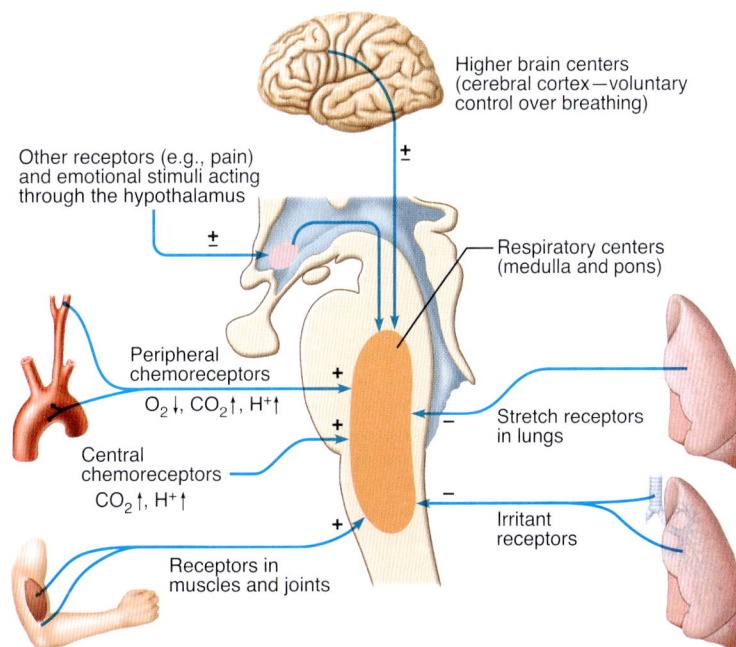

Higher brain centers (cerebral cortex—voluntary control over breathing)

Other receptors (e.g., pain) and emotional stimuli acting through the hypothalamus

±

Respiratory centers (medulla and pons)

Peripheral chemoreceptors
$O_2\downarrow$, $CO_2\uparrow$, $H^+\uparrow$

Stretch receptors in lungs

Central chemoreceptors
$CO_2\uparrow$, $H^+\uparrow$

Irritant receptors

Receptors in muscles and joints

Adapted from Marieb E, Hoehn K. Human anatomy and physiology. 4th ed. San Francisco: Pearson Benjamin Cummings; 2010, with permission.

cause accidental unconsciousness if the breath is held after hyperventilation. This phenomenon is well known amongst divers and is due to increasing levels of CO_2 as the primary trigger of breathing. If the CO_2 level is too low due to hyperventilation, the breathing reflex is not triggered until the level of oxygen has dropped below what is necessary to maintain consciousness.

Peripheral chemoreceptors also play a role in controlling ventilation, although to a lesser extent.[16] Located in the common carotid arteries and in the arch of the aorta, peripheral chemoreceptors detect changes in $PaCO_2$ and H^+ concentration/pH in arterial blood.[13] Peripheral chemoreceptors are sensitive to changes in PaO_2 and are the primary responders to hypoxaemia, stimulating the glossopharyngeal and vagus nerves and providing feedback to the medulla. In response to low PaO_2, such as below 70 mmHg (8 kPa),[11] they are stimulated and contribute to maintaining ventilation.

BOX 13.1

Patients with chronic respiratory conditions, including COPD, often exhibit signs of hypoxia and hypercarbia, particularly during an acute exacerbation of a chronic condition. There is a strongly held belief that patients who chronically retain CO_2 no longer have a central chemoreceptor response to increased $PaCO_2$ and their drive to breathe is in relation to peripheral chemoreceptor response, which detects hypoxia. However, the control of ventilation in such patients is highly complex and involves adaptations of the respiratory control system including changes to respiratory muscles, chemoreceptor signaling and central respiratory drive.[17] While it is true that an uncontrolled administration of oxygen to patients who chronically retain CO_2 results in hypercarbia, this is mainly because of reversal of hypoxic vasoconstriction and changes to ventilation and perfusion matching. To a lesser extent, arterial CO_2 increases because of a rightward shift in the CO_2 dissociation curve (the Haldane effect).[18]

Those patients most likely to develop hypercarbia associated with oxygen administration are also those with significant hypoxaemia. For patients who chronically retain CO_2 and are hypoxic, the hypoxia must be treated and should be tailored to the patient's clinical condition. Evidence suggests that aiming for oxygen saturation between 88% and 92% results in improved patient outcome.[19,20] For a more in-depth description of the physiological changes associated with COPD please refer to *Further reading* at the end of this chapter.

Other receptors include stretch receptors located in the lungs, which inhibit inspiration and protect the lungs from over-inflation (Hering-Breuer reflex), and in the muscles and joints (see Figure 13.7).

Pulmonary volumes and capacities

In healthy individuals, the lungs are readily distensible or compliant; when exposed to high expanding pressures or in disease states, compliance is increased or decreased. Ranges of lung volumes and capacities are illustrated in Figure 13.8. Tidal volume is the volume of air entering the lungs during a single inspiration and is normally equal to the volume leaving the lungs on expiration (around 500 mL). During inspiration, the tidal volume of inspired air is added to the 2400 mL of air already in the lungs. This remaining volume of air in the lungs after normal expiration is the functional residual capacity,[7] which:

- has an important role in keeping small alveoli open and avoiding atelectasis
- can be reduced during anaesthesia or neuromuscular blockade, most likely due to loss of muscle tone[21]
- if reduced, results in the smallest alveoli closing at the end of the expiration (the 'closing volume').

The closing volume plus the residual volume is called the 'closing capacity'. The closure of the smallest airways may occur because dependent areas of the lungs are compressed, although this is not the only mechanism as these airways also close in the weightlessness of space. The closing volume is dependent on patient age: in a young healthy person it is 10% of vital capacity while, for an individual aged 65 years, it increases to 40%, approximating total functional residual capacity (FRC).[11]

Alveolar ventilation

Minute volume represents the volume of gas inhaled or exhaled in one minute and is calculated by multiplying the tidal volume by respiratory frequency (e.g. 500 mL × 12 breaths per minute = 6000 mL). In this example only the first 350 mL of inhaled air in each breath reaches the alveolar exchange surface, with 150 mL remaining in the conducting airways, referred to as the 'anatomic dead space'. Alveolar ventilation is the amount of inhaled air that reaches the alveoli each minute (e.g. 350 mL × 12 = 4200 mL of alveolar ventilation).[12]

Work of breathing

At rest, the energy required to breathe is minimal (less than 5% of total O_2 consumption).[11] However, changes in airway resistance and lung compliance affect the work of breathing, resulting in increased oxygen consumption.[22] As noted earlier, the lungs are very distensible, expanding during inspiration. This expansion is called the elastic or compliance work and refers to the ease with which lungs expand under pressure. Lung compliance is often monitored when patients are mechanically ventilated, and is calculated by dividing the change in lung volume by the change in trans-pulmonary pressure.[6] For the lung to expand, it must overcome lung viscosity and chest wall tissue (called 'tissue resistance work'). Finally, there is airway resistance work − movement of air into the lungs via the airways. The work associated with resistance and compliance is easily overcome in healthy individuals but, in pulmonary disease, both resistance work and compliance work are increased.[6,23] During exertion, when increased muscle function heightens metabolic rate, oxygen

FIGURE 13.8 For lung volume measurements, all values are approximately 25% lower in women.[3] ERV = expiratory reserve volume; FRC = functional residual capacity; IC = inspiratory capacity; IRV = inspiratory reserve volume; RV = residual volume; TLC = total lung capacity; VC = vital capacity; V_T = tidal volume.

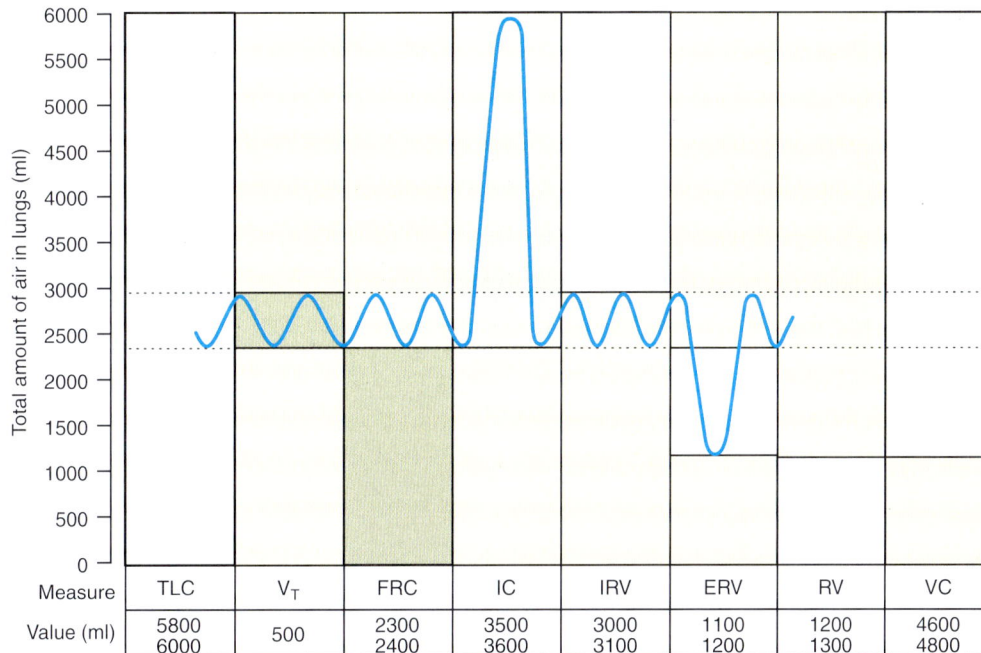

Measure	TLC	V_T	FRC	IC	IRV	ERV	RV	VC
Value (ml)	5800 6000	500	2300 2400	3500 3600	3000 3100	1100 1200	1200 1300	4600 4800

demand rises to match consumption and avoid anaerobic metabolism, and work of breathing is increased. The term 'work of breathing' is often used in critical illness, when basic respiratory processes are challenged and breathing consumes a far greater proportion of total energy.

Principles of gas transport and exchange in alveoli and tissues

Oxygen and CO_2 are transported in the bloodstream between alveoli and the tissue cells. Delivery of oxygen to tissues and transfer of CO_2 from the tissues to the capillaries occurs by diffusion and is therefore dependent on the pressure gradient between the capillary and the cell. Diffusion involves molecules moving from areas of high concentration to low concentration. Other determinants of the rate of diffusion include the thickness of the alveolar membrane, the surface area of the membrane available for gas transfer and the inherent solubility of the gas. CO_2 diffuses about 20 times more rapidly than oxygen, being much more soluble in blood.[11] At the most distal ends of the conducting airways lay an extensive network of approximately 300 million alveoli. The surface area of the lungs, if spread out flat, would be about 90 m^2 – about 40 times greater than the surface area of the skin.[7] Gas exchange occurs through the exceptionally thin alveolar membranes. Oxygen uptake takes place from the external environment via the lungs through to the blood in the adjacent alveolar capillary networks. Similarly, CO_2 diffuses from capillaries to the alveoli and is then expired.

Oxygen transport

In oxygenated blood transported by the pulmonary capillaries, there is 20 mL of oxygen in each 100 mL of blood. Oxygen is transported in two ways: dissolved in plasma (about 0.3 mL; 1.5%) with the remainder bound to haemoglobin.[12] Measured by arterial blood gases (ABGs), the 1.5% of oxygen dissolved in blood constitutes the PaO_2.[7] One gram of haemoglobin carries 1.34 mL of oxygen. The level of saturation within the total circulating haemoglobin can be measured clinically, by pulse oximetry. The amount of oxygen actually bound to haemoglobin compared with the amount of oxygen the haemoglobin can carry is commonly reported as arterial oxygen saturation or SaO_2. Oxygen is attached to the haemoglobin molecule at four haem sites. As the majority of oxygen transport is via haemoglobin, if all four sites are occupied by oxygen molecules the blood is determined to be 'fully saturated' (SaO_2 = 100%).[23]

A large reserve of oxygen is available if required, without the need for any increase in respiratory or cardiac workload. Oxygen extraction is the percentage of oxygen extracted and utilised by the tissues. At rest, just 25% of the total oxygen delivered to the tissue is extracted, although this amount does vary throughout the body, with some tissue beds extracting more and others taking less. Normally, the oxygen saturation of venous blood is 60–75%; values below this indicate that more oxygen than normal is being extracted by tissues. This can be due to a reduction in oxygen delivery to the tissues or to an increase in the tissue consumption of oxygen.[12,13]

Oxygen delivery and oxygen consumption are important considerations in the management of critically ill patients. Normal oxygen delivery in a healthy person at rest is approximately 1000 mL/min. Normal oxygen consumption is 200–250 mL/min,[13] but this can increase significantly during episodes of sepsis, fever, hypercatabolism and shivering.[23] The difference between normal delivery and normal consumption highlights the large degree of oxygen reserve available to the body.

Oxygen–haemoglobin dissociation curve

As blood is transported to the tissues and end-organs, the tendency of haemoglobin and oxygen to combine decreases, relative to the surrounding arterial oxygen tension. This relationship is illustrated by the oxygen–haemoglobin dissociation curve (see Figure 13.9). As oxygen is offloaded at the tissue level, CO_2 binds more readily with haemoglobin, to be transported back to the lungs for removal.[7]

The oxygen–haemoglobin dissociation curve relates the partial pressure of oxygen to the haemoglobin saturation in blood. While the initial part of the curve rises steeply, the latter part of the curve flattens representing the binding of oxygen to haemoglobin in the lungs. In the upper part of the curve (within the lungs), relatively large changes in the PaO_2 cause only small changes in haemoglobin saturation. Therefore, if the PaO_2 drops from 100 to 60 mmHg (14–8 kPa), the saturation of haemoglobin changes only 7% (from a normal 97% to 90%). As long as PaO_2 remains above 60 mmHg (7.8 kPa) haemoglobin will be more than 90% saturated. The minimal changes in O_2 binding within this substantial PO_2 range allow survival at high altitudes.[7,12,24]

The lower portion (steep component) of the oxygen–haemoglobin dissociation curve, between 40 and 60 mmHg (5–8 kPa), represents the release of oxygen from haemoglobin in tissue capillaries. At this point, a small drop in PaO_2 will cause a large increase in oxygen unloading. As haemoglobin is further de-saturated, larger amounts of oxygen are released for tissue use, ensuring an adequate oxygen supply to peripheral tissues, even when oxygen delivery is reduced. Oxygen saturation remains at 70–75%, leaving a significant amount of oxygen in reserve. Normally only 25% of bound oxygen is unloaded during one systemic circuit. However, during exercise when the muscles need more oxygen, the PaO_2 drops and more oxygen dissociates from haemoglobin for use by muscle cells without any complementary increase in respiratory rate or cardiac output.[7,12]

The relationship between the two axes of this curve assumes values for haemoglobin, pH, temperature, $PaCO_2$ and 2,3-bisphosphoglycerate (BPG), a product of the breakdown of red blood cells that binds reversibly with haemoglobin, are normal. Changes to any of these values will shift the curve to the right or left and therefore reflect different values for PaO_2 and SaO_2[12] (see Figure 13.9).

Both the binding and dissociation of oxygen to haemoglobin are reversible reactions depending on the surrounding tissue. When the curve shifts to the right

FIGURE 13.9 Shift of the oxygen–haemoglobin dissociation curve: (**A**) to the right and (**B**) to the left.[25]

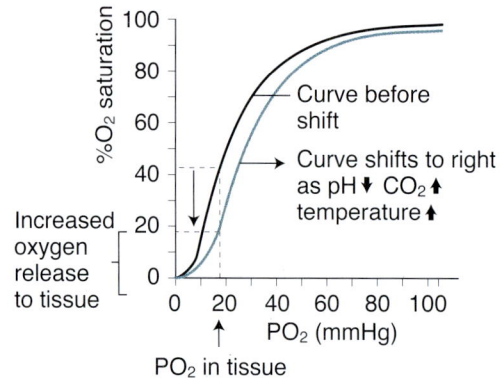

In the tissues, the oxygen–haemoglobin dissociation curve shifts to the right. As pH decreases, PCO_2 increases, or as temperature rises, the curve (black) shifts to the right (blue), resulting in an increased release of oxygen.

A

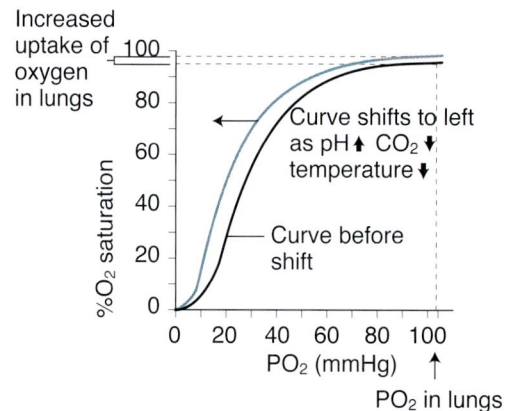

In the lungs, the oxygen–haemoglobin dissociation curve shifts to the left. As pH increases, PCO_2 decreases, or as temperature falls, the curve (black) shifts to the left (blue), resulting in an increased ability of haemoglobin to pick up oxygen.

B

Adapted from Seely R, Stephens T, Tate P. Anatomy and physiology. 7th ed. Boston: McGraw Hill; 2006.

there is a reduced capacity for oxygen binding to haemoglobin in the lungs but oxygen is more readily released to the tissues. At a local level, in active tissue such as working muscle that generates lactic acid, acid release lowers the pH resulting in release of oxygen from haemoglobin molecules to the surrounding tissue. The same process occurs when active skeletal muscle generates heat. The increase in local temperature leads to oxygen release for use by the surrounding muscle.[7,12]

As blood is transported to the tissues and end-organs, the binding affinity of haemoglobin and oxygen decreases relative to the surrounding arterial oxygen tension. As oxygen is offloaded at the tissue level, CO_2 binds more readily with haemoglobin, to be transported to the lungs for removal.[7]

Carbon dioxide transport

CO_2 is transported by blood in three forms: combined with water as carbonic acid (80–90%), dissolved (5%) or attached to plasma proteins (5–10%), including haemoglobin. The dissolved CO_2 constitutes $PaCO_2$ and is measured by ABGs. The greater solubility of CO_2 compared with oxygen results in its rapid diffusion across the capillary membranes, and its easy removal.[7] As a byproduct of cellular respiration, CO_2 is produced at a rate of 200 mL/min, with only minor differences in normal concentrations in arterial (480 mL/L) and venous (520 mL/L) blood.[13]

Relationship between ventilation and perfusion

Gas exchange is the key function of the lungs, and the unique anatomy of capillaries and alveoli facilitates this process. However, because of a number of physiological factors, the ventilation to perfusion ratio (V/Q) is not matched in a 1:1 relationship. As normal alveolar ventilation is about 4 L/min and pulmonary capillary perfusion is about 5 L/min, the normal V/Q is 0.8.[11] In addition, pressure in the pulmonary circulation is low relative to systemic pressure, and is influenced much more by gravity and hydrostatic pressure. In the upright position, lung apices receive less perfusion compared with the bases.[11] In the supine position, apical and basal perfusions are almost equal, but the posterior (dependent) portion of the lungs receives greater perfusion than the anterior lung area. Ventilation is also uneven throughout the lung, with the bases receiving more ventilation per unit volume than the apices.[11]

Pressure within the surrounding alveoli also influences blood flow through the pulmonary capillary network. The pressure gradients between the arterial and venous ends of a capillary network normally determine blood flow. However, alveolar pressure (P_A) can be greater than venous (P_v) and/or arterial (P_a) pressure, and therefore influences blood flow and gas exchange.

For a patient in an upright position, perfusion and ventilation vary as follows:

- Zone 1 (upper area of the lungs): alveolar pressure is generally greater than both arterial and venous capillary pressure [$P_A > P_a > P_v$], and blood flow is reduced, leading to alveolar dead space (alveoli ventilated but not adequately perfused).

- Zone 2 (middle portion of the lungs): perfusion and gas exchange are influenced more by pressure differences between arterial and alveolar pressures than by the usual difference between arterial and venous pressures [$P_a > P_A > P_v$], with a normal V/Q ratio.

- Zone 3 (lung bases): alveolar pressure is lower than both arterial and venous pressures [$P_a > P_v > P_A$], and ventilation is reduced, leading to intrapulmonary shunting (alveoli perfused but not adequately ventilated)[11] (see Figure 13.10).

FIGURE 13.10 The effects of gravity and alveolar pressure on pulmonary blood flow. Notice the three lung zones.[26] (published with permission).

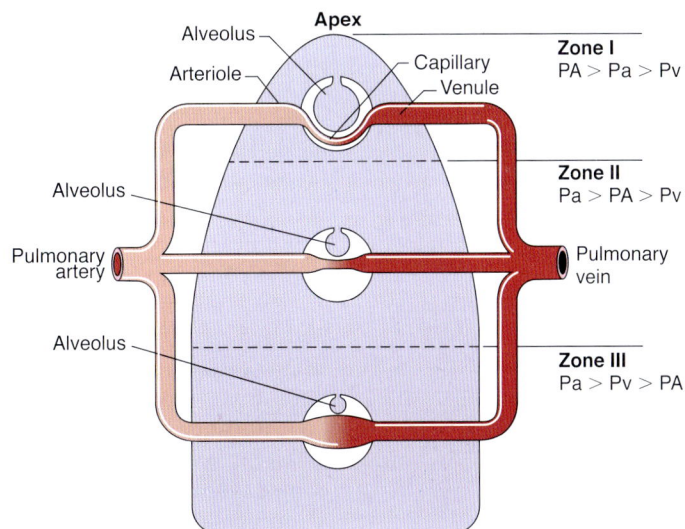

Adapted from Seely R, Stephens T, Tate P. Anatomy and physiology. 7th ed. Boston: McGraw Hill; 2006, with permission.

These physiological relationships are more complex in a critically ill patient when ventilation and/or lung perfusion is further compromised by disease processes and positive pressure ventilation, and the patient is in a supine or semi-recumbent position.[11]

Acid–base control: respiratory mechanisms

The respiratory system plays a vital role in acid–base balance. Changes in respiratory rate and depth can produce changes in body pH by altering the amount of carbonic acid (H_2CO_3) in the blood. The body has substantial control over acid–base balance by altering alveolar ventilation and the elimination of CO_2 through the lungs. The elimination of acid through the lungs is more than 100 times more efficient than the elimination of acid through the kidneys. If CO_2 in body water increases due to low alveolar ventilation, more H^+ will be produced because CO_2 combines with H_2O to form H_2CO_3. This breaks down to HCO_3^- and H^+ resulting in a decrease in pH.

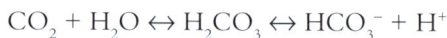

$$CO_2 + H_2O \leftrightarrow H_2CO_3 \leftrightarrow HCO_3^- + H^+$$

The strength of the dissociation is defined by the Henderson-Hasselbach equation, which describes the relationship between HCO_3^-, CO_2 and pH, and explains why an increase in dissolved CO_2 causes an increase in the acidity of the plasma, while an increase in HCO_3^- causes the pH to rise resulting in more alkaline plasma:

$$pH = 6.1 + \log \frac{(HCO_3^-)}{(CO_2)}$$

where 6.1 = the negative logarithm of the acid dissociation constant in plasma for carbonic acid.[11]

Respiratory acidosis is caused by CO_2 retention and increases the denominator in the Henderson-Hasselbach equation resulting in a decreased pH level. In a spontaneously breathing patient, this condition occurs due to hypoventilation from either shallow breaths and/or a low respiratory rate. In the acute state the body cannot compensate. If the patient develops chronic CO_2 retention over a long period, there will be a renal response to the increase in CO_2. The renal system retains HCO_3^- to return the pH to normal (i.e. respiratory acidosis is compensated).

Respiratory alkalosis occurs when a patient hyperventilates and alveolar ventilation is increased as a result of large, frequent breaths; CO_2 decreases in arterial blood and the pH rises. If this condition is maintained (e.g. walking at high altitude), the kidneys excrete HCO_3^- and the pH returns to normal (i.e. the respiratory alkalosis is compensated).[11]

Pathophysiology

Three common pathophysiological concepts that influence respiratory function in critically ill patients are hypoxaemia, inflammation and oedema. Related disease states including respiratory failure, pneumonia, acute respiratory distress syndrome, asthma and COPD are described in Chapter 14.

Hypoxaemia

Hypoxaemia describes a decrease in the PaO_2 of less than 60 mmHg (7.8 kPa).[7] This leads to less efficient anaerobic metabolism at the tissue and end-organ level, and compromised cellular function. Hypoxia is abnormally low PO_2 in the tissues, and can be due to:

- 'hypoxic' hypoxia – low PaO_2 in arterial blood due to pulmonary disease
- 'circulatory' hypoxia – reduction of tissue blood flow due to shock or local obstruction
- 'anaemic' hypoxia – reduced ability of the blood to carry oxygen due to anaemia or carbon monoxide poisoning
- 'histotoxic' hypoxia – a cellular environment that does not support oxygen utilisation due to tissue poisoning (e.g. cyanide poisoning).[11]

A hypoxic patient can show symptoms of fatigue and shortness of breath if the hypoxia has developed gradually. If the patient has severe hypoxia with rapid onset, they will have ashen skin and blue discolouration (cyanosis) of the oral mucosa, lips and nail beds. Confusion, disorientation and anxiety are other symptoms. In later stages, unconsciousness, coma and death occur.[27]

Acute respiratory failure is a common patient presentation in ICU that is characterised by decreased gas exchange with resultant hypoxaemia.[28] Two different mechanisms cause acute respiratory failure: Type I presents with low PaO_2 and normal $PaCO_2$; Type II presents with low PaO_2 and high $PaCO_2$[3] (see Chapter 14 for further discussion).

In general, impaired gas exchange results from alveolar hypoventilation, ventilation/perfusion mismatching and intrapulmonary shunting, each resulting in hypoxaemia. Hypercapnia may also be present depending on the underlying pathophysiology.[29]

Alveolar hypoventilation occurs when the metabolic needs of the body are not met by the amount of oxygen delivered and CO_2 removed from the alveoli. Alveolar hypoventilation causing hypoxaemia is usually extrapulmonary (e.g. altered metabolism, interruption to neuromuscular control of breathing/ventilation) and is associated with hypercapnia.[3,29]

V/Q mismatch results when areas of lung that are perfused are not ventilated (no participation in gas exchange) because alveoli are collapsed or infiltrated with fluid from inflammation or infection (e.g. pulmonary oedema, pneumonia). This results in an overall reduction in blood oxygen levels, which is usually countered by compensatory mechanisms.[3]

Intrapulmonary shunting is an extreme case of V/Q mismatch. Shunting occurs when blood passes alveoli that are not ventilated. If there is significant intrapulmonary shunting, there may be overwhelming reductions

FIGURE 13.11   Ventilation perfusion mismatch.[30]

FIGURE 13.11   Ventilation perfusion mismatch.[30]

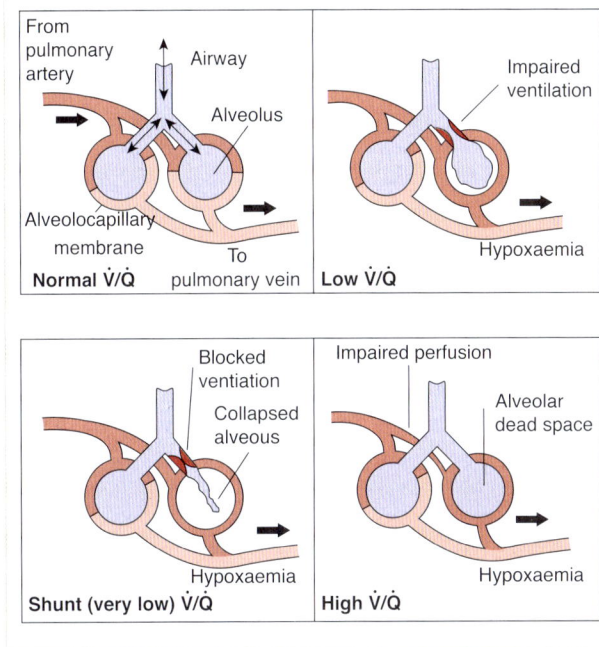

Changes to the oxygen–haemoglobin dissociation curve also occur in states related to hypoxia. The curve shifts to the right when there is acidosis and/or raised levels of $PaCO_2$ as commonly seen in respiratory failure. The shift in the oxygen–haemoglobin dissociation curve to the right means that, in the lung, fewer oxygen molecules attach to the haemoglobin molecule, resulting in a decrease in arterial oxygen saturation. However, what oxygen does attach to the haemoglobin molecule is more readily released at the tissue level.[11]

Compensatory mechanisms to optimise oxygenation

When PO_2 in the alveoli is reduced, regional hypoxic pulmonary vasoconstriction occurs, with contraction of smooth muscles in the small arterioles, directing blood flow away from the hypoxic area of the lung.[11] Peripheral chemoreceptors also detect hypoxaemia and initiate compensatory mechanisms to optimise cellular oxygen delivery. Initial responses are increased respiratory rate and depth, resulting in increased minute ventilation, and raised heart rate with possible vasoconstriction as the body attempts to maintain oxygen delivery and uptake. This overall upregulation cannot be sustained indefinitely, particularly in a person who is critically ill, and compensatory mechanisms begin to fail with worsening hypoxaemia and cellular and organ dysfunction. Unless the hypoxaemia is reversed and/or respiratory and cardiovascular support is provided, irreversible hypoxia and death will ensue.

in PaO_2.[30] CO_2 levels may still be normal but, depending on the onset and progression of respiratory pathophysiology, compensatory mechanisms may not be able to maintain homeostasis[3,13] (see Figure 13.11).

Tissue hypoxia

There are few physiological changes with mild hypoxaemia (when O_2 saturation remains at 90% despite a PaO_2 of 60 mmHg [8 kPa]), with only a slight impairment in mental state. If hypoxaemia deteriorates and the PaO_2 drops to 40–50 mmHg (5.3–6.7 kPa), severe tissue hypoxia ensues. Hypoxia at the central nervous system level manifests with headaches and somnolence. Compensatory mechanisms include catecholamine release, and a decrease in renal function results in sodium retention and proteinuria.[31]

Different tissues vary in their vulnerability to hypoxia, with the central nervous system and myocardium at most risk. Hypoxia in the cerebral cortex results in a loss of function within 4–6 seconds, loss of consciousness in 10–20 seconds and irreversible damage in 3–5 minutes. In an environment that lacks oxygen, cells function by anaerobic metabolism and produce much less energy. For example, with aerobic metabolism 38 molecules of adenosine triphosphate are generated compared with 2 molecules of adenosine triphosphate generated in anaerobic metabolism. During anaerobic metabolism, lactic acid also increases. With less available energy, the efficiency of cellular functions such as the sodium–potassium pump, nerve conduction, enzyme activity and transmembrane receptor function diminishes.[31] The overall effect of interruption to these vital cellular activities is a reduction in organ or tissue function, which in turn compromises system and body functions.

Inflammation

Inflammatory processes can occur at a local level (e.g. as a result of inhalation injuries, aspiration or respiratory infections) or are secondary to systemic events (e.g. sepsis, trauma). Damage to the pulmonary endothelium and type I alveolar cells appears to play a key role in the inflammatory processes associated with acute respiratory distress syndrome (ARDS).[32] Once triggered, inflammation results in platelet aggregation and complement release. Platelet aggregation attracts neutrophils, which release inflammatory mediators (e.g. proteolytic enzymes, oxygen free radicals, leukotrienes, prostaglandins and platelet-activating factor). Neutrophils also appear to play a key role in the perpetuation of ARDS.[3] As well as altering pulmonary capillary permeability, resulting in haemorrhage and leaking of fluid into the pulmonary interstitium and alveoli, mediators released by neutrophils and some macrophages precipitate pulmonary vasoconstriction. Resulting pulmonary hypertension leads to diminished perfusion to some lung areas, with dramatic alterations to both perfusion and ventilation leading to significant V/Q mismatch, and the subsequent signs and symptoms typically seen in patients with pulmonary inflammation/oedema.

Oedema

Pulmonary oedema also alters gas exchange, and results from abnormal accumulation of extravascular fluid in the lung. Two main reasons for this are an increase in hydrostatic or osmotic forces, as seen in left ventricular dysfunction or volume overload, and increased membrane permeability of the lung epithelium or endothelium, allowing accumulation of fluid. This is referred to as non-cardiogenic pulmonary oedema. ARDS may result from increased permeability of the epithelium. A more detailed discussion of ARDS is provided in Chapter 14.

Changes to respiratory function

During the early exudative phase of ARDS, tachypnoea, signs of hypoxaemia (apprehension, restlessness) and an increase in the use of accessory muscles are usually evident. These symptoms result from infiltration of fluid into the alveoli. With impaired production of surfactant during the proliferative phase, respiratory function deteriorates, and dyspnoea, agitation, fatigue and the emergence of fine crackles on auscultation are common.[3,31] Airway resistance is increased when oedema affects larger airways. Lung compliance is reduced as interstitial oedema interferes with the elastic properties of the lungs, and it may become challenging to adequately ventilate patients. Infiltration of type II alveolar cells into the epithelium may lead to interstitial fibrosis on healing,[33] causing chronic lung dysfunction.

Respiratory dysfunction: changes to work of breathing

Without reversal of respiratory compromise, significant increases to the work of breathing will result. Clinical manifestations include tachypnoea, tachycardia, dyspnoea, low tidal volumes and diaphoresis. Hypercapnia ensues, which further compromises respiratory muscle function and precipitates diaphragmatic fatigue. Oxygen consumption during breathing can be so great that reserve capacity is reduced. If patients with pre-existing COPD (who may breathe close to the fatigue work level) experience an acute exacerbation, this can easily tip them into a fatigued state. Early identification and management of respiratory compromise before these stages improves patient outcomes.[31]

Assessment

Respiratory insufficiency is a common reason for admission to ICU, for either a potential or an actual problem, so comprehensive and frequent respiratory assessments are an essential practice role. This section outlines history taking, physical examination, bedside monitoring and diagnostic testing focused on a critically ill patient with respiratory dysfunction.

Assessment is a systematic process comprising history taking of a patient's present and previous illnesses and physical examination of their thorax, lungs and related systems. History taking and physical examination can occur simultaneously if the patient is very ill. Related diagnostic findings inform an accurate and comprehensive assessment. A thorough assessment, followed by accurate ongoing monitoring, enables early detection of changes

in condition and the impact of treatment. Depending on a patient's situation, assessment can be either brief or detailed.

Patient history

History taking determines a patient's baseline respiratory status on ICU admission. If the patient is distressed only a few questions should be asked but, if the patient is able, a more comprehensive interview can be performed, focusing on four areas: the current problem, previous problems, symptoms and personal and family history. Question a family member or close friend if a patient is unable to provide their own history.

When introducing yourself, ask the patient's name, seek eye contact and create a rapport with the patient and the family. Ensure that the patient is in a comfortable position, ideally sitting up in bed. Provide privacy so that the interview is confidential. The physical examination should maintain the patient's dignity and modesty. To minimise distress for a patient who is acutely breathless, the use of short closed questions is preferable.

> **Practice tip**
>
> History taking by the nurse should be an interactive experience, especially the initial interview where both the patient and nurse learn a lot about each other. This knowledge has considerable influence on rapport building between patient and nurse.

Current respiratory problems

Begin by asking why the patient is seeking care. If possible, let the patient describe the respiratory problem in his or her own words. Be focused and listen actively. Ask for location, onset and duration of the respiratory symptoms.

Previous respiratory problems

Many respiratory disorders can be chronic and pulmonary diseases may recur (e.g. tuberculosis). New diseases can complicate existing ones.[34] Problems with breathing and chest problems, number of hospitalisations, treatments and childhood respiratory diseases should be discussed with the patient.

Symptoms

Assess the onset and duration, pattern, severity and episodic or continuous nature of presenting symptoms. Also ask about the patient's perception of their respiratory problem, their opinion about its cause and, if the symptoms cause fatigue, anxiety or stress. Ask specifically about dyspnoea, cough, sputum production, haemoptysis, wheezing, chest pain or other pain, sleep disturbances and snoring.

Dyspnoea (shortness of breath) is subjective and therefore difficult to grade. The mechanism that underlies the sensation of dyspnoea is poorly understood but it is extremely uncomfortable and frightening.[34] Assess the severity of dyspnoea by asking about breathing in relation to activities (e.g. breathlessness when dressing or walking across a room). Ask the patient how many pillows they need to sleep as this may indicate the severity of any *orthopnoea* (shortness of breath when lying flat). Orthopnoea can be a symptom of increased blood in the pulmonary circulation due to left ventricular failure, pulmonary oedema, bronchitis, asthma or obstructive sleep apnoea.

A cough can be dry or productive, episodic or continuous and, if exacerbated when the patient is lying flat, can imply heart failure. A cough can also be related to viral infections and allergies or may indicate intrathoracic disease. Ask the patient if they wake at night due to the cough, how long the cough has been present and if it is getting better or worse.

Sputum production should be considered for amount, colour or the presence of blood. Yellow or green sputum is typical in bacterial infection. Haemoptysis or sputum mixed with blood is a significant finding and can indicate tuberculosis or lung cancer. Wheezing can indicate vocal cord disorder or asthma.[34]

Chest pain can result from multiple causes; therefore appropriate assessment is essential. Chest pain that occurs during inspiration can be due to irritation or inflammation of the pleural surface. Pleural pain is experienced mostly on one side of the chest, is knifelike in character and occurs in pneumonia, pleurisy and pneumothorax. Chest pain also occurs with fractured ribs.

The most ominous chest pain occurs as a result of myocardial ischaemia, due to poor oxygen delivery to the coronary vessels. This pain is termed angina pectoris and can arise from chronic stable angina or acute coronary syndrome[34] (see Chapter 10 for further discussion).

Sleep disturbance and snoring may be related to obstructive sleep apnoea. If the patient complains about drowsiness in the daytime, ask how many hours of continuous sleep they have at night, and whether they take a nap during the day.

Personal and family history

Family history and environment can influence pulmonary presentations. The focus of this questioning is on: tobacco use, allergies, recent travel, occupational risk, home situation and family history. Use of tobacco, current or past, is important in evaluating pulmonary symptoms. Ask the patient to quantify the amount of cigarette packs per week and how many years they have smoked. The majority of smokers have reduced lung function. Tobacco smoking is responsible for 80–90% of the risk of developing COPD but only 10–15% of these patients will develop clinically significant symptoms.[35] Exposure to secondhand smoke may also be of interest, with evidence that extended exposure is a major cause of chronic bronchitis.[36] A history of recent travel increases possible exposure to infectious respiratory diseases.[37] Recent long flights increase the possibility of deep venous thrombosis, which can lead to pulmonary embolism.[38] An occupation with exposure to allergens and toxins is important to document as this can be associated with declining lung function.[39] Ask about the patient's home situation and whether they live with someone with an illness such as influenza or tuberculosis. Ask about

children who are close to the patient, as innocuous viral infections in small children may account for severe disease in adults.[34] Also check for a family history of cancer and heart or respiratory diseases.

Physical examination

The four activities of physical examination are inspection, palpation, percussion and auscultation. Prior to commencing the examination, prepare the patient as well as possible by providing privacy, warmth, good light and quiet surroundings. Explain that the examination is a standard procedure and you will use your eyes, hands and a stethoscope. Help the patient into a comfortable sitting position in the bed if possible and have all necessary equipment easily accessible.

Inspection

Inspection involves carefully observing the patient from head to toe for signs of respiratory problems. Focus on: patient position, chest wall inspection, respiratory rate and rhythm, respiratory effort, central or peripheral cyanosis and clubbing. Note what position appears preferable for the patient; whether they look comfortable in bed, have trouble breathing or appear anxious. Observe chest wall symmetry during the respiratory cycle, anatomical structures and for the presence of scars. The most important sign of respiratory distress is respiratory rate and rhythm. Count the rate for a 1-minute period. Normal respiratory rate for adults is 12–15 per minute.[7] Abnormal breathing patterns are noted in Table 13.1. Observe respiratory effort, in particular the use of accessory muscles, abdominal muscles, nasal flaring, body position and mouth-breathing.

Inspect the lips, tongue and sublingual area for central cyanosis (a late sign of hypoxia that is almost impossible to detect in a patient with anaemia).[3] Observe the extremities for oedema (can be a sign of heart failure), fingers and toes for peripheral cyanosis and clubbing of the nail beds. Peripheral cyanosis may indicate low blood flow to peripheral areas. Clubbing of finger or toe nail beds can be idiopathic or more commonly due to respiratory or circulatory diseases (e.g. chronic hypoxia in congenital heart disease).[23,34]

Note also if the patient requires oxygen and record the dose. If the patient is intubated and mechanically ventilated (monitoring is explained later in this chapter), ensure the airway is adequately secured. If the patient is orally intubated, observe the mouth for the presence of lesions or pressure on the oral mucosa and lips; and observe the size of the tube, the length at the lips or teeth margin and how it is secured. If the patient has a tracheostomy, observe the stoma for signs of infection or pressure areas, the type and size of tracheostomy tube, the length at the hub if it is a tracheostomy with an adjustable flange and the manner of securement.

Palpation

Palpate the patient's chest with warm hands, focusing on: areas of tenderness, tracheal position, presence of

TABLE 13.1

Description of different respiration patterns[23]

Pattern	Description	Pattern	Description
Normal	Regular and comfortable at a rate of 12–20 per minute	Air trapping	Increasing difficulty in getting breath out
Bradypnea	Slower than 12 breaths per minute	Cheyne-Stokes	Varying periods of increasing depth interspersed with apnea
Tachypnea	Faster than 20 breaths per minute	Kussmaul	Rapid, deep, labored
Hyperventilation (hyperpnea)	Faster than 20 breaths per minute, deep breathing	Biot	Irregularly interspersed periods of apnea in a disorganised sequence of breaths
Sighing	Frequently interspersed deeper breath	Ataxic	Significant disorganisation with irregular and varying depths of respiration

Adapted from: Morton P, Rempfer K. Patient assessment: respiratory system. In: Morton P, Fontaine D (eds). Critical care nursing: A holistic approach. 9th ed. Philadelphia: Wolters, Kluwer/Lippincott Williams & Wilkins; 2009.

subcutaneous emphysema and tactile fremitus. Assess for symmetry (left compared to right) and follow a systematic sequence of palpation over anterior and posterior surfaces (see Figure 13.12). Check the thorax for areas of tenderness or bony deformities and note symmetry of chest movement during breathing. Use the palm of your hand to assess skin temperature, noting clammy, hot or cold skin. To test for chest wall symmetry on inspiration, place both hands with thumbs together on the patient's posterior thorax and ask them to take a deep breath. Your thumbs should separate equally 3–5 cm during normal deep inspiration[1] (see Figure 13.13). Asymmetry can occur in pneumothorax, pneumonia or other lung disorders where inspiration is affected.

Palpation of the tracheal position is useful to detect a mediastinal shift; deviation of the trachea from midline may indicate a pulmonary problem such as large pneumothorax or previous pneumonectomy.[41] The presence of subcutaneous emphysema indicates air in the subcutaneous tissue and feels like crackling under your fingers due to air pockets in the tissue.[42] It most commonly occurs in the face, neck and chest after blunt or penetrating trauma to the chest (e.g. stabbing, gun shot, fractured ribs); facial fractures; tracheostomy; respiratory tract surgery; and in patients who are mechanically ventilated.

Palpation is also used to assess for tactile (vocal) fremitus, a normal palpable vibration. Place your hands on the patient's chest and ask them to vocalise repeatedly the term 'ninety-nine'. Fremitus is decreased (that is, impaired transmission of sounds) in pleural effusion and pneumothorax. Fremitus is increased over regions of lung where transmission is increased (e.g. pneumonia, consolidation).[34] In mechanically ventilated patients, fremitus can be detected when there are secretions in the airways.

Percussion

By tapping the chest with the bony structures of the hands, percussion can help to determine if the lung spaces are filled with air, fluid or sputum consolidation. Place your non-dominant hand with your middle finger extended over the area of chest to be examined. Using the middle finger of your dominant hand, tap on the distal knuckle of the finger resting on the chest wall. Starting from the upper chest wall and moving from side to side, following the same sequence as for auscultation (see Figure 13.12), compare one side to the other for variation in sound. Normally, the chest has a resonant percussion tone. A flat percussive note, soft and high-pitched, may indicate a large pleural effusion. A dull percussive note with medium intensity and pitch is heard in the presence of atelectasis, pulmonary oedema, pulmonary haemorrhage or pneumonia.[23]

FIGURE 13.12 Sequence of systematic movements for auscultation, percussion and palpation of the anterior and posterior chest. Comparison of the right and left sides of the chest should be performed by moving from side to side, beginning proximally and moving distally down the chest wall.[40]

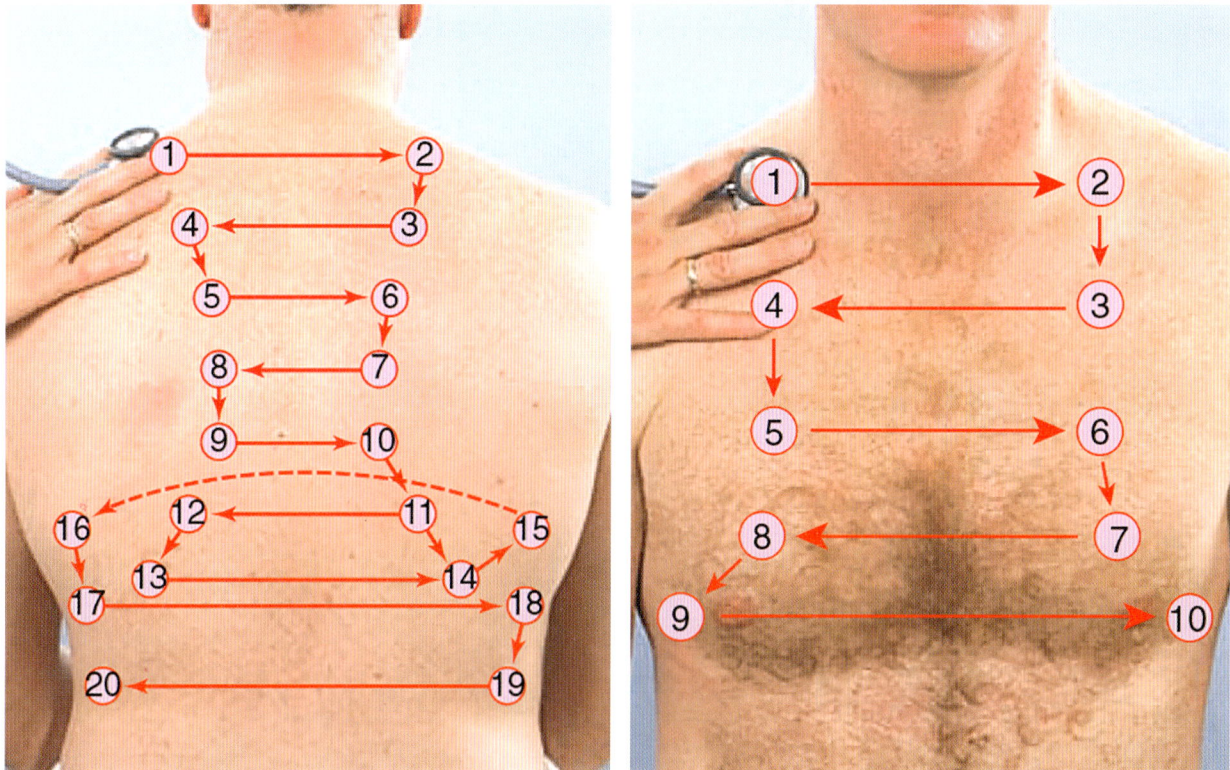

Adapted from Weber J, Kelly J. Health assessment in nursing. Philadelphia: Lippincott, Williams & Wilkins; 2010, with permission.

FIGURE 13.13 Assessment of thoracic expansion. **A** Exhalation. **B** Inhalation.[4] (Published with permission.)

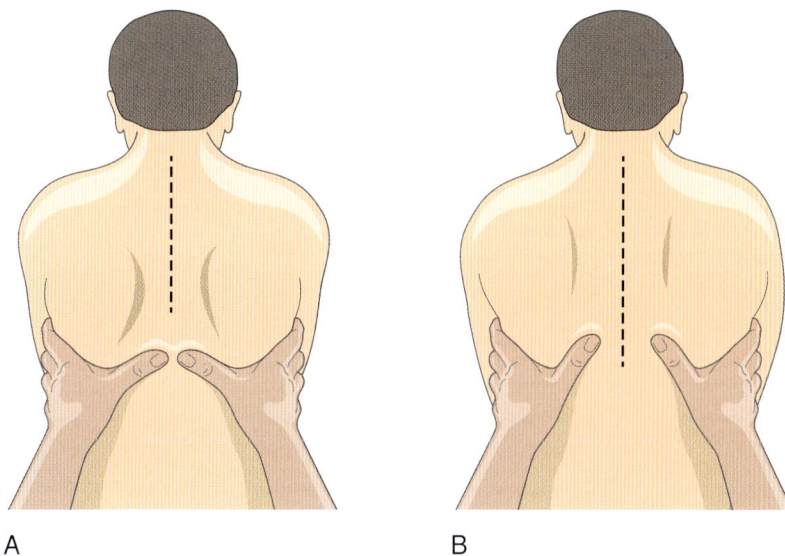

A   B

Practice tip

When performing palpation or percussion of the chest with your hand and auscultation of the chest with a stethoscope, the patient will appreciate the hand and stethoscope being warmed prior to placing them on the skin

Practice tip

When performing chest inspection, percussion and auscultation, always compare one side of the body with the other.

Auscultation

Careful interpretation of breath sounds and integration of this assessment data with other findings can provide important information about lung disorders. Use the diaphragm of the stethoscope and ensure full contact with the skin for optimal listening. For a spontaneously breathing patient, ask them to breathe through their mouth (nose breathing may alter the pitch of the breath sounds). Auscultation is performed in a systematic way so as to compare the symmetry of breath sounds (see Figure 13.12). Normal breath sounds reflect air movement through the bronchi, and sounds change as air moves from larger to smaller airways. Sounds also change when air passes though fluid or narrowed airways. Breath sounds therefore differ depending on the area auscultated. The three types of normal breath sounds are bronchial, bronchovesicular and vesicular breath sounds (see Table 13.2), and these should be heard only in the areas specific to their region.

TABLE 13.2
Characteristics of normal breath sounds

SOUND	CHARACTERISTICS
Vesicular	Heard over most of the lung field; low pitch; soft and short exhalation and long inhalation
Bronchovesicular	Heard over main bronchus area and over upper right posterior lung field; medium pitch; exhalation equals inhalation
Bronchial	Heard only over trachea; high pitch; loud and long exhalation

Adapted from: Urden L, Stacey K, Lough M. Critical care nursing: Diagnosis and management. 6th ed. St Louis: Mosby; 2010. Table 22.2.

Practice tip

Use an alcohol wipe to clean the earpieces on the stethoscope prior to use to protect yourself from infection.

Identify and become familiar with normal breath sounds before beginning to listen and identify abnormal breath sounds. Abnormal breath sounds are either continuous or discontinuous. Continuous sounds include wheezes and rhonchi, while discontinuous sounds include crackles (see Table 13.3). Stridor is an abnormal, loud, high-pitched breath sound caused by obstruction in the upper airways as a result of a foreign body, tissue or vocal cord swelling; this emergent condition requires immediate attention.[43] Absent or diminished breath sounds also require immediate treatment, indicating no airflow through that area of the lung.[34,44]

Practice tip

Respiratory rate is an early warning sign for respiratory distress. If the patient has a high respiratory rate it can be a sign of hypoxia as the patient attempts to compensate for low PaO_2.

Documentation and charting

Document the findings of your respiratory assessment in the patient's chart; if this is the first respiratory assessment, describe the patient's respiratory history carefully. Any abnormal findings including abnormal sounds and their characteristics should be described to enable subsequent re-assessment.[43]

Respiratory monitoring

A thorough and comprehensive assessment, with accurate ongoing monitoring, enables early detection of changes and assessment of responses to treatment for the critically ill. This section describes the main aspects of bedside respiratory monitoring and the instruments used to assess the efficiency of a patient's gas transfer mechanisms, including pulse oximetry, capnography, airway pressures and ventilator waveforms and loops.

Pulse oximetry

Pulse oximetry is a non-invasive device that measures the oxygen saturation of haemoglobin in a patient's arterial blood. The technology is common in critical and acute care areas. It is important to note that the device does not provide information on the patient's ventilatory state, but may determine oxygen saturation and detect hypoxaemia.[45] This prompt, non-invasive detection of hypoxaemia enables detection of clinical deterioration and more rapid treatment to avoid associated complications.[46]

Pulse oximetry works by emitting two wavelengths of light, red and infrared, that pass through a pulsatile flow of blood from a diode (positioned on one side of the probe) to a photodetector (positioned on the opposite side). The signal emitted is measured over five pulses, causing a slight delay when monitoring. Oxygenated blood absorbs light differently from deoxygenated blood; the oximeter measures the amount of light absorbed by the vascular bed and calculates the percentage of haemoglobin saturation in the capillaries.

Table 13.3

Description of abnormal breath sounds

ABNORMAL SOUND	DESCRIPTION	CONDITION
Absent breath sounds	No airflow to particular portion of lung	Pneumothorax Pneumonectomy Emphysematous blebs Pleural effusion Lung mass Massive atelectasis Complete airway obstruction
Diminished breath sounds	Little airflow to particular portion of lung	Emphysema Pleural effusion Pleurisy Atelectasis Pulmonary fibrosis
Displaced bronchial sounds	Bronchial sounds heard in peripheral lung fields	Atelectasis with secretions Lung mass with exudates Pneumonia Pleural effusion Pulmonary oedema
Crackles (rales)	Short, discrete popping or crackling sounds	Pulmonary oedema Pneumonia Pulmonary fibrosis Atelectasis Bronchiectasis
Rhonchi	Coarse, rumbling, low-pitched sounds	Pneumonia Asthma Bronchitis Bronchospasm
Wheezes	High-pitched, squeaking, whistling sounds	Asthma Bronchospasm
Pleural friction rub	Creaking, leathery, loud, dry, coarse sounds	Pleural effusion Pleurisy

Adapted from: Urden L, Stacey K, Lough M. Critical care nursing: Diagnosis and management. 6th ed. St Louis: Mosby; 2010, Table 22.3.

FIGURE 13.14 Common pulse oximetry waveforms.

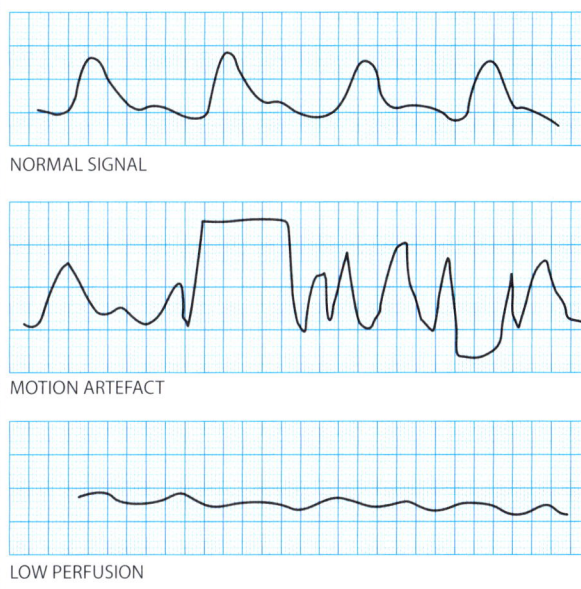

NORMAL SIGNAL

MOTION ARTEFACT

LOW PERFUSION

Practice tip

In cool environments, wrap the hand or foot that has the sensor attached. This may improve saturation readings.

It is important to understand that pulse oximetry measures the saturation of haemoglobin as an estimate of peripheral arterial oxygen saturation (SpO_2). SpO_2 differs from PaO_2. SaO_2 and PaO_2 are physiologically related and this relationship is illustrated by the two axes of the oxygen–haemoglobin dissociation curve (see Figure 13.9, and the previous physiology section for more discussion). A fit healthy adult with a normal haemoglobin level breathing room air would usually have an SpO_2 of 97–99%.[47]

Practice tip

Try to place the pulse oximeter on the finger of the opposite arm to where blood pressure is taken, particularly if you have no arterial line and are doing frequent non-invasive BPs.

Limitations of pulse oximetry

- Pulse oximetry in isolation does not provide all the necessary information to evaluate oxygenation, ventilation status or acid–base balance. ABG testing is required to assess other parameters.[48]
- Pulse oximetery readings are reasonably reliable when the SaO_2 is 90% or above; accuracy deteriorates when the SaO_2 falls to 80% or less.[46] When low SpO_2 readings occur and you are confident that the device is not influenced by artefact, formal ABG analysis should be conducted.

Indirect measurement of arterial oxygen saturation via the peripheral circulation using pulse oximetry is referred to as SpO_2 (the symbol 'p' denotes peripheral) and is displayed digitally on the monitor as a percentage, along with heart rate and a plethysmographic waveform. Interpreting this waveform is essential in distinguishing a true oximetry signal from one displaying dampening or artefact (see Figure 13.14). The probe is commonly placed on a finger, but can also be placed on the toe, earlobe or forehead. Change the probe position frequently to maintain adequate perfusion of the site and skin integrity.[45]

- Satisfactory arterial perfusion of the monitored tissue is required; low cardiac output states, vasoconstriction, peripheral vascular disease and hypothermia can cause inaccurate pulse signals and falsely low oxygen saturation readings. In such cases, confirm oxygen saturation with intermittent ABG testing.
- Cardiac arrhythmias can impair perfusion and flow, and so signal quality may be compromised (see Figure 13.14). In these cases, moving the probe to another location, such as the earlobe or forehead, can improve signal quality.
- Motion artefact (see Figure 13.14), caused by patient movement or shivering, is a significant cause of erroneously low readings and false alarms.[49] Keeping the patient warm (if not contraindicated) and encouraging them to minimise movement may limit this problem. Using an ear probe may also reduce motion artefact.
- There is conflicting evidence as to whether nail varnish or acrylic nails interfere with SpO_2 readings.[49] Blue, green and black nail varnishes are the most likely to affect SpO_2 accuracy. Placing the sensor probe sideways on the finger may avoid this effect. To ensure accuracy, it is recommended that nail varnish and acrylic nails be removed if possible. Newer technology pulse oximeters are less susceptible to these limitations.[46]
- As skin pigmentation allows a constant level of absorption, and pulse oximetry relies on the change in absorbance throughout the cardiac cycle,[50] theoretically darker skin should not affect the performance of the device. However, dark skin has been linked to falsely elevated SpO_2 values, especially saturation levels below 80%.[46]
- External light, especially fluorescent light and heat lamps, can lead to an over- or underestimation of SpO_2.[48] Covering the probe with an opaque barrier, such as a washcloth, can prevent this problem.
- Dyshaemoglobins, particularly carboxyhaemoglobin and methaemoglobin, render SpO_2 monitoring unreliable.[46] The pulse oximetry sensor cannot differentiate between oxyhaemoglobin, carboxyhaemoglobin and methaemoglobin, and therefore provides a false estimation of oxygen saturation.[48] An example of high levels of non-functioning haemoglobin is that of carbon monoxide poisoning; high carboxyhaemoglobin levels give a falsely high SpO_2 reading, leading to an overestimation of oxygenation.[51]
- In the presence of anaemia it is possible to have good oxygen saturation of available haemoglobin but poor tissue oxygenation due to a deficiency in the ability of the blood to transport oxygen. In anaemia, the pulse oximetry readings may be accurate, but it is the clinician's interpretation of these readings that is important. If we are looking at SpO_2 as a marker of oxygenation, a reduced amount of functioning haemoglobin may be well saturated with oxygen but is a poor reflection of tissue oxygenation.[51] Correction of anaemia is required to improve tissue oxygenation.

- Injection of intravenous dyes may lead to a false underestimation of SpO_2 for up to 20 minutes after their administration (methylene blue, indocyanine green, indigo carmine).[46]

Practice tip

Correlate the heart rate reading displayed in the pulse oximetry section of the monitor to the heart rate calculated by the ECG. If they don't correlate, this may indicate that not all pulsations are being detected and the pulse oximetry reading may not be accurate.

Practice tip

Patients with COPD who are hypoxic (SpO_2 <88%) should receive supplemental oxygen. The SpO_2 targets for patients with COPD are lower with SpO_2 generally maintained at >92% during an exacerbation if the patient is at risk of hypercapnia. It is important to frequently assess these patients receiving oxygen so that any compromise in breathing is noted and acted upon.

Capnography

Capnography, using infrared spectrometry, monitors expired CO_2 during the respiratory cycle and is referred to as end-tidal CO_2 ($PetCO_2$). The percentage of exhaled CO_2 at end-expiration is displayed on the monitor. A waveform, called a capnogram[3] is also produced (see Figure 13.15). Continuous capnography detects subtle changes in patients' lung dynamics (i.e. changes to physiological shunting or alveolar recruitment) and can be measured in both intubated and non-intubated patients.

FIGURE 13.15 Normal capnogram. (**A**) End inspiration; (**B**) expiratory upstroke; (**C**) expiratory plateau; (**D**) end-tidal carbon dioxide tension ($PetCO_2$).

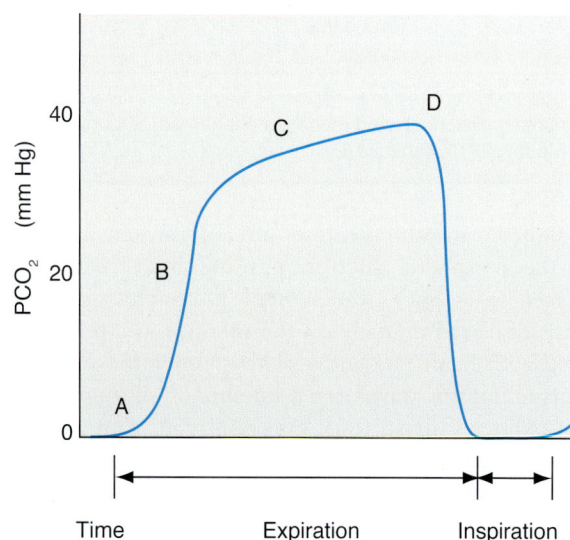

It can be used to estimate $PaCO_2$ levels in patients with a normal ventilation–perfusion ratio (usually 1–5 mmHg less than $PaCO_2$). Levels are, however, affected by conditions common in the critically ill (e.g. low cardiac output states, elevated alveolar pressures, sepsis, hypo/hyperthermia, pulmonary embolism), so use $PetCO_2$ to estimate $PaCO_2$ levels in these patients with caution.[50] Investigate any sudden changes in $PetCO_2$ levels with ABG analysis.

Despite this limitation, $PetCO_2$ monitoring has many uses in the critical care unit:

- indicating correct endotracheal tube (ETT) placement while awaiting CXR, assessing tube patency and detecting leaks or disconnection of the circuit
- monitoring ventilation status during and after weaning from mechanical ventilation
- assessing the effectiveness of cardiopulmonary resuscitation compressions and detecting return of spontaneous circulation
- monitoring ventilation continuously during sedation and anaesthesia
- assessing ventilation/perfusion status.[52,53]

Practice tip

The capnography monitoring line can fill with condensation, particularly if the patient has a humidified ventilator circuit. Regularly check for this and drain or replace the line as necessary. Condensation can interfere with the reading.

Capnography is recommended as a standard component of respiratory monitoring in mechanically ventilated patients in the ICU, during transport of critically ill patients and during anaesthesia.[54]

Ventilation monitoring

Mechanical ventilation is a common intervention for patients who require respiratory support in the ICU. Advances in ventilation technology have enhanced our ability to monitor many ventilator parameters. A detailed understanding of mechanical ventilation principles and functions enables patient data to be interpreted accurately and managed appropriately. Chapter 15 provides a detailed discussion of mechanical ventilation, including ventilation monitoring; airway pressures (peak airway pressure, plateau pressure and positive end–expiratory pressure); and waveforms and loop displays.

Bedside and laboratory investigations

Bedside and laboratory investigations add to available information about a patient's respiratory status and assist in diagnosis and treatment. This section focuses on common investigations used to assess a patient's respiratory status

and their response to treatment: ABG analysis; blood testing; and sputum and tracheal aspirates.

Arterial blood gases

ABGs are one of the most commonly performed laboratory tests in critical care. Therefore, accurate ABG interpretation is an important clinical skill. ABG measurements enable rapid assessment of oxygenation and ventilation, and all ICUs are recommended to have a blood gas analyser as a minimum standard.[55]

Blood for ABG analysis is sampled by arterial puncture or, more commonly in critically ill patients, from an arterial catheter usually sited in the radial or femoral artery. Both techniques are invasive and only allow for intermittent analysis. The advantage of the arterial catheter is that it facilitates ABG sampling without repeated arterial punctures. Continuous blood gas monitoring is possible using an in-line fibre optic sensor as part of the arterial line, but this practice is yet to have wide application in Australasia due to cost and accuracy concerns.[56] Questions also remain regarding the possibility for arteriovenous shunting, blood loss and infection risk with continuous systems.[57]

Sampling technique

A correct sampling technique is essential for accurate results. Prior to arterial sampling from the radial artery, a modified Allen's test should be performed. The patient should clench their fist tightly. Occlusive pressure is then applied to both the ulnar and radial arteries, to obstruct blood flow to the hand. While maintaining this pressure, ask the patient to relax their hand, and check whether the palm and fingers have blanched. Then release the occlusive pressure on the ulnar artery only. The modified Allen's test is positive if the hand flushes within 5–15 seconds, indicating that the ulnar artery has good blood flow and radial sampling is safe.[58]

Approximately 1 mL of arterial blood is collected anaerobically and aseptically using a premixed syringe containing dry heparin. If drawing the sample from an intra-arterial line, a portion of blood is discarded to prevent dilution and contamination of the sample from the saline in the flush line. The discard amount is twice the dead space volume to ensure clinically accurate ABG and electrolyte measurement, and to prevent unnecessary blood loss.[59] Dead space is defined as the priming volume from the sampling port to the catheter tip; this differs depending on the arterial line set-up used. Arterial blood exerts its own pressure, which is sufficient to fill the syringe to the required level; active negative pressure is to be avoided, as this causes frothing. Any excess air will cause inaccurate readings and is expelled before the syringe is capped with a hub, preventing further air contamination. The sample is analysed within 10 minutes if not packed in ice, or within 60 minutes if iced; delays cause degradation of the sample. Degradation also occurs if the sample is shaken; therefore gently roll the syringe/collection tube between your fingers to mix the sample with the heparin and prevent clotting.[60] The frequency of ABG sampling should be carefully considered and based on patient need. ABG sampling may lead to losses of up to 70 mL per day and the cumulative effect may worsen anaemia and increase the need for transfusion. This is particularly important in the paediatric population.[59]

Arterial blood gas analysis

ABG analysis includes measurement of the PaO_2, the $PaCO_2$, the H^+ concentration (pH) and the concentration of chemical buffer, HCO_3^-. Normal values for ABG parameters are listed in Table 13.4. Use a systematic approach when interpreting the results of ABG analysis (see Table 13.5).

Assessing oxygenation: when assessing oxygenation, hypoxaemia (PaO_2 <60 mmHg or <7.8 kilopascals or kPa) will be the most common abnormality and may indicate the need for supplemental oxygen to maintain adequate arterial oxygenation. Conversely, hyperoxia rarely occurs unless a patient is receiving supplemental oxygen therapy. Oxygen can be toxic to cells if delivered at high concentrations for a prolonged period.[61]

Assessing the pH: the body's acid–base balance is affected by both the respiratory and metabolic systems[61] and is evaluated by measuring the pH of arterial blood. On the pH scale of 1 to 14 (where 1 = the strongest acid and 14 = the strongest alkali), a pH of 7.4 is the middle of the normal range. Acidaemia is present with a pH of <7.35; alkalaemia is present with a pH of >7.45. The pH changes depending on the amount of H^+ or HCO_3^- in the blood with H^+ reflecting the acidic component and HCO_3^- the base or buffer.

Assessing for respiratory mechanisms: $PaCO_2$ indicates the effectiveness of ventilation and rises when ventilation is suboptimal. CO_2 combines with water to form carbonic acid (H_2CO_3), so can alter the pH of blood. Retention of CO_2 through hypoventilation or air trapping leads to increased H^+ ions resulting in a lower pH and development of respiratory acidosis. Alternatively, a loss of CO_2 through hyperventilation results in a higher pH and development of respiratory alkalosis.[62] A $PaCO_2$ of >45 mmHg (6 kPa) indicates alveolar hypoventilation, due to COPD, asthma, pulmonary oedema, airway obstruction, over-sedation, narcosis, drug overdose, pain, neurological deficit or permissive hypercapnia in mechanically ventilated patients.[63] Conversely, a $PaCO_2$ of

TABLE 13.5
Steps for arterial blood gas interpretation

STEP	INTERPRETATION
1	Assess oxygenation … PaO_2 <60 mmHg (<8 kPa) indicates hypoxaemia
2	Assess the pH level … <7.35 indicates acidosis, >7.45 indicates alkalosis
3	Assess $PaCO_2$ level … <35 mmHg (<4.7 kPa) indicates respiratory acidosis; >45 mmHg (>6.0 kPa) indicates respiratory alkalosis
4	Assess HCO_3^- level … <22 indicates metabolic acidosis; >32 indicates metabolic alkalosis
5	Assess pH, CO_2 and HCO_3^-. Is there an acid–base disturbance and is it fully compensated, partially compensated or uncompensated?
6	Assess other ABG results. Are they within normal limits for the patient?

TABLE 13.4
Arterial blood gas normal values*

BLOOD GAS MEASUREMENT	DESCRIPTION	NORMAL VALUE
Temperature (T)	Patient's body temperature. Analyser defaults to 37°C if not entered	37°C
Haemoglobin (Hb)	Samples should be fully mixed so should be constantly agitated until analysed	Females: 115–165 g/L Males: 130–180 g/L
Acid–base status (pH)	Overall acidity or alkalinity of blood	7.35–7.45 (36–44 nmol/L)
Carbon dioxide (CO_2)	Partial pressure of arterial CO_2. A potential acid	35–45 mmHg (4.7–6.0 kPa)
Oxygen (O_2)	Partial pressure of O_2. Varies with age	80–100 mmHg (10.7–13.3 kPa)
Bicarbonate (HCO_3^-)	Standardised HCO_3^- (actual HCO_3^- minus the HCO_3^- produced by respiratory dysfunction) estimates true metabolic function. An alkali or base	22–26 mmol/L
Base excess (BE)	Measures acid–base balance. The number of molecules of acid or base required to return 1 L of blood to the normal pH (7.4)	–3 to +3 mmol/L
Oxygen saturation (SaO_2)	Haemoglobin saturation by oxygen in arterial blood	94.5–98.2%

*Institutional norms may vary slightly.

<35 mmHg (4.7kPa) reflects alveolar hyperventilation, and can be due to hypoxia, pain, anxiety, pregnancy, permissive hypocapnia in mechanically ventilated patients or as a compensatory mechanism for metabolic acidosis.[63]

Assessing for renal mechanisms: HCO_3^- is regulated by the renal system. A $[HCO_3^-]$ of <22 mmol/L can lead to metabolic acidosis, caused by renal failure, ketoacidosis, lactic acidosis, diarrhoea or cardiac arrest. A HCO_3^- of >26 can lead to metabolic alkalosis, caused by severe vomiting, continuous nasogastric suction, diuretics, corticosteroids or excessive citrate administration from stored blood or renal replacement therapy.[63]

Base excess is an additional value included in the ABG report and it reflects the excess (or deficit) of base to acid in the blood. Normal base excess ranges from −2 to +2. If the base excess (BE) is +2 mmol/L, removal of 2 mmol of base per litre of blood is required to return the pH to 7.4. If the BE is −2 mmol/L (i.e. a base deficit), 2 mmol of base per litre of blood needs to be added to achieve a pH of 7.4. A BE greater than +3 indicates that there is more base than acid present and therefore alkalosis. A BE below −3 indicates that there is more acid than base. Understanding this concept is useful as it can determine how much treatment is necessary to restore a patient's pH to normal.[62,64,65]

Assessing for compensation: the final step of interpretation is to examine the pH, CO_2 and HCO_3^- levels collectively, to determine if the patient has either fully or partially compensated the primary dysfunction, or is in an uncompensated state. With the respiratory system regulating CO_2 and the metabolic system regulating HCO_3^-, restoration of normal acid–base balance and homeostasis is possible.[62] The ability of the body to achieve homeostasis and acid–base balance depends on the ability of the respiratory and renal systems to adjust to the underlying imbalance.

The degree of compensation depends on whether the pH returns to normal; full compensation results in a normal pH whereas, in partial compensation, the pH remains outside normal limits. In an uncompensated acid–base imbalance, there has been no attempt by the body to correct the acid–base imbalance and the pH, as well as either the CO_2 or HCO_3^-, is abnormal.

To assess compensation, pH, CO_2 and HCO_3^- are examined in the context of a patient's clinical presentation:

- In a fully compensated state, the pH is returned to within normal limits, but the other two parameters will be outside normal limits as the body has successfully manipulated CO_2 and HCO_3^- levels to restore the pH.

- In a partially compensated state, the pH is not within normal limits, and the other parameters will also be outside of normal limits but not enough to bring the pH back to normal.

- In a non-compensated state, the pH will be outside normal limits, and the primary disruption (either CO_2 or HCO_3^-) will also be outside normal limits while the remaining parameter has not compensated for this derangement and has stayed within normal limits.

It can be difficult to differentiate the patient's primary problem from their compensatory response. As a quick guide, if the CO_2 is moving in the opposite direction to pH, then the primary disruption is respiratory; if the HCO_3^- is moving in the same direction as pH, the disruption is metabolic.[65] Table 13.6 provides a guide to ABG findings for each acid–base disorder. Other parameters measured on the ABG sample, such as lactate, electrolytes, haemoglobin and glucose, are also considered in determining patient status.

TABLE 13.6

Arterial blood gas findings for acid–base disturbances

	PH	PaCO₂, MMHG (KPA)	HCO₃⁻, MMOL/L
RESPIRATORY ACIDOSIS			
Uncompensated	<7.35	>45 (6.0)	Within normal limits
Partially compensated	<7.35	>45 (6.0)	>26
Fully compensated	Within normal limits	>45 (6.0)	>26
RESPIRATORY ALKALOSIS			
Uncompensated	>7.45	<35 (4.7)	Within normal limits
Partially compensated	>7.45	<35 (4.7)	<22
Fully compensated	Within normal limits	<35 (4.7)	<22
METABOLIC ACIDOSIS			
Uncompensated	<7.35	Within normal limits	<22
Partially compensated	<7.35	<35 (4.7)	<22
Fully compensated	Within normal limits	<35 (4.7)	<22
METABOLIC ALKALOSIS			
Uncompensated	>7.45	Within normal limits	>26
Partially compensated	>7.45	>45 (6.0)	>26
Fully compensated	Within normal limits	>45 (6.0)	>26

The Stewart approach

As an adjunct to traditional ABG interpretation, Peter Stewart's seminal concepts on acid–base assessment[66] suggest that, in our body's fluids, pH and HCO_3^- are merely dependent variables that cannot be directly manipulated. Stewart was particularly interested in considering the influence of resuscitation fluid management on acid–base balance. He developed six equations to assist clinicians to analyse the physiological basis of acid–base shifts, considering the impacts of strong cations, the total concentration of weak acids and CO_2.[67] Stewart's intention was not to replace traditional methods of determining acid–base balance, but to extend their usefulness and to further explain the physiological basis of complex disorders.[67] An example of the utility of Stewart's work is evident in a recent study of 300 patients with abdominal sepsis. This report demonstrated that a modification of the Stewart approach was able to identify mixed acid–base disorders which would otherwise remain undetected.[68]

Stewart's complex equations have been made more user-friendly with the development of online calculators[69] where the clinician can enter patient chemistry data online to receive an online decision support related to complex acid/base disorders (see *Online resources*). Once patient data are entered, the site offers clinicians a breakup of the relative contributions to the overall disturbance in pH by its main controlling elements. When displayed graphically, this gives the user a sense of the severity of each contributing factor, and allows input of these individual factors into virtual scenarios to predict the possible impact of specific interventions.[67]

Oxygen tension-derived indices

The alveolar–arterial gradient is a marker of intrapulmonary shunting (i.e. blood flowing past collapsed areas of alveoli not involved in gas exchange). The index is calculated as $PAO_2 - PaO_2$ (where PAO_2 is the partial pressure of oxygen in the alveoli). PAO_2 is determined by a complex equation, the alveolar gas equation. PAO_2 and PaO_2 are equal when perfusion and ventilation are perfectly matched. The gradient increases with age but a value of 5–15 mmHg is normal up until approximately middle age. Despite questions about its clinical usefulness, particularly in the critically ill,[70] it is used in clinical practice as a trending tool to track intrapulmonary shunting. Simply put, the larger the gradient between PAO_2 and PaO_2, the larger the degree of intrapulmonary shunting.[71]

The ratio of PaO_2 to fraction of inspired oxygen (FiO_2), commonly referred to as the PaO_2/FiO_2 (or P/F) ratio, was introduced as a simple way of estimating pulmonary shunting, even though it does not formally measure alveolar partial pressure. A recent consensus paper outlines criteria known as the *Berlin Definition*[72] to define stages of ARDS. According to this definition, a PaO_2/FiO_2 ratio of 200–300 mmHg (≤39.9 kPa) indicates mild ARDS, a ratio of 100–200 mmHg (≤26.6 kPa) indicates moderate ARDS while a ratio of less than or equal to 100 mmHg

(<13.3 kPa) indicates severe ARDS. For example, in a patient receiving a FiO_2 of 0.65 who has a PaO_2 of 90 mmHg (12 kPa), their PaO_2/FiO_2 ratio would be 138.5 mmHg, indicating a moderate ARDS state. A diagnosis of ARDS also requires the above reductions in PaO_2/FiO_2 ratio to be present with the patient receiving at least 5 cmH_2O of positive end-expiratory pressure or continuous positive airway pressure. It requires this state to have developed within 1 week of a known clinical insult or worsening respiratory symptoms. A chest X-ray (CXR) should show bilateral opacities not fully explained by other causes and respiratory failure not fully explained by cardiac failure or fluid overload.[72]

Transcutaneous blood gas monitoring

A transcutaneous monitor provides an estimate of the PaO_2 and $PaCO_2$ by measuring these partial pressures at the skin surface. This form of monitoring is useful where arterial access is not obtainable, or there is a need to monitor continuous readings of oxygen and CO_2 with minimal drawing of blood. Transcutaneous monitoring is most appropriate to obtain continuous trend data; its use for intermittent readings is not appropriate.[73] Transcutaneous monitoring is a common approach with neonates because neonatal skin is particularly thin;[74] however, it may also prove useful for adult monitoring. Possible uses include evaluation of hypoventilation during management and weaning of mechanical ventilation, during bronchoscopy or other procedures requiring sedation, during sleep studies or pulmonary function studies, apnoea testing or titration of long-term oxygen therapy and to monitor tissue perfusion and revascularisation at the site of a wound. It is also useful to monitor a patient's response to therapy in diabetic ketoacidosis as transcutaneous measurement of CO_2 closely correlates with serum HCO_3^- levels.[73]

Transcutaneous monitoring devices increase the local skin temperature at the sensor site resulting in increased local capillary perfusion. This increases the metabolic rate of the skin and the solubility of CO_2, which in turn leads to local production of CO_2. A temperature correction then addresses the heightened local CO_2 production that results from heating the skin.[75]

The partial pressure of transcutaneous oxygen ($PtcO_2$) is measured using a Clark polarographic heated electrode.[74] The skin probe temperature needs to be 44°C to achieve an accurate $PtcO_2$ and this may lead to thermal injury, particularly if the skin is thin or damaged. Because of this risk, the site for transcutaneous electrodes should be observed and alternated every 4–6 hours[75] and as often as every 2 hours in small, premature neonates. $PtcO_2$ is an indirect measure of PaO_2 that is not reflective of oxygen content or delivery and requires a knowledge and consideration of both haemoglobin saturation and cardiac output.[73]

The partial pressure of transcutaneous CO_2 ($PtcCO_2$) is usually measured using a Severinghaus electrode. $PtcCO_2$ is much less reliant on a higher skin temperature. Accuracy may be achieved with skin probe temperatures as low as

37°C making longer probe dwell times possible. Although $PtcCO_2$ is an indirect measure of $PaCO_2$, it remains a useful assessment of ventilation.[73]

Skin preparation is important for accurate readings and should include removal of soaps, oils and dead skin cells. To secure the electrode, a sensor fixation ring should be placed in a highly vascularised location. In neonates and small children the upper chest is an ideal location. Alternative sites include the ear lobe, cheeks, forehead or over the zygomatic bone, the inner aspect of the thigh or forearm, the buttock or the lateral aspect of the abdomen.[73] Once the fixation device is secured, 1–2 drops of either normal saline or contact gel is placed inside the fixation ring to improve the diffusion of gases and, in turn, maximise the accuracy of the sensor. The sensor then snaps into place. A good seal should be sought between the sensor and fixation device as leaks or the formation of air bubbles can affect the accuracy of transcutaneous readings.[73]

A number of conditions should be documented in relation to transcutaneous monitoring results including the respiratory rate, the patient's position and level of activity; the fraction of inspired oxygen and the oxygen delivery device including ventilator mode and settings; the site, temperature and time of electrode placement; and the clinical appearance of the patient and the results of simultaneous ABGs, specifically PaO_2, $PaCO_2$ and pH.[73]

Limitations of transcutaneous monitoring

Following electrode placement 5–10 minutes should be allowed before taking transcutaneous readings. Poor calibration, trapped air or leaks in the fixation device or damage to the membranes can result in inaccurate readings. Generally speaking, $PtcO_2$ underestimates PaO_2 while $PtcCO_2$ overestimates $PaCO_2$. In addition, falsely elevated or diminished readings may occur due to:

- high arterial oxygen levels (PaO_2 >100 mmHg, 13.3 kPa) (overestimates $PtcO_2$)
- hypoperfusion (as in shock or acidosis) or vasoactive drug use (underestimates $PtcO_2$ and $PtcCO_2$); the use of more contemporary transcutaneous devices and placement of the sensor close to the carotid artery may limit this effect
- thickened or oedematous skin or subcutaneous tissue (underestimates $PtcO_2$ and $PtcCO_2$)
- poor skin preparation or poor electrode fixation (underestimates PtcO2 and $PtcCO_2$)
- distal placement of the electrode in the presence of vasoconstriction (underestimates $PtcO_2$ and $PtcCO_2$)
- active or passive patient movement causing increased capillary blood flow (overestimates $PtcO_2$ and $PtcCO_2$).

Transcutaneous oxygen and CO_2 readings should be validated by comparing them with simultaneous ABG results at baseline measurement and periodically thereafter.[73]

Practice tip

When comparing transcutaneous and arterial partial pressures of carbon dioxide, $PtCO_2$ is typically higher than $PaCO_2$. An acceptable range of agreement between arterial and transcutaneous measures is ± 7 mmHg.

Blood tests

Haematology and biochemistry investigations should inform treatment for patients with respiratory dysfunction. Full blood count, including a leukocyte differential count, can monitor white cell activity for patients with a confirmed or suspected infective process. When infections are severe, the full blood count will show a dramatic rise in the number of immature neutrophils. Blood cultures can also assist in diagnosis of bacterial or yeast infections and isolation of the causative organism. Viral studies may aid diagnosis for respiratory infections of unknown origin. Where pulmonary embolism is suspected, a D-dimer test can assist diagnosis of a thrombus. Routine measurement of urea and electrolytes can track renal function and acid–base status.[76]

Practice tip

Monitoring lactate levels is important as the levels can be used to assess the effectiveness and efficiency of resuscitative therapies. A persistently elevated lactate level is associated with higher morbidity and poorer patient outcomes.

Sputum, tracheal aspirates and nasopharyngeal aspirates

Colour, consistency and volume of sputum provide useful information in determining changes in a patient's respiratory status and progress. Regular cultures of tracheal sputum reveal colonisation by opportunistic organisms, and can identify the cause of an acute chest infection or sepsis. Many ICUs have routine (weekly or twice-weekly) surveillance monitoring of tracheal aspirates in long-term mechanically ventilated patients. In spontaneously breathing patients, sputum specimens can be collected in a sterile specimen receptacle. Specimens are best collected early in the morning and teeth cleaning prior to sample collection may reduce secondary contamination. In intubated patients, using a sputum trap between the suction catheter and suction tubing assists sputum collection. A sterile technique should be maintained to reduce sample contamination.[77]

If obtaining an adequate sputum specimen in non-intubated patients is difficult, there is evidence that administration of nebulised saline (isotonic or hypertonic) may assist sputum collection.[78] There is no evidence to support this among mechanically ventilated patients but, anecdotally, nebulised normal saline may assist sputum production by moistening the airways and thinning secretions. Physiotherapy[79] in the form of manual hyper-inflation and head-down tilt during therapy has been shown to increase sputum production for sample collection.[80,81]

Instilling normal saline in an ETT to facilitate clearance and/or collection of tenacious sputum remains a controversial issue. There is no evidence that instillation facilitates secretion clearance, while there is some evidence that it increases both patient discomfort and the risk of bacterial contamination of the lower airway. Therefore, this practice is not recommended.[82]

Nasopharyngeal aspirate or swabs may be necessary to diagnose viral respiratory infections. The nasopharyngeal aspirate is collected by inserting a fine, sterile suction catheter (8 or 10 F) attached to a sputum trap through the nare and back to the nasopharynx. Suction is applied while withdrawing and slowly rotating the catheter. The catheter is flushed through to the sputum trap with sterile normal saline or transport medium if available. A nasopharyngeal swab is collected by inserting a specially designed swab to the back of the nasopharynx and rotating for 5–10 seconds. The swab is then withdrawn slowly and placed in the plastic vial containing transport medium. As close contact with the patient is necessary, and the procedure can generate aerosols and droplets, personal protective equipment should be worn.[83]

Diagnostic procedures

Assessment and monitoring of the respiratory status of a critically ill patient may rely on various medical imaging

tests and bronchoscopy to determine the cause and severity of the illness episode, relevant comorbidities and the patient's response to treatment.

Medical imaging

A range of imaging techniques may be available for supporting care of a critically ill patient with a respiratory dysfunction, depending on the level of broader health service resources available. This sub-section describes X-ray, ultrasound, computerised tomography, magnetic resonance imaging and ventilation/perfusion scan techniques.

Chest X-ray

Chest radiography is a common diagnostic tool used for respiratory examination of critically ill patients. CXR allows basic information regarding abnormalities in the chest to be obtained relatively quickly. The image provides information about lung fields and other thoracic structures as well as the placement of invasive lines and tubes.[84,85] In the ventilated patient, serial CXRs also enable sequential assessment of lung status in relation to therapy.[85]

In-unit X-rays of patients using portable equipment are inferior to those taken using a fixed camera in the radiology department. Patient preparation is therefore important to optimise the quality of the film. Patients should ideally be positioned sitting or semi-erect; CXRs using a supine position are less effective at revealing gravity-related abnormalities such as haemothorax. Lateral view CXRs may assist identification of lesions in

FIGURE 13.16 Chest X-ray, PA view.

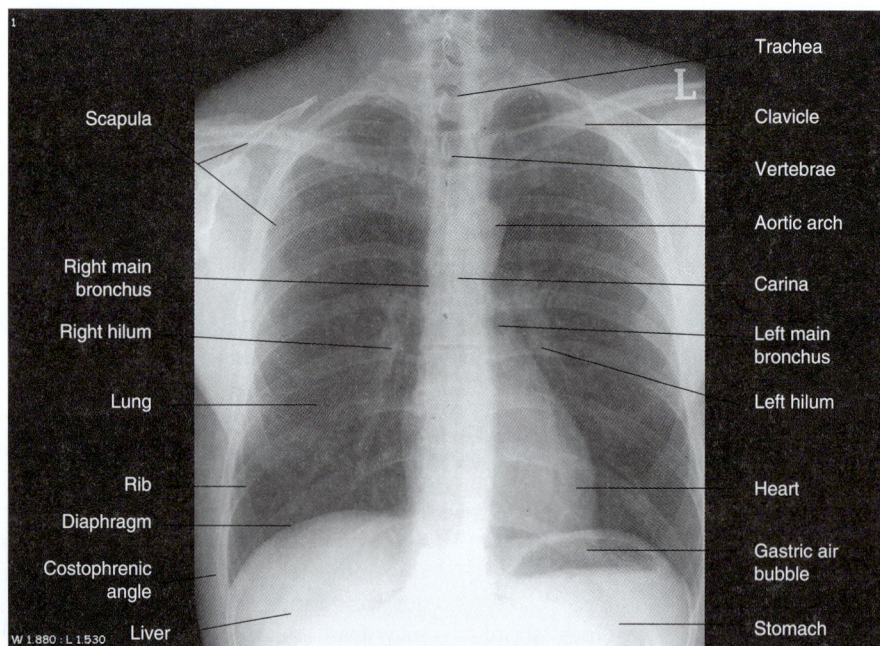

Published with permission, University of Auckland Faculty of Medical and Health Sciences.

TABLE 13.7

Guide to normal chest X-ray interpretation[84]

Technical issues	• Check X-ray belongs to correct patient; note date and time of film • Ensure you are viewing X-ray correctly (i.e. right and left markings correspond to thoracic structures) • Determine whether X-ray was taken supine or erect, and whether PA or AP • Check X-ray was taken at full inspiration (posterior aspects of 9th/10th ribs and anterior aspects of 5th/6th ribs should be visible above diaphragm) • Note the penetration of the film: dark films are overpenetrated and may require a strong light to view; white films are underpenetrated; good penetration will allow visualisation of the vertebrae behind the heart
Bones	• Check along each rib from vertebral origin, looking for fractures • Ensure clavicles and scapulas are intact
Mediastinum	• Check for presence of trachea and identify carina (approximately level of 5th–6th vertebrae) • Check width of mediastinum: should not be more than 8 cm
Apex	• Ensure blood vessels are visible in both apices, particularly looking to rule out pneumothoraces that present as clear black shading on the X-ray. Erect X-rays are essential to facilitate visibility of pneumothoraces
Hilum	• Check for prominence of vessels in this region: it generally indicates vascular abnormalities such as pulmonary oedema or pulmonary hypertension, or congestive heart failure
Heart	• Cardiac silhouette should be not more than 50% of the diameter of the thorax, with {1/3} of heart shadow to the right of the vertebrae and {2/3} of shadow to the left of the vertebrae; this positioning helps to rule out a tension pneumothorax. It should be noted that, post-cardiac surgery, if the mediastinum is left open the heart may appear wider than this; also in AP films this may be the case due to the plate being further away from the heart
Lung	• Identify the lobes of the lungs and determine if infiltrate or collapse is present in one or more of them. Lobes are approximately located as follows: —left upper lobe occupies upper half of lung —left lower lobe occupies lower half of lung —right lower lobe occupies costophrenic portion of lung —right middle lobe occupies cardiophrenic portion of lung —right upper lobe occupies upper portion of lung
Diaphragm	• Check levels of diaphragm: right diaphragm will normally be 1–2 cm above the left diaphragm to accommodate the liver
Gastric	Check for pneumoperitoneum and dilated loops of bowel
Catheters and lines	• Identify distal end of endotracheal tube and ensure above the carina (i.e. not in the right main bronchus) • Trace nasogastric tube along length and ensure tip is in stomach, or below stomach if nasoenteric tube • Check position of intra-aortic balloon pump and ensure it is in the descending thoracic aorta • Trace all central catheters and ensure distal tip is in correct location • Identify other lines (e.g. intercostal catheters, pacing wires) and note location

PA = posteroanterior; AP = anteroposterior.

Adapted from: Lareau C, Wootton J. The "frequently" normal chest x-ray. Can J Rural Med 2004;9(3):183–6.

the thorax. Film plate location against the patient's thorax determines the view: for posteroanterior (PA) the plate is positioned against the anterior thorax (see Figure 13.16) while the anteroposterior (AP) view has the plate against the patient's back. For mobile CXRs, the AP view is used. The AP view can magnify thoracic structures and can be less distinct or even distorted, so interpret findings with caution, particularly if comparing them with previous PA images.[86]

CXR interpretation follows a systematic process designed to identify common pathophysiological processes and the locations of lines and other items. Table 13.7 provides a comprehensive guideline for viewing and interpreting a CXR.

Common abnormalities that can be detected by CXR include:

- Lobar collapse or atelectasis: loss of lung volume, displacement of fissures and vascular markings and/or diaphragmatic elevation on the affected side.
- Pneumothorax: lack of pulmonary vascular markings on the affected side so the lung field appears black. There will be mediastinal and possible tracheal shift away from the affected side in tension pneumothorax.

Practice tip

When preparing your patient for a CXR, minimise the number of monitoring leads and unnecessary equipment in the CXR field to optimise the image.

- Pleural effusion: in the dependent areas of the pleural spaces, costophrenic angles are blunted by fluid and there may be a mediastinal shift away from a large effusion. Effusions are best visualised with the patient upright, and will only be evident on an AP image with 200–400 mL of fluid in the pleural space.
- Pulmonary oedema: lung fields, particularly central and perihilar areas, appear white. Kerley B lines (small horizontal lines <2 cm long) may be present in the lung periphery near the costophrenic angles.
- Pulmonary embolism: although not the optimal diagnostic tool, areas of infarction may be visualised on CXR and may be mistaken for collapse or consolidation.
- Pneumoperitoneum: free air under the diaphragm elevates the diaphragm.[86,87]

Ultrasound

Ultrasound imaging (sonography) is a useful bedside diagnostic tool for a select group of critically ill patients[88] and can add to the diagnostic information provided by CXR and computerised tomography (CT) scanning. Ultrasound uses high-frequency sound waves which, when probed on the body, reflect and scatter. The advantages are that the procedure can take place within the ICU, and it is radiation-free. Ultrasound is most useful for patients with fluid in the pleural space (i.e. pleural effusion, haemothorax or empyema), and provides more detailed diagnostic information than CXR alone.[89] Ultrasound allows an estimate of the volume and exact location of the fluid present and reduces the potential for serious complications during aspiration of fluid or chest tube insertion.[90]

Computed tomography

CT is a diagnostic investigation that provides greater specificity in chest anatomy and pathophysiology than a plain CXR, using multiple beams in a circle around the body. These beams are directed to a specific body area and provide detailed, consecutive cross-sectional slices of the scanned regions. CT scans can be performed with or without intravenous contrast.[91] Contrast improves diagnostic precision but is used with caution in patients with renal impairment; renal failure may preclude a patient from receiving contrast. CT scanning is useful in the detection and diagnosis of pulmonary, pleural and mediastinal disorders (e.g. pleural effusion, empyema, haemothorax, atelectasis, pneumonia, ARDS).[92] CT pulmonary angiography produces a detailed view of blood vessels and is therefore the most definitive method for diagnosing pulmonary embolism.[93]

A significant limitation of CT scanning is that the patient is transported away from the ICU. Transport increases the risks for critically ill patients and usually requires at least two appropriately trained staff to accompany the patient. Detailed planning by the healthcare team (including imaging staff) includes ventilator support, monitoring requirements and maintenance of infusions during scanning. Portable CT scanners are available in some centres, and may reduce the risks associated with transportation of critically ill patients to fixed CT scanners.[94] See Chapter 6 for discussion of in-hospital transfers, and Chapter 23 for inter-hospital transport.

Magnetic resonance imaging

Magnetic resonance imaging (MRI) uses radiofrequency waves and a strong magnetic field rather than X-rays to provide high contrast, detailed pictures of internal organs and soft tissues that are clearer than those generated by X-ray or CT scans. The strong magnetic field around the scanner means that ferromagnetic objects containing material that can be attracted by magnets, such as iron or steel, can become potentially fatal projectiles. MRI scans may therefore be unsuitable for some patients. American[95] and European guidelines[96] discourage the use of MRI where permanent pacemakers and implantable defibrillators are in situ; however, recent research suggests MRIs may be safe for many of these patients.[97,98] Some types of neurostimulation devices[99] and intracranial aneurysm clips[100] have been designed for safe use in MRI but careful screening should precede MRI to determine patient and device-specific risks. Dental fillings, braces and retainers are usually safe but may distort images of the face or brain.[101] MRI in people with such devices should be used where the potential benefit clearly outweighs the risks. The strong magnetic fields also have the potential to interfere with ventilators, infusion pumps and monitoring equipment.[102]

Ventilation/perfusion scan

A V/Q scan is indicated when a mismatch of lung ventilation and perfusion is suspected, most commonly for pulmonary embolism. The ventilation scan is performed with the patient inhaling a radioisotopic gas, while the perfusion scan is performed using an intravenous radioisotope that reveals the distribution of blood flow in the pulmonary vessels.[103] These two scans are then compared, seeking mismatches between perfusion and ventilation. In larger centres, the V/Q scan has been superseded by the CT pulmonary angiogram for detection of pulmonary embolism.

Bronchoscopy

Bronchoscopy is a bedside technique used for both diagnostic and therapeutic purposes. The bronchoscope can be either rigid or flexible, with the flexible fibre optic bronchoscope most widely used in critical care. A flexible fibre optic bronchoscope allows direct visualisation of respiratory mucosa and thorough examination of the upper airways and tracheobronchial tree. The scope is passed into the trachea via the oropharynx or nares. In mechanically ventilated patients, the scope can be passed quickly and easily down the ETT or tracheostomy tube using a specially adapted valve that allows passage of the scope without disconnection of mechanical ventilation.[104]

During bronchoscopy, supplemental oxygen can be administered in non-intubated patients and FiO_2 can be increased in intubated patients. Accurate continuous monitoring during the procedure includes continuous pulse oximetry, electrocardiography, respiratory rate, heart rate and blood pressure. Equipment for advanced airway management, suctioning, cardiac defibrillation and advanced life support medications is immediately available.[105] In intubated patients, one person is responsible for security of the airway to reduce the risk of displacement during the procedure.

When performed by an experienced operator, fibre optic bronchoscopy is a relatively safe procedure in critically ill patients. In mechanically ventilated patients, the correct diameter of bronchoscope relative to the endotracheal tube diameter is important to avoid decreases in tidal and minute volumes,[104] decreased PaO_2 and increased $PaCO_2$. Serious complications such as bleeding, bronchospasm,

arrhythmia, pneumothorax and pneumonia occur rarely.[106] Patient preparation may include CXR; haemoglobin and coagulation profile, particularly if a biopsy is to be performed; baseline ABGs; and fasting or cessation of feeds for 4–6 hours prior.

Diagnostic indications for bronchoscopy include further investigation of poor gas exchange; evaluation of haemoptysis; collection of specimens (e.g. bronchoalveolar lavage, bronchial washings, bronchial brushings, lung biopsy); diagnosis of infection, interstitial lung disease, rejection post lung transplantation, malignancy; and diagnosis of airway injury due to burns, aspiration or chest trauma. Therapeutic indications include removal of mucous plugs; removal of foreign bodies; treatment of atelectasis; assistance during tracheostomy; airway dilation and stenting for tracheobronchomalacia and tracheobronchial stenosis; and lung volume reduction for emphysema.[107,108]

Summary

In this chapter a comprehensive overview of assessment and monitoring of a patient with respiratory dysfunction to aid clinical decision making is provided. Acute respiratory dysfunction is a major cause for admission to a critical care unit. Whether due to a primary or secondary condition, compromise of the respiratory system can be a life-threatening situation. This chapter outlines related respiratory physiology, pathophysiology, assessment and respiratory monitoring, bedside laboratory investigations and medical imaging:

- Critical care nurses are in a prime position to provide systematic and dynamic bedside assessments of a patient's respiratory status including past and presenting respiratory history, and physical examination of the thorax and lungs using inspection, palpation and auscultation techniques.

- Monitoring a patient's respiratory function includes pulse oximetry and capnography. Bedside and laboratory investigations including ABG analysis, blood tests and sputum and tracheal aspirates add to available information and assists in both diagnosis and treatment. ABG testing is common and ABG interpretation is an important clinical skill for critical care nurses.

- CXR is the most common diagnostic imaging tool in the ICU. CXR interpretation follows a systematic process to identify common pathologies and to locate lines and other items. Bronchoscopy is a useful bedside diagnostic and therapeutic device. CT provides greater specificity than CXR. Ultrasound imaging is useful to diagnose fluid in the pleural space. MRI and V/Q scans are more sophisticated diagnostic tools.

Careful patient assessment is essential, as respiratory dysfunction can be immediately life-threatening. Contemporary critical care practice involves comprehensive clinical assessment skills and use of a range of monitoring devices and diagnostic procedures. This challenges critical care nurses to be adaptable and willing to embrace new skills and knowledge.

Case study

Presenting history: Max is a 63-year-old man who presented to the emergency department with a 3–4 week history of shortness of breath and a dry cough, worsening over the past week. Max weighs 122 kg and has a body mass index of 42.

Past medical history: Max had atrial fibrillation, obstructive sleep apnoea and hypertension and was an ex-smoker of 25 packet-years.

Medications: warfarin, digoxin, diltiazem and atenolol.

Social history: Max works as a taxi driver, lives at home with his wife and walks independently.

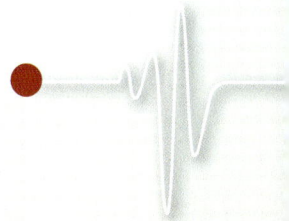

ON ADMISSION

Inspection: on arrival to the emergency department Max was speaking in short sentences. Respiratory rate was 32 breaths per minute, temperature 38°C and SpO_2 74% on room air. Max appeared to have an increased respiratory effort. It was difficult to assess his use of accessory muscles of respiration due to excess adipose tissue. He reported no chest pain.

Palpation: Max's apex beat was 92 beats per minute and irregular and BP was 107/79 mmHg. The nurse noted grade II bilateral pedal oedema with chronic skin changes. His peripheries were warm and pink and capillary refill time less than 2 seconds. Vocal fremitus was difficult to determine and chest wall expansion slightly diminished on the right side.

Percussion: there appeared to be dullness over the bases; however percussion was difficult to assess due to excessive adipose tissue.

Auscultation: bilateral bronchial breath sounds over the bases and a mild expiratory wheeze.

Initial management: non-invasive ventilation, serial electrocardiograms (ECGs) and cardiac enzymes were ordered. Bilevel positive airway pressure was commenced. Medical staff documented a target SpO_2 range of 88–92%.

Other assessment findings: ECG showed atrial fibrillation, rate 94 beats per minute. With no prior ECG for comparison, the poor R wave progression in the precordial leads and non-specific T wave changes in the context of raised cardiac enzymes suggested the possibility of a non-ST-elevation acute coronary syndrome. High sensitivity troponin-T was elevated at 22 ng/mL. An echocardiogram showed mild left ventricular hypertrophy with normal left ventricular ejection fraction. Right ventricular pressure was slightly elevated. The white cell count was 4.00 ($\times 10^9$ L).

Arterial blood gases: PaO_2 = 67 mmHg (8.9 kPa), pH = 7.44, $PaCO_2$ = 44 mmHg (5.9 kPa), BE= 5, SaO_2 = 93%. The pH and $PaCO_2$ are in the upper range of normal and the BE is abnormally high indicating a mixed disorder that needs monitoring and consideration within the patient's broader clinical picture.

Chest X-ray: bilateral fluffy interstitial opacities were noted, though they were more evident on the right side. Costophrenic angles were visible indicating there was no effusion.

Assessment plan: sputum culture, urine specimen for pneumococcal antigens, a nasopharyngeal swab for respiratory viruses, serial ECG and troponins, hourly urine measure and daily weight.

Management plan: Max had multifactorial Type 1 respiratory failure, including community-acquired pneumonia and a likely component of congestive cardiac failure. IV antibiotics azithromycin and cefotaxime, IV magnesium sulfate, IV hydrocortisone and nebulised salbutamol were prescribed and a respiratory and ICU consult were organised. Max was transferred to the high dependency unit. IV Lasix 40 mg daily, a 1500-mL fluid restriction and regular salbutamol via metered-dose inhaler with spacer were prescribed.

DAY 1

Inspection: Max became drowsy. He was able to follow simple commands but was irritable when roused. His respiratory rate was 28–38 breaths per minute and an increased work of breathing was noted despite increasing non-invasive ventilation support.

Vital signs: temperature 39.2°C, atrial fibrillation rate 128 bpm and BP 134/69 mmHg.

Palpation: grade II pitting oedema to mid calves. Calf compressors applied.

Auscultation: loud bi-basal crackles, widespread wheeze and reduced air entry.

Management plan: Max was considered at high risk for further deterioration and was predicted to have a difficult airway to manage under those circumstances. He was transferred to ICU.

On admission to ICU: ABG results were PaO_2 58 mmHg (7.7 kPa), pH 7.33, $PaCO_2$ 68 mmHg (9 kPa) and BE 7.8, indicating hypoxia and a partially compensated respiratory acidosis. Max's doctor explained the situation and received Max's verbal consent for endotracheal intubation.

ONGOING PROGRESS

Max managed well on pressure support ventilation. He was repositioned regularly, including in a high sitting position. He received frequent physiotherapy. His peripheral oedema reduced. Over time, nurses were able to reduce Max's FiO_2. His PaO_2 and $PaCO_2$ began to normalise. After 4 days, Max was extubated and, after a further week on the ward, he returned home. Follow-up was arranged with respiratory and cardiology doctors and a dietician and arrangements were made for home continuous positive airway pressure therapy at night.

DISCUSSION POINTS

- Obesity increases the prevalence of respiratory failure and augments the risk of conditions such as obstructive sleep apnoea, pulmonary embolism and pulmonary hypertension. Impaired lung mechanics in obese patients can facilitate the development of pneumonia and, when mechanically ventilated, they have reduced respiratory compliance.[109,110]
- The reverse Trendelenburg position can improve oxygenation and functional residual capacity.[109]
- Vocal fremitus is easier to feel over a thin chest wall. The vibrations produced in vocal fremitus are dampened in patients who are obese or heavily muscled.[111] Breath sounds are diminished in obese patients, losing strength as they travel through adipose tissue.[112]

CASE STUDY QUESTIONS

1 If a nurse anticipated Max might have areas of pulmonary consolidation, what changes would he/she expect to *feel* with vocal fremitus and *hear* using percussion compared to normal areas of lung?

2 What indicates partially compensated respiratory acidosis in Max's final ICU ABG prior to intubation? (PaO_2 58 mmHg [7.7 kPa], pH 7.33, $PaCO_2$ 68.3 mmHg [9.1 kPa], BE 7.8)

3 Consider the challenges that Max's high BMI creates for respiratory assessment and the mechanics of breathing while nursed in bed.

RESEARCH VIGNETTE

Lavelle C, Dowling M. The factors which influence nurses when weaning patients from mechanical ventilation: findings from a qualitative study. Intensive Crit Care Nurs 2011;27:244–52

Abstract

The aim of the study was to describe the factors that influence critical care nurses when deciding to wean patients from mechanical ventilation. The study adopted a qualitative methodology, using semi-structured interviews and a vignette. An invited sample of critical care nurses (n = 24) from one Irish intensive care unit was employed. Each nurse was interviewed once and a vignette was used to structure the interview questioning. The findings were analysed using thematic content analysis. Six major themes influencing nurses' decision to wean emerged: physiological influences; clinical reassessment and decision making; the nurse's experience, confidence and education; the patient's medical history and current ventilation; the intensive care working environment; and use of protocols. The findings highlight the complex nature of weaning patients from mechanical ventilation and the major role of the nurse in this process.

Critique

This study is relevant to the area of respiratory assessment and monitoring because it explores the way critical care nurses apply their assessment and monitoring skills to inform their decisions on weaning patients from mechanical ventilation.

The authors situate the relevance of this work in the acknowledged role of critical care nurses in the weaning process and the complexity of the process, despite the use of protocols. The role of nurses in weaning decisions is described as evolving from the domain of the intensivist, extending through the addition of what were previously seen as medical tasks and expanding through the growth of nursing knowledge. The critical nature of readiness for weaning and its commencement as soon as appropriate is justified through discussion of the complications associated with mechanical ventilation. These include increased mortality from ventilator-associated lung injury and ventilator-associated pneumonia, along with an increased need for sedation and neuromuscular blockade. Weaning that is undertaken too soon is discussed in terms of fatigue of respiratory muscles and cardiovascular instability. The authors cite previous studies that demonstrate nurse involvement in weaning can improve patient care and reduce weaning times. They note that, while in many countries nurses have a high level of autonomy and decision making and may also work collaboratively with medical colleagues on the decision to extubate, there are variations internationally in the nature and processes of nurse involvement. They draw attention, in particular, to the USA where ventilation management is the role of respiratory therapists.

The authors used the Critical Appraisal Skills Programme (CASP) criteria for qualitative research appraisal, a useful tool for considering methodological rigour, particularly in non-traditional qualitative methodologies. The aim and significance of this study were clearly stated: to explore and describe the involvement of nurses in decisions relating to weaning from mechanical ventilation in Ireland. The rationale was the lack of previous research on this topic in the Irish context and it was inferred that previous work in the UK using a similar approach was limited by its small sample of seven nurses.

The chosen method was a qualitative design that employed use of a patient case vignette. This approach was selected because it can provide insight into how participants might behave in a situation that could be difficult to observe in real life and so reduced the need for lengthy interviews or questionnaires. A three-step model to enhance the internal validity was utilised. This included grounding the vignette on the literature from case histories and weaning from mechanical ventilation, review and modification of the vignette by an expert panel made up of senior medical and nurse clinicians and pilot testing of the vignette with intensive care nurses.

The research setting, including the number of beds, typical APACHE 11 score and typical duration of ventilation, was explained. The study was undertaken in a single setting. This reduces the transferability of the findings as it is difficult to determine which findings might be attributed to the essential experiences of nurses working in critical care units in Ireland and which are determined by the local workplace culture. Qualitative research frequently uses purposive sampling that seeks the participants who can best illuminate the study question, rather than using probability methods more often seen in positivist studies. These researchers have employed a more objective approach to sampling; 57 possible participants were stratified into three levels of years of experience, and participants were randomly chosen by a person who was not involved in the research drawing names from a hat. This method may have been appropriately chosen to reduce the potential selection bias as at least one of the researchers knew and worked with the participants. The relationship with participants was not discussed in detail other than to say one of the researchers was a colleague of the participants and not working in a managerial role. It was not clear how this relationship was managed to reduce coercion or reduce the influence on the answers given by participants. The stratification of participants according to level of experience strengthened the research design and responses were examined for relationship to the years of experience.

Twenty-five nurses were subsequently invited to participate in the research and all agreed. The authors note that one participant had to withdraw for health reasons. They report the number of participants that were female, their level of experience in other intensive care units and experience with weaning but do not comment on how these sample characteristics compare with critical care nurses generally. Addressing this could help to inform the transferability of the results.

The authors did not examine their own role in the research setting and the potential for bias or influence. There was no reflexive statement about their personal motivations or opinions on the phenomenon under study. There was no statement as to how previous working relationships might influence or be subsequently altered by the study.

The 24 semi-structured interviews were audiotaped and transcribed verbatim. The analytical method of Burnard's content analysis was described in detail and seemed appropriate to the study question and aims. To increase the external validity, an independent expert nurse was brought in to independently recode the data to check for similarities in theme choice. Member checking is sometimes used by qualitative researchers to allow participants the opportunity to challenge the researcher's perceptions or to confirm the accuracy of their preliminary results. Although member checking is often viewed critically by interpretative qualitative researchers because of the nature of interpretative analysis that co-creates meaning between researcher and participant, in descriptive methods such as content analysis it is viewed as an important component of rigour. Member checking was used in this study, with three of the participants asked to identify main points from their own transcribed interviews with the intention of comparing these to the eventual themes and categories from the research analysis. Beyond noting that, due to the complexity of vignette and the weaning process, there were no right or wrong answers in this member checking, it was not made clear how the process influenced the researchers' final analysis or decision making.

While a solid number of participants had been recruited and the sample appeared reasonably homogeneous, the issue of data saturation was not discussed. It was therefore unclear how well developed these reported themes were within the participant interviews. This can sometimes be addressed by noting how many of the participants experienced this theme under discussion or how many participants were required to experience the main themes before interviewing would be stopped.

The results are important as they highlight the way nurses synthesise their respiratory assessment findings into a general clinical picture. They note the importance of an assessment of oxygenation and oxygen requirements to the nurses' understanding of readiness for weaning. Key aspects of continuous reassessment were ABGs, markers of respiratory distress, changes in cardiovascular status and 'the patient'. These were incorporated into decision making and were mediated by the nurses' experience and confidence. Findings are discussed and confirmed in relation to contemporary literature. The value of the research is that it suggests weaning protocols are useful for junior nurses, whereas senior nurses are more likely to use a more complex synthesis of respiratory assessment and clinical judgement to inform their weaning decisions. In conclusion, this is a well-conducted qualitative study that used the novel approach of a patient vignette to describe the factors that influence critical care nurses when deciding to wean patients from mechanical ventilation. International readers should consider their local ICU culture and the level of training and autonomy of their ICU nurses in relation to ventilation decisions when considering the transferability of these findings.

Learning activities

1 Describe what coarse crackles and wheezes sound like and the pathophysiological mechanisms that may lead to reduced air entry when these abnormal sounds are heard.

2 Outline the correct sampling technique for drawing an ABG from an arterial line.

3 Define Type 1 and Type 2 respiratory failure.

Online resources

Acidbase.org, www.acidbase.org

American Association for Respiratory Care, www.aarc.org

ARDS Network, www.ardsnet.org

Asian Pacific Society of Respirology, www.apsresp.org

Australian & New Zealand Society of Respiratory Science, www.anzsrs.org.au

Australian Lung Foundation, www.lungnet.org.au

Basic Lung Sounds Tutorial, http://solutions.3m.com/wps/portal/3M/en_EU/3M-Littmann-EMEA/stethoscope/littmann-learning-institute/heart-lung-sounds/lung-sounds/#rhonchi-low-pitched

Become an expert in spirometry, www.spirxpert.com

Capnography: a comprehensive educational website, www.capnography.com

Chest X-rays, www.learningradiology.com

Critical Care Medicine Tutorials, www.ccmtutorials.com

European Respiratory Journal, erj.ersjournals.com

Lung Health Promotion Centre, The Alfred Hospital, Victoria, www.lunghealth.org

Respiratory Care online, www.rcjournal.com

Respiratory Research, http://respiratory-research.com

Thoracic Society of Australia and New Zealand, www.thoracic.org.au

Thorax: An International Journal of Respiratory Medicine, http://thorax.bmj.com

World Health Organization, www.who.int/en

Further reading

Abdo WF, Heunks LMA. Oxygen-induced hypercapnia in COPD: myths and facts. Crit Care 2012:16:323.

Dempsey JA, Smith CA. Pathophysiology of human ventilator control. Eur Respir J 2014;44:495–512.

Higginson R, Jones B. Respiratory assessment in critically ill patients: airway and breathing. Br J of Nurs 2009;18(8):458–61.

Jacono FJ. Control of ventilation in COPD and lung injury. Respir Physiol Neurobiol 2013;189:371–6.

Robinson TD, Freiberg DB, Regnis JA, Young IH. The role of hypoventilation and ventilation–perfusion redistribution in oxygen-induced hypercapnia during acute exacerbations of chronic obstructive pulmonary disease. Am J Resp Crit Care Med 2000;161:1524–9.

Siela D. Chest radiograph evaluation and interpretation. AACN Adv Crit Care 2008;19(4):444–73.

Spiegel J. End-tidal carbon dioxide: the most vital of vital signs. Anesthesiology News, October 2013, <http://www.anesthesiologynews.com/download/Capnography_ANSE13_WM.pdf>; [accessed 30.07.14].

UK Resuscitation Council. Arterial blood gas analysis workshop, <http://www.resus.org. uk/pages/alsabgGd.pdf2012>; [accessed 30.07.14].

Valdez-Lowe C, Ghareeb SA, Artinian NT. Pulse oximetry in adults. Am J Nurs 2009;109(6):52–9.

Van Gestel AJR, Steier J. Autonomic dysfunction in patients with chronic obstructive pulmonary disease (COPD). J Thorac Dis 2010;2:215–22.

References

1 Wunsch H, Angus D, Harrison D, Linde-Zwirble W, Rowan K. Comparison of medical admissions to intensive care units in the United States and United Kingdom. Am J Respir Crit Care 2011;183:1666–73.

2 Hillman K, Bristow PJ C, Daffurn K, Jacques T, Norman S, Bishop G et al. Duration of life-threatening antecedents prior to intensive care admission. Intensive Care Med 2002;28:1629–34.

3 Urden LD, Stacy KM, Lough ME. Critical care nursing: Diagnosis and management. 7th ed. St Louis: Mosby; 2013.

4 Urden L, Stacy K, Lough M. Critical care nursing: Diagnosis and management. 6th ed. St Louis: Mosby; 2010.

5 Martini FH, Timmons MJ, Tallitsch RB. Human anatomy, International edition. 5th ed. San Francisco: Pearson Benjamin Cummings; 2006.

6 Fox S. Human physiology. 13th ed. New York: McGraw Hill; 2012.

7 Marieb E, Hoehn K. Human anatomy and physiology. 4th ed. San Francisco: Pearson Benjamin Cummings; 2010.

8 Shier D, Butler J, Lewis R. Hole's human anatomy and physiology. 13th International ed. New York: McGraw Hill; 2013.

9 Tadie JM, Behm E, Lecuyer L, Benhmamed R, Hans S, Brasnu D et al. Post-intubation laryngeal injuries and extubation failure: a fiberoptic endoscopic study. Intensive Care Med 2010;36(6):991-8.

10 Thompson J, McFarland G, Hirsch J, Tucker S. Mosby's clinical nursing. 5th ed. St Louis: Mosby; 2002.

11 West J. Pulmonary physiology: the essentials. 8th ed. Philadelphia: Lippincott Williams & Wilkins; 2012.

12 Martini F, Nath J. Fundamentals of anatomy and physiology. 9th ed. San Francisco: Pearson Benjamin Cummins; 2011.

13 Widmaier E, Raff H, Strang K. Vander's human physiology 10th ed. New York: McGraw-Hill International edition; 2006.

14 Enhorning G. Surfactant in airway disease. Chest 2008;133(4):975-80.

15 West J. Respiratory physiology: the essentials. 8th ed. Philadelphia: Lippincott, Williams & Wilkins; 2008.

16 Brashers V. Structure and function of the pulmonary system. Pathophysiology: the biologic basis for disease in adults and children. 6th ed. St Louis: Mosby; 2009.

17 Jacono F. Control of ventilation in COPD and lung injury. Respir Physiol Neurobiol 2013;189:371-6.

18 Abdo W, Heunks L. Oxygen-induced hypercapnia in COPD: myths and facts. Critical Care 2012;16:323.

19 Austin M, Willis K, Blizzard L, Walters E, Wood-Baker R. Effect of high flow oxygen on mortality in chronic obstructive pulmonary disease patients in prehospital setting: randomised controlled trial. BMJ 2010;341:c5462.

20 O'Driscoll B, Howard L, Davidson A. BTS guideline for emergency oxygen use in adult patients. Thorax 2008;63(Suppl 6):vi1-68.

21 Ayas N, Zankynthinos SR, Pare P. Respiratory system mechanics and energetics. In: Mason R, Broaddus C, Martin TR, King TE, Schaufnadel DE, eds. Murray and Nadel's textbook of respiratory medicine [Internet]. 5th ed. Philadelphia: Elsevier Saunders; 2010.

22 Guton A, Hall J. Gyton and Hall's textbook of medical physiology. 12th ed. Philadelphia: Elseveir Saunders; 2011.

23 Morton P, Rempher K. Patient assessment: respiratory system. In: Morton PG, Fontaine DK, eds. Essentials of critical care nursing: A holistic approach. [Internet]. 10th ed. Philadelphia: Wolters Kluwer/Lippincott Williams & Wilkins; 2013.

24 Lynne M, Johnson K. Anatomy and physiology of the respiratory system. In: Morton PG, Fontaine DK, eds. Essentials of critical care nursing: An holistic approach [Internet]. 9th ed. Philadelphia: Wolters Kluwer / Lippincott Williams & Wilkins; 2010.

25 Seely R, Stephens T, Tate P. Anatomy and physiology. 7th ed. Boston: McGraw Hill; 2006.

26 Urden LD, Stacey K, Lough ME. Thelan's critical care nursing: Diagnosis and management. St Louis: Mosby Elsevier; 2006.

27 Luks A, Schoene R, Swenson E. High altitude. In: Mason R, Broaddus C, Martin TR, King TE, Schaufnadel DE, eds. Murray and Nadel's textbook of respiratory medicine [Internet]. 5th ed. Philadelphia: Elsevier Saunders; 2010.

28 Oliveira R, Trece M, Chagas N, Teles J. Epidemiology and clinical characterization of patients with acute respiratory failure admitted to a general ICU. Crit Care 2009;13(Suppl 3):42.

29 Hill N, Schmidt G. Acute ventilatory failure. In: Mason R, Broaddus C, Martin T, King T, Schraufnagel D, eds. Murray and Nadel's textbook of respiratory medicine. 5th ed. Philadelphia: Saunders Elsevier; 2010.

30 Baumgartner L. Acute respiratory faliure and acute lung injury. In: Carlson K, ed. Advanced critical care nursing. St Louis: Saunders Elsevier; 2009.

31 West J. Pulmonary physiology and pathophysiology: An integrated, case-based approach. 2nd ed. Baltimore: Lippincott Williams & Wilkins; 2007.

32 Sakka S. Extravascular lung water in ARDS patients. Minerva Anestesiologica 2013;79(3):274-84.

33 Matthay M, Martin T. Pulmonary edema and acute lung injury. In: Mason R, Broaddus C, Martin TR, King TE, Schaufnadel DE, eds. Murray and Nadel's textbook of respiratory medicine [Internet]. 5th ed. Philadelphia: Saunders Elsevier; 2010.

34 Schraufnagel D, Murray J. History and physical examinations. In: Mason R, Broaddus C, Martin T, King T, Schraunadel D, eds. Murray and Nadel's textbook of respiratory medicine. 5th ed. Philadelphia: Saunders Elsevier; 2010.

35 Shapiro S, Reilly J, Rennard S. Chronic bronchitis and emphysema. In: Mason R, Broaddus C, Martin T, King T, Schraufnagel D, eds. Murray and Nadel's textbook of respiratory medicine. 5th ed. Philadelphia: Saunders Elsevier; 2010.

36 Wu CF, Feng NH, Chong IW, Wu KY, Lee CH, Hwang JJ et al. Second-hand smoke and chronic bronchitis in Taiwanese women: a health-care based study. BMC Public Health 2010;10:44.

37 Jauréguiberry S, Boutolleau D, Grandsire E, Kofman T, Deback C, Aït-Arkoub Z et al. Clinical and microbiological evaluation of travel-associated respiratory tract infections in travelers returning from countries affected by pandemic A(H1N1) 2009 influenza. J Travel Med 2012;19(1):22-7.

38 Cannegieter SC. Travel-related thrombosis. Best Pract Res Clin Haematol 2012;25(3):345-50.

39 Rushton L. Occupational causes of chronic obstructive pulmonary disease. Rev Environ Health 2007;22(3):195-212.

40 Weber J, Kelly J. Health assessment in nursing. Philadelphia: Lippincott, Williams & Wilkins; 2010.

41 Light R, Lee G. Pneumothorax, chylothorax, hemothorax, and fibrothorax. In: Mason R, Broaddus C, Martin T, King T, Schraufnagel D, eds. Murray and Nadel's textbook of respiratory medicine. 5th ed. Philadelphia: Saunders Elsevier; 2010.

42 Park DVE. Pneumomediastinum and mediastinitis. In: Mason R, Broaddus C, Martin T, King T, Schraufnagel D, eds. Murray and Nadel's textbook of respiratory medicine. 5th ed. Philadelphia: Saunders Elsevier; 2010.

43 Hunter J, Rawlings-Anderson K. Respiratory assessment. Nurs Stand 2008;22(41):41-3.

44 McGhee S. Evidence-based physical diagnosis. 3rd ed. Philadelphia: Elsevier Saunders; 2012.

45 Moore T. Respiratory assessment in adults. Nurs Stand 2007;21(49):48-56; quiz 8.

46 Fouzas S, Priftis K, Anthracopoulos M. Pulse oximetry in pediatric practice. Pediatrics 2011;128(4):740-52.

47 Clark AP, Giuliano K, Chen HM. Pulse oximetry revisited: "but his O(2) sat was normal!". Clin Nurse Spec 2006;20(6):268-72.

48 Callahan JM. Pulse oximetry in emergency medicine. Emerg Med Clin North Am 2008;26(4):869-79, vii.

49 Valdez-Lowe C, Ghareeb SA, Artinian NT. Pulse oximetry in adults. Am J Nurs 2009;109(6):52-9; quiz 60.

50 Mannheimer P. The light-tissue interaction of pulse oxymetry. Anesth Analg 2007;105:S10-7.

51 World Health Organization. Pulse oximetry training manual 2011, <http://www.who.int/patientsafety/safesurgery/pulse_oximetry/who_ps_pulse_oxymetry_training_manual_en.pdf>.

52 Zwerneman K. End-tidal carbon dioxide monitoring: a VITAL sign worth watching. Crit Care Nurs Clin North Am 2006;18(2):217-25, xi.

53 Joint Faculty of Intensive Care Medicine. Minimum standards for transport of critically ill patients. Melbourne: Joint Faculty of Intensive Care Medicine; 2010.

54 Australian and New Zealand College of Anaesthetists. Monitoring during anaesthesia. Review PS18. Melbourne: Australian and New Zealand College of Anaesthetists; 2008.

55 Joint Faculty of Intensive Care Medicine. Minimum standards for intensive care units. Review IC-1. Melbourne: Joint Faculty of Intensive Care Medicine; 2010.

56 Umegaki T, Kikuchi O, Hirota K, Adachi T. Comparison of continuous intraarterial blood gas analysis and transcutaneous monitoring to measure oxygen partial pressure during one-lung ventilation. J Anesth 2007;21(1):110-1.

57 Gelsomino LR, Livi U, Romagnoli S, Romano S, Carella R, Luca F et al. Assessment of a continuous blood gas monitoring system in animals during circulatory stress. BMC Anesthesiol 2011;11(1), <http://www.biomedcentral.com/1471-2253/11/1>.

58 World Health Organization. WHO guidelines on drawing blood: Best practices in phlebotomy. Geneva: WHO; 2010.

59 Rickard CM, Couchman BA, Schmidt SJ, Dank A, Purdie DM. A discard volume of twice the deadspace ensures clinically accurate arterial blood gases and electrolytes and prevents unnecessary blood loss. Crit Care Med 2003;31(6):1654-8.

60 Siemens. Arterial blood gas analysis: Preanalytical concerns. Siemens Healthcare Diagnostics Inc; 2011. Available from, <http://www.siemens.com/diagnostics>.

61 Martin D. Oxygen therapy in critical illness. Crit Care Med 2013;41(2):423-32.

62 Rogers K, McCutcheon K. Understanding arterial blood gases. J Perioper Pract 2013;23(9):191-7.

63 Morgan TJ. Acid-base balance and disorders. In: Bersten AD, Soni N, eds. Oh's intensive care manual. 6th ed. Philadelphia: Butterworth Heinemann; 2009, pp 949-61.

64 Coggon JM. Arterial blood gas analysis 1: understanding ABG reports. Nurs Times 2008;104(18):28-9.

65 Coggon JM. Arterial blood gas analysis 2: compensatory mechanisms. Nurs Times 2008;104(19):24-5.

66 Stewart P. How to understand acid-base. In: Stewart PA, ed. A quantitative acid-base primer for biology and medicine. New York: Elsevier; 1981.

67 Morgan T. The Stewart approach – one clinician's perspective. Clin Biochem Rev 2009;30(2):41-54.

68 Ahmed SM, Maheshwari P, Agarwal S, Nadeem A, Singh L. Evaluation of the efficacy of simplified Fencl-Stewart equation in analyzing the changes in acid base status following resuscitation with two different fluids. Int J Crit Illn Inj Sci 2013;3(3):206-10.

69 Elbers P, Gatz R. Acidbase.org: Bringing Stewart to the bedside. Amsterdam: VU University Medical Centre; N.D., <http://www.acidbase.org/>; [accessed 23.07.14].

70 Doorduin J, Haans A, van der Hoeven J, Heunks L. Difficult weaning: principles and practice of a structured diagnostic approach. Netherlands J Crit Care 2013;17(4):11-15.

71 Maiden J. Pulmonary diagnostic procedures. In: Urden L, Stacy K, Lough M, eds. Critical care nursing: Diagnosis and management. 7th ed. St Louis: Mosby; 2014, pp 505-13.

72 The ARDS Definition Taskforce. Acute respiratory distress syndrome: the Berlin definition. JAMA 2012;307(23):2526-33.

73 American Association of Respiratory Care. AARC clinical practice guideline: transcutaneous monitoring of carbon dioxide and oxygen: 2012. National Guideline Clearinghouse: Agency for Healthcare Research and Quality; 2012.

74 Jubran A, Tobin M. Non-invasive respiratory monitoring. In: Parillo J, Dellinger R, eds. Critical care medicine: Principles of diagnosis and management in the adult. 4th ed. Philadelphia: Elsevier; 2014, pp 190-201.

75 Restrepo R, Hirst K, Wittnebel R. AARC clinical practice guideline: transcutaneous monitoring of carbon dioxide and oxygen: 2012. Respir Care 2012;57(11):1955-62.

76 The Royal College of Pathologists of Australia. RCPA manual. 6th ed. Sydney: The Royal College of Pathologists of Australia, <http://rcpamanual.edu.au/index.php?option=com_pttests&task=show_test&id=268&Itemid=77&msg=425>; 2009 [accessed 16.07.10].

77 The Joanna Briggs Institute. Evidence based recommended practices: Sputum specimen. Adelaide: The Joanna Briggs Institute; 2010.

78 Wai Y, Joliffe D, Islam K, Greiller C, Martineau A. Safety and efficacy of sputum induction in COPD patients. Eur Respir J 2013;42(Suppl 57):1381.

79 McCool FD, Rosen MJ. Nonpharmacologic airway clearance therapies: ACCP evidence-based clinical practice guidelines. Chest 2006; 129(1 Suppl):250S-9S.

80 Paulus F, Binnekade J, Vroom M, Schultz M. Benefits and risks of manual hyperinflation in intubated and mechanically ventilated intensive care unit patients: a systematic review. Crit Care [Internet]. 2014;16:[R145 p.], <http://www.biomedcentral.com/content/pdf/cc11457.pdf>.

81 Waqas M, Malik A, Javed M. Effectiveness of conventional chest physiotherapy versus manual hyperinflation during postural drainage of ventilated COPD patients. RMJ 2014;39(1):32-4.

82 Pedersen CM, Rosendahl-Nielsen M, Hjermind J, Egerod I. Endotracheal suctioning of the adult intubated patient – what is the evidence? Intensive Crit Care Nurs 2009;25(1):21-30.

83 World Health Organization. WHO guidelines for the collection of human specimens for laboratory diagnosis of avian influenza infection, <http://www.who.int/csr/disease/avian_influenza/guidelines/humanspecimens/en/>; 2005 [accessed 18.07.10].

84 Lareau C, Wootton J. The "frequently" normal chest x-ray. Can J Rural Med 2004;9(3):183-6.

85 Siela D. Chest radiograph evaluation and interpretation. AACN Adv Crit Care 2008;19(4):444-73; quiz 74-5.

86 Raoof S, Feigin D, Sung A, Raoof S, Irugulpati L, Rosenow E. Interpretation of plain chest roentgenogram. Chest 2012;141(2):545-58.

87 Tarrac SE. A systematic approach to chest x-ray interpretation in the perianesthesia unit. J Perianesth Nurs 2009;24(1):41-7; quiz 7-9.

88 Padley SPG. Imaging the chest. In: Bersten AD, Soni N, eds. Oh's intensive care manual. 6th ed. Philadelphia: Butterworth Heinemann; 2009, pp 451-70.

89 Chen HJ, Yu YH, Tu CY, Chen CH, Hsia TC, Tsai KD et al. Ultrasound in peripheral pulmonary air-fluid lesions. Color Doppler imaging as an aid in differentiating empyema and abscess. Chest 2009;135(6):1426-32.

90 Havelock TR, Laws D, Gleeson F. Pleural procedures and thoracic ultrasound: British Thoracic Society pleural disease guideline 2010. Thorax 2010;65(Suppl 2):ii61-ii76.

91 Revell MA, Pugh M, Smith TL, McInnis LA. Radiographic studies in the critical care environment. Crit Care Nurs Clin North Am 2010;22(1):41-50.

92 Hill JR, Horner PE, Primack SL. ICU imaging. Clin Chest Med 2008;29(1):59-76, vi.

93 Davies AR, Pilcher DV. Pulmonary embolism. In: Bersten AD, Soni N, eds. Oh's intensive care manual. 6th ed. Philadelphia: Butterworth Heinemann; 2009, pp 387-98.

94 Rumbolt Z, Huda W, All J. Review of portable CT with assessment of a dedicated head CT scanner. Am J Neuroradiol 2009;30:1630-6.

95 Levine G, Gomes A, Arai A, Bluemke D, Flamm S, Kanal E et al. Safety of magnetic resonance imaging in patients with cardiovascular devices: an American Heart Association scientific statement from the Committee on Diagnostic and Interventional Cardiac Catheterization. Circulation 2007;116(24):2878-91.

96 Rogiuin A, Schwitter J, Vahlhaus C, Lombardi M, Brugada J, Vardas P et al. Magnetic resonance imaging in individuals with cardiovascular implantable electronic devices. Europace 2008;10:336-46.

97 Beinart R, Nazarian S. Magnetic resonance imaging in patients with ICDs and pacemakers. Cardiac Rhythm Management [Internet]. August 2014, <http://crm.cardiosource.org/Learn-from-the-Experts/2012/10/MRI-in-Patients-with-ICDs-and-Pacemakers.aspx>.

98 Arbelo E, Brugada J. Cardiac rhythm management devices: when regulatory agencies "over-regulate". J Am CollCardiol 2014;63(17):1776-7.

99 Shellock F. MRI guidelines for InterStim therapy neurostimulation systems. MRIsafetycom [Internet]. July 2014, <http://www.mrisafety.com/SafetyInfov.asp?SafetyInfoID=236>.

100 Brain Aneurysm Foundation. Understanding: Treatment options. [Internet], <http://www.bafound.org/ treatment-options>; [accessed 08.03.15].

101 American College of Radiology and the Radiological Society of North America. Magnetic resonance imaging (MRI). RadiologyInfoorg [Internet], <http://www.radiologyinfo.org/en/safety/index.cfm?pg=sfty_mr>; 2013 [accessed August 2014].

102 Everest E, Munford B. Transport of the critically ill. In: Bersten AD, Soni N, eds. Oh's intensive care manual. 6th ed. Philadelphia: Butterworth Heinemann; 2009, pp 31-42.

103 Dugdale D. Pulmonary ventilation/perfusion scan. Medline Plus [Internet]. 2012, <http://www.nlm.nih.gov/medlineplus/ency/article/003828.htm>.

104 Estella A. Bronchoscopy in mechanically ventilated patients. 2012. In: Global Perspectives on Bronchoscopy [Internet]. Rijeka: InTech, <http://cdn.intechopen.com/pdfs-wm/37333.pdf>; [accessed August 014].

105 Taylor DL. Bronchoscopy: what critical care nurses need to know. Crit Care Nurs Clin North Am 2010;22(1):33-40.

106 Nseir S. Could fiberoptic bronchoscopy and CT lung scan differentiate ventilator-associated tracheobronchitis from ventilator-associated pneumonia? Chest 2009;136(4):1187–8.

107 Turner JS, Willcox PA, Hayhurst MD, Potgieter PD. Fiberoptic bronchoscopy in the intensive care unit – a prospective study of 147 procedures in 107 patients. Crit Care Med 1994;22(2):259-64.

108 Murgu SD, Pecson J, Colt HG. Bronchoscopy during noninvasive ventilation: indications and technique. Respir Care 2010;55(5):595-600.

109 Kaw R, Bae C, Jaber W. Challenges in pulmonary risk assessment and perioperative management in bariatric surgery patients. Obesity Surg 2008;18:134-38.

110 Schachter L. Respiratory assessment and management in bariatric surgery. Respirology 2012;17(7):1039-47.

111 Quizlet. Health assessment. Chapter 18, NUR314. Quizlet LLC, <http://quizlet.com/10775005/ch-18-nur-314-health-assessment-flash-cards/>; 2014 [accessed 30.07.14].

112 Shank Coviello J. Absent and diminished breath sounds. Auscultation skills: Breath and heart sounds. 5th ed. Philadelphia: Wolters Kluwer/Lippincott Williams & Wilkins; 2014, pp 174.

Chapter 14

Respiratory alterations and management

Sharon Wetzig, Bronagh Blackwood, Judy Currey

Learning objectives

After reading this chapter, you should be able to:

- describe the pathophysiological mechanisms of acute respiratory failure and key principles of patient management
- differentiate between failure to oxygenate (hypoxaemic/type I) and failure to ventilate (hypercapnoeic/type II) respiratory failure
- outline the incidence of respiratory alterations in the critical care context
- discuss the aetiology, pathophysiology, clinical manifestations and management of common respiratory disorders managed in intensive care, specifically pneumonia, pandemic respiratory infections, asthma, chronic obstructive pulmonary disease, acute lung injury, pneumothorax and pulmonary embolism
- describe the evidence base for key components of nursing and collaborative practice involved in the management of patients with acute respiratory failure in the intensive care unit
- outline the principles and immediate postoperative management for lung transplant recipients.

Introduction

The most common reason why patients require admission to an intensive care unit (ICU) is for support of the respiratory system. Use of mechanical ventilation is high with almost half of all patients admitted to ICU requiring this level of support.[1] Failure or inadequate function of the respiratory system occurs as a result of direct or indirect pathophysiological conditions. The process of mechanical ventilation may also injure a patient's lungs, further impacting functioning of the respiratory system. Preventing or minimising ventilator-associated lung injury is therefore also a primary goal of patient care.

In chapter 13 the relevant assessment and monitoring practices for a patient with life-threatening respiratory dysfunction were described. In this chapter the incidence, pathophysiology, clinical manifestations and management of common respiratory disorders that result in acute respiratory failure are described. Specific conditions such as pneumonia, pandemic respiratory infections, asthma, chronic obstructive pulmonary disease (COPD), acute lung injury (ALI), pneumothorax and lung transplantation are discussed. Respiratory support strategies including oxygenation and ventilation to support respiratory function during a critical illness are presented in Chapter 15.

Incidence of respiratory alterations

Respiratory diseases are common and affect significant numbers of people. They are among the leading causes of death worldwide. Lung infections (primarily pneumonia and tuberculosis), lung cancer and COPD together accounted for 17% of global deaths in 2008. These diseases also accounted for one-tenth of the disability-adjusted life years lost worldwide in the same year.[2] Respiratory diseases are also the most common illnesses responsible for emergency admissions to hospital and visits to general practitioners and represent the most frequently reported long-term illnesses in children.[3]

Infective processes, such as influenza and pneumonia, COPD and asthma represent the three largest groups of presentations requiring hospital admission. Conditions such as ALI, pneumothorax, pulmonary embolus and pulmonary oedema are relatively small groups. It should be noted, however, that these conditions often evolve throughout the course of an illness and may not, therefore, be included as the reason for admission.[3] Common respiratory alterations managed in ICU are discussed in the following sections.

Respiratory failure

Respiratory failure occurs when there is a reduction in the body's ability to maintain either oxygenation or ventilation, or both. It may occur acutely, as observed in pneumonia and ALI, or it may persist in chronic form, as observed in asthma and COPD.

Aetiology of respiratory failure

For the respiratory system to function effectively, the rate and depth of breathing has to be controlled appropriately by the brain, the chest wall must expand adequately, air needs to flow easily through the airways and effective exchange of gases needs to occur at the alveolar level. Conditions that impact on one or more aspects of normal physiological functioning of the respiratory system can cause respiratory failure, for example:

- decreased respiratory drive may be caused by brain trauma, drug overdose or anaesthesia/sedation
- decreased respiratory muscle strength may be caused by Guillain-Barré syndrome, poliomyelitis, myasthenia gravis or spinal cord injury
- decreased chest wall expansion may be caused by postoperative pain, rib fractures or a pneumothorax
- increased airway resistance may be caused by asthma or COPD
- increased metabolic oxygen requirements may be caused by severe sepsis
- decreased capacity for gas exchange may be caused by impairment in either ventilation (e.g. pulmonary oedema, pneumonia, ALI, COPD) or pulmonary perfusion (e.g. pulmonary embolism), or a combination of the two.

Importantly, respiratory failure can be an acute or chronic condition. Whereas acute respiratory failure is characterised by life-threatening alterations in function, the manifestations of chronic respiratory failure are more subtle and potentially more difficult to diagnose. Patients with chronic respiratory failure often experience acute exacerbations of their disease, also resulting in the need for intensive respiratory support.[3]

Pathophysiology

Respiratory failure occurs when the respiratory system fails to achieve one or both of its essential gas exchange functions – oxygenation or elimination of carbon dioxide – and can be described as either type I, which is primarily a failure of oxygenation, or type II, which is primarily a failure of ventilation.[3]

Type I respiratory failure – failure to oxygenate

A patient with type I or 'hypoxaemic' respiratory failure presents with a low partial pressure of oxygen (PaO_2) and a normal or low partial pressure of carbon dioxide ($PaCO_2$). Hypoxaemic respiratory failure may be caused by a reduction in inspired oxygen pressure as might occur at extreme altitude, hypoventilation, impaired diffusion or ventilation–perfusion mismatch. Most major respiratory alterations cause type I respiratory failure, usually as a result of hypoventilation due to alveolar collapse or consolidation, or a perfusion abnormality.

When there is mismatch between ventilation and perfusion in the lungs, exchange of gases is impaired and hypoxaemia ensues (see Figure 14.1).[3]

In some cases, there may be reduced ventilation to a certain area of lung tissue (e.g. pulmonary oedema, pneumonia, atelectasis, ALI). A severe form of mismatch known as intrapulmonary shunting occurs when adequate perfusion exists but there are sections of lung tissue that are not ventilated. In these alveoli, the oxygen content is similar to that of the mixed venous blood and the carbon dioxide is elevated. In other instances, ventilation may be adequate but perfusion is impaired (e.g. pulmonary embolus). In its severe form, this is known as dead space ventilation as the lungs continue to be ventilated but there is limited or no perfusion, and therefore no gas exchange. In this situation, the alveolar oxygen content is similar to that of the inspired gas mixture and the carbon dioxide is minimal (see Chapter 13 for further discussion).

Type II respiratory failure – failure to ventilate

A patient with type II respiratory or 'hypercapnoeic/hypoxaemic' failure presents with a high $PaCO_2$ as well as a low PaO_2. This failure is caused by alveolar hypoventilation, where the respiratory effort or minute ventilation is insufficient to allow adequate exchange of oxygen and carbon dioxide. This may be caused by conditions that affect respiratory drive such as neuromuscular diseases, chest wall abnormalities or severe airways disease (e.g. asthma or COPD).

FIGURE 14.1 Ventilation–perfusion mismatches.[3] Ventilation-perfusion (V/Q) ratio displays the normal balance (*star*) between alveolar ventilation and vascular perfusion allowing for proper oxygenation. When ventilation is reduced, the V/Q ratio decreases, in the most extreme case resulting in pure shunt, where V/Q = 0. When perfusion is reduced, the V/Q ratio increases, in the most extreme case resulting in pure dead space, where V/Q = infinite (∞).

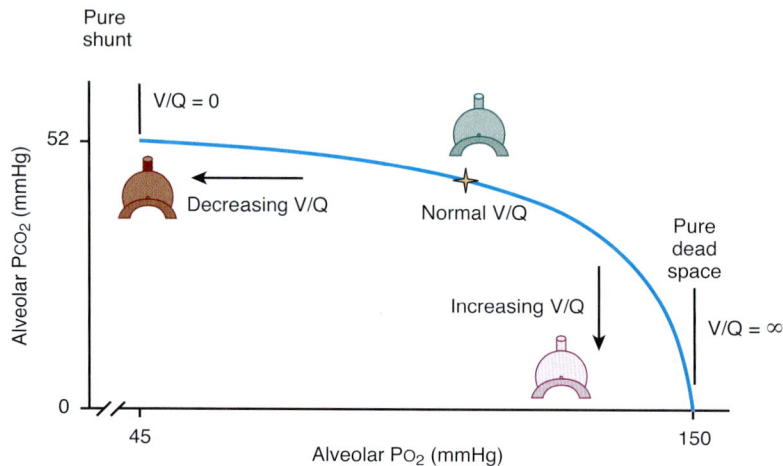

Adapted, with permission, from Mason R, Broaddus V, Martin T, King T, Schraufnagel D, Murray J, Nadel J, eds. Murray and Nadel's textbook of respiratory medicine. 5th ed. Philadelphia: Saunders; 2010.

Clinical manifestations

Patient presentations in acute respiratory failure can be quite diverse and are dependent on the underlying pathophysiological mechanism, the specific aetiology and any comorbidities that may exist.[3] Specific clinical manifestations for the disorders discussed in this chapter are provided in each section. Dyspnoea is the most common symptom associated with acute respiratory failure; this is often accompanied by an increased rate and reduced depth of breathing and the use of accessory muscles. Patients may also present with cyanosis, anxiety, confusion and/or sleepiness.[4]

A systematic approach to clinical assessment and management of patients with acute respiratory failure is crucial, given the large number of possible causes. Clinical investigations to assess the cause of respiratory failure vary depending on the suspected underlying aetiology and the progression of disease. Continuous monitoring of oxygen saturation using pulse oximetry, arterial blood gas (ABG) analysis and analysis of chest X-rays (CXR) are used in almost all cases of respiratory failure. Other more specialised tests such as computed tomography (CT) of the chest and microbiological cultures may be used in specific circumstances.[5] With ABG analysis, the measurement of PaO_2, $PaCO_2$, alveolar–arterial PO_2 difference and patient response to supplemental oxygen are key elements in determining the cause of acute respiratory failure[5] (see Chapter 13).

Patient management

The primary survey (airway, breathing and circulation) and immediate management form initial routine practice.[6] Frequent assessment and monitoring of respiratory function, including a patient's response to supplemental oxygen and/or ventilatory support, is the focus. Patient comfort and compliance with the ventilation mode, ABG analysis and pulse oximetry guide any titration of respiratory support. The key goals of management are to treat the primary cause of respiratory failure, maintain adequate gas exchange and prevent or minimise the potential complications of positive pressure mechanical ventilation.[3]

Comorbidities add to the complexity of managing a patient's primary condition and increase the risk of additional organ dysfunction or failure. Chronic respiratory conditions can have a significant impact on the severity of respiratory infections, while cardiovascular and renal diseases impact on disease severity and the management of many respiratory alterations. Other factors such as smoking and alcohol use, living conditions and lifestyle impact on the predisposition and clinical course of an illness.[2]

Maintaining oxygenation

The therapeutic aim is to titrate the fraction of inspired oxygen (FiO_2) to achieve a PaO_2 of 65–70 mmHg and to maintain minute ventilation to achieve $PaCO_2$ within normal limits where possible.[3] Nursing staff in ICU are commonly responsible for titration of oxygen therapy to maintain a specific PaO_2 or SpO_2 and the alteration of respiratory rate and/or tidal volume to maintain a specified $PaCO_2$. One concern that often arises, particularly with patients who require high concentrations of oxygen, is the risk of oxygen toxicity. The link between prolonged periods of oxygen concentrations approaching 100% and oxidant injuries in airways and lung parenchyma has been established, although mostly from animal research.[3] Although it remains unclear how these data apply to human populations, most consensus groups have argued that FiO_2 values less than 0.4 are safe for prolonged periods of time and that FiO_2 values of greater than 0.8 should be avoided if possible[3] (see Chapter 15 for further detail on assessment and management of oxygenation).

Supporting ventilation

Ventilator-associated lung injury is also a concern when managing patients with acute respiratory failure. A lung can be injured when it is stretched excessively as a result of tidal volume settings that generate high pressures, often referred to as barotrauma or volutrauma. The most common injury is that of alveolar rupture and/or air in the pleural space resulting in a pneumothorax. An approach known as 'lung protective ventilation' aims to minimise over-distension of the alveoli through careful monitoring of tidal volumes and airway pressures. This method should be considered for all ventilated patients. The approach may result in tolerance of higher $PaCO_2$ than normal in patients presenting with acute lung injury[3] (see Chapter 15 for further discussion).

Development of ventilator-associated respiratory muscle weakness has been reported as a significant issue when the respiratory muscles are rendered inactive through adjustment of ventilator settings and administration of pharmacotherapy. While it is not yet possible to provide precise recommendations for interventions to avoid this, clinicians are advised to select ventilator settings that provide for some respiratory muscle use.[7]

Prevention or minimisation of complications associated with positive pressure mechanical ventilation remains a major focus of nursing practice. These complications may relate to the patient–ventilator interface (artificial airway and ventilator circuitry), infectious complications or complications associated with sedation and/or immobility. Some common complications and the appropriate management strategies are briefly outlined in Table 14.1[3,8,9,10] and are discussed further in Chapter 15.

A patient with acute respiratory failure requires extensive multidisciplinary collaboration between nurses,

---

TABLE 14.1

Complications of mechanical ventilation and associated management strategies[3,8,9,10]

PATIENT–VENTILATOR INTERFACE COMPLICATION	MANAGEMENT STRATEGIES
Airway dislodgement/disconnection	Endotracheal tube or tracheostomy tube is secured to optimise ventilation and prevent airway dislodgement or accidental extubation
Circuit leaks	Cuff pressure assessment Circuit checks Exhaled tidal volume measurement
Airway injury from inadequate heat/humidity	Maintain humidification of the airway using either a heat–moisture exchanger or a water-bath humidifier
Obstructions from secretions	Assess the need for suctioning regularly and suction as required
Tracheal injury from the artificial airway	Assessment of airway placement and cuff pressure (minimal occlusion method)
INFECTIOUS COMPLICATION	**MANAGEMENT STRATEGIES**
Ventilator-associated pneumonia (VAP)	Alcohol-based hand hygiene Appropriate antibiotic therapy Oral decontamination Selective digestive decontamination Semi-recumbent positioning, 30–45° Daily sedation holds Peptic ulcer disease prophylaxis Minimising interruptions to ventilator circuit (e.g. closed suctioning technique) Use of oropharyngeal vs nasopharyngeal feeding tubes Drainage of sub-glottic secretions Small bowel feeding rather than gastric feeding Aerosolised antibiotics for patients who are colonised Weaning and discontinuation of ventilatory support as soon as possible, including using nurse-led weaning protocols Early tracheostomy Prophylactic probiotics
COMPLICATION ASSOCIATED WITH IMMOBILITY/SEDATION	**MANAGEMENT STRATEGIES**
Gastrointestinal dysfunction	Prokinetic medication Constipation – bowel therapy regimen
Muscle atrophy	Passive limb movements, foot splints (see Chapter 6) and early activity/mobility (see Chapter 4)
Pressure injuries	Pressure-relieving mattresses, regular repositioning Assessment of risks and management of pressure injuries by wound care specialists, nutrition advice

physiotherapists, specialist medical staff, speech and occupational therapists, dieticians, social workers, radiologists and radiographers, pharmacists and microbiologists. Patients may require intervention to improve capacity for oxygen delivery through an adequate haemoglobin level and a cardiac output sufficient to supply oxygenated blood to the tissues.[3] At times this may require blood transfusion and/or the use of vasoactive medications (see Chapters 11 and 21).

Chest physiotherapy is a routine activity for managing patients with acute respiratory failure. This involves positioning, manual hyperinflation, percussion and vibration and suctioning. The evidence base for these techniques is limited, however, with a systematic review reporting no improvement in mortality for patients with pneumonia.[8] Guidelines for physiotherapy assessment have enabled identification of patient characteristics for treatments to be prescribed and modified on an individual basis. Table 14.2[3,8,11] provides an outline of management interventions for patients with respiratory failure, particularly those who may require prolonged mechanical ventilation.

Medications

Medications commonly prescribed in respiratory failure include inhalation/intravenous steroids and bronchodilators, antibiotic therapy, analgesia and sedation to maintain patient–ventilator synchrony, but may also involve nitric oxide, glucocorticoid or surfactant administration. A patient's condition, comorbidities and the above-mentioned pharmacological therapy may also be supported with inotropic and other resuscitation therapies (see Chapters 11 and 21). As the use of medications will vary depending on the underlying cause of respiratory failure, these are discussed separately in the sections below.

Practice tip

Respiratory failure in pregnancy

Respiratory physiology and the respiratory tract itself are altered during pregnancy; this may result in exacerbation of pre-existing respiratory disease or increased susceptibility to disease (see Chapter 28). Upper airway mucosal oedema may increase the likelihood of upper respiratory tract infection. Lung function and lung volume are also altered, compensated by an increase in respiratory drive and minute ventilation. The impact on the fetus of infection, hypoxia and drug therapy is an important consideration.[3]

Practice tip

Respiratory failure in the elderly

The elderly have ageing organs and systems and other comorbidities that may exacerbate their respiratory dysfunction. Drug metabolism and excretion is slowed, complicating drug dosing and response.[150] Metabolism of anaesthetic agents is slower due to the diminished physiology of ageing organs. Common comorbidities may also be present, including obesity, heart disease, diabetes and renal impairment or muscle wasting.[3]

TABLE 14.2

Long-term patient management in respiratory failure[3,8,11]

MANAGEMENT	BEST PRACTICE
Timing of tracheostomy insertion	Where mechanical ventilation is expected to be 10 days or more, tracheostomy should be performed as soon as identified. Early tracheostomy is associated with less nosocomial pneumonia, reduced ventilation time and shorter ICU stay
Weaning protocols	Specific plan is patient dependent; better outcomes are achieved when there is an agreed and well communicated weaning plan (see Chapter 15)
Nutrition	Consider adequate nutrition for physiological needs – important to not overfeed as this increases CO_2 production – and the need to have a balance of vitamins and minerals
Swallow assessment	Assess for dysphagia
Mobilisation	Sitting out of bed, mobilising (see Chapter 4)
Communication	Communication aids, speaking valves
Activities	Activity plan/routine, entertainment (TV/films), visitors, outings
Sleep	Clustering cares, reducing stimuli to promote sleep (see Chapter 7)
Family support	Importance of providing physical, emotional and/or spiritual support to family members (see Chapter 8)
Tracheostomy follow-up	Outreach team: follow-up care by nurses experienced in tracheostomy care can prevent complications and improve outcomes
End-of-life decisions in acute respiratory failure	See Chapter 5

Pneumonia

Pneumonia is infection of the lung. Depending on the type and severity of the infection and the overall health of the person, it may result in acute respiratory failure. Pneumonia can be caused by most types of microorganisms, but is most commonly a result of bacterial or viral infection. In critical care the key distinctions in assessing and managing a patient with pneumonia relate to the specific aetiology or causative organism. This section reviews the pathophysiology, aetiology, clinical presentation and management of two types of pneumonia:

1 community-acquired pneumonia (CAP)
2 ventilator-associated pneumonia (VAP) and ventilator-associated events (VAE).

As a result of the complexity and ambiguity associated with previous definitions of VAP, there has been a significant shift towards measuring VAE as a way of monitoring ventilator-associated complications more broadly.[12] A VAE is said to have occurred when a decline in respiratory function occurs (defined by a significant increase in FiO_2 or positive end-expiratory pressure [PEEP]) in a ventilated patient after a period of initial stability. Patients who are identified as having had a VAE are then reviewed to determine if clinical signs and symptoms meet the criteria for an infective ventilator-associated complication. Further investigation of microbiological culture results then determines if the definition of VAP applies.[13]

Pathophysiology

The normal human lung is sterile, unlike the gastrointestinal tract and upper respiratory tract, which have resident bacteria. A number of defence mechanisms exist to prevent microorganisms entering the lungs, such as particle filtration in the nostrils, sneezing and coughing to expel irritants and mucus production to trap dust and infectious organisms and move particles out of the respiratory system. Infection occurs when one or more of these defences are not functioning adequately or when an individual encounters a large amount of microorganisms at once and the defences are overwhelmed.[3] An invading pathogen provokes an immune response in the lungs, resulting in the following pathophysiological processes:

* alteration in alveolar capillary permeability that leads to an increase in protein-rich fluid in the alveoli; this impacts on gas exchange and causes the patient to breathe faster in an effort to increase oxygen uptake and remove carbon dioxide
* mucus production increases and mucous plugs may develop that block off areas of the lung, further reducing capacity for gas exchange
* consolidation occurs in the alveoli, which fill with fluid and debris; this occurs particularly with bacterial pneumonia where debris accumulates from the large number of white blood cells involved in the immune response.[3]

Aetiology

Pneumonia is caused by a variety of microorganisms, including bacteria, viruses, fungi and parasites. In many cases, the causative organism may not be known and current practice in many cases is to initiate antimicrobial treatment as soon as possible, based on symptoms and patient history, rather than waiting for microorganism culture results.[14] The true incidence of pneumonia is not well known as many patients do not require hospitalisation. Different ages and characteristics of patients are often associated with different causative organisms. Viral pneumonias, especially influenza, are most common in young children, while adults are more likely to have pneumonia caused by bacteria such as *Streptococcus pneumoniae* and *Haemophilus influenzae*.[3]

> ### Practice tip
>
> **Pneumonia in the elderly**
>
> Pneumonia is a particular concern among elderly adults as they experience an increase in the frequency and severity of pneumonia. This is largely due to the decline in immune system response that is associated with age and with the presence of comorbid disease, such as cardiac and respiratory disease. CAP is a major cause of morbidity and mortality in elderly patients. *Streptococcus pneumoniae* is the most common causative organism, with an increase in drug-resistance being reported more widely in the over-65 age group. Immunisation with pneumococcal and influenza vaccines is beneficial in the prevention of pneumonia in elderly patients.[3]

Community-acquired pneumonia

The International CAP Collaboration Cohort study[15] provides information from a pooled multicentre data set of patients with CAP. This study reports that around 30% of patients with CAP require hospital admission and up to 20% require ICU admission. The causative organism is frequently unidentified.

Clinical assessment, especially patient history, is important in distinguishing the aetiology and likely causative organism in patients with CAP. Specific information regarding exposure to animals, travel history, nursing home residency and any occupational or unusual exposure may provide the key to diagnosis.[14] Personal habits such as smoking and alcohol consumption increase the risk of developing pneumonia and should be explored. Many patients admitted to hospital with CAP have comorbidities, suggesting that those who are chronically ill have an increased risk of developing acute respiratory failure. The most common chronic illnesses involved are respiratory disease, including smoking history, COPD and asthma, congestive cardiac failure and diabetes mellitus. Table 14.3 outlines aspects of the clinical history associated with particular causative organisms in CAP.[3,16,17]

TABLE 14.3

Clinical history/comorbidities associated with particular causative organisms in community-acquired pneumonia[3,16,17]

CONDITION	CAUSATIVE ORGANISMS
INDIVIDUAL FACTORS	
Alcoholism	*S. pneumoniae* (including penicillin-resistant), anaerobes, gram-negative bacilli (possibly *K. pneumoniae*), tuberculosis
Poor dental hygiene	Anaerobes
Elderly	Group B streptococci, *M. catarrhalis*, *H. influenzae*, *L. pneumophila*, gram-negative bacilli, *C. pneumoniae* and polymicrobial infections
Smoking (past or present)	*S. pneumoniae*, *H. influenzae*, *M. catarrhalis*, *Aspergillus* spp.
IV drug use	*S. aureus*, anerobes, *M. tuberculosis*, *S. pneumoniae*
COMORBIDITIES	
COPD	*S. pneumoniae*, *H. influenzae*, *M. catarrhalis*, *Aspergillus* spp.
Post influenza pneumonia	*S. pneumoniae*, *S. aureus*, *H. influenzae*
Structural disease of lung (e.g., bronchiectasis, cystic fibrosis)	*P. aeruginosa*, *P. cepacia* or *S. aureus*
Sickle cell disease, asplenia	Pneumococccus, *H. influenzae*
Previous antibiotic treatment and severe pulmonary comorbidity, (e.g. bronchiectasis, cystic fibrosis, and severe COPD)	*P. aeruginosa*
Malnutrition-related diseases	Gram-negative bacilli
ENVIRONMENTAL EXPOSURE	
Air conditioning	*L. pneumophila*
Residence in nursing home	*S. pneumoniae*, gram-negative bacilli, *H. influenzae*, *S. aureus*, *C. pneumoniae*; consider *M. tuberculosis*; consider anaerobes, but less common
Homeless population	*S. pneumoniae*, *S. aureus*, *H. influenzae*, *C. gattii*: caused by inhalation of spores while sleeping, associated with red gum trees (Australia, Southeast Asia, South America)
Suspected bioterrorism	Anthrax, tularaemia, plague
ANIMAL EXPOSURE	
Bat exposure	*H. capsulatum*
Bird exposure	*C. psittaci*, *C. neoformans*, *H. capsulatum*
Rabbit exposure	*F. tularensis*
Exposure to farm animals or parturient cats	*C. burnetii* (Q fever)
TRAVEL HISTORY	
Travel to southwestern USA	Coccidioidomycosis; hantavirus in selected areas
Travel to southeast Asia	Severe acute respiratory syndrome (coronavirus), *M. tuberculosis*, melioidosis
Residence or travel to rural tropics	Melioidosis (*B. pseudomallei*)
Travel to area of known epidemic	Avian influenza (H5N1), swine influenza (H1N1) and severe acute respiratory syndrome (coronavirus)

COPD = chronic obstructive pulmonary disease; IV = intravenous. *B. pseudomallei* = *Burkholderia pseudomallei*; *C. burnetii* = *Coxiella burnetii*; *C. gattii* = *Cryptococcus gattii*; *C. neoformans* = *Cryptococcus neoformans*; *C. pneumoniae* = *Chlamydophila pneumoniae*; *C. psittaci* = *Chlamydia psittaci*; *F. tularensis* = *Francisella tularensis*; *H. capsulatum* = *Histoplasma capsulatum*; *H. influenzae* = *Haemophilus influenzae*; *K. pneumoniae* = *Klebsiella pneumoniae*; *L. pneumophila* = *Legionella pneumophila*; *M. catarrhalis* = *Moraxella catarrhalis*; *M. tuberculosis* = *Mycobacterium tuberculosis*; *P. aeruginosa* = *Pseudomonas aeruginosa*; *P. cepacia* = *Pseudomonas cepacia*; *S. aureus* = *Staphylococcus aureus*; *S. pneumoniae* = *Streptococcus pneumoniae*.

Diagnosis

Routine screening of patients with suspected pneumonia continues to rely on microscopy and culture of lower respiratory tract specimens, blood cultures, detection of antigens in urine and serology. Methods for detection of antigens are now widely available for several pneumonia pathogens, particularly *S. pneumoniae, Legionella* and some respiratory viruses. Culture of respiratory secretions may be limited due to difficulty in obtaining sputum samples. For this reason, nasopharyngeal aspirates or swabs may be taken as part of the routine screening for CAP.[18]

Severity assessment scoring

International guidelines recommend a severity-based approach to management of CAP, in relation to the initial site of treatment (e.g. home, hospital ward, ICU), and appropriate level of intervention, including antibiotic therapy.[15] Several severity scores have been developed and validated; however, to date there is no agreement on the optimal tool or an agreed definition of the term 'severe pneumonia'.[19] CUR65/CURB65 and the Pneumonia Severity Index are the most widely recommended systems that produce scores and assess severity based on patient demographics, risk factors, comorbidities, clinical presentation and laboratory results. Recent evaluation of these tools found no significant differences in their ability to predict mortality in hospitalised patients.[20]

The Australian CAP Collaboration team devised and validated the SMART-COP scoring system for predicting the need for intensive respiratory or vasopressor support in patients with CAP. The acronym relates to the factors: low **S**ystolic blood pressure, **M**ultilobar involvement, low **A**lbumin level, high **R**espiratory rate, **T**achycardia, **C**onfusion, poor **O**xygenation and low arterial **p**H.[21]

Hospital-acquired and ventilator-associated pneumonia (VAP)

Hospital-acquired pneumonia is defined as pneumonia occurring more than 48 hours after hospital admission.[16] It is the second most common nosocomial infection and the leading cause of death from infection acquired in-hospital. VAP is a form of hospital-acquired pneumonia that occurs in patients who are mechanically ventilated. The incidence of VAP is reported at 10–30% among patients who require mechanical ventilation for greater than 48 hours.[22]

Critically ill ventilated patients commonly experience chest colonisation as a result of translocation of bacteria from the mouth to the lungs via the endotracheal tube (ETT) or via contamination of the ventilator circuit. This may lead to clinical signs of infection, or the patient may remain colonised without an infective process. The patient's severity of disease, physiological reserve and comorbidity influence the development of infection.[3] Most cases of VAP are associated with infection involving gram-negative bacilli such as *Pseudomonas aeruginosa* and *Acinetobacter* spp. A high number of cases are associated with gram-positive *Staphylococcus aureus*. Many cases of

---

BOX 14.1

Severity scoring in CAP

CURB65/CUR65[19]

The score is an acronym for each of the risk factors measured. One point is allocated for each risk factor present, with maximum scores of 5 and 4, respectively:

- C – **c**onfusion: a new onset of confusion, defined as an abbreviated mental test score of 8 or less
- U – **u**rea: blood urea nitrogen level >19 mg/dL
- R – **r**espiratory rate: ≥30 breaths per minute
- B – **b**lood pressure: ≤90 mmHg systolic or ≤60 mmHg diastolic (not measured as part of CUR65 scoring system)
- 65 – age: ≥**65** years

Pneumonia Severity Index[20]

The PSI considers a range of patient characteristics, comorbid diseases, signs and symptoms and laboratory findings with the intent of classifying the severity of a patient's pneumonia at a risk level ranging from I to V, with V being the most severe. An online PSI calculator (see *Online resources* for link) is available to assist clinicians in applying the scoring system.

- PSI risk class I – patient can be sent home on oral antibiotics
- PSI risk class II–III – patient should be treated with IV antibiotics and may need to be monitored in hospital for 24 hours
- PSI risk class IV–V – patient should be hospitalised for treatment

Adapted from Singanayagam A, Chalmers JD, Hill AT. Severity assessment in community-acquired pneumonia: a review. QJM 2009;6:379–88, with permission.

VAP are associated with multiple organisms. As in CAP, the presence of comorbidities and other risk factors influences the causative organism.[3]

Diagnosis

VAP can be difficult to diagnose, as clinical features can be non-specific and other conditions may cause infiltrates on CXR. In addition to this, ambiguity in the definition of VAP has led to inconsistencies in interpretation and application of the definition, which has meant that comparison of incidence and/or treatment effects has been difficult. The current definition used by the Centres for Disease Control in the USA focuses on more objective data.[13] VAP is suspected when additional support is required to maintain oxygenation, such as increased FiO_2 or higher PEEP, clinical signs of infection begin to develop, including new onset of pyrexia or raised white blood cell counts, or when indicated by microbiological culture.[13] Specific risk factors associated with increased mortality in VAP have been identified over the past decade. The most widely-recognised risk-minimisation factor is the provision of appropriate antibiotic treatment, which has reduced mortality and the rate of complications. Timeliness of antibiotic administration is an independent risk factor for mortality – mortality was increased where administration of antibiotics was delayed for more than 24 hours after diagnosis.[22]

When VAP is suspected there are two treatment strategies that are commonly used, and a systematic review of these strategies was not able to demonstrate any differences in patient outcome measures including mortality, length of ICU stay or length of ventilation period:[23]

1 Clinical strategy: involves treatment of patients with new antibiotics, based on patient risk factors and the local microbiological and resistance patterns. Therapy is adjusted based on culture results and the patient's response to treatment.

2 Invasive strategy: involves collection and quantitative analysis of respiratory secretions from samples obtained by bronchoalveolar lavage to confirm the diagnosis and causative organism. Antibiotic therapy is then guided by specific protocols.

Clinical manifestations

Symptoms for pneumonia are both respiratory and systemic. Common characteristics include fever, sweats, rigours, cough, sputum production, pleuritic chest pain, dyspnoea, tachypnoea, pleural rub, inspiratory crackles on auscultation, plus radiological evidence of infiltrates or consolidation.[3] Cough is the most common finding in CAP and is present in up to 80% of all patients.[16]

Patient management

VAP prevention strategies

Prevention of VAP is a key emphasis in the care of all mechanically ventilated patients and involves a number of interventions. One approach in encouraging the implementation of VAP prevention was the combination of key aspects of patient management into an evidence-based guideline, the *Ventilator Care Bundle*, which advocates semi-recumbent positioning, sedation holds, peptic ulcer disease prophylaxis and deep vein thrombosis prophylaxis.[24] A number of different VAP bundles, clinical guidelines or checklists have been reported. A VAP prevention bundle used in Scotland, which included head elevation, oral care with chlorhexidine, sedation interruptions and a ventilator weaning protocol, demonstrated a reduced VAP rate in a before-and-after study.[25] A Canadian VAP prevention bundle demonstrating a reduction in VAP rate included preferential use of oral versus nasal tubes for access to the trachea or stomach and subglottic secretion drainage, in addition to semi-recumbent positioning and sedation holds.[26]

Further evaluation of the effectiveness of these strategies and the issues associated with implementation has been performed. However, differences in the definitions used for VAP/VAE, combined with a limited impact on patient outcome measures, have made interpretation of these data complex. In addition, the high mortality reported to be associated with VAP has also been questioned,[27] leading clinicians to debate the benefit of implementing interventions that reduce the incidence of VAP but may not impact on patient outcome measures.

Effective oral hygiene care has been recommended in ventilated patients, especially when performed with chlorhexidine as this is associated with a 40% reduction in the odds of developing VAP. Despite this reduction, there is no evidence of it influencing other outcome measures such as mortality, duration of mechanical ventilation or duration of ICU stay.[28]

The Surviving Sepsis Campaign Guidelines[29] recommend that selective oral decontamination and selective digestive decontamination be introduced and investigated as a method to reduce the incidence of VAP. The aim of selective digestive decontamination is to prevent or eradicate the abnormal colonisation of potentially pathogenic microorganisms, such as gram-negative aerobic microorganisms and methicillin-sensitive *Staphylococcus aureus* and yeasts, from the oropharyngeal and intestinal tracts. Although this strategy has been shown to be effective in reducing morbidity and mortality[30], with antibiotic resistance being controlled, it is yet to be widely adopted in clinical practice.[31] Recent review of nursing considerations for administration of selective digestive decontamination highlights the importance of a comprehensive education program and an implementation plan that considers patient safety issues as well as the impact on nursing practice.[32]

Several other new strategies have been suggested and evaluated for their effectiveness in reducing VAP rates. These include: specialised ETTs that allow for aspiration of subglottic secretions; continuous maintenance of appropriate ETT cuff inflation pressures; modified shape of ETT cuff; ETTs that have an external silver/antimicrobial coating; and administration of probiotics. These have been shown to be effective, but need evaluation in large randomised clinical trials before practice recommendations can be made.[33]

Management

Early recognition of pneumonia, timely administration of appropriate antibiotic therapy and supportive care are key aspects in pneumonia management. Supportive ventilation is a key focus for managing patients with pneumonia. In some instances this may include increased oxygen delivery and PEEP to maintain oxygenation and prevent alveolar collapse. Chest physiotherapy remains a key component of management of all ventilated patients. However, its contribution towards improving mortality in patients with pneumonia is unclear.[8] Upright positioning and early mobilisation are important elements of both prevention and management of pneumonia. The evidence supporting use of additional strategies, such as beds with a continuous lateral rotation or a vibration function, is limited and has been associated with complications, so recommendations for their use cannot be made.[33] See Chapter 15 for further discussion.

Medications

Antibiotic administration is fundamental to a patient's clinical progress. As noted earlier, the importance of accurate and timely administration of antibiotics directly impacts on patient outcome. In particular, the first dose of antibiotics is required as soon as possible after the diagnosis of pneumonia has been made.[29] Antibiotic cover for pneumonia depends on the causative organism and sensitivity to drugs (see Table 14.4[3]).

> ### Practice tip
>
> **Pneumonia during pregnancy**
>
> Pneumonia is a leading cause of maternal and fetal morbidity and mortality. It also increases the likelihood of the complications of pneumonia, including requirement for mechanical ventilation. Bacterial pneumonia is the most common type experienced in pregnancy although diagnosis is often delayed as a result of the reluctance to obtain a CXR. Management is similar to a non-pregnant patient with antibiotic therapy adjusted to consider the impact on the fetus.[3]

Respiratory pandemics

Serious outbreaks of respiratory infections that spread rapidly on a global scale are termed pandemics. Their spread is rapid because the infection is usually associated with the emergence of a new virus where the majority of the population has no immunity. These infections are characterised by extremely rapid 'transmission with concurrent outbreaks throughout the globe; the occurrence of disease outside the usual seasonality, including during the summer months; high attack rates in all age groups, with high levels of mortality particularly in healthy young adults; and multiple waves of disease immediately before and after the main outbreak'.[14]

Several severe respiratory infections have progressed to become pandemics in recent years; these have been associated with the coronavirus and influenza viruses. Prediction of the interval between pandemics is difficult, but occurrence is likely to continue and therefore requires that the healthcare community be well prepared. The InFACT H1N1 Research Collaborative is a global initiative aimed at reducing the mortality associated with H1N1 through clinical research groups and professional

TABLE 14.4
Preferred antimicrobial agents in pneumonia[3]

TYPE OF INFECTION	PREFERRED AGENT(S)
COMMUNITY-ACQUIRED PNEUMONIA	
Streptococcus pneumoniae	Penicillin-susceptible organisms: penicillin G, amoxicillin, clindamycin, doxycycline, telithromycin Penicillin-resistant organisms: cefotaxime, ceftriaxone, vancomycin, fluoroquinolone
Mycoplasma	Doxycycline, macrolide
Chlamydophila pneumoniae	Doxycycline, macrolide
Legionella	Azithromycin, fluoroquinolone (including ciprofloxacin), erythromycin (rifampicin)
Haemophilus influenzae	Second- or third-generation cephalosporin, clarithromycin, doxycycline, beta-lactam/beta-lactamase inhibitor, trimethoprim/sulfamethoxazole, azithromycin, telithromycin
Moraxella catarrhalis	Second- or third-generation cephalosporin, trimethoprim–sulfamethoxazole, macrolide doxycycline, beta-lactam–beta-lactamase inhibitor
Neisseria meningitidis	Penicillin
Streptococci (other than *S. pneumoniae*)	Penicillin, first-generation cephalosporin
Anaerobes	Clindamycin, beta-lactam–beta-lactamase inhibitor, beta-lactam + metronidazole
Staphylococcus aureus Methicillin-susceptible Methicillin-resistant	Oxacillin, nafcillin, cefazolin; all + rifampin or gentamicin Vancomycin, rifampicin or gentamicin
Klebsiella pneumoniae and other *Enterobacteriaceae* (excluding *Enterobacter* spp.)	Third-generation cephalosporin or cefepime (all + aminoglycoside), carbapenem
HOSPITAL-ACQUIRED INFECTIONS	
Enterobacter spp.	Carbapenem, beta-lactam–beta-lactamase inhibitor, cefepime, fluoroquinolone, all + aminoglycoside in seriously ill patients
Pseudomonas aeruginosa	Anti-pseudomonal beta-lactam + aminoglycoside, carbapenem + aminoglycoside
Acinetobacter	Aminoglycoside + piperacillin or a carbapenem

organisations working together to gain a rapid understanding of the epidemiology and clinical presentation of the disease, and the identification of effective management strategies.[34]

Aetiologies of severe acute respiratory syndrome and influenza

In 2002–03 an outbreak of a novel coronavirus occurred in China and rapidly spread throughout the world. The infection was highly virulent with over 8000 cases reported and a mortality rate of 11%. The infection was called severe acute respiratory syndrome (SARS) due to the severity of the disease, characterised by diffuse alveolar infiltrates, resulting in about 20% of patients requiring respiratory support. The outbreak provoked a rapid and intense public health response coordinated by the World Health Organization, resulting in a cessation of disease transmission within 10 months.[14]

Epidemics of influenza occur regularly and are associated with high morbidity and mortality. Incidence is usually highest in the young, while mortality is highest in the elderly population. Those with pre-existing respiratory conditions such as asthma or COPD experience particularly high morbidity and mortality. In contrast, when influenza occurs on a pandemic scale it has been shown to affect greater numbers of younger and otherwise healthy people.

A feature of the influenza virus that explains why it continues to be associated with epidemic and pandemic disease is its high frequency of antigenic variation. This occurs in two of the external glycoproteins and is referred to as antigenic drift or antigenic shift, depending on the extent of the variation. The result of this is that new viruses are introduced into the population and, due to the absence of immunity to the virus, a pandemic of influenza results.[3]

Pandemics of influenza were observed a number of times in the twentieth century, and were believed to have involved viruses circulating in humans that originated from influenza A viruses in birds. The 'Spanish influenza' pandemic of 1918–19 resulted in the deaths of over 50 million people worldwide and remains unprecedented in its severity.[14]

The first reported infection of humans with avian influenza viruses occurred in Hong Kong in 1997, with six recorded fatalities. The increased virulence of this disease was observed in the acuity of those affected by the outbreak of the highly pathogenic avian influenza virus (H5N1) in 2004–05.[14] Most patients presented with non-specific symptoms of fever, cough and shortness of breath. In many patients this progressed rapidly to acute respiratory failure requiring ventilation and other supportive measures. The majority of people affected (90%) were less than 40 years of age with case fatality rates highest in the 10–19-year-old age group.[35]

The most recent influenza pandemic was declared by the World Health Organization in 2009 when a novel H1N1 influenza A virus emerged in Mexico and the USA. This virus contained genes from avian, human and swine influenza viruses and affected millions of people worldwide. Patients typically presented with nonspecific flu-like symptoms; however, in a quarter of patients this was accompanied by diarrhoea and vomiting. The disease spread globally with millions of cases reported and resulted in over 16,000 deaths by March 2010.[36]

Australian and New Zealand communities had a high proportion of cases of H1N1 influenza A infection, with 856 patients being admitted to ICU, 15 times the incidence of influenza A in other recent years. Infants (aged 0–1 years) and adults aged 25–64 years were at particular risk; others at increased risk were pregnant women, adults with a body mass index over 35 and indigenous Australian and New Zealand populations. Australian and New Zealand Intensive Care Society investigators prepared a report based on the Australian and New Zealand experience to assist those in the northern hemisphere to better prepare for their winter influenza season.[37]

The emergence of a novel swine-origin influenza A virus was not anticipated and it is unlikely, given the limitations of current knowledge, that future pandemics can be predicted. The threat of pandemic disease from avian influenza remains high with the rapid evolution of H5N1 viruses; however, the direction this will take is unpredictable. Priorities for prevention and management of future influenza pandemics therefore involve development of an international surveillance and response network for early detection and containment of the disease, local preparation for controlling the spread of the infection and further development of vaccines and antiviral agents.[36]

Patient management

Vaccination

Influenza vaccines are formulated annually based on current and recent viral strains. Success in protecting an individual against influenza requires that the virus strains included in the vaccine are the same as those currently circulating in the community. Vaccines are commonly effective in preventing influenza in 70–90% of healthy adults younger than 65 years of age. Efficacy appears lower in elderly persons. Healthcare workers are a key target group for the influenza vaccine, at the very least to reduce absenteeism over what is often the busiest period for most hospitals and health services and to reduce the risk of nosocomial influenza in hospitals.[14]

Isolation precautions and personal protective equipment

Key aspects of infection control in an epidemic or pandemic situation focus on limiting opportunities for nosocomial spread and the protection of healthcare workers. Guidelines for institutional management of these infections involve designing and implementing appropriate isolation procedures and recommending appropriate personal protective equipment. The importance of adequate personal protective equipment was highlighted particularly during the SARS epidemic where there was overrepresentation of healthcare workers who became patients infected with the virus.[14]

Specific infection control guidelines are usually developed for individual institutions, based on government recommendations for management of staff, appropriate personal protective equipment and isolation procedures. This topic is covered in detail in Chapter 6.

Acute lung injury/acute respiratory distress syndrome

ALI is a generic term that encompasses conditions causing physical injury to the lungs. Acute respiratory distress syndrome (ARDS) is a severe form of ALI resulting from bilateral and diffuse alveolar damage due to an acute insult, and is the predominant form of ALI observed in ICU.[3]

Aetiology

ARDS is a characteristic inflammatory response of the lung to a wide variety of insults. Epidemiological studies show a variable incidence of ARDS. For example, estimates of incidence from studies conducted in the USA range from 64 to 79 cases per 100,000 person-years, whereas estimates from other areas are substantially lower with Northern Europe reporting 17 cases per 100,000, Spain reporting 7.2 cases per 100,000 and Australia/New Zealand reporting 34 cases per 100,000. Reasons for this variation may include differences in demographics, healthcare delivery systems and clinical coding practices.[38] Regardless of the variations in incidence, ARDS remains a syndrome of significant impact with an in-hospital mortality rate of approximately 40%.[39]

Clinical disorders that are commonly associated with ARDS can be separated into those that directly or indirectly injure the lung[16] (see Table 14.5).

The most common cause of indirect injury resulting in ALI/ARDS is sepsis, followed by severe trauma and haemodynamic shock states. Transfusion-related ALI is not common but is observed in ICU. ARDS arising from direct injury to the lung is most commonly seen in

patients with pneumonia. The risk of developing ARDS increases significantly when more than one predisposing factor is present.[38]

Pathophysiology

Inflammatory damage to alveoli from locally or systemically released inflammatory mediators causes a change in pulmonary capillary permeability, with resulting fluid and protein leakage into the alveolar space and pulmonary infiltrates. Dilution and loss of surfactant causes diffuse alveolar collapse and a reduction in pulmonary compliance and may also impair the defence mechanisms of the lungs. Intrapulmonary shunt is confirmed when hypoxaemia does not improve despite supplemental oxygen administration. The characteristic course of ARDS is described as having three phases:[39]

1   Oedematous phase: involves an early period of alveolar damage and pulmonary infiltrates resulting in hypoxaemia. This phase is characterised by migration of neutrophils into the alveolar compartment, releasing a variety of substances including proteases, gelatinases A and B and reactive nitrogen and oxygen species that damage the alveoli. Further damage is caused by resident alveolar macrophages and release of proinflammatory cytokines that amplify the inflammatory response in the lung. Significant ventilation–perfusion (intrapulmonary shunt) mismatch evolves, causing hypoxaemia.

2   Proliferative phase: begins after 1–2 weeks as pulmonary infiltrates resolve and fibrosis and remodelling occur. This phase is characterised by reduced alveolar ventilation and pulmonary compliance and ventilation–perfusion mismatch. Reduced compliance causes further atelectasis in the mechanically ventilated patient as alveoli are damaged by increased volume and/or pressure on inspiration.

3   Fibrotic phase: the final phase where alveoli become fibrotic and the lung is left with emphysema-like alterations.

Diagnosis

A standardised definition of ARDS was first described in 1988, with three clinical findings; 1) hypoxia, 2) decreased pulmonary compliance and 3) diffuse infiltrates observed on CXR. The Murray Lung Injury Score was developed as a method for clarifying and quantifying the existence and severity of the disease.[40] The American-European Consensus Conference on ARDS provided the following definition: acute onset of arterial hypoxaemia (PaO_2/FiO_2 ratio <200) and bilateral infiltrates on CXR without evidence of left atrial hypertension or congestive cardiac failure. The spectrum of disease was also acknowledged and the term ALI was introduced to describe patients with a less severe but clinically similar form of respiratory failure (PaO_2/FiO_2 ratio <300).[41]

TABLE 14.5

Direct and indirect causes of acute lung injury[16]

DIRECT LUNG INJURY	INDIRECT LUNG INJURY
Pneumonia	Sepsis
Aspiration of gastric contents	Multiple trauma
Pulmonary contusion	Cardiopulmonary bypass
Fat, amniotic fluid or air embolus	Drug overdose
	Acute pancreatitis
Near drowning	Transfusion of blood products
Inhalational injury (chemical or smoke)	
Reperfusion pulmonary oedema	

Recent review of the American-European Consensus Conference definition and drafting of the Berlin definition of ARDS[42] have resulted in a definition that is feasible, reliable and prognostic. Major changes include:

- replacing the term ALI with three levels of ARDS severity, based on PaO_2/FiO_2 measured with at least 5 cmH_2O of applied PEEP
- defining 'acute' as less than 7 days from the predisposing clinical insult
- eliminating pulmonary wedge pressure cut-off values that discriminate ARDS from cardiogenic pulmonary oedema.

Clinical manifestations

Although no specific test exists to determine whether a patient has ARDS, it should be considered in any patient with a predisposing risk factor who develops severe hypoxaemia, reduced compliance and diffuse pulmonary infiltrates on CXR.[38] ARDS usually occurs 1–2 days following onset of a presenting condition and is characterised by rapid clinical deterioration. Common symptoms include severe dyspnoea, dry cough, cyanosis, hypoxaemia requiring rapidly escalating amounts of supplemental oxygen and persistent coarse crackles on auscultation.[3]

Assessment

A patient with ARDS requires ongoing monitoring of oxygenation and ventilation through pulse oximetry and ABG analysis, especially $PaCO_2$ to monitor permissive hypercapnia. Monitoring of ventilatory pressures and volumes ensures that additional lung injury is prevented. As many patients with ARDS require cardiovascular support, assessment of haemodynamics and peripheral perfusion is important to ensure oxygen delivery to cells is achieved.[3]

Patient management

The key principles of management are treatment of the precipitating cause and providing supportive care during the period of respiratory failure. The most significant advances in the supportive care of ARDS patients have been associated with improved ventilator management. Several clinical trials have shown that a large number of pharmacological strategies have not been effective in reducing mortality.[43]

Other strategies include cautious fluid management, adequate nutrition, prevention of ventilator-associated pneumonia, prophylaxis for deep vein thrombosis and gastric ulcers, weaning of sedation and mechanical ventilation as early as possible and physiotherapy and rehabilitation. Management involves a coordinated collaborative approach including supportive ventilation, patient positioning and medication administration.

Ventilation strategies

The key focus of ventilation in ARDS is the prevention of refractory hypoxaemia rather than its reversal after development. The use of small tidal volumes and adequate levels of PEEP, along with careful attention to fluid status and patient–ventilator synchrony, may be sufficient to maintain oxygenation at an appropriate level while minimising further damage from barotrauma and nosocomial pneumonia.[44]

The use of rescue therapies, when refractory hypoxaemia does occur, is controversial. Ideally, such therapies should improve oxygenation but also improve survival, and need to be considered safe and effective regardless of the particular patient issues.

Some therapies have demonstrated improved oxygenation, which may be an important goal in many patients who experience severe hypoxaemia. The key focus of rescue ventilatory strategies is alveolar recruitment. An evidence-based approach is likely to involve lung-protective ventilation (volume and pressure limitation with modest PEEP) requiring permissive hypercapnia and permissive hypoxaemia.[44,45] Strategies to support gas exchange, such as the use of extracorporeal membrane oxygenation, may also be used for patients with ARDS. This strategy is described in more detail in Chapter 15.

The recently reported findings that high-frequency oscillatory ventilation in patients with ARDS resulted in an increased mortality (most likely due to the elevated mean airway pressures affecting venous return and venous resistance) has meant that this therapy is no longer used as a rescue strategy.[46]

Prone positioning

Use of prone positioning in patients with ARDS was described almost 30 years ago as a means of improving oxygenation. This improvement is largely due to the effect that the prone position has on chest wall and lung compliance. The result is a more homogeneous ventilation of the lungs and improved ventilation–perfusion matching.[16] For many years, investigation into the effectiveness of this as a therapy in ARDS has noted improvement in oxygenation, but no corresponding improvement in mortality. However, a recent clinical trial found that use of prone positioning can improve survival in patients with ARDS and severe hypoxaemia when applied early and for relatively long periods.[47] See Chapter 15 for further discussion.

Medications

A number of non-ventilatory strategies may form part of the treatment of patients with ARDS. Neuromuscular blocking agents are used to promote patient–ventilator synchrony, especially when non-conventional modes of ventilation are used. Improvements in oxygenation are usually observed and may be attributed to reduction in oxygen consumption and improved chest wall compliance. However, as the use of neuromuscular blocking agents is also associated with an increased risk of myopathy, demonstration of a clinically significant improvement in oxygenation with one dose prior to continuous administration is recommended.[48]

Inhaled nitric oxide therapy may be used to improve oxygenation through selective vasodilation of the pulmonary blood vessels, promoting improvement in ventilation–perfusion matching. Improvement in oxygenation should be observed within the first hour of treatment to support its ongoing use.[48] Some groups have reported the use of inhaled nitric oxide to be harmful, especially to renal function, and recommend that it not be used,[49] given the lack of evidence demonstrating reduction in mortality.[50] A similar effect, in terms of pulmonary vasodilation, has been achieved using inhaled prostacyclins, which remains under investigation as an alternative therapy.[51]

A number of drug therapies continue to be investigated to treat ARDS in acute and subacute exudative phases. These include agents that target the disrupted surfactant system (exogenous surfactant therapy), oxidative stress and antioxidant activity (antioxidants), neutrophil recruitment and activation, activation of the coagulation cascade (immune-modulating agents, heparin, aspirin and statins), microvascular injury and leak (beta-2-agonists, ACE inhibitors), and tissue regeneration (growth factors, stem cell therapy). To date, however, the advantages that have been observed in initial investigations have not been shown in human trials.[52,53,54] Although an improvement in oxygenation has been reported, improvements in other outcomes such as duration of mechanical ventilation, length of ICU stay or improved survival have not been shown.[54] The use of low-dose corticosteroids has been associated with improved outcomes for patients with ARDS, although its use remains controversial and further investigation is ongoing.

Asthma and chronic obstructive pulmonary disease

Asthma is a chronic respiratory condition where airflow limitation may be fully or partially reversible either spontaneously or with treatment.[55,56] COPD is a chronic respiratory condition where airflow limitation is progressive and not fully reversible, although there may be some reversibility of airflow limitation with bronchodilators. The partial airflow responsiveness to therapy in COPD results in a clinical overlap between COPD and asthma, as well as chronic bronchitis and emphysema. A non-proportional Venn diagram (see Figure 14.2), originally used by the American Thoracic Society[57] and now in the Australian and New Zealand expert guidelines,[58] depicts this overlap between conditions. It is not uncommon for people with an obstructive lung disease to share clinical characteristics for more than one respiratory condition, although the dominant clinical symptom is usually indicative of the underlying condition.[59] It is, however, important to differentiate between COPD and asthma as they have different management and illness trajectories.

Asthma affects approximately 150 million adults and children worldwide, with Australia, New Zealand and the UK having the highest incidences.[59] In the majority of cases, asthma is well controlled; however, there are approximately 180,000 deaths worldwide each year. Most deaths occur in the pre-hospital setting although, in the USA, 2–20% of admissions to ICU are attributed to severe asthma[60] with a 10–20% mortality rate in intubated patients.[61]

Pathophysiology

Asthma is a complex syndrome of unknown aetiology. However, it is known to be influenced by genetic, immunological and environmental factors, and epidemiological studies show strong associations with respiratory pathogens.[62] The factors that contribute to asthma lead to infection and allergic responses, inflammation and smooth airway muscle contraction resulting in wheezing, breathlessness and coughing. The pathophysiology of life-threatening asthma involves constriction of the bronchioles and subsequent air trapping in the alveoli beyond the constriction, leading to hyperinflation and generation of intrinsic positive end-expiratory pressure. This is exacerbated by increased resistance in expiratory gas flow due to a loss of elastic recoil and rapid respiratory rates. The patient increases the work of breathing, becomes rapidly fatigued and anxious and there is diminished gas exchange. These factors reduce carbon dioxide elimination while increasing its production and eventually will progress to respiratory failure and hypoxaemia.[63]

In 2014, the International European Respiratory Society/American Thoracic Society published new guidelines on the definition, evaluation and treatment of severe asthma targeted mainly to respiratory specialists. In common with previous guidelines, they do not address issues of management in intensive care. In this respect, the *Australian Asthma Handbook* and the British Thoracic Society are more specific in their recommendations, recommending admission to ICU or a high dependency unit for deteriorating respiratory function, oxygenation and reduced level of consciousness.[64]

In contrast to asthma, COPD is a preventable and treatable disease associated with an inflammatory response to harmful gases or particles. Inflammation causes significant airflow narrowing that results in a permanent and progressive condition. Smoking (both active and passive) is the cardinal risk factor and continuation is the most significant determinant for disease progression.[65,66] However, only 25% of smokers actually develop clinically significant COPD,[67,68] suggesting that other factors are also involved including environmental and occupational pollutants, genetic predisposition, hyper-responsive airways and respiratory infections.[69,70] Disease progression in susceptible individuals is most likely to be dependent on the synergistic effects of these factors. It is estimated that approximately 210 million people worldwide have COPD[71] and, despite public health effects, the World Health Organization has predicted that by 2030 it will be the third most common cause of death.[72]

The airflow limitation characterised in COPD may be a result of three different pathological mechanisms.

First, chronic inflammation leads to fibrosis of the small airways. Second, loss of elastic support and recoil leads to airway collapse because the small airways close on expiration. Third, the mucous and plasma exudate from the inflammation obstructs the airway lumen. These mechanisms lead to air trapping and lung hyperinflation, which consequently produces dyspnoea and exercise limitation for the patient.[73]

Perfusion abnormalities arise from hypoxaemia-induced vasoconstriction of the capillary beds. Pulmonary ventilation/perfusion abnormalities and hyperinflation contribute to increased pulmonary vascular resistance, and respiratory muscle fatigue.[74] Increased pulmonary vascular resistance and hypoxaemia require the right side of the heart to work harder and may lead to right ventricular hypertrophy, dysfunction and failure (cor pulmonale).[75] The incidence of right ventricular hypertrophy is approximately 40% for patients with moderate levels of COPD (i.e. FEV_1 <1000 mL).[55] The left ventricle may also be compromised by hyperinflation, which generates increased afterload. Pulmonary hypertension, coronary artery disease and arrhythmias are therefore a frequent concomitant condition with COPD[76] (see Chapter 11 for further discussion). Impaired ventilation and perfusion leads to hypoxaemia and mechanical dysfunctions, with the primary cause of adverse lung mechanics being hyperinflation.

COPD is not just a disease of the lungs. COPD and systemic inflammation have been widely studied and inflammation has been considered an important key linking the disease and systemic manifestations. It has been established that systemic inflammation is present during both stable phases and acute exacerbations of COPD. Increased numbers of leucocytes, acute phase response proteins, cytokines and tumour necrosis factor are found in the blood of COPD patients.[77] COPD is associated with quite significant systemic abnormalities including kidney and hormonal imbalances, malnutrition, muscle-wasting, osteoporosis and anaemia. What is not clear, however, is if the systemic abnormalities are a consequence of the pulmonary disorder or if COPD is a systemic disease.[78]

Clinical manifestations

With asthma and COPD, a patient may present with wheeze, cough and/or dyspnoea. History and physical assessment are fundamental to determining the severity of presentation. Presence of diminished or silent breath sounds, central cyanosis, an inability to speak, an altered level of consciousness, an upright posture and diaphoresis indicate a life-threatening case.[56] Chest pain or tightness may be present. Underestimation of severity is associated with higher mortality.[56] Large longitudinal datasets for Australia and New Zealand, the UK and Saudi Arabia[79] show hospital survival rates ranging from 90% to 100%, largely due to the reversibility of the condition. Conversely, the largest epidemiological study of COPD in Europe showed that hospital mortality of patients admitted to ICU due to COPD was double that of patients without COPD

(32% versus 16%) and that COPD was associated with prolonged mechanical ventilation and prolonged weaning. The authors also reported that the use of non-invasive ventilation within the COPD cohort more than doubled during the study period, and that this was associated with a reduction in mortality.[80]

Assessment and diagnostics

Communication with patients that builds trust, through honesty and effective intervention, contributes considerably to the de-escalation of panic and fear in patients presenting with hypoxaemia. Creating a calm and trusting environment is paramount for those struggling for breath. Forward-planning for potential deterioration and constant assessment of respiratory, cardiovascular and neurological systems are fundamental in determining optimal clinical progress for these patients. Diagnostic tests and procedures involve peak flow monitoring, spirometry, radiology and ABGs.[56]

The 'gold standard' for diagnosing COPD is spirometry.[69,81,82,83] Although there is no gold standard in the diagnosis of asthma, spirometry is the lung function test of choice.[81] Respiratory function tests are usually performed according to standard principles.[84] Values obtained are expressed at body temperature, ambient pressure, saturated with water vapour, in absolute units (L or L/s) and as a percentage of predicted normal values. The carbon monoxide pulmonary diffusing capacity may be measured using the single breath technique modified by Krogh.[84] Diffusing capacity indicates the available surface area for gas exchange, and is reduced with emphysema but can be normal with asthma.[85] The carbon monoxide pulmonary diffusing capacity can be a directly measured value or expressed as a percentage of predicted normal for age, sex, height and weight. A number of reference tables of predicted normal values enable comparison with population norms.[85] A continuing lack of consensus remains for differentiating asthma and COPD. The most commonly used criterion in Australia and New Zealand is airway reversibility in response to bronchodilator therapy: <15% reflects COPD; >15% reflects asthma.[70]

Patient management

Contemporary management of asthma follows an asthma management plan, to minimise acute exacerbation and any subsequent respiratory arrest. Many presentations will be managed in the emergency department (see Chapter 23 for further discussion). For patients requiring ventilatory support, they are better managed with non-invasive ventilation, as mechanical ventilation is associated with significant mortality and morbidity[80] from hyperinflation and aggravation of bronchospasm.[60] Contemporary management of COPD has advocated a care plan for patients in the community setting. This has an effect on prompting patients to recognise a change in their symptoms and seek appropriate care. However, improving symptom recognition does not reduce healthcare utilisation.[86] Patients with acute exacerbations of COPD managed with non-invasive ventilation in a timely manner have a reduced need for endotracheal intubation and reduced mortality rate.[87,88] In patients with COPD who are mechanically ventilated, a weaning strategy that includes non-invasive ventilation has been shown to reduce mortality and VAP without increasing the risk of re-intubation or weaning failure. There are published guidelines on the prevention, identification and management of asthma[60] and COPD.[65]

Medications

Administration of oxygen and beta-agonists (salbutamol) are first-line therapies. Nebulised salbutamol is the preferred route, with intravenous administration considered for patients not responding to nebulised medication. See Table 14.6[60] for key medications used in the treatment of asthma.

Pneumothorax

Pneumothorax describes air that has escaped from a defect in the pulmonary tree and is trapped in the potential space between the two pleura. A pneumothorax can be classified as spontaneous, traumatic or iatrogenic and can be life-threatening. A spontaneous pneumothorax can be primary (in persons without lung disease) or secondary (in persons with lung disease). A pneumothorax is traumatic if caused by a blunt or penetrating injury or iatrogenic if caused by complications from diagnostic or therapeutic interventions.[89]

In some cases, the amount of air trapped increases markedly if the defect in the pulmonary tree functions as a one-way valve. In this case, air enters the pleural cavity on inspiration but is unable to exit on expiration, leading to increasing intrapleural pressure. This is termed a tension pneumothorax. A patient with tension pneumothorax can present with symptoms similar to asthma, including respiratory distress, wheeze, tachycardia, tachypnoea, desaturation, hyper-expansion, agitation and decreased air entry.[90] Fortunately, tension pneumothorax is a far less common condition, and the patient is more likely to report additional chest pain. The actual incidence of tension pneumothorax is relatively unexamined, but it is more likely to occur in a ventilated patient where a pneumothorax has been missed on assessment.[91]

Pathophysiology

Tension pneumothorax occurs when a one-way valve forms, allowing air to flow into the pleural space but stopping air from flowing out. The volume of intrapleural air increases with each inspiration. Consequently, pressure rises within the thoracic cavity, the lung collapses and hypoxaemia ensues. Further pressure causes a mediastinal shift that subsequently compresses the lung (causing further hypoxaemia) and the superior and inferior vena cava entering the right atrium of the heart (causing compromised venous return). Untreated, the hypoxaemia, metabolic acidosis and decreased cardiac output lead to cardiac arrest and death.[91]

Clinical manifestations

Severe presentations are identified by history and clinical examination (respiratory distress, cyanosis, tachycardia, tracheal shift and unilateral movement of the chest). They are also detected on CXR with a translucent appearance of the air and absence of lung markings[92] (see Chapter 13 for information on CXR interpretation).

Patient management

It is essential to check airway, breathing and circulation in all patients with chest trauma. Upright positioning may

---

TABLE 14.6

Key medications in an acute episode of asthma[60]

TYPE OF DRUG	GENERIC MEDICATION	ACTION	NURSING CONSIDERATIONS
Beta-agonist	salbutamol	Produces relaxation of bronchial smooth muscle by action at beta-2-receptors	Metered-dose inhaler – one to two puffs (100–200 mcg) 4-hourly and as required. Also continuous nebulisation via ultrasonic nebuliser and intravenous administration
Steroids	hydrocortisone	Starts effect 6–12 hours after administration Increases beta-responsiveness of airway smooth muscle	Glucocorticoid dramatically reduces inflammation by its profound effects on concentration, distribution and function of peripheral leucocytes and a suppressive effect on inflammatory cytokines and chemokines
	methyl-prednisolone	Decreases inflammatory response Decreases mucus secretion	A synthetic adrenal steroid with similar glucocorticoid activity, but considerably less severe sodium and water retention effects than those of hydrocortisone
Xanthine	aminophylline	Bronchodilator Inhibits the inflammatory phase in asthma Stimulates the medullary respiratory centre	Administration can be in oral or intravenous form. The half-life is variable dependent on age, liver and thyroid function. This is a drug now used with decreasing frequency

be beneficial if there is no contraindication. Penetrating wounds should be covered immediately with an occlusive or pressure bandage. If a tension pneumothorax is suspected, a thin needle can be used to relieve the pressure and allow the lung to re-inflate. If this is unsuccessful, insertion of a thoracic underwater seal drain will allow the collapsed lung to re-expand. If a haemothorax is present, suction on the underwater seal drain (20–60 mmHg) will expedite drainage and re-expansion of the lung.[93] There are no reported differences in short- and long-term health outcomes between insertion of an underwater seal drainage system and simple aspiration of the air for patients with a spontaneous primary pneumothorax.[92] Pain management and facilitation of respiratory care with oxygen therapy, non-invasive or invasive ventilation, positioning and deep breathing and coughing, and the monitoring of the chest tube and drainage for the presence of air leak and serous drainage, are key to recovery without development of further complications.[94] Chapter 12 discusses chest tube management in more detail.

Medications

Management of pain associated with chest trauma is guided by the presence of comorbidities. Epidural or intravenous opioids are the most effective pain management strategies (see Table 14.7).[95]

Pulmonary embolism

Deep vein thrombosis and pulmonary embolism (PE) are two aspects of the disease process known as venous thromboembolism. Certain factors lead to higher incidence, immobilisation (due to long bone, pelvic and spinal fractures) and closed head injury in particular (see Table 14.8 for a list of risk factors).[96]

In addition, critically ill patients have many additional risk factors, such as the need for surgery, catheters, immobility and use of sedatives and paralytic agents.[97] Most PEs originate in the lower limbs, pelvic veins or inferior vena cava.

Three predisposing risk factors for thrombosis are venous stasis, vein wall injury and hypercoagulability of blood. Clinical risk factors are immobility, surgery, trauma, malignancy, pregnancy or thrombophilia. PE may have no clinical consequence or it may be catastrophic, causing sudden death. Terms such as 'massive', 'sub-massive' and 'non-massive' are often found in the literature, although they are ambiguous.[98] Outcomes from PE vary substantially depending on patient characteristics; for example, a non-massive PE may be associated with a high risk for complications in a patient with COPD or congestive heart failure.[99] International registries maintained over two decades affirm that hypotension and cardiac arrest

---

TABLE 14.7

Common medications prescribed with chest injury: pneumothorax[95]

TYPE OF DRUG	GENERIC MEDICATION	ROUTE / ACTIONS	NURSING CONSIDERATIONS
Opioids	morphine	Intravenous Activates opioid receptors in the brain and spinal cord Depresses respiratory centre and cough reflex Alters pain perception and CNS modulation of painful stimuli	Sedative effect with respiratory depression, decreased cough reflex, bradycardia Histamine release may lead to flushing of face or hypotension, nausea and vomiting Reduces gastrointestinal motility Reversed by naloxone
	fentanyl	Epidural and intravenous A synthetic phenylpiperidine derivative Pharmacological actions are similar to those of morphine, but action is more prompt and less prolonged, and fentanyl appears to have less emetic activity	Sedative effect with respiratory depression Can obscure the clinical course of patients with head injury Slow intravenous injection reduces the risk of respiratory muscle rigidity Use with caution in patients with renal and hepatic impairment, as action will be prolonged Respiratory depression can be reversed by naloxone Bradycardia can be reversed by atropine
Antibiotic	cephalosporin (1st generation) for 24 hours	Intravenous Bactericidal as a result of inhibition of bacterial cell wall synthesis	Active against a wide range of gram-positive and gram-negative bacilli. Highly active against *Staphylococcus aureus*, including strains resistant to penicillin

Adapted from Adrales G, Huynh T, Broering B, Sing RF, Miles W, Thomason MH et al. A thoracostomy tube guideline improves management efficiency in trauma patients. J Trauma 2002;52(2):210–16, with permission.

TABLE 14.8

Risk factors for venous thromboembolism[96]

Individual	Age
	Pregnancy and the puerperium
	Active or occult malignancy
	Previous venous thromboembolism
	Varicose veins
	Marked obesity
	Prolonged severe immobility (bed rest, long haul flights)
	Oestrogen-containing hormone replacement therapy or oral contraceptives
	Inherited or acquired thrombophilia
Medical	Acute or acute on chronic chest infection
	Heart failure
	Myocardial infarction
	Stroke with immobility
	Some forms of cancer chemotherapy
	Acute inflammatory bowel disease
Surgical	All surgical procedures, especially abdominal, pelvic, thoracic, orthopaedic
	Leg injury that requires surgery or prolonged immobilisation
ICU	Presence of central venous catheters
	Mechanical ventilation
	Pharmacological paralysis
	Acquired coagulation disorders

Adapted from National Health and Medical Research Council (NHMRC). Clinical practice guideline for the prevention of venous thromboembolism in patients admitted to Australian hospitals. Melbourne: NHMRC, <https://www.nhmrc.gov.au/_files_nhmrc/publications/attachments/guideline_prevention_venous_thromboembolism.pdf>; 2009 [accessed 09.07.14].

are associated with increased mortality in acute PE. The International Cooperative Pulmonary Embolism Registry reported the 90-day mortality rate of patients with acute PE and a systolic blood pressure <90 mmHg as 52% in comparison with 15% for normotensive patients.[100] The Management Strategy and Prognosis of Pulmonary Embolism Registry reported in-hospital mortality rates of 8.1% for haemodynamically stable patients versus 25% for those with cardiogenic shock and 65% for those requiring cardiopulmonary resuscitation.[101] A number of international clinical practice guidelines have been published to address this significant health issue.[102,103] They address risks and benefits of treatment for medical, surgical and oncology patients.

Clinical manifestations

In most cases, PE is a consequence of deep vein thrombosis, therefore clinical manifestations should be considered together. The risk of venous thromboembolism is highest during the first 2 weeks after surgery and remains high for 2–3 months. In patients with a symptomatic deep vein

thrombosis, 40–50% may progress to develop a PE. PE occurs 3–7 days after the onset of deep vein thrombosis and in 10% of cases may be fatal within 1 hour after symptoms develop.[102]

The consequences of acute PE are primarily haemodynamic. Pulmonary artery obstruction causes release of vasoactive agents from accumulating platelets, with subsequent raised pulmonary vascular resistance and acute pulmonary hypertension. The arterial obstruction causes severe shunting and life-threatening hypoxaemia. Early recognition is of utmost importance, but may be difficult in the ICU setting. In the mechanically ventilated patient, difficulty to wean or sudden incidences of hypotension, tachycardia and hypoxia may be a consequence of an undetected PE.[104] In 90% of cases, PE is suspected if patients develop dyspnoea (most common), pleuritic chest pain and haemoptysis. Physical signs of tachypnoea, fever, tachycardia and right ventricular dysfunction may also be present. If a massive PE has occurred, the patient exhibits hypotension with pale, mottled skin and peripheral and/or central cyanosis.[105]

Assessment and diagnostics

Several clinical prediction scoring tools to estimate the probability of PE have been developed. The two most validated are the Modified Wells Scoring System[106] and the Revised Geneva Scoring System.[107] These tools are based on a list of criteria of known risk factors and clinical signs: points are assigned to each criterion to produce a score indicating clinical probability of a PE. Evidence-based literature supports the practice of using these tools before proceeding to diagnostic testing. Diagnostic investigations include compression ultrasonography for a suspected deep vein thrombosis, pathology test for elevated levels of D-dimer in plasma and a ventilation–perfusion isotope scan, CT and pulmonary angiography (helical CT) scan for PE.[96]

Patient management

Due to the high risk of venous thromboembolism in the critically ill, ICUs should have a policy for thromboembolic prophylaxis.[108] It is recommended that patients undergo a risk assessment prior to initiating preventative therapies. Recommended prophylactic interventions include anticoagulant-based prophylaxis or, for patients with a high risk of bleeding, mechanical prophylaxis with either graduated anti-embolic compression stockings alone or stockings combined with intermittent pneumatic compression devices. Combined pharmaceutical and mechanical prophylaxis has been shown to significantly reduce the incidence of deep vein thrombosis, but it has not been studied in the ICU setting.[109]

The management of PE in the ICU can be complex, hence the need for an ongoing risk assessment. For example, multisystem organ failure (particularly of the liver and kidney) and the need for invasive procedures or surgery may complicate decisions on anticoagulant therapy. Providing there are no contraindications, the first line of treatment is subcutaneous or intravenous heparin or non-heparin based anticoagulant therapy. If anti-coagulation therapy is absolutely contraindicated or has failed, surgical pulmonary embolectomy or percutaneous catheter embolectomy can be used in high-risk patients. A further technique that can be used if thrombolysis is contraindicated is the deployment of a filter in the inferior vena cava.[105]

Medications

Medications commonly prescribed in PE include inotropes, analgesics, thrombolytic and anticoagulant therapy. Supportive treatment of acute right ventricular failure and hypotension is vital. Inotropic drugs such as adrenaline, noradrenaline and dobutamine need to be carefully administered because of associated peripheral vasodilation, which may exacerbate the problem.[96] In general, antico-agulation treatment plays the major role in patient therapy. Rapid anticoagulation is achieved with intravenous unfractionated heparin, subcutaneous low-molecular weight heparin or subcutaneous fondaparinux, a synthetic

anticoagulant similar to low-molecular weight heparin.[110] In high-risk PE with cardiogenic shock, thrombolytic therapy, for example recombinant tissue plasminogen activator or streptokinase, is the first line of treatment.[111] Table 14.9[112] outlines some of the key medications recom-mended and prescribed for patients with PE.

Lung transplantation

Transplantation is a life-saving and cost-effective form of treatment that enhances the quality of life for people with chronic respiratory disease. Lung transplantation is facili-tated by organ donation from patients with brain death or donation after cardiac death. Donation after cardiac death significantly increased the number of organs available for lung transplantation.[113,114] Encouragingly, results of a large multicentre study demonstrate early and intermedi-ate patient outcomes for patients with transplants arising from organ donation after cardiac death are equivalent to outcomes for donation after brain death.[115] In 1985, 13 lung transplant procedures were reported worldwide.

TABLE 14.9
Medications for pulmonary embolism[112]

TYPE OF DRUG	GENERIC MEDICATION	ACTION	NURSING CONSIDERATIONS
Opioid	morphine	Pain relief	See Table 14.7
Anticoagulant	unfractionated heparin	A strongly acidic mucopolysaccharide with rapid anticoagulant effects. Inhibits thrombin and potentiates naturally occurring inhibitors of coagulation, antifactor X (Xa) and antithrombin III. No effect on existing thrombi. Standard heparin has a molecular weight of 5000–30,000 daltons	Prophylaxis and treatment of venous thromboembolism, PE and disseminated intravascular coagulopathy. To prevent clotting in extracorporeal blood circuits (e.g. renal dialysis or intravascular catheters). Prophylaxis of arterial thrombosis (e.g. after vascular surgery, interventional radiology or after thrombolysis for an acute myocardial infarction)
	Low-molecular-weight (LMW) heparin	LMW heparin ranges from 1000–10,000 daltons, resulting in distinct properties. LMW-heparin binds less strongly to protein, has enhanced bioavailability, interacts less with platelets and yields a very predictable dose response, eliminating the need to monitor aPPT	Administered subcutaneously
Acetyl salicylic acid	aspirin	Preventive: inhibits thromboxane A$_2$ (platelet agonist), prevents formation of thrombi and arterial vasoconstriction	The aspirin antiplatelet effect lasts 8–10 days (the life of a platelet in general); aspirin should be stopped 1 week before surgery
Thrombolysis	recombinant tissue-type plasminogen activator (rt-PA) alteplase, urokinase and streptokinase	Massive pulmonary embolism, where restoration of pulmonary arterial flow is urgently required due to right ventricular failure	The risks of therapy include haemorrhage. Safety and monitoring of the patient's clinical state are paramount

Adapted from Pastores SM. Management of venous thromboembolism in the intensive care unit. J Crit Care 2009;24(2):185–9, with permission.

In the 2013 report, the number of recipients worldwide has steadily increased to be in excess of 3640 annually.[116] Patients have received lung transplants in Australasia since the early 1990s. Lung transplantation can be either single or double, depending on a patient's underlying disease state. In the postoperative period, clinicians need to carefully balance fluid management to optimise respiratory function without causing haemodynamic compromise or renal dysfunction. As severe pain, particularly for transverse thoracotomy incisions, can compromise recovery significantly, effective analgesic regimens to facilitate physiotherapy are critical.

Indications

The two generally accepted criteria for lung transplantation in patients with end-stage pulmonary or pulmonary vascular disease are a poor prognosis (less than 50% chance of surviving 2 years) and poor quality of life.[117] About a third of recipients suffer from COPD, with idiopathic pulmonary fibrosis and cystic fibrosis the next most common indications.[118] In terms of quality of life, prospective lung transplant recipients usually struggle to perform activities of daily living, may be oxygen-dependent and have New York Heart Association functional class III or IV symptoms. As a result, most patients presenting for surgery are at risk of being debilitated and may be malnourished or over-nourished, and therefore require specific interventions by health team members. A recent study found that, although no specific nutritional deficit was predictive of long-term adverse outcomes, preoperative hypoalbuminaemia as a marker of malnutrition (and critical illness) was associated with poorer survival and postoperative infections; thus optimising nutritional state is critical.[119]

Description

The four possible forms of lung transplantation, indications for each form of surgery and salient nursing implications are outlined in Table 14.10.[120] Currently, lung transplantation takes two main forms: bilateral sequential

TABLE 14.10

Comparison of the four standard lung replacement techniques, including their common indicators[120]

	HEART–LUNG	BILATERAL SEQUENTIAL LUNG	SINGLE LUNG	LIVE DONOR LOBAR
Incision	Midline sternotomy	Transverse sternotomy, i.e. horizontal 'clam shell'	Lateral thoracotomy	Transverse sternotomy, i.e. horizontal 'clam shell'
Anastomoses	Tracheal Right atrial Aortic	Left and right bronchial 'Double' left atrial Right and left pulmonary artery	Bronchial Left atrial Pulmonary artery	Lobar bronchus to bronchus Lobar vein to superior pulmonary vein Lobar artery to main pulmonary artery
Advantages	Airway vascularity All indications	Access to pleural space No cardiac allograft Less cardiopulmonary bypass	Easiest procedure Increases recipients	Increases donors Can be performed 'electively'
Disadvantages	Cardiac allograft Organ 'consumption'	Airway complications Postoperative pain severe	Airway complications Poor reserve	Complex undertaking Donor morbidity
Common indications	Congenital heart disease with pulmonary hypertension Heart and lung disease Primary pulmonary hypertension	Cystic fibrosis Bullous emphysema Primary pulmonary hypertension bronchiectasis	Emphysema COPD Pulmonary fibrosis Primary pulmonary hypertension	Cystic fibrosis Pulmonary fibrosis Primary pulmonary hypertension
Nursing considerations	Recipients may be malnourished and debilitated Rarely performed due to use of three organs. If native heart from heart–lung recipient is transplanted into another patient ('domino'), it is judicious to have relatives in separate waiting rooms during surgery (i.e. complex issues may arise)	Pain must be optimally managed to facilitate physiotherapy and timely recovery Postoperative management requires careful optimisation of haemodynamic, respiratory and renal function	Risk of pulmonary dynamic hyperinflation in obstructive disorders Complex ventilatory issues Postoperative management requires careful optimisation of haemodynamic, respiratory and renal function	Complex ethical issues

COPD = chronic obstructive pulmonary disease.

Adapted from Williams TJ, Snell GI. Lung transplantation. In: Albert RK, Spiro SG, Jett JR, eds. Clinical respiratory medicine. St. Louis: Mosby; 2004, pp 831–45, with permission.

lung transplantation (BSLTx) and single-lung transplantation (SLTx). BSLTx is the most common form of lung transplantation and has a survival advantage over and above SLTx. However, the advantage of SLTx over BSLTx is that twice as many people receive life-saving surgery. For SLTx recipients with COPD, there is an increase in the complexity of postoperative respiratory management and, for this reason, some centres may perform BSLTx for patients with COPD. SLTx is also utilised for patients with idiopathic pulmonary fibrosis and other forms of interstitial lung disease who have a high waiting list mortality.[120]

Clinical manifestations

Postoperative management of all lung transplant recipients involves intensive clinical monitoring similar to that required for heart transplant recipients, with a focus on the stabilisation and optimisation of haemodynamic, respiratory and renal status. Great skill by clinicians is required to manage this complex interplay. Respiratory dysfunction can develop due to severe dysfunction of the transplanted lung resulting from ischaemia–reperfusion injury, pulmonary oedema, hyperacute rejection and pulmonary venous or arterial anastomotic obstruction. Other major complications in the early postoperative period that affect respiratory management include severe pain, diaphragmatic dysfunction, acute rejection and infection. Patients who receive an SLTx for COPD are at risk of developing pulmonary dynamic hyperinflation, requiring independent lung ventilation. Haemodynamic function can be compromised in the early postoperative phase due to cardiac and respiratory problems; renal and gastrointestinal dysfunction is also prevalent. Long-term respiratory complications include airway anastomotic problems (stricture and dehiscence), suboptimal exercise performance and chronic rejection manifesting as bronchiolitis obliterans syndrome.[116]

Respiratory dysfunction

Respiratory dysfunction within the first 24–48 hours postoperatively is usually caused by primary graft dysfunction (PGD), a syndrome characterised by non-specific alveolar damage, lung oedema and hypoxaemia.[121] PGD may be aggravated by factors associated with the donor (e.g. trauma, mechanical ventilation, aspiration, pneumonia and hypotension), cold ischaemic storage[120] or inadequate preservation and disruption of pulmonary lymphatics. Clinical signs of PGD range from mild hypoxaemia with infiltrates on CXR to severe ARDS requiring high-level ventilatory support, pharmacological support and extracorporeal membrane oxygenation.[122] Australian researchers have shown a decrease in the severity and incidence of PGD following the implementation of an evidence-based guideline for managing patients' respiratory and haemodynamic status postoperatively.[123] The guideline directs clinicians to minimise crystalloid fluids, use vasopressors as the first-line treatment to maintain blood pressure if cardiac output is adequate and use lung-protective ventilation strategies.[122,124] Respiratory dysfunction beyond

72 hours is likely to be due to infection or hemidiaphragm paralysis secondary to phrenic nerve damage. Although BSLTx is usually performed without cardiopulmonary bypass, for those patients who require cardiopulmonary bypass for surgery, it is recognised that there is a higher incidence of PGD.

Patient management

Severity of allograft dysfunction is assessed by ABG analysis, respiratory function and patient comfort, CXR, bronchoscopy and haemodynamic parameters. A careful balance in the management of haemodynamic, respiratory and renal status is vital in the first 12 hours, and their optimisation should be achieved with inotropes (e.g. adrenaline, noradrenaline) and judicious use of colloids to ensure adequate end-organ perfusion without causing pulmonary overload. Fluid management should aim to keep filling pressures low to normal in light of a recent retrospective review that found a high CVP (>7 mmHg) was associated with prolonged mechanical ventilation and high mortality. Importantly, there was no evidence of renal complications associated with these low filling pressures. Fluid resuscitation should include products to correct anaemia and preoperative low plasma protein levels.[125]

For patients who have required intraoperative cardiopulmonary bypass, high doses of inotropes are often needed to overcome a transient relative hypovolaemia. Additionally, gentle rewarming measures are needed to re-establish normothermia in order to prevent haematological and peripheral perfusion impairments associated with hypothermia. Gentle rewarming, and close monitoring of cardiac output/index and pulmonary haemodynamics should minimise the development of pulmonary oedema at this time. For patients with allograft dysfunction accompanied by high pulmonary pressures, inhaled nitric oxide is useful in decreasing high pulmonary pressures and reducing intrapulmonary shunting.[126,127] Continuous monitoring of cardiac output, haemodynamic parameters and urine output assists in guiding haemodynamic therapeutic interventions (see Chapter 9).

To assess the causes and progress of allograft dysfunction, CXR provides vital information about line placement, ETT position, lung expansion, lung size, position of the diaphragm and mediastinum and the presence of pneumothorax, oedema and atelectasis.[128] Allograft dysfunction due to ischaemia–reperfusion injury appears on CXR as a rapidly developing diffuse alveolar pattern of infiltration that is greater in the lower regions,[129] most commonly seen on the first postoperative day but may occur up to 72 hours following surgery. The presence of rapidly worsening pulmonary infiltrates (especially if associated with low cardiac indices) should, however, prompt urgent echocardiography to assess cardiac function and pulmonary venous anastomosis patency.[129] Beyond 72 hours, alveolar and interstitial infiltration may indicate either acute rejection or an infective process. This information is combined with other respiratory and haemodynamic data to inform appropriate collaborative interventions.

Commonly, ventilatory settings and respiratory weaning are guided by pH rather than $PaCO_2$ levels. A modest degree of hypercarbia is anticipated postoperatively and resolves over time. Given that lung-protective ventilation has been shown to have a positive impact on recovery and long-term outcomes in patients with ARDS,[130] it is now recommended that SLTx and BSLTx recipients receive similar ventilator settings.[131] In SLTx recipients, ventilation/perfusion mismatches can also be improved by inhaled nitric oxide and by positioning patients regularly with the allograft uppermost.

Allograft dysfunction can develop in SLTx recipients with a remaining native COPD lung who are ventilated via a single-lumen ETT, due to gas trapping in the over-distensible native lung, a condition known as pulmonary dynamic hyperinflation (PDH) (see Figure 14.2). Any condition that lowers the compliance of the allograft can lead to PDH in these patients. Nurses need to be aware of the patients who can potentially develop PDH and to remain hypervigilant, as early signs and opportunities to stabilise patients' haemodynamic and respiratory status quickly can be easily missed. Initial presentation of PDH is usually an ABG showing inadequate ventilation (hypercapnoea) and oxygenation (hypoxaemia). For many critically ill patients the response to this clinical presentation might be to increase respiratory rate, tidal volume or PEEP. However, in the patient who has received a lung transplant and exhibits PDH, these actions will exacerbate the degree of native lung hyperinflation. A more appropriate strategy would be to reduce minute ventilation.[131]

Other common presenting cues of PDH include a haemodynamic profile of cardiac tamponade, tracheal deviation, obvious hyperinflation of the native lung with or without mediastinal shift on CXR, decreased air entry to the allograft on auscultation and pneumothorax. The early stages of PDH in a patient with a left SLTx for COPD can be seen on the CXR in Figure 14.3.

Immediate management of the condition requires attempts to minimise hyperinflation with altered ventilatory settings and bronchodilators. If this fails, insertion of a dual-lumen ETT is required. Precise positioning and secure placement of the tube is vital, to avoid slight movement of the position and consequent displacement of correct cuff placement (see Figure 14.4 for correct positioning of a dual-lumen ETT).

FIGURE 14.3 Chest X-ray of a patient with left single lung transplant for COPD who has developed PDH.

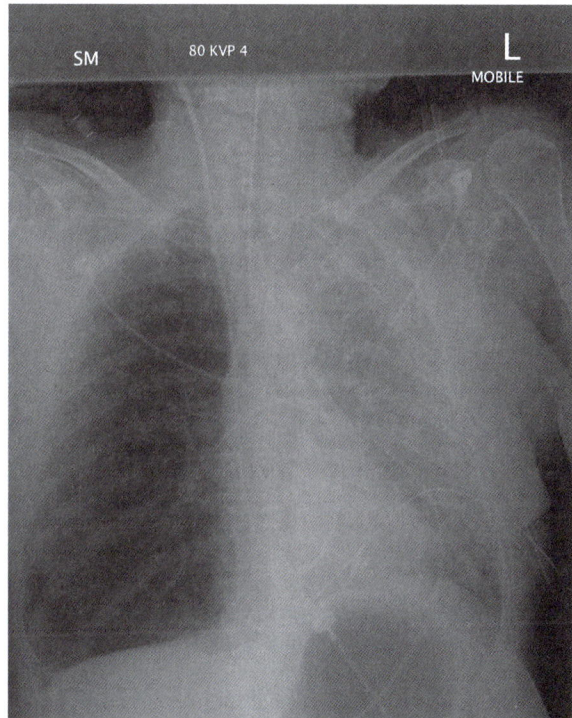

FIGURE 14.2 Mechanism of pulmonary dynamic hyperinflation: distribution of inspiratory gas.

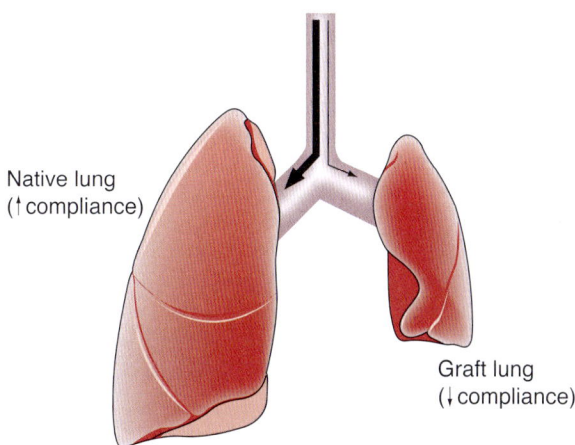

FIGURE 14.4 Correct positioning of a double-lumen endotracheal tube for pulmonary dynamic hyperinflation.

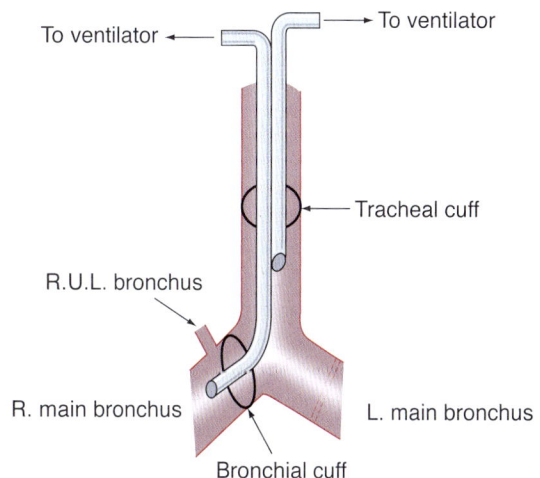

Independent lung ventilation is then established to ensure that the native lung receives no PEEP and a minimal tidal volume and rate.[132] The allograft may require high levels of PEEP to provide adequate oxygenation. Ongoing assessment of respiratory function determines the timing of weaning independent lung ventilation (i.e. replacement of the dual-lumen ETT with a single-lumen ETT) and return to standard ventilatory practice. If PDH is not recognised until the patient has a cardiac arrest, the single-lumen ETT should be pushed into the bronchus of the transplanted lung in order to selectively ventilate the allograft until the patient's condition is stable and a dual-lumen ETT can be safely inserted.

Patients with allograft dysfunction are always assessed for the emergence of rejection and pulmonary infection using transbronchial biopsy and bronchoalveolar lavage in critical care. Evidence of rejection will be treated with changes in the immunosuppression regimen and appropriate ventilatory and haemodynamic support. Many patients with rejection in the immediate postoperative period may not exhibit classic signs of rejection such as abrupt onset of dyspnoea, cough and chest tightness while mechanically ventilated. Subtle changes in respiratory effort, gas exchange and minute ventilation may be the only signs to alert the nurse to respiratory dysfunction secondary to rejection or infection during mechanical ventilation.

Classic clinical signs of pulmonary infection include a low-grade fever, increasing dyspnoea and sputum production, cough and infiltrates on a CXR. Hypotension, a reduced cardiac index and subtle changes in respiratory parameters during mechanical ventilation noted above may also be present. Pulmonary infections may be acquired through nosocomial, community or donor means, with recipient-colonised and opportunistic infections prevalent. Regardless of the means of acquisition, all infections are treated promptly with specific antibiotic, antifungal or antiviral therapies. The risk of developing cytomegalovirus and *Pneumocystis carinii* in lung transplant recipients is somewhat higher than in heart transplant recipients, so prophylactic therapies for both infections are provided. Clinicians play an important role in preventing the transmission of infection between patients and cross-contamination within patients. Meticulous hand washing between patients and between procedures as well as minimising traffic into and out of patient care areas are important measures in reducing infection rates.[133]

Pain

All recipients of lung transplantation can experience severe pain afterwards due to the incisions and chest drains. However, recipients of BSLTx in particular experience extremely severe postoperative pain secondary to the transverse sternotomy (clam-shell incision) and presence of four chest tubes. The recent use of a minimally invasive thoracotomy rather than transverse sternotomy for patients with obstructive respiratory illnesses may also reduce the postoperative pain experienced by recipients. Ideally, all lung transplant recipients should receive epidural analgesia;

however, the insertion of an epidural catheter at the time of surgery may be contraindicated due to preoperative anticoagulation therapy. In these circumstances, epidural analgesia should be instituted as soon as appropriate after surgery. Higher failure rates of transition from epidural to oral analgesia have been reported in lung transplant recipients than in other thoracotomy patients,[134] and it is not uncommon for BSLTx recipients to require opiate analgesia for a month after surgery in order to perform activities of daily living and physiotherapy.

Patient management

Consultation with pain services to ensure that patients receive optimal analgesic regimens should be an integral component of patients' postoperative management (see Chapters 7 and 26). Paracetamol is beneficial in relieving mild-to-moderate pain, and may be used as an adjunct to centrally-acting analgesics for moderate-to-severe pain.[134] The use of non-steroidal anti-inflammatory drugs should be avoided, due to their detrimental effects on renal and gastrointestinal function.[135]

The nursing management of intercostal chest tubes is similar to that for cardiac surgical patients (see Chapter 12), with a few additional considerations. Recipients of SLTx have one apical and one basal chest tube, whereas BSLTx recipients have four chest tubes: two apical and two basal. Both BSLTx and SLTx recipients have one pleural space, so the amount and consistency of drainage from basal tubes will vary depending on patient positioning. Apical chest tubes are removed prior to basal tubes. Once lung expansion is optimal and any pneumothoraces have resolved, the apical tubes are removed. Basal chest tubes are removed once drainage is considered minimal in volume (approximately 250 mL/day) and serous in nature.[136]

Haemodynamic instability

As noted earlier, all lung transplant patients can experience haemodynamic compromise and renal impairment postoperatively as a result of managing respiratory function. Potential causes of a low cardiac output are outlined in Table 14.11. Patients with pulmonary hypertension must be carefully managed in the early postoperative period because of impaired cardiac output and changes in right ventricular dynamics. Prior to surgery, prolonged periods of a high right ventricular afterload lead to right ventricular thickening and stiffness, accompanied by limited wall motion of the left ventricle.[137]

Patient management

During arousal from anaesthesia and patient activity, fluctuations in oxygenation and systemic and pulmonary pressures exacerbate haemodynamic instability.[138,139] When weaning from mechanical ventilation, as ventilation pressures fall, increases in preload may precipitate acute pulmonary oedema, even days after surgery.[138] Conversely, if the patient is hypovolaemic at the time of weaning, right ventricular outflow obstruction may

TABLE 14.11

Possible causes of low cardiac output in the first week after lung transplantation[137]

CARDIOVASCULAR

Hypovolaemia

Haemorrhage

Hypothermia

Acute myocardial infarction

Pulmonary venous or arterial anastomosis obstruction (embolism, clot, stitch, torsion)

Pulmonary embolism (thrombus or air)

Non-specific left ventricular dysfunction

Arrhythmias

Coronary artery air embolism

PULMONARY

Pulmonary dynamic inflation of native lung in single-lung transplantation

Pneumothorax

Oversized pulmonary allograft

OTHER

Sepsis/infection (especially line or occult gut)

Sedatives

Analgesics (especially epidural)

Transfusion reaction

Anaphylaxis

Hyperacute rejection (rare)

Adapted from Birsan T, Kranz A, Mares P, Artemiou O, Taghavi S, Zuckermann A et al. Transient left ventricular failure following bilateral lung transplantation for pulmonary hypertension. J Heart Lung Transpl 1999;18(1):4–9, with permission.

occur.[125] These potential events confirm that careful titration of fluid and inotropic therapies, guided by frequent, accurate monitoring of invasive haemodynamic parameters, is required in patients with preoperative pulmonary hypertension.

Renal and gut dysfunction

Reasons for renal dysfunction in lung transplant recipients in the early postoperative period are similar to those for heart recipients. The situation is, however, compounded in lung recipients due to aminoglycoside and non-steroidal anti-inflammatory drug use preoperatively, the high number of patients with diabetes and a requirement

for 'dry' lungs postoperatively. Fortunately, the use of interleukin-2 receptor antibody drugs can assist in lowering the doses of calcineurin inhibitor agents to offer some early protection to the kidneys without inducing acute rejection.[140]

Patient management

Routine management of gut function is an important aspect of nursing practice, including the prevention of constipation (see Chapter 6). For patients receiving surgery for cystic fibrosis, pancreatic enzyme supplements are required postoperatively. As these patients are invariably debilitated preoperatively, enteral feeds that do not require pancreatic enzyme supplements should be commenced as soon as possible after surgery, as these supplements cannot be administered via enteral feeding tubes. Further specific information on managing patients with cystic fibrosis is available.[141]

Psychosocial care

In the early postoperative period, corticosteroids, sedatives, sleep deprivation and persistent pain contribute to acute organic brain syndrome[117] (see Chapter 7). Rejection episodes can be emotionally demanding, and the requirement for higher doses of corticosteroids can lead to irritability, insomnia, profound depression, mania or psychosis.[117]

Although lung transplantation offers recipients relief from shortness of breath and increased exercise tolerance, many patients have to continue managing other aspects of their underlying disease (e.g. cystic fibrosis). Thus, the burden of living with a chronic illness remains. Conversely, some recipients experience wellness for the first time in their life, and this can alter family and relationship dynamics. In circumstances where lung function deteriorates after initial success, patients and families experience feelings of devastation and hopelessness. Counselling services are essential in both the preoperative and the postoperative phase.[142,143]

Long-term sequelae

Long-term sequelae for lung transplant recipients include renal impairment, hypertension and increased risk of malignancies, similar to those with heart transplantations. Further information about long-term complications specific to lung transplantation, such as bronchiolitis obliterans syndrome and other non-pulmonary complications, is available.[144,145]

Summary

Respiratory alterations, whether a primary condition or a secondary complication of comorbidity, are a common reason for ICU admission. Vigilant assessment, monitoring and provision of a rapid response to a deteriorating state are central to critical care nursing practice. Contemporary approaches to respiratory support focus on preserving a patient's respiratory function, including use of non-invasive ventilation, using less controlled ventilation when appropriate and consideration of weaning from mechanical ventilation at the earliest opportunity. The current evidence base supports strategies to prevent VAP, using daily checklists or care bundles.

Case study

A 69-year-old man is admitted to the hospital because of a productive cough. The patient has a history of alcohol abuse and is a 20 pack-year smoker. He has been in good health until 5 days ago when he developed a cough, productive of yellow sputum. The cough is associated with fever and chills. He also has dyspnoea with minimal exertion. He denies weight loss, night sweats and previous exposure to tuberculosis. He periodically sees a general practitioner and is being treated for hypertension, increased cholesterol and ischaemic heart disease. His current medications include captopril 6.25 mg twice daily, metoprolol 50 mg twice daily and anginine as required.

On presentation he had mild respiratory distress and could only talk in short sentences. His clinical observations were: GCS 15/15, temperature 38.5°C, respiratory rate 34 breaths/min, heart rate 110 beats/min, blood pressure 150/80 mmHg, SpO_2 (room air) 92%.

On physical examination crackles were audible on auscultation and percussion of the chest revealed dullness over the right lower chest. Blood was taken and testing revealed normal serum electrolyte values, haematocrit and platelet count, but his white blood cell count was elevated. A chest radiograph was taken and showed a right pleural effusion and alveolar infiltrate involving the right middle and lower lobes.

Blood and expectorated sputum were obtained for gram-stain and culture. The patient was started on erythromycin and vancomycin. Results of the blood cultures were negative but the sputum grew *Streptococcus pneumoniae*, which is sensitive to penicillin, and appropriate changes to antibiotic therapy were made.

The patient continued to have difficulty breathing and arterial blood gas analysis provided the following results: pH 7.29, $PaCO_2$ 55 mmHg, HCO_3^- 23 mmol/L, PaO_2 47 mmHg, SaO_2 86%. As a result of the hypoxaemia demonstrated in this result, the patient was commenced on supplemental oxygen via a venturi mask with FiO_2 of 0.50.

Further clinical assessment revealed: pale, cool, dry skin; dry, cracked lips; decreased urine output (voided once in 8 hours – volume 150 mL); history of poor food/fluid intake over the past 5 days; BGL 9.0 mmol/L.

DISCUSSION

The patient presents with signs of a lower respiratory tract infection including an increased respiratory rate and difficulty breathing, low oxygen saturation, temperature and increased white cell count. Chest X-ray and physical examination reveal involvement of the right middle and lower lobes of the lung. His history includes increased alcohol intake and smoking, which are risk factors for developing respiratory infections.

Alveolar infiltrate will decrease ventilation relative to perfusion and this will contribute to decreased amounts of oxygen in the arterial blood as evidenced through the SpO_2 of 92%. The alveolar infiltrate and presence of pleural effusion will increase the patient's work of breathing. Supplemental oxygen is required as the PaO_2 and SaO_2 have both decreased. The patient also has increased carbon dioxide in the arterial blood despite a significant increase in his respiratory rate, suggesting that ventilation perfusion mismatch is significant and preventing adequate carbon dioxide removal.

The decreased oxygen present in the arterial blood is of particular concern given the patient has a history of ischaemic heart disease and angina. His increased heart rate will be increasing the myocardial work and myocardial oxygen demand and may predispose him to cardiac ischaemia.

Treating the underlying infection will be important in improving oxygenation and minimising the physiological stress. As the patient already shows signs of sepsis, preventing transmission from the respiratory system to the blood is paramount. Management of his apparent sepsis will involve fluid administration and other evidence-based therapies, so the nurse must be vigilant to ongoing assessment of the patient's response and averting progression to full septic shock.

CASE STUDY QUESTIONS

1 There are several severity scoring systems that can be used in CAP (see Box 14.1) to determine the severity of the patient's condition and predict his need for further intervention and support. Using the information provided in the case study, describe the severity of this patient's presentation according to one or more of the scoring systems outlined.

2 Interpret the results from the patient's arterial blood gas analysis and outline the likely management strategies that would be considered priorities in this situation.

3 Explain whether the ventilation–perfusion mismatch in this patient is due to alveolar hypoventilation, intrapulmonary shunting, dead-space ventilation or a combination of these factors.

RESEARCH VIGNETTE

Burns KEA, Meade MO, Premji A, Adhikari NKJ. Non-invasive positive-pressure ventilation as a weaning strategy for intubated adults with respiratory failure. Cochrane Database Syst Rev 2013;12:CD004127

Abstract

Background: Non-invasive positive-pressure ventilation (NPPV) provides ventilatory support without the need for an invasive airway. Interest has emerged in using NPPV to facilitate earlier removal of an endotracheal tube and to decrease complications associated with prolonged intubation.

Objectives: We evaluated studies in which invasively ventilated (IPPV) adults with respiratory failure of any cause (chronic obstructive pulmonary disease [COPD], non-COPD, postoperative, non-operative) were weaned by means of early extubation followed by immediate application of NPPV or continued IPPV weaning. The primary objective was to determine whether the non-invasive positive-pressure ventilation (NPPV) strategy reduced all-cause mortality compared with invasive positive-pressure ventilation (IPPV) weaning. Secondary objectives were to ascertain differences between strategies in proportions of weaning failure and ventilator-associated pneumonia (VAP), intensive care unit (ICU) and hospital length of stay (LOS), total duration of mechanical ventilation, duration of mechanical support related to weaning, duration of endotracheal mechanical ventilation (ETMV), frequency of adverse events (related to weaning) and overall quality of life. We planned sensitivity and subgroup analyses to assess (1) the influence on mortality and VAP of excluding quasi-randomized trials, and (2) effects on mortality and weaning failure associated with different causes of respiratory failure (COPD vs mixed populations).

Search methods: We searched the Cochrane Central Register of Controlled Trials (The Cochrane Library, Issue 5, 2013), MEDLINE (January 1966 to May 2013), EMBASE (January 1980 to May 2013), proceedings from four conferences, trial registration websites and personal files; we contacted authors to identify trials comparing NPPV versus conventional IPPV weaning.

Selection criteria: Randomized and quasi-randomized trials comparing early extubation with immediate application of NPPV versus IPPV weaning in intubated adults with respiratory failure.

Data collection and analysis: Two review authors independently assessed trial quality and abstracted data according to pre-specified criteria. Sensitivity and subgroup analyses assessed (1) the impact of excluding quasi-randomized trials, and (2) the effects on selected outcomes noted with different causes of respiratory failure.

Main results: We identified 16 trials, predominantly of moderate-to-good quality, involving 994 participants, most with COPD. Compared with IPPV weaning, NPPV weaning significantly decreased mortality. The benefits for mortality were significantly greater in trials enrolling exclusively participants with COPD (risk ratio [RR] 0.36, 95% confidence interval [CI] 0.24 to 0.56) versus mixed populations (RR 0.81, 95% CI 0.47 to 1.40). NPPV significantly reduced weaning failure (RR 0.63, 95% CI 0.42 to 0.96) and ventilator-associated pneumonia (RR 0.25, 95% CI 0.15 to 0.43); shortened length of stay in an intensive care unit (mean difference [MD] −5.59 days, 95% CI −7.90 to −3.28) and in hospital (MD −6.04 days, 95%CI −9.22 to −2.87); and decreased the total duration of ventilation (MD −5.64 days, 95% CI −9.50 to −1.77) and the duration of endotracheal mechanical ventilation (MD −7.44 days, 95% CI −10.34 to −4.55) amidst significant heterogeneity. NPPV weaning also significantly reduced tracheostomy (RR 0.19, 95% CI 0.08 to 0.47) and reintubation (RR 0.65, 95% CI 0.44 to 0.97) rates. NPPV weaning had no effect on the duration of ventilation related to weaning. Exclusion of a single quasi-randomized trial did not alter these results. Subgroup analyses suggest that the benefits for mortality were significantly greater in trials enrolling exclusively participants with COPD versus mixed populations.

Authors' conclusions: Summary estimates from 16 trials of moderate-to-good quality that included predominantly participants with COPD suggest that a weaning strategy that includes NPPV may reduce rates of mortality and ventilator-associated pneumonia without increasing the risk of weaning failure or reintubation.

Critique

Focus: Minimising the duration of mechanical ventilation is an important goal because of the risk of VAP resulting in increased morbidity and mortality. This systematic review is clearly focused on evaluating the impact of weaning for critically ill adults (population) using NPPV (intervention) versus IPPV (comparator) on mortality and VAP (outcomes).

Methodological quality: The review has good methodological quality. The authors reported transparent processes demonstrating robustness in meeting the PRISMA checklist standards.[146] The search strategy was fairly comprehensive, but somewhat geographically constrained because the authors searched the conference proceedings of the top four USA and European meetings for unpublished research. It is possible that unpublished conference abstracts of studies presented at top Australian, Asian or South American meetings may have been missed, resulting in potential publication bias. Selection, data extraction and quality assessment of included studies were undertaken by two authors independently; furthermore, all analyses were determined a priori and there was no deviation from the review protocol. These practices demonstrate a reliable process and reflect high standards in conducting the review.

Characteristics and methodological quality of included studies: Characteristics related to study settings (i.e. country; nurse- and doctor-to-patient ratios; presence of sedation or ventilator weaning protocols) were poorly described in the review. This is an important omission as it minimises the ability to generalise to one's own clinical setting. The quality of the majority of studies was judged as moderate, yet more than 50% failed to report their methods of generating and concealing randomisation. This means we cannot reliably determine the level of selection bias in these trials. If clinicians had prior knowledge of group allocation, recruitment to the NPPV group may be compromised because of clinician-perceived clinical assessment of risk.

Interpretation of results: Nine of the 16 studies exclusively studied patients with COPD, and the impact of NPPV in this patient population was significantly more beneficial than IPPV weaning for all outcomes (except duration of ventilator weaning and arrhythmias). While this is very encouraging, the strength of this conclusion is somewhat limited because of the reported variability in weaning methods employed in both NPPV and IPPV groups; the low event rate for deaths and VAP; and variability in selecting and reporting continuous outcomes. Variability is not a new phenomenon and the extent of the problem has been reported elsewhere.[147] Furthermore, we are unsure of the contexts in which these trials were conducted. Knowledge of the presence or absence of particular ICU contextual factors (i.e. staffing, workload, usual weaning processes, expertise with NPPV) is essential when considering if this intervention could be implemented and sustained in clinical practice.[148] The authors proposed further research before recommending the routine use of NPPV as an adjunct for weaning and a multicentre trial is currently underway in the UK.[149]

Learning activities

1 A patient has severe ARDS following aspiration pneumonia. His FiO_2 is 1.0 and PaO_2 is 60 mmHg. Core temperature is 40°C and the only medications are antibiotics. Any activity including suctioning causes profound desaturation. What additional measures could be implemented to minimise this effect?

2 Assess the next five patients that you look after against current criteria for ARDS and see how many patients are categorised as having mild, moderate or severe ARDS.

3 List the interventions required for a nurse to safely care for a patient with a provisional diagnosis of H1N1 influenza.

4 Describe and compare the differences between a simple, persistent and reoccurring pneumothorax.

5 Outline the clinical manifestations that may be present in a mechanically ventilated patient with a pulmonary embolism.

Online resources

American Association for Respiratory Care, www.aarc.org

ARDS Network, www.ardsnet.org

Asthma Foundation, www.asthmaaustralia.org.au

Australian and New Zealand Society of Respiratory Science, www.anzsrs.org.au

Australian Lung Foundation, www.lungnet.org.au

Become an expert in spirometry, www.spirxpert.com

British Thoracic Society, www.brit-thoracic.org.uk

Centers for Disease Control and Prevention, www.cdc.gov

Critical Care Medicine Tutorials, www.ccmtutorials.com

InFACT, www.infactglobal.org

Lung Health Promotion Centre, The Alfred Hospital, Victoria – resources, www.lunghealth.org

Organ and Tissue Authority: Donate Life Australia, www.donatelife.gov.au/discover/facts-and-statistics

Pneumonia Severity Index Calculator, http://pda.ahrq.gov/clinic/psi/psicalc.asp

Respiratory Care online, www.rcjournal.com

Respiratory Research, http://respiratory-research.com

Thoracic Society of Australia and New Zealand, www.thoracic.org.au

World Health Organization, www.who.int/en

Further reading

Fuller J, Fisher A. An update on lung transplantation. Breathe 2013;9(3):189–200.

George E, Guttendorf J. Lung transplant. Crit Care Nurs Clin N Am 2011;23(3):481–503.

Lawrence P, Fulbrook P. The ventilator care bundle and its impact on ventilator-associated pneumonia: a review of the evidence. Nurs Crit Care 2011;16(5):222–34.

Rose L, Nelson S. Issues in weaning from mechanical ventilation: literature review. J Adv Nurs 2006;54(1):73–85.

Shi Z, Xie H, Wang P, Zhang Q, Wu Y, Chen E et al. Oral hygiene care for critically ill patients to prevent ventilator associated pneumonia. Cochrane Database Syst Rev 2013;CD008367.

References

1 Wunsch H, Linde-Zwirble WT, Angus DC, Hartman ME, Milbrandt EB, Kahn JM. The epidemiology of mechanical ventilation use in the United States. Crit Care Med 2010;38(10):1947–53.

2 Gibson GJ, Loddenkemper R, Lundback B, Sibille Y. Respiratory health and disease in Europe: the new European Lung White Book. European Respiratory Society, <http://www.erswhitebook.org/chapters/the-burden-of-lung-disease/>; 2013 [accessed 20.06.14].

3 Mason R, Broaddus V, Martin T, King T, Schraufnagel D, Murray J, Nadel J, eds. Murray and Nadel's textbook of respiratory medicine. 5th ed. Philadelphia: Saunders; 2010.

4 Partridge M. Understanding respiratory medicine: a problem orientated approach. London: Manson Publishing; 2006.

5 West J. Respiratory physiology: the essentials. 9th ed. Baltimore: Lippincott Williams & Wilkins; 2011.

6 Nettina SM, ed. Lippincott manual of nursing practice. 10th ed. Philadelphia: Lippincott, Williams & Wilkins; 2013.

7 Tobin M, Laghi F, Jubran A. Narrative review: ventilator-induced respiratory muscle weakness. Ann Intern Med 2010;153(4):240–5.

8 Yang M, Yan Y, Yin X, Wang BY, Wu T, Li JG et al. Chest physiotherapy for pneumonia in adults. Cochrane Database Syst Rev 2013;(2):CD006338.

9 Morris AC, Hay AW, Swann DG, Everingham K, McCulloch C, McNulty J et al. Reducing ventilator-associated pneumonia in intensive care: impact of implementing a care bundle. Crit Care Med 2011;39:2218–24.

10 Kalanuria AA, Zai W, Mirski M. Ventilator-associated pneumonia in the ICU. Crit Care 2014;18:208.

11 Engels P, Bagshaw S, Meier M, Brindley P. Tracheostomy: from insertion to decannulation. Can J Surgery 2009;52(5):427–33.

12 Wunderink RG.Ventilator-associated complications, ventilator-associated pneumonia, and Newton's third law of mechanics. Am J Resp Crit Care Med 2014;189(8):882-3.

13 Centers for Disease Control. Ventilator-Associated Events, Device-Associated Module. January 2014, <http://www.cdc.gov/nhsn/PDFs/pscManual/10-VAE_FINAL.pdf>; [accessed 21.06.14].

14 Mandell GL, Bennett GE, Dolin R, eds. Principles and practice of infectious diseases. 7th ed. Philadelphia: Churchill Livingstone: 2010.

15 Myint PK, Kwok CS, Majumdar SR, Eurich D, Clarke A, Espana P et al. The International Community-Acquired Pneumonia (CAP) Collaboration Cohort (ICCC) study: rationale, design and description of study cohorts and patients. BMJ Open 2012;2(3). Pii: e001030.

16 Fink M, Abraham E, Vincent JL, Kochanek P, eds. Textbook of critical care. 6th ed. London: Elsevier; 2011.

17 King J, DeWitt M. Cryptococcosis. eMedicine Specialties-Infectious Diseases-Fungal Infections, <http://emedicine.medscape.com/article/215354-overview>; 2014 [accessed 20.06.14].

18 Murdoch D, O'Brien K, Scott J, Karron R, Bhat N, Driscoll A et al. Breathing new life into pneumonia diagnostics. J Clin Micro 2009;47(11):3405–8.

19 Singanayagam A, Chalmers JD, Hill AT. Severity assessment in community-acquired pneumonia: a review. QJM 2009;6:379-88.

20 Chalmers J, Singanayagam A, Akram A, Mandal P, Short P, Choudhury G et al. Severity assessment tools for predicting mortality in hospitalised patients with community-acquired pneumonia: systematic review and meta-analysis. Thorax 2010;65(10):878–83.

21 Charles P, Wolfe R, Whitby M, Fine J, Fuller A, Stirling R et al. SMART-COP: a tool for predicting the need for intensive respiratory or vasopressor support in community acquired pneumonia. Clin Infect Dis 2008;47(3):375–84.

22 Torres A, Ferrer M, Badia J. Treatment guidelines and outcomes of hospital-acquired and ventilator-associated pneumonia. Clin Infect Dis 2010;51(Suppl 1):S48–53.

23 Berton D, Kalil A, Cavalcanti M, Teixeira P. Quantitative versus qualitative cultures of respiratory secretions for clinical outcomes in patients with ventilator-associated pneumonia. Cochrane Database Syst Rev 2011;(4):CD006482.

24 Wip C, Napolitano L. Bundles to prevent ventilator-associated pneumonia: how valuable are they? Current Opin Infect Dis 2009;22(2):159–66.

25 Morris AC, Hay AW, Swann DG, Everingham K, McCulloch C, McNulty J et al. Reducing ventilator-associated pneumonia in intensive care: impact of implementing a care bundle. Crit Care Med 2011;39:2218-24.

26 Esmail R, Duchscherer G, Giesbrecht J, King J, Ritchie P, Zuege D. Prevention of ventilator-associated pneumonia in the Calgary health region: a Canadian success story! Health Care Quarterly 2008;11(SI):129-36.

27 Bekaert M, Timsit JF, Vansteelandt S, Depuydt P, Vesin A, Garrouste-Orgeas M et al. Attributable mortality of ventilator associated pneumonia: a reappraisal using causal analysis. Am J Resp Crit Care Med 2011;184:1133-9.

28 Shi Z, Xie H, Wang P, Zhang Q, Wu Y, Chen E et al. Oral hygiene care for critically ill patients to prevent ventilator associated pneumonia. Cochrane Database Syst Rev 2013;CD008367.

29 Dellinger RP, Levy MM, Rhodes A, Annane D, Gerlach H, Opal S et al. Surviving Sepsis Campaign: International guidelines for management of severe sepsis and septic shock: 2012. Crit Care Med 2013;41:580-637.

30 Daneman N, Sarwar S, Fowler RA, Cuthbertson BH (SuDDICU Canadian Study Group). Effect of selective decontamination on antimicrobial resistance in intensive care units: a systematic review and meta-analysis. Lancet Infect Dis 2013;13(4):328-41.

31 Cuthbertson B, Campbell M, MacLennan G, Duncan EM, Marshall AP, Wells EC et al. Clinical stakeholders' opinions on the use of selective decontamination of the digestive tract in critically ill patients in intensive care units: an international Delphi study. Crit Care 2013;17:R266.

32 Marshall AP, Weisbrodt L, Rose L, Duncan E, Prior M, Todd L et al. Implementing selective digestive tract decontamination in the intensive care unit: a qualitative analysis of nurse-identified considerations. Heart Lung 2014;43(1):13-8.

33 Coppadoro A, Bittner E, Berra L. Novel preventive strategies for ventilator-associated pneumonia. Crit Care 2012;16:210.

34 InFACT Global H1N1 Collaboration. InFACT: a global critical care research response to H1N1. Lancet 2010;375(9708):11-3.

35 Neumann G, Noda T, Kawaoka Y. Emergence and pandemic potential of swine-origin H1N1 influenza virus. Nature 2009;459(7249):931–9.

36 Taubenberger J, Morens D. Influenza: the once and future pandemic. Public Health Report 2010;125(Suppl3):16–26.

37 ANZICS Influenza Investigators. Critical care services and 2009 influenza in Australia and New Zealand. New Eng J Med 2009;361(20):1925–34.

38 Walkey A, Summer R, Ho V, Alkana P. Acute respiratory distress syndrome: epidemiology and management approaches. Clin Epidemiol 2012;4:159-69.

39 Villar J, Blanco J, Anon JM, Santos-Bouza A, Blanch L, Ambrós A et al. The ALIEN study: incidence and outcome of acute respiratory distress syndrome in the era of lung protective ventilation. Intensive Care Med 2011;37(12):1932–41.

40 Murray J, Matthay M, Luce J, Flick M. An expanded definition of the adult respiratory distress syndrome. Am Rev of Resp Dis 1988;138(3): 720–23.

41 Bernard G, Artigas A, Brigham K, Carlet J, Falke K, Hudson L et al. The American–European Consensus Conference on ARDS. Definitions, mechanisms, relevant outcomes, and clinical trial coordination. Am J Respiratory Crit Care Med 1994;149(3Pt1):818–24.

42 The ARDS Definition TaskForce. Acute respiratory distress syndrome: the Berlin definition. JAMA 2012;307(23):2526-33.

43 Johnson E, Matthay M. Acute lung injury: epidemiology, pathogenesis and treatment. J Aerosol Med Pulm Drug Deliv 2010;23(4):234-52.

44 Donohoe M. Acute respiratory distress syndrome: a clinical review. Pulm Circ 2011;1(2):192-211.

45 Esan A, Hess D, Raoof S, George L, Sessler C. Severe hypoxaemic respiratory failure: part 1: ventilatory strategies. Chest 2010;137(5):1203–16.

46 Ferguson ND, Cook DJ, Guyatt GH, Mehta S, Hand L, Austin P et al for the OSCILLATE Trial Investigators and the Canadian Critical Care Trials Group. High-frequency oscillation in early acute respiratory distress syndrome. N Engl J Med 2013;368:795-805.

47 Guerin C, Reignier J, Richard JC, Beuret P, Gacouin A, Boulain T et al. Prone positioning in severe acute respiratory distress syndrome. N Engl J Med 2013;368:2159-68.

48 Raoof S, Goulet K, Esan A, Hess D, Sessler C. Severe hypoxaemic respiratory failure: part 2: nonventilatory strategies. Chest 2010;137(6): 1437–48.

49 Afshari A, Brok J, Moller A, Wetterslev J. Inhaled nitric oxide for acute respiratory distress syndrome (ARDS) and acute lung injury in children and adults. Cochrane Database Syst Rev 2010;(7):CD002787.

50 Adhikari NK, Dellinger RP, Lundin S, Payen D, Vallet B, Gerlach H et al. Inhaled nitric oxide does not reduce mortality in patients with acute respiratory distress syndrome regardless of severity: systematic review and meta-analysis. Crit Care Med 2014;42(2):404-12.

51 Puri N, Dellinger R. Inhaled nitric oxide and inhaled prostacyclin in acute respiratory distress syndrome: what is the evidence? Crit Care Clin 2011;27(3):561-87.

52 Bosma K, Taneja R, Lewis J. Pharmacotherapy for prevention and treatment of acute respiratory distress syndrome: current and experimental approaches. Drugs 2010;70(10):1255–82.

53 Dushianthan A, Grocott MP, Postle AD, Cusack R. Acute respiratory distress syndrome and acute lung injury. Postgrad Med J 2011;87(1031): 612-22.

54 Boyle A, MacSweeney R, McAuley D. Pharmacological treatments in ARDS; a state-of-the-art update. BMC Med 2013;11:166.

55 National Asthma Council Australia. The Australian asthma handbook. Version 1.0, <http://www.asthmahandbook.org.au/>; 2014 [accessed 10.07.14].

56 Tuxen D, Naughton M. Acute severe asthma. In: Bersten AD, Soni N, eds. Oh's intensive care manual. 7th ed. Oxford: Elsevier; 2014, pp 401-13.

57 American Thoracic Society. Standards for the diagnosis and care of patients with chronic obstructive pulmonary disease. Am J Respir Crit Care Med 1995;152(Supp):S77–120.

58 Abramson M, Crockett AJ, Dabscheck E, Frith PA, George J, Glasgow N et al, on behalf of Lung Foundation Australia and the Thoracic Society of Australia and New Zealand. The COPD-X Plan: Australian and New Zealand guidelines for the management of chronic obstructive pulmonary disease. V2.36, 2013, <http://www.copdx.org.au/home>; 2013 [accessed July 2014].

59 World Health Organization. Bronchial asthma fact sheet No. 206, <http://www.who.int/mediacentre/ factsheets/fs206/en/>; [accessed 09.07.14].

60 McFadden ER Jr. Acute severe asthma. Am J Respir Crit Care Med 2003;168:740–59.

61 Shapiro JM. Intensive care management of status asthmaticus. Chest 2001;120:1439–41.

62 Edwards MR, Bartlett NW, Hussell T, Openshaw P, Johnston SL. The microbiology of asthma. Nat Rev Microbiol 2012; 10:459-71, <http://www.nature.com/nrmicro/journal/v10/n7/pdf/nrmicro2801.pdf>; [accessed 09.07.2014]

63 Stanley D, Tunnicliffe W. Management of life-threatening asthma in adults. Contin Educ Anaesth Crit Care Pain 2008; 8 (3): 95-9.

64 British Thoracic Society. British guideline on the management of asthma, <https://www.brit-thoracic.org.uk/document-library/clinical-information/ asthma/btssign-guideline-on-the-management-of-asthma/>; revised 2012 [accessed 09.07.14].

65 Abramson M, Brown J, Crockett AJ, Dabscheck E, Frith P, George J et al. The COPD-X plan: Australian and New Zealand guidelines for the management of chronic obstructive pulmonary disease, <http://www.copdx.org.au/home>; 2010 [accessed 14.07.14].

66 Diaz-Guzman E, Mannino DM. Epidemiology and prevalence of chronic obstructive pulmonary disease. Clin Chest Med 2014;35:7–16.

67 Lokke A, Lange P, Scharling H, Fabricius P, Vestbo J. Developing COPD: A 25 year follow up study of the general population. Thorax 2006;61:935-9.

68 Tan WC, Seale P, Ip M, Shim YS, Chiang CH, Ng TP et al. Trends in COPD mortality and hospitalizations in countries and regions of Asia-Pacific. Respirology 2009;14(1):90-7.

69 Raherison C, Girodet PO. Epidemiology of COPD. Eur Resp Rev 2009;18(114):213-2.

70 Regional COPD working group. COPD prevalence in 12 Asia-Pacific countries and regions: projections based on the COPD prevalence estimation model. Respirology 2003;8:192–8.

71 Bousquet J, Kiley J, Bateman ED, Viegi G, Cruz A, Khaltaev N et al. Prioritised research agenda for prevention and control of chronic respiratory diseases. Eur Respir J 2010;36(5):995–1001.

72 World Health Organization. Chronic respiratory diseases, COPD, <http://www.who.int/whosis/whostat/ EN_WHS08_Part1.pdf?ua=1>; 2008 [accessed 09.07.14].

73 Barnes PJ, Rennard SI. Pathophysiology of COPD. In: Barnes PJ, Drazen JM, Rennard SI, Thomson NC, eds. Asthma and COPD: basic mechanisms and clinical management. 2nd ed. San Diego: Elsevier; 2009, pp 425-42.

74 Gronkiewicz C, Borkgren-Okonek M. Acute exacerbations of COPD: nursing application of evidenced based guidelines. Crit Care Nurs Q 2004: 27(4):336–52.

75 Hunninghake D. Cardiovascular disease in chronic obstructive pulmonary disease. Proc Am Thorac Soc 2005;2:44–9.

76 Huiart L, Ernst P, Suissa S. Cardiovascular morbidity and mortality in COPD. Chest 2005;128(4):2640–66.

77 Gan WQ, Man SF, Senthilselvan A, Sin DD. Association between chronic obstructive pulmonary disease and systemic inflammation: a systematic review and a meta-analysis. Thorax 2004;59:574-80.

78 Huertas A, Palange P. COPD: a multifactorial systemic disease. Ther Adv Respir Dis 2011;5:217-24.

79 Gibbeson B, Griggs K, Mukherjee M, Sheikh A. Ten years of asthma admissions to adult critical care units in England and Wales. BMJ Open 2013;3:e003420.

80 Funk GC, Bauer P, Burghuber OC, Fazekas A, Hartl S, Hochrieser H et al. Prevalence and prognosis of COPD in critically ill patients between 1998 and 2008. Eur Respir J 2013;41:792–9.

81 Gjevre JA, Hurst TS, Taylor-Gjevre RM, Cockcroft DW. The American Thoracic Society's spirometric criteria alone is inadequate in asthma diagnosis. Can Respir J 2006;13(8):433–7.

82 Pauwels RA, Buist AS, Ma P, Jenkins CR, Hurd SS. Global strategy for the diagnosis, management, and prevention of chronic obstructive pulmonary disease: National Heart, Lung, and Blood Institute and World Health Organization Global Initiative for Chronic Obstructive Lung Disease (GOLD): executive summary. Respir Care 2001;46(8):798–825.

83 Halbert RJ, Isonaka S, George D, Iqbal A. Interpreting COPD prevalence estimates: what is the true burden of disease? Chest 2003;123(5):1684–92.

84 Miller MR, Hankinson J, Brusasco V, Burgos F, Casaburi R, Coates A et al. Standardisation of spirometry. Eur Resp J 2005;26:319-38.

85 Hughes J, Pride N. Lung function tests: physiological principles and clinical applications. London: Saunders; 2000.

86 Williams T, Tuxen D, Scheinkestel C, Czarny D, Bowes G. Risk factors for morbidity in mechanically ventilated patients with acute severe asthma. Am Rev Respir Dis 1992;146(3):607–15.

87 Keenan SP, Sinuff T, Cook DJ, Hill NS. Which patients with acute exacerbations of COPD benefit from noninvasive positive-pressure ventilation? A systematic review. Ann Int Med 2003;138:861–70.

88 Peter JV, Moran JL, Phillips-Hughes J, Warn D. Noninvasive ventilation in acute respiratory failure: a meta-analysis update. Crit Care Med 2002;30:555–62.

89 Matthys H. Spontaneous pneumothorax. Multidisciplinary Respir Med 2011;6:6-7, <http://www.mrmjournal.com/content/6/1/6>; [accessed 05.09.14].

90 Roberts DJ, Leigh-Smith S, Faris PD, Ball CG, Robertson HL, Blackmore C et al. Clinical manifestations of tension pneumothorax: protocol for a systematic review and meta-analysis. Syst Rev 2014;3:3, <http://www.systematicreviewsjournal.com/content/3/1/3>; [accessed 05.09.14].

91 Sharma A, Jindall P. Principles of diagnosis and management of traumatic pneumothorax. J Emerg Trauma Shock 2008;1(1):34–41.

92 Padley SPG. Imaging the chest. In: Berstern N, Soni N, eds. Oh's intensive care manual. 7th ed. Oxford: Elsevier; 2014, pp 445-60.

93 Leigh-Smith S, Christey G. Tension pneumothorax in asthma. Resuscitation 2006;69(3):525–7.

94 Amin R, Noone PG, Ratjen F. Chemical pleurodesis versus surgical intervention for persistent and recurrent pneumothoraces in cystic fibrosis. Cochrane Database Syst Rev 2009;CD007481.

95 Adrales G, Huynh T, Broering B, Sing RF, Miles W, Thomason MH et al. A thoracostomy tube guideline improves management efficiency in trauma patients. J Trauma 2002;52(2):210–16.

96 National Health and Medical Research Council (NHMRC). Clinical practice guideline for the prevention of venous thromboembolism in patients admitted to Australian hospitals. Melbourne: NHMRC, <https://www.nhmrc.gov.au/_files_nhmrc/publications/attachments/guideline_prevention_venous_thromboembolism.pdf>; 2009 [accessed 09.07.14].

97 Geerts W, Cook DJ, Selby R, Etchells E. Venous thromboembolism and its prevention in critical care. J Crit Care 2002;17:95–104.

98 Goldhaber SZ. Thrombolysis for pulmonary embolism. N Engl J Med 2002;347:1131–2.

99 Aujesky D, Obrosky DS, Stone RA, Auble TE, Perrier A, Cornuz J et al. Derivation and validation of a prognostic model for pulmonary embolism. Am J Respir Crit Care Med 2005;172:1041–6.

100 Kucher N, Rossi E, De Rosa M, Goldhaber SZ. Massive pulmonary embolism. Circulation 2006;113:577–82.

101 Kasper W, Konstantinides S, Geibel A, Olschewski M, Heinrich F, Grosser KD et al. Management strategies and determinants of outcome in acute major pulmonary embolism: results of a multicenter registry. J Am Coll Cardiol 1997;30:1165–71.

102 Torbicki A, Perrier A, Konstantinides S, Agnelli G, Galiè N, Pruszczyk P et al. Guidelines on the diagnosis and management of acute pulmonary embolism: the Task Force for the Diagnosis and Management of Acute Pulmonary Embolism of the European Society of Cardiology (ESC). Eur Heart J 2008; 9:2276–315.

103 Kearon C, Kahn SR, Agnelli G, Goldhaber S, Raskob GE, Comerota AJ; American College of Chest Physicians. Antithrombotic therapy for venous thromboembolic disease: American College of Chest Physicians Evidence-Based Clinical Practice Guidelines (8th Edition) [published correction appears in Chest 2008;134:892]. Chest 2008;133(suppl):454S-545S.

104 Cook D, Meade M, Guyatt G, Griffith L, Granton J, Geerts W et al, and the Canadian Critical Care Trials Group. Clinically important deep vein thrombosis in the intensive care unit: a survey of intensivists. Crit Care 2004;8(3):R145–R152.

105 Schuerer D, Whinney E, Robb R, Freeman B, Nash J, Prasad S et al. Evaluation of the applicability, efficacy and safety of a thromboembolic event prophylaxis guideline designed for quality improvement of the traumatically injured patient. Trauma 2005;58(4):731–9.

106 Douma RA, Gibson NS, Gerdes VE, Büller HR, Wells PS, Perrier A et al. Validity and clinical utility of the simplified Wells rule for assessing clinical probability for the exclusion of pulmonary embolism. Thromb Haemost 2009;101(1):197-200.

107 Klok FA, Mos IC, Nijkeuter M, Righini M, Perrier A, Le Gal G et al. Simplification of the revised Geneva score for assessing clinical probability of pulmonary embolism. Arch Intern Med 2008;168(19):2131-6.

108 Barrera LM, Perel P, Ker K, Cirocchi R, Farinella E, Morales Uribe CH. Thromboprophylaxis for trauma patients. Cochrane Database Syst Rev 2013;Issue 3:Art. No.: CD008303.

109 Young T, Tang H, Hughes R. Vena caval filters for the prevention of pulmonary embolism. Cochrane Database Syst Rev 2010;CD006212.

110 Geerts WH, Bergqvist D, Pineo GF, Heit JA, Samama CM, Lassen MR et al. Prevention of venous thromboembolism. American College of Chest Physicians Evidence-Based Clinical Practice Guidelines (8th Edition). Chest 2008;133:381S-453S.

111 Watson L, Armon M. Thrombolysis for acute deep vein thrombosis. Cochrane Database Syst Rev 2004;CD002783.

112 Pastores SM. Management of venous thromboembolism in the intensive care unit. J Crit Care 2009;24(2):185-9.

113 Cypel M. Favorable outcomes of donation after cardiac death in lung transplantation: a multicentre study. J Heart Lung Transplant 2013;32(4):S15.

114 Levvey BJ, Harkess M, Hopkins P, Chambers D, Merry C, Glanville AR et al. Excellent clinical outcomes from a National Donation-After-Determination-of-Cardiac-Death Lung Transplant Collaborative. Am J Transplant 2012;12(9):2406-13.

115 Snell GI, Levvey BJ, Oto T, McEgan R, Pilcher D, Davies A et al. Early lung transplantation success utilizing controlled donation after cardiac death donors. Am J Transpl 2008;8:1282–9.

116 Lund LH, Edwards LB, Kucheryavaya AY, Dipchand AI, Benden C, Christie JD et al. The Registry of the International Society for Heart and Lung Transplantation: Thirtieth Adult Lung and Heart-Lung Transplant Report – 2013; Focus theme: age. J Heart Lung Transplant 2013;32(10):965-78.

117 Hertz MI, Aurora P, Christie JD, Dobbels F, Edwards LB, Kirk R et al. Scientific registry of the International Society for Heart and Lung Transplantation: Introduction to the 2010 annual reports. J Heart Lung Transpl 2010;29(10):1083–141.

118 Kotloff R, Thabut G. Lung transplantation. Am J Respir Crit Care Med 2011;184(2):159-71.

119 Chamogeorgakis T, Mason DP, Murthy SC, Thuita L, Raymond DP, Pettersson GB et al. Impact of nutritional state on lung transplant outcomes. J Heart Lung Transplant 2013;32(7):693-700.

120 Williams TJ, Snell GI. Lung transplantation. In: Albert RK, Spiro SG, Jett JR, eds. Clinical respiratory medicine. St. Louis: Mosby; 2004, pp 831–45.

121 Keating D, Levvey B, Kotsimbos T, Whitford H, Westall G, Williams T et al. Lung transplantation in pulmonary fibrosis: challenging early outcomes counterbalanced by surprisingly good outcomes beyond 15 years. Transplant Proc 2009;41(1):289–91.

122 de Perrot M, Liu M, Waddell TK, Keshavjee S. Ischemia-reperfusion-induced lung injury. Am J Resp Crit Care Med 2003;167(4):490–51.

123 King RC, Binns OA, Rodriguez F, Kanithanon RC, Daniel TM, Spotnitz WD et al. Reperfusion injury significantly impacts clinical outcome after pulmonary transplantation. Ann of Thor Surg 2000;69(6):1681–5.

124 Currey J, Pilcher DV, Davies A, Scheinkestel C, Botti M, Bailey M et al. Implementation of a management guideline aimed at minimizing the severity of primary graft dysfunction following lung transplantation. J Thor and Card Surg 2010;139(1):154–61.

125 Pilcher DV, Scheinkestel CD, Snell GI, Davey-Quinn A, Bailey MJ, Williams TJ. High central venous pressure is associated with prolonged mechanical ventilation and increased mortality after lung transplantation. J Thor and Card Surg 2005;129(4):918.

126 Snell GI, Klepetko W. Lung transplant perioperative management. ERS monograph on lung transplantation. 2003;26:130–43.

127 Ardehali A, Hughes K, Sadeghi A, Esmailian F, Marelli D, Moriguchi J et al. Inhaled nitric oxide for pulmonary hypertension after heart transplantation. Transplantation 2001;72(4):638–41.

128 Thabut G, Brugiere O, Leseche G, Stern JB, Fradi K, Herve P et al. Preventive effect of inhaled nitric oxide and pentoxifylline on ischemia/reperfusion injury after lung transplantation. Transplantation 2001;71(9):1295–300.

129 Van Breuseghem I, De Wever W, Verschakelen J, Bogaert J. Role of radiology in lung transplantation. JBR-BTR 1999;82(3):91–6.

130 Ward S, Muller NL. Pulmonary complications following lung transplantation. Clin Rad 2000;55(5):332–9.

131 Brower RG, Matthay MA, Morris A, Schoenfeld D, Thompson BT, Wheeler A. Ventilation with lower tidal volumes as compared with traditional tidal volumes for acute lung injury and the acute respiratory distress syndrome. The Acute Respiratory Distress Syndrome Network. New Eng J Med 2000;342(18):1301–8.

132 Weill D, Torres F, Hodges TN, Olmos JJ, Zamora MR. Acute native lung hyperinflation is not associated with poor outcomes after single lung transplant for emphysema. J Heart Lung Transpl 1999;18(11):1080–87.

133 Walsh TR, Guttendorf J, Dummer S, Hardesty RL, Armitage JM, Kormos RL et al. The value of protective isolation procedures in cardiac allograft recipients. Ann of Thor Surg 1989;47(4):539–44.

134 Richard C, Girard F, Ferraro P, Chouinard P, Boudreault D, Ruel M et al. Acute postoperative pain in lung transplant recipients. Ann of Thor Surg 2004;77(6):1951–5.

135 National Health and Medical Research Council (NHMRC). Acute pain management: scientific evidence. Canberra: NHMRC; 1998.

136 Charnock Y, Evans D. Nursing management of chest drains: a systematic review. Aust Crit Care 2001;14(4):156–60.

137 Birsan T, Kranz A, Mares P, Artemiou O, Taghavi S, Zuckermann A et al. Transient left ventricular failure following bilateral lung transplantation for pulmonary hypertension. J Heart Lung Transpl 1999;18(1):4–9.

138 Mendeloff EN, Meyers BF, Sundt TM, Guthrie TJ, Sweet SC, de la Morena M et al. Lung transplantation for pulmonary vascular disease. Ann of Thor Surg 2002;73(1):209–17.

139 Simpson KP, Garrity ER. Perioperative management in lung transplantation. Clin Chest Med 1997;18(2):277–84.

140 Garrity ER Jr, Villanueva J, Bhorade SM, Husain AN, Vigneswaran WT. Low rate of acute lung allograft rejection after the use of daclizumab, an interleukin 2 receptor antibody. Transplantation 2001;71(6):773–7.

141 Egan JJ, Woodcock AA, Webb AK. Management of cystic fibrosis before and after lung transplantation. J Royal Soc of Med 1997;90:47–58.

142 Burker EJ, Evon DM, Sedway JA, Egan T. Appraisal and coping as predictors of psychological distress and self-reported physical disability before lung transplantation. Prog Transpl 2004;14(3):222–32.

143 Collins TJ. Organ and tissue donation: a survey of nurses' knowledge and educational needs in an adult ITU. Intensive Crit Care Nurs 2005;21(4):226–33.

144 Ruiz LG, Garrity ER. Lung transplantation. In: Albert RK, Spiro SG, Jett JR, eds. Clinical respiratory medicine. 3rd ed. Philadelphia: Mosby; 2008, pp 955-76.

145 Kotloff R, Thabut G. Lung transplantation. Am J Resp Crit Care Med 2011;184(2):159-71.

146 PRISMA. Transparent reporting of systematic reviews and meta-analyses, <http://www.prisma-statement.org/>; [accessed 09.07.14].

147 Blackwood B, Clarke M, McAuley DF, McGuigan P, Marshall JC, Rose L. How ventilation outcomes are defined in clinical trials in the intensive care unit. Am J Resp Crit Care Med 2014;189:8, 886-93.

148 Jordan J, Rose L, Noyes J, Dainty KN, Blackwood B. Factors that impact on protocolized weaning from mechanical ventilation in critically ill adults and children: a Cochrane qualitative synthesis (Protocol). Cochrane Database Syst Rev 2012;Issue 5, 16 May.

149 ISRCTN [Internet]. London: Current Controlled Trials, c/o BioMed Central. 2012. Identifier ISRCTN15635197. Protocolised trial of invasive and non-invasive weaning off ventilation (The 'Breathe' study): a pragmatic randomised controlled open multi-centre effectiveness trial, <http://www.controlled-trials.com/ISRCTN15635197>; [accessed 09.07.14].

150 Bagshaw S, Webb S, Delaney A, George C, Pilcher D, Hart G et al. Very old patients admitted to intensive care in Australia and New Zealand: a multi-centre cohort analysis. Crit Care 2009;13(2):R45.

Chapter 15

Ventilation and oxygenation management

Louise Rose, Rand Butcher

Learning objectives

After reading this chapter, you should be able to:

- describe complications associated with oxygen therapy and management priorities
- state nursing priorities for airway management strategies including laryngeal masks, endotracheal tubes and tracheostomy tubes
- summarise current knowledge on the physiological benefits, indications for use, associated monitoring priorities, complications, modes, settings and interfaces for non-invasive ventilation
- state the indications for use, associated monitoring priorities, complications, classification framework, modes and settings for invasive mechanical ventilation
- outline the weaning continuum and current evidence for optimising safe and efficient weaning from mechanical ventilation
- discuss ventilation management strategies for refractory hypoxaemia
- discuss ventilation management strategies for severe airflow limitation.

Introduction

Support of oxygenation and ventilation are two of the most common interventions in intensive care; in 2012–13, approximately 41% of patients in Australian and New Zealand intensive care units (ICUs) received invasive mechanical ventilation and 8% received non-invasive ventilation (NIV).[1] Similar numbers of critically ill patients receive ventilation in the UK,[2] whereas in the USA reported numbers range from 21% to 39%.[3] The technology available for supporting oxygenation and ventilation is complex, ranging from simple interventions such as nasal cannulae through to invasive mechanical ventilation and extracorporeal support. Additionally, the meaning of ventilator terminology is often unclear and terms may be used interchangeably. Critical care nurses must have a strong knowledge of the underlying principles of oxygenation and ventilation that will facilitate an understanding of respiratory support devices, associated monitoring priorities and risks.

KEY WORDS

artificial airway
mechanical ventilation
non-invasive ventilation
oxygen therapy
weaning

Oxygen therapy

Oxygen is required for aerobic cellular metabolism and ultimately for human survival, with some cells, such as those in the brain, being more sensitive to hypoxia than others. Refer to Chapter 13 for a discussion of oxygen delivery and consumption, the oxygen–haemoglobin dissociation curve, hypoxaemia and tissue hypoxia; this material provides rationales for clinical decisions regarding the administration of oxygen therapy or ventilation strategies. Oxygen therapy should be considered for patients with a significant reduction in arterial oxygen levels, irrespective of diagnosis and especially if the patient is drowsy or unconscious.

Indications

Indications for oxygen therapy include:

- cardiac and respiratory arrest
- type I respiratory failure
- type II respiratory failure
- chest pain or acute coronary syndrome with hypoxia (i.e. SpO_2 <93%) or evidence of shock[4]
- low blood pressure, cardiac output
- increased metabolic demands
- carbon monoxide poisoning.

Complications

Administration of oxygen, regardless of the delivery device, has potential adverse effects. High concentrations of oxygen cause nitrogen washout, resulting in absorption atelectasis.

Hypoventilation and CO_2 narcosis

High-dose oxygen therapy may lead to hypoventilation, hypercapnia and CO_2 narcosis in a small proportion of patients with chronic obstructive pulmonary disease (COPD). The processes underpinning these physiological changes are described in Chapter 13. These patients require close monitoring of $PaCO_2$ levels when oxygen therapy is instituted or increased. Although COPD patients frequently may have a lower baseline SpO_2 (88–94% compared to 96–100% in patients with no lung pathology), treatment of hypoxia is still essential, and oxygen should not be withheld or withdrawn while hypoxia remains, even if hypercapnia worsens.[5,6]

> **Practice tip**
>
> Oxygen should not be withheld or withdrawn while hypoxia remains, even if hypercapnia worsens.

Oxygen toxicity

Administration of high oxygen concentrations may lead to oxygen toxicity; symptoms include non-productive cough, substernal pain, reduced lung compliance, interstitial oedema, and pulmonary capillary haemorrhage. These

symptoms may be mistakenly attributed to the underlying illness, especially in a sedated and ventilated patient. Many of the symptoms abate once the fraction of inspired oxygen (FiO_2) is reduced, although irreversible pulmonary fibrosis may occur (see Box 15.1). The concentration and duration of oxygen exposure that induces oxygen toxicity varies between patients;[7] the lowest possible FiO_2 should therefore be used to achieve the target partial pressure of oxygen in arterial blood (PaO_2) or peripheral oxygen saturation (SpO_2).

> **BOX 15.1**
>
> **Signs and symptoms of oxygen toxicity**
>
> Central nervous system:
> - Nausea and vomiting
> - Anxiety
> - Visual changes
> - Hallucinations
> - Tinnitus
> - Vertigo
> - Hiccups
> - Seizures
>
> Pulmonary:
> - Dry cough
> - Substernal chest pain
> - Shortness of breath
> - Pulmonary oedema
> - Pulmonary fibrosis

Oxygen administration devices

Initial management of hypoxia in a spontaneously-breathing patient with an intact airway is low-flow oxygen via nasal cannulae (up to 6 L/min) or face mask (up to 15 L/min). Although oxygen devices have traditionally had FiO_2 ascribed to specific flow rates, the FiO_2 delivered to the alveoli is influenced by:

- patient factors – inspiratory flow rate, respiratory rate, tidal volume (V_T), respiratory pause
- oxygen device factors – oxygen flow rate, volume of mask/reservoir, air vent size, tightness of fit.

Normal inspiratory flow in a healthy adult ranges between 25 and 35 L/min. Patients with respiratory failure tend to increase their flow demand from 50 up to 300 L/min. Patients in respiratory distress are characterised by high respiratory rates and low V_T[7,8] that can significantly decrease the FiO_2 available via an oxygen delivery device, depending on the type in use.

All oxygen delivery devices use some type of reservoir to support oxygen delivery and prevent CO_2 rebreathing. For face masks, the reservoir is the mask; for nasal cannulae, it is the patient's pharynx. Patients with high inspiratory flow demand will deplete the reservoir faster than it can be replenished, resulting in air entrainment and dilution of the oxygen concentration.

Variable flow devices

Various low- or variable-flow oxygen delivery devices are available. These devices range from nasal cannulae and oxygen masks with different features, through to bag–mask ventilation.

Low-flow nasal cannulae

Traditional low-flow nasal cannulae sit at the external nares and deliver 3–4 L/min of oxygen. Higher flows may cause discomfort and damage from the drying effect on respiratory mucosa. Increased flow demand with respiratory distress dilutes the oxygen, reducing the FiO_2 to the alveoli.

High-flow nasal cannulae

High-flow nasal cannulae have slightly larger prongs that facilitate oxygen flow of up to 60 L/min, leading to less air entrainment than with other oxygen delivery systems.[8,9] High-flow nasal cannulae generate low levels of end-expiratory pressure, though this is dependent on the flow rate, trachea size and mouth closing,[10] and can therefore reduce tachypnoea and work of breathing.[11,12] The high gas flow may flush CO_2 from the anatomical dead space preventing CO_2 rebreathing and thereby decreasing $PaCO_2$, although this is not well supported by the literature.[13,14] These systems are generally well-tolerated, but must be used with heated humidification to avoid drying the respiratory mucosa.[12] High-flow nasal cannulae are now used frequently in clinical practice to avoid, or as an alternative to,[15] more invasive therapies but there is limited high-quality evidence on their use in adults and children other than neonates.[16]

Oxygen masks

Loose-fitting oxygen masks include simple (Hudson) face masks, aerosol masks used in combination with heated humidification and nebuliser treatments, tracheostomy masks and face tents. All are considered low-flow or variable-flow devices, with the delivered FiO_2 varying with patient demand. Flow rates ≥ 5 L/min minimise CO_2 rebreathing. The addition of 'tusks' to a Hudson mask may increase the oxygen reservoir[17] but does not guarantee a consistent FiO_2 and has probably been superseded by high-flow systems.[18]

Partial rebreather and non-rebreather masks have an attached reservoir bag that enables delivery of higher levels of FiO_2. Both mask types have a one-way valve precluding expired gas entering the reservoir bag. A non-rebreather mask has two one-way valves preventing air entrainment.[19] The maximum FiO_2 delivery with non-rebreather masks is 0.85 with low flow demand, with a steep decline in alveolar oxygen concentration as minute volume increases. Non-rebreather masks may perform worse than a Hudson mask without a reservoir bag.[8]

Venturi systems

Venturi systems use the Venturi effect to entrain gas via a narrow aperture via a side port increasing gas speed and augmenting kinetic energy. FiO_2 concentration can be altered by widening or narrowing the Venturi device aperture to a maximum FiO_2 of 0.6. The FiO_2 concentration using a Venturi system is less affected by changes in respiratory pattern and demand compared to other low-flow oxygen devices.[8]

Bag–mask ventilation

Bag–mask ventilation with a self-inflating bag (and reservoir), non-return valve and mask delivers assisted ventilation at an FiO_2 of 1.0. Addition of a positive end-expiratory pressure (PEEP) valve will improve oxygenation. Manual ventilation requires a good seal between the patient's face and the mask; this may be difficult to achieve as a single operator. One person should hold the mask and lift the patient's chin, while another squeezes the bag. Effective bag–mask ventilation is confirmed when the chest visibly rises as the bag is squeezed and oxygen saturations improve.[20] Bag–mask ventilation may cause gastric insufflation, increasing the risk of vomiting and subsequent aspiration.

Practice tip

Transparent face masks are recommended for bag–mask ventilation as they allow immediate recognition if a patient vomits.

Airway support

The most common cause of partial airway obstruction in an unconscious patient is loss of oropharyngeal muscle tone, particularly of the tongue. This may be alleviated by tilting the head slightly back and lifting the chin, or thrusting the jaw forward. The head-tilt/chin-lift manoeuvre is not used if cervical spine injury is suspected.[21] The jaw-thrust manoeuvre may require two hands to maintain.[22] If more prolonged support is required, an oro- or nasopharyngeal airway can be used, which may also facilitate bag–mask ventilation.

Oro- and nasopharyngeal airways

The Guedel oropharyngeal airway is available in various sizes (a medium-sized adult requires a size 4). The airway is inserted into the patient's mouth past the teeth, with the end facing up into the hard palate, then rotated 180°, taking care to bring the tongue forward and not push it back. Oropharyngeal airways are poorly tolerated in conscious patients and may cause gagging and vomiting.[20]

A nasopharyngeal airway (see Figure 15.1) is inserted through the nares into the oropharynx; it can be difficult to insert and requires generous lubrication to minimise trauma. This type of airway should not be used for patients with a suspected head injury. As well as opening the airway,

FIGURE 15.1 Nasopharyngeal airways.

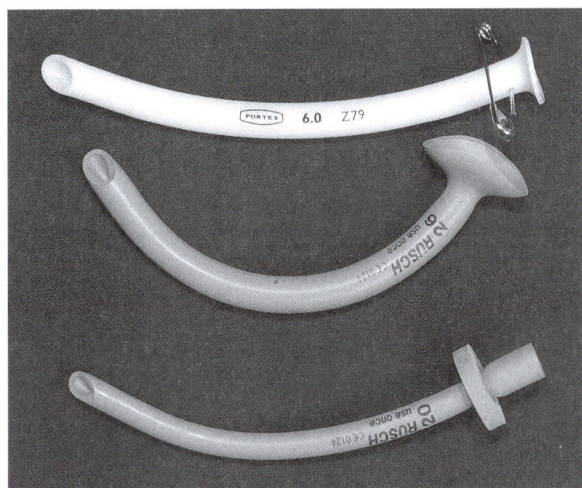

suction catheters can be passed to facilitate secretion clearance. Once inserted, these airways are better tolerated than an oropharyngeal airway.

Laryngeal mask airway and insertion

The classic laryngeal mask airway (cLMA) (see Figure 15.2) is positioned blindly into the pharynx to form a low-pressure seal against the laryngeal inlet. It is easier and quicker to insert than an endotracheal tube, and is particularly useful for operators with limited airway skills; the cLMA does not carry the same potentially fatal complications such as oesophageal intubation although the risk of aspiration remains.[23]

Mechanical ventilation can be delivered with low-airway pressures (<20 cmH$_2$O) via a cLMA. This device is widely used in elective general anaesthesia,[21] and can be used in critical care as an alternative to bag–mask ventilation[23] or endotracheal intubation when initial attempts at intubation have failed.[24] The 'intubating' LMA

is most commonly used when a difficult intubation is anticipated or encountered. This device has a handle and is more rigid, wider and curved than the cLMA, enabling passage of a purpose-made endotracheal tube.[23]

Combitube

The combitube is more widely used in North America for emergency situations than in Australia and the UK.[21] It is a dual-lumen, dual-cuff oesophageal–tracheal airway that enables ventilation if inserted into either the oesophagus or trachea. Inexperienced operators may find a combitube more difficult to insert correctly than a cLMA.[25] Complications may occur in up to 40% of patients and include aspiration pneumonitis, pneumothorax, airway injuries and bleeding, oesophageal laceration and perforation and mediastinitis.[26]

Endotracheal tubes

Endotracheal intubation is the 'gold standard' for airway support, providing airway protection in the presence of airway oedema, absent gag, cough or swallow reflex. Intubation facilitates mechanical ventilation and pulmonary secretion clearance.[22]

Endotracheal tubes (ETT) have common design characteristics, are generally made from polyvinyl chloride, are available with internal diameters ranging from 2–10 mm (common adult sizes are 7–9 mm) and are up to 30 cm long. A longitudinal radio-opaque line allows visualisation of tube placement on a chest X-ray. Markings at 1-cm intervals indicate the length from the distal end, a design feature that facilitates the ability to gauge insertion depth and monitor tube movement.[27] Tubes are available with and without a distal cuff, an inflatable balloon that seals the trachea, facilitates positive pressure ventilation and prevents aspiration of oropharyngeal contents. Cuffs come in a range of profiles and volumes, but are commonly high-volume, low-pressure enabling application of a safe pressure over a larger surface area (see Figure 15.3). A smaller inflatable balloon, attached to the cuff via a pilot line, provides a tactile gauge of cuff pressure and a small air reservoir to prevent minor changes in cuff pressure.[28]

FIGURE 15.2 Laryngeal mask airways.

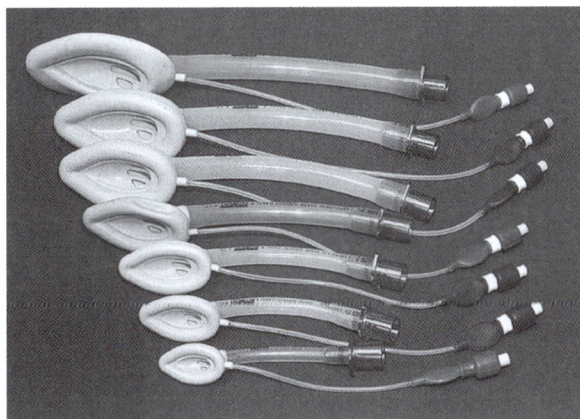

FIGURE 15.3 Endotracheal tubes.

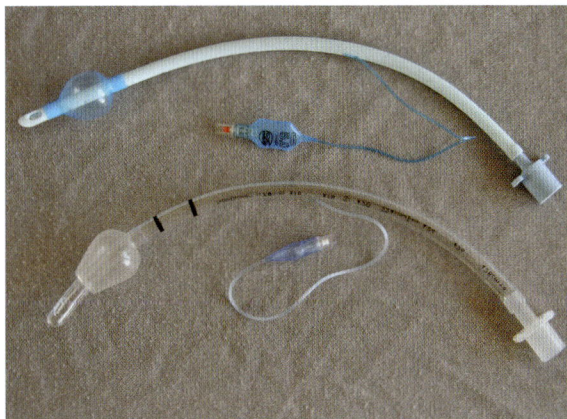

Endotracheal tubes reinforced with a wire coil embedded within the plastic along the entire tube length prevent kinking and occlusion. These tubes are more commonly used in the operating room.[29] The wire coils can be irreversibly compressed by a strong bite occluding the airway. Reinforced tubes also increase the risk of tracheal damage and should be replaced with a standard ETT on ICU arrival. Most ETTs have a 'Murphy eye', an oval-shaped hole in the side of the tube between the cuff and the tube end that provides a patent aperture if the distal opening is occluded.[30]

Preparation for intubation

Adequate preparation of the patient, equipment and environment, as well as knowledge of emergency procedures, is important to ensure safe and efficient intubation. Up to 50% of patients undergoing endotracheal intubation in the ICU experience complications; 28% will have a serious complication, including hypoxaemia, circulatory collapse, cardiac arrhythmia, cardiac arrest, oesophageal intubation, aspiration and death.[31]

Patient preparation

If appropriate, and time permits, explain the procedure to the patient and family. Prepare the patient with:

- reliable intravenous access established to allow rapid fluid and drug administration
- accurate blood pressure monitoring (preferably intra-arterial)
- continuous oxygen saturation and ECG monitoring
- nasogastric tube (if in situ) aspirated and placed on free drainage
- positioning supine in the 'sniff' position.

Equipment and drugs

All equipment should be available and checked immediately prior to intubation, including:

- oxygen supply
- suction supply, with a range of Yankauer and y-suction catheters/closed suction device
- laryngoscope blades and compatible holder, with a functioning light
- appropriately-sized face mask
- manual ventilation (Ambu bag™) attached to oxygen supply
- ETT cuff inflated in sterile water to ensure no leaks and even inflation
- water-based lubricant applied to tube and cuff (while maintaining sterility)
- capnography (chemical CO_2 detectors are often used in emergency situations)
- ventilator and circuit
- emergency/resuscitation trolley at bedside
- gloves, eye protection
- drugs (sedative and muscle relaxant).

> **Practice tip**
>
> During intubation, know who to call for help, and do not hesitate to do so.

Procedure

The patient is preoxygenated to minimise desaturation during apnoea and laryngoscopy, commonly via bag and mask, although other methods such as non-invasive ventilation have been suggested.[32] The practice of apnoeic oxygenation during endotracheal intubation through the administration of 15 litres per minute via nasal cannula has become very popular in emergency departments. To date, there is insufficient evidence to recommend its routine use during endotracheal intubation in the critically ill. Intubation in ICU is usually performed via laryngoscopy with insertion of an oral ETT. Intubation may be performed using a fibre optic bronchoscope when difficulty is encountered, or for nasal intubation.

Oral vs nasal intubation

Oral intubation is preferred unless there are specific indications for nasal intubation. Oral intubation is easier to perform and allows use of a larger diameter ETT. While nasal intubation provides better splinting for the ETT and facilitates oral hygiene, it can damage nasal structures, is contraindicated in skull fractures and increases the risk of maxillary sinusitis and ventilator-associated pneumonia (VAP).[33]

Cricoid pressure

The cricoid cartilage, situated below the thyroid prominence, is a closed tracheal ring which, when compressed, closes the oesophagus while the trachea remains open. Cricoid pressure is performed by placing the thumb on one side of the patient's trachea, middle finger on the other side and index finger directly on the cricoid.[34] Although widely used, its efficacy is questionable as technique is frequently poor,[35] and there is wide anatomical variation in the exact orientation of the oesophagus in relation to the trachea.[36]

Backwards, upwards, rightward pressure manoeuvre

The backwards, upwards, rightward pressure (BURP) manoeuvre on the thyroid cartilage was introduced in the mid-1990s to improve visualisation during difficult laryngoscopy. The patient's jaw is thrust forward, so the head is in the 'sniffing' position. The thumb and third finger are placed on either side of the thyroid cartilage and the index finger on top. Pressure is applied in the sequence **b**ackwards (towards the spine), **u**pwards (towards the head), **r**ightward (towards the patient's right side). This is easier to perform following administration of muscle relaxants.

Cuff management

Endotracheal and tracheostomy tube cuffs prevent airway contamination by pharyngeal secretions and gastric contents and loss of V_T during mechanical ventilation. The cuff does not secure the tube in the trachea.

Confirmation of tube position

The correct position of the ETT distal end is 3–5 cm above the carina. A lip level of 20 cm for women and 22 cm for men should prevent endobronchial intubation, with the proximal end fixed at either the centre or side of the mouth.[37] Confirmation of the ETT position is required immediately following intubation and at regular intervals thereafter as tube movement can occur.

Chest auscultation and observation of chest expansion to confirm ETT position is unreliable, as the chest may appear to rise with oesophageal intubation. Conversely, the chest may not rise with a correctly positioned tube if the patient is obese or has a rigid chest wall. Patients with left main bronchus intubation may exhibit bilateral breath sounds.[38] End-tidal CO_2 monitoring is the 'gold standard' method for confirming ETT placement (see Chapter 13 for further information on end-tidal CO_2 monitoring). Disposable devices that change colour in the presence of CO_2 are inexpensive and easy to use, but may be inaccurate during cardiopulmonary resuscitation, or if contaminated. Capnography is the most reliable technique to identify ETT placement in both arrest and non-arrest situations.[24] Continuous end-tidal CO_2 monitoring during intubation is recommended as a minimum standard by the College of Intensive Care Medicine of Australia and New Zealand (CICM).[39]

Practice tip

Always ensure there is someone who is skilled at intubation immediately available when extubating a patient.

Tracheostomy

Tracheostomy may be required for upper airway obstruction, although it is most commonly performed for ICU patients requiring prolonged mechanical ventilation. The advantages of tracheostomy over endotracheal intubation include: decreased risk of laryngeal damage and subglottic stenosis; reduced airway resistance and dead space, which decreases the work of breathing and therefore supports weaning;[40] and improved patient tolerance enabling sedation reduction. The optimum time to perform tracheostomy remains contentious, and is often influenced by patient diagnosis.[41]

Procedure

Tracheostomy can be performed using a surgical or percutaneous dilatational technique. Percutaneous dilatation is contraindicated in patients with anatomical anomalies of the neck and serious bleeding disorders, and should be undertaken with caution in patients who are obese, have a cervical spine injury, coagulopathy, difficult airway or require high levels of ventilatory support.[42] Percutaneous dilatation is more commonly performed than the surgical technique in Australian and New Zealand ICUs.[42]

A variety of tracheostomy tubes are available that facilitate secretion clearance, communication and differing patient anatomy. Inner cannulae (re-usable or disposable) prevent secretion build up on the tracheostomy tube, while fenestrated and talking tracheostomies facilitate communication, as do one-way speaking valves, such as the Passy-Muir® valve, used with the cuff deflated.

Tracheostomy care

The aim of tracheostomy care is to keep the stoma free of infection, and prevent tube blockage or dislodgement. The stoma is cleaned with normal saline and fixation devices are changed at least 12-hourly with two nurses required to safely perform changes.[43] Velcro tapes are easier to change and more comfortable than cotton tape.[44] Lint-free or superabsorbent foam dressings are used under the flange to absorb secretions. Adequate humidification and suctioning will usually prevent tube obstruction (see later in this chapter). The use of inner cannulae has obviated the need for frequent tracheostomy tube changes. Single lumen (no inner cannula) tracheostomy tubes should be changed every 7–10 days.[43]

Complications of endotracheal intubation and tracheostomy

Tube blockage, tube dislodgement and aspiration are major complications. Partial ETT or tracheostomy tube dislodgement can cause greater harm than complete removal because of delays in diagnosis and resultant aspiration and worsening gas exchange. Tube dislodgement is most likely to occur when turning the patient, in agitated patients or when nursing staff are distracted or on breaks.[45] While physical restraint may be considered to prevent tube dislodgement, multiple studies noted patients were restrained when self-extubation or device removal occurred.[46–51] Appropriate levels of analgesia and sedation are therefore required for minimising self-extubation risk.

Complications during, and immediately after, endotracheal intubation and tracheostomy include cardiovascular compromise, bleeding, tracheal wall injury, vocal cord damage, pneumothorax, pneumomediastinum and subcutaneous emphysema. Late complications of tracheostomy include tracheal stenosis, tracheomalacia and tracheo-oesophageal fistula and infection. As noted earlier, damage to the trachea is exacerbated by high cuff pressures.[52] Percutaneous tracheostomy results in fewer wound infections, decreased incidence of bleeding and reduced mortality compared to surgical tracheostomy.[53]

Managing endotracheal and tracheostomy tubes

Tracheal suction

Patients with an ETT or tracheostomy tube require tracheal suction to remove pulmonary secretions that can lead to atelectasis or airway obstruction and impair gas exchange.[54] Suction should be performed as clinically indicated, with assessment of visible or audible secretions, rising inspiratory pressure, decreasing V_T or increased work of breathing.[55] A sawtooth pattern on the flow–volume waveform may also indicate the need for suction.[56]

Preoxygenation using a FiO_2 of 1.0 for approximately 60 seconds prior to suctioning is commonly performed though not supported by strong evidence unless the patient is experiencing hypoxia or has compromised cerebral circulation.[57] Preoxygenation of patients without hypoxia should be avoided as it may cause harm associated with oxygen toxicity. If a patient's oxygen saturation declines to an unacceptable level during suctioning, the FiO_2 should be increased to 1.0. Manual hyperinflation should be discouraged due to the risk of haemodynamic compromise, derecruitment and barotrauma and lack of evidence of benefit.[58] Similarly, installation of saline is not supported due to increased risk of flushing pathogens into distal lung regions.[59]

Methods

The three methods of suctioning are:

1 Open suction: a suction catheter is passed under aseptic technique directly into the ETT/tracheostomy after disconnection from the ventilator circuit. Disadvantages include loss of PEEP resulting in alveolar derecruitment and increased risk of transmission of infective organisms. A surgical mask and protective eyewear should be worn.[60]

2 Semi-closed suction: a suction catheter is passed through a swivel connector with a self-sealing rubber flange.

3 Closed suction: an in-line system is attached between the ETT/tracheostomy tube and the ventilator circuit where the suction catheter is contained in an integrated plastic sleeve. Alveolar derecruitment occurs to a lesser degree than with open suction.

There is no difference between techniques in relation to development of VAP and quantity of secretions removed.

The suction catheter diameter should not be greater than half the airway diameter, using the formula: suction catheter size [French] = (ETT size [mm] − 1) × 2. The suction catheter should be inserted to the carina, then withdrawn 2 cm before suction is applied to prevent damage. Suction should only last 15 seconds, using continuous, rather than intermittent, suction. Suction pressure should be set as low as possible with <150 mmHg recommended for adults and <100 mmHg for neonates.[59] Use of ETTs or tracheostomy tubes with integrated subglottic suction ports may assist in preventing VAP, especially when performed with other prevention strategies such as semirecumbant positioning and good cuff seal management.

Adverse effects

Adverse effects of suctioning include hypoxaemia, introduction of infective organisms, tracheal trauma, bradycardia,

hypertension and increased intracranial pressure. Tracheal suctioning causes discomfort, and should therefore be performed only when clinically indicated, such as audible presence of secretions, desaturation and when a sawtooth pattern is observed on the flow–time scalar and flow/volume loop.[57,58]

Securing endotracheal and tracheostomy tubes

The purpose of ETT and tracheostomy tube fixation is to maintain the tube in the correct position, prevent unintended extubation or dislodgement and facilitate mechanical ventilation while maintaining skin integrity and oral hygiene.[61] ETT fixation methods include:

- tying cotton tape around the tube, then around the neck
- taping the tube to the face using medical adhesive tape
- commercial tube holders of varying designs.

There is no evidence supporting a preferred method[62] with each having specific strengths and weaknesses. A manikin study comparing cotton tapes with the Thomas™ Endotracheal Tube Holder demonstrated less ETT movement with the commercial tube holder.[63] Two nurses are required to prevent ETT dislodgement during fixation. Although there is also no evidence recommending a preferred frequency, ETT fixation is generally changed at least daily, to allow assessment of the underlying skin with particular attention to the ears and corners of the mouth and to facilitate oral hygiene.[61] The ETT position in the mouth is alternated at this time.

> **Practice tip**
>
> Adhesive devices may become dislodged as facial hair grows under them.

Cuff pressure management

Cuff inflation pressures should be maintained at 20–30 cmH_2O (15–22 mmHg). Tracheal wall damage may occur if cuff pressure exceeds tracheal capillary perfusion pressure (27–40 cmH_2O/20–30 mmHg). Cuff inflation pressures ≤20 cmH_2O (≤15 mmHg) are associated with an increased risk of aspiration and a 2.5-fold increase in VAP.[64]

There are four methods for assessing cuff inflation:

1 minimal occluding volume
2 minimal leak test
3 cuff pressure measurement
4 palpation.

In Australia and New Zealand, cuff pressure measurement is most commonly used,[65] in contrast to the UK[66] and North America[67] where it is used less frequently. Cuff pressure measurement requires a manometer attached to the pilot balloon. Cuff pressure varies with head and body position, tube position and airway pressures.[68,69]

The optimum frequency of cuff pressure monitoring is unclear; at a minimum it should be done post-intubation, on arrival in ICU and once per nursing shift. Recently, continuous cuff pressure measurement has been shown to reduce VAP.[70] Even with appropriate cuff inflation, micro-aspiration occurs via the longitudinal folds in the cuff.[71]

If performing minimal occluding volume and minimal leak tests, aspiration should be prevented by semirecumbent positioning, suctioning the back of the mouth (as far back as tolerated), aspiration of the nasogastric tube and discontinuation of feeds before cuff deflation.

Subglottic secretion management

For the intubated patient, oropharyngeal secretions drain into the subglottic space, pool above the cuff and gradually leak via the longitudinal cuff folds to the lungs increasing the risk of pneumonia. Subglottic secretion drainage, a dedicated lumen within the ETT dorsal wall that exits above the cuff, enables removal of subglottic secretions either continuously via low pressure suction or intermittently via suction or a syringe.[27] A recent systematic review and meta-analysis found subglottic secretion drainage reduced the risk of VAP by 48% though there was no evidence of effect on ICU or hospital mortality or duration of ventilation.[72]

Managing emergencies associated with endotracheal and tracheostomy tubes

Pilot tube

If the pilot tube for the ETT or tracheostomy tube is accidentally cut or a hole is suspected in the tubing or balloon, cannulate the tubing with a 23- or 24-gauge needle to reinflate the cuff and clamp the tubing. If using a clamp with serrations, place gauze between the tube and the clamps to avoid further damage to the pilot tube.

Cuff herniation

ETT cuff herniation occurs infrequently with low pressure high volume cuffs, may be difficult to diagnose, but can cause life-threatening bronchial obstruction.[73] If cuff herniation is suspected (profound desaturation, loss of breath sounds), deflate and reinflate the cuff, checking the cuff pressure is within normal range. If the problem persists the tube will need changing.

Persistent cuff leaks

Cuff leaks may be categorised as leaks around an intact cuff or those due to structural damage to the cuff.[74] Structural damage generally requires replacement of the tube, particularly if leaks are large and ventilation is ineffective.

> **Practice tip**
>
> A persistent cuff leak as indicated by bubbling or other noises suggestive of gas leak and loss of V_T or cuff pressures of ≥30 cmH$_2$O (≥22 mmHg) indicating failure to generate a seal should be reviewed. Check ETT position for migration and refer to medical staff.

Extubation

Following successful weaning from mechanical ventilation (see later in this chapter), assessment of the patient prior to extubation should indicate adequate gas exchange, respiratory rate and work of breathing on minimal support; respiratory muscle strength; the ability to cough and clear secretions spontaneously; and a stable haemodynamic status and mental status.[75] Serious post-extubation complications of laryngospasm and stridor cannot be reliably predicted,[76] so the ease/grade of intubation should be considered prior to extubation and provision made for immediate reintubation.[77]

Mechanical ventilation

The most recent international study of mechanical ventilation practices, reporting data from 4968 patients in 349 ICUs and 23 countries, found the median duration of ventilation was 4 days (interquartile range 2–8 days).[78] In this patient cohort the three most common reasons for mechanical ventilation were postoperative respiratory failure, coma and pneumonia. This international report did not include data from Australia and New Zealand. As stated in the introduction, 41% of patients in Australian and New Zealand ICUs received invasive mechanical ventilation and 8% received NIV in 2012–13.[1] The median duration of invasive mechanical ventilation for these patients was 2.5 days. A study describing ventilation and weaning practices of 55 ICUs in Australia and New Zealand in 2005 reported a similar profile as international studies for the most common indications for mechanical ventilation.[79]

Principles of mechanical ventilation

Mechanical ventilation describes the application of positive or negative pressure breaths using non-invasive or invasive techniques. Indications for initiation of mechanical ventilation are discussed below. Table 15.1 lists the patient parameters typically observed in acute and chronic respiratory failure that may influence the decision to ventilate. During positive pressure ventilation, the type of ventilation used most commonly in critical care, the ventilator delivers a flow of gas into the lungs during inspiration using a pneumatic system. Expiration is passive.

The equation of motion

The equation of motion for the respiratory system is a mathematical model that relates pressure, volume and flow during breath delivery, with the pressure required to deliver a volume of gas determined by the elastic and resistive properties of the respiratory system[80] (see Table 15.2).

Compliance and elastance

Compliance refers to the ease with which lung units distend. Elastance is the tendency of the lung units to return to their original form once stretched. Compliance is defined as the change in volume that occurs due to a change in pressure and is expressed as $C = \Delta V/\Delta P$.

TABLE 15.1

Physiological indications suggesting the need for mechanical ventilation

PARAMETER	NORMAL VALUES	ARF	CRF	ASSOCIATED SIGNS AND SYMPTOMS
Respiratory rate	12–20	≥28	≥30	Dyspnoea, increased activation of accessory muscles and active expiration
pH	7.35–7.45	<7.30 No compensatory changes	7.35–7.40 May be normal due to metabolic compensation	Failure to adequately ventilate: elevated $PaCO_2$, acidic pH, headache, confusion or other mental status change, tachypnoea (RR >30), flushed skin
$PaCO_2$	35–45 mmHg	>50 mmHg and rising	>50 mmHg and rising	
PaO_2	80–100 mmHg	<65 mmHg and falling	<50 mmHg and falling Hb/HCT elevated as compensatory mechanism	Failure to adequately oxygenate: decreased PaO_2 and SpO_2, tachycardia, hyper- or hypotension, dyspnoea, gasping, nasal flaring, use of accessory muscles, anxiety, agitation and altered mental status, cyanosis
HCO_3^-	22–26 mmol/L	Within normal limits	If chronic hypercapnia, then HCO_3^- >26 mmol/L is a compensatory mechanism If CRF is primarily failure to oxygenate, then HCO_3^- will be within normal limits	

ARF = acute respiratory failure; CRF = chronic respiratory failure; HCT = haematocrit; RR = respiratory rate.

TABLE 15.2

Equation of motion

EQUATION:

$$P_T (P_{AIRWAY} + P_{MUSCLE}) = V_T/C + V_T/T_I \times R + PEEP_T$$

Abbreviations	P_T = total pressure – the sum of the pressure in the proximal airway and the pressure generated by the respiratory muscles V_T = tidal volume C = compliance T_I = inspiratory time R = resistance $PEEP_T$ = total positive end-expiratory pressure – alveolar pressure at the end of expiration and is the sum of PEEP applied by the ventilator and any intrinsic (auto) PEEP
Notes	V_T/C: describes the elastic properties of the respiratory system V_T/T_I: reflects flow in the system $V_T/T_I \times R$: resistance of the respiratory system

Lung tissue and the surrounding thoracic structures contribute to respiratory compliance. Normal compliance for a mechanically ventilated patient ranges from 35 to 50 mL/cmH$_2$O.[81]

Resistance

Resistance refers to the forces that oppose airflow. Resistance in the airways is affected by their diameter and length (including the artificial airway), the gas flow rate and the density and viscosity of the inspired gas. During mechanical ventilation, bronchospasm, airway oedema, endotracheal tube lumen size, increased secretions and inappropriate setting of flow rates can influence airway resistance. Normal resistance for intubated patients is 6 cmH$_2$O/(L/s).[81]

Ventilator graphics

Analysis of ventilator graphics provides clinicians with the ability to assess patient–ventilator interaction, appropriateness of ventilator settings and lung function.

Scalars: Pressure/time, flow/time, volume/time

Many ventilators now offer integrated graphic displays as waveforms that plot one of three parameters, pressure, flow or volume, on the vertical (y) axis against time, measured in seconds, on the horizontal (x) axis referred to as scalars. Examination of scalars can assist with assessment of patient–ventilator synchrony, patient triggering, appropriateness of inspiratory/expiratory times, presence of gas trapping, appropriateness and adequacy of flow, lung compliance and airway resistance and circuit leaks.[82, 83]

Pressure vs time scalar

The morphology of this waveform depends on the control variable (volume or pressure), breath type (mandatory or spontaneous) and whether the breath is initiated by the ventilator or the patient's inspiratory effort.[84] Pressure–time waveforms reflect airway pressure (P_{aw}) during inspiration and expiration and can be used to evaluate peak and plateau inspiratory pressures and end-expiratory pressures, inspiratory and expiratory times and appropriateness of flow (see Figure 15.4). The peak pressure represents the maximum pressure achieved during inspiration. The plateau pressure is measured during an inspiratory hold and represents the pressure applied to the small airways and alveoli. The expiratory pressure is the pressure measured once the patient has expired. Pressure–time scalars vary in appearance depending on the control variable (volume vs pressure). In *volume-control breaths* (see Figure 15.4) the inspiratory waveform continues to rise until peak inspiratory pressure is achieved according to V_T set. If an inspiratory hold is applied a plateau pressure will be generated. As the patient expires airway pressure will drop back to the set PEEP level. *In pressure control breaths*, the inspiratory waveform reaches its peak at the beginning of inspiration and remains at this elevation until cycling to expiration.

FIGURE 15.4 Pressure, flow, volume and time waveforms.

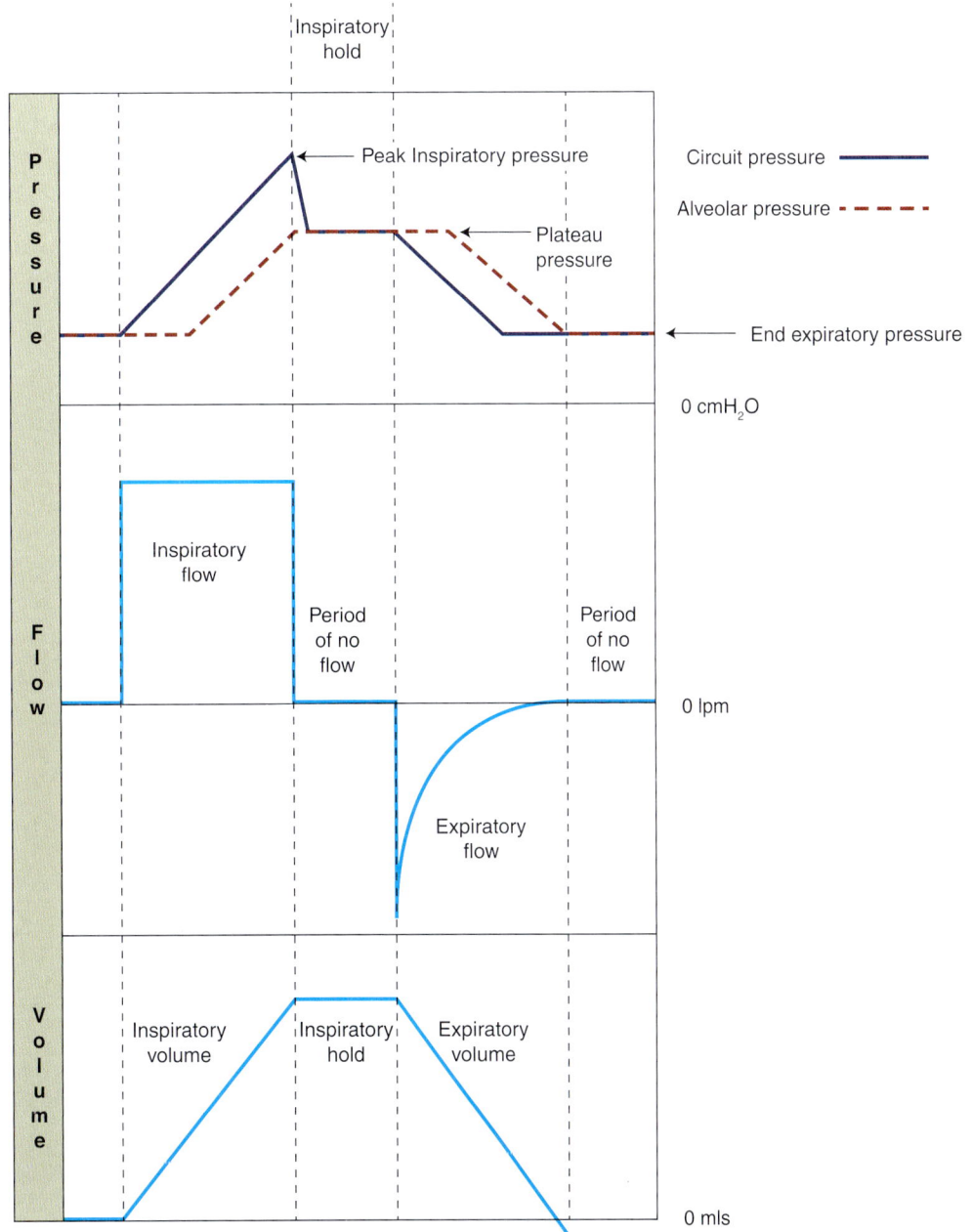

When interpreting the pressure waveform it is important to recognise that the graphic waveforms display circuit pressure, which does not always represent alveolar pressure. Periods of no flow (inspiratory and expiratory holds/pauses) are required to estimate alveolar pressure. The plateau pressure is a more reliable estimate of inspiratory alveolar pressure than the peak inspiratory pressure. An expiratory hold is required to determine end-expiratory alveolar pressure. Estimating alveolar pressure may be useful to assess the patient's respiratory resistance and compliance. Comparing the difference between the peak inspiratory pressure and plateau pressure can give an indication of the patient's inspiratory resistance. Comparing the difference between the plateau pressure and the end-expiratory pressure can provide information about the patient's compliance. A large difference between peak and plateau pressures indicates high airway resistance. An elevated plateau pressure indicates reduced compliance.

Spontaneous triggering of ventilation can be identified by examination of the pressure–time scalar at the beginning of inspiration. A small negative deflection indicates patient effort. When pressure-triggering is used, a breath is triggered when the pressure drops below baseline. The depth of the deflection is proportional to patient effort required to trigger inspiration (see Figure 15.5). A flow-triggered breath occurs when the flow rises above baseline, although this is frequently accompanied by a small negative deflection in the pressure–time scalar. Patient inspiratory attempts that fail to trigger the ventilator can also be identified as negative deflections in the pressure waveform without corresponding responses from the ventilator.[85] Appropriateness of flow can be detected from the pressure–time scalar. If the flow is set too high or the rise time is too short this can be seen as a sharp peak in the waveform (see Figure 15.5). Conversely, if flow is inadequate or the rise time is too long, the incline of the inspiratory portion of the pressure waveform may be dampened or even negative.[82]

Flow vs time scalar

The flow–time scalar presents the inspiratory phase above the horizontal axis and the expiratory phase below (see Figure 15.6). The shape of the inspiratory flow waveform is influenced by the selection of flow pattern (constant, decelerating, sinusoidal) in volume-control breaths or the variable and decelerating flow waveform associated with pressure-control breaths. The inspiratory flow waveform of spontaneous breaths, those triggered and cycled by the patient, is influenced by the presence or absence of pressure support and the expiratory sensitivity.[82]

Evaluation of the expiratory limb of the flow–time scalar assists with detection of gas trapping and the patient's response to bronchodilators. In the absence of gas trapping, the expiratory limb drops sharply below baseline then gradually returns to zero before the next breath. Failure to return to baseline indicates gas trapping whereby the inspired gas is not totally expired. Gas trapping results in development of intrinsic or 'auto-PEEP'. This can adversely affect a patient's haemodynamic

FIGURE 15.5 Triggering and rise time.

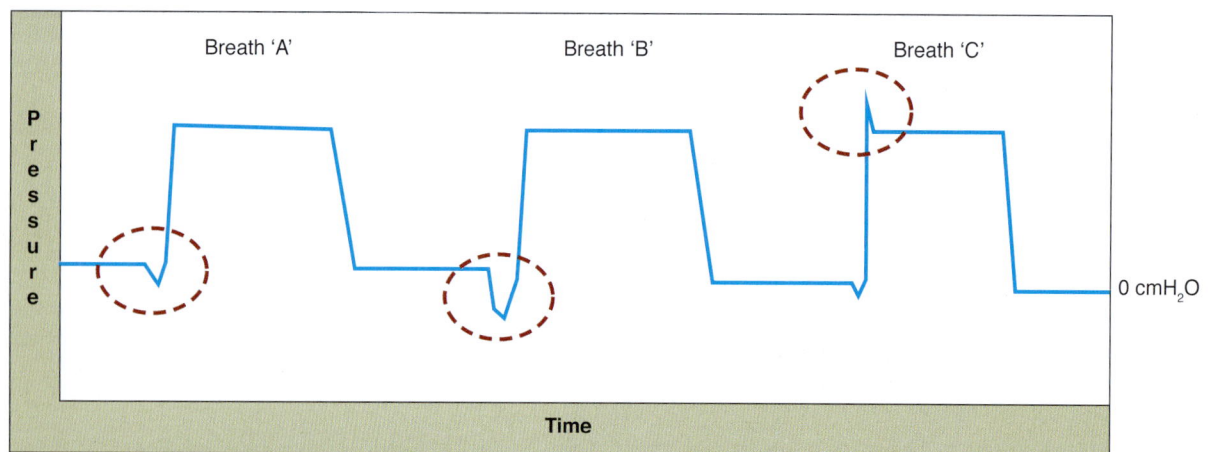

Pressure time scalar demonstrating:

1) how negative dips in pressure prior to the breath are indicative of patient effort required to trigger inspiration. Compare the drop in pressure in breath 'A' to breath 'B'. The greater drop in pressure in breath 'B' indicates a greater patient effort to trigger gas flow.

2) the effect on the pressure time scalar when the rise time is set too short. Note the 'overshoot' in the pressure waveform on breath 'C'. This sometimes occurs in patients with a high airway resistance (e.g. acute severe asthma) and a short rise time. It is questionable whether this pressure overshoot has any effect on the patient but it can trigger the high-pressure alarm and compromise ventilation.

FIGURE 15.6 Flow vs time waveform.

Unbel	Flow wave pattern	Description
(Rectangular, square)	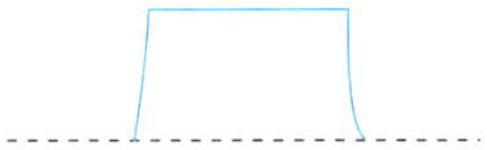	Peak flow rate is delivered immediately at the onset of inspiration, maintained throughout the inspiratory phase, and abruptly terminated at the onset of expiration.
		Common default pattern with volume-targeted modes.
Sinusoidal	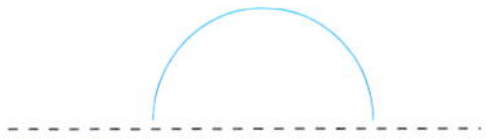	Inspiratory flow rate gradually accelerates to peak flow and then tapers off.
		Believed to mimic spontaneous inspiratory patterns.
		May increase peak inspiratory pressure (PIP).
Accelerating (ascending ramp)	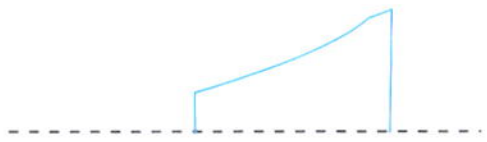	Flow gradually accelerates in a linear fashion to the set peak flow rate.
Decelerating (descending ramp)	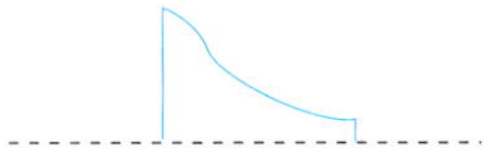	Flow is at peak at onset of inspiration and gradually decelerates throughout inspiratory phase.
		Flow ceases and ventilator cycles to expiratory phase when flow decays to a percentage of peak flow, usually 25% but varies by ventilator model. Terminal flow criteria may be adjustable in some newer ventilators.
		Rapid intial flow raises mean airway pressure and may assist in alveolar recruitment.
		May improve the distribution of gases when there is inhomogeneity of alveolar ventilation.
		Decreases dead space, increases arterial oxygen tension, and reduces PIP.

status and cause patient–ventilator asynchrony.[86] Gas trapping may occur in patients with airflow limitation such as those with COPD and asthma. Consequences of gas trapping include dynamic hyperinflation, reduced respiratory compliance and respiratory muscle fatigue.[87] Evaluation of the expiratory flow waveform also enables evaluation of the effects of bronchodilator therapy as, if efficacious, the expiratory flow waveform will return to baseline (see Figure 15.7).[86] Patient–ventilator asynchrony can be detected in the flow waveform as abrupt decreases in expiratory flow in the expiratory limb and abrupt increases in flow in the inspiratory limb.[85]

Volume vs time scalar

The volume–time waveform originates from the functional residual capacity (baseline), rises as inspiratory flow is delivered to reach the maximum inspiratory V_T then returns to baseline during expiration. The volume waveform is useful in troubleshooting circuit leaks (see Figure 15.8) as it will fail to return to baseline if a leak in the circuit–patient interface is present.

Loops: Pressure/volume, flow/volume

Most contemporary critical care ventilators allow for monitoring of pressure, flow and volume parameters integrated into graphic loops enabling measurement of airway resistance, chest wall and lung compliance.

Pressure–volume loops

The two parameters, P_{aw} and V_T are plotted against each other, with P_{aw} on the x axis. For mandatory breaths, the loop is drawn counterclockwise (see Figure 15.9). Spontaneous (triggered and cycled) breaths are drawn in a clockwise fashion. When low gas flow is delivered and the patient is unable to initiate ventilation, pressure–volume loops may be used to identify the lower and upper inflection points. The lower inflection point begins near the beginning of inspiration as the P_{aw} starts to rise with little change in V_T. As P_{aw} continues to rise, the V_T increases exponentially as alveoli are recruited, resulting in a marked increase in the inspiratory limb slope. This point represents alveolar recruitment and is referred to

FIGURE 15.7 AutoPEEP and gas trapping.

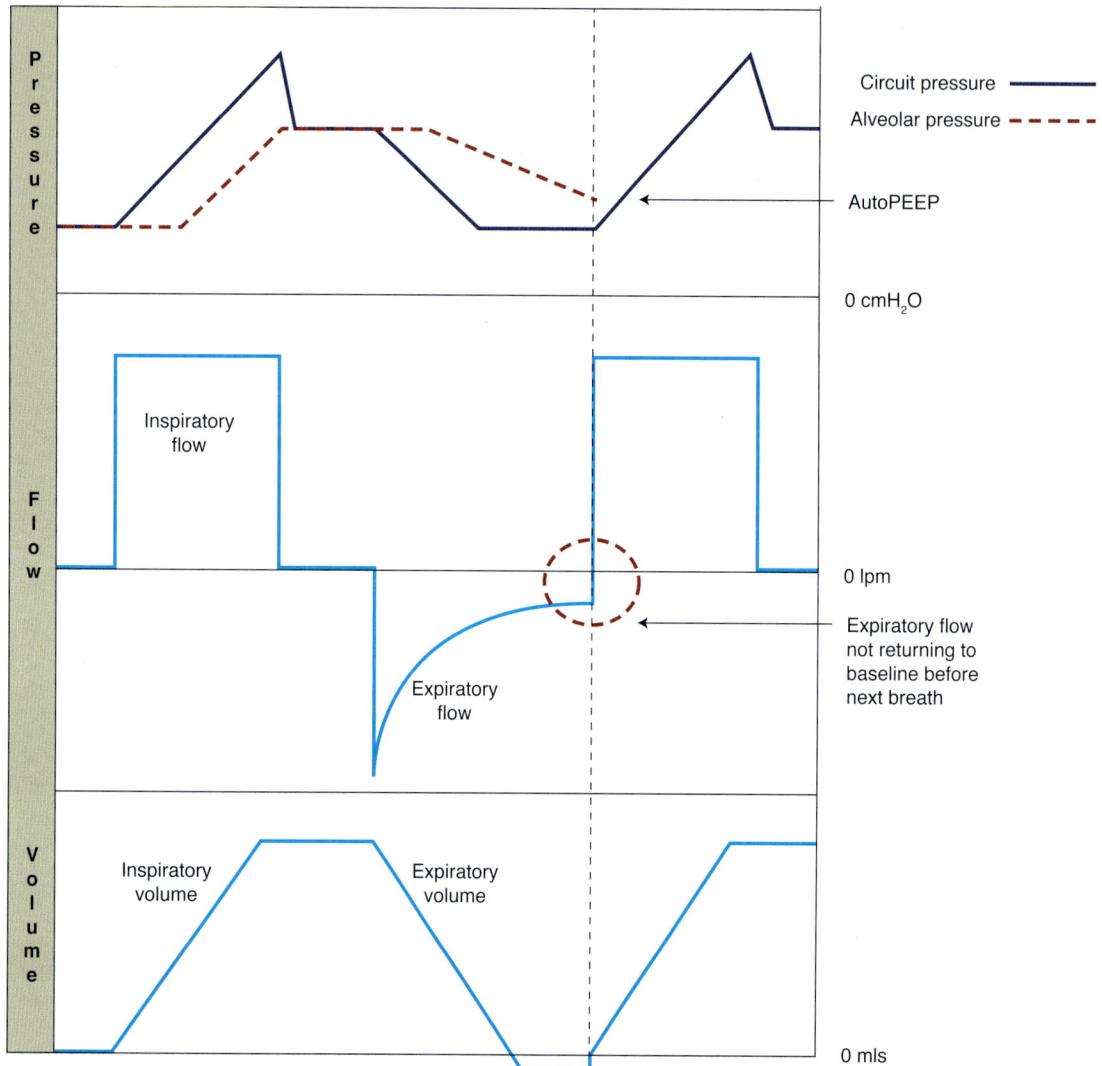

Circuit pressure ————
Alveolar pressure – – – –

AutoPEEP

0 cmH$_2$O

Inspiratory flow

Expiratory flow

0 lpm

Expiratory flow not returning to baseline before next breath

Inspiratory volume

Expiratory volume

0 mls

This diagram demonstrates the use of the flow pressure scalar to identify the presence of autoPEEP. In the area highlighted by the circle with the dashed line the expiratory flow has not returned to zero before the onset of the next breath. This indicates that gas trapping has occurred and the pressure in the alveoli is greater than the pressure in the ventilator circuit. This indicates the presence of 'autoPEEP' or inadvertent PEEP.

FIGURE 15.8 Tidal volume vs time, with and without leak.

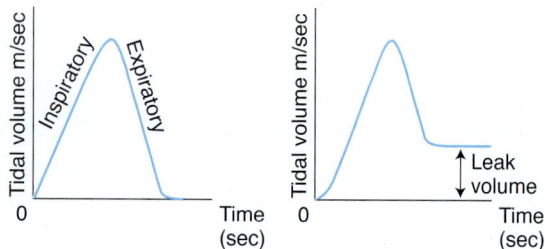

as the lower inflection point, and may be used to guide PEEP selection.[88,89] The inspiratory limb continues until peak inspiratory pressure and maximal V$_T$ are achieved. The bend in the inspiratory limb towards the end of inspiration is referred to as the upper inflection point, and denotes the point at which small volume increases produce large pressure increases indicating lung overdistension.[88] The expiratory limb represents lung derecruitment and is also useful in guiding PEEP selection.[90,91]

For patient-triggered mandatory breaths, the initial part of the loop occurs to the left of the *y* axis and flows

FIGURE 15.9 Pressure–volume loop.

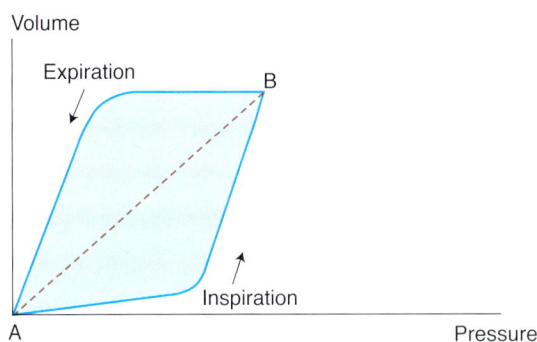

Adapted from Dräegerwerk AG & Co. Available from: http://www.draeger.com/sites/assets/Publixhingimages/Products/savina-300/UK/9097421-Fibel-Curves_Loops-en.pdf, p 26, with permission.

in a clockwise fashion, reflecting patient effort. The loop then shifts to the right of the *y* axis and moves in a counterclockwise fashion as the ventilator assumes the work of breathing.[81] Pressure–volume loops reflect dynamic compliance between the lungs and the ventilator circuit. Decreased compliance requires greater pressure to achieve V_T and is reflected in a flattened pressure–volume loop.[92] The area between the loops represents the resistance to inspiration and expiration, known as hysteresis. As resistance increases, less V_T is delivered resulting in a shorter and wider loop; conversely, as resistance decreases, a longer, wider loop is generated (see Figure 15.10).[93]

Flow–volume loops

Flow–volume loops recorded during positive pressure ventilation depict inspiration above the baseline and expiration below it. These loops are useful in determining response to bronchodilators and examining changes in airway resistance.

FIGURE 15.10 Pressure–volume loop representing resistance changes.

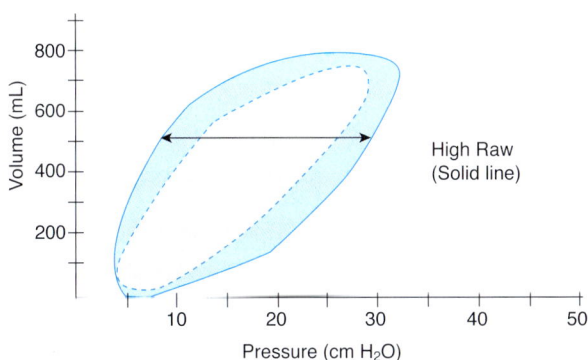

*Dashed line depicts normal Raw

Ventilator circuits

Delivery of mechanical ventilation requires a ventilator circuit to transport gas flow to the patient. To prevent condensation from cooling of warm humidified gas, inspired gas is heated via a wire inside the circuit wall in either the inspiratory limb alone or both the inspiratory and expiratory limbs.[94] Historically, ventilator circuits were changed frequently (48–72 hours) to decrease the risk of VAP.[95] Current guidelines for VAP prevention found evidence that the frequency of ventilator circuit changes had no relationship to the VAP incidence and, therefore, recommended routine circuit changes were not necessary and circuits should only be changed when soiled or damaged.[96]

Humidification

Humidification warms and moistens gas to facilitate cilia action and mucus removal as well as to prevent drying and irritation of respiratory mucosa and solidification of secretions. During endotracheal intubation and mechanical ventilation, the normal humidification processes of the nasopharynx are bypassed. This, in combination with the use of dry medical gas at high flow rates, means alternative methods of humidification are required. The best conditions for mucosal health and function over prolonged periods are when inspired gas is warmed to core body temperature and is fully saturated with water.[97]

Absolute and relative humidity

Absolute humidity refers to the amount of water vapour in a given volume of gas at a given temperature. Absolute humidity rises with increasing temperature; during mechanical ventilation gas is heated to increase the amount of water vapour it will hold. Relative humidity is expressed as a percentage, and is the actual amount of water vapour in a gas compared to the maximum amount this gas can hold (ratio of absolute to maximal humidity). Ideal humidification is achieved when the:

1 inspired gas delivered into the trachea is at 37°C with a water content of 30–43 g/m^3 (relative humidity is 100% at 37°C in the bronchi)

2 set temperature remains constant without fluctuation

3 humidification and temperature are unaffected by large or differing types of gas flow

4 device is simple to use

5 humidifier can be used with spontaneously breathing and ventilated patients

6 safety alarms prevent overheating, overhydration and electrocution

7 resistance, compliance and dead space characteristics do not adversely affect spontaneous breathing modes

8 sterility of the inspired gas is not compromised.[98]

Humidification is applied using either a heat–moisture exchanger (HME) or a heated water bath reservoir device in combination with a heated ventilator circuit.

Heat–moisture exchanger

HMEs conserve heat and moisture during expiration enabling inspired gas to be heated and humidified. Two types of HMEs exist: hygroscopic and hydrophobic. Hygroscopic HMEs absorb moisture onto a chemically impregnated foam or paper material and have been shown to be more effective than hydrophobic HMEs.[99] HMEs are placed distally to the circuit Y-piece in line with the ETT and increase dead space by an amount equal to their internal volume.[100] HMEs should be changed every 24 hours or when soiled with secretions and are usually reserved for short-term humidification.

Heated humidification

Generally, heated humidification is used for patients requiring more than 24 hours of mechanical ventilation. Various models of heater bases and circuits are on the market and we recommend their use in accordance with manufacturer instructions. A recent systematic review and meta-analysis reported no overall effect on artificial airway occlusion, mortality, pneumonia or respiratory complications when HMEs were compared to heated humidification, although it noted that the $PaCO_2$ and minute ventilation were increased and body temperature was lower with the use of HMEs.[101]

Non-invasive ventilation

NIV is an umbrella term describing the delivery of mechanical ventilation without the use of an invasive airway, via an interface such as an oronasal, nasal or full-face mask or helmet. NIV techniques include both negative and positive pressure ventilation, although in critical care positive pressure ventilation is primarily used.

Terminology

Positive pressure NIV can be further categorised as non-invasive positive pressure ventilation (NIPPV) or continuous positive airway pressure (CPAP). NIPPV is the provision of inspiratory pressure support, also referred to as inspiratory positive airway pressure (IPAP), usually in combination with positive end-expiratory pressure (PEEP). PEEP is also referred to as expiratory positive airway pressure (EPAP). CPAP does not actively assist inspiration but provides a constant positive airway pressure throughout inspiration and expiration.[102]

The terms biphasic (or bilevel) positive airway pressure (BiPAP®) and non-invasive pressure support ventilation (NIPSV) are also used to refer to NIPPV.[103] The acronym BiPAP® is registered to Respironics (Murrayville, PA), a company that produces non-invasive ventilators including the BiPAP® Vision, which is commonly used in the ICU. The acronym NIPSV is primarily used in European descriptions of NIPPV.

Physiological benefits

The efficacy of NIV in patients with acute respiratory failure is, at least in part, related to avoidance of inspiratory

muscle fatigue through the addition of inspiratory positive pressure, thus reducing inspiratory muscle work.[104] Application of positive pressure during inspiration increases transpulmonary pressure, inflates the lungs, augments alveolar ventilation and unloads the inspiratory muscles.[105] Augmentation of alveolar ventilation, demonstrated by an increase in V_T, increases CO_2 elimination and reverses acidaemia. High levels of inspiratory pressure may also relieve dyspnoea.[106]

The main physiological benefit in patients with congestive heart failure (CHF) is attributed to the increase in functional residual capacity associated with the use of PEEP that reopens collapsed alveoli and improves oxygenation.[107] Increased intrathoracic pressure associated with the application of positive pressure also may improve cardiac performance by reducing myocardial work and oxygen consumption through reductions to ventricular preload and left ventricular afterload.[107–109] NIV also preserves the ability to speak, swallow, cough and clear secretions, and decreases risks associated with endotracheal intubation.[110]

Indications for NIV

The success of NIV treatment is dependent on appropriate patient selection.[111] Table 15.3 outlines indications and contraindications to NIV.

Acute respiratory failure

Evidence supporting the role of NIV in patients with hypoxaemic respiratory failure is limited and conflicting.[107] For patients with community-acquired pneumonia, NIV has been shown to reduce intubation rates, ICU length of stay and 2-month mortality but only in the subgroup of patients with COPD.[112] Pneumonia also has been identified as a risk factor for NIV failure.[113]

Acute exacerbation of COPD and CHF

Strong evidence exists to support the use of NIV for patients with acute exacerbation of COPD and CHF. Three meta-analyses have shown a reduction in intubation rates, hospital length of stay and mortality for COPD patients managed with NIPPV compared to standard medical treatment.[114–116] COPD patients most likely to respond favourably to NIPPV include those with an unimpaired level of consciousness, moderate acidaemia, a respiratory rate of <30 breaths/minute and who demonstrate an improvement in respiratory parameters within 2 hours of commencing NIPPV.[104,117]

Early use of NIV in combination with standard therapy for patients with CHF has also been shown to reduce intubation rates and mortality when compared to standard therapy alone.[118–120] The most recent meta-analysis including 32 trials found NIV reduced hospital mortality and reintubation rates by nearly 50% compared to standard medical care and no increased risk of acute myocardial infarction.[121] The authors recommended CPAP may be considered as the first option for NIV due to more robust evidence for its effectiveness, safety and lower cost compared with NIPPV.[121] Practice surveys indicate CPAP may be the preferred method of NIV for patients with CHF in Australia and internationally.

NIV in weaning

NIV may be used as an adjunct to weaning to reduce the duration of invasive ventilation and associated complications.[122] Patients are extubated directly to NIV and then weaned to standard oxygen therapy. This use of NIV differs from its role in preventing reintubation in patients that develop, or who are at high risk of, post-extubation respiratory failure.[123] A recent systematic review and meta-analysis of 16 trials with 994 participants (mostly COPD) using NIV immediately after extubation reported reductions in mortality, weaning failure, VAP, tracheostomy, reintubation, ICU and hospital lengths of stay and total duration of ventilation.[124] Conversely, the effectiveness of NIV for postextubation respiratory failure is not so clear. The largest study of NIV use in postextubation respiratory failure reported worsened survival rates hypothesised to be as a result of delayed reintubation.[125] A subsequent meta-analysis suggested NIV may have a role in preventing the development of respiratory failure postextubation for those at risk, but should be used with caution once respiratory failure has developed and should not delay the decision to reintubate.[106]

Other indications

Other indications for NIV include:

- asthma[126,127]
- pulmonary infiltrates in immunocompromised patients
- neuromuscular disorders (e.g. muscular dystrophy, amyotrophic lateral sclerosis)
- fractured ribs
- obesity and central hypoventilation syndromes
- palliation.[128]

Patient selection

Selection of patients to receive NIV depends on the presence of an indication listed above as well as bedside observations and gas exchange parameters found in Table 15.3.

Interfaces and settings

NIV requires an interface that connects the patient to a ventilator, portable compressor or flow generator with a CPAP valve. The selection of an appropriate interface can influence NIV success or failure. Oronasal masks cover both the mouth and nose and are the preferred mask type for the management of acute respiratory failure.[129] Nasal masks enable speech, eating and drinking, and therefore are employed more frequently for long-term NIV use. An oronasal mask enables delivery of higher ventilation

---

TABLE 15.3

Indications and contraindications for non-invasive ventilation

	INDICATIONS
Bedside observations	Increased dyspnoea; moderate-to-severe tachypnoea: >24 breaths per min [obstructive] >30 breaths per min [restrictive] Signs of increased work of breathing, accessory muscle use and abdominal paradox
Gas exchange	Acute or acute-on-chronic ventilatory failure (best indication), $PaCO_2$ >45 mmHg, pH <7.35 Hypoxaemia (use with caution), PaO_2/FiO_2 ratio <200
	CONTRAINDICATIONS
Absolute	Respiratory arrest Unable to fit mask
Relative	Medically unstable: hypotensive shock, uncontrolled cardiac ischaemia or arrhythmia, uncontrolled upper gastrointestinal bleeding Agitated, uncooperative Unable to protect airway Swallowing impairment Excessive secretions not managed by secretion clearance techniques Multiple (i.e. two or more) organ failure Recent upper airway or upper gastrointestinal surgery

$PaCO_2$ = partial pressure of carbon dioxide in arterial blood; PaO_2 = partial pressure of oxygen in arterial blood; PaO_2/FiO_2 = ratio of partial pressure of oxygen in arterial blood to fraction of inspired oxygen.

pressures with less leak and greater comfort for the patient.[130] Other interfaces include full-face masks[130] that seal around the perimeter of the face and cover the eyes as well as the nose and mouth, nasal pillows, mouthpieces that are placed between the patient's lips and helmets that cover the whole head and consist of a transparent plastic hood attached to a soft neck collar. These alternative interfaces may increase patient tolerance by reducing pressure ulceration, air leaks and patient discomfort.[131]

Initiation and monitoring priorities

Successful initiation of NIV is dependent on patient acceptance and tolerance. Patient acceptance may be aided by a brief explanation of the procedure and its benefits. Strategies to enhance patient tolerance include: use of an interface that fits the patient's facial features, commencing with low pressure levels, holding the mask gently in position prior to securing with the straps/headgear and ensuring straps prevent major leaks but are not so tight they increase discomfort. Once NIV is commenced, the patient should be monitored for respiratory and haemodynamic stability, response to NIV treatment, ongoing tolerance and presence of air leaks (Table 15.4). Arterial blood gas analysis should be performed at baseline and within the first 1 to 2 hours of commencement.[132] During the initiation and stabilisation period, patients should be monitored using a nurse-to-patient ratio of 1:1 with ongoing coaching to promote NIV tolerance throughout the early stabilisation period.

Practice tip

NIV tolerance may be promoted with a simple explanation of the therapy, reassurance and constant monitoring for your patient. During initiation, allow them to take short breaks from the mask if they are in discomfort or experiencing claustrophobia.

Potential complications

Masks need to be tight-fitting to reduce air leaks; however, this contributes to pressure ulceration on the bridge of the nose or above the ears (due to mask straps/headgear). Air leaks may cause conjunctival irritation and the high flow of dry medical gas results in nasal congestion, oral or nasal dryness and insufflation of air into the stomach. Claustrophobia associated with the NIV interface may also lead to agitation, reducing the efficacy of NIV treatment due to poor coordination of respiratory cycling between the patient and NIV unit.[104] More serious, yet infrequent, complications include aspiration pneumonia, haemodynamic compromise associated with increased intrathoracic pressures and pneumothorax.[105]

Detecting NIV failure

Failure to respond to NIV within 1–2 hours of commencement is demonstrated by unchanged or worsening gas exchange, as well as ongoing or new onset of rapid shallow breathing and increased haemodynamic instability.[130] Decreased level of consciousness may be indicative of imminent respiratory arrest.

Weaning from NIV

Existing guidelines provide little guidance on weaning of NIV.[133] In many cases, NIV may be simply withdrawn as opposed to weaned.[132] Those commencing on high levels of IPAP and/or EPAP may need weaning based on ongoing assessment of dyspnoea and chest wall movement, as well as ventilation and oxygenation parameters. Another weaning method may be progressive extension of time off NIV, while monitoring tolerance.

Invasive mechanical ventilation

Critically ill patients with persistent respiratory insufficiency (hypoxaemia and/or hypercapnia), due to drugs, disease or other conditions, may require intubation and mechanical ventilation to support oxygenation and ventilatory demands. Clinical criteria for intubation and ventilation should be based on individual patient assessment and patient response to measures aimed at reversing hypoxaemia.

TABLE 15.4
Monitoring priorities for non-invasive ventilation

PRIORITY	ASSESSMENT
Patient comfort	Restlessness Mask tolerance Anxiety level Dyspnoea score Pain score
Conscious level	Glasgow Coma Score
Work of breathing	Chest wall motion Accessory muscle activation Respiratory rate
Gas exchange parameters	Continuous SpO_2 Arterial blood gas analysis (baseline and 1–2 hourly subsequently) Patient colour
Haemodynamic status	Continuous heart rate Intermittent blood pressure
Ventilator parameters	Air leak around mask Adequacy of pressure support (V_T, pH, $PaCO_2$) Adequacy of peak end-expiratory pressure (SpO_2, PaO_2)

$PaCO_2$ = partial pressure of carbon dioxide in arterial blood; PaO_2 = partial pressure of oxygen in arterial blood; SpO_2 = saturation of peripheral oxygen; V_T = tidal volume.

Adapted from Rose L, Gerdtz M. Use of non-invasive ventilation in Australian emergency departments. Int J Nurs Stud 2009;46(5):617–23, with permission.

Indications

Indications for intubation and mechanical ventilation include:

- apnoea
- inability to protect airway; e.g. loss of gag/cough reflex; decreased Glasgow Coma Scale score
- clinical signs indicating respiratory distress; e.g. tachypnoea,[134] activation of accessory and expiratory muscles, abnormal chest wall movements,[135] tachycardia and hypertension
- inability to sustain adequate oxygenation for metabolic demands; e.g. cyanosis, SpO_2 <88%, with supplemental FiO_2 ≥0.5
- respiratory acidosis (e.g. acute decrease in pH <7.25)
- postoperative respiratory failure
- shock.

The goals of mechanical ventilation are to achieve and maintain adequate pulmonary gas exchange, minimise the risk of lung injury, reduce patient work of breathing and optimise comfort.

Mechanical ventilators

Contemporary ventilators use sophisticated microprocessor controls with sensitive detection, response and control of pressure and gas flow characteristics. These ventilators are more sensitive to patient ventilatory demands, enabling improved patient–ventilator synchrony during

---

BOX 15.2

Mechanical ventilation of the elderly patient

- Elderly survivors of mechanical ventilation may have a greater increase in disability than those hospitalised and not requiring ventilation;[136] this is information that should be shared with patients and family members when considering treatment options.
- Frail elderly are at increased risk of delirium resulting in prolonged mechanical ventilation.[137]

---

both inspiratory and expiratory breath phases. Parameters commonly manipulated during mechanical ventilation are detailed in Table 15.5. Parameters often observed and documented are discussed below.

Phases of breath delivery

The respiratory cycle comprises both inspiratory and expiratory phases (see Figure 15.11). Pressure, flow, volume and time are parameters used to describe or classify mechanical ventilator breaths during the phases of inspiration. Ventilator breaths are classified by: 1) the mechanism (ventilator or patient) that 'triggers' the start of inspiration; 2) the parameter that is 'targeted' (also referred to as 'controlled' or 'limited') during inspiration; and 3) the parameter that 'cycles' the breath from inspiration to expiration.[138]

TABLE 15.5

Set ventilator parameters

PARAMETER	DESCRIPTION
Fraction of inspired oxygen (FiO_2)	The fraction of inspired oxygen delivered on inspiration to the patient
Tidal volume (V_T)	Volume (mL) of each breath
Set breath rate (f)	The clinician-determined set rate of breaths delivered by the ventilator (bpm)
Inspiratory trigger or sensitivity	Mechanism by which the ventilator senses the patient's inspiratory effort. May be measured in terms of a change in pressure or flow
Inspiratory pressure (P_{insp}, P_{high})	Clinician-determined pressure that is targeted during inspiration
Inspiratory time (T_{insp})	The duration of inspiration (s)
Inspiratory : expiratory ratio (I:E)	The ratio of the inspiratory time to expiratory time
Flow ($\dot{V}$)	The speed gas travels during inspiration (L/min)
Pressure support (PS)	The flow of gas that augments a patient's spontaneously initiated breath to a clinician-determined pressure (cmH_2O)
Positive end-expiratory pressure (PEEP)	Application of airway pressure above atmospheric pressure at the end of expiration (cmH_2O)
Rise time	Time to achieve maximal flow at the onset of inspiration for pressure-targeted breaths
Expiratory sensitivity	During a spontaneous breath, the ventilator cycles from inspiration to expiration once flow has decelerated to a percentage of initial peak flow
Minute volume (V_E)	Generally not set directly but is determined by V_T and f settings. Tidal volume multiplied by the respiratory rate over one minute (L/min)
Airway pressure (P_{aw})	The pressure measured in cmH_2O by the ventilator in the proximal airway
Plateau pressure (P_{plat})	The pressure, measured in cmH_2O, applied to the small airways and alveoli. P_{plat} is not set but can be measured by performing an inspiratory hold manoeuvre

FIGURE 15.11 Phases of breath delivery.

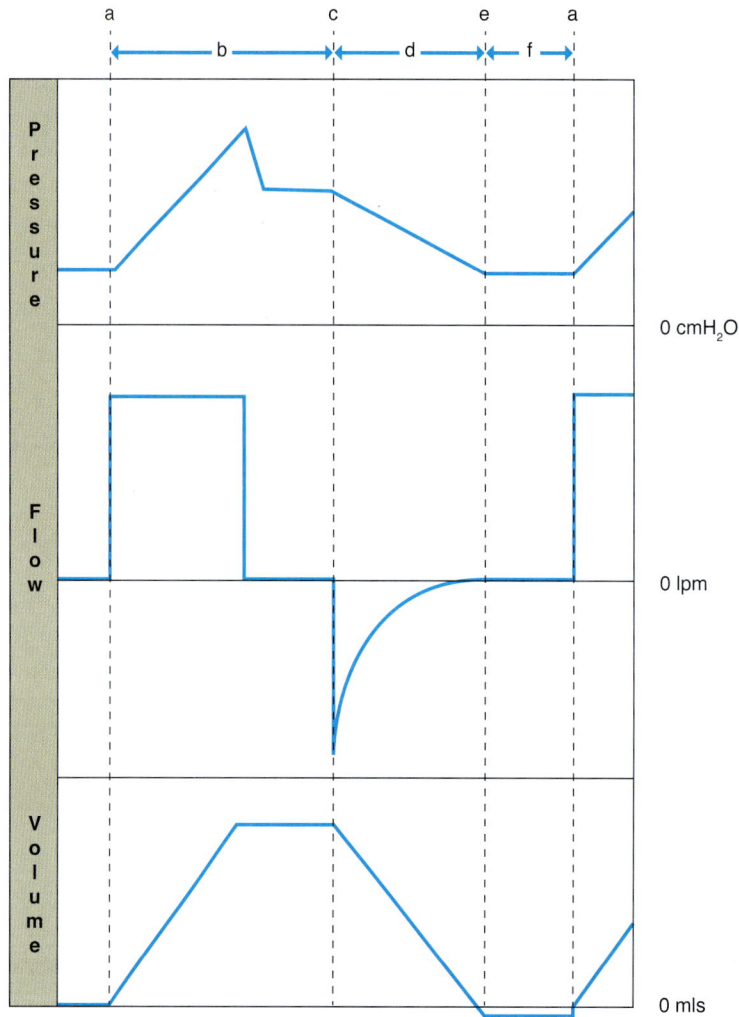

a) start of ventilator inspiration
b) inspiration
c) cycle from inspiration to expiration
d) expiration
e) end of expiration
f) between inspiration and expiration

Pressure vs volume delivery

Traditionally, clinicians have favoured volume control ventilation (VCV) due to the ability to regulate minute ventilation (V_E) and CO_2 elimination with straightforward manipulation of respiratory rate and V_T.[139] VCV provides consistent V_T delivery, independent of lung mechanics. The set V_T and flow rates used in VCV mean that the ventilator is unable to increase volume or flow rates in response to the patient's inspiratory demands during mandatory breaths. This inability to respond to the patient's

inspiratory flow requirements can lead to dyssynchrony. Another disadvantage of VCV is the lack of control over peak airway pressure that changes in response to altered compliance and resistance. Elevated plateau pressure may cause alveolar overdistension, barotrauma and haemodynamic effects such as reduced venous return and cardiac output resulting in hypotension and thus decreased organ perfusion.[140] Clinicians need to carefully monitor ventilation to avoid injurious pressures. In VCV the peak airway pressure is achieved towards the end of inspiration, and only for a short duration; therefore, distribution of gas may not be optimised and shearing stress can occur.[141] This can be overcome with the use of a decelerating waveform and an inspiratory time that produces an inspiratory hold.

Pressure controlled ventilation (PCV) allows control over the peak inspiratory pressure and inspiratory time. Clinicians must monitor minute ventilation and gas exchange due to the lack of a guaranteed V_T and possible changes in respiratory compliance and resistance. The variable flow and V_T mean that there is the potential for greater interaction between patient efforts and ventilator breaths than is present in volume controlled ventilation. The variable and decelerating inspiratory gas flow pattern of PCV enables rapid alveolar filling and more even gas distribution compared to the constant flow pattern that may be used with volume control. This decelerating flow pattern also results in improved gas exchange, decreased work of breathing and prevention of overdistension in healthy alveoli.[142–145] During PCV, the set inspiratory pressure is achieved at the beginning of the inspiratory cycle and maintained for the set inspiratory time. This promotes recruitment of alveoli with high opening pressures and long time-constants.

Ventilator parameters

Fraction of inspired oxygen

The FiO_2 is expressed as a decimal, between 0.21 and 1.0, when supplemental oxygen is applied. Room air has an oxygen content of 0.21 (21%). Ventilation is commonly commenced on a high FiO_2 setting but, as noted earlier, clinicians should consider the risks of oxygen toxicity, which include disruption to the alveolar-capillary membrane and alveolar wall fibrosis.[146]

Tidal volume

V_T is the volume, measured in mL, of each breath. Set or targeted V_T is calculated using the patient's ideal body weight using height and gender-specific tables[147] to achieve 6–8 mL/kg (see Table 15.6). Strong evidence indicates

TABLE 15.6

ARDSnet tables for predicted body weight for females and males

PBW AND TIDAL VOLUME FOR FEMALES					HEIGHT, CENTIMETRES	PBW AND TIDAL VOLUME FOR MALES					
PBW	4 ML	5 ML	6 ML	7 ML	8 ML	(INCHES)	PBW	4 ML	5 ML	6 ML	7 ML	8 ML
31.7	127	159	190	222	254	137 (54)	36.2	145	181	217	253	290
34	136	170	204	238	272	140 (55)	38.5	154	193	231	270	308
36.3	145	182	218	254	290	142 (56)	40.8	163	204	245	286	326
38.6	154	193	232	270	309	145 (57)	43.1	172	216	259	302	345
40.9	164	205	245	286	327	147.5 (58)	45.4	182	227	272	318	363
43.2	173	216	259	302	346	150 (59)	47.7	191	239	286	334	382
45.5	182	228	273	319	364	152.5 (60)	50	200	250	300	350	400
47.8	191	239	287	335	382	155 (61)	52.3	209	262	314	366	418
50.1	200	251	301	351	401	157.5 (62)	54.6	218	273	328	382	437
52.4	210	262	314	367	419	160 (63)	56.9	228	285	341	398	455
54.7	219	274	328	383	438	162.5 (64)	59.2	237	296	355	414	474
57	228	285	342	399	456	165 (65)	61.5	246	308	369	431	492
59.3	237	297	356	415	474	167.5 (66)	63.8	255	319	383	447	510
61.6	246	308	370	431	493	170 (67)	66.1	264	331	397	463	529
63.9	256	320	383	447	511	172.5 (68)	68.4	274	342	410	479	547
66.2	265	331	397	463	530	175 (69)	70.7	283	354	424	495	566
68.5	274	343	411	480	548	178 (70)	73	292	365	438	511	584
70.8	283	354	425	496	566	180 (71)	75.3	301	377	452	527	602
73.1	292	366	439	512	585	183 (72)	77.6	310	388	466	543	621
75.4	302	377	452	528	603	185.5 (73)	79.9	320	400	479	559	639
77.7	311	389	466	544	622	188 (74)	82.2	329	411	493	575	658
80	320	400	480	560	640	190.5 (75)	84.5	338	423	507	592	676
82.3	329	412	494	576	658	193 (76)	86.8	347	434	521	608	694
84.6	338	423	508	592	677	195.5 (77)	89.1	356	446	535	624	713
86.9	348	435	521	608	695	198 (78)	91.4	366	457	548	640	731

PBW = predicted body weight.

The formulae, when using height in centimetres, are:

- Females = 45.5 + 0.91 × (height in cm − 152.4)
- Males = 50 + 0.91 × (height in cm − 152.3).

Adapted from information courtesy of ARDSnet. Further information available at http://www.ardsnet.org/node/77460.

a mortality benefit for using 6 mL/kg in patients with acute respiratory distress syndrome (ARDS).[148,121] Increasingly, evidence indicates protective lung ventilation using 6 mL/kg as a target for patients without ARDS is associated with improved clinical outcomes.[149-151] While further studies are required, clinicians should consider aiming for 6–8 mL/kg in all ventilated patients.

Respiratory rate

Mandatory frequency (f) or respiratory rate (RR) is set with consideration of the patient's own respiratory effort, anticipated ventilatory requirements and the effect on the I:E ratio. Use of high doses of sedation with or without neuromuscular blockade requires setting a mandatory rate that facilitates adequate gas exchange and meets oxygenation requirements. A lower frequency can be set for a patient able to breathe spontaneously in modes such as synchronised intermittent mandatory ventilation (SIMV) and assist control (A/C) (see below) to enable spontaneous triggering. Physiologically normal respiratory rates are 12–20 breaths per minute. Patients with hypoxaemic respiratory failure generally breathe 20–30 breaths per minute.[152]

Triggering of inspiration

Depending on the ventilation mode, breaths are triggered by the ventilator or patient in various sequences. A breath may be triggered by the ventilator in response to time elapsed in modes with clinician-determined set frequency, such as controlled mandatory ventilation (CMV), and in A/C and SIMV in the absence of spontaneous effort. Patient triggering requires the ventilator to sense the patient's inspiratory effort. Most modern ventilators now use flow triggering, as evidence indicates that flow triggering may be more responsive to patient effort than pressure triggering.[153] Pressure triggering requires the patient to create a negative pressure within the ventilator circuit of sufficient size to enable the ventilator to sense the effort and commence flow of gas. Flow triggering is sometimes used in conjunction with a predetermined flow of gas, usually 5–10 L/min, referred to as the bias (or base) flow, that travels continuously through the ventilator circuit. When the patient makes an inspiratory effort, they divert flow, which is sensed by the ventilator. If the flow diversion reaches a clinician-determined set value, a breath is initiated.[154] The flow trigger is usually set at 1–3 L/min (1 L/min represents less patient effort and 3 L/min represents greater patient effort). Despite advances in ventilator technology, various studies continue to identify missed patient triggers that contribute to patient–ventilator asynchrony.[155] Conversely, 'auto-triggering' is ventilator triggering in the absence of spontaneous inspiratory effort. Auto triggering is sometimes observed in patients with an increased cardiac output, such as those fulfilling brain death criteria.

Rise time

The rise time controls how quickly the ventilator reaches the clinician-determined inspiratory pressure (P_{insp}) for mandatory breaths and pressure support for spontaneous breaths. Reducing the rise time to its lowest value will enable the ventilator to reach target pressure in the shortest time frame resulting in a more rapid delivering of flow in the early phase of inspiration. This reduces work of breathing and improves synchrony. In patients with a high airway resistance (e.g., severe asthma), a short inspiratory time may cause oscillation and overshoot of the pressure waveform. The clinical relevance of this is questionable but it produces an abnormal pressure waveform and results in alarm violations. Increasing the rise time may alleviate this problem. In other patients, an increased rise time may unnecessarily increase their work of breathing.[156]

Inspiratory time and inspiratory-to-expiratory ratio

The total time available for each mandatory breath is determined by the set inspiratory time and breath frequency. Normal inspiratory time is 0.8 to 1.2 seconds. Total breath time comprises the inspiratory and expiratory time, which is expressed as the I:E ratio. In normal spontaneous breathing, expiratory time is approximately twice the inspiratory time (1:2 ratio). Gas flow also influences inspiratory time, with higher gas flows resulting in decreased time to achieve the target V_T. The I:E ratio can be manipulated to create an inverse relationship (1:1, 2:1, 4:1) with the goal of increased mean airway pressure resulting in alveolar recruitment and improved oxygenation. Prolonging the inspiratory time beyond normal or using inverse ratio ventilation in any mode can result in patient ventilator dyssynchrony and increased risk of barotrauma.[157]

Inspiratory flow and flow pattern

The flow rate refers to the speed of gas, is measured in litres per minute (L/min) and generally delivered at speeds of 30–60 L/min. Higher flow rates cause turbulent gas flow, resulting in increased peak airway pressures. Lower flow rates result in laminar flow, increased inspiratory time, improved gas distribution and lower peak airway pressures.[158] The flow of inspiratory gas can be delivered in three styles: constant or square wave, decelerating ramp and sinusoidal pattern (see Figure 15.6). In a constant flow pattern, the peak flow is achieved at the beginning of inspiration and is held constant throughout the inspiratory phase. This may result in higher peak airway pressures. Using a decelerating ramp, the gas flow is highest at the beginning of inspiration and tapers throughout the inspiratory phase. Sinusoidal gas flow resembles spontaneous ventilation.

Peak airway pressure

Airway pressures vary across the respiratory cycle with a number of pressures identifiable (e.g. peak inspiratory, end-expiratory). The airway pressure (P_{aw}) is an important parameter in assessing respiratory compliance and patient–ventilator synchrony, and will vary depending on V_T, RR, ventilator flow pattern, dynamic compliance and airway resistance. In pressure-targeted modes the peak inspiratory pressure is equivalent to the P_{insp}. In volume-targeted modes the peak inspiratory pressure is determined by the set V_T and patient compliance and resistance.

Positive end-expiratory pressure

PEEP is the pressure applied at the end of the expiratory cycle to prevent alveolar collapse. PEEP increases residual lung volume thereby recruiting collapsed alveoli, improving ventilation/perfusion match and enhancing movement of fluid out of the alveoli.[159,160] PEEP was originally introduced by Ashbaugh and colleagues[161] in the 1960s as a technique for treating refractory hypoxaemia in patients with ARDS. Animal studies suggest ventilator-associated lung injury may be prevented using PEEP by recruiting atelectic alveoli and bronchioles and preventing cyclic opening and closing of alveoli.[162–165] PEEP may be beneficial, however, only if the lung is recruitable such as in collapsed, as opposed to consolidated, lung.[159] Selection of optimal PEEP remains controversial. Low PEEP levels have been shown to be associated with higher mortality for ARDS patients in several studies.[166–169] Two randomised, controlled trials comparing low tidal volume ventilation and conventional PEEP to low tidal volume ventilation and high PEEP, with and without additional recruitment manoeuvres (40 cmH$_2$O applied for 40 s),[170, 171] did not demonstrate a reduction in hospital[170] or 28-day[171] mortality.

Pressure support

When triggered by the patient, the ventilator delivers flow to achieve the clinician-determined set pressure support. The flow is variable, depending on the patient demand. The V_T achieved with pressure support is dependent on chest and lung compliance as well as airway and ventilator resistance. Pressure support is generally set at 5–20 cmH$_2$O. Increasing the level of pressure support will result in increased V_T and improvements in gas exchange if compliance and resistance remain constant.

Expiratory sensitivity

Expiratory sensitivity describes the percentage of decay in peak flow reached during the inspiratory phase that signals the ventilator to cycle to expiration for spontaneous breaths. In some ventilator models this is predetermined at 25%, while others allow clinician selection. Premature termination of a breath will increase inspiratory muscle workload whereas delayed breath termination increases expiratory muscle load.[172] Reducing the expiratory sensitivity in patients with COPD may prolong the inspiratory time, thereby increasing the V_T and reducing the respiratory rate and gas trapping.[173]

Practice tip

The P_{insp} setting reflects a different value on different ventilators. P_{insp} equals total pressure including PEEP on some ventilators and P_{insp} above PEEP on others. Use the pressure–time scalar to confirm.

Ventilator modes

The mode of ventilation describes inspiratory phase variables; how the ventilator controls pressure, volume and flow during a breath; as well as describing how breaths are sequenced. All breaths have trigger, limit and cycle inspiratory phase variables.[174] Each breath is triggered (started) either by the patient or by the ventilator. During inspiration, the breath is limited to a set target of pressure, volume or flow. This target cannot be exceeded during each breath. The cycling variable determines the end of the inspiratory phase. Again this variable may be pressure, flow, volume or time. Gas delivery during each breath is described by the control variable. There are five control variables: pressure, volume, flow, time and dual control (such as used in the mode pressure-regulated volume control). Breath sequencing refers to the sequence of mandatory and spontaneous breath. A spontaneous breath is one during which inspiration is both started (triggered) and stopped (cycled) by the patient. Spontaneous breaths may be assisted, as with pressure support, or unassisted. Mandatory breaths are either triggered or cycled by the ventilator.[175] A complete mode description should include: 1) the control variable; 2) the breath sequence; and 3) the targeting scheme (limit variable).

Commonly employed ventilation modes

Contemporary ventilators now provide a range of modes to facilitate mechanical ventilation. See Table 15.7.

Controlled mandatory ventilation

CMV is a mandatory mode, and is the original and most basic mode of ventilation.[176] CMV delivers all breaths at a clinician-determined set frequency (rate); the patient's spontaneous effort is not acknowledged by the ventilator.[81] VCV requires clinician selection of the frequency, PEEP, FiO$_2$, tidal volume, flow waveform, peak inspiratory flow and either the inspiratory time or I:E ratio. PCV requires clinician selection of rate, PEEP, FiO$_2$, inspiratory pressure, as opposed to tidal volume, and inspiratory time or I:E ratio depending on the ventilator type. Peak inspiratory flow and the flow waveform are manipulated by the ventilator, to achieve the clinician-selected inspiratory pressure within the set inspiratory time. The inability to breathe spontaneously during CMV contributes to diaphragm muscle dysfunction and atrophy, which may result in difficulty weaning from the ventilator.[177]

Assist control

In A/C the patient can trigger the ventilator; however, unlike SIMV, every patient-initiated breath is assisted to the same clinician-determined V_T (volume targeted) or inspiratory pressure (pressure targeted). All breaths are cycled by the ventilator irrespective of being patient- or ventilator-triggered. In the absence of spontaneous breathing, A/C resembles CMV.

TABLE 15.7

Ventilator modes

MODE	DESCRIPTION	CLINICAL IMPLICATIONS
Controlled mandatory ventilation (CMV)	All breaths are mandatory, no patient triggering is enabled. Also called volume controlled ventilation (volume targeted) (VCV) and pressure controlled ventilation (pressure targeted) (PCV)	Patients with respiratory effort require sedation and neuromuscular blockade Potential for respiratory muscle atrophy due to disuse
Assist-control (A/C)	Breaths may be either machine or patient triggered but all are cycled by the ventilator. Assist control may be delivered as volume (AC-VC) or pressure (AC-PC) targeted	Activation of the diaphragm with patient triggering Potential for respiratory alkalosis if tachypnoea develops
Synchronised intermittent mandatory ventilation (SIMV)	Mandatory breaths are delivered using a set rate and volume (SIMV-VC) or pressure (SIMV-PC). Mandatory breaths are synchronised with patient triggers within a timing window. Between mandatory breaths the patient can breathe spontaneously	Reduced need for sedation Activation of the diaphragm with patient triggering
Pressure support ventilation (PSV)	All breaths are patient triggered and cycled. Pressure applied by the ventilator during inspiration (pressure support) augments patient effort	Reduced need for sedation Facilitates ventilator weaning Level of PS can be adjusted to achieve desired V_T Sustains respiratory muscle tone and decreases work of breathing
Continuous positive airway pressure (CPAP)	All breaths are patient triggered and cycled. Positive pressure is applied throughout inspiratory and expiratory phases of the respiratory cycle	Requires intact respiratory drive and patient ability to maintain adequate tidal volumes
Volume support (VS)	Spontaneous mode with clinician preset target tidal volume delivery achieved with the lowest inspiratory pressure	Requires intact respiratory drive
Pressure-regulated volume control (PRVC)	Mandatory rate and target tidal volume are set, and the ventilator then delivers the breaths using the lowest achievable pressure	Dual control of volume and pressure enables guarantee of volume and pressure
Airway pressure release ventilation (APRV)	Ventilator cycles between 2 preset pressure levels for defined time periods. I:E ratio is inverse, often with a prolonged inspiratory time (4 s) and shortened expiratory time (0.8 s). Patient can breathe spontaneously at both pressure levels	Reduced need for sedation Activation of the diaphragm with patient triggering Promotes alveolar recruitment Considered a rescue mode in ARDS when used with extreme inverse ratio
Biphasic positive airway pressure (BiPAP/ BILEVEL/ Bivent)	As with APRV, the ventilator cycles between 2 preset pressure levels for defined time periods and the patient can breathe spontaneously at both pressure levels. The inspiratory time is generally shorter than, or the same length, as the expiratory time	Reduced need for sedation Activation of the diaphragm with patient triggering Promotes alveolar recruitment
Mandatory minute ventilation (MMV)	The patient's spontaneous minute ventilation is monitored by the ventilator. When the minute ventilation falls below the clinician-determined target, the ventilator increases the mandatory rate or size of tidal volumes to regain the desired minute ventilation	Guarantees minute ventilation for patients with fluctuating respiratory drive and muscle innervation such as patients awakening from anaesthesia and those with Guillain–Barré
Proportional assist ventilation (PAV)[269]	Delivers positive pressure throughout inspiration in proportion to patient generated effort, and dependent on the set levels of flow assist (offsets resistance) and volume assist (offsets elastance)[268]	Requires intact respiratory drive Patients with high respiratory drive as the ventilator may over-assist and continue to apply support when the patient has stopped inspiration[269]
Proportional assist ventilation (PAV+™)	Clinician only sets a percentage of work for the ventilator. The ventilator assesses total work of breathing by randomly measuring compliance and resistance every 4–10 breaths	Requires intact respiratory drive Decreases work of breathing and improves patient ventilator synchrony Potential for use as a weaning mode
Adaptive support ventilation (ASV)	Automatic adaptation of respiratory rate and pressure levels based on a clinician-set desired percentage of minute ventilation[270]	Automatically sets all ventilator settings except PEEP and FiO_2 Potential for use as a weaning mode
Volume assured pressure support (VAPS)	The ventilator switches from pressure control to volume control, or pressure support to volume control during inspiration	Enables maintenance of a preset minimum V_T and reduces work of breathing

Synchronised intermittent mandatory ventilation

SIMV delivers breaths at a set frequency (rate), and can be either pressure- or volume-targeted. Setting of the ventilator is similar to setting VCV or PCV. The availability of patient triggering with SIMV facilitates provision of gas flow in recognition of a patient's spontaneous effort. SIMV uses a timing window to deliver mandatory breaths in synchrony with patient inspiratory effort.[178] Additional spontaneous breaths occurring outside of the timing window may be assisted with pressure support to augment the patient's spontaneous effort to a pre-set pressure level.

Pressure support ventilation

Pressure support ventilation (PSV) is a spontaneous mode in which the patient initiates and cycles all breaths, with support of the patient's inspiratory effort by the ventilator using rapid acceleration of flow to achieve a preset level of inspiratory pressure. Unlike CMV, SIMV or A/C, PSV does not require setting of ventilator (mandatory) breaths. PSV is usually employed with PEEP, which maintains partial inflation of alveoli during the expiratory phase to promote alveolar recruitment and oxygenation.

Continuous positive airway pressure

CPAP applies a set baseline positive pressure throughout the inspiratory and expiratory phases. In this spontaneous breathing mode, unlike PSV, no additional positive pressure is provided to the patient during inspiration. Due to nomenclature used on some ventilator models, PSV is frequently misrepresented as CPAP.

Volume-targeted pressure control breaths

A number of hybrid ventilator modes are commercially available that use an algorithm to target a set V_T by regulating the inspiratory pressure during pressure-controlled breaths based on the patient's resistance, compliance and inspiratory effort. Examples include pressure-regulated volume control, available on the Servo 300 and Servo I (Maquet, Solna, Sweden) and SIMV with autoflow (Dräger, Lübeck, Germany). On initiation of these modes the ventilator delivers a number of breaths during a 'learning period' to establish an estimate of the pressure required to achieve the targeted V_T. The patient's resistance, compliance and inspiratory effort continue to influence the pressure and flow delivered to attain the targeted V_T. The ventilator constantly regulates inspiratory pressure based on the pressure/volume calculation of the previous breaths and the clinician-determined target tidal volume.

Airway pressure release ventilation and biphasic positive airway pressure

Airway pressure release ventilation (APRV) and BIPAP are ventilator modes that allow unrestricted spontaneous breathing independent of ventilator cycling, using an active expiratory valve that allows patients to exhale even in the inspiratory phase.[140,141,179,180] Both modes are pressure-limited and time-cycled. In the absence of spontaneous breathing, these modes resemble conventional pressure-limited, time-cycled ventilation.[181] In North America the acronym BiPAP® is registered to Respironics non-invasive ventilators (Murrayville, PA). Therefore ventilator companies have developed brand names such as BiLevel (Puritan Bennett, Pleasanton, CA, GE Healthcare, Madison, WI) Bivent (Maquet, Solna, Sweden), DuoPaP (Hamilton Medical, Rhäzüns, Switzerland), PCV+ (Dräger Medical, Lübeck, Germany) or BiPhasic (Viasys, Conshocken, PA) to describe essentially equivalent modes. Ambiguity exists in the criteria that distinguish APRV and BIPAP. When applied with the same I:E ratio, no difference exists between the two modes. APRV, as opposed to BIPAP, however, is more frequently described with an extreme inverse ratio and advocated as a method to improve oxygenation in refractory hypoxemia.[182]

Automatic tube compensation

Automatic tube compensation is active during spontaneous breaths and compensates for the work of breathing associated with ETT resistance via closed-loop control of continuously calculated tracheal pressure.[183,184] During spontaneous inspiration, a pressure gradient exists between the proximal and distal ends of the ETT due to resistance created by the tube. A reduced pressure at the proximal end of the tube means a patient needs to produce a greater inspiratory force (greater negative pressure) to generate an adequate V_T.[185] Higher flow rates generate larger pressure gradients and greater resistance. Automatic tube compensation requires the airway type and size to be selected as well as a percentage of automatic tube compensation to be applied. It appears to have most use in reducing the work of breathing for patients with high respiratory drive who require high inspiratory flow.[186]

Neurally adjusted ventilatory assist

Neurally adjusted ventilatory assist is available on the Servo-I ventilator (Maquet, Solna, Sweden) and uses the electrical activity of the diaphragm to control patient–ventilator interaction.[187] Electrical activity of the diaphragm, measured using an oesophageal catheter, should result in optimal patient–ventilator synchrony as it represents the end point of neural output from the respiratory centres, and thus is the earliest signal of patient inspiratory trigger and expiratory cycling. Pressure delivered to the airways is proportional to inspiratory diaphragmatic electrical activity using a clinician-determined proportionality factor set on the ventilator.[188] Neurally adjusted ventilatory assist provides breath-by-breath assist in synchrony with, and in proportion to, respiratory demand.[189] Although clinical data on neurally adjusted ventilatory assist are currently limited,[188,190–192] this mode shows promise for improving patient–ventilator synchrony.

Managing the mechanically ventilated patient

Management of refractory hypoxaemia

Refractory hypoxaemia may require strategies in addition to conventional lung-protective mechanical ventilation.[148] These include recruitment manoeuvres (RMs), high frequency oscillatory ventilation (HFOV), extracorporeal membrane oxygenation (ECMO) and nitric oxide (NO).

Recruitment manoeuvres

RMs refer to brief application of high levels of PEEP to raise the transpulmonary pressure to levels higher than achieved during tidal ventilation with the goals of opening collapsed alveoli, recruiting slow opening alveoli, preventing alveolar derecruitment and reducing shearing stress.[193–195] The most common RM is elevation of PEEP to achieve a peak pressure of 40 cmH_2O for a sustained period of 40 s, although studies report peak pressure elevations ranging from 25–50 cmH_2O for durations ranging from 20–40 s.[196] The best method in terms of pressure, duration and frequency has yet to be determined.[197] RMs in humans have not produced consistent results in clinical studies,[198,199] with a recent systematic review demonstrating no mortality benefit despite transient increases in oxygenation.[196] Effective recruitment may be difficult to assess with the potential for either alveolar overdistension or failure to recruit.[169] Once the RM is terminated, derecruitment may occur rapidly. Serious adverse effects have been noted during RMs due to increased intrathoracic and intrapulmonary pressures resulting in reductions in venous return and cardiac output, cardiac arrest and increased risk of barotrauma.[195,200]

High frequency oscillatory ventilation

HFOV requires a specialised ventilator and manipulation of four variables: mean airway pressure (cmH_2O), frequency (Hz), inspiratory time and amplitude (or power [ΔP]).[201] Alveolar overdistension is limited through the use of sub-dead space tidal volumes whereas alveolar cyclic collapse is prevented by maintenance of high end-expiratory lung pressures.[202,203] High frequency (between 3 and 15 Hz) oscillations at extremely fast rates (300–420 breaths/min) create pressure waves enabling CO_2 elimination.[162,204] Oxygenation is facilitated through application of a constant mean airway pressure via the bias flow (rate of fresh gas).[204,205] In adults, recommendations for the initiation of HFOV state mean airway pressure should be set 5 cmH_2O above the peak airway pressure achieved with conventional ventilation.[206] The recommended frequency range is 3–10 Hz with 5 Hz conventionally used to initiate HFOV. Inspiratory time is set at 33% and the amplitude setting is determined by adequate CO_2 elimination.[162] Increased CO_2 elimination is achieved by lowering the frequency and increasing the amplitude.

HFOV is generally considered a rescue mode for adult patients with ARDS experiencing refractory hypoxaemia and failing conventional ventilation.[207,208] A recent large, multicentre, randomised controlled trial of HFOV was stopped early for harm with increased mortality in the HFOV arm.[209] A contemporaneous trial conducted in the UK found no effect for HFOV compared to usual ventilatory care on 30-day mortality in patients undergoing mechanical ventilation for ARDS.[210]

Extracorporeal membrane oxygenation

ECMO improves total body oxygenation using an external (extracorporeal) oxygenator, while allowing intrinsic recovery of lung pathophysiology by resting the lung. Indications for ECMO include acute severe cardiac or respiratory failure such as severe ARDS and refractory shock or as a bridge to transplantation.[211] Due to the need for rescue treatment with ECMO during the 2009 H1N1[212] outbreak and a randomised clinical trial indicating a survival benefit with venous–venous ECMO compared to conventional ventilation,[213] ECMO is being used more frequently for refractory respiratory failure. Bleeding as a complication of anticoagulation is a major risk of ECMO, with cerebral bleeds being the most catastrophic.[214] Another serious complication is limb ischaemia when the femoral artery is used.

ECMO consists of three key components:

1 a blood pump (either a simple roller or centrifugal force pump)

2 a membrane oxygenator (bubble, membrane or hollow fibre)

3 a countercurrent heat exchanger, where the blood is exposed to warmed water circulating within metal tubes.

In addition, essential safety features include: bubble detectors that detect gas in the arterial line and shut the pump off; arterial line filters between the heat exchanger and arterial cannula, to trap air thrombi and emboli; pressure monitors placed before and after the oxygenator that measure the pressure within the circuit and detect rising circuit pressures commonly caused by thrombus or circuit or cannulae occlusion; and continuous venous oxygen saturation and temperature monitoring. On commencement of ECMO the circuit is primed with fresh blood. The acid–base balance and blood gas of the primer is adjusted to ensure that the pH is within the normal range (7.35–7.45) and PaO_2 is adequate. ECMO can be delivered via venoarterial access, which requires cannulation of an artery. This method bypasses the pulmonary circulation while providing cardiac support to the systemic circulation and achieves a higher PaO_2 with lower perfusion rates. The alternative is veno-venous access, used for patients in respiratory failure with adequate cardiac function as there is no support of systemic circulation. Perfusion rates are higher, the mixed venous PO_2 is elevated and the PaO_2 is lower.[214]

Nitric oxide

NO is an endothelial smooth muscle relaxant. Inhaled NO is effective for dilation of pulmonary arteries resulting in reduced pulmonary shunting and reduced right ventricular afterload due to reduced pulmonary artery tone. Pulmonary shunting refers to failure of uptake of alveolar gas by the pulmonary vascular bed due to vascular constriction or interstitial oedema. Inhaled NO has a role in the management of pulmonary hypertension and was previously thought to have a role in management of refractory hypoxaemia for patients with ARDS. However, the most recent systematic review and meta-analysis of NO in ARDS comprising 14 RCTs and 1303 participants reported no effect on overall mortality despite a statistically significant improvement in oxygenation in the first 24 hours.[215]

Positioning

Regular repositioning of critically ill patients is essential for lung recruitment, prevention of atelectasis and maintenance of skin integrity (see Chapter 6).

Head-of-bed elevation

Supine positioning has been associated with aspiration of abnormally colonised oropharyngeal and gastric contents[216–218] and increased incidence of VAP compared to a semirecumbent position, defined as backrest elevation at 45°.[219] Guidelines and care bundles for VAP prevention recommend semirecumbent positioning for all mechanically ventilated patients.[96,220,221] A more recent trial has, however, questioned the feasibility of 45° semirecumbent positioning as this backrest elevation was only achieved for 15% of study observations.[222] There was also no difference in VAP incidence between the supine and semirecumbent group. Contraindications to backrest elevation include:

- suspected or existing spinal injury
- intracranial hypertension (for 45° elevation)
- unstable pelvic fractures
- prone positioning
- haemodynamic support devices (intra-aortic balloon pumps, left ventricular assist devices and ECMO)
- femoral catheterisation for continuous renal replacement therapy
- large abdominal wounds
- following femoral sheath removal.

As some degree of semirecumbent positioning is preferable to supine positioning, patients with suspected or existing spinal injury, pelvic fractures or being managed with prone positioning can have the head elevated by tilting the whole bed. Patients with femoral cannulation and large abdominal wounds can usually achieve 25–30° positioning.

Clinical practice audits conducted internationally and in Australia and New Zealand indicate that compliance with a 45° semirecumbent position rarely occurs, even when taking into consideration contraindications.[223–227] Similarly, interventions to improve compliance failed to demonstrate adherence to the 45° semirecumbent position that can be sustained by the patient over time.[228,229] Due to uncertainty over compliance with 45° semirecumbency in the original trial conducted by Drakulovic,[219] and the lack of difference in VAP rates despite difficulty achieving compliance with semirecumbency in the van Niewenhoven study,[222] new studies are required to confirm the equivalence or lack of inferiority of lower degrees of backrest elevation to the strict 45° semirecumbent position.

Practice tip

Backrest elevation is difficult to estimate accurately. Use an objective measurement device such as an inclinometer or protractor.

BOX 15.3

Mechanical ventilation and the bariatric patient
- Bariatric patients are at increased risk of atelectasis and have decreased chest wall compliance due to the weight of the abdomen.
- Avoid the supine position as this will further decrease lung volumes.
- Bariatric patients may require higher airway pressures to generate adequate tidal volumes.
- Recruitment manoeuvres may improve oxygenation.[230]
- Frail elderly may experience difficult weaning due to the presence of comorbidities such as CHF, ischaemic heart disease and COPD.

Lateral positioning

Patients with unilateral lung disease experience a mismatch of ventilation to perfusion if the consolidated or atelectic lung is placed in the dependent position.[231] Temporary and early positioning of the affected lung in the dependent position, amongst other strategies such as avoiding manual hyperinflation, for patients with unilateral pneumonia or following aspiration may be beneficial in preventing the movement of bacteria or acidic gastric contents into the non-affected lung.[232] This theory has been coined 'propagation prevention'. While appealing, as yet there have been no adequately powered randomised controlled trials to support its use. Continuous lateral rotational therapy is a positioning therapy advocated for the prevention and management of respiratory complications associated with immobility.[233] The most recently reported multicentre randomised controlled trial found a significant reduction in VAP and shorter durations of ventilation and ICU stay.[234] Continuous lateral rotation therapy requires a special bed system enabling rotation of the upper part of the body to a maximum angle of 90°.

Prone positioning

Prone positioning has been shown to improve oxygenation and intrapulmonary shunt fraction when compared with rotational turning during the first 72 hours of ARDS[235] and in patients with multiorgan failure.[236] Prone positioning may also decrease the risk of VAP due to improved bronchial secretion drainage, limitation of colonisation of distal lung, decreased atelectasis and increased alveolar recruitment but may increase the spread of pathogens in the lung and may increase the risk of aspiration.[237–240]

Prone positioning results in changes to the distribution of ventilation and pulmonary blood flow. Pleural pressures are lower in non-dependent regions and higher in dependent regions due to gravitational forces, the weight of the overlying lung and mismatch between the local physical structures of the lung and chest wall.[241] The weight of the overlying lung increases in ARDS due to parenchymal oedema and fluid within the alveoli.[242] This gradient in pleural pressures means transpulmonary pressure is higher in non-dependent lung regions, compared to dependent regions.[242] Perfusion also increases from previously non-dependent to dependent lung regions resulting in optimal matching of ventilation and perfusion to promote gas exchange.

Increased pleural pressure in the dependent dorsal regions in the supine position can result in airway closure, atelectasis and hypoxaemia.[241] The difference in pleural pressures from non-dependent and dependent lung regions is greater in the supine compared to the prone position. In the supine position, the heart and abdominal contents also compress lung bases and decrease functional residual capacity, whereas in prone positioning, the weights of these structures are lifted from the lung.

The benefits of prone positioning continue to be debated. Although oxygenation improves in 70–80% of patients turned from supine to prone,[243] a mortality benefit has not been shown in all trials. The most recent systematic review and meta-analysis that included 11 randomised controlled trials[244] found reduced mortality and improved oxygenation for patients with ARDS managed with protective lung ventilation. Adverse events related to prone positioning were increased risk of decubitus ulcer formation, endotracheal obstruction and thoracotomy tube dislodgement.

Implementing prone positioning requires forward planning to ensure eye care and protection, mouth care, wound dressings and tracheal suction are attended to before positioning the patient prone. Intravenous lines, electrocardiogram leads, urinary catheter drainage, chest drains and ostomy bags need to be secured and repositioned appropriately once the patient is positioned.[245] Prone positioning can be achieved by manual handling of the patient, requiring up to five staff, although commercial devices are available that facilitate the turning and positioning.[245]

Complications of mechanical ventilation

Physiological complications associated with mechanical ventilation include ventilator-associated lung injury and nosocomial infection, including VAP.[178,246] Ventilator-associated lung injury occurs through alveolar over-distension and cyclic opening and closing of alveoli resulting in diffuse alveolar damage, increased permeability, pulmonary oedema, cell contraction and cytokine production.[149,159,165,247–249] VAP substantially increases the duration of ICU stay and is associated with an attributable mortality of 5.8–8.5%.[250–252] Additional complications associated with mechanical ventilation are listed in Table 15.8. Complications can occur due to inappropriate application of mechanical ventilation. This may result in extra-alveolar gas causing pneumothoraces or subcutaneous emphysema due to high peak P_{insp}, and alveolar stretch and oedema formation as a result of large V_T.[81]

Weaning from mechanical ventilation

Weaning traditionally occurs via clinician-directed adjustments to the level of support provided by the ventilator, culminating in a spontaneous breathing trial (SBT) comprising either low level pressure support or a T piece trial.

Current recommendations

No ventilation strategy is more lung-protective than the timely and appropriate discontinuation of mechanical ventilation. Weaning refers to the transition from ventilatory support to spontaneous breathing.[253] Evidence-based consensus guidelines published for weaning in 2001[178] and 2007[254] emphasise the importance of preventing unnecessary delays in the weaning process, early recognition of a patient's ability to breathe spontaneously and the use of a systematic method to identify the potential for extubation.

Weaning predictors

Clinician judgement regarding prediction of weaning readiness is known to be imperfect, with unnecessary prolongation of ventilation[255] or high rates of reintubation as resultant consequences, both of which are associated with adverse outcomes.[256,257] An evidence-based review evaluating over 50 objective physiological measurements for determining readiness for weaning and extubation found most had only a modest relationship with weaning outcome; no single factor or combination of factors demonstrated superior accuracy.[258] Of all predictors studied, the respiratory frequency to tidal volume ratio (f/V_T) appears to be most accurate.[259] However, inclusion of the f/V_T as part of a weaning protocol was found in one randomised study to increase, as opposed to decrease, the duration of weaning.[260] At present, consensus guidelines[254] do not recommend routine inclusion of weaning predictors.

Weaning methods

Various studies have attempted to identify the best weaning method. Two of the most frequently-cited

TABLE 15.8

Complications of mechanical ventilation

ITEM	COMPLICATION(S)
Barotrauma	Pneumothorax Pneumomediastinum Pneumopericardium Pulmonary interstitial emphysema Subcutaneous emphysema
Volutrauma	Shearing stress, endothelial and epithelial cell injury, fluid retention and pulmonary oedema, perivascular and alveolar haemorrhage, alveolar rupture
Biotrauma	Activation of systemic and local inflammatory mechanisms
Ventilation/perfusion mismatch	Alveolar distension causes compression of the adjacent pulmonary capillaries resulting in dead space ventilation
↓ Cardiac ouput	Resulting in hypotension, ↓ cerebral perfusion pressure (CPP), ↓ renal and hepatic blood flow
↑ Right ventricular afterload	Due to ↑ intrathoracic pressure may result in ↓ left ventricular compliance and preload
↓ Urine output	Due to ↓ glomerular filtration rate, ↑ sodium reabsorption and activation of the renin–angiotensin–aldosterone system
Fluid retention	Due to above renal factors as well as ↑ antidiuretic hormone and ↓ atrial natriuretic peptide
Impaired hepatic function	Due to ↑ pressure in the portal vein, ↓ portal venous blood flow, ↓ hepatic vein blood flow
↑ Intracranial pressure	Due to ↓ cerebral venous outflow
Oxygen toxicity	Alterations to lung parenchyma similar to those found in ARDS
Pulmonary emboli and deep vein thrombosis	Due to immobility
Ileus, diarrhoea	Due to alterations in gastric motility
Gastrointestinal haemorrhage	Gastritis and ulceration may occur due to stress, anxiety and critical illness
ICU-acquired weakness	Neuropathies and myopathies develop in association with critical illness, corticosteroids and neuromuscular blockade
Psychological issues	Delirium, anxiety, depression, agitation and post-traumatic stress disorder may be experienced by critically ill ventilated patients in the acute and recovery phases

studies have produced conflicting results. Brochard and colleagues[261] compared PSV, T piece trials and SIMV, and concluded that PSV reduced the duration of mechanical ventilation compared with the other methods. Esteban and colleagues[262] compared PSV, T piece trials, CPAP and progressive reduction of SIMV support, and found a once-daily T piece trial led to extubation three times more quickly than SIMV and nearly twice as quickly as PSV. A recent systematic review comparing trials of PSV and T piece found no clear evidence of a difference between these weaning strategies for weaning success.[263] Failure to produce consistent results favouring a single weaning style suggests it is not the mode that is important but rather the application of a systematic process.[264]

Spontaneous breathing trials

SBTs incorporate a focused assessment of a patient's capacity to breathe prior to extubation[265] and are recommended as the major diagnostic test to determine extubation readiness.[254] SBTs can be conducted using either a T piece or low levels of pressure support[266] and should need to last only 30 minutes.[267] This method of weaning is less common in Australia and New Zealand, in contrast to international findings.[78,79]

Weaning protocols

Implementation of various organisational strategies such as weaning teams and non-physician-led weaning protocols may assist in the timely recognition of weaning and extubation readiness.[268–272] Coupling of a sedation and weaning protocol was found to result in a three-day reduction in the duration of ventilation compared to standard care in four North American hospitals.[273] A systematic review and meta-analysis of 11 weaning protocol trials including 1971 patients demonstrated a reduction in the duration of mechanical ventilation.[274] However, the authors cautioned that the effect of weaning protocols may vary according to ICU organisational characteristics such as an intensivist-led ICU model, high levels of physician staffing, structured ward rounds, collaborative discussion and more frequent medical review; all are characteristics reported for ICUs in Australia and New Zealand.[275,276]

Automated weaning

Automated computerised systems potentially enable more efficient weaning by providing improved adaptation of ventilatory support through continuous monitoring and real-time intervention.[277] One such system, SmartCare™/PS, monitors three respiratory parameters, f, V_T and end-tidal carbon dioxide concentration, every 2 or 5 minutes and periodically adapts PS.[277,278] SmartCare™/PS establishes a respiratory status diagnosis, based on evaluation of the three parameters, and may either decrease or increase PS, or leave it unchanged to maintain the patient in a defined 'respiratory zone of comfort'.[279,280] Once SmartCare™/PS has successfully minimised the level of PS, a 1-hour observation period occurs. For patients who remain within the respiratory zone of comfort throughout the observation period, SmartCare™/PS recommends to 'consider separation', indicating the patient's respiratory status now suggests the patient will tolerate extubation.

A recent meta-analysis of automated weaning systems has shown that SmartCare™/PS may reduce the duration of weaning, total ventilation and ICU length of stay when compared to protocolised or usual care weaning.[281]

The difficult-to-wean patient

International reports indicate patients that require mechanical ventilation for ≥21 days account for less than 10% of all mechanically ventilated patients, but occupy 40% of ICU bed days and accrue 50% of ICU costs.[282,283] A recommendation from the National Association for Medical Direction of Respiratory Care states that prolonged mechanical ventilation should be defined as '≥21 consecutive days of ventilation required for ≥6 hours per day'.[254] Prolonged weaning has been defined as >7 days of weaning after the first SBT or more than three SBTs.[254] Little evidence defines the optimal method for managing the difficult-to-wean patient. One trial found no difference in weaning duration or success when comparing tracheostomy trials to low-level pressure support in patients with COPD experiencing weaning difficulty.[284] A recent randomised controlled trial demonstrated increased weaning success with use of a once daily progressive tracheostomy mask trial compared to pressure support weaning.[285] These patients are most likely to benefit from an individualised and structured approach to weaning using progressive lengthening of tracheostomy trials with supportive ventilation in between in combination with early physical therapy.

Practice tip

Tachypnoea and decreased V_T during weaning are indicators that a patient is not ready for extubation.

Summary

Support of oxygenation and ventilation during critical illness are key activities for nurses in ICU. Oxygen therapy promotes aerobic metabolism but has adverse effects that need to be considered. Various oxygen delivery devices provide low or variable flows of oxygen.

Strong evidence supports the use of NIV for COPD and CHF, but caution is required when it is used for other diagnoses such as pneumonia. NIV success is dependent on patient tolerance, with common complications including pressure ulcers, conjunctival irritations, nasal congestion, insufflation of air into the stomach and claustrophobia.

Airway support can be provided with oro- or nasopharyngeal airways, LMAs and endotracheal intubation; oral intubation is the preferred method. For a patient with an ETT, the key points for practice are:

- ETT placement should be confirmed with end-tidal CO_2 monitoring
- The aim of endotracheal cuff management is to prevent airway contamination and enable positive pressure ventilation
- Closed suctioning reduces alveolar derecruitment compared to open suctioning
- Instillation of normal saline is not recommended during routine tracheal suctioning.

The optimal timing of tracheostomy remains uncertain; however, tracheostomy should be considered for patients experiencing weaning difficulty.

The goals of mechanical ventilation are to promote gas exchange, minimise lung injury, reduce work of breathing and promote patient comfort:

- Despite its life-saving potential, mechanical ventilation carries the risk of serious physical and psychological complications.
- Humidification of dry medical gas is required during mechanical ventilation to prevent drying of secretions, mucous plugging and airway occlusion.
- The pressure required to deliver a volume of gas into the lungs is determined by elastic and resistive forces.
- Contemporary ventilators now provide a range of modes to facilitate mechanical ventilation.
- Analysis of ventilator graphics provides clinicians with the ability to assess patient–ventilator interaction, appropriateness of ventilator settings and lung function.
- Semirecumbent positioning at 45° elevation has been shown to reduce VAP but compliance is poor.
- RMs, HFOV, ECMO and prone positioning are strategies that may facilitate management of refractory hypoxaemia.

Case study

A 60-year-old female, Martha, was admitted to the ICU with acute respiratory failure due to community-acquired pneumonia. Martha was morbidly obese (190 kg) with extensive central obesity and a body mass index of 74.2. She had a history of COPD but was not prescribed steroids and had not been investigated for sleep apnoea.

Martha was commenced on broad spectrum antibiotic cover in the emergency department. On arrival to the ICU, Martha was placed in an isolation room, and respiratory isolation using droplet precautions for possible H1N1 were initiated. The patient was commenced on oral oseltamivir at 150 mg twice a day. Martha had a trial of NIV with FiO_2 0.7, PEEP 7 cmH_2O (EPAP 7 cmH_2O) and pressure support 5 cmH_2O (IPAP 12 cmH_2O) to reduce her work of breathing and improve gas exchange. The NIV trial was discontinued as Martha's dyspnoea was unrelieved, and hypoxia and hypercapnia persisted. She was intubated with a size 7 oral ETT and a bronchial alveolar lavage was performed to obtain samples for bacterial and viral screening. Nasopharyngeal swabs were also obtained. Ventilator settings following intubation were A/C, FiO_2 1.0, respiratory rate 16, P_{insp} 30 cmH_2O, PEEP 15 cmH_2O and inspiratory time of 1.1 seconds. Initial blood gases were as follows: pH 7.07, PaO_2 71 mmHg, $PaCO_2$ 71 mmHg, HCO_3^- 16.4 mmol, base excess −9.5, sodium 123 mmol, chloride 94 mmol, lactate 0.7, SpO_2 94% and PaO_2/FiO_2 (PF) ratio 71. Dynamic compliance was 25.6 mL/cmH_2O, resistance was 8.6 $cmH_2O/(L/s)$. A chest X-ray showed bilateral pulmonary infiltrates and a lobular pneumonia. Chest auscultation revealed bilateral crackles, late in the inspiratory phase.

Nursing assessment indicated the following issues:

1 notable audible cuff leak on inspiration despite a cuff pressure of 30 cmH_2O

2 atelectasis as evidenced by decreased air entry in lung bases, reduced compliance, diminished gas exchange and obliteration of costophrenic angles on the chest X-ray.

To address the cuff leak, nursing staff connected rigid manometer tubing between the cuff pressure gauge and the ETT pilot tube to enable continuous cuff pressure measurement. Cuff pressure did not decrease over time indicating that the ETT cuff was intact. Therefore, the audible air leak was not caused by a leaking ETT cuff but was due to an air leak around the cuff. On careful examination of the chest X-ray the ETT cuff was found to be above the level of the vocal cords and therefore needed repositioning.

To address the atelectasis, Martha was repositioned in a high semi-Fowler position (≥45° HOB elevation). This change in positioning resulted in an immediate improvement in compliance from a baseline of 25.6 to 38.4 mL/cmH_2O. V_T also increased from 300 mL to 400 mL. These improvements enabled rapid downward titration of FiO_2 to 0.7 while maintaining SpO_2 >90%. An RM using 40 cmH_2O for 40 seconds was performed with further improvement of Martha's oxygenation indicating her lungs were responsive to this strategy. The ventilator mode was changed to APRV with a P_{insp} of 27 cmH_2O for 6 seconds and an expiratory pressure of 5 cmH_2O for 0.4 seconds. Further improvements in oxygenation were noted (PaO_2 180 mmHg and PF ratio 225).

DISCUSSION

A cuff leak may be assumed to be secondary to a hole in either the cuff or pilot tube; however, this is relatively rare. Audible cuff leaks are more frequently due to a malpositioned ETT. It is important to note that each time cuff pressure is measured, a small volume of gas leaves the cuff to pressurise the pressure gauge. Repeated cuff pressure measurement may cause reduced cuff pressure over time, which may be falsely assumed to indicate the cuff is losing volume due to other causes. Attaching rigid tubing between the cuff and pressure gauge eliminates this problem and facilitates continuous cuff pressure measurement. This is a useful strategy for assessing cuff leak problems. In this case scenario, careful troubleshooting averted the need for ETT replacement and avoided unnecessary risk to the patient.

Patient positioning is extremely important in managing the bariatric patient. Central obesity causes cephalic displacement of the diaphragm resulting in a positive pleural pressure and subsequent alveolar collapse. Inspiratory crackles late in the inspiratory phase indicate late alveolar opening and an increased potential for lung injury due to cyclic alveolar inflation and deflation. Positive pleural pressure decreases transpulmonary pressure and often necessitates the use of higher levels of PEEP to prevent collapse. Positioning in the high semi-Fowler position can have a dramatic and positive effect on lung mechanics for these patients evidenced by the increase in compliance in this case study. RMs typically have a limited period of effectiveness, i.e. derecruitment generally occurs following the manoeuvre. APRV maintains the higher level of pressure for a prolonged time thus sustaining alveolar recruitment. In this case study APRV and position changes appeared to promote recruitment and improved oxygenation enabling downwards titration of the FiO_2. When considering extubation for the bariatric patient, maintaining PEEP at a high level prior to extubation and using CPAP following extubation may prevent alveolar derecruitment.

CASE STUDY QUESTIONS

1 In this case study Martha received relatively low levels of PEEP and pressure support prior to intubation. What are the potential advantages and disadvantages of increasing these parameters for this patient?

2 What is the rationale for using oxygen therapy in patients with COPD and low SpO_2?

3 Explain why Martha's lung compliance increased when positioning was changed from the supine to high semi-Fowler position.

RESEARCH VIGNETTE

Guérin C, Reignier J, Richard JC, Beuret P, Gacouin A, Boulain T et al. Prone positioning in severe acute respiratory distress syndrome. N Engl J Med 2013;368(23):2159–68

Abstract

Background: Previous trials involving patients with the ARDS have failed to show a beneficial effect of prone positioning during mechanical ventilatory support on outcomes. We evaluated the effect of early application of prone positioning on outcomes in patients with severe ARDS.

Methods: In this multicenter, prospective, randomized, controlled trial, we randomly assigned 466 patients with severe ARDS to undergo prone-positioning sessions of at least 16 hours or to be left in the supine position. Severe ARDS was defined as a ratio of the partial pressure of arterial oxygen to the FiO_2 of less than 150 mmHg, with a FiO_2 of at least 0.6, a positive end-expiratory pressure of at least 5 cmH_2O, and a tidal volume close to 6 mL per kilogram of predicted body weight. The primary outcome was the proportion of patients who died from any cause within 28 days after inclusion.

Results: A total of 237 patients were assigned to the prone group, and 229 patients were assigned to the supine group. The 28-day mortality was 16.0% in the prone group and 32.8% in the supine group (P<0.001). The hazard ratio for death with prone positioning was 0.39 (95% confidence interval [CI], 0.25 to 0.63). Unadjusted 90-day mortality was 23.6% in the prone group versus 41.0% in the supine group (P<0.001), with a hazard ratio of 0.44 (95% CI, 0.29 to 0.67). The incidence of complications did not differ significantly between the groups, except for the incidence of cardiac arrests, which was higher in the supine group.

Conclusion: In patients with severe ARDS, early application of prolonged prone-positioning sessions significantly decreased 28-day and 90-day mortality.

Critique

This well conducted randomised controlled trial has a number of strengths. Patients with severe ARDS (defined as a PF ratio of <150 mmHg, with an FiO2 of ≥0.6, PEEP of ≥5 cmH_2O and a V_T of approximately 6 mL per kilogram of predicted body weight) were recruited early (within 36 hours of ventilation) ensuring the intervention was applied in the early phase of ARDS and not as a rescue measure. Patients were assessed for 12 to 24 hours prior to randomization, thus confirming the presence of severe ARDS. All patients received standardised protective lung ventilation thereby removing the style of ventilation as a potential confounder. In the intervention arm, all patients were proned within 1 hour of randomisation and proning sessions extended for at least 16 consecutive hours, thereby producing maximal effects of proning. Considerations for translation of this research into practice are as follows. All participating centres had extensive (greater than 5 years) experience with proning. The study found no difference in adverse event rates between the prone and supine groups. This finding may not be generalisable to centres without this level of experience. Additionally, the notable reduction in 28-day mortality found in this study with proning applies to patients with severe ARDS. Again, the findings are not generalisable to patients with mild-to-moderate ARDS.

Learning activities

1 Describe how the terms IPAP and EPAP used on some NIV ventilators correlate with the more generic terms of PEEP and pressure support.

2 Why is it important to consider the patient's respiratory rate and tidal volume when using a low flow (variable flow) oxygen delivery device?

3 How do increasing PEEP and recruitment manoeuvres increase oxygenation?

4 Identify some of the potential risks of recruitment manoeuvres and the nursing observations to detect signs of deterioration.

5 Explain how a reduction in the FiO_2 from 1.0 to 0.8 can increase the SpO_2.

Online resources

American Association for Respiratory Care, www.aarc.org/resources

American Thoracic Society, www.thoracic.org/statements

Anaesthesia UK, www.frca.co.uk/default.aspx

Australian and New Zealand Intensive Care Society, www.anzics.com.au

ARDS network, www.ardsnet.org/

Canadian Society of Respiratory Therapists, Respiratory Resource, www.respiratoryresource.ca

College of Intensive Care Medicine of Australia and New Zealand (CICM), www.cicm.org.au

Covidien education resources, www.nellcor.com/educ/OnlineEd.aspx

Critical Care Medicine Tutorials, www.ccmtutorials.com

Department of Anaesthesia and Intensive Care, Chinese University of Hong Kong, http://aic-server4.aic.cuhk.edu.hk/web8

Fisher and Paykel Resource Centre, www.fphcare.com/respiratory-acute-care/resource-library.html

Intensive Care Coordination and Monitoring Unit, http://intensivecare.hsnet.nsw.gov.au

NHS Institute for Innovation and Improvement, www.institute.nhs.uk/safer_care/general/human_factors.html

Thoracic Society of Australia and New Zealand, www.thoracic.org.au

Vent World, www.ventworld.com

Further reading

Branson RD, Gomaa D, Rodriquez D Jr. Management of the artificial airway. Respir Care 2014;59(6):974–89.

Canadian Critical Care Trials Group/Canadian Critical Care Society Noninvasive Ventilation Guidelines Group. Clinical practice guidelines for the use of noninvasive positive-pressure ventilation and noninvasive continuous positive airway pressure in the acute care setting. CMAJ 2011;183(3):E195–214.

Chatburn RL, Khatib ME, Mireles-Cabodevila E. A taxonomy for mechanical ventilation: 10 fundamental maxims. Respir Care 2014;59(11):1747–63.

Ferrer M, Sellares J, Torres A. Noninvasive ventilation in withdrawal from mechanical ventilation. Semin Respir Crit Care Med 2014;35(4):507–18.

Jiang JR, Yen SY, Chien JY, Liu HC, Wu YL, Chen CH. Predicting weaning and extubation outcomes in long-term mechanically ventilated patients using the modified Burns Wean Assessment Program scores. Respirol 2014;19(4):576–82.

Suzumura EA, Figueiró M, Normilio-Silva K, Laranjeira L, Oliveira C, Buehler AM et al. Effects of alveolar recruitment maneuvers on clinical outcomes in patients with acute respiratory distress syndrome: a systematic review and meta-analysis. Intensive Care Med 2014;40(9):1227–40.

References

1 Australian and New Zealand Intensive Care Society Centre for Outcome and Resource Evaluation (ANZICS CORE) Annual Report 2012–13. Melbourne: Australian and New Zealand Intensive Care Society; 2014.

2 Shahin J, Harrison D, Rowan K. Is the volume of mechanically ventilated admissions to UK critical care units associated with improved outcomes? Intensive Care Med 2014;40(3):353–60.

3 Wunsch H, Wagner J, Herlim M, Chong D, Kramer A, Halpern S. ICU occupancy and mechanical ventilator use in the United States. Crit Care Med 2013;41(12): 712-9.

4 Chew D, Aroney C, Aylward P, Kelly A, White H, Tideman PA et al. 2011 Addendum to the National Heart Foundation of Australia/Cardiac Society of Australia and New Zealand Guidelines for the management of acute coronary syndromes (ACS) 2006. Heart Lung Circ 2011;20(8):487-502.

5 Celli B, MacNee W, ATS/ERS Taskforce. Standards for the diagnosis and treatment of patients with COPD: a summary of the ATS/ERS position paper. Eur Respir J 2004;23(6):932-46.

6 Naughton M, Tuxen D. Acute respiratory failure in chronic obstructive pulmonary disease. In: Bersten A, Soni N, eds. Oh's intensive care manual. 6th ed. Philadelphia: Butterworth, Heineman, Elsevier; 2009, pp 343-54.

7 Wagstaff A. Oxygen therapy. In: Bersten A, Soni N, editors. Oh's intensive care manual. 6th ed. Philadelphia: Butterworth, Heineman, Elsevier; 2009, pp 316-26.

8 Wagstaff T, Soni N. Performance of six types of oxygen delivery devices at varying respiratory rates. Anaesthesia 2007;62(5):492-503.

9 Sim M, Dean P, Kinsella J, Black R, Carter R, Hughes M. Performance of oxygen delivery devices when the breathing pattern of respiratory failure is simulated. Anaesthesia 2008;63(9):938-40.

10 Chanques G, Riboulet F, Molinari N, Carr J, Jung B, Prades A et al. Comparison of three high flow oxygen therapy delivery devices: a clinical physiological cross-over study. Minerva Anestesiol 2013;79(12):1344-55.

11 Groves N, Tobin A. High flow nasal oxygen generates positive airway pressures in adult volunteers. Aust Crit Care 2007;20(4):126-31.

12 Kernick J, Magary J. What is the evidence for the use of high flow nasal cannula oxygen in adult patients admitted to critical care units? A systematic review. Aust Crit Care 2010;23(2):53-70.

13 Fisher and Paykel Healthcare New Zealand. Respiratory and acute care, nasal high flow. Auckland: Fisher and Paykel Healthcare New Zealand, <http://www.fphcare.com/rsc/adult-care/nasal-high-flow.html>; 2010 [accessed 26.09.10].

14 Dysart K, Miller T, Wolfson M, Shaffer T. Research in high flow therapy: mechanisms of action. Respir Med 2009;103(10):1400-5.

15 Peters S, Holets S, Gay P. High-flow nasal cannula therapy in do-not-intubate patients with hypoxemic respiratory distress. Respir Care 2013;58(4):597-600.

16 Mayfield S, Jauncey-Cooke J, Hough J, Schibler A, Gibbons K, Bogossian F. High-flow nasal cannula therapy for respiratory support in children. Cochrane Database Syst Rev 2014;3(CD009850).

17 Hnatiuk O, Moores L, Thompson J, Jones M. Delivery of high concentrations of inspired oxygen via tusk mask. Crit Care Med 1998;26(6):1032-5.

18 Peruzzi W, Smith B. Oxygen delivery: tusks versus flow. Crit Care Med 1998;26(6):986.

19 Boumphrey S, Morris E, Kinsella S. 100% Inspired oxygen from a Hudson mask – a realistic goal? Resuscitation 2003;57(1):69-72.

20 Anesthesiology Rotation and Elective. Understanding equipment. Charlottesville: University of Virginia School of Medicine, <http://www.health system.virginia.edu/Internet/Anesthesiology-Elective/airway/equipment.cfm>; 2004 [accessed 17.02.11].

21 Cook T, Hommers C. New airways for resuscitation? Resuscitation 2006;69(3):371-87.

22 Joynt G. Airway management and acute upper-airway obstruction. In: Bersten A, Soni N, eds. Oh's intensive care manual. 6th ed. Philadelphia: Butterworth, Heineman, Elsevier; 2009, pp 327-41.

23 Lavery G, McCloskey B. The difficult airway in adult critical care. Crit Care Med 2008;36(7):2163-73.

24 Nolan JP, Hazinski MF, Billi JE, Boettiger BW, Bossaert L, de Caen AR et al. Part 1: Executive summary: 2010 International consensus on cardiopulmonary resuscitation and emergency cardiovascular care science with treatment recommendations. Resuscitation 2010;81(1):e1-e25.

25 Wahlen B, Roewer N, Lange M, Kranke P. Tracheal intubation and alternative airway management devices used by healthcare professionals with different level of pre-existing skills: a manikin study. Anaesthesia 2009;64(5):549-54.

26 Vézina M-C, Trépanier C, Nicole P, Lessard M. Complications associated with the Esophageal-Tracheal Combitube® in the pre-hospital setting. Can J Anesth 2007;54(2):124-8.

27 Haas C, Eakin R, Konkle M, Blank R. Endotracheal tubes: old and new. Respir Care 2014;59(6):933-52.

28 Haas CF, Branson RD, Folk LM, Campbell RS, Wise CR, Davis K Jr et al. Patient-determined inspiratory flow during assisted mechanical ventilation. Respir Care 1995;40(7):716-21.

29 Ball J, Platt S. Obstruction of a reinforced oral tracheal tube. Brit J Anaesthesia 2010;105(5):699-700.

30 Davies R. The importance of a Murphy eye. Anaesthesia 2001;56(9):906-24.

31 Jaber S, Amraoui J, Lefrant J-Y, Arich C, Cohendy R, Landreau L. Clinical practice and risk factors for immediate complications of endotracheal intubation in the intensive care unit: a prospective, multiple-center study. Crit Care Med 2006;34(9):2355-61.

32 Weingart S. Preoxygenation, reoxygenation, and delayed sequence intubation in the emergency department. J Emerg Med 2010;40(6):661-7

33 Holzapfel L, Chastang C, Demingeon G, Bohe J, Piralla B, Coupry A. A randomized study assessing the systematic search for maxillary sinusitis in nasotracheally mechanically ventilated patients. Influence of nosocomial maxillary sinusitis on the occurrence of ventilator-associated pneumonia. Am J Resp Crit Care Med 1999;159(3):695-701.

34 Beavers R, Moos D, Cuddeford J. Analysis of the application of cricoid pressure: implications for the clinician. J PeriAnesth Nurs 2009;24(2):92-102.

35 Brisson P, Brisson M. Variable application and misapplication of cricoid pressure. J Trauma 2010;69(5):1182-4.

36 Priebe H. Cricoid pressure: an expert's opinion. Minerva Anestesiol 2009;75(12):710-4.

37 Sitzwohl C, Langheinrich A, Schober A, Krafft P, Sessler D, Herkner H et al. Endobronchial intubation detected by insertion depth of endotracheal tube, bilateral auscultation, or observation of chest movements: randomised trial. BMJ 2010;341:c5943.

38 Rudraraju P, Eisen L. Confirmation of endotracheal tube position: a narrative review. J Intensive Care Med 2009;24(5):283-92.

39 College of Intensive Care Medicine of Australia and New Zealand (CICM). IC-1 Minimum standards for intensive care units, <http://www.cicm. org.au/policydocs.php>; 2010 [accessed 17.02.11].

40 Mallick A, Bodenham A. Tracheostomy in critically ill patients. Eur J Anaesthesiol 2010;27(8):676–82.

41 De Leyn P, Bedert L, Delcroix M, Depuydt P, Lauwers G, Sokolov Y et al. Tracheotomy: clinical review and guidelines. Eur J Cardiothorac Surg 2007;32(3):412-21.

42 Australian and New Zealand Intensive Care Society. Percutaneous dilatational tracheostomy consensus statement, <http://www.anzics.com.au/ safety-quality?start=2>; 2010 [accessed January 2011].

43 Russell C. Providing the nurse with a guide to tracheostomy care and management. Brit J Nurs 2005;14(8):428-33.

44 Dennis-Rouse M, Davidson J. An evidence-based evaluation of tracheostomy care practices. Crit Care Nurs Q 2008;31(5):150-60.

45 Thomas A, McGrath B. Patient safety incidents associated with airway devices in critical care: a review of reports to the UK National Patient Safety Agency. Anaesthesia 2009;64(4):358–65.

46 Happ MB. Treatment interference in acutely and critically ill adults. Am J Crit Care 1998;7(3):224-35.

47 Curry K, Cobb S, Kutash M, Diggs C. Characteristics associated with unplanned extubations in a surgical intensive care unit. Am J Crit Care 2008;17(1):45-51.

48 Mion LC, Minnick AF, Leipzig R, Catrambone CD, Johnson ME. Patient-initiated device removal in intensive care units: a national prevalence study. Crit Care Med 2007;35(12):2714-20.

49 Birkett KM, Southerland KA, Leslie GD. Reporting unplanned extubation. Intensive Crit Care Nurs 2005;21(2):65-75.

50 Tung A, Tadimeti L, Caruana-Montaldo B, Atkins PM, Mion LC, Palmer RM et al. The relationship of sedation to deliberate self-extubation. J Clin Anesth 2001;13(1):24-9.

51 Atkins PM, Mion LC, Mendelson W, Palmer RM, Slomka J, Franko T. Characteristics and outcomes of patients who self-extubate from ventilatory support: a case-control study. Chest 1997;112(5):1317-23.

52 Engels P, Bagshaw S, Meier M, Brindley P. Tracheostomy: from insertion to decannulation. Can J Surg 2009;52(5):427-33.

53 Delaney A, Bagshaw S, Nalos M. Percutaneous dilatational tracheostomy versus surgical tracheostomy in critically ill patients: a systematic review and meta-analysis. Crit Care 2006;10(2):R55.

54 Fernandez M, Piacentini E, Blanch L, Fernandez R. Changes in lung volume with three systems of endotracheal suctioning with and without pre-oxygenation in patients with mild-to-moderate lung failure. Intensive Care Med 2004;30(12):2210-5.

55 Intensive Care Coordination and Monitoring Unit. Suctioning an adult with a tracheal tube. NSW Health Statewide Guidelines for Intensive Care, <http://intensivecare.hsnet.nsw.gov.au/state-wide-guidelines>; 2007 [accessed January 2011].

56 Overend T, Anderson C, Brooks D, Cicutto L, Keim M, McAuslan D et al. Updating the evidence base for suctioning adult patients: a systematic review. Can Respir J 2009;16(3):e6-17.

57 Chaseling W, Bayliss S-L, Rose K, Armstrong L, Boyle M, Caldwel J et al. Suctioning an adult ICU patient with an artificial airway, version 2. Chatswood, NSW: Agency for Clinical Innovation NSW Government; 2014.

58 Paulus F, Binnekade J, Vroom M, Schultz M. Benefits and risks of manual hyperinflation in intubated and mechanically ventilated intensive care unit patients: a systematic review. Crit Care 2012;16(4):R145.

59 AARC. AARC Clinical Practice Guidelines. Endotracheal suctioning of mechanically ventilated patients with artificial airways. Respir Care 2010;55(6):758-64.

60 National Health and Medical Research Council (NHMRC). Australian Guidelines for the Prevention and Control of Infection in Healthcare. Canberra: NHMRC; 2010.

61 Intensive Care Coordination and Monitoring Unit. Stabilisation of an endotracheal tube for the adult intensive care patient. NSW Health statewide guidelines for intensive care, <http://intensivecare.hsnet.nsw.gov.au/state-wide-guidelines>; 2007 [accessed January 2011].

62 Gardner A, Hughes D, Cook R, Osborne S, Gardner G. Best practice in stabilisation of oral endotracheal tubes: a systematic review. Aust Crit Care 2005;18(4):158-65

63 Murdoch E, Holdgate A. A comparison of tape-tying versus a tube-holding device for securing endotracheal tubes in adults. Anaesth Intensive Care 2007;35(5): 30-5.

64 Rello J, Sonara R, Jubert P, Artigas A, Rue M, Valles J. Pneumonia in intubated patients: role of respiratory airway care. Am J Respir Crit Care Med 1996;154(1):111-5.

65 Rose L, Redl L. Survey of cuff management practices within Australia and New Zealand. Am J Crit Care 2008;17(5):428-35

66 Vyas D, Inweregbu K, Pittard A. Measurement of tracheal tube cuff pressure in critical care. Anaesthesia 2002;57(3):275-7.

67 Sole M, Byers J, Ludy J, Zhang Y, Banta C, Brummel K. A multisite survey of suctioning techniques and airway management practices. Am J Crit Care 2003;12(3):220-30.

68 Sole M, Penoyer D, Su X, Jimenez E, Kalita S, Poalillo E et al. Assessment of endotracheal cuff pressure by continuous monitoring: a pilot study. Am J Crit Care 2009;18(2):133-43

69 Lizy C, Swinnen W, Labeau S, Poelaert J, Vogelaers D, Vandewoude K et al. Cuff pressure of endotracheal tubes after changes in body position in critically ill patients treated with mechanical ventilation. Am J Crit Care 2014;23(1):e1-8

70 Lorente L, Lecuona M, Jiménez A, Lorenzo L, Roca I, Cabrera J et al. Continuous endotracheal tube cuff pressure control system protects against ventilator-associated pneumonia. Crit Care 2014;18(2):R77.

71 Fernandez J, Levine S, Restrepo M. Technologic advances in endotracheal tubes for prevention of ventilator-associated pneumonia. Chest 2012;142(1):231-8.

72 Frost S, Azeem A, Alexandrou E, Tam V, Murphy J, Hunt L et al. Subglottic secretion drainage for preventing ventilator associated pneumonia: a meta-analysis. Aust Crit Care 2013;26(4):180-8.

73 Bitgani M, Madineh H. Intraoperative atelectasis due to endotracheal tube cuff herniation: a case report. Acta Medica Iranica 2012;50(9):652-4.

74 El-Orbany M, Salem M. Endotracheal tube cuff leaks: causes, consequences, and management. Anesth Analg 2013;117:428-34.

75 AARC. AARC clinical practice guideline: removal of the endotracheal tube 2007 revision & update. Respir Care 2007;52(6):81-93.

76 Antonaglia V, Vergolini A, Pascotto S, Bonini P, Renco M, Peratoner A et al. Cuff-leak test predicts the severity of post extubation acute laryngeal lesions: a preliminary study. Eur J Anaesthesiol 2010;27(6):534–41.

77 Cormack R, Lehane J. Difficult tracheal intubation in obstetrics. Anaesthesia 1984;39(11):1105-11.

78 Esteban A, Ferguson N, Meade M, Frutos-Vivar F, Apezteguia C, Brochard L et al. Evolution of mechanical ventilation in response to clinical research. Am J Respir Crit Care Med 2008;177(2):170-7.

79 Rose L, Presneill J, Johnston L, Nelson S, Cade J. Ventilation and weaning practices in Australia and New Zealand. Anaeth Intensive Care 2009;37(1):99-107.

80 Hess D. Ventilator waveforms and the physiology of pressure support ventilation. Respir Care 2005;50(2):166-86.

81 Pilbeam S, Cairo J. Mechanical ventilation: physiological and clinical applications. 4th ed. St Louis: Mosby Elsevier; 2006.

82 Burns S. Working with respiratory waveforms: how to use bedside graphics. AACN Clin Issues 2003;14(2):133-44.

83 Rittner F, Doring M. Curves and loops in mechanical ventilation. Hong Kong: Draeger Medical Asia Pacific.

84 Tobin M. Monitoring of pressure, flow, and volume during mechanical ventilation. Respir Care 1992;37(9):1081-96.

85 Nilsestuen J, Hargett K. Using ventilator graphics to identify patient–ventilator asynchrony. Respir Care 2005;50(2):202-34.

86 Yang S, Yang S. Effects of inspiratory flow waveforms on lung mechanics, gas exchange, and respiratory metabolism in COPD patients during mechanical ventilation. Chest 2002;122(6):2096-104.

87 Blanch L, Bernabé F, Lucangelo U. Measurement of air trapping, intrinsic positive end-expiratory pressure, and dynamic hyperinflation in mechanically ventilated patients. Respir Care 2005;50(1):110-23.

88 Lu Q, Rouby J-J. Measurement of pressure–volume curves in patients on mechanical ventilation: methods and significance. Crit Care 2000;4(2):91–100.

89 Bonetto C, Calo M, Delgado M, Mancebo J. Modes of pressure delivery and patient–ventilator interaction. Respir Care Clin N Am 2005; 11(2):247–63.

90 Maggiore S, Jonson B, Richard J, Jaber S, Lemaire F, Brochard L. Alveolar derecruitment at decremental positive end-expiratory pressure levels in acute lung injury: comparison with the lower inflection point, oxygenation, and compliance. Am J Respir Crit Care Med 2001;164(5):795-801.

91 Hickling K. Best compliance during a decremental, but not incremental, positive end-expiratory pressure trial is related to open-lung positive end-expiratory pressure: a mathematical model of acute respiratory distress syndrome lungs. Am J Respir Crit Care Med 2001;163(1):69-78.

92 Banner MJ, Jaeger MJ, Kirby RR. Components of the work of breathing and implications for monitoring ventilator-dependent patients. Crit Care Med 1994;22(3):515-23.

93 Lucangelo U, Bernabé F, Blanch L. Respiratory mechanics derived from signals in the ventilator circuit. Respir Care 2005;50(1):55-65.

94 Nishida T, Nishimura M, Fujino Y, Mashimo T. Performance of heated humidifiers with a heated wire according to ventilatory settings. J Aerosol Med 2001;14(1):43-51.

95 Branson R. The ventilator circuit and ventilator-associated pneumonia. Respir Care 2005;50(6):774-85.

96 Muscedere J, Dodek P, Keenan S, Fowler R, Cook D, Heyland D. Comprehensive evidence-based clinical practice guidelines for ventilator-associated pneumonia: prevention. J Crit Care 2008;23(1):126-37.

97 Kilgour E, Rankin N, Ryan S, Pack R. Mucociliary function deteriorates in the clinical range of inspired air temperature and humidity. Intensive Care Med 2004;30(7):1491-4.

98 Bersten A. Humidification and inhalation therapy. In: Bersten A, Soni N, Oh T, eds. Oh's intensive care manual. 5th ed. Oxford: Butterworth-Heinemann; 2003.

99 Branson R, Davis K. Evaluation of 21 passive humidifiers according to the ISO 9360 standard: moisture output, dead space, and flow resistance. Respir Care 1996;41:736-43.

100 Iotti G, Olivei M, Braschi A. Mechanical effects of heat-moisture exchangers in ventilated patients. Crit Care 1999;3(5):R77-82.

101 Kelly M, Gillies D, Todd D, Lockwood C. Heated humidification versus heat and moisture exchangers for ventilated adults and children. Cochrane Database Syst Rev 2010;(4):CD004711.

102 Nava S, Hill N. Non-invasive ventilation in acute respiratory failure. Lancet 2009;374(9685):250-9.

103 Rose L, Gerdtz M. Review of non-invasive ventilation in the emergency department: clinical considerations and management priorities. J Clin Nurs 2009;18(23):3216-24.

104 Mehta S, Hill N. Noninvasive ventilation: state of the art. Am J Respir Crit Care Med 2001;163(2):540-77.

105 Hill N. Noninvasive positive pressure ventilation. In: Tobin M, ed. Principles and practice of mechanical ventilation. 2nd ed. New York: McGraw-Hill; 2006.

106 L'Her E, Deye N, Lellouche F, Taille S, Demoule A, Fraticelli A et al. Physiologic effects of noninvasive ventilation during acute lung injury. Am J Respir Crit Care Med 2005;172(9):1112-8.

107 Hill N, Brennan J, Garpestad E, Nava S. Noninvasive ventilation in acute respiratory failure. Crit Care Med 2007;35(10):2402-7.

108 Naughton M, Rahman M, Hara K, Floras J, Bradley T. Effect of continuous positive airway pressure on intrathoracic and left ventricular transmural pressures in patients with congestive heart failure. Circulation 1995;91(6):1725-31.

109 Kaye D, Mansfield D, Naughton MT. Continuous positive airway pressure decreases myocardial oxygen consumption in heart failure. Clin Sci 2004;106(6):599-603.

110 Pladeck T, Hader C, Von Orde A, Rasche K, Wiechmann H. Non-invasive ventilation: comparison of effectiveness, safety, and management of acute heart failure syndromes and acute exacerbations of chronic obstructive pulmonary disease. J Physiol Pharmacol 2007;58(5suppl, Pt2):539-49.

111 Caples S, Gay P. Noninvasive positive pressure ventilation in the intensive care unit: a concise review. Crit Care Med 2005;33(11):2651-8.

112 Confalonieri M, Potena A, Carbone G, Della Porta R, Tolley E, Meduri G. Acute respiratory failure in patients with severe community-acquired pneumonia. Am J Respir Crit Care Med 1999;160(5, Pt 1):1585-91.

113 Antonelli M, Conti G, Moro M, Esquinas A, Gonzalez-Diaz G, Confalonieri M et al. Predictors of failure of noninvasive positive pressure ventilation in patients with acute hypoxemic respiratory failure; a multi-center study. Intensive Care Med 2001;27(11):1718-28.

114 Keenan S, Sinuff T, Cook D, Hill N. Which patients with acute exacerbation of chronic obstructive pulmonary disease benefit from noninvasive positive pressure ventilation? A systematic review of the literature. Ann Int Med 2003;138(11):861-70.

115 Lightowler JV, Wedzicha JA, Elliott MW, Ram FS. Non-invasive positive pressure ventilation to treat respiratory failure resulting from exacerbations of chronic obstructive pulmonary disease: Cochrane systematic review and meta-analysis. BMJ 2003;326(7382):185.

116 Ram FS, Picot J, Lightowler J, Wedzicha JA. Non-invasive positive pressure ventilation for treatment of respiratory failure due to exacerbations of chronic obstructive pulmonary disease. Cochrane Database Syst Rev 2004 (1):CD004104.

117 Confalonieri M, Garuti G, Cattaruzza M, Osborn J, Antonelli M, Conti G et al.. A chart of failure risk for noninvasive ventilation in patients with COPD exacerbation. Eur Respir J 2005;25(2):348-55.

118 Masip J, Roque M, Sanchez B, Ferandez R, Subirana M, Exposito J. Noninvasive ventilation in acute cardiogenic pulmonary edema. JAMA 2005;294(24):3124-30.

119 Peter JV, Moran JL, Phillips-Hughes J, Graham P, Bersten AD. Effect of non-invasive positive pressure ventilation (NIPPV) on mortality in patients with acute cardiogenic pulmonary oedema: a meta-analysis. Lancet 2006;367(9517):1155-63.

120 Winck JC, Azevedo LF, Costa-Pereira A, Antonelli M, Wyatt JC. Efficacy and safety of non-invasive ventilation in the treatment of acute cardiogenic pulmonary edema – a systematic review and meta-analysis. Crit Care 2006;10(2):R69.

121 Vital F, Ladeira M, Atallah A. Non-invasive positive pressure ventilation (CPAP or bilevel NPPV) for cardiogenic pulmonary oedema. Cochrane Database Syst Rev 2013;(5):CD005351.

122 Udwadia Z, Santis G, Steven M, Simonds A. Nasal ventilation to facilitate weaning in patients with chronic respiratory insufficiency. Thorax 1992;47(9):715-8.

123 Agarwal R, Aggarwal A, Gupta D, Jindal S. Role of noninvasive positive-pressure ventilation in postextubation respiratory failure: a meta-analysis. Respir Care 2007;52(11):1472-9.

124 Burns K, Meade MO, Premji A, Adhikari NK. Non-invasive positive pressure ventilation as a weaning strategy for intubated patients with respiratory failure. Cochrane Database Syst Rev 2013(12):CD004127

125 Esteban A, Frutos F, Ferguson ND, Arabi Y, Apezteguia C, González M et al. Noninvasive positive pressure ventilation for respiratory failure after extubation. N Engl J Med 2004;350(24):2452-60.

126 Ram FS, Wellington S, Rowe BH, Wedzicha JA. Non-invasive positive pressure ventilation for treatment of respiratory failure due to severe acute exacerbations of asthma. Cochrane Database Syst Rev 2005(1):CD004360.

127 Pallin M, Naughton M. Noninvasive ventilation in acute asthma. J Crit Care 2014;29(4):586-93.

128 Quill C, Quill T. Palliative use of noninvasive ventilation: navigating murky waters. J Palliat Med 2014;17(6):657-61.

129 Maheshwari V, Paioli D, Rothaar R, Hill N. Utilization of noninvasive ventilation in acute care hospitals: a regional survey. Chest 2006;129(5): 1226-33.

130 Evans TW. International Consensus Conferences in Intensive Care Medicine: Non-invasive positive pressure ventilation in acute respiratory failure. Intensive Care Med 2001;27(1):166-78.

131 Chiumello D. Is the helmet different than the face mask in delivering noninvasive ventilation. Chest 2006;129(6):1402-3.

132 British Thoracic Society Standards of Care Committee. Non-invasive ventilation in acute respiratory failure. Thorax 2002;57(3):192-211.

133 Keenan S, Sinuff T, Burns K, Muscedere J, Kutsogiannis J, Mehta S et al. Clinical practice guidelines for the use of noninvasive positive-pressure ventilation and noninvasive continuous positive airway pressure in the acute care setting. CMAJ 2011;183(3):E195-214.

134 Laghi F, Tobin M. Indications for mechanical ventilation. In: Tobin M, ed. Principles and practice of mechanical ventilation. 2nd ed. New York: McGraw-Hill; 2006.

135 Tobin M, Guenther S, Perez W, Lodato R, Mador M, Allen SJ et al. Konno-Mead analysis of ribcage-abdominal motion during successful and unsuccessful trials of weaning from mechanical ventilation. Am Rev Respir Dis 1987;135(8):1320-8.

136 Barnato A, Albert S, Angus D, Lave J, Degenholtz H. Disability among elderly survivors of mechanical ventilation. Am J Respir Crit Care Med 2011;183(8):1037-42.

137 Vasilevskis E, Han J, Hughes C, Ely E. Epidemiology and risk factors for delirium across hospital settings. Best Pract Res Clin Anaesthesiol 2012;26(3):277-87.

138 Chatburn R, Volsko T, Hazy J, Harris L, Sanders S. Determining the basis for a taxonomy of mechanical ventilation. Respir Care 2012;57(4): 514-24.

139 Rose L. Advanced modes of mechanical ventilation: implications for practice. AACN Adv Crit Care 2006;17(2):145-58.

140 Kuhlen R, Rossaint R. The role of spontaneous breathing during mechanical ventilation. Respir Care 2002;47(3):296-303.

141 Habashi N. Other approaches to open-lung ventilation: airway pressure release ventilation. Crit Care Med 2005;33(3Suppl):S228-40.

142 Marik P, Krikorian J. Pressure-controlled ventilation in ARDS: a practical approach. Chest 1997;112(4):1102-6.

143 Esteban A, Alia I, Gordo F, de Pablo R, Suarez J, Gonzalez G et al. Prospective randomized trial comparing pressure-controlled ventilation and volume-controlled ventilation in ARDS. Chest 2000;117(6):1690-6.

144 Campbell R, Davis B. Pressure-controlled versus volume-controlled ventilation: does it matter? Respir Care 2002;47(4):416-26.

145 Brochard L, Pluskwa F, Lemaire F. Improved efficacy of spontaneous breathing with inspiratory pressure support. Am Rev Respir Dis 1987;32(2):1110-6.

146 Davis W, Rennard S, Bitterman P, Crystal R. Pulmonary oxygen toxicity – early reversible changes in human alveolar structures induced by hyperoxia. N Engl J Med 1983;309(15):878-83.

147 Diacon A, Koegelenberg C, Klüsmann K, Bolliger C. Challenges in the estimation of tidal volume settings in critical care units. Intensive Care Med 2006;32(10):1670-1.

148 ARDSnet. Ventilation with lower tidal volumes compared with traditional tidal volumes for acute lung injury and the acute respiratory distress syndrome. N Engl J Med 2000;342(18):1301-8.

149 Gajic O, Saqib I, Mendez J, Adesanya A, Festic E, Caples SM et al. Ventilator-associated lung injury in patients without acute lung injury at the onset of mechanical ventilation. Crit Care Med 2004;32(9):1817-24.

150 Determann R, Royakkers A, Wolthuis E, Vlaar A, Choi G, Paulus F et al. Ventilation with lower tidal volumes as compared with conventional tidal volumes for patients without acute lung injury: a preventive randomized controlled trial. Crit Care Med 2010;14(1):R1.

151 Serpa Neto A, Cardoso S, Manetta J, Pereira V, Espósito D, Pasqualucci Mde O et al. Association between use of lung-protective ventilation with lower tidal volumes and clinical outcomes among patients without acute respiratory distress syndrome: a meta-analysis. JAMA 2012;308(16):1651-9.

152 Holets S, Hubmayr R. Setting the ventilator. In: Tobin M, ed. Principles and practice of mechanical ventilation. 2nd ed. New York: McGraw-Hill; 2006.

153 Goulet R, Hess D, Kacmarek R. Pressure vs flow triggering during pressure support ventilation. Chest 1997;111(6):1649-53.

154 Hill L, Pearl R. Flow triggering, pressure triggering, and autotriggering during mechanical ventilation. Crit Care Med 2000;28(2):579-81.

155 Kondili E, Akoumianaki E, Alexopoulou C, Georgopoulos D. Identifying and relieving asynchrony during mechanical ventilation. Expert Rev Respir Med 2009;3(3):231-43.

156 Chiumello D, Pelosi P, Taccone P, Slutsky A, Gattinoni L. Effect of different inspiratory rise time and cycling off criteria during pressure support ventilation in patients recovering from acute lung injury. Criti Care Med 2003;31(11):2604-10.

157 Amato M, Marini J. Pressure-controlled and inverse-ratio ventilation. In: Tobin M, ed. Principles and practice of mechanical ventilation. 2nd ed. New York: McGraw-Hill; 2006, pp 251-72.

158 Pierce L. Management of the mechanically ventilated patient. 2nd ed. St Louis: Saunders: Elsevier; 2007.

159 Gattinoni L, Caironi P, Carlesso E. How to ventilate patients with acute lung injury and acute respiratory distress syndrome. Curr Opin Crit Care 2005;11(1):69-76.

160 Kallet R. Evidence-based management of acute lung injury and acute respiratory distress syndrome. Respir Care 2004;49(7):793-809.

161 Ashbaugh D, Bigelow D, Petty T, Levine B. Acute respiratory distress in adults. Lancet 1967;2(7511):319-23.

162 Hemmila M, Napolitano LM. Severe respiratory failure: advanced treatment options. Crit Care Med 2006;34(9):S278-S90.

163 Ferguson ND, Frutos-Vivar F, Esteban A, Anzueto A, Alia I, Brower RG et al. Airway pressures, tidal volumes and mortality in patients with acute respiratory distress syndrome. Crit Care Med 2005;33(1):21-30.

164 Muscedere J, Mullen J, Gan K, Slutsky A. Tidal ventilation at low airway pressures can augment lung injury. Am J Respir Crit Care Med 1994;149(5):1327-34.

165 Tremblay L, Valenza F, Ribeiro S, Li J, Slutsky AS. Injurious ventilatory strategies increase cytokines and c-fos m-RNA expression in an isolated rat lung model. J Clin Invest 1997;99(5):944-52.

166 Amato M, Barbas C, Medeiros D, Magaldi R, Schettino G, Lorenzi-Filho G et al. Effect of a protective-ventilation strategy on mortality in the acute respiratory distress syndrome. N Engl J Med 1998;338(6):347-54.

167 Grasso S, Fanelli V, Cafarelli A, Anaclerio R, Amabile M, Ancona G et al. Effects of high versus low positive end-expiratory pressure in acute respiratory distress syndrome. Am J Respir Crit Care Med 2005;171(9):1002-8.

168 Brower RG, Lanken PN, MacIntyre N, Matthay MA, Morris A, Ancukiewicz M et al. Mechanical ventilation with higher versus lower positive end-expiratory pressures in patients with acute lung injury and acute respiratory distress syndrome. N Engl J Med 2004;351(4):327-36.

169 Suarez-Sipmann F, Bohm S, Tusman G, Pesch T, Thamm O, Reissmann H et al. Use of dynamic compliance for open lung positive end-expiratory pressure titration in an experimental study. Crit Care Med 2007;35(1):214-21.

170 Meade M, Cook D, Guyatt G, Slutsky A, Arabi Y, Cooper DJ et al.. Ventilation strategy using low tidal volumes, recruitment maneuvers, and high positive end-expiratory pressure for acute lung injury and acute respiratory distress syndrome: a randomized controlled trial. JAMA 2008;299(6):637-45.

171 Mercat A, Richard J-CM, Vielle B, Jaber S, Osman D, Diehl JL et al. Positive end-expiratory pressure setting in adults with acute lung injury and acute respiratory distress syndrome: a randomized controlled trial. JAMA 2008;299(6):646-55.

172 Hess D, Kacmarek R. Essentials of mechanical ventilation. 2nd ed. New York: McGraw-Hill; 2002.

173 Chiumello D, Polli F, Tallarini F, Chierichetti M, Motta G, Azzari S et al. Effect of different cycling-off criteria and positive end-expiratory pressure during pressure support ventilation in patients with chronic obstructive pulmonary disease. Crit Care Med 2007;35(11):2547-52.

174 Chatburn R. Classification of ventilator modes: update and proposal for implementation. Respir Care 2007;52(3):301-23.

175 Chatburn R. Understanding mechanical ventilators. Expert Rev Respir Med 2010;4(6):809-19.

176 Chen K, Sternbach G, Fromm R, Varon J. Mechanical ventilation: past and present. J Emerg Med 1998;16(3):435-60.

177 Haitsma J. Diaphragmatic dysfunction in mechanical ventilation. Curr Opin Anaesthesiol 2011;24(2):435-60

178 MacIntyre NR. Evidence-based guidelines for weaning and discontinuing ventilatory support. Chest 2001;120(6):375S-95S.

179 Hormann C, Baum M, Putensen C, Mutz N, Benzer H. Biphasic positive airway pressure (BIPAP) – a new mode of ventilatory support. Eur J Anaesthesiol 1994;11(1):37-42.

180 McCunn M, Habashi NM. Airway pressure release ventilation in the acute respiratory distress syndrome following traumatic injury. Int Anesthesiol Clin 2002;40(3):89-102.

181 Putensen C, Wrigge H. Airway pressure-release ventilation. In: Tobin M, ed. Principles and practice of mechanical ventilation. 2nd ed. New York: McGraw-Hill; 2006.

182 Rose L, Hawkins M. Airway pressure release ventilation and biphasic positive airway pressure: a systematic review of definitional criteria. Intensive Care Med 2008;34(10):1766-73.

183 Mols G, von Ungern-Sternberg B, Rohr E, Haberthur C, Geiger K, Guttman J. Respiratory comfort and breathing pattern during volume proportional assist ventilation and pressure support ventilation: a study on volunteers with artificially reduced compliance. Crit Care Med 2000;28(6):1940-6.

184 Guttmann J, Bernhard H, Mols G, Benzing A, Hofmann P, Haberthür C et al. Respiratory comfort of automatic tube compensation and inspiratory pressure support in conscious humans. Intensive Care Med 1997;23(11):1119-24.

185 Unoki T, Serita A, Grap M. Automatic tube compensation during weaning from mechanical ventilation: evidence and clinical implications. Crit Care Nurse 2008;28(4):34-42.

186 Fabry B, Haberthur C, Zappe D, Guttmann J, Kuhlen R, Stocker R. Breathing pattern and additional work of breathing in spontaneously breathing patients with different ventilatory demands during inspiratory pressure support and automatic tube compensation. Intensive Care Med 1997;23(5):545-52.

187 Branson R, Johannigman J. Innovations in mechanical ventilation. Respir Care 2009;54(7):933-47.

188 Sinderby C, Navalesi P, Beck J, Skrobik Y, Comtois N, Friberg S et al. Neural control of mechanical ventilation in respiratory failure. Nat Med 1999;5(12):1433-6.

189 Brander L, Sinderby C, Lecomte F, Leong-Poi H, Bell D, Beck J et al. Neurally adjusted ventilatory assist decreases ventilator-induced lung injury and non-pulmonary organ dysfunction in rabbits with acute lung injury. Intensive Care Med 2009;35(11):1979-89.

190 Spahija J, de Marchie M, Albert M, Bellemare P, Delisle S, Beck J et al. Patient–ventilator interaction during pressure support ventilation and neurally adjusted ventilatory assist. Crit Care Med 2010;38(2):518-26.

191 Piquilloud L, Vignaux L, Bialais E, Roeseler J, Sottiaux T, Laterre PF et al. Neurally adjusted ventilatory assist improves patient–ventilator interaction. Intensive Care Med 2011;37(2):263-71.

192 Coisel Y, Chanques G, Jung B, Constantin J, Capdevila X, Matecki S et al. Neurally adjusted ventilatory assist in critically ill postoperative patients: a crossover randomized study. Anesthesiol 2010;113(4):925-35.

193 Gattinoni L, Caironi P, Cressoni M, Chiumello D, Ranieri V, Quintel M et al. Lung recruitment in patients with the acute respiratory distress syndrome. N Engl J Med 2006;354(17):1775-86.

194 Hinz J, Moerer O, Neumann P, Dudykevych T, Hellige G, Quintel M. Effect of positive end-expiratory pressure on regional ventilation in patients with acute lung injury evaluated by electrical impedance tomography. Eur J Anaesthesiol 2005;22(11):817-25.

195 Brower R, Morris A, MacIntyre N, Matthay M, Hayden D, Thompson T et al.. Effects of recruitment maneuvers in patients with acute lung injury and acute respiratory distress syndrome ventilated with high positive end-expiratory pressure. Crit Care Med 2003;31(11):2592-7.

196 Hodgson C, Keating J, Holland A, Davies A, Smirneos L, Bradley S. Recruitment manoeuvres for adults with acute lung injury receiving mechanical ventilation. Cochrane Database Syst Rev 2009:CD006667.

197 Fan E, Needham D, Stewart T. Ventilatory management of acute lung injury and acute respiratory distress syndrome. JAMA 2005;294(22):2889-96.

198 ARDSnet. Effects of recruitment maneuvers in patients with acute lung injury and acute respiratory distress syndrome ventilated with high positive end-expiratory pressure. Crit Care Med 2003;31:2592-7.

199 Foti G, Cereda M, Sparacini M, de Marchi L, Villa F, Pesenti A. Effects of periodic lung recruitment maneuvers on gas exchange and respiratory mechanics in mechanically ventilated acute respiratory distress syndrome (ARDS) patients. Intensive Care Med 2000;26(5):501-7.

200 Odenstedt H, Aneman A, Kárason S, Stenqvist O, Lurdin S. Acute hemodynamic changes during lung recruitment in lavage and endotoxin-induced ALI. Intensive Care Med 2005;31(1):112-20.

201 Rose L. Clinical application of ventilation modes: ventilatory strategies for lung protection. Aus Crit Care 2010;23(2):71-80.

202 Mehta S, Grabton J, MacDonald R, Bowman D, Meatte-Martyn A, Bachman T et al. High-frequency oscillatory ventilation in adults: the Toronto experience. Chest 2004;126(2):518-27.

203 Singh J, Stewart T. High-frequency mechanical ventilation principles and practices in the era of lung-protective ventilation strategies. Respir Care Clin N Am 2002;8(2):247-60.

204 Singh J, Stewart T. High-frequency oscillation ventilation in adults with acute respiratory distress syndrome. Curr Opin Crit Care 2003;9(1):28-32.

205 Krishnan J, Brower R. High-frequency ventilation for acute lung injury and ARDS. Chest 2000;118(3):795-807.

206 Mehta S, Lapinsky SE, Hallett DC, Merker D, Groll R, Cooper AB et al. A prospective trial of high frequency oscillatory ventilation in adults with acute respiratory distress syndrome. Crit Care Med 2001;29(7):1360-9.

207 Mehta S, MacDonald R. Implementing and troubleshooting high-frequency oscillatory ventilation in adults in the intensive care unit. Respir Care Clin N Am 2001;7(4):683-95.

208 Higgins J, Estetter B, Holland D, Smith B, Derdak S. High-frequency oscillatory ventilation in adults: respiratory therapy issues. Crit Care Med 2005;33(3(suppl)):S196-S203.

209 Ferguson N, Cook D, Guyatt G, Mehta S, Hand L, Austin P et al. High-frequency oscillation in early acute respiratory distress syndrome. N Engl J Med 2013;368(9):795-805.

210 Young D, Lamb S, Shah S, MacKenzie I, Tunnicliffe W, Lall R et al., OSCAR Study Group. High-frequency oscillation for acute respiratory distress syndrome. N Engl J Med 2013;368(9):806-13.

211 Rossaint R, Slama K, Lewandowski A, Streich R, Henin P, Hopfe T et al. Extracorporeal lung assist with heparin-coated systems. Int J Artificial Organs 1992;15:29–34.

212 Davies A, Jones D, Bailey M, Beca J, Bellomo R, Blackwell N et al. Extracorporeal membrane oxygenation for 2009 influenza A(H1N1) acute respiratory distress syndrome. JAMA 2009;302(17):1888-95.

213 Peek G, Mugford M, Tiruvoipati R, Wilson A, Allen E, Thalanany M et al., CESAR trial collaboration. Efficacy and economic assessment of conventional ventilatory support versus extracorporeal membrane oxygenation for severe adult respiratory failure (CESAR): a multicentre randomised controlled trial. Lancet 2009;374(9698):1351-63.210.

214 Iwahashi H, Yuri K. Development of the oxygenator: past, present, and future. Artificial Organs 2004;7(3):111–20.

215 Afshari A, Brok J, Møller A, Wetterslev J. Inhaled nitric oxide for acute respiratory distress syndrome (ARDS) and acute lung injury in children and adults. Cochrane Database Syst Rev 2010:CD002787.

216 Orozco-Levi M, Torres A, Ferrer M, Piera C, el-Ebiary M, de la Bellacasa JP et al. Semirecumbent position protects from pulmonary aspiration but not completely from gastroesophageal reflux in mechanically ventilated patients. Am J Respir Crit Care 1995;152 (4Pt1):1387-90.

217 Torres A, Serra-Battlles J, Ros E, Piera C, Puig de la Bellacasa J, Cobos A et al. Pulmonary aspiration of gastric contents in patients receiving mechanical ventilation: the effect of body position. Ann Int Med 1992;116(7):540-3.

218 Ibanez J, Penafiel A, Raurich J, Marse P, Jorda R, Mata F. Gastroesophageal reflux in intubated patients receiving enteral nutrition: effect of supine and semirecumbent positions. J Parenter Enteral Nutr 1992;16(5):419-22.

219 Drakulovic M, Torres A, Bauer T, Nicolas J, Nogue S, Ferrer M. Supine body position as a risk factor for nosocomial pneumonia in mechanically ventilated patients: a randomised trial. Lancet 1999;354(9193):1851-8.

220 American Thoracic Society. Guidelines for the management of adults with hospital-acquired, ventilator associated, and healthcare associated pneumonia. Am J Respir Crit Care Med 2005;171(4):388-416.

221 Tablan O, Anderson L, Besser R, Bridges C, Hajjeh R. Guidelines for prevention of health care-associated pneumonia, 2003: recommendations of the CDC and the Healthcare Infection Control Practices Advisory Committee. MMWR Recomm Rep 2004;53(3):1-36.

222 van Nieuwenhoven C, Vandenbroucke-Grauls C, van Tiel F, Joore H, van Schijndel RJ, van der Tweel I et al. Feasibility and effects of the semirecumbent position to prevent ventilator-associated pneumonia: a randomized study. Crit Care Med 2006;34(2):396-402.

223 Evans D. The use of position during critical illness: current practice and review of the literature. Aust Crit Care 1994;7(3):16-21.

224 Reeve B, Cook D. Semirecumbency among mechanically ventilated ICU patients: a multicentre observational study. Clin Intensive Care 1999;10(6):241-4.

225 Heyland D, Cook D, Dodek P. Prevention of ventilator-associated pneumonia: current practice in Canadian intensive care units. J Crit Care 2002;17(3):161-7.

226 Grap M, Munro C, Bryant S, Ashanti B. Predictors of backrest elevation in critical care. Intensive Crit Care Nurs 2003;19(2):68-74.

227 Rose L, Baldwin I, Crawford T, Parke R. A multicenter, observational study of semirecumbent positioning in mechanically ventilated patients. Am J Crit Care 2010;19(6):e100-e8.

228 Helman D, Sherner J, Fitzpatrick T, Callendar M, Shorr A. Effect of standardized orders and provider education on head-of-bed positioning in mechanically ventilated patients. Crit Care Med 2003;31(9):2285-90.

229 Rose L, Baldwin I, Crawford T. The use of bed-dials to maintain recumbent positioning for critically ill mechanically ventilated patients (The RECUMBENT study): multicentre before and after observational study. Int J Nurs Studies 2010;47(11):1425-31.

230 Sprung J, Whalen F, Comfere T, Bosnjak Z, Bajzer Z, Gajic O et al. Alveolar recruitment and arterial desflurane concentration during bariatric surgery. Anesth Analg 2009;108(1):120-7.

231 Remolina C, Khan A, Santiago T, Edelman N. Positional hypoxemia in unilateral lung disease. N Engl J Med 1981;304(9):523-5.

232 Marini J, Gattinoni L. Propagation prevention: a complementary mechanism for "lung protective" ventilation in acute respiratory distress syndrome. Crit Care Med 2008;36(12):3252-8.

233 Choi S, Nelson L. Kinetic therapy in critically ill patients: combined results based on meta-analysis. J Crit Care 1992;7(1):57-62.

234 Staudinger T, Bojic A, Holzinger U, Meyer B, Rohwer M, Mallner F et al. Continuous lateral rotation therapy to prevent ventilator-associated pneumonia. Crit Care Med 2010;38(2):486-90.

235 Staudinger T, Kofler J, Müllner M, Locker G, Laczika K, Knapp S et al. Comparison of prone positioning and continuous rotation of patients with adult respiratory distress syndrome: results of a pilot study. Crit Care Med 2001;29(1):51-6.

236 Hering R, Wrigge H, Vorwerk R, Brensing K, Schröder S, Zinserling J et al. The effects of prone positioning on intraabdominal pressure and cardiovascular and renal function in patients with acute lung injury. Anesth Analg 2001;92(5):1226-31.

237 Guerin C, Badet M, Rosselli S, Heyer L, Sab J, Langevin B et al. Effects of prone position on alveolar recruitment and oxygenation in acute lung injury. Intensive Care Med 1999;25(11):1222-30.

238 van Kaam A, Lachmann R, Herting E, De Jaegere A, van Iwaarden F, Noorduyn LA et al. Reducing atelectasis attenuates bacterial growth and translocation in experimental pneumonia. Am J Respir Crit Care Med 2004;169(9):1046-53.

239 Gattinoni L, Tognoni G, Pesenti A, Taccone P, Mascheroni D, Labarta V et al. Effect of prone positioning on the survival of patients with acute respiratory failure. N Engl J Med 2001;345(8):568-73.

240 Schortgen F, Bouadma L, Joly-Guillou M, Ricard J, Dreyfuss D, Saumon G. Infectious and inflammatory dissemination are affected by ventilation strategy in rats with unilateral pneumonia. Intensive Care Med 2004;30(4):693-701.

241 Fessler H, Talmor D. Should prone positioning be routinely used for lung protection during mechanical ventilation? Respir Care 2010;55(1):88-99.

242 Pelosi P, Brazzi L, Gattinoni L. Prone position in acute respiratory distress syndrome. Eur Respir J 2002;20(4):1017-28.

243 Gattinoni L, Carlesso E, Taccone P, Polli F, Guérin C, Mancebo J. Prone positioning improves survival in severe ARDS: a pathophysiologic review and individual patient meta-analysis. Minerva Anestesiol 2010;76(6):448-54.

244 Sud S, Friedrich J, Adhikari N, Taccone P, Mancebo J, Polli F et al. Effect of prone positioning during mechanical ventilation on mortality among patients with acute respiratory distress syndrome: a systematic review and meta-analysis. CMAJ 2014;186(10):E381-90.

245 Vollman K. Prone positioning in the patient who has acute respiratory distress syndrome: the art and science. Crit Care Nurs Clin North Am 2004;16(3):319-36.

246 Burns SM, Ryan B, Burns JE. The weaning continuum use of Acute Physiology and Chronic Health Evaluation III, Burns Wean Assessment Program, Therapeutic Intervention Scoring System, and Wean Index scores to establish stages of weaning. Crit Care Med 2000;28(7):2259-67.

247 Gajic O, Lee J, Doerr C, Berrios J, Myers J, Hubmayr R. Ventilator-induced cell wounding and repair in the intact lung. Am J Respir Crit Care Med 2003;167:1057-63.

248 Gajic O, Saqib I, Mendez J, Adesanya A, Festic E, Caples SM et al. Ventilator-associated lung injury in patients without acute lung injury at the onset of mechanical ventilation. Crit Care Med 2004;32(9):1817-24.

249 Ranieri VM, Suter P, Tortorella C, deTullio R, Dayer J, Brienza A et al. Effect of mechanical ventilation on inflammatory mediators in patients with acute respiratory distress syndrome. JAMA 1999;282(1):54-61.

250 Heyland D, Cook D, Griffith L, Keenan S, Brun-Buisson C. The attributable morbidity and mortality of ventilator-associated pneumonia in the critically ill patient Am J Respir Crit Care Med 1999;159(4Pt1):1249-56.

251 Vallés J, Pobo A, García-Esquirol O, Mariscal D, Real J, Fernández R. Excess ICU mortality attributable to ventilator-associated pneumonia: the role of early vs late onset. Intensive Care Med 2007;33(8):1363-8.

252 Muscedere J, Martin C, Heyland D. The impact of ventilator-associated pneumonia on the Canadian health care system. J Crit Care 2008; 23(1):5-10.

253 Mancebo J. Weaning from mechanical ventilation. Eur Respir J 1996;9(9):1923-31.

254 Boles J-M, Bion J, Connors A, Herridge M, Marsh B, Melot C et al. Weaning from mechanical ventilation. Eur Respir J 2007;29(5):1033-56.

255 Stroetz RW, Hubmayr RD. Tidal volume maintenance during weaning with pressure support. Am J Respir Crit Care Med 1995;152(3):1034-40.

256 Epstein SK, Ciubotaru RL, Wong JB. Effect of failed extubation on the outcome of mechanical ventilation. Chest 1997;112(1):186-92.

257 Esteban A, Alia I, Gordo F, Fernandez R, Solsona JF, Vallverdú I et al. Extubation outcome after spontaneous breathing trials with T-tube or pressure support ventilation. The Spanish Lung Failure Collaborative Group. Am J Respir Crit Care Med 1997;156(2Pt1):459-65.

258 Meade M, Guyatt G, Cook D, Griffith L, Sinuff T, Kergl C et al. Predicting success in weaning from mechanical ventilation. Chest 2001;120 (6 Suppl):400S-24S.

259 Yang KL, Tobin MJ. A prospective study of indexes predicting the outcome of trials of weaning from mechanical ventilation. N Engl J Med 1991;324(21):1445-50.

260 Tanios M, Nevins M, Hendra K, Cardinal P, Allan J, Naumova EN et al. A randomized, controlled trial of the role of weaning predictors in clinical decision making. Crit Care Med 2006;34(10):2530-5.

261 Brochard L, Rauss A, Benito S, Conti G, Mancebo J, Rekik N et al. Comparison of three methods of gradual withdrawal from ventilatory support during weaning from mechanical ventilation. Am J Respir Crit Care Med 1994;150(4):896-903.

262 Esteban A, Frutos F, Tobin MJ, Alia I, Solsona JF, Valverdú I et al. A comparison of four methods of weaning patients from mechanical ventilation. Spanish Lung Failure Collaborative Group. N Engl J Med 1995;332(6):345-50.

263　Ladeira M, Vital F, Andriolo R, Andriolo B, Atallah A, Peccin M. Pressure support versus T-tube for weaning from mechanical ventilation in adults. Cochrane Database Syst Rev 2014(5):CD006056.

264　Kollef MH, Horst HM, Prang L, Brock WA. Reducing the duration of mechanical ventilation: three examples of change in the intensive care unit. New Horizons 1998;6(1):52-60.

265　Robertson T, Mann H, Hyzy R, Rogers A, Douglas I, Waxman AB et al. Multicenter implementation of a consensus-developed, evidence-based, spontaneous breathing trial protocol. Crit Care Med 2009;36(10):2753-62.

266　Matic I, Majeric-Kogler V. Comparison of pressure support and T-tube weaning from mechanical ventilation: randomized prospective study. Croat Med J 2004;45(2):162-6.

267　Esteban A, Alia I, Tobin MJ, Gil A, Gordo F, Vallverdú I et al. Effect of spontaneous breathing trial duration on outcome of attempts to discontinue mechanical ventilation. Spanish Lung Failure Collaborative Group. Am J Respir Crit Care Med 1999;159(2):512-8.

268　Hughes MR, Smith CD, Tecklenburg FW, Habib DM, Hulsey TC, Ebeling M. Effects of a weaning protocol on ventilated pediatric intensive care unit (PICU) patients. Topics Health Inform Manage 2001;22(2):35-43.

269　Burns SM, Earven S. Improving outcomes for mechanically ventilated medical intensive care unit patients using advanced practice nurses: a 6 year experience. Crit Care Nurs Clin N Am 2002;14(3):231-43.

270　Marelich GP, Murin S, Battistella F, Inciardi J, Vierra T, Roby M. Protocol weaning of mechanical ventilation in medical and surgical patients by respiratory care practitioners and nurses: effect on weaning time and incidence of ventilator-associated pneumonia. Chest 2000;118(2):459-67.

271　Ely EW, Baker AM, Dunagan DP, Burke HL, Smith AC, Kelly PT et al. Effect on the duration of mechanical ventilation of identifying patients capable of breathing spontaneously. N Engl J Med 1996;335(25):1864-9.

272　Kollef MH, Shapiro SD, Silver P, St John RE, Prentice D, Sauer S et al. A randomized, controlled trial of protocol-directed versus physician-directed weaning from mechanical ventilation. Crit Care Med 1997;25(4):567-74.

273　Girard T, Kress J, Fuchs B, Thomason J, Schweickert W, Pun BT et al. Efficacy and safety of a paired sedation and ventilator weaning protocol for mechanically ventilated patients in intensive care (Awakening and Breathing Controlled trial): a randomised controlled trial. Lancet 2008;371(9607):126-34.

274　Blackwood B, Alderdice F, Burns K, Cardwell C, Lavery G, O'Halloran P. Protocolized versus non-protocolized weaning for reducing the duration of mechanical ventilation in critically ill adult patients. Cochrane Database Syst Rev 2010;5:CD006904.

275　Bellomo R, Stow P, Hart G. Why is there such a difference in outcome between Australian intensive care units and others? Curr Opin Anaesthesiol 2007;20(2):100-5.

276　Rose L, Nelson S, Johnston L, Presneill J. Workforce profile, organisation structure and role responsibility for ventilation and weaning practices in Australia and New Zealand intensive care units. J Clin Nur 2008;17(8):1035-43.

277　Dojat M, Harf A, Touchard D, Laforest M, Lemaire F, Brochard L. Evaluation of a knowledge-based system providing ventilatory management and decision for extubation. Am J Respir Crit Care Med 1996;153(3):997-1004.

278　Rose L, Presneill J, Cade J. Update in computer-driven weaning from mechanical ventilation. Anaesth Intensive Care 2007;35(2):213-21.

279　Dojat M, Brochard L, Lemaire F, Harf A. A knowledge-based system for assisted ventilation of patients in intensive care units. Int J Clin Monit Comput 1992;9(4):239-50.

280　Dojat M, Harf A, Touchard D, Lemaire F, Brochard L. Clinical evaluation of a computer-controlled pressure support mode. Am J Respir Crit Care Med 2000;161(4):1161-6.

281　Rose L, Schultz M, Cardwell C, Jouvet P, McAuley D, Blackwood B. Automated versus non-automated weaning for reducing the duration of mechanical ventilation for critically ill adults and children. Cochrane Database Syst Rev 2014 (6):CD009235.

282　Carson SS. Outcomes of prolonged mechanical ventilation. Curr Opin Crit Care 2006;12(5):405-11.

283　Iregui M, Malen J, Tutleur P, Lynch J, Holtzman M, Kollef M. Determinants of outcome for patients admitted to a long-term ventilator unit. South Med J 2002;95(3):310-7.

284　Vitacca M, Vianello A, Colombo D, Clini E, Porta R, Bianchi L et al. Comparison of two methods for weaning patients with chronic obstructive pulmonary disease requiring mechanical ventilation for more than 15 days. Am J Respir Crit Care Med 2001;164(2):225-30.

285　Jubran A, Grant BJ, Duffner LA, Collins EG, Lanuza DM, Hoffman LA et al. Effect of pressure support vs unassisted breathing through a tracheostomy collar on weaning duration in patients requiring prolonged mechanical ventilation: a randomized trial. JAMA 2013;309(7):671-7.

Chapter 16

Neurological assessment and monitoring

Diane Chamberlain, Leila Kuzmiuk

KEY WORDS

afferent neuron

autonomic nervous
system

central nervous
system

decerebrate
(extensor)

decorticate (flexor)

efferent neuron

Glasgow Coma
Scale

intracranial pressure

neurological
assessment

parasympathetic
nervous system

post-traumatic
amnesia

peripheral nervous
system

sympathetic
nervous system

Learning objectives

After reading this chapter, you should be able to:

- describe the anatomy and physiology of the nervous system
- differentiate between the central and peripheral nervous systems
- describe the techniques used for neurological assessment
- identify the distinction between normal and abnormal findings
- state the determinants of intracranial pressure and describe compensatory mechanisms
- explain the importance and process of continuous neurological assessment in the brain-injured patient
- relate the procedures of selected neurodiagnostic tests to nursing implications for patient care.

Introduction

The nervous system is the major controlling, regulating and communicating system in the body. It accounts for a mere 3% of total body weight, yet it is the most complex organ system. It is the centre of all mental activity, including thought, learning and memory. Together with the endocrine and immune systems, the nervous system is responsible for regulating and maintaining homeostasis. Through its receptors, the nervous system keeps in touch with the environment, both external and internal. Diseases of the nervous system are common in the critical care unit, both as primary processes and as complications of multiple organ failure in the critically ill patient. An understanding of basic neurophysiology is important if these disorders are to be recognised and treated. This chapter provides an overview of the anatomy and physiology, and describes and details neurological assessment.

Neurological anatomy and physiology

All the sensory details that incorporate a body's own information systems are related to neurological anatomy and physiology. Composed of central and peripheral components, with the brain as the command centre, the nervous system is responsible for the body's most fundamental activities. Nerves, which are made up of bundles of fibres, deliver impulses to various parts of the body, including the brain. The brain translates the information delivered by the impulses, which then enables the person to react. This section discusses the main components of the nervous system starting from neurons and nervous system transmission. Then the central nervous system and the peripheral nervous system are examined and related to neurological assessment.

Components of the nervous system

The central nervous system (CNS) consists of the spinal cord and the brain and is responsible for integrating, processing and coordinating sensory data and motor commands[1] (see Figure 16.1).

The CNS is linked to all parts of the body by the peripheral nervous system (PNS), which transmits signals to and from the CNS. The PNS is composed of 43 pairs of spinal nerves that issue in orderly sequence from the spinal cord, and 12 pairs of cranial nerves that emerge from the base of the brain. All branch and diversify prolifically as they distribute to the tissues and organs of the body. The peripheral nerves carry input to the CNS via their sensory afferent fibres and deliver output from the CNS via the efferent fibres. Specific physiology of the CNS and PNS is discussed in detail later in the chapter. First, however, neuron cell anatomy and physiology are examined.

Neurons

Neurons are specialised cells in the nervous system; each is comprised of a dendrite, cell body (soma) and axon.[2] Each neuron uses biochemical reactions to receive, process and transmit information. Most synaptic contacts between neurons are either axodendritic (excitatory) or axosomatic (inhibitory). A neuron's dendritic tree is connected to many neighbouring neurons and receives positive or negative charges from other neurons. The input is then passed to the soma (cell body). The primary role of the soma and the enclosed nucleus is to perform the

---

FIGURE 16.1 The functional divisions of the nervous system.[1]

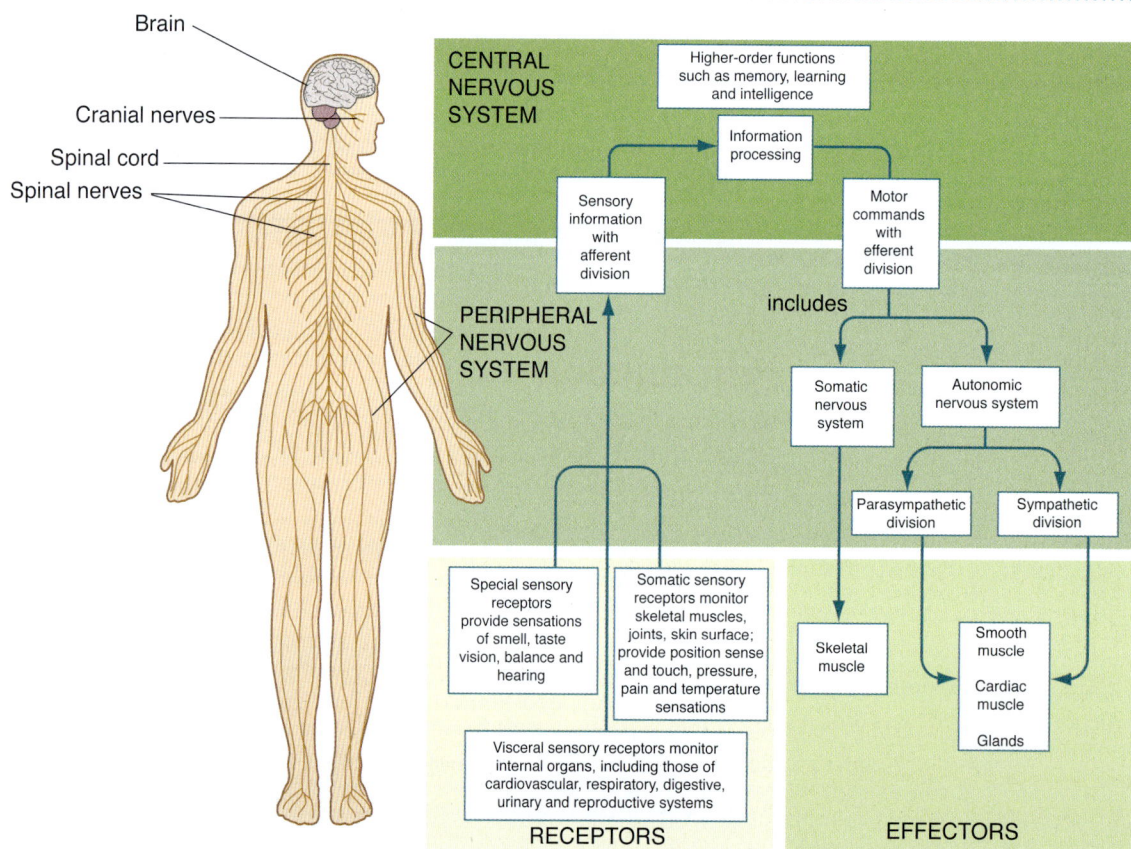

Adapted from Martini F, Nath J, Bartholomew E. Anatomy and physiology. 9th ed. San Francisco: Pearson Benjamin Cummings; 2011, with permission.

continuous maintenance required to keep the neuron functional. Most neurons lack centrioles, important organelles involved in the organisation of the cytoskeleton and the movement of chromosomes during mitosis. As a result, typical CNS neurons cannot divide and cannot be replaced if lost to injury or disease. The fuel source for the neuron is glucose; insulin is not required for cellular uptake in the CNS.[2]

A myelin sheath, consisting of a lipid–protein casing, covers the neuron and provides protection to the axon and speeds the transmission of impulses along nerve cells from node to node[3] (see Figure 16.2b). Myelin is not a continuous layer but has gaps called nodes of Ranvier (see Figure 16.2a).

Each synaptic knob contains mitochondria, portions of the endoplasmic reticulum and thousands of vesicles filled with neurotransmitter molecules. Breakdown products of neurotransmitter released at the synapse are reabsorbed and reassembled at the synaptic knob. The synaptic knob also receives a continuous supply of neurotransmitter synthesised in the cell body, along with enzymes and lysosomes.[2] The movement of materials between the cell body and synaptic knobs is called axoplasmic transport. Some materials travel slowly, at rates of a few millimetres per day. This transport mechanism is known as the 'slow stream'. Vesicles containing neurotransmitter move much more rapidly, travelling in the 'fast stream' at 5–10 mm per hour, which increases synaptic activity. Axoplasmic transport occurs in both directions. The flow of materials from the cell body to the synaptic knob is anterograde flow. At the same time, other substances are being transported towards the cell body in retrograde flow ('retro' meaning backward). If debris or unusual chemicals appear in the synaptic knob, retrograde flow soon delivers them to the cell body. The arriving materials may then alter the activity of the cell by turning appropriate genes on or off. Retrograde flow is the means of transport for viruses,

FIGURE 16.2 **A** Afferent and **B** efferent neurons, showing the soma or cell body, dendrites and axon. Arrows indicate the direction for conduction of action potentials.[3]

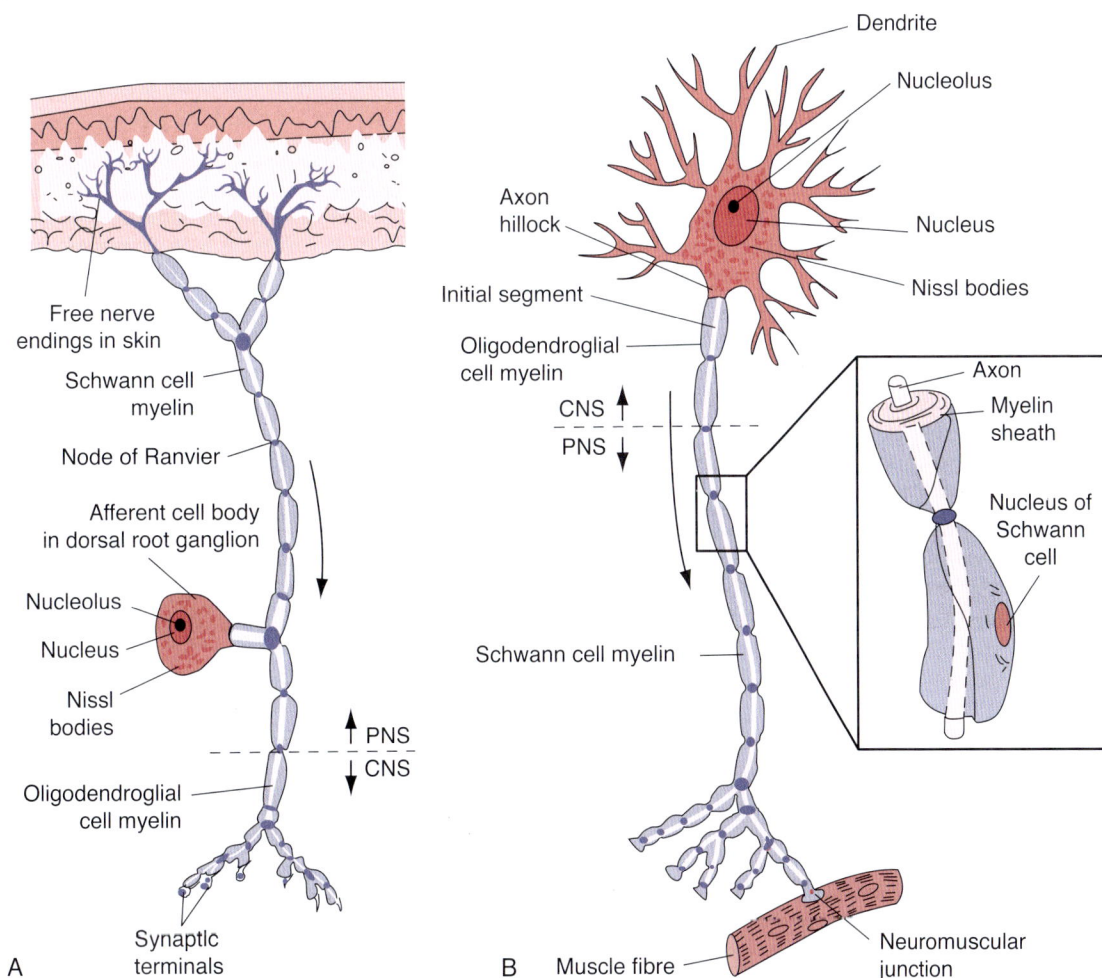

Adapted from Porth C. Pathophysiology concepts of altered health states. 9th ed. Philadelphia: Lippincott, Williams & Wilkins; 2013, with permission.

pathogenic bacteria, heavy metals and toxins to the CNS, with resulting disease such as tetanus, viral encephalitis and lead intoxication. Defective anterograde transport seems to be involved in certain neuropathies, including critical illness neuropathies.[4]

Synapses

The human brain contains at least 100 billion neurons, each with the ability to influence many other cells.[2] Although there are many kinds of synapses within the brain, they can be divided into two general classes: electrical synapses and chemical synapses. Electrical synapses permit direct, passive flow of electrical current from one neuron to another in the form of an action potential; they are described in Table 16.1. The current flows through gap junctions, which are specialised membrane channels that connect the two cells. Chemical synapses, in contrast, enable cell-to-cell communication via the secretion of neurotransmitters; the chemical agents released by the presynaptic neurons produce secondary current flow in postsynaptic neurons by activating specific receptor molecules[5] (see Figure 16.3).

Myelin increases conduction velocity. Demyelination of peripheral nerves, as occurs in Guillain-Barré syndrome, slows conduction and may result in conduction block, which manifests clinically as weakness. Consequently,

chronically demyelinated axons become vulnerable, with axon loss being a major cause of disability. In time, remyelination may occur, requiring the generation of myelin-competent oligodendrocytes, but most often it does not fully recapitulate developmental myelination.[5]

Neurotransmitters

A neurotransmitter is a chemical messenger used by neurons to communicate in one direction with other neurons.[2] Unidirectional transmission is required for multineuronal pathways, for example to and from the brain. Neurons communicate with each other by recognising specific neuroreceptors.

Chemically, there are four classes of neurotransmitters:

1 acetylcholine (ACh): the dominant neurotransmitter in the peripheral nervous system, released at neuromuscular junctions and synapses of the parasympathetic division
2 biogenic amines: serotonin, histamine and the catecholamines dopamine and noradrenaline
3 excitatory amino acids: glutamate and aspartate; and the inhibitory amino acids: gamma–aminobutyric acid (GABA), glycine and taurine
4 neuropeptides: over 50 are known, amino acid neurotransmitters being the most numerous.

TABLE 16.1
Generation of action potentials (nervous tissue)

STEP 1: Depolarisation
- A graded depolarisation brings an area of excitable membrane to threshold (–60 mV)

STEP 2: Activation of sodium channels and rapid depolarisation
- The voltage-regulated sodium channels open (sodium channel activation)
- Sodium ions, driven by electrical attraction and the chemical gradient, flood into the cell
- The transmembrane potential goes from –60 mV, the threshold level, towards +30 mV

STEP 3: Repolarisation: inactivation of sodium channels and activation of potassium channels
- The voltage-regulated sodium channels close (sodium channel inactivation occurs) at +30 mV
- The voltage-regulated potassium channels are now open, and potassium ions diffuse out of the cell
- Repolarisation begins

STEP 4: Return to normal permeability
- The voltage-regulated sodium channels regain their normal properties in 0.4–1.0 ms. The membrane is now capable of generating another action potential if a larger-than-normal stimulus is provided
- The voltage-regulated potassium channels begin closing at –70 mV. Because they do not all close at the same time, potassium loss continues, and a temporary hyperpolarisation to approximately –90 mV occurs
- At the end of the relative refractory period, all voltage-regulated channels have closed, and the membrane is back to its resting state

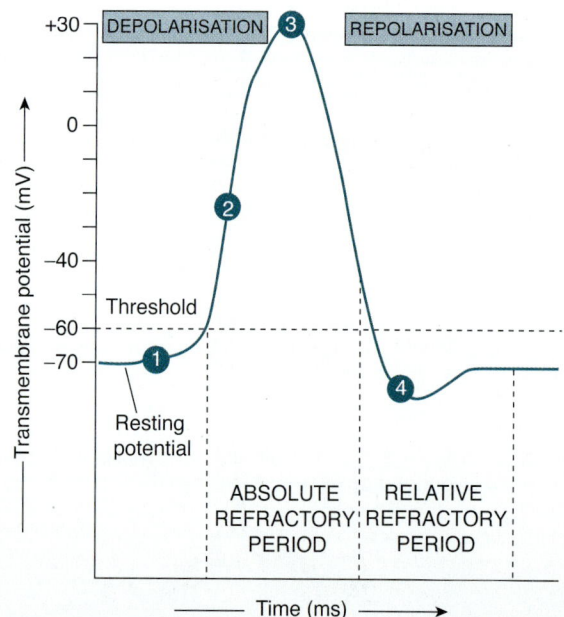

FIGURE 16.3 Sequence of events involved in transmission at a typical chemical synapse.[84]

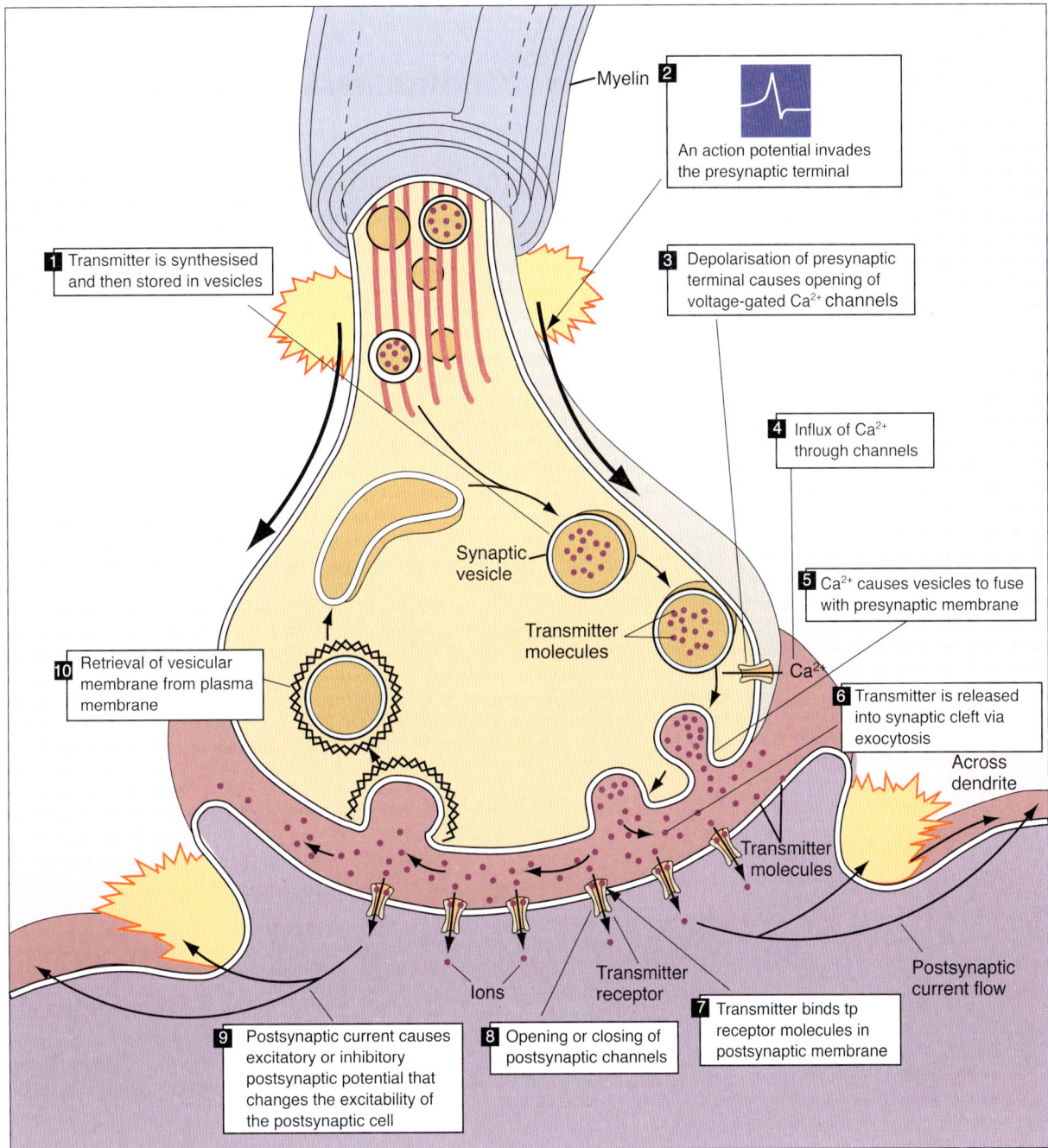

1 Transmitter is synthesised and then stored in vesicles

2 An action potential invades the presynaptic terminal

3 Depolarisation of presynaptic terminal causes opening of voltage-gated Ca^{2+} channels

4 Influx of Ca^{2+} through channels

5 Ca^{2+} causes vesicles to fuse with presynaptic membrane

6 Transmitter is released into synaptic cleft via exocytosis

7 Transmitter binds tp receptor molecules in postsynaptic membrane

8 Opening or closing of postsynaptic channels

9 Postsynaptic current causes excitatory or inhibitory postsynaptic potential that changes the excitability of the postsynaptic cell

10 Retrieval of vesicular membrane from plasma membrane

Myelin

Synaptic vesicle

Transmitter molecules

Ca^{2+}

Transmitter molecules

Across dendrite

Postsynaptic current flow

Ions

Transmitter receptor

Adapted from Purves D, Augustine G, Hall W, LaMantia A, McNamara J, White L. Neuroscience. 5th ed. New York: Sinauer Associates; 2012, with permission.

In 2009, it was discovered that there is also more than one neurotransmitter per synapse; these are called co-transmitters. For example, neuropeptide Y (NPY) and adenosine triphosphate (ATP) are co-transmitters of noradrenaline; they are released together and mediate their function by activation of α- and β-adrenoceptors, and regulate renovascular resistance.[6] Similarly, receptors are an important control point for the effectiveness of synapses. Neurotransmitters are the common denominator between the nervous, endocrine and immune systems. Many neurotransmitters are endocrine analogues and acetylcholine, the main parasympathetic neurotransmitter, interacts with immune cells such as macrophages through the anti-inflammatory cholinergic pathway.[7]

Neuroglia

Neuroglia are the non-neuronal cells of the nervous system and are 10–50 times more prevalent than neurons.[1] They are divided into macroglia (astrocytes, oligodendroglia and Schwann cells) and microglia, and are described in Table 16.2. They not only provide physical support but also respond to injury, regulate the ionic and chemical composition of the extracellular milieu, participate in the blood–brain and blood–retina barriers, form the myelin insulation of nervous pathways, guide neuronal migration during development and exchange metabolites with neurons.[8] The CNS has a greater variety of neuroglia. Unlike neurons, neuroglia continue to multiply throughout life. Because of their capacity to reproduce, most tumours of the nervous system are tumours of neuroglial tissue and not of nervous tissue itself.[9]

Central nervous system

The CNS is composed of the brain and spinal cord (see Figure 16.4).[5] The primary purpose is to acquire, coordinate and disseminate information about the body and its environment. This section describes the anatomy and physiology of the brain and spinal cord.

TABLE 16.2

Neuroglia, their location and role as supporting nervous tissue

CELL TYPE	LOCATION	MAIN FUNCTION
Astrocytes	CNS: the largest and most numerous neuroglial cells in the brain and spinal cord	• Astrocytes are considered as important as the neuron in communication and brain regulation • They regulate communication, extracellular ionic and chemical environments between neurons • They respond to injury and have an important role in cerebral oedema
Ependymal cells	CNS: line the ventricular system of the brain and central cord of the spinal canal	• Transport of CSF and brain homeostasis • Phagocytotic defence against pathogens • Store glycogen for brain tissue
Microglia	CNS: located within the brain parenchyma behind the blood–brain barrier	• Wander between the peripheral immune system and the CNS as a defence to infection • Displace synaptic input in injured neurons
Oligodendrocytes	CNS: spiral around an axon to form a multilayered lipoprotein coat in both the white and grey matter in the brain and spinal cord PNS: Schwann cells are the supporting cells of the PNS	• Responsible for the formation of myelin sheaths surrounding axons • Oligodendrocytes wrap themselves around numerous axons at once • Schwann cells wrap themselves around peripheral nerve axons • Unlike oligodendrocytes, a single Schwann cell makes up a single segment of an axon's myelin sheath

FIGURE 16.4 The subdivisions and components of the central nervous system.[84]

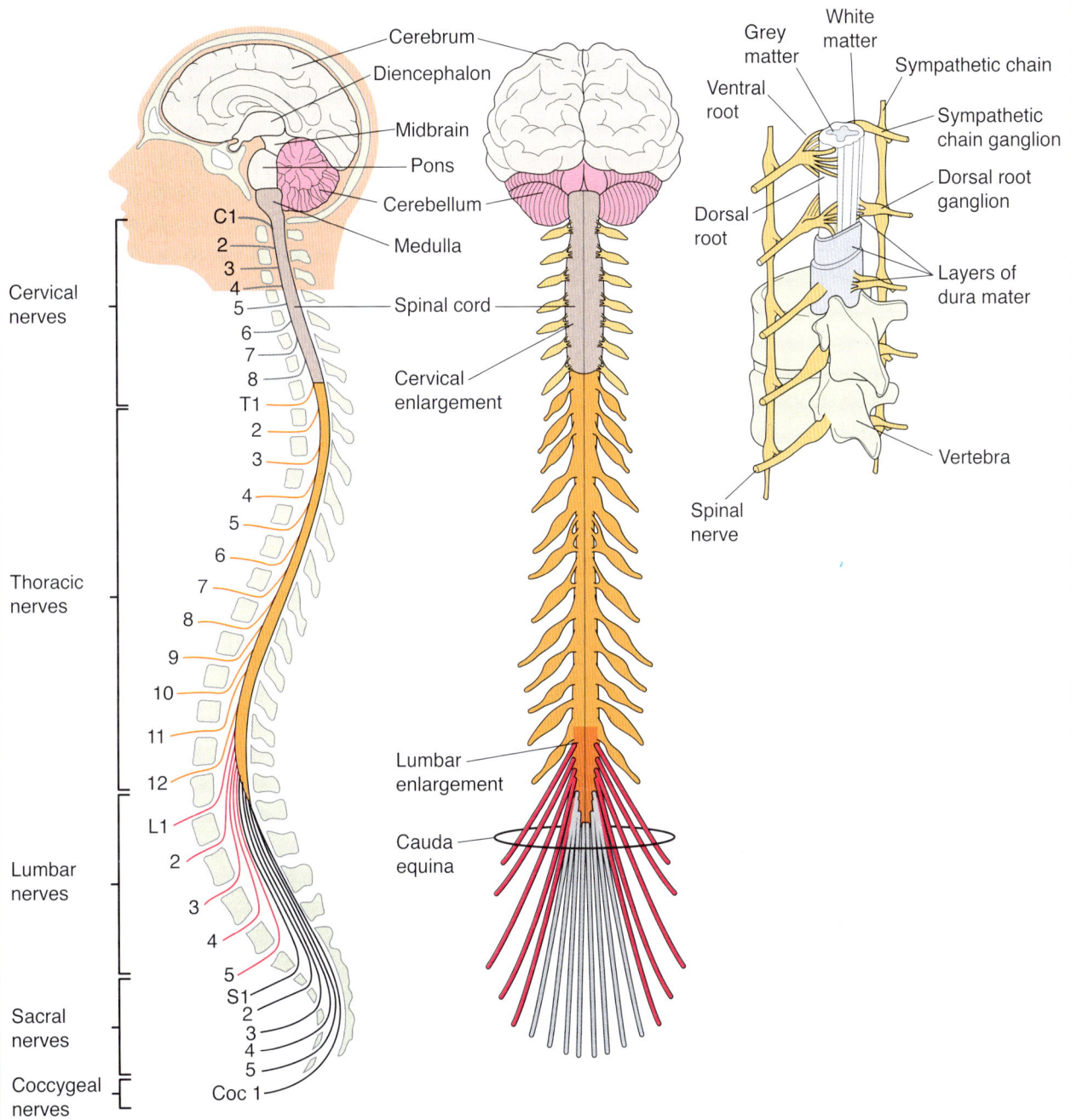

Adapted from Purves D, Augustine G, Hall W, LaMantia A, McNamara J, White L. Neuroscience. 5th ed. New York: Sinauer Associates; 2012, with permission.

Practice tip

The brain consists of three major divisions: 1) the massive paired hemispheres of the cerebrum; 2) the brainstem, consisting of the thalamus, hypothalamus, epithalamus, subthalamus, midbrain, pons and medulla oblongata; and 3) the cerebellum.

Brain

The brain is divided into three regions: forebrain, midbrain and hindbrain, as described in Table 16.3. The forebrain, which consists of two hemispheres and is covered by the cerebral cortex, contains central masses of grey matter, the basal ganglia, the neural tube and the diencephalon with its adult derivatives: the thalamus and hypothalamus.[1] Midbrain structures include two pairs of

TABLE 16.3

Organisation of the brain

DIVISION	DESCRIPTION	FUNCTIONS
FOREBRAIN		
Cerebrum	Largest and uppermost portion of the brain. Divided into two hemispheres, each subdivided into the frontal, parietal, temporal and occipital lobes	Cortex (outer layer) is the site of conscious thought, memory, reasoning and abstract mental functions, all localised within specific lobes
Diencephalon	Between the cerebrum and the brainstem. Contains the thalamus and hypothalamus	Thalamus sorts and redirects sensory input; hypothalamus controls visceral, autonomic, endocrine and emotional function, and the pituitary gland. Contains some of the centres for coordinated parasympathetic and sympathetic stimulation, temperature regulation, appetite regulation, regulation of water balance by antidiuretic hormone (ADH) and regulation of certain rhythmic psychobiological activities (e.g. sleep)
Brain stem	Anterior region below the cerebrum: the medulla, pons and midbrain compose the brainstem	Connects cerebrum and diencephalon with spinal cord
MIDBRAIN		
Midbrain	Below the centre of the cerebrum	Has reflex centres concerned with vision and hearing; connects cerebrum with lower portions of the brain. It contains sensory and motor pathways and serves as the centre for auditory and visual reflexes
Basal ganglia or corpus striatum	The mass of grey matter in the midbrain beneath the cerebral hemispheres. Borders the lateral ventricles and lies in proximity to the internal capsule	An important role in planning and coordinating motor movements and posture. Complex neural connections link the basal ganglia to the cerebral cortex. The major effect of these structures is to inhibit unwanted muscular activity; disorders of the basal ganglia result in exaggerated, uncontrolled movements
Pons	Anterior to the cerebellum	Connects the cerebellum with other portions of the brain; contains motor and sensory pathways; helps to regulate respiration; axons from the cerebellum, basal ganglia, thalamus and hypothalamus; portions of the pons also control the heart, respiration and blood pressure. Cranial nerves V–VIII connect the brain in the pons
Hindbrain	Contains a portion of the pons, the medulla oblongata and the cerebellum	
Reticular activation system (RAS)	The reticular formation networks run through the brainstem core, known as the tegmentum	Activity of the cerebral cortex is dependent on both specific sensory input and non-specific activating impulses from the RAS, and is critical to the existence of the conscious state, states of alertness and arousal
Medulla oblongata	Between the pons and the spinal cord	The medulla oblongata contains motor fibres from the brain to the spinal cord and sensory fibres from the spinal cord to the brain. Most of these fibres cross at this level. Cranial nerves IX–XII connect to the brain in the medulla, which has centres for control of vital functions, such as respiration and the heart rate
Cerebellum	Below the posterior portion of the cerebellum. Divided into two hemispheres	Coordinates voluntary muscles; maintains balance and muscle tone; has both excitatory and inhibitory actions. It also controls fine movement, balance, position sense and integration of sensory input

dorsal enlargements, the superior and inferior colliculi. The medulla, pons and midbrain compose the brainstem.[1] The hindbrain includes the medulla oblongata, the pons and its dorsal outgrowth, the cerebellum.

Nervous tissue has a high rate of metabolism. Although the brain constitutes only 3% of the body's weight, it receives approximately 15% of the resting cardiac output and consumes 20% of its oxygen.[1] Despite its substantial energy requirements, the brain can neither store oxygen nor effectively engage in anaerobic metabolism. An interruption in the blood or oxygen supply to the brain rapidly leads to clinically observable signs and symptoms. Without oxygen, brain cells continue to function for approximately 10 seconds. Glucose is virtually the sole energy substrate for the brain, and it is entirely oxidised.[10] The brain can be seen as an almost exclusive glucose-processing machine, producing water (H_2O) and carbon dioxide (CO_2). Glucose also provides the carbon backbone for regeneration of the neuronal pool of glutamate. This process results from close astrocyte–neuron cooperation.[11]

Cerebral cortex

The forebrain contains the cerebral cortex and the subcortical structures rostral (sideways) to the diencephalon. The cortex, or outermost surface of the cerebrum, makes up about 80% of the human brain. The cerebral cortex varies in thickness from 2 mm to 4 mm. It contains the cell bodies and dendrites of neurons or grey matter that receive, integrate, store and transmit information. Conscious deliberation and voluntary actions also arise from the cerebral cortex. White matter lies beneath the cerebral cortex and is composed of myelinated nerve fibres. The cortex is involved in the processing of both sensory information from the body and the delivery of motor commands. These occur in specific areas of the brain and can be mapped. Topographically, the cerebral cortex is divided into areas of specialised functions, including the primary sensory areas for vision (occipital cortex), hearing (temporal cortex), somatic sensation (postcentral gyrus), and primary motor area (precentral gyrus).[5] As shown in Figure 16.5,[1] these well-defined areas comprise only a small fraction of the surface of the cerebral cortex.

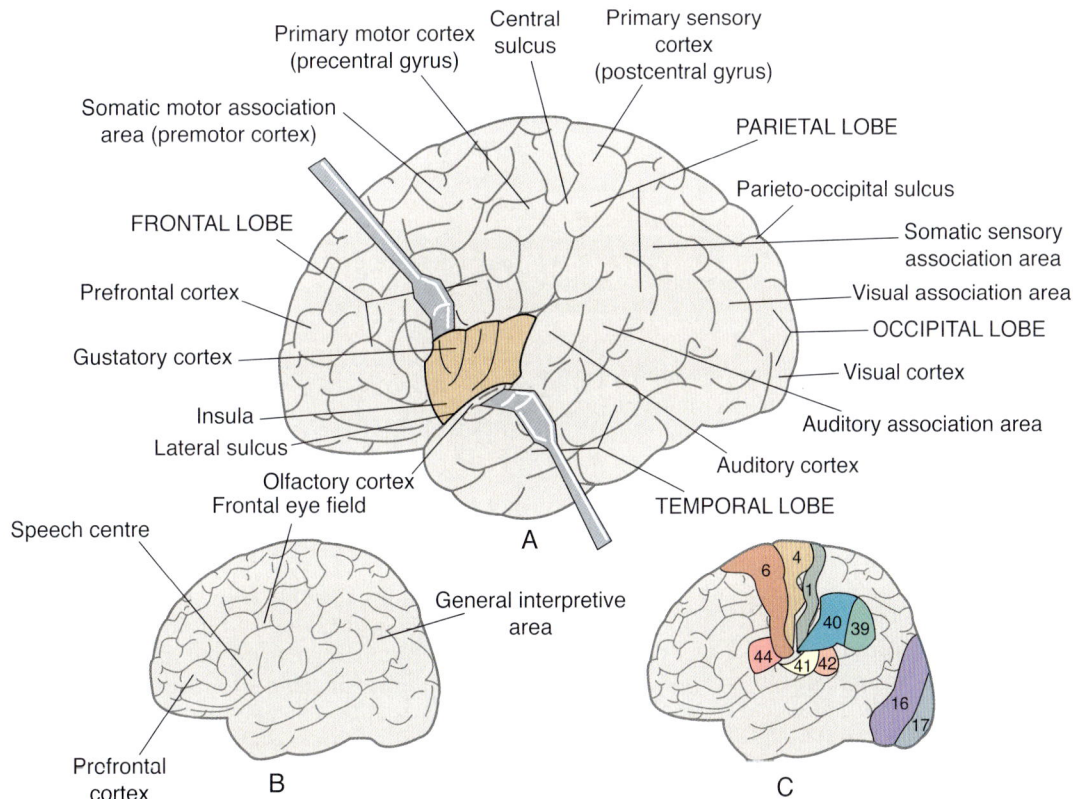

FIGURE 16.5 **A** Major anatomical landmarks on the surface of the left cerebral hemisphere. The lateral sulcus has been pulled apart to expose the insula. **B** The left hemisphere generally contains the general interpretive area and the speech centre. The prefrontal cortex of each hemisphere is involved with conscious intellectual functions. **C** Regions of the cerebral cortex as determined by histological analysis. Several of the 47 regions described by Brodmann are shown for comparison with the results of functional mapping.[1]

Adapted from Martini F, Nath J, Bartholomew E. Anatomy and physiology. 9th ed. San Francisco: Pearson Benjamin Cummings; 2011, with permission.

The majority of the remaining cortical area is known as the association cortex, where the processing of extensive and sophisticated neural information is performed.[12] The association areas are also sites of long-term memory, and they control human functions such as language acquisition, speech, musical ability, mathematical ability, complex motor skills, abstract thought, symbolic thought and other cognitive functions. Association areas interconnect and integrate information from the primary sensory and motor areas via intra-hemispheric connections.[5] The parietal–temporal–occipital association cortex integrates neural information contributed by visual, auditory and somatic sensory experiences. The prefrontal association cortex is extremely important as the coordinator of emotionally motivated behaviours, by virtue of its connections with the limbic system.

In addition, the prefrontal cortex receives neural input from the other association areas and regulates motivated behaviours by direct input to the premotor area, which serves as the association area of the motor cortex. Sensory and motor functions are controlled by cortical structures in the contralateral hemisphere. Particular cognitive functions or components of these functions may be lateralised to one side of the brain.[12]

The cerebral cortex receives sensory information from many different sensory organs and processes the information. The two hemispheres receive the information from the opposite sides of the body. Sensory information is relayed to the cortex by the thalamus. Parts of the cortex that receive this information are called primary sensory areas and cross at various points in the sensory pathway, because the cerebral cortex operates on a contralateral basis.[13] The discriminative touch system crosses high, in the medulla. The pain system crosses low, in the spinal cord. The proprioceptive sensory system that guards balance and position goes to the cerebellum, which works ipsilaterally and therefore does not cross. Almost every region of the body is represented by a corresponding region in both the primary motor cortex and the somatic sensory cortex.[14]

The homunculus (see Figure 16.6) visualises the connection between different areas of the body and areas in brain hemispheres.[15] The body on the right side is the motor homunculus and on the left the sensory homunculus. Representations of parts of the body that exhibit fine motor control and sensory capabilities occupy a greater amount of space than those that exhibit less precise motor or sensory functions.

Basal ganglia and cerebellum

The basal ganglia play an important role in movement, as evidenced by the hypokinetic/rigid and hyperkinetic disorders seen with lesions of related nuclei. Their role in the initiation and control of movement cannot be isolated from the motor activities of the cortex and brainstem centres discussed previously. Procedural memories for motor and other unconscious skills depend on the integrity of the premotor cortex, basal ganglia and cerebellum.[16] The cerebellum plays a more obvious role in coordinating movements by giving feedback to the motor cortex, as well as by providing important influences on eye movements through brainstem connections, and on postural activity through projections down the spinal cord.

Brainstem

The brainstem is composed of the midbrain, the pons and the medulla oblongata.[1] These structures connect the cerebrum and diencephalon with the spinal cord. Brainstem centres are organised into medial, lateral and aminergic systems. Collectively, these integrate vestibular, visual and somatosensory inputs for the control of eye movements and, through projections to the spinal cord, provide for postural adjustments. For example, these centres keep the images on matching regions of the retinas when the head moves by causing conjugate eye movements in the opposite direction to which the head is turned. This is the basis for the 'doll's eyes' test in neurological assessment, in which the head is rapidly turned and the eyes move conjugately in the opposite direction, demonstrating the integrity of much of the brainstem.[15] The sequence of sleep states is governed by a group of brainstem nuclei that project widely throughout the brain and spinal cord.[17]

The midbrain, inferior to the centre of the cerebrum, forms the superior part of the brainstem. It contains the reticular formation (which collects input from higher brain centres and passes it on to motor neurons), the substantia nigra (which regulates body movements – damage to the substantia nigra causes Parkinson's disease) and the ventral tegmental area (which contains dopamine-releasing neurons that are activated by nicotinic acetylcholine receptors).[18] White matter at the anterior of the midbrain conducts impulses between the higher centres of the cerebrum and the lower centres of the pons, medulla, cerebellum and spinal cord. The midbrain contains the autonomic reflex centres for pupillary accommodations to light, which constrict the pupil and accommodate the lens. The fibres travel in cranial nerve III, so damage to that nerve will also produce a dilated pupil.[3] It also contains the ventral tegmental area, packed with dopamine-releasing neurons that synapse deep within the forebrain and seem to be involved in pleasure: amphetamines and cocaine bind to the same receptors that it activates, and this may account at least in part for their addictive qualities.

The medulla oblongata lies between the pons and the spinal cord and looks like a swollen tip to the spinal cord. Running down the ventral aspect of the medulla are the pyramids, which contain corticospinal fibres. The function of the medulla oblongata is to control automatic functions (e.g. breathing and heart rate) and to relay nerve messages from the brain to the spinal cord. Processing of interaural time differences for sound localisation occurs in the olivary nuclei. The neurons controlling breathing have mu (μ) receptors, the receptors to which opiates bind.[5] This accounts for the suppressive effect of opiates on breathing. Impairment of any of the vital functions or reflexes involving these cranial nerves suggests medullary damage.[19]

The pons Varolii is the part of the brainstem that lies between the medulla oblongata and the mesencephalon.

FIGURE 16.6 Somatosensory and motor homunculi. Note that the size of each region of the homunculi is related to its importance in sensory or motor function, resulting in a distorted-appearing map.[15]

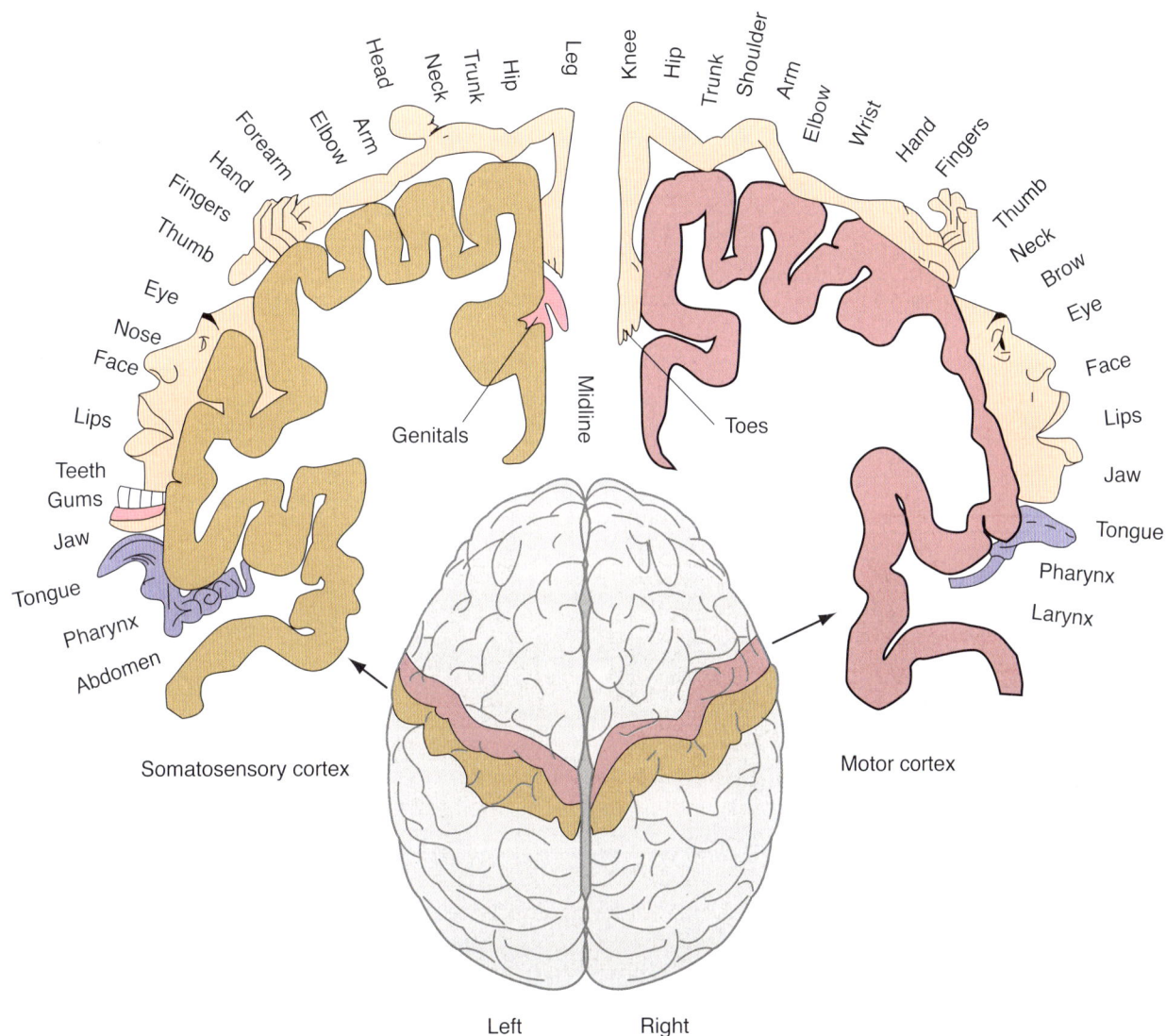

Adapted from Blumenfeld H. Neuroanatomy through clinical cases. New York: Sinauer Associates; 2010, with permission.

It contains pneumotaxic and apneustic respiratory centres and fibre tracts connecting higher and lower centres, including the cerebellum.[2] The pons seems to serve as a relay station, carrying signals from various parts of the cerebral cortex to the cerebellum. Nerve impulses coming from the eyes, ears and touch receptors are sent on to the cerebellum. The pons also participates in the reflexes that regulate breathing. Table 16.4 contains a description of the cranial nerves including their type of tract, their function and location of origin.

Hypothalamus and limbic system

The hypothalamus, the cingulate gyrus of the cortex, the amygdala and hippocampus in the temporal lobes and the septum and interconnecting nerve fibre tracts among these areas comprise the limbic system. The hypothalamus and limbic system, which are closely linked to homeostasis, act to regulate endocrine secretion and the autonomic nervous system, and to influence behaviour through emotions and drives.[1] The hypothalamus integrates information from the forebrain, brainstem, spinal cord and various endocrine systems. This area of the brain also contains some of the centres for coordinated parasympathetic and sympathetic stimulation, as well as those for temperature regulation, appetite regulation, regulation of water balance by antidiuretic hormone (ADH) and regulation of certain rhythmic psychobiological activities (e.g. sleep). The release of stored serotonin from axon terminals in the diencephalon, medulla, thalamus and a small forebrain area (DMTF) results in inactivation of the

TABLE 16.4

The cranial nerves, their locations and functions

CRANIAL NERVE	TRACT(S)	FUNCTION	LOCATION OF ORIGIN
I Olfactory	Sensory	Sense of smell	Diencephalon
II Optic	Sensory	Vision	Diencephalon
III Oculomotor	Parasympathetic	Muscles that move the eye and lid, pupillary constriction, lens accommodation	Midbrain
	Motor	Elevation of upper eyelid and four of six extraocular movements	
IV Trochlear	Motor	Downward, inward movement of the eye (superior oblique)	Midbrain
V Trigeminal	Motor	Muscles of mastication and opening jaw	Pons
	Sensory	Tactile sensation to the cornea, nasal and oral mucosa and facial skin	
VI Abducens	Motor	Lateral deviation of eye (lateral rectus)	Pons
VII Facial	Parasympathetic	Secretory for salivation and tears	Pons
	Motor	Movement of the forehead, eyelids, cheeks, lips, ears, nose and neck to produce facial expression and close eyes	
	Sensory	Tactile sensation to parts of the external ear, auditory canal and external tympanic membrane	
		Taste sensation to the anterior two-thirds of the tongue	
VIII Vestibulocochlear	Sensory	Vestibular branch: equilibrium Cochlear branch: hearing	Pons
IX Glossopharyngeal	Parasympathetic	Salivation	Medulla
	Motor	Voluntary muscles for swallowing and phonation	
	Sensory	Sensation to pharynx, soft palate and posterior one-third of tongue	
		Stimulation elicits gag reflex	
X Vagus	Parasympathetic	Autonomic activity of viscera of thorax and abdomen	Medulla
	Motor	Voluntary swallowing and phonation	
		Involuntary activity of visceral muscles of the heart, lungs and digestive tract	
	Sensory	Sensation to the auditory canal and viscera of the thorax and abdomen	
XI Spinal accessory	Motor	Sternocleidomastoid and trapezius muscle movements	Medulla
XII Hypoglossal	Motor	Tongue movements	Medulla

reticular activating system (RAS) and activation of the DMTF. DMTF activity results in the four stages of sleep.[17] The hypothalamus contains a plethora of neurotransmitters. These are found in the terminals of axons that originate from neurons outside the hypothalamus, but most are synthesised within the hypothalamus itself. The list of putative neurotransmitters includes the 'classic' transmitters ACh, GABA, glutamate, serotonin, dopamine and noradrenaline, as well as literally dozens of peptides that have been identified in recent years.[20]

Protection and support of the brain

The brain occupies the cranial cavity and is covered by membranes, fluid and the bones of the skull. The delicate tissues of the brain are protected from mechanical forces by 1) the bones of the cranium, 2) the cranial meninges and 3) cerebrospinal fluid. In addition, the neural tissue of the brain is biochemically isolated from the general circulation by the blood–brain barrier.

Practice tip

Openings in the fourth ventricle permit cerebrospinal fluid to enter subarachnoid spaces surrounding both the brain and the spinal cord.

Cerebral spinal fluid

Cerebral spinal fluid (CSF) is an ultrafiltrate of blood plasma composed of 99% water with other constituents, making it close to the composition of the brain extracellular fluid.[1] Approximately 500 mL of CSF is secreted each day, but only approximately 150 mL is in the ventricular system at any one time, meaning that the CSF is continuously being absorbed. The CSF produced in the ventricles must flow through the interventricular foramen, the third ventricle, the cerebral aqueduct and the fourth ventricle to exit from the neural tube.[21] Three openings, or foramina, allow the CSF to pass into the subarachnoid space (see Figure 16.7).[1] Approximately 30% of the CSF passes down into the subarachnoid space that surrounds the spinal cord, mainly on its dorsal surface, and moves back up to the cranial cavity along its ventral surface. Reabsorption of CSF into the vascular system occurs, through a pressure gradient. The normal CSF pressure is approximately 10 mmHg in the lateral recumbent position, although it may be as low as 5 mmHg or as high as 15 mmHg in healthy persons. The microstructure of the arachnoid villi is such that, if the CSF pressure falls below approximately 3 mmHg, the passageways collapse and reverse flow is blocked. Arachnoid villi function as one-way valves, permitting CSF outflow into the blood but not allowing blood to pass into the arachnoid spaces. The pressure in the CSF manifests as normal intracranial pressure (ICP).[3]

Blood–brain–cerebral spinal fluid barrier

The CNS is richly supplied with blood vessels that bring oxygen and nutrients to its cells. However, many substances cannot easily be exchanged between blood and brain because the endothelial cells of the vessels and the astrocytes of the CNS form extremely tight junctions, collectively referred to as the blood–brain barrier (BBB).[1] In particular, small non-charged, lipid-soluble molecules can cross the BBB with ease. Evidence suggests that the BBB maintains the chemical environment for neuronal function and protects the brain from harmful substances.[22] Substances in the blood that gain rapid entry to the brain include glucose, the important source of energy, certain ions that maintain a proper medium for electrical activity

FIGURE 16.7 Circulation of the cerebrospinal fluid: **A** sagittal section indicating the sites of formation and routes of circulation of cerebrospinal fluid (arrows); **B** orientation of the arachnoid granulations.[1]

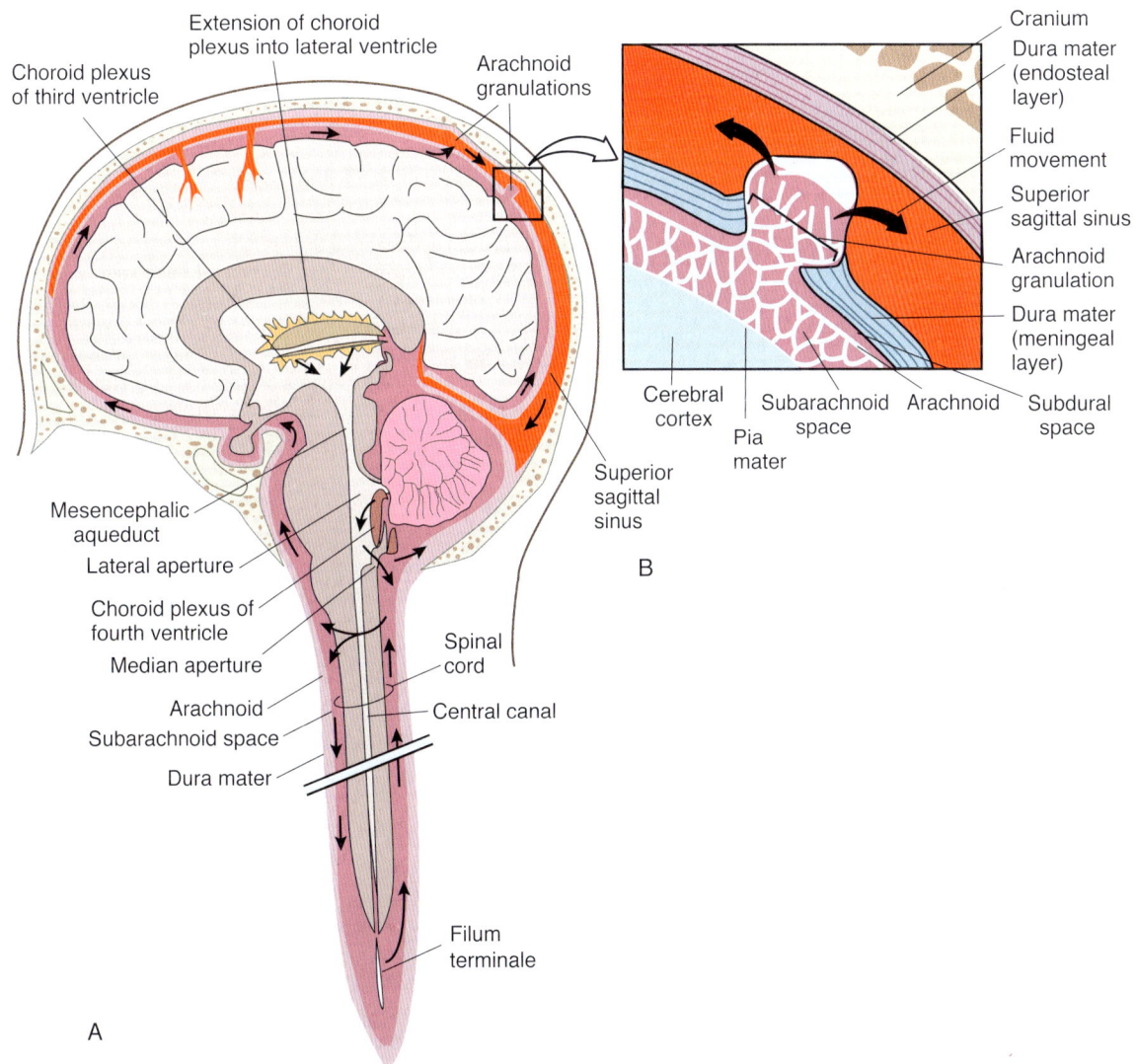

Adapted from Martini F, Nath J, Bartholomew E. Anatomy and physiology. 9th ed. San Francisco: Pearson Benjamin Cummings; 2011, with permission.

and oxygen for cellular respiration. Small fat-soluble molecules, like ethanol, pass through the BBB. Some water-soluble molecules pass into the brain carried by special proteins in the plasma membrane of the endothelial cells. Excluded molecules include proteins, toxins, most antibiotics and monoamines (e.g. neurotransmitters). Some of these unwanted molecules are actively transported out of the endothelial cells. When injured (by force or infection or oxidative processes), the permeability of the BBB is disrupted, allowing a proliferation of various chemicals and molecules – even bacteria – into the brain parenchyma, with at times devastating consequences.[3]

Cerebral circulation

The brain must maintain a constant flow of blood in order for brain activity to occur. The arterial blood flow to the brain consists of approximately 20% of the cardiac output (see Figure 16.8).[5] Normal cerebral blood flow is 750 mL/min. The brain autoregulates blood flow over a wide range of blood pressure by vasodilation or vasoconstriction of the arteries.[1] In response to decreased arterial flow, the circle of Willis can act as a protective mechanism by shunting blood from one side to the other or from the anterior to posterior portions of the brain.

FIGURE 16.8 The major arteries of the brain: **A** ventral view: the enlargement of the boxed area showing the circle of Willis; **B** lateral and **C** mid-sagittal views showing anterior, middle and posterior cerebral arteries; **D** idealised frontal section showing the course of middle cerebral artery.[84]

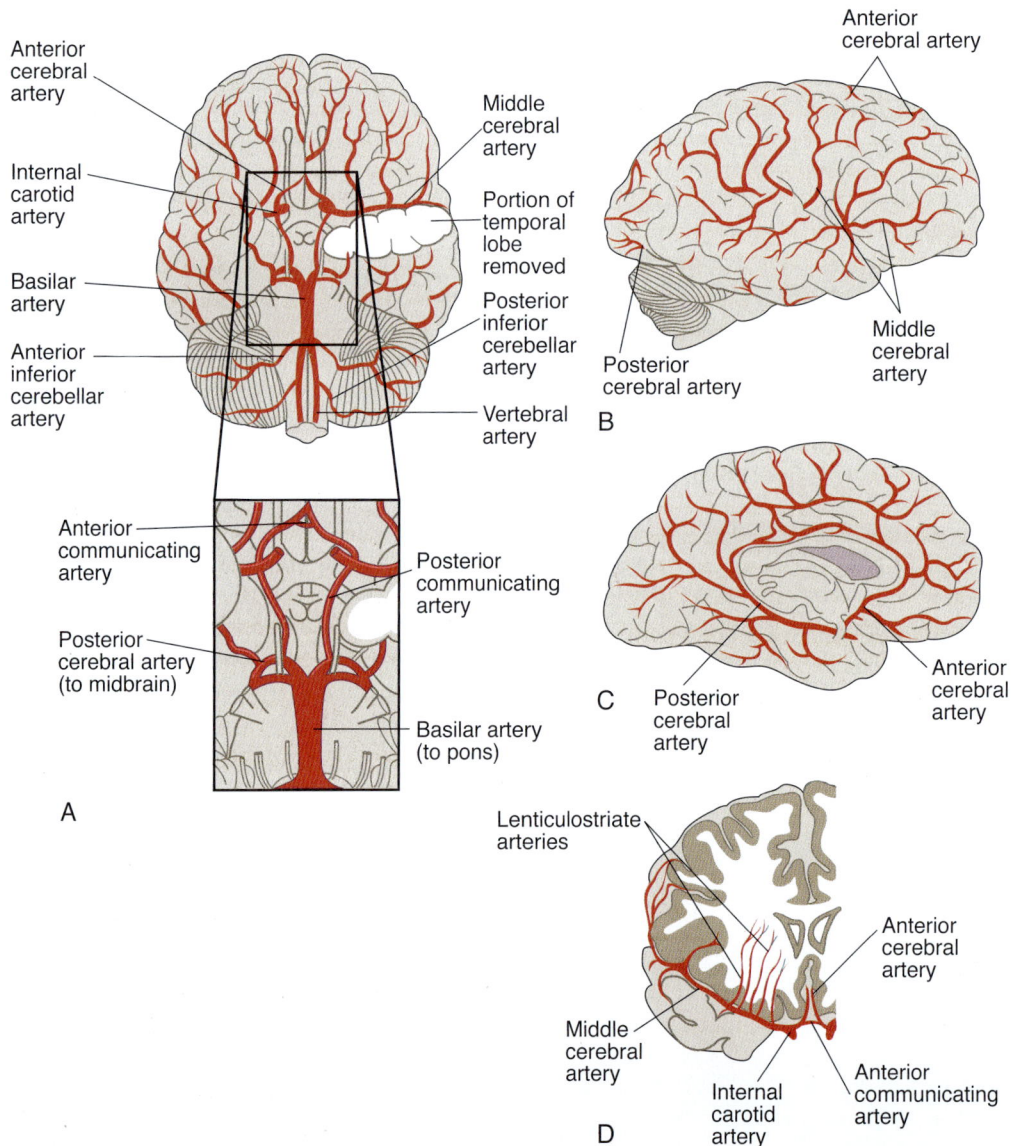

Adapted from Purves D, Augustine G, Hall W, LaMantia A, McNamara J, White L. Neuroscience. 5th ed. New York: Sinauer Associates; 2012, with permission.

This compensatory mechanism delays neurological deterioration in patients.[3]

The cerebral veins drain into large venous sinuses and then into the right and left internal jugular veins (see Figure 16.9).[23] The venous sinuses are found within the folds of the dura mater. The veins and sinuses of the brain do not have valves, so the blood flows freely by gravity.[1] The face and scalp veins can flow into the brain venous sinuses; therefore, infection can easily be spread into the dural venous sinuses and then enter the brain.

Patient position can prevent or promote venous drainage from the brain. Head turning and tilting may kink the jugular vein and decrease or stop venous flow from the brain, which will then raise the pressure inside the cranial vault.

Cerebral blood flow (CBF) is the cerebral perfusion pressure (CPP) divided by cerebrovascular resistance (CVR). CVR is the amount of resistance created by the cerebral vessels, and it is controlled by the autoregulatory mechanisms of the brain. Specifically, vasoconstriction (and vasospasm) will increase CVR, and vasodilation will decrease CVR.[1] It is influenced by the inflow pressure (systole), outflow pressure (venous pressure), cross-sectional diameter of cerebral blood vessels and intracranial pressure (ICP).[1] CVR is similar to systemic vascular resistance but, due to the lack of valves in the venous system of the brain, cerebral venous pressure also influences the CVR. An important characteristic of the cerebral circulation is its ability to autoregulate, that is, the ability to maintain constant cerebral blood flow despite variations in perfusion pressure (see Table 16.5). This is important in protecting the brain from both ischaemia during hypotension and haemorrhage during hypertension.

TABLE 16.5

Changes in cerebrovascular and cerebrometabolic parameters when various cerebral variables are reduced with and without intact autoregulation

PRIMARY REDUCTION IN THESE VARIABLES	CBF	CBV (ICP)	AVDO$_2$
CMRO$_2$	↑	↓	–
CPP (autoregulation intact)	–	↑	–
CPP (autoregulation defective)	↓	↓	↑
Blood viscosity (autoregulation intact)	–	↓	–
Blood viscosity (autoregulation defective)	↑	–	↓
PaCO$_2$	↓	↓	↑
Conductive vessel diameter (vasospasm above ischaemic threshold)	↓	↑	↑

AVDO$_2$ = arteriovenous O$_2$ difference; CBF = cerebral blood flow; CBV = cerebral blood volume; ICP = intracranial pressure; CMRO$_2$ = cerebral metabolic rate of oxygen; CPP = cerebral perfusion pressure; PaCO$_2$ = arterial CO$_2$ tension; ↑ = increase; ↓ = decrease; – = no change.

FIGURE 16.9   Cerebral venous drainage.[23]

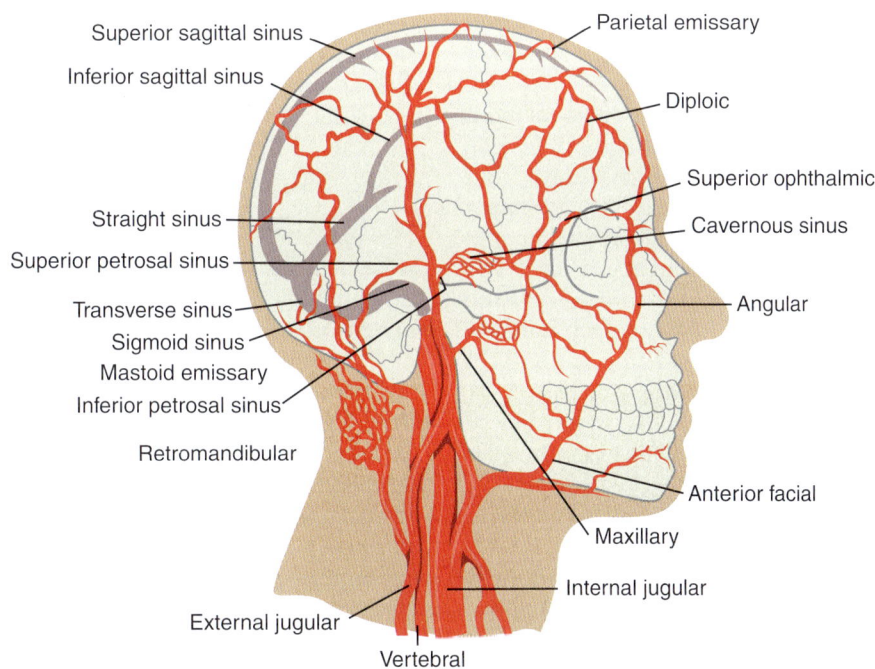

Adapted from Martini F, Nath J, Bartholomew E. Anatomy and physiology. 9th ed. San Francisco: Pearson Benjamin Cummings; 2011, with permission.

CBF is affected by extrinsic and intrinsic factors.[1] Extrinsic factors include systemic blood pressure, cardiac output, blood viscosity and vascular tone. The body responds to these demands with changes in blood flow. Aerobic metabolism is critically dependent on oxygen in order to process glucose for normal energy production, and the brain does not store energy. Therefore, without a constant source of oxygen and energy, its supply from CBF can be exhausted within 3 minutes. Intrinsic factors include $PaCO_2$ (pH), PaO_2 and ICP. The vessels dilate with increases in $PaCO_2$ (hypercarbia) or low pH (acidosis) and with decreases in PaO_2 (hypoxia). This vasodilation increases CBF. The vessels constrict with decreases in $PaCO_2$ or high pH and with increases in local PaO_2.[1] This vasoconstriction will decrease the CBF. In addition, intrinsic factors can change the extrinsic factors by altering the metabolic mechanisms. These changes can lead to an alteration in the CBF. For example, there can be a change from aerobic to anaerobic metabolism, which increases the concentrations of other end-products such as lactic acid, pyruvic acid and carbonic acid, which causes a localised acidosis. These end-products result in a high pH that will cause an increase in CBF. Other factors that can affect CBF include pharmacological agents (anaesthetic agents and some antihypertensive agents), rapid-eye-movement sleep, arousal, pain, seizures, elevations in body temperature and cerebral trauma.

Spinal cord

The spinal cord is the link between the peripheral nervous system and the brain. The spinal cord has a small, irregularly shaped internal section of grey matter (unmyelinated tissue) surrounded by a larger area of white matter (myelinated axons). The internal grey matter is arranged so that it extends up and down dorsally in a column, one on each side; another column is found in the ventral region on each side (see Figure 16.10).[1]

The spinal cord is an essential component of both the sensory and motor divisions of the nervous system. The first of the primary functions of the spinal cord is to transmit sensory impulses along the ascending tracts to the brain as well as to transmit motor impulses down the descending tracts away from the brain.[24] The second primary function of the spinal cord is to house and regulate spinal reflexes. Receipt of sensory impulses may cause a reaction anywhere in the body; alternatively, the signal might be stored in the memory to be used at some stage in the future. Within the motor division of the nervous system the spinal cord helps to control the various bodily activities, including skeletal muscle activity, smooth muscle activity and secretion by both endocrine and exocrine glands.

Sensory neurons from all over the skin, except for the skin of the face and scalp, feed information into the spinal cord through the spinal nerves. The skin surface can be mapped into distinct regions that are supplied by a single spinal nerve[19] (see Figure 16.11).[25]

Each of these regions is called a dermatome. Sensation from a given dermatome is carried over its corresponding spinal nerve. This information can be used to identify the spinal nerve or spinal segment that is involved in an injury. In some areas, the dermatomes are not absolutely distinct. Some dermatomes may share a nerve supply with neighbouring regions. For this reason, it is necessary to numb several adjacent dermatomes to achieve successful anaesthesia.

The blood supply to the spinal cord arises from branches of the vertebral arteries and spinal radicular arteries.[19] The mid-thoracic region, at approximately T4–T8, lies between the lumbar and vertebral arterial supplies and is a vulnerable zone of relatively decreased perfusion. This region is most susceptible to infarction during periods of hypotension, thoracic surgery or other conditions, causing decreased aortic pressure and potentially leading to ischaemic spinal injury with devastating consequences.[19]

Peripheral nervous system

The PNS consists of 12 pairs of cranial nerves and 31 pairs of spinal nerves, and includes all neural structures lying outside the spinal cord and brainstem. The cranial nerves have previously been discussed regarding their role in brainstem function. The PNS has both motor and sensory components. The former includes the motor neuron cell body in the anterior horn of the spinal cord and its peripheral axonal process travelling through the ventral root and eventually the peripheral nerve. The motor nerve terminal, together with the muscle endplate and the synapse between the two, comprises the neuromuscular junction. The peripheral sensory axon, beginning at receptors in cutaneous and deep structures, as well as muscle and tendon receptors, travels back through peripheral nerves to its cell body located in the dorsal root ganglion. Its central process, travelling through the dorsal root, enters the spinal cord in the region of the dorsal horn. All commands for movement, whether reflexive or voluntary, are ultimately conveyed to the muscles by the activity of the lower motor neurons.

Motor control

Movements can be divided into three main classes: voluntary activity, rhythmic motor patterns and reflex responses. The highest-order activity is voluntary movement, which allows for expression of the will and a purposeful response to the environment (e.g. reading, speaking, performing calculations).[1] Such activity is goal-directed and largely learned, and improves with practice. In rhythmic motor patterns, the initiation and termination may be voluntary, but the rhythmic activity itself does not require conscious participation (e.g. chewing, walking, running). Reflex responses are simple, stereotyped responses that do not involve voluntary control (e.g. deep tendon reflexes or withdrawal of a limb from a hot surface). Motor control is carried out in a hierarchical yet parallel fashion in the cerebral cortex, the brainstem and the spinal cord. Modulating influences are provided by the basal ganglia and cerebellum through the thalamus.[1]

FIGURE 16.10 The spinal cord and spinal meninges: **A** posterior view of the spinal cord, showing the meningeal layers, superficial landmarks and distribution of grey matter and white matter; **B** sectional view through the spinal cord and meninges, showing the peripheral distribution of spinal nerves.[1]

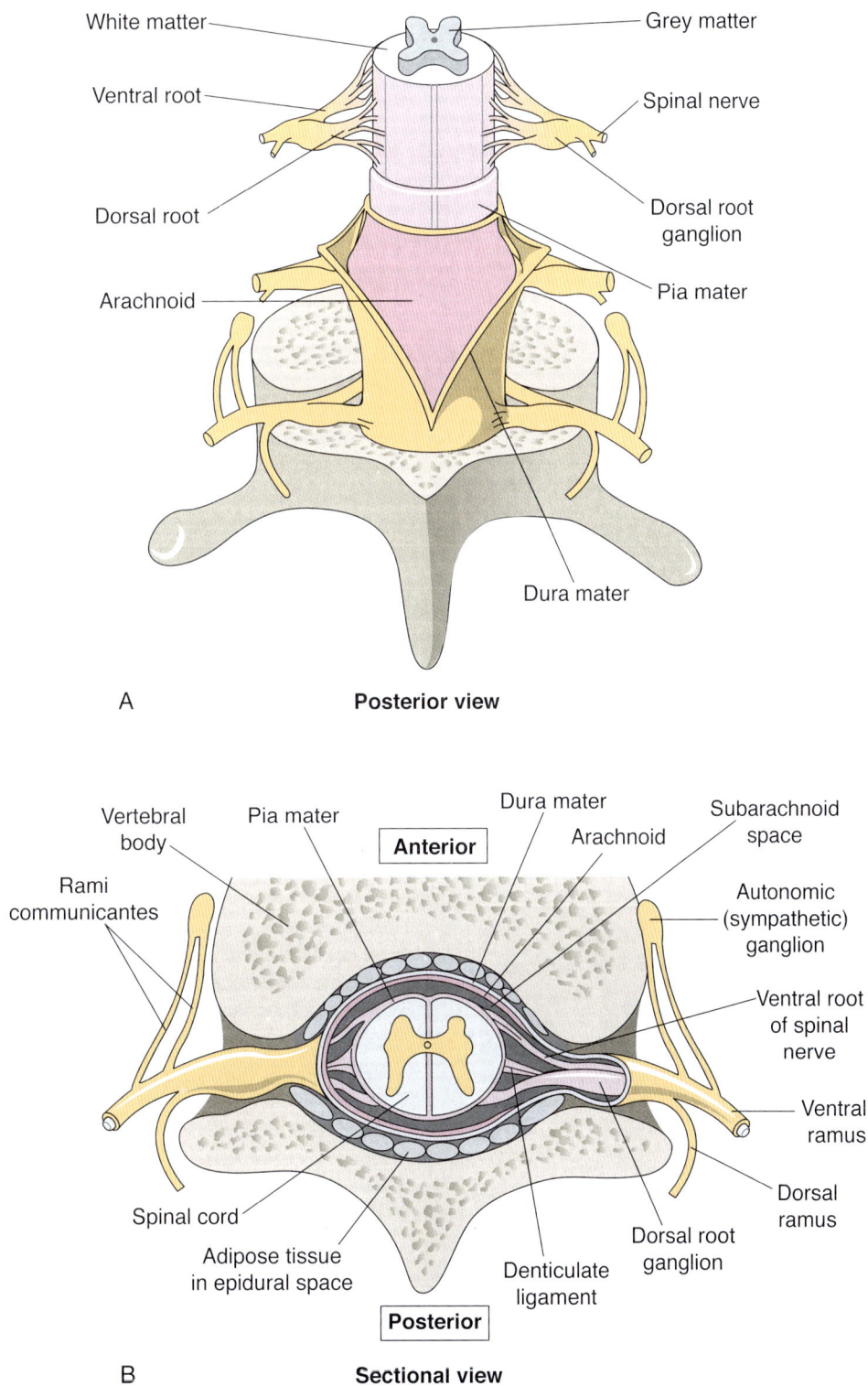

A   **Posterior view**

B   **Sectional view**

Adapted from Martini F, Nath J, Bartholomew E. Anatomy and physiology. 9th ed. San Francisco: Pearson Benjamin Cummings; 2011, with permission.

FIGURE 16.11 **A** Anterior and **B** posterior distributions of dermatomes on the surface of the skin.[25]

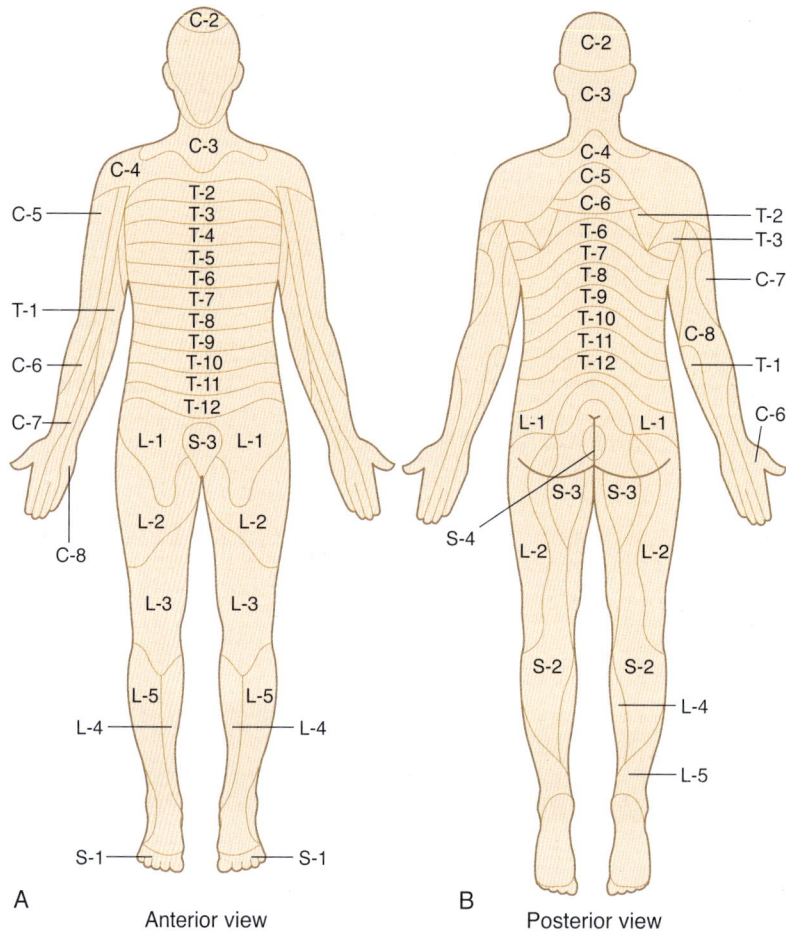

Anterior view

Posterior view

Adapted from Cohen B, Taylor J. Memmler's human body in health and disease. 12th ed. Philadelphia: Lippincott, Williams & Wilkins; 2012, with permission.

Sensory control

The somatic sensory system has two major components: a subsystem for the detection of mechanical stimuli (e.g. light touch, vibration, pressure, cutaneous tension) and a subsystem for the detection of painful stimuli and temperature.[1] Together, these subsystems provide the ability to identify the shapes and textures of objects, to monitor the internal and external forces acting on the body at any moment and to detect potentially harmful circumstances. Mechanosensory processing of external stimuli is initiated by the activation of a diverse population of cutaneous and subcutaneous mechanoreceptors at the body surface that relay information to the central nervous system for interpretation and ultimately for action. Additional receptors located in muscles, joints and other deep structures monitor mechanical forces generated by the musculoskeletal system, and are called proprioceptors. Mechanosensory information is carried to the brain by several ascending pathways that run in parallel through the spinal cord, brainstem and thalamus to reach the primary somatic sensory cortex in the postcentral gyrus of the parietal lobe.[1] The primary somatic sensory cortex projects in turn to higher-order association cortices in the parietal lobe, and back to the subcortical structures involved in mechanosensory information processing.

Autonomic nervous system

The autonomic nervous system, with its three major divisions (sympathetic, parasympathetic and enteric), is largely an involuntary system and is part of the efferent division, as shown in Figure 16.1. It allows the body to adjust to rapidly changing external events (the 'flight or fight' response of the sympathetic division) and to regulate internal activities (blood pressure, temperature, airway and breathing, urinary function, digestion by the parasympathetic and enteric divisions).[1] Whereas the major controlling centres for somatic motor activity are the primary and secondary motor cortices in the frontal lobes and a variety of related brainstem nuclei, the major locus of central control in the visceral motor system is the hypothalamus and the complex circuitry that it controls in the brainstem tegmentum and spinal cord.[1] The status of both divisions of the visceral motor system is modulated by descending pathways from these centres to preganglionic neurons in the brainstem and spinal cord, which in turn determine the activity of the primary visceral motor neurons in autonomic ganglia. The postganglionic neurons of the sympathetic system,

with few exceptions, act on their effectors by releasing the neurotransmitter adrenaline and the related compound noradrenaline. This system is therefore described as adrenergic, which means 'activated by adrenaline'.[1] The autonomic regulation of several organ systems of particular importance in clinical practice is illustrated in Figure 16.12.[15]

FIGURE 16.12 (Sympathetic and parasympathetic divisions of the autonomic nervous system. Sympathetic outputs (**left**) arise from thoracolumbar spinal cord segments and synapses in paravertebral and prevertebral ganglia. Parasympathetic outputs (**right**) arise from craniosacral regions and synapses in ganglia in or near effector organs.[15]

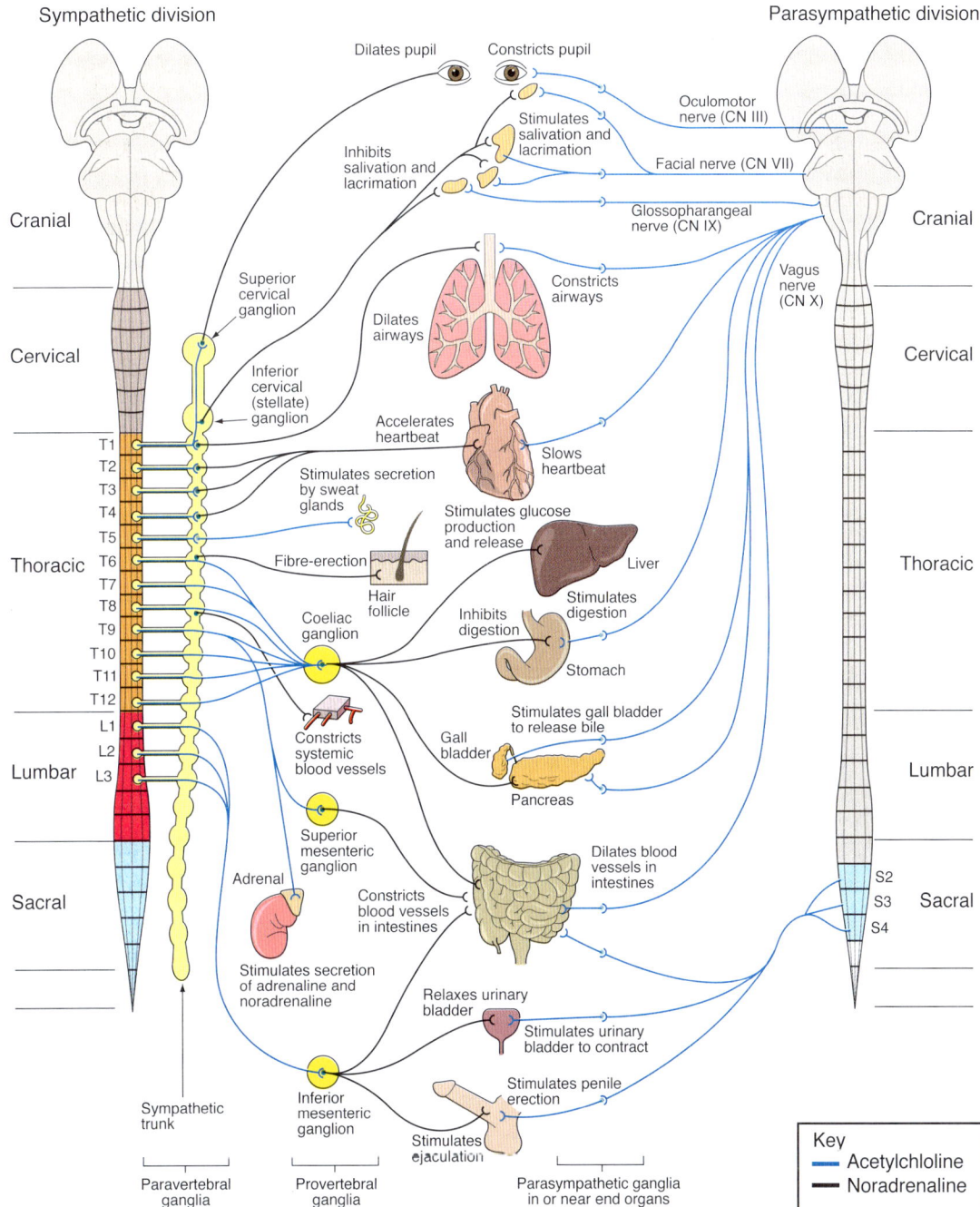

Adapted from Blumenfeld H. Neuroanatomy through clinical cases. New York: Sinauer Associates; 2010, with permission.

Neurological assessment and monitoring

This section explores the complex issues surrounding cerebral haemodynamics and assessment. The objective of assessment is to determine the extent of neurological injury, recognise fluctuations in condition and imminent deterioration and assist in maintaining cerebral perfusion as part of multimodal monitoring.

Physical examination

The neurological physical exam begins at the onset of patient contact, and the priorities are defined by a primary survey and vital signs. The patient's history and contact with family can inform the clinical examination and should include the patient's normal baseline status, medications and other substance use and past neurological symptoms such as syncope or seizures.

Specific areas tested during the initial physical exam include level of consciousness, general behaviour, memory, attention and concentration, abstract thought and judgement. Not every aspect of the examination will be relevant in all critical care situations and therefore may not be tested. Nevertheless, the clinician should understand how all components are integrated and how they influence priority decision making for patient care. At change of shift, performing a physical examination with the incoming nurse ensures clear communication of the patient's previous status. The patient's ability to perform should be taken into consideration, as it may be necessary to modify assessment techniques. For example, intubated patients who are otherwise awake and aware may gesture or write answers to questions instead of verbalising them. In addition, when patients are the recipients of very frequent neurological assessment over an extended period of time (including arousal and awareness, pupil and motor response), sleep and sensory rest deprivation is common. Sleep deprivation and sensory overload will confound assessment accuracy. Therefore, careful consideration needs to be given in regard to the priorities of assessment and rest; a plan needs to implemented to promote rest as neurological injury requires rest and sleep for restoration. See *Online resources* for links to a full neurological assessment and physical examination protocol.

> **Practice tip**
>
> Evaluation of the level of consciousness and mentation are the most important parts of the neurological examination. A change in either is usually the first clue to CNS dysfunction.

Conscious state

Arousal and awareness are the fundamental constituents of consciousness and should be evaluated and documented repeatedly for trend analysis. Changes in the conscious state are the first to occur in deterioration.

Arousal assessment

The evaluation of arousal focuses on the ability to be able to respond to a variety of stimuli and can be described using the Awake, Verbal, Pain, Unresponsive (AVPU) scale or terms such as disorientated, lethargic or obtunded. The advanced trauma life support course[26] recommends an initial assessment during initial resuscitation based on the response to stimulation: **A**wake, **V**erbal, **P**ain, **U**nresponsive (AVPU). Observe the patient's response (verbal or motor). If there is no response to voice or light touch, painful stimulus is needed to assess neurological status. Central pain should be used first and applied with care. Sternal rub, supraorbital pressure (least used), trapezius pinch (most used) or pinching the fleshy portion of the upper arm near the axilla are methods for introducing central pain. Hand grasp is a reflex and is a poor test for motor strength. If the patient does not respond to verbal stimulus but moves spontaneously in a purposeful manner (picks at linen, pulls at tubes), the patient is localising. Painful stimulus is not required if spontaneous localisation has been observed. Watch for symmetry. Localising is purposeful and intentional movement intended to eliminate a noxious stimulus, whereas withdrawal is a 'smaller' movement used to 'get away from' noxious stimulus. Abnormal flexion differs from withdrawal in that the flexion is rigid and abnormal looking. Abnormal extension is a rigid movement with extension of the limbs.

> **Practice tip**
>
> When a patient opens their eyes when you call their name, it is an indication that their reticular activating centre (brainstem) functioning is intact but it does not tell you if they are awake or aware.

> **Practice tip**
>
> Awareness means that the cerebral cortex is working in conjunction with the reticular activating system (arousal) and that the patient can interact with and interpret their environment.

Assessment of awareness

If arousable, progress to assessment of awareness using the Glasgow Coma Scale (GCS). Teasdale and Jennett[27] designed the GCS to establish an objective, quantifiable measure to describe the prognosis of a patient with a brain injury and include scoring of separate subscales related to eye opening, verbal response and motor response (Table 16.6). Originally, the GCS was developed as three separate response areas and reported as such. Contemporary use of the GCS automatically adds the three best response scores and easily loses the information given from the separate response areas. Reporting the GCS as three numbers and then the total gives a broader assessment interpretation.

TABLE 16.6

Glasgow Coma Scale

The Glasgow Coma Scale is scored between 3 and 15, 3 being the worst, and 15 the best. It comprises three parameters: best eye response, best verbal response and best motor response. The definition of these parameters is given below.

THE GLASGOW COMA SCALE FOR ADULTS	PAEDIATRIC VERSION OF THE GLASGOW COMA SCALE
Best eye response (4)	Best eye response (4)
1 No eye opening	1 No eye opening
2 Eye opening to pain	2 Eye opening to pain
3 Eye opening to verbal command	3 Eye opening to verbal command
4 Eyes open spontaneously	4 Eyes open spontaneously
Best verbal response (5)	Best verbal response (5)
1 No verbal response	1 No vocal response
2 Incomprehensible sounds	2 Occasionally whimpers and/or moans
3 Inappropriate words	3 Cries inappropriately
4 Confused	4 Less than usual ability and/or spontaneous irritable cry
5 Orientated	5 Alert, babbles, coos, words or sentences to usual ability
Best motor response (6)	Best motor response (6)
1 No motor response	1 No motor response to pain
2 Extension to pain	2 Abnormal extension to pain (decerebrate)
3 Flexion to pain	3 Abnormal flexion to pain (decorticate)
4 Withdrawal from pain	4 Withdrawal to painful stimuli
5 Localising pain	5 Localises to painful stimuli or withdraws to touch
6 Obeys commands	6 Obeys commands or performs normal spontaneous movements

The advantage of the GCS is that it allows rapid serial comparisons and categorisation of basic neurological function over time. However, it has several recognised weaknesses, including poor prediction of outcome beyond survival, poor inter-rater reliability and inconsistent use in the prehospital and hospital settings. GCS accuracy will be affected if the patient is receiving anaesthetic agents or sedation and noxious stimuli should be avoided. Furthermore, the rare event of a *locked-in syndrome*, where a patient is neurologically aware and awake but not responding, is poorly represented by the GCS. Also, interpretation of response in regard to language used or a previous communication disability is important for assessment accuracy. See *Online resources* for a link to a full GCS procedure.

The **F**ull **O**utline of **U**n**r**esponsiveness (FOUR) scale is an accurate predictor of outcome in traumatic brain injury (TBI) patients. It is easy to learn, remember and administer. It has some advantages over GCS: for example,

all its components can be rated in intubated patients, it gives all components equal weight and it allows the examiner to localise lesions and diagnose a locked-in state.[28] The FOUR score assesses four variables: eye response, motor response, brainstem reflexes and respiration pattern. This assesses respirations as: 1) spontaneous regular or irregular, 2) Cheyne-Stokes, 3) intubated but independently breathing above the ventilator or 4) absent. If all four categories are graded at zero, brain death testing is suggested.[29]

The administration of the FOUR offers a few specific advantages over utilising the GCS.[28] The FOUR adds to the eye opening of the GCS by testing eye tracking, thus incorporating midbrain and pontine functions. It allows for testing of afferent language processing and remains testable regardless of endotracheal intubation, aphasia, aphonia or trauma to the vocal apparatus. It adds to the motor score of the GCS, incorporating hand gestures into the evaluation. The bulk of the motor score is similar to the GCS except that no difference is delineated between flexor posturing and normal flexion to pain. Specific testing of brainstem reflexes via pupillary, corneal and cough reflexes further allows the clinician to localise lesions and track progression of cerebral injury, specifically by addressing unilateral fixed mydriasis, a sign alerting to uncal herniation.[29]

Eye and pupil assessment

Pupillary responses, including pupil size and reaction to light, are important neurological observations and localise cerebral disease to a specific area of the brain. The immediate constriction of the pupil when light is shone into the eye is referred to as the direct light reflex. Withdrawal of the light should produce an immediate and brisk dilation of the pupil. Introduction of the light into one eye should cause a similar constriction to occur in the other pupil (consensual light reaction).[30]

Other points to consider when conducting pupillary observations include the following:[31]

- Pinpoint non-reactive pupils are associated with opiate overdose.
- Non-reactive pupils may also be caused by local damage.
- Atropine will cause dilated pupils.
- One dilated or fixed pupil may be indicative of an expanding or developing intracranial lesion, compressing the oculomotor nerve on the same side of the brain as the affected pupil.
- A sluggish pupil may be difficult to distinguish from a fixed pupil and may be an early focal sign of an expanding intracranial lesion and raised intracranial pressure. A sluggish response to light in a previously reacting pupil must be reported immediately.

Assessment of pupillary function focuses on three areas: 1) estimation of pupil size and shape; 2) evaluation of pupillary reaction to light; and 3) assessment of eye movements. Metabolic disturbances rarely cause pupillary changes, so abnormal pupillary findings are usually due to a nervous system lesion.[32] Irregular-sized pupils are normal for some people and eye prostheses are common; it is important to establish and document these findings so a trend can be established to distinguish normal from altered states.

> ### Practice tip
>
> Localising is purposeful and intentional movement intended to eliminate a noxious stimulus, whereas withdrawal is a 'smaller' movement used to 'get away from' noxious stimulus.

Eye and eyelid movements

Patients who are comatose will exhibit no eye opening. In patients with bilateral thalamic damage, there may be normal consciousness, but an eye opening apraxia (i.e. non-paralytic motor abnormality characterised by difficulty initiating the act of lid elevation after lid closure) may mimic coma. If the patient's eyes are closed, the clinician should gently raise and release the eyelids. Brisk opening and closing of the eyes indicates that the pons is grossly intact. If the pons is impaired, one or both eyelids may close slowly or not at all. In the patient with intact frontal lobe and brainstem functioning, the eyes, when opened, should be pointed straight ahead and at equal height. If there is awareness, the patient should look towards stimuli after eye opening. Eye deviation indicates either a unilateral cerebral or brainstem lesion. If the eyes deviate laterally, gently turn the head to see if the eyes will cross the midline to the other side. A pattern of spontaneous, slow and random movements (usually laterally) is termed roving-eye movements. This indicates that the brainstem oculomotor control is intact but awareness is significantly impaired.[33]

Limb movement

Assessment of extremities and body movement (or motor response) provides valuable information about the patient with a decreased level of consciousness.[34] The clinician must observe the patient's spontaneous movements, muscle tone and response to tactile stimuli. Decorticate (flexor) posturing is seen when there is involvement of a cerebral hemisphere and the brain stem. It is characterised by adduction of the shoulder and arm, elbow flexion and pronation and flexion of the wrist while the legs extend. In terms of the GCS motor score, the *withdrawal flexor* scores higher (4/6) than a *spastic flexor* movement (3/6). Decerebrate (extensor) posturing is seen with severe metabolic disturbances or upper brainstem lesions. It is characterised by extension and pronation of the arm(s) and extension of the legs. Patients may have an asymmetrical response and may posture spontaneously or to stimuli.

Motor tone is first assessed by flexing the limbs and noting increased or absent tone.[33] If no tone is present, the hand is lifted approximately 30 cm above the bed and carefully dropped while protecting the limb from injury.

The test is repeated with all extremities. Typically, the lower the level of consciousness, the closer to flaccid the limb(s) will be. An asymmetrical examination may indicate a lesion in the contralateral hemisphere or brainstem.

The next assessment, *peripheral reflex response*, is response to tactile stimuli peripherally and usually elicits a reflex response rather than a central or brain response. It is important to apply stimuli in a progressive manner, using the least noxious stimuli necessary to elicit a response. If there is no response to light or firm pressure, the clinician must use noxious stimuli. Each extremity is assessed individually. The typical technique for peripheral noxious stimuli involves pressure on the nail beds for asserting a peripheral stimulus. The triple-flexion response is a withdrawal of the limb in a straight line with flexion of the wrist–elbow–shoulder or the ankle–knee–hip. This response is considered a spinal reflex and is not an indication of brain involvement in the movement. The triple-flexion response is common in patients with severe neurological impairment. It is not uncommon in patients who have become brain dead, and great care must be taken to avoid confusion between brain and spinal-mediated responses. If the patient has any other motor activity to peripheral extremity noxious stimuli, it is an indication of higher brain function.[35]

If a noxious stimulus is applied *centrally* through a sternal rub, trapezius pinch or supraorbital nerve pressure and the patient moves an extremity, it is an indication of brain involvement in the movement and not a spinal reflex.[36] The movement should be noted as normal, decorticate (flexor: either withdrawal or spastic) or decerebrate (extensor) and documented accordingly. It should be noted that careful consideration should be given to the choice of noxious stimuli with trapezius pinch the preferred choice as both sternal rub and supraorbital nerve pressure can be traumatic when applied. In ventilated patients, endotracheal suction can also be a substitute for a central noxious stimulus, but the choice of stimulus needs to be consistent.

> ### Practice tip
>
> The ability to cough with suctioning can be tested in an intubated patient and implies an intact cranial nerve X.

Facial symmetry

Facial symmetry is often difficult to appreciate in, for example, severely ill patients due to oedema, endotracheal tube tape and nasogastric tubes. An asymmetric response is indicative of a lesion of cranial nerve (CN) VII. Complete hemi-facial involvement is typically seen in peripheral dysfunction (Bell's palsy), whereas superior division (forehead) sparing weakness indicates a pontine/medullary (central) involvement. It is important to refrain from supraorbital pressure until after pupillary responses have been assessed because this noxious stimulation may cause alteration in pupillary reactivity (hence one reason for the lack of preference for its use).

Corneal reflexes

The corneal reflex is assessed by holding the patient's eye open and lightly stimulating the cornea.[37] The stimuli should result in a reflexive blink, best seen in the lower eyelid. The traditional assessment technique involves using a wisp of cotton, lightly brushed along the lower aspect of the cornea. An alternative, and less potentially traumatic, method is to gently instil isotonic eye drops or saline irrigation ampoules onto the cornea. This reflex is dependent upon CN V for its sensation and CN VII for its motor response. Loss of this reflex is indicative of lower brainstem damage, but it may be absent due to trauma, surgery or long-term contact lens usage.

Oropharyngeal reflexes

The oropharyngeal reflexes are controlled by CN IX and CN X.[38] The gag reflex is elicited by lightly stimulating the soft palate with a suction catheter or tongue blade. Clinicians should always avoid stimulating a gag reflex by wiggling the endotracheal tube because doing so may result in an inadvertent extubation. A gag reflex is a forceful, symmetrical lowering of the soft palate. The cough reflex is usually assessed only in patients with an endotracheal tube. This reflex is elicited by gently passing a suction catheter through the tube and stimulating a cough. Loss of these reflexes is indicative of lower brainstem damage.[39]

> **Practice tip**
>
> Sluggish pupils are found in conditions that compress the third cranial nerve, such as cerebral oedema and herniation.

Post-traumatic amnesia scale

Post-traumatic amnesia (PTA) is a disorder after brain injury that is classified as a traumatic delirium and may even be found in patients who rate a GCS of 15.[40] The incidence of delirium after a brain injury event is high especially with severe injuries and loss of consciousness. Delirium is discussed in detail in Chapter 7; however, traumatic delirium historically has been referred to in the literature as post-traumatic amnesia. Post-traumatic amnesia is defined as the 'time elapsed from injury until recovery of full consciousness and the return of ongoing memory'.[41,p.841] It is the initial stage of recovery from brain injury and is characterised by anterograde (formation of new memory) and retrograde (memory before injury) amnesia, disorientation and rapid forgetting. Brief periods of PTA can occur after minor concussion and may be the only clinical sign of any brain injury. This is when PTA is useful for defining the severity of injury and alerting the clinician in regard to greater surveillance and investigation as described in Table 16.7. Patients often progress directly from coma into delirium without a clearly-defined stupor stage, so using a tool to measure PTA can be useful to gauge the actual condition of the patient in the delirium state. Duration of PTA is extremely variable, ranging from

TABLE 16.7

PTA scale used to determine severity of brain injury

PTA SCORE	SEVERITY
1–4 hours	Mild brain injury
≤1 day	Moderate brain injury
2–7 days	Severe brain injury
1–4 weeks	Very severe brain injury
1–6 months	Extremely severe brain injury
>6 months	Chronic amnesia state

minutes to months. Although the early stages of PTA are easily recognised, identifying the end point is difficult and complex.[42]

The duration of PTA is the best indicator of the extent of cognitive and functional deficits after TBI. The two most common means of assessing PTA are the Galveston Orientation and Amnesia Test (GOAT) and the Westmead PTA scale.[43] GOAT features ten questions that assess temporal and spatial orientation, biographical recall and memory. The test consists of 10 items that involve the recall of events that occurred right before and after the injury, as well as questions about disorientation. Scores of 75 or more on this scale (out of a total possible score of 100) correspond to the termination of the PTA episode. In the Westmead PTA scale, four pictures, one with the examiner's face and name, are to be recalled by the patient on the next day. Those with severe PTA will have difficulty completing such short-term memory tasks. Often, patients will have a GCS of 15 but have moderate-to-severe PTA and can be overlooked by inexperienced clinicians who fail to watch for secondary insults. The duration of PTA correlates well with the extent of diffuse axonal injury and with functional outcomes. For example, one study found that 80% of patients with PTA duration of less than 2 weeks had a good recovery, compared with 46% for those with PTA duration between 4 and 6 weeks.[44] A person is said to be absolved of PTA if they can achieve a perfect score for three consecutive days.

Assessment of the injured brain

The primary aim of managing patients with acute brain injury in the critical care unit is to maintain cerebral perfusion and oxygenation.[45] There is little that can be done to reverse the primary damage caused by an insult. Secondary insults may be subtle and can remain undetected by routine systemic physiological monitoring. Continuous monitoring of the central nervous system in the ICU serves three functions:[46]

1. determination of the extent of the primary injury
2. early detection of secondary cerebral insults so that appropriate interventions can be instituted
3. monitoring of therapeutic interventions to provide feedback.

Although serial cranial imaging such as computerised tomography (CT) or functional magnetic resonance imaging (fMRI) provides useful information, these are neither continuous nor can they be undertaken at the bedside. Continuous invasive arterial blood pressure monitoring in addition to pulse oximetry, temperature, end-tidal carbon dioxide and urine output should be included as part of standard general monitoring of brain-injured patients. In addition, techniques specific to the CNS are required. The commonest and most easily performed clinical assessment tool is the GCS. Brain-specific methods of monitoring reflect pressure in the cranial cavity, changes in brain oxygenation and metabolism (brain oxygen saturation) and include jugular venous oxygen saturation, near-infrared spectroscopy, brain tissue monitoring, cerebral haemodynamics (transcranial Doppler) and electrical activity of the CNS (EEG).

Brain imaging techniques

Computed tomography

CT is the primary neuroimaging technique in the initial evaluation of the acute brain injury patient and uses a computer to digitally construct an image based upon the measurement of the absorption of X-rays through the brain. Table 16.8 generally summarises the white to black intensities seen for selected tissues in CT. The advantages of CT are: 1) it is rapidly performed, which is especially important in neurological emergencies; 2) it clearly shows acute and subacute haemorrhages into the meningeal spaces and brain; and 3) it is less expensive than an MRI.[47] Disadvantages include: 1) it does not clearly show acute or subacute infarctions or ischaemia, or brain oedema, but only shows injury; 2) it does not differentiate white from grey matter as clearly as an MRI; and 3) it exposes the patient to ionising radiation. Despite these limitations it is still the most prevalent form of neurological imaging.[48]

Magnetic resonance imaging

The tissues of the body contain proportionately large amounts of protons (nuclei of hydrogen atoms) that function like tiny spinning magnets. Normally, these protons are arranged randomly in relation to each other

due to the constantly fluctuating magnetic field produced by the associated electrons. However, when placed in a superconducting magnet, the magnetic moments of the protons will tend to align along the direction of this external field. Magnetic resonance imaging (MRI) uses this characteristic of protons to generate images of the brain and body. The advantages of MRI are: 1) it can be manipulated to visualise a wide variety of abnormalities within the brain; and 2) it can show a great deal of detail of the brain in normal and abnormal states.[49] The disadvantages of MRI are: 1) it does not show acute or subacute haemorrhage into the brain in any detail; 2) the time frame and enclosed space required to perform and prepare a patient for the procedure are not advantageous for neurological emergencies; 3) it is relatively more expensive compared to CT; 4) the loud noise of the procedure needs to be considered in patient management; and 5) equipment for life support and monitoring needs to be non-magnetic due to the magnetic nature of the procedure.[50]

Functional magnetic resonance imaging

Functional magnetic resonance imaging (fMRI) is similar to MRI but uses deoxyhaemoglobin as an endogenous contrast, which serves as the source of the magnetic signal for fMRI. It can determine precisely which part of the brain is handling critical functions such as thought, speech, movement and sensation; help assess the effects of stroke, trauma or degenerative disease on brain function; monitor the growth and function of brain tumours; and guide the planning of surgery or radiation therapy for the brain.[51]

Cerebral angiography

Cerebral angiography involves cannulation of cerebral vessels and the administration of intra-arterial contrast agents and medications for conditions involving the arterial circulation of the brain. This procedure also has the benefit of using non-invasive CT or MRI with or without contrast to guide the accuracy of the procedure. For example, intracranial aneurysms and arteriovenous malformations can be accurately diagnosed and repaired without surgical intervention.[52]

Cerebral perfusion imaging techniques

Numerous imaging techniques have been developed and applied to evaluate brain haemodynamics, perfusion and blood flow. The main imaging techniques dedicated to brain haemodynamics are positron emission tomography (PET), single photon emission computed tomography (SPECT), xenon-enhanced computed tomography (XeCT), dynamic perfusion computed tomography (PCT), MRI dynamic susceptibility contrast (DSC) and arterial spin labelling (ASL). All of these techniques give similar information about brain haemodynamics in the form of parameters such as CBF or CBV.[53] They use different tracers and have different technical requirements. Some are feasible at the bedside and others not (see Table 16.9). The duration of

---

TABLE 16.8

The brain and related structures in CT

STRUCTURE/FLUID/SPACE	GREY SCALE
Bone, acute blood	Very white
Enhanced tumour	Very white
Subacute blood	Light grey
Muscle	Light grey
Grey matter	Light grey
White matter	Medium grey
Cerebrospinal fluid	Medium grey to black
Air, fat	Very black

TABLE 16.9

A comparison of various imaging techniques for assessing brain structure haemodynamics

IMAGING TECHNIQUE	BEDSIDE USE	SPATIAL RESOLUTION	TEMPORAL RESOLUTION	SCOPE OF USE	EASE OF INTERPRETATION
CEEG	excellent	good	excellent	excellent	poor
Evoked potentials	good	fair	fair	fair	poor
Transcranial Doppler	good	fair	fair	fair	poor
MRI	poor	excellent	poor	good	fair
Functional MRI	poor	excellent	good	poor	poor
CT	poor	excellent	poor	good	fair
Xenon CT	poor	good	poor	fair	poor
ICP monitoring	excellent	poor	good	fair	good

CEEG, continuous EEG; CT, computed tomography; ICP, intracranial pressure; MRI, magnetic resonance imaging.

data acquisition and processing varies from one technique to the other. Brain perfusion imaging techniques also differ in quantitative accuracy, brain coverage and spatial resolution.[54]

Practice tip

The fixed volume of brain parenchyma, CSF and intravascular blood contained within the rigid, non-expandable cranium determines ICP. Brain tissue accounts for 80% of this volume whereas blood and CSF each account for about 10%. An expansion of any one of these components must occur at the expense of another (Monro-Kellie hypothesis).

Intracranial pressure monitoring

Invasive measures for monitoring intracranial pressure (ICP) are commonly used in patients with a severe head injury or after neurological surgery. Normal ICP varies with age, body position and clinical condition. The normal ICP is 7–15 mmHg in a supine adult, 3–7 mmHg in children and 1.5–6 mmHg in term infants. The definition of intracranial hypertension depends on the specific pathology and age, although ICP >15 mmHg is generally considered to be abnormal. Increased ICP causes a critical reduction in CPP and CBF and may lead to secondary ischaemic cerebral injury. A number of studies have shown that high ICP is strongly associated with poor outcome, particularly if the period of intracranial hypertension is prolonged.[55] ICP is not a static pressure and varies with arterial pulsation, with breathing and during coughing and straining. Each of the intracranial constituents occupies a certain volume and, being essentially liquid, is incompressible. ICP cannot be reliably estimated from any specific clinical feature or CT finding and must actually be measured. Different methods of monitoring ICP have been described but two methods are commonly used in clinical practice: intraventricular catheters and intraparenchymal fibre optic

microtransducer systems. The reference point for the transducer is the foramina of Monro (the duct joining the lateral and third ventricle that is in alignment with the middle of the ear) although, in practical terms, the external auditory meatus is often used.

For many years ventriculostomy has been recognised as the most accurate (although the intraparenchymal fibre optic system is now similar in accuracy), cost-effective and reliable method of monitoring ICP and is associated with low infection risks if the duration of placement is less than 72 hours.[56] The ventriculostomy catheter is part of a system that includes an external drainage system and a transducer. The drainage system and transducer are primed on insertion with preservative-free saline. The transducer can easily be calibrated or zeroed against a known pressure. Advantages of using an indwelling ventricular catheter include allowing CSF drainage to effectively decrease ICP and using the catheter as a way to instil medications. Access to CSF drainage allows serial laboratory tests of CSF and determination of volume–pressure relationships. Disadvantages of ventriculostomy include risk of infection, which is higher than that associated with other ICP-monitoring techniques.[57] In addition, the catheter may become occluded with blood or tissue debris, interfering with CSF drainage or ICP monitoring. Also, if significant cerebral oedema is present, locating the lateral ventricle for insertion of the ventriculostomy catheter may be difficult. Importantly, bleeding or ventricular collapse may occur if CSF is drained too rapidly.[58] For this last reason, many clinicians set the ventriculostomy drainage system to drain CSF when the ICP is greater than 15–20 mmHg by adjusting the height of the drip chamber. In addition, limiting ventricular drainage per hour using gravity and three-way taps to 5–10 mL/h has been used to avoid excessively rapid CSF drainage. Using a ventriculostomy may allow life-saving CSF drainage and control of intracranial hypertension and secondary injury.[59]

While routine ICP monitoring is widely accepted as a mandatory monitoring technique for management of patients with severe head injury and is a guideline suggested by the Brain Trauma Foundation, there is some debate over its efficacy in improving outcome from severe TBI.[60] A review of neurocritical care and outcome from TBI suggested that ICP/CPP-guided therapy may benefit patients with severe head injury, including those presenting with raised ICP in the absence of a mass lesion and also patients requiring complex interventions.[61]

Pulse waveforms

Interpretation of waveforms that are generated by the cerebral monitoring devices is important in the clinical assessment of intracranial adaptive capacity (the ability of the brain to compensate for rises in intracranial volume without raising the ICP).[62] Brain tissue pressure and ICP increase with each cardiac cycle and, thus, the ICP waveform is a modified arterial pressure wave (see Figure 16.13). The cardiac waves reach the cranial circulation via the choroid plexus and resemble the waveforms transmitted by arterial catheters, although the amplitude is lower.

There are three distinct peaks seen in the ICP waveform:[63]

- P1, the percussion wave, which is sharp and reflects the cardiac pulse as the pressure is transmitted from the choroid plexus to the ventricle

- P2, the tidal wave, which is more variable in nature and reflects cerebral compliance and increases in amplitude as compliance decreases

- P3, which is due to the closure of the aortic valve and is known as the dicrotic notch. Of recent importance is that the elevation of P3 may indicate low global cerebral perfusion.[64]

It is important that the waveform be continuously observed, as changes in mean pressure or in waveform shape usually require immediate attention. In acute states such as head injury and subarachnoid haemorrhage, the value of ICP depends greatly on the link between monitoring and therapy, so close inspection of the trend in the ICP and the details derived from the waveform is extremely important. Simple ongoing visual assessment of the ICP waveform for increased amplitude, elevated P2 and rounding of the waveform provides non-specific information suggestive of decreased intracranial adaptive capacity and altered intracranial dynamics.[65]

Assessment of cerebral perfusion

CPP is calculated as the mean arterial pressure minus the ICP and represents the pressure gradient across the vessel that drives CBF:

$$CPP = MAP - ICP$$

CPP is a pressure-based indicator of oxygen and metabolite delivery. There is no evidence for the optimum level of CPP, but 70–80 mmHg is probably the critical

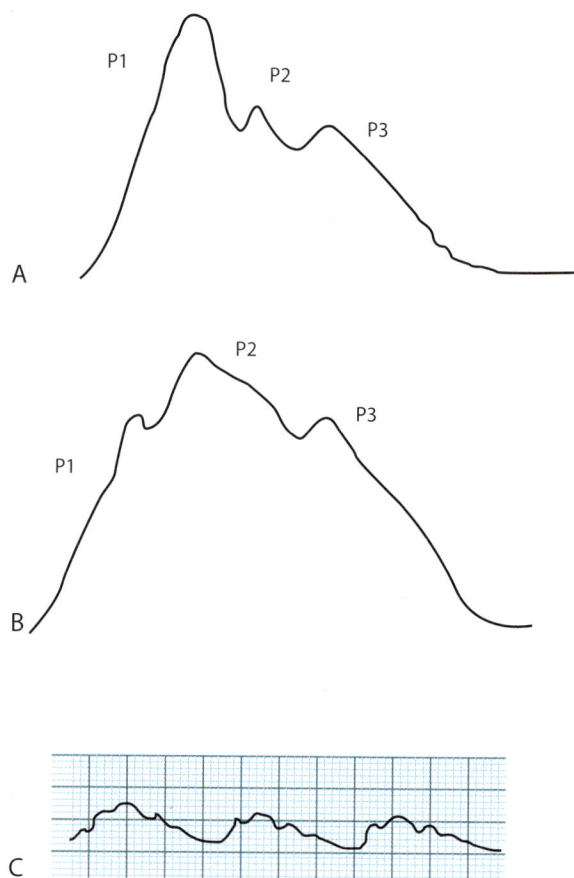

FIGURE 16.13   The intracranial pressure waveforms. **A** Depicts the situation of a compliant system; **B** a high pressure wave recorded from a non-compliant system in which P2 exceeds the level of the P1 waveform, due to a marked decrease in cerebral compliance. The lower tracing **C** is an example of an ICP waveform from a patient monitoring system in which can be identified the three distinct components, as indicated in the text.

threshold in adults, especially those who are pressure-active (i.e. ICP varies inversely with mean arterial pressure [MAP]).[63] Higher CPP has been associated with increased lung water and acute respiratory distress syndrome. Furthermore, mortality rises approximately 20% for each 10 mmHg loss of CPP. In those studies where CPP was maintained above 70 mmHg, the reduction in mortality was as much as 35% for those with severe head injury.[66] The Brain Trauma Foundation recommends a CPP goal of 50–70 mmHg despite the lack of definitive data, such as from randomised controlled trials and intention-to-treat clinical trials.[67] In the paediatric population a CPP >40 mmHg is the recommended guideline.[68,69] Utilising cerebral oxygenation monitoring in combination with pressure has been associated with better outcomes for brain-injured patients, and is part of the multimodal assessment for brain injury.

Assessment of cerebral oxygenation

The three main factors determining cerebral oxygenation are cerebral blood flow, arterial oxygen content and cerebral metabolic rate of oxygen consumption. In clinical practice monitoring of arterial blood gas tensions is routine in most critically ill patients. Measurement of cerebral metabolic rate of oxygen consumption is not commonplace as it is technically difficult and cumbersome. Therefore, the predominant monitoring strategy in clinical practice has relied on measurements of cerebral blood flow and its surrogates. This section will outline those modalities.

Jugular venous oximetry

Jugular venous catheterisation is used for deriving oxygen-based variables.[70] It facilitates the assessment of jugular venous oxygenation ($SjvO_2$), cerebral oxygen extraction (CEO_2) and arteriovenous difference in oxygen ($AVDO_2$). All of these variables indicate changes in cerebral metabolism and blood flow, and therefore the catheter generates continuous data that reflect the balance between supply and demand of cerebral oxygen.

The catheter is inserted in the right jugular vein, as it is slightly larger than the left and provides readings that are more representative of overall brain function. The catheter tip is advanced so that the tip sits in the bulb of the internal jugular vein.

The normal requirement for cerebral oxygen delivery is consumption at 35–40% of available oxygen, giving a normal SjvO2 of 60–65%. Changes in $SjvO_2$ reflect changes in cerebral metabolic rate and cerebral blood flow; however, as it is a global measure, it does not detect regional ischaemia. A high $SjvO_2$ is indicative of increased cerebral blood flow, reduced oxygen consumption and hyperventilation. Low $SjvO_2$ levels suggest that cerebral perfusion is reduced, with levels below 40% indicative of global cerebral ischaemia.[71] However, caution must be used when interpreting values generated using this method, as high values might also imply an increase in arteriovenous shunting secondary to vasoconstriction, maldistribution of blood flow or lack of oxygen consumption as in brain death. Because $SjvO_2$ monitoring is a global measure of cerebral oxygenation,[72] smaller areas of ischaemia are not detected unless these are of sufficient magnitude to affect global brain saturation. $SjvO_2$ requires special care such as frequent recalibration to ensure accurate measurements, observing for catheter migration that interferes with signal quality and, often, medical intervention to reposition the catheter. The position of the patient also affects signal quality and, ideally, the patient should be nursed supine with a head elevation of 10–15° and at least a neutral head alignment. It is important that measurement errors be excluded when abnormal readings are noted; algorithms have been developed to assist nurses when caring for patients with jugular bulb oximetry.[73]

Partial brain tissue oxygenation monitoring

Changes in ICP values alone do not accurately depict poor cerebral blood flow or oxygenation deficits to brain tissue.

Consequently, brain tissue hypoxaemia is often observed during the first 24 hours after injury despite controlled brain pressures. Monitoring partial pressure of oxygen in brain tissue ($PbtO_2$) can be used to collect more accurate and timely information about cerebral oxygen delivery and demand than ICP allows.[74] A tissue oxygen value of less than 10 mmHg for more than 10 minutes carries a higher risk of death. Normal brain oxygen levels ($PbtO_2$ between 20 and 25 mmHg) emerge as a critical determinant of outcome, with values below 20 mmHg carrying a higher risk of poor outcomes.[71]

Regardless of ICP, brain tissue oxygenation falls with a decrease in cerebral blood flow below an ischaemic threshold of 18 mL/100 g/min. ICP may respond to the changes but often several hours later when the damage cannot be reversed. Alterations in cerebral metabolic rate can also change tissue oxygen levels. Reducing the patient's energy consumption via reduced noise and/or distractions, and increasing their protein caloric intake to complement their increased stress state, can improve tissue oxygenation.[73]

Microdialysis

Cerebral microdialysis (using a catheter ideally placed in the frontal lobe) is a tool for investigating the metabolic status of the injured brain and is part of multimodal monitoring. The microdialysis probe is inserted into the cerebral tissue where substances in the extracellular fluid surround the semipermeable membrane at the tip of the catheter. Following equilibration of the tissue metabolites with the perfusion fluid, the dialysate can be analysed for concentrations of products of energy metabolism (glucose, lactate, pyruvate) as indicators of hypoxia and ischaemia. In addition, interstitial glycerol can be determined, which is a parameter of lipolysis and/or cell membrane damage. In theory, the microdialysis catheter acts like a blood capillary.[75] Thereby, it is proposed that microdialysis provides information regarding events that take place in the tissue before any chemical events are reflected by changes in systemic blood levels of indicator substances.[76] These molecules diffuse across the membrane part of the catheter and equilibrate with the perfusion fluid, which is pumped through the probe at very low rates of flow. Changes in the concentration of a substrate in the surrounding milieu are reflected by subsequent changes in the dialysate.[77] Rather than inserting an instrument into the tissue, microdialysate is extracted and later analysed in the laboratory or clinically at the patient's bedside.

Non-invasive assessment

Most of the invasive methods of measuring cerebral blood flow and oxygenation can be associated with complications. Because of this, many patients with low- or moderate-grade TBI are not monitored. Patients benefit from noninvasive means of detecting episodes of cerebral hypoxia and ischaemia that could lead to poor outcomes, and these are detailed in the following section.

Transcranial Doppler

Transcranial Doppler (TCD) ultrasound has proved to be a safe, reliable and relatively inexpensive technology for measuring cerebrovascular blood velocities and evaluating cerebral circulation and haemodynamics. Pulses of ultrasound are directed using a handheld transducer towards the vascular formations in the base of the skull. Velocities from the cerebral arteries, the internal carotids, the basilar and the vertebral arteries can be sampled by altering the transducer location, angle and the instrument's depth setting. The commonest windows in the cranium are located in the orbit (of the eye) and in the temporal and suboccipital regions. TCD measures systolic, diastolic and mean middle cerebral artery (MCA) flow velocities and a derived value, the pulsatility index (PI). Changes in the PI can be used to identify the threshold of autoregulation or cerebral perfusion pressure break point in individual patients. In subarachnoid haemorrhage (SAH) and TBI this may be due to vasospasm or impaired autoregulation or abnormal intracranial compliance. TCD is a simple, portable and non-invasive tool, well suited to serial monitoring, that can be used at the bedside to detect relative changes in CBF in brain-injured patients.[78]

Continuous electroencephalography

Electroencephalography (EEG) is the recording by sensors along the scalp of electrical activity produced by the firing of neurons within the brain. Continuous EEG (cEEG) has the advantage of being continuous and noninvasive and carries the potential to detect alterations in brain physiology at a reversible stage, which may trigger treatment before permanent brain injury occurs. The invention of digital EEG has made cEEG monitoring feasible for ICU patients.[79] Currently, the main applications of cEEG are diagnosing non-convulsive status epilepticus, monitoring and guiding the treatment of status epilepticus and detecting delayed cerebral ischaemia from vasospasm in subarachnoid haemorrhage patients. Other applications may include monitoring of reperfusion after tissue plasminogen activator administration in acute stroke patients and detection of intracranial hypertension. Clinically unrecognised electrographic seizures and periodic epileptiform discharges have been shown to be frequent and associated with poor outcome in patients with severe brain injury from different aetiologies, including TBI, ischaemic and haemorrhagic strokes and CNS infection.[80]

The EEG becomes substantially abnormal (suppressed) when cerebral blood flow declines to 20–30 mL/100 g/min. More subtle abnormalities accompany lesser degrees of hypoperfusion, including initial loss of beta activity, slowing to the theta range and then to the delta range. Irreversible injury to brain tissue occurs at cerebral flows of about 10–12 mL/100 g/min. Thus, EEG sensitivity to ischaemia allows its use in situations where cerebral perfusion is at risk.[81] Changes over time in these quantitative EEG (qEEG) parameters can trigger remote reading, focused neurological examination, imaging studies and early treatment. Subtle EEG changes may be difficult to interpret in isolation, but may be better understood when interpreted in concert with other components of a multimodality monitoring paradigm, which may include microdialysis, brain tissue oxygen and cerebral perfusion pressure.

Near-infrared spectroscopy

Near-infrared spectroscopy (NIRS) is a non-invasive method of monitoring continuous trends of cerebral oxygenated and deoxygenated haemoglobin by utilising an infrared light beam transmitted through the skull. Oxygenated and deoxygenated haemoglobin moieties have different absorption spectra, and cerebral oxygenation and haemodynamic status can be determined by their relative absorption of near-infrared light. NIRS allows interrogation of the cerebral cortex using reflectance spectroscopy via optodes, light transmitting and detecting devices, placed on the scalp. Normal saturation is 70%. Because NIRS interrogates arterial, venous and capillary blood within the field of view, the derived saturation represents regional tissue oxygenation (rSO_2) measured from these three compartments and can be used to identify tissue hypoxia and ischaemia in the brain cortex.

The clinical and bedside use of NIRS is constrained by potential sources of error, which include contamination of the signal by the extracerebral circulation (such as in the scalp), extraneous light and the presence of extravascular blood arising from subarachnoid or subdural haemorrhage.[82] In a recent study in patients with subarachnoid haemorrhage, episodes of angiographic cerebral vasospasm were strongly associated with reduction in trend in the ipsilateral NIRS signal.[83] Furthermore, the degree of spasm (especially more than 75% vessel diameter reduction) was associated with a greater reduction in same-side NIRS signal, demonstrating real-time detection of intracerebral ischaemia.

Summary

This chapter provides an overview of anatomy and physiology in the context of and as applied to neurological assessment of the critically ill. Priorities of clinical assessment are described. Imaging techniques and assessment incorporate the therapeutics of intracranial pressure, cerebral perfusion pressure and partial brain tissue oxygenation monitoring, cEEG, transcranial Doppler and cerebral perfusion imaging. The research vignette reports a systematic review and meta-analysis of the effectiveness of hypertonic saline in reducing intracranial pressure. The clinical case demonstrates neurological assessment priorities in an unstable, traumatic brain injury patient. Clinical, non-invasive and invasive assessment techniques are described within the context of this patient's care.

Case study

On the 26th April a 68-year-old male, Jonathan, was on the roof of his house cleaning the leaves from the gutters. He was found some time later by his wife unconscious, lying on his back on the ground. She immediately called ambulance emergency services. At the scene Jonathan was conscious with a GCS of 13. He was verbally repetitive with diminished orientation to time and place. His pupils were 3 mm in diameter and were equal and reacting to light. An occipital scalp haemotoma and contusion was noted. His lung air entry was equal with diminished rise and fall of the chest. No obvious motor, neural, abdominal or thorax injures were seen.

Intravenous access was obtained and ondansetron 4 mg administered. Oxygen 8 L via a Hudson mask was administered and Jonathan was transferred to the nearest trauma tertiary centre by helicopter.

EMERGENCY DEPARTMENT

The transport team arrived 30 minutes later to the emergency department (ED) and bypassed triage. Jonathan was admitted to the resuscitation area where the trauma team conducted primary and secondary surveys. On presentation, Jonathan's vital signs were: heart rate 68 beats/min, respirations 16 breaths/min, blood pressure 166/78 mmHg, SpO$_2$ 97%, temperature 35.3°C, GCS 13.

Primary survey

Jonathon's primary survey revealed the following details.

- Airway: upper airway cleared. Cervical spine: status unknown, Philadelphia collar in situ.
- Breathing: spontaneously breathing on 6 L/min at 20 breaths/min, equal air entry, decreased bilaterally, no tracheal deviation.
- Circulation: brief episodes of bradycardia, hypertensive and normovolaemic; pulses present on palpation, temperature centrally warm, well perfused, skin pink in colour, peripherally cold and pale; capillary refill >4 seconds.
- Disability: he was alert but agitated and confused, GCS 13; pupils equal and reactive, size 4 mm. Mobile trauma series performed – chest and pelvis X-ray.

Secondary survey

The secondary survey revealed the following details.

- Head: large posterior occipital haemotoma present. CT revealed extensive acute subdural and subarachnoid haemorrhages with an occipital communicated fracture and basilar skull fracture into the carotid canal. Basal cisterns were moderately effaced.
- Face: no oedema, rhinorrhoea or otorrhoea.
- Neck: Philadelphia neck collar left in situ; no obvious lacerations observed around neck area; no evidence of tracheal deviation. Cervical spine CT reported no bony injury, spine not cleared.
- Chest: abdomen – firm, no abnormal distension. IDC insertion revealed haematuria.
- Pelvis: bruising bilaterally with no obvious deformity.
- Back: marked flank bruising, no lacerations, right perinephric haemotoma on CT; rectal tone present.
- Upper limbs: X-ray revealed right radial and ulna fractures, lacerations and bruising present; pulses present.
- Lower limbs: all pulses present, no obvious injuries present.

EMERGENCY SURGERY

Jonathan's GCS decreased to 9 and he was electively intubated. A repeat CT brain scan was performed and revealed an extension of the left-sided subdural haemorrhage and a new left frontal haemotoma.

Jonathan was transferred to operating theatre within 30 minutes for a craniectomy and evacuation of the acute subdural and frontal haemorrhages and insertion of an external ventricular drain (EVD). The EVD insertion was unsuccessful and left as a subdural monitor. A Jackson Pratt drain was inserted and intraoperatively drained 500 mL.

Following surgery, he was admitted to the intensive care unit (ICU) for further management (Table 16.10).

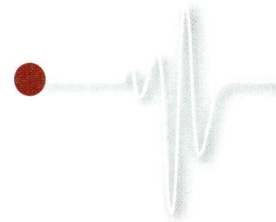

TABLE 16.10

Overview of Jonathan's clinical parameters and assessment, days 1–6

	DAY OF ADMISSION					
PARAMETER	1	2	3	4	5	6
Pupils (mm)						
Right	3+	2S	2S	3+	3+	3+
Left	3+	2S	2S	3+	3+	3+
GCS	3 T (E1V1(T)M1)	3 T (E1V1(T)M1)	3 T (E1V1(T)M1)	3 T (E1V1(T)M1)	4 T (E2V1(T)M1)	5 T (E2V1(T)M3)
CSF drainage (mL/24 h)	Nil	26	38	30	25	18*
ICP range (mmHg)	6–25	9–21	16–25	12–26	12–22	11–18
Sedation infusion	Morphine/ midazolam	Fentanyl/ midazolam	Fentanyl/ midazolam Propofol	Fentanyl/ midazolam Propofol	Fentanyl/ midazolam Propofol	Fentanyl/ midazolam Propofol
Paralysing agent	Vecuronium intermittent	Vecuronium intermittent	Vecuronium intermittent	Vecuronium intermittent	Vecuronium intermittent	
Noradrenaline (mcg/min)	5–18	5–20	2–13	3–10	3–6	Nil
Heart rate range (bpm)	60–108	58–80	57–88	58–95	60–90	58–88
MAP range (mmHg)	65–100	75–92	72–88	85–98	85–98	78–92
CPP range (mmHg)	59–92	64–79	61–72	60–78	62–81	63–90*

CPP = cerebral perfusion pressure; CSF = cerebrospinal fluid; E = eye opening; GCS = Glasgow Coma Scale; ICP = intracranial pressure; M = motor; MAP = mean arterial pressure; V = verbal; (T) = intubated; * = ICP external ventricular drain removed.

ICU MANAGEMENT

Day 1

On arrival to the ICU, Jonathan's condition was critical. His vital signs were: heart rate 115 beats/min; intubated and mechanically ventilated at 22 breaths/min, Vt 500 mL, FiO_2 0.4, PEEP 8 cmH_2O; blood pressure 132/85 mmHg (MAP 100) with noradrenaline support for a CPP of 65; SaO_2 98%; temperature 37.5°C; pupils 3/3 mm (R/L), sluggish sequential reaction. He was heavily sedated and unresponsive with a Glasgow Coma Score (GCS) of 3T (eye opening 1, verbal 1 [T = intubated], motor 1). His subdural monitor displayed a surrogate ICP of 8 mmHg. He required paralysis with intermittent boluses of vecuronium and with the need for increasing levels of sedation, noradrenaline and hypertonic saline bolus to control his ICP and CPP. Normal saline was infused for maintenance fluid. Pain stimulation for neurological assessment under these conditions was only performed during endotracheal suction.

Days 2–7

Jonathan's clinical parameters and assessment are depicted in Table 16.10. His condition remained variable and on day 2 he returned to the operating theatre for insertion of an intraventricular catheter and external ventricular drainage system. His ICP and CPP were unstable with increasing need for sedation and intermittent paralysis. Bolus doses of hypertonic saline were administered and increased drainage from the EVD (38 mL in 24 hours) was noted. Jonathan's serum sodium levels elevated to hypernatraemic state with a sodium (Na^+) range of 144–154 mmol/L (normal range is 136–144 mmol/L). He was administered free water boluses of 300 mL by orogastric tube.

A repeat CT determined no significant change. The ventricles were effaced but not compressed. After stabilising on day 5, Jonathan's noradrenaline and sedation infusions were reduced for neurological assessment. His GCS was 5 (E2, V1[T], M3) with normal flexion to pain and remained unchanged up until day 7. Despite an increased GCS it was difficult to assess his verbal response while intubated. The EVD was removed on day 6 and he remained sedated and ventilated. Jonathan continued to slowly recover.

CASE STUDY QUESTIONS

1 Indicate whether the following factors increase or decrease cerebral blood flow: a) $PaCO_2$ of 30 mmHg; b) PaO_2 of 45 mmHg; c) decreased MAP; d) increased ICP; e) arterial blood pH of 7.
2 Explain the physiological mechanism for dilated (size 5), non-reactive pupils.

RESEARCH VIGNETTE

Lazaridis C, Neyens R, Bodle J, DeSantis S. High-osmolarity saline in neurocritical care: systematic review and meta-analysis. Crit Care Med 2013;41(5):1353–60

Abstract

Background and purpose: Intracranial hypertension and cerebral edema are known contributors to secondary brain injury and to poor neurologic outcomes. Small volume solutions of exceedingly high osmolarity, such as 23.4% saline, have been used for the management of intracranial hypertension crises and as a measure to prevent or reverse acute brain tissue shifts. We conducted a systematic literature review on the use of 23.4% saline in neurocritically ill patients and a meta-analysis of the effect of 23.4% saline on intracranial pressure reduction.

Design: We searched computerized databases, reference lists, and personal files to identify all clinical studies in which 23.4% saline has been used for the treatment of neurocritical care patients. Studies that did not directly involve either effects on cerebral hemodynamics or the treatment of patients with clinical or radiographic evidence of intracranial hypertension and/or cerebral swelling were eliminated.

Measurements and main results: We identified 11 clinical studies meeting eligibility criteria. A meta-analysis was performed to evaluate the percent decrease in intracranial pressure and the 95% confidence intervals, from baseline to 60 minutes or nadir from the six studies from which this information could be extracted. A fixed effects meta-analysis estimated that the percent decrease in intracranial pressure from baseline to either 60 minutes or nadir after administration of 23.4% saline was 55.6% (se 5.90; 95% confidence interval, 43.99–67.12; $p < 0.0001$).

Conclusions: Highly concentrated hypertonic saline such as 23.4% provides a small volume solution with low cost and an over 50% reduction effect on raised intracranial pressure. Side effects reported are minor overall in view of the potentially catastrophic event that is being treated. High quality data are still needed to define the most appropriate osmotherapeutic agent, the optimal dose, the safest and most effective mode of administration and to further elucidate the mechanism of action of 23.4% saline and of osmotherapy in general.

Critique

This review found that, across a broad range of acute brain injury syndromes, ICP reduction was greater with hypertonic saline (HTS) 23.4% compared with mannitol (in most instances), at 60 minutes or nadir. While 11 studies were included in the systematic review, only six were used in the meta-analysis. Meta-analysis should only be used if studies are similar in terms of interventions and outcomes, thus it seemed reasonable to not include all studies. However, the authors do acknowledge that some of the studies they did include in the meta-analysis had differing interventions in terms of dosing of the saline. This fact may make the results less meaningful. Prior to undertaking a meta-analysis, it is important to assess the extent to which studies are similar (i.e. homogeneous), to determining if it is reasonable to pool the data from these studies. If studies are very different, then pooling the data is not appropriate. There are several statistical tests to determine the extent to which studies are 'heterogeneous', but the one used in this study (Cochran's Q) has several limitations. Given the small number of studies there may have been a more appropriate test, such as the I^2 statistic. In terms of the systematic review process, there was no a priori research question published on a publicly accessible website such as PROSPERO (http://www.crd.york.ac.uk/PROSPERO/), usually in the form of a protocol. Grey literature was not included in the search strategy, accounting for the lack of inaccessible papers, a general fault in the systematic process. The flow sheet did not conform to the Preferred Reporting Items for Systematic Reviews and Meta-Analyses (see http://www.prisma-statement.org) guidance for systematic reviews, and there was absence of a measure of trial quality for each study. In regard to the studies' findings, improvements in ICP percent decrease outcome did not always lead to improvements in patient-oriented outcomes such as symptoms, morbidity, quality of life or mortality. Further, in many of the studies, equimolar hypertonic comparison was not made, making a reliable conclusion about the efficacy of HTS difficult. However, the results were encouraging for HTS. ICP reduction was greatest with HTS, and there were limited but encouraging serious adverse event data.

Learning activities

The first three activities refer to the research vignette.

1   What are the theoretical side effects and complications associated with hypertonic saline therapy administration?

2   Discuss the physiological effects of how hypertonic 23.4% saline reduces ICP.

3   What effect would decreasing the concentration of extracellular potassium ions have on the transmembrane potential of a neuron?

4   Which brain structure coordinates endocrine and nervous system activities?

5   Which component of the brain controls the cardiac centres, the vasomotor centres and the respiratory rhythm centre?

6   What information does the GCS provide? What does the GCS predict?

7   During the testing of motor response a noxious stimulus is applied to the nail bed of the middle finger. The unconscious patient elicits a flexion withdrawal response of the wrist, arm and shoulder. Explain what this response means in terms of central or peripheral response.

8   What is the pathophysiological basis for the rise in ICP? How would this manifest on the ICP waveform?

9   A patient recovering from a subarachnoid haemorrhage cannot remember events prior to the haemorrhage event. What type of amnesia is this?

Online resources

Adult Neurological Observation Chart: Education Package, www.aci.health.nsw.gov.au/__data/assets/pdf_file/0018/201753/AdultChartEdPackage.pdf

American Association of Neuroscience Nurses (AANN), www.aann.org

Australasian Neuroscience Nurses' Association, www.anna.asn.au

Brain Explorer, www.brainexplorer.org

Brain Injury Association of America, www.biausa.org

FOUR score for Neuro Assessments, http://w3.rn.com/News/clinical_insights_details.aspx?Id=29828

GCS Part 1, www.youtube.com/watch?v=T93Ah9ZkurI&feature=player_detailpage

GCS Part 2, www.youtube.com/watch?v=_jTTPjZ_ruE&feature=player_detailpage

Neurocritical Care Society, www.neurocriticalcare.org

Neurological Exam, www.neuroexam.com/neuroexam

Neurological Foundation of New Zealand, www.neurological.org.nz

Neuroscience tutorials, http://thalamus.wustl.edu/course

Official Journal of the American Academy of Neurology (AAN), http://neurology.org

Physical Examination and Neurological Assessment, www.neurologyexam.com

Post-traumatic amnesia protocol, www.psy.mq.edu.au/pta

Rural Neurotrauma Assessment, www.racs.edu.au/media/16138/PUB_090824_-_Neurotrauma_(Standard_Version).pdf

Society for Neuroscience, http://web.sfn.org

The Brain Trauma Foundation, www.braintrauma.org

World Health Organization Neurotrauma, www.who.int/violence_injury_prevention/road_traffic/activities/neurotrauma/en

Further reading

Allen BB, Chiu YL, Gerber LM, Ghajar J, Greenfield JP. Age-specific cerebral perfusion pressure thresholds and survival in children and adolescents with severe traumatic brain injury. Pediatr Crit Care Med 2014;15(1):62–70.

Crossley S, Reid J, McLatchie R, Hayton J, Clark C, MacDougall M et al. A systematic review of therapeutic hypothermia for adult patients following traumatic brain injury. Crit Care 2014;18(2):R75.

Kumar R, Singhi S, Singhi P, Jayashree M, Bansal A, Bhatti A. Randomized controlled trial comparing cerebral perfusion pressure-targeted therapy versus intracranial pressure-targeted therapy for raised intracranial pressure due to acute CNS infections in children. Crit Care Med 2014;42(8):1775–87.

Lazaridis C, Neyens R, Bodle J, Desantis SM. High-osmolarity saline in neurocritical care: systematic review and meta-analysis. Crit Care Med 2013;41(5):1353–60.

Le Roux P, Menon D, Citerio G, Vespa P, Bader M, Brophy G et al. Consensus summary statement of the International Multidisciplinary Consensus Conference on Multimodality Monitoring in Neurocritical Care. Intensive Care Med 2014; 40(9):1189–209.

Manno EM. Update on intracerebral hemorrhage. CONTINUUM Lifelong Learning in Neurology 2012;18(3):598–610.

Sharshar T, Citerio G, Andrews PD, Chieregato A, Latronico N, Menon D et al. Neurological examination of critically ill patients: a pragmatic approach. Report of an ESICM expert panel. Intensive Care Med 2014;40(4):484–95.

References

1 Martini F, Nath J, Bartholomew E. Anatomy and physiology. 9th ed. San Francisco: Pearson Benjamin Cummings; 2011.

2 Guyton A, Hall J. Textbook of medical physiology. 12th ed. Philadelphia: Elsevier Saunders; 2010.

3 Porth C. Pathophysiology concepts of altered health states. 9th ed. Philadelphia: Lippincott, Williams & Wilkins; 2013.

4 Perlson E, Maday S, Fu MM, Moughamian AJ, Holzbaur EL. Retrograde axonal transport: pathways to cell death? Trends Neuroscience 2010; 33(7):335–44.

5 Purves D, Augustine G, Hall W, LaMantia A, McNamara J, White L. Neuroscience. 5th ed. New York: Sinauer Associates; 2012.

6 Byku M, Macarthur H, Westfall TC. Inhibitory effects of angiotensin-(1–7) on the nerve stimulation-induced release of norepinephrine and neuropeptide Y from the mesenteric arterial bed. Am J Physiol Heart Circ Physiol 2010;298(2):457–65.

7 Rosas-Ballina M, Tracey KJ. Cholinergic control of inflammation. J Intern Med 2009;265(6):663–79.

8 Parkhurst C, Gan W. Microglia dynamics and function in the CNS. Curr Opin Neurobiol 2010;20(4):474–80.

9 Graeber MB, Streit WJ. Microglia: biology and pathology. Acta Neuropathol 2010;119(1):89–105.

10 Dziedzic T, Metz I, Dallenga T, König FB, Müller S, Stadelmann C et al. Wallerian degeneration: a major component of early axonal pathology in multiple sclerosis. Brain Pathol 2010;20(5):976–85.

11 Hoffman-Kim D, Mitchel JA, Bellamkonda RV. Topography, cell response, and nerve regeneration. Annu Rev Biomed Eng 2010;15(12):203–31.

12 Tavor I, Yablonski M, Mezer A, Rom S, Assaf Y, Yovel G. Separate parts of occipito-temporal white matter fibers are associated with recognition of faces and places. Neuroimage 2014;86:123-30.

13 Willems RM, Toni I, Hagoort P, Casasanto D. Neural dissociations between action verb understanding and motor imagery. J Cogn Neurosci 2010;22(10):2387–400.

14 Guillery RW. Anatomical pathways that link perception and action. Prog Brain Res 2005;149(28):235–56.

15 Blumenfeld H. Neuroanatomy through clinical cases. New York: Sinauer Associates; 2010.

16 Elliott D, Khan MA. Vision and goal-directed movement: neurobehavioral perspectives. Champaign, IL: Human Kinetics; 2010.

17 Szymusiak R. Hypothalamic versus neocortical control of sleep. Curr Opin Pulm Med 2010;16(6):530–35.

18 Bostan AC, Strick PL. The cerebellum and basal ganglia are interconnected. Neuropsychol Rev 2010;20(3):261–70.

19 Strominger N, Demarest R, Laemle L. Brainstem: medulla, pons, and midbrain. In: Noback's human nervous system. 7th ed. New York: Humana Press; 2012, pp 217-238.

20 Ley S, Weigert A, Brüne B. Neuromediators in inflammation – a macrophage/nerve connection. Immunobiology 2010;215(9–10):674–84.

21 Veening JG, Barendregt HP. The regulation of brain states by neuroactive substances distributed via the cerebrospinal fluid; a review. Cerebrospinal Fluid Res 2010;6(7):1.

22 Abbott NJ, Patabendige AA, Dolman DE, Yusof SR, Begley DJ. Structure and function of the blood–brain barrier. Neurobiol Dis 2010;37(1):13–25.

23 Urden L, Stacy K, Lough M. Thelan's critical care nursing, diagnosis and management. 7th ed. Philadelphia: Mosby Elsevier; 2014.

24 Varma AK, Das A, Wallace IV G, Barry J, Vertegel AA, Ray SK et al. Spinal cord injury: a review of current therapy, future treatments, and basic science frontiers. Neurochem Res 2013;38(5):895-905.

25 Cohen B, Taylor J. Memmler's human body in health and disease. 12th ed. Philadelphia: Lippincott, Williams & Wilkins; 2012.

26 Deakin CD, Nolan JP, Soar J, Sunde K, Koster RW, Smith GB et al. European Resuscitation Council Guidelines for Resuscitation 2010. Section 4. Adult advanced life support. Resuscitation 2010;81(10):1305–52.

27 Teasdale G, Jennett B. Assessment of coma and impaired consciousness. A practical scale. Lancet 1974;2(7872):81–4.

28 Johnson VD, Whitcomb J. Neuro/trauma intensive care unit nurses' perception of the use of the full outline of unresponsiveness score versus the Glasgow Coma Scale when assessing the neurological status of intensive care unit patients. Dimens Crit Care Nurs 2013;32(4):180-3.

29 Chen B, Grothe C, Schaller K. Validation of a new neurological score (FOUR score) in the assessment of neurosurgical patients with severely impaired consciousness. Acta Neurochir 2013;155(11):2133-9.

30 Zuercher M, Ummenhofer W, Baltussen A, Walder B. The use of Glasgow Coma Scale in injury assessment: a critical review. Brain Injury 2009;23(5):371–84.

31 Oddo M, Villa F, Citerio G. Brain multimodality monitoring: an update. Curr Opin Crit Care 2012;18(2):111-8.

32 Jevon P. Neurological assessment part 2 – pupillary assessment. Nurs Times 2008;104(28):26–7.

33 Bajekal R. Eye signs in anaesthesia and intensive care medicine. Anaesthes Intens Care Med 2014;15(1):37-9.

34 Kung W, Tsai S, Chiu W, Hung K, Wang SP, Lin JW et al. Correlation between Glasgow Coma Score components and survival in patients with traumatic brain injury. Injury 2011;42 (9):940-4.

35 Healey C, Osler TM, Rogers FB, Healey MA, Glance LG, Kilgo PD et al. Improving the Glasgow Coma Scale score: motor score alone is a better predictor. J Trauma 2003;54(4):671–8.

36 Seel RT, Sherer M, Whyte J, Katz DI, Giacino JT, Rosenbaum AM et al. Assessment scales for disorders of consciousness: evidence-based recommendations for clinical practice and research. Arch Phys Med Rehabil 2010;91(12):1795–813.

37 Pullen RL Jr. Testing the corneal reflex. Nursing 2005;35(11):68.

38 Lang IM. Brain stem control of the phases of swallowing. Dysphagia 2009;24(3):333–48.

39 Widdicombe JG, Addington WR. Cough in patients after stroke. Eur Respir J 2011;37(1):218.

40 Kosch Y, Browne S, King C, Fitzgerald J, Cameron I. Post-traumatic amnesia and its relationship to the functional outcome of people with severe traumatic brain injury. Brain Injury 2010;24(3):479–85.

41 Tate RL, Pfaff A, Baguley IJ, Marosszeky JE, Gurka JA, Hodgkinson AE et al. A multicentre, randomised trial examining the effect of test procedures measuring emergence from post-traumatic amnesia. J Neurol Neurosurg Psych 2006;77:841–9.

42 Sherer M, Struchen MA, Yablon SA, Wang Y, Nick TG. Comparison of indices of traumatic brain injury severity: Glasgow Coma Scale, length of coma and post-traumatic amnesia. J Neurol Neurosurg Psych 2008;79(6):678–85.

43 Marshman L, Jakabek D, Hennessy M, Quirk F, Guazzo EP. Post-traumatic amnesia. J Clin Neurosci 2013;20(11):1475-81.

44 Formisano R, Carlesimo GA, Sabbadini M, Loasses A, Penta F, Vinicola V et al. Clinical predictors and neuropsychological outcome in severe traumatic brain injury patients. Acta Neurochir 2004;146(5):457–62.

45 Chestnut RM, Marshall SB, Piek J, Blunt BA, Klauber MR, Marshall LF. Early and late systemic hypotension as a frequent and fundamental source of cerebral ischemia following severe brain injury in the Traumatic Coma Data Bank. Acta Neurochir (Wien) 1993;59(Suppl):121–5.

46 Bhatia A, Gupta AK. Neuromonitoring in the intensive care unit. I. Intracranial pressure and cerebral blood flow monitoring. Intensive Care Med 2007;33(7):1263–71.

47 Bremmer R, De Jong BM, Wagemakers M, Regtien JG, Van Der Naalt J. The course of intracranial pressure in traumatic brain injury: relation with outcome and CT-characteristics. Neurocritical Care 2010;12(3):362–8.

48 Downer JJ, Pretorius PM. Symmetry in computed tomography of the brain: the pitfalls. Clin Radiol 2009;64(3):298–306.

49 Hillary FG, Biswal BB. Automated detection and quantification of brain lesions in acute traumatic brain injury using MRI. Brain Imaging Behavior 2009;3(2):111–22.

50 Mannion RJ, Cross J, Bradley P, Coles JP, Chatfield D, Carpenter A et al. Mechanism-based MRI classification of traumatic brainstem injury and its relationship to outcome. J Neurotrauma 2007;24(1):128–35.

51 Leitch JK, Figley CR, Stroman PW. Applying functional MRI to the spinal cord and brainstem. Magn Reson Imaging 2010;28(8):1225–33.

52 Greenberg ED, Gold R, Reichman M, John M, Ivanidze J, Edwards AM et al. Diagnostic accuracy of CT angiography and CT perfusion for cerebral vasospasm: a meta-analysis. Am J Neuroradiol 2010;31(10):1853–60.

53 Vespa PM. Imaging and decision-making in neurocritical care. Neurol Clin 2014;32(1):211-24.

54 Kannan S, Balakrishnan B, Muzik O, Romero R, Chugani D. Positron emission tomography imaging of neuroinflammation. J Child Neurol 2009;24(9):1190–9.

55 Vik A, Nag T, Fredriksli OA, Skandsen T, Moen KG, Schirmer-Mikalsen K et al. Relationship of "dose" of intracranial hypertension to outcome in severe traumatic brain injury. J Neurosurg 2008;109(4):678–84.

56 Koskinen LO, Olivecrona M. Clinical experience with the intraparenchymal intracranial pressure monitoring Codman MicroSensor system. Neurosurgery 2005;56(4):693–8.

57 Harrop JS, Sharan AD, Ratliff J, Prasad S, Jabbour P, Evans JJ et al. Impact of a standardized protocol and antibiotic-impregnated catheters on ventriculostomy infection rates in cerebrovascular patients. Neurosurgery 2010;67(1):187–91.

58 Adelson PD, Bratton SL, Carney NA, Chesnut RM, du Coudray HE, Goldstein B et al. Guidelines for the acute medical management of severe traumatic brain injury in infants, children, and adolescents. Chapter 7, Intracranial pressure monitoring technology. Pediatr Crit Care Med 2003;4(3 Suppl):S28-30.

59 Hoffmann J, Goadsby PJ. Update on intracranial hypertension and hypotension. Curr Opin Neurol 2013;26(3):240-7.

60 Brain Trauma Foundation. Guidelines for the management of severe traumatic brain injury. VIII. Intracranial pressure thresholds. J Neurotrauma 2007;24(Supp 1):S55–8.

61 Tzeng Y, Ainslie P. Blood pressure regulation. IX: Cerebral autoregulation under blood pressure challenges. Eur J Appl Physiol 2014;114(3):545-59.

62 Di Ieva A, Schmitz E, Cusimano M. Analysis of intracranial pressure: past, present, and future. Neuroscientist 2013;19(6):592-603.

63 Kasprowicz M, Asgari S, Bergsneider M, Czosnyka M, Hamilton R, Hu X. Pattern recognition of overnight intracranial pressure slow waves using morphological features of intracranial pressure pulse. J Neurosci Methods 2010;190(2):310–8.

64 Hu X, Glenn T, Scalzo F, Bergsneider M, Sarkiss C, Martin N et al. Intracranial pressure pulse morphological features improved detection of decreased cerebral blood flow. Physiol Meas 2010;31(5):679–95.

65 Howells T, Elf K, Jones PA, Ronne-Engstrom E, Piper I, Nilsson P et al. Pressure reactivity as a guide in the treatment of cerebral perfusion pressure in patients with brain trauma. J Neurosurg 2005;102(2):311–7.

66 Johnston AJ, Steiner LA, Coles JP, Chatfield DA, Fryer TD, Smielewski P et al. Effect of cerebral perfusion pressure augmentation on regional oxygenation and metabolism after head injury. Crit Care Med 2005;33:189–95.

67 Brain Trauma Foundation Guidelines IX. Cerebral perfusion thresholds. J Neurotrauma 2007;24(Supp 1):S59–64.

68 Brain Trauma Foundation Guidelines, Ch 5. Cerebral perfusion pressure thresholds: Guidelines for the acute medical management of severe traumatic brain injury in infants, children, and adolescents. Paediat Crit Care Med 2012;13(1):S1–82.

69 Ragan D, McKinstry R, Benzinger T, Leonard J, Pineda J. Udomphorn Y et al. Alterations in cerebral oxygen metabolism after traumatic brain injury in children. J Cereb Blood Flow Metab 2013;33(1):48-52.

70 Chieregato A, Calzolari F, Trasforini G, Targa L, Latronico N. Normal jugular bulb oxygen saturation. J Neurol Neurosurg Psych 2003;74(6):784–6.

71 Bratton SL, Chestnut RM, Ghajar J, McConnell Hammond FF, Harris OA, Hartl R et al. Guidelines for the management of severe traumatic brain injury. X. Brain oxygen monitoring and thresholds. J Neurotrauma 2007;24(S1):S65–70.

72 Rabinstein AA. Elucidating the value of continuous brain oxygen monitoring. Neurocritical Care 2010;12(1):144–5.

73 Leal-Noval SR, Cayuela A, Arellano-Orden V, Marín-Caballos A, Padilla V, Ferrándiz-Millón C et al. Invasive and noninvasive assessment of cerebral oxygenation in patients with severe traumatic brain injury. Intensive Care Med 2010;36(8):1309–17.

74 Maloney-Wilensky E, Gracias V, Itkin A, Hoffman K, Bloom S, Yang W et al. Brain tissue oxygen and outcome after severe traumatic brain injury: a systematic review. Crit Care Med 2009;37(6):2057–63.

75 Kawai N, Kawakita K, Yano T, Tamiya T, Abe Y, Kuroda Y. Use of intracerebral microdialysis in severe traumatic brain injury. Neurol Surg 2010;38(9):795–809.

76 Chefer VI, Thompson AC, Zapata A, Shippenberg TS. Overview of brain microdialysis. Curr Prot in Neuroscience 2009;7.1.1–7.1.28.

77 Uehara T, Sumiyoshi T, Itoh H, Kurata K. Lactate production and neurotransmitters; evidence from microdialysis studies. Pharm Bio Behav 2008;90(2):273–81.

78 Bouzat, P, Francony G, Fauvage B, Payen J. Transcranial Doppler pulsatility index for initial management of brain-injured patients. Neurosurgery 2010;67(6):E1863–4.

79 White DM, Van Cott AC. EEG artifacts in the intensive care unit setting. Am J Elect Tech 2010;50(1):8–25.

80 Kurtz P, Hanafy KA, Claassen J. Continuous EEG monitoring: is it ready for prime time? Curr Opin Crit Care 2009;15(2):99–109.

81 Guérit J. Neurophysiological testing in neurocritical care. Curr Opin Crit Care 2010;16(2):98–104.

82 Murkin JM, Arango M. Near-infrared spectroscopy as an index of brain and tissue oxygenation. Br J Anaesth 2009;103 (Suppl 1):i3–13.

83 Bhatia R, Hampton T, Malde S, Kandala NB, Muammar M, Deasy N et al The application of near-infrared oximetry to cerebral monitoring during aneurysm embolization: a comparison with intraprocedural angiography. J Neurosurg Anesthesiol 2007;19:97–104.

84 Purves D, Augustine G, Hall W, LaMantia A, McNamara J, White L. Neuroscience. 5th ed. New York: Sinauer Associates; 2012.

Chapter 17

Neurological alterations and management

Diane Chamberlain, Elaine McGloin

Learning objectives

After reading this chapter, you should be able to:

- differentiate cerebral hypoxia from cerebral ischaemia and focal from global ischaemia
- differentiate between primary and secondary brain insults due to brain injury
- relate the procedures of selected neurodiagnostic tests to nursing implications for patient care
- discuss the rationale for medical and nursing management in the care of the brain-injured patient.

Introduction

Numerous conditions encountered in critical care areas relate to serious neurological dysfunction. While most are associated with critical illness, or are at least well defined, several others are very infrequent and not addressed extensively in this chapter. One problem arises in that the onset of an abrupt neurological complication is frequently obscured by the effects of the primary illness. For example, a metabolic disorder producing encephalopathy can delay recognition of an intracerebral haemorrhage, or do so because of its treatment, such as using sedation to allow better synchrony with a mechanical ventilator. Neurological alterations are generally defined by problems that derive from the acute aspects of diseases such as stroke, brain and spinal cord injury and status epilepticus. This chapter discusses the concepts that underlie neurological abnormalities and addresses current management techniques and modalities.

Neurological dysfunction

This section discusses the concepts of neurological dysfunction including altered levels of consciousness, motor and sensory function and cerebral metabolism and perfusion.

Alterations in consciousness

In critical illness, impaired consciousness is often the first sign of a severe pathological process. Consciousness is defined as recognition of self and the environment, which requires both arousal and awareness. Depressed consciousness can range from mild depression to coma, the most severe form of absolute unconsciousness.

Altered cognition and coma

Coma is a state of unresponsiveness from which the patient, who appears to be asleep, cannot be aroused by verbal and physical stimuli to produce any meaningful response. Therefore, the diagnosis of coma implies the absence of both arousal and content of consciousness.[1] Coma must be considered a symptom with numerous causes, different natural modes and several management modes. Stupor is a state of unconsciousness from which the patient can be awakened to produce inadequate responses to verbal and physical stimuli. Somnolence is a state of unconsciousness from which the patient can be fully awakened.

Although there are many specific causes of unconsciousness, the sites of cerebral affection are either the bilateral cerebral cortex or the brainstem reticular activating system. The commonest causes of bilateral cortical disease are deficiencies of oxygen, metabolic disorders, physical injury, toxins, post-convulsive coma and infections.[2] The reticular activating system maintains the state of wakefulness through continuous stimulation of the cortex. Any interruption may lead to unconsciousness. The reticular activating system can be affected in three principal ways: by supratentorial pressure, by infratentorial pressure and by intrinsic brainstem lesions. Supratentorial and infratentorial lesions produce impaired consciousness by enlarging and displacing tissue. Lesions that affect the brainstem itself damage the reticular activating system directly.

> ### Practice tip
>
> The first principle of management of a person found unconscious is to keep the patient alive by maintaining the airway and the circulation.

Recently acquired confusion, severe apathy, stupor or coma implies dysfunction of the cerebral hemispheres, the diencephalon and/or the upper brainstem.[3] Focal lesions in supratentorial structures may damage both hemispheres, or may produce swelling that compresses the diencephalic activating system and midbrain, causing transtentorial herniation and brainstem damage. Primary infratentorial (brainstem or cerebellar) lesions may compress or directly damage the reticular formation anywhere between the level of the mid-pons and (by upward pressure) the diencephalon. Metabolic or infectious diseases may depress brain functions by a change in blood composition or the presence of a direct toxin. Impaired consciousness may also be due to reduced blood flow (as in syncope or severe heart failure) or a change in the brain's electrical activity (as in epilepsy). Concussion, anxiolytic drugs and anaesthetics impair consciousness without producing detectable structural changes in the brain.

Many of the enzymatic reactions of neurons, glial cells and specialised cerebral capillary endothelium in the brain must be catalysed by the energy-yielding hydrolysis of adenosine triphosphate to adenosine diphosphate and inorganic phosphate. Without a constant and generous supply of adenosine triphosphate, cellular synthesis slows or stops, neuronal functions decline or cease, and cell structures quickly fall apart.[4] The use of lactate for oxidative metabolism becomes prominent when extracellular brain lactate concentration increases to supraphysiological levels, inducing a sparing of cerebral glucose. The brain depends entirely on the process of glycolysis and respiration within its own cells to provide its energy needs. Even a short interruption of blood flow, and thereby of the oxygen and glucose supply, threatens tissue vitality.

Seizures

A seizure is an uninhibited, abrupt discharge of ions from a group of neurons resulting in epileptic activity.[5] The majority of patients experiencing seizures in the ICU do not have pre-existing epilepsy, and their chances of developing epilepsy in the future are usually more dependent on the cause than on the number or intensity of seizures that they experience. However, because of the other deleterious neuronal and systemic effects of seizures, their rapid diagnosis and suppression during a period of critical illness is necessary.

Seizures are classified depending on how they start as: 1) partial or focal seizures, 2) generalised or full body seizures involving both cerebral hemispheres or 3) partial seizures with secondary generalisation. Patients may be conscious during a partial seizure whereas during generalised seizures they are not. As partial seizures may not always progress to tonic–clonic movement or alteration in consciousness, partial seizure represents one of the most elusive diagnoses in neurology and is often misdiagnosed. One of the most helpful points in the history of a partial seizure patient is the pre-epileptic event, the aura. The patient will describe the aura as a virtually identical sensation every time.

Seizures may either prompt the patient's admission to ICU (because of status epilepticus) or develop as a complication of another illness.[6] Seizures can be due to vascular, infectious, neoplastic, traumatic, degenerative, metabolic, toxic or idiopathic causes. Factors influencing the development of post-traumatic epilepsy include an early post-traumatic seizure, depressed skull fracture, intracranial haematoma, dural penetration, focal neurological deficit and post-traumatic amnesia over 24 hours with the presence of a skull fracture or haematoma. Seizures in critically ill patients are most commonly due to drug effects; metabolic, infectious or toxic disorders; or intracranial mass lesions, although they may be due to trauma or neoplasm.[7] Conditions producing seizures tend either to increase neuronal excitation or to impair neuronal inhibition. A few generalised disorders (e.g. non-ketotic hyperglycaemia) may produce partial or focal seizures.

Alterations in motor and sensory function

Alterations in motor and sensory function include skeletal muscle weakness and paralysis. They result from lesions in the voluntary motor and sensory pathways, including the upper motor and sensory neurons of the corticospinal and corticobulbar tracts, or the lower motor and sensory neurons that leave the central nervous system (CNS) and travel by way of the peripheral nerves to the muscle and sensory receptors.

Muscle tone, which is a necessary component of muscle movement, is a function of the muscle spindle (myotatic) system and the extrapyramidal system, which monitors and buffers input to the lower motor neurons by way of the multisynaptic pathways.[8] Upper motor neuron lesions produce spastic paralysis, and lower motor neuron lesions produce flaccid paralysis. Damage to the upper motor and sensory neurons of the corticospinal, corticobulbar and spinothalamic tracts is a common component of stroke.[9] Polyneuropathies involve multiple peripheral nerves and produce symmetrical sensory, motor and mixed sensori-motor deficits:

- Lesions of the corticospinal and corticobulbar tracts result in weakness or total paralysis of predominantly distal voluntary movement, Babinski's sign (i.e. dorsiflexion of the big toe and fanning of the other toes in response to stroking the outer border of the foot from heel to toe) and often spasticity (increased muscle tone and exaggerated deep tendon reflexes).

- Disorders of the basal ganglia (extrapyramidal disorders) do not cause weakness or reflex changes. Their hallmark is involuntary movement (dyskinesia), causing increased movement (hyperkinesias) or decreased movement (hypokinesia) and changes in muscle tone and posture.

- Cerebellar disorders cause abnormalities in the range, rate and force of movement. Strength is minimally affected.

Autonomic nerve dysfunction

Dysfunctions of the autonomic nervous system (ANS) or autonomic dysreflexia are recognised by the symptoms that result from failure or imbalance of the sympathetic or parasympathetic components of the ANS such as: 1) increased (>120/min) or decreased (<50/min) heart rate, 2) increased respiratory rate (>24/min), 3) raised temperature (>38.5°C), 4) increased (>160 mmHg) or decreased (<85 mmHg) systolic blood pressure, 5) increased muscle tone, 6) decerebrate (extensor) or decorticate (flexor) posturing and 7) profuse sweating. For example, in spinal injury the presence of a noxious stimulus can be transmitted from the periphery to the spinal cord and activate a dysfunctional sympathetic response.

There are numerous interactions among the CNS, peripheral nervous system (both sympathetic and parasympathetic branches), the endocrine system and the immune system, hence ANS dysfunction is related to this complex triad.[10] Autonomic nerve dysfunction ranges from alterations in the sympathetic–parasympathetic balance to almost complete cessation of activity as occurs in spinal cord injury. As the ANS controls organ function autonomic nerve dysfunction is related to all-organ alteration and failure. The immune system is connected to the nervous system through the ANS with many patients with infections, systemic inflammatory response and multi-organ failure exhibiting autonomic nerve dysfunction. Autonomic nerve dysfunction is assessed by time and spectral domain heart rate variability and is currently being researched as a neurological assessment technique.[11]

Alterations in cerebral metabolism and perfusion

Neuronal cell death occurs in both high and low oxygenated states during injury. Cerebral metabolism and perfusion are compromised by diverse injury processes and biochemical patterns of ischaemia and mitochondrial dysfunction, forming the basis of secondary brain injury processes.[12]

Cerebral ischaemia and mitochondrial dysfunction

Ischaemia is the inadequate delivery of oxygen, the inadequate removal of carbon dioxide from the cell and an increase in the production of intracellular lactic acid. Ischaemia can be caused by an increase in nutrient utilisation by the brain in a hyperactive state, a decrease in delivery related to either cerebral or systemic complications and/or a mismatch between delivery and demand.[13] The ischaemic cascade is described in Figure 17.1. Inflammation together with oxidative stress, excitotoxicity, failure of ionic homeostasis including disrupted calcium, sodium and potassium homeostasis and energy failure are the key pathological changes in ischaemic brain damage.[14] There is a significant inflammatory response in the ischaemic brain with significant changes in the peripheral immune system.[15] When cerebral blood flow (CBF) falls to about 40% of normal, EEG slowing occurs. When CBF falls below 10 mL/100 g/min (20%), the function of ionic pumps fails, which leads to membrane depolarisation. Cerebral ischaemia and reperfusion injury contribute to the cascade of physiological events that is termed secondary brain injury.[16]

Mitochondrial dysfunction occurs in the secondary phase of brain injury and is often associated with normal oxygen levels after reperfusion in the brain. Mitochondria are sensitive to the high levels of free glutamate that are the product of injury and reperfusion. Free calcium and nitrous oxide promote excessive production of reactive oxygen species and mitochondrial membrane permeability. Degradation of deoxyribonucleic acid and essential proteins follows and results in neuronal cell death.[17]

FIGURE 17.1 Ischaemic cascade. In cerebral ischaemia, energy failure causes depolarisation of the neuronal membrane, and excitatory neurotransmitters such as glutamate are released together. A marked influx of Ca^{2+} into neurons then occurs, which provokes the enzymatic process leading to irreversible neuronal injury. Inflammation is also a contributing factor in the development of ischaemic damage.

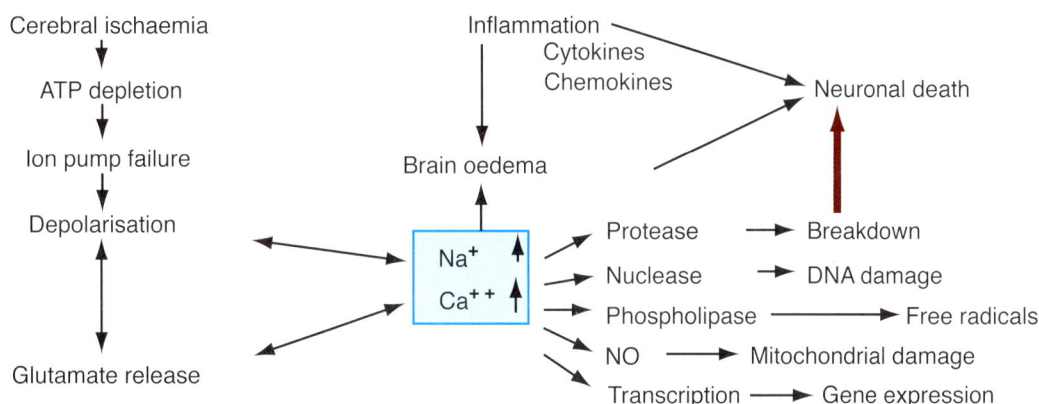

Cerebral oedema

Cerebral oedema is defined as increased brain water content. The brain is particularly susceptible to injury from oedema because of its confined space and limitation of expansion. There are no lymphatic pathways within the CNS to carry away the fluid that accumulates. The Monro–Kellie hypothesis states that the contents of the cranium, which is about 80% brain tissue, 10% blood and 10% cerebral spinal fluid (CSF), are incompressible and thus an increase in volume in one of the components without a corresponding decrease in another component causes a rise in pressure.[18] After brain injury, alterations in ionic gradients lead to a stepwise progression from what is known as cytotoxic (cellular) oedema to ionic oedema, and finally to vasogenic oedema. Ischaemia leads to the cessation of primary active transport via the sodium–potassium pump. As a result co-transporters (secondary active transport) and passive transporters (via ion channels) attempt to maintain cellular processes.[19] By doing so, neurons and neuroglia accumulate active solutes that cause cellular swelling and eventually passage of fluid into the extracellular space. The primary basis for the formation of cytotoxic oedema is the intracellular accumulation of sodium. Eventually, endothelial and neuroglial dysfunction impairs the ability to maintain the integrity of the blood–brain barrier and vasogenic oedema ensues. Historical conventions that characterise oedematous states into 'cytotoxic' or 'vasogenic' categories are fading, as a better understanding of the pathophysiological processes that underlie oedema formation in brain-injured states develop.

Cytotoxic oedema

Cellular swelling, usually of astrocytes in the grey matter, is generally seen after cerebral ischaemia caused by cardiac arrest or minor head injury.[19] The blood–brain barrier (BBB) is intact and capillary permeability is not impaired.

The cause of cytotoxic oedema, also termed intracellular oedema, is anoxia and ischaemia; it is usually not clinically significant, and is reversible in its early phases.

Vasogenic oedema

Vasogenic oedema, sometimes termed extracellular oedema, involves increased capillary permeability, and had been termed 'BBB breakdown'.[20] Rises in brain water content with extracellular oedema are often quite dramatic because the fluid that results from increased capillary permeability is usually rich in proteins, resulting in the spread of oedema and brain ischaemia. This can lead to cytotoxic oedema, and to the progressive breakdown of both astrocytes and neurons.[19] While the classification of oedema is useful to define specific treatments, it is somewhat arbitrary, as cytotoxic and vasogenic oedema often occur concurrently. In fact, each of these processes may cause the other. Ultimately, these changes can lead to raised intracranial pressure (ICP) and herniation.

Interstitial oedema

Interstitial oedema occurs as a result of hydrocephalus, when the pressure within the ventricles is higher than the capacity of the ependymal cells to confine the CSF within the ventricles. The ventricular ependymal lining ruptures allowing CSF into the extracellular space, most commonly the periventricular white matter. Various causes of interstitial oedema include obstructing masses, meningitis, subarachnoid hemorrhage and normal pressure hydrocephalus.[21]

Hydrocephalus

Hydrocephalus is the result of an imbalance between the formation and drainage of CSF. Reduced absorption most often occurs when one or more passages connecting the ventricles become blocked, preventing movement of CSF to its drainage sites in the subarachnoid space just inside the skull.[21] This type of hydrocephalus is called 'non-communicating'. Reduction in absorption rate, called 'communicating hydrocephalus', can be caused by damage to the absorptive tissue. Both types lead to an elevation of the CSF pressure in the brain. A third type of hydrocephalus, 'normal pressure hydrocephalus', is marked by ventricle enlargement without an apparent rise in CSF pressure, which mainly affects the elderly. The presenting symptoms are cognitive decline, gait disturbances and urinary incontinence.

Hydrocephalus may be caused by congenital brain defects, haemorrhage in either the ventricles or the subarachnoid space, CNS infection (syphilis, herpes, meningitis, encephalitis or mumps) or tumours. Irritability is the commonest sign of hydrocephalus in infants and, if untreated, may lead to lethargy. Bulging of the fontanelle, the soft spot between the skull bones, may also be an early sign. Hydrocephalus in infants prevents fusion of the skull bones, and causes expansion of the skull. Symptoms of normal pressure hydrocephalus include dementia, gait abnormalities and incontinence.[22] Treatment includes ventriculostomy drainage of CSF in the short term or a surgical shunt for those with chronic conditions. Either is predisposed to blockage and infection.

Intracranial hypertension

ICP is the pressure exerted by the contents of the brain within the confines of the skull and the BBB. ICP incurs changes to the compensatory reserve and pulse amplitude, as illustrated in Figure 17.2.[23] Normal ICP is 0–10 mmHg, and a sustained pressure of >15 mmHg is termed intracranial hypertension, with implications for CBF.[24] Areas of reduced CBF and focal ischaemia appear when ICP is >20 mmHg and global ischaemia occurs at >50 mmHg. The ICP waveform contains valuable information about the nature of cerebrospinal pathophysiology. Both autoregulation of CBF and compliance of the cerebrospinal system are reflected in the ICP waveform.[25] Waveform analysis of ICP is described in Chapter 16.

Initially, intracranial compliance allows compensation for rises in intracranial volume due to autoregulation. During a slow continuous rise in volume, the ICP rises to a plateau level at which the increased level of CSF absorption keeps pace with the rise in volume with

FIGURE 17.2 The volume–ICP curve relationship.

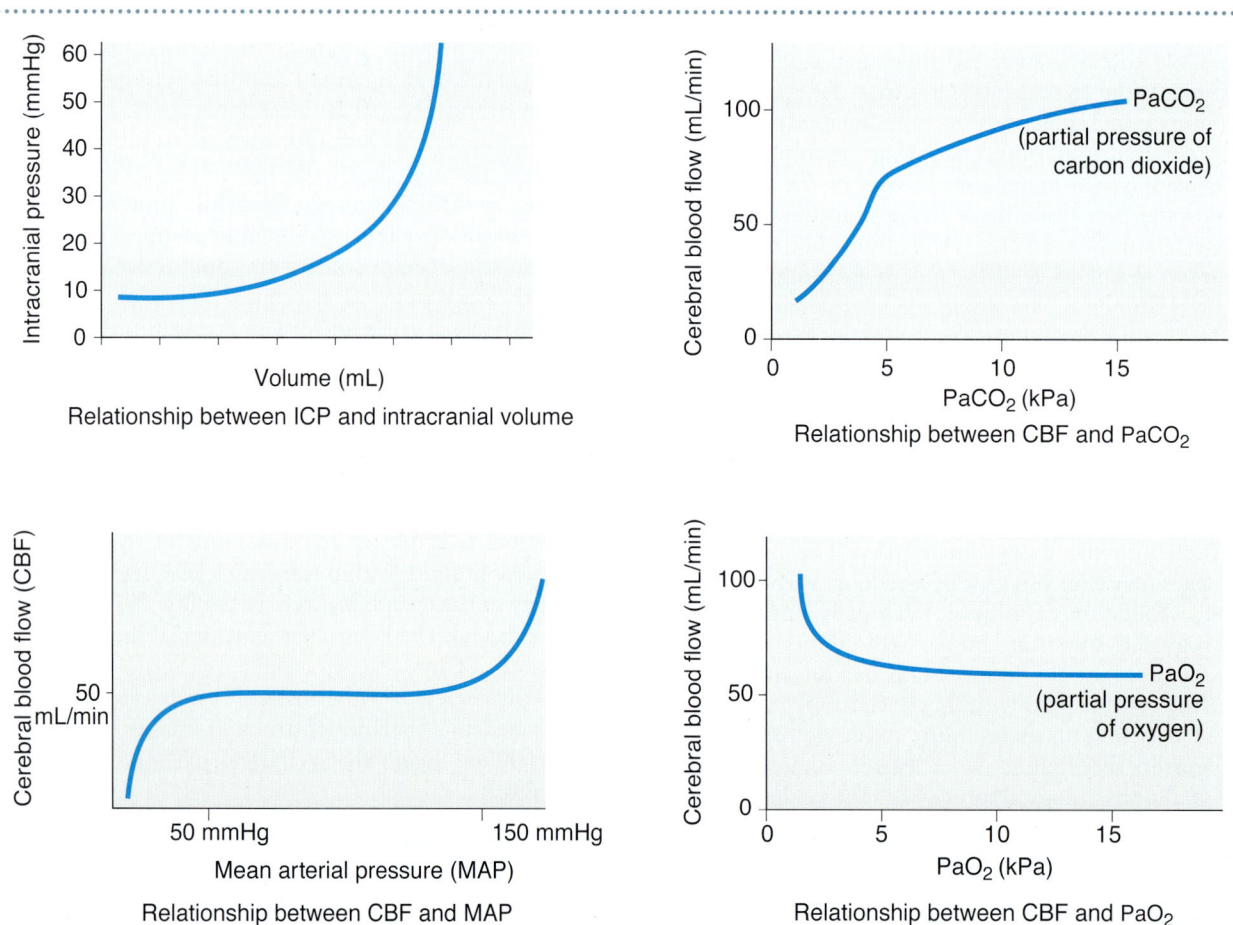

Relationship between ICP and intracranial volume

Relationship between CBF and $PaCO_2$

Relationship between CBF and MAP

Relationship between CBF and PaO_2

Adapted from McLeod A. Traumatic injuries to the head and spine, 2: nursing considerations. Br J Nurs 2004;13(17):1041–9, with permission.

ample compensatory reserve. This is expressed as an index, as shown in Figure 17.3.[26] Intermittent expansion causes only a transient rise in ICP at first. When sufficient CSF has been absorbed to accommodate the volume, the ICP returns to normal. The ICP finally rises to the level of arterial pressure, which itself begins to rise, accompanied by bradycardia or other disturbances of heart rhythm, termed the Cushing's response. This is accompanied by dilation of the small pial arteries and some slowing of venous flow, which is followed by pulsatile venous flow.

The respiratory changes associated with increased ICP depend on the level of brainstem involved. A midbrain involvement results in Cheyne-Stokes respiration. When the midbrain and pons are involved, there is sustained hyperventilation. There are rapid and shallow respirations with upper medulla involvement, with ataxic breathing in the final stages (see Figure 17.4).[27]

Often, neurogenic pulmonary oedema may occur due to increased sympathetic activity as a result of the effects of elevated ICP on the hypothalamus, medulla or cervical spinal cord. The causes of intracranial hypertension are classified as acute or chronic. Acute causes include brain trauma, ischaemic injury and intracerebral haemorrhage. Infections such as encephalitis or meningitis may also lead to intracranial hypertension. Chronic causes include many intracranial tumours, such as ependymomas, or subdural bleeding that may gradually impinge on CSF pathways and interfere with CSF outflow and circulation. As the ICP continues to increase, the brain tissue becomes distorted, leading to herniation and additional vascular injury.[28]

FIGURE 17.3 In a simple model, pulse amplitude of intracranial pressure (ICP) (expressed along the *y*-axis on the right side of the panel) results from pulsatile changes in cerebral blood volume (expressed along the *x*-axis) transformed by the pressure–volume curve. This curve has three zones: a flat zone, expressing good compensatory reserve; an exponential zone, depicting poor compensatory reserve; and a flat zone again, seen at very high ICP (above the 'critical' ICP), depicting derangement of normal cerebrovascular responses. The pulse amplitude of ICP is low and does not depend on mean ICP in the first zone. The pulse amplitude increases linearly with mean ICP in the zone of poor compensatory reserve. In the third zone, the pulse amplitude starts to decrease with rising ICP. RAP = index of compensatory reserve.

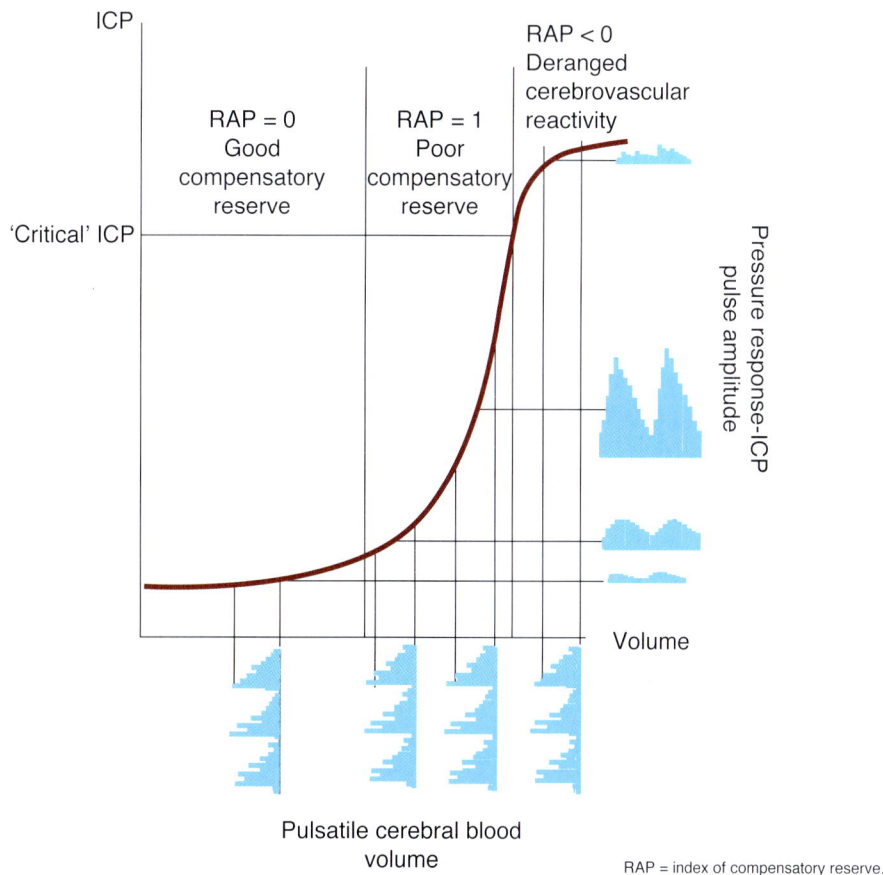

Adapted from Czosnyka M, Pickard J. Monitoring and interpretation of intracranial pressure. J Neurol Neurosurg Psychiat 2004;75(6): 813–21, with permission.

FIGURE 17.4 Injury to the brainstem can result in various abnormal respiratory patterns.[27]

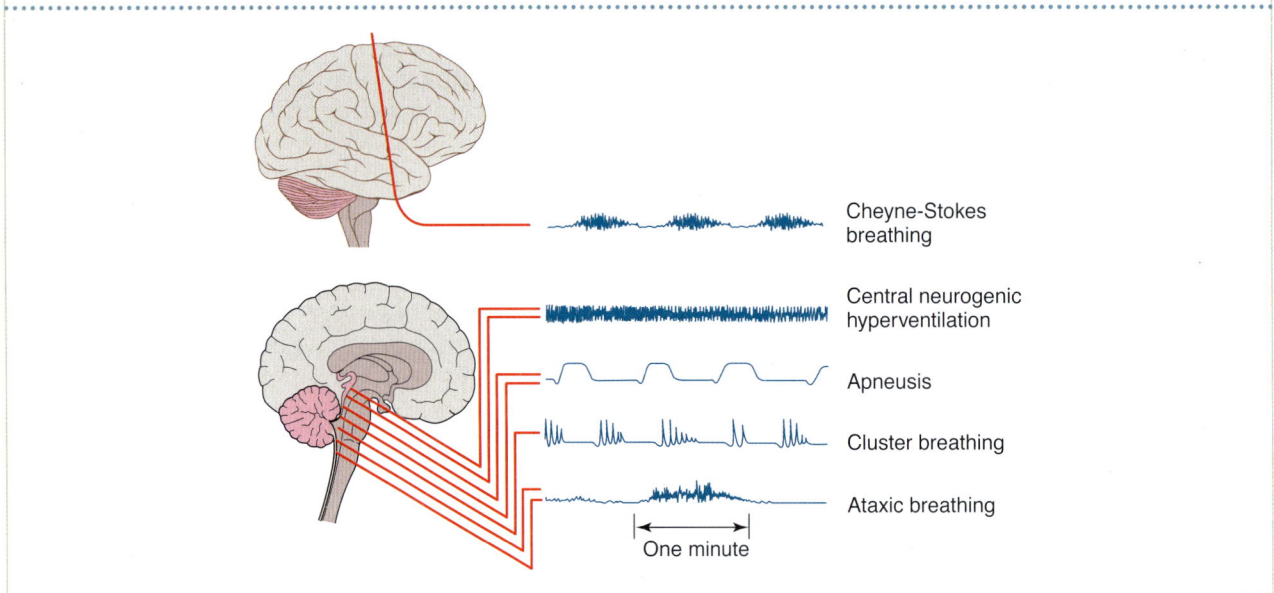

Cheyne-Stokes breathing

Central neurogenic hyperventilation

Apneusis

Cluster breathing

Ataxic breathing

One minute

Neurological therapeutic management

This section explores cerebral perfusion, oxygenation and assessment. The objective of assessment is to identify and then initiate strategies in an attempt to prevent secondary insults and ischaemia. ICP monitoring is discussed in terms of therapeutic management.

Optimising cerebral perfusion and oxygenation

Intracranial hypertension and cerebral ischaemia are the two most important secondary injury processes that can be anticipated, monitored and treated in the ICU. This applies to all aetiologies of brain injury including trauma. This section discusses the modalities of neuroprotection, including the management of intracranial hypertension, vasospasm and cerebral ischaemia. Nursing interventions for the prevention of secondary insults and promotion of cerebral perfusion are described in Table 17.1. Importantly, the aims of nursing management are based on published guidelines and are directed at optimising cerebral perfusion and metabolism by various initiatives.

Management of cerebral oxygenation and perfusion

Cerebral monitoring in brain-injured patients has focused on the prevention of secondary injury to the brain. There are currently four techniques that can be used to assess cerebral oxygenation: jugular venous oxygen saturation, positron emission tomography, near-infrared spectroscopy and brain tissue oxygenation ($PbtO_2$) monitoring.[29] Brain oxygen monitoring is useful in a variety of clinical situations in which secondary brain injury may occur, and some studies suggest that $PbtO_2$ complements ICP monitoring. Episodes of brain hypoxia are common and may occur even when ICP and cerebral perfusion pressure (CPP) are normal,[30] emphasising the potential value of multimodal monitoring that integrates data from several physiological monitors. A strong relationship is observed between $PbtO_2$ and several drivers of brain perfusion, such as mean arterial pressure, CPP and end-tidal CO_2.[31] This observation can help clinicians to better understand the complex pathophysiology of the brain after an acute insult, evaluate autoregulation and identify optimal physiological targets and the utility of therapeutic interventions. The selection among these forms of oxygenation monitoring is focused on the appropriateness of focal or global monitoring, the location of the monitor in relation to the injury and the intermittent or continuous nature of the monitoring.

Jugular venous oxygen saturation (SjO_2) is representative of global cerebral oxygen metabolism, but technically it is difficult to obtain reproducible results. Cerebral tissue oxygenation values of <20 mmHg are targeted for intervention based on Brain Trauma Foundation (BTF) guidelines but this is based on lower quality evidence.[32] $PbtO_2$ can be increased by increasing the FiO_2/PaO_2 ratio and by reducing cerebral metabolic requirements for oxygen ($CMRO_2$) using brain temperature control with active cooling and metabolic rate control with sedation and adequate feeding. Additional interventions such as volume infusion, transfusion and inotropic support directed at improving cardiac output can also be used to increase oxygen delivery.[33]

Cerebral microdialysis has been used extensively in traumatic brain injury, measuring concentrations reflecting biochemical changes in the brain after injury.[33] Cerebral microdialysis measurements are focused on metabolites

TABLE 17.1

Nursing interventions for the promotion of cerebral perfusion in acute brain injury

AIM	GOAL	INTERVENTIONS
Maintain oxygenation	SaO_2 98%, PaO_2 100 mmHg, PaO_2/FiO_2 ratio >350 $PbtO_2$ >20	• Maintain airway • Use 100% O_2 during initial resuscitation phase • Intubate as soon as possible for Glasgow Coma Scale <8 or diaphragmatic respiratory insufficiency (C-spine number) • Obtain arterial blood gas and manipulate set FiO_2 to meet parameter goal • Suction patient as needed • Consider need for kinetic therapy, e.g. rotation/percussion therapy bed within spinal precautions. Use frequent subglottal suctioning, and maintain head of bed elevation at 30° or more to prevent VAP • In recovery: assess for upper airway weakness and reflex (prevent aspiration), sputum retention and atelectasis
Maintain $PaCO_2$	$PaCO_2$ 35–40 mmHg	• ABG assessment • Adjust ventilator settings to obtain $PaCO_2$ of 35–40 mmHg • Ensure optimal $PaCO_2$ for your patient: observe $PbtO_2$ and ICP during manipulation of $PaCO_2$ • Monitor end-tidal CO_2 continuously • Observe for hypoventilation
Maintain mean arterial pressure (MAP)	MAP 90 mmHg	• Maintain euvolaemia • Give IV volume as prescribed to maintain CVP and PCWP within parameters • Use noradrenaline once euvolaemic in order to optimise MAP • Observe $PbtO_2$ for sedation-induced hypotension • Transfuse to haematocrit 33% or haemoglobin content 80–100 g/L • Stroke: thrombolytic, embolic and ICH, MAP 90–120 mmHg with modest reduction and CPP ≥60 mmHg
Maintain cerebral perfusion pressure 50–70 mmHg	CPP 50–70 mmHg	• Effectively reduce ICP while preserving or improving CPP • Position body with neck straight and no knee elevation in order to maintain venous outflow • Make sure cervical collar and endotracheal tube ties are not too tight, especially behind the neck • If patient has a ventriculostomy, drain per prescription
Maintain intracranial pressure (CP) <20 mmHg	ICP <20 mmHg	• Elevate head of bed above the level of the heart to obtain optimal level of ICP and CPP. Monitor ICP, CPP and $PbtO_2$ to ensure optimal level for your patient (15–30°) • Sedate using propofol, morphine, fentanyl and/or lorazepam/midazolam • Hypertonic saline prescription *or* • Mannitol prescription at 0.25–1.0 g/kg IV for ICP sustained at <20 mmHg (watch serum osmolality and consider holding for values >320 mOsmol/kg) • Consider paralytics if positioning, cooling, sedation and mannitol does not resolve increased ICP • Maintain the brain temperatures at 36–37°C, using cooling measures; prevent shivering (increases cerebral metabolic demands) • Prepare for surgical craniotomy if indicated
Maintain environment/reduce stimulation	SjO_2 50–75% $PbtO_2$ >20	• Group necessary interventions in a timely manner to allow for rest periods • Screen visitors • Minimise noise and lighting • Avoid stimulation and prioritise interventions if ICP precarious • Sedation as prescribed

TABLE 17.1 *continued*

AIM	GOAL	INTERVENTIONS
Maintain cerebral blood flow	PbtO$_2$ <20	• Optimise CPP to prescribed levels (60–70 mmHg) • Optimise PaCO$_2$ as indicated to increase CBF • Optimise sedation and consider paralytics • Consider barbiturate prescription if above measures are not successful • PaO$_2$FiO2 ratio >350 • Maintain CVP of 5–10 mmHg, and a PCWP of 10–15 mmHg • Administer normal saline and/or colloids as prescribed to maintain parameters • Transfuse to haematocrit of 33% or haemoglobin content 80–100 g/L (prescription to correct coagulopathies) • Monitor closely for signs and symptoms of neurogenic pulmonary oedema, especially in patients with cardiac history • Maintenance of brain temperature at 36–37°C, with active cooling if necessary • Transcranial Doppler image to check for vasospasm • Non-traumatic aSAH, administer IV nimodipine infusion to prevent vasospasm as prescribed; consider components of HH therapy • Ischaemic stroke, administer tPA within 3 hours of event • ICH, prevent rebleeding; administer prescribed haemostatic medications, reduce hypertension
Maintain nutrition		• Ensure early enteric feeding • Oral enteric feeding tube (nasogastric contradicted in TBI) • Dietitian referral for metabolic requirements

ABG = arterial blood gas; aSAH = aneurysmal subarachnoid haemorrhage; CBF = cerebral blood flow; CPP = cerebral perfusion pressure; CVP = central venous pressure; FiO$_2$ = fraction of inspired oxygen; HH = hypervolaemic hypertensive; ICH = intracerebral haemorrhage; ICP = intracranial pressure; IV = intravenous; MAP = mean arterial pressure; PaCO$_2$ = partial pressure of alveolar carbon dioxide; PaO$_2$ = partial pressure of alveolar oxygen; PbtO$_2$ = brain tissue oxygenation; PCWP = pulmonary capillary wedge pressure; SaO$_2$ = arterial oxygen saturation; SjO$_2$ = jugular venous oxygen saturation; TBI = traumatic brain injury; tPa = tissue plasminogen activator; VAP = ventilator-associated pneumonia.

(glucose, lactate, pyruvate) and neurotransmitters (acetylcholine, dopamine, glutamate) and certain ions (Ca^{2+}, K$^+$, Na$^+$). Cerebral microdialysis glucose levels are reduced in patients with severe TBI, and consistently low concentrations (<0.66 mmol/L) are associated with poor outcome. Similarly, reduced cerebral microdialysis glucose, including that associated with intensive insulin therapy, is associated with mortality in aneurysmal subarachnoid haemorrhage (aSAH). Very low brain glucose may be observed during severe hypoxia or ischaemia after TBI and aSAH. However, the determinants of cerebral microdialysis glucose concentration are complex, and in some patients a reduced cerebral microdialysis glucose may result from a large increase in glucose consumption rather than reduced supply of glucose and oxygen.

Practice tip

Cerebral perfusion pressure (CPP) = mean arterial pressure (MAP) − ICP. So, if ICP is increased (common in moderate/severe TBI), MAP must be increased to maintain CPP.

Management of intracranial hypertension

Raised ICP is treated by removing mass lesions and/or increasing the volume available for expansion of injured tissue. This may be achieved by reducing one of the other available intracranial fluid volumes:

1 CSF by ventricular drainage (as discussed previously)
2 cerebral blood volume by hyperventilation, osmotic diuretic therapy or hypothermia
3 brain tissue water content by osmotic diuretic therapy
4 removing swollen and irreversibly injured brain
5 increasing cranial volume by craniotomy decompression.

The application of these concepts to the following therapeutic strategies is important in the management of intracranial hypertension.[34]

Practice tip

In brain injury, position the patient at 45° head-up to maximise the balance between cerebral perfusion and minimise cerebral oedema.

Hyperventilation

Hyperventilation reduces $PaCO_2$ and will reduce ICP by vasoconstriction induced by alkalosis, but it also decreases CBF.[35] The fall in ICP parallels the fall in cerebral blood volume. Hyperventilation decreases regional blood flow to hypoperfused areas of the brain. Thus, generally $PaCO_2$ should be maintained in the low normal range of about 35 mmHg. Hyperventilation should be utilised only when ICP elevations are refractory to other methods and when brain tissue oxygenation is in the normal range.[36] The BTF Guidelines recommend hyperventilation therapy only for brief periods when there is no neurological deterioration or for longer periods when ICP is refractory to other therapies and not within the acute phase (i.e. 24–48 hours).[32]

Osmotherapy

Acute administration of an osmotic such as mannitol or hypertonic saline produces a potent anti-oedema action, primarily on undamaged brain regions with an intact BBB. This treatment causes the movement of water from the interstitial and extracellular space into the intravascular compartment, thereby improving intracranial compliance or elastance. In addition to causing 'dehydration' of the brain, osmotic agents have been shown to exert beneficial non-osmotic cerebral effects, such as augmentation of CBF (by reducing blood viscosity, resulting in enhanced oxygen delivery), free radical scavenging and diminishing CSF formation and enhancing CSF reabsorption.[37]

Intravenous hypertonic saline increases cerebral perfusion and decreases brain swelling and inflammation more effectively than conventional resuscitation fluids. Hypertonic saline behaves like 20% mannitol in acute cerebral oedema but maintains haemodynamic status. However, unlike hypertonic saline, mannitol induces a diuresis, which is relatively contraindicated in patients with both TBI and hypovolaemia as it may worsen intravascular volume depletion and decrease cerebral perfusion.[38] A systemic review found that hypertonic saline given as either a bolus or continuous infusion can be more effective than mannitol in reducing episodes of elevated ICP.[39]

The BTF has recommended that therapy to reduce ICP should begin at pressures >20 mmHg. The recommendation of the use of hypertonic saline therapy over mannitol lies in the fact the hypertonic saline pulls water intravascularly, increasing blood pressure and maintaining cerebral perfusion. Mannitol has the unfortunate result of diuresis and potential decrease in blood pressure, decreasing cerebral perfusion pressure. Current BTF guidelines show that reasonably good quality evidence exists to avoid hypotension (systolic blood pressure [SBP] <90 mmHg). The BTF refers to mannitol as the mainstay of treatment in the management of intracranial hypertension, but hypertonic saline is the preferred option since the guidelines were developed.

Normothermia

Hyperthermia occurs in up to 40% of patients with ischaemic stroke and intracerebral haemorrhage and in 40–70% of patients with severe TBI or aneurysmal subarachnoid haemorrhage. Hyperthermia is independently associated with increased morbidity and mortality after ischaemic and haemorrhagic stroke and, in subarachnoid haemorrhage and TBI patients, temperature elevation has been linked to raised intracranial pressure.[40] Temperature elevations as small as 1–2°C above normal can aggravate ischaemic neuronal injury and exacerbate brain oedema.[41] Mild hypothermia protects numerous tissues from damage during ischaemic insult. The use of paracetamol, cooling blankets, ice packs, evaporative cooling and new cooling technologies may be useful in maintaining normothermia. Hyperaemia (increased blood flow) may occur during rewarming, resulting in acute brain swelling and rebound intracranial hypertension.[42]

Maintenance of body temperature at 35°C may be optimal.[43] Intracranial pressure falls significantly at brain temperatures below 37°C but no difference was observed at temperatures below 35°C. Cerebral perfusion pressure peaks at 35–36°C and decreases with further falls in temperature.[44] At temperatures below 35°C, both oxygen delivery and oxygen consumption decrease. Cardiac output decreases progressively with hypothermia.[45] Therefore, cooling to 35°C may reduce intracranial hypertension and maintain sufficient CPP without associated cardiac dysfunction or oxygen debt.[46] As the temperature is lowered from 34°C to 31°C, the volume of IV fluid infusion and inotrope requirements increase substantially and, despite such interventions, mean arterial pressure decreases. At 31°C serum potassium, white blood cell count and platelet counts are diminished.[47] Thus, it seems that hypothermia to 35°C may be optimal.

Corticosteroids

Excessive inflammation has been implicated in the progressive neurodegeneration that occurs in multiple neurological diseases, including cerebral ischaemia. The efficacy of glucocorticoids is well established in ameliorating oedema associated with brain tumours and in improving the outcome in subsets of patients with bacterial meningitis. Despite encouraging experimental results, clinical trials of glucocorticoids in ischaemic stroke, intracerebral haemorrhage, aneurysmal subarachnoid haemorrhage and traumatic brain injury have not shown a definite therapeutic effect. Furthermore, the CRASH (**c**orticosteroid **r**andomisation **a**fter **s**ignificant **h**ead injury) trial reported that risk of death was higher in the treatment group than in the control group (26% vs 22%; p<0·0001).[48] Thus, high-dose steroids are not indicated for use in severe traumatic brain injury. However, anterior pituitary insufficiency is an under-recognised problem in patients with severe traumatic brain injury, particularly in elderly people or those who have diffuse axonal injury and skull base fracture. In these instances, administration of hydrocortisone in physiological doses and endocrine follow-up are indicated.

Barbiturates and sedatives

The BTF Guidelines state that high-dose barbiturate therapy may be considered in haemodynamically-salvageable severe

TBI patients with intracranial hypertension refractory to maximal medical and surgical interventions.[49] The utilisation of barbiturates for the prophylactic treatment of ICP has not been indicated. Barbiturates exert cerebral protective and ICP-lowering effects through alteration in vascular tone, suppression of metabolism and inhibition of free radical-mediated lipid peroxidation. Barbiturates may effectively lower CBF and regional metabolic demands. The lower metabolic requirements decrease CBF and cerebral volume. This results in beneficial effects on ICP and global cerebral perfusion. The BTF Guidelines for barbiturates are included under the heading of 'Anaesthetics, analgesics and sedatives'. These guidelines recommend that barbiturates are beneficial to minimise painful or noxious stimuli as well as agitation as they may potentially contribute to elevations in ICP. Therefore, propofol is recommended for the control of ICP, but does not improve mortality or 6-month outcome.[49]

Surgical interventions

The European TBI Guidelines suggest that operative management be considered for large intracerebral lesions within the first 4 hours of injury. The use of unilateral craniectomy after the evacuation of a mass lesion, such as an acute subdural haematoma or traumatic intracerebral haematoma, is accepted practice. Surgery is also recommended for open compound depressed skull fractures that cause a mass effect.[50] Mass effect on CT scan is defined as distortion, dislocation or obliteration of the fourth ventricle; compression or loss of visualisation of the basal cisterns or the presence of obstructive hydrocephalus.

Decompressive craniectomy for refractory intracranial hypertension has been performed since 1977, with a significant reduction in ICP for both TBI[50] and ischaemic stroke.[51] In 2011 a multicentre trial of early decompressive craniectomy in patients with severe TBI, called DECRA, reported that, in adults with severe diffuse traumatic brain injury and refractory intracranial hypertension, an early bifrontotemporoparietal decompressive craniectomy decreased ICP and the length of stay in the ICU but was associated with more unfavorable outcomes at both 6 and 12 months.[52] This finding has resulted in controversy about the technique, timing and selection of patients for decompressive craniectomy. The **r**andomised **e**valuation of **s**urgery with **c**raniectomy for **u**ncontrollable **e**levation of intracranial pressure (RESCUEicp) trial is a continuing randomised trial of decompressive craniectomy.[53] This trial has a higher intracranial pressure threshold for decompressive craniectomy than did the DECRA trial, and includes patients with mass lesions and unilateral or bilateral decompressive craniectomy.

Prevention of delayed cerebral ischaemia and cerebral vasospasm

Delayed cerebral ischaemia is defined as the occurrence of focal neurological impairment (such as hemiparesis, aphasia, apraxia, hemianopia or neglect) or a decrease of at least 2 points on the Glasgow Coma Scale (GCS) (either on the total score or one of its individual components [eye, motor on either side, verbal]). This should last for at least 1 hour, and is not apparent immediately after aneurysm occlusion and cannot be attributed to other causes by means of clinical assessments, cerebral CT or MRI scanning, and appropriate laboratory studies.[54] It occurs in about 30% of patients surviving the initial haemorrhage, mostly between days 4 and 10 after aSAH. The known clinical symptoms, such as decrease in the level of consciousness and focal signs such as aphasia and hemiparesis, may be reversible or otherwise progress to cerebral infarction resulting in an unfavourable outcome or even death. Clinical deterioration attributable to delayed cerebral ischaemia is a diagnosis after exclusion of other causes (such as infection, hypotension, hyponatraemia and others), and it is especially difficult to diagnose in patients who are comatose or sedated.[55] The latter are typically patients with a high grade on the World Federation of Neurosurgical Societies scale (grade 4–5), which represent approximately 40–70% of the patient population with ruptured aneurysms.[56] Early brain injury and cell death, blood–brain barrier disruption and initiation of an inflammatory cascade, microvascular spasm, microthrombosis, cortical spreading depolarisations and failure of cerebral autoregulation have all been implicated in the pathophysiology of delayed cerebral ischaemia.

Cerebral vasospasm is a self-limited vasculopathy that develops 4–21 days after aSAH and/or TBI (see Figure 17.6 later). Oxyhaemoglobin, a product of haemoglobin (Hb) breakdown, probably initiates vasoconstriction, leading to smooth-muscle proliferation, collagen remodelling and cellular infiltration of the vessel wall. The resulting vessel narrowing can lead to delayed cerebral ischaemia. The initial pro-inflammatory effect elicited by Hb and Hb-bound cells initiates an inflammatory cascade and cortical spreading depolarisation involving an increase of cytokines, leukocytes and cell adhesion molecules characterising the inflammatory process. The symptoms are poorly localised and develop gradually over hours, suggesting a progressing, global disease process. aSAH patients develop cerebral vasospasm, and about one-third develop symptomatic vasospasm, which is associated with neurological signs and symptoms of ischaemia. Post TBI cerebral vasospasm occurs in approximately 10–15% of patients.

Calcium antagonists, such as nimodipine, have not been effective in TBI subarachnoid haemorrhage with vasospasm, and studies have suggested that calcium antagonists even prevent neurogenesis after TBI. Nimodipine has demonstrated effectiveness in the treatment of vasospasm in aSAH and is now the only drug for which high quality evidence exists, reducing the incidence of delayed cerebral ischaemia and poor outcome by 40%, without ameliorating vasospasm. An initial study of nimodipine in patients with TBI demonstrated no difference in outcome, and a Cochrane systematic review supports this conclusion.[57]

In aSAH, the outdated 'Triple H' therapy (hypervolaemia, hypertension, haemodilution) was aimed at increasing cerebral perfusion. Despite its widespread use as a mainstay therapy for cerebral vasospasm, there are no randomised controlled trials to support the intervention. While no benefit was shown for cerebral vasospasm, CBF or clinical outcome, clinical studies revealed that hypervolaemia resulted in pulmonary oedema, as well as haemodilution, and with it a decrease in arterial oxygen and oxygen carrying capacity. Anaemia has been associated with a worse outcome after aSAH. These studies achieved the elimination of haemodilution from 'Triple-H' therapy and a change from hypervolaemia target to euvolaemia. These changes, along with the established hypertensive therapy, are the mainstays in clinical practice as recommended in the Neurocritical Care Society aSAH guidelines.[58]

In aSAH, endovascular therapies should be considered in patients at risk for vasospasm-related ischaemia prior to the development of delayed cerebral ischaemia. The literature on this intervention is limited to only a few prospective studies. Prophylactic angioplasty done without the presence of angiographic arterial narrowing exposes patients to risk of vessel rupture and death without clear benefit in outcome.[58] Thus, routine prophylactic cerebral angioplasty is not recommended in the Neurocritical Care Society aSAH guidelines.

Central nervous system disorders

CNS disorders include brain and/or spinal injury from trauma, infection or immune conditions. The pathophysiology and aetiology of these disorders are discussed here, including management of these conditions.

Traumatic brain injury

Head injury is a broad classification that includes injury to the scalp, skull or brain. TBI is the most serious form of head injury. The range of severity of TBI is broad, from concussion through to post coma unresponsiveness. The incidence rates of TBI are increasing worldwide, though estimates vary considerably between countries.[59] In the USA, rates of TBI-related hospitalisations and emergency department visits were approximately 90 per 100,000 population and 715 per 100,000 population, respectively, in 2010.[60] A systematic review of studies from 23 European countries reported an overall average TBI incidence rate range of 150–300 per 100,000 population.[61] This is comparable to the 2004/5 Australian age-standardised incidence rate of about 150 per 100,000 population.[62,63] Reviewers of the global literature agree that the incidence of TBI is highest in countries of low to middle income.[59, 64] Males have a higher incidence of TBI across all age groups in all regions[61,65,66] with the highest rates reported in those aged 15–25 years. Rates in older populations (over 65 years) are increasing[65,66] and this group is at highest risk of TBI. In the very young (0–4 years), TBI rates have declined significantly over the past decade. Quality outcome data from long-term follow-up of TBI cohorts are limited but physical complaints, disabilities and neuropsychological difficulties appear common and it is estimated that there are 13 million people living with TBI-related disability in the USA and the European Union.[59] An Australian and New Zealand epidemiological study of TBI[67] found that the mean age was 41.6 years; 74% were men; 61% were due to vehicular trauma, 24% were falls in elderly patients and 57% had severe TBI (Glasgow Coma Scale score ≤8). Twelve-month mortality was 26% in all patients and 35% in patients with severe TBI.

Aetiology of TBI

Falls are the leading cause of TBI among all age groups (35.2%), followed by motor vehicle collisions or traffic accidents (17.3%), being struck by/against an object (16.5%) and assaults (10%).[64,68] However, causes of TBI fatalities are slightly different. Among all causes of injury, road traffic accidents lead to the most TBI fatalities (31.6%). As another example, the lethality of gunshot wounds to the head is approximately 90%. Because of this, gunshot wounds are a much higher percentage of TBI fatalities than the overall incidence would suggest.[69] Sporting accidents and falls account for a far greater percentage of mild injuries. Infants and toddlers up to 4 years of age, older adolescents aged 15–19 years and adults older than 65 years of age are the highest risk age groups for TBI.[70] This trimodal distribution has been demonstrated for most ethnic and racial groups studied, as well as in global studies of TBI.[64] Most studies have found that the highest age-specific incidence is in the young adult years. Injury and debility in this age group also carries significant morbidity, with many more years of potential life lost and lost productivity for injuries incurred in young people. For every age group studied, males are more likely to suffer TBI than females. Among young people, males are up to seven times more likely to suffer a TBI. People of colour and those of lower socioeconomic strata also suffer rates of TBI 30% to 50% higher than majority individuals. Alcohol is involved in 50% of cases of TBI, either because of intoxicated drivers or pedestrians, increased risk of falls, suicide attempts or interpersonal violence.[64,67]

The transfer of energy to the brain tissue actually causes the damage and is a significant determinant in the severity of injury. In the past 10 years, the introduction of safer car designs, airbags and other road traffic initiatives (e.g. redesigning hazardous intersections, driver education campaigns, random breath testing and reducing speed limits) have decreased the overall number of road fatalities; improvements in retrieval, neurosurgery and intensive care in the past few decades have enabled many people to survive injuries that would previously have been fatal.[66,67]

Pathophysiology of TBI

TBI is a heterogeneous pathophysiological process (see Figure 17.5). The mechanisms of injury forces inflicted on the head in TBI produce a complex mixture of diffuse and focal lesions within the brain.[71] Damage resulting from an injury can be immediate (primary) or secondary in nature. Secondary injury results from disordered autoregulation and other pathophysiological changes within the brain in the days immediately after injury. Urgent neurosurgical intervention for intracerebral, subdural or extradural haemorrhages can mitigate the extent of secondary injury. Scalp lesions can bleed profusely and quickly lead to hypovolaemic shock and brain ischaemia. Cerebral oedema, haemorrhage and biochemical response to injury, infection and increased ICP are among the commonest physiological responses that can cause secondary injury. Tissue hypoxia is also of major concern and airway obstruction immediately after injury contributes significantly to secondary injury. Poor CBF, as a result of direct (primary) vascular changes or damage, can lead to ischaemic brain tissue, and eventually neuronal cell death.[72] Systemic changes in temperature, haemodynamics and pulmonary status can also lead to secondary brain injury (Figure 17.6). In moderate-to-severe, and occasionally in mild, injury CBF is altered in the initial 2–3 days, followed by a rebound hyperaemic stage (days 4–7) leading to a precarious state (days 8–14) of cerebral vessel unpredictability and vasospasm.[73] More than 30% of TBI patients have autonomic nerve

dysfunction characterised by episodes of increased heart rate, respiratory rate, temperature, blood pressure, muscle tone, decorticate or decerebrate posturing and profuse sweating.[74] Lack of insight into these processes and implementing early weaning of supportive therapies can lead to significant secondary insults.

Focal injury

Because of the shape of the inner surface of the skull, focal injuries are most commonly seen in the frontal and temporal lobes, but they can occur anywhere. Contact phenomena or a local blow to the head or the head coming into contact with another item with force are commonly superficial and can generate contusional haemorrhages through coup and contrecoup mechanisms.[75] Cerebral contusions are readily identifiable on CT scans, but may not be evident on day 1 scans, becoming visible only on days 2 or 3. Deep intracerebral haemorrhages can result from either focal or diffuse damage to the arteries.

FIGURE 17.5 Pathophysiology of traumatic brain injury.

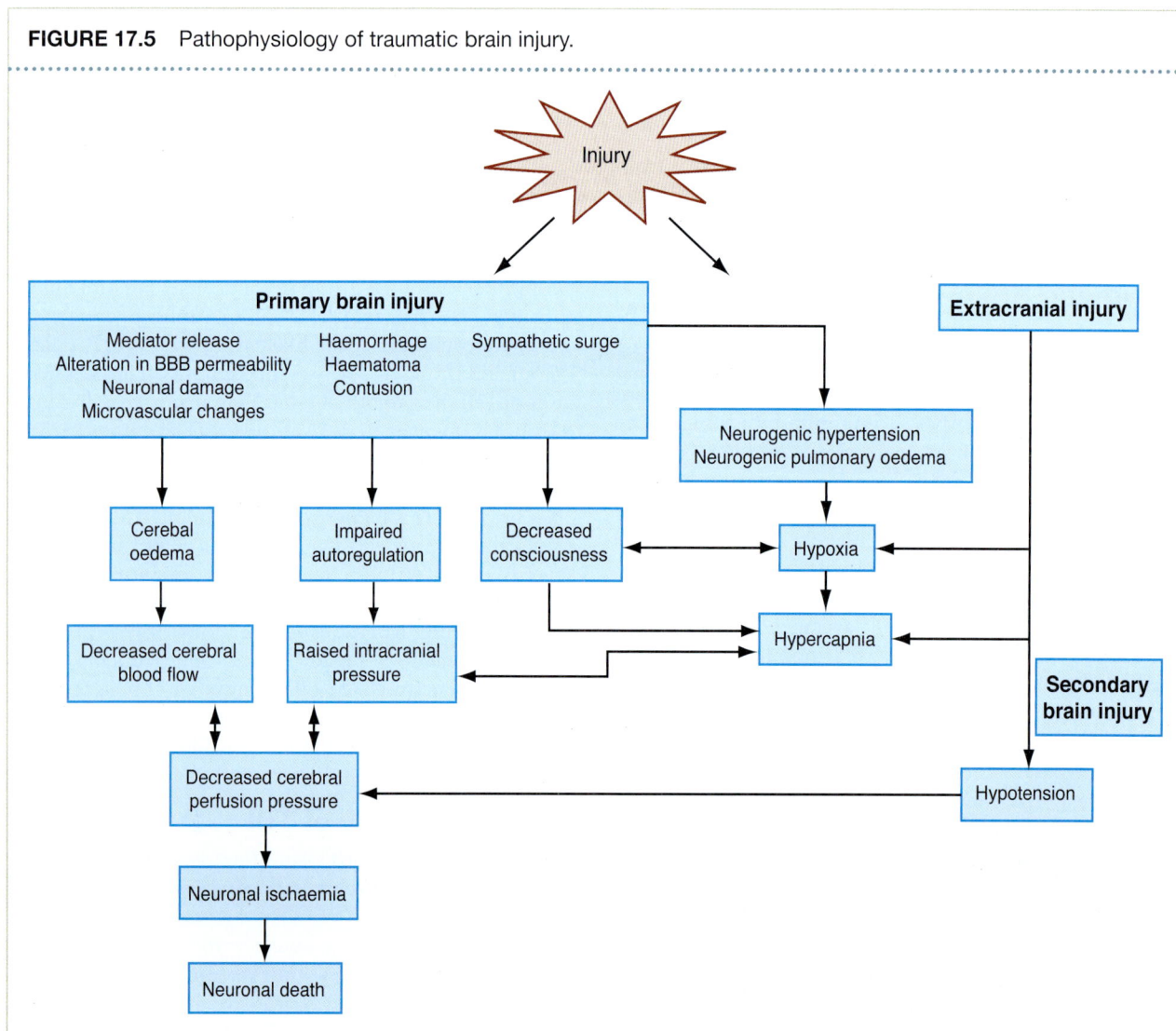

FIGURE 17.6 Conceptual changes in cerebral blood flow and intracranial pressure (ICP) over time following traumatic brain injury: (**A**) cytotoxic oedema; (**B**) vasogenic oedema; (**C**) cerebral blood flow. CPP = cerebral perfusion pressure; MAP = mean arterial pressure.

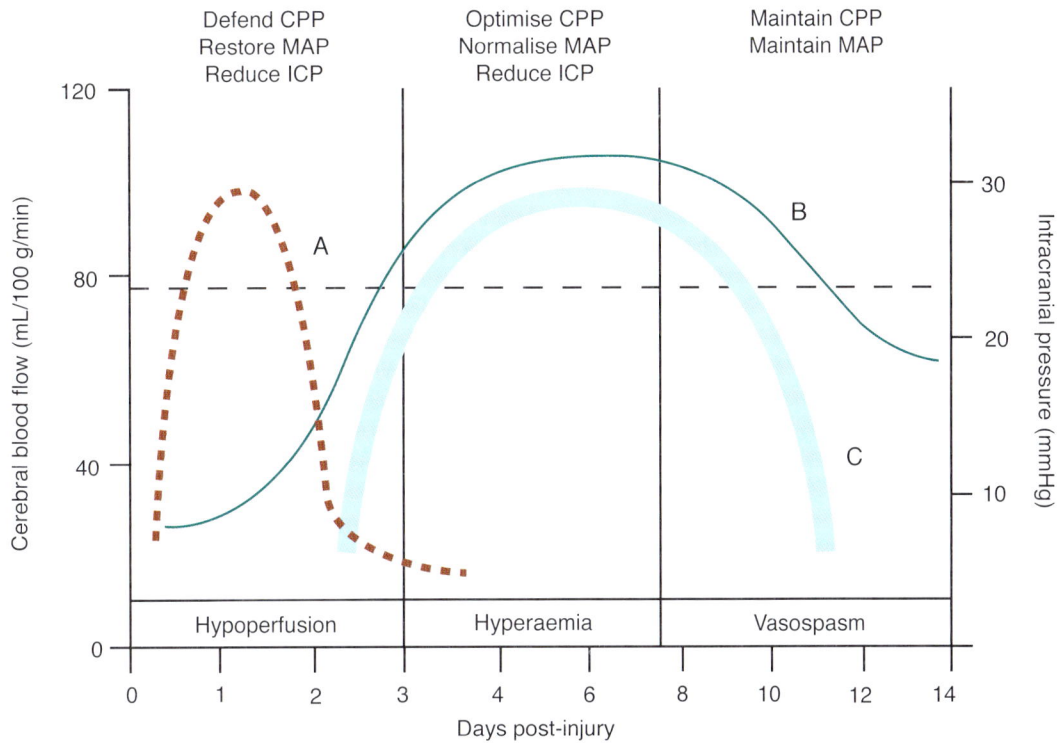

Diffuse injury

Diffuse (axonal) injury refers to the shearing of axons and supporting neuroglia; it may also traumatise blood vessels and can cause petechial haemorrhages, deep intracerebral haematomas and brain swelling.[75] Diffuse injury results from the shaking, shearing and inertial effects of a traumatic impact. Mechanical damage to small venules as part of the BBB can also trigger the formation of haemorrhagic contusions. This vascular damage may increase neuronal vulnerability, causing post-traumatising perfusion deficits and the extravasation of potentially neurotoxic blood-borne substances. The most consistent effect of diffuse brain damage, even when mild, is the presence of altered consciousness. The depth and duration of coma provide the best guide to the severity of the diffuse damage. The majority of patients with diffuse injury will not have any CT evidence to support the diagnosis. Other clinical markers of diffuse injury include the high speed or force strength of injury, absence of a lucid interval and prolonged retrograde and anterograde amnesia. Figure 17.7 contrasts CT scans with haematoma formation and diffuse axonal injury.

Mild TBI

Mild TBI often presents as a component of multitrauma or sports injury and can be overlooked at the expense of other peripheral injuries. Risk factors such as vomiting,

FIGURE 17.7 Extradural haematoma and a subtle subdural haematoma (**left**), subdural haematoma (**middle left**), diffuse axonal injury (**middle right**) and combination injuries (**right**).

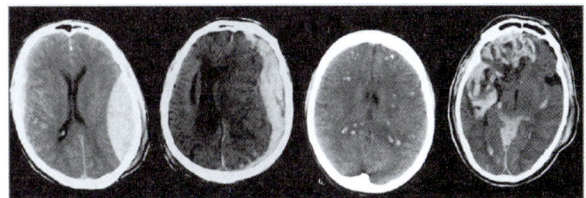

dizziness, facial and skull fractures, including the loss of CSF from the nose or the ear, will categorise those needing further surveillance. Routine head CT and assessment of post-traumatic amnesia are recommended to exclude mass lesions and diffuse axonal injury. Diagnosis and management in the acute phase of mild TBI are as crucial to functional outcome and rehabilitation as in moderate-to-severe TBI.[76]

Skull fractures

Skull fractures are present on CT scans in about two-thirds of patients after TBI. Skull fractures can be linear, depressed or diastatic, and may involve the cranial vault or skull base.

In depressed skull fractures the bone fragment may cause a laceration of the dura mater, resulting in a cerebrospinal fluid leak.[73] Basal skull fractures include fractures of the cribriform plate, frontal bones, sphenoid bones, temporal bone and occipital bones. The clinical signs of a basal skull fracture may include: CSF otorrhoea or rhinorrhoea, haemotympanum or presence of blood in the tympanic cavity of the middle ear, postauricular ecchymoses, periorbital ecchymoses and injury to the cranial nerves – VII (weakness of the face), VIII (loss of hearing), olfactory (loss of smell), optic (vision loss) and VI (double vision).

Patient management

The surveillance and prevention of secondary injury is the key to improving morbidity and mortality outcomes[73]

(see Table 17.1). Interventions are targeted at maintaining adequate CBF and minimising oxygen consumption by the brain in order to prevent ischaemia. In a post hoc analysis of the use of saline in critically ill patients with TBI, fluid resuscitation with albumin was associated with higher mortality rates than was resuscitation with saline.[77] The anticipation and prevention of systemic complications are also crucial. Assessment is vital to establish priorities in care and is discussed in Chapter 16.

Nursing management of the neurologically impaired, immobilised, mechanically ventilated patient is described in Table 17.2 and is an adaptation of the current guidelines[32] (see Table 17.3) to clinical practice (see *Online resources* for TBI-related protocols). In all TBI multitrauma patients, disability and exposure/environmental

---

TABLE 17.2

Nursing management of the neurologically impaired, immobilised, mechanically-ventilated patient

NURSING DOMAIN	NURSING OUTCOME	NURSING INTERVENTIONS
Ventilation and oxygenation	• Airway patent • Arterial pH, PaO_2, $PbtO_2$, SaO_2 within normal range • $PaCO_2$ and $ETCO_2$ within normal range • Lungs clear to auscultation • No evidence of atelectasis or aspiration • Chest X-ray clear of pathology	• Assess ventilation parameters: ensure ET patency and position • Assess bilateral chest movement: listen for airway obstruction or ET cuff leak; auscultate for air entry. • Assess chest X-ray • Adequate sedation and ventilation to maintain $PbtO_2$, ICP, CPP • Suction only as necessary: preoxygenate, avoid prolonged coughing; effective technique. • Avoid ICP complications of PEEP • Position to avoid aspiration • Provide meticulous oral hygiene
Mobility/safety	• Cerebral blood flow uncompromised • Minimal and transient changes in $PbtO_2$–ICP–CPP and return to desired parameters within 5 min of nursing intervention • Patient integument maintained and infection free: skin, mucous membranes, cornea, wounds, invasive lines • Complications of immobility prevented: deep vein thrombosis, pneumonia, muscle strength • Patient safety enabled, preventing nosocomial infection, secondary brain injury, self-harm • Nutrition prescribed according to patient need • Healing defined and uneventful	• Haemodynamic stability maintained. Brain ischaemia and intracranial hypertension controlled • Nursing interventions planned for minimal disturbance; efficient intervention • Pressure-relieving mattress: allows minimal position changes for integument protection, with minimal cerebral oxygen consumption, sequential compression device for venous return • Hygiene maintained: assess integument, assess cornea, assess mucous membranes • Maintain infection control interventions with invasive devices and wounds • Administer preventive plan of treatment with vigilance and prediction • Enable communication with other health professionals • Chemical and physical restraint applied per assessment and prescription, within institutional policy
Psychological/family	• Family and significant others informed and supported • Psychological wellbeing of patient in recovery • The patient will feel safe	• Refer and coordinate information and service provision from other health professionals • The provision of quality, informed and inclusive care to the patient provides family and significant others with the confidence that the nurse advocates for the patient in their place • Ensure psychological assessment and administer prescribed therapy for delirium and post-traumatic stress • Nursing interventions planned to allow for rest and recovery • Administer coordinated rehabilitation strategies

CPP = cerebral perfusion pressure; $ETCO_2$ = end tidal carbon dioxide; ICP = intracranial pressure; $PaCO_2$ = partial pressure of alveolar carbon dioxide; PaO_2 = partial pressure of alveolar oxygen; $PbtO_2$ = brain tissue oxygenation; PEEP = positive end-expiratory pressure; SaO_2 = arterial oxygen saturation.

TABLE 17.3

Summary of guidelines of the management of severe traumatic brain injury from the Brain Trauma Foundation

ITEM	LEVEL I	LEVEL II	LEVEL III
Blood pressure and oxygenation	None	Blood pressure should be monitored and hypotension (SBP <90 mmHg) avoided	Oxygenation should be monitored and hypoxia (PaO_2 <60 mmHg or O_2 saturation <90%) avoided
Hyperosmolar therapy	None	Mannitol is effective for control of raised intracranial pressure at doses of 0.25 gm/kg to 1 g/kg body weight. Arterial hypotension (SBP <90 mmHg) should be avoided Hypertonic saline evidence is limited on the use, concentration and method of administration for the treatment of traumatic intracranial hypertension	Restrict mannitol use prior to ICP monitoring to patients with signs of transtentorial herniation or progressive neurological deterioration not attributable to extracranial causes
Prophylactic hypothermia	Insufficient data	Insufficient data	Prophylactic hypothermia is not significantly associated with decreased mortality Prophylactic hypothermia is associated with significant higher Glasgow Outcome Scale scores
Infection prophylaxis	Insufficient data	Periprocedural antibiotics for intubation should be administered to reduce the incidence of pneumonia – but does not change length of stay or mortality	Routine ventricular catheter or prophylactic antibiotic use for ventricular catheter placement is not recommended to reduce infection
		Early tracheostomy – reduces mechanical ventilation days	Early extubation in qualified patients, without increased risk of pneumonia
Deep vein thrombosis prophylaxis	Insufficient data	Insufficient data	Graduated compression stockings or intermittent pneumatic compression stockings until ambulatory Low-molecular-weight heparin or low unfractionated heparin in combination with above. Risk of expansion of intracranial haemorrhage
Indications for ICP monitoring	Insufficient data	ICP monitoring recommended for patients with GCS score of 3–8 with abnormal CT	Normal CT with 2 or more of the following: • Age 40+ years • Motor posturing • SBP <90 mmHg • GCS score 9–15 with abnormal CT at prescription discretion
ICP monitoring technology	Insufficient data	Insufficient data	Insufficient data The ventricular catheter with external strain gauge, most accurate low-cost, reliable ICP device Can also be recalibrated in situ Parenchymal ICP cannot be recalibrated. Negligible drift
ICP treatment threshold	Insufficient data	Treatment initiated ICP above 20 mmHg	A combination of ICP values, clinical and brain CT should be used to determine the need for treatment
Cerebral perfusion	Insufficient data	Aggressive attempts to maintain CPP above 70 mmHg with fluids and pressors due to risk of ARDS	CPP of <50 mmHg should be avoided The CPP value to target lies within the range of 50–70 mmHg Patients with intact pressure autoregulation tolerate higher CPP values Ancillary monitoring of cerebral parameters that include blood flow, oxygenation or metabolism facilitates CPP management
Brain oxygen monitoring and thresholds	Insufficient data	Insufficient data	Jugular venous oxygenation (<50%) or brain tissue oxygen tension (<15 mmHg) are treatment thresholds and are to be avoided
Anaesthetics, analgesics and sedatives	Insufficient data	Manage pain and agitation High-dose barbiturate may be used in haemodyamically stable patients refractory to other ICP treatments. Propofol for the control of ICP. High-dose propofol can produce significant morbidity	None advised

TABLE 17.3 *continued*

ITEM	LEVEL I	LEVEL II	LEVEL III
Nutrition	Insufficient data	Full caloric replacement by day 7 post injury	None advised
Antiseizure prophylaxis	Insufficient data	Phenytoin or valproate is not recommended for preventing late post-traumatic seizures Anticonvulsants are indicated to decrease the incidence of early post-traumatic seizures	None advised
Hyperventilation	Insufficient data	Prophylactic hyperventilation ($PaCO_2$ <25 mmHg) is not recommended	Use hyperventilation for temporary reduction of elevated ICP Hyperventilation should be avoided during the first 24 hours after injury when CBF is often critically reduced If hyperventilation used; SjO_2 or $PbrO_2$ measures recommended to monitor oxygen delivery
Steroids	Not recommended	None advised	None advised

ARDS = acute respiratory distress syndrome; CBF = cerebral blood flow; CPP = cerebral perfusion pressure; CT = computerised tomography (scan); GCS = Glasgow Coma Scale; ICP = intracranial pressure; $PaCO_2$ = partial pressure of alveolar carbon dioxide; PaO_2 = partial pressure of alveolar oxygen; $PbrO_2$ = brain tissue oxygenation; SBP = systolic blood pressure; SjO_2 = jugular venous oxygen saturation.

Adapted from Brain Trauma Foundation, American Association of Neurological Surgeons, Joint Section on Neurotrauma and Critical Care. Guidelines for management of severe head injury. New York: Brain Trauma Foundation; 2007, with permission.

control assessment includes further investigations with complete CT scans. The management of TBI should include spinal precautions until spinal injury is definitively excluded.

Spinal cord trauma

A 2014 report summarising the epidemiology of traumatic spinal cord injury (SCI) estimated a global-incident rate of 23 cases per million of the population.[78,79] This translates to almost 180,000 cases per year. Traffic-related accidents are the leading cause of traumatic SCI in developed countries, accounting for one-third to one-half of cases.[80] Falls are the next most common cause of traumatic SCI, with rates increasing in the elderly in particular. In developing countries, traumatic SCI is most often caused by falls at home or in the workplace, with rates as high as 63%.[79] The highest proportion of violence-related traumatic SCI occurs in areas of armed conflict or high availability of weapons. Recreational injuries occur most often with snowboarding, rugby and diving accidents. A systematic review of 13 studies from around the world indicated that in most regions there are peak rates of traumatic SCI in young adults (15–29 years) and that in older age groups the incidence rate increased steadily with increasing age. A predominance of males is also evident in cases from all regions.[81,82]

Of all SCI cases, 51% resulted in complete tetraplegia (loss of function in the arms, legs, trunk and pelvic organs). The predominant risk factors for SCI include age, gender, and alcohol and drug use. The vertebrae most often involved in SCI are the 5th, 6th and 7th cervical (neck), the 12th thoracic and the 1st lumbar. These vertebrae are the most susceptible because there is a greater range of mobility in the vertebral column in these areas.[83] Damage to the spinal cord ranges from transient concussion or stunning (from which the patient fully recovers) to contusion, laceration and compression of the cord substance (either alone or in combination) to complete transection of the cord (which renders the patient paralysed below the level of the injury).

Mechanisms of injury

Cervical injury can occur from both blunt and penetrating trauma but, in reality, is a combination of different mechanisms of acceleration and deceleration with and without rotational forces and axial loading.[78] An illustrative example is a diving injury, caused by a direct load through the head and cervical spine. Cervical trauma is produced by a combination of the mechanisms listed below.

- Hyperflexion: usually results from forceful deceleration and is often seen in patients who have sustained trauma from a head-on motor vehicle collision or diving accident. The cervical region is most often involved, especially at the C5–C6 level.

- Vertical compression or axial loading: typically occurs when a person lands on the feet or buttocks after falling or jumping from a height. The vertebral column is compressed, causing a fracture that results in damage to the spinal cord.

- Hyperextension: is the most common type of injury. Hyperextension injuries can be caused by a fall, a rear-end motor vehicle collision or hit on the head (e.g. during a boxing match). Hyperextension of the head and neck may cause contusion and ischaemia of the spinal cord without vertebral column damage. Whiplash injuries are the result of hyperextension. Violent hyperextension with fracture of the pedicles of C2 and forward movement of C2 on C3 produces the 'Hangman's fracture'.

- Extension–rotation: rotational injuries result from forces that cause extreme twisting or lateral flexion of the head and neck. Fracture or dislocation of vertebrae may also occur. The spinal canal is narrower in the thoracic segment relative to the width of the cord so, when vertebral displacement occurs, it is more likely to damage the cord. Until the age of 10, the spine has increased physiological mobility due to lax ligaments, which affords some protection against acute SCI. Elderly patients are at a higher risk due to osteophytes and narrowing of the spinal canal.

Classification of spinal cord injuries

SCIs can be broadly classified as complete or incomplete.[78] The diagnosis of complete SCI cannot be made until spinal cord shock resolves. There are four incomplete SCI syndromes as follows:

- Anterior cord syndrome: injury to the motor and sensory pathways in the anterior parts of the spine; thus patients are able to feel crude sensation, but movement and detailed sensation are lost in the posterior part of the spinal cord. Clinically, the patient usually has complete motor paralysis below the level of injury (corticospinal tracts) and loss of pain, temperature and touch sensation (spinothalamic tracts), with preservation of light touch, proprioception and position sense. The prognosis for anterior cord syndrome is the worst of all the incomplete syndrome prognoses.

- Posterior cord syndrome: this is usually the result of a hyperextension injury at the cervical level and is not commonly seen. Position sense, light touch and vibratory sense are lost below the level of the injury.

- Central cord syndrome: injury to the centre of the cervical spinal cord, producing weakness, paralysis and sensory deficits in the arms but not the legs. Hyperextension of the cervical spine is often the mechanism of injury, and the damage is greatest to the cervical tracts supplying the arms. Clinically, the patient may present with paralysed arms but with no deficit in the legs or bladder.

- Brown-Séquard syndrome: this involves injury to the left or right side of the spinal cord. Movements are lost below the level of injury on the injured side, but pain and temperature sensation are lost on the side opposite the injury. The clinical presentation is one in which the patient has either increased or decreased cutaneous sensation of pain, temperature and touch on the same side of the spinal cord at the level of the lesion. Below the level of the lesion on the same side, there is complete motor paralysis. On the patient's opposite side, below the level of the lesion, there is loss of pain, temperature and touch because the spinothalamic tracts cross soon after entering the cord.

Pathophysiology

SCIs can be separated into two categories: primary injuries and secondary injuries. Primary injuries are the result of the initial insult or trauma, and are usually permanent. The force of the primary insult produces its initial damage in the central grey matter of the cord. Secondary injuries are usually the result of a contusion or tear injury, in which the nerve fibres begin to swell and disintegrate. Secondary neural injury mechanisms include ischaemia, hypoxia and oedema, cellular and molecular inflammatory injury and cell death. Ischaemia, the most prominent post SCI event, may occur up to 2 hours post injury and is intensified by the loss of autoregulation of the spinal cord microcirculation.[84] This will decrease blood flow, which is then dependent on the systemic arterial pressure in the presence of hypotension or vasogenic spinal shock. Oedema develops at the injured site and spreads into adjacent areas. Hypoxia may occur as a result of inadequate airway maintenance and ventilation. Immune cells, which normally do not enter the spinal cord, engulf the area after a spinal cord injury and release regulatory chemicals, some of which are harmful to the spinal cord. Highly reactive oxidising agents (free radicals) are produced, which damage the cell membrane and disrupt the sodium–potassium pump.

Free radical production and the formation of reactive oxygen and nitrogen species or lipid peroxidation lead to vasoconstriction, increased endothelial permeability and increased platelet activation. A secondary chain of events produces ischaemia, hypoxia, oedema and haemorrhagic lesions, which in turn result in the destruction of myelin and axons. Autoregulation of spinal cord blood flow may be impaired in patients with severe lesions or substantial oedema formation. These secondary reactions, believed to be the principal causes of spinal cord degeneration at the level of injury, are now thought to be reversible 4–6 hours after injury. Therefore, if the cord has not suffered irreparable damage, early intervention is needed to prevent partial damage from developing into total and permanent damage.[85]

Spinal shock occurs with physiological or anatomical transection or near-transection of the spinal cord; it occurs immediately or within several hours of a spinal cord injury and is caused by the sudden cessation of impulses from the higher brain centres.[86] It is characterised by the loss of motor, sensory, reflex and autonomic function below the level of the injury, with resultant flaccid paralysis. Loss of bowel and bladder function also occurs. In addition, the body's ability to control temperature is lost (i.e. poikilothermia) and the patient's temperature tends to equilibrate with that of the external environment.

Neurogenic spinal shock occurs as a result of mid- to upper-level cervical injuries and is the result of sympathetic vascular denervation and peripheral vasodilation. The loss of spinal cord vasculature autoregulation occurs, causing the blood flow to the spinal cord to be dependent on the systemic blood pressure. Signs and symptoms include hypotension, severe bradycardia and loss of the ability to sweat below the level of injury. The same clinical findings pertaining to disruption of the sympathetic transmissions in spinal shock occur in neurogenic shock.[78]

Systemic effects of spinal cord injury

The traumatic insult causing the spinal cord injury is associated with an immediate stimulation of central and peripheral sympathetic tone. Initially, the elevated sympathetic activity raises systemic arterial blood pressure and induces cardiac arrhythmias. At the stage of spinal shock with loss of neuronal conduction, the sympathetic excitation is closely followed by decreases in systemic vascular resistance, arterial hypotension and venous pooling. Lesions above the level of T5 additionally present with severe bradycardia and cardiac dysfunction. The decreases in cardiac output combined with systemic hypotension further aggravate spinal cord ischaemia in tissues with defective autoregulation.[85]

Spinal cord injury may produce respiratory failure. The extent of respiratory complications is related to the level of the injured segments. Injuries above the level of C4–C5 produce complete paralysis of the diaphragm, with substantial decreases in tidal volume and consecutive hypoxia. With lesions below C6, the function of the diaphragm is maintained and there is incomplete respiratory failure due to paralysed intercostal and abdominal musculature. As a consequence, arterial hypoxia and hypercapnia occur, both of which promote neuronal and glial acidosis, oedema and neuroexcitation.[86]

Patient management

Spinal cord injury should be suspected in patients with neck pain, sensory and motor deficits, unconsciousness, intoxication, spondylitis or rheumatoid arthritis, all major trauma, distracting injuries, head injury and facial fractures. Prior to admission, if spinal cord injury is suspected or cannot be excluded, the patient must be placed on a spine board with the head and neck immobilised in a neutral position using a rigid collar to reduce the risk of neurological deterioration from repeated mechanical insults. Spinal injury patients are susceptible to pressure injuries (see Chapter 6), so time must be considered when hard surfaces are used for immobilisation. Total neck immobilisation should not interfere with maintenance of the airway, and inadequate respiratory function must be avoided.[82]

Resuscitation

Initial treatment aims for decompression of the spinal cord and reversal of neurogenic shock and respiratory failure.

Spinal shock is associated with decreases in systemic vascular resistance, arterial hypotension, venous pooling, severe bradycardia and decreased myocardial contractility. Consequently, treatment of neurogenic shock includes fluid replacement using crystalloid solutions to maintain arterial blood pressure, circulatory volume, renal function and tissue oxygenation. Lower-limb compression assists with venous return. Infusion of free water must be avoided, as this decreases plasma osmolarity and promotes spinal cord oedema. Atropine may be administered to reverse bradycardia and increase cardiac output. Administration of vasopressors (e.g. noradrenaline) prior to correction of the intravascular volume status may increase systemic vascular resistance (left ventricular afterload) and further impair myocardial contractility. Therefore, careful volume replacement is the first step, and administration of vasopressors the second step, in the treatment of arterial hypotension and low cardiac output after acute cervical spinal cord injury.[8]

The major early cause of death in patients with acute cervical SCI is respiratory failure. Tracheal intubation may be indicated in unconscious patients, during shock, in patients with other major associated injuries and during cardiovascular and respiratory distress. It is also indicated in conscious patients presenting with the following criteria: maximum expiratory force below +20 cmH$_2$O, maximum inspiratory force below −20 cmH$_2$O, vital capacity below 1000 mL and presence of atelectasis, contusion and infiltrate.[85]

Investigations and alignment

Following the initial assessment of the patient, detailed CT diagnostic radiography defines the bone damage and compression of the spinal cord. Cervical spine fractures occur predominantly at two levels, at the level of C2 and at the level of C6 or C7. Unfortunately, 20–30% of these fractures can be missed on plain radiographs. Current data and the American College of Radiology Appropriateness Criteria recommend use of multidetector-row computed tomography as the initial screening examination in suspected cervical trauma instead of radiographs. Specific radiological procedures such as cervical myelography, high-resolution CT scan or magnetic resonance imaging will identify fractures, dislocation of bony fragments and spinal cord contusion.[83] In patients with a dislocated cervical fracture, decompression and anatomical bony realignment may be achieved with traction forces applied manually, or with halo or Gardner–Wells systems under radiological control. If the anatomical bony alignment procedures and traction forces fail to decompress the cord, surgical intervention to remove the lesion is required. The timing of surgical intervention remains controversial. While urgent surgical decompression or internal stabilisation should be performed in all patients with deteriorating neurological status, some centres tend to defer surgical treatment in patients with spinal cord injury who have stable neurological deficits.[87]

Neuroprotection and regeneration

There is robust experimental and some clinical evidence that hypothermia may be beneficial in acute SCI.[88] Most other neuroprotective agents have not been successful, which has been attributed to attempting to block only one molecular pathway of a complex range of SCI molecular mechanisms. There has been renewed interest in regeneration, which involves stem cell transplantation or similar restorative approaches designed to optimise spontaneous axonal growth and myelination, but it is still in its infancy in some countries due to limiting legislation in regard to stem cell research.

Collaborative management

Patients with acute cervical spinal cord injury require ICU monitoring, observation and support of ventilation, a nasogastric tube to reduce abdominal distension and risk of aspiration, a urinary catheter and thermal maintenance.

- Tracheostomy is indicated in high cervical spine injury and ischaemia, sometimes only while the early oedema is resolving.
- Spinal alignment and immobilisation requires careful positioning with dedicated neck support by experienced clinicians.
- Shoulder and lumbar support pillows are often prescribed. Pressure-relief mattresses must be suitably designed for spine immobilisation and, when prescribed, can be tilted to facilitate ventilation.
- Meticulous integument and bowel care is indicated with daily protocols for regular stool softeners and peristaltic stimulants essential for the prevention of autonomic dysreflexia (i.e. strong sensory input from the bowel to the spinal cord that evokes a massive reflex sympathetic surge) and autonomic nerve dysfunction.
- Early nutritious feeding is essential, whether oral or enteric; however, aspiration must be prevented. The supplementation of feeding with high-energy protein fluids to match the catabolic state assists with recovery (see Chapter 19).
- Hyperglycaemia is associated with increased inflammation and must be controlled to less than 10 mmol/L, avoiding hypoglycaemia.[89]
- The concepts of pain relief and sedation in patients with spinal cord injury are based on the maintenance of coupling between metabolism and spinal cord blood flow while achieving hypnosis, analgesia and a 'relaxed cord'. These concepts include maintenance of normal to high systemic perfusion pressures, normoxia and normocapnia.
- Psychological and empathetic support is essential and appropriate referral for grieving and stress is paramount. Rehabilitation counselling and planning starts at the acute stage in order to give the family unit some future focus and hope.

See *Online resources* for specific protocols related to spinal injury.

Cerebrovascular disorders

Cerebral vascular disorders include cerebrovascular disease and cerebral vascular accidents (stroke). A stroke (acute brain injury of vascular origin) may be either ischaemic or haemorrhagic and is defined as an interruption of the blood supply to any part of the brain, resulting in damaged brain tissue.

Stroke

According to World Health Organization (WHO) estimates, one in every 10 deaths is caused by stroke; thus, it is the third most common cause of death in developed countries, exceeded only by coronary heart disease and cancer.[89] Worldwide, 15 million people suffer a stroke each year; one-third die and one-third are left permanently disabled. The prevalence of stroke in the USA is about 7 million (3.0%).[90] China has one of the highest rates of mortality (19.9% of all deaths in China), along with Africa and parts of South America. In Europe, the incidence of stroke varies from 101.1 to 239.3 per 100,000 in men and 63.0 to 158.7 per 100,000 in women.[91] Stroke is the primary cerebrovascular disorder in Australia and New Zealand and is still the third-leading cause of death. Every year approximately 40,000 people in Australia are admitted to hospital with a diagnosis of stroke.[92] The prevalence of stroke is higher among men than women. Almost 60% of people who have had a stroke are aged 65 years and over, while 18% are under the age of 55 years. Stroke can be divided into two major categories: ischaemic (85%), in which vascular occlusion and significant hypoperfusion occur; and haemorrhagic (15%), in which there is extravasation of blood into the brain. Although there are some similarities between the two broad types of stroke, the aetiology, pathophysiology, medical management, surgical management and nursing care differ.

Aetiology

Hypertension is the leading risk factor for stroke. Other risk factors include diabetes, cardiac disease, previous cerebrovascular disease (transient ischaemic attack or stroke or myocardial infarction), age, sex, lipid disorders, excessive ethanol ingestion, elevated hematocrit, elevated fibrinogen and cigarette smoking. Cerebral arteriosclerosis predisposes individuals to both ischaemic and haemorrhagic stroke. Smoking is the strongest risk factor for aSAH. Atrial fibrillation, endocarditis and medications containing supplemental oestrogen are risk factors for embolic stroke. Seizures develop in approximately 10% of cases, usually appearing in the first 24 hours and more likely to be focal than generalised. Occurrence of seizures within 24 hours of stroke is associated with higher 30-day mortality, which may be a reflection of severe neuronal damage.[93]

Ischaemic stroke

Ischemic stroke compromises blood flow and energy supply to the brain, which triggers mechanisms that lead to cell death. Infarction occurs rapidly in the region of most severe ischaemia (termed ischaemic penumbra) and expands at the expense of the surrounding hypoxic tissue, from the centre to the periphery. Therapeutic strategies in acute ischaemic stroke are based on the concept of arresting the transition of the penumbral region into infarction, thereby limiting ultimate infarct size and improving neurological and functional outcome. Ischaemic stroke can be further categorised as middle cerebral artery occlusion, acute basilar occlusion and cerebellar infarcts.[94]

Practice tip

For consideration of ischaemic stroke lysis, the timing of the onset of symptoms needs to be very clearly defined. In particular, if a patient wakes from sleep with stroke symptoms, the timing of onset must be assumed to be when they were last well – that is, the time when they went to sleep.

The management of an ischaemic stroke comprises four primary goals: restoration of CBF (reperfusion), prevention of recurrent thrombosis, neuroprotection and supportive care. The timing of each element of clinical management needs to be implemented in a decisive manner.

For eligible patients, IV tissue plasminogen activator should be administered intravenously with a dose of 0.9 mg/kg (maximum of 90 mg), with 10% of the total dose administered as an initial bolus and the remainder infused over 60 minutes, provided that treatment is initiated within 4.5 hours of clearly defined symptom onset.[95] The recommendation assumed a relatively higher value on long-term functional improvement and a relatively lower value on minimising the risk of intracerebral hemorrhage in the immediate peristroke period.[96]

Table 17.4 shows the classification and treatment strategies, and the *Online resources* reflect specific ischaemic stroke protocols.

Intracerebral haemorrhage

Intracerebral haemorrhage (ICH) comprises 10–15% of all strokes with an incidence of 24.6 per 100,000 person-years, with a growing incidence associated with the use of anticoagulation, antiplatelet agents and an ageing population.[97] Despite this, ICH remains the last stroke type without a definitive treatment and contributes to significant morbidity and mortality. Up to half of patients die within 30 days, often despite extensive stays in the ICU. Moreover, those who survive have a high degree of long-term disability.[98] Ideally, patients with acute ICH should be admitted to an ICU based on the need for close monitoring of neurological and haemodynamic condition and the risk for early deterioration from haematoma expansion, cerebral oedema, hydrocephalus or airway compromise. Many ICHs continue to grow and expand over several hours after onset of symptoms.[99]

As with all emergency management, initial assessment of airway, breathing and circulation is critical. Until the diagnosis of ICH is made from neuroimaging, overall

---

TABLE 17.4

Classification and type of ischaemic stroke and treatment options

CLASSIFICATION	TREATMENT OPTIONS
Middle cerebral artery occlusion	Intravenous or intra-arterial tissue plasminogen activator (tPA) Exclusion criteria: >3 hours elapsed from stroke onset and widespread early infarct changes on CT scan Tolerate autoprotective hypertension for perfusion of the ischaemic penumbra
Acute basilar occlusion	Anticoagulation with intravenous heparin Thrombolysis up to 12 hours after onset
Cerebellar infarcts	May be difficult to recognise because of the slow evolution of brainstem and cerebellar signs Aspirin, antihypertensives and conventional cerebral oedema strategies

---

airway and haemodynamic management proceeds in a common pathway with other stroke subtypes. Because many ICH patients are obtunded or comatose, airway management (specifically the need for intubation for airway protection) should be considered throughout the early treatment course. Following the diagnosis of ICH, immediate consideration should be given to the need for 1) acute control of elevated blood pressure, 2) correction of coagulopathy because of medications or underlying medical conditions and 3) the need for urgent surgical haematoma evacuation.

Over 90% of patients have acute hypertension exceeding 160/100 mmHg, whether or not there is a history of pre-existing hypertension. It remains unclear whether this response is adaptive (to maintain perfusion to an ischemic penumbra surrounding the haematoma) or potentially harmful (resulting in rebleeding, peri-haematoma oedema expansion, or both).[100] Presently, based on the existing incomplete evidence, American Heart Association/American Stroke Association guidelines recommend that, for patients with SBP of >200 mmHg or mean arterial pressure (MAP) of >150 mmHg, continuous intravenous infusion to reduce the blood pressure should be applied, with monitoring every 5 minutes. For SBP of >180 mmHg or MAP of >130 mmHg in patients with a likelihood of ICP elevation, reducing blood pressure while simultaneously maintaining a cerebral perfusion pressure of ≥60 mmHg is recommended. If there is no evidence of elevated ICP, a modest reduction of blood pressure (e.g., MAP of 110 mmHg or a target BP of 160/90 mmHg) with a re-examination every 15 minutes is recommended.[101]

Antithrombotic medications are a risk factor for the occurrence of ICH, as well as for haematoma expansion if an ICH occurs. As there is a broad range of antithrombotic medications, including warfarin, heparin, antiplatelet agents such as aspirin and clopidogrel and newer agents such as dabigatran and rivaroxaban, the specific risks and interventions to reverse coagulopathy vary. Also, coagulopathies may be due to underlying medical conditions, such as liver disease or haematological malignances.[102] Most of the brain injury and swelling that happens in the days after ICH is the result of inflammation caused by thrombin and other coagulation end-products. Dysautonomia, in the form of central fever, hyperventilation, hyperglycaemia and tachycardia or bradycardia, is also common. Hyperglycaemia at the time of hospital admission is associated with early mortality and poor outcome in ICH patients.[103]

Subarachnoid haemorrhage

Admission to the ICU is indicated for aSAH Hunt Hess Severity Scale III (see Table 17.5) or the World Federation of Neurosurgical Societies Scale grade 4. This level of severity is at greater risk of systemic complications and clinical deterioration.[104] Resuscitation is directed towards maintaining cerebral perfusion pressure by ensuring adequate arterial blood pressure (often with the use of inotropes to produce relative hypertension although reactive hypertension is often present), ensuring euvolaemia and producing relative haemodilution.[105]

Hypovolaemia occurs in 30–50% of patients, as does hyponatraemia in 30% of patients. In the first 6 days, plasma volume decreases of greater than 10% can occur following aSAH, thus increasing the risk of delayed cerebral ischaemia and vasospasm.[106] Women have been found to have more significant drops in blood volume than men following aSAH. 'Third space' loss, insensible losses and blood loss account for this drop in fluid volume, as well as electrolyte disturbances.[107]

TABLE 17.5

Hunt-Hess scale for aneurysmal subarachnoid haemorrhage (aSAH)

SCORE	DESCRIPTION
0	Unruptured; asymptomatic discovery
I	Asymptomatic or minimal headache with slight nuchal rigidity
II	Moderate-to-severe headache, nuchal rigidity; no neurological deficit other than cranial nerve deficit
III	Drowsiness, confusion or mild focal deficit (e.g. hemiparesis), or a combination of these findings
IV	Stupor, moderate-to-severe deficit, possibly early decerebrate rigidity and vegetative disturbances
V	Deep coma, decerebrate rigidity, moribund appearance

Practice tip

Fever is the most common medical complication in patients suffering from aSAH and is associated with neurological deterioration.

Other aspects of management in the acute stages include suitable analgesia, seizure control and treatment with nimodipine to prevent delayed cerebral ischaemia and vasospasm. Vasospasm often occurs 4–21 days after initial haemorrhage when the clot undergoes lysis (dissolution), increasing the chances of rebleeding. It is believed that early open surgical clipping or wrapping and endovascular coil embolisation prevent rebleeding and that removal of blood from the basal cisterns around the major cerebral arteries may prevent vasospasm.[108] (See previous section on *Prevention of delayed cerebral ischaemia and cerebral vasospasm*.) The management of acute hydrocephalus secondary to aSAH is usually managed by external ventricular drainage (EVD) and is associated with neurological improvement. ICP monitoring and drainage of CSF via ventriculostomy is indicated in aSAH.[109]

Increased sympathetic activation from the presence of haemoglobin in the subarachnoid space results in elevated catecholamine levels. This is characterised by hypothalamically mediated changes including increased sympathetic and parasympathetic activity that causes cardiac and pulmonary complications (neurogenic pulmonary oedema).[110] Manifestations include electrocardiographic changes, arrhythmias, impaired cardiac contractility, elevated troponin levels and myocardial necrosis. Cardiac and pulmonary complications are associated with delayed cerebral ischaemia and poor outcome after aSAH. As cardiac function is one of the determinants for adequate CBF, it is essential to identify such occurrences early and treat them accordingly.

Hyponatraemia occurs from alterations in atrial natriuretic factor in response to sympathetic nervous system activation. The syndrome of inappropriate secretion of antidiuretic hormone is primarily responsible for hyponatraemia in those with aSAH, as is cerebral salt-wasting syndrome; however, both mechanisms are still relatively misunderstood.[109]

Cerebral venous thrombosis

Compared to cerebral infarctions from arterial sources, cerebral venous infarctions are less common. The ratio of venous strokes to arterial stroke is reported as 1:62.5. Cerebral venous thrombosis is particularly important to recognise because there is general consensus that early anticoagulation can result in good clinical outcomes.[111] Magnetic resonance and CT vascular imaging has made it easier to establish the diagnosis, but close monitoring of the patient is essential, as late deterioration can occur.

Patient management

Expected outcomes for patients with acute ischaemic and haemorrhagic stroke include prevention of secondary injury and of airway and respiratory complications, and maintenance of haemodynamic stability. Timely assessment and intervention are paramount in the management of ischaemic stroke, especially regarding interventional pharmacology and prevention of cerebral haemorrhage.[104] See *Online resources* for specific protocols related to stroke.

Atrial fibrillation and deep vein thrombosis prevention (in ischaemic stroke) requires anticoagulation control. In haemorrhagic stroke, a sequential compression device and stockings are indicated for deep vein thrombosis prophylaxis as anticoagulants are a risk factor for rebleeding.[102] Maintenance of bowel and bladder function and prevention of integument complications, malnutrition, seizures and increasing neurological deficits are important goals. Environmental precautions are implemented to provide a non-stimulating environment, preventing rises in ICP and further bleeding.

Sensory perceptual and motor alterations need to be assessed in regard to effective communication and pain management. Rehabilitation and psychological support for the patient and significant others are integrated into the acute care phase for a smooth transition.[104]

Infection and inflammation

The CNS infections of major interest in the ICU are divided into those that affect the meninges (meningitis) and those that affect the brain parenchyma (encephalitis). They may be viral or bacterial in aetiology. There are also numerous medical conditions that may produce an encephalopathic illness that may mimic viral encephalitis. In patients recently returning from abroad, particular vigilance must be paid to the possibility of such non-viral infections as cerebral malaria, which may be rapidly fatal if not treated early. A number of metabolic conditions, including liver and renal failure and diabetic complications, may also cause confusion due to the manifestation of cerebral oedema. The possible role of alcohol and drug ingestion must always be considered.

Meningitis

Meningitis is inflammation of the pia and arachnoid layers of the meninges. Acute community-acquired meningitis can develop within hours to days and is usually viral or bacterial. Viral meningitis usually has a good prognosis, whereas bacterial meningitis is associated with significant rates of morbidity and death, so it is critical to recognise and differentiate them promptly.[112] The incidence, mortality and morbidity from acute community-acquired meningitis have decreased significantly, especially in high-income countries, probably as a result of vaccination and better antimicrobial and adjuvant therapy, but the disease still has a high toll. The incidence of bacterial meningitis has declined from 3–5 per 100,000 per year a few decades ago to 1.3–2 per 100,000 per year currently.[112]

The incidence of disease caused by *Neisseria meningitidis* remains an issue of public health concern in Australia and New Zealand. The introduction of a publicly funded program of selective vaccination with conjugate serogroup C meningococcal vaccine in 2004 has resulted in a significant reduction in the number of cases of meningococcal disease.[113] The policy of giving antibiotics prior to hospital admission in Australia, implemented in 1995, reduced the case-fatality rate for those receiving antibiotics. The onset of meningococcal disease varies seasonally, rising in June and peaking in late spring each year.[114] The highest incidence of meningococcal disease is for children aged 4 years and under. A secondary peak in the incidence of meningococcal disease is seen in adolescents and young adults. During the 2009 H1N1 influenza epidemic there were several cases of H1N1 influenza-related meningitis. Table 17.6 has the CSF profiles for acute meningitis and encephalitis and Table 17.7 has the classification, treatment and clinical presentation of meningitis.

Complications of meningitis vary according to the aetiological organism, the duration of symptoms prior to

---

TABLE 17.6

Typical profiles of cerebrospinal fluid in acute meningitis and encephalitis

| INVESTIGATION | REFERENCE RANGE | MENINGITIS | | ENCEPHALITIS |
		BACTERIAL	VIRAL	BACTERIAL/VIRAL
Opening pressure	<30 mmH$_2$O	Raised	Normal	Raised
White cells				
Total count	<5 × 10^6/L	Greatly raised	Moderately raised	Moderately raised
Differential	Lymphocytes (60–70%), monocytes (30–50%), no neutrophils or red blood cells	Neutrophils predominate	Lymphocytes predominate	Lymphocytes predominate
Glucose concentration	2.8–4.4 mmol/L	Lowered	Normal	Normal
CSF: serum glucose ratio	>60%	Lowered	Normal	Normal
Protein concentration	<0.45 g/L	Raised	Normal or slightly raised	Normal or slightly raised

TABLE 17.7

Classification of acute meningitis

ACUTE MENINGITIS	BACTERIAL – NOTIFIABLE DISEASE	VIRAL
Aetiology	*Neisseria* meningitis • Serogroups A, B, C – 90% invasive isolates • Serogroup B – most disease • Serogroup A – epidemic disease and indigenous haemophilus influenzae type B streptococcus pneumoniae listeria monocytogenes	Enteroviruses: 85–95% of cases Herpes simplex 1 and 2 Varicella zoster Cytomegalovirus Epstein–Barr HIV infection can also present as aseptic meningitis Post infectious encephalomyelitis: may occur following a variety of viral infections, usually of the respiratory tract. *Cryptococcus neoformans* Fungal isolates
Pathophysiology	Rapid recognition and diagnosis of meningitis is imperative Quick and insidious progress of disease Colonisation of mucosal surfaces (nasopharynx) Haematogenous or contiguous spread Specific antibodies important defence Bacterial invasion of meninges: inflammatory response, breakdown of the BBB, cerebral oedema, intracranial hypertension Vasculitis, spasm and thrombosis in cerebral blood vessels	The physical signs are not so marked and the illness is not as severe and prolonged as bacterial meningitis Viral infection of mucosal surfaces of respiratory or gastrointestinal tract Virus replication in tonsillar or gut lymphatics Viraemia with haematogenous dissemination to the CNS Meningeal inflammation, BBB breakdown, cerebral oedema, vasculitis and spasm
Clinical presentation and progression	Presents with sepsis: headache, fever, photophobia, vomiting, neck stiffness, alteration of mental status Meningococcaemia is characterised by an abrupt onset of fever (with petechial or purpuric rash) Progresses to purpura fulminans, associated with the rapid onset of hypotension, acute adrenal haemorrhage syndrome and multi-organ failure Kernig's sign Brudzinski's sign Cranial nerve palsy (III, IV, VI, VII) uncommon and develop after several days Focal neurological signs in 10–20% cases Seizures in 30% of cases Signs of intracranial hypertension: coma, altered respiratory status Leads to hypertension and bradycardia before herniation, or brain death, leads to irreversible septic shock	Presents with non-specific symptoms, viral respiratory illness, diarrhoea, fever, headache, photophobia, vomiting, anorexia, rash, cough and myalgia Occurs in summer or late autumn Enteroviral, pleurodynia, chest pain, hand-foot-mouth disease HSV-2: acute genital herpes
Treatment	If meningococcal infection is suspected, the best way to reduce mortality is to administer empirical IV therapy immediately Ceftriaxone 2 g IV 12-hourly or cefatoxime 2 g IV 6-hourly or immediately Consequent dose, times and type of antibiotic need to be modified after full investigation and a detailed examination have taken place Dexamethasone may be prescribed: needs to be at same time as antibiotic as outcome neurologically is reduced if given after antibiotic. Reduces BBB permeability Supportive treatment and resuscitation Management of intracranial hypertension/ischaemia	Administer intravenous aciclovir Dexamethasone may be prescribed: reduces BBB permeability Supportive treatment and resuscitation Management of intracranial hypertension/ischaemia

BBB = blood–brain barrier; CNS = central nervous system

initiation of appropriate therapy and the age and immune status of the patient.[114] Temporary problems include development of haemodynamic instability and disseminated intravascular coagulopathy, particularly in meningococcal infection, syndrome of inappropriate secretion of antidiuretic hormone or other dysregulation of the hypothalamic–pituitary axis (e.g. diabetes insipidus), and an acute rise in ICP.

> ### Practice tip
>
> CSF concentrations of most antimicrobial drugs are considerably less than in the serum due to poor penetration of the blood–CSF barrier. Thus, the dose for treating meningitis is usually higher than the regular dose.

Focal neurological signs may develop in the early stages of meningitis, but are more common later. The development of subdural empyema, brain abscess and acute hydrocephalus may require surgical intervention. Bacterial meningitis with accompanying bacteraemia can lead to a marked systemic inflammatory response with septic shock and acute respiratory distress syndrome.

Encephalitis

Encephalitis implies inflammation of the brain substance (parenchyma), which may coexist with inflammation of the meninges (meningoencephalitis) or spinal cord (encephalomyelitis). Encephalitis may be mild and self-limited, or may produce devastating illness.

Herpes simplex virus encephalitis is the most common sporadic viral encephalitis worldwide, with an annual incidence of 1 in 250,000–500,000.[115] It is the commonest cause of non-seasonal encephalitis in Australia. Without treatment, herpes simplex virus encephalitis is fatal in up to 80% of cases, and leaves up to 50% of survivors with long-term sequelae.[116]

- In the absence of particular risk factors, other common causes are enteroviruses, influenza virus and *Mycoplasma pneumoniae*. However, the likely pathogens in encephalitis are dramatically influenced by geographical location, history of travel and animal exposure and vaccination.
- Murray Valley encephalitis virus causes seasonal epidemics of encephalitis at times of high regional rainfall. This arthropod-borne virus is the commonest flavivirus to cause encephalitis in Australia.
- Since 2005, the distribution of Japanese B encephalitis virus has expanded into Australia via the Torres Strait Islands.[117] It causes disease clinically similar to Murray Valley encephalitis. In addition, two novel encephalitis viruses were recently identified in Australia, the Hendra virus and Australian bat lyssavirus. These should be considered if there is a history of animal exposure, or if no other pathogen can be implicated.

- *Mycobacterium tuberculosis*, the yeast *Cryptococcus neoformans* and *Treponema pallidum* (syphilis) may also affect the brain parenchyma but usually produce chronic or subacute meningitis in such circumstances.

In the majority of encephalitis cases, the offending organism finds access to the brain via the nasopharyngeal epithelium and the olfactory nerve system. Arboviruses are transmitted from infected animals to humans through bite of infected animals.[117] The cytokine storm results in neural cell damage, as well as the apoptosis of astrocytes. The disruption of the blood–brain barrier progresses to septic shock, disseminated intravascular coagulopathy and multi-organ failure. Encephalitis may present with progressive headache, fever and alterations in cognitive state (confusion, behavioural change, dysphasia) or consciousness. Focal neurological signs (paresis) or seizures (focal or generalised) may also occur. Upper motor signs (hyperreflexia and extensor–plantar responses) are often present, but flaccid paralysis and bladder symptoms may occur if the spinal cord is involved.[118] Associated movement disorders or the inappropriate secretion of antidiuretic hormone may be seen. The most sensitive type of imaging for diagnosis of encephalitis is MRI; in HSV encephalitis, CT scans may initially appear normal, but MRI usually shows involvement of the temporal lobes and thalamus.[119] Examination of CSF can assist in differential diagnosis. Refer to Table 17.6 for CSF profiles. Electroencephalography is less sensitive but may be helpful if it shows characteristic features (e.g. lateralising periodic sharp and slow-wave patterns).

Patient management

Neurological derangement often coexists with circulatory insufficiency, impaired respiration, metabolic derangement and seizures. Protecting the patient from injury secondary to raised ICP and seizure activity is essential. Prevention of complications associated with immobility, such as decubitus and pneumonia, is required. It is important to institute droplet infection control precautions in those attending the patient until 24 hours after the initiation of antibiotic therapy (oral and nasal discharge is considered infectious). See *Online resources* for infection control protocols relating specifically to meningitis.

Support in an ICU is often required in encephalitis to maintain ventilation, protect the airway and manage complications, such as cerebral oedema. The management of acute viral encephalitis includes aggressive airway, ventilation, sedation, seizure, haemodynamic and fluid and nutritional support. Clinical deterioration is usually the result of severe cerebral oedema with diencephalic herniation or systemic complications, including generalised sepsis and multiple organ failure. The use of ICP monitoring in acute encephalitis remains controversial but should be considered if there is a rapid deterioration in the level of consciousness, and if imaging suggests raised ICP. Prolonged sedation may be necessary. Decompressive craniotomy may be successful in cases where there is rapid swelling of a non-dominant temporal lobe, as poor outcome is otherwise likely.[119]

Neuromuscular alterations

Generalised muscle weakness can manifest in several disorders that require ICU admission or complicate the clinical course of patients. These may involve motor neuron disease, disorders of the neuromuscular junction, peripheral nerve conduction and muscular contraction. These disorders manifest as Guillain–Barré syndrome, myasthenia gravis and critical illness polyneuropathy and myopathy.

Guillain–Barré syndrome

Guillain–Barré syndrome (GBS) is an immune-mediated disorder resulting from generation of autoimmune antibodies and/or inflammatory cells that cross-react with epitopes on peripheral nerves and roots, leading to demyelination or axonal damage or both, and autoimmune insult to peripheral nerve myelin. Estimates of GBS incidence range from 0.8 to 1.9 cases per 100,000 person-years, are higher in males and increase with age.[120] In Australia, Guillain–Barré has an average incidence of about 1.5 per 100,000, in men slightly higher than in women.[120] Of all patients, 85% recover with minimal residual symptoms; severe residual deficits occur in up to 10%. Residual deficits are most likely in patients with rapid disease progression, those who require mechanical ventilation or those 60 years of age or over. Death occurs in 3–8% of cases, resulting from respiratory failure, autonomic dysfunction, sepsis or pulmonary emboli.[121]

Aetiology

The diagnosis of GBS is confirmed by the findings of cytoalbuminological dissociation (elevation of the CSF protein without concomitant CSF pleocytosis), and by neurophysiological findings suggestive of an acute (usually demyelinating) neuropathy. These abnormalities may not be present in the early stages of the illness.[120] There are two forms of GBS. The demyelinating form, the more common one, is characterised by demyelination and inflammatory infiltrates of the peripheral nerves and roots. In the axonal form the nerves show Wallerian degeneration (the fatty degeneration of a nerve fiber after it has been severed from its cell body) with an absence of inflammation. Discrimination between the axonal and demyelinating forms relies mainly on electrophysiological methods. There is a close association between GBS and a preceding infection, suggesting an immune basis for the syndrome. The commonest infections are due to *Campylobacter jejuni*, cytomegalovirus and Epstein–Barr virus.

Pathophysiology

GBS is the result of a cell-mediated immune attack on peripheral nerve myelin proteins. The Schwann cell is spared, allowing for remyelination in the recovery phase of the disease. With the autoimmune attack there is an influx of macrophages and other immune-mediated agents

that attack myelin, cause inflammation and destruction and leave the axon unable to support nerve conduction. This demyelination may be discrete or diffuse, and may affect the peripheral nerves and their roots at any point from their origin in the spinal cord to the neuromuscular junction. The weakness of GBS results from conduction block and concomitant or primary axonal injury in the affected motor nerves. Pain and paraesthesias are the clinical correlates of sensory nerve involvement.

Clinical manifestations

Onset is rapid, and approximately 20% of cases lead to total paralysis, requiring prolonged intensive therapy with mechanical ventilation. The therapeutic window for GBS is short, and the current optimal treatment with whole plasma exchange or immunoglobulin therapy lacks immunological specificity and only halves the severity of the disease.[120] GBS has three phases – acute, plateau and recovery – each stage lasting from days to weeks and in recovery to months and years. The patient presents with:

- symmetrical weakness, diminished reflexes and upward progression of motor weakness; a history of a viral illness in the previous few weeks suggests the diagnosis
- changes in vital capacity and negative inspiratory force, which are assessed to identify impending neuromuscular respiratory failure.

Indications for ICU admission include the following: ventilatory insufficiency, severe bulbar weakness threatening pulmonary aspiration, autonomic instability or coexisting general medical factors,[122] and often a combination of factors, are present. About 30% of patients have respiratory failure that requires mechanical ventilation.

> **Practice tip**
>
> In Guillian–Barré syndrome vital capacity less than 20 mL/kg is a sign of respiratory fatigue requiring early intubation and leads to earlier extubation and a better prognosis.

Ventilatory failure is primarily caused by inspiratory muscle weakness, although weakness of the abdominal and accessory muscles of respiration, retained airway secretions leading to pulmonary aspiration and atelectasis are all contributory factors. The associated bulbar weakness and autonomic instability reinforce the need for control of the airway and ventilation.

Acute motor and sensory axonal neuropathy, the acute axonal form of GBS, usually presents with a rapidly developing paralysis developing over hours and a rapid development of respiratory failure requiring tracheal intubation and ventilation. $PaCO_2$ may remain constant until just before intubation, emphasising the importance of not relying purely on arterial blood gas analysis to make decisions regarding intubation.

Recently, sensory involvement in relation to pain has been studied asserting the clinical observation of pain ranging from mild to severe in the acute and rehabilitant phases. Chronic pain is often present in survivors of GBS.[123]

There may be total paralysis of all voluntary muscles of the body, including the cranial musculature, the ocular muscles and the pupils. Prolonged paralysis and incomplete recovery are more likely, and prolonged ventilatory support may be necessary. Walgaard and colleagues found that GBS patients who experience rapid disease progression, bulbar dysfunction, bilateral facial weakness or autonomic nerve dysfunction were more likely to require mechanical ventilation.[124] Tracheostomy is usually performed within 2 weeks, and mechanical ventilation is delivered in a supportive mode with minimal yet adequate sedation and pain management.

Patient management

Assessment and understanding of neuromuscular weakness through motor and sensory neurological assessment is vital in the acute care and rehabilitation of GBS patients:

- Comprehensive respiratory assessment (level of overall patient comfort, frequency and depth of breathing, forced vital capacity, use of accessory muscles, presence of paradoxical respiration and integrity of upper airway reflexes), ABG data and chest radiography determine levels of fatigue in both the acute stage (for intubation and ventilation) and rehabilitation (weaning) stage. Long-term ventilation increases the risk of ventilator-associated pneumonia (VAP), and routine surveillance for VAP is vital.

- Cardiovascular assessment is important, as serious tachyarrhythmias and bradyarrhythmias and destabilising fluctuations in blood pressure caused by autonomic impairment are prevalent. This feature is common during fatigue, sleep and states of dehydration. Often, autonomic dysfunction is worst in the early stages of a nosocomial infection.[125]

- Cranial nerve assessment and dermatome (for sensory) and muscle strength assessment assist in mapping the progression, severity and rehabilitation of the disease and determining the risk of aspiration. Pain (especially neuropathic) is particularly common in GBS during changes in myelination, and can be difficult to treat.[126] Assessment will include all aspects as indicated for the long-term immobile, intubated, ventilated and neuromuscular-impaired patient.

When caring for a neuromuscular-impaired patient, a structured care plan is essential for continuity of care and should involve the patient and family. This is of particular importance in the long-term recovery phase, where the provision of sleep, good nutrition and prevention of the complications of immobility (nosocomial infections, deep vein thrombosis, integument and muscular weakening, adequate nutrition and constipation) are important:

- Endotracheal and pharyngeal suction can be demanding (weakened upper airway reflexes), and sputum plugging and retention requires frequent repositioning and physiotherapy.

- Routine daily gentle exercise as part of a flexible program improves wellbeing and strength.

- Fatigue must be avoided, as autonomic nerve dysfunction, deafferent pain syndromes, muscle pain and depression can be exacerbated.

- Suctioning, coughing, bladder distension, constipation and the Valsalva manoeuvre can also aggravate autonomic nerve dysfunction instability.

- Therapeutic massage, warm and cold packs and careful positioning contribute to comfort and pain management.

- The patient's surroundings should be pleasant and presentable, especially during long recovery.

- Communication techniques need to be refined to prevent fatigue and frustration.

- Patience, tolerance, empathy, humour and family involvement assist the patient in psychological resilience and recovery.

In the acute phase, accurate diagnosis and timely ventilatory support are provided by effective communication between primary and in-hospital care providers. Patients who require mechanical ventilation typically present with rapidly progressive weakness and fatigue.

The side effects of intravenous immunoglobulin administration include low-grade fever, chills, myalgia, diaphoresis, fluid imbalance, neutropenia, nausea and headaches, and at times acute tubular necrosis. Administration and assessment require adherence to transfusion protocols. Plasmapheresis is performed by transfusion nurse specialists in collaboration with the patient care nurse. Multidisciplinary case management is utilised after stabilisation in the acute phase, especially when the level of severity is determined. Recovery and rehabilitation process information is provided to the patient and family so that consultation and communication are effective in recovery.

Myasthenia gravis

Myasthenia gravis is an autoimmune disorder caused by autoantibodies against the nicotinic acetylcholine receptor on the postsynaptic membrane at the neuromuscular junction. It is characterised by weakness and fatigability of the voluntary muscles. It peaks in the third and sixth decades of life. Its prevalence in Western countries is 14.2/100,000.[127] Prevalence rates have been rising steadily over recent decades, probably due to decreased mortality, longer survival and higher rates of diagnosis. The development of respiratory failure, progressive bulbar weakness leading to failure of airway protection and severe limb and truncal weakness causing extensive paralysis, as in a myasthenic crisis, all may result in admission to ICU.

Aetiology

Myasthenic crisis occurs when weakness from acquired myasthenia gravis becomes severe enough to necessitate intubation for ventilatory support or airway protection.

At some point in their illness, usually within 2–3 years after diagnosis, 12–16% of myasthenic patients experience crisis. This occurrence is most likely in patients whose history includes previous crisis, oropharyngeal weakness or thymoma. Possible triggers include infections, aspiration, physical and emotional stress and changes in medications.[128] Most antibiotics have a trigger effect and should be carefully prescribed by an informed doctor. Median duration of hospitalisation for crisis is 1 month. The patient usually spends half of this time intubated in the ICU. About 25% of patients are extubated on hospital day 7, 50% by hospital day 13, and 75% by hospital day 31. The mortality rate during hospitalisation for crisis has fallen from nearly 50% in the early 1960s to between 3% and 10% today. With the incidence of crisis remaining stable over the past 30 years, this fall in mortality rates probably reflects improvements in the intensive care assessment and management of these patients.[129]

Pathophysiology

In myasthenia gravis both structural changes in the architecture of the neuromuscular junction and dynamic alterations in the turnover of acetylcholine receptors erode the safety margin and efficiency of neuromuscular transmission. Of all patients with myasthenia gravis, 80–85% have an identifiable and quantifiable antibody found in the immunoglogulin G fraction of plasma, which is responsible for blocking receptors to the action of acetylcholine at the neuromuscular junction.[128] Therefore, successful neuromuscular transmission is markedly affected by small and subtle changes in acetylcholine release and other triggers (as above), and this gives rise to the decrement in transmission with repetitive stimulation and the characteristic fatigable muscle weakness. Pharmacological management for myasthenia gravis includes the use of anticholinesterases (pyridostigmine), steroids, azathioprine and cyclophosphamide. Thymectomy reduces the antibodies responsible for acetylcholine blockade and is often performed early in the disease.[129] Plasmapheresis and intravenous immunoglobulin are used in the short term for myasthenic crisis and are especially useful for preventing respiratory collapse or assisting with weaning.

Clinical manifestations

In a myasthenic crisis, vital capacity falls, cough and sigh mechanisms deteriorate, atelectasis develops and hypoxaemia results.[130] Ultimately, fatigue, hypercarbia and ventilatory collapse occur. Commonly, superimposed pulmonary infections lead to increased morbidity and mortality. Assessment for triggers begins with a careful review of systems, with attention to recent fevers, chills, cough, chest pain, dysphagia, nasal regurgitation of liquids and dysuria. Detailed history taking should note any trauma, surgical procedures and medication use. General assessment includes vital signs; ear, nose and throat inspection; chest auscultation; and abdominal check. In addition to supportive care and the removal of triggers, management of myasthenic crisis includes treatment of the underlying myasthenia gravis. An experienced neurologist, who will ultimately provide the patient's care outside the ICU, should be part of the care team. Options for treatment during crisis include: use of acetylcholinesterase inhibitors, plasma exchange, IV immunoglobulins and immunosuppressive drugs, including corticosteroids.[131]

Patient management

Careful and accurate assessment by the nurse in the presenting myasthenic crisis patient determines the triggers of the event and incorporates a history, including infections and prescribed medications. These medications can exacerbate acetylcholine receptor blockade, and respiratory demand proves too much for the myasthenic patient. Awareness by the nurse of trigger medications ensures advocacy for the patient when the prescription is uncertain.[128]

- Respiratory and cardiovascular assessment incorporates upper and lower airway muscle weakness. ABGs are a poor marker for intubation and ventilation because these values change late in the decompensation cycle. Being able to recognise fatigue (inability to speak, poor lung expansion, VC below 1 L, shoulder and arm weakness) in patients with neuromuscular weakness and air hunger is important.[130]

- Non-invasive ventilation can be difficult to administer safely, with the potential for aspiration due to insidious upper airway weakness; however, the option should be considered with careful assessment of gag, swallow and cough reflexes in order to prevent intubation.[129]

- Neuromuscular blockade should be avoided (residual long-term paralysis), with the use of glottal local anaesthetic spray for emergency intubation and ventilation.

- Placement of small-bore duodenal tubes decreases the risk of aspiration and may be more comfortable than regular nasogastric tubes for the patient.

- Tracheostomy is generally not needed, as the duration of intubation is often less than 2 weeks.

- Cardiac assessment needs to include assessment for arrhythmias of both atrial and ventricular origin due to autonomic nerve dysfunction.[128] These can be insidious and can be provoked by subtle changes in electrolytes.

- Nursing care will relate to the needs of long-term immobilised, intubated, ventilated patients with neuromuscular alterations.

Myasthenia gravis patients have similar care needs to those of patients with GBS (refer to *Patient management* for GBS). Fatigue and the structure and timing of care are very important. Flexibility of care is important, as energy fluctuates on an hourly basis.[130] Despite having a shorter recovery time than GBS, weaning and recovery in myasthenia gravis is still a slow process and impulsive extubation is discouraged.[131] Therapy should be tailored on an individual basis using best clinical judgement.

Status epilepticus

Status epilepticus (SE) has been generally defined as enduring seizure activity that is not likely to stop spontaneously. The traditional SE definition is 30 minutes of continuous seizure activity (which has been updated due to neurological alteration to 5 minutes only) or two or more seizures without full recovery of consciousness between the seizures.[132] There are as many types of SE as there are types of seizures. The distinction between convulsive and non-convulsive SE depends on clinical observation and on a clear understanding of several SE types. Estimates of the overall incidence of SE have varied from 10 to 60 per 100,000 person-years, depending on the population studied and the definitions used.[133] Over half the cases of SE are acute symptomatic, emphasising the importance in management of identifying an acute precipitant. Infections with fever are the major cause of SE, accounting for 52% of cases, while in adults low antiepileptic drug levels, cerebrovascular accident, hypoxia, metabolic causes and alcohol represent the main acute causes. The mortality in status epilepticus is about 20%; most patients die of the underlying condition rather than the status epilepticus itself. SE can result in permanent neurological and mental deterioration, particularly in young children; the risks of morbidity greatly increase with longer duration of the status epilepticus episode. SE in the intensive care setting falls into two main groups: those transferred to the ICU because of uncontrolled SE (refractory SE) and those who are admitted to the ICU for another reason and have SE as an additional finding.[134]

Pathophysiology

At a cellular level, status epilepticus results from a failure of normal inhibitory pathways, primarily mediated by gamma-aminobutyric acid acting via gamma-aminobutyric acid A receptors. This loss of inhibitory drive allows the activation of excitatory feedback loops, leading to repetitive, synchronous firing of large groups of neurons. As seizure activity continues, there is further decline in gamma-aminobutergic inhibitory tone that counterbalances neuronal excitation function. Continued excitatory input mediated primarily by glutamate leads to neuronal cell death.[134]

Clinical manifestations

Convulsive SE is a medical emergency. The initial consequence of a prolonged convulsion is a massive release of plasma catecholamines, which results in a rise in heart rate, blood pressure and plasma glucose. During this stage cardiac arrhythmias are often seen, and may be fatal. CBF is greatly increased, and thus glucose delivery to active cerebral tissue is maintained. As the seizure continues, hyperthermia above 40°C with lactic and respiratory acidosis continues to intensify, especially without adequate resuscitation and control of the seizure.[135]

The SE may then enter a second, late phase in which cerebral and systemic protective measures progressively fail. The main characteristics of this phase are: a fall in blood pressure; a loss of cerebral autoregulation, resulting in the dependence of CBF on systemic blood pressure; and hypoglycaemia due to the exhaustion of glycogen stores and increased neurogenic insulin secretion. Intracranial pressure can rise precipitously in SE. The combined effects of systemic hypotension and intracranial hypertension may result in a compromised cerebral circulation and cerebral oedema. Intracranial pressure monitoring is advisable in prolonged severe SE when raised intracranial pressure is suspected. Further complications that can occur include rhabdomyolysis leading to acute tubular necrosis, hyperkalaemia and hyponatraemia.[135]

Patient management

The following patient management should be considered.

Resuscitation

SE requires control of the seizure and then investigation regarding the cause. Airway protection is often difficult in the seizing patient, so the first line of treatment includes basic life-support measures followed by the administration of IV propofol, midazolam or, in refractory cases, phenytoin. Neuromuscular blockade will be required to facilitate intubation in patients who continue to have tonic–clonic seizure activity despite these pharmacological interventions. Rocuronium (1 mg/kg), a short-acting, non-depolarising muscle relaxant that is devoid of significant haemodynamic effects and does not raise intracranial pressure, is the preferred agent. Succinylcholine should be avoided if possible, as the patient may be hyperkalaemic as a consequence of possible rhabdomyolysis. Prolonged neuromuscular blockade should be avoided as it only stops the motor response, hence masking the altered neuronal activity.[131] Once the seizures are controlled, intubation and ventilation can protect the airway and potentially reverse the acidosis. In the patient who already has an airway secured, urgent IV administration of propofol, midazolam or phenytoin is indicated.[132]

> ### Practice tip
>
> The three most crucial factors determining the outcome from status epilepticus are the underlying aetiology, the speed of anti-seizure treatment and the age of the person. Older aged individuals with status epilepticus frequently have a symptomatic cause, possess a more limited reserve to recover due to comorbidities and have a higher mortality rate.

Specific post SE patient assessment

Post SE, the patient remains intubated, ventilated and sedated. Neurological assessment is limited in the sedated patient. Pupillary response is usually sluggish and reflects the medication prescribed. Routine monitoring in an ICU is essential, with CT and MRI to exclude mass lesions. Blood glucose level should be checked immediately by bedside testing. Blood should be tested for electrolytes, magnesium, phosphate, calcium, liver and renal function, haematocrit, white blood cell count, platelet count, anti-epileptic drug levels, toxic drugs and substances (particularly salicylates) and alcohol.

EEG monitoring in the ICU for refractory SE is essential, as a patient may enter a drug-induced coma with little outward sign of convulsions yet have ongoing electrographic epileptic activity. Furthermore, continuous recording will give an indication of worsening of generalised convulsive status epilepticus regardless of the presence or absence of sedating drugs or paralysing agents. This can be monitored only by EEG and manifests as bilateral EEG ictal discharges. Deeper sedation and anaesthesia is then indicated and can be titrated to EEG results.[136]

Pharmacological patient management

Because only a small fraction of seizures go on to become SE, the probability that a given seizure will proceed to SE is small at the start of the seizure and increases with seizure duration. The goal of pharmacological therapy is to achieve the rapid and safe termination of the seizure, and to prevent its recurrence without adverse effects on the cardiovascular and respiratory systems or without altering the level of consciousness. Diazepam, lorazepam, midazolam, phenytoin and phenobarbitone have all been used as first-line therapy for the termination of SE.[102] The antiseizure activity of phenytoin is complex; however, its major action appears to block the voltage-sensitive, use-dependent sodium channels. Once SE is controlled, attention turns to preventing its recurrence. The best regimen for an individual patient will depend on the cause of the seizure and any history of antiepileptic drug therapy. A patient who develops SE in the course of alcohol withdrawal may not need antiepileptic drug therapy once the withdrawal has run its course. In contrast, patients with new, ongoing epileptogenic stimuli (e.g. encephalitis or trauma) may require high doses of antiepileptic medication to control their seizures.

Summary

This chapter provides a description and application of neurological alterations and their management. The chapter launches with an overview of neurological dysfunction, specifically pathophysiological alterations of consciousness, alterations in motor and sensory function and alterations in cerebral perfusion and metabolism. Cerebral oedema is related to intracranial pressure preceding the therapeutic management of these conditions. Intracranial hypertension is discussed in association with cerebral perfusion and metabolic events. Delayed cerebral ischaemia and vasospasm are applied to brain injury in general but, more specifically, aneurysmal subarachnoid haemorrhage. Central nervous system disorders include traumatic brain and spinal injury, their aetiology, clinical pathophysiology and management. Cerebrovascular disorders focus on ischaemic stroke, intracerebral haemorrhage and aneurysmal subarachnoid haemorrhage. The research vignette reports on a randomised controlled trial of blood pressure reduction in ischaemic stroke in a highly prevalent Chinese population. Meningitis and encephalitis are included in the section on infection and inflammation with Guillain–Barré syndrome, myasthenic crisis and status epilepticus in the neuromuscular alterations component. A traumatic brain injury case is presented with learning activities.

Case study

Luke, a 25-year-old male, was standing outside a pub on a Friday night and became involved in a verbal altercation with another man. Without warning Luke was punched in the left side of his head, causing him to fall backwards and strike his head on the concrete pavement. As the attack was sudden, Luke did not have time to break his fall with his hands and his head took the full impact. It was about 10 minutes before a passerby recognised that Luke was unconsciousness.

An ambulance was called and arrived approximately 6 minutes later. On initial assessment Luke's GCS was 7: eye opening response = 2, verbal response = 2 and motor response = 3. His limbs: extension in the right and abnormal flexion in the left to pain. His vital signs: heart rate 85 beats per minute and regular, respirations 12 per minute and regular. Blood pressure was 135/89 mmHg. A hard C spine collar was applied and spinal precautions were applied. As the officers were carrying out this initial assessment, Luke's GCS dropped to 4 (eye opening response = 1, verbal response = 1 and motor response = 2). His pupils were unequal, the left pupil was noted to be unresponsive and size 6 and his right pupil was briskly reactive and size 3. At the same time his breath rate dropped to 8 per minute and his blood pressure rose to 168/98 mmHg. The ambulance officers inserted a wide bore antecubital fossa cannula and administered mannitol 100 mL immediately stat. Luke was intubated and hand ventilated with a size 7.5 endotracheal tube and transferred to a major tertiary hospital approximately 500 metres away. The time from the 000 phone call being logged to 'time off stretcher' in the emergency department was 37 minutes.

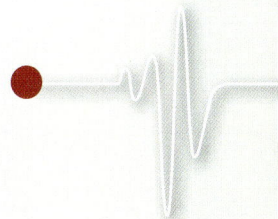

On arrival into the emergency department Luke was attached to a ventilator. His GCS remained as 4, but his vital signs were unremarkable. A full primary trauma survey was performed together with a CT scan of his head and cervical spine. The CT scan of his head indicated an acute left-sided extradural haematoma, 13 mm in depth overlying the left temporal lobe with effacement of the left lateral ventricle and 3 mm midline shift to the right. The CT of the cervical spine confirmed no abnormality. Luke was transferred to the operating theatre where a left-sided craniotomy and evacuation of a large extradural haematoma was performed. An EVD was inserted into the right lateral ventricle. There was significant swelling of the brain tissue during surgery, so that the bone flap was unable to be replaced at the end of surgery. The neurosurgeons prescribed an ICP below 20 mmHg and CPP greater than 65 mmHg. Luke was then transferred to the ICU.

INTENSIVE CARE

In the ICU Luke was connected to the ventilator and monitor. EtCO$_2$ continuous monitoring was in progress. At that time his ICP increased to 28 mmHg. In response, the EVD system was opened to drain CSF and Luke was placed in a reverse Trendelenburg position with neutral alignment while maintaining spinal precautions. IV propofol and fentanyl infusions were commenced. Luke's vital signs on admission to the ICU were: GCS 3; left pupil remained fixed and dilated, size 6, right pupil size 3 and sluggishly reactive; core temperature 37.9°C; heart rate 62 beats per minute; sinus rhythm; blood pressure 117/54, MAP 69 mmHg. Noradrenaline infusion was commenced through a central venous catheter commencing at 0.567 mcg/kg/min to maintain a CPP greater than 65 mmHg.

Luke's core body temperature was actively cooled to between 35°C and 36°C. To prevent shivering, an IV cisaturcurium infusion was commenced. In response to a high PaCO$_2$ of 43 mmHg his respiratory rate on the ventilator was increased to 16 breaths per minute. After these interventions Luke's ICP reduced to 19 mmHg.

Luke's parents finally arrived and a meeting was arranged for them to speak with the neurosurgeons and the intensive care specialist. During this meeting Luke's prognosis was described as very poor due to the nature of his injury. Also, the pupillary changes, changes in vital signs and fact that his brain appeared to be non-pulsatile at the end of surgery were indicators of a very poor prognosis.

DAY 2

Over the next 24 hours, Luke's condition remained critical. A progress CT scan was performed and showed evolving petechial haemorrhages in the pons located in the brain stem. He remained heavily sedated and neuromuscular blockade was continued. The ICP continued to fluctuate, ranging between 17 mmHg and 26 mmHg. The spikes in ICP were treated with IV boluses of propofol and fentanyl. At one occasion in response to rising ICP, a Cushing's triad response was noted. The heart rate dropped to 48 beats per minute, and the systolic blood pressure increased to 187 mmHg despite the noradrenaline infusion being titrated to 0 mL/hour. In response, IV mannitol 100 mL was administered. The prescribed CPP of greater than 65 mmHg was maintained by titrating high doses of IV noradrenaline with regular IV fluid boluses. The EVD height was initially set at 15 cmH$_2$O and on free drainage but, with the rises in ICP, this was lowered to 10 cmH$_2$O. This was to allow for a greater drainage of CSF to reduce the pressure and volume within the brain. The ventilator settings were adjusted to maintain a PaCO$_2$ between 35 and 40 mmHg. Active cooling continued, maintaining core temperature between 35°C and 36°C. Heart rate ranged from 63–72 beats per minute. Central venous pressure varied from 6 to 13 mmHg.

Luke's IV fluid intake included IV infusions of 0.9% normal saline, propofol, fentanyl, cisaturcurium infusions and noradrenaline. An IV crystalloid fluid bolus of 250 mL was administered on two occasions due to increasing noradrenaline requirements, large urinary output and low central venous pressure measurements. Luke was also commenced on enteral feeding via a nasogastric tube. Luke's hourly urinary output varied between 40 and 195 mL/hour. Given the seriousness of Luke's condition, his parents, siblings and close friends were in attendance throughout the day and night and they were given regular updates in regard to Luke's progress and condition by the nursing and medical teams.

DAY 3

At 04:26 Luke's ICP increased suddenly to 31 mmHg. His core temperature and PaCO$_2$ were within the prescribed target limits. Luke's heart rate initially increased to 145 beats per minute and then slowed to 39 beats per minute and his blood pressure rose to 194 mmHg. During this time his right pupil had become unreactive and increased to size 5. A further bolus of mannitol 100 mL was given immediately stat and the EVD height was lowered to 5 cmH$_2$0. Over the next 20 minutes Luke's ICP fell to 22 mmHg. Despite this, Luke remained bradycardic (rate 48 beats per minute) and noradrenaline requirements increased to 1.11 mcg/kg/min. Soon after, Luke's hourly urinary output measure increased to 480 mL of dilute urine, which was attributed to the mannitol. In the subsequent hour the urinary output increased to 680 mL and serum and urine osmolality samples were sent to the laboratory. The results were consistent with diabetes insipidus. A fluid bolus was administered to counteract the diuresis and 1 mcg of desmopressin intravenously was prescribed and administered with effect.

Later that morning the neurosurgeons and intensive care staff specialist requested to meet with Luke's family. As with all meetings between the medical teams and family, the bedside nurse was in attendance. They were informed that Luke was showing signs consistent with severe brain damage and possibly even brain death. The decision was made to reduce the sedation and the neuromuscular blockade and, if the ICP remained at 20 mmHg or below, to cease it altogether to allow the medical team to assess Luke's neurological condition and to carry out cranial nerve testing. Although devastated by the outcome of the meeting, the family appeared to understand the progression of Luke's condition. During the course of the afternoon, sedation and neuromuscular blockade were reduced and finally ceased altogether without a correlating rise in ICP. Overnight, haemodynamics were maintained within acceptable parameters with the support of noradrenaline, fluid bolus and further desmopressin administration. The family stayed with Luke overnight. The next day Luke was declared brain dead after extensive brain death tests. The medical and nursing team met with the family to inform them that Luke had died. At this stage the family broached the topic of organ donation as they had discussed this amongst themselves overnight. They felt that Luke would have wanted to donate his organs. A meeting was set up with the organ donation coordinator who then started the process. Following the donation of his organs, Luke's family, in a follow-up with the coordinator, stated that they found much solace from the fact that he had donated his organs and so had improved the lives of others.

CASE STUDY QUESTIONS

1 With a brain injury to the left side of the brain, what deficits would you expect to see in your patient? What potential communication problems may be encountered and why?

2 From your reading of the *Case study*, explain the rationale for why pupil dysfunction is ipsilateral while limb movement is contralateral.

3 What clinical signs are indicative of a fractured base of skull?

4 Explain the compensatory mechanisms used by the body to help control intracranial pressure.

5 What is the basis for PaCO$_2$ control in a patient with a traumatic brain injury?

RESEARCH VIGNETTE[137]

He J, Zhang Y, Xu T, Zhao Q, Wang D, Chen CS et al; CATIS Investigators. Effects of immediate blood pressure reduction on death and major disability in patients with acute ischemic stroke: the CATIS randomized clinical trial. JAMA 2014;311(5):479–89

Abstract

Importance: Although the benefit of reducing blood pressure for primary and secondary prevention of stroke has been established, the effect of antihypertensive treatment in patients with acute ischemic stroke is uncertain.

Objective: To evaluate whether immediate blood pressure reduction in patients with acute ischemic stroke would reduce death and major disability at 14 days or hospital discharge.

Design, setting, and participants: The China Antihypertensive Trial in Acute Ischemic Stroke, a single-blind, blinded end-points randomized clinical trial, conducted among 4071 patients with nonthrombolysed ischemic stroke within

48 hours of onset and elevated systolic blood pressure. Patients were recruited from 26 hospitals across China between August 2009 and May 2013.

Interventions: Patients (n = 2038) were randomly assigned to receive antihypertensive treatment (aimed at lowering systolic blood pressure by 10% to 25% within the first 24 hours after randomization, achieving blood pressure less than 140/90 mmHg within 7 days, and maintaining this level during hospitalization) or to discontinue all antihypertensive medications (control) during hospitalization (n = 2033).

Main outcomes and measures: Primary outcome was a combination of death and major disability (modified Rankin Scale score ≥3) at 14 days or hospital discharge.

Results: Mean systolic blood pressure was reduced from 166.7 mmHg to 144.7 mmHg (–12.7%) within 24 hours in the antihypertensive treatment group and from 165.6 mmHg to 152.9 mmHg (–7.2%) in the control group within 24 hours after randomization (difference, –5.5% [95% CI, –4.9 to –6.1%]; absolute difference, –9.1 mmHg [95% CI, –10.2 to –8.1]; P < 0.001). Mean systolic blood pressure was 137.3 mmHg in the antihypertensive treatment group and 146.5 mmHg in the control group at day 7 after randomization (difference, –9.3 mm Hg [95% CI, –10.1 to –8.4]; P < 0.001). The primary outcome did not differ between treatment groups (683 events [antihypertensive treatment] vs 681 events [control]; odds ratio, 1.00 [95% CI, 0.88 to 1.14]; P = 0.98) at 14 days or hospital discharge. The secondary composite outcome of death and major disability at 3-month posttreatment follow-up did not differ between treatment groups (500 events [antihypertensive treatment] vs 502 events [control]; odds ratio, 0.99 [95% CI, 0.86 to 1.15]; P = 0.93).

Conclusion and relevance: Among patients with acute ischemic stroke, blood pressure reduction with anti-hypertensive medications, compared with the absence of hypertensive medication, did not reduce the likelihood of death and major disability at 14 days or hospital discharge.

Critique

This is the first randomised trial with sufficient statistical power to test the effect of immediate blood pressure reduction on adverse clinical outcomes in patients with acute ischaemic stroke. One of the major unresolved management issues in stroke care is how to manage this early elevation of blood pressure in patients with cerebral ischaemia. Despite the large sample size, blood pressure reduction with antihypertensive medications, compared with the absence of hypertensive medication, did not reduce the likelihood of death and major disability at 14 days or hospital discharge.

This study reflects the population and clinical practice of China. Compared with white populations, Chinese have a higher age-adjusted incidence of stroke, a lower mean age of stroke onset and a higher proportion of strokes attributable to ICH.[138] Enrolled patients were substantially younger, smoked more often and received concomitant acute anticoagulation therapy more often than typical Western stroke cohorts.

The CATIS design and implementation has some limitations. The open-label intervention where both the researchers and participants know which treatment is being administered left outcome assessments vulnerable to rater bias and may have influenced the results. Also, the entry stroke severity was relatively mild, with a median National Institutes of Health Stroke Scale score of 4. This degree of severity parallels the average severity of ischaemic stroke in clinical practice but is substantially less than other clinical trials because of the high rate of good outcomes expected with mild deficits at presentation. As a result, two-thirds of enrolled patients in the control group achieved the primary outcome (alive and not disabled), reducing opportunities for the intervention to demonstrate benefit. As well, patients treated with intravenous thrombolytic therapy at baseline were excluded because of different requirements for blood pressure reduction, excluding another group of greater severity. The remaining unanswered question in blood pressure management in early ischaemic stroke involves the acute period, within the first few hours after stroke onset, when there is still substantial penumbral, at-risk tissue and if blood pressure modification has a role in improving outcome.

Learning activities

1   What are the different types of cerebral oedema that can occur?

2   What are the main therapeutic management strategies used to minimise vasospasm post clipping of a ruptured aneurysm?

3   A child is taken to the emergency room with lethargy, fever and a stiff neck on examination.

    a) What findings on initial lumbar puncture indicate bacterial versus viral meningitis? b) In the case of bacterial meningitis, what are the most likely organisms?

4   Your patient had symptoms of an ischaemic stroke approximately 2 hours ago and is undergoing a confirmatory CT scan in 30 minutes. You know tPA must be administered within 3 hours of the symptoms. What actions would you take? What is your rationale for these actions?

Online resources

Academy Spinal Cord Injury Nurses (ASCIP), www.academyscipro.org

Australian Institute of Health and Welfare publication: Stroke and its management in Australia: an update, www.aihw.gov.au/publication-detail/?id=60129543613

Brain Injury Association of America, www.biausa.org

Brain Trauma Foundation, www.braintrauma.org

Centers for Disease Control: Traumatic Brain Injury, www.cdc.gov/traumaticbraininjury

Cervical collars, www.youtube.com/watch?v=cYxnp6ml8mE

Cervical traction, www.alfredhealth.org.au/Assets/Files/SpinalClearanceManagementProtocol_External.pdf

CSF drainage and ICP monitoring system, www.youtube.com/watch?v=MPpH8MnXhb8&list=PLH9gpVKlHL6p09M1Pz8Upo qggfwLsfxzA

Ethical guidelines for the care of people in post-coma unresponsiveness, www.nhmrc.gov.au/_files_nhmrc/file/publications/synopses/e81.pdf

External ventricular drain, www.aann.org/uploads/AANN11_ICPEVDnew.pdf

Hypertonic Saline Protocol, https://ambulance.qld.gov.au/docs/cpm_dtp_combined_040514_b.pdf

Meningitis, http://netsvic.org.au/clinicalguide/cpg.cfm?doc_id=5179

Model of Stroke Care Western Australia, www.healthnetworks.health.wa.gov.au/modelsofcare/docs/Stroke_Model_of_Care.pdf

National Resource Centre for Traumatic Brain Injury, www.brainlink.org.au

National Stroke Foundation of Australia publication, www.strokefoundation.com.au

Sports injuries: head and spine, www.injuryupdate.com.au/injury-head-neck-spinal.php

Stroke Management Guidelines, http://strokefoundation.com.au/site/media/clinical_guidelines_stroke_managment_2010_interactive.pdf

Stroke Thrombolytic Protocol, www.health.wa.gov.au/circularsNew/attachments/556.pdf

Traumatic Brain Injury National Data Centre, www.tbindc.org

World Health Organization Neurological Disorders, www.who.int/mental_health/.../neurological_disorders_report_web.pdf

Further reading

Anaesth Intensive Care Med 2014;15(4):141–208. Special edition on neurosurgical anaesthesia and physiology, <http://www.sciencedirect.com/science/journal/14720299/15/4>; [accessed 11.14].

Crlt Care Clin 2014;30(4).657–842. Special edition on neurocritical care, <http://www.sciencedirect.com/science/journal/07490704/30/4>; [accessed 11.14].

Gibson CL. Cerebral ischemic stroke: is gender important? J Cereb Blood Flow Metab 2013;33(9):1355–61. Open Access, <http://www.nature.com/jcbfm/journal/v33/n9/full/jcbfm2013102a.html>; [accessed 11.14].

Schweizer S, Meisel A, Marschenz S. Epigenetic mechanisms in cerebral ischemia. J Cereb Blood Flow Metab 2013; 33(9):1335–46. Open Access, <http://www.nature.com/jcbfm/journal/v33/n9/full/jcbfm201393a.html>; [accessed 11.14].

References

1 Cavanna AE, Shah S, Eddy CM, Williams A, Rickards H. Consciousness: a neurological perspective. Behav Neurol 2011;24(1):107–16.

2 Duffau H. Does post-lesional subcortical plasticity exist in the human brain? Neurosci Res 2009;65(2):131–5.

3 Cavanna AE, Cavanna SL, Servo S, Monaco F. The neural correlates of impaired consciousness in coma and unresponsive states. Discov Med 2010;9(48):431–8.

4 Strosznajder RP, Czubowicz K, Jesko H, Strosznajder JB. Poly(ADP-ribose) metabolism in brain and its role in ischemia pathology. Mol Neurobiol 2010;41(2–3):187–96.

5 Huff JS, Fountain NB. Pathophysiology and definitions of seizures and status epilepticus. Emerg Med Clin North Am 2011;29(1):1-13.

6 Varelas PN, Spanaki MV, Mirski MA. Status epilepticus: an update. Curr Neurol Neurosci Rep 2013;13(7):357.

7 Veening JG, Barendregt HP. The regulation of brain states by neuroactive substances distributed via the cerebrospinal fluid; a review. Cerebrospinal Fluid Res 2010;6(7):1.

8 Winhammar J, Rowe D, Henderson R, Kiernan M. Assessment of disease progression in motor neuron disease. Lancet Neurol 2005;4(4):229–38.

9 Di Pino G, Pellegrino G, Assenza G, Capone F, Ferreri F, Formica D. Modulation of brain plasticity in stroke: a novel model for neurorehabilitation. Nat Rev Neurol 2014;10(10):597-608.

10 Silverman MN, Heim CM, Nater UM, Marques AH, Sternberg EM. Neuroendocrine and immune contributors to fatigue. PM&R 2010;2(5):338-46.

11 Thayer JF, Ahs F, Fredrikson M, Sollers JJ 3rd, Wager TD. A meta-analysis of heart rate variability and neuroimaging studies: implications for heart rate variability as a marker of stress and health. Neurosci Biobehav Rev 2012;36(2):747-56.

12 Bulstrode H, Nicoll JAR, Hudson G, Chinnery PF, Di Pietro V, Belli A. Mitochondrial DNA and traumatic brain injury. Ann Neurol 2014;75(2):186-95.

13 Trendelenburg G. Molecular regulation of cell fate in cerebral ischemia: role of the inflammasome and connected pathways. J Cereb Blood Flow Metab 2014; advance online publication, September 17, 2014; doi:10.1038/jcbfm.2014.159.

14 Kumar VSS, Gopalakrishnan A, Nazıroğlu M, Rajanikant GK. Calcium ion – the key player in cerebral ischemia. Curr Med Chem 2014;21(18):2065-75.

15 Smith CJ, Lawrence CB, Rodriguez-Grande B, Kovacs KJ, Pradillo JM, Denes A. The immune system in stroke: clinical challenges and their translation to experimental research. J Neuroimmune Pharmacol 2013;8(4):867–87.

16 Bhattarai S, Ning Z, Tuerxun T. EEG and SPECT changes in acute ischemic stroke. J Neurol Neurophysiol 2014;5:190.

17 Giacino JT, Fins JJ, Laureys S, Schiff ND. Disorders of consciousness after acquired brain injury: the state of the science. Nature Reviews Neurology 2014;10(2):99-114.

18 Partington T, Farmery A. Intracranial pressure and cerebral blood flow. Anaesthesia & Intensive Care Medicine 2014;15(4):189-94.

19 Iffland P, II, Grant G, Janigro D. Mechanisms of cerebral edema leading to early seizures after traumatic brain injury. In: Lo EH, Lok J, Ning M, Whalen MJ, eds. Vascular mechanisms in CNS trauma. Springer Series in Translational Stroke Research 5. New York: Springer; 2014, pp 29-45.

20 Strbian D, Durukan A, Pitkonen M, Marinkovic I, Tatlisumak E, Pedrono E et al. The blood–brain barrier is continuously open for several weeks following transient focal cerebral ischemia. Neuroscience 2008;153(1):175–81.

21 Fukuda AM, Badaut J. Aquaporin 4: a player in cerebral edema and neuroinflammation. J Neuroinflammation 2012;9:279.

22 Kiefer M, Unterberg A. The differential diagnosis and treatment of normal-pressure hydrocephalus. Dtsch Arztebl Int 2012;109(1-2):15–26.

23 McLeod A. Traumatic injuries to the head and spine, 2: nursing considerations. Br J Nurs 2004;13(17):1041–9.

24 Cummings BM, Yager PH, Murphy SA, Kalish B, Bhupali C, Bell R et al. Managing edema and intracranial pressure in the intensive care unit. In: Lo EH, Lok J, Ning MM, Whalen MJ, eds. Vascular mechanisms in CNS trauma. New York: Springer; 2014, pp 363-78.

25 Di Ieva A, Schmitz EM, Cusimano MD. Analysis of intracranial pressure: past, present, and future. Neuroscientist 2013;19(6):592-603.

26 Czosnyka M, Pickard J. Monitoring and interpretation of intracranial pressure. J Neurol Neurosurg Psychiat 2004;75(6):813–21.

27 Porth C, Martin G. Essentials of pathophysiology: concepts of altered health states. 3rd ed. Philadelphia: Lippincott, Williams & Wilkins; 2011.

28 Latronico N. The relationship between the intracranial pressure–volume index and cerebral autoregulation. Appl Physiol Intensive Care Med 1: Physiological Notes-Technical Notes-Seminal Studies in Intensive Care. 2013;1:153.

29 Martini RP, Deem S, Treggiari MM. Targeting brain tissue oxygenation in traumatic brain injury. Respir Care 2013;58(1):162-72.

30 Oddo M, Levine JM, Mackenzie L, Frangos S, Feihl F, Kasner SE et al. Brain hypoxia is associated with short-term outcome after severe traumatic brain injury independently of intracranial hypertension and low cerebral perfusion pressure. Neurosurgery 2011;69(5):1037-45.

31 Jaeger M, Dengl M, Meixensberger J, Schuhmann MU. Effects of cerebrovascular pressure reactivity-guided optimization of cerebral perfusion pressure on brain tissue oxygenation after traumatic brain injury. Crit Care Med 2010;38(5):1343–7.

32 Brain Trauma Foundation, American Association of Neurological Surgeons, Joint Section on Neurotrauma and Critical Care. Guidelines for management of severe head injury. New York: Brain Trauma Foundation; 2007.

33 Le Roux P. Physiological monitoring of the severe traumatic brain injury patient in the intensive care unit. Curr Neurol Neurosci Rep 2013;13(3):1-16.

34 Stocchetti N, Maas AI. Traumatic intracranial hypertension. N Engl J Med 2014;370(22):2121-30.

35 Curley G, Kavanagh BP, Laffey JG. Hypocapnia and the injured brain: more harm than benefit. Crit Care Med 2010;38(5): 1348–59.

36 Fletcher JJ, Bergman K, Blostein PA, Kramer AH. Fluid balance, complications, and brain tissue oxygen tension monitoring following severe traumatic brain injury. Neurocrit Care 2010;13(1):47–56.

37 Kheirbek T, Pascual J. Hypertonic saline for the rreatment of intracranial hypertension. Curr Neurol Neurosci Rep 2014;14(9):1-6.

38 Diringer MN, Scalfani MT, Zazulia AR, Videen TO, Dhar R, Powers WJ. Effect of mannitol on cerebral blood volume in patients with head injury. Neurosurgery 2012;70(5):1215-8.

39 Mortazavi MM, Romeo AK, Deep A, Griessenauer CJ, Shoja M, Tubbs RS et al. Hypertonic saline for treating raised intracranial pressure: literature review with meta-analysis: a review. J Neurosurg 2012;116(1):210-21.

40 Dietrich WD, Bramlett HM. The evidence for hypothermia as a neuroprotectant in traumatic brain injury. Neurotherapeutics 2010;7(1):43–50.

41 Yenari MA, Colbourne F, Hemmen TM, Han HS, Krieger D. Therapeutic hypothermia in stroke. Stroke Res Treat 2011;2011:157969. doi: 10.4061/2011/157969.

42 Povlishock JT, Wei EP. Posthypothermic rewarming considerations following traumatic brain injury. J Neurotrauma 2009;26(3):333–40.

43 Dietrich WD, Bramlett H. Vascular actions of hypothermia in brain trauma. In: Lo EH, Lok J, Ning MM, Whalen MJ, eds. Vascular mechanisms in CNS trauma. Springer Series in Translational Stroke Research 5. New York: Springer; 2014, pp 223-35.

44 Zhao Q-J, Zhang X-G, Wang L-X. Mild hypothermia therapy reduces blood glucose and lactate and improves neurologic outcomes in patients with severe traumatic brain injury. J Crit Care 2011;26(3):311-5.

45 Akbari Y, Mulder M, Razmara A, Geocadin R. Cool down the inflammation: hypothermia as a therapeutic strategy for acute brain injuries. In: Chen J, Hu X, Stenzel-Poore M, Zhang JH, eds. Immunological mechanisms and therapies in brain injuries and stroke. Springer Series in Translational Stroke Research 6. New York: Springer; 2014, pp 349–75.

46 Saxena M, Andrews PJ, Cheng A, Deol K, Hammond N. Modest cooling therapies (35°C to 37.5°C) for traumatic brain injury. Cochrane Database Syst Rev 2014;8:CD006811.

47 Marion DW, Regasa LE. Revisiting therapeutic hypothermia for severe traumatic brain injury... again. Crit Care 2014;18(3):160.

48 Lauzier F, Turgeon AF, Boutin A, Shemilt M, Côté I, Lachance O et al. Clinical outcomes, predictors, and prevalence of anterior pituitary disorders following traumatic brain injury: a systematic review. Crit Care Med 2014;42(3):712-21

49 Brain Trauma Foundation. Anesthetics, analgesics, and sedatives. J Neurotrauma 2007;24(Supp 1):S71–76.

50 Li LM, Timofeev I, Czosnyka M, Hutchinson PJ. Review article: the surgical approach to the management of increased intracranial pressure after traumatic brain injury. Anesth Analg 2010;111(3):736–48.

51 Vibbert M, Mayer SA. Early decompressive hemicraniectomy following malignant ischemic stroke: the crucial role of timing. Curr Neurol Neurosci Rep 2010;10(1):1–3.

52 Cooper JD, Rosenfeld JV, Murray L, Arabi YM, Davies AR, D'Urso P et al. Decompressive craniectomy in diffuse traumatic brain injury. N Engl J Med 2011;364(16):1493–502.

53 Bohman L-E, Schuster JM. Decompressive craniectomy for management of traumatic brain injury: an update. Curr Neurol Neurosci Rep 2013;13(11):1-8.

54 de Rooij NK, Rinkel GJ, Dankbaar JW, Frijns CJ. Delayed cerebral ischemia after subarachnoid hemorrhage: a systematic review of clinical, laboratory, and radiological predictors. Stroke 2013;44(1):43-54

55 Brathwaite S, Macdonald RL. Current management of delayed cerebral ischemia: update from results of recent clinical trials. Transl Stroke Res 2014;5(2):207-26

56 Sarrafzadeh AS, Vajkoczy P, Bijlenga P, Schaller K. Monitoring in neurointensive care – the challenge to detect delayed cerebral ischemia in high grade aSAH. Frontiers in Neurology 2014;5:34 Published online Jul 21, 2014.

57 Dorhout Mees SM, Rinkel GJ, Feigin VL, Algra A, van den Bergh WM, Vermeulen M et al. Calcium antagonists for aneurysmal subarachnoid haemorrhage. Cochrane Database Syst Rev 2007;3:CD000277.pub3.

58 Diringer MN, Bleck TP, Claude Hemphill J 3rd, Menon D, Shutter L, Vespa P et al. Neurocritical Care Society. Critical care management of patients following aneurysmal subarachnoid hemorrhage: recommendations from the Neurocritical Care Society's Multidisciplinary Consensus Conference. Neurocritical Care 2011;15:211–40.

59 Roozenbeek B, Maas AIR, Menon DK. Changing patterns in the epidemiology of traumatic brain injury. Nat Rev Neurol 2013;9(4):231–6.

60 National Center for Injury Prevention and Control. Rates of TBI-related emergency department visits, hospitalizations, and deaths – United States, 2001–2010. Atlanta: Centers for Disease Control and Prevention; 2014.

61 Tagliaferri F, Compagnone C, Korsic M, Servadei F, Kraus J. A systematic review of brain injury epidemiology in Europe. Acta Neurochir (Wien) 2006;148(3):255-68.

62 Australian Institute of Health and Welfare (AIHW). Australian hospital statistics 2008–09. Health Services Series no. 34. AIHW cat. no. HSE 37. Canberra: AIHW; 2010.

63 Helps Y, Henley G, Harrison JE. Hospital separations due to traumatic brain injury, Australia 2004–05. Injury research and statistics series number 45. Cat no. INJCAT 116. Adelaide: AIHW; 2008.

64 Corrigan JD, Selassie AW, Orman JA. The epidemiology of traumatic brain injury. J Head Trauma Rehabil 2010;25(2):72-80.

65 National Center for Injury Prevention and Control. Rates of TBI-related hospitalizations by sex – United States, 2001–2010. Atlanta: Centers for Disease Control and Prevention; 2014.

66 Rance L. Disability in Australia: acquired brain injury. Cat. no. AUS 96. Canberra: AIHW; 2007.

67 Myburgh JA, Cooper DJ, Finfer SR, Venkatesh B, Jones D, Higgins A et al. Epidemiology and 12-month outcomes from traumatic brain injury in Australia and New Zealand. J Trauma-Injury Infect Crit Care 2008;64(4):854–62.

68 National Center for Injury Prevention and Control. Rates of TBI-related hospitalizations by age group – United States, 2001–2010 [online]. Atlanta: Centers for Disease Control and Prevention; 2014.

69 Luukinen H, Viramo P, Herala M, Kervinen K, Kesaniemi YA, Savola O et al. Fall-related brain injuries and the risk of dementia in elderly people: a population-based study. Eur J Neurol 2005;12(2):86–92.

70 Namjoshi DR, Good C, Cheng WH, Panenka W, Richards D, Cripton PA et al. Towards clinical management of traumatic brain injury: a review of models and mechanisms from a biomechanical perspective. Dis Model Mech 2013;6(6):1325-38.

71 Soustiel JF, Sviri GE, Mahamid E, Shik V, Abeshaus S, Zaaroor M. Cerebral blood flow and metabolism following decompressive craniectomy for control of increased intracranial pressure. Neurosurgery 2010;67(1):65–72.

72 Badruddin A, Taqi MA, Abraham MG, Dani D, Zaidat OO. Neurocritical care of a reperfused brain. Curr Neurol Neurosci 2011;11(1):104–10.

73 Choi HA, Jeon S-B, Samuel S, Allison T, Lee K. Paroxysmal sympathetic hyperactivity after acute brain injury. Curr Neurol Neurosci Rep 2013;13(8):1-10.

74 Zakharova N, Kornienko V, Potapov A, Pronin I. Mapping of cerebral blood flow in focal and diffuse brain injury. In: Zakharova N, Kornienko V, Potapov A, Pronin I. Neuroimaging of traumatic brain injury. Switzerland: Springer International Publishing; 2014, pp 107-23.

75 Rabinowitz AR, Li X, Levin HS. Sport and nonsport etiologies of mild traumatic brain injury: similarities and differences. Annu Rev Psychol 2014;65:301-31.

76 SAFE Study Investigators; Australian and New Zealand Intensive Care Society Clinical Trials Group; Australian Red Cross Blood Service; George Institute for International Health, Myburgh J, Cooper DJ, Finfer S, Bellomo R, Norton R et al. Saline or albumin for fluid resuscitation in patients with traumatic brain injury. N Engl J Med 2007;357(9):874–84.

77 Kirshblum SC, Biering-Sorensen F, Betz R, Burns S, Donovan W, Graves DE et al. International standards for neurological classification of spinal cord injury: cases with classification challenges. J Spinal Cord Med 2014;37(2):120-7.

78 Lee BB, Cripps RA, Fitzharris M, Wing PC. The global map for traumatic spinal cord injury epidemiology; update 2011, global incidence rate. Spinal Cord 2014;52(2):110-6.

79 Wilson JR, Cho N, Fehlings MG. Acute traumatic spinal cord injury: epidemiology, evaluation, and management. In: Patel VV, Patel AP, Harrop JS, Burger E, eds. Spine surgery basics. Berlin: Springer-Verlag; 2014, pp 399-409.

80 Jazayeri SB, Beygi S, Shokraneh F, Hagen EM, Rahimi-Movaghar V. Incidence of traumatic spinal cord injury worldwide: a systematic review. Eur Spine J 2014:1-14.

81 Norton L. Spinal cord injury, Australia 2007–08. Injury research and statistics series no. 52. Cat. no. INJCAT 128. Canberra: Australian Institute of Health and Welfare; 2010.

82 Silva NA, Sousa N, Reis RL, Salgado AJ. From basics to clinical: A comprehensive review on spinal cord injury. Prog Neurobiol 2014;114:25-57.

83 Gupta R, Bathen ME, Smith JS, Levi AD, Bhatia NN, Steward OJ. Advances in the management of spinal cord injury. Am Acad Orthop Surg 2010; 18(4): 210–22.

84 Evans LT, Lollis SS, Ball PA. Management of acute spinal cord injury in the neurocritical care unit. Neurosurg Clin N Am 2013; 24(3):339-47.

85 Lo V, Esquenazi Y, Han MK, Lee K. Critical care management of patients with acute spinal cord injury. J Neurosurg Sci 2013; 57(4):281-92.

86 Pimentel L, Diegelmann L. Evaluation and management of acute cervical spine trauma. Emerg Med Clin North Am 2010; 28(4): 719–38.

87 Plemel JR, Yong VW, Stirling DP. Immune modulatory therapies for spinal cord injury–Past, present and future. Exp Neurol 2014;258:91-104.

88 Godoy DA, Di Napoli M, Rabinstein AA. Treating hyperglycemia in neurocritical patients: benefits and perils. Neurocrit Care 2010; 13(3): 425–38.

89 Kim AS, Johnston SC. Global variation in the relative burden of stroke and ischemic heart disease. Circulation 2011; 124(3):314-23.

90 Finegold JA, Asaria P, Francis DP. The global burden of ischemic heart disease in 1990 and 2010: the Global Burden of Disease 2010 study. Int J Cardiol 2013 30;168(2):934-45.

91 EROS Investigators. Incidence of stroke in Europe at the beginning of the 21st century. Stroke 2009;40:1557-1563.

92 Australian Institute of Health and Welfare 2013. Stroke and its management in Australia: an update. Cardiovascular disease series no. 37. Cat. no. CVD 61. Canberra: AIHW.

93 Chung JM. Seizures in the acute stroke setting. Neurol Res 2014;36(5):403-6.

94 Jauch EC, Saver JL, Adams HP, Bruno A, Demaerschalk BM, Khatri P. Guidelines for the early management of patients with acute ischemic stroke, a guideline for healthcare professionals from the American Heart Association/American Stroke Association. Stroke 2013;44(3):870-947.

95 Saver JL, Fonarow GC, Smith EE, Reeves MJ, Grau-Sepulveda MV, Pan W et al. Time to treatment with intravenous tissue plasminogen activator and outcome from acute ischemic stroke. JAMA 2013;309(23):2480-8.

96 Ciccone A, Valvassori L, Nichelatti M, Sgoifo A, Ponzio M, Sterzi R. Endovascular treatment for acute ischemic stroke. N Engl J Med 2013;368(10):904-13.

97 Van Asch CJ, Luitse MJ, Rinkel GJ, van der Tweel I, Algra A, Klijn CJ. Incidence, case fatality, and functional outcome of intracerebral haemorrhage over time, according to age, sex, and ethnic origin: a systematic review and meta-analysis. Lancet Neurol 2010;9:167–176.

98 Maas MB, Rosenberg NF, Kosteva AR, Bauer RM, Guth JC, Liotta EM. Surveillance neuroimaging and neurologic examinations affect care for intracerebral hemorrhage. Neurology 2013;81(2):107-12.

99 Langhorne P, Fearon P, Ronning OM, Kaste M, Palomaki H, Vemmos K. Stroke unit care benefits patients with intracerebral hemorrhage: systematic review and meta-analysis. Stroke 2013;44(11):3044-9.

100 Zhou Y, Wang Y, Wang J, Anne Stetler R, Yang Q-W. Inflammation in intracerebral hemorrhage: from mechanisms to clinical translation. Prog Neurobiol 2014;115:25-44.

101 Morgenstern LB, Hemphill JC, Anderson C, Becker K, Broderick JP, Connolly ES. Guidelines for the management of spontaneous intracerebral hemorrhage: a guideline for healthcare professionals from the American Heart Association/American Stroke Association. Stroke 2010;41(9):2108-29.

102 Steiner T, Al-Shahi Salman R, Beer R, Christensen H, Cordonnier C, Csiba L et al. European Stroke Organisation guidelines for the management of spontaneous intracerebral hemorrhage. Int J Stroke 2014;9(7):840-55.

103 Tan X, He J, Li L, Yang G, Liu H, Tang S et al. Early hyperglycaemia and the early-term death in patients with spontaneous intracerebral haemorrhage: a meta-analysis. Internal Med J 2014;44(3):254-60.

104 Helbok R, Kurtz P, Vibbert M, Schmidt MJ, Fernandez L, Lantigua H et al. Early neurological deterioration after subarachnoid haemorrhage: risk factors and impact on outcome. J Neurol Neurosurg Psychiatry 2013;84(3):266-70.

105 Connolly ES, Rabinstein AA, Carhuapoma JR, Derdeyn CP, Dion J, Higashida RT et al; American Heart Association Stroke Council; Council on Cardiovascular Radiology and Intervention; Council on Cardiovascular Nursing; Council on Cardiovascular Surgery and Anesthesia; Council on Clinical Cardiology. Guidelines for the management of aneurysmal subarachnoid hemorrhage: a guideline for healthcare professionals from the American Heart Association/American Stroke Association. Stroke 2012;43(6):1711-37.

106 Tagami T, Kuwamoto K, Watanabe A, Unemoto K, Yokobori S, Matsumoto G. Effect of Triple-h prophylaxis on global end-diastolic volume and clinical outcomes in patients with aneurysmal subarachnoid hemorrhage. Neurocrit Care 2014;21(3):462-9.

107 Hamdan A, Barnes J, Mitchell P. Subarachnoid hemorrhage and the female sex: analysis of risk factors, aneurysm characteristics, and outcomes. J Neurosurg 2014;121(6):1367-73.

108 Sandström N, Yan B, Dowling R, Laidlaw J, Mitchell P. Comparison of microsurgery and endovascular treatment on clinical outcome following poor-grade subarachnoid hemorrhage. J Clin Neurosci 2013;20(9):1213-8.

109 Wang X, Chen J-X, Mao Q, Liu Y-H, You C. Relationship between intracranial pressure and aneurysmal subarachnoid hemorrhage grades. J Neurol Sci 2014;346(1-2):284-7.

110 Moussouttas M, Lai EW, Huynh TT, James J, Stocks-Dietz C, Dombrowski K. Association between acute sympathetic response, early onset vasospasm, and delayed vasospasm following spontaneous subarachnoid hemorrhage. J Clin Neurosci 2014;21(2):256-62.

111 Einhaupl K, Stam J, Bousser MG, De Bruijn SF, Ferro JM, Martinelli I et al. EFNS guideline on the treatment of cerebral venous and sinus thrombosis in adult patients. Eur J Neurol 2010;17(10):1229-35.

112 Kasanmoentalib ES, Brouwer MC, van de Beek D. Update on bacterial meningitis: epidemiology, trials and genetic association studies. Curr Opin Neurol 2013;26(3):282-8.

113 Communicable Diseases Network Australia, Meningococcal Disease Sub-Committee. Guidelines for the early clinical and public health management of meningococcal disease in Australia 2007, <http://www.health.gov.au/internet/main/ publishing.nsf/Content/4DFF673115 F66413CA257BF00020630F/$File/meningococcal-guidelines.pdf>; [accessed 10.14].

114 Markey PG, Davis JS, Harnett GB, Williams SH, Speers DJ. Meningitis and a febrile vomiting illness caused by echovirus type 4, Northern Territory, Australia. Emerg Infect Dis 2010;16(1):63–8.

115 Kennedy PG, Steiner I. Recent issues in herpes simplex encephalitis. J Neurovirol 2013;19(4):346-50.

116 Huppatz C, Durrheim DN, Levi C, Dalton C, Williams D, Clements MS et al. Etiology of encephalitis in Australia, 1990–2007. Emerg Infect Dis 2009;15(9):1359–65.

117 Hills SL, Weber IB, Fischer M. Japanese encephalitis. CDC Health Information for International Travel 2014: The Yellow Book. 2013;60(33):212.

118 Middleton D, Pallister J, Klein R, Feng Y-R, Haining J, Arkinstall R. Hendra virus vaccine, a one health approach to protecting horse, human, and environmental health. Emerg Infect Dis 2014;20(3):372.

119 Rozenberg F. Acute viral encephalitis. Handb Clin Neurol 2013;112:1171–81.

120 Vellozzi C, Iqbal S, Stewart B, Tokars J, DeStefano F. Cumulative risk of Guillain–Barré syndrome among vaccinated and unvaccinated populations during the 2009 H1N1 influenza pandemic. Am J Public Health 2014;104(4):696-701.

121 Hughes RAC, Swan AV, van Doorn PA. Intravenous immunoglobulin for Guillain–Barré syndrome. Cochrane Database Syst Rev 2012;7:CD002063.

122 Bhagat H, Dash HH, Chauhan RS, Khanna P, Bithal PK. Intensive care management of Guillain–Barré syndrome: a retrospective outcome study and review of literature. Journal of Neuroanaesthesiology and Critical Care 2014;1(3):188.

123 Ruts L, Drenthen J, Jongen JLM, Hop WCJ, Visser GH, Jacobs BC et al. Pain in Guillain–Barré syndrome: a long-term follow-up study. Neurology 2010;75(16):1439–47.

124 Walgaard C, Lingsma HF, Ruts L, Drenthen J, van Koningsveld R, Garssen MJ et al. Prediction of respiratory insufficiency in Guillain–Barré syndrome. Ann Neurol 2010;67(6):781–7.

125 Yuki N, Hartung H-P. Guillain–Barré syndrome. N Engl J Med 2012;366(24):2294-304.

126 van den Berg B, Walgaard C, Drenthen J, Fokke C, Jacobs BC, van Doorn PA. Guillain–Barré syndrome: pathogenesis, diagnosis, treatment and prognosis. Nature Rev Neurol 2014;10(8):469-82.

127 Hohlfeld R, Wekerle H, Marx A. The immunopathogenesis of myasthenia gravis. Myasthenia Gravis and Myasthenic Disorders 2012;81:60.

128 Sakaguchi H, Yamashita S, Hirano T, Nakajima M, Kimura E, Maeda Y et al. Myasthenic crisis patients who require intensive care unit management. Muscle Nerve 2012;46(3):440-2.

129 Bhagat H, Grover V, Jangra K. What is optimal in patients with myasthenic crisis: invasive or non-invasive ventilation? J Neuroanaesth Crit Care 2014;1(2):116.

130 Elsais A, Wyller VB, Loge JH, Kerty E. Fatigue in myasthenia gravis: is it more than muscular weakness? BMC Neurol 2013;13(1):132.

131 Cabrera Serrano M, Rabinstein A. Usefulness of pulmonary function tests and blood gases in acute neuromuscular respiratory failure. Eur J Neurol 2012;19(3):452-6.

132 Huff JS, Fountain NB. Pathophysiology and definitions of seizures and status epilepticus. Emerg Med Clin North Am 2011;29(1):1–13.

133 Neligan A, Sander JW. Epidemiology of seizures and epilepsy. Epilepsy 2013:28-32.

134 Hocker S, Wijdicks EF, Rabinstein AA. Refractory status epilepticus: new insights in presentation, treatment, and outcome. Neurol Res 2013;35(2):163-8.

135 Fernandez A, Claassen J. Refractory status epilepticus. Curr Opin Crit Care 2012;18(2):127-31.

136 Claassen J, Taccone FS, Horn P, Holtkamp M, Stocchetti N, Oddo M. Recommendations on the use of EEG monitoring in critically ill patients: consensus statement from the neurointensive care section of the ESICM. Intensive Care Med 2013;39(8):1337-51.

137 He J, Zhang Y, Xu T, Zhao Q, Wang D, Chen CS et al; CATIS Investigators. Effects of immediate blood pressure reduction on death and major disability in patients with acute ischemic stroke: the CATIS randomized clinical trial. JAMA 2014 5;311(5):479-89.

138 Yong H, Foody J, Linong J, Dong Z, Wang Y, Ma L. A systematic literature review of risk factors for stroke in China. Cardiol Rev 2013;21(2):77-93.

Chapter 18

Support of renal function

Ian Baldwin, Gavin Leslie

Learning objectives

After reading this chapter, you should be able to:

- summarise the physiology of urine production
- describe the most likely causes of kidney injury in the critically ill adult
- differentiate between acute and chronic renal failure
- outline treatment approaches in managing acute kidney injury in critical illness
- appreciate historical developments in dialysis
- describe the indications for renal replacement therapy in critical care
- understand the principles and challenges associated with nursing management of continuous renal replacement therapy in critical care.

Introduction

Sudden deterioration of kidney function as a result of physiological injury, to the point where there is retention of nitrogenous wastes, referred to as acute renal failure (ARF), is a common manifestation of critical illness and is often associated with failure of other organs. Acute renal failure is a syndrome with numerous causes, including glomerulonephritis, prerenal azotaemia, urinary tract obstruction and vasculitis. Acute tubular necrosis (ATN) is a collective term commonly used in the past to describe acutely deteriorating renal function, reflecting pathological changes from various renal insults of a nephrotoxic or ischaemic origin. Factors that cause renal function to deteriorate are not, however, always ischaemic or necrotic in origin, and a syndrome with degrees of deterioration prior to failure is often evident. Therefore, a consensus definition and classification system has been established that focuses on incremental organ injury rather than end-stage organ failure.[1] This approach describes staging of ARF severity and embraces the concept of acute kidney injury (AKI) where, like other organs of the body, a dynamic spectrum is found, from small indiscrete changes in function that are immediately reversible through to gross signs and irreversible organ failure.[2] With this change of conceptual focus in recent years new consensus guidelines have been released in an effort to better guide clinical understanding and decision making, the most comprehensive being from the Kidney Disease: Improving Global Outcomes (K-DIGO) group.[3] Acute kidney injury is defined

KEY WORDS

acute kidney injury

acute renal failure

continuous renal replacement therapy

dialysis history

urine production

by a rapid deterioration in renal function (hours to days), which is easily detected by commonly measured markers of kidney performance, including blood urea nitrogen and serum creatinine, with inability to adequately regulate electrolytes, sodium and water balance.[4,5] While generally reversible, AKI can be life-threatening in the critically ill patient if acid–base imbalance, abnormal electrolyte levels (particularly potassium) or fluid overloads are not effectively diagnosed and managed.

The preferred serum marker of renal function is the serum creatinine level.[3] The exact level of serum creatinine that is considered excessive is disputed; however, an increase in magnitude of 1.5 or more of the baseline serum creatinine is commonly agreed on as being indicative of AKI.[3] Urine output is also a key factor in determining the severity of ARF. It is well established that oliguric renal failure, that is, a urine output of less than 0.5 mL/kg/h in adults and 1 mL/kg/h in infants, is associated with poorer patient outcome than the non-oliguric form.[6]

AKI is reported to occur in more than 60% of intensive care patient admissions, much higher than the broader hospital rate of 5%.[7,8] In critical care, AKI often forms part of the multiple organ dysfunction syndrome, whose cause has often been associated with sepsis, trauma, pneumonia or cardiovascular dysfunction (see Chapter 22). Mortality in intensive care AKI is high, with those patients requiring renal replacement therapy (RRT) having worse outcomes than patients who can be managed without this intervention.[9]

This chapter focuses on the underlying causes and management of AKI in critical care, with particular emphasis on nursing perspectives for managing patients with this life-threatening organ system dysfunction.

Related anatomy and physiology

The renal system has a number of functions, including regulation and maintenance of fluid and electrolyte balance, clearance of metabolic and other waste products, an indirect role in the maintenance of blood pressure, acid–base balance and an endocrine function. In critical care, an appreciation of renal function in relation to fluid management, blood pressure, electrolyte and acid–base functions is essential.

Regulation and maintenance of the extracellular fluid and electrolyte constituents occur principally via the process of filtration and reabsorption. The kidneys receive approximately 25% of the cardiac output each minute, and excrete approximately 180 L/day of glomerular filtrate. Fortunately, tubular reabsorption accounts for approximately 178.5 L/day of the original filtrate, allowing for a modest daily fluid intake of 1.5 L to achieve fluid balance. During this process of filtration and reabsorption, metabolic byproducts and electrolyte and other wastes (including many drugs) are also excreted and maintained in balance. As with all body organ systems, an adequate blood pressure and supply of oxygen to the kidneys is paramount in maintaining the fluid and electrolyte regulatory role.

Anatomy of the kidney, nephron and urinary drainage system

The functional anatomy of the renal system includes the two kidneys, ureters, bladder and urethra (see Figure 18.1). The ureters, bladder and urethra collect, drain and

FIGURE 18.1 Kidney and urinary drainage system.

Organs and structures of the urinary system

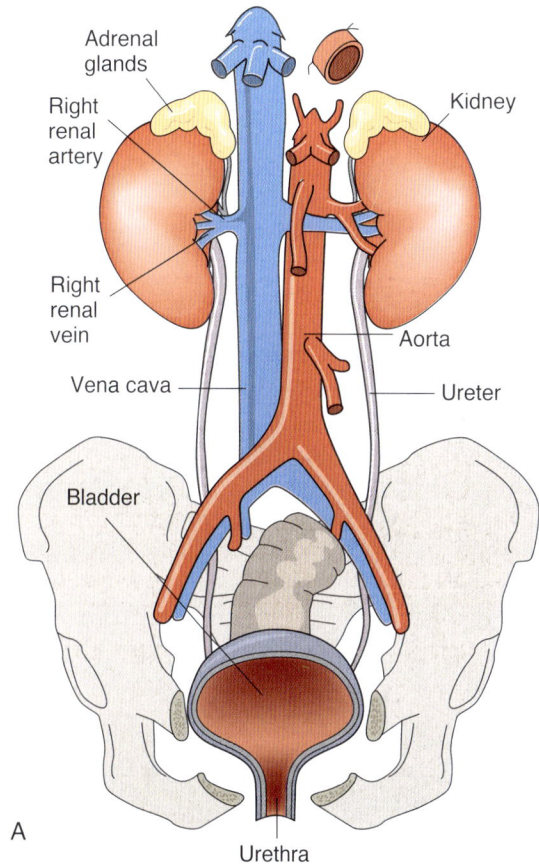

A

Frontal section of kidney

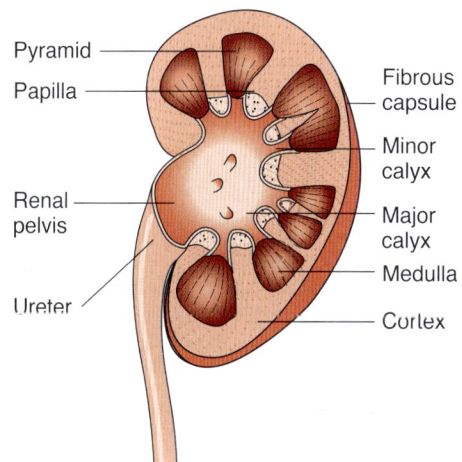

B

temporarily store the urine produced from each kidney.[10] While important in providing the conduit for the final excretion of urine, the kidney is the primary organ of interest in the renal system, particularly in critical care practice, and hence will be described in more detail from the anatomical and physiological perspectives.

The kidneys are located in the retroperitoneal space on the posterior wall of the abdominal cavity, encased in a protective combination of the ribs, muscle, fat, tendon and the renal capsule. Each adult kidney weighs approximately 140 g. The kidneys may develop a different anatomical appearance, or vary in number and location from the classic description provided here. The functional unit of the kidney is the nephron, which consists of a filtrate-collecting device (the Bowman's capsule), a convoluted tubule that varies in length and diameter, finally attaching to a common filtrate-collecting tubule and duct (see Figure 18.2). Within the Bowman's capsule rests the glomerulus, a tuft of interlaced capillaries that arise from the afferent arteriole. The efferent arteriole then drains from the glomerulus, via a closely entwined network called the peritubular capillaries, until these collect in the venous network of the kidney.

The glomeruli and nephrons lie in the cortical area of the kidney, while the collecting ducts gather together into the renal pyramids, which lie in the medulla of the kidney. The pyramids drain into the calyces of the kidney, which then drain into the renal pelvis where urine is gathered to drain into the ureter. The major blood vessels of the kidney, the renal artery and veins also enter the renal capsule through the pelvis of the kidney.[10]

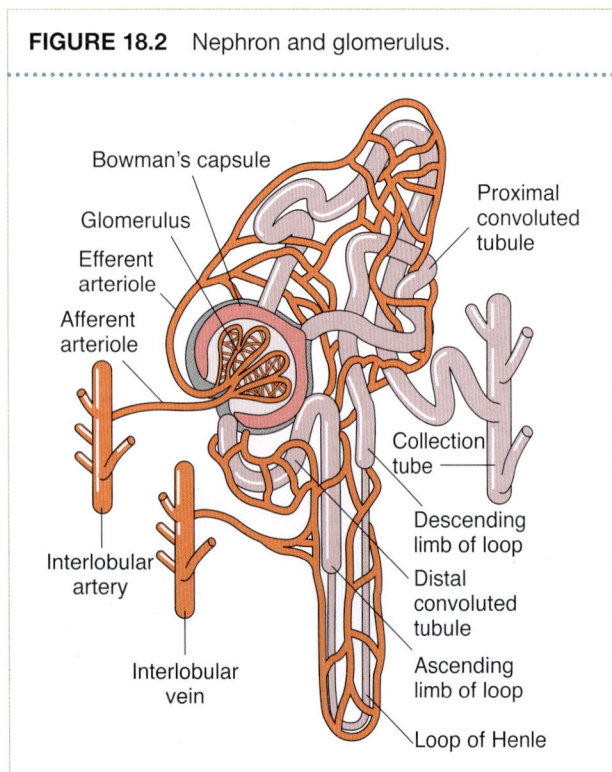

FIGURE 18.2 Nephron and glomerulus.

Urine production, regulation of GFR and filtrate reabsorption in the nephron

Urine production consists of a three-stage process, which occurs in the nephron: glomerular filtration, tubular reabsorption and tubular secretion (see Figure 18.3). As previously noted, the production of urine is highly dependent on delivery of blood under pressure to the glomerulus. This results in the first step of the urine production process, glomerular filtration. The glomerular filtration rate (GFR) is about 125 mL/min under normal conditions. Changes in the diameter of the afferent and efferent arteriole help regulate glomerular blood flow, but this is unable to compensate for large variations of mean blood pressure; hence, filtration rates may rise or fall markedly over the course of a day.[11]

As the filtrate transgresses the glomerulus it is collected into the Bowman's capsule and delivered into the proximal convoluted tubule, loop of Henle and then the distal convoluted tubule, where a number of processes result in the reabsorption of about 99% of the glomerular filtrate. The remaining fluid within the tubule drains into the collecting tubule to form urine. This fluid has substantially different properties from the original glomerular filtrate, as fluid and many electrolytes and glucose are reabsorbed by the peritubular capillaries.[11]

Along with blood pressure, the sodium content of the extracellular fluid is critical in maintaining fluid balance, as it constitutes the major electrolyte and osmotic agent of the glomerular filtrate. It is imperative that sodium intake and loss are equally balanced, as excessive losses will result in associated fluid loss and excessive intake will result in fluid retention. If sodium balance is not maintained, other compensations such as a rise in blood pressure may result to restore fluid balance. As blood pressure rises, the excretion of sodium also increases by way of additional glomerular filtrate. In this way, water and sodium balance are inextricably linked.[11]

Hormonal and neural regulation of renal function

Various feedback mechanisms exist that assist in precisely adjusting the final amount of fluid and electrolyte to be excreted from the kidney. These include the sympathetic nervous system response, angiotension II, aldosterone, antidiuretic hormone and atrial natriuretic peptide. All these mechanisms work in synchrony with blood pressure and sodium balance in ensuring a highly regulated circulating and extracellular fluid volume.[11]

Sympathetic nervous system

Stimulation of the sympathetic nervous system by loss of blood volume occurs by reflex via the low-pressure volume sensors in the pulmonary and venous circulations. This is complemented by further stimulation if arterial pressure falls. The sympathetic nervous system widely innervates

FIGURE 18.3   Urine formation: filtration, reabsorption and excretion.

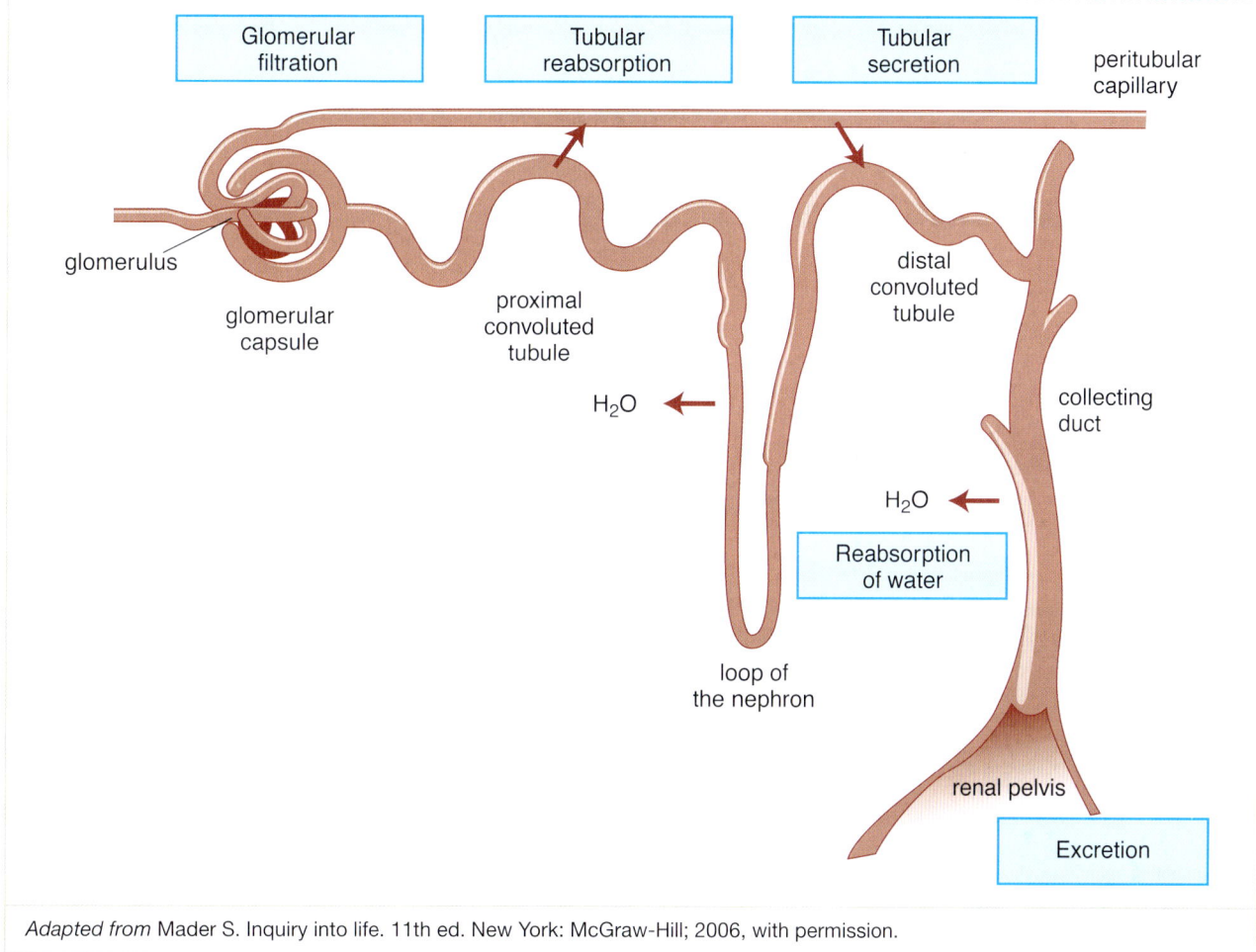

Adapted from Mader S. Inquiry into life. 11th ed. New York: McGraw-Hill; 2006, with permission.

the kidney and is able to reduce the filtration rate by constricting the afferent arteriole of the glomerulus, thus inhibiting blood flow and pressure necessary to create the glomerular filtration rate. This stimulation of the sympathetic nervous system also increases the reabsorption of salt and water in the tubule and stimulates the release of renin.

Antidiuretic hormone

The antidiuretic hormone is excreted from the pituitary gland under regulation of hypothalamic osmoreceptors (thirst centre), and reduces kidney diuresis (the excretion of water). By enhancing the kidney's ability to concentrate urine, it ensures that the excretory functions of waste products and electrolytes continue while limiting fluid loss. Antidiuretic hormone is essential to surviving limited periods of fluid deprivation and fine-tuning the urine volume production on a continuous basis.

Renin–angiotensin–aldosterone system

Renin is the chemical trigger that initiates a cascade system resulting in two powerful hormones acting on the kidney to significantly influence sodium and water excretion

(see Figure 18.4). Renin is produced and released from the juxtaglomerular apparatus, a collection of cells in the macula densa of the distal tubule, and the adjacent afferent arteriole next to the glomerulus, which monitors blood sodium concentration. When released, renin stimulates the activation of angiotensin I from angiotensinogen. Under the influence of coenzyme A, angiotensin I converts to angiotensin II, a potent vasoconstrictor and stimulus to reabsorb sodium and water. The vasoconstrictor effect raises blood pressure and flow to the glomerulus, inhibiting further renin release (a negative feedback mechanism) as perfusion pressure normalises. This allows the return of natriuresis (sodium excretion) and diuresis. This response is essential in assisting with retaining fluid in the event of falling blood pressure, or boosting fluid excretion as blood pressure rises. It also responds effectively to a rise in sodium intake by reducing angiotensin II formation and allowing a larger natriuresis, resulting in maintenance of sodium balance, a key to tissue fluid distribution and balance.[11]

Aldosterone is a mineralocorticoid excreted from the adrenal cortex in response to angiotensin II. Aldosterone

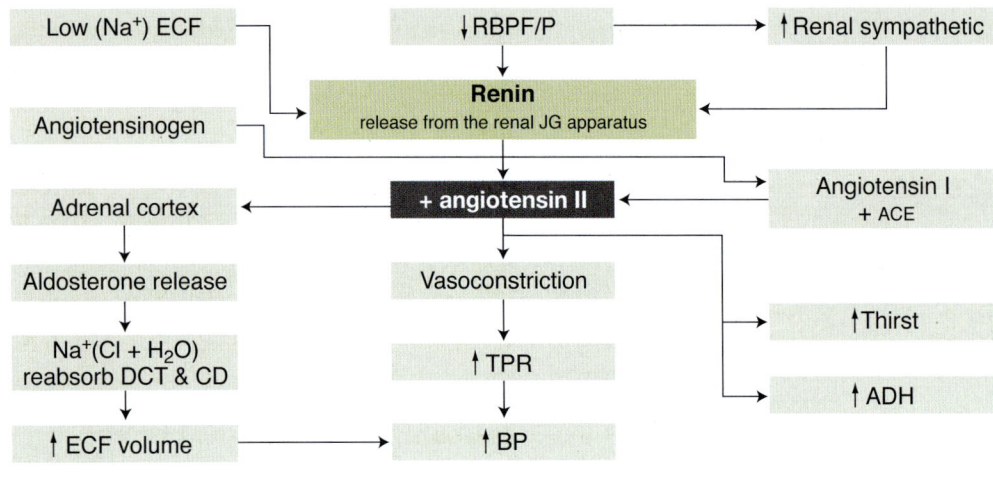

FIGURE 18.4 Renin–angiotensin–aldosterone system (RAAS).

Abbreviations

ACE = angiotension-converting enzyme
ADH = antidiurectic hormone
BP = blood pressure
CD = collecting duct
DCT = distal collecting duct

ECF = extracellular fluid
JG = juxtaglomerular
RBF/P = renal blood flow/pressure
TPR = total peripheral resistance

increases the reabsorption of sodium, and hence water, in the cortical collecting tubules and increases the rate of potassium excretion. This has a dual effect of regulating sodium balance and extracellular fluid volume. As fluid volume accumulates, the rise in glomerular filtration rate self-limits the volume effect by increasing both diuresis and natriuresis.

Atrial natriuretic peptide

Atrial natriuretic peptide is a hormone released from the atria of the heart in response to atrial stretching during periods of increased circulating fluid volume. Atrial natriuretic peptide is therefore often described as having an antagonising effect to the renin–angiotensin–aldosterone system (which acts primarily to preserve sodium and water). These natriuretic, and hence diuretic, effects are mild and self-limiting, and occur in response to mild rises in GFR and reductions in sodium reabsorption. As blood pressure falls, the drop in GFR compensates for the effect of atrial natriuretic peptide, ensuring that excessive loss of sodium and water does not occur.[11]

Regulation of acid–base and electrolyte balance

The kidney assists in the management of body pH by regulation of the excretion of hydrogen (H^+) and bicarbonate (HCO_3^-) ions. While the renal response to alkalosis or acidosis is slow in comparison with plasma buffers and respiratory regulation (see Chapter 13), it does result in a net loss of H^+ ions or recovery of HCO_3^- ions, which are the basis of human pH balance (see Figure 18.5). During

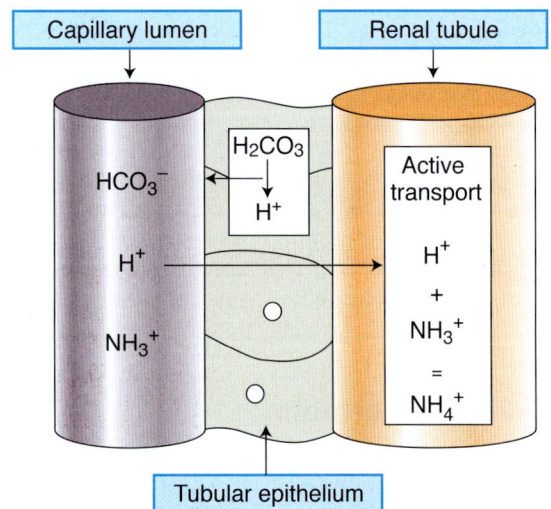

FIGURE 18.5 Hydrogen ion regulation in the kidney.

acidosis the kidney raises H^+ secretion by active transport to combine with ammonia in the renal tubule to form ammonium, which is unable to be reabsorbed. Coincidentally, raised H^+ excretion increases the reabsorption of sodium, which increases the alkalotic ion, bicarbonate (HCO_3^-). Conversely, during alkalosis the reabsorption of hydrogen ions is increased. These changes in hydrogen ion concentration in the renal filtrate alter the pH of the urine down to a maximum level of four.[6] The buffering of H+ with ammonia reduces the acidifying effect of the hydrogen ions, particularly as some ammonium combines with chloride to form ammonium chloride.[11]

Role as an endocrine organ

The kidney has two homeostatic roles as an endocrine organ. Although neither has effects relevant to acute illness, patients with chronic renal dysfunction often need supplementation to overcome the loss of renal endocrine support. Erythropoietin is important in stimulating the generation of new red blood cells and is released from the kidney in response to a sustained drop in arterial blood oxygen levels. Calcitriol helps regulate the absorption of calcium from the gut, which in turn promotes bone resorption of calcium and the reabsorption of calcium in the kidney. The kidney also acts to convert vitamin D to its active form, which is necessary for the maintenance of body calcium levels.[11]

Pathophysiology and classification of renal failure

Diseases of the kidneys affect the structure and therefore the function of the nephrons in some way. Pathology such as this, if untreated, may not cause complete loss of renal function (i.e. ARF), but is dependent on the amount of nephron damage or 'injury' occurring at the time of the illness, and whether the patient has had any previous illness that resulted in undetected kidney damage.[12] By focusing on factors that resulted in kidney injury, both individually and collectively, more serious damage that

may result in failure can be averted. This concept is more clearly described in the later section on ATN and AKI, which includes the RIFLE Criteria (see Figure 18.6).[1,2]

The conventional classification of ARF is based on the perceived causative mechanisms:[5,13]

- prerenal
- intrarenal (intrinsic)
- postrenal.

However, irrespective of causative mechanism, should kidney injury progress to failure the same renal replacement therapies are suitable to treat this.

Prior to considering whether a critically ill patient has suffered acute injury, it has been recommended the effects of intra-abdominal hypertension be considered.[14] As it is possible up to half of mechanically ventilated patients will have this to some degree, measures to relieve the pressure should be considered as changes in renal function can result due to either direct pressure on the kidney and/or drainage system or increased pressure within the venous circulation of the kidney. Intra-abdominal hypertension also clouds the assessment of haemodynamic parameters and cardiovascular performance, making it difficult to assess fluid needs and responsiveness to fluid resuscitation.[15] For a more detailed discussion of intra-abdominal hypertension, please refer to Chapter 20.

Prerenal causes

Prerenal factors affecting blood supply to the kidneys, such as hypovolaemia, cardiac failure or hypotension/shock, can cause AKI. The mechanism and outcome are

FIGURE 18.6 Criteria for diagnosis of acute renal failure: the risk, injury and failure criteria with outcomes of loss and end-stage renal disease (RIFLE).[32]

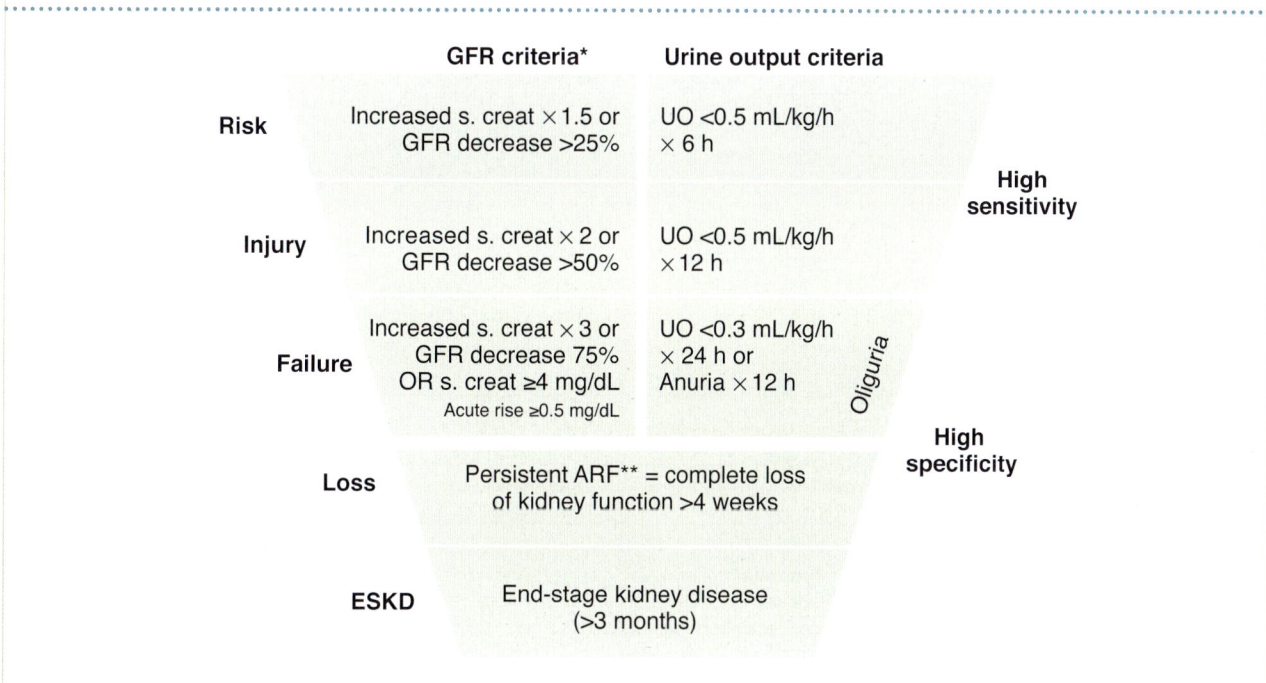

easily related. As blood flow to the kidneys is reduced, less glomerulofiltration occurs, urine production diminishes and wastes accumulate. This state can be reversed by restoration of blood volume or blood pressure. In the short term (1–2 hours), nephrons remain structurally normal and respond by limiting fluid lost by urine production while concentrating the excretion of waste products. The physiological process combines the neuroendocrine control of the hypothalamus and the sympathomimetic response, which then regulates both antidiuretic hormone secretion and the stimulation of the renin–angiotensin–aldosterone system (see Figure 18.7). This process is highly influenced by any pre-existing illness or concurrent factors such as diabetes and systemic infection.[13]

Intrarenal (intrinsic) causes

Intrinsic damage to the nephron structure and function can be due to infective or inflammatory illness, toxic drugs, toxic wastes from systemic inflammation in sepsis, vascular obstructive thrombus or emboli. In differentiating this type of ARF, a process of elimination has been suggested where failure of kidney function persists after the restoration of adequate perfusion (blood flow), or where no loss of perfusion has occurred, and there is no obstruction to urine flow.[16] Diagnosis is made by exclusion of other causes. The common causes of this type of ARF, glomerulonephritis, nephrotoxicity and chronic vascular insufficiency, are discussed below.

Glomerulonephritis

This condition is caused by either an infective or a non-infective inflammatory process damaging the glomerular membrane or a systemic autoimmune illness attacking the membrane.[16] Either cause results in a loss of glomerular membrane integrity, allowing larger blood components such as plasma proteins and white blood cells to cross the glomerular basement membrane. This causes a loss of blood protein, tubular congestion and failure of normal nephron activity. Resolution is based on treating the cause, such as an infection or autoimmune inflammatory illness.[17]

Nephrotoxicity

Nephrotoxicity occurs as a result of damage to nephron cells from a wide range of agents, including many drugs used in critical care (e.g. antibiotics, anti-inflammatory agents, cancer drugs, radio-opaque dyes). Toxic products of

FIGURE 18.7 Neuroendocrine response to shock, resulting in oliguria.

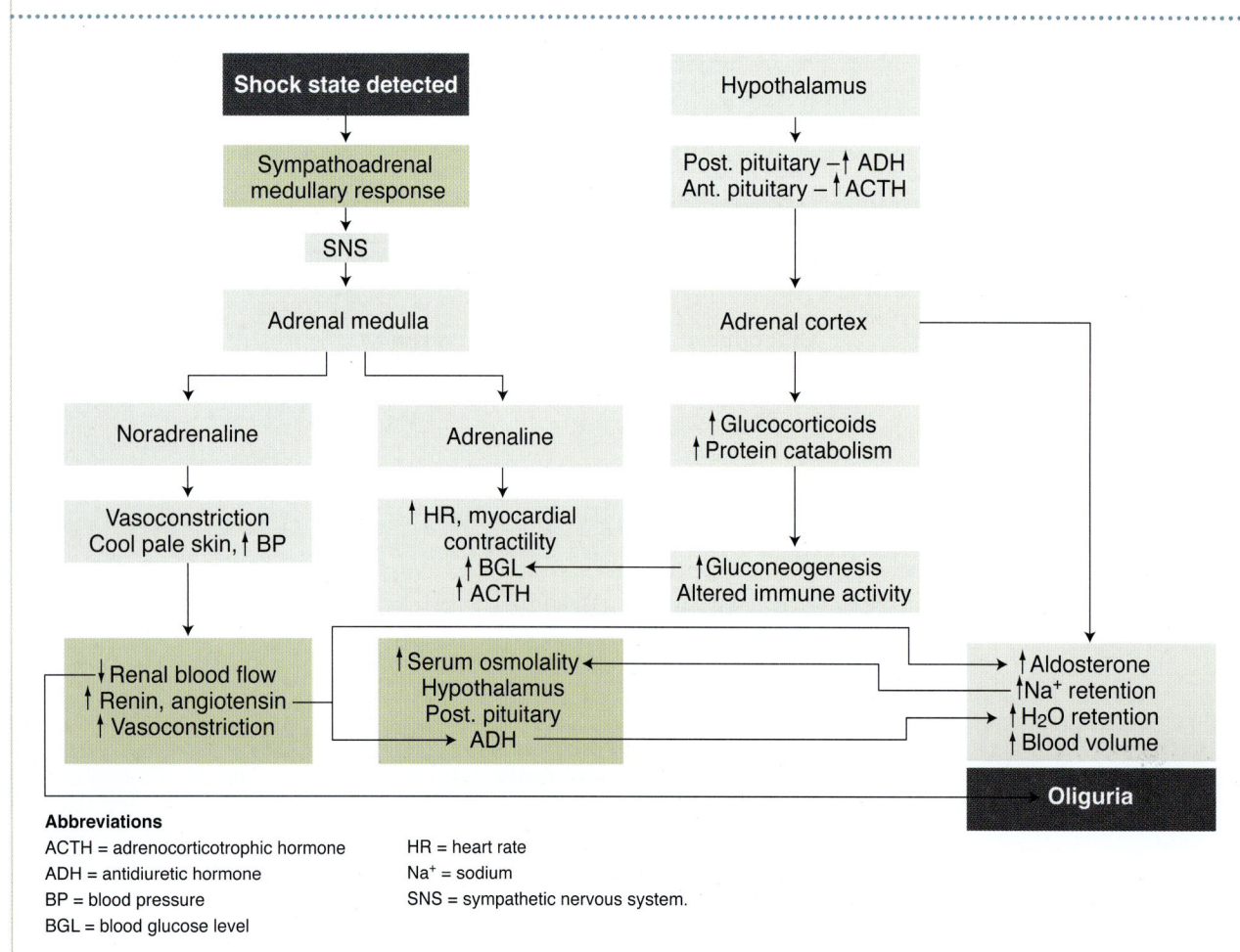

Abbreviations

ACTH = adrenocorticotrophic hormone
ADH = antidiuretic hormone
BP = blood pressure
BGL = blood glucose level
HR = heart rate
Na⁺ = sodium
SNS = sympathetic nervous system.

muscle breakdown in severe illness and trauma, commonly called rhabdomyolysis (see Chapter 23),[6,13] blood product administration reactions and blood cell damage associated with major surgery are also causative agents.[18] As these agents may often be given concurrently, a cumulative effect, along with intermittent falls in renal perfusion, may result in the development of intrinsic ARF.

Vascular insufficiency

One-third of patients who develop ARF in the intensive care unit (ICU) have chronic renal dysfunction.[19] This chronic dysfunction may be undiagnosed prior to the critical illness, and may be related to diabetes, the ageing process and/or long-term hypertension. These factors create a reduction in both large and microvasculature blood flow into and within the kidney, therefore reducing glomerular filtration activity and affecting the reabsorption and diffusive process of the nephron. This reduction in blood flow is exacerbated by degenerative vessel obstruction with atheromatous plaque, particularly pronounced in diabetic patients due to ineffective glucose metabolism. Diabetic patients are more likely to develop ARF associated with medical care in hospital from what may otherwise seem to be a relatively trivial insult to the kidneys in a younger, healthy patient. The event may be enough to move the patient from kidney injury to ARF, as they lack any degree of 'renal reserve' or tolerance to events such as low blood pressure or administration of nephrotoxic drugs normally filtered by the kidneys.[13]

Postrenal causes

Urinary tract obstruction is the primary postrenal cause of ARF, and is uncommon in the critical care setting as it is rarely associated with acute onset renal failure.[13] Postrenal obstruction is more common in the community and is associated with urological disorders such as prostate gland enlargement in males, urinary tract tumours and renal calculi formation impairing urine outflow. It is essential that blockage of any urinary drainage device be excluded in the critically ill patient when undertaking an assessment of apparent oliguria.

Acute tubular necrosis and acute kidney injury

Intrinsic ARF (described above) is often associated with typical microscopic changes on pathology examination of kidney tissue. This pathology is termed ATN, and possibly explains how and why, in the acute setting, kidneys can fail abruptly to minimal to no function (no urine output and therefore no waste clearance), and can then after a period of time, with artificial support, recover to normal function in many patients.[20] This is now a contentious issue amongst leading researchers who are cautioning against the widespread adoption of the term ATN to explain the pathophysiological changes and disruption of kidney function seen as kidney injury develops.[3,5] Current opinion suggests renal dysfunction is possibly attributable to a functional rather than structural derangement, more likely explained through an imbalance in energy generation sufficient to support renal function combined with a renal protective 'shutdown' at a cellular level.[5,21]

ATN describes damage to the tubular portion of the nephron and may range from subtle metabolic changes to total dissolution of cell structure, with tubular cells 'defoliating' or detaching from the tubule basement membrane.[22] Most AKI in ICU patients is multifactorial in origin and may involve more than one causative mechanism and is not always an ischaemic or necrotic event.[16] In critical illness, the most common combination causing ARF is the administration of nephrotoxic agents in association with prolonged hypoperfusion or ischaemia.[22] This type of tubular necrosis can be further mediated by infection, blood transfusion reactions, drugs, ingested toxins and poisons, or be a complication of heart failure or major cardiovascular surgery. The initial insult can also be compounded by metabolic disturbances and subsequent systemic infection.

While ATN is reported as the causative mechanism for up to 30% of acute kidney failure in the intensive care setting, the precise causative pathology is not easily identifiable in critically ill patients with multiple comorbidities, for example diabetes, advanced age, investigations requiring radio-opaque dye administration, potent and nephrotoxic drug administration or major surgery with an inflammatory state due to an underlying infection. This is the context of critical illness and AKI where, despite modulation of the cause and support with artificial renal replacement therapies, mortality ranges from 28–90% depending on diagnostic criteria or definition.[4,23]

This type of kidney damage is of particular importance, as it is abrupt in onset and causes a rapid cessation of normal nephron function, a picture typical of any critical illness and failure of other body organs.[4] As this failure is commonly mediated by a loss in total or regional blood flow to the kidney,[24] it is more pronounced in the kidney medulla or outer regions sensitive to reduced blood flow. The cause of this loss in blood flow may be multifactorial but is commonly associated with shock and consequent low blood pressure (see Figure 18.7). Tubular cells suffer an ischaemic insult, causing a shedding of the cells from the nephron basement membrane. This shedding of cells has an initial loss of cell polarity, and then cell death, with a 'patchy' occurrence along the tubule basement membrane.[22] In addition, some cells detach themselves before death in a response known as apoptosis (cell self-death)[22] (see Chapter 22). The response is aimed at organ survival, with some individual cells 'sacrificing' themselves during a period of crisis. This protective response reduces oxygen demand by initiating cell death in some tubules, while others differentiate and/or proliferate for repair, and allows continuation of some normal function. If the causative process abates, remaining cells regenerate by differentiation and proliferation, tissue repair occurs with restoration of normal epithelium in some tubules and nephron function returns.

During this period cellular 'debris' collects in the tubule loops, causing obstruction of tubular flow, with backleak of filtrate occurring through the 'patchy' exposed tubular membrane surface. An inflammatory process is also stimulated due to release of cell adhesion factors and leucocyte activation,[25] which in turn causes further vasoconstriction and ischaemia[26] in the acute stage. The backleakage and static tubular fluid creates a concentrate that, by diffusion, raises blood levels of wastes such as urea, creatinine and other toxins. Along with the cessation of urine flow, toxicity occurs due to high serum levels of wastes such as urea, creatinine, potassium and undefined toxins.[25] This is the clinical state associated with the pathology of AKI that better describes the total 'picture' of pre-illness status, immediate causative events and degree of injury determined by patient serum creatinine or urine output.[1,2]

In the past authors have often employed the term ATN to describe ARF,[11] using it as a surrogate for ARF in the acute setting, as it focuses on the pathophysiology of tubular damage, recognising this damage as a final outcome of all causative factors. However, more recently, with the development of a consensus definition for ARF describing stages of illness severity, the term AKI is now used reflecting pathophysiology, the outcome of many causative factors and the clinical context where small derangements may be evident with reversibility of dysfunction and recovery, through to irreversible damage with kidney failure.[1-3]

The kidneys are vital human body organs essential to sustaining life. An important interrelationship of the kidneys and other body organs exists, with the brain, heart, liver and lungs dependent on receiving 'clean' blood to function. As toxins and fluid rapidly accumulate due to AKI during critical illness these changes contribute to organ dysfunction,[27,28] although many of these interrelationships (e.g. with the liver) are poorly understood.[29]

Acute kidney injury: Clinical and diagnostic criteria for classification

Clinical assessment

Clinical assessment of the patient with impending renal failure can involve myriad tests and investigations; however, the majority of these are not used to assess the critically ill patient. The clinical history is important in differentiating pre-existing renal disease and cataloguing the numerous factors already discussed that can contribute to AKI. The key assessments used in monitoring renal function are urine output, serum creatinine and urea levels, combined with more general measures including heart rate, blood pressure, fluid balance and daily weight. These measures are essential for the critically ill patient, and alterations provide the diagnostic key. They also link into the wider assessment of fluid and electrolyte balance, as described in Chapters 9 and 21.

Uraemic complications

Uraemic complications are influenced by the rate of urea accumulation and vary from patient to patient. As serum urea levels rise rapidly (i.e. over the course of a few days), above 20 mmol/L blood coagulation can be affected. A rash and related itchiness can occur. As blood levels continue to rise, neurological function can be affected and level of consciousness will deteriorate. In some cases high levels of urea can result in encephalopathy.[30]

Cardiovascular alterations

Cardiovascular alterations can occur as a result of acute kidney injury[31] as a result of direct effects on the myocardium but also because of fluid accumulation and electrolyte disturbance. The greatest concern is fluid overload as a consequence of failure to excrete the excess quantities of fluid used in resuscitating critically ill patients and the necessity to provide adequate nutrition in the form of parenteral or enteral nutrition.[32] Without appropriate management heart failure and pulmonary oedema can develop. Electrolyte disturbances are numerous in the patient with severe AKI, but of paramount concern is hyperkalaemia to the extent that cardiac rhythm disturbance can occur. As potassium levels rise the cardio-electric cycle becomes 'dampened', eventually deteriorating to a sign wave with no concurrent cardiac pumping action. Please refer to Chapter 11 for a more detailed discussion of cardiac arrhythmias associated with electrolyte disturbances.

Respiratory alteration

As noted earlier, fluid accumulation will invariably result in inadequate clearance of the pulmonary interstitial space by the pulmonary lymphatics, resulting firstly in interstitial oedema and moving on to overt pulmonary oedema and serious impairment of pulmonary gas exchange. Respiratory rate may also increase as patients develop metabolic acidosis both through renal injury and associated critical illness.

Haematological alterations

The primary haematological concern in AKI is related to the anti-coagulatory effects of rapidly increasing serum urea. While the kidney accounts for 90% of circulating erythropoietin production,[12] the acute nature of severe AKI does not influence anaemia to the extent of more common causes such as haemorrhage related to trauma or surgery or even iatrogenic blood loss.

Neurological alterations

Changes to central nervous system function can be related to accumulating urea, fluid and disruption of sodium balance. In the most severe form these can result in loss of consciousness and fitting.

Diagnosis

The management of AKI begins with the diagnosis, based on the patient's presenting signs and symptoms linked to a patient history. A long-term history of renal disease involving urinary tract infections, diabetes, cardiac failure and systemic inflammatory illnesses are all highly relevant.[12] Immediate history of presentation to a hospital involving surgery or any life-threatening illness with associated shock is also highly relevant in association with reduced urine output volumes over time.

Nurses in the critical care setting, who measure urine output hourly, readily recognise a key sign of impending renal dysfunction. Oliguria in the absence of catheter obstruction should be responded to quickly, as this suggests inadequate kidney blood flow and, to some extent, is a delayed observation considering the continual moderation of kidney function producing urine output. Persisting oliguria or the onset of anuria with associated rises in blood creatinine defines the injury phase of AKI. This sequence of events can be identified in the collective criteria known as the 'RIFLE' criteria – **r**isk, **i**njury, **f**ailure, and outcome criteria of **l**oss and **e**nd-stage disease – which provides the basis for a widely-accepted approach to diagnosing and classifying AKI.[3]

Consensus definition: the RIFLE criteria

The RIFLE criteria are shown in Figure 18.6, and use rising creatinine and falling urine output as highly sensitive and specific indicators for a continuum of renal failure. This is a useful classification system to grade loss of kidney function, reflecting stages of injury to the kidney before failure occurs. Without this, the small but important losses of kidney function before the failure state are not adequately considered.[1] This approach provides a consensus definition for loss of kidney function that is useful for clinical practice and research into this area, with clinicians all talking the same 'language' when comparing patients and/or results from clinical trials. The shape of the diagram indicates that more people will develop symptoms of ARF linked to kidney 'injury' and be considered 'at risk' (high sensitivity) than those at the bottom of the definition, who are fewer in number but need to fulfil strict criteria (high specificity).

To better understand the RIFLE criteria in a clinical care context, the following discussion is useful to consider in association with a review of Figure 18.6. In a hospital setting, those patients with a risk of renal injury would be identified by a low urine output of less than 0.5 mL/kg/h for 6 hours. In this situation their creatinine would be expected to rise, indicating a concurrent reduction in glomerular filtration rate. Reducing renal risk requires basic measures such as ensuring an adequate fluid intake and continuing to closely monitor urine output, while reviewing the patient's medications, haemodynamic state, signs of infection and possible other causes of injury in order to prevent further deterioration.

In the event that urine output decreases further, or was worse than this when first identified, to less than 0.5 mL/kg/h or a creatinine increase of twice the normal value occurs, renal injury is likely, with these clinical changes proposed as being highly sensitive towards injury having occurred. At this stage the above measures would be appropriate and further investigation as to possible causes is warranted. With treatment of the underlying cause, close monitoring, support of haemodynamics and fluid administration, most patients should not progress further in the failure continuum.

The next progression in clinical deterioration is oliguria, or urine output being less than 0.5 mL/kg/h for 24 hours or anuria for 12 hours. The creatinine increase is now proposed as being three times the normal level and, with minimal to no urine output, renal 'failure' is proposed as a clinical diagnosis using this criterion. It is at this stage when renal replacement therapy would need to be considered and, if not already attended to, patients should be transferred to ICU. A continuous therapy, or continuous renal replacement therapy (CRRT), is recommended. This term is more specific for the modes of treatment commonly applied in the ICU. Renal replacement therapy (RRT) refers to any treatment that replaces renal function and includes intermittent haemodialysis and peritoneal dialysis (PD). It is also important to understand that, in the setting of an acute illness, many patients progress through these stages of renal dysfunction to the failure stage quickly or the problem is unidentified until the failure stage is met. The timing for taking a blood sample to measure creatinine or when a urine catheter is passed to measure urine output also influences this identification. The diagnosis may be made only at the failure stage, without any identifiable period of risk or injury as proposed by the RIFLE criteria. With a critical illness, serum values of creatinine, urea, pH and potassium are readily available in the ICU and are used for diagnosis in association with the RIFLE definition. Daily monitoring of these values as a minimum is necessary for diagnosis and monitoring during CRRT in the ICU. The normal laboratory values for these biochemical markers are essential knowledge for nurses to understand AKI and management.

Treatment with CRRT may not be implemented until failure is evident, by anuria and uraemia, or until patients meet the RIFLE definition criteria. However, in some patients, CRRT may be commenced earlier, in anticipation of failure and as a strategy to prevent further kidney damage or complications of functional renal deterioration.

Practice tip

Reducing urine output is an important sign of impending AKI; however, checking a catheter for blockage is also important. A bladder scanner may also reveal a full bladder where no catheter is in place.

Management of the patient with acute kidney injury

Reducing further insults to the kidneys

After diagnosis, the next management principle is to remove or modify any cause that may exacerbate the pathological process associated with AKI. Further interventions and investigations are performed in relation to the findings from the history and presentation. These may include:[13]

- further intravenous fluid resuscitation (despite an oligo-anuric state) and restoration of blood pressure using inotropic/vasoactive drugs
- physical or diagnostic assessment for renal outflow obstruction and alleviation if present
- avoiding contrast-enhanced radiological investigations
- ceasing or modifying the dose of any nephrotoxic drugs or agents and treating infection with alternative, less toxic antibiotics.

Initial management strategies for the early stages of ARF remain conservative, with careful management of fluid (once adequate circulating volume is assured) and haemodynamics, encouraging diuresis if present, monitoring blood profiles for changes in urea and electrolytes and limiting or reformulating the administration of agents that may contribute to the accumulation of urea and electrolytes (e.g. enteral or intravenous nutritional supplements). The use of agents such as mannitol, dopamine and frusemide, while popular in practice, have not been shown to be of any value in improving outcome in patients at risk of ARF.[13,20]

Despite these efforts, life-threatening biochemistry may arise in ARF, such as severe acidosis and hyperkalaemia (pH of <7.1 and serum potassium >6.5 mmol/L), that requires immediate treatment and is an indication for beginning RRT without elevation of serum creatinine and oliguria and fluid overload.[33]

Fluid balance

As oliguria and anuria are key diagnostic and clinical signs of renal dysfunction, reducing fluid intake is necessary to prevent intravascular overload and tissue oedema until renal recovery begins or a renal replacement therapy is started. Reducing or restricting fluid intake can be a challenge in the critically ill as it is not uncommon for these patients to be administered 3 L of fluid in 24 hours.[34] A balance state for this degree of fluid administration suggests a urine output at 125 mL/h without considering other insensible losses. Strategies can be considered to minimise fluid intake such as preparing drug infusions without diluent and in a concentrated version of the usual preparation. Pharmacists may assist with this requirement and offer advice for drug preparation and delivery. Restriction of oral fluids can be implemented and

monitored using a fluid chart, with the aim of adhering to the prescribed volume. Nutrition therapy is important for optimising patient outcome but can also contribute to increased fluid intake. Enteral feeding is preferred for most critically ill patients and standard enteral feeding formulas can contribute about 1.5 L of fluid intake per day in an adult.[35] Nutrition is very important in the patient experiencing ARF where growth and repair is needed with damaged kidney cells and protein depletion avoided.[36] Calorie dense enteral feeding formulas (2 kcal/mL) can be considered as a strategy to minimise fluid intake associated with enteral feeding (see Chapter 19 for further discussion on nutrition in critical illness). Fluid balance charting and a clear understanding of the maximum fluid intake per day is vital for managing AKI at this stage, and a maximum intake of 1.5 L per day is a common target in the adult patient.[35] An inability to prevent a positive fluid balance, largely due to meeting nutritional requirements, is often the reason CRRT is initiated.[37]

Electrolyte balance

Managing serum electrolytes, in particular potassium, is essential for patient stability as low or high levels are more likely to be associated with life-threatening arrhythmias.[38] However, phosphate, calcium and sodium may also be abnormal and require strategies to reduce, supplement or control the serum level away from toxicity. Hyponatraemia, for example, may be associated with altered mental state, impaired consciousness and even seizures.[39]

Acid–base balance

Control of the acid–base balance is another essential function of the healthy kidneys and, with failure, metabolic acidosis will develop due to decreased buffering and accumulation of many acids not excreted.[39] An increased minute ventilation may be observed in the patient, representing a physiological attempt to control acidaemia. This requires additional energy and caloric consumption and is another indication that RRT should be implemented using bicarbonate fluids to control the acidaemia.[39]

Pharmacotherapy and altered pharmacokinetics

The modification of drug regimens to effect changes to excretion and volume of distribution is a further aspect of clinical management during the onset of ARF. Drugs are excreted from the body after hepatic and other organ metabolism, which converts them to a water soluble form such that they appear in the urine. Therefore, modification of dose (through reduction or frequency of administration) and monitoring for serum levels helps to prevent further renal insult while ensuring the desired clinical effect.[40]

Aminoglycosides are a key group of antibiotics requiring adjustment and monitoring in AKI, if not ceasing and substituting for another appropriate but less nephrotoxic antibiotic.[40] Other drugs administered in the ICU that warrant attention include narcotics, histamine-2 receptor antagonists and beta blockers. Pharmacy product information attached with packaging and/or local pharmacy information usually provides helpful suggestions and guidelines for relevant drug use in AKI. If RRT is started, and is functioning continuously with efficiency, the clearance and toxicity of drugs is of less concern and dosing may resume to normal for some drugs with close monitoring continuing.[40]

If conservative measures fail, the ongoing management of the patient with ARF requires RRT. This enables control of blood biochemistry, prevents toxin accumulation, and allows removal of fluids so that adequate nutrition can be achieved. The criteria and indications for initiating RRT are listed in Box 18.1. One indication is sufficient to initiate RRT, while two or more make RRT urgent. Combined derangements can create the necessity to commence therapy before individually-defined limits have been reached. Early initiation of treatment is widely advocated and may confer more rapid renal recovery.

BOX 18.1

Proposed criteria for the initiation of renal replacement therapy in adult critically ill patients[14]

- Oliguria (urine output <200 mL/12 h)
- Anuria/extreme oliguria (urine output <50 mL/12 h)
- Hyperkalaemia (K^+ >6.5 mmol/L)
- Severe acidaemia (pH <7.1)
- Azotaemia (urea >30 mmol/L)
- Clinically significant organ (esp lung) oedema
- Uraemic encephalopathy
- Uraemic pericarditis
- Uraemic neuropathy/myopathy
- Severe dysnatraemia (Na^+ >160 or <115 mmol/L)
- Hyperthermia
- Drug overdose with dialysable toxin

Approaches to renal replacement therapy

A brief review of the historical perspectives associated with the development of modern day dialysis and RRT provided in the ICU is helpful in understanding key concepts and methods of CRRT, including PD.

History

Dialysis is a term describing RRT and refers to the purification of blood through a membrane by diffusion of waste substances.[41] Table 18.1 outlines historical events during the development of dialysis in Europe and the USA. The Kolff rotating drum kidney, one of the earliest attempts at RRT (illustrated in Figure 18.8), used cellulose tubing rolled around a wooden skeleton built

FIGURE 18.8 Kolff dialyser.

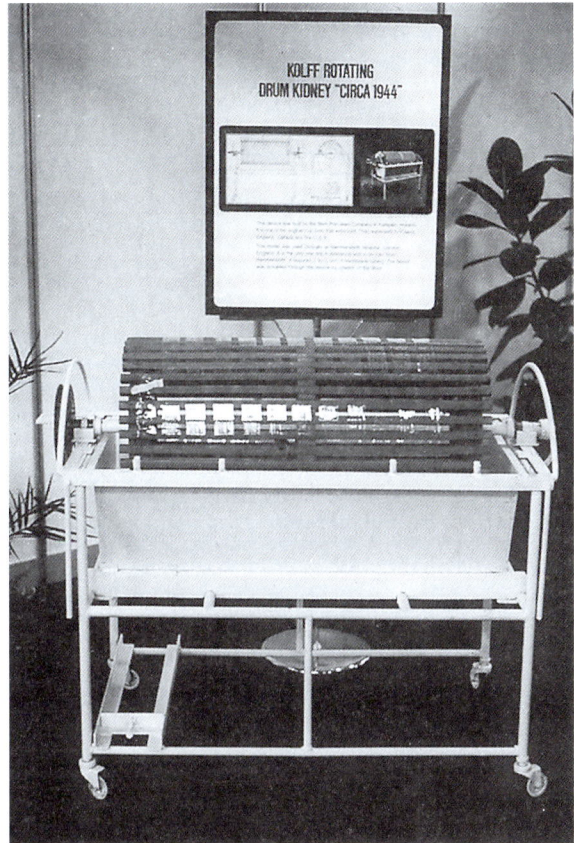

Reproduced from Thomas N. Haemodialysis. In: Thomas N, ed. Renal nursing. 2nd ed. London: Baillière Tindall; 2002.

as a large, drum-styled cage. The drum with the blood-filled cellulose tubing was immersed in a bath of weak salt solution and, as blood passed through, the rotating cellulose tubing allowed waste exchange to occur by diffusion.

The Kolff rotating drum kidney provided limited effective waste clearance and prompted design and development of a new membrane for solute exchange that had a greater surface area and required less blood volume. This led to the development of the hollow-fibre filter membrane structure in the 1960s, which became the 'artificial kidney'.[42]

The combination of an extracorporeal circuit (EC), blood pump and filter membrane and the associated nursing management are now commonly known as haemodialysis. With industrial and scientific developments, such as plastics moulding and electronics, current dialysis techniques are safe, effective and a life-sustaining treatment for the millions of people who suffer acute and chronic kidney failure.[43,44]

Key to the application of these technical and scientific developments has been the role of nurses, who have made a substantial contribution to the safety and efficiency of dialysis.[45] Nursing of dialysis patients has developed

TABLE 18.1

Historical events in the development of dialysis

TIME PERIOD AND DEVELOPER	DESCRIPTION
1854: Thomas Graham, Scottish chemist	First used the term 'dialysis' to describe the transport of solutes through an ox bladder, which drew attention to the concept of a membrane for solute removal from fluid
1920s: George Haas, German physician	First human dialysis was carried out, performing six treatments on six patients. Haas failed to make further progress with the treatment but is recognised as an early pioneer of dialysis
1920–30s	Synthetic polymer chemistry allowed development of cellulose acetate, a membrane integral to the further development of dialysis treatments
1940s: Willem Kolff, Dutch physician	The discovery of heparin, an anticoagulant, enabled further development of dialysis during World War II, the Kolff rotating drum kidney
1940–50s: Kolff and Allis-Chalmers, USA	Further modification of the Kolff dialyser and the development of improved machines
1950s: Fredrik Kiil, Norway	Developed the parallel plate dialyser made of a new cellulose, Cuprophane. This required a pump to push the blood through the membrane and return the blood to the patient
1950–60s	Dialysis began to be widely used to treat kidney failure
1960s: Richard Stewart and Dow Chemical, USA	The hollow-fibre membrane dialyser used a membrane design of a cellulose acetate bundle, with 11,000 fibres providing a surface area of 1 m²
1970s	Use of the first CAVH circuits for diuretic resistant oedema by Kramer
1980s	First continuous therapies using blood pump and intravenous pumps to control fluid removal and substitution: Australia and New Zealand led the way
1990s	New purpose-built machines used; Gambro Prisma, Baxter BM 11 + 14 to provide pump-controlled therapies with integrated automated fluid balance using scales to measure fluids. Cassette circuits, automated priming; new membranes
2000	Further purpose-built machines using direct measurement for waste and substitution fluids via Hygieia–Kimal machine. Introduction of high fluid exchange rates for sepsis treatment. Introduction of dialysis-based machines in ICU for daily 'hybrid' treatments: SLEDD and SLEDDf
2010	Multiple CRRT machines; more advanced graphics interface and smart alarms. Waste disposal systems. High flux, porous membranes

CAVH = continuous arteriovenous haemofiltration; CRRT = continuous renal replacement therapy; SLEDD = sustained low-efficiency daily dialysis; SLEDDf = sustained low-efficiency daily diafiltration.

into a specialist field of knowledge and skill, with nurses combining their holistic view of patient management with the specialist needs of patients with renal failure, from the outpatient setting to the ICU, including a collaborative approach to further adaptations of dialysis best suited to the critically ill.[46–48]

Development of renal replacement therapy in critical care

Improvements in many fields of health care, including resuscitation and treatment for shock, and the growing number of patients undergoing and surviving extensive surgery and trauma, have led to developments and challenges in critical care practice. Many patients who would previously have died from an acute illness now survive, but develop ARF as a complication.

Historically, ARF was treated in the ICU with the use of PD, which did not require specialist nurses or doctors. This simple technique removes wastes by infusing a dialysis fluid into the abdomen, allowing diffusion and osmosis to occur between the peritoneum and fluid before draining out again in repeated cycles.[49] This was performed by the ICU nurse and prescribed by ICU doctors, but was inadequate in its clearance of waste and fluid volume, and was associated with infection, limitation of respiratory function and exacerbated glucose intolerance.[16,49]

In 1977 Peter Kramer, a German ICU doctor, developed a new dialytic technique called continuous arteriovenous haemofiltration (CAVH). It was later renamed slow continuous ultrafiltration (SCUF), as it enabled the removal of plasma water in addition to dissolved wastes (convective clearance of solutes) at a flow rate of 200–600 mL/h by passive drainage from the membrane as blood flowed through it.[50] This marked the beginning of continuous RRT in the ICU as an intervention prescribed and managed by ICU nurses and doctors for patients with ARF.

Refinement of renal replacement therapy

Although CAVH as developed by Kramer was useful in removing excessive body water and some wastes, a dialysis blood pump enabled a much more efficient technique for therapeutic benefit in the ICU patient with ARF. The use of roller blood pumps to generate pressure and a reliable flow of blood, thus eliminating the need for arterial puncture and access, was introduced. This approach, termed continuous veno-venous haemofiltration (CVVH), could reliably pump blood at a constant rate and achieve ultrafiltration volumes of 1000 mL/h. With further modifications to the circuit and filter set-up, a diffusive component was added to the therapy by running a dialysate volume through the haemofilter, flowing between the membrane fibres and countercurrent to blood flow. This was termed continuous veno-venous haemodiafiltration (CVVHDf).[51]

Principles of peritoneal dialysis

PD relies on the simple physical processes of osmosis and diffusion to achieve the goal of adequate fluid and toxic metabolite removal and electrolyte balance in the patient who can no longer sustain this through deteriorating renal function. Unlike extracorporeal approaches for renal replacement, PD uses the abdominal peritoneum as the membrane through which filtration and diffusion occur. The peritoneum provides simple access to the circulating blood and is highly permeable to the range of electrolytes and metabolites that are the target of therapeutic exchange for any renal replacement approach.[52]

By introducing a solution that has a mix of electrolytes and osmotic components formulated to create both a diffusion and osmotic gradient to the peritoneal cavity, then allowing sufficient dwell time for equilibration between the solution and peritoneal blood supply to occur, then draining off the fluid, both solute and fluid removal can occur. By repeating this simple process of instilling between 1 and 3 L of fluid in a regular cycle of between 30 to 60 minutes (instillation/dwell/drain), fluid balance and metabolic control can be achieved for the patient with AKI.[53,54] PD is a gentle but effective form of dialysis if repeated regularly over days and can bridge the gap between failure of the kidneys to adequately perform their function to the point where they then recover sufficient function to again control patient fluid and metabolite balance with or without medication and dietary manipulation.

Numerous formulations and combinations of solutions and constituents have been used (Table 18.2). Variations in the osmotic component of the solutions (often a glucose-based element expressed as percentage) will increase or decrease the rate of fluid removal along with the frequency and duration of cycle time. Likewise, the absence or relative concentration of electrolytes in the solution will determine the removal or addition of substances such as potassium from or into the circulation.

TABLE 18.2

Typical fluid constituents for peritoneal dialysis

	BAXTER (TOONGABBIE, NSW, AUSTRALIA) DIANEAL® PD-4	FRESENIUS (FMC, JAPAN, FUKUOKA) STAY SAFE® BALANCE
Volume, mL	2000	2000
Glucose	2.5 %	2.3 %
Sodium mmol/L	132	134
Calcium mmol/L	1.25	1.25
Magnesium mmol/L	0.25	0.5
Lactate mmol/L	40	35
Glucose, g	25	25
Osmolarity, mOsm/kg	395	399

A solution component to assist in managing acid–base balance is also necessary. Originally, acetate was incorporated in solutions to counter the acidosis seen in renal failure; more recently lactate has been used. Both of these components are stable in solution and, when exchanged at the peritoneal interface, will be metabolised in the patient's liver while contributing to neutralisation of excessive H^+ accumulation. However, critically ill patients often have impaired liver function that limits the effectiveness of these agents in controlling excess acidity. The use of HCO_3^- as an acid buffer is preferential but represents challenges due to its instability in solution and higher production cost.

Management of peritoneal dialysis

The management of PD, apart from the peritoneal cannula insertion and dose prescription, is largely a nursing responsibility. Running PD for a critically ill patient with AKI might be considered when resource limitations (equipment, power or fluids) or expertise to use extracorporeal CRRT is not available. The process of PD can be particularly demanding due to the regular cycling of fluid required to manage the hypermetabolic state often seen in these patients. Major management considerations include cannula care, fluid formulation and fluid cycling in and out. Frequent monitoring of the patient's blood profile is necessary to determine the impact and identify untoward effects of the treatment. Common problems associated with PD include:

- heat loss due to instillation of inadequately warmed fluids
- raised intra-abdominal pressure, impinging on respiratory and bowel function
- infection introduced through the cannula at insertion, or during treatment, or PD fluid contamination.

Cannula care

Soft polyurethane cannulas are preferred in PD as they are more comfortable for the patient, less likely to perforate abdominal anatomy and easier to manage.[53,54] The cannula breaches the abdominal wall and floats in the peritoneal space (see Figure 18.9) providing an entry point for infection. While specific research on cannula care for acute insertion is limited, the same principles used in managing intravascular devices should be applied. Care needs to be taken to ensure the cannula remains straight so flow and effectiveness of the treatment are maintained. Repositioning the patient should prompt review of the catheter position.[55]

A single cannula may be used for both inflow and outflow of dialysate solution; a dual-lumen device allows both inflow and outflow to occur simultaneously as does placement of two cannulas.[54] During cannula insertion a catheter may cause trauma or a build-up of fibrin and connective tissue may occur with time. Instillation of heparin has been suggested to help avoid clotting and blockage of the cannula; if used, monitoring of subsequent bleeding within the abdominal cavity is required.

Fluid selection

Fluid selection will be based on specific treatment goals with higher glucose concentrations prescribed to increase the osmotic gradient and fluid removal over the cycle length. These solutions can be absorbed to the systemic circulation through the peritoneum, so regular monitoring of patient blood glucose levels is necessary, particularly in the diabetic patient. Careful assessment of blood glucose

levels is also required when reducing, increasing or ceasing the glucose load in the dialysate solution for systemic rebound effects.[55]

Potassium may be entirely absent from the solution in order to allow its removal from the circulation as would normally occur in the functioning kidney. Once potassium levels normalise it can then be added to prevent ongoing loss. The use of an H^+ ion buffer is also needed; if bicarbonate is used ensure it is added at the time of administration to retain a useful level in solution. The nature of the peritoneum and the crystalloid-based infused fluids means significant protein losses in the outflow fluid can be anticipated. This may require additional nutritional supplementation and problems with hypoalbuminaemia.

All of these additions to the solution require careful concentration calculation to ensure the correct dose is delivered in a physiologically stable solution. Consulting with a pharmacist is recommended if regular additions to dialysate solutions are to occur. Pre-formulation can assist in ensuring both correct solution and the sterility of the solution are maintained.

Circuit design and management

PD circuit configurations vary from simple to more complex (see Figure 18.10). Through a closed circuit, a machine can be used to deliver 24-hourly cycles of multiple bags. Using a machine to deliver PD minimises nursing time and maintains a closed circuit, reducing infection risk. Of course, using a cycler increases the complexity of the circuit and introduces the need for a power source, two of the claimed benefits of PD.

Modern PD offers a realistic alternative for uncomplicated AKI despite its many limitations. No RRT is without its problems and PD is possibly underrated as a treatment alternative. This could be particularly the case in paediatric patients. In underdeveloped countries it may be the preferred option of RRT due to its simplicity of operation and low cost. In disaster areas where high numbers of victims with injury-induced AKI are likely it may also offer a treatment that can be instituted on site and can be a life-saving proposition until more specific treatment can be accessed.

Principles of extracorporeal CRRT

Both intermittent haemodialysis and CRRT require a machine to pump blood and fluids; pressure and flow devices to monitor treatment; a tubing and filter membrane set that together create an extracorporeal circuit (EC) (outside the body blood pathway); and a catheter connecting the patient's circulation to the circuit (see Figure 18.11). This catheter enables blood to be drawn from and returned to the patient (known as 'access'). Access can be achieved by three different techniques:

- temporary catheters inserted via a skin puncture into an artery for drawing blood and a vein to return the blood (AV access)

FIGURE 18.9 PD cannula example.

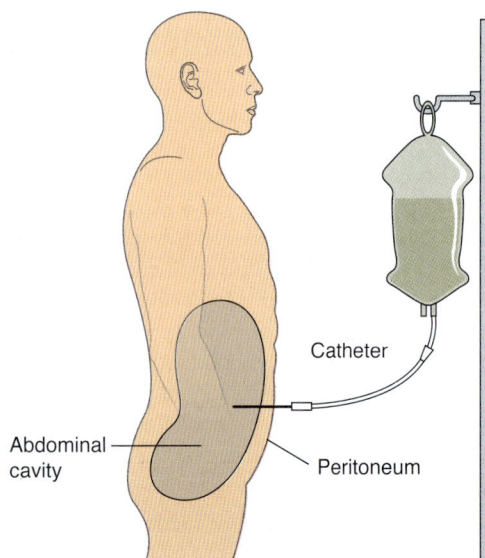

Catheter

Abdominal cavity

Peritoneum

Adapted from National Kidney and Urologic Diseases Information Clearinghouse website, http://kidney.niddk.nih.gov/KUDiseases/pubs/peritoneal/index.aspx, with permission.

FIGURE 18.10 PD circuit example.

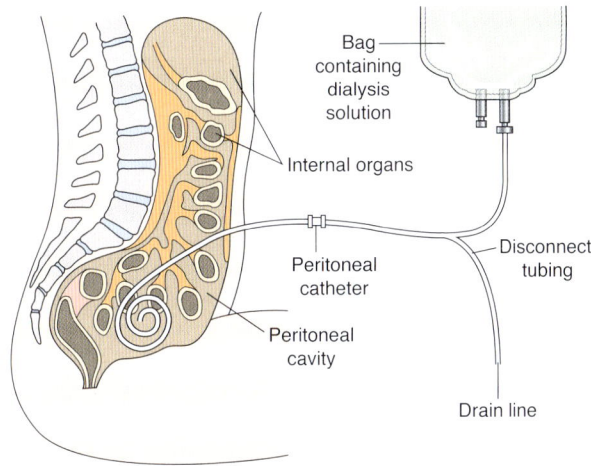

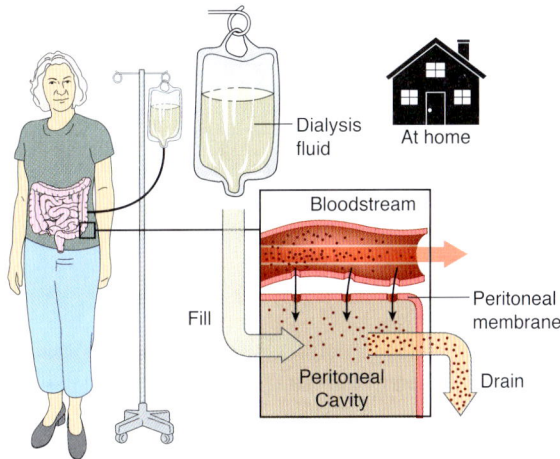

Adapted from National Kidney and Urologic Diseases Information Clearinghouse website, http://kidney.niddk.nih.gov/KUDiseases/pubs/peritoneal/index.aspx, with permission.

- a surgical joining of an artery and vein (usually in the forearm), making a large vessel that is punctured with needles to both draw and return the blood (AV fistula)

- a catheter with two lumens to draw and return blood via a large central vein (a dual veno-venous access catheter).

In the acute renal failure setting and where temporary treatment is anticipated, the two-lumen catheter is recommended.[56,57]

Haemodialysis, haemofiltration and haemodiafiltration

Haemodialysis, haemofiltration and haemodiafiltration are three common techniques used to achieve artificial kidney support in ARF. The basic blood path or circuit for these therapies is indicated in Figure 18.11 and is useful to

FIGURE 18.11 Renal replacement therapy blood path circuit common to all approaches.

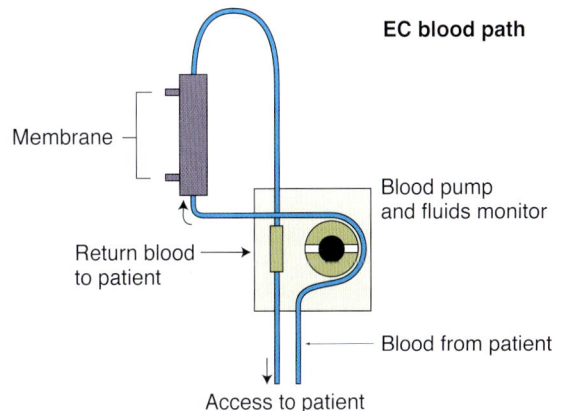

TABLE 18.3

Abbreviations describing modes of renal replacement therapy

TIMING OF THERAPY	ROUTE OF ACCESS	MECHANISM OF SOLUTE REMOVAL
I = intermittent	A = arterial	H (or HF) = haemofiltration – convection
C = continuous	V = venous	D (or HD) = haemodialysis – dialysis
S = slow	AV = arteriovenous	HDF = haemodiafiltration – diffusion and convection
	VV = veno-venous	UF = ultrafiltration – plasma water removal

review to understand each therapy and where the RRT fluids are then applied to the circuit, differentiating them as techniques.

The extracorporeal component is a common factor in all these different circuit designs. The difference between treatments is how the solutes such as urea, creatinine and other waste products and the solvent or plasma water are removed from the blood as it passes through the filter membrane (artificial kidney), and the intermittent versus continuous prescription of the therapy. The three physical mechanisms of fluid and solute management are convection, diffusion and ultrafiltration. Table 18.3 lists the commonly used abbreviations to describe the timing of treatment, blood access for the therapy and mode of solute removal.

Convection

Convection is the process whereby dissolved solutes are removed with plasma water as it is filtered through the dialysis membrane. The word is derived from the Latin *convehere*, meaning 'to remove or to carry along with'.[58] This process is similar to that occurring in the native kidney glomerulus, as plasma water is filtered across the nephron tubule via the Bowman's capsule. In RRT, the plasma water with the dissolved wastes is discarded; the deficit is then replaced with manufactured artificial plasma water in equal or slightly lower amounts to achieve a desired fluid balance. This blood purification process is commonly known as haemofiltration. When applied on a continuous basis in the ICU, haemofiltration can adequately replace essential renal functions, and is particularly effective in managing fluid balance.[33,59] Figure 18.12 illustrates the circuit and set-up for continuous veno-venous hemofiltration.

Diffusion

Diffusion refers to the physical movement of solutes across a semipermeable membrane from an area of high concentration to that of a relatively low concentration; that is, solutes move across a concentration gradient.[60] A higher concentration gradient results in a greater rate of diffusive clearance. As blood passes through the dialysis membrane, dialysate fluid, reflecting normal blood chemistry, is exposed to the blood on the opposing side of the membrane fibre. Diffusive clearance is continuous as solute exchange occurs with the dialysate fluid and the blood continually moving in and out of the membrane. As waste-laden blood enters the hollow membrane fibre

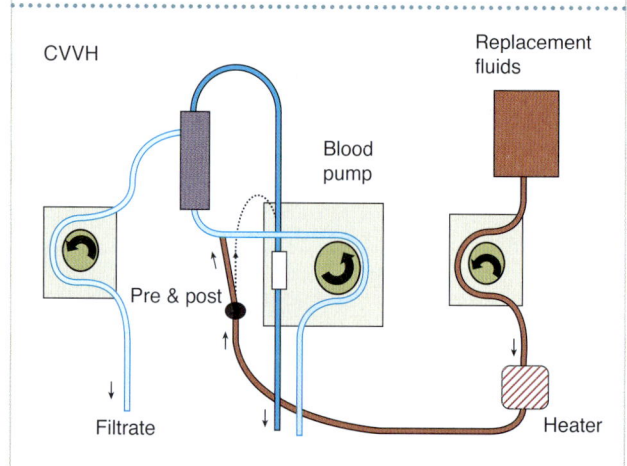

FIGURE 18.12 Continuous veno-venous haemofiltration (CVVH) circuit.

and fresh dialysate is in continuous supply, this process performs an effective waste-removal function. Blood and dialysate are established in a countercurrent or opposing flow to each other to maximise the diffusive process, mimicking the normal nephron function of the kidneys.[61]

A diffusive clearance technique can be performed with increasing intensity and effect by making the blood and dialysate flow faster, with technical problems associated with delivering the high fluid and blood flow being the main limiting factor increasing clearance. The two flows need to be maintained in relation to each other; for the diffusive clearance to be efficient the dialysate flow must always equal or exceed the blood flow. A common setting for an intermittent dialysis treatment would be a blood flow and dialysate fluid flow of 300 mL/min each. A faster blood flow is not useful unless dialysate flow is also increased, as more waste solutes will not be cleared if the dialysate fluid and blood are in diffusive equilibrium. The technique of solute removal using diffusion alone is termed dialysis; when used with blood, the process is termed haemodialysis. When applied on an intermittent basis, as is normal for patients receiving RRT for chronic renal failure, it is called intermittent haemodialysis.[62] Figure 18.13 illustrates the circuit set-up for intermittent haemodialysis.

Ultrafiltration

Ultrafiltration is the process that allows plasma water to leave the blood, achieving body fluid or water loss.[61]

FIGURE 18.13 Intermittent haemodialysis circuit. RO = reverse osmosis 'treated water'.

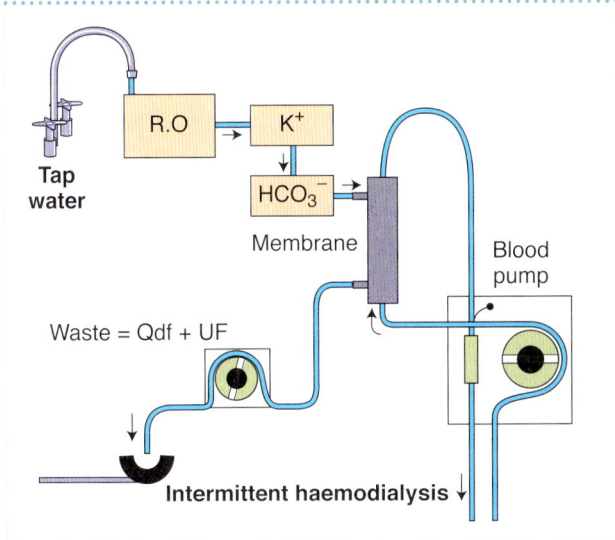

FIGURE 18.14 Continuous veno-venous haemodiafiltration (CVVHDf) circuit.

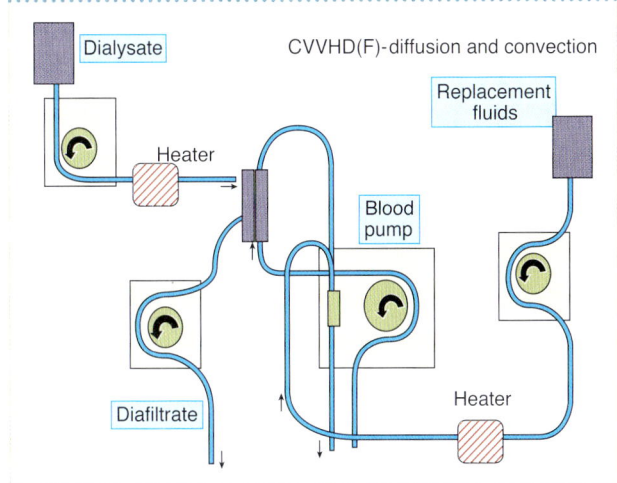

Dialysis nurses measure a fluid loss by weighing the patient before and after a treatment. This process is primarily used to achieve fluid balance, an important function of the kidneys. The only difference between this process and the convective clearance of solutes is that this fluid is not replaced, and it is therefore not considered an adequate solute management method. Ultrafiltration cannot be undertaken in large amounts without fluid replacement, as it would cause hypovolaemia. It is implemented during a dialysis period by removing small amounts each hour (e.g. 250 mL/h for 4 hours) during the intermittent treatment cycle.

There are different therapeutic effects from each form of RRT and different operational prescriptions of blood and fluid flow. Combinations of convection and diffusion can be used, known as CVVHDf.[62] An increase in the diffusive component (i.e. raising the dialysate flow rate in CVVHDf) will increase the removal of small-molecular-weight substances such as potassium and assist with hydrogen ion exchange via buffer solution. This can also be achieved via increasing filtration fluid flow (convective clearance), which will also add an increase in clearance of larger molecules, for example those associated with severe infection and systemic inflammation or sepsis. Figure 18.14 illustrates the circuit and set-up for CVVHDf.

Delivering CRRT

To correctly understand the different variants of RRT, how each achieves waste removal and fluid balance along with knowledge of how to 'troubleshoot' the machine providing RRT, nurses must have a clear understanding of the major circuit components and their functions.

Membranes

The filter or haemofilter (blood filter) is the primary functional component of the RRT system, responsible for

separating plasma water from the blood and/or allowing the exchange of solutes across the membrane by diffusion. The filter is made of a plastic casing, containing a synthetic polymer inner structure arranged in longitudinal fibres. A schematic diagram of a haemofilter is shown in Figure 18.15. The fibres are hollow and have pores along their length with a size of 15,000–30,000 daltons. This allows plasma water to pass through, carrying dissolved wastes out of the blood (most of which have a molecular weight <20,000 daltons), while larger plasma proteins and blood cells (at least 60–70,000 daltons) are retained.[58] Plasma water separated from the blood in this way is carried away from the filter by a side exit port and a pump, where it is measured and directed into a collection bottle or bag as waste; this convective clearance of solutes is similar to urine produced by the normal kidneys. The plasma water loss is replaced in equal volume with a commercially manufactured plasma water substitute, either after the 'filtered' blood exits the haemofilter (postdilution) or prior to the blood entering the haemofilter (predilution), or both at the same time. The plasma water replacement contains no metabolic wastes and achieves blood purification as it is continuously replaced.[63]

Filter membrane polymers are made of different materials: AN69 (acrylonitrile/sodium methallyl sulfonate), PAN (polyacrylonitrile) or PA (polyamide) and polysulfone;[63] however, all demonstrate similar artificial kidney effects and are generally chosen according to the supplier circuit provided or, when this is not fixed, by the vendor or doctor preference.[46] The most important characteristics of filters used in continuous modes of therapy are: 1) a high plasma water clearance rate at low blood flow rates and circuit pressures; and 2) high permeability to middle-sized molecular weight substances (500–15,000 daltons, e.g. inflammatory cytokines), which are often encountered in critical illness.

FIGURE 18.15 Haemofilter (dialysis membrane). Cross-sectional view indicating longitudinal synthetic fibres conveying blood into and out of the plastic casing outer structure. Plasma water is removed via the side ultrafiltrate port during CVVH applying convective clearance. In CVVHDf, the blood is exposed to fluid via the membrane fibres so that diffusive clearance can occur.

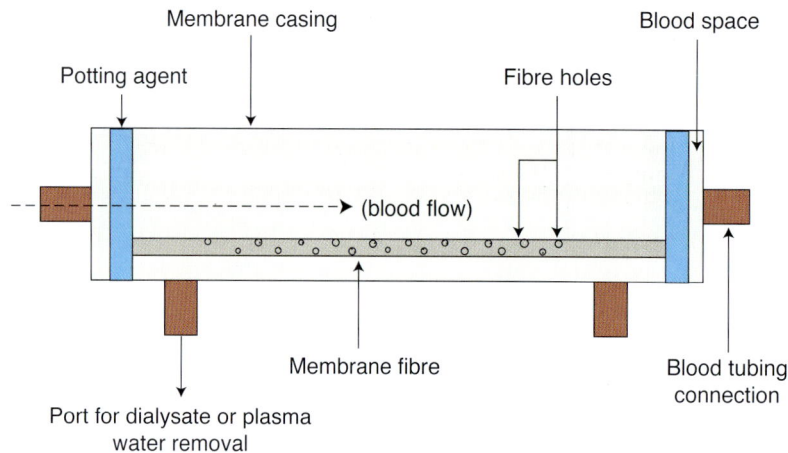

Vascular access

As previously noted, in order to establish CRRT it is necessary to create a blood flow outside the body using the EC. Blood is most commonly accessed from the venous circulation of the critical care patient via a catheter placed in a central vein (e.g. femoral). Blood is both withdrawn from the vein and returned to the same vein – that is, veno-venous (VV) access by means of a double (dual)-lumen catheter. When the same procedure is carried out by accessing the blood from the patient's systemic circulation via an artery and returning it to a vein, the term arteriovenous (AV) is used.[57,64] In this system there is no mechanical blood pump required, as the patient's arterial blood pressure provides a flow of blood in the EC. Veno-venous haemofiltration (CVVH) has the advantages of requiring only a single venipuncture, a reliable blood flow delivered from a blood pump and alternative venous access sites if site infection or access is difficult.[57] While it is easy to establish flow within AV-driven circuits and no complex system of blood pumps and pressure sensors is necessary, this method is susceptible to flow problems associated with low patient arterial blood pressure and high venous pressures, a common occurrence in critically ill patients.

The dual-lumen catheter used for veno-venous access has an internal diameter of 1.5–3 mm and the ends of the catheter are sufficiently separated from each other in the patient's vein to prevent filtered blood from mixing with unfiltered blood when used in the recommended sequence.[64] This ensures that filtered blood does not simply pass back through the artificial kidney, where there would be minimal waste clearance compared with 'fresh' unfiltered blood; this design is illustrated in Figure 18.16(A). The catheter must be small enough to place into

a vein but large enough to provide blood flow of at least 200 mL/min for an adult CRRT circuit. Catheters are made with different arrangement of the lumens revealing variation in their cross-section profile (see Figure 18.16B). There is no evidence to suggest which profile is better, but the larger the internal diameter, the less likely flow will be obstructed during patient care with CRRT. After a catheter is threaded into a vein, the blood flow may be adequate, but later during patient care it may obstruct due to different nursing interventions and patient movement, which may alter blood flows within the low pressure venous system.[65]

Insertion sites may be affected by nursing care interventions. Placement of the catheter is usually in the femoral or subclavian vein, and occasionally in the internal jugular vein.[64] Anecdotally, the subclavian position is more easily managed for dressing and securing, continuous observation and patient comfort, but is more problematic in terms of flow reliability. Intrathoracic pressure changes associated with physiotherapy or spontaneous patient coughing and breathing, coupled with the upright position of patients, may hinder blood flow from the subclavian-sited access catheter. While these issues are not encountered with a femoral-placed catheter, flow problems can arise due to side lying and flexion at the groin or hip.[65]

The flow performance of any vascular-access catheter can be affected by the patient's position in bed, spontaneous movement and repositioning activities as part of routine nursing care in the critically ill for pressure-area prevention. Catheter lumen outlet or inlet obstruction can be due to contact with the vessel wall, or to the formation of a sharp bend due to the patient's movement. These factors contribute to compromising blood flow in the EC,[65,66] and have been identified by an ultrasound Doppler flow probe attached to the circuit tubing.[65]

FIGURE 18.16 **A** Vascular access catheters for CRRT. Dual-lumen, Bard® Niagara™ and Gambro Dolphin Protect™ catheters; **B** concept diagram of catheter lumen profiles used for dual-lumen CRRT catheters.

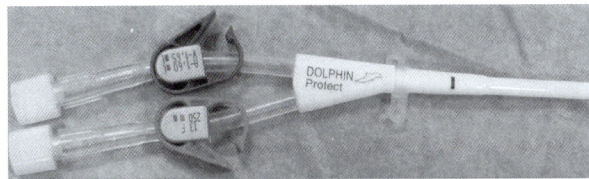

1.

Gambro Dolphin Protect®

2.

3.

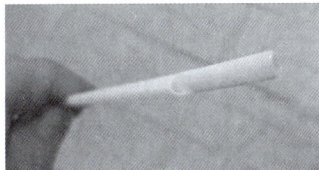

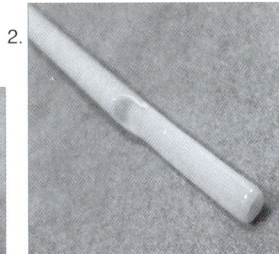

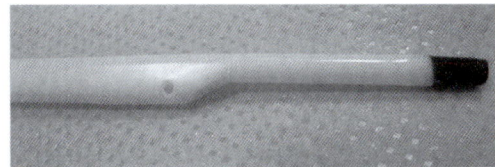

4.

Bard Niagara Vas-cath®

5.

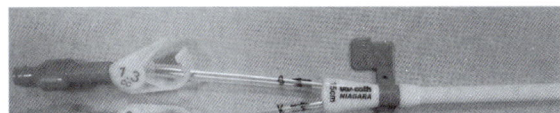

A

CRRT vascular access catheter
lumen design profiles

Double 'D' design or 'D' and 'O': one
lumen extended longer for return blood

Inner and outer lumen: 'Coaxial' with
side holes at tip for drawing blood into
outer lumen

Side by side: Double 'O': one
lumen extended longer for return blood

B

Practice tip

If CRRT circuits clot or fail, remember, if this is associated with failure of the access catheter, restarting a new treatment is also likely to fail unless the catheter is changed or re-sited. The solution is not to increase anticoagulant dose.

Blood pump

In veno-venous modes, a pump component is essential as part of the patient's blood volume flows externally to the body via the EC. Blood flow is maintained by a 'roller pump' (see Figure 18.17), which propels the blood along the tubing in a peristaltic fashion (milking along by compression of the tubing), compressing the blood-filled tubing but having no contact with the blood itself. This roller rotates at a rate providing a flow of fresh unfiltered blood to the haemofilter, enabling it to clear metabolic waste products.

The roller pump has a central anticlockwise rotating shaft driving two roller wheels inside a rigid housing. Blood-filled tubing sits stationary inside the housing and is compressed by the outer surface of the roller wheels during 180° (half) of their rotation through the pump housing. This means that one of the two wheels is almost continuously compressing the tubing, moving blood forward out of the roller housing. The compression is not absolutely continuous, as there is a short time (<0.5 s) when there is no compression to allow the tubing to refill with fresh blood. The compressed tubing re-expands behind the rotating roller and fills with fresh blood from the access and will be compromised if the catheter is obstructed in any way.

FIGURE 18.17 Roller pump for RRT.

Blood-filled tubing fits inside outer housing and is compressed
by two cams to milk blood along, creating flow.

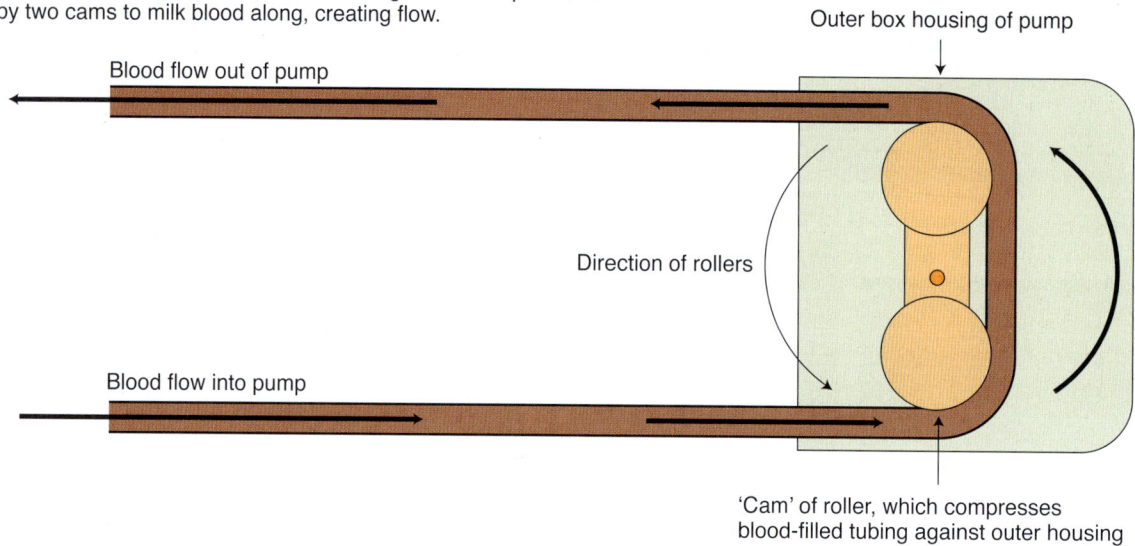

Outer box housing of pump

Blood flow out of pump

Direction of rollers

Blood flow into pump

'Cam' of roller, which compresses
blood-filled tubing against outer housing

Venous return line bubble trap chamber

The purpose of the bubble trap chamber is to prevent
any gas bubbles in the EC from entering the patient's
circulation by allowing them to rise to the top of a small,
vertically positioned collection reservoir (see Figure
18.18). Venous pressure is commonly measured via a
tubing connection into the top of the venous chamber,
and additional intravenous fluids can be administered
into this chamber via a secondary tube connection. The
level of the blood in the chamber must be below the
top, to prevent spillage into the pressure monitoring
line. It is advised that the blood level be adjusted to
near full but allow for visual inspection of incoming
blood flow and to ensure that any air or gas bubbles
are trapped here.[67] As this creates a gas–blood interface
within the venous chamber there is a potential source of
venous chamber clotting and hence circuit failure.[46,66,67]
Addition of replacement fluids into this chamber when
using post-dilution fluid administration can cause a
plasma fluid layer to develop above the blood level
and may reduce clotting by stopping blood foaming
on its surface and eliminates air or gas contact with
the blood.[68]

Anticoagulation

There are several different drugs utilised to prevent blood
clotting in the EC; heparin, prostacyclin and sodium citrate
have been used separately or in various combinations (see
Table 18.4).[69–71] As blood comes into contact with the
plastic tubing and the polymer fibres of the filter, various
clotting systems are activated. This is a normal action of
blood when exposed to non–biological surfaces. The aim

FIGURE 18.18 Schematic of typical venous bubble trap design.

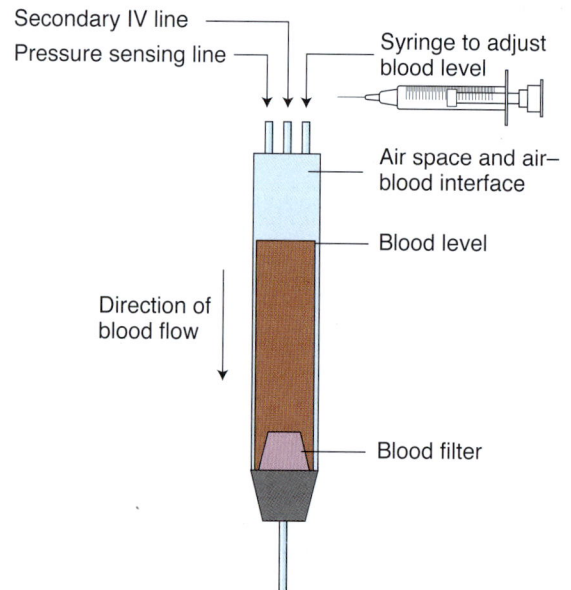

Secondary IV line
Pressure sensing line

Syringe to adjust
blood level

Air space and air–
blood interface

Blood level

Direction of
blood flow

Blood filter

of anti-clotting drugs is to delay clot formation while
the blood is outside the body, particularly when within
the densely-packed fibres of the filter. As calcium, blood
platelet cells and thrombin are vital in clot formation,[66]
these drugs are targeted to one of these elements. This
targeting must not be too pronounced, as the patient may
begin to bleed when the blood returns from the EC to
the body.[66]

TABLE 18.4

Commonly used anti-clotting agents for CRRT

DRUG	BENEFITS	PRECAUTIONS
Heparin	Inexpensive, wide experience, easily reversed, easily monitored, short half-life	Sensitivity reactions, heparin-induced thrombocytopenia, to be effective means increased risk of bleeding systemically
Low-molecular-weight heparin (LMWH)	Moderately inexpensive, increasing experience, less likely to result in sensitivity reactions	Difficult to monitor, not easily reversed, longer half-life, dosing varies between types of LMWH
Prostacyclin	Very short-acting, has a physiological role in inhibiting platelet activity, does not exacerbate other drug reactions	Expensive, no measure of effectiveness, narrow dose range with associated hypotension, individual patients sensitive to haemodynamic effects, unstable in solution
Citrate-based solutions	Limit anticlotting effect to extracorporeal circuit (EC) – 'regional anticoagulation'; results suggest very effective in prolonging circuit life	Substantial metabolic effect if not adequately managed (serum ionised calcium must be monitored closely); requires additions to EC to administer and reverse and use of specialised replacement/dialysate solutions Not useful when liver failure present, citrate is converted to bicarbonate by the liver providing the necessary buffer for renal replacement therapy (RRT). Acidosis may occur in liver failure
No anti-clotting agent (with saline flushes)	No side effects, no exacerbation of unstable haematological status, liver failure	May encounter very short circuit life that consumes remaining haematological components, risk of fluid overload if saline flushes not part of fluid balance. No evidence saline flushes have any benefit

Heparin is the most commonly-used agent for the prevention of clotting, as it is inexpensive, widely available and easily reversed by another drug, protamine.[69] Heparin is usually administered into the EC before the blood enters the filter, although the optimal place to administer any anticoagulant drug during CRRT is not agreed upon.[72,73] A bolus is often given prior to circuit connection, either in the circuit prime or via the venous access catheter. A maintenance dose (5–15 units/kg/h) is then adjusted against the relevant laboratory tests and a visual inspection for clotting in the EC is undertaken, particularly noting the venous bubble trap.

Citrate is another popular anticoagulant for CRRT as an alternative to heparin. Citrate buffers pH and chelates calcium, inducing anticoagulation of blood by reducing serum ionised calcium level. For anticoagulation, the dose and dose rate of citrate are commonly set to achieve a reduction in the CRRT circuit blood ionised calcium level to <0.3 mmol/L.[74,75] As ionised calcium is essential for the progression of the coagulation cascade to form a stable clot, an anticoagulant effect is achieved when the calcium is bound or chelated.[75] A continuous infusion of citrate is administered into the CRRT circuit, as patient blood enters the circuit, similar to heparin administration. A new approach in Australia includes citrate as an additive to commercially prepared CRRT replacement fluids. When circuit blood returns to the patient circulation, it mixes with systemic blood and the calcium concentration is restored to normal; free citrate not binding to calcium is metabolised by the liver to provide carbon dioxide and

bicarbonate as a necessary buffer.[74,75] However, citrate-bound calcium is lost in the waste fluid removed and requires replacement by a separate calcium infusion to maintain serum calcium levels to normal, at 1.0–1.3 mmol/L.[74] With this method, the circuit is anticoagulated, but the patient is not (also called a 'regional' method of anticoagulation) as the patient blood calcium level is restored to normal, making this approach safer compared to heparin use; it can be applied in auto-anticoagulated patients where premature circuit clotting continues to occur.[76,77] Due to the complex nature of the citrate-based anticoagulation approach a number of different protocols have been proposed to aid in management.[78] Not all methods will be applied in the one ICU, and local expertise development of one method and an alternative is common. Recent reviews provide a good synopsis of each method as they are different depending on CVVH or CVVHDF mode.[79]

Normal clotting time, a laboratory test designed to measure the time taken for blood to clot under laboratory conditions, is used as a reference to determine a suitable therapeutic range of the anti-clotting drug during CRRT. Different tests are applicable to different medications and their site of action in the clotting cascade. When using any anti-clotting agent, a balance is required between the benefits of increased coagulation suppression and the higher risk of patient systemic bleeding. In each patient this risk may vary, depending on illness, accompanying liver failure and administration of concurrent anti-clotting agents.

Fluids and fluid balance

Fluid used during any form of CRRT is a commercially manufactured product with an electrolyte composition similar to blood plasma.[80] This provides a solution useful as a replacement solution for plasma water removed in convective mode (CVVH), or as a dialysate solution in diffusive mode or CVVHD(f).These respective applications allow for plasma water replacement with 'clean' and buffered plasma water following toxin laden plasma water removal or, during CVVHD(f), for plasma water to be exposed to the whole blood across the membrane fibres so that toxins and molecules will diffusively exchange from the blood into the fluid. The additives or recipe for three commonly used commercial fluids are listed in Table 18.5 together with saline solution and normal blood plasma chemistry for comparative analysis. The key additives of note in the commercial fluids are the elevated level of bicarbonate and the variable concentration of potassium (no potassium option also), providing an effective buffer for the acidaemia and hyperkalaemia associated with AKI.

Throughout the course of a continuous treatment with CRRT, hypokalaemia may occur and a higher potassium added solution may be required to correct and maintain normal serum levels. First-generation commercial fluids used lactic acid as the buffer additive, requiring liver metabolism to produce bicarbonate in vivo.[80,81] This preparation is now not used in favour of a bicarbonate added fluid, prepared just prior to use using a two-compartment bag (see Figure 18.19) as the two fluids are unstable in long-term storage. The higher cost, problems with reconstituting bicarbonate solution bags and manual handling of large (5 L) fluid bags has increased interest in 'online'

fluid production from tap-water at the bedside. This approach can be less expensive, requires no bag changing or reconstituting by nurses,[82] but does require the installation of a complex and expensive reverse osmosis machine, the cost of which would be offset if large volumes of fluid were then consumed from this online manufacture. This approach is used in some centres for these reasons, and is applied as ICU daily dialysis (EDDf) or extended dialysis modes (SLED) are the therapy of choice.

Fluid balance monitoring and adjustment to machine settings is a key nursing responsibility in managing a patient treated with CRRT.[57] This requires an operator of the machine to enter a rate of fluid removal each hour, or for a longer set time period, and the machine is intended to achieve this target for the set time. It is important to remember this volume of fluid removed is simply the machine-prescribed loss of fluid removed, commonly determined by electronic scales in the machine, and does not equate to the overall fluid balance of the patient.[83] The patient may have substantial fluid inputs and outputs from other sources such as surgical drains and all amounts must be considered to determine the desired fluid balance for the day. Therefore, the machine setting to achieve a desired fluid state must be determined in context for the entire clinical status of a patient where verbal communication and written prescribing orders must be clear to differentiate 'machine loss – setting' from patient net 'loss' or balance per hour.[57] Despite simple software and screen interface for setting the desired fluid loss or removal per hour during treatment, mistakes and errors occur.[83] In some cases, particularly in small children and babies, this can be fatal.[84,85] Most machines now provide

---

TABLE 18.5

Blood plasma chemistry compared with commonly used commercial CRRT fluids

	BLOOD – PLASMA[a]	SALINE (BAXTER, TOONGABBIE, AUSTRALIA)	BAXTER ACCUSOL	GAMBRO HEMOSOL BO (GAMBRO, LUND, SWEDEN)	BAXTER HAEMOFILTRATION CITRATE SOLUTION (BAXTER, TOONGABBIE, AUSTRALIA)
Sodium (mmol/L)	136–145	150	140	140	152
Chloride (mmol/L)	98–07	150	113.5	109.5	99
Potassium (mmol/L)	3.5–5.1	0	4.0 or 2.0	4.0 or 2.0	5
Bicarbonate (mmol/L)	22–29	0	35	32	0
Calcium	2.15–2.55	0	1.75	1.75	0
Magnesium	0.66–1.07	0	0.5	0.5	0
Citrate	0	0	0	0	90
Lactate	0.5–2.2		0	3.0	0.0
pH (range)	7.35–7.45	4.0–7.0	7.4	7.0–8.5	5–6.5
mOsm/kg (listed or estimated)	280–300	300	300.3	287	270

[a]Adult ranges reproduced with permission from: plasmahttp://www.austinpathology.org.au/test-directory.

FIGURE 18.19 Two-compartment bicarbonate bag.

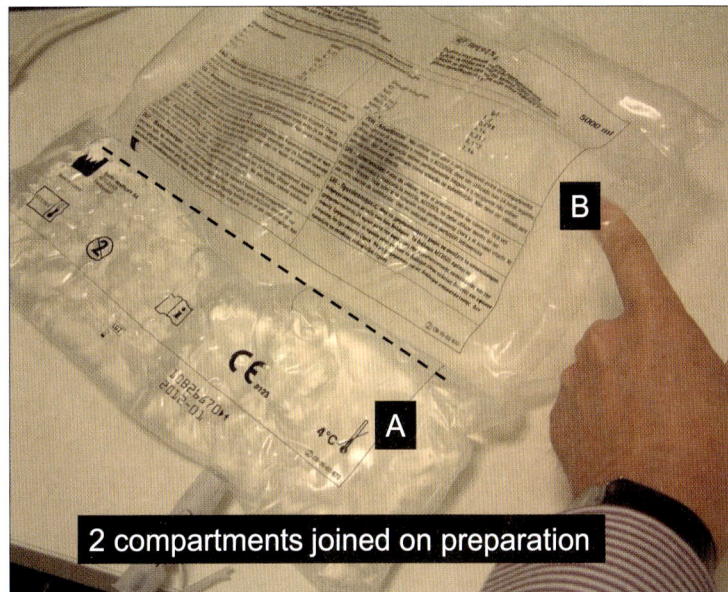

Bicarbonate CRRT fluid
Main bag – bicarbonate – B
Small bag – electrolytes – A

K+ of 0 or K+ of 4
No glucose

2 compartments joined on preparation

limits for the amount of accumulative fluid balance error (+ve or −ve) before an alarm will sound with a display message to advise the nurse. Such errors can occur due to fluid bags remaining clamped, or fluid pathway lines kinked or clamped. Logically, the machine is removing or infusing fluid but the machine scales are not detecting a weight change. The fluids infused as replacement or removed as waste plus additional fluid for a loss are usually all recorded on a fluid balance chart at the bedside. This is presented as traditional inputs and outputs charting, with the difference between these amounts understood as the balance; usually a negative in the context of a patient with AKI, anuric and in the ICU setting, is commonly set for a negative balance overall. Where anticoagulation infusions are used in the CRRT circuit, this volume may be recorded into the CRRT calculations as 'input' and contribute to the balance determined. This is all achieved easily with recent electronic fluid charts included in ICU clinical information and patient management systems. See Figure 18.20 as an example of such a spread sheet chart from a bedside computer.

Irrespective of patient acuity, when CRRT is used, individual patient assessment for fluid status must occur at least twice a day. Subtle temperature changes in the patient, surgical drain losses, diarrhoea and variable absorption of feed may all contribute fluid losses not included in routine fluid maintenance. Similarly, fluid boluses, transducer flush volumes and drugs administered may together create a positive fluid balance. If sustained this clinical state is reported as a contributor to delayed renal recovery and increased mortality in the ICU.[86] Regular weighing of patients may assist in assessing this situation, in addition to regular physical and clinical assessment

of the patient. Electrolyte disturbances may also occur despite use of balanced replacement solutions. Particular attention should focus on regular assessment of fluid and electrolytes, especially potassium, sodium, phosphate and magnesium levels.

> **Practice tip**
>
> Fluid removal during CRRT is prescribed by doctors and usually to a time frame. The nurse needs to calculate the rate per hour and must also include a recalculation of the treatment if it is off for long periods.

Patient management

Nursing protocols have previously been focused on machine priming, patient preparation and use of a CRRT system as this was the essential training pathway for nurses learning the operator–machine–patient interface.[87] Current CRRT machines are highly automated and have advanced software with instructional on-screen coloured pictures, circuit diagrams and text prompts providing a sequential step-by-step approach for priming, patient connection and key alarms. This has often made bedside e-policies and paper documents redundant, with nurses learning the machine preparation sequence without the need to follow any paper instruction booklet or on-screen pictures. Nonetheless, the clinical knowledge, psychomotor skills and the responsibility for managing an extracorporeal circuit to efficiently and safely treat a critically ill patient should not be understated. The nurse-to-patient ratio for CRRT is commonly 1:1 worldwide, acknowledging the attention and focus required despite

FIGURE 18.20　Screen dump of a bedside e-fluid balance chart.

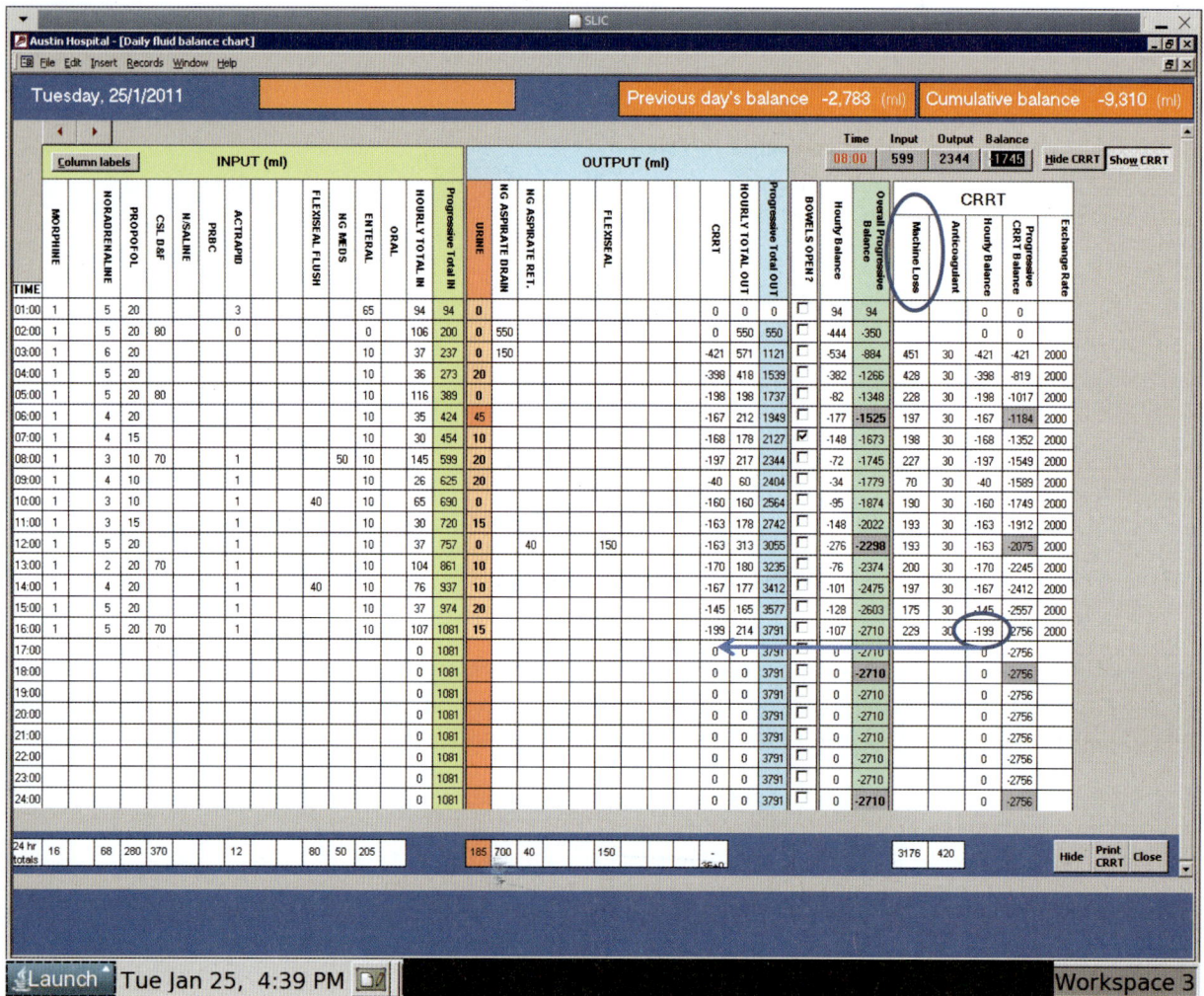

SLIC

Austin Hospital - [Daily fluid balance chart]

File Edit Insert Records Window Help

Tuesday, 25/1/2011　　Previous day's balance -2,783 (ml)　Cumulative balance -9,310 (ml)

	Time	Input	Output	Balance	
	08:00	599	2344	1745	Hide CRRT Show CRRT

Column labels — INPUT (ml) — OUTPUT (ml) — CRRT

TIME	MORPHINE	NORADRENALINE	PROPOFOL	CSL D&F	N/SALINE	PRBC	ACTRAPID	FLEXISEAL FLUSH	NG MEDS	ENTERAL	ORAL	HOURLY TOTAL IN	Progressive Total IN	URINE	NG ASPIRATE DRAIN	NG ASPIRATE RET.	FLEXISEAL	CRRT	HOURLY TOTAL OUT	Progressive Total OUT	BOWELS OPEN?	Hourly Balance	Overall Progressive Balance	Machine Loss	Anticoagulant	Hourly Balance	Progressive CRRT Balance	Exchange Rate
01:00	1	5	20				3			65		94	94	0				0	0	0	☐	94	94			0	0	
02:00	1	5	20	80			0			0		106	200	0	550			0	550	550	☐	-444	-350			0	0	
03:00	1	6	20							10		37	237	0	150			-421	571	1121	☐	-534	-884	451	30	-421	-421	2000
04:00	1	5	20							10		36	273	20				-398	418	1539	☐	-382	-1266	428	30	-398	-819	2000
05:00	1	5	20	80						10		116	389	0				-198	198	1737	☐	-82	-1348	228	30	-198	-1017	2000
06:00	1	4	20							10		35	424	45				-167	212	1949	☐	-177	-1525	197	30	-167	-1184	2000
07:00	1	4	15							10		30	454	10				-168	178	2127	☑	-148	-1673	198	30	-168	-1352	2000
08:00	1	3	10	70					50	10		145	599	20				-197	217	2344	☐	-72	-1745	227	30	-197	-1549	2000
09:00	1	4	10				1			10		26	625	20				-40	60	2404	☐	-34	-1779	70	30	-40	-1589	2000
10:00	1	3	10				1		40	10		65	690	0				-160	160	2564	☐	-95	-1874	190	30	-160	-1749	2000
11:00	1	3	15				1			10		30	720	15				-163	178	2742	☐	-148	-2022	193	30	-163	-1912	2000
12:00	1	5	20				1			10		37	757	0		40	150	-163	313	3055	☐	-276	-2298	193	30	-163	-2075	2000
13:00	1	2	20	70			1			10		104	861	10				-170	180	3235	☐	-76	-2374	200	30	-170	-2245	2000
14:00	1	4	20				1		40	10		76	937	10				-167	177	3412	☐	-101	-2475	197	30	-167	-2412	2000
15:00	1	5	20				1			10		37	974	20				-145	165	3577	☐	-128	-2603	175	30	-145	-2557	2000
16:00	1	5	20	70			1			10		107	1081	15				-199	214	3791	☐	-107	-2710	229	30	-199	-2756	2000
17:00												0	1081	0				0	0	3791	☐	0	-2710			0	-2756	
18:00												0	1081	0				0	0	3791	☐	0	-2710			0	-2756	
19:00												0	1081	0				0	0	3791	☐	0	-2710			0	-2756	
20:00												0	1081	0				0	0	3791	☐	0	-2710			0	-2756	
21:00												0	1081	0				0	0	3791	☐	0	-2710			0	-2756	
22:00												0	1081	0				0	0	3791	☐	0	-2710			0	-2756	
23:00												0	1081	0				0	0	3791	☐	0	-2710			0	-2756	
24:00												0	1081	0				0	0	3791	☐	0	-2710			0	-2756	
24 hr totals	16	68	280	370			12		80	50	205			185	700	40	150					3176	420					

Launch　Tue Jan 25, 4:39 PM　Workspace 3

Hide　Print CRRT　Close

the advances in machine automation.[88] This is a reasonable approach as CRRT in the ICU is very different to the use of dialysis for chronic renal failure where a nurse may oversee three or four patients on dialysis under their care and with different start times (overlapping) for a 3–4-hour treatment in each case. In the ICU these patients are usually in a multi-organ failure state, are intubated and require mechanical ventilation, cardiovascular support, enteral feeding, need many intravenous drugs and infusions and have reduced neurological function with or without sedation. This is a picture mandating both technical and cognitive tasks in addition to comprehensive nursing care, including full hygiene and all care for the bedridden, unconscious patient.

Monitoring correct machine function for reliable flow of blood, continuous changing of bags as substitution fluids empty and waste bags fill, adjustment and constant review for stability with anticoagulation agents and the overall monitoring and response to other parameters of patient metabolic stability with electrolyte, acid–base and temperature management represent some of the work associated with the nursing care required.[57,68] Machine and circuit preparation, connection and, when required, stopping and disconnecting a treatment are further skill and knowledge sets for ICU nurses. Consideration of all these factors represents why nurses are particularly concerned that a new treatment, when started, is stabilised, then functions continuously for as long as possible. This perspective is an additional consideration to the medical aims of treatment ensuring solute, acid–base and fluid balance are controlled. It is the key interest of both doctors and nurses in the ICU that the treatment be 'continuous' as frequent stopping and restarting is a lot of work for nurses and may cause instability in the patient.[89]

In Table 18.6 a summary of key nursing practice and interventions for bedside use is provided making this information a suitable reference for nursing knowledge and skills associated with CRRT use in the ICU.

TABLE 18.6

Trouble-shooting guide: key nursing practice and interventions for CRRT

	POTENTIAL PROBLEM (NUMBERED LIST)	KEY NURSING INTERVENTIONS REQUIRED, REFERENCED TO LISTED NUMBER
Patient and machine/system preparation before use	1 Machine alarms and technical failure on starting treatment 2 Air entrainment during prime 3 Fluid setting errors 4 Fluids/electrolytes incorrect 5 Machine and patient too far apart or machine placed out of staff view	1 Machine self-test and/or checklist completed 2 Double-check all circuit lines around circuit, particularly for clamps ON or OFF as required 3 Treatment orders cross-checked with settings 4 Double-check fluids used, e.g. any additives required 5 Position machine according to access catheter site: at feet for femoral line, at bedside for sub-clavian and at bed head for jugular with screen faced to staff desk or charts/computer Recommendation: • Have your own pre-start check routine (paper document list)
Connection to the system and initiation of therapy	1 Access catheter obstruction/failure 2 Hypotension on start	1 Prepare access connections with antiseptic, aspirate any instilled drug and test easy flush return (venous) lumen and aspirate outflow (arterial) lumen 2 Connect both circuit lines to access catheter administering priming volume to patient (a) Increase vasoactive drugs if necessary to increase MAP (b) Start blood pump slowly with small increases until blood fills all of the circuit Recommendations: • Use two nurses for connection routine. Start fluid replacement and removal only after blood circuit is full and at prescribed speed, stay with patient until stable ~ first 15 min • Patient in bed, supine position and MAP >70 mmHg, stable
In-use troubleshooting alarms and maintenance, fluid balance	1 Excessive negative pressure >−100 mmHg: 'arterial alarm' 2 High pressure > +100 mmHg: 'venous alarm' 3 High TMP alarm 4 Air detected alarm 5 Hypothermia 6 Fluid balance errors 7 Electrolyte imbalance	1 & 2 Maintain access catheter alignment, preventing kinks in access and circuit lines 1 & 2 Do not place extra connections or taps between access catheter and circuit lines 3 Suggests filter clotting or blood flow too slow for fluids settings 4 Ensure venous chamber full high with blood, bubbles removed regularly, prescribe post-dilution fluid into the chamber 5 Heater set to 37°C or greater to compensate for heat loss from extracorporeal circuit 6 Use fluids charting or similar to account for all fluid inputs including anticoagulant volume. Clarify orders to set machine 'loss' in respect of this. Commonly a net negative. Orders and settings should not be prescribed to administer fluid – no net positive 7 Potassium additive to CRRT fluid is often required after 24–48 h of treatment; some patients are hypokalaemic despite acute renal failure. Phosphate monitoring and correction is important Recommendations: • Assess and reset fluid balance settings hourly, particularly in unstable patients and for inexperienced staff • Fluid gain or positive fluid balance using CRRT should be considered an adverse event or complication of use
Monitoring and adjustment to anticoagulation	1 Premature clotting in circuit and filter	1 Check and monitor effect of anticoagulant therapy according to local policy. With heparin use this could be after first 6 h and then daily (a) Maintain adequate dose to therapeutic range (b) Use predilution fluid administration (c) Use blood flow greater than 150 mL/min (d) Use large-bore access catheter and take care not to obstruct or kink catheter (e) Keep blood pump operating: minimise stops >30 s Recommendation: • If frequent failure (clotting <4 h), always check for blood flow obstruction before more, or alternative anticoagulation; e.g. review to consider change or replacement of access catheter

TABLE 18.6 *continued*

	POTENTIAL PROBLEM (NUMBERED LIST)	KEY NURSING INTERVENTIONS REQUIRED, REFERENCED TO LISTED NUMBER
Access care and dressings	1 Access dislodgement 2 Access catheter infection 3 Access catheter obstruction	1 Ensure catheter sutured in place and well secured with dressing; single or double ('sandwich' technique) biofilm–polyurethane (see Figure 18.22) 2 Use asepsis when flushing or connecting to access catheter; monitor site for infection and patient for suspected line sepsis. Use catheter site alcohol patch, e.g. Biopatch™ 3 Use heparin to fill catheter dead-space when not in use for >4 h and label accordingly Recommendation: • Use flexible dressing with application to both sides along catheter allowing movement away off skin surface, preventing obstruction during patient care/positioning and lifting or tearing off dressing.
Vital sign monitoring	1 Arrhythmias, hypotension, temperature	1 Monitor vital signs hourly, consider any links between changes, and use of RRT; e.g. low CVP and excessive fluid removal, temperature fluctuations when CRRT OFF and ON Recommendation: • CVP readings should be performed 2–4-h during CRRT; CVP can be used as a target for daily fluid loss prescription. Weigh the patient if possible. Do frequent blood gas and electrolytes commonly associated with ICU care
Assessment of filter function and patency	1 Filter clotting abruptly with inability to return circuit blood to the patient 2 Inadequate solute removal	1 If trans-membrane pressure (TMP) or pre-filter pressure (P-IN) >250 mmHg is diagnostic of filter clotting; consider electively returning blood by crystalloid infusion into outflow limb of circuit and ceasing treatment – follow local policy (a) Observe for venous chamber clot development. If excessive and venous pressure >150 mmHg, consider electively returning blood – cease treatment 2 Assess patient's solute levels: urea and creatinine should be reducing or stable Recommendations: • Predicting circuit or filter clotting can be difficult. TMP and P-IN can rise quickly after being stable or within normal range. If there is a trend upwards reflecting diagnosis of clotting, cease treatment electively to avoid blood flow 'standstill' and a failure to restart and blood loss • Nurses may document these pressures hourly or check the machine frequently, but they must respond quickly to cease treatment
Cessation of treatment and disconnection from the extracorporeal circuit	1 Blockage and/or clotting in access catheter 2 Inadvertent blood loss 3 Infectious risk	1 Use concentrated heparin (other anticoagulant) to fill dead-space of catheter when not in use >4 h. Use heparin 1000 IU/mL and follow manufacturer's specifications for volume required 2 Always attempt to cease a circuit before it clots and always return patient blood if possible 3 Use asepsis for disconnection procedure Recommendation: • Access catheter should not be used for other purposes/infusions when RRT is not connected
Temporary disconnection for procedures	1 Maintenance of circuit before reconnection 2 Infection 3 Inadvertent fluid administration	1 Flush out any excess blood residue in circuit, keep blood pump operational with saline (prime) in circuit 2 Circuits in use for >24 h before disconnection or not restarted after 6 hours following temporary disconnection, consider discarding 3 After restarting circuit, increase fluid loss to remove fluid used to re-establish RRT Recommendation: • Re-use of circuits in this context is not desirable and with prior planning should be avoidable. E.g. plan for radiology, surgery etc when circuit off or restart new circuit around these interventions. If this is done, consider adding heparin 5000 IU to circuit when temporarily disconnected unless contraindicated, but flush this out with 200–300 mL prime solution before reconnection; always use additive label indicating heparin added

CRRT = continuous renal replacement therapy; CVP = central venous pressure; MAP = mean arterial pressure; TMP = trans-membrane pressure.

Practice recommendations are also included. This information is general to any CRRT machine, and does not include a detailed anticoagulation protocol. Anticoagulation technique for CRRT usually dominates any policy and is viewed more frequently in comparison to the psychomotor skills component for machine preparation, connection and fluids bags management. Nursing practice policies can also be supplemented with machine-specific and quick reference 'one page' lists for shift check or

anticoagulation method. See Figure 18.21 as an example of a shift checklist.

Continuous renal replacement machines

There are many machines available for CRRT in the ICU. How to identify the machine that a particular ICU should use or purchase is a common question from nurses, and there is limited literature available to guide this decision; however, literature providing comparisons of their

FIGURE 18.21 Shift checklist for CRRT at Austin Health, Melbourne, Australia.

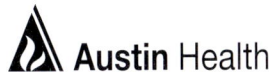

Austin Health

Shift check list CRRT as CVVH: Infomed HF 440

Check	Rationale
Machine position relative to patient with blood lines not too tight - stretched	Patient movement could cause excess drag on vascath site and securing tape
Brakes ON	Machine must have brakes on to prevent inadvertent movement and risk of above
Fluids: correct for K^+ and both bags hanging from same point – height, both line clamps open	Fluids should empty at similar rate, minimise mixing, scales and balance alarms more likely if the bags hanging at different heights
Flush line connected, correct fluid, clamped as close to blood path as possible. Date this bag.	Fluid to return patient blood; this may be required any time. Clamp close to blood path prevent blood tracking back up this line and clotting, only to be flushed in with use
Waste bottle hanging stable and waste pump hose with end plug ready, coiled on machine holder.	This bottle will weigh > 16 Kg on full. Needs to hang with stability to prevent scales alarms. Hose ready for use with end cap to prevent drips
Venous – bubble chamber full and inspect for clot	Adjust this up slowly, with syringe attached. Keep full to trap gas / air and allow for the level to fall during use with gas entry associated with bicarbonate fluids (CO_2) when heated
Luer syringe (10 ml), 3 way tap and dead end cap(red) in line - for chamber adjustment	Luer syringe will not fall / slip off during use; red cap blocks pathway between venous blood chamber and UF pathway if 3 way tap was accidently opened to both chambers.
Screen settings & Alarms	
Blood flow - speed	200 mls/min. standard
UF flow	2000 ml/hr standard CVVH
Manual Pre-dilution %	50:50 for CVVH (Citrate use 70% pre)
'Weight loss' – Fluid loss rate ml/hr	Check orders – fluid loss target
Next intervention (hr:min)	Time until fluids bag change or bottle empty
Temperature setting	Default at 37°, maybe ↑↓ to patient need
Venous +10 ---- + 150 mmHg (influenced by blood flow rate and chamber clotting, access function – blue lumen)	This pressure always positive, measured on the return limb of circuit. ~ 50 – 100 mmHg
Arterial -150 ---- -10 mmHg (influenced by blood flow rate and access function – red lumen)	This pressure always negative, measured on the outflow limb of circuit. ~ -50 – -100 mmHg
Trans-membrane pressure (TMP) (Pin + Pv)/2 - Puf	Indicative of clotting / clogging in the membrane. Set at 200 mmHg initially. When 250+ mmHg, usually terminate treatment.
Anticoagulation and Prescription orders	Check drug dose and orders correct

TABLE 18.7

Machine design and build approaches

MACHINE TYPE	WASTE COLLECTION	MEMBRANE	CIRCUIT	PRESSURE MEASUREMENT	PRIMING PREPARATION AND SOFTWARE OPTION(S)
A	One 5-L or 10-L bag, empty when full, change bag(s)	AN69, prefitted, not changeable	Cartridge kit-based, multipurpose; all modes	In-line pressure transducers	Fully automated, software for management of citrate anticoagulation
B	One 5-L or 2 bags, empty when full, change bags	Different membranes possible – polyethersulfone or others	Cartridge kit-based, multipurpose; all modes	In-line pressure transducers	Fully automated, Intelligence software for fluid management

technical characteristics is limited.[90,91] Table 18.7 outlines the major differences in machines or system approaches. Two machines adopting common design features from Table 18.7 are shown in Figures 18.22 (Prismaflex; Hospal, Lyon, France) and 18.23 (Aquarius, Nikkiso, Sydney, Australia), each highlighting the major technical differences in how CRRT machines are presented and used.

FIGURE 18.22 Prismaflex CRRT Machine.

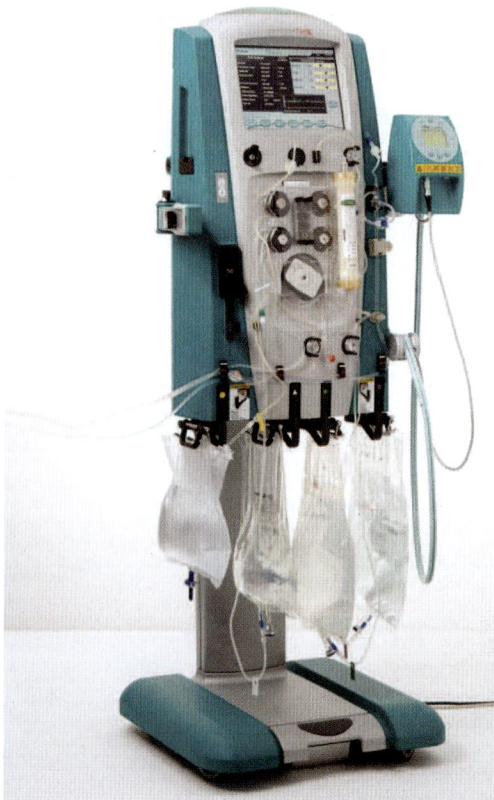

Courtesy Gambro Australia

FIGURE 18.23 Aquarius CRRT Machine, Nikkiso, Sydney, Australia.

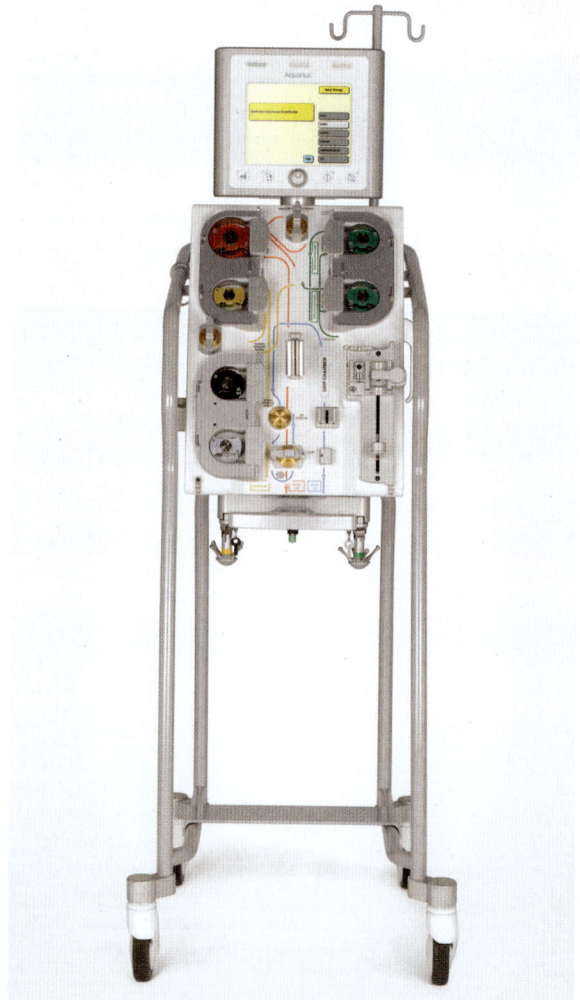

Image courtesy of Nikkiso, Sydney, Australia.

Teaching and training CRRT

Since introduction of CRRT to the ICU in the 1980s and early 90s, medical companies as machine vendors have developed and expanded their offerings for teaching and training nurses in the use of CRRT machines and the broader aspects of acute kidney injury and patient care. Depending upon the hospital, training and education may be conducted for small groups or entire ICU staffing cohorts associated with a new machine fleet installation or when CRRT is introduced without any previous experience with artificial renal support. More commonly, where CRRT is imbedded in use for many years, the education focus is with smaller groups teaching new procedures and

methods, updates, orientation for new staff and specialist training in association with postgraduate certification. Figure 18.24 provides a list of suggested education topics in sequence for a local teaching and training activity. These didactic session topics may be scheduled in the sequence and over several weeks to become more powerful when supplemented with simulation activities linked to live patient care and bedside clinical support.[46,88] A recent report suggests that, when simulation is added to didactic CRRT education programs, an improvement in CRRT functional time (filter 'life') is observed – a direct benefit to users, lessening cost and better for patients.[92]

Refer to Figure 18.25 for a CRRT demonstration or simulation set-up.

FIGURE 18.24 List of suggested education topics for CRRT.

Topic	Key areas
A.R.F. and critical illness	Kidney physiology, AKI diagnosis, definitions, ICU care, shock, sepsis.
Theory of solvent and solute removal	Diffusion and convection; basic chemistry. Artificial kidney concepts.
Techniques for CRRT	Nomenclature, circuits for different modes, key terms for set up.
Fluids and fluid balance	Fluid composition—additives, prescribing and administration of fluids, charting, key terms.
Anticoagulation	Coagulation physiology, different drugs and methods for anticoagulation, monitoring.
Machines and E.C. Circuit	Practical: Key machine design, sensors and alarms, circuit assembly, priming & prep.
Patient care	Connection of circuit and machine to patient, management during treatment, monitoring common problems, cease treatment.

FIGURE 18.25 CRRT demonstration or simulation set-up.

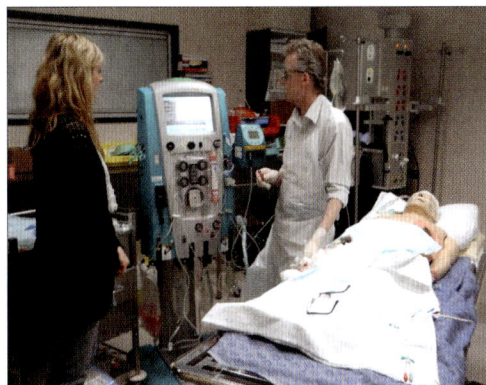

Simulating CRRT

- Use a basic resus doll
- Add food dye to a saline bag to create red fluid
- Insert a vascular access catheter into the bag and seal tight with a cable tie
- Place the bag into the doll with access visible e.g. femoral site
- Prepare an unsterile / old circuit
- Demonstrate or simulate common procedures
- Prismaflex (Hospal Gambro, Lyon, France) shown here

The key to successful CRRT education and training is to develop nurses with clinical experience managing CRRT regularly in the ICU and encouraging these experts to teach others around them when they can. This may require a nurse being allocated to this role formally, such as a clinical nurse specialist role dedicated to teaching within the ICU, or assigning these experienced nurses close to those learning CRRT during a shift. Such educators may already be in place for broader aspects of ICU education and postgraduate trainees but, for any staffing structure with or without dedicated teaching roles, identifying a small number of nurses as CRRT 'champions' for training and ongoing support when CRRT is in progress is a common and successful approach[47,87,88] to provide learning for others over the 24/7 context in ICU.

Quality and measures of success

Maintaining quality and nursing expertise for CRRT in the ICU will be related to the frequency of use and the size of the user group. When there are long periods between CRRT use, and/or when the ICU has a large staff number, ensuring competency may be challenging. Regular competency checks and staff assessments can be performed[88] depending upon resource allocation for this task but, where CRRT is in frequent use with several patients treated continuously, such checks may not be done suggesting that continual experience with CRRT in itself provides the competency process. Shift allocation of the nurse to a patient with AKI and treatment with CRRT care may benefit from predetermined skill sets as a guide to best match the individual nurse's competency with the CRRT-treated patient and ensure safety.[47,88] The most useful measure for quality when using CRRT is the progressive 'life' of the circuit or filter.[57] This data point may be recorded on bedside charts alongside hourly observations (see Figure 18.26) or electronically into an ICU clinical information system and provides an instant audit for each circuit used and throughout the patient treatment. This variable is most commonly used to compare efficacy of different anticoagulation techniques, but may also be considered a measure of access catheter and blood flow reliability, machine technical function and staff user competence.[93] Circuit or filter life (these terms are used interchangeably) is reported widely in the literature and, despite lacking a clear bedside definition, published data indicate that a median life of 21 hours is common.[94,95] Poor circuit life at 4–6 hours reflects clinical problems and an interprofessional review before the next treatment begins is warranted.

Special considerations

Paediatrics: babies and small children of 3–30-kg body weight

The use of dialysis and haemofiltration in babies and small children is a specialty area; however, many aspects of adult CRRT apply, particularly for those patients >15 kg.[96] Key differences, depending on size and weight, for this patient group are: 1) a smaller membrane surface area (size), and smaller circuit tubing to reduce priming and circuit volume; 2) a smaller access catheter (<7 Fr) depending on body weight and often placed in

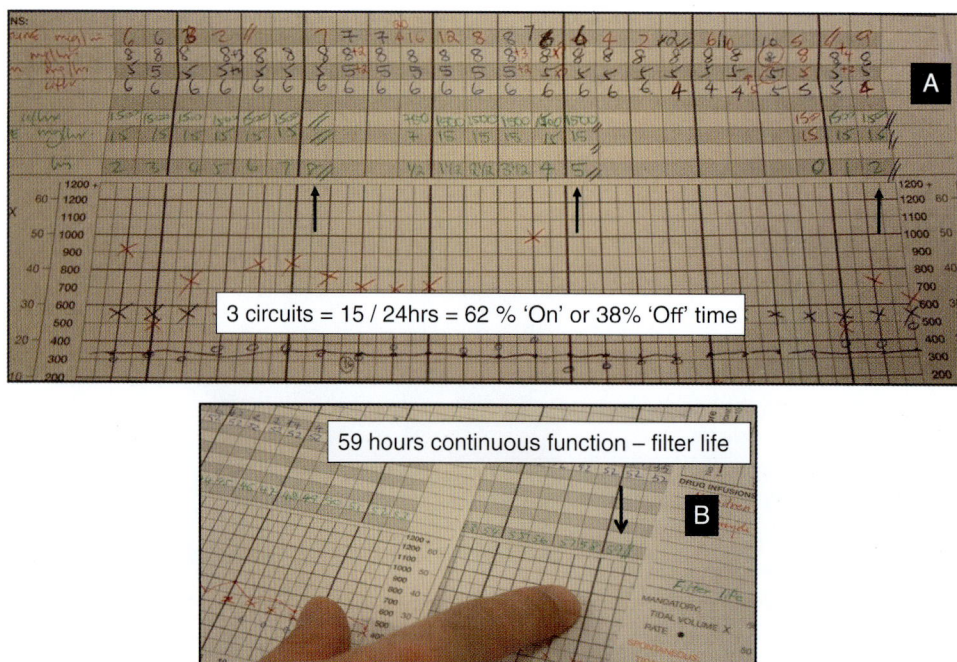

FIGURE 18.26 Bedside charts with consecutive filter life hours.

3 circuits = 15 / 24hrs = 62 % 'On' or 38% 'Off' time

59 hours continuous function – filter life

the femoral vein; 3) blood flow rate 3–5 mL/kg/min; 4) fluids flow (dialysate or substitution) rates – variable depending on mode but 2 L/1.73 m²/h is common; 5) increased prevention of hypothermia as this problem is exacerbated in babies and small infants.[97] Anticoagulation is the same as for adults but with reduced drug doses for the size of the infant or child.[97]

Extracorporeal membrane oxygenation

Increasingly, extracorporeal membrane oxygenation (ECMO) is applied for those with refractory hypoxaemia in association with respiratory failure or used in the context of right heart failure and combined heart-lung failure.[98] These critically ill patients frequently have AKI and require CRRT.[98] It is convenient and often necessary to connect the CRRT circuit into the ECMO circuit as the patient may have other access sites used for multiple cannulation. In any case, the high blood flow associated with ECMO and the placement of the circuit tubing allows for a connection of the CRRT circuit at many places. The only limiting factor is the positive pressure in the ECMO circuit, which is not compatible with the

normally negative access pressure when using venous access with a CRRT machine. Some machines provide a software option to select access pressure +ve, allowing this use with ECMO, others do not and may require some alarm override or restrictive device to create negative pressure for the outflow from the ECMO into the CRRT line. The anticoagulation provided for the use of ECMO is a convenient state for the successful use of the CRRT and much of this is usually controlled by a perfusionist or a cardiac anaesthetist overseeing the ECMO support.[99]

Operating theatre

There are some circumstances when CRRT is useful in the operating theatre. This is in association with any prolonged surgical case where AKI exists in association with a critical illness and specific surgery such as hepatic transplant. Local factors related to ICU staffing, and the surgical and anaesthetic teams' working relationship with the ICU, will influence exactly how this is achieved. The literature in this area is sparse; however, retrospective and small data sets reflect that CRRT in the operating theatre is achievable and safe.[100,101]

Summary

In this chapter a review of the important physiological functions of the kidney is provided and the context of kidney failure is also defined as an injury, or AKI. Management of patients with AKI is discussed and includes prevention of further injury, fluid and electrolyte balance and aspects of nutrition and pharmacy before consideration of an artificial support or RRT. There are now established criteria for stages of AKI indicating when an artificial kidney support should begin replacing the functions of the kidney. This support is broadly termed dialysis but is provided in the many variants of RRT, including PD, and as a continuous therapy in the ICU setting, by CRRTs. The history of dialysis is relevant as nurses have always played an important role in providing this treatment that, when integrated into the care of the critically ill, requires substantial knowledge and skills. The machine and circuit for CRRT are useful to understand as this assists preparation, connection to the patient and then troubleshooting during use. The major failing of CRRT is clotting of the extracorporeal circuit and anticoagulation approaches are the key preventative strategy. Teaching CRRT and quality review are very important for a successful program in the ICU. Finally, the use of CRRT in special considerations is briefly discussed and includes use in the operating theatre, with small children and use with ECMO.

Case study

Ms S is a 46-year-old woman transferred to the ICU from a regional hospital following a paracetamol overdose associated with an alcohol 'binge'. Her past history is unremarkable, but she is a heavy drinker of alcohol, which has increased since her recent divorce.

Current medications include pantoprazole and atorvastatin. Ms S had been suffering with a heavy cold in the last few days and reported taking 1–2 g of paracetamol every 4–6 hours. However, it appears that she had ingested approximately 20 g in a short time period suggesting a suicide attempt.

On arrival to ICU she was intubated, ventilated and unconscious, sedated with propofol. Prior to intubation her GCS was 7. Cardiac and blood pressure monitoring was instituted. A CVC, nasogastric tube and urinary catheter were inserted. Oliguria was noted on arrival. A brain CT revealed cerebral oedema.

She had elevated AST and ALT. An initial diagnosis of paracetamol overdose with associated acute liver failure was made.

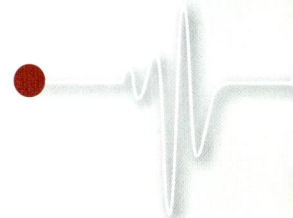

Her blood profile was as follows (normal values in brackets):

- pH 7.32 (7.35 to 7.45)
- potassium 5.9 mmol/L (3.5 to 5 mmol/L)
- lactate 4.8 mmol/L (0.5 to 1.6 mmol/L)
- INR 5.2 (0.9 to 1.2)
- ammonia 83 micromol/L (20 to 65 micromol/L)
- arterial bicarbonate 14 mmol/L (18 to 23 mmol/L)
- WCC 20.4 $\times$ 10^4 (3.5 to 9.0 $\times$ 10^9/L)
- urea 5.9 mmol/L (3 to 7 mmol/L)
- creatinine 165 micromol/L (60 to 90 micromol/L)
- panadol level 220 micromol/L (commonly considered toxic if >100 micromol/L in chronic alcoholics).

She was unconscious and intubated and ventilated with minute volume of 10.8 L/min and FiO$_2$ of 0.6. Her heart rate was 112 beats per minute with normal sinus rhythm, blood pressure was 95/45 mmHg while receiving noradrenalin at 18 mcg/min. She was slightly febrile (temperature 37.8°C) with cool peripheries. Urine output was 20 mL over the past 6 hours. Her body weight is estimated at 80 kg.

TREATMENT

Key primary treatments were to provide some further fluid resuscitation with 1.5 L of 4% albumin solution, evaluate the CXR and commence antibiotics, followed by the local ICU policy of 'H' therapy: hypothermia (active cooling), hypernatraemia (hypertonic saline infusion commenced) and haemodiafiltration at 4 L/h, hyperventilation and head of bed elevation. An infusion of the drug N-acetylcystein was started to protect the liver following paracetamol overdose.

Two hours after ICU admission a femoral vein access catheter was inserted for haemodiafiltration to manage acute kidney injury and oliguric acute renal failure. The patient's serum biochemistry (elevated K$^+$, creatinine and urea) and developing metabolic acidosis (raised ammonia and lactate, pH <7.35) in addition to the neurotoxicity associated with an elevated ammonia indicated the need to provide RRT. Other benefits of renal support are to remove some of the toxic metabolites of paracetamol and allow for fluid removal and a negative fluid balance for cerebral oedema.

Haemodiafiltration provides a combination of convective and diffusive clearance for all solutes and toxins; however some doctors may also prescribe haemofiltration as CVVH utilising pure convective removal for these solutes. The dose or intensity of treatment is controlled by the number of litres per hour of fluid removed in relation to the body weight and this is achieved by the combination of plasma water substitution fluid and dialysate fluid. In this case a dose of 50 mL/kg/h was prescribed with a body weight of 80 kg (4 L/h). This is considered 'high dose' treatment and is preferred for this acute toxic state until stabilisation. Fluid loss is achieved with fluid removal and the filtrate volume may exceed 4 L/h.

The patient was not prescribed any anticoagulation as the INR was elevated. If any gastrointestinal bleeding were to occur, this would aggravate the toxin load into the failing liver, in particular ammonia. Bicarbonate buffered fluid is preferred where acidosis is present and particularly where liver impairment is present. No potassium should be added until the serum level has decreased. The treatment would also provide cooling and the desired reduction in body temperature.

In 24 hours Ms S stabilised and was starting to awaken with limb movements and eye opening, and started to breathe spontaneously. The dose for noradrenalin was then 4 mcg/min. The ammonia level was 62 mmol/L and other biochemistry normalised. The dose prescription was reduced to 3 L/h and the circuit continued to function well without anticoagulation. A negative fluid balance was achieved slowly over this time and the loss setting was then prescribed as 'patient even'; only inputs were included in the setting for fluid removal. This was at 100 mL/h over 24 hours to avoid excessive fluid removal and hypovolaemia.

Ms S continued to improve and after 4 days RRT was ceased. She was producing urine at >60 mL/h and had normal acid–base balance, biochemistry and low ammonia levels. Ms S was extubated on day 5 after resolution of a lung infection. Her mild fever had receded (temperature 35.5°C) and the RRT machine fluids heater was adjusted to maintain a temperature of 36°C. The RRT access catheter was left in place in the event that RRT was needed again, but her full recovery looked promising.

CASE STUDY QUESTIONS

1 Consider the RIFLE criteria outlined in this chapter and Ms S's presentation to the ICU and her subsequent management with CRRT. Which stage of the criteria was met in the context of RIFLE for Ms S?

2 Review 10 patients in your ICU who are prescribed CRRT and observe which stage or RIFLE criteria they satisfy before beginning CRRT. This may be useful and help you better understand AKI, diagnosis and initiation of CRRT.

3 From the case describing Ms S's management, a femoral access catheter was placed for CRRT. This is usually because central line access is in place via the jugular or subclavian site. Review the placement of access for CRRT in your ICU. Is there a preference for this? Correlate the site used (femoral, jugular vein or subclavian) with the filter or circuit 'life' for the different access sites used. Is there any relationship reflecting an association between access site and filter life? Your finding may be compared to the literature; also see key references in the *Further reading* section.

RESEARCH VIGNETTE

RENAL Replacement Therapy Study Investigators. Bellomo R, Cass A, Cole L, Finfer S, Gallagher M, Lo S et al. Intensity of continuous renal-replacement therapy in critically ill patients. N Engl J Med 2009;361:1627–38

Abstract

Background: The optimal intensity of continuous renal-replacement therapy remains unclear. We conducted a multicenter, randomized trial to compare the effect of this therapy, delivered at two different levels of intensity, on 90-day mortality among critically ill patients with acute kidney injury.

Methods: We randomly assigned critically ill adults with acute kidney injury to continuous renal-replacement therapy in the form of postdilution continuous venovenous hemodiafiltration with an effluent flow of either 40 mL per kilogram of body weight per hour (higher intensity) or 25 mL per kilogram per hour (lower intensity). The primary outcome measure was death within 90 days after randomization.

Results: Of the 1508 enrolled patients, 747 were randomly assigned to higher-intensity therapy, and 761 to lower-intensity therapy with continuous venovenous hemodiafiltration. Data on primary outcomes were available for 1464 patients (97.1%): 721 in the higher-intensity group and 743 in the lower-intensity group. The two study groups had similar baseline characteristics and received the study treatment for an average of 6.3 and 5.9 days, respectively (P = 0.35). At 90 days after randomization, 322 deaths had occurred in the higher-intensity group and 332 deaths in the lower-intensity group, for a mortality of 44.7% in each group (odds ratio, 1.00; 95% confidence interval [CI], 0.81 to 1.23; P = 0.99). At 90 days, 6.8% of survivors in the higher-intensity group (27 of 399), as compared with 4.4% of survivors in the lower-intensity group (18 of 411), were still receiving renal-replacement therapy (odds ratio, 1.59; 95% CI, 0.86 to 2.92; P = 0.14). Hypophosphatemia was more common in the higher-intensity group than in the lower-intensity group (65% vs 54%, P < 0.001).

Conclusions: In critically ill patients with acute kidney injury, treatment with higher-intensity continuous renal-replacement therapy did not reduce mortality at 90 days. (Clinical Trials gov number, NCT00221013)

Critique

This seminal study was conducted as a prospective, randomised, controlled trial across 35 intensive care units (ICU) in Australia and New Zealand over a 3-year period in an effort to assess what level of treatment 'intensity' might influence mortality in critically ill patients with severe acute kidney injury. Participants were offered either a higher dose of treatment, which was an effluent rate of 40 mL/kg/h, with the lower dose intensity at 25 mL/kg/h. The principal outcome measure was patient survival at 90 days after study entry, with numerous other outcomes including various death points, lengths of ICU and hospital stay, return of renal function or deterioration of other organ systems.

The undertaking of this study was driven by clinical equipoise over what the preferred dose of treatment should be in continuous renal replacement therapy in terms of patient outcome. This question had been prompted by a number of reports that increasing the dose might be beneficial and outweigh the risks associated with higher intensity treatments. These risks include hypothermia, electrolyte disturbances, nutrient loss, altered drug levels and additional cost. The process of treatment dosing for continuous therapies is inherently different to intermittent treatment for chronic renal failure (CRF) so, while there is some precedent in terms of the benefits of early initiation and balanced regimens with CRF, the context and approach to therapy demanded a more specific approach for dosing CRRT.

The RENAL study enrolled 1508 participants who received a standardised CRRT treatment based on post dilutional continuous veno-venous haemodiafitration. The predetermined sample size was met and patients were assigned to one of the two treatment intensity groups, although subsequent issues left 1464 participants in the final study analysis. Both groups were similar in terms of patient characteristics and were seriously ill with almost three-quarters ventilated and just under half with severe sepsis. In terms of dose delivery, as would be expected, the higher intensity group had lower creatinine and urea levels as treatment progressed, but used more circuits.

In terms of the principal outcome of 90-day mortality the same proportion (44.7%) of patients died in both groups. There were no statistically different outcomes for other mortality measures with the vast majority of those surviving recovering renal function by day 90. Serious therapy-related events were low in both groups. The only appreciable difference was hypophosphataemia, which occurred in 65% of high intensity cases versus 54% of low intensity, as would be expected. The study was conducted using the mode of therapy most commonly used in Australia and New Zealand, albeit the use of post-dilutional replacement solution differs from many who deliver this in a predilution approach. Prescribed treatment dose was under-delivered in both groups because of treatment interruptions and highlighted findings from many studies that 'continuous' is not in fact continuous in terms of the delivery of these treatments.

While no improvement in survival was found by increasing the dose of therapy in this study, this does not translate to dose not being important. Outcomes were consistent in this study and better than many others reported from around the world so it is appropriate to conclude a minimum dose, possibly around 25 mL/kg/h, is necessary to achieve good survival in severe acute kidney injury. It is worth noting that measures focusing on ensuring the continuity of treatment are important if the prescribed dose is to be achieved. This study tended to consider clearance of metabolites associated with renal function as a measure of treatment performance, but it is equally important to emphasise that good fluid balance control is critical when supporting patients with oliguric renal failure.

Learning activities

1   Review the serum creatinine and the urine output preceding the commencement of CRRT for a patient in your care. Which of the RIFLE criteria did they meet at this time?

2   Review the medications prescribed for a patient managed with CRRT and check the available information for clearance with renal failure. Are the prescribed doses modified in this patient?

3   Review the 'filter life' in your ICU and compare to the data cited from large multicentre trials associated with CRRT. How does the experience from your ICU compare?

Online resources

Acute Dialysis Quality Initiative, www.ADQI.org

Continuous renal replacement therapies, www.CRRTonline.com

Pediatric continuous renal replacement therapy, www.pcrrt.com

Further reading

Dunn W, Shyamala S. Filter lifespan in critically ill adults receiving continuous renal replacement therapy: the effect of patient and treatment-related variables. Crit Care Resusc 2014;16(3):225–31.

Legrand M, Darmon M, Joannidis M, Payen D. Management of renal replacement therapy in ICU patients: an international survey. Intensive Care Med 2013;39:101–8.

References

1 Kellum JA, Bellomo R, Ronco C. Definition and classification of acute kidney injury. Nephron Clin Prac 2008;109:c182–7.

2 Kellum JA, Bellomo R, Ronco C. The concept of acute kidney injury and the RIFLE criteria. In: Ronco C, Bellomo R, Kellum J, eds. Contributions to nephrology. Vol 156. Basel: Karger; 2007, pp 10–6.

3 Kidney Disease: Improving Global Outcomes (KDIGO) Acute Kidney Injury Work Group. KDIGO clinical practice guideline for acute kidney injury. Kidney Inter Suppl 2012;2:1–138.

4 Esson ML, Schrier RW. Diagnosis and treatment of acute tubular necrosis. Ann Intern Med 2002;137:744–52.

5 Bellomo R, Kellum JA, Ronco C. Acute kidney injury. Lancet 2012;380: 756-66.

6 Myers BD, Moran SM. Haemodynamically mediated acute renal failure. N Engl J Med 1986;314:97–105.

7 Bellomo R, Mehta R. Acute renal replacement in the intensive care unit: now and tomorrow. New Horizons 2005;3(4):760–7.

8 Hoste EA, Clermont G, Kersten A, Venkataraman R, Angus DC, De Bacquer D et al. RIFLE criteria for acute kidney injury are associated with hospital mortality in critically ill patients: a cohort analysis. Crit Care 2006;10:R73.

9 Silvester W, Bellomo R, Cole L. Epidemiology, management, and outcome of severe acute renal failure of critical illness in Australia. Crit Care Med 2001;29:1910–5.

10 Gray's anatomy of the human body: the Bartleby.com edition, <http://www.bartleby.com/107/253.html>; [accessed 08.14].

11 Unit V: The kidneys and body fluids. In: Guyton AC, Hall JE, eds. Textbook of medical physiology. 11th ed. Philadelphia: WB Saunders; 2006.

12 Endre ZH. Acute renal failure. In: Whitworth JA, Lawrence JR, Kincaid-Smith P, eds. Textbook of renal disease. 2nd ed. Edinburgh: Churchill Livingstone; 1994.

13 Bellomo R. Acute renal failure. In: Bersten A, Soni N, eds. Oh's intensive care manual. 6th ed. Elsevier: Butterworth-Heinemann; 2009.

14 Chalkias A, Xanthos T. Acute kidney injury (Letter). Lancet 2012;380:1904.

15 Hendenstierna G, Larsson A. Influence of abdominal pressure on respiratory and abdominal organ function. Curr Opin Crit Care 2012;18:80-5.

16 Bellomo R. Renal replacement therapy. In: Bersten A, Soni N, eds. Oh's intensive care manual. 6th ed. Elsevier: Butterworth-Heinemann; 2009.

17 Cumming AD. Acute renal failure: definitions and diagnosis. In: Ronco C, Bellomo R, eds. Critical care nephrology. Dordrecht: Kluwer Academic; 1998.

18 Iaina A, Peer G. Post surgery/polytrauma and acute renal failure. In: Ronco C, Bellomo R, eds. Critical care nephrology. Dordrecht: Kluwer Academic; 1998.

19 Endre ZH. Post cardiac surgery acute renal failure in the 1990s. Aust J Med 1997;25:278–9.

20 Cole L, Bellomo R, Silvester W, Reeves JH. A prospective, multicenter study of the epidemiology, management and outcome of severe acute renal failure in a 'closed' ICU system. Am J Respir Crit Care Med 2000;162:191–6.

21 Rudiger A, Singer M. Acute kidney injury (Letter). Lancet 2012;380:1904.

22 Sheridan A, Bonventre J. Pathophysiology of ischaemic acute renal failure. Contrib Nephrol 2001;132:7–21.

23 Consentino F, Chaff C, Piedmonte M. Risk factors influencing survival in ICU acute renal failure. Nephrol Dial Transplant 1994;9:179–82.

24 Schiffle H, Lang SM, Fischer R. Daily hemodialysis and the outcome of acute renal failure. N Engl J Med 2002;346:305–10.

25 Bonventre JV. Pathophysiology of ischemic acute renal failure. Inflammation, lung-kidney cross talk, and biomarkers. Contrib Nephrol 2004;144:19–30.

26 Bonventre JV. Dedifferentiation and proliferation of surviving epithelial cells in acute renal failure. J Am Soc Nephrol 2003;14(Suppl 1):S55–61.

27 Sheridan AM, Bonventre JV. Cell biology and molecular mechanisms of injury in ischaemic acute renal failure. Curr Opin Nephrol 2000;9(4):427–34.

28 Kellum JA, Hoste EA. Acute renal failure in the critically ill: impact on morbidity and mortality. Contrib Nephrol 2004;144:1–11.

29 Chun C-C, Landon KS, Rabb H. Mechanisms underlying combined acute renal failure and acute lung injury in the intensive care unit. Contrib Nephrol 2004;144:53–62.

30 Seifter JL, Samuels MA. Uremic encephalopathy and other brain disorders associated with renal failure. Semin Neurol 2011;31(2):139-43.

31 Gams ME, Rabbs H. The distal organ effect of acute kidney injury. Kidney Int 2012;81:942–48; doi:10.1038/ki.2011.241.

32 Schrier RW. Fluid administration in critically ill patients with acute kidney injury. Clin J Am Soc Nephrol 2010;5(4):733-9.

33 Bellomo R, Ronco C, Kellum J, Mehta R, Palevsky P; ADQI working group. Acute renal failure: definition, outcome measures, animal models, fluid therapy and information technology needs: the Second International Consensus Conference of the Acute Dialysis Quality Initiative (ADQI) Group. Crit Care 2004;8(4):R204–12.

34 Finfer S, Norton R, Bellomo R, Boyce N, French J, Myburgh J, on behalf of the SAFE Study Investigators. The SAFE study: saline versus albumin for fluid resuscitation in the critically ill patient. Vox Sang 2004;87(Suppl 2):S123–S31.

35 The RENAL Replacement Therapy Study Investigators. An observational study for fluid balance and patient outcomes in the randomized evaluation of normal vs. augmented level of replacement therapy trial. Crit Care Med 2012;40:1753-60.

36 Peake SL, Chapman MJ, Davies AR, Moran JL, O'Connor S, Ridley E et al; George Institute for Global Health; Australian and New Zealand Intensive Care Society Clinical Trials Group. Enteral nutrition in Australian and New Zealand intensive care units: a point-prevalence study of prescription practices. Crit Care Resusc 2012;14(2):148-53.

37 Fiaccadori E, Cremaschi E, Regolisti G. Semin Dial Nutritional assessment and delivery in renal replacement therapy patients. 2011;24(2):169-75.

38 Bellomo R, Ronco C. Indications and criteria for initiating renal replacement therapy in the intensive care unit. Kidney Int 1998;53:S66, pp. s106–9.

39 Ostermann M, Dickie H, Tovey L, Treacher D. Management of sodium disorders during continuous haemofiltration. Crit Care 2010;14:418.

40 Choi G, Gomersall CD, Tain Q, Joynt GM, Freebairn RC, Lipman J. Principles of antibacterial dosing in continuous real replacement therapy. Crit Care Med 2009;37:2268–82.

41 Medline Plus. Online Medical Dictionary, <http://www.nim.nih.gov/medlineplus/mplusdictionary.html>; [accessed 12.15].

42 Vienken J, Diamantoglou M, Henne W, Nederlof B. Artificial dialysis membranes: from concept to large scale production. Am J Nephrol 1999; 19:355–62.

43 Cameron JS. Practical haemodialysis began with cellophane and heparin: the crucial role of William Thalhimer (1884–1961). Nephrol Dial Transplantat 2000;15:1086–91.

44 Ronco C, La Greca G. The role of technology in hemodialysis. Contrib Nephrol 2002;137:1–12.

45 Coleman B, Merrill JP. The artificial kidney. Am J Nurs 1952;52(3):327–9.

46 Baldwin I, Elderkin T. Continuous hemofiltration: nursing perspectives in critical care. New Horizons 1995;3(4):738–47.

47 Martin R, Jurschak J. Nursing management of continuous renal replacement therapy. Semin Dial 1996;9(2):192–9.

48 Mehta R, Martin R. Initiating and implementing a continuous renal replacement therapy program. Semin Dial 1996;9(2):80–7.

49 Wild J. Peritoneal dialysis. In: Thomas N, ed. Renal nursing. 2nd ed. London: Baillière Tindall; 2002.

50 Kramer P, Wigger W, Rieger J, Matthaei D, Scheler F. Arteriovenous haemofiltration: a new and simple method for treatment of overhydrated patients resistant to diuretics. Klin Wochenschr 1977;55:1121–2.

51 Ronco C, Brendolan A, Bellomo R. Current technology for continuous renal replacement therapies. In: Ronco C, Bellomo R, eds. Critical care nephrology. Dordrecht: Kluwer Academic; 1998.

52 Teschner M, Heidland A. George Ganter – a pioneer of peritoneal dialysis and his tragic and academic demise at the hands of the Nazi regime. J Nephrol 2004;17(Suppl 3):457-60.

53 Burdmann E, Chakravarthi R. Peritoneal dialysis in acute kidney injury: lessons learned and applied. Semin Dial 2011;24:149-56.

54 Lamiere N. Principles of peritoneal dialysis and its application in acute renal failure. In: Ronco C, Bellomo R (eds). Critical care nephrology. Dordrecht: Kluwer Academic; 1998, pp 1357-71.

55 Goel S, Saran R, Nolph KD. Indications, contraindications and complications of peritoneal dialysis in the critically ill. In: Ronco C, Bellomo R (eds). Critical care nephrology. Dordrecht: Kluwer Academic; 1998, pp 1373-81.

56 Baldwin I, Fealy N. Nursing for renal replacement therapies in the intensive care unit: historical, educational, and protocol review. Blood Purification 2009;27:174–81.

57 Davenport A, Mehta S. The acute dialysis quality initiative – Part VI: access and anticoagulation in CRRT. Adv Renal Replace Ther 2002;9(4):273–81.

58 Ofsthun NJ, Colton CK, Lysaght MJ. Determinants of fluid and solute removal rates during hemofiltration. In: Henderson LW, Quellhorst G, Baldamus CA, Lysaght MJ, eds. Hemofiltration. Berlin: Springer-Verlag; 1986.

59 Baldwin I and Fealy N. Clinical nursing for the application of renal replacement therapies in the intensive vare unit. Semin Dial 2009;22(2):189–93.

60 Thomas N. Haemodialysis. In: Thomas N, ed. Renal nursing. 2nd ed. London: Baillière Tindall; 2002.

61 Ronco C, Bellomo R. Basic mechanisms and definitions for continuous renal replacement therapies. Int J Artificial Organs 1996;19:95–9.

62 Bellomo R, Ronco C, Mehta R. Technique of continuous renal replacement therapy: nomenclature for continuous renal replacement therapies. Am J Kidney Dis 1996;28(5 Supp 3):s2–7.

63 Relton S, Greenberg A, Palevsky P. Dialysate and blood flow dependence of diffusive solute clearance during CVVHD. ASAIO J 1992;38(3):M691–6.

64 Kox WJ, Rohr U, Wauer H. Practical aspects of renal replacement therapy. Int J Artificial Organs 1996;19(2):100–5.

65 Baldwin I, Bellomo R, Koch B. A technique for the monitoring of blood flow during continuous hemofiltration. Intens Care Med 2002;28:1361–4.

66 Webb AR, Mythen MG, Jacobsen D, Mackie IJ. Maintaining blood flow in the extracorporeal circuit: haemostasis and anticoagulation. Intens Care Med 1995;21:84–93.

67 Dirkes S. How to use the new CVVH renal replacement systems. Am J Nurs 1994;94:67–73.

68 Baldwin I. Factors affecting circuit patency and filter life. In: C Ronco, Bellomo R, Kellum J, eds. Contributions to nephrology, Vol 156. Basel: Karger; 2007, pp 178–84.

69 Gretz N, Quintel M, Ragaller M, Odenwalder W, Bender HJ, Rohmeiss SM. Low-dose heparinization for anticoagulation in intensive care patients on continuous hemofiltration. Contrib Nephrol 1995;116:130–5.

70 Langeneker SA, Felfernig M, Werba A, Meuller CM, Chiari A, Zinpfer M. Anticoagulation with prostacyclin and heparin during continuous venovenous hemofiltration. Crit Care Med 1994;22(11):1774–81.

71 Cassina T, Mauri R, Engeler A, Giannini O. Continuous veno-venous haemofiltration with regional citrate anticoagulation: a four year single center experience. Int J Artificial Organs 2008;31(11):937–43.

72 Baldwin I, Tan HK, Bridge N, Bellomo R. Possible strategies to prolong circuit life during hemofiltration: three controlled studies. Renal Failure 2002;24(6):839–48.

73 Leslie G, Jacobs I, Clarke G. Proximally delivered high volume heparin does not improve circuit life in continuous venovenous haemodiafiltration (CVVHD). Intensive Care Med 1996;22:1261–4.

74 Monchi M, Berghmans D, Ledoux D, Canivet JL, Dubois B, Damas P. Citrate vs. heparin for anticoagulation in continuous venovenous hemofiltration: a prospective randomized study. Intensive Care Med 2004;30(7):260–5.

75 Tolwani A, Campbell R, Schenk M, Allon M, Warnock D. Simplified citrate anticoagulation for continuous renal replacement therapy. Kidney Int 2001;60(1):370–4.

76 Naka T, Egi M, Bellomo R, Cole L, French C, Botha J et al. Commercial low citrate anticoagulation haemofiltration in high risk patients with frequent filter clotting. Anaesth Intensive Care 2005;33(5):601–8.

77 Mehta R, McDonald B, Aguilar M, Ward D. Regional citrate anticoagulation in continuous arteriovenous hemodialysis in critically ill patients. Kidney Int 1990;38:976–81.

78 Davies H, Morgan D, Leslie GD. A regional citrate anticoagulation protocol for pre-dilutional CVVHDf: the 'Alabama concept'. Aust Crit Care 2008;21(3):154–6.

79 Tolwani AJ, Wille K. Anticoagulation for continuous renal replacement therapy. Semin Dial 2009;22(2):141–5.

80 Aucella F, Di Paolo S, Gesualdo L. Dialysate and fluid composition for CRRT. Contrib Nephrol 2007;156:287–96.

81 Davenport A. Replacement and dialysate fluids for patients with acute renal failure treated by continuous veno-venous haemofiltration and/or haemodiafiltration. Contrib Nephrol 2004;144:317–28.

82 Baldwin I, Bellomo R. Sustained low efficiency dialysis in the ICU. Int J Intensive Care 2002;Winter:177–87.

83 Ronco C, Ricci Z, Bellomo R, Baldwin I, Kellum J. Management of fluid balance in CRRT: a technical approach. Int J Artif Organs 2005;28(8):765-76.

84 Barletta JF, Barletta G-M, Brophy PD, Maxvold NJ, Hackbarth RM, Bunchman TE. Medication errors and patient complications with continuous renal replacement therapy. Pediatr Nephrol 2006;21(6):842-5.

85 Sutherland SM, Zappitelli M, Alexander SR, Chua AN, Brophy PD, Bunchman TE et al. Fluid overload and mortality in children receiving continuous renal replacement therapy: the prospective pediatric continuous renal replacement therapy registry. Am J Kidney Dis 2010;55: 316-25.

86 Bouchard J, Soroko SB, Chertow GM, Himmelfarb J, Ikizler TA, Paganini E et al, and the PICARD group. Fluid accumulation, survival and recovery of kidney function in critically ill patients with acute kidney injury. Kidney Int 2009;76:422-7.

87 Baldwin I. Training management and credentialling for CRRT in critical care. Am J Kidney Dis 1997;30(5):S112–6.

88 Graham P, Lischer E. Nursing issues in renal replacement therapy: organization, manpower assessment, competency evaluation and quality improvement processes. Semin Dial 2011;24(2):183-7.

89 Fealy N, Baldwin I, Bellomo R. The effect of circuit down time on uraemic control during continuous veno-venous haemofiltration. Crit Care Resusc 2002;4:266–70.

90 Cruz D, Bobek I, Lentini P, Soni S, Chionh CY, Ronco C. Machines for continuous renal replacement therapy. Semin Dial 2009;22(2):123–32.

91 Ronco C. Machines used for continuous renal replacement therapy. In: Kellum J, Bellomo R, Ronco C, eds. Continuous renal replacement therapy. New York: Oxford University Press; 2010.

92 Mottes T, Owens T, Niedner M, Juno JS, Thomas P, Heung M. Improving delivery of continuous renal replacement therapy: impact of a simulation-based educational intervention. Pediatr Crit Care Med 2013;14(8):747-54.

93 Boyle M, Baldwin I. Understanding the continuous renal replacement therapy circuit for acute renal failure support; a quality issue in the intensive care unit. AACN 2010;21(4):365-75.

94 RENAL Replacement Therapy Investigators. Intensity of renal support in critically ill patients with acute kidney injury. N Engl J Med 2009;361(17):1627-38.

95 VA/NIH Acute Renal Failure Trail Network. Intensity of renal support in critically ill patients with acute kidney injury. N Engl J Med 2008;359(1):7-20.

96 Ronco C, Garzotto F, Ricci Z. CA.R.PE.DI.E.M. (cardio-renal pediatric dialysis emergency machine): evolution of continuous renal replacement therapies in infants. A personal journey. Pediatr Nephrol 2012;27:1203-11.

97 Askenazi DJ, Goldstein SL, Koralkar R, Fortenberry J, Baum M, Hackbarth R et al. Continuous renal replacement therapy for children ≤10 kg: a report from the prospective pediatric continuous renal replacement therapy registry. J Pediatric 2013;162(3):587-92.e3.

98 Combesa A, Bacchettab M, Brodieb D, Müllerc T, Pellegrino V. Extracorporeal membrane oxygenation for respiratory failure in adults. Curr Opin Crit Care 2012;18(1):99–104.

99 Combes A, Brodie D, Bartlett R, Brochard L, Brower R, Conrad S et al. Position paper for the Organization of Extracorporeal Membrane Oxygenation Programs for Acute Respiratory Failure in Adult Patients. Am J Respir Crit Care Med 2014;190(5):488-96. doi: 10.1164/rccm.201404-0630CP.

100 Parmar A, Bigam D, Meeberg G, Cave D, Townsend DR, Gibney RT et al. An evaluation of intraoperative renal support during liver transplantation: a matched cohort study. Blood Purification 2011;32(3):238-48.

101 Douthitt L, Bezinover D, Uemura T, Kadry Z, Shah RA, Ghahramani N et al. Perioperative use of continuous renal replacement therapy for orthotopic liver transplantation. Transplant Proc 2012;44(5):1314-7.

Chapter 19

Nutrition assessment and therapeutic management

Andrea Marshall, Teresa Williams

Learning objectives

After reading this chapter, you should be able to:

- describe the changes in metabolism associated with critical illness
- describe the consequences of malnutrition and how they influence recovery from critical illness
- identify appropriate nutrition assessment strategies and critique methods of determining nutritional requirements in critical illness
- apply theoretical knowledge of nutritional requirements, assessment of and potential for malnutrition in critical illness
- rationalise selected nutritional support strategies for specific clinical conditions
- critically analyse the role of glycaemic control in the context of critical illness.

KEY WORDS
....
anabolism
catabolism
enteral nutrition
glycaemic control
hypermetabolism
total parenteral
  nutrition

Introduction

Critical illness is associated with increased catabolism that occurs at a time when oral intake may be difficult or impossible. Failure to provide adequate nutrition during this time will result in an accumulated energy deficit, muscle wasting and decreased lean body mass, which are associated with adverse outcomes. During critical illness optimising protein and calorie intake is important because inadequate nutrition, which results in an overall nutrition deficit, is associated with increases in morbidity and mortality. Enteral nutrition (EN) is the preferred method of nutrition therapy for the critically ill although some patients might require parenteral nutrition (PN) or a combination of EN and PN.

As part of the interdisciplinary team, nurses play an important role in achieving optimal nutrition and are responsible for monitoring achievement of nutrition goals and implementing strategies to optimise nutrition intake. In this chapter an overview of metabolism and the consequences of malnutrition are provided. This is followed by discussion of nutritional assessment and delivery strategies where an emphasis is placed on nutrition therapy through the provision of EN. Tailoring nutrition to specific disease states is also included in this chapter. Lastly, we discuss the importance of glycaemic control in critical illness.

Metabolism

The body requires energy in order to support normal body and cellular function. Energy is derived from the metabolism of macronutrients including carbohydrate, protein and fat. Following consumption of food, carbohydrates are broken down and stored as glycogen in the liver and skeletal muscle, and fat, stored in adipose tissue, is available for long-term energy requirements. Proteins and amino acids, however, are not stored and reduced protein intake can result in catabolism of body protein.[1]

The breakdown of food to produce energy is carried out in three phases. The first phase is where protein, carbohydrates and fats are broken down through the process of digestion into the subunits of amino acids, simple sugars and fatty acids. The second phase is the further breakdown of these subunits, within the cytoplasm of the cell. The most important part of the second phase is glycolysis, where a molecule of the simple sugar glucose is split and two molecules of adenosine triphosphate are produced. In the final phase of catabolism the majority of adenosine triphosphate is created within the citric acid cycle and the process of oxidative phosphorylation[1] (see Figure 19.1).

FIGURE 19.1 Three phases of catabolism.

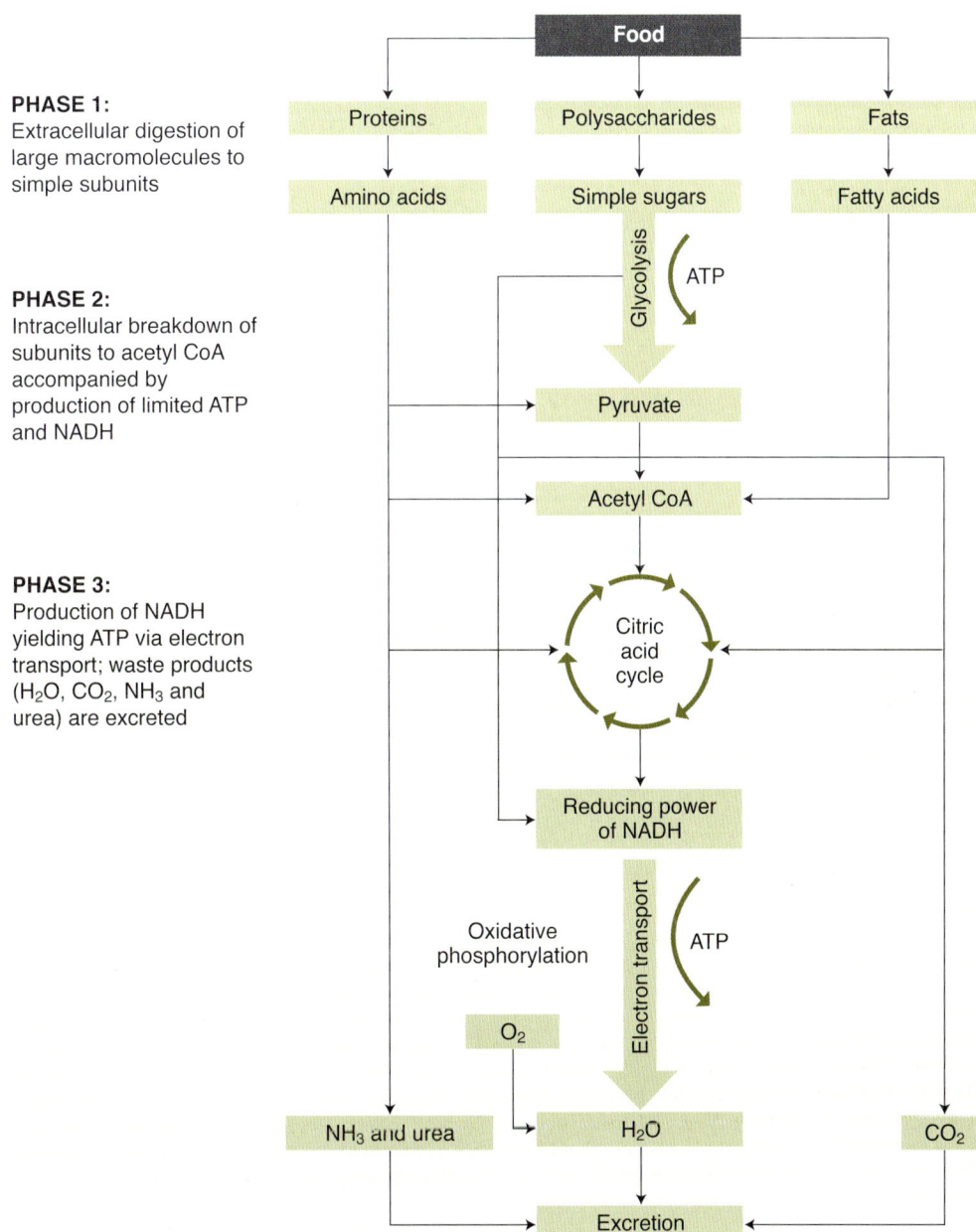

PHASE 1:
Extracellular digestion of large macromolecules to simple subunits

PHASE 2:
Intracellular breakdown of subunits to acetyl CoA accompanied by production of limited ATP and NADH

PHASE 3:
Production of NADH yielding ATP via electron transport; waste products (H_2O, CO_2, NH_3 and urea) are excreted

Adapted from McCance KL, Huether SE, Brashers VL, Rote NS, eds. Pathophysiology: The biologic basis for disease in adults and children. 6th ed. Maryland Heights, MI: Mosby Elsevier; 2010, Figure 1-22, p 24, with permission.

Effect of critical illness on metabolism

The stress and injury associated with critical illness triggers the hypothalamus, sympathetic nervous system and adrenal medulla to initiate a response that results in hyper-catabolism.[2] An increased release of cytokines including interleukin-1, interleukin-6 and tumor necrosis factor-α and production of counter-regulatory hormones such as catecholamines, cortisol, glucagon and growth hormone induce catabolism and oppose the anabolic effects of insulin.[3] Hypercatabolism occurs with the imbalance between anabolism and catabolism. To compensate for the altered metabolic regulation, neuroendocrine stimulation increases the mobilisation and consumption of nutrients, such as glycogen and protein, from existing body stores. As the metabolic rate rises, nutritional requirements in critical illness are increased, characterised by a rise in resting energy expenditure and oxygen consumption which, in some critically ill patients, can be increased by over 50%.[4] Depletion of body energy stores results from alterations in protein, carbohydrate and fat metabolism. In addition to the rise in metabolic demands, patients who are critically ill often experience a concomitant fall in nutritional intake. The metabolic and nutrition alterations vary with the stress level, severity of illness, type of injury, organ dysfunction and nutrition status.[4]

> **Practice tip**
>
> Metabolic rate fluctuates throughout an episode of critical illness and can vary significantly between patients. Generally, the sicker a patient is the higher their metabolic rate.

To maintain normal cellular function, body cells require adequate amounts of the six basic nutrients: carbohydrates, fats and proteins to provide energy, and vitamins, minerals and water to catalyse metabolic processes. Unlike normal metabolism, which preferentially uses carbohydrates and fats for energy, the hypermetabolic state associated with critical illness consumes proportionally more fats and proteins than carbohydrates to generate energy.[5] As a consequence of the gluconeogenesis and the synthesis of acute-phase proteins, there is a decrease in lean body mass and negative nitrogen balance.

Malnutrition

Malnutrition in critical illness is an important consideration with an estimated 50% of critically ill patients affected.[6] In the critically ill patient malnutrition can be pre-existing and the result of chronic starvation without inflammation being present or associated with chronic disease with mild-to-moderate degrees of inflammation. Malnutrition can also occur as the result of recent and acute disease with marked inflammatory response.[7] Determining the extent of pre-existing malnutrition in critical care is challenging because of the heterogeneous patient populations and use of different criteria to characterise malnutrition.[8]

In addition to disease-related malnutrition, critically ill patients are also at risk of developing iatrogenic or hospital-acquired malnutrition. There are a number of contributing factors to the development of hospital-acquired malnutrition related to both the prescription and delivery of nutrition, highlighting the importance of accurate assessment of nutritional requirements and strategies to ensure the prescribed nutrition is delivered. The patient's clinical presentation can also have an impact on nutritional adequacy with surgical patients receiving less nutrition than medical patients.[9]

> **Practice tip**
>
> Critically ill patients, particularly the elderly, can present to the ICU with existing malnutrition. Obtaining information on pre-admission nutrition status can help guide nutrition therapy.

Consequences of malnutrition

When adequate and timely nutrition support is not provided, body energy and protein depletion can occur with negative consequences on patient outcome.[10] Critically ill patients require adequate nutrition to limit muscle wasting, respiratory and gastrointestinal dysfunction and alterations in immunity, all of which are associated with malnutrition. Respiratory support is often necessary during critical illness, and decreased respiratory muscle function and ventilatory drive may contribute to an increase in the number of ventilator days.[11] Furthermore, infection rates may be increased in malnourished critically ill patients. The decrease in lean body mass and negative nitrogen balance are associated with delayed wound healing and a higher risk of infection.[12]

These complications are associated with an increased length of stay, cost, morbidity and mortality,[13] although the extent to which the provision of artificial nutrition ameliorates these complications is unclear.[14] The degree of critical illness and hypercatabolism varies between patients and is often difficult to determine. For this reason it is necessary to assess, as accurately as possible, the nutritional requirements of each individual patient.

> **Practice tip**
>
> Malnourished patients are more susceptible to developing infection.

Nutritional assessment

Not all critically ill patients have the same nutritional needs[15,16] with protein and energy requirements influenced by the degree and type of critical illness. Nutritional assessment is required to determine the most appropriate nutrition therapy for each patient and should incorporate patient history, clinical diagnosis, physical examination, anthropometric data, laboratory tests, dietary assessment and functional outcomes.[17,18] The degree of acute or chronic inflammation is an important contributing factor to the development of malnutrition and can also influence the effectiveness of nutrition therapy.[17]

Not all critically ill patients are alike and energy expenditure varies from 22 to 34 kcal/kg/day.[2] Assessing which patients might be at greatest nutritional risk is important. Existing nutrition screening tools for hospitalised patients are often not used in routine clinical practice and have not been validated for use in the critically ill.[19] Recently, a novel scoring tool, The NUTritional Risk in the Critically ill (NUTRIC) score[20], was developed based on the recent definitions of malnutrition, which incorporate concepts of inflammation.[7] The conceptual basis for the NUTRIC score incorporates variables related to acute and chronic starvation, acute and chronic inflammation, age and severity of illness. To test this, model data were collected during a multicentre observational study of 597 critically ill patients. While individual variables (Table 19.1), with the exception of body mass index (BMI), had a statistically significant relationship with mortality and ventilator-free days, not all were included in the final model with oral intake, recent weight loss, C-reactive protein and procalcitonin excluded as they did not improve model fit. Interleukin-6 improved model fit but not in a clinically or statistically significant way so, where interleukin-6 is not routinely collected, it is suggested that this too can be dropped from the score. The resulting NUTRIC score includes six variables (Table 19.1). Despite the proposed model being described as 'adequate' the data did show that patients with a worse NUTRIC score also had poorer clinical outcomes.[20] Further work is needed to refine this or other tools to identify nutrition risk in critically ill patients so we can determine which patients are most likely to benefit from nutrition therapy.

Determining nutritional requirements

Determining caloric requirements is largely dependent on energy expenditure, influenced by patient activity, stage of illness, type of injury and previous nutritional status.[4] Resting energy expenditure (REE) is the primary consideration when prescribing energy intake because it is the largest component of total energy expenditure for hospitalised patients.[21] Determining REE can be done through direct measurement using indirect calorimetry or can be estimated using one of many different predictive equations. While no randomised controlled studies have compared patient outcome according to measured (using indirect calorimetry) versus predicted energy expenditure, data from two recent observational studies suggest the need to monitor changes in energy expenditure and adjust nutrient intake accordingly.[22,23] Both approaches are used in intensive care units and have advantages and limitations.

TABLE 19.1

Conceptual model and variables included in the NUTritional Risk in the Critically ill (NUTRIC) score[20]

CONCEPTS	PROPOSED VARIABLES	VARIABLES RETAINED IN FINAL SCORE
Acute starvation	Decreased oral intake over the last week	No
	Pre-ICU hospital admission	Yes
Chronic starvation	Weight loss over the last 6 months	No
	BMI <20	No
Acute inflammation	IL-6	Yes
	PCT	No
	CRP	No
Chronic inflammation	Comorbid illness	Yes
Severity of illness	Age	Yes
	APACHE II score	Yes
	SOFA score	Yes

APACHE = Acute physiology and chronic health evaluation; BMI = body mass index; CRP = C-reactive protein; IL-6 = interleukin-6; PCT = procalcitonin; SOFA = sequential organ failure assessment.

> **Practice tip**
>
> For severely malnourished patients improving nutrition support can cause refeeding syndrome to occur. In this syndrome metabolic disturbances occur that are characterised by electrolyte disorders, particularly hypophosphataemia.

Indirect calorimetry

Indirect calorimetry is the 'gold standard' and most precise way of determining energy expenditure in critical illness.[21,24] Despite this, it is infrequently used because of high equipment costs and resources constraints.[25] Through indirect calorimetry energy expenditure is calculated using oxygen consumption and carbon dioxide production.[26] Accuracy of these measurements can be affected by many factors including instrument performance,[27] ambient temperature[21] and volume leaks that might occur through the calorimeter, endotracheal tube or through chest drains.[24] Patient-related factors also can influence the measurement of REE, such as physical activity, food consumption and physiological stress such as pain. To obtain the most accurate measurement of REE it is recommended that these measurements be taken under steady-state conditions,[28] that is where there is at least a 5-minute period with ≤10% coefficient of variance in the oxygen consumption and carbon dioxide production.[29] It is recognised that metabolic equilibrium is not well defined and lacks consensus so there is variation in how steady state is determined and implemented in both clinical practice and research.[29] Comprehensive discussions of practical aspects of indirect calorimetry are published elsewhere.[26,28]

Predictive equations

Because indirect calorimetry is not available in many intensive care units, it is common practice to predict energy expenditure using one of many predictive equations (Table 19.2). Many predictive equations are based on requirements for healthy humans and then are adjusted to account for added stress or injury.[30] The accuracy of predictive equations is poor compared to measurement of REE using indirect calorimetry; however, some predictive equations perform better in critical illness than do others. Some equations use only static variables (such as height, weight, age and sex) to predict resting energy expenditure. Others use more dynamic variables (such as body temperature, minute ventilation, heart rate) in an attempt to account for the metabolic variation that occurs in critical illness.[31]

Some work has been done to validate the accuracy of predictive equations used in critical care. The largest of these studies compared predicted energy expenditure

to indirect calorimetry in 202 mechanically ventilated critically ill patients.[32] In this study 17 predictive equations were evaluated against an accuracy benchmark of 10% of the measured energy expenditure. The Penn State equation was the most accurate (67%) except for older obese patients where the accuracy fell to 53%.[32] The predictive equations that performed with less than 50% accuracy were the Harris-Benedict equation (34%) and the American College of Chest Physicians equation (35%). Accuracy of these equations did not surpass 50% following adjustment for body weight (American College of Chest Physicians equation 46%) or activity factor of 1.5 (Harris-Benedict equation 46%).[32]

While most predictive equations are likely to underestimate measured energy expenditure in the critically ill wide variations in predicted energy expenditure have been reported, which suggest that the use of predictive equations can contribute to both over and under feeding.[25] The extent to which these equations accurately predict energy expenditure is also influenced by factors such as BMI,[32] sex[25] and age.[33]

Although predictive equations may not be as accurate as indirect calorimetry in determining energy expenditure, they may nevertheless provide some guidance for nutrition prescription in the absence of this technology.

TABLE 19.2
Predictive equations for estimating energy expenditure in critically ill patients

American College of Chest Physicians	25 × weight If BMI 16–25 kg/m² use usual body weight If BMI > 25 kg/m² use ideal body weight If BMI <16 kg/m² use existing body weight for the first 7×10 days then ideal body weight
Harris-Benedict equation	Men: 66.4730 + (13.7516 × weight) + (5.0033 × height) – (6.7550 × age) Women: 655.0955 + (9.5634 × weight) + (1.8496 × height) – (4.6756 × age)
Ireton-Jones 1992 equation	1.925 – (10 × age) + (5 × weight) + (281 for males) + (292 if trauma present) + (851 if burns present)
Ireton-Jones 1997 equation	(5 × weight) – (11 × age) + (244 for males) + (239 if trauma present) + (840 if burns present) + 1,784
Penn State 1998	(1.1 × value from Harris-Benedict equation) + (140 × Tmax) + (32 × VE) – 5340
Penn State 2003	(0.85 × value from Harris-Benedict equation) + (175 × Tmax) + (33 × VE) – 6433
Swinamer 1990	(945 × body surface area) – (6.4 × age) + (108 × temperature) + 24.2 × respiratory rate) + (817 × V$_T$) – 4349

BMI = body mass index.

Adapted from Walker RN, Heuberger RA. Predictive equations for energy needs for the critically ill. Respir Care 2009;54(4):509-21, with permission.

Nutrition support

Optimal nutritional support in the critically ill aims to prevent, detect and correct malnutrition, optimise the patient's metabolic state, reduce morbidity and improve recovery. Metabolic response to stress is decreased, oxidative cellular injury restricted and the immune response moderated in patients receiving adequate nutrition.[34,35] EN is the preferred method of feeding for patients who are not able to take food and fluids orally. PN alone or combined with EN may be used for those patients where oral intake is not possible.[36,37]

Enteral nutrition

EN has benefits beyond simply the supply of nutrients to the body.[38] Any amount of nutrition administered to the gut is beneficial. EN increases gastric mucosal blood flow, stimulates brush border enzymes, preserves epithelial tight cell junctions and provides gut-derived mucosal immunity.[35] Major effects of EN are: preservation of intestinal epithelium,[39] mucosal mass and microvilli height;[40] prevention of bacterial translocation; and a positive effect on the gut-associated lymphoid tissue, the source of most mucosal immunity in humans.[41] Septic complications are decreased when EN is provided.[42,43] Stimulating and improving gastrointestinal immune function is an important goal of early EN.[44]

Early or delayed enteral nutrition?

Early EN (within 48 hours) is recommended[36,45] but the definition of 'early' has not been established and study results are inconsistent. Meta-analyses have shown early

EN was associated with decreased mortality.[46,47] However, the methodological quality of the studies included in the meta-analyses was questionable and heterogeneity was high, making interpretation of the results difficult. Other studies[48,49] have also found improved outcomes but evidence from large, high-quality, randomised, controlled trials that compare timing of EN in critically ill patients is needed to define the optimal time for commencing EN.[50,51]

Hypocaloric intake in the critically ill

A significant number of hospitalised patients receiving enteral nutrition do not have their nutritional needs met.[52] Hypocaloric feeding in the first few days of critical illness is controversial.[53] In several observational studies[10,13,54,55] the reduced provision of energy and protein were associated with worse outcomes. However, observational studies may be confounded by many factors including severity of illness, where patients who were less sick and tolerated enteral nutrition better were more likely to be adequately fed and have better outcomes.[34] In a recent randomised controlled trial (the EDEN study), conducted in 1000 patients with acute lung injury who required mechanical ventilation, trophic feeding was compared with administration of full enteral feeding for the first 6 days a patient was in the ICU.[56] Initial trophic enteral feeding did not improve ventilator-free days, 60-day mortality, infectious complications or have an effect on physical and cognitive performance.[56,57] The patients enrolled in this study were reasonably young (mean age 52 years) and were moderately obese (BMI 30).[56] Moderate obesity can be protective during critical illness – the obesity paradox.[58] The findings of the EDEN study may not be generalisable to all critically ill patients, especially those who are malnourished or grossly obese. The results of the EDEN trial are similar to those of Arabi et al,[59] who demonstrated similar patient outcomes when permissive underfeeding was compared to targeted full feeding in a randomised controlled trial but outcomes were similar. Despite these results, current evidence-based guidelines do not recommend the use of trophic feeding because of a lack of high quality research to support this approach.[36]

In most cases, hypocaloric feeding is unnecessary and avoidable.[60,61] Factors that contribute to unintentional hypocaloric feeding include staffing shortages, unavailability of feeds/equipment, low priorities for feeding, fasting for clinical investigations, blockages in feeding tubes and variations in feed prescriptions.[62,63] Delivery issues, such as elective interruption for investigative procedures or operations, contributed to hypocaloric feeding with only 76% of prescribed feeds delivered to critically ill patients.[64] Similar results were observed in mechanically-ventilated patients,[65] where more than 36% of patients received less than 90% of their caloric requirements.

The concept that the bowel should be rested is questionable because bowel function is not inhibited by starvation. Starvation actually depresses splanchnic blood flow. Marik[34] likens bowel rest to resting the heart by inducing asystole! Enteral nutrition, and in particular lipid- and protein-rich formulae, has anti-inflammatory effects on the gut–brain immune axis of the gastrointestinal mucosa.[34,66] Outcomes of gastrointestinal disorders traditionally treated with bowel rest are improved with enteral nutrition.[34]

Patients can receive enteral nutrition while vasopressors are being administered,[34,36] although the evidence for the effect of vasopressors on gastric tolerance and patient outcomes is weak and inconsistent.[67] Splanchnic perfusion is reduced in critical illness but enteral nutrients improve gut blood flow enabling the bowel to absorb nutrients during vasopressor therapy.[68,69] The administration of vasopressors in patients with sepsis and shock, however, is associated with both improved and diminished perfusion. Mentec et al[70] reported gastric intolerance was higher in patients receiving vasopressor therapy while others found patients tolerated enteral nutrition.[71,72] Khalid et al[68] reported improved outcomes for patients receiving early rather than late enteral nutrition in patients requiring vasopressors.

Patients should not have enteral nutrition withheld if they have absent bowel sounds, postoperative ileus[34,45] or after gastrointestinal surgery. The risk of anatomic leaks and fistulas in patients who have had bowel surgery and also receive early enteral nutrition is lower compared to delayed feeding or parenteral nutrition.[34] Enteral nutrition following gastrointestinal surgery is associated with a significantly lower risk of infection and reduced hospital length of stay.[73,74]

> ### Practice tip
>
> Nurses should regularly assess for barriers to achieving daily nutritional goals and work with the interdisciplinary team to ensure nutrition intake is optimised.

Enteral nutrition protocols

Enteral nutrition protocols improve the delivery of enteral feeds[64] and have been shown to improve clinical outcomes.[75,76] Protocols vary widely between units and institutions[37,77] mainly because of the lack of robust research in the management of enteral nutrition. In the absence of strong research evidence, rituals are embraced and rarely challenged.[78] Furthermore, the implementation and sustainability of guidelines are influenced by multiple factors such as clinician preference, patient population, clinical contexts and content of guidelines.[79,80]

Management of enteral feeding

Routes of enteral feeding

Wide-bore nasogastric or orogastric tubes are most commonly used in the critically ill in the early stages of enteral nutrition. Should prolonged enteral nutrition be anticipated (longer than 1 month), or where patients have gastric intolerance then gastrostomy, duodenostomy or jejunostomy tubes may be used.[81]

Postpyloric feeding is useful if patients are not tolerating gastric feeding[82] but has not been shown to be superior to gastric feeding.[83,84] A randomised, controlled trial[83] was conducted in 17 multidisciplinary ICUs to test the hypothesis that early nasojejunal feeding would improve outcomes for mechanically ventilated adults with mildly elevated gastric residual volumes who were already receiving enteral nutrition through a nasogastric tube. There was no difference in the proportion of targeted energy delivered from enteral nutrition or incidence of ventilator-associated pneumonia. The study investigators recommended that routine placement of nasojejunal tubes in such patients should not be performed. Patients may also have a gastric tube inserted to aspirate the contents of the stomach.

For some critically ill patients, gastric secretions may increase when small bowel feeding is initiated.[85] A double-lumen tube is available, one lumen for gastric aspiration and decompression and the second for simultaneous jejunal feeding, but these tubes are not widely used in the clinical setting.[86]

Assessment of enteral feeding tube placement

The correct placement of enteral feeding tubes is crucial to promote adequate nutrition and avoid adverse events. The correct insertion of enteral feeding tubes in the critically ill can be challenging because these patients often have a reduced cough reflex, altered sensorium and receive sedative and narcotic medications.[87,88] Misplacement of the feeding tube into the tracheobronchial tree is an important complication of tube insertion.[89] Additional complications such as infusion of tube feedings, pneumothorax, pneumonitis, hydropneumothorax, bronchopleural fistula, empyema and pulmonary haemorrhage have also been reported.[90] Confirmation of tube placement is routinely done with radiography (Figure 19.2). However, assessment of nasogastric tube placement on X-ray does not prevent

---

FIGURE 19.2 Correct placement of a nasogastric tube.[92]

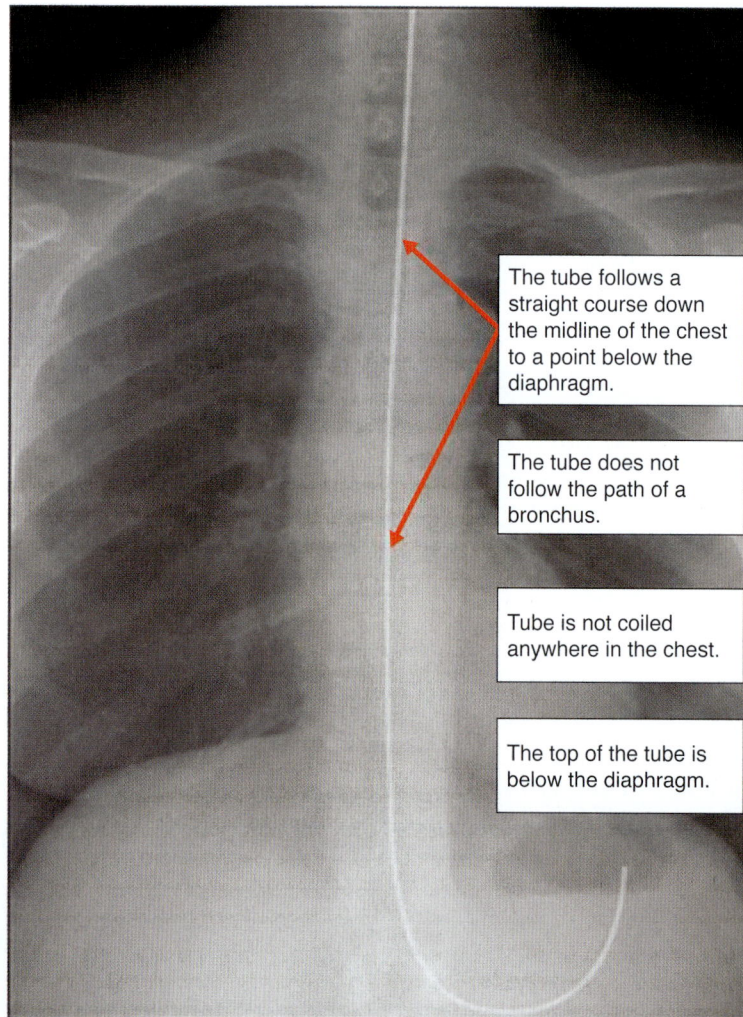

The tube follows a straight course down the midline of the chest to a point below the diaphragm.

The tube does not follow the path of a bronchus.

Tube is not coiled anywhere in the chest.

The top of the tube is below the diaphragm.

Reproduced from Patient Safety Authority. Confirming feeding tube placement: old habits die hard. PA PSRA Patient Saf Advis 2006;3(4):23-30, with permission.

incorrect placement occurring during insertion. Less reliable methods of confirming tube placement include the use of pH, observation of the colour of gastric aspirates and auscultation and other novel methods such as capnography.[87,91]

Assessment of feeding tube placement by auscultation of air insufflated into the stomach remains a common clinical practice although auscultation should NOT be used as the sole method to determine placement of the gastric tube because it is unreliable. Other important points are:

- Nasogastric aspirate from critically ill patients who receive continuous feedings may have the appearance of unchanged formula, regardless of the site of the feeding tube; therefore this method should not be used.[93]

- Analysis of the pH of gastric secretions is not reliable. A pH of 0–5 may be used to indicate gastric placement of enteral feeding tubes, although this technique may be problematic for patients receiving histamine-2-receptor antagonists or proton pump inhibitors. If the aspirated fluid has a low pH, it may be assumed that the fluid originated in the stomach but the pH of fluid from an infected pleural space can also be acidic;[94] therefore pH testing as a sole method to determine tube placement is not recommended.

- Capnometry and capnography use end-tidal carbon dioxide detectors to evaluate enteral tube placement where respiratory placement is indicated by the presence of a capnogram that suggests an increase in measured carbon dioxide.[95] Although not routinely used in clinical practice there is emerging evidence that this strategy might be useful in assessing placement of nasogastric tubes in mechanically ventilated patients.[96] It is important to recognise that this technique does not help differentiate oesophageal, gastric or intestinal placement.

- Measuring the concentrations of pepsin and trypsin in feeding tube aspirates can be used as a method of predicting tube placement; however, methods to measure pepsin and trypsin at the bedside are currently unavailable.[97]

Ongoing assessment of feeding tube placement is essential, as feeding tubes may migrate after initial placement. Marking the feeding tube at the point where it exits the nose and measurement of tube length protruding from the anterior nares will facilitate detection of migration of the enteral tube. Radio-opaque tubes have markers to enable accurate measurement and documentation of tube position. They should be used with the methods previously described for ongoing assessment.

In the absence of X-ray, several approaches should be used in combination to verify tube position. Metheny et al[93] found measuring: 1) length of tubing extending from the insertion site, 2) volume of aspirate from the feeding tube, 3) appearance of the aspirate and 4) pH of the aspirate were able to correctly differentiate between gastric and bowel tube placement during continuous feedings in 81% of predictions.

> **Practice tip**
>
> Radiographic assessment of feeding tube placement is gold standard. When this is not available feeding tube placement should be confirmed using more than one method.

Feeding regimens

Once the enteral feeding tube is successfully placed, administration of the feeding solution can begin using a variety of methods, including bolus, intermittent and continuous enteral feeding (see Table 19.3). Bolus enteral feeding is rarely used in ICU. It is less clear whether intermittent or continuous feeding is more beneficial.[98] Concerns about increased risk of aspiration with intermittent enteral feeding has not been substantiated in the literature; however, the research in this area is limited in both quantity and quality. Because of inconclusive evidence regarding feeding regimens, decisions are based on individual patient assessment and the clinician's clinical judgement.

Commencing enteral nutrition

The appropriate starting rate for enteral nutrition is controversial and there are no empirical data on which to base the decision. Feeding is often started at 30 mL/h, but may range from 10 to 100 mL/h. Increasing the

TABLE 19.3
Methods of feed delivery[98]

METHOD	DESCRIPTION
Bolus	• Delivery of a large volume of tube feed into the stomach over a short period of time (>100 mL) • Associated with complications, such as aspiration and vomiting
Intermittent	• A several-hour infusion a few times a day (e.g. 150 mL/h for 3 hours, three times per day), or delivered over a longer period (12–16 hours) with an 8–12-hour rest period • Allows gastric acidity and therefore limits bacterial overgrowth • Requires a higher hourly rate to meet caloric requirements
Continuous	• The delivery of small amounts of formula per hour over a 24-hour period • May make caloric requirements more achievable • Continuous dilution of gastric acid may contribute to bacterial overgrowth

rate of enteral feeding is equally variable, but strategies to progress patients towards meeting their daily caloric requirements should be employed. When a patient has experienced a prolonged period of starvation or total parenteral nutrition, the approach to enteral feeding is somewhat more reserved as the risk of refeeding syndrome is increased.[99] Although not common, this syndrome is associated with severe derangement in fluid and electrolyte levels (particularly hypophosphataemia, hypomagnesaemia and hypokalaemia), and may result in significant morbidity and mortality.[100]

Managing complications of enteral nutrition

Once enteral nutrition is established, it is important to assess for such complications as feeding intolerance that can result in gastric distension, vomiting, diarrhoea and increased gastric residual volume.[101] Pulmonary aspiration, hyperglycaemia, hypercarbia, electrolyte imbalances and feed contamination are also complications that should be monitored and interventions implemented to minimise their occurrence.

Critically ill patients exhibit elevated gastric residual volume for a variety of reasons including feeding intolerance[102] and reduced gastric motility.[103] Monitoring tolerance to enteral nutrition through the measurement of gastric residual volume has always been viewed as an important aspect of nursing management, although consensus on what constitutes a high gastric residual and any recommendations for interventions remain controversial.[104] High gastric residual volumes do not necessarily predict aspiration, and low gastric residual volumes do not mean that aspiration will not occur. Studies[105,106] have shown no difference in risk for pulmonary aspiration between low and high gastric residual volume groups. It is assumed that measuring gastric residual volume is accurate and useful but gastric residual volume does not correlate with clinical or radiological abdominal findings.[107]

In addition to gastrointestinal function there are other important factors associated with the accuracy of measurement of gastric residual volume such as tube diameter, tube position, type of gastric access and the patient's position.[34] The amount of gastric residual volume considered excessive in clinical practice varies. The Canadian Clinical Guidelines recommend 250 to 500 mL as the cut-off because there are insufficient data to make a recommendation for a specific gastric residual volume threshold.[36] After aspiration of gastric residual volume the gastric aspirate is either returned or discarded. The evidence for discarding gastric aspirate is weak,[108] and refeeding gastric residual volumes up to a maximum of 250 mL or discarding gastric residual volumes may be acceptable.[36] Enteral feeding is interrupted when the gastric residual volume exceeds a prescribed threshold for acceptable gastric residual volume; however, there are no data to support this practice. Ceasing feeds in response to gastric residual volume is questionable,[105] particularly as a balanced enteral diet in itself has a prokinetic effect.[109,110]

> ### Practice tip
>
> In determining feeding intolerance, a single high gastric residual volume in the absence of physical examination or radiographic findings should not result in the cessation of enteral feeding. Persisting with enteral feeding has demonstrated benefits.

> ### Practice tip
>
> When evaluating gastric residual volume in relation to the rate of enteral feeding, remember to take into account the production of gastric secretion, which can be as much as 2500 mL/day.

Development of diarrhoea is another complication for enterally fed patients,[111] and is a common reason why enteral feeding is reduced or ceased.[112] Diarrhoea may contribute to fluid and electrolyte disorders, patient (and nursing) distress and a higher cost of patient care.[113] Unfortunately, defining diarrhoea is problematic, as it is a subjective assessment that relies on nursing interpretation rather than on quantifiable assessment of stool weight.[114] Enteral feeding should not be considered a primary cause of diarrhoea. There are many reasons for diarrhoea in critically ill patients who receive enteral nutrition, often occurring simultaneously, including:

- underlying disease[115]
- medications including antibiotics due to their side effects, toxicity and disruption to gut microbiota[3]
- hypoalbuminaemia[116]
- use of histamine-2-receptor antagonists[117]
- contamination of enteral feeding solution.[118]

Current evidence-based nutrition guidelines suggest that probiotics be considered for critically ill patients.[36] Human lactoferrin and probiotic derivatives may be helpful in reducing diarrhoea in tube-fed patients, but more research is needed.[119] Probiotic (*Saccharomyces boulardii*) administration was reported to limit the development of diarrhoea in a multicentre, randomised, double-blind placebo-controlled study[120] but reports from studies are inconsistent. No difference was found in the occurrence of diarrhoea in a double-blind, randomised, controlled trial of 167 adults who were mechanically ventilated for more than 48 hours and received probiotics or placebo enterally until successful weaning from mechanical ventilation.[121] Subgroup analysis of these data demonstrated a decrease in 28-day mortality among patients with severe sepsis in the probiotic group; however, mortality was higher for those in a non-severe septic group who also received probiotics.[121]

Fermentable oligosaccharides, disaccharides, monosaccharides and polyols, which are common in commercial enteral nutrition formulas, have been found to reduce the likelihood of diarrhoea in patients receiving enteral nutrition.[122] Randomised controlled trials with human patients are needed to evaluate the effect of fermentable oligosaccharides, disaccharides, monosaccharides and polyols and other probiotics on enteral nutrition-associated diarrhoea in the critically ill.[115,123]

> **Practice tip**
>
> Nurses may be tempted to stop enteral nutrition in the presence of diarrhoea but there is no evidence to support withholding enteral feeding in critically ill patients. The only exception may be if there are significant disturbances in fluid and/or electrolyte balance.

Enteral feeding solutions present an excellent medium for the growth of microorganisms and bacterial contamination of enteral feeds is common.[124] Infection control programs are important. Strategies to limit bacterial contamination of enteral feeding solutions include:

- meticulous preparation of feeding solutions and equipment[125]
- commercially prepared formula used in preference to decanted feeds[126]
- use of closed feeding systems[37]
- limiting the time feeding solution is kept at room temperature once opened and hang times[127]
- meticulous attention to hand washing and limiting manipulation of the enteral nutrition bags and delivery system at the bedside.[124]

Prevention of pulmonary aspiration

An important complication of enteral feeding is the development of pulmonary aspiration and nosocomial pneumonia. Determining whether aspiration has occurred is difficult, even for experienced clinicians. High gastric residual volumes have been linked to the potential for pulmonary aspiration, although this has not been shown in research.[105] Oropharyngeal secretions can contribute to nosocomial pneumonia and subglottic aspiration has improved outcomes.[128] Nursing strategies to improve gastric emptying include elevation of the head of the bed 30–45° (unless otherwise contraindicated), because the likelihood of gastro-oesophageal reflux is likely to be reduced;[129,130] however, this recommendation is based on weak evidence. A small single-centre randomised controlled trial (47 patients)[131] demonstrated lower frequency of clinically suspected ventilator-associated pneumonia in 39 intubated patients randomised to the semirecumbent (45°) group compared to the supine position. The study was stopped early after a very large treatment effect in favour of the 45° elevation was shown in an interim analysis. Two earlier studies[132,133] showed similar results. Based on this weak evidence, elevating the head of bed to 30–45° position became standard of care.[134,135]

More recently, two randomised controlled trials[136,137] and an observational study[138] did not support these results. In a randomised controlled trial with 221 patients no difference was found in outcomes including no increased risk for ventilator-associated pneumonia.[136] A systematic review of research examining the effect of semi-upright position in ventilated patients including three studies[131,136,137] was the basis for developing consensus-based recommendations for clinical practice.[139] The panel recommended the head of the bed of mechanically ventilated patients be elevated 20° to 45°, preferably ≥30°, as long as there were no risks or it did not conflict with other nursing tasks, medical interventions or with patients' wishes. Marik[34] suggests that clinical judgement should be exercised when using semi-upright positioning in the critically ill because the evidence to support this practice is not compelling and the balance between benefits and harms is unknown. Nursing patients semi-recumbent at 45° can be difficult because the patient often slides down and the position can be uncomfortable for the patient. Experimental models also suggest that the semi-recumbent position may enhance the flow of mucous into the lungs with an increased risk of bacterial colonisation and pneumonia.[140] Until further evidence is available to guide practice decisions, patient positioning should be at the discretion of clinicians.

Prokinetic agents, such as erythromycin and metoclopramide, can improve gastric emptying and feeding tolerance, and avoid gastro-oesophageal reflux and pulmonary aspiration.[141] These prokinetic agents do, however, have undesirable effects. Use of erythromycin is associated with the development of bacterial resistance, and metoclopramide is associated with numerous systemic side effects. Erythromycin is more effective than metoclopramide in treating gastric intolerance among patients receiving enteral nutrition. However, combination therapy with erythromycin and metoclopramide is more effective than erythromycin alone in improving the delivery of enteral nutrition.[142,143]

Assessment of pulmonary aspiration

Despite preventive strategies, pulmonary aspiration may still occur in some patients, and accurate assessment is essential. Common methods that can be performed easily at the bedside to determine whether a patient has experienced aspiration of gastric contents and/or enteral feeding formula follow:

- The dye method previously was commonly used to assess aspiration of enteral feeds but should not be standard practice because of safety concerns. The efficacy of this method is questionable as blue dye is poorly standardised and has a low sensitivity in detecting microaspiration.[144] There have been case reports of blue dye absorption describing discolouration of the skin, urine, serum and organs,[145] and refractory hypotension and severe acidosis, suggesting poisoning by a mitochondrial toxin.[146] These safety concerns, coupled with minimal benefits, have resulted in the recommendation that the practice of using blue food colouring in enteral feeding solutions be abandoned.[145,147]

- Measurement of glucose in tracheobronchial secretions is another method to detect pulmonary aspiration.[148] As these secretions normally contain <5 mg/dL glucose, higher amounts of glucose may indicate the aspiration of glucose-rich enteral feeding formula. Differences in enteral feeding solutions affect the sensitivity of this method, with low glucose solutions being more difficult to detect. Also, patients not receiving enteral feeding can have detectable glucose in aspirates.[149] This is further confounded by the presence of blood, which is closely associated with glucose values >20 mg/dL; consequently, any blood in the respiratory tract could contribute to a false-positive result. These findings led to the consensus that glucose monitoring in respiratory secretions should also be abandoned.[147]

- Measurement of pepsin in tracheobronchial secretions has been used in an animal study that suggested that the detection of pepsin, a component of gastric secretions, may be useful in determining pulmonary aspiration.[150] Further investigation in acutely ill patients receiving enteral feeding is necessary.

- Electromagnetic tube placement device technology enables tracking gastric tube insertion electromagnetically on a monitoring screen. The stylet within the gastric tube transmits an electromagnetic signal that is detected over the patient's epigastric region by a receiver. Metheny and Meert[151] reviewed reports from 2007 to 2012 of the electromagnetic tube placement device technology and concluded that there is sufficient room for error with this method and recommend assessment of feeding tube placement through radiographic confirmation.

> **Practice tip**
>
> Nursing patients with the head of bed elevated is common in ICU; however, more evidence is needed to demonstrate that this practice prevents pulmonary aspiration.

Parenteral nutrition

EN is the preferred method of nutritional support because it has physiological advantages, and is associated with fewer infectious and metabolic complications. EN as a nutrition therapy is also less expensive than PN and the use of PN in the context of critical illness remains controversial. PN bypasses the gastrointestinal system and the crucial role that hormones and nutrients play in regulating gut function, metabolic pathways and hepatic function.[34] In addition there are metabolic, immunological, endocrine and infective complications from infusing solutions of high glucose concentration and fat globules intravenously.[152] Grau et al[153] found a strong association of PN and the development of liver dysfunction, whereas early EN was protective. PN impairs humoral and cellular immunological defences and the association of PN with increased free radical formation may be important for patients who are critically ill.[34]

Studies report conflicting results on the benefit of PN for the nutrition support of critically ill patients. A meta-analysis of PN versus no nutritional support in critically ill patients reported a two-fold increased risk of death in the PN group.[154] A retrospective cohort study compared patients with severely injured blunt trauma who received PN within 7 days after injury with a control group that did not. In these critically ill trauma patients who were able to tolerate at least some EN, early PN administration contributed to increased infectious morbidity and worse clinical outcomes.[155] A growing trend is to supplement EN with PN in patients who cannot commence early EN or until target nutrition goals are achieved.[156] Four studies examined the effect of supplemental PN and found no improvement in patient outcomes,[42,157–159] and none was able to demonstrate a clear benefit to critically ill patients when PN was administered.[34] The lack of quantity and quality of data on the use of PN in the critically ill means that this strategy is not recommended in current evidence-based nutrition guidelines.[36,160,161]

In the patient who is not tolerating adequate EN, the data are insufficient and clinicians will have to weigh the safety and benefits of initiating PN on an individual case-by-case basis.[36] The American Society for Parenteral and Enteral Nutrition and Society of Critical Care Medicine clinical guidelines[160] recommend PN be initiated after 1 week, unless the patient is severely malnourished, and the European Society of Enteral and Parenteral guidelines[161] recommend consideration of EN supplemented by PN after 2–3 days in the ICU if enteral nutrition alone is insufficient at that time.

PN solutions contain carbohydrates, lipids, proteins, electrolytes, vitamins and trace elements. PN, whether supplementary or complete, provides daily allowances of nutrients and minerals. The components of PN are listed in Table 19.4. The addition of vitamins and trace elements to PN solutions is necessary, particularly as water-soluble vitamins and trace elements are rapidly depleted (see Table 19.5).[162] Standardised PN formulations, although as effective as custom-made PN in providing caloric requirements, are less likely to achieve estimated protein requirements and have been noted to be associated with hyponatraemia.[163] Glucose is the primary energy source in PN solutions. Concentrations of 10–70% glucose may be used in PN solutions although the final concentration of the solution should be no more than 35%. The high concentration of PN solutions can cause thrombosis so PN is normally infused via a central venous catheter. Catheter insertion, ongoing care and replacement are similar to that with any other central venous catheter. A dedicated central venous catheter, or lumen of a multilumen catheter, should be used for PN.[164] Manipulation of the catheter and tubing should be avoided to minimise infection of the catheter. Peripheral administration can be considered when the final solution concentration is 10–12%,[165] but is not usually used in the context of critical illness because high volumes of PN would be required to meet caloric requirements.[166]

TABLE 19.4

Components of PN solutions

COMPONENT	RECOMMENDATION	GRADE*
Carbohydrate	The minimal amount of carbohydrate required is about 2 g/kg of glucose per day	B
	Hyperglycemia (glucose >10 mmol/L) contributes to death in the critically ill patient and should also be avoided to prevent infectious complications	B
	Reductions and increases in mortality rates have been reported in ICU patients when blood glucose is maintained between 4.5 and 6.1 mmol/L. No unequivocal recommendation on this is therefore possible at present	C
	There is a higher incidence of severe hypoglycemia in patients treated to the tighter limits	A
Lipids	Lipids should be an integral part of PN for energy and to ensure essential fatty acid provision in long-term ICU patients	B
	Intravenous lipid emulsions (LCT, MCT or mixed emulsions) can be administered safely at a rate of 0.7 g/kg up to 1.5 g/kg over 12 to 24 h	B
	The tolerance of mixed LCT/MCT lipid emulsions in standard use is sufficiently documented. Several studies have shown specific clinical advantages over soybean LCT alone but require confirmation by prospective controlled studies	C
	Olive oil-based parenteral nutrition is well tolerated in critically ill patients	B
	Addition of EPA and DHA to lipid emulsions has demonstrable effects on cell membranes and inflammatory processes. Fish oil-enriched lipid emulsions probably decrease length of stay in critically ill patients	B
Amino acids	When PN is indicated, a balanced amino acid mixture should be infused at approximately 1.3–1.5 g/kg ideal body weight/day in conjunction with an adequate energy supply	B
	When PN is indicated in ICU patients the amino acid solution should contain 0.2–0.4 g/kg/day of L-glutamine (e.g. 0.3–0.6 g/kg/day alanyl-glutamine dipeptide)	A
Micronutrients	All PN prescriptions should include a daily dose of multivitamins and of trace elements	C

*Grade of recommendation – the grade of recommendation is based on the quality of the evidence where A is high, B is moderate, C is low and D is very low (as quoted in Guyatt GH, Oxman AD, Vist GE, Kunz R, Falck-Ytter Y, Alonso-Coello P et al. GRADE: an emerging consensus on rating quality of evidence and strength of recommendations. BMJ 2008; 336:924–6).

DHA = docosahexaenoic acid; EPA = eicosapentaenoic acid; LCT = long chain triglycerides; MCT = medium chain triglycerides.

Adapted from Singer P, Berger MM, Van den Berghe G, Biolo G, Calder P, Forbes A et al. ESPEN Guidelines on Parenteral Nutrition: intensive care. Clin Nutr 2009;28(4):387-400, with permission.

TABLE 19.5

Trace elements in TPN[162]

TRACE ELEMENT	ACTION
Zinc	Wound healing
Iron	Haemoglobin synthesis
Copper	Erythrocyte maturation and lipid metabolism
Manganese	Calcium and phosphorus metabolism
Cobalt	Essential constituent of vitamin B12
Iodine	Thyroxine synthesis
Chromium	Glucose utilisation

Practice tip

PN solutions are high in glucose and therefore require vigilance in preventing catheter-related infection.

Routine monitoring of the patient's fluid balance, glucose, biochemical profile, full blood count, triglycerides, trace elements and vitamins is necessary. The patient is also assessed for signs of complications associated with the administration of PN (see Table 19.6).

Transition to oral diet and fluids

The patient's condition, length of stay in ICU and their ability to swallow will influence when and how quickly oral nutrition can commence. Accurate identification of swallowing disorders in ICU patients is crucial to determine the safety and type of oral nutrition. Dysphagia that occurs in ICU patients following extubation is usually an ICU-acquired disorder,[167] although it is also possible for patients to have an undiagnosed swallowing disease. The prevalence of swallowing disorders in patients with acute respiratory failure who are extubated is unknown. The estimated prevalence of dysphagia ranges between 3% and 62% for patients recovering from critical illnesses.[168] Six potential mechanisms can cause patients in the ICU to develop

TABLE 19.6

Short-term metabolic complications associated with total parenteral nutrition

COMPLICATION	CAUSE	DETECTION AND TREATMENT
Hyperosmolar coma	Occurs acutely if a rapid infusion of hypertonic fluid is administered. Infusion can cause severe osmotic diuresis, resulting in electrolyte abnormalities, dehydration and malfunction of the central nervous system	Daily blood samples, accurate measurements of fluid balance, routine blood samples Reduce infusion rate, correct electrolyte imbalances
Electrolyte imbalance	Disturbances in serum electrolytes, particularly sodium potassium, urea and creatinine, may occur early in the treatment of TPN. Electrolyte imbalances can be caused by the patient's underlying medical condition; requirements vary with individual patients' needs. Can be caused by inadequate or excessive administration of intravenous fluids	Daily blood samples taken early in treatment to detect abnormalities Replacement fluid as required, extra intravenous fluids may be required during the stabilisation period
Hyperglycaemia	Critically ill patients may be resistant to insulin because of the secretion of ACTH and adrenaline. This promotes the secretion of glycogen, which inhibits the insulin response to hyperglycaemia	Monitor the patient's blood sugar 4-hourly after commencement of treatment or as required. Monitor daily urinalysis for glucose and ketones An insulin infusion may be required to keep blood sugar levels within prescribed limits
Rebound hypoglycaemia	May occur on discontinuation of TPN because hyperinsulinism may occur after prolonged intravenous nutrition. A rise in serum insulin occurs with infusion, and thus sudden cessation of infusion can result in hypoglycaemia	Glucose infusion rate should be gradually reduced over the final hour of infusion before discontinuing. Some patients may receive a 10% glucose solution after cessation of TPN
Hypophosphataemia	Glucose infusion results in the continuous release of insulin, stimulating anabolism and resulting in rapid influx of phosphorus into muscle cells. The greatest risk is to malnourished patients with overzealous administration of feeding. Patients who are hyperglycaemic, who require insulin therapy during TPN or who have a history of alcoholism or chronic weight loss may require extra phosphate in the early stages of treatment	Monitor phosphate levels daily. Hypophosphataemia will usually appear after 24–48 hours of feeding Reduce the carbohydrate load and give phosphate supplementation
Lipid clearance	Lipids are broken down in the bloodstream with the aid of lipoprotein lipase found in the epithelium of capillaries in many tissues. A syndrome known as fat overload syndrome can occur when infusion of lipid is administered that is beyond the patient's clearing capacity, resulting in lipid deposits in the capillaries	Blood samples should be taken after the first infusion commences (within 6 hours) to observe for lipid in the blood
Side effects of lipid infusion	Some patients suffer symptoms either during or after an infusion of lipid mix parenteral nutrition. The exact cause is unknown. The patient may complain of headache, nausea or vomiting, and generally feels unwell	Treat mild symptoms. If tolerated, the TPN solution of non-protein calories can be given in the form of glucose. However, it is essential that the regimen includes some fat to prevent the development of fatty acid deficiency
Anaphylactic shock	This is a rare complication but may occur as a reaction to the administration of a lipid	It may be necessary to administer adrenaline and/or steroids, and to provide supportive therapy as required
Glucose intolerance	TPN using glucose as the main source of calories is associated with a rise in oxygen consumption and CO_2 production. The workload imposed by the high CO_2 production may precipitate respiratory distress in susceptible patients, particularly those requiring mechanical ventilation	Observe patients for signs of respiratory distress. Provide non-protein calories in the form of glucose lipid mix. Slow initial rate of infusion
Liver function	Abnormalities with liver function can be associated with TPN. May be attributable to hepatic stenosis with moderate hepatomegaly; patients may also develop jaundice. Liver function tests often return to normal after cessation of therapy; however, TPN can lead to severe hepatic dysfunction in neonates	Monitor liver function tests twice weekly. There are several factors that may contribute to development of abnormal liver function tests. These most often occur after a period of time and appear to be more of a problem when there is an excess calorie intake or in glucose-based regimens

ACTH = adrenocorticotrophic hormone; TPN = total parenteral nutrition.

dysfunctional swallowing. Endotracheal and tracheostomy tubes can cause direct trauma, focal ulceration and inflammation.[167] Neuromyopathy resulting in muscular weakness can also cause postextubation dysphagia.[169] The third mechanism for dysphagia is the development of dysfunctional oropharyngeal and laryngeal sensation. Sensation abnormalities can result from either critical illness polyneuropathy or local oedema.[170] Swallowing dysfunction in critical illness can be related to impaired sensorium as a result of ICU-acquired delirium, underlying critical illness or the effects of sedating medications.[171] Gastro-oesophageal reflux is disordered swallowing in critically ill patients and some of the pathophysiological processes responsible for gastro-oesophageal reflux are likely to continue in the immediate postextubation period.[167]

Swallowing dysfunction can also occur because of dyssynchronous breathing and swallowing in patients with underlying respiratory impairment and tachypnoea. The study of those factors that increase the risk for impaired swallowing in awake, recently extubated patients without strokes or neuromuscular diseases is less advanced. Specific risk factors for this type of postextubation dysphagia have been reported in a few epidemiology studies.[168,172,173] Lower preadmission functional status has been independently associated with postextubation dysphagia in a cohort of 84 elderly patients but there is conflicting evidence on the association of age, intubation duration, diabetes mellitus, renal failure, postoperative pulmonary complications and tracheostomy as potential risk factors for postextubation dysphagia.[174] Comparisons of studies are limited by biased patient selection, heterogeneous study populations and differing diagnostic protocols.

The most common diagnostic test to evaluate for postextubation dysphagia is a bedside swallow evaluation performed by a speech language pathologist. Although the components of this examination are not standardised and can vary by practitioner,[167] patients usually undergo an interview, a structural and functional evaluation of their mouth and their cough response and an assessment of swallowing function with different food textures and liquid thicknesses. The bedside swallow evaluation has been criticised for poor sensitivity as well as poor inter- and intra-rater reliability.[175] Despite not being validated against gold standard tests, a seven-point scale that incorporates the perceived aspiration risk and subsequent dietary recommendations is often used to grade the severity of dysphagia.[176] Additional tests may be ordered to assist in the diagnosis of postextubation dysphagia. A videofluoroscopic swallow study, often referred to as a modified barium swallow, is highly sensitive and specific for aspiration.[168] The other gold standard instrumental procedure to evaluate for postextubation dysphagia is a fibre optic endoscopic swallow study.

Patients who are being weaned from nutrition support may have oral nutrition slowly introduced. For longer stay patients, particularly those who have ICU-acquired weakness, weaning from enteral or parenteral nutrition onto oral nutrition may commence with a trial of oral feeding by day supplemented by nutrition support at night.

Nutrition in specific clinical conditions

Not all critically ill patients are equal. Age, severity of illness, BMI and specific clinical presentations can each influence nutritional requirements and therefore the nutrition approach used.[177] Some general approaches to nutrition therapy may be similar regardless of clinical presentation, such as the timing and route of feeding and techniques used to monitor nutritional status and tolerance of nutrition. However, every patient should be individually assessed and nutrition therapy approaches targeted to their specific clinical condition. There are some general recommendations for specific clinical presentations that can serve as a guide for selecting optimal nutrition in some patient groups.

Obesity

As the proportion of the population with obesity increases so too does the number of obese patients admitted to critical care areas. The key difference for obese patients is the accumulation of body fat. There can also be an increase in muscle mass because of the effort of carrying extra body weight.[178] However, increased muscle mass is not uniformly present in all obese patients and those whose movement is severely restricted, are older or who have chronic illness may have loss of skeletal muscle mass.[179]

As most predictive equations of energy expenditure are weight-based it is necessary to adjust to ideal body weight so as to avoid overfeeding.[180] It is important to recognise that, although body weight increases, the energy expenditure does not increase to the same extent.[181] When the BMI is >40 the increase in energy expenditure is only 14%, less than those patients with a BMI <30 or between 30 and 40 where the increase is approximately 25%.

Understanding how obesity influences energy expenditure can help guide nutrition prescription. Attention has been given to hypocaloric feeding for critically ill obese patients as a strategy to improve outcome.[182] This is based on the premise that nitrogen balance does not deteriorate during hypocaloric feeding[183] and that energy expenditure is more difficult to accurately determine in obese patients – so overfeeding is more likely. Overfeeding can also contribute to increased carbon dioxide production and therefore increase ventilator load, which is less efficient in the critically ill obese patient.[184] Despite these physiological rationales there is a lack of evidence to suggest hypocaloric feeding of the critically ill patient is beneficial.

> **Practice tip**
>
> Effective monitoring of nutrition therapy is essential in the critically ill obese patient to avoid complications such as hyperglycaemia, dyslipidaemia, hypercapnia, fluid overload and hepatic stenosis.

Protein requirements are another important consideration for the critically ill obese patient. In critical illness protein requirements are usually increased[185] and most recommendations are for 1.2–1.5 g/kg/day protein although these recommendations can be as high as 2.0 g protein/kg ideal body weight.[45] A recent systematic review of protein provision in critical illness highlights the limited quantity and quality of research in this area but suggests that provision of 2.0–2.5 g protein/kg/day could be optimum.[185] For the critically ill obese patient protein prescription should be based on ideal body weight with adjustments for increasing body weight.[45] Whether other specific nutrients, such as arginine, glutamine and leucine, are beneficial for the critically ill obese patient is unclear.[186]

> **Practice tip**
>
> Obese critically ill patients might have increased gastric residual volumes because of increased intra-abdominal pressure, which inhibits gastric emptying.

Sepsis

The incidence of sepsis is on the increase worldwide and, although mortality rates have improved in recent years, these can still be high.[187,188] Sepsis results in an overwhelming cytokine-mediated, proinflammatory response to the presence of infection and is characterised by widespread inflammation, vasodilation, leukocyte accumulation and increased microvascular permeability.[189]

Few literature reports specifically address the nutritional needs of patients with sepsis;[190] however, multiple randomised trials and large observational studies of heterogeneous critically ill patients suggest that optimising enteral nutrition is beneficial.[36] However, the current recommendations within the Surviving Sepsis Guidelines suggest mandatory full caloric feeding should be avoided in favour of low-dose EN during the first 7 days in ICU.[191] There are no contraindications to administering EN in patients with sepsis and shock; however, it is recommended that initial resuscitation be accomplished before EN is commenced.[192] A clear approach for how nutrition support might be provided is lacking because studies using different methodologies and different patient populations have produced conflicting results.[193]

Renal failure

Critically ill patients with renal failure have widely variable metabolic patterns and nutritional requirements, making decisions about patient-specific nutritional requirements and goals challenging. The optimal nutrition requirements for patients with acute kidney injury are unclear and assessment of nutritional requirements is complicated not only by fluctuating fluid balance and body weight[194] but also by the underlying disease and type and intensity of renal replacement therapy.[195] For critically ill patients who require renal replacement therapy, there can be additional loss of glucose, amino acids, proteins, trace elements and vitamins that are water soluble and have a low molecular weight.[196] These losses can be pronounced when highly efficient renal replacement therapy such as continuous veno-venous haemofiltration or prolonged intermittent strategies such as sustained low-efficiency dialysis are used.[197]

Although each patient requires nutritional assessment and tailored nutritional prescription, it is suggested that a calorie intake of 25–30 kcal/kg/day is required for patients with renal failure.[198] Because protein catabolism and a sustained negative nitrogen balance are often present in acute kidney injury[198] protein supplementation becomes important to prevent lean muscle loss. Optimal intake of proteins and amino acids for the patient with acute kidney injury who may require renal replacement therapy is often hotly debated. Recommendations range from 1.4 g/kg/day[195] up to 2.5 g/kg/day.[199] In addition to protein and calorie replacement, the use of pharmaconutrients with anti-inflammatory effects, such as glutamine and omega-3 fatty acids, might play a role preventing further deterioration of renal function and assisting with improvement in renal function following acute kidney injury, although there are insufficient data at present that demonstrate such an approach improves outcomes in these patients.[194]

Pancreatitis

Severe acute pancreatitis is a disease associated with increased morbidity and mortality.[200] Severe acute pancreatitis causes both local and systemic complications and results in increased catabolism and hypermetabolism, although the severity of clinical presentations can vary widely.

Traditionally, patients with pancreatitis have been fasted and provided nutrition parenterally[201] with the aim of 'resting' the pancreas.[34] Early enteral nutrition is now encouraged in pancreatitis as significant reductions in morbidity and mortality have been demonstrated.[202] Compared to PN, EN significantly reduces infection, hospital length of stay, organ failure, need for surgical intervention and mortality.[203] The beneficial effects of EN as compared to PN are also observed when enteral nutrition is commenced early (within 48 hours).[204] Despite clear recommendations from evidence-based guidelines, adherence to these recommendations can be poor[205] and highlights an area where evidence could be further integrated into clinical practice.

Recommendations for managing nutrition therapy for the critically ill patient with pancreatitis are clear and, unlike other areas of nutrition therapy, there is consensus within recommendations from different professional organisations.[206] A summary of the key recommendations is provided in Table 19.7 At present, there are no data to support the use of pharmaconutrition supplements,[207] except for parenteral glutamine administration.[200]

Trauma and surgery

Nutritional recommendations for trauma patients are generally the same as those for all critically ill patients. Like data from more heterogeneous critically ill patients, early enteral nutrition has a demonstrated mortality benefit.[46] Nasogastric feeding is suitable for most trauma patients although small bowel feeding might be required for those patients who require longer periods of nutrition support.[208]

Critically ill surgical patients do require special attention because they are at the highest risk of hospital-acquired malnutrition.[9] Prolonged periods of inadequate oral nutrition are associated with higher mortality and, even for those patients who are well nourished at time of surgery, should they be unable to eat for more than 7 days, nutritional support is indicated.[208]

Postoperative patients may, however, continue to receive little or no nutrition following surgery. Postoperative ileus is often a concern, which means some clinicians do not provide enteral nutrition. Instead, gastric aspiration is implemented and the patient is given intravenous fluids. However, studies of gut motility demonstrate that small bowel peristalsis returns within hours following a laparotomy.[34] Therefore, interruption of nutritional intake is not necessary following surgery, even for patients who have undergone gastrointestinal surgery. A meta-analysis of 15 studies that included 1240 patients demonstrated that early postoperative nutrition was associated with significant reductions in complications and there was no evidence of negative outcomes that commonly concern clinicians, including anastomotic dehiscence.[73]

TABLE 19.7
Recommendations for nutrition therapy in severe acute pancreatitis[206]

RECOMMENDATION	GRADE OF EVIDENCE
Pancreatitis patients are at nutritional risk and should be screened	B
For mild-to-moderate disease, analgesics, intravenous fluids and nothing by mouth with a gradual advancement to diet within 3–4 days is recommended	C
Nutrition therapy is generally not needed for mild-to-moderate disease unless complications arise	A
Nutrition therapy should be considered in any patient regardless of disease severity if the anticipated duration of being nil by mouth is >5–7 days	B
Nutrition therapy is needed in mild-to-moderate disease when the patient has been nil by mouth for 5–7 days	B
Early nutrition therapy is indicated for severe pancreatitis	A
Nutrition therapy is useful in the management of patients who develop complications of surgery	B
EN is generally preferred over PN, or at least EN should, if feasible, be initiated first	A
EN may be used in the presence of pancreatic complications such as fistulas, ascites and pseudocysts	C
Continuous EN infusion is preferred over cyclic or bolus administration	B
Nasogastric tubes may be used for administration of EN. Postpyloric placement is not always required	B
For EN, consider a small peptide-based medium-chain triglyceride oil formula to improve tolerance	B
Use PN if nutrition therapy is indicated, when EN is contraindicated or not well tolerated	A
Intravenous fat emulsions are generally safe and well tolerated as long as baseline triglycerides are below 400 mg/dL (4.4 mmol/L) and there is no previous history of hyperlipidemia	B
Glucose is the preferred carbohydrate source with metabolic control of glucose as close to normal as possible	C
Consider use of glutamine (0.30 g/kg Ala-Gln dipeptide)	C
No specific complications of PN are unique to patients with pancreatitis. Avoid overfeeding	C

Grades of evidence:
A: guideline statement meeting the criteria for high grade of evidence with uniform consensus across multiple societal reports
B: guideline statement that meets the criteria for low/intermediate grade of evidence or where there is lack of consensus across societal reports (at least one societal report is in disagreement)
C: guideline statement meeting the criteria for high grade of evidence, published only in a single societal report (consensus not applicable in this case).

Enteral feeding may often be withheld in those patients with abdominal compartment syndrome who have a decompressive celiotomy because of the concerns about bowel dysfunction.[34] However, early enteral nutrition has been shown to be feasible in these situations and is associated with improved outcomes.[209,210]

Existing malnutrition can be a significant concern for surgical patients because of the association with complication rates, delayed recovery and longer ICU and hospital stay.[208] Preconditioning may be required and is usually best delivered by the enteral route.

Burns

Shortly after injury severe burns are associated with a high degree of hypermetabolism and hypercatabolism.[211] Burns can also result in destruction of skeletal muscle.[212] The hypermetabolic and hypercatabolic response to severe burn injury can result in significant caloric deficits and weight loss that may lead to immune dysfunction, decreased wound healing, severe infections and death.[211] Comprehensive nutritional assessment is important for patients with severe burns and helps to inform nutrition therapy strategies (Table 19.8). Assessing caloric requirements can be challenging and, as for all critically ill patients, indirect calorimetry is the preferred method of determining resting energy expenditure. When this equipment is unavailable, predictive equations that are specific for patients with burns can be used. Many formulas were developed before improvements to burn management, which reduce the hypermetabolic response, were implemented and can result in an overestimation of requirements.[213] Of the predictive equations used in burns, the Toronto Formula is the most complicated and likely difficult within a busy clinical setting (Table 19.9).

Early and aggressive nutrition therapy, along with other interventions, is necessary for improvements in patient outcome.[214] Early EN, that is nutrition provided within 24 hours of injury, is recommended for the severely burned patient and can help to modulate the hypermetabolic response.[215] There are several benefits to early and continuous EN including a decreased hypermetabolic response; decreased levels of circulating catecholamines, cortisol and glucagon;[216] preservation of gut mucosal blood flow and mucosal integrity; and improved gut motility.[211] High protein delivery of 1.5–3.0 g/kg ideal body weight may be required for burn patients.[213] Administering specific micronutrients may improve immune function and positively influence septic morbidity and mortality.[217] Many pharmconutrients have been studied in the context of nutrition support for the patient with burns[218] although their benefit is yet to be clearly demonstrated.[219,220]

Glycaemic control in critical illness

Hyperglycaemia and increased insulin resistance are characteristics of the body's stress response and activation of the sympathetic and adrenal and hypothalamic–pituitary–adrenal (HPA) axis responses to critical illness.[221] Hyperglycaemia has been considered a beneficial adaptive response to stress to provide energy substrate to the organs involved in the 'fight or flight' response.[222] There is some,

---

TABLE 19.8

Comprehensive nutrition assessment in the patient with severe burns[211]

HISTORY AND PHYSICAL EXAMINATION	PRE-EXISTING MALNUTRITION
	Malabsorption
	Paralytic ileus
	Severe shock
	Bowel obstruction
	Diffuse peritonitis
Laboratory measurements	Serum albumin and prealbumin
	Nitrogen balance
	Tests for immune function
Clinical examination	Anthropometric measurements
	Fluid intake and output
Metabolic assessment	Indirect calorimetry

TABLE 19.9

Predictive equations for estimating caloric requirements in patients with burns[211]

AGE, Y	NAME	FORMULA
0–1	Galveston Infant	2100 kcal/m² + 1000 kcal/m² burn
1–11	Galveston Revised	1800 kcal/m² + 1300 kcal/m² burn
12–16	Galveston Adolescent	1500 kcal/m² + 1500 kcal/m² burn
16–59	Curreri formula	25 kcal/kg body weight + (40) TBSA
	Toronto formula	−4343 + (10.5 × TBSA) + (0.23 × CI) + (0.84 × HBE) + (114 × T) − (4.5 × PBD)
≥60	Curreri formula	20 kcal/kg body weight + 65 (TBSA)

CI = total calorie intake the previous day; HBE = Harris-Benedict estimates; PBD = number of postburn days to the day preceding the estimation; T = average of core temperatures (°C) the previous day; TBSA = burn size in total body surface area.
Reproduced from Rodriguez NA, Jeschke MG, Williams FN, Kamolz LP, Herndon DN. Nutrition in burns: Galveston contributions. JPEN J Parenter Enteral Nutr 2011;35(6): 704-14, Table 1, with permission.

although inconsistent, evidence of an association of hyperglycaemia with high mortality and morbidity.[223–227]

The complexity of the physiological processes associated with hyperglycaemia in critical illness and the sophisticated research required to generate valid information render clinical decision making related to glycaemic control challenging. Nevertheless, the concept of tight glycaemic control is accepted but a 'gold standard' for the range of acceptable values for glucose levels is not available. Multiple randomised trials have been conducted in a variety of ICU patient groups, health care settings and using different study methods.[223,228,229] The meta-analyses do not provide clear resolution of the issue of glycaemic control with differing results reported by Griesdale et al,[230] who found that intensive insulin therapy was beneficial in surgical ICU patients, and Friedrich et al,[231] who were unable to demonstrate a benefit from intensive insulin therapy for surgical patients. The inconsistent results, even from those studies that appear to have used similar methods, has continued to fuel the debate on tight glycaemic control with some experts urging caution and others seeing tight glycaemic control as a marker of quality practice.[232] The discrepancies in these studies have been attributed to many factors including the variability in target ranges for blood glucose, methods of blood glucose measurement, difficulty for some studies to achieve separation of the treatment and control groups, compliance with the therapy and employment of different nutritional strategies.[233]

Insulin protocols for blood glucose levels often have an upper target blood glucose level of 10.0 mmol/L (180 mg/dL) or less based on the NICE-SUGAR study protocol,[223] although different targets of insulin therapy are reported where the glucose is ≤6.1 mmol/L or ≤8.3 mmol/L.[230] Several consensus statements for glycaemic control of hospitalised patients have been published[234–237] that do include a lower threshold other than hypoglycaemia and recommend avoidance of hyperglycaemia, hypoglycaemia and wide swings in glucose levels. Data from several studies indicate that the risk of hypoglycaemia is increased with intensive insulin therapy and that there is no overall mortality benefit conferred when this therapy is used in critically ill patients.[230]

Insulin infusions are used to control high blood glucose levels and nurses have an integral role in the management of these patients. The Canadian Clinical Guidelines recommend blood glucose values be monitored every 1–2 hours until glucose values and insulin infusion rates are stable, then every 4 hours thereafter.[36] The continuation of insulin infusions in patients who have their enteral nutrition decreased or ceased requires more frequent blood glucose monitoring because of the risk for hypoglycaemia.[229] Reports from studies suggest variability in glucose levels over time is an important determinant of mortality[238,239] but is not associated with increased mortality rates in diabetic patients when compared to non-diabetic patients.[238,240]

The use of intravenous insulin for tight glycaemic control can contribute to rapidly changing blood glucose levels; therefore vigilant monitoring is required. The time and frequency of blood glucose measurement that may be required for some patients may impact on the provision of patient care, and inability to perform the testing as often as required may contribute to underdetection of hypoglycaemia. Another potentially important factor that may contribute to underdetection of hypoglycaemia is fatigue in nurses caring for the critically ill. Louie et al[241] reported the results of a single-centre study that found the increased number of antecedent shifts worked by bedside nurses was associated with an increased incidence of hypoglycaemia.

The validity of blood glucose measurement is also an important consideration. Formal laboratory testing is considered 'gold standard' for blood glucose measurement but point-of-care testing of blood glucose is common in the critical care setting. Blood glucose may be sampled from arterial, venous and capillary blood. The use of capillary blood in testing blood glucose may be problematic, particularly in those patients for whom hypoperfusion is an issue.[191] It is recommended that point-of-care testing using capillary blood be interpreted with caution because the measurements may not accurately estimate arterial blood or plasma glucose values.[36]

It is clear that hyperglycaemia should be avoided. However, the inconsistencies in published studies mean that an agreed specified target for blood glucose in the critically ill patient population is difficult to achieve.[233] The optimal target blood glucose level is unknown and may differ depending on the patient's clinical presentation.[191]

Summary

Critically ill patients are at increased risk of malnutrition because of increased metabolic requirements coupled with challenges in delivering prescribed nutrition. Critical care nurses play a pivotal role in ensuring nutritional adequacy and are well positioned to coordinate interdisciplinary collaboration to optimise nutrition therapy. Optimising nutrition in critical illness is assisted by accurate assessment of nutritional requirements and prescribing nutrition that closely matches the patient's individual needs. Delivery of prescribed nutrition is the role of the nurse and attention should be given to minimising interruptions to nutrition therapy. During recovery from critical illness and when the patient resumes oral intake, nutritional risk can be increased because of factors that impact on the patient's ability to eat. Assessment of the ability to safely resume oral intake might be necessary for those patients at risk of dysphagia. Attention to nutritional requirement should commence on admission to the ICU and extend beyond both ICU and hospital discharge.

Case study

Peter was admitted to ICU following clinical deterioration on the ward. He was originally admitted with acute abdominal pain, suspected to be caused by pancreatitis. He was morbidly obese and had a medical history of hypertension. Peter lived independently before admission to hospital.

On arrival to ICU the patient was tachycardic, tachypnoeic and hypotensive. He was intubated and mechanically ventilated and required moderate doses of noradrenaline and vasopressin to correct hypotension. He had acute kidney injury with a creatinine of 177 micromol/L and metabolic acidosis requiring continuous renal replacement therapy. His bilirubin was elevated at 24 micromol/L on admission.

On arrival to ICU a nasogastric tube was inserted and Peter was commenced on enteral feeding at 10 mL/h of a concentrated enteral feeding solution of 2 kcal/mL. EN was supplemented with standard total PN at 40 mL/h for the first 24 hours Peter was in ICU. On day 2 of ICU admission enteral feeding was increased to 37 mL/h and the PN was ceased. Peter tolerated EN well and had minimal aspirates from the nasogastric tube.

The patient continued to be dialysed for the next 16 days and had a tracheostomy tube inserted on day 7 for a slow respiratory wean from mechanical ventilation. Peter was decannulated 2 days prior to being transferred to the ward.

DISCUSSION

Critically ill patients often have increased nutritional requirements either as a result of pre-existing malnutrition or because of decreased nutritional intake that is insufficient to meet the increased energy expenditure that is typical in critical illness. There are a number of key issues relating to nutritional status and the provision of nutrition that are central to this case study. These include pre-existing obesity, hypotension and shock requiring vasopressors, presence of pancreatitis and renal failure.

Obesity: It can be challenging to accurately determine nutritional requirements for critically ill patients and this is particularly the case in the context of obesity. While obese patients do accumulate increased body fat they can also have an increased amount of muscle mass because of the need to carry extra body weight. Most ICUs do not have the benefit of a metabolic cart to measure energy expenditure so predictive equations are often used to determine caloric requirements. Most of these equations are weight based; therefore, adjustment needs to be made so ideal body weight is used in the equation, otherwise overfeeding might result. Some clinicians believe that hypocaloric feeding is optimal in obese critically ill patients because overfeeding can result in increased carbon dioxide production and ventilator load – a challenging situation for the obese patient. There is, however, a lack of evidence to support this approach in obese critically ill patients. In this case study Peter was fed at goal rate, based on his ideal body weight. It is possible that the estimation of Peter's energy expenditure could have led to either over- or underfeeding. Indirect calorimetry, where available, could assist with more accurate measures of energy expenditure and caloric requirements.

Hypotension: Hypotension and the use of vasopressors can reduce splanchnic perfusion and is sometimes perceived as a contraindication to EN. Enteral nutrients have been shown to increase gut blood flow, which allows the bowel to absorb nutrients during vasopressor therapy. There is insufficient evidence to suggest whether EN should continue or be withheld when vasopressors are being administered with the results from a limited number of studies being inconsistent. Individual patient assessment is required to guide clinical practice in this area. In this case study EN was commenced despite vasopressor therapy and the patient did not exhibit any signs of gastric intolerance.

Pancreatitis: It has been commonly thought that patients with pancreatitis should not ingest food or fluid orally. In such cases, nutrition is often provided parenterally with the aim of allowing the gut to rest. Current research now suggests that EN should be provided, even in the context of acute severe pancreatitis, and can contribute to significant reductions in morbidity and mortality. In this case study the patient was commenced on EN on ICU admission but at a low rate (even for a concentrated EN solution), which was unlikely to address metabolic requirements so EN was supplemented with PN. Within 24 hours of admission the patient was able to receive EN alone, which raises a question as to whether PN could have been avoided initially.

Renal failure: Optimal nutrition requirements in renal failure are unclear and assessment of nutritional requirements is complicated by shifting fluid balance and body weight. In this case study actual body weight should not be used as a factor in determining nutrition intake so fluctuations in fluid balance are unlikely to confound decisions. It is important, however, to consider the potential loss of glucose, amino acids, proteins, trace elements and vitamins that can occur in the setting of renal replacement therapy. An additional consideration is the provision of adequate amounts of protein because of protein catabolism and sustained negative nitrogen balance that occurs in renal failure. The recommendations for protein for patients with renal failure do vary considerably from 1.4 g/kg/day up to 2.5 g/kg/day.

CASE STUDY QUESTIONS

1   On admission, what information might you request from the family to help you to assess whether Peter was nutritionally at risk prior to admission?

2   In the case study the patient presented with pancreatitis and was also morbidly obese. Discuss how these two factors might influence tolerance of enteral nutrition.

3   During the course of recovery from critical illness Peter had a tracheostomy but was eventually decannulated. Discuss the implication of this treatment on nutritional intake and recovery after ICU discharge.

RESEARCH VIGNETTE

Needham D, Dinglas VD, Morris PE, Jackson JC, Hough CL, Mendez-Tellez PA et al, for the HIH NHLBI ARDS Network. Physical and cognitive performance of patients with acute lung injury 1 year after initial trophic versus full enteral feeding: EDEN Trial Follow-up. Am J Respir Crit Care Med 2013;188(5):567–76

Rationale: We hypothesized that providing patients with acute lung injury two different protein/calorie nutritional strategies in the intensive care unit may affect longer-term physical and cognitive performance.

Objectives: To assess physical and cognitive performance 6 and 12 months after acute lung injury, and to evaluate the effect of trophic versus full enteral feeding, provided for the first 6 days of mechanical ventilation, on 6-minute-walk distance, cognitive impairment, and secondary outcomes.

Methods: A prospective, longitudinal ancillary study of the ARDS Network EDEN trial evaluating 174 consecutive survivors from 5 of 12 centers. Blinded assessments of patients' arm anthropometrics, strength, pulmonary function, 6-minute-walk distance, and cognitive status (executive function, language, memory, verbal reasoning/concept formation, and attention) were performed.

Measurements and main results: At 6 and 12 months, respectively, the mean (SD) percent predicted for 6-minute-walk distance was 64% (22%) and 66% (25%) ($P = 0.011$ for difference between assessments), and 36% and 25% of survivors had cognitive impairment ($P = 0.001$). Patients performed below predicted values for secondary physical tests with small improvement from 6 to 12 months. There was no significant effect of initial trophic versus full feeding for the first 6 days after randomization on survivors' percent predicted for 6-minute-walk distance, cognitive impairment status, and all secondary outcomes.

Conclusions: EDEN trial survivors performed below predicted values for physical and cognitive performance at 6 and 12 months, with some improvement over time. Initial trophic versus full enteral feeding for the first 6 days after randomization did not affect physical and cognitive performance.

Critique

The EDEN follow-up study did not show any difference in physical and cognitive performance of patients with acute lung injury at 1 year. Sample size was small and consequently there may have been insufficient patients to demonstrate a statistical difference. Nevertheless, the results of this study are consistent with the patient-reported outcomes from 525 patients with acute lung injury from 11 of 12 EDEN study centres evaluated via telephone survey.[242] They are also consistent with the findings of other follow-up studies of survivors of acute lung injury.[243–245] The multicentre study was conducted in the USA. Engaging multiple centres enables a larger sample size and improves interpretation of the results but generalisability may be threatened if conducted in different health care settings to your clinical practice.

The study used a comprehensive battery of physical and cognitive tests and demonstrated impairments across multiple aspects of physical and cognitive performance. The impairments may have existed prior to the episode of critical illness but Needham et al[57] argue that the patient group was relatively young and 93% were living independently without assistance before admission.

The longitudinal study design was an appropriate method to follow up patients over time but loss to follow-up can be problematic.[246] In this follow-up study half of the patients from 12 EDEN study hospitals were included; 20% died before hospital discharge, 6% died after discharge but before follow-up and 24% who met exclusion criteria were excluded.[57] The study used several strategies to minimise loss to follow-up, including conducting research visits at patients' homes or healthcare facilities for those who were unable to attend the research clinic.[247,248] In addition, the validated cognitive performance tests were completed by telephone if a personal visit was not feasible.[249] To promote consistency in data collection, research personnel underwent in-person training and annual in-person quality assurance reviews for conducting the physical and cognitive performance tests in this study. In addition, staff also conducted validated and reliable daily assessments of sedation and delirium status at study sites that did not routinely assess for delirium. Post-hoc analyses and their inherent bias were avoided by deciding subgroup analyses *a priori*.

Long-term sequelae to critical illness are common. This study did not find a difference in outcomes between those who received initial trophic enteral nutrition to those receiving full enteral nutrition. The patients in this study had acute lung injury, were relatively young and well-nourished and it is unknown if the results of this study (and the EDEN study) can be extrapolated to older and less well-nourished patients. The investigators acknowledge that caution should be taken in interpreting the results of the study before considering changes in clinical practice because there are no other randomised controlled trials examining the effects of this feeding strategy on outcomes, and our understanding of anabolism and catabolism during critical illness and its effect on long-term functional outcomes is limited.[250,251] Further research is needed.

Learning activities

1 Review your patients' notes and calculate what their total daily caloric intake was for the previous day. Once you have obtained this figure, compare this to the prescribed intake. If patients have not received their total daily caloric intake, consider what factors may have contributed to this and how these might be overcome in future.

2 What strategies can be used to minimise the risk of aspiration pneumonia in enterally fed, critically ill patients?

3 Should critically ill patients who have had gastrointestinal surgery not receive enteral nutrition postoperatively?

4 Tight glycaemic control can increase the incidence and severity of hypoglycaemia. Consider what factors might contribute to wide fluctuations in blood glucose levels.

Online resources

American Society for Parenteral and Enteral Nutrition, www.nutritioncare.org
Australasian Society for Parenteral and Enteral Nutrition, www.auspen.org.au
Critical Care Nutrition, www.criticalcarenutrition.com
The European Society for Clinical Nutrition and Metabolism, www.espen.org

Further reading

Canada T, Crill C, Guenter P, eds. A.S.P.E.N. Parenteral nutrition handbook. Maryland: The American Society for Parenteral and Enteral Nutrition; 2009.

Farber P, Siervo M. Nutrition in critical care. Cambridge: Cambridge University Press; 2014.

Merritt R, ed. The A.S.P.E.N. Nutrition support practice manual. 2nd ed. Maryland: The American Society for Parenteral and Enteral Nutrition; 2005.

Singer P. Nutrition in intensive care medicine: Beyond physiology. In: Koletzko B. World review of nutrition and dietetics, Vol 105. Basel: Karger; 2013.

References

1 McCance KL. Cellular biology. In: McCance KL, Huether SE, Brashers VL, Rote NS, eds. Pathophysiology: The biologic basis for disease in adults and children. 6th ed. Maryland Heights, MI: Mosby Elsevier; 2010, pp 1–45.

2 Singer P. From mitochondrial disturbances to energy requirements. In: Singer P, ed. Nutrition in intensive care medicine: Beyond physiology. World Rev Nutr Diet 105. Basel, Switzerland: Karger; 2013, pp 1–11.

3 Btaiche IF, Chan LN, Pleva M, Kraft MD. Critical illness, gastrointestinal complications, and medication therapy during enteral feeding in critically ill adult patients. Nutr Clin Pract 2010;25(1):32–49.

4 Fontaine E, Muller MJ. Adaptive alterations in metabolism: practical consequences on energy requirements in the severely ill patient. Curr Opin Clin Nutr Metab Care 2011;14(2):171–5.

5 Cartwright MM. The metabolic response to stress: a case of complex nutrition support management. Crit Care Nurs Clin North Am 2004;16(4):467-87.

6 Sriram K, Mizock BA. Critical care nutrition: are the skeletons still in the closet? Crit Care Med 2010;38(2):690-1.

7 Jensen GL, Mirtallo J, Compher C, Dhaliwal R, Forbes A, Grijalba RF et al. Adult starvation and disease-related malnutrition: a proposal for etiology-based diagnosis in the clinical practice setting from the International Consensus Guideline Committee. JPEN J Parenter Enteral Nutr 2010;34(2):156-9.

8 Jensen GL, Bistrian B, Roubenoff R, Heimburger DC. Malnutrition syndromes: a conundrum vs continuum. JPEN J Parenter Enteral Nutr 2009;33(6):710-6.

9 Drover JW, Cahill NE, Kutsogiannis J, Pagliarello G, Wischmeyer P, Wang M et al. Nutrition therapy for the critically ill surgical patient: we need to do better! JPEN J Parenter Enteral Nutr 2010;34(6):644-52.

10 Weijs PJ, Stapel SN, de Groot SD, Driessen RH, de Jong E, Girbes AR et al. Optimal protein and energy nutrition decreases mortality in mechanically ventilated, critically ill patients: a prospective observational cohort study. JPEN J Parenter Enteral Nutr 2012;36(1):60-8.

11 de Souza Menezes F, Leite HP, Kochogueira PC. Malnutrition as an independent predictor of clinical outcome in critically ill children. Nutrition 2012;28(3):267-70.

12 Marik PE, Zaloga GP. Immunonutrition in high-risk surgical patients: a systematic review and analysis of the literature. JPEN J Parenter Enteral Nutr 2010;34(4):378-86.

13 Alberda C, Gramlich L, Jones N, Jeejeebhoy K, Day AG, Dhaliwal R et al. The relationship between nutritional intake and clinical outcomes in critically ill patients: results of an international multicenter observational study. Intensive Care Med 2009;35(10):1728-37.

14 Schetz M, Casaer MP, Van den Berghe G. Does artificial nutrition improve outcome of critical illness? Crit Care 2013;17(1):302.

15 Wischmeyer PE. Malnutrition in the acutely ill patient: is it more than just protein and energy? S Afr J Clin Nutr 2011;24(3):S1-27.

16 Heyland DK, Cahill N, Day AG. Optimal amount of calories for critically ill patients: depends on how you slice the cake! Crit Care Med 2011; 39(12):2619-26.

17 Jensen GL, Wheeler D. A new approach to defining and diagnosing malnutrition in adult critical illness. Curr Opin Crit Care 2012;18(2):206-11.

18 White JV, Guenter P, Jensen G, Malone A, Schofield M; Academy of Nutrition and Dietetics Malnutritiion Work Group; A.S.P.E.N. Malnutrition Task Force; A.S.P.E.N. Board of Directors. Consensus statement of the Academy of Nutrition and Dietetics/American Society for Parenteral and Enteral Nutrition: characteristics recommended for the identification and documentation of adult malnutrition (undernutrition). J Acad Nutr Diet 2012;112(5):730-8.

19 van Bokhorst-de van der Schueren MA, Guaitoli PR, Jansma EP, de Vet HC. Nutrition screening tools: does one size fit all? A systematic review of screening tools for the hospital setting. Clin Nutr 2014;33(1):39-58.

20 Heyland DK, Dhaliwal R, Jiang X, Day AG. Identifying critically ill patients who benefit the most from nutrition therapy: the development and initial validation of a novel risk assessment tool. Crit Care 2011;15(6):R268.

21 Schoeller DA. Making indirect calorimetry a gold standard for predicting energy requirements for institutionalized patients. J Am Diet Assoc 2007;107(3):390-2.

22 Dvir D, Cohen J, Singer P. Computerized energy targeting adapted to the clinical conditions balance and complications in critically ill patients: an observational study. Clin Nutr 2003;25:37-44.

23 Singer P, Anbar R, Cohen J, Shapiro H, Shalita-Chesner M, Lev S et al. The tight calorie control study (TICACOS): a prospective, randomized, controlled pilot study of nutritional support in critically ill patients. Intensive Care Med 2011;37(4):601-9.

24 McClave SA, Martindale RG, Kiraly L. The use of indirect calorimetry in the intensive care unit. Curr Opin Clin Nutr Metab Care 2013;16(2):202-8.

25 Kross EK, Sena M, Schmidt K, Stapleton RD. A comparison of predictive equations of energy expenditure and measured energy expenditure in critically ill patients. J Crit Care 2012;27(3):321 e5-12.

26 Haugen HA, Chan LN, Li F. Indirect calorimetry: a practical guide for clinicians. Nutr Clin Pract 2007;22(4):377-88.

27 Sundstrom M, Tjader I, Rooyackers O, Wernerman J. Indirect calorimetry in mechanically ventilated patients. A systematic comparison of three instruments. Clin Nutr 2013;32(1):118-21.

28 Compher C, Frankenfield D, Keim N, Roth-Yousey L, Evidence Analysis Working Group. Best practice methods to apply to measurement of resting metabolic rate in adults: a systematic review. J Am Diet Assoc 2006;106(6):881-903.

29 McClave SA, Spain DA, Skolnick JL, Lowen CC, Kieber MJ, Wickerham PS et al. Achievement of steady state optimizes results when performing indirect calorimetry. JPEN J Parenter Enteral Nutr 2003;27(1):16-20.

30 Walker RN, Heuberger RA. Predictive equations for energy needs for the critically ill. Respir Care 2009;54(4):509-21.

31 Cooney RN, Frankenfield DC. Determining energy needs in critically ill patients: equations or indirect calorimeters. Curr Opin Crit Care 2012;18(2):174-7.

32 Frankenfield DC, Coleman A, Alam S, Cooney RN. Analysis of estimation methods for resting metabolic rate in critically ill adults. JPEN J Parenter Enteral Nutr 2009;33(1):27-36.

33 Siervo M, Bertoli S, Battezzati A, Wells JC, Lara J, Ferraris C et al. Accuracy of predictive equations for the measurement of resting energy expenditure in older subjects. Clin Nutr 2014;33(4):613-9.

34 Marik PE. Enteral nutrition in the critically ill: myths and misconceptions. Crit Care Med 2014;42(4):962-9.

35 Hermsen JL, Sano Y, Kudsk KA. Food fight! Parenteral nutrition, enteral stimulation and gut-derived mucosal immunity. Langenbecks Arch Surg 2009;394(1):17-30.

36 Dhaliwal R, Cahill N, Lemieux M, Heyland DK. The Canadian critical care nutrition guidelines in 2013: an update on current recommendations and implementation strategies. Nutr Clin Pract 2014;29(1):29-43.

37 Bankhead R, Boullata J, Brantley S, Corkins M, Guenter P, Krenitsky J et al. Enteral nutrition practice recommendations. JPEN J Parenter Enteral Nutr 2009;33(2):122-67.

38 McClave SA, Heyland DK. The physiologic response and associated clinical benefits from provision of early enteral nutrition. Nutr Clin Pract 2009;24(3):305-15.

39 Hadfield RJ, Sinclair DG, Houldsworth PE, Evans TW. Effects of enteral and parenteral nutrition on gut mucosal permeability in the critically ill. Am J Respir Crit Care Med 1995;152(5 Pt 1):1545-8.

40 Hernandez G, Velasco N, Wainstein C, Castillo L, Bugedo G, Maiz A et al. Gut mucosal atrophy after a short enteral fasting period in critically ill patients. J Crit Care 1999;14(2):73-7.

41 McClure RJ, Newell SJ. Randomised controlled study of clinical outcome following trophic feeding. Arch Dis Child Fetal Neonatal Ed 2000;82(1):F29-33.

42 Heidegger CP, Berger MM, Graf S, Zingg W, Darmon P, Costanza MC et al. Optimisation of energy provision with supplemental parenteral nutrition in critically ill patients: a randomised controlled clinical trial. Lancet 2013;381(9864):385-93.

43 Marik P, Hooper M. Supplemental parenteral nutrition in critically ill patients. Lancet 2013;381(9879):1716.

44 Kudsk KA. Beneficial effect of enteral feeding. Gastrointest Endosc Clin N Am 2007;17(4):647-62.

45 McClave SA, Martindale RG, Vanek VW, McCarthy M, Roberts P, Taylor B et al. Guidelines for the provision and assessment of nutrition support therapy in the adult critically ill patient: Society of Critical Care Medicine (SCCM) and American Society for Parenteral and Enteral Nutrition (A.S.P.E.N.). JPEN J Parenter Enteral Nutr 2009;33(3):277-316.

46 Doig GS, Heighes PT, Simpson F, Sweetman EA. Early enteral nutrition reduces mortality in trauma patients requiring intensive care: a meta-analysis of randomised controlled trials. Injury 2011;42(1):50-6.

47 Doig GS, Heighes PT, Simpson F, Sweetman EA, Davies AR. Early enteral nutrition, provided within 24 h of injury or intensive care unit admission, significantly reduces mortality in critically ill patients: a meta-analysis of randomised controlled trials. Intensive Care Med 2009;35(12):2018-27.

48 van Schijndel RJS, Weijs PJ, Koopmans RH, Sauerwein HP, Beishuizen A, Girbes AR. Optimal nutrition during the period of mechanical ventilation decreases mortality in critically ill, long-term acute female patients: a prospective observational cohort study. Critical Care 2009;13(4):R132.

49 Ibrahim EH, Mehringer L, Prentice D, Sherman G, Schaiff R, Fraser V et al. Early versus late enteral feeding of mechanically ventilated patients: results of a clinical trial. JPEN J Parenter Enteral Nutr 2002;26(3):174-81.

50 Casaer MP, Van den Berghe G. Nutrition in the acute phase of critical illness. N Engl J Med 2014;370(25):2450-1.

51 Heighes PT, Doig GS, Sweetman EA, Simpson F. An overview of evidence from systematic reviews evaluating early enteral nutrition in critically ill patients: more convincing evidence is needed. Anaesth Intensive Care 2010;38(1):167-74.

52 Engel JM, Muhling J, Junger A, Menges T, Karcher B, Hempelmann G. Enteral nutrition practice in a surgical intensive care unit: what proportion of energy expenditure is delivered enterally? Clin Nutr 2003;22(2):187-92.

53 Berger MM, Chiolero RL. Hypocaloric feeding: pros and cons. Curr Opin Crit Care 2007;13(2):180-6.

54 Allingstrup MJ, Esmailzadeh N, Wilkens Knudsen A, Espersen K, Hartvig Jensen T, Wiis J et al. Provision of protein and energy in relation to measured requirements in intensive care patients. Clin Nutr 2012;31(4):462-8.

55 Faisy C, Llerena MC, Savalle M, Mainardi J-L, Fagon J-Y. Early ICU energy deficit is a risk factor for *Staphylococcus aureus* ventilator-associated pneumonia. Chest 2011;140(5):1254-60.

56 The National Heart Lung and Blood Institute. Initial trophic vs full enteral feeding in patients with acute lung injury: the EDEN randomized trial. JAMA 2012;307(8):795.

57 Needham DM, Dinglas VD, Morris PE, Jackson JC, Hough CL, Mendez-Tellez PA et al. Physical and cognitive performance of patients with acute lung injury 1 year after initial trophic versus full enteral feeding. EDEN trial follow-up. Am J Respir Crit Care Med 2013;188(5):567-76.

58 Marik PE. The paradoxical effect of obesity on outcome in critically ill patients. Crit Care Med 2006;34(4):1251-3.

59 Arabi YM, Tamim HM, Dhar GS, Al-Dawood A, Al-Sultan M, Sakkijha MH et al. Permissive underfeeding and intensive insulin therapy in critically ill patients: a randomized controlled trial. Am J Clin Nutr 2011;93(3):569-77.

60 Marshall AP, Cahill NE, Gramlich L, MacDonald G, Alberda C, Heyland DK. Optimizing nutrition in intensive care units: empowering critical care nurses to be effective agents of change. Am J Crit Care 2012;21(3):186-94.

61 O'Meara D, Mireles-Cabodevila E, Frame F, Hummell AC, Hammel J, Dweik RA et al. Evaluation of delivery of enteral nutrition in critically ill patients receiving mechanical ventilation. Am J Crit Care 2008;17(1):53-61.

62 Cahill NE, Day AG, Cook D, Heyland DK, Canadian Critical Care Trials G. Development and psychometric properties of a questionnaire to assess barriers to feeding critically ill patients. Implement Sci 2013;8:140.

63 Williams TA, Leslie GD, Leen T, Mills L, Dobb GJ. Reducing interruptions to continuous enteral nutrition in the intensive care unit: a comparative study. J Clin Nurs 2013;22(19-20):2838-48.

64 Adam S, Batson S. A study of problems associated with the delivery of enteral feed in critically ill patients in five ICUs in the UK. Intensive Care Med 1997;23(3):261-6.

65 McClave SA, Lowen CC, Kleber MJ, Nicholson JF, Jimmerson SC, McConnell JW et al. Are patients fed appropriately according to their caloric requirements? JPEN J Parenter Enteral Nutr 1998;22(6):375-81.

66 Lubbers T, de Haan JJ, Luyer MD, Verbaeys I, Hadfoune M, Dejong CH et al. Cholecystokinin/cholecystokinin-1 receptor-mediated peripheral activation of the afferent vagus by enteral nutrients attenuates inflammation in rats. Ann Surg 2010;252(2):376-82.

67 Allen JM. Vasoactive substances and their effects on nutrition in the critically ill patient. Nutr Clin Pract 2012;27(3):335-9.

68 Khalid I, Doshi P, DiGiovine B. Early enteral nutrition and outcomes of critically ill patients treated with vasopressors and mechanical ventilation. Am J Crit Care 2010;19(3):261-8.

69 Berger MM, Berger-Gryllaki M, Wiesel PH, Revelly JP, Hurni M, Cayeux C et al. Intestinal absorption in patients after cardiac surgery. Crit Care Med 2000;28(7):2217-23.

70 Mentec H, Dupont H, Bocchetti M, Cani P, Ponche F, Bleichner G. Upper digestive intolerance during enteral nutrition in critically ill patients: frequency, risk factors, and complications. Crit Care Med 2001;29(10):1955-61.

71 Seguin P, Laviolle B, Guinet P, Morel I, Malledant Y, Bellissant E. Dopexamine and norepinephrine versus epinephrine on gastric perfusion in patients with septic shock: a randomized study [NCT00134212]. Crit Care 2006;10(1):R32.

72 McClave SA, Chang WK. Feeding the hypotensive patient: does enteral feeding precipitate or protect against ischemic bowel? Nutr Clin Pract 2003;18(4):279-84.

73 Osland E, Yunus RM, Khan S, Memon MA. Early versus traditional postoperative feeding in patients undergoing resectional gastrointestinal surgery: a meta-analysis. JPEN J Parenter Enteral Nutr 2011;35(4):473-87.

74 Barlow R, Price P, Reid TD, Hunt S, Clark GW, Havard TJ et al. Prospective multicentre randomised controlled trial of early enteral nutrition for patients undergoing major upper gastrointestinal surgical resection. Clin Nutr 2011;30(5):560-6.

75 Doig GS, Simpson F, Finfer S, Delaney A, Davies AR, Mitchell I et al. Effect of evidence-based feeding guidelines on mortality of critically ill adults: a cluster randomized controlled trial. JAMA 2008;300(23):2731-41.

76 Heyland DK, Dhaliwal R, Day A, Jain M, Drover J. Validation of the Canadian clinical practice guidelines for nutrition support in mechanically ventilated, critically ill adult patients: results of a prospective observational study. Crit Care Med 2004;32(11):2260-6.

77 Kreymann KG, Berger MM, Deutz NE, Hiesmayr M, Jolliet P, Kazandjiev G et al. ESPEN Guidelines on Enteral Nutrition: intensive care. Clin Nutr 2006;25(2):210-23.

78 Marshall A, West S. Nutritional intake in the critically ill: improving practice through research. Aust Crit Care 2004;17(1):6-8, 10-5.

79 Cahill NE, Murch L, Cook D, Heyland DK, Canadian Critical Care Trials G. Improving the provision of enteral nutrition in the intensive care unit: a description of a multifaceted intervention tailored to overcome local barriers. Nutr Clin Pract 2014;29(1):110-7.

80 Jones NE, Suurdt J, Ouelette-Kuntz H, Heyland DK. Implementation of the Canadian Clinical Practice Guidelines for Nutrition Support: a multiple case study of barriers and enablers. Nutr Clin Pract 2007;22(4):449-57.

81 Levy H. Nasogastric and nasoenteric feeding tubes. Gastrointest Endosc Clin N Am 1998;8(3):529-49.

82 Berger MM, Soguel L. Feed the ICU patient 'gastric' first, and go post-pyloric only in case of failure. Crit Care 2010;14(1):123.

83 Davies AR, Morrison SS, Bailey MJ, Bellomo R, Cooper DJ, Doig GS et al. A multicenter, randomized controlled trial comparing early nasojejunal with nasogastric nutrition in critical illness. Crit Care Med 2012;40(8):2342-8.

84 White H, Sosnowski K, Tran K, Reeves A, Jones M. A randomised controlled comparison of early post-pyloric versus early gastric feeding to meet nutritional targets in ventilated intensive care patients. Crit Care 2009;13(6):R187.

85 Chendrasekhar A. Jejunal feeding in the absence of reflux increases nasogastric output in critically ill trauma patients. Am Surg 1996;62(11):887-8.

86 Gentilello LM, Cortes V, Castro M, Byers PM. Enteral nutrition with simultaneous gastric decompression in critically ill patients. Crit Care Med 1993;21(3):392-5.

87 Metheny NA, Meert KL, Clouse RE. Complications related to feeding tube placement. Curr Opin Gastroenterol 2007;23(2):178-82.

88 Booker KJ, Niedringhaus L, Eden B, Arnold JS. Comparison of 2 methods of managing gastric residual volumes from feeding tubes. Am J Crit Care 2000;9(5):318-24.

89 Metheny NA. Preventing respiratory complications of tube feedings: evidence-based practice. Am J Crit Care 2006;15(4):360-9.

90 Burns SM, Carpenter R, Blevins C, Bragg S, Marshall M, Browne L et al. Detection of inadvertent airway intubation during gastric tube insertion: capnography versus a colorimetric carbon dioxide detector. Am J Crit Care 2006;15(2):188-95.

91 Metheny NA, Davis-Jackson J, Stewart BJ. Effectiveness of an aspiration risk-reduction protocol. Nurs Res 2010;59(1):18-25.

92 Patient Safety Authority. Confirming feeding tube placement: old habits die hard. PA PSRA Patient Saf Advis 2006;3(4):23-30.

93 Metheny NA, Schnelker R, McGinnis J, Zimmerman G, Duke C, Merritt B et al. Indicators of tubesite during feedings. J Neurosci Nurs 2005; 37(6):320-5.

94 Gharib AM, Stern EJ, Sherbin VL, Rohrmann CA. Nasogastric and feeding tubes. The importance of proper placement. Postgrad Med 1996;99(5):165-8, 74-6.

95 Elpern EH, Killeen K, Talla E, Perez G, Gurka D. Capnometry and air insufflation for assessing initial placement of gastric tubes. Am J Crit Care 2007;16(6):544-9.

96 Chau JP, Lo SH, Thompson DR, Fernandez R, Griffiths R. Use of end-tidal carbon dioxide detection to determine correct placement of nasogastric tube: A meta-analysis. Int J Nurs Stud 2011;48(4):513-21.

97 Metheny NA, Stewart BJ, Smith L, Yan H, Diebold M, Clouse RE. pH and concentrations of pepsin and trypsin in feeding tube aspirates as predictors of tube placement. JPEN J Parenter Enteral Nutr 1997;21(5):279-85.

98 Aguilera-Martinez R, Ramis-Ortega E, Carratalá-Munuera C, Fernández-Medina JM, Saiz-Vinuesa MD, Barrado-Narvión J. Effectiveness of continuous enteral nutrition versus intermittent enteral nutrition in intensive care patients: a systematic review. JBI Database Syst Rev Implement Rep 2014;12(1):281-317.

99 Khan LU, Ahmed J, Khan S, Macfie J. Refeeding syndrome: a literature review. Gastroenterol Res Pract 2011;2011 pii: 410971. doi: 10.1155/2011/410971.

100 Owers EL, Reeves AI, Ko SY, Ellis AK, Huxtable SL, Noble SA et al. Rates of adult acute inpatients documented as at risk of refeeding syndrome by dietitians. Clin Nutr 2015;34(1):134-9.

101 Blaser AR, Starkopf J, Kirsimagi U, Deane AM. Definition, prevalence, and outcome of feeding intolerance in intensive care: a systematic review and meta-analysis. Acta Anaesthesiol Scand 2014;58(8):914-22.

102 DeLegge MH. Managing gastric residual volumes in the critically ill patient: an update. Curr Opin Clin Nutr Metab Care 2011;14(2):193-6.

103 Deane A, Chapman MJ, Fraser RJ, Bryant LK, Burgstad C, Nguyen NQ. Mechanisms underlying feed intolerance in the critically ill: implications for treatment. World J Gastroenterol 2007;13(29):3909-17.

104 Dhaliwal R, Madden SM, Cahill N, Jeejeebhoy K, Kutsogiannis J, Muscedere J et al. Guidelines, guidelines, guidelines: what are we to do with all of these North American guidelines? JPEN J Parenter Enteral Nutr 2010;34(6):625-43.

105 McClave SA, Lukan JK, Stefater JA, Lowen CC, Looney SW, Matheson PJ et al. Poor validity of residual volumes as a marker for risk of aspiration in critically ill patients. Crit Care Med 2005;33(2):324-30.

106 Reignier J, Mercier E, Le Gouge A, Boulain T, Desachy A, Bellec F et al. Effect of not monitoring residual gastric volume on risk of ventilator-associated pneumonia in adults receiving mechanical ventilation and early enteral feeding: a randomized controlled trial. JAMA 2013;309(3):249-56.

107 Landzinski J, Kiser TH, Fish DN, Wischmeyer PE, MacLaren R. Gastric motility function in critically ill patients tolerant vs intolerant to gastric nutrition. JPEN J Parenter Enteral Nutr 2008;32(1):45-50.

108 Juve-Udina ME, Valls-Miro C, Carreno-Granero A, Martinez-Estalella G, Monterde-Prat D, Domingo-Felici CM et al. To return or to discard? Randomised trial on gastric residual volume management. Intensive Crit Care Nurs 2009;25(5):258-67.

109 Metheny NA, Schallom ME, Edwards SJ. Effect of gastrointestinal motility and feeding tube site on aspiration risk in critically ill patients: a review. Heart Lung 2004;33(3):131-45.

110 Kesek DR, Akerlind L, Karlsson T. Early enteral nutrition in the cardiothoracic intensive care unit. Clin Nutr 2002;21(4):303-7.

111 Bishop S, Young H, Goldsmith D, Buldock D, Chin M, Bellomo R. Bowel motions in critically ill patients: a pilot observational study. Crit Care Resusc 2010;12(3):182-5.

112 Jack L, Coyer F, Courtney M, Venkatesh B. Diarrhoea risk factors in enterally tube fed critically ill patients: a retrospective audit. Intensive Crit Care Nurs 2010;26(6):327-34.

113 Bowling TE, Silk DB. Enteral feeding – problems and solutions. Eur J Clin Nutr 1994;48(6):379-85.

114 Guenter PA, Sweed MR. A valid and reliable tool to quantify stool output in tube-fed patients. JPEN J Parenter Enteral Nutr 1998;22(3):147-51.

115 Chang SJ, Huang HH. Diarrhea in enterally fed patients: blame the diet? Curr Opin Clin Nutr Metab Care 2013;16(5):588-94.

116 Tan M, Zhu JC, Yin HH. Enteral nutrition in patients with severe traumatic brain injury: reasons for intolerance and medical management. Br J Neurosurg 2011;25(1):2-8.

117 Buendgens L, Bruensing J, Matthes M, Duckers H, Luedde T, Trautwein C et al. Administration of proton pump inhibitors in critically ill medical patients is associated with increased risk of developing Clostridium difficile-associated diarrhea. J Crit Care 2014;29(4):696 e11-5.

118 Guenter P. Safe practices for enteral nutrition in critically ill patients. Crit Care Nurs Clin North Am 2010;22(2):197-208.

119 Barrett JS, Shepherd SJ, Gibson PR. Strategies to manage gastrointestinal symptoms complicating enteral feeding. JPEN J Parenter Enteral Nutr 2009;33(1):21-6.

120 Bleichner G, Blehaut H, Mentec H, Moyse D. Saccharomyces boulardii prevents diarrhea in critically ill tube-fed patients. A multicenter, randomized, double-blind placebo-controlled trial. Intensive Care Med 1997;23(5):517-23.

121 Barraud D, Blard C, Hein F, Marcon O, Cravoisy A, Nace L et al. Probiotics in the critically ill patient: a double blind, randomized, placebo-controlled trial. Intensive Care Med 2010;36(9):1540-7.

122 Halmos EP, Muir JG, Barrett JS, Deng M, Shepherd SJ, Gibson PR. Diarrhoea during enteral nutrition is predicted by the poorly absorbed short-chain carbohydrate (FODMAP) content of the formula. Aliment Pharmacol Ther 2010;32(7):925-33.

123 Ochoa TJ, Chea-Woo E, Baiocchi N, Pecho I, Campos M, Prada A et al. Randomized double-blind controlled trial of bovine lactoferrin for prevention of diarrhea in children. J Pediatr 2013;162(2):349-56.

124 Roy S, Rigal M, Doit C, Fontan JE, Machinot S, Bingen E et al. Bacterial contamination of enteral nutrition in a paediatric hospital. J Hosp Infect 2005;59(4):311-6.

125 Patchell CJ, Anderton A, Holden C, MacDonald A, George RH, Booth IW. Reducing bacterial contamination of enteral feeds. Arch Dis Child 1998;78(2):166-8.

126 Mathus-Vliegen EM, Bredius MW, Binnekade JM. Analysis of sites of bacterial contamination in an enteral feeding system. JPEN J Parenter Enteral Nutr 2006;30(6):519-25.

127 Neely AN, Mayes T, Gardner J, Kagan RJ, Gottschlich MM. A microbiologic study of enteral feeding hang time in a burn hospital: can feeding costs be reduced without compromising patient safety? Nutr Clin Pract 2006;21(6):610-6.

128 Muscedere J, Rewa O, McKechnie K, Jiang X, Laporta D, Heyland DK. Subglottic secretion drainage for the prevention of ventilator-associated pneumonia: a systematic review and meta-analysis. Crit Care Med 2011;39(8):1985-91.

129 Metheny NA, Frantz RA. Head-of-bed elevation in critically ill patients: a review. Crit Care Nurse 2013;33(3):53-66; quiz 7.

130 Schallom M, Orr J, Metheny N, Pierce J. Gastroesophageal reflux in critically ill patients. Dimens Crit Care Nurs 2013;32(2):69-77.

131 Drakulovic MB, Torres A, Bauer TT, Nicolas JM, Nogue S, Ferrer M. Supine body position as a risk factor for nosocomial pneumonia in mechanically ventilated patients: a randomised trial. Lancet 1999;354(9193):1851-8.

132 Ibanez J, Penafiel A, Raurich JM, Marse P, Jorda R, Mata F. Gastroesophageal reflux in intubated patients receiving enteral nutrition: effect of supine and semirecumbent positions. JPEN J Parenter Enteral Nutr 1992;16(5):419-22.

133 Torres A, Serra-Batlles J, Ros E, Piera C, Puig de la Bellacasa J, Cobos A et al. Pulmonary aspiration of gastric contents in patients receiving mechanical ventilation: the effect of body position. Ann Intern Med 1992;116(7):540-3.

134 Tablan OC, Anderson LJ, Besser R, Bridges C, Hajjeh R, CDC, et al. Guidelines for preventing health-care-associated pneumonia, 2003: recommendations of CDC and the Healthcare Infection Control Practices Advisory Committee. MMWR Recomm Rep 2004;53(RR-3):1-36.

135 Institute of Health Care Improvement. Implement the IHI Ventilator Bundle, <http://www.ihi.org/resources/Pages/Changes/Implementthe VentilatorBundle.aspx>; [accessed 11.11].

136 van Nieuwenhoven CA, Vandenbroucke-Grauls C, van Tiel FH, Joore HC, van Schijndel RJS, van der Tweel I et al. Feasibility and effects of the semirecumbent position to prevent ventilator-associated pneumonia: a randomized study. Crit Care Med 2006;34(2):396-402.

137 Keeley L. Reducing the risk of ventilator-acquired pneumonia through head of bed elevation. Nurs Crit Care 2007;12(6):287-94.

138 Grap MJ, Munro CL, Hummel RS, 3rd, Elswick RK, Jr., McKinney JL, Sessler CN. Effect of backrest elevation on the development of ventilator-associated pneumonia. Am J Crit Care 2005;14(4):325-32; quiz 33.

139 Niël-Weise BS, Gastmeier P, Kola A, Vonberg RP, Wille JC, van den Broek PJ. An evidence-based recommendation on bed head elevation for mechanically ventilated patients. Crit Care 2011;15(2):R111.

140 Bassi GL, Zanella A, Cressoni M, Stylianou M, Kolobow T. Following tracheal intubation, mucus flow is reversed in the semirecumbent position: possible role in the pathogenesis of ventilator–associated pneumonia. Crit Care Med 2008;36(2):518-25.

141 Aderinto-Adike AO, Quigley EM. Gastrointestinal motility problems in critical care: a clinical perspective. J Dig Dis 2014;15(7):335-44.

142 Ridley EJ, Davies AR. Practicalities of nutrition support in the intensive care unit: the usefulness of gastric residual volume and prokinetic agents with enteral nutrition. Nutrition 2011;27(5):509-12.

143 Nguyen NQ, Chapman MJ, Fraser RJ, Bryant LK, Holloway RH. Erythromycin is more effective than metoclopramide in the treatment of feed intolerance in critical illness. Crit Care Med 2007;35(2):483-9.

144 Metheny NA, Dahms TE, Stewart BJ, Stone KS, Edwards SJ, Defer JE et al. Efficacy of dye-stained enteral formula in detecting pulmonary aspiration. Chest 2002;122(1):276-81.

145 Maloney JP, Ryan TA, Brasel KJ, Binion DG, Johnson DR, Halbower AC et al. Food dye use in enteral feedings: a review and a call for a moratorium. Nutr Clin Pract 2002;17(3):169-81.

146 Clay AS, Behnia M, Brown KK. Mitochondrial disease: a pulmonary and critical-care medicine perspective. Chest 2001;120(2):634-48.

147 McClave SA, DeMeo MT, DeLegge MH, DiSario JA, Heyland DK, Maloney JP et al. North American Summit on Aspiration in the Critically Ill Patient: consensus statement. JPEN J Parenter Enteral Nutr 2002;26(6 Suppl):S80-5.

148 Metheny NA, St John RE, Clouse RE. Measurement of glucose in tracheobronchial secretions to detect aspiration of enteral feedings. Heart Lung 1998;27(5):285-92.

149 Metheny NA, Clouse RE. Bedside methods for detecting aspiration in tube-fed patients. Chest 1997;111(3):724-31.

150 Metheny NA, Dahms TE, Chang YH, Stewart BJ, Frank PA, Clouse RE. Detection of pepsin in tracheal secretions after forced small-volume aspirations of gastric juice. JPEN J Parenter Enteral Nutr 2004;28(2):79-84.

151 Metheny NA, Meert KL. Effectiveness of an electromagnetic feeding tube placement device in detecting inadvertent respiratory placement. Am J Crit Care 2014;23(3):240-7; quiz 8.

152 Marik PE, Flemmer M, Harrison W. The risk of catheter-related bloodstream infection with femoral venous catheters as compared to subclavian and internal jugular venous catheters: a systematic review of the literature and meta-analysis. Crit Care Med 2012;40(8):2479-85.

153 Grau T, Bonet A, Rubio M, Mateo D, Farre M, Acosta JA et al. Liver dysfunction associated with artificial nutrition in critically ill patients. Crit Care 2007;11(1):R10.

154 Heyland DK, MacDonald S, Keefe L, Drover JW. Total parenteral nutrition in the critically ill patient: a meta-analysis. JAMA 1998;280(23):2013-9.

155 Sena MJ, Utter GH, Cuschieri J, Maier RV, Tompkins RG, Harbrecht BG et al. Early supplemental parenteral nutrition is associated with increased infectious complications in critically ill trauma patients. J Am Coll Surg 2008;207(4):459-67.

156 Heidegger CP, Romand JA, Treggiari MM, Pichard C. Is it now time to promote mixed enteral and parenteral nutrition for the critically ill patient? Intensive Care Med 2007;33(6):963-9.

157 Doig GS, Simpson F, Sweetman EA, Finfer SR, Cooper DJ, Heighes PT et al. Early parenteral nutrition in critically ill patients with short-term relative contraindications to early enteral nutrition: a randomized controlled trial. JAMA 2013;309(20):2130-8.

158 Casaer MP, Mesotten D, Hermans G, Wouters PJ, Schetz M, Meyfroidt G et al. Early versus late parenteral nutrition in critically ill adults. N Engl J Med 2011;365(6):506-17.

159 Casaer MP, Wilmer A, Van den Berghe G. Supplemental parenteral nutrition in critically ill patients. Lancet 2013;381(9879):1715.

160 Martindale RG, McClave SA, Vanek VW, McCarthy M, Roberts P, Taylor B et al. Guidelines for the provision and assessment of nutrition support therapy in the adult critically ill patient: Society of Critical Care Medicine and American Society for Parenteral and Enteral Nutrition: Executive Summary. Crit Care Med 2009;37(5):1757-61.

161 Singer P, Berger MM, Van den Berghe G, Biolo G, Calder P, Forbes A et al. ESPEN Guidelines on Parenteral Nutrition: intensive care. Clin Nutr 2009;28(4):387-400.

162 Strachan S. Trace elements. Curr Anaesthesia Crit Care 2010;21(1):44-8.

163 Blanchette LM, Huiras P, Papadopoulos S. Standardized versus custom parenteral nutrition: impact on clinical and cost-related outcomes. Am J Health Syst Pharm 2014;71(2):114-21.

164 Mirtallo J, Canada T, Johnson D, Kumpf V, Petersen C, Sacks G et al. Safe practices for parenteral nutrition. JPEN J Parenter Enteral Nutr 2004;28(6):S39-70.

165 Worthington PH, Gilbert KA. Parenteral nutrition: risks, complications, and management. J Infus Nurs 2012;35(1):52-64.

166 Ziegler TR. Parenteral nutrition in the critically ill patient. N Engl J Med 2009;361(11):1088-97.

167 Macht M, Wimbish T, Bodine C, Moss M. ICU-acquired swallowing disorders. Crit Care Med 2013;41(10):2396-405.

168 Skoretz SA, Flowers HL, Martino R. The incidence of dysphagia following endotracheal intubation: a systematic review. Chest 2010;137(3):665-73.

169 Goldsmith T. Evaluation and treatment of swallowing disorders following endotracheal intubation and tracheostomy. Int Anesthesiol Clin 2000; 38(3):219-42.

170 Hermans G, De Jonghe B, Bruyninckx F, Van den Berghe G. Clinical review: critical illness polyneuropathy and myopathy. Crit Care 2008;12(6):238.

171 Leder SB, Suiter DM, Lisitano Warner H. Answering orientation questions and following single-step verbal commands: effect on aspiration status. Dysphagia 2009;24(3):290-5.

172 Rousou JA, Tighe DA, Garb JL, Krasner H, Engelman RM, Flack JE, 3rd et al. Risk of dysphagia after transesophageal echocardiography during cardiac operations. Ann Thorac Surg 2000;69(2):486-9; discussion 9-90.

173 Hogue CW, Jr, Lappas GD, Creswell LL, Ferguson TB, Jr, Sample M, Pugh D et al. Swallowing dysfunction after cardiac operations. Associated adverse outcomes and risk factors including intraoperative transesophageal echocardiography. J Thorac Cardiovasc Surg 1995;110(2):517-22.

174 Romero CM, Marambio A, Larrondo J, Walker K, Lira MT, Tobar E et al. Swallowing dysfunction in nonneurologic critically ill patients who require percutaneous dilatational tracheostomy. Chest 2010;137(6):1278-82.

175 Ramsey DJ, Smithard DG, Kalra L. Early assessments of dysphagia and aspiration risk in acute stroke patients. Stroke 2003;34(5):1252-7.

176 Mullen R. Evidence for whom?: ASHA's National Outcomes Measurement System. J Commun Disord 2004;37(5):413-7.

177 Magnuson B, Peppard A, Auer Flomenhoft D. Hypocaloric considerations in patients with potentially hypometabolic disease states. Nutr Clin Pract 2011;26(3):253-60.

178 Muller MJ, Bosy-Westphal A, Kutzner D, Heller M. Metabolically active components of fat-free mass and resting energy expenditure in humans: recent lessons from imaging technologies. Obes Rev 2002;3(2):113-22.

179 Gallagher D, DeLegge M. Body composition (sarcopenia) in obese patients: implications for care in the intensive care unit. JPEN J Parenter Enteral Nutr 2011;35(5 Suppl):21S-8S.

180 Frankenfield DC. Obesity. In: Singer P, ed. Nutrition in intensive care medicine: Beyond physiology. Basel: Switzerland; 2013.

181 Frankenfield DC, Ashcraft CM. Estimating energy needs in nutrition support patients. JPEN J Parenter Enteral Nutr 2011;35(5):563-70.

182 McClave SA, Kushner R, Van Way CW, 3rd, Cave M, DeLegge M, Dibaise J et al. Nutrition therapy of the severely obese, critically ill patient: summation of conclusions and recommendations. JPEN J Parenter Enteral Nutr 2011;35(5 Suppl):88S-96S.

183 Frankenfield DC, Smith JS, Cooney RN. Accelerated nitrogen loss after traumatic injury is not attenuated by achievement of energy balance. JPEN J Parenter Enteral Nutr 1997;21(6):324-9.

184 Porhomayon J, Papadakos P, Singh A, Nader ND. Alteration in respiratory physiology in obesity for anesthesia-critical care physician. HSR Proc Intensive Care Cardiovasc Anesth 2011;3(2):109-18.

185 Hoffer LJ, Bistrian BR. Appropriate protein provision in critical illness: a systematic and narrative review. Am J Clin Nutr 2012;96(3):591-600.

186 Martindale RG, DeLegge M, McClave S, Monroe C, Smith V, Kiraly L. Nutrition delivery for obese ICU patients: delivery issues, lack of guidelines, and missed opportunities. JPEN J Parenter Enteral Nutr 2011;35(5 Suppl):80S-7S.

187 Kaukonen KM, Bailey M, Suzuki S, Pilcher D, Bellomo R. Mortality related to severe sepsis and septic shock among critically ill patients in Australia and New Zealand, 2000–2012. JAMA 2014;311(13):1308-16.

188 Levy MM, Dellinger RP, Townsend SR, Linde-Zwirble WT, Marshall JC, Bion J et al. The Surviving Sepsis Campaign: results of an international guideline-based performance improvement program targeting severe sepsis. Crit Care Med 2010;38(2):367-74.

189 Cinel I, Dellinger RP. Advances in pathogenesis and management of sepsis. Curr Opin Infect Dis 2007;20(4):345-52.

190 Aitken LM, Williams G, Harvey M, Blot S, Kleinpell R, Labeau S et al. Nursing considerations to complement the Surviving Sepsis Campaign guidelines. Crit Care Med 2011;39(7):1800-18.

191 Dellinger RP, Levy MM, Rhodes A, Annane D, Gerlach H, Opal SM et al. Surviving sepsis campaign: international guidelines for management of severe sepsis and septic shock: 2012. Crit Care Med 2013;41(2):580-637.

192 Cohen J, Chin WDN. Nutrition and sepsis. In: Singer P, ed. Nutrition in intensive care medicine: Beyond physiology. Basel, Switzerland: Karger; 2013.

193 Elke G, Heyland DK. Enteral nutrition in critically ill septic patients – less or more? JPEN J Parenter Enteral Nutr 2014 Apr 21.

194 Fiaccadori E, Regolisti G, Maggiore U. Specialized nutritional support interventions in critically ill patients on renal replacement therapy. Curr Opin Clin Nutr Metab Care 2013;16(2):217-24.

195 Druml W. The renal failure patient. In: Singer P, ed. Nutrition in intensive care medicine: Beyond physiology. Basel, Switzerland: Karger; 2013, pp 126-35.

196 Wiesen P, Van Overmeire L, Delanaye P, Dubois B, Preiser JC. Nutrition disorders during acute renal failure and renal replacement therapy. JPEN J Parenter Enteral Nutr 2011;35(2):217-22.

197 Cano NJ, Aparicio M, Brunori G, Carrero JJ, Cianciaruso B, Fiaccadori E et al. ESPEN guidelines on parenteral nutrition: adult renal failure. Clin Nutr 2009;28(4):401-14.

198 Fiaccadori E, Cremaschi E, Regolisti G. Nutritional assessment and delivery in renal replacement therapy patients. Semin Dial 2011;24(2): 169-75.

199 Lopez Martinez J, Sanchez-Izquierdo Riera JA, Jimenez Jimenez FJ, Metabolism, Nutrition Working Group of the Spanish Society of Intensive Care M, Coronary u. Guidelines for specialized nutritional and metabolic support in the critically-ill patient: update. Consensus SEMICYUC-SENPE: acute renal failure. Nutr Hosp 2011;26 Suppl 2:21-6.

200 Bordeje Laguna L, Lorencio Cardenas C, Acosta Escribano J, Metabolism, Nutrition Working Group of the Spanish Society of Intensive Care M, Coronary u. Guidelines for specialized nutritional and metabolic support in the critically-ill patient: update. Consensus SEMICYUC-SENPE: severe acute pancreatitis. Nutr Hosp 2011;26 Suppl 2:32-6.

201 Andersson R, Sward A, Tingstedt B, Akerberg D. Treatment of acute pancreatitis: focus on medical care. Drugs 2009;69(5):505-14.

202 McClave SA, Chang WK, Dhaliwal R, Heyland DK. Nutrition support in acute pancreatitis: a systematic review of the literature. JPEN J Parenter Enteral Nutr 2006;30(2):143-56.

203 Jafri NS, Mahid SS, Gopathi SK, Hornung CA, Galandiuk S, McClave SA. Enteral nutrition is superior to parenteral nutrition in severe acute pancreatitis: a systematic review and meta-analysis. Gastro 2008:A 141.

204 Petrov MS, Loveday BP, Pylypchuk RD, McIlroy K, Phillips AR, Windsor JA. Systematic review and meta-analysis of enteral nutrition formulations in acute pancreatitis. Br J Surg 2009;96(11):1243-52.

205 Davies AR, Morrison SS, Ridley EJ, Bailey M, Banks MD, Cooper DJ et al. Nutritional therapy in patients with acute pancreatitis requiring critical care unit management: a prospective observational study in Australia and New Zealand. Crit Care Med 2011;39(3):462-8.

206 Mirtallo JM, Forbes A, McClave SA, Jensen GL, Waitzberg DL, Davies AR et al. International consensus guidelines for nutrition therapy in pancreatitis. JPEN J Parenter Enteral Nutr 2012;36(3):284-91.

207 Al Samaraee A, McCallum IJ, Coyne PE, Seymour K. Nutritional strategies in severe acute pancreatitis: a systematic review of the evidence. Surgeon 2010;8(2):105-10.

208 Weimann A. The surgical/trauma patient. In: Singer P, ed. Nutrition in intensive care medicine: Beyond physiology. Basel, Switzerland: Karger; 2013, pp 106-15.

209 Tsuei BJ, Magnuson B, Swintosky M, Flynn J, Boulanger BR, Ochoa JB et al. Enteral nutrition in patients with an open peritoneal cavity. Nutr Clin Pract 2003;18(3):253-8.

210 Moore EE, Jones TN. Benefits of immediate jejunostomy feeding after major abdominal trauma – a prospective, randomized study. J Trauma 1986;26(10):874-81.

211 Rodriguez NA, Jeschke MG, Williams FN, Kamolz LP, Herndon DN. Nutrition in burns: Galveston contributions. JPEN J Parenter Enteral Nutr 2011;35(6):704-14.

212 Garcia de Lorenzo y Mateos A, Ortiz Leyba C, Sanchez SM, Metabolism, Nutrition Working Group of the Spanish Society of Intensive Care M, Coronary u. Guidelines for specialized nutritional and metabolic support in the critically-ill patient: update. Consensus SEMICYUC-SENPE: critically-ill burnt patient. Nutr Hosp 2011;26 Suppl 2:59-62.

213 NSW Statewide Burn Injury Service. Clinical practice guidelines: nutrition burn patient management. 2nd ed. Chatswood, NSW: Agency for Clinical Innovation; 2011.

214 Latenser BA. Critical care of the burn patient: the first 48 hours. Crit Care Med 2009;37(10):2819-26.

215 Dominioni L, Trocki O, Fang CH, Mochizuki H, Ray MB, Ogle CK et al. Enteral feeding in burn hypermetabolism: nutritional and metabolic effects of different levels of calorie and protein intake. JPEN J Parenter Enteral Nutr 1985;9(3):269-79.

216 McDonald WS, Sharp CW, Jr., Deitch EA. Immediate enteral feeding in burn patients is safe and effective. Ann Surg 1991;213(2):177-83.

217 Jacobs DG, Jacobs DO, Kudsk KA, Moore FA, Oswanski MF, Poole GV et al. Practice management guidelines for nutritional support of the trauma patient. J Trauma 2004;57(3):660-78; discussion 79.

218 Heyland D, Dhaliwal R. Immunonutrition in the critically ill: from old approaches to new paradigms. Intensive Care Med 2005;31(4):501-3.

219 Levy J, Turkish A. Protective nutrients. Curr Opin Gastroenterol 2002;18(6):717-22.

220 Hayashi N, Tashiro T, Yamamori H, Takagi K, Morishima Y, Otsubo Y et al. Effect of intravenous omega-6 and omega-3 fat emulsions on nitrogen retention and protein kinetics in burned rats. Nutrition 1999;15(2):135-9.

221 Van Cromphaut SJ. Hyperglycaemia as part of the stress response: the underlying mechanisms. Best Pract Res Clin Anaesthesiol 2009;23(4):375-86.

222 Robinson LE, van Soeren MH. Insulin resistance and hyperglycemia in critical illness: role of insulin in glycemic control. AACN Clin Issues 2004;15(1):45-62.

223 Investigators N-SS, Finfer S, Chittock DR, Su SY, Blair D, Foster D et al. Intensive versus conventional glucose control in critically ill patients. N Engl J Med 2009;360(13):1283-97.

224 Arabi YM, Dabbagh OC, Tamim HM, Al-Shimemeri AA, Memish ZA, Haddad SH et al. Intensive versus conventional insulin therapy: a randomized controlled trial in medical and surgical critically ill patients. Crit Care Med 2008;36(12):3190-7.

225 De La Rosa Gdel C, Donado JH, Restrepo AH, Quintero AM, Gonzalez LG, Saldarriaga NE et al. Strict glycaemic control in patients hospitalised in a mixed medical and surgical intensive care unit: a randomised clinical trial. Crit Care 2008;12(5):R120.

226 Capes SE, Hunt D, Malmberg K, Gerstein HC. Stress hyperglycaemia and increased risk of death after myocardial infarction in patients with and without diabetes: a systematic overview. Lancet 2000;355(9206):773-8.

227 Weir CJ, Murray GD, Dyker AG, Lees KR. Is hyperglycaemia an independent predictor of poor outcome after acute stroke? Results of a long-term follow up study. BMJ 1997;314(7090):1303-6.

228 Investigators CS, Annane D, Cariou A, Maxime V, Azoulay E, D'Honneur G et al. Corticosteroid treatment and intensive insulin therapy for septic shock in adults: a randomized controlled trial. JAMA 2010;303(4):341-8.

229 Preiser JC, Devos P, Ruiz-Santana S, Melot C, Annane D, Groeneveld J et al. A prospective randomised multi-centre controlled trial on tight glucose control by intensive insulin therapy in adult intensive care units: the Glucontrol study. Intensive Care Med 2009;35(10):1738-48.

230 Griesdale DE, de Souza RJ, van Dam RM, Heyland DK, Cook DJ, Malhotra A et al. Intensive insulin therapy and mortality among critically ill patients: a meta-analysis including NICE-SUGAR study data. CMAJ 2009;180(8):821-7.

231 Friedrich JO, Chant C, Adhikari NK. Does intensive insulin therapy really reduce mortality in critically ill surgical patients? A reanalysis of meta-analytic data. Crit Care 2010;14(5):324.

232 Padkin A. How to weigh the current evidence for clinical practice. Best Pract Res Clin Anaesthesiol 2009;23(4):487-96.

233 Mesotten D, Van den Berghe G. Clinical benefits of tight glycaemic control: focus on the intensive care unit. Best Pract Res Clin Anaesthesiol 2009;23(4):421-9.

234 Jacobi J, Bircher N, Krinsley J, Agus M, Braithwaite SS, Deutschman C et al. Guidelines for the use of an insulin infusion for the management of hyperglycemia in critically ill patients. Crit Care Med 2012;40(12):3251-76.

235 Peberdy MA, Callaway CW, Neumar RW, Geocadin RG, Zimmerman JL, Donnino M et al. Part 9: post-cardiac arrest care: 2010 American Heart Association Guidelines for Cardiopulmonary Resuscitation and Emergency Cardiovascular Care. Circulation 2010;122(18 Suppl 3):S768-86.

236 Qaseem A, Humphrey LL, Chou R, Snow V, Shekelle P, Clinical Guidelines Committee of the American College of Physicians. Use of intensive insulin therapy for the management of glycemic control in hospitalized patients: a clinical practice guideline from the American College of Physicians. Ann Intern Med 2011;154(4):260-7.

237 Moghissi ES, Korytkowski MT, DiNardo M, Einhorn D, Hellman R, Hirsch IB et al. American Association of Clinical Endocrinologists and American Diabetes Association consensus statement on inpatient glycemic control. Diabetes Care 2009;32(6):1119-31.

238 Egi M, Bellomo R, Stachowski E, French CJ, Hart GK, Hegarty C et al. Blood glucose concentration and outcome of critical illness: the impact of diabetes. Crit Care Med 2008;36(8):2249-55.

239 Mackenzie IM, Whitehouse T, Nightingale PG. The metrics of glycaemic control in critical care. Intensive Care Med 2011;37(3):435-43.

240 Krinsley JS. Glycemic variability: a strong independent predictor of mortality in critically ill patients. Crit Care Med 2008;36(11):3008-13.

241 Louie K, Cheema R, Dodek P, Wong H, Wilmer A, Grubisic M et al. Intensive nursing work schedules and the risk of hypoglycaemia in critically ill patients who are receiving intravenous insulin. Qual Saf Health Care 2010;19(6):e42.

242 Needham DM, Dinglas VD, Bienvenu OJ, Colantuoni E, Wozniak AW, Rice TW et al. One year outcomes in patients with acute lung injury randomised to initial trophic or full enteral feeding: prospective follow-up of EDEN randomised trial. BMJ 2013;346:f1532.

243 Carlson CG, Huang DT. The Adult Respiratory Distress Syndrome Cognitive Outcomes Study: long-term neuropsychological function in survivors of acute lung injury. Crit Care 2013;17(3):317.

244 Mikkelsen ME, Christie JD, Lanken PN, Biester RC, Thompson BT, Bellamy SL et al. The adult respiratory distress syndrome cognitive outcomes study: long-term neuropsychological function in survivors of acute lung injury. Am J Respir Crit Care Med 2012;185(12):1307-15.

245 Bienvenu OJ, Colantuoni E, Mendez-Tellez PA, Dinglas VD, Shanholtz C, Husain N et al. Depressive symptoms and impaired physical function after acute lung injury: a 2-year longitudinal study. Am J Respir Crit Care Med 2012;185(5):517-24.

246 Williams TA, Leslie GD. Challenges and possible solutions for long-term follow-up of patients surviving critical illness. Aust Crit Care 2011;24(3):175-85.

247 Robinson KA, Dennison CR, Wayman DM, Pronovost PJ, Needham DM. Systematic review identifies number of strategies important for retaining study participants. J Clin Epidemiol 2007;60(8):757-65.

248 Tansey CM, Matte AL, Needham D, Herridge MS. Review of retention strategies in longitudinal studies and application to follow-up of ICU survivors. Intensive Care Med 2007;33(12):2051-7.

249 Christie JD, Biester RC, Taichman DB, Shull WH, Jr., Hansen-Flaschen J, Shea JA et al. Formation and validation of a telephone battery to assess cognitive function in acute respiratory distress syndrome survivors. J Crit Care 2006;21(2):125-32.

250 Iwashyna TJ. Trajectories of recovery and dysfunction after acute illness, with implications for clinical trial design. Am J Respir Crit Care Med 2012;186(4):302-4.

251 Batt J, dos Santos CC, Cameron JI, Herridge MS. Intensive care unit-acquired weakness: clinical phenotypes and molecular mechanisms. Am J Respir Crit Care Med 2013;187(3):238-46.

Gastrointestinal, metabolic and liver alterations

Andrea Marshall, Christopher Gordon

Learning objectives

After reading this chapter, you should be able to:

- describe the changes in gastrointestinal physiology and metabolism associated with critical illness
- identify patients at risk for the development of stress ulcers and rationalise therapeutic interventions for their prevention
- identify patients at risk for the development of intra-abdominal hypertension and abdominal compartment syndrome and suggest management strategies to decrease intra-abdominal pressure
- describe the physiological changes that occur during diabetic ketoacidosis and rationalise assessment and treatment strategies
- discuss the effects of critical illness on hepatic function and evaluate the consequences of liver dysfunction
- describe the treatment of liver failure, including liver support therapies and transplantation.

Introduction

During episodes of critical illness, patients often experience disturbance in their metabolic and/or endocrine function. In the previous chapter, the changes to metabolism that occur during critical illness and the role of the gastrointestinal system in nutrition were outlined. The gastrointestinal system is also involved in many other important functions including immunity and protection.

Effective gastrointestinal function requires an adequate blood supply to ensure oxygen and nutrients are available at the cellular level. However, in critical illness splanchnic circulation may be compromised without overt signs being evident. This alteration in regional blood flow and tissue oxygen delivery can compromise normal metabolic and endocrine function.

In this chapter the effect of gastrointestinal physiology on critical illness is discussed. Gastrointestinal dysfunction, including the development of stress-related mucosal diseases and development of increased intra-abdominal pressure, is discussed. A major component of this chapter is dedicated to the assessment and management of liver dysfunction, including liver transplantation. An overview of the assessment and management of diabetic ketoacidosis is also provided.

Gastrointestinal physiology

As described in Chapter 19, digestion and absorption of nutrients such as carbohydrates, amino acids, minerals and water are key functions of the gastrointestinal system. Another important role of the gastrointestinal tract is immunity. Part of this immunity is the established barrier between the gastrointestinal tract and the blood supply. There are a number of different mechanisms by which the gastrointestinal system prevents the movement of substances (other than nutrients, water and electrolytes) into the systemic circulation and these are outlined in Table 20.1. In the setting of critical illness, gastrointestinal hypoperfusion may be present, resulting in decreased oxygen and nutrient delivery at the cellular level, and this in turn can lead to decreased effectiveness of these protective functions.

Alterations to normal gastrointestinal physiology in critical illness

During critical illness, there are a number of alterations that can occur to gastrointestinal physiology. The digestion and absorption of nutrients may be altered, as alterations to glucose absorption.[7,8] Changes can also occur with gastric acid production, which is commonly thought to increase in critical illness. There is some evidence to suggest that many critically ill patients do not hypersecrete gastric acid[9] with increased gastric pH being observed in some critically ill patients, even in the absence of pharmacological inhibition of gastric acid secretion.[10] The ability of the small intestine to absorb nutrients can be impaired during critical illness,[11] although most critically ill patients appear to be able to tolerate enteral nutrition, making the clinical significance of impaired absorption unclear.

Some alterations to normal gastrointestinal physiology in critical illness relate to hypoperfusion and decreased oxygenation in this area and have high metabolic demands.[12] Historically, gastrointestinal dysfunction in critical illness was described in relation to symptoms, such as gastrointestinal bleeding, mechanical obstruction and pancreatitis[13] resulting from ischaemia.[14] However, the presence of covert ischaemia has resulted in a heightened interest in the prevention and early detection of gastrointestinal ischaemia in the critically ill, in an attempt to minimise ischaemia-related dysfunction.

TABLE 20.1
Protective mechanisms of the gastrointestinal system and impacts of critical illness

MECHANISM	ACTION
Motility	Propels bacteria through the GI tract. In critical illness, motility may be altered because of enteric nerve impairment and altered smooth muscle function, inflammation (mediated by cytokines and nitric oxide), gut injury, hypoperfusion, medications (opioids, dopamine), electrolyte disturbances, hyperglycaemia, sepsis and increased intracranial pressure[1]
Hydrochloric acid secretion	Reduces gastric acidity and destroys bacteria. Parietal cells in the stomach produce hydrochloric acid and keep the intragastric environment relatively acidic (pH approx 4.0). An acidic pH has bactericidal and bacteriostatic properties,[2] thus limiting overgrowth in the stomach
Bicarbonate	Bicarbonate ions bind with hydrogen ions to form water and carbon dioxide, preventing the hydrogen ions (acid) from damaging the duodenal wall[6]
Bile salts	Bile salts provide protection against bacteria by breaking down the liposaccharide portion of endotoxins, thereby detoxifying gram-negative bacteria in the gastrointestinal tract. The deconjugation of bile salts into secondary bile acids inhibits the proliferation of pathogens and may destroy their cell walls[3]
Mucin production	Prevents the adhesion of bacteria to the wall of the GI tract. Mucous cells secrete large quantities of very thick, alkaline mucus (approximately 1 mm thick in the stomach). Glycoproteins present in the mucus prevent bacteria from adhering to and colonising the mucosal wall[4]
Epithelial cell shedding	Limits bacterial adhesion. The mucosal lining of the entire gastrointestinal tract is composed of epithelial cells that create a physical barrier to bacterial invasion. These cells are replaced approximately every 3–5 days,[4] limiting bacterial colonisation
Zona occludens (tight junctions surrounding each cell in the epithelial sheet)	The junctions between epithelial cells provide a barrier to microorganisms. Intermediate junctions (zonula adherens) function primarily in cell–cell adhesion, while the tight junctions (zonula occludens) limit the movement of bacteria and toxins across the gut wall[5]
Gut-associated lymphoid tissue	Protection against bacterial invasion is provided by gut-associated lymphoid tissue, capable of cell-mediated and humoral-mediated immune responses[4]
Kupffer cells	Kupffer cells in the liver and spleen provide a back-up defence against pathogens that cross the barrier of the gastrointestinal wall and enter the systemic circulation

Gastrointestinal mucosal hypoperfusion

The gastrointestinal system is particularly susceptible to alterations in regional blood flow and oxygen delivery because it has a higher critical oxygen delivery than the rest of the body. Splanchnic vasoconstriction is also proportionally greater than in other vascular beds and the countercurrent oxygen exchange between vessels within the villi further contributes to decreased regional oxygen delivery.[4]

During shock states, decreased blood flow due to vasoconstriction occurs in this region first. It is the last place where blood flow is restored following successful resuscitation.[15] In shock states, the gastrointestinal system attempts to maintain adequate cellular oxygenation by increasing the amount of oxygen extracted from the blood. This increase in oxygen extraction may prevent serious compromise of tissue oxygenation even in the presence of reduced oxygen delivery.[16]

Practice tip

Remember, assessment of arterial blood pressure, heart rate and urine output provides information about the haemodynamic and oxygenation status of the whole body. A reduction in regional perfusion and oxygenation may occur despite conventional clinical assessment findings being normal.

During periods of ischaemia and hypoxia, oxygen free radicals are generated as byproducts of anaerobic metabolism. With successful resuscitation of the gastrointestinal tract, blood flow and oxygen delivery are restored but the oxygen free radicals are liberated, contributing to the microvascular and mucosal changes characteristic of ischaemia and reperfusion of the gut mucosa.[17]

Consequences of gastrointestinal hypoperfusion

The consequences of gastrointestinal hypoperfusion are significant, and include disruption of the physical barrier to pathogens; disruption of chemical control of bacterial overgrowth; decreased peristalsis; and reduced immunological activities of gastrointestinal-associated lymphoid tissue. In health, all of these mechanisms work efficiently to contain bacteria within the gastrointestinal tract. During critical illness, however, reduced oxygenation contributes to decreased cellular function and failure of the protective mechanisms described in Table 20.1. Consequently, bacterial proliferation and translocation from the gastrointestinal tract to the systemic circulation may occur.[17] Changes in gastrointestinal perfusion also have the capacity to affect hepatic perfusion, oxygenation and function. In approximately 50% of critically ill patients, ischaemic hepatitis or 'shock liver' occurs, which is evidenced by jaundice, elevation of liver function tests or overt hepatic dysfunction.[18] Ischaemic hepatitis can vary from a mild elevation of serum aminotransferase and

bilirubin levels in septic patients, to an acute elevation following haemodynamic shock. Ischaemic hepatic injury influences morbidity and mortality but remains underdiagnosed, probably because the clinical signs become apparent long after hypoperfusion has occurred. Physiological changes contributing to ischaemic hepatitis include changes to the portal and arterial blood supply as well as hepatic microcirculation. The degree to which the liver is damaged is directly related to the severity and duration of hypoperfusion, and both anoxic and reperfusion injury can damage hepatocytes and the vascular endothelium.[18]

Stress-related mucosal damage

The reported incidence of stress-related mucosal damage is variable[19] and complicated by definitions of end points, difficulty in measuring the end points and the heterogeneity of patient populations.[20] It is estimated that between 74% and 100% of critically ill patients have evidence of stress-related mucosal erosion and subepithelial haemorrhage on endoscopy at their first day of admission to the intensive care unit (ICU).[20] With occult bleeding (drop in haemoglobin level or positive stool occult blood test) as an end point, it is estimated that 15–50% of critically ill patients would be reported to have stress-related mucosal damage.[21] Reported incidence is reduced to 25% or less when haematemesis or nasogastric lavage positive for bright red blood is used as an end point to describe clinically overt bleeding.[19,22] The incidence of clinically significant bleeding, that is bleeding associated with hypotension, tachycardia and a drop in haemoglobin level necessitating transfusion, is estimated to be 3–4%.[23] Over time the incidence of stress-related mucosal damage has continued to decrease and this is largely attributed to overall advances and improvements in the management of critically ill patients, particularly optimal resuscitation and targeted nutritional therapy.[24]

Factors influencing the development of stress-related mucosal damage include splanchnic hypoperfusion, which may influence mucosal ischaemia and reperfusion injury.[25] The mucus–bicarbonate gel layer[26] and decreased prostaglandin levels, which impair mucus replenishment, and increased nitric oxide synthase contribute to reperfusion injury and cell death.[27] The protective mechanisms and factors that promote injury are detailed in Table 20.2.

Risk factors for stress-related mucosal damage

A number of risk factors are associated with the development of stress-related mucosal damage, including respiratory failure requiring at least 48 hours of mechanical ventilation and coagulopathy,[38] acute hepatic failure, hypotension, chronic renal failure, prolonged nasogastric tube placement, alcohol abuse, sepsis and an increased serum concentration of anti-*Helicobacter pylori* immunoglobulin A.[39]

Although the reported prevalence of overt gastrointestinal bleeding is reported to be between 0.6% and 4%,[40,41]

TABLE 20.2

Factors contributing to stress-related mucosal disease[206]

FACTORS	MECHANISM	ACTION
Protective mechanisms	Mucosal prostaglandins	Protect the mucosa by stimulating blood flow, mucus and bicarbonate production[28] Stimulate epithelial cell growth and repair
	Mucosal bicarbonate barrier	Forms a physical barrier to acid and pepsin, preventing injury to the epithelium[29]
	Epithelial restitution and regeneration	Epithelial cells rapidly regenerate but the process is highly metabolic and may be impaired by physiological stress[29]
	Mucosal blood flow	Mucosal blood flow helps remove acid from the mucosa, supplies bicarbonate and oxygen to the mucosal epithelial cells[30]
	Cell membrane and tight junctions	Tight junctions between mucosal epithelial cells prevent the back diffusion of hydrogen ions[31]
Factors promoting injury	Acid	Acid is a key issue in the pathogenesis of stress-related mucosal injury but not all critically ill patients hypersecrete acid.[31] However, small amounts of acid may still cause injury and the prevention of acid secretion has led to a reduction in injury[32]
	Pepsin	May cause direct injury to the mucosa[33] Facilitates the lysis of clots[22]
	Mucosal hypoperfusion	Reduced mucosal blood flow results in reduced oxygen and nutrient delivery, making epithelial cells susceptible to injury[31] Contributes to mucosal acid–base imbalances Results in the formation of free radicals
	Reperfusion injury	Nitric oxide, which causes vasodilation and hyperaemia, is released during hypoperfusion and results in an increase in cell-damaging cytokines
	Intramucosal acid–base balance	The mucus layer protects the epithelium and traps bicarbonate ions that neutralise acid, thus a decrease in bicarbonate secretion results in intramucosal acidosis and local injury[29]
	Systemic acidosis	Results in increased intramucosal acidity[30]
	Free oxygen radicals	Generated as a result of tissue hypoxia, free oxygen radicals cause oxidative injury to the mucosa[34]
	Bile salts	Bile salts reflux from the duodenum into the stomach and may have a role in stress-related damage although the exact mechanism is uncertain[35]
	Helicobacter pylori	Conflicting results about the role of *H. pylori* as a cause of stress-induced mucosal disease in the critically ill[36,37]

Reproduced with permission from Marshall AP. The gut in critical illness. In: Carlson K, ed. AACN Advanced critical care nursing. Philadelphia: Elsevier; 2009, Table 29-3.

when this occurs mortality rates approximate 50%.[42] Consequently, there is a strong imperative to implement stress-ulcer prophylaxis, particularly in those patients who are considered at risk.

Preventing stress-related mucosal damage

Prophylaxis for stress-related mucosal damage is often part of the care of the critically ill, although evidence demonstrating an added benefit when this therapy is applied to those patients who are not identified as at risk for developing stress-related mucosal damage is limited in both quantity and quality.[43,44] A positive impact on mortality and intensive care length of stay associated with stress ulcer prophylaxis is also yet to be established.[45]

It is common for the majority of critically ill patients to receive some form of stress-ulcer prophylaxis during their episode of critical illness, likely because of recommendations from influential groups such as the Surviving Sepsis Campaign.[46] With the risk for clinical substantial bleeding being low, it is important to consider whether stress-ulcer prophylaxis is always warranted, especially considering the pharmacological therapy is not risk-free and is associated with economic consequences.[47,48] There are a variety of pharmacological strategies that can be used to prevent stress ulcers from developing and, most commonly, histamine-2-receptor antagonists (H_2RAs) and proton pump inhibitors (PPIs) are used as first-line therapy[20] although sucralfate can be used if neither of these agents is suitable.[49]

Histamine-2-receptor antagonists

H$_2$RAs inhibit the production of gastric acid by binding to the histamine-2 receptor on the basement membrane of the parietal cell.[20] However, gastric acid secretion may also occur through stimulation of the acetylcholine or gastrin receptors present in parietal cells;[50] therefore, complete blocking of gastric acid production does not occur when H$_2$RAs are used. Further limitations of H$_2$RAs are that tachyphylaxis can occur quickly[20] and tolerance may develop within 72 hours of administration.[51,52] Nevertheless, this pharmacological strategy to prevent stress-related mucosal disease remains commonplace in critical care.[53] The decrease in gastric acidity as a result of H$_2$RA use may be beneficial from the perspective of preventing stress-related mucosal disease, but changes in gastric pH could lead to bacterial overgrowth in the stomach, micro-aspiration and, consequently, an increase in the incidence of nosocomial pneumonia,[54] although there is some research that does not support this notion.[55]

Proton pump inhibitors

PPIs have a greater ability to maintain an increased intra-gastric pH than H$_2$RAs. These drugs work by irreversibly binding to the proton pump, effectively blocking all three receptors responsible for gastric acid secretion by the parietal cell.[56,57] PPIs are also able to limit vagally-mediated gastric acid secretion.[58]

PPIs are more effective than H$_2$RAs in reducing clinically important bleeding and do not appear to increase the risk of nosocomial pneumonia.[41] Clinical evaluation of the efficacy of PPIs is, however, somewhat limited; few studies have specifically studied the prophylactic use of PPIs for stress-related mucosal damage and many have methodological limitations.[55] PPIs are similar to H$_2$RAs in their ability to raise the gastric pH above 4, a level considered adequate to prevent stress ulceration, and the use of PPIs is not associated with the development of tolerance, such that is seen with the use of H$_2$RAs.[20] PPIs are also more likely to maintain the pH at greater than 6, which may be necessary to maintain clotting in those patients at risk of re-bleeding from peptic ulcer.[57] However, the administration of PPIs is associated with an increased risk of developing *Clostridium difficile*-associated diarrhoea.[59]

PPIs that may be administered intravenously include omeprazole, esomeprazole and pantoprazole. Omeprazole has the highest potential for drug interactions and interferes with the metabolism of some drugs commonly used in intensive care, including cyclosporine, diazepam, phenytoin and warfarin.[27] Pantoprazole has the lowest potential for drug interactions.[58]

> **Practice tip**
>
> Stress-ulcer prophylaxis is still commonly used in critical illness. Histamine-2-receptor antagonists, such as ranitidine, are effective at reducing clinically important bleeding but patients can develop resistance to these drugs within 72 hours of commencement.

Sucralfate

Sucralfate provides protection against stress-related mucosal disease through a number of mechanisms. Sucralfate provides a protective barrier on the surface gastric epithelium, stimulates mucus and bicarbonate secretion, stimulates epithelial renewal, improves mucosal blood flow and enhances prostaglandin release.[21] Given orally or via a nasogastric tube, sucralfate is well tolerated but appears to be less effective than H$_2$RAs in decreasing clinically significant bleeding.[20] Earlier reports comparing sucralfate with ranitidine showed a decrease in the development of pneumonia in those patients receiving sucralfate; however, these findings were not supported in a subsequent level I randomised controlled trial.[32]

Enteral nutrition

It is postulated that enteral nutrition has a role in stress-ulcer prophylaxis because its administration can buffer gastric acid and increase intragastric pH,[20] improves gastric mucosal blood flow[60] and promotes the release of protective substances such as prostaglandins and mucus.[61] In critically ill patients, enteral nutrition administration is more effective at increasing intragastric pH than either H$_2$RAs or PPIs.[62] In a recent systematic review, stress-ulcer prophylaxis with H$_2$RAs reduced the risk of gastrointestinal bleeding (odds ratio 0.47; 95% confidence interval, 0.29–0.76) but this was only observed in a subgroup of patients who did not receive enteral nutrition[63] suggesting that, for patients receiving enteral nutrition, stress-ulcer prophylaxis may not be warranted. The lack of well-designed prospective studies examining the role of enteral nutrition in stress-ulcer prophylaxis prevents the use of this therapy as a sole therapeutic agent for this purpose.

Intra-abdominal hypertension and abdominal compartment syndrome

Intra-abdominal hypertension (IAH) and abdominal compartment syndrome have received increased attention in recent years and clinical research in this area is on the increase. IAH occurs in nearly half of all intensive care patients and is associated with significant morbidity and mortality. The development of IAH is not isolated to surgical patients or those with abdominal injury, and is an important consideration for medical patients without abdominal conditions.

Aetiology

IAH and abdominal compartment syndrome can and do occur in a variety of patient populations.[64] Factors associated with IAH include body mass index, fluid resuscitation, multiple transfusions, total sepsis-related organ failure score and respiratory, renal and coagulation sepsis-related organ failure sub-scores. However, only blood transfusion and the rate of fluid resuscitation are significantly correlated with IAH.[65] There are a number of different risk factors for the development of IAH with large volume crystalloid resuscitation, respiratory status and hypotension being factors that were associated with IAH and abdominal compartment syndrome.[66] Risk factors that are more specific to critically ill patients include obesity, sepsis, abdominal surgery and ileus. Abdominal compartment syndrome is potentially fatal. Consequently, it is imperative that all clinicians be aware of the underlying physiological changes, assessment and management in at-risk patients.

Practice tip

The critically ill obese patient is at higher risk of developing intra-abdominal hypertension and abdominal compartment syndrome and may benefit from intra-abdominal pressure monitoring.

Pathophysiology

Increased intra-abdominal pressure (IAP) results from an increase in pressure within the confined anatomic space of the abdominal cavity.[64] When IAP rises in this closed anatomic space, blood flow may be reduced and tissue viability threatened.[67]

This increase in pressure may result from causes such as intraperitoneal bleeding, peritonitis, ascites or distention of the gas-filled bowel. Clinical data show that increases in IAP result in physiological changes in vital organ function.[68] Early detection of increases in IAP can be challenging, and

it is a sustained increase in abdominal pressure or the development of IAH that affects regional blood flow and impairs tissue perfusion, contributing to the development of multiple organ failure.[69] The pathophysiological consequences occur as a direct result of increased pressure within the abdominal cavity, resulting in vascular compression, direct compression of the organs and elevation of the diaphragm,[70] which can falsely elevate intracardiac pressures. A summary of the physiological changes associated with abdominal compartment syndrome is provided in Table 20-3.

Normal intra-abdominal pressure

In the spontaneously breathing patient, IAP is normally either atmospheric or subatmospheric. Mechanical ventilation, however, causes the IAP to increase near end-inspiration. After abdominal surgery, IAP may be increased slightly. The patient's clinical context must be considered when evaluating IAP. The most recent grading system for IAP is provided in Table 20.4.[79]

Because IAP is variable between patients, it has been suggested that abdominal perfusion pressure be calculated by subtracting IAP from mean arterial pressure. It appears that the calculation of abdominal perfusion pressure may be a more clinically useful resuscitation end point and is statistically superior in predicting survival from IAH and abdominal compartment syndrome than either mean arterial pressure or IAP;[80] however, further well-designed research is needed in this area.

TABLE 20.3

Physiological changes associated with abdominal compartment syndrome

SYSTEM	PHYSIOLOGICAL EFFECTS
Respiratory	Cephalad deviation of diaphragm leads to decreased lung and chest wall compliance[71] Peak inspiratory pressures increase[64] Functional residual volume and lung capacity are reduced, resulting in ventilation/perfusion mismatching Hypoxia and hypercarbia may result, necessitating mechanical ventilation Pulmonary vascular resistance increases[72]
Cardiovascular	Inferior vena cava and portal vein compression results in decreased venous return Decreased left ventricular compliance[68] Artificially increased right atrial pressure, pulmonary artery occlusion pressure[73] Decreased cardiac index[74] Elevated systemic vascular resistance from arteriolar vasoconstriction and increased intra-abdominal pressure (IAP)[72]
Renal	Oliguria (IAP 15–20 mmHg)[75] Anuria (IAP >30 mmHg) May be a consequence of decreased cardiac output, compression of renal vessels, increased renal vascular resistance or redistribution of blood flow to renal medulla[71]
Gastrointestinal	Decreased splanchnic perfusion and tissue hypoxia Increased GI mucosal acidosis[76] Reduced hepatic blood flow[64] Abnormalities in normal gut mucosal barrier function that may permit bacterial translocation[72] Decreased abdominal wall blood flow[68] Increased pressure on oesophageal varices may result in bleeding[77]
Neurological	Increased intracranial pressure because of impaired venous return[78]

Reproduced with permission from Marshall AP. The gut in critical illness. In: Carlson K, ed. AACN Advanced critical care nursing. Philadelphia: Elsevier; 2009, Table 29-4.

TABLE 20.4

Intra-abdominal Hypertension Grading System[79]

GRADE	BLADDER PRESSURE (MMHG)
I	12–15
II	16–20
III	21–25
IV	>25

Adapted from Kirkpatrick AW, Roberts DJ, De Waele J, Jaeschke R, Malbrain ML, De Keulenaer B et al. Intra-abdominal hypertension and the abdominal compartment syndrome: updated consensus definitions and clinical practice guidelines from the World Society of the Abdominal Compartment Syndrome. Intensive Care Med 2013;39(7): 1190–206, with permission.

Measurement of intra-abdominal pressure

Clinical assessment of the abdomen is not a sensitive or accurate technique for detecting increased IAP.[81] Measurement of pressure within the bladder has been validated as closely approximating IAP[82] and is the recommended standard approach for the measurement of intra-abdominal pressure.[79] This technique can, however, be influenced by the measurement technique. For example, air bubbles in the system and changes in transducer positions may influence pressure measurement, with wide variations in IAP being noted.[83] There is also little consistency in the amount of fluid used to prime the bladder; this may result in overestimates of IAP.[84,85]

There are a variety of techniques for measuring IAP described in the literature[86,87] and the direct peritoneal catheter measurement is the most ideal but not the most practical. IAP measurements should be performed when patients exhibit one or more of the risk factors and the trans-bladder technique is the measurement technique recommended by the World Society of the Abdominal Compartment Syndrome.[79] The reliability of other methods, such as intragastric measurement, is not well demonstrated in clinical practice.[88] Continuous measurement of IAP is becoming more common.[89]

Practice tip

The trans-bladder technique is the most common method used for measuring intra-abdominal pressure. Attention should be given to consistent and accurate measurement to track trends.

IAP measurement should be accurate and reproducible. There are a number of commercial devices now available to aid the measurement of IAP; however, these are not required and a measurement system can easily be created from existing equipment normally available

TABLE 20.5

Key principles for measuring intra-abdominal pressure (IAP)

	RECOMMENDATION
Measurement techniques	• IAP should be measured in mmHg • Measurement should be recorded at end-expiration • The transducer should be zeroed at the mid-axillary line at the level of the iliac crest[90] • Determine measurement 60 seconds after instillation of saline to allow bladder detrusor muscle to relax[91]
Instillation volume	• A maximum of 25 mL sterile saline should be used as the instillation volume in adults • In children the volume instilled should be 3 mL/kg[92]
Patient position	• IAP should be measured in supine position, where possible[90] • IAP is significantly increased when the head of bed is elevated more than 20° • If head-of-bed elevation is required, consider the reverse Trendelenberg position during IAP measurement to minimise compression of the abdomen by the chest

in most intensive care units. The procedures for IAP measurement techniques may differ; however, the key principles for performing measurements are outlined in Table 20.5.

Management of intra-abdominal hypertension and abdominal compartment syndrome

Surveillance for IAH and abdominal compartment syndrome requires close observation of the patient to identify potential risk factors and relevant changes to physiological parameters. For those patients who are at risk, close monitoring of IAP is required and pre-emptive measures are instituted. For example, a decision may be made to delay closure of the abdomen or to use an alternative means of abdominal content coverage. For the nonsurgical patient, optimal resuscitation may be important in preventing IAH; over-resuscitation needs to be avoided. The approach to managing the patient with IAH or abdominal compartment syndrome is dependent on their clinical presentation. The World Society of the Abdominal Compartment Syndrome has developed evidence-based management algorithms that are useful in guiding clinical management (see Figures 20.1 and 20.2).

FIGURE 20.1   Intra-abdominal hypertension and abdominal compartment syndrome management algorithm.[79]

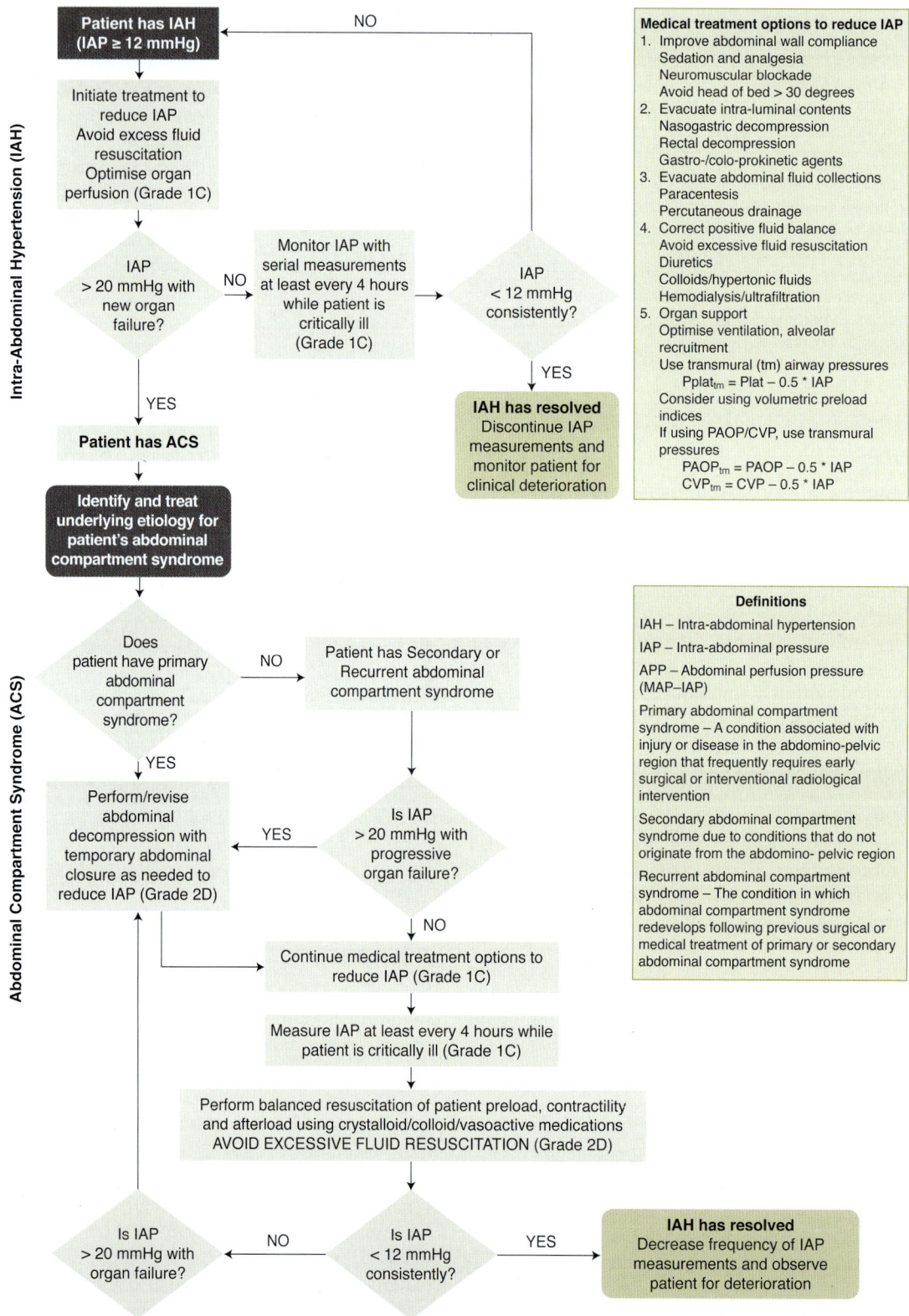

Medical treatment options to reduce IAP
1. Improve abdominal wall compliance
   Sedation and analgesia
   Neuromuscular blockade
   Avoid head of bed > 30 degrees
2. Evacuate intra-luminal contents
   Nasogastric decompression
   Rectal decompression
   Gastro-/colo-prokinetic agents
3. Evacuate abdominal fluid collections
   Paracentesis
   Percutaneous drainage
4. Correct positive fluid balance
   Avoid excessive fluid resuscitation
   Diuretics
   Colloids/hypertonic fluids
   Hemodialysis/ultrafiltration
5. Organ support
   Optimise ventilation, alveolar recruitment
   Use transmural (tm) airway pressures
   $Pplat_{tm} = Plat - 0.5 * IAP$
   Consider using volumetric preload indices
   If using PAOP/CVP, use transmural pressures
   $PAOP_{tm} = PAOP - 0.5 * IAP$
   $CVP_{tm} = CVP - 0.5 * IAP$

Definitions

IAH – Intra-abdominal hypertension

IAP – Intra-abdominal pressure

APP – Abdominal perfusion pressure (MAP–IAP)

Primary abdominal compartment syndrome – A condition associated with injury or disease in the abdomino-pelvic region that frequently requires early surgical or interventional radiological intervention

Secondary abdominal compartment syndrome due to conditions that do not originate from the abdomino- pelvic region

Recurrent abdominal compartment syndrome – The condition in which abdominal compartment syndrome redevelops following previous surgical or medical treatment of primary or secondary abdominal compartment syndrome

Reproduced with permission from Kirkpatrick AW, Roberts DJ, De Waele J, Jaeschke R, Malbrain ML, De Keulenaer B et al. Intra-abdominal hypertension and the abdominal compartment syndrome: updated consensus definitions and clinical practice guidelines from the World Society of the Abdominal Compartment Syndrome. Intensive Care Med 2013;39(7):1190–206, Figure 1.

FIGURE 20.2 Intra-abdominal hypertension and abdominal compartment syndrome medical management algorithm.[79]

IAH/ACS medical management algorithm

- The choice (and success) of the medical management strategies listed below is strongly related to both the etiology of the patient's IAH/abdominal compartment syndrome and the patient's clinical situation. The appropriateness of each intervention should always be considered prior to implementing these interventions in any individual patient.
- The interventions should be applied in a stepwise fashion until the patient's intra-abdominal pressure (IAP) decreases.
- If there is no response to a particular intervention, therapy should be escalated to the next step in the algorithm.

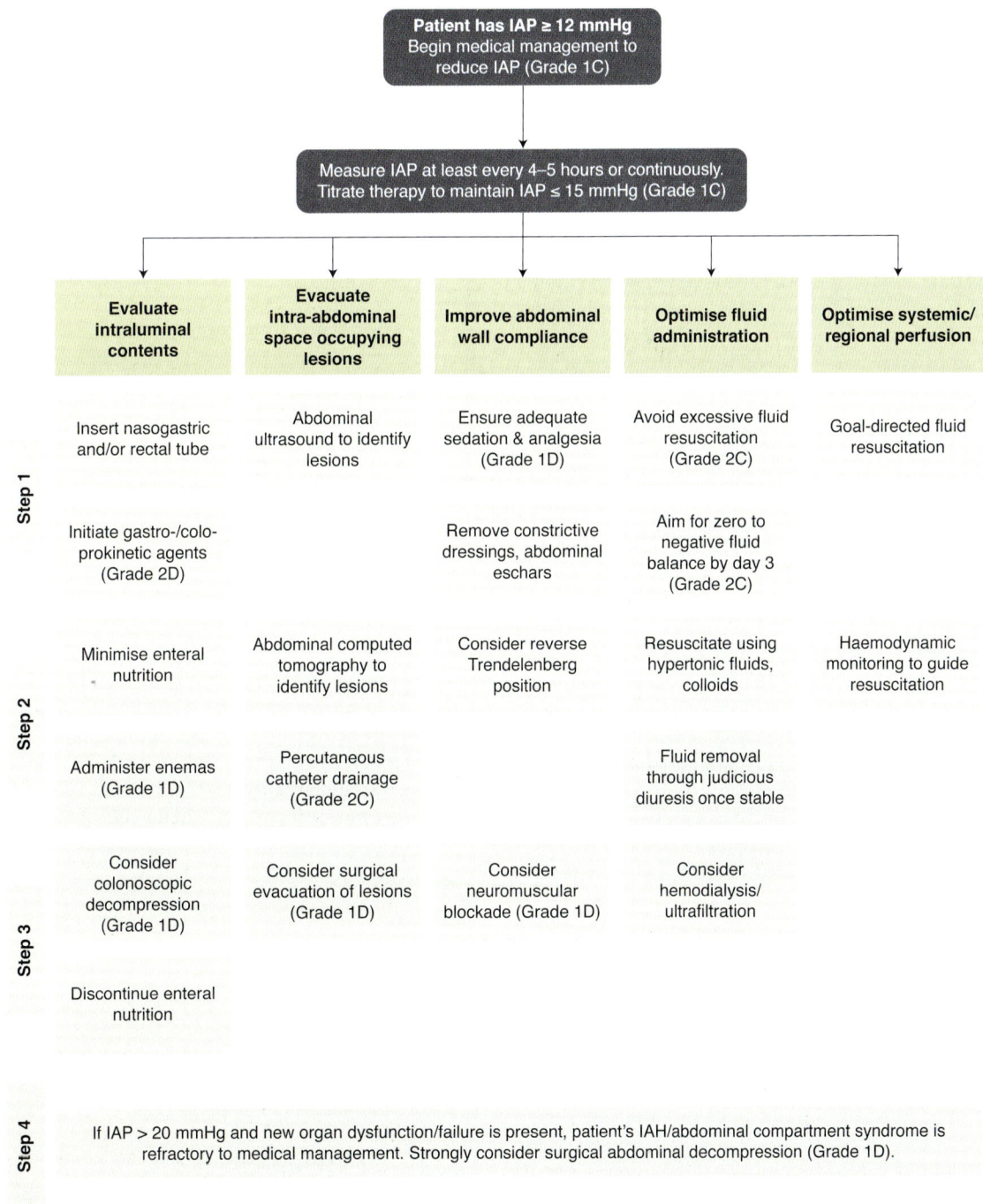

Patient has IAP ≥ 12 mmHg
Begin medical management to reduce IAP (Grade 1C)

Measure IAP at least every 4–5 hours or continuously. Titrate therapy to maintain IAP ≤ 15 mmHg (Grade 1C)

	Evaluate intraluminal contents	Evacuate intra-abdominal space occupying lesions	Improve abdominal wall compliance	Optimise fluid administration	Optimise systemic/ regional perfusion
Step 1	Insert nasogastric and/or rectal tube	Abdominal ultrasound to identify lesions	Ensure adequate sedation & analgesia (Grade 1D)	Avoid excessive fluid resuscitation (Grade 2C)	Goal-directed fluid resuscitation
	Initiate gastro-/colo-prokinetic agents (Grade 2D)		Remove constrictive dressings, abdominal eschars	Aim for zero to negative fluid balance by day 3 (Grade 2C)	
Step 2	Minimise enteral nutrition	Abdominal computed tomography to identify lesions	Consider reverse Trendelenberg position	Resuscitate using hypertonic fluids, colloids	Haemodynamic monitoring to guide resuscitation
	Administer enemas (Grade 1D)	Percutaneous catheter drainage (Grade 2C)		Fluid removal through judicious diuresis once stable	
Step 3	Consider colonoscopic decompression (Grade 1D)	Consider surgical evacuation of lesions (Grade 1D)	Consider neuromuscular blockade (Grade 1D)	Consider hemodialysis/ ultrafiltration	
	Discontinue enteral nutrition				
Step 4	If IAP > 20 mmHg and new organ dysfunction/failure is present, patient's IAH/abdominal compartment syndrome is refractory to medical management. Strongly consider surgical abdominal decompression (Grade 1D).				

Reproduced with permission from Kirkpatrick AW, Roberts DJ, De Waele J, Jaeschke R, Malbrain ML, De Keulenaer B et al. Intra-abdominal hypertension and the abdominal compartment syndrome: updated consensus definitions and clinical practice guidelines from the World Society of the Abdominal Compartment Syndrome. Intensive Care Med 2013;39(7):1190–206, Figure 2.

The critically ill patient with diabetes

Diabetes is a major cause of morbidity and mortality worldwide.[93] The prevalence of diabetes internationally is rising and follows a global trend.[94] Reasons for this include an increase in the rates of obesity, physical inactivity, the ageing population, better detection of diabetes and longer survival of affected individuals.[95] The prevalence of diagnosed diabetes continues to increase worldwide, in adults as well as youth.[96] In 2013, a reported 382 million people worldwide had diabetes and this number is projected to increase to 592 million by the year 2035.[97] Worryingly, reports of undiagnosed diabetes are on the increase with type 2 diabetes remaining undetected for many years, particularly in developing countries.[98]

Aetiology of diabetes

Diabetes mellitus is a disorder of metabolism that is characterised by glucose intolerance. Diabetes is not a single disease per se, but a group of heterogeneous disorders where the aetiology of glucose disturbance is multifactorial. Ongoing effect of poor glycaemic control can ultimately contribute to the development of end-organ damage. In the long term, diabetes is associated with increased morbidity and mortality but acute complications of diabetes, such as diabetic ketoacidosis and hyperosmolar hyperglycaemic state, may necessitate patient management in the intensive care unit.

Acute complications of diabetes

Diabetic ketoacidosis (DKA) and hyperosmolar hyperglycaemic state (HHS) are two extremes of what can occur when a deficiency in insulin is present.[99] DKA is a metabolic derangement resulting from a relative or absolute insulin deficiency, characterised by hyperglycaemia (>11.1 mmol/L), metabolic acidosis (pH <7.3) and ketosis (raised blood ketone bodies or ketonuria).[100] It is usually precipitated, in insulin- and non-insulin-dependent diabetics, by infection or the omission (or inadequate dosing) of insulin.[101] It may also be the cause of the first presentation in new-onset diabetes. Additionally, DKA is increasingly being identified in patients with type 2 diabetes.[102]

HHS is seen more often in older patients with type 2 diabetes, and is characterised by hyperglycaemia and the pathological consequences of extreme dehydration. Unlike DKA, where there is insufficient insulin, in HHS insulin excretion is maintained, so lipolysis and ketoacidosis do not feature. Although DKA and HHS are considered separate entities, DKA and HHS may coexist in about a third of cases, especially among older patients.[103]

While these are often considered two distinct states, they can present simultaneously.[104] DKA usually occurs much more quickly with the onset of HHS being more insidious. Both complications are characterised by polyuria, polydipsia and weight loss. Patients with DKA can also present with nausea and vomiting.[105] A comparison of DKA with HHS is provided in Table 20.6.

TABLE 20.6

Comparison of presentation and electrolyte deficits in DKA and HHS[105]

PRESENTATION	DKA	HHS
Prodromal illness	Days	Weeks
Coma	++	+++
Blood glucose	++	+++
Ketone	+++	0 or +
Acidaemia	+++	0 or +
Anion gap	++	0 or +
Osmolality	++	+++
TYPICAL DEFICITS		
Total water (litres)	6	9
Water (mL/kg)	100	100–200
Na^+ (mmol/kg)	7–10	5–13
Cl^- (mmol/kg)	3–5	5–15
K^+ (mmol/kg)	3–5	4–6
PO_4 (mmol/kg)	5–7	3–7
Mg^{2+} (mmol/kg)	0.5–1.0	0.5–1.0
Ca^{2+} (mmol/kg)	0.5–1.0	0.5–1.0

Adapted with permission from Keays RT. Diabetic emergencies. In: Bersten AD, Soni N, eds. Oh's intensive care manual. 6th ed. Philadelphia: Elsevier; 2009, pp 613–20.

Pathophysiology

The metabolic profile seen in DKA is similar to that seen in the fasting state, with substrate utilisation shifting from glucose to fat in insulin-sensitive tissues (fat, liver, muscles). The brain is insulin-insensitive, and requires a continuous supply of glucose to support metabolism even in a fasting state or DKA.[106]

Inadequate production (or administration) of insulin to meet metabolic need (or a rise in metabolic demand resulting from the stress of infection, trauma or surgery, for instance) is associated with a rise in the secretion of the counter-regulatory hormones glucagon, the catecholamines and cortisol.[107] The effects of the counter-regulatory hormones are presented in Box 20.1.

BOX 20.1

Effects of counter-regulatory hormones in DKA[108,109]
- Catecholamines:
  - Promote lipolysis, resulting in the production of FFA and glycerol; FFA and glycerol used as precursors for gluconeogenesis
- Glucagon:
  - Stimulates gluconeogenesis
- Cortisol:
  - Promotes lipolysis
  - Promotes protein breakdown and release of amino acids
  - Promotes hepatic gluconeogenesis

DKA = diabetic ketoacidosis; FFA = free fatty acids.

Hyperglycaemia results from increased gluconeogenesis (glucose production from precursors other than carbohydrates, e.g. amino acids), the conversion of glycogen stores to glucose (glycogenolysis) and the reduced uptake of glucose resulting from insulin deficiency.[107] Free fatty acids and glycerol are produced by the breakdown of triglycerides that results from increased catecholamine secretion.[107] Metabolism of free fatty acids results in accumulation of ketone bodies or ketoacids (acetone, beta-hydroxybutyrate, acetoacetate).[107] These compensatory mechanisms are ultimately responsible for the pathophysiological effects seen in DKA (see Table 20.7). The pathophysiology of DKA is illustrated in Figure 20.3.

Management of diabetic ketoacidosis and hyperosmolar hyperglycaemic state

Management of DKA involves rehydration and electrolyte replacement, insulin administration, correction of acidosis and treatment of the precipitating factor.[106,112] Although historically the approach to managing DKA

has been variable, there is evidence to suggest that a standardised approach can have a positive impact on patient outcome.[113,114]

Management of HHS is similar to that for DKA, and includes: respiratory support; fluid replacement; insulin treatment to turn off ketogenesis and the accompanying metabolic derangement; electrolyte replacement; correction of acidosis (in DKA); monitoring for and prevention of complications of hypoglycaemia, hypokalaemia, hyperglycaemia and fluid volume overload; and patient teaching and support.[100,115,116] Assessment of blood glucose levels is essential.

Effectiveness of treatment is usually assessed by resolution of the acidosis and the control of hyperglycaemia. Regular testing of arterial blood gases, blood sugar and electrolytes (especially potassium) is vital until the blood sugar has stabilised and the ketosis and acidosis resolves.[105] Considering that fewer patients are now admitted to ICU with DKA and HHS, understanding the management of these patients is vital and protocols have been developed to guide practice.[115,116]

FIGURE 20.3 Pathophysiology of diabetic ketoacidosis.[106,108]

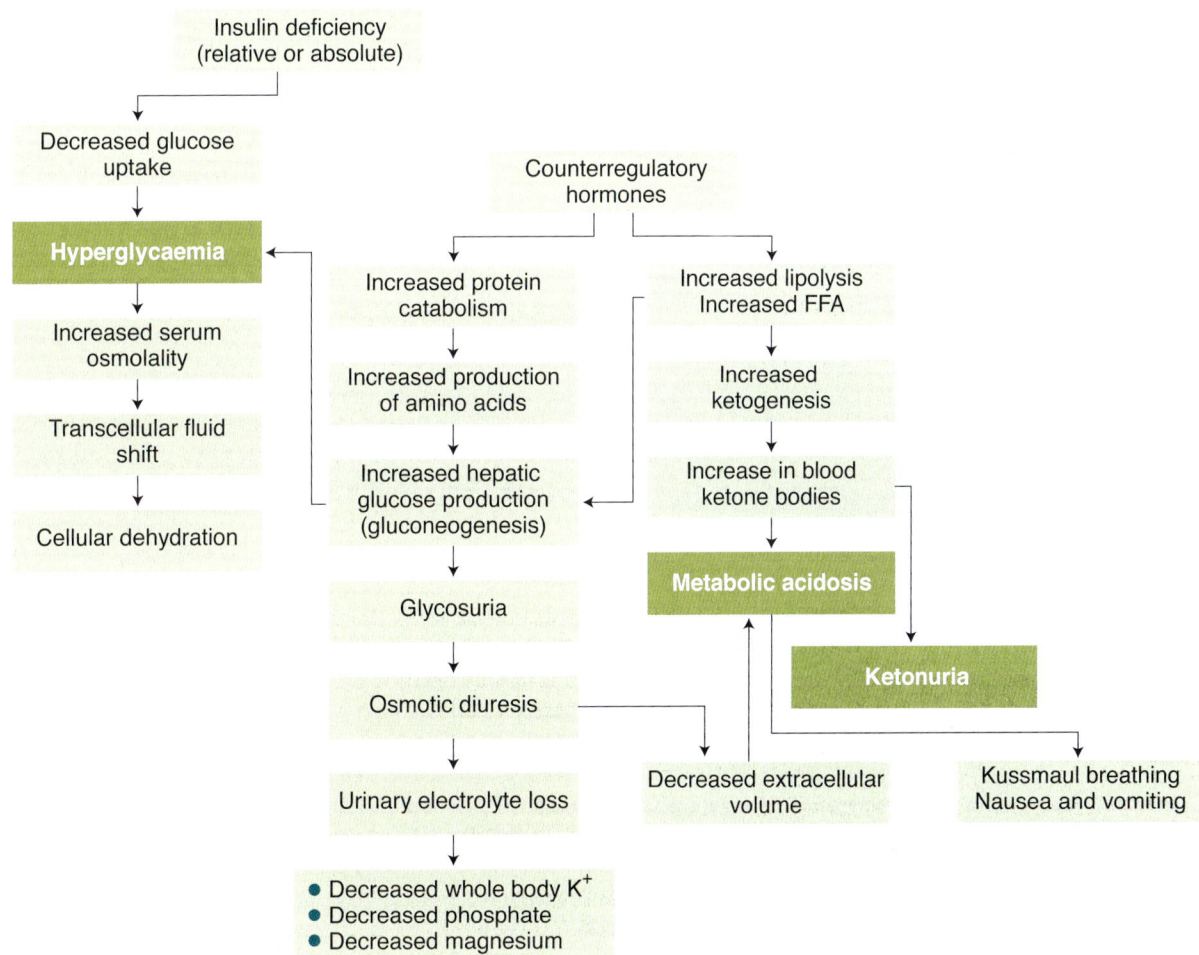

TABLE 20.7

Pathological effects of diabetic ketoacidosis (DKA)

MECHANISM	ACTION
Cellular dehydration and intravascular volume depletion	• Hyperglycaemia increases the extracellular fluid osmolality and results in water movement from the cell • Osmotic diuresis results from obligatory excretion of glucose in the urine • Osmotic diuresis results in reduction of total body water and severe dehydration
Metabolic acidosis	• Ketoacids are fully dissociated at physiological pH (strong acids). Because of the complete dissociation, acetoacetate and beta-hydroxybutyrate are strong ions (anions)[108] • The metabolic acidosis is explained by extracellular (and intracellular) buffering of the dissociated H⁺, resulting in a decrease in bicarbonate. Alternatively, the acidosis can be explained by accumulation of strong anions (acetoacetate and beta-hydroxybutyrate) with resulting reduction of the strong ion difference, causing an increased H⁺ dissociation from plasma water and thus a metabolic acidosis[110,111] • The presence of ketone bodies widens the anion gap, strong ion gap and base excess gap. These 'gaps' can be used to assess the degree of ketonaemia. As ketosis resolves, acidosis caused by high chloride relative to sodium levels is often seen and probably results from administration of normal saline in the initial resuscitation, especially in the setting of decreased renal function where the ability to excrete chloride is reduced
Electrolyte imbalances	• The osmotic diuresis results in potassium, phosphate and magnesium loss • Total body potassium losses are particularly significant, as potassium shifts from the intracellular to the extracellular space in concert with the osmotically driven water shift. Acidosis and lack of insulin exacerbates the potassium shift. The final pathway for potassium loss is via the urine[108]

Blood ketones (beta-hydroxybutyrate) can now easily be measured using blood from a finger prick with a bedside handheld monitor. It has been suggested that blood ketone monitoring allows for insulin titration with reference to ketones in addition to usual blood sugar monitoring.[117] An outline of the treatment of DKA and HHS is presented in Table 20.8.

TABLE 20.8

Treatment of DKA and HHS[105,106]

ISSUE	TREATMENT CONSIDERATIONS
Dehydration and sodium loss	• Intravenous fluid is initially given to restore intravascular volume. Isotonic fluid such as normal saline or a colloid solution may be used. Solutions containing sodium are used in order to replace sodium lost as a result of the osmotic diuresis • Assessment of volume status is undertaken using basic clinical assessment, such as heart rate, blood pressure, urine output (allowing for the possibility of continuing osmotically-driven diuresis) or invasive haemodynamic monitoring • Hypotonic solutions are added after the initial fluid resuscitation to correct the total body water deficit • Adequate resuscitation and rehydration reduces the effect of the counter-regulatory hormones
Insulin therapy	• A soluble insulin is usually administered via continuous infusion to allow rapid titration of dose • Blood glucose levels and blood chemistry should be regularly monitored • Care is taken to prevent too rapid a change in blood sugar level, as this will cause a rapid reduction in the extracellular fluid osmolarity. This rapid reduction would result in fluid shift from the extracellular space to the intracellular space, which may result in cerebral oedema • There is a risk of hypoglycaemia resulting from insulin therapy. Sympathetic activation accompanies a low blood glucose level and results in sweating, tremor, tachycardia and anxiety. Reduced blood glucose levels also cause global central nervous system depression and result in decreased level of consciousness and possibly fitting. Severe hypoglycaemia with a blood glucose level <2 mmol/L is a medical emergency and is treated with administration of 50 mL 50% glucose
Electrolytes	• Intravenous potassium replacement will be required • Plasma potassium levels will fall rapidly as a result of commencement of insulin therapy and, to a lesser extent, with rehydration. Insulin causes the lowering of plasma potassium by mediating the re-entry of potassium into the intracellular compartment • Phosphate and magnesium replacement may be required

Liver dysfunction

The liver is responsible for a vast array of metabolic functions. It performs the vital functions of controlling metabolic pathways, participating in digestion, immunological protection, detoxifying chemicals and clearing toxins and drugs. This means that alterations to normal liver function can have broad-ranging consequences, from changes in metabolic processes (such as glucose homeostasis), failure to produce clotting factors (with resultant severe haemorrhage) to other organ effects such as brain, lung and kidney impairment and injury. Accordingly, liver dysfunction can impact substantially on the nursing care needs of the critically ill patient.

Related anatomy and physiology

The liver is the largest internal organ, weighing approximately 1200 to 1600 g in the adult. It receives approximately 25% of total cardiac output through a dual vascular supply consisting of the hepatic artery and portal vein. Approximately 75% of all hepatic blood flow arises from the portal vein with the remaining 25% from the hepatic artery. Anatomically, the liver consists of four lobes: the major left and right lobes and the minor caudate and quadrate lobes. The right lobe is considerably larger than the left. Functionally, the liver is divided into eight segments each with their own inflow and outflow blood supply and biliary drainage. Hepatic lobules, or liver *acinus*, are small units consisting of a single or double layer of hepatocytes arranged in plates interspersed with capillaries (sinusoids) that receive inflowing blood from the portal and hepatic pathways. To protect the systemic circulation from the toxins absorbed from the intestines, the sinusoids are lined with macrophages known as Kupffer cells. The hepatic vein then drains effluent blood from the liver into the general circulation.

The liver is responsible for the synthesis and drainage system for bile (used in the breakdown and absorption of lipids from the intestine). Biliary salts are formed from multiple enzymatic reactions in the hepatocytes. Bile drains from the hepatocytes into bile ducts and then into the common hepatic duct, before passing into the gall bladder via the common bile duct.[118]

The arrangement of the circulation to the liver with its rich vascular architecture enables it to perform the vital functions of carbohydrate, fat and protein metabolism; production of bile to aid in digestion; production, conjugation and elimination of bilirubin; immunological and inflammatory responses; glycogen storage; and detoxification of toxins and drugs. As the kidneys are responsible for clearance of water-soluble toxins from the body, the liver clears protein (largely albumin)-bound toxins and excretes them into the gastrointestinal tract for elimination, or reabsorption in water-soluble form for subsequent renal excretion.[118]

Mechanisms of liver cell injury

Liver cell injury and death can occur either as a direct result of injury to the cell, resulting in cell necrosis, or as a result of cellular stress and the triggering of apoptotic pathways, leading to programmed cell death. Major factors for the triggering of the apoptotic pathway are hypoxia causing ischaemia and reperfusion; reactive oxygen metabolites resulting from alcohol or drug ingestion; accumulation of bile acids resulting from cholestasis; and inflammatory cytokines such as tumour necrosis factor alpha (TNF-α).[119] The apoptotic pathway results in the deconstruction of the cellular structure from the inside out, while necrosis results in cell rupture and release of cellular contents. Although these processes may overlap, it is thought that the apoptotic pathway is a way of preventing the inflammatory response that is triggered with cell necrosis. The activation of the inflammatory response results in secondary liver cell injury and contributes to the multiple organ dysfunction seen in liver failure.[119,120]

The degree and time course of liver cell damage from viral hepatitis depends on the immune response. Immune recognition and destruction of infected cells may result in either clearance of the virus or ongoing inflammation, cell death and fibrosis if the virus is not cleared. This process may progress over 20–40 years to cirrhosis and hepatocellular carcinoma.[121] Chronic excessive alcohol intake may also result in a slower chronic course of liver injury that eventually results in cirrhosis, liver failure or hepatocellular carcinoma.[122]

Liver cells may also be injured by the toxic effects of drugs or their metabolites, as in paracetamol overdose, or by therapeutic doses of drugs such as non-steroidal anti-inflammatory drugs, phenytoin or antimalarial agents. Other poisoning from the ingestion of mushrooms (e.g. *Amanita phalloides*) and from the use of recreational drugs such as ecstasy and amphetamines may result in liver cell death and liver failure.[123–125] Diseases of the biliary system such as primary biliary cirrhosis and primary sclerosing cholangitis also result in liver dysfunction and failure.[126,127]

The liver has a remarkable regenerative capacity. After injury and necrosis, liver cells rapidly regenerate around areas of surviving cells to restore the lost tissue while maintaining homeostasis during hepatic regeneration.[128,129] However, with chronic injury, fibrosis or scarring occurs, resulting in the loss of the functional architecture and cell mass and ultimately in cirrhosis. Cirrhosis results in destruction of the normal liver vasculature, increased resistance to blood flow and back pressure into the portal circulation. Dilation of the venous system leading into the liver results in the formation of varices.[130]

Liver cell injury may occur to such a degree that a critical amount of hepatic necrosis results in the failure of the liver to maintain metabolic, synthetic and clearance functions leading to death. Liver cell injury may also occur more slowly, giving rise to chronic liver injury.[131]

Epidemiology of viral hepatitis

Worldwide, the incidence of hepatitis B and C is estimated to be 390 million.[121,132–135] This has led to a high mortality rate from hepatitis accounting for approximately 1.3 million deaths worldwide annually.[136,137] In Australia and New Zealand, chronic hepatitis B and hepatitis C viral infections are the major cause of hepatic dysfunction that may lead to cirrhosis and hepatocellular carcinoma. While the prevalence of hepatitis B in Australia and New Zealand is generally low, newly diagnosed infection rates are predominantly related to people with a recent history of injecting drug use.[138] In Australia in 2013, approximately 230,000 people were living with chronic hepatitis C infection, with 58,000 in the moderate-to-severe liver disease category.[138] It should be noted, however, that approximately 25% of people with hepatitis C virus exposure have cleared the virus and are not chronically infected. Also, many patients can be cured of hepatitis C virus due to newer therapies; however, lack of access to antiviral therapy may limit the number of people who can be successfully treated and reducing newer infections is a major focus of health organisations.[139]

Liver dysfunction/failure

Liver dysfunction can be acute or chronic. Chronic liver disease is usually associated with cirrhosis and can develop from viral (hepatitis B and C), drug (alcohol), metabolic (Wilson's disease) or autoimmune (primary biliary cirrhosis) conditions. Acute liver failure (ALF) is an uncommon condition associated with rapid liver dysfunction leading to jaundice, hepatic encephalopathy and coagulopathy.[140] Terminology for acute liver failure is not standardised and several terms have been proposed, including acute hepatic failure and fulminant hepatic failure. Historically, fulminant hepatic failure was used to refer to the rapid onset of liver failure accompanied by hepatic encephalopathy within 8 weeks of diagnosis in the absence of pre-existing liver disease.[141] Unfortunately, this was problematic because determining the onset of jaundice and encephalopathy is often difficult and coagulation results, such as INR, are more reliable indicators of liver failure. It has also been proposed that 'hyperacute', 'acute' and 'subacute' liver failure should be used instead,[142] with hyperacute referring to the development of encephalopathy within 7 days of the onset of jaundice, acute related to 8–28 days from jaundice to encephalopathy and subacute liver failure when encephalopathy occurs within 5–12 weeks of the onset of jaundice.[142] It has further been proposed that acute and subacute hepatic failure should be used;[143] however, universal acceptance of these terms has not occurred with clinical use of all of the above terms.

Acute liver failure without pre-existing liver disease can result from drug reactions, toxins or viral infection, or from the effect on inflammatory mediators released in response to tissue injury. Liver failure can also occur as an acute decompensation of chronic liver disease, described as acute-on-chronic liver failure (AoCLF), or as an end-stage decompensation in chronic liver failure. AoCLF can be precipitated by bacterial or viral infection, bleeding or intoxication, and results in the same clinical syndrome as seen in ALF.[140]

End-stage decompensation of chronic liver failure represents irreversible deterioration with inadequate residual function to maintain homeostasis, and liver transplantation is the only viable treatment. However, in AoCLF, the function of the residual liver cell mass may be adequate to maintain hepatic homeostasis if the precipitating event can be treated.

Liver dysfunction is also a common consequence of critical illness, and may be caused by inadequate perfusion leading to ischaemic injury or as a result of the inflammatory response in sepsis. Given the number of drugs that critically ill patients receive, the possibility of liver injury as a result of drug reactions and toxicity should always be considered.

Consequences of liver failure

The consequences of liver failure manifest as a syndrome of hepatic encephalopathy (HE), hepatorenal syndrome (HRS), oesophageal and gastric varices, ascites, respiratory compromise, haemodynamic instability, susceptibility to infection, coagulopathy and metabolic derangement.[140]

Hepatic encephalopathy

Hepatic encephalopathy is a reversible neuropsychiatric complication due to metabolic dysfunction associated with liver disease.[144] The cerebral effects of liver failure may manifest as an altered sleep–wake cycle, mild confusion/disorientation, asterixis and coma. Patients with AoCLF may develop a mild degree of cerebral oedema, while a differential feature of ALF is the risk of death from cerebral oedema and raised intracranial pressure.[145]

The exact mechanisms responsible for the development of hepatic encephalopathy are unknown, although raised ammonia levels resulting from the failure of the liver urea cycle are thought to be central to the pathogenesis. The raised ammonia levels disrupt the blood–brain barrier, which leads to the development of cerebral oedema. Ammonia levels also seem to be related to the disruption of neurotransmission, resulting in decreased cerebral function.[145,146] In addition, reactive oxidative species causing oxidative stress and inflammatory cytokine release have been suggested; however, the exact pathophysiology is yet to be fully elucidated.[147]

Hepatic encephalopathy is usually classified using the West Haven criteria,[148] a four-stage scale, according to the severity of clinical signs and symptoms (Table 20.9). Although used in clinical practice, the West Haven criteria have poor sensitivity and no inherent metric component. For instance, in patients with grades III–IV encephalopathy, the Glasgow Coma Scale (GCS) is probably a more sensitive tool for neurological assessment.[145] Accordingly, other grading criteria have been proposed but are yet to be validated in large clinical trials.[149,150]

Hepatorenal syndrome

Hepatorenal syndrome (HRS) is the development of renal failure in patients with severe liver disease (acute or chronic), in the absence of any other identifiable cause of renal dysfunction. HRS that develops rapidly in the setting of ALF or AoCLF is classified as type 1 HRS, while

TABLE 20.9

West Haven grading of hepatic encephalopathy[148]

GRADE	CHARACTERISTICS
I	Trivial lack of awareness Euphoria or anxiety Shortened attention span Impaired performance of simple tests, e.g. addition
II	Lethargy or apathy Subtle personality changes Inappropriate behaviour
III	Somnolence to semi-stupor, but unresponsive to verbal stimuli Confusion Gross disorientation
IV	Coma: unresponsive to verbal or painful stimuli

type 2 HRS is slowly progressing and is usually associated with diuretic-resistant ascites.[151]

The pathophysiological features of HRS appear to be caused by an inflammatory response from the injured liver, resulting in upregulation of nitric oxide production that results in splanchnic vasodilation.[152,153] Splanchnic vasodilation results in redistribution of circulating blood volume and a lowered mean arterial pressure. The reduction in perfusion pressure results in an enhanced sympathetic nervous system response and local renal autoregulatory responses. The net result of these effects is a reduction in renal blood flow and increased activity of the renin–angiotensin–aldosterone system, resulting in sodium (aldosterone) and water retention (arginine vasopressin; see Chapter 18).

Practice tip

Avoid using lactate- or citrate-buffered substitution/dialysis fluid for renal replacement therapy in patients with liver dysfunction, as they will be unable to metabolise the lactate or citrate and will develop an increasing metabolic acidosis.

Varices and variceal bleeding

The development of varices and variceal bleeding arises from portal hypertension. This manifests when blood flowing from an area of high pressure (i.e. the cirrhotic liver) to areas of lower pressure (i.e. the collateral circulation, involving veins of the oesophagus, spleen, intestines and stomach) causes the tiny, thin-walled vessels to become engorged and dilated, forming varices that are vulnerable to gastric secretions, resulting in rupture and haemorrhage.[154] Variceal haemorrhage is a major cause of acute decompensation and a reason for admission to the ICU. It is an acute clinical event characterised by severe gastrointestinal haemorrhage presenting as haematemesis, with or without melaena, and haemodynamic instability (tachycardia and hypotension).[155]

Practice tip

Coagulation state and the risk of trauma to varices should be carefully considered before insertion of nasogastric or orogastric tubes, or suctioning of the upper airway. Trauma may result in epistaxis with significant bleeding or variceal bleeding.

Ascites

Ascites is usually present in patients with chronic liver disease. In the ICU setting it becomes an issue when abdominal pressures rise, resulting in reduced cardiac output due to decreased venous return and renal impairment. Pressure on the diaphragm causes loss of lung volume, resulting in increased work of breathing and compromised oxygenation.

Respiratory compromise

Patients with liver failure may have poor oxygen exchange, fluctuating GCS that requires intubation for airway protection and hepatopulmonary syndrome. Hepatopulmonary syndrome is found in 15–20% of patients with cirrhosis.[156] It is defined as pulmonary microvascular dilation resulting in impaired oxygenation, and it is generally assumed that vascular production of vasodilators, specifically nitric oxide, underlies the vasodilation in hepatopulmonary syndrome. It has also been hypothesised that the mechanisms that trigger hepatopulmonary syndrome are the same as those that result in the hyperdynamic circulation (low systemic vascular resistance and high cardiac output) seen in liver failure.[156] Other factors, such as pleural effusions or severe ascites, may impinge on ventilation.

Haemodynamic instability, susceptibility to infection, coagulopathy and metabolic derangement

A hyperdynamic, low vascular resistance picture, similar to that associated with sepsis, is seen in liver dysfunction. This probably results from the production of vasodilator substances (nitric oxide) from the inflammatory response of the injured liver cells.[157] Sepsis may also be a complication of liver dysfunction because of the failure of the liver to produce acute-phase proteins and the impaired function of Kupffer cells.[158]

Hepatocyte damage leads to a decreased production of the majority of clotting factors and, therefore, haemostasis. Hence, the risk of bleeding is elevated.[159] Disordered metabolic function and failure of synthetic function can manifest as unstable blood glucose levels.

Practice tip

Patients in ALF or AoCLF are at risk of hypoglycaemia, and blood glucose levels should be measured routinely.

Patient management

Early signs of the patient presenting with ALF are malaise, loss of appetite, fatigue, nausea, jaundice, bruising, bleeding, inflamed/enlarged liver, possibly epigastric and right-upper-quadrant pain, deranged liver function tests, fluctuating GCS due to cerebral oedema and high or low blood glucose levels.[140] Fluctuating blood glucose levels may require close monitoring, at least every 4 hours; patients may require insulin infusion or 10–50% dextrose infusion to maintain normoglycaemia. If acute liver failure is suspected, admission to an ICU is recommended to monitor for further deterioration, and provide supportive management and airway protection. The patient presenting with AoCLF will have similar symptoms but will present with other unique characteristics. Cirrhosis and portal hypertension will often lead to oesophageal and gastric varices, ascites, hepatorenal and hepatopulmonary syndrome, malnutrition, bone disease, sepsis, palmar erythema, spider naevi and feminisation in males.[122] If liver failure is suspected, investigating ingestion of hepatotoxic substances, such as paracetamol, steroids and ethanol, oral or intravenous recreational drug use and any recent travel that might have exposed the patient to viral infections is required.

Neurological considerations

Cerebral oedema is present in 80% of patients with grade IV encephalopathy and is the leading cause of death due to brain herniation.[160] Patients with cerebral oedema and raised intracranial pressure due to ALF are managed primarily as patients with acute head injury (see Chapter 17).

Assessment of liver function

Patients presenting with ALF require a careful history to establish the cause of liver injury. The well-known signs of chronic liver disease (e.g. palmar erythema, spider naevi and ascites) may not be present. Biochemical and haematological tests determine whether liver cell injury is occurring, with liver synthesis and clearance functions assessed by albumin level and prothrombin time, and bilirubin level, respectively.[161] These measures have been incorporated into a scoring system to determine liver dysfunction and prognostic information for liver transplantation suitability (model for end-stage liver disease [MELD], see later in this chapter under *Liver transplantation*).[162] Liver function test values and indications are listed in Table 20.10.

TABLE 20.10
Liver function tests[163]

BLOOD TEST	NORMAL VALUE	DESCRIPTION
Alanine aminotransferase (ALT) and aspartate aminotransferase (AST)	ALT: <35 U/L AST: <40 U/L	• ALT and AST are enzymes that indicate liver cell damage; they are produced within the liver cells (hepatocytes) and leak out into the general circulation when the liver cells are damaged • ALT is a more specific indication of liver inflammation • In acute liver injury, ALT and AST may be elevated to the high 100s, even 1000s, of U/L • In chronic liver damage, such as hepatitis or cirrhosis, there may be mild-to-moderate elevation (100–300 U/L) • ALT and AST are commonly used to measure the course of chronic hepatitis and the response to treatments
Alkaline phosphatase (ALP) and gamma-glutamyl-transpeptidase (GGT)	ALP: 25–100 U/L GGT: males <50 U/L; females <30 U/L	• These are enzymes that indicate obstruction to the biliary system • They are produced in the liver, or within the larger bile channels outside the liver • GGT is used as the supplementary test to be sure that a rise in ALP is indeed coming from the liver or biliary tree • A rise in GGT but normal ALP may indicate liver enzyme changes induced by alcohol or medications, causing no injury to the liver • ALP and GGT are commonly used to measure bile flow obstructions due to disorders such as gallstones, a tumour blocking the common bile duct, biliary tree damage, alcoholic liver disease or drug-induced hepatitis
Bilirubin	< 20 micromol/L	Results from the breakdown of red blood cells. Thus bilirubin is protein-bound and circulates in the blood in an unconjugated form. The liver processes bilirubin to a water-soluble conjugated form that is excreted in the urine and faeces. • Liver injury or cholestasis results in an elevated bilirubin level • Raised unconjugated bilirubin without an accompanying rise in conjugated bilirubin is consistent with red blood cell destruction (haemolysis) • Raised bilirubin levels result in jaundice • In cases of chronic liver disease, bilirubin levels usually remain normal until significant damage occurs and cirrhosis develops • In cases of acute liver failure (ALF), bilirubin levels will rise rapidly and result in marked jaundice; the degree of rise is indicative of the severity of illness
Albumin	32–45 g/L	• Albumin is a major protein formed by the liver; it provides a gauge of liver synthetic function (i.e. albumin levels are lowered in liver disease)

Treatment

ALF or AoCLF therapy often involves the support and treatment of the consequences of liver failure, such as sepsis, encephalopathy, renal failure and coagulopathy (see Table 20.11). Treatments are usually directed to supportive therapy, depending on the severity of manifestation; however, liver transplantation is used according to selection criteria in acute liver failure and several different liver support systems have been trialled without long-term survival benefits.[164]

Oesophageal balloon tamponade and transjugular intrahepatic portosystemic stent/shunt

There are two types of balloon tamponade devices available on the market: the Sengstaken-Blakemore tube and the Linton tube. The Sengstaken-Blakemore is a four-lumen tube with oesophageal and gastric balloons, and oesophageal and gastric aspiration ports. The benefit of this tube is that direct pressure can be applied to gastric and oesophageal varices by balloon inflation and traction.[166] The Linton tube has one lumen for inflation of the pear-shaped gastric balloon and two additional lumens for oesophageal and gastric aspiration.

Prior to insertion (oral or nasal), balloons are lubricated, checked for leakage and the distance to the cardio-oesophageal junction is estimated (nose to ear, then to xiphisternum). Once inserted, the gastric balloon is inflated with 50 mL air and pulled back until resistance is felt. Position (lying compressed against the cardio-oesophageal junction) is confirmed by X-ray. Then, the gastric balloon is inflated according to the manufacturer's instructions and

TABLE 20.11

Treatment of liver failure complications

CONDITION	TREATMENT
Hepatic encephalopathy	• Treatment revolves around general supportive therapy until liver function recovers or liver transplant is undertaken[145,146] • Cerebral oedema and raised intracranial pressure are treated as for an acute head injury (see Chapter 17) • Reduce production and absorption of ammonia by preventing/controlling upper gastrointestinal bleeding and gastrointestinal administration of non-absorbable disaccharides such as lactulose or lactitol to remove protein derived from dietary intake or bleeding[165]
Hepatorenal syndrome (HRS)	• Liver transplant is the primary treatment for type 1 HRS in patients with cirrhosis • If transplant is contraindicated or delayed, vasoconstrictors (e.g. terlipressin) may be effective in constricting the dilated splanchnic arterial bed, thus improving renal perfusion pressure and renal function. Vasoconstrictors may be given in association with intravenous albumin in order to increase intravascular volume[152,153]
Variceal bleeding	A successful outcome, as in all cases of gastrointestinal haemorrhage, hinges on prompt resuscitation, haemodynamic support and correction of haemostatic dysfunction, preferably in the intensive care setting. • The patient is intubated for airway protection • Adequate intravenous access in inserted, preferably large, wide-bore cannulas for rapid fluid resuscitation • Haemodynamic instability is corrected with volume expanders initially and then blood products • The source of bleeding is identified by endoscope, and varices are banded/ligated (latex bands placed around the varices to 'strangle' the vessel), or sclerotherapy or diathermy (heat used to cauterise bleeding vessel) is used • Terlipressin and octreotide infusions may be used to reduce portal circulation pressure • If bleeding is uncontrollable, a balloon tamponade device is inserted
Ascites	Salt and water restrictions along with diuretic therapy are methods that have been used to control ascites in the preliminary phases of end-stage liver failure; however, in the intensive care setting these measures are impractical and usually unsuccessful. • Paracentesis is very effective at reducing ascites and is a simple procedure to remove fluid and an aid in diagnosis • Correction of coagulopathy or thrombocytopenia should be considered when the INR is greater than 2.5 or the platelet count is markedly reduced • Paracentesis may aid in determining the cause of ascites (ascites-serum albumin gradient, ascitic cytology, microscopy and culture for acid-fast bacilli, chylous ascites) and in establishing or excluding primary or secondary peritonitis in patients with ascites (ascitic white cell and neutrophil count, culture) • Litres of ascites are normally removed, and the volume is replaced with IV concentrated albumin to prevent fluid shifts and hypotension • Mean arterial pressures, central venous pressures, heart rate and urine output are carefully monitored during the procedure

traction is applied using a weight (500 or 1000 mL IV fluid bag) attached to rope; traction is applied via a pulley and IV pole at the foot of the bed. Nursing care of patients involves:

- sedation for comfort
- head of the bed raised at least 30° to facilitate gastric emptying and prevent aspiration
- ensuring that gastric/oesophageal ports are on free drainage, with regular monitoring of type and amount of drainage
- ensuring that correct traction is maintained, with regular checking of tube migration and checking position at nares/lips at regular intervals (4/24 hours).[166]

Tamponade is generally maintained for 24–48 hours, then traction is removed and the balloon deflated to assess for further bleeding. If the patient is stabilised, endoscopy can be performed. If bleeding persists, the balloon(s) is/are reinflated and traction reapplied.[166]

Once the patient has been stabilised, a transjugular intrahepatic portosystemic stent/shunt, also known as TIPS, may be considered to control variceal haemorrhage. TIPS is a metal expandable stent inserted to decompress the portal venous system.[167]

Extracorporeal liver support

The aim of extracorporeal liver support therapy is to allow time for liver recovery or to provide support until a liver transplant is possible.[149,168,169] There are two main types of extracorporeal liver support therapy, namely artificial and bioartificial devices. The artificial devices are cell-free systems that use a combination of dialysis, mainly using albumin, and plasma exchange.[170] These systems aim to reduce toxins and have been shown to reduce bilirubin and improve hepatic encephalopathy.[171–173] In contrast, bioartificial extracorporeal liver support devices are biological systems utilising either porcine hepatocytes or a human hepatoblastoma cell line to sustain temporary hepatic function; however the construction and use of these devices is complex and has been limited to specialist centres. There are continuing challenges with extracting viable hepatic cells and incorporation into the bioreactors with which the extracorporeal circuits interface, thereby limiting their use.[168,170]

Despite much research, the clinical use of extracorporeal liver support therapies has been difficult due to a lack of clinical guidelines about when to institute and which types of patients should be selected, and technical considerations, such as flow rate and duration of therapy, have yet to be elucidated.[149,169,171] In many cases, the definitive treatment for severe ALF is liver transplantation when irreversible liver injury has occurred;[161] however, extracorporeal liver support systems may provide sufficient liver support until transplantation is available.[169] To date, evidence suggests that there may be a reduction in mortality in ALF using extracorporeal liver support, yet the number and size of the randomised controlled trials limits clinical efficacy.[172] In patients presenting with AoCLF, there has been little evidence to warrant the use of these liver support systems.[169]

Liver transplantation

Liver transplantation is the definitive treatment for patients suffering acute and chronic end-stage liver failure when other supportive critical care therapies have been exhausted.[161,174] Over the past 20 years, survival after liver transplantation has improved, which has been related to better pre-transplant and postoperative therapies and increases in intraoperative surgical refinement and management.[175] This has also reduced time in critical care and reduced overall hospital length of stay. Survival rates of all patients who have undergone liver transplantation exceed 80% at 1 and 5 years,[176,177] with children having superior survival rates to adults.[176] Acute liver failure patients accounted for 7% in the USA and 8% in Europe of all liver transplantations with lower survival rates (68% at 5 years) compared to all liver transplants.[175]

Indications for transplantation

Indications for liver transplantation are patients with severe liver disease in whom alternative treatments have been exhausted. Categories consist of acute liver failure, end-stage liver disease, metabolic liver disease and primary liver cancer.[178] Timing and patient selection is of critical importance, as this has contributed to the success of transplantation. Re-transplantation for any disorder is considered only in patients with acceptable predicted survival.[179]

Contraindications for transplantation

Patients with extrahepatic malignancy and uncontrolled systemic infection where high-dose immunosuppressive therapy is contraindicated are not suitable for transplantation. In addition, patients with alcoholic liver disease with social instability and patients with inadequate or absent social support are relative contraindications due to increased risk of non-adherence to immunosuppressive therapy.[180]

Recipient selection

Recipient selection for liver transplantation is of critical importance as it affects mortality, especially when determining patients with ALF. There are a variety of prognostic indicators and selection scoring systems, including the Kings College, Clichy, Child-Turcotte-Pugh and model for end-stage liver disease (MELD) classification systems.[161] While there are different systems, most incorporate the severity of hepatic encephalopathy and coagulation status. In Australia and New Zealand, the MELD and paediatric end-stage liver disease (PELD) scoring systems are used for liver transplantation eligibility.[180,181] The MELD score is a mathematical model that includes bilirubin, creatinine and the international normalised ratio (INR), which was originally devised to predict survival after TIPS.[182] The MELD/PELD score is an excellent predictor of mortality, especially in ALF (Figure 20.4).[162,181]

Once the need for transplantation is established, the decision to allocate a donor liver to a patient is based on donor and recipient blood group; donor size and size of

FIGURE 20.4   The model for end-stage liver disease (MELD/PELD) calculation.[162,181]

MELD

$(3.78 \times \log_e [\text{serum bilirubin*}]) + 11.20[\log_e \text{INR}] + 9.57[\log_e \text{serum creatinine*}]$
$+ 6.43 \text{ (constant for liver disease aetiology)}$

PELD

$(0.436 \times \text{age†}) - (0.687 \times \log [\text{albumin\#}]) + (0.480 \times \log [\text{bilirubin*}])$
$+ (1.857 \times \log [\text{INR}]) + (0.667 \times \text{growth failure‡})$

*   measured in mg/dL
\#   measured in g/dL
†   Age < 1 year = 1; all others = 0
‡   Values > 2 standard deviations from the norm = 1; all others = 0

recipient; suitability of donor liver for splitting; severity of disease; matching of functional status of donor with severity of liver disease; and hepatitis B and C status of donor and recipient. Extensive testing and consultation is part of the liver transplant process. Clinical consultation occurs with hepatologists, clinical nurse consultants, social workers, dietitians, psychiatrists, psychologists and drug and alcohol professionals if required.

Surgical techniques

Orthotopic liver transplantation

Orthotopic liver transplantation is the replacement of the diseased liver. It was pioneered in the 1960s and has been improved considerably due to technical aspects of the surgery itself and enhanced haemodynamic stability during the procedure.[183]

Two main techniques are used for orthotopic liver transplantation: portal bypass or the piggyback technique. Portal bypass occurs where an internal temporary portocaval shunt or external veno-venous bypass is used.[184] In the piggyback technique, the recipient's inferior vena cava (IVC) is left and the donor IVC is piggybacked onto the recipient's IVC. The advantages of this technique include haemodynamic stability during the anhepatic phase, reduced operating times and reduced use of blood products, enabling a shorter length of hospital stay.[185]

Split-liver transplantation

The disparity between the increasing number of people on transplant waiting lists and the shortage of donor livers available has led to several innovative strategies. Split-liver transplantation occurs when the donated organ is divided for two recipients, with the larger right segment to an adult and the smaller left lobe to a child.[186] The complication rate is higher in split-liver than whole-liver transplants due to biliary leaks and anastomosis strictures. This technique has significantly reduced the number of children waiting for liver transplantation, although little impact has been made on adult waiting lists.[186]

Adult living donor liver transplantation

Living donor liver transplantation is an established option for paediatric patients with end-stage liver disease.[187]

This technique involves removal of the left lobe from the live donor, usually the recipient's parent, which is then transplanted into the child. It is a relatively straightforward procedure, with little risk to the donor.[187,188]

Postoperative management

Initial management and nursing care

The initial postoperative care of liver transplant patients on return to critical care involves stabilisation, management of positive pressure ventilation, continuous haemodynamic monitoring and physical assessment, as with all critically ill surgical patients. It is common for patients to be hypertensive post-surgery, displaying systolic blood pressure above 160 mmHg with a mean arterial pressure of 110 mmHg. Aggressive treatment is required due to the risk of stroke, which is compounded by low platelet counts and abnormal clotting. Once pain is controlled and excluded as a cause of hypertension, clonidine or hydralazine is considered. Oliguria is commonly related to intraoperative fluid losses and fluid shifts.

Once initial stabilisation is achieved, treatment is governed by clinical progress. Typically, the critical care stay for a routine postoperative liver transplantation does not exceed 24–48 hours; as long as physiological systems are maintained, discharge to the ward can be anticipated. An abdominal CT scan may be considered at 7–10 days postoperatively or when clinically indicated.

The initial postoperative care is similar for all liver transplant patients. However, progress, stability and discharge from critical care can be affected by the patient's preoperative condition and severity of liver failure. The unique pathophysiology inherent in the liver failure patient will predispose to varying effects on coagulopathy, cardiopulmonary, neurological, haemodynamic and metabolic functions.[140,161,189]

Blood loss and coagulopathy

The major risk during and post-surgery is massive blood loss, due to a combination of factors. The surgical process itself involves anastomosis of major arteries and veins, predisposing the patient to bleeding and hypovolaemia during surgery and anastomotic leaks post-surgery.[190] Patients are likely to be coagulopathic from hepatic synthetic dysfunction, leading to failure of synthetic clotting factors.[191] Correction of coagulopathy with blood products such as fresh frozen plasma, platelets, cryoprecipitate and factor VIIa may control minor postoperative bleeding, but if bleeding continues an exploratory laparotomy may be required. Conversely, it is not desirable to overcorrect coagulopathy, due to the potential for vascular complications such as hepatic artery thrombosis. Careful monitoring is required to identify and manage hypotension, tachycardia, excessive blood loss from drains, falling haemoglobin, abdominal swelling and oozing from insertion sites. Thrombocytopenia is a common postoperative problem, with platelet counts often falling in the first week post-transplant. If platelet counts are low, a platelet transfusion may be necessary, especially prior to removal of drains, lines, cannulae and sheaths.

Cardiovascular

Haemodynamic instability in the early postoperative period may be due to hypovolaemia or haemorrhage. Treatment includes fluid boluses to increase preload and the initiation of inotropes may be necessary. The patient may present with a hyperdynamic profile including a high cardiac output, low systemic vascular resistance and low mean arterial pressure,[192] although this usually reverses 1 week after transplantation.

Neurological

The most frequent neurological complications relate to patients with pre-existing hepatic encephalopathy. In ALF patients, cerebral oedema with raised intracranial pressure is common and, after liver transplantation, cerebral oedema may take up to 48 hours to subside. Therefore, continuation of preoperative measures to reduce intracranial pressure is necessary. These include elevating the head of the bed 30°; ensuring head, neck and body alignment; maintaining endotracheal tapes so they are not constrictive to allow venous return and prevent cerebral congestion; reducing neurological stimuli; and timing activities to prevent spikes in intracranial pressure (see Chapter 17).[192,193]

Respiratory

Pre-existing pulmonary complications associated with liver disease can affect postoperative recovery and need to be considered when weaning ventilation and maintaining adequate oxygenation. Patients post-transplant often experience bi-basal collapse and consolidation, and are prone to infection, similar to other critical care patients who undergo complex surgical procedures that are extended.[194] Incentive spirometry, chest physiotherapy, early mobilisation and adequate pain relief are recommended, with early extubation the most effective in reducing pulmonary complications.[194,195]

Gastrointestinal

Patients with end-stage liver disease often have malnutrition and bone disease, which may influence postoperative management. Fluid overload and ascites can quite often mask signs of malnutrition. Early nutrition is imperative in the postoperative period, and enteral feeding can supplement caloric needs (see Chapter 19). If caloric intake is inadequate, consultation with a dietitian will assist with enteral supplementation. Total parenteral nutrition is rarely required.[196]

Renal

Renal dysfunction is a significant post-transplantation problem.[197] Risk factors include pre-existing renal disease or hepatorenal syndrome, intraoperative hypotension, extensive transfusion of blood products, nephrotoxic drugs such as cyclosporin and tacrolimus, sepsis and graft dysfunction.[189] Hepatorenal syndrome is reversible post-transplantation. Patients who are receiving renal support such as continuous renal replacement therapy usually require continuation of renal support postoperatively for a period of time until recovery of kidney function is evident (see Chapter 18).

Graft dysfunction and rejection

Acute graft rejection was the most challenging obstacle in the early years of transplantation but, with the development of current immunosuppressive therapy, acute rejection can be avoided, resulting in improved success rates of transplantation.[198] Immunosuppressive therapy has improved with the use of newer drugs and patients are most commonly placed on a combination of tacrolimus or cyclosporine and steroids.[199,200]

Allograft dysfunction occurs within 48 hours of transplantation, and is characterised by varying degrees of coma, renal failure, worsening coagulopathy, poor bile production and marked elevation in the liver enzymes (AST, ALT) and worsening acidosis. The cause of allograft dysfunction is not always known; possible causes are injury to the liver, either before or during the donor operation procedure, ischaemic-reperfusion injury or graft stenosis. Acute rejection is generally evident in the second week post-transplant, and is generally suspected with an elevation in liver enzymes, a decline in bile quality (only if a T tube is present), occasional fever and tachycardia.

Primary graft non-function is defined as failure of the graft to function in the first postoperative week. It is manifested by failure to regain consciousness, sustained elevated transaminases, increasing coagulopathy, acidosis and poor bile production. Causes include massive haemorrhagic necrosis, ischaemia-reperfusion injury and hepatic artery thrombosis.

Management of late complications

Readmission to critical care after liver transplantation is not uncommon. Factors include cardiopulmonary dysfunction from infection or fluid overload, respiratory failure from collapse and consolidation, tachypnoea, recipient age, preoperative liver function, bilirubin, the amount of blood products administered intraoperatively, graft dysfunction, severe sepsis and postoperative surgical complications such as bleeding and biliary anastomotic leaks.[201] Outcomes are affected by intraoperative and postoperative complications, renal failure, advanced liver disease and malnutrition.[202]

Summary

The gastrointestinal system can become significantly compromised during critical illness. Alterations in the gastrointestinal system can also cause critical illness. The gastrointestinal system involves not just the gastrointestinal tract but also organs that support digestion including the pancreas and liver. Disruptions to the gastrointestinal system and normal gastrointestinal physiology can be altered during critical illness because of redistribution of blood flow away from the gut and other abdominal organs. Specifically, the gastrointestinal system can become hypoperfused and normal physiological processes responsible for digestion, absorption, immunity and protection become compromised.

Critically ill patients can be at risk of developing stress-related mucosal disease although incidence of clinically important bleeding remains relatively low. Nevertheless, it remains common practice to provide stress-ulcer prophylaxis to critically ill patients, particularly for those patients considered at high risk. During critical illness patients may also be at risk for the development of IAH, with approximately half of all ICU patients having increased IAP. Recognising potential risk factors for the development of IAH is essential so that monitoring can be commenced and treatment initiated where necessary.

Critical illness can also result from the inability of the body to effectively use glucose in energy production. An increasing number of people worldwide have diabetes and when illness occurs this can precipitate significant alterations in blood glucose and result in the development of DKA or HHS. Because of the ensuing physiological derangements these patients often need to be admitted to a critical care area for close monitoring and treatment until they are stabilised.

Liver dysfunction causing hepatocellular injury and death can occur due to direct injury or cellular stress. This can be mediated via several avenues, such as metabolic disturbances, ischaemia, inflammatory processes or reactive oxygen metabolites from drug and alcohol ingestion. Acute failure can be acute or preceded by a chronic dysfunction. In Australia and New Zealand, high rates of hepatitis B and C predispose individuals to chronic liver dysfunction that can lead to acute hepatic decompensation. While acute liver failure is uncommon, patients who present are often critically ill. In addition, liver failure causes major disturbances in other body systems often resulting in coagulopathy, cerebral oedema (hepatic encephalopathy), sepsis, renal failure and metabolic derangement. Therapy is usually directed at multi-organ support as extracorporeal liver support therapies have not sufficiently developed to sustain liver function during the acute phase.

Liver transplantation remains the definitive treatment option for acute and chronic liver failure patients when supportive multi-organ therapy is not sustainable. Pre-existing hepatic dysfunction and liver transplantation surgery can lead to a high risk of haemorrhage and coagulopathy postoperatively. Careful haematological management is required to control postoperative bleeding. Clinicians must ensure that patients receive appropriate haemodynamic management for hyperdynamic states and that measures to avoid rises in intracranial pressure are implemented.

Case study

A 56-year-old woman was admitted to the ICU after presenting to the emergency department with icterus and confusion and a history of alcoholism. She was emaciated and dehydrated with renal failure, hyponatraemia, hypokalaemia, tachycardia and tachypnoea. In the emergency department she received thiamine 300 mg, flucloxacillin 2 g, gentamicin 320 mg, ceftriaxone 1 g, acyclovir 400 mg and vitamin K 1 mg. She also received 2 L of normal saline for fluid resuscitation.

On arrival in ICU she became very agitated. She was intubated and sedated and had a central line and arterial line placed and nasogastric tube inserted, through which enteral nutrition was commenced at 20 mL/h. A diagnosis of acute hepatitis was made and an abdominal ultrasound revealed hepatomegaly. She remained mechanically ventilated for 3 days and was then successfully weaned to spontaneous ventilation and extubated. Laboratory tests in ICU revealed disseminated intravascular coagulation (DIC) with an increased INR of 2.2, which decreased to 1.5 by day 4. Following extubation oral intake was poor and to avoid dehydration a central line remained in place in the event parenteral nutrition was required.

The day after extubation the patient deteriorated and showed signs of hepatic encephalopathy. She was highly agitated and confused. She was unable to swallow and had a poor cough. Korsacoff's encephalopathy was diagnosed. She developed left side pneumonitis as a result of aspiration. In consultation with the family treatment limitations were initiated and palliative management was commenced. The patient's condition continued to worsen – resulting in death within 24 hours.

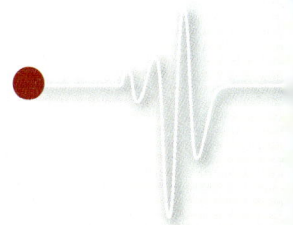

DISCUSSION

Alcoholism results in about 2.5 million deaths worldwide each year and, although it is associated with many diseases, mortality is usually associated with alcoholic liver disease. The development of alcoholic liver disease is dose dependent with the risk of developing the disease increased for both men and women who consume more than 30 g of alcohol per day (a standard drink contains approximately 14 g of alcohol). Women are, however, at increased risk of developing alcoholic liver disease because of differences in the way that they metabolise ethanol.[203]

The spectrum of alcoholic liver disease includes alcoholic fatty liver, alcoholic hepatitis and alcoholic cirrhosis. Alcoholic steatosis is characterised by microvesicular and macrovesicular fat accumulation in the hepatocytes and is often reversible with abstinence. Patients might have elevated liver enzymes and the INR and albumin levels tend to be normal. Alcoholic hepatitis is an inflammatory process with neutrophil infiltration. Clinical findings are similar to what was observed in this case study and include jaundice, pyrexia, unintentional weight loss, malnutrition and a tender, enlarged liver. Liver enzymes are usually moderately elevated. Ascites and encephalopathy might be present.

Alcoholic cirrhosis is less common and present in about 15% of patients with alcoholic liver disease. Patients present with the stigmata of chronic liver disease including gynaecomastia, palmar erythema, spider angiomata, testicular atrophy, parotid gland enlargement and signs of portal hypertension, including caput medusa. There are multiple complications as a result of alcoholic cirrhosis. Patients can exhibit low albumin, increased bilirubin, thrombocytopenia and alterations in coagulation including prolonged prothrombin time and increased INR, as demonstrated in this case study.

Malnutrition is common in alcoholic liver disease and can negatively influence outcomes for critically ill patients (see Chapter 19). This patient was emaciated on admission suggesting prolonged malnutrition. While early nutrition support is important, when long periods of malnutrition have been present it is important to commence enteral nutrition slowly to avoid refeeding syndrome. Refeeding syndrome is associated with severe derangement in fluid and electrolyte levels that may result in significant morbidity and mortality. During commencement of enteral nutrition this patient should have been monitored closely for signs for hypophosphataemia, hypomagnesaemia and hypokalaemia. In this case study, the patient had feeds commenced on admission to ICU but only at 20 mL/h, which would not have met her nutritional requirements. Addition of parenteral nutrition to support nutrition therapy can be implemented alongside enteral nutrition to help match nutrition intake with requirements.

During the ICU admission the patient had DIC. The main feature of DIC is intravascular clotting in the microcirculation, which can contribute to the development of multiple organ failure. Platelets and coagulation factors were also depleted and these cannot be quickly replaced by the liver and bone marrow. Consequently, this microvascular formation of clots occurs alongside the inability to form clots where needed, resulting in bleeding.

As the patient's condition continued to deteriorate a decision was made with the family to limit treatment.

CASE STUDY QUESTIONS

1   What management might you expect for this patient specific to the diagnosis of DIC?
2   Following extubation all critically ill patients are at risk for decreased nutritional intake. What strategies might be useful in ensuring adequate nutrition in this case study?
3   Describe the nursing management of a patient with hepatic encephalopathy.

RESEARCH VIGNETTE

Hunt L, Frost SA, Hillman K, Newton PJ, Davidson PM. Management of intra-abdominal hypertension and abdominal compartment syndrome: a review. J Trauma Manag Outcomes 2014;8(1):2

Patients in the intensive care unit (ICU) are at risk of developing of intra-abdominal hypertension (IAH) and abdominal compartment syndrome (ACS).

Aim: This review seeks to define IAH and ACS, identify the aetiology and presentation of IAH and ACS, identify IAP measurement techniques, identify current management and discuss the implications of IAH and ACS for nursing practice. A search of the electronic databases was supervised by a health librarian. The electronic databases Cumulative Index of Nursing and Allied Health Literature (CINAHL), Medline, EMBASE and the World Wide Web were searched from 1996 to January 2011 using MeSH and key words that included but were not limited to: abdominal compartment syndrome, intra-abdominal hypertension, intra-abdominal pressure in adult populations. Articles that met the search criteria were reviewed by three authors using a critical appraisal tool. Data derived from the retrieved material are discussed under the following themes: 1) aetiology of intra-abdominal hypertension; 2) strategies for measuring intra-abdominal pressure; 3) the manifestation of abdominal compartment syndrome; and 4) the importance of nursing assessment, observation and interventions. Intra-abdominal pressure (IAP) and abdominal compartment syndrome (ACS) have the potential to alter organ perfusion and compromise organ function.

Critique

This integrative review provides a summary of the literature on IAH and abdominal compartment syndrome, including measurement techniques, and goes beyond other reviews[79,204] by providing a discussion of the implications for nursing practice. The methodology provides a description of the databases searched and keywords used in the search. The search terms used, however, aren't described in a way that would permit replication of the search as the way in which search terms have been combined and the databases to which they are applied are not clear. The omission of medical subject headings (MeSH) could have resulted in some relevant papers being omitted from the search results. The search is strengthened by the inclusion of hand searching relevant reference lists for additional publications, although no further publications were identified through this method.

In total 514 articles were retrieved, although it is not clear from the flow diagram which databases yielded the most results. According to the flow diagram 374 papers were excluded. It is not clear how many of these papers were duplicates. The reasons for exclusion of papers are provided but confusing. Specifically, they refer to papers being excluded because they were 'not culture related' , were 'ICU practice culture' or 'other discipline practice culture'; this is confusing and it is difficult to see how these exclusion criteria related to the stated aim of the paper.

Although the authors indicate that papers meeting the aim of the review were included the inclusion/exclusion criteria were not clearly articulated so the decision path is not clear. Whether all manuscript types were included or only those based on primary research is not stated although review of the reference list suggests that opinion pieces and/or discussion papers might have been included. Figure 1 in the article provides an overview of the flowchart for the study selection process and indicates that a total of 53 papers were included in the review. The data from papers included in this review are summarised according to key areas including: diagnosis of IAH; aetiology of IAH; IAP measurement; definition of abdominal compartment syndrome; indications for IAP monitoring; and implications for nursing practice.

As a summary paper, this integrative review provides a broad overview of IAH and abdominal compartment syndrome and includes important aspects of nursing practice. Aspects of nursing practice that are highlighted in this paper include vigilance in monitoring IAH or abdominal compartment syndrome, assessing organ function, pain management, vital signs, lower extremity perfusion and assessment of wound drainage.

Although not a systematic review, this paper would have been strengthened methodologically by following the Preferred Reporting Items for Systematic Reviews and Meta-Analyses (PRISMA) recommendations.[205] Specifically, articulating the selection criteria for the papers and addressing limitations of the research included in this review would be helpful, particularly as there seems to be a mix of research articles and opinion pieces. Despite the limitations of this publication, this integrative review provides a useful summary of the literature and incorporates clear messages for nursing practice that can be readily implemented in the intensive care unit. Directions for future research are also included and highlight opportunities for nursing and interdisciplinary research.

Learning activities

1 On your next clinical shift, identify what stress-ulcer prophylaxis your patient is receiving (if any) and whether they have risk factors for the development of stress-related mucosal disease.

2 When you are next in the clinical area, consider the clinical presentations of the patients in the ICU and identify which patients might most benefit from intra-abdominal pressure monitoring.

3 Compare and contrast the physiological changes that occur in DKA and HHS. How do these differences influence the management strategy for restoring normoglycaemia?

4 Liver transplantation can be considered in patients with alcoholic liver disease. What would make liver transplantation in this group most successful?

Online resources

Australian Diabetes Council, www.australiandiabetescouncil.com

European Association for the Study of the Liver, www.easl.eu

National Diabetes Education Program, http://ndep.nih.gov

Online MELD Calculator, http://optn.transplant.hrsa.gov/resources/professionalResources.asp?index=8

The Australia and New Zealand Liver Transplant Registry, www.anzltr.org

The Transplantation Society of Australia and New Zealand, www.tsanz.com.au

World Society of the Abdominal Compartment Syndrome, www.wsacs.org

Further reading

Holt RIG, Cockram C, Flyvbjerg A, Goldstein BJ. Textbook of diabetes. 4th ed. Hoboken: Wiley Blackwell; 2010.

Lee WE, Williams R. Acute liver failure. Cambridge: Cambridge University Press; 2011.

References

1 Ukleja A. Altered GI motility in critically ill patients: current understanding of pathophysiology, clinical impact, and diagnostic approach. Nutr Clin Pract 2010;25(1):16–25.

2 Husebye E. The pathogenesis of gastrointestinal bacterial overgrowth. Chemotherapy 2005;51 Suppl 1:1-22.

3 Floch MH, Binder HJ, Filburn B, Gershengoren W. The effect of bile acids on intestinal microflora. Am J Clin Nutr 1972;25(12):1418-26.

4 Puleo F, Arvanitakis M, Van Gossum A, Preiser JC. Gut failure in the ICU. Semin Respir Crit Care Med 2011;32(5):626-38.

5 Wells CL, Erlandsen SL. Bacterial translocation: intestinal epithelial permeability. In: Rombeau JL, Takala J, eds. Gut dysfunction in critical illness. Berlin: Springer; 1996.

6 Takeuchi K, Kita K, Hayashi S, Aihara E. Regulatory mechanism of duodenal bicarbonate secretion: roles of endogenous prostaglandins and nitric oxide. Pharmacol Ther 2011;130(1):59-70.

7 Deane AM, Rayner CK, Keeshan A, Cvijanovic N, Marino Z, Nguyen NQ et al. The effects of critical illness on intestinal glucose sensing, transporters, and absorption. Crit Care Med 2014;42(1):57-65.

8 Dive A. Impaired glucose and nutrient absorption in critical illness: is gastric emptying only a piece of the puzzle? Crit Care 2009;13(5):190.

9 Fennerty MB. Rationale for the therapeutic benefits of acid-supression therapy in the critically ill patient. Medscape Gastroenterology [Internet]. 2004; 6(2).

10 Higgins D, Mythen MG, Webb AR. Low intramucosal pH is associated with failure to acidify the gastric lumen in response to pentagastrin. Intensive Care Med 1994;20(2):105-8.

11 Nguyen NQ, Besanko LK, Burgstad C, Bellon M, Holloway RH, Chapman M et al. Delayed enteral feeding impairs intestinal carbohydrate absorption in critically ill patients. Crit Care Med 2012;40(1):50-4.

12 Derikx JP, Poeze M, van Bijnen AA, Buurman WA, Heineman E. Evidence for intestinal and liver epithelial cell injury in the early phase of sepsis. Shock 2007;28(5):544-8.

13 Marshall JC. Clinical markers of gastrointestinal dysfunction. In: Rombeau JL, Takala J, eds. Gut dysfunction in critical illness. Berlin: Springer; 1996, pp 114-30.

14 Haglund U. Gut ischaemia. Gut 1994;35(1 Suppl):S73-6.

15 Vallet B, Neviere R, Chagon J-L. Gastrointestinal mucosal ischaemic. In: Rombeau JL, Takala J, eds. Gut dysfunction in critical illness. Berlin: Springer; 1996, pp 233-45.

16 Antonsson JB, Engstrom L, Rasmussen I, Wollert S, Haglund UH. Changes in gut intramucosal pH and gut oxygen extraction ratio in a porcine model of peritonitis and hemorrhage. Crit Care Med 1995;23(11):1872-81.

17 Gatt M, Reddy BS, MacFie J. Review article: bacterial translocation in the critically ill – evidence and methods of prevention. Aliment Pharmacol Ther 2007;25(7):741-57.

18 Strassburg CP. Gastrointestinal disorders of the critically ill. Shock liver. Best Pract Res Clin Gastroenterol 2003;17(3):369-81.

19 Mutlu GM, Mutlu EA, Factor P. GI complications in patients receiving mechanical ventilation. Chest 2001;119(4):1222-41.

20 Plummer MP, Blaser AR, Deane AM. Stress ulceration: prevalence, pathology and association with adverse outcomes. Critical Care 2014;18:213.

21 Duerksen DR. Stress-related mucosal disease in critically ill patients. Best Pract Res Clin Gastroenterol 2003;17(3):327-44.

22 Fennerty MB. Pathophysiology of the upper gastrointestinal tract in the critically ill patient: rationale for the therapeutic benefits of acid suppression. Crit Care Med 2002;30(6 Suppl):S351-5.

23 Choung RS, Talley NJ. Epidemiology and clinical presentation of stress-related peptic damage and chronic peptic ulcer. Curr Mol Med 2008;8(4):253-7.

24 Faisy C, Guerot E, Diehl JL, Iftimovici E, Fagon JY. Clinically significant gastrointestinal bleeding in critically ill patients with and without stress-ulcer prophylaxis. Intensive Care Med 2003;29(8):1306-13.

25 Marik PE, Vasu T, Hirani A, Pachinburavan M. Stress ulcer prophylaxis in the new millennium: a systematic review and meta-analysis. Crit Care Med 2010;38(11):2222-8.

26 Laine L, Takeuchi K, Tarnawski A. Gastric mucosal defense and cytoprotection: bench to bedside. Gastroenterology 2008;135(1):41-60.

27 Spirt MJ, Stanley S. Update on stress ulcer prophylaxis in critically ill patients. Crit Care Nurse 2006;26(1):18-20, 2-8; quiz 9.

28 Hawkey CJ, Rampton DS. Prostaglandins and the gastrointestinal mucosa: are they important in its function, disease, or treatment? Gastroenterology 1985;89(5):1162-88.

29 Beejay U, Wolfe MM. Acute gastrointestinal bleeding in the intensive care unit. The gastroenterologist's perspective. Gastroenterol Clin North Am 2000;29(2):309-36.

30 Durham RM, Shapiro MJ. Stress gastritis revisited. Surg Clin North Am 1991;71(4):791-810.

31 Goldin GF, Peura DA. Stress-related mucosal damage. What to do or not to do. Gastrointest Endosc Clin N Am 1996;6(3):505-26.

32 Cook D, Guyatt G, Marshall J, Leasa D, Fuller H, Hall R et al. A comparison of sucralfate and ranitidine for the prevention of upper gastrointestinal bleeding in patients requiring mechanical ventilation. Canadian Critical Care Trials Group. N Engl J Med 1998;338(12):791-7.

33 Schiessel R, Feil W, Wenzl E. Mechanisms of stress ulceration and implications for treatment. Gastroenterol Clin North Am 1990;19(1):101-20.

34 Bhattacharyya A, Chattopadhyay R, Mitra S, Crowe SE. Oxidative stress: an essential factor in the pathogenesis of gastrointestinal mucosal diseases. Physiol Rev 2014;94(2):329-54.

35 Ritchie WP, Jr, Mercer D. Mediators of bile acid-induced alterations in gastric mucosal blood flow. Am J Surg 1991;161(1):126-30.

36 Waldum HL, Hauso O, Fossmark R. The regulation of gastric acid secretion – clinical perspectives. Acta Physiol (Oxf) 2014;210(2):239-56.

37 Robertson MS, Cade JF, Clancy RL. *Helicobacter pylori* infection in intensive care: increased prevalence and a new nosocomial infection. Crit Care Med 1999;27(7):1276-80.

38 Cook DJ, Fuller HD, Guyatt GH, Marshall JC, Leasa D, Hall R et al. Risk factors for gastrointestinal bleeding in critically ill patients. Canadian Critical Care Trials Group. N Engl J Med 1994;330(6):377-81.

39 Ellison RT, Perez-Perez G, Welsh CH, Blaser MJ, Riester KA, Cross AS et al. Risk factors for upper gastrointestinal bleeding in intensive care unit patients: role of *Helicobacter pylori*. Federal Hyperimmune Immunoglobulin Therapy Study Group. Crit Care Med 1996;24(12):1974-81.

40 Cook CA, Booth BM, Blow FC, McAleenan KA, Bunn JY. Risk factors for AMA discharge from VA inpatient alcoholism treatment programs. J Subst Abuse Treat 1994;11(3):239-45.

41 Alhazzani W, Alenezi F, Jaeschke RZ, Moayyedi P, Cook DJ. Proton pump inhibitors versus histamine 2 receptor antagonists for stress ulcer prophylaxis in critically ill patients: a systematic review and meta-analysis. Crit Care Med 2013;41(3):693-705.

42 Cook DJ, Griffith LE, Walter SD, Guyatt GH, Meade MO, Heyland DK et al. The attributable mortality and length of intensive care unit stay of clinically important gastrointestinal bleeding in critically ill patients. Crit Care 2001;5(6):368-75.

43 Barkun AN, Bardou M, Martel M. Controversies in stress ulcer bleeding prophylaxis arise from differences in the quality of the evidence. Anaesth Intensive Care 2013;41(2):269-70.

44 Reveiz L, Guerrero-Lozano R, Camacho A, Yara L, Mosquera PA. Stress ulcer, gastritis, and gastrointestinal bleeding prophylaxis in critically ill pediatric patients: a systematic review. Pediatr Crit Care Med 2010;11(1):124-32.

45 Bardou M, Barkun AN. Stress ulcer prophylaxis in the ICU: who, when, and how? Crit Care Med 2013;41(3):906-7.

46 Dellinger RP, Levy MM, Rhodes A, Annane D, Gerlach H, Opal SM et al. Surviving Sepsis Campaign: international guidelines for management of severe sepsis and septic shock, 2012. Intensive Care Med 2013;39(2):165-228.

47 Barletta JF, Sclar DA. Use of proton pump inhibitors for the provision of stress ulcer prophylaxis: clinical and economic consequences. Pharmacoeconomics 2014;32(1):5-13.

48 Barkun AN, Adam V, Martel M, Bardou M. Cost-effectiveness analysis: stress ulcer bleeding prophylaxis with proton pump inhibitors, H_2 receptor antagonists. Value Health 2013;16(1):14-22.

49 Cook DJ, Reeve BK, Guyatt GH, Heyland DK, Griffith LE, Buckingham L et al. Stress ulcer prophylaxis in critically ill patients. Resolving discordant meta-analyses. JAMA 1996;275(4):308-14.

50 Pisegna JR. Pharmacology of acid suppression in the hospital setting: focus on proton pump inhibition. Crit Care Med 2002;30(6 Suppl): S356-61.

51 Netzer P, Gaia C, Sandoz M, Huluk T, Gut A, Halter F et al. Effect of repeated injection and continuous infusion of omeprazole and ranitidine on intragastric pH over 72 hours. Am J Gastroenterol 1999;94(2):351-7.

52 Merki HS, Wilder-Smith CH. Do continuous infusions of omeprazole and ranitidine retain their effect with prolonged dosing? Gastroenterology 1994;106(1):60-4.

53 Quenot JP, Thiery N, Barbar S. When should stress ulcer prophylaxis be used in the ICU? Curr Opin Crit Care 2009;15(2):139-43.

54 Miano TA, Reichert MG, Houle TT, MacGregor DA, Kincaid EH, Bowton DL. Nosocomial pneumonia risk and stress ulcer prophylaxis: a comparison of pantoprazole vs ranitidine in cardiothoracic surgery patients. Chest 2009;136(2):440-7.

55 Krag M, Perner A, Wetterslev J, Wise MP, Hylander Moller M. Stress ulcer prophylaxis versus placebo or no prophylaxis in critically ill patients. A systematic review of randomised clinical trials with meta-analysis and trial sequential analysis. Intensive Care Med 2014;40(1):11-22.

56 ASHP therapeutic guidelines on stress ulcer prophylaxis. ASHP Commission on Therapeutics and approved by the ASHP Board of Directors on November 14, 1998. Am J Health Syst Pharm 1999;56(4):347-79.

57 Ali T, Harty RF. Stress-induced ulcer bleeding in critically ill patients. Gastroenterol Clin North Am 2009;38(2):245-65.

58 Sesler JM. Stress-related mucosal disease in the intensive care unit: an update on prophylaxis. AACN Adv Crit Care 2007;18(2):119-26; quiz 27-8.

59 Buendgens L, Bruensing J, Matthes M, Duckers H, Luedde T, Trautwein C et al. Administration of proton pump inhibitors in critically ill medical patients is associated with increased risk of developing *Clostridium difficile*-associated diarrhea. J Crit Care 2014;29(4):696.

60 Kozar RA, Hu S, Hassoun HT, DeSoignie R, Moore FA. Specific intraluminal nutrients alter mucosal blood flow during gut ischemia/reperfusion. JPEN J Parenter Enteral Nutr 2002;26(4):226-9.

61 Ephgrave KS, Kleiman-Wexler RL, Adair CG. Enteral nutrients prevent stress ulceration and increase intragastric volume. Crit Care Med 1990;18(6):621-4.

62 Bonten MJ, Gaillard CA, van Tiel FH, van der Geest S, Stobberingh EE. Continuous enteral feeding counteracts preventive measures for gastric colonization in intensive care unit patients. Crit Care Med 1994;22(6):939-44.

63 Chanpura T, Yende S. Weighing risks and benefits of stress ulcer prophylaxis in critically ill patients. Crit Care 2012;16(5):322.

64 Morken J, West MA. Abdominal compartment syndrome in the intensive care unit. Curr Opin Crit Care 2001;7(4):268-74.

65 Malbrain ML, Chiumello D, Pelosi P, Wilmer A, Brienza N, Malcangi V et al. Prevalence of intra-abdominal hypertension in critically ill patients: a multicentre epidemiological study. Intensive Care Med 2004;30(5):822-9.

66 Holodinsky JK, Roberts DJ, Ball CG, Blaser AR, Starkopf J, Zygun DA et al. Risk factors for intra-abdominal hypertension and abdominal compartment syndrome among adult intensive care unit patients: a systematic review and meta-analysis. Crit Care 2013;17(5):R249.

67 Schein M, Wittmann DH, Aprahamian CC, Condon RE. The abdominal compartment syndrome: the physiological and clinical consequences of elevated intra-abdominal pressure. J Am Coll Surg 1995;180(6):745-53.

68 Moore AF, Hargest R, Martin M, Delicata RJ. Intra-abdominal hypertension and the abdominal compartment syndrome. Br J Surg 2004;91(9):1102-10.

69 Oda J, Ivatury RR, Blocher CR, Malhotra AJ, Sugerman HJ. Amplified cytokine response and lung injury by sequential hemorrhagic shock and abdominal compartment syndrome in a laboratory model of ischemia–reperfusion. J Trauma 2002;52(4):625-31; discussion 32.

70 Fritsch DE, Steinmann RA. Managing trauma patients with abdominal compartment syndrome. Crit Care Nurse 2000;20(6):48-58.

71 Hunter JD, Damani Z. Intra-abdominal hypertension and the abdominal compartment syndrome. Anaesthesia 2004;59(9):899-907.

72 Bailey J, Shapiro MJ. Abdominal compartment syndrome. Crit Care 2000;4(1):23-9.

73 Ridings PC, Bloomfield GL, Blocher CR, Sugerman HJ. Cardiopulmonary effects of raised intra-abdominal pressure before and after intravascular volume expansion. J Trauma 1995;39(6):1071-5.

74 McNelis J, Marini CP, Simms HH. Abdominal compartment syndrome: clinical manifestations and predictive factors. Curr Opin Crit Care 2003;9(2):133-6.

75 Sugrue M, Jones F, Deane SA, Bishop G, Bauman A, Hillman K. Intra-abdominal hypertension is an independent cause of postoperative renal impairment. Arch Surg 1999;134(10):1082-5.

76 Ivatury RR, Porter JM, Simon RJ, Islam S, John R, Stahl WM. Intra-abdominal hypertension after life-threatening penetrating abdominal trauma: prophylaxis, incidence, and clinical relevance to gastric mucosal pH and abdominal compartment syndrome. J Trauma 1998;44(6):1016-21; discussion 21-3.

77 Malbrain ML. Is it wise not to think about intraabdominal hypertension in the ICU? Curr Opin Crit Care 2004;10(2):132-45.

78 Bloomfield GL, Ridings PC, Blocher CR, Marmarou A, Sugerman HJ. A proposed relationship between increased intra-abdominal, intrathoracic, and intracranial pressure. Crit Care Med 1997;25(3):496-503.

79 Kirkpatrick AW, Roberts DJ, De Waele J, Jaeschke R, Malbrain ML, De Keulenaer B et al. Intra-abdominal hypertension and the abdominal compartment syndrome: updated consensus definitions and clinical practice guidelines from the World Society of the Abdominal Compartment Syndrome. Intensive Care Med 2013;39(7):1190-206.

80 Cheatham ML, White MW, Sagraves SG, Johnson JL, Block EF. Abdominal perfusion pressure: a superior parameter in the assessment of intra-abdominal hypertension. J Trauma 2000;49(4):621-6; discussion 6-7.

81 Kirkpatrick AW, Brenneman FD, McLean RF, Rapanos T, Boulanger BR. Is clinical examination an accurate indicator of raised intra-abdominal pressure in critically injured patients? Can J Surg 2000;43(3):207-11.

82 Fusco MA, Martin RS, Chang MC. Estimation of intra-abdominal pressure by bladder pressure measurement: validity and methodology. J Trauma 2001;50(2):297-302.

83 Pouliart N, Huyghens L. An observational study on intraabdominal pressure in 125 critically ill patients. Crit Care 2002;6(Suppl 1):S3.

84 De Waele JJ, De Laet I, De Keulenaer B, Widder S, Kirkpatrick AW, Cresswell AB et al. The effect of different reference transducer positions on intra-abdominal pressure measurement: a multicenter analysis. Intensive Care Med 2008;34(7):1299-303.

85 Gudmundsson FF, Viste A, Gislason H, Svanes K. Comparison of different methods for measuring intra-abdominal pressure. Intensive Care Med 2002;28(4):509-14.

86 Ejike JC, Bahjri K, Mathur M. What is the normal intra-abdominal pressure in critically ill children and how should we measure it? Crit Care Med 2008;36(7):2157-62.

87 Malbrain ML. Different techniques to measure intra-abdominal pressure (IAP): time for a critical re-appraisal. Intensive Care Med 2004;30(3):357-71.

88 Becker V, Schmid RM, Umgelter A. Comparison of a new device for the continuous intra-gastric measurement of intra-abdominal pressure (CiMon) with direct intra-peritoneal measurements in cirrhotic patients during paracentesis. Intensive Care Med 2009;35(5):948-52.

89 Balogh Z, De Waele JJ, Malbrain ML. Continuous intra-abdominal pressure monitoring. Acta Clinica Belgica 2007;62(Supplement 1):26-32.

90 McBeth PB, Zygun DA, Widder S, Cheatham M, Zengerink I, Glowa J et al. Effect of patient positioning on intra-abdominal pressure monitoring. Am J Surg 2007;193(5):644-7; discussion 7.

91 Chiumello D, Tallarini F, Chierichetti M, Polli F, Li Bassi G, Motta G et al. The effect of different volumes and temperatures of saline on the bladder pressure measurement in critically ill patients. Crit Care 2007;11(4):R82.

92 De Waele J, Pletinckx P, Blot S, Hoste E. Saline volume in transvesical intra-abdominal pressure measurement: enough is enough. Intensive Care Med 2006;32:455-59.

93 The global challenge of diabetes. The Lancet 2008;371(9626):1723.

94 Shi Y, Hu FB. The global implications of diabetes and cancer. Lancet 2014;383(9933):1947-8.

95 Oggioni C, Lara J, Wells JCK, Soroka K, Siervo M. Shifts in population dietary patterns and physical inactivity as determinants of global trends in the prevalence of diabetes: an ecological analysis. Nutr Metab Cardiovasc Dis 2014;24(10):1105-11.

96 Dabelea D, Mayer-Davis EJ, Saydah S, Imperatore G, Linder B, Divers J et al. Prevalence of type 1 and type 2 diabetes among children and adolescents from 2001 to 2009. JAMA 2014;311(17):1778-86.

97 Guariguata L, Whiting DR, Hambleton I, Beagley J, Linnenkamp U, Shaw JE. Global estimates of diabetes prevalence for 2013 and projections for 2035. Diabetes Res Clin Pract 2014;103(2):137-49.

98 Beagley J, Guariguata L, Weil C, Motala AA. Global estimates of undiagnosed diabetes in adults. Diabetes Res Clin Pract 2014;103(2):150-60.

99 Kitabchi AE, Nyenwe EA. Hyperglycemic crises in diabetes mellitus: diabetic ketoacidosis and hyperglycemic hyperosmolar state. Endocrinol Metab Clin North Am 2006;35(4):725-51, viii.

100 Noble-Bell G, Cox A. Management of diabetic ketoacidosis in adults. Nurs Times 2014;110(10):14-7.

101 Brenner ZR. Management of hyperglycemic emergencies. AACN Clin Issues 2006;17(1):56-65; quiz 91-3.

102 Newton CA, Raskin P. Diabetic ketoacidosis in type 1 and type 2 diabetes mellitus: clinical and biochemical differences. Arch Intern Med 2004;164(17):1925-31.

103 Yared Z, Chiasson JL. Ketoacidosis and the hyperosmolar hyperglycemic state in adult diabetic patients. Diagnosis and treatment. Minerva Med 2003;94(6):409-18.

104 Magee MF, Bhatt BA. Management of decompensated diabetes. Diabetic ketoacidosis and hyperglycemic hyperosmolar syndrome. Crit Care Clin 2001;17(1):75-106.

105 Keays RT. Diabetic emergencies. In: Bersten AD, Soni N, eds. Oh's intensive care manual. 6th ed. Philadelphia: Elsevier; 2009, pp 613-20.

106 Kitabchi AE, Umpierrez GE, Miles JM, Fisher JN. Hyperglycemic crises in adult patients with diabetes. Diabetes Care 2009;32(7):1335-43.

107 Schmitz K. Providing the best possible care: an overview of the current understanding of diabetic ketoacidosis. Aust Crit Care 2000;13(1):22-7.

108 Bardsley JK, Want LL. Overview of diabetes. Crit Care Nurs Q 2004;27(2):106-12.

109 Dunstan DW, Zimmet PZ, Welborn TA, De Courten MP, Cameron AJ, Sicree RA et al. The rising prevalence of diabetes and impaired glucose tolerance: the Australian Diabetes, Obesity and Lifestyle Study. Diabetes Care 2002;25(5):829-34.

110 Boyle M, Lawrence J. An easy method of mentally estimating the metabolic component of acid/base balance using the Fencl-Stewart approach. Anaesth Intensive Care 2003;31(5):538-47.

111 Hardern RD, Quinn ND. Emergency management of diabetic ketoacidosis in adults. Emerg Med J 2003;20(3):210-3.

112 Maletkovic J, Drexler A. Diabetic ketoacidosis and hyperglycemic hyperosmolar state. Endocrinol Metab Clin North Am 2013;42(4):677-95.

113 Thuzar M, Malabu UH, Tisdell B, Sangla KS. Use of a standardised diabetic ketoacidosis management protocol improved clinical outcomes. Diabetes Res Clin Pract 2014;104(1):e8-e11.

114 Hara JS, Rahbar AJ, Jeffres MN, Izuora KE. Impact of a hyperglycemic crises protocol. Endocr Pract 2013;19(6):953-62.

115 De Beer K, Michael S, Thacker M, Wynne E, Pattni C, Gomm M et al. Diabetic ketoacidosis and hyperglycaemic hyperosmolar syndrome – clinical guidelines. Nurs Crit Care 2008;13(1):5-11.

116 Bull SV, Douglas IS, Foster M, Albert RK. Mandatory protocol for treating adult patients with diabetic ketoacidosis decreases intensive care unit and hospital lengths of stay: results of a nonrandomized trial. Crit Care Med 2007;35(1):41-6.

117 Wallace TM, Matthews DR. Recent advances in the monitoring and management of diabetic ketoacidosis. QJM 2004;97(12):773-80.

118 Arias IM, Alter HJ, Boyer JL, Cohen DE, Fausto N, Shafritz DA et al. The liver: Biology and pathobiology. 5th ed. West Sussex: Wiley-Blackwell; 2009.

119 Tacke F, Luedde T, Trautwein C. Inflammatory pathways in liver homeostasis and liver injury. Clin Rev Allergy Immunol 2009;36(1):4-12.

120 Guicciardi ME, Gores GJ. Apoptosis: a mechanism of acute and chronic liver injury. Gut 2005;54(7):1024-33.

121 Perz JF, Armstrong GL, Farrington LA, Hutin YJ, Bell BP. The contributions of hepatitis B virus and hepatitis C virus infections to cirrhosis and primary liver cancer worldwide. J Hepatol 2006;45(4):529-38.

122 Asrani SK, O'Leary JG. Acute-on-chronic liver failure. Clin Liver Dis 2014;18(3):561-74.

123 Hodgman MJ, Garrard AR. A review of acetaminophen poisoning. Crit Care Clin 2012;28(4):499-516.

124 Brok J, Buckley N, Gluud C. Interventions for paracetamol (acetaminophen) overdose. Cochrane Database Syst Rev 2006;2:CD003328.

125 Santi L, Maggioli C, Mastroroberto M, Tufoni M, Napoli L, Caraceni P. Acute liver failure caused by *Amanita phalloides* poisoning. Int J Hepatol 2012;2012:487-80.

126 Lammers WJ, Kowdley KV, van Buuren HR. Predicting outcome in primary biliary cirrhosis. Ann Hepatol 2014;13(4):316-26.

127 Williamson KD, Chapman RW. Primary sclerosing cholangitis. Dig Dis 2014;32(4):438-45.

128 Subba Rao M, Sasikala M, Nageshwar Reddy D. Thinking outside the liver: induced pluripotent stem cells for hepatic applications. World J Gastroenterol 2013;19(22):3385-96.

129 Duncan AW, Soto-Gutierrez A. Liver repopulation and regeneration: new approaches to old questions. Curr Opin Organ Transplant 2013; 18(2):197-202.

130 Mehta G, Gustot T, Mookerjee RP, Garcia-Pagan JC, Fallon MB, Shah VH et al. Inflammation and portal hypertension – the undiscovered country. J Hepatol 2014;61(1):155-63.

131 Rosselli M, MacNaughtan J, Jalan R, Pinzani M. Beyond scoring: a modern interpretation of disease progression in chronic liver disease. Gut 2013;62(9):1234-41.

132 Mohd Hanafiah K, Groeger J, Flaxman AD, Wiersma ST. Global epidemiology of hepatitis C virus infection: new estimates of age-specific antibody to HCV seroprevalence. Hepatology 2013;57(4):1333-42.

133 World Health Organization. Hepatitis B Fact Sheet No. 204. Geneva: World Health Organisation; 2014, Contract No.: July.

134 World Health Organization. Hepatitis C Fact Sheet No. 164. Geneva: World Health Organisation; 2014.

135 World Health Organization. Prevention and control of viral hepatitis infection: framework for global action. Geneva: World Health Organisation; 2012.

136 World Health Organization. Hepatitis. Geneva: World Health Organisation; 2014.

137 Cowie BC, MacLachlan JH, eds. The global burden of liver disease attributable to hepatitis B, hepatitis C, and alcohol: increasing mortality, differing causes. 64th Annual Meeting of the American Association for the Study of Liver Diseases (AASLD 2013). Washington, DC, November 1–5, 2013. Abstract 23.

138 The Kirby Institute. HIV, viral hepatitis and sexually transmissible infections in Australia Annual Surveillance Report 2013. The Kirby Institute, The University of New South Wales, Sydney, 2013.

139 Ageing DoHa. Third National Hepatitis C Strategy 2010–2013. Canberra, Australia: Australian Government; 2010.

140 Bernal W, Auzinger G, Dhawan P, Wendon J. Acute liver failure. Lancet 2010;376(9736):190-201.

141 Trey D, Davidson C. The management of fulminant hepatic failure. In: Popper H, Schaffner Fe, eds. Progress in liver disease. New York: Grune and Stratton; 1970, pp 292-8.

142 O'Grady JG, Schalm SW, Williams R. Acute liver failure: redefining the syndromes. Lancet 1993;342(8866):273-5.

143 Tandon BN, Bernauau J, O'Grady J, Gupta SD, Krisch RE, Liaw YF et al. Recommendations of the International Association for the Study of the Liver Subcommittee on nomenclature of acute and subacute liver failure. J Gastroenterol Hepatol 1999;14(5):403-4.

144 Bismuth M, Funakoshi N, Cadranel JF, Blanc P. Hepatic encephalopathy: from pathophysiology to therapeutic management. Eur J Gastroenterol Hepatol 2011;23(1):8-22.

145 Vaquero J, Chung C, Cahill ME, Blei AT. Pathogenesis of hepatic encephalopathy in acute liver failure. Semin Liver Dis 2003;23(3):259-69.

146 Frontera JA. Management of hepatic encephalopathy. Curr Treat Options Neurol 2014;16(6):297.

147 Haussinger D, Schliess F. Pathogenetic mechanisms of hepatic encephalopathy. Gut 2008;57(8):1156-65.

148 Conn HO, Leevy CM, Vlahcevic ZR, Rodgers JB, Maddrey WC, Seeff L et al. Comparison of lactulose and neomycin in the treatment of chronic portal-systemic encephalopathy. A double blind controlled trial. Gastroenterology 1977;72(4 Pt 1):573-83.

149 Hassanein TI, Schade RR, Hepburn IS. Acute-on-chronic liver failure: extracorporeal liver assist devices. Curr Opin Crit Care 2011;17(2):195-203.

150 Ortiz M, Cordoba J, Doval E, Jacas C, Pujadas F, Esteban R et al. Development of a clinical hepatic encephalopathy staging scale. Aliment Pharmacol Ther 2007;26(6):859-67.

151 Lata J. Hepatorenal syndrome. World J Gastroenterol 2012;18(36):4978-84.

152 Gines P, Guevara M, Arroyo V, Rodes J. Hepatorenal syndrome. Lancet 2003;362(9398):1819-27.

153 Dagher L, Moore K. The hepatorenal syndrome. Gut 2001;49(5):729-37.

154 Rajoriya N, Tripathi D. Historical overview and review of current day treatment in the management of acute variceal haemorrhage. World J Gastroenterol 2014;20(21):6481-94.

155 Cat TB, Liu-DeRyke X. Medical management of variceal hemorrhage. Crit Care Nurs Clin North Am 2010;22(3):381-93.

156 Fallon MB. Mechanisms of pulmonary vascular complications of liver disease: hepatopulmonary syndrome. J Clin Gastroenterol 2005;39 (4 Suppl 2):S138-42.

157 Liu H, Lee SS. Acute-on-chronic liver failure: the heart and systemic hemodynamics. Curr Opin Crit Care 2011;17(2):190-4.

158 Bauer M, Press AT, Trauner M. The liver in sepsis: patterns of response and injury. Curr Opin Crit Care 2013;19(2):123-7.

159 Mahajan A, Lat I. Correction of coagulopathy in the setting of acute liver failure. Crit Care Nurs Clin North Am 2010;22(3):315-21.

160 Wendon J, Lee W. Encephalopathy and cerebral edema in the setting of acute liver failure: pathogenesis and management. Neurocrit Care 2008;9(1):97-102.

161 Wang DW, Yin YM, Yao YM. Advances in the management of acute liver failure. World J Gastroenterol 2013;19(41):7069-77.

162 Kamath PS, Kim WR, Advanced Liver Disease Study G. The model for end-stage liver disease (MELD). Hepatology 2007;45(3):797-805.

163 Australasia RCoP. RCPA Manual Surrey Hills: Royal College of Pathologists Australasia; 2011 [updated 22 August 2011; cited 2014 3 August].

164 Castaldo ET, Chari RS. Liver transplantation for acute hepatic failure. HPB (Oxford) 2006;8(1):29-34.

165 Sharma BC, Sharma P, Agrawal A, Sarin SK. Secondary prophylaxis of hepatic encephalopathy: an open-label randomized controlled trial of lactulose versus placebo. Gastroenterology 2009;137(3):885-91, 91 e1.

166 Christensen T. The treatment of oesophageal varices using a Sengstaken-Blakemore tube: considerations for nursing practice. Nurs Crit Care 2004;9(2):58-63.

167 Colombato L. The role of transjugular intrahepatic portosystemic shunt (TIPS) in the management of portal hypertension. J Clin Gastroenterol 2007;41(Suppl 3):S344-51.

168 Zhao LF, Pan XP, Li LJ. Key challenges to the development of extracorporeal bioartificial liver support systems. Hepatobiliary Pancreat Dis Int 2012;11(3):243-9.

169 Stange J. Extracorporeal liver support. Organogenesis 2011;7(1):64-73.

170 Carpentier B, Gautier A, Legallais C. Artificial and bioartificial liver devices: present and future. Gut 2009;58(12):1690-702.

171 Leckie P, Davies N, Jalan R. Albumin regeneration for extracorporeal liver support using prometheus: a step in the right direction. Gastroenterology 2012;142(4):690-2.

172 Rademacher S, Oppert M, Jorres A. Artificial extracorporeal liver support therapy in patients with severe liver failure. Expert Rev Gastroenterol Hepatol 2011;5(5):591-9.

173 Kortgen A, Rauchfuss F, Gotz M, Settmacher U, Bauer M, Sponholz C. Albumin dialysis in liver failure: comparison of molecular adsorbent recirculating system and single pass albumin dialysis – a retrospective analysis. Ther Apher Dial 2009;13(5):419-25.

174 Liou IW, Larson AM. Role of liver transplantation in acute liver failure. Semin Liver Dis 2008;28(2):201-9.

175 O'Grady J. Liver transplantation for acute liver failure. Best Pract Res Clin Gastroenterol 2012;26(1):27-33.

176 Lynch SV, Balderson GA. ANZLT Registry Report 2012. Brisbane, QLD, Australia: ANZLT; 2012.

177 Thuluvath PJ, Guidinger MK, Fung JJ, Johnson LB, Rayhill SC, Pelletier SJ. Liver transplantation in the United States, 1999–2008. Am J Transplant 2010;10(4 Pt 2):1003-19.

178 O'Leary JG, Lepe R, Davis GL. Indications for liver transplantation. Gastroenterology 2008;134(6):1764-76.

179 Yoo PS, Umman V, Rodriguez-Davalos MI, Emre SH. Retransplantation of the liver: review of current literature for decision making and technical considerations. Transplant Proc 2013;45(3):854-9.

180 Transplantation Society of Australia and New Zealand. Organ transplantation from deceased donors: Consensus statement on eligibility criteria and allocation protocols. Canberra, Australia: TSANZ; 2010.

181 Trotter JF, Osgood MJ. MELD scores of liver transplant recipients according to size of waiting list: impact of organ allocation and patient outcomes. JAMA 2004;291(15):1871-4.

182 Llado L, Figueras J. Techniques of orthotopic liver transplantation. HPB (Oxford) 2004;6(2):69-75.

183 Agopian VG, Petrowsky H, Kaldas FM, Zarrinpar A, Farmer DG, Yersiz H et al. The evolution of liver transplantation during 3 decades: analysis of 5347 consecutive liver transplants at a single center. Ann Surg 2013;258(3):409-21.

184 Sizer E, Wendon J. Liver transplantation. In: Bersten AD, Soni N, eds. Oh's intensive care manual. 6th ed. Oxford: Butterworth Heinemann; 2009.

185 Reddy KS, Johnston TD, Putnam LA, Isley M, Ranjan D. Piggyback technique and selective use of veno-venous bypass in adult orthotopic liver transplantation. Clin Transplant 2000;14(4 Pt 2):370-4.

186 Renz JF, Yersiz H, Reichert PR, Hisatake GM, Farmer DG, Emond JC et al. Split-liver transplantation: a review. Am J Transplant 2003;3(11):1323-35.

187 Crawford M, Shaked A. The liver transplant operation. Graft 2003;6(2):98-109.

188 Russo MW, Brown RS, Jr. Adult living donor liver transplantation. Am J Transplant 2004;4(4):458-65.

189 Razonable RR, Findlay JY, O'Riordan A, Burroughs SG, Ghobrial RM, Agarwal B et al. Critical care issues in patients after liver transplantation. Liver Transpl 2011;17(5):511-27.

190 Perera T, Bramhall S. Surgical aspects of liver transplantation. In: Neuberger J, Ferguson J, Newsome PN, eds. Liver transplantation: Clinical assessment and management. West Sussex: John Wiley & Sons; 2014.

191 Esmat Gamil M, Pirenne J, Van Malenstein H, Verhaegen M, Desschans B, Monbaliu D et al. Risk factors for bleeding and clinical implications in patients undergoing liver transplantation. Transplant Proc 2012;44(9):2857-60.

192 Larsen FS, Strauss G, Knudsen GM, Herzog TM, Hansen BA, Secher NH. Cerebral perfusion, cardiac output, and arterial pressure in patients with fulminant hepatic failure. Crit Care Med 2000;28(4):996-1000.

193 Živković SA. Neurologic complications after liver transplantation. World J Hepatology 2013;5(8):409-18.

194 Feltracco P, Carollo C, Barbieri S, Pettenuzzo T, Ori C. Early respiratory complications after liver transplantation. World J Gastroenterol 2013;19(48):9271-81.

195 Mandell MS, Stoner TJ, Barnett R, Shaked A, Bellamy M, Biancofiore G et al. A multicenter evaluation of safety of early extubation in liver transplant recipients. Liver Transpl 2007;13(11):1557-63.

196 Weimann A, Ebener C, Holland-Cunz S, Jauch KW, Hausser L, Kemen M et al. Surgery and transplantation – guidelines on parenteral nutrition, Chapter 18. Ger Med Sci 2009;7:Doc10.

197 Barri YM, Sanchez EQ, Jennings LW, Melton LB, Hays S, Levy MF et al. Acute kidney injury following liver transplantation: definition and outcome. Liver Transpl 2009;15(5):475-83.

198 Dienstag JL, Cosimi AB. Liver transplantation – a vision realized. N Engl J Med 2012;367(16):1483-5.

199 Gotthardt DN, Bruns H, Weiss KH, Schemmer P. Current strategies for immunosuppression following liver transplantation. Langenbecks Arch Surg 2014:DOI: 10.1007/s00423-014-1191-9.

200 Choudray NS, Saijal S, Shukla R, Kotecha H, Saraf N, Soin AS. Current status of immunosuppression in liver transplantation. J Clin Exper Hepatol 2013;3(2):150-8.

201 Seehofer D, Eurich D, Veltzke-Schlieker W, Neuhaus P. Biliary complications after liver transplantation: old problems and new challenges. Am J Transplant 2013;13(2):253-65.

202 Bilbao I, Armadans L, Lazaro JL, Hidalgo E, Castells L, Margarit C. Predictive factors for early mortality following liver transplantation. Clin Transplant 2003;17(5):401-11.

203 Jaurigue MM, Cappell MS. Therapy for alcoholic liver disease. World J Gastroenterol 2014;20(9):2143-58.

204 Bjorck M, Wanhainen A. Management of abdominal compartment syndrome and the open abdomen. Eur J Vasc Endovasc Surg 2014;47(3):279-87.

205 Moher D, Liberati A, Tetzlaff J, Altman DG, Group P. Preferred reporting items for systematic reviews and meta-analyses: the PRISMA statement. J Clin Epidemiol 2009;62(10):1006-12.

206 Marshall AP. The gut in critical illness. In: Carlson K, ed. AACN Advanced critical care nursing. Philadelphia: Elsevier; 2009.

Chapter 21

Pathophysiology and management of shock

Margherita Murgo, Ruth Kleinpell

Margherita Murgo, Ruth Kleinpell

KEY WORDS

anaphylactic shock

cardiogenic shock

distributive shock

hypovolaemic shock

neurogenic shock

obstructive shock

sepsis

septic shock

severe sepsis

systemic
inflammatory
response
syndrome

Learning objectives

After reading this chapter, you should be able to:

- describe the clinical manifestations of shock
- distinguish between the various shock states
- describe general principles of shock management
- discuss end points of resuscitation
- identify appropriate monitoring for a patient with shock
- review and evaluate care for a patient with a specific shock type.

Introduction

It is a bad symptom when the head, hands, and feet are cold, while the belly and sides are hot, but it is a very good symptom when the whole body is equally hot.

THE BOOK OF PROGNOSTICS BY HIPPOCRATES, 400 BC[1]

Shock is an altered physiological state that affects the functioning of every cell and organ system in the body. It is a complex syndrome reflecting changing blood flow to body tissues with accompanying cellular dysfunction and eventual organ failure. Shock presents as a result of impaired nutrient delivery to the tissue:

- when compensatory mechanisms can no longer respond to decreases in tissue perfusion[2]
- when nutrient uptake is impaired at the cellular level.

While the cause of shock may be multifactorial, treatment focuses on optimising tissue perfusion and oxygen delivery. Shock is often classified according to the primary underlying mechanism: a disruption of intravascular blood volume, impaired vasomotor tone or altered cardiac contractility.[3] The shock syndrome is one of the most pervasive manifestations of critical illness present in intensive care patients.

Early detection and management of shock to reverse pathological processes improves patient outcomes.[4] Although the traditional hallmark of shock is hypotension – where the systolic blood pressure is <90 mmHg – this can be a late or misleading sign and is considered a medical emergency.[5] It is therefore critical that other signs and symptoms are identified early by frequent observations to detect a patient's deteriorating state and respond before irreversible shock ensues.[6] No single vital sign is adequate in determining the level or extent of shock[4] nor is there a specific laboratory test that diagnoses the shock syndrome.

In this chapter an overview of the pathophysiology of shock, the commonly described categories and associated pathologies, along with appropriate monitoring and interventions for managing a patient in shock are provided.

Pathophysiology

Shock is classified by aetiology: hypovolaemic, cardiogenic, distributive[2,7,8] and obstructive (Figure 21.1).[9] Each type has a specific mechanism of action that leads to altered tissue perfusion and oxygen and nutrient uptake at the cellular level (see Table 21.1). In practice, it is common for different shock types to be existent in the

FIGURE 21.1 Types of shock.

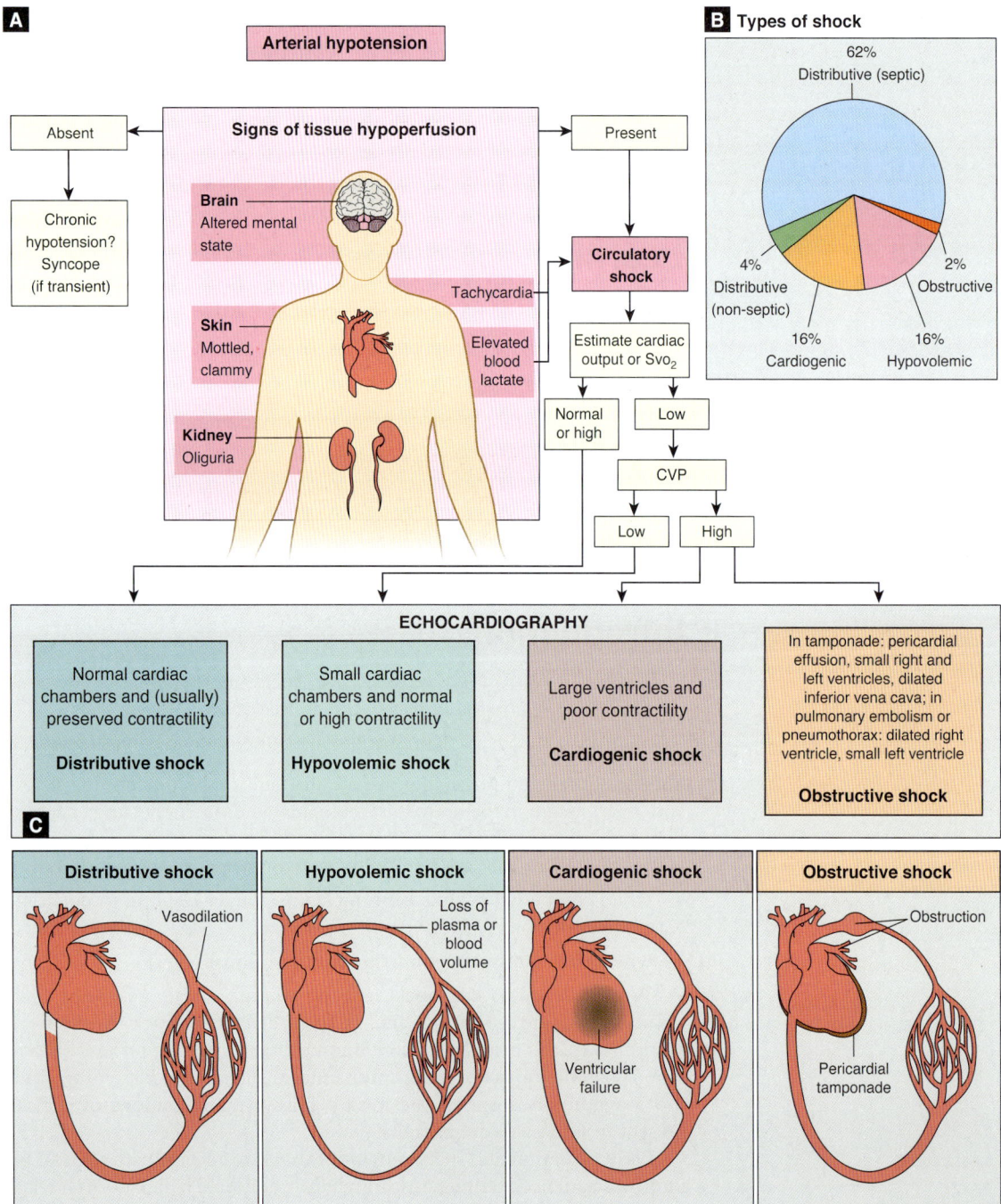

Adapted from Vincent J-L, De Backer D. Circulatory shock. New Engl J Med 2013;369:1726–34, with permission.

TABLE 21.1

Shock types

SHOCK TYPE	MAIN CHARACTERISTIC
Hypovolaemic	A reduction in circulating blood volume through haemorrhage or dehydration or plasma fluid loss
Cardiogenic	Pump failure (impaired cardiac contractility) usually as a result of myocardial infarction
Obstructive	Characterised by blockage of circulation to the tissues by impedance of outflow or filling in the heart (e.g. due to cardiac tamponade or pulmonary emboli)
Distributive	A maldistribution of circulation from sepsis, anaphylaxis or neurogenic injury

Adapted from Manji RA, Wood KE, Kumar A. The history and evolution of circulatory shock. Crit Care Clin 2009;25:1–29, with permission.

same presentation, for example a patient with septic shock might also be hypovolaemic and/or have myocardial dysfunction.

Shock occurs when there is an inability of the body to meet metabolic demands of the tissues; hypoperfusion (decreased blood flow to the tissues) results in cellular dysfunction, as there is homeostatic imbalance between nutrient supply and demand, and adaptive responses can no longer accommodate circulatory changes.[2,10] These adaptive responses are moderated via numerous 'sensors' throughout the thorax and large vessels in particular, which detect subtle changes in pressure (baroreceptors) or biochemical changes (chemoreceptors). These receptors feed back to the hypothalamus, which regulates, through the pituitary gland and adrenal cortex, the release of a number of hormones including antidiuretic hormone and adrenocorticotrophic hormone to target organs such as the kidney. The adrenal cortex mediates the mineral and glucocorticoid response to counter the developing effects of shock. This concurrent direct feedback stimulates the sympathetic nervous system to act on blood vessel tone, particularly the arterioles, and organs such as the adrenal gland and kidney to respond via the release of endogenous catecholamines (adrenaline and noradrenaline), mineral and glucocorticoids (aldosterone, cortisol) and the renin–angiotensin–aldosterone system. Activation of the renin–angiotensin–aldosterone system results in synthesis of angiotensin II, a powerful vasoconstrictor that further potentiates the reduction in peripheral blood vessel capacity.

Collectively, these responses form a sympatho–endocrine–adrenal axis that moderates the systemic response to shock. The axis maintains circulation to the vital organ system and combines with the inflammatory response to limit local and systemic tissue damage and ultimately confer a survival advantage. Combined responses include profound vasoconstriction, oligoanuria

(fluid retention), redirection of blood flow to vital organs, hyperglycaemia, immunomodulation and procoagulation. This universal response to impending shock is particularly effective in compensating for loss of circulating blood volume, but may be counterproductive when pump failure occurs or is 'uncoupled' in distributive shock states.

As adaptive responses fail, cardiac output becomes insufficient to provide adequate organ perfusion despite increasing tissue oxygen consumption (see Chapters 9 and 10). When oxygen is 'supply dependent', oxygen delivery is decreased and, to compensate, increased extraction occurs to enable continued tissue oxygen consumption. However, when oxygen delivery falls below a critical threshold, and extraction demand rises above the available blood oxygen levels, this compensation mechanism fails and oxygen debt results.[4,11]

Hypoperfusion may also exist despite a relatively normal cardiac output, and may not be immediately clinically evident.[4] This results in maldistribution of blood flow to some tissues while other areas receive more blood flow than needed[2,5,10,11] and is often referred to as distributive shock. This response is typical of the shock types that affect vasomotor tone, for example septic, neurogenic and anaphylactic shock. Maldistribution may leave some organ systems ischaemic for long periods leading to persistent organ dysfunction and failure.[4] There is also evidence supporting the presence of cytopathic hypoxia as a result of excessive production of cellular proinflammatory mediators such as nitric oxide and tumour necrosis factor-alpha. Adenosine triphosphate (ATP) stores become depleted due to this impaired mitochondrial oxygen utilisation[11–13] interfering with electron transport and metabolism. Nitric oxide is associated with vascular relaxation and is a major contributor to alterations in microvasculature and capillary leak in sepsis.[14]

Organ systems have varying responses in shock and are not measured directly. Often surrogate markers of global hypoperfusion are used to indicate the severity of shock. Lactate and acid–base disturbances, such as an increase in strong ion gap, have been suggested as early markers of mitochondrial dysfunction and cellular hypoperfusion.[6,9,15] These 'surrogate' biochemical markers of hypoperfusion (pH, serum lactate and standard base excess) assess acidaemia and provide some insight into the degree of shock.[16] Lactate, a strong anion with basal production of approximately 1300 mmol/day,[17] is a product of metabolism. Increased levels are present in tissue hypoxia, hypermetabolism, decreased lactate clearance, inhibition of pyruvate dehydrogenase and activation of inflammatory cells, all characteristics of developing shock (Table 21.2). Increased lactate production is a warning sign of impending organ failure, as it is indicative of anaerobic metabolism. Blood lactate levels have been directly linked to deteriorating patient outcomes in shock.[16,18]

Serum concentrations greater than 5 mmol/L in the setting of metabolic acidosis are indicative of high mortality.[17]

As the shock state deteriorates and the body fails to compensate, organ systems begin to fail. This is

TABLE 21.2

Hyperlactataemia due to tissue hypoxia

MECHANISMS	SERUM LEVELS	CAUSES
Increased glycolysis Decreased clearance	Lactate >5 mmol/L and pH <7.35 (normal lactate <2 mmol/L)	Hypoxaemia Anaemia Hypoperfusion Shock Sepsis

Adapted from Phypers B, Pierce JT. Lactate physiology in health and disease. Continuing Education in Anaesthesia, Crit Care Pain 2006;6:128–32, with permission.

complicated by a systemic inflammatory response (SIRS), which can be a direct cause of the shock state or develop as a consequence of protracted shock. SIRS results in 'capillary leak' or increased microvascular permeability that leads to interstitial oedema due to alterations to the vascular endothelium. Many immune mediators including circulating cytokines, oxygen free radicals and activated neutrophils alter the structure of the endothelial cells, creating space to allow larger intra-vascular molecules to cross into the extravascular space,[19] with proteins and water moving from the intravascular space into the interstitium.[20] This response mechanism improves the supply of nutrient-rich fluid to the site of injury; however, systemically, fluid shifts lead to hypo-volaemia, impaired organ function and development of acute organ injury such as acute kidney injury.[20] This developing organ injury is the precedent to organ failure (see Chapter 22).

The next sections of this chapter describe the general assessment and management of shock, different classifi-cations of shock and specific management principles to avoid or limit tissue injury and the eventual progression to organ failure.

Patient assessment

Critically ill patients often exhibit signs of tissue hypoxia as a result of cardiovascular disturbances.[21] Table 21.3 provides an overview of the physiological changes in shock. Therapy is targeted to maintain oxygen delivery to vital organs to prevent ischaemia and cell death.[21,22] Ideally, organ systems and tissues should be monitored individually;[21] however global measures, such as perfusion pressure, cardiac output and oxygen delivery, are commonly used as surrogates to assist in treatment decision making.[23] Patient assessment and haemo-dynamic monitoring, including calculation of cardiac output, are used to differentiate shock states and assess progress in relation to treatment.[22,24,25] Cardiac output is seen by many clinicians as an important assessment of shock patients as it is a major determinant of oxygen delivery.[21,22] Critically ill patients are frequently assessed clinically, although cardiac output estimations from physical examination alone are generally unreliable and patient status may change quickly.[26] Therefore, invasive techniques are most commonly used in critical care to measure cardiac output (see also Chapter 9).

Non-invasive assessment

Perfusion status is determined clinically using gross organ function such as mental status, urine output and peripheral warmth and colour.[4,9] Basic physical assessment of cardiovas-cular, central nervous system and renal function is essential when assessing a patient at risk of shock. Subtle changes in mentation, urine output, heart rate and capillary refill are all signs of physiological compensation in response to altered tissue perfusion associated with shock. Regular tracking of these vital signs and trend monitoring through careful docu-mentation can alert clinicians to impending deterioration in the shock state. Level of consciousness may deteriorate; an early sign may be anxiety, and progress to restlessness, agitation or coma. Other assessment findings include cool, clammy skin, postural hypotension, tachycardia and decreased urine output.[8,9] The reliability of these measures is questionable, particularly where multiple assessments by

TABLE 21.3

Physiological changes in shock

SHOCK CLASSIFICATION	PHYSIOLOGICAL CHANGE				
	CARDIAC OUTPUT	SYSTEMIC VASCULAR RESISTANCE	CAPILLARY CIRCULATION	PULMONARY CAPILLARY PRESSURE	PULMONARY VASCULAR RESISTANCE
Hypovolaemic	↓	↑	↓	↓	↑
Cardiogenic	↓	↑	↓	↑	↑
Distributive:					
• septic	↑	↓	↓	↓	↑
• anaphylactic	↓	↓	↓	↓	↓
• neurogenic	↓/NC	↓	↓	↓	↑
Obstructive	↓	↓	↓	↑	↑

↑ = increase; ↓ = decrease; NC = no change.

Adapted from Weil M. Personal commentary on the diagnosis and treatment of circulatory shock states. Curr Opin Crit Care 2004; 10:246–9, with permission.

different clinicians are performed. In the intensive care unit (ICU) continuous electrocardiograph monitoring and invasive monitoring techniques are employed to assist in the objective assessment of changes in cardiovascular state. Although estimation of cardiac output based on physical assessment findings is unreliable, physical examination using an estimation of vascular resistance has shown reasonable accuracy.[28] Clinical assessment may determine cardiac output using the rearranged equation where the systemic vascular resistance equals the mean arterial pressure minus the central venous pressure/cardiac output.[28] A reliable and accurate non-invasive clinical assessment technique of estimating cardiac output would be clinically useful,[24] allowing assessment of patients without invasive monitoring, or used to verify accuracy of invasive devices. While a number of non-invasive cardiac output measuring devices are available, further research and refinement is required before widespread application in critical care.[29] New technologies hold promise in aiding clinician assessment of haemodynamic status using non-invasive methods. Clinical ultrasound is being used with increasing frequency with assessment of inferior vena cava (IVC) collapsibility during respiration to assess volume status. A meta-analysis of studies comparing IVC diameter in hypotensive versus normotensive individuals demonstrated a trend towards a decreased IVC size in the hypotensive group compared to the control group. However, measures such as cardiac output or stroke volume variation were not consistently examined to assess for clinical changes based on increased IVC diameter. Additional research is warranted to evaluate the clinical application of clinical ultrasound using IVC.[30]

Invasive assessment

Continuous assessment of heart rate and blood pressure by an intra-arterial catheter also enables circulatory access for frequent blood sampling to assess serum lactate levels, electrolytes and blood gas estimation, including pH and lactate levels.

The indicator dilution method using a thermal (thermodilution) signal (cold or hot) is the customary clinical standard for measuring cardiac output in ICU.[22] This has been achieved by placement of a pulmonary artery catheter, or a central line, in conjunction with a thermistor-tipped arterial cannula (transpulmonary aortic thermodilution). Other invasive techniques measure cardiac output continuously using pulse contour or arterial pressure analysis and ultrasound Doppler methods using an oesophageal probe. All methods have degrees of invasiveness, can be time-consuming to yield measurements of acceptable accuracy,[31] may be expensive and are not without risk of complications.[24,32] The pulmonary artery catheter is a controversial assessment tool[22,25,32] due to the risk associated with the invasive device versus benefits for the measurement of cardiac output.[33] This has led to decreased use and increased interest in less or non-invasive measures of cardiac output.

A further invasive assessment approach is the continuous estimation of mixed venous oxygen saturation using a light-emitting sensor in a pulmonary artery catheter. As tissue oxygen delivery fails to meet demand and oxygen extraction rises, the residual oxygen content of blood returning to the lungs will fall; in effect, this is a surrogate indicator of failure to meet body tissue oxygen demand. This technology was used in the landmark study by Rivers and colleagues[34] to monitor early deterioration of septic shock patients presenting to the emergency department in need of resuscitation and was part of a goal-directed approach to managing patients. This single-centre study was the subject of much interest for its claimed improvement in patient outcome, with this goal-directed approach being assessed in a number of major multicentre studies to verify findings within an international context and varying approaches to critical care delivery.[35] The recent publication of the ProCESS[36] and ARISE[37] trials has further impacted this approach and will be discussed later in the chapter.

Management principles

Managing a patient in shock focuses on treating the underlying cause, and restoration and optimisation of perfusion and oxygen delivery; this includes relevant activities using the acronym VIP.[27] It is also suggested that giving critically ill patients a daily 'FASTHUG', to ensure daily assessment and interventions in priority areas, improves the quality of care for patients in ICU[38] (see Practice tips below). Specific management of patients with different types of shock is discussed separately below.

Practice tip

'VIP' acronym
- **V**entilation, including airway, added oxygen and ventilation
- **I**nfusion of appropriate volume expanders
- Improved heart **P**umping with drug therapy such as antiarrhythmics, inotropes, diuretics and vasodilators

Adapted from Weil M. Personal commentary on the diagnosis and treatment of circulatory shock states. Curr Opin Crit Care 2004;10:246–9, with permission.

Practice tip

'FASTHUG' mnemonic

Feeding (prevent malnutrition, promote adequate caloric intake)

Analgesia (reduce pain, improve physical and psychological wellbeing)

Sedation (titrate to the 3Cs – calm, cooperative, comfortable)

Thromboembolic prophylaxis (prevent DVT)

Head of bed elevated (up to 45° to reduce reflux and VAP)

Ulcer prophylaxis (to prevent stress ulceration)

Glycaemic control (to maintain normal blood glucose levels)

Adapted from Vincent J-L. Give your patient a fast hug (at least) once a day. Crit Care Med 2005;33:1225–9, with permission.

Hypovolaemic shock

Hypovolaemia is a common primary cause of shock and also a factor in other shock states. Insufficient circulating blood volume is the underlying mechanism, leading to decreased cardiac output and altered perfusion.[39,40] Death related to haemorrhage is most likely in the first few hours after injury.[40] The most obvious cause is direct injury to vessels leading to haemorrhage, but there are more insidious causes such as dehydration from prolonged vomiting or diarrhoea, sepsis and burns.[41] Hypovolaemic shock is classified as mild, moderate or severe, depending on the amount of volume loss (see Table 21.4). As the shock state worsens, associated compensatory mechanisms will be more pronounced,[8] and hypovolaemic shock may deteriorate to multiple organ dysfunction syndrome if poor oxygen delivery is prolonged[39] (see Chapter 22).

Clinical manifestations

Symptoms of haemorrhage may not be present until more than 15–30% of blood volume is lost, and will deteriorate as the shock state worsens.[8,41] Estimating blood or plasma loss is difficult and dilutional effects of resuscitation fluids may be evident when assessing haemoglobin and hematocrit.[41] As the body compensates for the reduced circulating volume, widespread vasoconstriction occurs in most body systems apart from the heart and central nervous system; systemic vascular resistance rises markedly in an attempt to retain a viable circulatory system; this accounts for many of the signs and symptoms associated with circulatory compensation. However, as tissues are starved of oxygen and nutrients over a prolonged ischaemic time, local mediators are released as part of the inflammatory responses, leading to organ microvasculature vasodilation, and capillaries re-open to maintain oxygen delivery and reduce hypoxia.[41] This is a hallmark of developing multiple organ dysfunction syndrome.

Patient management

Clinical management of hypovolaemia focuses on minimising fluid loss and restoration of circulating blood volume[41] once the airway and breathing are secure. More than one large-bore intravenous cannulae are usually inserted and lost circulating volume is replaced by colloids, isotonic crystalloids or blood products to achieve haemodynamic end points, such as a mean arterial pressure >65 mmHg. Body heat can be lost rapidly due to blood loss, the rapid infusion of room temperature fluids and exposure in the pre-hospital setting or during repeated physical examination. It is therefore important to institute measures to maintain patient temperature >35°C to avoid coagulopathies and loss of thermoregulation.[42] The aim is to ameliorate the lethal triad of anaemia, coagulopathy and hypothermia, which can lead to worsening hemorrhage and eventual death (see Figure 21.2).[40–42]

Critical care nurses must be efficient and practised at initial patient assessment to establish the degree of compensation occurring in a hypovolaemic patient. Figure 21.2 highlights clinical manifestations of haemorrhage. Careful consideration of a patient's clinical picture will establish a hierarchy and priority of needs. Many hospitals have some level of track and trigger response that escalates care to appropriate levels such as medical emergency teams or rapid response teams. However, nurses are in a position to institute first-line management, such as establishing intravenous access, if this is a core skill. There are also many

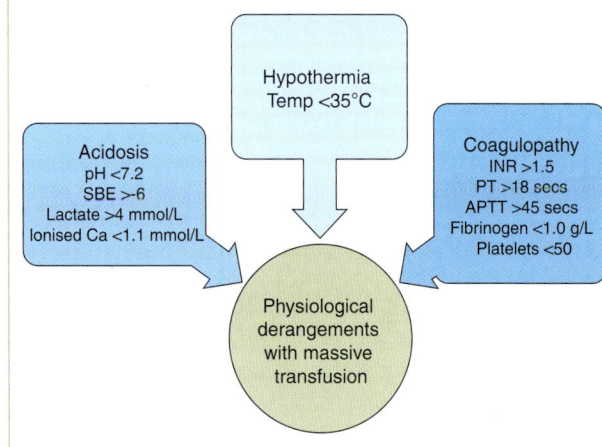

FIGURE 21.2 Physiological derangements during haemorrhage/massive transfusion

TABLE 21.4

Signs and symptoms of hypovolaemic shock

PARAMETER	MILD (15–30% LOSS)	MODERATE (30–40% LOSS)	SEVERE (>40% LOSS)
Blood pressure	No change	Lowered	Hypotensive
Pulse (beats/min)	≥100	≥120	≥140
Respirations (breaths/min)	>20	>30	>40
Neurological	Normal to slightly anxious	Mildly anxious to confused	Confused, lethargic
Urine output (mL/h)	>30	20–30	5–15, negligible
Capillary refill	Normal	Reduced, >4 s	Reduced, >4 s

Adapted from Kelley D. Hypovolemic shock: an overview. Crit Care Nurs Q 2005;28:2–19, with permission.

protocols and guidelines available to guide initial fluid resuscitation where a patient has indications of inadequate circulating blood volume. Although such guidelines might vary slightly, they aim to restore circulating blood volume through the administration of fluid boluses. Up to 20 mL/kg of colloid or 30–40 mL/kg crystalloid may be recommended. Critical bleeding and massive transfusion protocols (see Figure 21.3) should also be available to guide patient management. BloodSafe Australia (https://www.bloodsafelearning.org.au) has lessons available on this issue.

Fluid resuscitation

Fluid resuscitation is a first-line treatment for hypovolaemic shock; providing fluid volume increases preload and therefore cardiac output and organ perfusion. A related principle is that the fluid infused should reflect fluid loss. For example, in burns, plasma replacement might be warranted or, in massive haemorrhage, fresh blood may be indicated. It has been suggested that fluid therapy should be managed in the same way as prescribing medication after consideration of the risks and benefits of a selected fluid.[44] Giving a fluid challenge is not always appropriate; the determining factors will be assessment of volume responsiveness, and whether the infusion will not be deleterious, causing overload, fluid shifts and perpetuating inflammatory responses.[4] The fluid type, volume, rate and targeted end points should be documented;[41] and often this is structured as a bolus dose in volume/kg to achieve a measured haemodynamic variable. See Table 21.5 for a list of some of the frequently used resuscitation fluids and their compositions. When massive transfusion is required, attention should be given to product selection and this should be guided by an evidence-based protocol.

Practice tip

Fluid bolus in high risk groups
- Care should be taken when administering fluid bolus to all patients with particular attention to high risk groups such as the elderly.
- Assess regularly for signs of fluid overload and pulmonary oedema including: shortness of breath, orthopnoea, bibasal auscultation of fine end-inspiratory crackles, oedema, increased central venous pressure. Escalate signs of distress immediately for medical review.

Minimum volume resuscitation

The use of high ratios of blood products and low fluid volume during damage control resuscitation confers a survival benefit.[45] Much of the knowledge around major trauma and haemorrhage has come from military research and management of 'field trauma'.[46] Maintaining a systolic blood pressure of approximately 90 mmHg may be beneficial as clotting factors are not diluted and remaining blood volume retains its viscosity.[47] Selection

of the appropriate fluid for surgical management and 'permissive hypotension' (deliberate limiting or minimising resuscitation until after adequate surgical control of haemorrhage)[40,42] will be assessed by the multidisciplinary team. This restrictive fluid regimen is a process linked to damage control surgery.[47] The goal of this management strategy is to maintain the systolic blood pressure end point using blood products in an effort to limit coagulopathy[47] and stopping the haemorrhage through direct pressure, tamponade devices and other techniques.[46]

Debate surrounds early surgical intervention prior to aggressive fluid resuscitation.[40] The premise is that allowing a lower perfusion pressure prior to achieving haemostasis with controlled or no fluid infusion results in less blood loss, as the compensatory mechanisms described earlier in this chapter are not as profound.[40] Use of medications such as factor IVa and erythropoietin also remains controversial in the setting of critical haemorrhage.[42] Guidelines for 'massive transfusion' released by the Australian National Blood Authority do not recommend use of factor IVa beyond licensed indications, although there may be an indication when conventional therapy has failed to secure haemostasis following massive blood loss and transfusion of blood products.[43] The current debate also includes dosage and thromboembolic complications associated with its use.[42]

Crystalloids versus colloids

The scientific rationale for using colloids over crystalloids is to preserve plasma oncotic pressure so as to retain intravascular fluid and minimise oedema. Colloids may also attenuate the inflammatory response.[15] This scientific rationale has not been supported by the research. The recently published CRISTAL study has not improved understanding around which fluid is most suitable in hypovaolaemic shock as no treatment benefit between crystalloids and colloids was identified.[48] This unblinded multicentre randomised controlled trial was conducted over a decade and enrolled nearly 3000 patients. The primary outcome was 28-day mortality.[48] The colloid versus crystalloid fluid resuscitation debate will continue as other large trials have also been unable to demonstrate outcome benefits except in some subsets of patients.[49–51]

If moderate-to-severe hypovolaemia is suspected, blood is often used to improve oxygen-carrying capacity. Further dilution of blood by volume expanders increases hypoxia, otherwise known as isovolaemic anaemia, and red cells are usually required. Use of isotonic saline as a volume expander is common, although resuscitation with large volumes of saline solutions can be associated with hyperchloraemic acidosis[40] and haemodilution.[46] Blood and blood components are usually considered necessary where patients exhibit signs of moderate-to-severe haemorrhage. There is no perfect resuscitation fluid, and selection is guided by patient condition and the type of fluid lost.

Blood and blood products

There are a number of factors to consider when administering large amounts of blood products. Massive

TABLE 21.5
Resuscitation fluids

VARIABLE	HUMAN PLASMA	4% ALBUMIN	COLLOIDS — HYDROXYETHYL STARCH						4% SUCCINYLATED MODIFIED FLUID GELATIN	3.5% UREA-LINKED GELATIN	CRYSTALLOIDS — 0.9% SALINE	COMPOUNDED SODIUM LACTATE	BALANCED SALT SOLUTION
			10% (200/0.5)	6% (450/0.7)	6% (130/0.4)			6% (130/0.42)					
Trade name		Albumex	Hemohes	Hextend	Voluven	Volulyte	Venofundin	Tetraspan	Gelofusine	Haemaccel	Normal saline	Hartmann's or Ringer's lactate	PlasmaLyte
Colloid source		Human donor	Potato starch	Maize starch	Maize starch	Maize starch	Potato starch	Potato starch	Bovine gelatin	Bovine gelatin			
Osmolarity (mOsm/L)	291	250	308	304	308	286	308	296	274	301	308	280.6	294
Sodium (mmol/L)	135-145	148	154	143	154	137	154	140	154	145	154	131	140
Potassium (mmol/L)	4.5-5.0			3.0		4.0		4.0		5.1		5.4	5.0
Calcium (mmol/L)	2.2-2.6			5.0				2.5		6.25		2.0	
Magnesium (mmol/L)	0.8-1.0			0.9		1.5		1.0					3.0
Chloride (mmol/L)	94-111	128	154	124	154	110	154	118	120	145	154	111	98
Acetate (mmol/L)						34		24					27
Lactate (mmol/L)	1-2			28								29	
Malate (mmol/L)								5					
Gluconate (mmol/L)													23
Bicarbonate (mmol/L)	23-27												
Octanoate (mmol/L)		6.4											

Note: to convert the values for potassium to milligrams per decilitre, divide by 0.2558. To convert the values for calcium to milligrams per decilitre, divide by 0.250. To convert the values for magnesium to milligrams per decilitre, divide by 0.4114.

Adapted from Myburgh JA, Mythen MG. Resuscitation fluids. New Engl J Med 2013;369:1243–51, with permission.

transfusion is defined as replacement of a patient's total blood volume in less than 24 hours. This equates to approximately 10 units of packed red blood cells,[46,52,53] although there are inconsistent descriptions in the literature.[53] A number of complications following massive transfusion can be evident such as transfusion reactions, coagulopathies, hypothermia and sepsis.[8] Massive transfusion is also associated with high mortality.[53]

Patients receiving massive blood transfusions require careful monitoring for signs of metabolic derangements, hypothermia, citrate toxicity, hyperkalaemia and coagulopathies because clotting factors are often depleted. Dilution and clotting factor consumption cause microvascular bleeding, often manifesting as oozing from multiple sites even after surgical correction.[52,53] Massive transfusion of stored blood with high oxygen affinity adversely affects oxygen delivery to the tissues. It is therefore preferable to transfuse blood cells that are less than 1 week old; 2,3-diphosphoglycerate levels rise rapidly after transfusion, and normal oxygen affinity is usually restored within a few hours of transfusion.[52] Current research is underway by the Australian and New Zealand Intensive Care Society Clinical Trials Group to determine if fresher blood decreases 90-day mortality (TRANSFUSE ClinicalTrials.gov identifier: NCT01638416 – see *Online resources*).

Each unit of blood contains approximately 3 g of citrate, which binds to ionised calcium. A healthy adult liver metabolises 3 g of citrate every 5 minutes. If blood is transfused rapidly or liver function is impaired, citrate toxicity and hypocalcaemia may develop. The patient should therefore be monitored for signs of tetany, hypotension and electrocardiographic evidence of hypocalcaemia.[52] As stored blood ages, plasma potassium levels rise (possibly to over 30 mmol/L). Hypokalaemia may be more common as red cells begin active metabolism and intracellular uptake of potassium restarts with transfusion.[52]

Acid–base disturbances may also be evident due to the stored blood lactic acid levels and the citric acid. Citrate is metabolised to bicarbonate, and metabolic alkalosis may result from massive blood transfusion. As hypothermia causes reduced citrate and lactic acid metabolism, an increase in the affinity of haemoglobin to oxygen, platelet dysfunction and an increased tendency for cardiac dysrhythmias,[52] the patient and the blood transfused should be warmed to avoid complications.

Leucocyte depletion occurs during donation in many countries. This decreases upregulation of the inflammatory immune response associated with transfusion. Internationally, there are a number of organisations that produce guidelines for blood transfusion. The Council of Europe has published a high level guide on the preparation of and quality assurance on the use of blood components. The Australian National Blood Authority has published four comprehensive and easy-to-use clinical practice guidelines (see Practice tip).

Practice tip

Blood product usage

Keep up to date and download abbreviated recommendations and tools for use at the bedside from the National Blood Authority (Australia) website as they are completed (see *Online resources*). Always refer back to your local policies and guidelines before patient intervention.

The Australian National Blood Authority Critical Bleeding/Massive Transfusion guideline makes clear recommendations about blood product use during haemorrhage. See Figure 21.3 for the Massive Transfusion Protocol template.

The use of tranexamic acid, an antifibrinolytic agent, is on the increase for patients in need of massive transfusion.[54] Mortality was reduced in a large randomised controlled trial of more than 20,000 trauma patients in those patients that received tranexamic acid.[55] The survival benefit in this study was greatest when treatment occurred in the first hour. This effect was all but lost if administered more than 3 hours after injury. Even though a large sample, these results have given rise to significant debate about including the use of tranexamic acid in guidelines due to insufficient evidence.[56]

Cardiogenic shock

Cardiogenic shock manifests as circulatory failure from cardiac dysfunction,[57] and is reflected in a low cardiac output (cardiac index <2.1 L/min/m^2), hypotension (systolic blood pressure <90 mmHg), severe pulmonary congestion and high central vascular filling pressures (pulmonary artery occlusion pressure >18 mmHg).[58] Additional parameters obtained through invasive monitoring include intrathoracic blood volume index >850 mL/m^2, global end-diastolic volume >700 mL/m^2 and extravascular lung volume index >10 mL/kg.[59,60] Cardiogenic shock is commonly associated with acute myocardial infarction and manifests when 40% or more of the left ventricle is ischaemic. It is also related to mechanical disorders such as acute cardiac valvular dysfunction or septal defects, deteriorating cardiomyopathies or congestive cardiac failure,[61] and trauma. Cardiogenic shock can also occur as a result of obstruction or inhibition of left ventricular ejection, also referred to as obstructive shock, such as occurs in pulmonary embolus, dissecting aneurysm or cardiac tamponade[27,61] (see Chapter 10). Myocardial depression from non-cardiac causes such as sepsis, acidosis, myocardial depressant factor, hypocalcaemia or drug impact[62] may be so severe as to present as cardiogenic shock.

Incidence has been estimated at 3% of patients presenting with acute myocardial infarction. Mortality remains high (50–80%)[63] given death from acute myocardial infarction overall is 7%. This increased mortality occurs despite treatment advances such as emergency

FIGURE 21.3 Massive transfusion protocol.

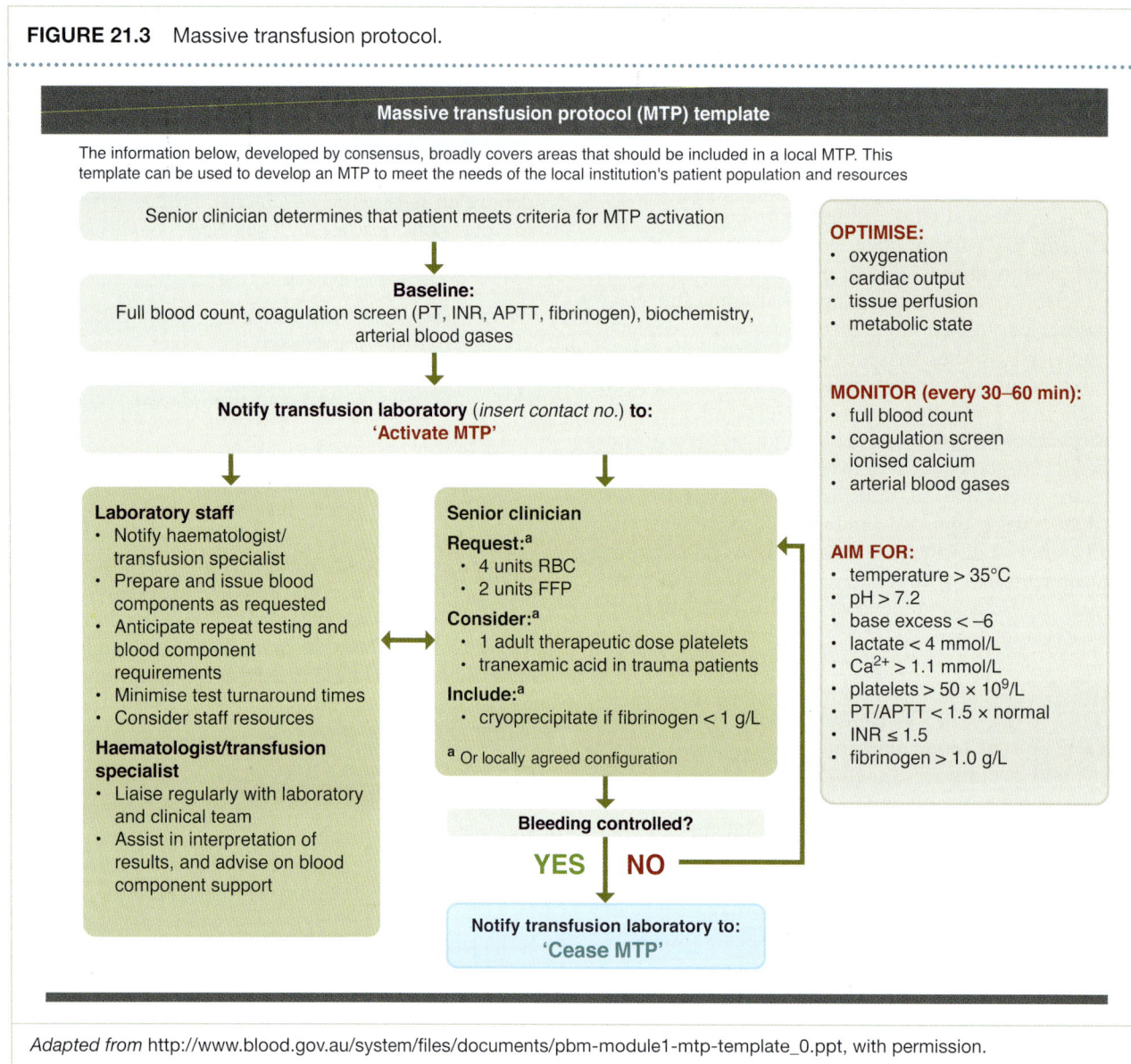

Massive transfusion protocol (MTP) template

The information below, developed by consensus, broadly covers areas that should be included in a local MTP. This template can be used to develop an MTP to meet the needs of the local institution's patient population and resources

Senior clinician determines that patient meets criteria for MTP activation

Baseline:
Full blood count, coagulation screen (PT, INR, APTT, fibrinogen), biochemistry, arterial blood gases

Notify transfusion laboratory (*insert contact no.*) **to:**
'Activate MTP'

Laboratory staff
- Notify haematologist/transfusion specialist
- Prepare and issue blood components as requested
- Anticipate repeat testing and blood component requirements
- Minimise test turnaround times
- Consider staff resources

Haematologist/transfusion specialist
- Liaise regularly with laboratory and clinical team
- Assist in interpretation of results, and advise on blood component support

Senior clinician
Request:[a]
- 4 units RBC
- 2 units FFP

Consider:[a]
- 1 adult therapeutic dose platelets
- tranexamic acid in trauma patients

Include:[a]
- cryoprecipitate if fibrinogen < 1 g/L

[a] Or locally agreed configuration

Bleeding controlled?

YES | **NO**

Notify transfusion laboratory to:
'Cease MTP'

OPTIMISE:
- oxygenation
- cardiac output
- tissue perfusion
- metabolic state

MONITOR (every 30–60 min):
- full blood count
- coagulation screen
- ionised calcium
- arterial blood gases

AIM FOR:
- temperature > 35°C
- pH > 7.2
- base excess < −6
- lactate < 4 mmol/L
- Ca^{2+} > 1.1 mmol/L
- platelets > 50×10^9/L
- PT/APTT < 1.5 × normal
- INR ≤ 1.5
- fibrinogen > 1.0 g/L

Adapted from http://www.blood.gov.au/system/files/documents/pbm-module1-mtp-template_0.ppt, with permission.

revascularisation.[64,65] Wider distribution of interventional cardiac revascularisation services has likely improved outcome for patients who present early in the course of their acute disease. Current timing recommendations for treating myocardial infarction with ST elevation with primary percutaneous coronary intervention include a door-to-balloon time of 90 minutes or less to improve outcomes.[66]

Clinical signs include poor peripheral perfusion, tachycardia and other signs of organ dysfunction such as confusion, agitation, oliguria, cool extremities and dyspnoea, many of which are present in hypovolaemic shock.[57] Compensatory mechanisms are conflicting, as cardiac workload is increased on an already-failing heart yet cardiac muscle oxygen delivery may be compromised. A careful but rapid assessment of the clinical history is helpful in differentiating the precipitant cause of this shock.

Because of similar clinical presentation, obstructive shock is at times described as cardiogenic shock. Obstructive shock is not as common as other types of shock[9] and is associated with a low cardiac output due to extra cardiac processes inhibiting circulatory flow. The two main types are associated with impedance to cardiac filling from causes such as tension pneumothorax and cardiac tamponade and factors that increase afterload such as aortic dissection or massive pulmonary embolus.[67] Examples of conditions that can lead to obstructive shock are provided in Table 21.6. Obstructive shock may be temporarily treated by maintaining preload with fluid resuscitation until definitive intervention to remove the obstruction to forward blood flow.

Managing patients with heart failure as a result of cardiogenic shock can be challenging and is often undertaken simultaneously with preparation for definitive treatment. Maintaining perfusion is difficult, as compensatory

TABLE 21.6

Obstructive shock types

TYPE	DESCRIPTION	SIGNS	AETIOLOGY	TYPICAL MANAGEMENT
Cardiac tamponade	Acute circulatory failure secondary to compression of the heart chambers by a pericardial effusion	Anxiety, hypotension, chest pain, tachypnoea, pulsus paradoxus, tachycardia, high CVP	Pericardial injury, aortic dissection, trauma, post cardiac surgery and rarely infective causes Symptoms include right sided diastolic collapse	Pericardial drainage
Tension pneumothorax	Progressive build-up of air within the pleural space by allowing air in but not out; pressure in the pleural space pushes the mediastinum to the opposite side, obstructing venous return to the heart	Deviated trachea away from the affected side, hyperexpansion on the side of the pneumothorax with little air movement and distended neck veins	Penetrating chest injury, blunt trauma, hospital procedures such as insertion or removal of central lines, lung biopsy	Needle thoracostomy as soon as possible (large cannula inserted to the 2nd intercostal space at the mid-clavicular line); however this procedure is not without complications and it has been suggested that the diagnosis should be confirmed on X-ray prior to the procedure, and a pleural drain will be required after
Pulmonary embolism	Thrombotic occlusion of a pulmonary artery	Increases right-sided afterload, enlarges RV and deviates septum to left, thus decreasing left ventricular volume and compliance	Shortness of breath, chest pain, haemoptysis	Thrombolysis or surgical embolectomy

CVP = central venous pressure; RV = right ventricle.

Adapted from Bodson L, Bouferrache K, Vieillard-Baron A. Cardiac tamponade. Curr Opin Crit Care 2011;17:416–24, with permission.

mechanisms usually cause further harm to the heart. While judicious administration of fluid is considered in terms of optimising remaining cardiac function, administration of pharmacological agents that reduce cardiac workload and improve function is paramount: dobutamine for inotropic and afterload-reducing effects via vasodilation and morphine to reduce pain, improve coronary perfusion and reduce oxygen demand. Treatment of the underlying cause is critical and may include surgery to repair obstruction to flow or percutaneous resolution of a coronary artery blockage. See Chapter 10 for a more detailed discussion of the management of acute myocardial infarction and heart failure.

Clinical manifestations

The clinical features of cardiogenic shock are reflective of congestive cardiac failure, although with greater severity[58,59] (see Box 21.1). Other symptoms consistent with the cause of the cardiogenic shock may also be present, including chest pain and ST-segment changes, murmurs, features of pericardial tamponade and arrhythmias.

BOX 21.1

Clinical features of cardiogenic shock:

- low cardiac output and hypotension
- poor peripheral perfusion – pale, cool, clammy peripheries
- oliguria
- altered mentation, restlessness and anxiety
- tachycardia and arrhythmias
- pulmonary congestion with widespread inspiratory crackles and hypoxaemia (perhaps with frank pulmonary oedema)
- dyspnoea and tachypnoea
- respiratory alkalosis (hyperventilation) or acidosis (respiratory fatigue)
- lactic acidosis
- distended neck veins, elevated jugular venous pressure.

In the absence of invasive monitoring, the profile of hypotension, peripheral hypoperfusion and severe pulmonary and venous congestion is evident although this 'classic' profile is not universal. On initial examination, approximately 30% of patients with shock of left ventricular aetiology will have no pulmonary congestion and an estimated 9% will have no hypoperfusion.[69]

Based on the underlying pathology of an acute left ventricular myocardial infarction, the structural or contractile abnormality impairs systolic performance resulting in incomplete left ventricular emptying.[58] This results in subsequent progressive congestion of first the left atrium, then the pulmonary circulation, right ventricle, right atrium and finally the venous circulation.[58,70,71] When invasive haemodynamic monitoring is available, changes that may be observed include decreased cardiac output and increased systemic resistance and myocardial oxygen demand (see Figure 21.4).

A patient with cardiogenic shock is also assessed and monitored for their oxygen delivery and tissue oxygen requirements. Systemic oxygen delivery falls in proportion to a declining cardiac output, and is further exacerbated as hypoxaemia develops with pulmonary oedema. Initially, oxygen consumption may be sustained by an increase in tissue oxygen extraction ratio.[72] A quarter of delivered oxygen is extracted by tissues but, as delivery falls, tissues extract proportionally more oxygen to meet metabolic needs. Oxygen consumption can therefore be sustained until the severity of oxygen delivery deficit exceeds the ability to increase extraction. Maximal extraction is approximately 50%, and consumption falters when oxygen delivery falls to around 500–600 mL/min (cardiac index <2.2 L/min/m²).[72,73] While use of a pulmonary artery catheter is a well-described measure of severity in cardiogenic shock (as with hypovolaemic shock), evidence of improved patient outcome is unclear.[25,33]

Once oxygen consumption falls, subsequent anaerobic metabolism leads to lactic acidosis.[21,58] Progressive tissue ischaemia and injury ensues, along with worsening metabolic acidosis unless oxygen delivery can be restored.

FIGURE 21.4 Sequence of haemodynamic changes in cardiogenic shock.

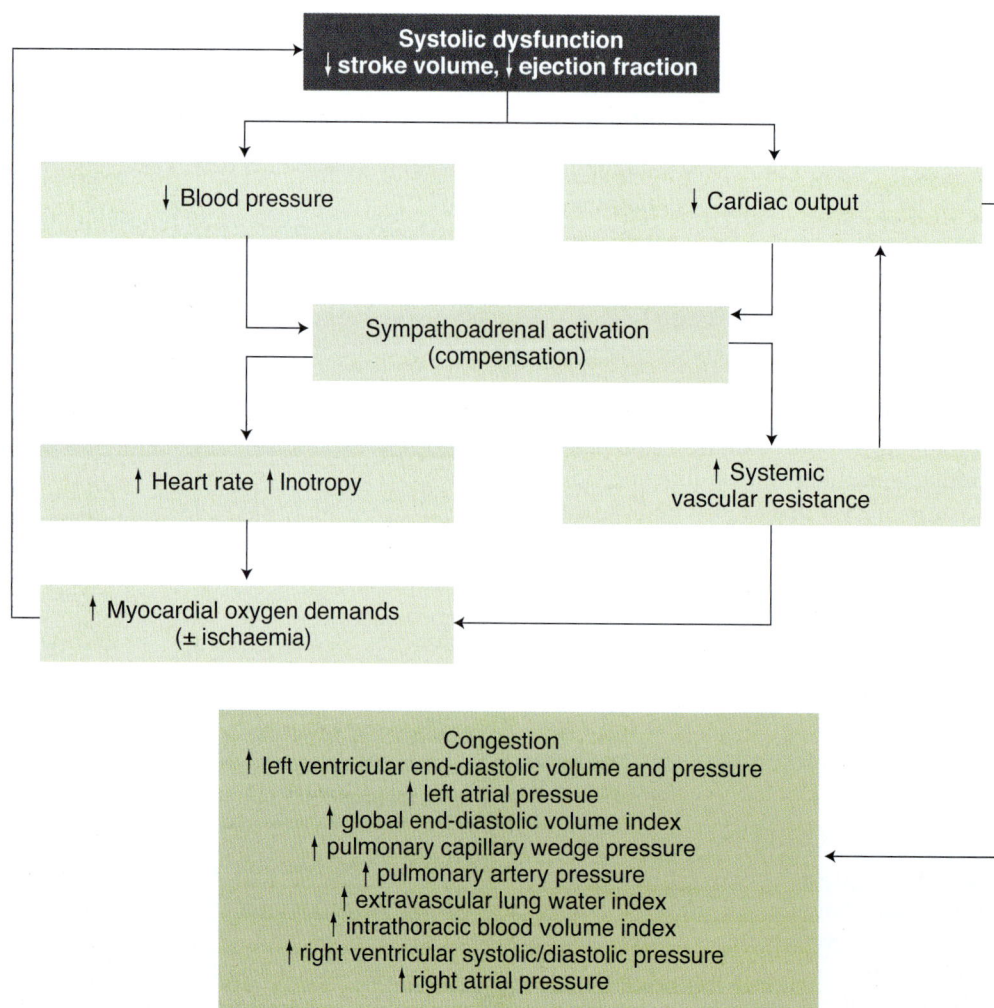

Myocardial contractile performance continues to deteriorate when myocardial ischaemia develops or when existing ischaemia or infarction extends, leading to a vicious cycle of ischaemia and dysfunction.[72]

Compensatory responses effective in hypovolaemic shock are initially advantageous, but may ultimately be counterproductive when cardiogenic shock is due to myocardial infarction:

- Tachycardia offsets low stroke volume but increases myocardial oxygen consumption and decreases diastolic duration, reducing coronary perfusion time.

- Vasoconstriction limits the severity of hypotension but increases resistance to left ventricular emptying and may contribute to worsening of the cardiac output, in particular when cardiogenic shock is due to contractile dysfunction.

- An increase in cardiac workload to overcome the rise in systemic afterload increases myocardial oxygen demand, which cannot be met due to coronary artery occlusion.

- Developing pulmonary congestion is no longer contained within the pulmonary capillary and moves into the alveolar capillary space, creating pulmonary oedema, further impeding oxygen delivery to the circulation.

Patient management

Treatment of cardiogenic shock includes haemodynamic management, respiratory and cardiovascular support, biochemical stabilisation and reversal or correction of the underlying cause. This complex presentation requires a coordinated approach to the multiple aspects of care of a patient with cardiogenic shock.

A rapid response to impending deterioration associated with cardiogenic shock includes repeated assessment and measures to optimise oxygen supply and demand. Frequent, thorough assessment of the patient's status is essential, and should focus on:

1 identification of patients at risk of clinical deterioration
2 assessment of the severity of shock and identification of organ or system dysfunction
3 assessment of the impact of treatment
4 identification of complications of treatment.

Assessment follows a systematic approach and is conducted as often as indicated by the patient's condition, centring on the cardiovascular system as well as related systems that cardiac function influences, including respiratory, renal, neurological and integumentary systems.

Typical treatment regimens require preload reduction, augmentation of contractility with intravenous inotropes and afterload manipulation. These aspects are undertaken concurrently due to the potential severity of cardiogenic shock. Endotracheal intubation with mechanical ventilation is implemented if necessary, but the need for mechanical ventilation is associated with an increase in mortality.[74]

Optimising oxygen supply and demand

As cardiogenic shock is associated with an imbalance of oxygen supply and demand throughout the body, measures to optimise this balance by increasing oxygen supply and decreasing demand are essential (see Box 21.2).

BOX 21.2

Managing oxygen supply and demand

Strategies to increase oxygen supply include:

- positioning the patient upright to promote optimum ventilation by reducing venous return and lessening pulmonary oedema; this strategy may contribute to hypotension

- administering oxygen, continuous positive airway pressure and bi-level positive airway pressure support as required.[75]

Strategies to reduce oxygen demand include:

- limiting physical activity

- implementing measures to reduce patient anxiety, including communication, explanation and analgesic and sedative medications. Avoid those medications that are cardio-depressive.

Preload management

Preload reduction relieves pulmonary congestion, reduces myocardial workload and improves contractility, which is in part impaired by overstretched ventricles. Careful assessment of patient fluid status is necessary prior to either the administration of small aliquots of fluid to enhance deteriorating myocardial function or enhanced diuresis to reduce circulating blood volume. Any fluid offloading is balanced against the risk of excessive blood volume depletion and depression of cardiac output and blood pressure. Desired end points of therapy may include a reduction in right atrial, pulmonary artery and pulmonary artery occlusion pressures, or improvements in

---

Practice tip

Measures to reduce preload include:

- sitting a patient up with their legs either hanging over the side of the bed or in a dependent position

- IV diuretics such as frusemide[1] usually administered as an intermittent bolus or if necessary as a continuous infusion

- venodilation (glyceryl trinitrate infusions at 10–200 mcg/min titrated to blood pressure)[3]

- ultrafiltration (may be considered to rapidly reduce circulating volume)

- respiratory support with continuous positive airway pressure (indicated for pulmonary relief, with the additional benefit of reducing venous return).

intrathoracic blood volume, global end-diastolic volume and extravascular lung water, depending on available monitoring equipment.

Additional measures to reduce pulmonary hypertension may be employed. Morphine is useful to lessen anxiety and oxygen demands during cardiogenic shock, and may offer additional benefits by reducing pulmonary artery pressure and pulmonary oedema.[76] Other treatment options include correction of hypercapnoea, if present, and nitric oxide by inhalation.

Inotropic therapy

Intravenous positive inotropes promote myocardial contractility to improve cardiac output and blood pressure.

Currently available inotropes are not uniform in their beneficial effect on cardiac output and blood pressure because of additional vasoactive actions (either vasodilation or constriction) (see Table 21.7). Selection of an inotropic agent is therefore partly based on inotropic potency as well as the desired effect on vascular resistance:

- vasodilation in addition to inotropy (inodilator effect) favours cardiac output, but may compromise blood pressure[76]
- vasoconstriction in addition to inotropy (inoconstrictor effect) improves blood pressure, but may at times compromise left ventricular emptying and cardiac output.

TABLE 21.7
Vasoactive agents

DRUG	ACTIONS	DOSE RANGE	PHYSIOLOGICAL EFFECTS	NURSING CONSIDERATIONS
dobutamine	Synthetic adrenergic agonist β_1-agonist β_2-agonist	100–200 mcg/min	Inotropy Vasodilation ↑↑ Cardiac output ↑Blood pressure ↑Heart rate	CVC administration Arrhythmia risk Excess dilation may cause hypotension
dopamine	Dopaminergic β_1-agonist α-agonist (at higher doses)	'Inotropic' dose: 5–10 mcg/kg/min 'High' dose: 10–20 mcg/kg/min	Mainly inotropic ↑Blood pressure ↑Cardiac output Vasoconstriction dominates ↑↑Blood pressure	CVC administration Tachycardia Arrhythmia risk Risk peripheral vascular compromise
levosimendan	Calcium sensitiser	Loading: 6–12 mcg/kg over 10 min Infusion: 0.05–0.2 mcg/kg/min (max 24–48 hours use)	Inotropy Vasodilation ↑↑Cardiac output	Tachycardia Arrhythmia risk Risk hypokalaemia Risk Q-T prolongation Excess dilation may cause hypotension Half-life: 5 days
adrenaline	Sympathomimetic α-agonist β_1-agonist β_2-agonist	1–20 mcg/min or higher	Potent inotrope and constrictor ↑Cardiac output ↑↑Blood pressure ↑↑Heart rate	Tachycardia common Arrhythmia risk Risk peripheral vascular compromise Myocardial work
milrinone	Phosphodiesterase inhibitor	Loading: 50–75 mcg/kg Infusion: 0.375–0.75 mcg/kg/min	Inotropy Potent vasodilator ↑↑Cardiac output ↓Blood pressure	Vasodilation may be marked Observe for hypotension
noradrenaline	Sympathomimetic α-agonist β_1-agonist Little effect on β_2-receptors	1–20 mcg/min or higher	Potent inotrope and constrictor ↑↑Blood pressure ↑Coronary artery blood flow	Reflex bradycardias Arrhythmia risk Risk peripheral vascular compromise
vasopressin	Vascular (V-1) receptors Renal (V-2) receptors	0.1–0.4 mcg/min	Inotropy ↑SVR ↑Vasoconstriction	Check liver function

CVC = central venous catheter; SVR = systemic vascular resistance; ↑ = increase; ↓ = decrease.
Adapted from: Lampard JG, Lang E. Vasopressors for hypotensive shock. Ann Emerg Med 2013;61:351–2 Magder SA. The highs and lows of blood pressure: toward meaningful clinical targets in patients with shock. Crit Care Med 2014;42:1241–51.

All inotropes present a paradox in the treatment of cardiogenic shock, as they have the potential to increase heart rate and myocardial oxygen demands, and increase the frequency of arrhythmias. Monitoring is used to identify heart rate, rhythm and the development of ST-segment or T-wave changes. The best regimen for cardiogenic shock has not been established. There is controversy about using drug combinations with opposing effects; however, there is evidence that using dilators and pressors together is superior to the use of inopressors alone.[80] The vasodilation seen with inodilator agents may reduce both preload and afterload, leading to more effective myocardial pumping and an increased cardiac output. The effect on blood pressure is variable, as the opposing actions of increased contractility and vasodilation are not uniform in potency, and occur with differing effects between patients. By reducing afterload, left ventricular emptying is favoured with a reduction in cardiac contractility, reducing myocardial oxygen demand.[81–83] In a large study of more than 900 patients with cardiogenic shock requiring a vasopressor agent to maintain perfusion, short-term mortality was improved when a dilator was part of the medication regimen.[80]

Inoconstrictors constrict the vasculature, resulting in increased preload and afterload while also increasing myocardial contractility.[77] These increases, particularly in afterload, generally result in a raised blood pressure, but the impact on cardiac output is less predictable. An increase in cardiac output is often seen with these agents, but the increase in afterload may become limiting to left ventricular emptying when there is significant contractile impairment. Inoconstrictors are therefore generally selected when the afterload and resultant blood pressure are more severely compromised than the cardiac output. Vasoconstriction also further increases myocardial work and myocardial oxygen demand, and may worsen ischaemia.[80]

Dobutamine has traditionally been the inodilator of choice,[84] although accumulating evidence for levosimendan, a calcium-sensitising agent, suggests improved outcomes.[81,83] The slow onset of action time of levosimendan (hours) makes it a less suitable drug for acute resuscitation; other inotropes are therefore currently used initially and, if required, levosimendan is introduced later. The long half-life (>5 days) of levosimendan confers a lasting impact on contractility after cessation of the infusion. Milrinone is also an effective inodilator,[77] but excessive vasodilation may contribute to significant hypotension; in practice, a concurrent vasoconstrictor (e.g. noradrenaline) may be administered. Close management of intravascular fluid volume is critical when using these agents.

Dopamine and adrenaline are the major agents in the inoconstrictor class, and are more effective at raising blood pressure than inodilators. Both agents also increase cardiac output, but when there is significant impairment of contractility the increase in afterload may cause cardiac output to suffer. Importantly, inoconstrictors increase myocardial work and oxygen demands, raise heart rate and increase the risk of tachyarrhythmias; these impacts are stronger with adrenaline than for dopamine.

Afterload control

Specific management of afterload, independent of contractility, is sometimes necessary, although caution is needed as the maintenance of blood pressure often provides little scope for further afterload reduction. Arteriodilators such as sodium nitroprusside reduce afterload and increase cardiac output, although with limitations due to hypotension.[85] The introduction of oral angiotensin-converting enzyme inhibitors is recommended as soon as possible after stabilisation of the patient with infarct-related cardiogenic shock.[86,87]

Adjunctive therapies

A range of adjunctive therapies is available for refractory shock, when first-line treatments are ineffective, and can include insertion of an intra-aortic balloon pump (IABP), extracorporeal membrane oxygenation (ECMO), initiation of mechanical ventilation and correction of metabolic disturbances. These strategies are discussed below in relation to cardiogenic shock.

Intra-aortic balloon pumping

Low cardiac output, pulmonary congestion, reduced mean arterial pressure and myocardial ischaemia from cardiogenic shock may all be improved by the introduction of IABP therapy (see Chapter 12). Balloon inflation during diastole raises mean arterial pressure and promotes coronary and systemic blood flow, while balloon deflation in advance of systole reduces afterload. This afterload reduction improves cardiac output and reduces left ventricular systolic pressure, lessening the oxygen demands of the ischaemic ventricle by reducing the necessary contractile force of the left ventricle. In a large trial database, IABP did not impart a survival benefit at 12 months in an open label trial comparing outcomes from patients with early revascularisation and optimal medical management.[88]

Extracorporeal membrane oxygenation

ECMO is an accepted treatment of cardiac failure when persistent shock is evident despite adequate fluid resuscitation and administration of vasopressors and inotropes. ECMO is defined as the temporary use of a modified cardiopulmonary bypass circuit for support of patients with potentially reversible cardiac and/or respiratory failure.[89] ECMO provides a mechanism for gas exchange as well as cardiac support thereby allowing for recovery from existing disease. This therapy is complex and should be provided in centres where adequate facilities and human resources are available to ensure optimal implementation.[90]

Management of the patient receiving ECMO is complex. Often, more than one nurse is required to provide support in the first 24 hours. Large bore catheters are used to ensure adequate extracorporeal circulation. Apart from the infective risk, disconnection poses a risk of rapid exsanguination. While ECMO provides cardiac support and gas exchange it is vital to continue to promote recovery by maintaining cardiac function and reducing the risk of complications.

Respiratory support

Varying degrees of pulmonary oedema accompany cardiogenic shock, causing hypoxaemia due to intrapulmonary shunt, decreased compliance and increased work of breathing. Hyperventilation with respiratory alkalosis may initially compensate for hypoxaemia and lactic acidosis, but fatigue during this increased work of breathing may cause patient progression to hypoventilation and respiratory acidosis. Oxygen is administered for hypoxaemia, but the response may be limited as the primary gas exchange defect is an intrapulmonary shunt. Non-invasive ventilatory approaches may be sufficient, but intubation and mechanical ventilation may be required in the acute phase of treatment. Continuous positive airway pressure at conventional levels of 5–15 cmH$_2$O is well established as a support for the spontaneously breathing patient with pulmonary oedema.[91] This respiratory support strategy improves hypoxaemia, decreases work of breathing, reduces left ventricular afterload and provides additional benefit by impeding venous return, an effect that may lessen pulmonary congestion. These benefits are weighed against the potential for hypotension.

If hypoventilation and dyspnoea continue despite the use of continuous positive airway pressure, non-invasive bi-level positive airway pressure may be considered. Additional pressure support is applied during inspiration, above existing baseline pressure, improving inspiratory efficiency, with increased tidal volume and reduced work of breathing.[92,93] Endotracheal intubation and ventilation should be undertaken when neither strategy results in improvement, or when the patient continues to deteriorate or tire. Many clinicians prefer to intubate and ventilate early, even in the absence of a specific respiratory need, to decrease the cardiovascular demands of the greater ventilatory effort. However, this approach is controversial as mechanical ventilation is associated with poorer patient outcomes[93] and disturbs cardiovascular balance as it exerts changes to intrathoracic pressures, particularly at inspiratory initiation.

Ventilation strategies largely reflect those for other compliance disorders such as adult respiratory distress syndrome and are described in more detail in Chapter 15. Initially, full mechanical ventilation with little or no contribution from the patient is appropriate to correct arterial blood gases and lessen the cardiovascular demands of the ventilatory burden. Subsequent reduction of ventilatory support, as the patient's respiratory ability improves, follows conventional processes.

Biochemical normalisation

Frequent biochemistry measurement is necessary to detect and monitor the following aspects of care:

- arterial blood gases to identify the adequacy of ventilation and oxygenation and the presence of metabolic acidosis
- lactic acid measurement to assess the level of shock and changes in patient response to treatment

- hypokalaemia or hypomagnesaemia due to aggressive diuretic use
- hyperkalaemia due to severe acidosis, especially in the presence of renal failure
- hyperglycaemia due to the stress response to acute illness, and in response to sympathomimetic administration
- decline in bicarbonate levels due to pH buffering, although replacement therapy is not routinely undertaken unless the arterial pH is life-threatening
- urea and creatinine to detect the onset of acute renal failure due to renal hypoperfusion.

Renal replacement therapies may be used for fluid and electrolyte control when renal function suffers or as a strategy for unloading fluid from the circulation (see Chapter 18).

Sepsis and septic shock

Severe sepsis and septic shock is a leading cause of admission to ICU and has an associated high mortality. The terms 'severe sepsis' and 'septic shock' were defined and then refined during international consensus meetings that also described the systemic inflammatory response syndrome.[95] The incidence of severe sepsis in the European Union has been estimated at 90.4 cases per 100,000 population and the estimated annual rate worldwide is 1.8 million cases.[96] Accuracy of this figure is likely hampered by the ongoing worldwide issues with recognition. The incidence of severe sepsis in Australia and New Zealand was 11.8% of ICU admissions, with median ICU and hospital stays of 6 days and 18 days, respectively, and corresponding mortality rates of 32% at 28 days and an in-hospital mortality of 40%.[97] Recent Australian data show mortality remaining relatively high but in decline.[35,98] In fact, between 2000 and 2012 a retrospective observation study showed a mortality decrease of 16.1% over the time period.[99] The consequence of early reports of such high mortality focused attention on sepsis and its associated sequelae in the critical care literature, and led to a worldwide campaign in 2002 to reduce the mortality from sepsis.

The Surviving Sepsis Campaign

The Surviving Sepsis Campaign is an international collaborative formed after the Barcelona Declaration in 2002 to reduce the mortality of sepsis by 25% over a 5-year period. The aims included increasing awareness and developing treatment guidelines for severe sepsis and shock, including a comprehensive list of graded recommendations (now in its third version).[100–102] Worldwide Sepsis Day occurs on September 13 each year to continue the push for improving outcomes. Although the first version of the sepsis guidelines was supported by many countries, the second and much expanded version was not endorsed in Australia,[98] as many of the recommendations were based on research involving non-ICU and/or non-sepsis patients.

The most recent update of the 'Surviving Sepsis Campaign Guidelines' was published in 2013 and outlines evidence-based recommendations for the management of severe sepsis and septic shock. Various recommendations were combined to form 'care bundles', which are interventions or care elements implemented together to achieve better outcomes.[103] Bundles have been introduced to change processes of care and as quality or benchmarking measures (see Chapter 3). Further research and evaluation is needed as mortality benefits of 'care bundles' may be a result of increased clinician awareness rather than the impact of treatment changes.[104] In a recent meta-analysis of the 6- and 24-hour sepsis bundles, the better treatment effect was seen with the 6-hour bundle.[105] Current bundles can be found on the Surviving Sepsis website and include the 3- and 6-hour bundle. The current suggested sepsis bundles appear in Box 21.3.

Some bundles were developed then refuted, so it is important for critical care nurses to continuously update knowledge as further evidence becomes available. An example of a refuted bundle relates to tight glycaemic control. The recommendation in the Surviving Sepsis guidelines supported tight glycaemic control in earlier versions.[107,108] The NICE-SUGAR study subsequently concluded that measures to maintain blood glucose level of ≤10 mmol/L increased mortality, particularly in relation to severe hypoglycaemia.[109] A meta-analysis of 26 ICU-related 'tight glycaemic control' studies suggested that the practice could increase risk to ICU patients.[110] The more pragmatic approach of maintaining blood glucose levels close to normal without inducing hypoglycaemia and other metabolic imbalances is therefore appropriate.[107] The Surviving Sepsis guideline was modified in 2009 to maintain currency. The 2012 version recommends a protocolised approach to instituting insulin to manage hyperglycaemia when two consecutive measurements are greater than 10 mmol/L with blood glucose measured every 1–2 hours until stable and then 4-hourly, preferably using arterial sampling to target an upper blood glucose ≤180 mg/dL (10 mmol/L).[101]

Clinical manifestations

Septic shock results when infectious agents or infection-induced mediators in the bloodstream produce haemodynamic compromise. Primarily a form of distributive shock, it is characterised by ineffective tissue oxygen delivery and extraction associated with inappropriate peripheral vasodilation, despite preserved or increased cardiac output.[70] Hypovolaemia is also associated with septic shock due to the characteristic increased vasodilation. This presents a clinical picture of a warm, pink and apparently well-perfused patient in early stages of septic shock with an elevated cardiac output, in contrast to that seen in hypovolaemic or cardiogenic shock patients.

Unchecked, cellular dysfunction in the presence of a failing compensatory process leads to cellular membrane damage, loss of ion gradients, leakage of lysosomal enzymes, proteolysis due to activation of cellular proteases and reductions in cellular energy stores that may result in cell death. Once enough cells from vital organs have reached this stage, shock becomes irreversible and death can occur despite eradication of the underlying septic focus. About half of patients who succumb to septic shock die of failure of multiple organs.[70]

The effect of sepsis and septic shock on the cardiovascular system is profound; the haemodynamic hallmark is generalised arterial vasodilation with an associated decrease in systemic vascular resistance. Arterial vasodilation is mediated in part by cytokines that upregulate the expression of inducible nitric oxide synthase in the vasculature. Vascular response to the vasodilatory effect of nitric oxide and the activation of ATP-sensitive potassium channels combine to cause closure of the voltage-gated calcium channels in the cell membrane. As the vasoconstrictor effect of noradrenaline and angiotensin II depends on open calcium channels, lack of response to these pressor hormones that are central to compensatory mechanisms in shock can occur with the inevitable failure of delivery of oxygen to the functional mitochondria, resulting in lactic acidosis in patients with sepsis.[111] With high circulating levels of endogenous vasoactive hormones during sepsis, downregulation of their receptors occurs.

Severe sepsis and septic shock includes four different phenotypes, when using lactate level and blood pressure[112]

BOX 21.3

Types of sepsis bundles

Resuscitation bundle (now called the 3-hour bundle):

1 Measure lactate.

2 Culture prior to administration of antimicrobials.

3 Administer empirical (broad spectrum) antimicrobials as soon as possible.

4 Volume-load as appropriate. (Administer 30 mL/kg crystalloid for hypotension or lactate ≥4 mmol/L.)

Sepsis management bundle (now called the 6-hour bundle):

1 Use vasopressors for persisting hypotension or apply vasopressors (for hypotension that does not respond to initial fluid resuscitation) to maintain a mean arterial pressure ≥65 mmHg.

2 In the event of persistent arterial hypotension despite volume resuscitation (septic shock) or initial lactate ≥4 mmol/L (36 mg/dL):

   a maintain adequate central venous pressure

   b maintain adequate central venous oxygen saturation

   c re-measure lactate if initial lactate was elevated.

Adapted from Barochia A, Cui X, Vitberg D, Suffredini AF, O'Grady NP, Banks SM et al. Bundled care for septic shock: an analysis of clinical trials. Crit Care Med 2010;38:668–78, with permission.

as clinical indicators: severe sepsis without hyperlactataemia (where hyperlactataemia is defined as lactate >4 mmol/L) and normotension (systolic blood pressure at least 90 mmHg); vasoplegic shock, persistent hypotension without hyperlactataemia; dysoxia with hypotension and hyperlactataemia; and cryptic shock, defined as a hyperlactataemia and normotension.[112] There are increasing numbers of studies comparing these profiles. Cryptic shock and overt shock (vasoplegic and dysoxic profile), defined as hypotension (systolic blood pressure lower than 90mmHg), had a similar mortality in one study.[113] This research is still evolving and the results from studies are equivocal; for example, another study was only able to demonstrate cryptic shock and vasoplegic shock had similar outcomes.[114] The learning from these studies is the importance of vigilance in checking the haemodynamic profile of a patient and the biochemical results to ensure deterioration is not overlooked.

Early identification and diagnosis

Where a patient is able to respond cogently during history and physical assessment, timelines of the infective process should be documented. Sites considered as infective sources include decubitus ulcers, invasive lines, drains, wounds, sinuses, ears, teeth, throat, chest, blood, lungs, back, abdomen, perianal, genital/urinary tract, bones and joints. More invasive sampling may include bronchioalveolar lavage, cerebral spinal fluid, pleural fluid, abdominal collections or biopsy of other sites as clinically appropriate. X-rays, computerised tomography scans and surgical consultation will also be a priority.

Patient management

As with other forms of shock, initial management includes not only acting to correct physiological deterioration by initiating fluid management and frequent observation and assessment, but also addressing the underlying cause of sepsis through source (of infection) control. Goal-directed therapy includes prevention of tissue hypoxia, typically through rigorous fluid resuscitation with either crystalloids or colloids to achieve specific haemodynamic end points, such as a central venous pressure of 8–12 mmHg, mean arterial pressure of >65 mmHg, and urine output >0.5 mL/kg/h. Vasopressor and inotropic therapy may then be added to maintain adequate perfusion pressure; noradrenaline is the vasopressor of choice because of vasoconstrictor effects.[115]

Initial resuscitation

The 2012 sepsis guidelines recommend a protocolised approach for resuscitation for sepsis-induced shock, defined as tissue hypoperfusion where hypotension persists after initial fluid challenge or where there is a blood lactate concentration ≥4 mmol/L. Measuring surrogate markers of preload as an indicator of volume status is a contentious issue, as central venous pressure as a measure of preload is not a good marker of volume responsiveness.[31,116] While central venous pressure was used in sepsis trials

of early goal-directed therapy (EGDT) protocols[34,117–119] and is an often-documented end point of resuscitation, EGDT has been widely discussed and criticised in the literature. Australian data indicate that the incidence of patients meeting the criteria and mortality is lower than the treatment group in the original EGDT trial.[35] EGDT was the focus of the ProCESS trial,[36] the ARISE trial in Australia and New Zealand[37] and the ProMISe trial.[120]

The ProCESS trial showed no significant outcome difference between three resuscitation groups including two protocol-based approaches, EGDT and standard resuscitation, and the third group of 'usual care'.[36] Of note, mortality rates were 18+% in all three groups, including the control group. ARISE results showed no significant difference in all-cause mortality at 90 days between EGDT and usual care. At the time of randomisation (median 2.8 hours), over 2.5 litres of fluid had been given to patients and time to antibiotics after arrival in emergency department was <70 minutes. Similarly, mortality rates were 18.6% in the EGDT and 18.8% in the usual care group.

The EGDT group in the ARISE trial received more fluid in the first 6 hours and was more likely to receive vasopressors, red cell transfusions and dobutamine.[37] Study critiques have identified the potential role that sepsis identification and treatment in patients prior to randomisation may have played, along with notable lower mortality rates in both study groups. However, there is a plan to pool the data from the three trials to perform a meta-analysis. It seems likely, given the results to date, the Surviving Sepsis guidelines recommendations related to EGDT may need to be reconsidered. Additionally, the role of non-invasive evaluation using ultrasound assessment of volume status and fluid infusion responsiveness and echocardiography evaluation of cardiac contractility will need further consideration based on additional clinical trial data. The current statement available on the Surviving Sepsis website regarding EGDT indicates that the evidence is under review and that the guidelines will be updated pending this review process.

The ProMISe trial conducted in the UK was a pragmatic randomised controlled trial of 1260 patients who received either EGDT or usual care. Despite patients in the EGDT group receiving more intravenous fluids, vasoactive drugs and red-cell transfusions there was no difference between the two groups in terms of 90-day mortality.[120]

Minimum continuous monitoring includes electrocardiogram, blood pressure, pulse oximetry and other measures to assess preload and volume responsiveness, along with regular assessment of lactate, oxygenation and markers of inflammation and coagulation.

Source control and antimicrobial therapy

Identifying and removing the source of infection and treating the infection with appropriate antimicrobial therapy are the mainstays of therapy for a patient with sepsis. Research indicates that in the ICU setting the most prevalent site of primary infection is pulmonary, followed by abdominal, together accounting for approximately 70% of cases.[97,121,122]

To provide patients with appropriate antimicrobial treatment for targeting the infecting organism, obtaining appropriate samples prior to instigating antimicrobial therapy is the clinical standard, although any prescribed treatment should not be delayed as time to antibiotic administration is important in severe sepsis.[123] The Surviving Sepsis guidelines recommend that, to optimise identification of causative organisms, at least two blood cultures should be obtained before antimicrobial therapy with at least one drawn percutaneously and one drawn through each vascular access device.[101] In a large retrospective study, every additional hour to effective antimicrobial initiation in the first 6 hours after onset of hypotension was associated with >7% decrease in survival.[123,124] Optimising dosage to achieve a therapeutic concentration is also important. Current practice depends on the mechanism of action of the antibiotic. For example glycopeptides are often continuously infused to maintain a serum concentration above the minimum inhibitory concentration and therefore kill microbes more effectively. More recently there has been evidence that beta-lactams should also be infused.[125] Beta-lactams are time dependent and the concentration needs to be 4 times above the minimum inhibitory concentration in order to have efficacy.[126] Aminoglycosides have an effect through rapid administration to reach target concentrations and have a 'post-antibiotic effect'.

Recently, a paradigm shift has been suggested in relation to antimicrobial therapy: to get it right the first time with high doses, while limiting the duration of therapy and the potential to increase resistance.[127] Regardless, empirical therapy should be de-escalated as soon as microbiology results support directed therapy.

Haemodynamic support and adjunctive therapy

A range of drug therapies aimed at supporting and ameliorating the signs and symptoms of septic shock is available and, while inotropes in particular provide an important adjunct in managing the acute shock phase, other drug therapies remain controversial.

Fluid therapy in sepsis

Fluid resuscitation with crystalloid or colloid has long been controversial in the critical care literature. The landmark Saline versus Albumin Fluid Evaluation (SAFE) study[49] demonstrated that, in the adult intensive care patient population, albumin can be considered safe, without demonstrating any clear advantage over sodium chloride 0.9%. In the study, 6997 patients were randomised to receive either saline ($n = 3500$) or albumin ($n = 3497$). No significant differences were noted between the two treatment groups for 28-day all-cause mortality, days in intensive care, days in hospital, days on mechanical ventilation and days of renal replacement therapy.[49] In a pre-defined subgroup analysis of severe sepsis patients in this study, the adjusted

odds ratio for death for albumin versus saline was 0.71.[128] There have been a number of landmark studies published since SAFE but the fluid of choice remains controversial. CHEST[129] compared 0.9% sodium chloride with 6% hydroxyethyl starch and showed that fluid resuscitation of all-comers requiring fluid resuscitation had no significant outcome difference at 90 days but higher levels of renal injury. Nearly 29% of patients in the study were septic.[130] Hydroxyethyl starch is not recommended for patients with sepsis. This study, along with the retraction of many research papers related to prior research,[131] led to changes globally in the recommendations for use of hydroxyethyl starch. More recently, the ProCESS trial showed no significant outcome difference between three resuscitation groups including two protocol-based approaches, EGDT and standard resuscitation, and the third group of 'usual care'.[36] A 2013 Cochrane review of eligible randomised trials in critically ill patients supports the use of crystalloids for resuscitation given the lack of clear outcome benefit of other fluids.[132]

The Surviving Sepsis Campaign response to ProCESS and ARISE maintains its 2012 guideline. The guidelines do not advocate a preferred resuscitation fluid but support fluid challenge in volume responsive patients.[101] Crystalloids are recommended as the initial fluid choice (up to 30 mL/kg). Albumin is suggested when patients require a substantial fluid resuscitation.[101]

Irrespective of fluid selection, the disruption of the vascular bed in early septic shock through widespread vasodilatation results in increased capillary permeability and rapidly developing interstitial oedema. Large amounts of fluid can be administered without seemingly improving oxygen delivery while adding to developing generalised oedema that further impairs cellular delivery of oxygen and nutrients. Fluid resuscitation alone is therefore of limited value in septic shock and other measures must be considered.

Inotropes and vasopressors

A goal of maintaining mean arterial pressure greater than 65 mmHg is common, with inotropes and vasopressors commenced when fluid resuscitation is considered adequate. Administration of these drugs requires continuous blood pressure monitoring and enables effective titration to meet the treatment goal. The Surviving Sepsis guidelines recommend noradrenaline for its specific alpha-receptor effects as the first choice vasopressor, with use of adrenaline (added or substituted) when an additional agent is needed, with the use of vasopressin 0.03 units/min added to or substituted for noradrenaline.

Dobutamine (2.5–10 mcg/kg) may be added to support patients with myocardial dysfunction to increase myocardial contractility and oxygen delivery to the tissues.[101] Refractory hypotension, resistant to vasopressors, has been linked to downregulation of receptors. Vasopressin (0.4–0.6 units/h) has been shown to reduce the requirements of other vasopressor agents.[133]

Administration of vasopressin in vasodilatory shock may help maintain blood pressure despite the relative ineffectiveness of other vasopressor hormones.[111] Specifically, arginine vasopressin (AVP) may inactivate the KATP channels and thereby lessen vascular resistance to noradrenaline and angiotensin II. It also decreases the synthesis of nitric oxide (as a result of a decrease in the expression of nitric oxide synthase) as well as cyclic guanosine monophosphate signalling by nitric oxide.[111] The sites of major arterial vasodilation in sepsis – the splanchnic circulation, the muscles and the skin – are vascular beds that contain abundant arginine vasopressin (AVP) receptors. In sepsis, vasopressin stores are quickly depleted. Administration of exogenous arginine vasopressin (0.04–0.06 units/min) can raise blood pressure by 25–50 mmHg by returning plasma concentrations of antidiuretic hormones to their earlier high levels.[111]

Steroids

The use of steroid therapy in severe sepsis remains controversial. At times, steroid replacement therapy may be used when patients display resistance to increasing doses of adrenergic agonists, as might occur in adrenal insufficiency. Some research indicates that patients with septic shock who are unable to increase cortisol levels in response to a challenge may benefit from administration of low-dose corticosteroids[134] (see Chapter 22). The Surviving Sepsis guidelines recommend not using intravenous hydrocortisone to treat adult septic shock patients if adequate fluid resuscitation and vasopressor therapy are able to restore haemodynamic stability. Where this is not achievable, the use of intravenous hydrocortisone alone at a dose of 200 mg per day is recommended.[101]

Supportive therapy

The Surviving Sepsis guidelines outline several areas of supportive therapy including blood product administration, renal replacement therapy, stress ulcer prophylaxis, deep vein thrombosis prophylaxis and nutritional support. Red blood cell transfusion is recommended when the haemoglobin concentration decreases to <7.0 g/dL to target a haemoglobin concentration of 7.0 to 9.0 g/dL in adults. In patients with severe sepsis, platelets are recommended to be administered prophylactically when counts are ≤10,000/mm³ in the absence of apparent bleeding, as well as when counts are ≤20,000/mm³ if the patient has a significant risk of bleeding.[101]

The Surviving Sepsis guidelines recommend continuous renal replacement therapies or intermittent haemodialysis to facilitate the management of fluid balance in haemodynamically unstable septic patients. The guidelines also recommend that patients with severe sepsis receive daily pharmacoprophylaxis against venous thromboembolism and that a combination of pharmacological therapy and intermittent pneumatic compression devices be used.[101] Translocation of gut bacteria due to splanchnic hypoperfusion and increased permeability is a factor in secondary septic insults and stress ulceration.[135] Stress ulcer prophylaxis using an H₂ blocker or proton pump inhibitor is therefore recommended for patients who have bleeding risk factors[100] (see Chapter 20). The new guidelines address nutritional

support for the first time. Adequate nutritional support with oral or enteral feeding to offset high caloric and protein demands is preferred to fasting or parenteral glucose administration. Chapter 19 provides further discussion of the nutrition support relevant to patients with sepsis. Equally important to patient-specific measures is institution of diligent infection control practices in ICU.[136]

As the patient with severe sepsis and shock has a high mortality rate, addressing goals of care is an additional area of focus recommended in the guidelines. The guidelines outline that the prognosis for achieving goals of care and the level of certainty for the prognosis be discussed with patients and families; that treatment plans should incorporate palliative care principles and, as appropriate, end-of-life care planning; and that goals of care be addressed as early as feasible but no later than within 72 hours of ICU admission.[101] As critical care nursing promotes patient- and family-centred care, addressing the needs of families and providing ongoing information and support are essential. A modified Delphi study using a group of international nurses used the Surviving Sepsis guidelines as the basis of making 63 consensus recommendations for sepsis care.[137] Recommendations relate to prevention and management, particularly in relation to recognition and management of deterioration. Paediatric recommendations are also included (see *Further reading*).

Symptom management of fever is prevalent in hospitals. Treatment with medicines that have an antipyretic effect has been considered a standard of care without the support of good evidence. Fever is an adaptive response to infection and is beneficial in activating various immune responses. A study in progress is the HEAT trial,[138] which aims to explore if permissive hyperthermia through avoidance of paracetamol in known or suspected infection in ICU improves survival to 28 days. In the absence of good evidence around the benefit of reducing temperature in sepsis and the potential harm from inhibiting normal immune responses, the pragmatic approach of supporting patient comfort seems reasonable when considering measures to normalise temperature.

Anaphylaxis

Anaphylaxis is the most severe, potentially life-threatening form of an allergic or hypersensitivity reaction,[139–143] and is mostly immunoglobulin E mediated.[144] Food-induced anaphylaxis has been defined by the National Institute of Allergy and Infectious Diseases (NIAID) as a serious allergic reaction that is rapid in onset, typically mediated by immunoglobulin E, involving systemic mediator release from sensitive mast cells and basophils.[145] Food-induced anaphylaxis is being increasingly studied due to increasing prevalence because of both genetic and unspecified environmental factors.[146] Food anaphylaxis has the same mechanism and clinical manifestations as other allergens with sensitised mast cells and basophils. Exercise-induced anaphylaxis, where a reaction depends on the temporal association of allergen ingestion and exercise, has also been described.[145]

Allergies are common; however, anaphylaxis appears rare.[141] Although data are sporadic in the literature, 0.01–0.02% of the general population is affected.[144] Anaphylaxis appears more common in Western countries with a rising incidence,[145,147,148] but this may be related to better reporting mechanisms. The prevalence of allergy with anaphylaxis has been documented to be as high as 7% in an Australian study of children, with insect stings, oral medications or food the most often cited causes. However, in this study, less than 1% of the population actually suffered an anaphylactic reaction manifesting with generalised multisystem allergic reaction, including evidence of airway involvement, rashes, gastrointestinal and cardiovascular dysfunction.[149] The published American prevalence is based on large population surveys and estimates that anaphylaxis affects 1.6% of the population.[150] There have been more than 100 food allergens identified but there are a few responsible for most reactions and this differs based on geographical location[147,148] and cannot always be explained by genetic factors.[146] The International Collaboration in Asthma, Allergy and Immunology are developing consensus guidelines to support management.[147]

Three criteria have been established in order to rapidly diagnose anaphylaxis as set out in Box 21.4.[145] There are currently no recommended biomarkers to support clinical diagnosis although histamine and tryptase are sometimes used.[151]

Clinical manifestations

The allergic response is via a host mast-cell reaction mediated by immunoglobulin E,[139] and antibody produced in response to the allergen that is attached to basophils (mast cells). Once sensitised to an allergen, subsequent exposure may lead to an anaphylactic reaction in affected individuals. One suggested mechanism is that subsequent exposure leads to mast-cell–allergen complexes and the release of histamine.[152] Reactions to an allergen cannot be predicted, however, and subsequent exposure may lead to either an amplified or lesser response.[140] There may be an initial reaction, which subsides with treatment over about 24 hours, but there has been described a second or rebound reaction up to 8–10 hours after initial exposure to an allergen.[139]

Exposure to an allergen causes release of histamine and other mediators, with subsequent vasodilation and increased microvascular permeability – a distributive form of shock. Histamine peaks at 5–10 minutes and is metabolised rapidly, returning to baseline within 60 minutes. Other mediators have a sustained effect.[144] This makes histamine a poor clinical biomarker for anaphylaxis. The antigen–antibody reaction may directly damage vascular walls, while release of vasoactive mediators such as histamine, serotonin, bradykinins and prostaglandins triggers a systemic response, resulting in vasodilation

---

BOX 21.4

Diagnostic criteria for anaphylaxis

1 Acute onset of an illness (over minutes to several hours) involving skin, mucosal tissue or both (for example, generalised hives, pruritus or flushing, swollen lips/tongue/uvula),

   plus either

   a Respiratory compromise (for example, dyspnoea, wheeze/bronchospasm, stridor, reduced peak expiratory flow rate, hypoxaemia)

   b Reduced blood pressure (BP) or associated symptoms of end-organ dysfunction (for example, hypotonia [circulatory collapse], syncope, incontinence)

   or

2 **Two** or more of the following that occur rapidly after exposure to a likely allergen for that patient (minutes to several hours):

   a Involvement of the skin/mucosal tissue (for example, generalised hives, itch/flush, swollen lips/tongue/uvula)

   b Respiratory compromise (for example, dyspnoea, wheeze/bronchospasm, stridor, reduced peak expiratory flow rate, hypoxaemia)

   c Reduced BP or associated symptoms of end-organ dysfunction (for example, hypotonia, syncope, incontinence)

   d Persistent GI symptoms (for example, crampy abdominal pain, vomiting)

   or

3 Age-related decrease in systolic blood pressure or a greater than 30% decrease from baseline after exposure to a known allergen for that patient (minutes to several hours):

   a 1 month to 1 year: systolic blood pressure of less than 70 mmHg

   b 1–10 years old: systolic blood pressure of less than (70 mmHg plus twice the age)

   c 11 years to adult: systolic blood pressure of less than 90 mmHg or greater than 30% decrease from baseline

....

Adapted with permission from Sampson HA, Munoz-Furlong A, Campbell RL, Adkinson NF Jr, Bock SA, Branum A et al. Second symposium on the definition and management of anaphylaxis: summary report – Second National Institute of Allergy and Infectious Disease/Food Allergy and Anaphylaxis Network Symposium. [Reprint in Ann Emerg Med. 2006 Apr;47(4):373-80; PMID: 16546624]. J Allergy Clin Immunol 2006;117:391-7.

and increased capillary permeability, with widespread loss of fluid into the interstitial space and hypovolaemia. Blood pressure and cardiac output/index may fall with a compensatory rise in heart rate. Severe bronchospasm may also occur from mediator-induced bronchial oedema and pulmonary smooth muscle contraction.[7] Abdominal pain is thought to be due to the inflammation of Peyer's patches, which are clusters of lymphatic tissue containing B lymphocytes, located in the mucosa and submucosa of the small intestine.[152]

A list of signs and symptoms for anaphylaxis appears in Table 21.8. It is thought that anaphylaxis is sometimes misdiagnosed because up to 20% of presentations do not have obvious cutaneous signs.[145] Anaphylaxis should be considered when there are two or more organ systems involved.[150] There is a high mortality in patients with asthma and those on beta-blocker or ACE inhibitor medications;[140,153] these medications may limit the effectiveness of adrenaline therapy. Age and pre-existing lung disease are the most important factors in relation to severity; older people and those with asthma or airways disease have a higher risk of a life-threatening reaction.[152]

Patient management

Initial management

Diagnosis of an anaphylactic reaction requires an appropriate assessment and history, including acute onset, history of allergic reaction and initial measures instituted to support airway, breathing and circulation. Removal of the causative agent, if possible, and treatment within 30 minutes of exposure to an allergen result in improved outcomes.

The Australian and New Zealand Anaesthetic Allergy Group have produced a consensus guideline (see *Online resources*) and devised a number of useful resources to support management of anaphylaxis during anaesthesia.[154] These guidelines are broadly applicable in critical care units. See Practice tip below for a list of suggested anaphylaxis emergency equipment.

Practice tip

Anaphylaxis emergency box

- Adrenaline 1:1000 (consider adrenaline autoinjector availability in rural locations for initial administration by nursing staff)
- 1-mL syringes; 21 gauge needles
- Oxygen
- Airway equipment, including nebuliser and suction
- Defibrillator
- Manual blood pressure cuff
- Intravenous access equipment (including large bore cannulae)
- Pressure sleeve (aids rapid infusion of fluid under pressure)
- At least 3 litres of normal saline

TABLE 21.8

Symptoms of allergic reactions

ORGAN SYSTEM	IMMEDIATE SYMPTOMS	DELAYED SYMPTOMS
Cutaneous	Erythema, Pruritus, Urticaria, Morbilliform eruption, Angioedema	Erythema, Flushing, Pruritus, Morbilliform eruption, Angio-oedema, Eczematous rash
Ocular	Pruritus, Conjunctival erythema, Tearing, Periorbital oedema	Pruritus, Conjunctival erythema, Tearing, Periorbital oedema
Upper respiratory	Nasal congestion, Pruritus, Rhinorrhoea, Sneezing, Laryngeal oedema, Hoarseness, Dry staccato cough	
Lower respiratory	Cough, Chest tightness, Dyspnoea, Wheezing, Intercostal retractions, Accessory muscle use	Cough, dyspnoea, wheezing
GI (oral)	Angio-oedema of the lips, tongue or palate, Oral pruritus, Tongue swelling	
GI (lower)	Nausea, Colicky abdominal pain, Reflux, Vomiting, Diarrhoea	Nausea, Abdominal pain, Reflux, Vomiting, Diarrhoea, Haematochezia, Irritability and food refusal with weight loss (young children)
Cardiovascular	Tachycardia (occasionally bradycardia in anaphylaxis), Hypotension, Dizziness, Fainting, Loss of consciousness	
Miscellaneous	Uterine contractions, Sense of 'impending doom'	

Adapted from Sampson HA, Munoz-Furlong A, Campbell RL, Adkinson NF Jr, Bock SA, Branum A et al. Second symposium on the definition and management of anaphylaxis: summary report – Second National Institute of Allergy and Infectious Disease/Food Allergy and Anaphylaxis Network Symposium. [Reprint in Ann Emerg Med. 2006 Apr;47(4):373-80; PMID: 16546624]. J Allergy Clin Immunol 2006;117:391–7, with permission.

Measures to assess and support airway, breathing and circulation are important, considering the rapid impact of circulating mediators and potential decline in respiratory and cardiovascular function. Securing the airway and providing high oxygen concentration is vital as most anaphylactic-related deaths are due to asphyxiation.[144] Adrenaline is recommended as first-line drug treatment[140,144,152] and in a recent systematic review the evidence suggested prompt use of adrenaline to reduce the risk of death.[143] Administration is usually via intramuscular injection (to the vastus lateralis muscle or mid-outer thigh) as it leads to a more rapid increase in plasma concentration than subcutaneous administration.[143] The first dose is often given using the patient's own injecting device (e.g. Epipen or Anapen) for common food and venom allergies as they are more likely to occur out of hospital. Subsequent doses are usually required once a patient is in hospital. The Australasian Society of Clinical Immunology and Allergy Incorporated suggest intramuscular adrenaline in the doses suggested in Table 21.9.[155]

Intravenous doses of adrenaline depend on the severity and condition of the patient. If the patient is unresponsive and life support algorithms are in play, the dose of adrenaline is 1 mg as per the International Liaison Committee on Resuscitation Guidelines and the algorithms for cardiopulmonary resuscitation are followed for subsequent dosing. The dose of adrenaline administered in anaphylaxis for patients that have not been managed with Advanced Life Support algorithms is more controversial. When a continuous infusion is required for ongoing symptom management it is suggested an adrenaline infusion be prepared and administered at a dose of 0.1 mcg/kg/min with titration to maintain the desired blood pressure. The same monitoring as for any patient on an adrenaline infusion should be used including continuous blood pressure.[154,155]

Aggressive fluid resuscitation (20 mL/kg) is also usually required[154,155] as the intravascular blood volume may quickly be depleted by up to 70%. The type of fluid used in resuscitation can vary and, if a colloid is being administered to the patient and there is no known other trigger for the reaction, the colloid should cease as it may be responsible.[154] A maximum of 50 mL/kg in the first 30 minutes is suggested for persistent hypotension.[154,155]

Airway management

Early elective intubation is recommended for patients with airway oedema, stridor or any oropharyngeal swelling. Patients with airway swelling and/or angio-oedema are at high risk for rapid deterioration and respiratory compromise.[154] Late presentation to hospital or delayed intubation when airway swelling is present may mean that intubation and other emergency airway procedures may be extremely difficult. Multiple attempts at intubation increase laryngeal oedema or cause trauma to the airway. Early recognition of the potentially difficult airway allows planning for alternative airway management by experts in difficult airways.

Adjunctive support

Adjunctive drugs include H_1- and H_2-antagonists, antihistamines, corticosteroids and other beta-2-agonists for airway symptoms. The H_2-antagonists are competitive antagonists of histamine at the parietal cell histamine-2 receptor. A systematic review assessed the evidence related to efficacy of H_2-antihistamines. The review did not find any studies based on the inclusion criteria and made no specific treatment recommendation.[142] However, it seems at this stage that it is likely to be beneficial to block both H_1 and H_2 receptors when urticaria is present.[143] H_1-antihistamines are also helpful to reduce pruritus.[143] It is important to note the use of antihistamines is not recommended for anaphylaxis crisis management.[155]

Corticosteroids (1 mg/kg up to 200 mg)[155] may be beneficial for persistent bronchospasm, asthma and severe cutaneous reactions but not in acute management,[154,155] and their use remains unproven.[155] Glucagon and noradrenaline may be required for patients on beta-blockers who may have resistant severe hypotension and bradycardia.[156] Glucagon exerts positive inotropic and chronotropic effects, independently of catecholamines, while atropine

TABLE 21.9

Adrenaline doses

AGE (YEARS)	WEIGHT (KG)	VOLUME OF ADRENALINE 1:1000	ADRENALINE AUTOINJECTORS
<1	5–10	0.05–0.1 mL	
1–2	10	0.1 mL	
2–3	15	0.15 mL	10–20 kg (~1–5 years): 0.15 mg (green-labelled) device
4–6	20	0.2 mL	
7–10	30	0.3 mL	
10–12	40	0.4 mL	>20 kg (~>5 years): 0.3 mg (yellow-labelled) device
>12 and adults	>50	0.5 mL	

Adapted with permission from Australasian Society of Clinical Immunology and Allergy Inc. Acute management of anaphylaxis guidelines, <http://www.allergy.org.au/health-professionals/papers/acute-management-of-anaphylaxis-guidelines>; 2013.

may reverse bradycardia. Vasopressin and other vasopressors such as metaraminol are suggested where shock is refractory to adrenaline.[144] Given that a second reaction (biphasic) may occur after the initial allergic response, monitoring should continue for up to 48 hours.[144]

Preventative care

There is no current cure for anaphylaxis.[147] Individuals with known allergies are taught avoidance of allergens as a first line, and then to have a management plan for inadvertent exposure including the use of emergency kits with adrenaline for intramuscular injection (Epipen).[141,147,152,157] Antihistamines are also used in food allergy to manage non-severe reactions and immune-modulating pharmacological agents are a probable future direction for management.[145] Desensitisation therapy may also reduce severity of symptoms and therefore improve quality of life.

Neurogenic/spinal shock

Neurogenic shock is a form of distributive shock caused by loss of vasomotor (sympathetic) tone from disruption to or inhibition of neural output. Characteristics include a systolic blood pressure <90–100 mmHg and a heart rate <80 beats per minute without other obvious causes.[158] Note that the heart rate is within otherwise accepted normal limits. Most often it is described as a triad of hypotension, bradycardia and hypothermia. However, the precise mechanisms are unknown.[159] The primary cause is a spinal cord injury above T6, secondary to disruption of sympathetic outflow from T1–L2 and to unopposed vagal tone, leading to decreased vascular resistance and associated vascular dilation.[160] It may also develop after anaesthesia, particularly spinal, cerebral medullary ischaemia or when there is spinal cord complete or partial injury above the mid-thoracic region (thoracic outflow tract).

Spinal shock is a subclass of neurogenic shock, with a transient physiological (rather than anatomical) reflex depression of cord function below the level of injury and associated loss of sensorimotor functions. Incidence has been reported at 14% of patients presenting to the emergency department within 2 hours of injury and predominantly affects patients with cervical damage.[158] Spinal shock can also occur with a spinal cord laceration or contusion, and is associated with varying degrees of motor and sensory deficit (see also Chapters 17 and 23). Trauma is frequently the reason for primary injury,[158] with traffic accidents, assault, falls at work and sport the most common causes and a 4:1 ratio of males to females.[161] Simultaneous injuries may also be responsible for haemodynamic compromise,[158] and neurogenic shock with hypotension may have multiple aetiologies.[159] Haemorrhagic shock in combination with neurogenic shock has a poor outcome.

Clinical manifestations

Inhibited sympathetic outflow results in dominance of the parasympathetic nervous system, with a reduction in systemic vascular resistance and lowered blood pressure. Preload to the right heart is reduced, which lowers stroke volume and subsequent cardiac output/index. The usual response to reduction in cardiac output (a raised heart rate) does not occur due to the parasympathetic nervous system and blockage of sympathetic compensatory responses, and the patient may be bradycardic and hypotensive,[160] with their skin warm and dry.

In spinal shock there may be an initial rise in blood pressure due to release of catecholamines, followed by hypotension,[160] which usually resolves within 24 hours.[161] Flaccid areflexic paralysis,[161] including that of the bladder and bowel, is observed and sustained priapism may also develop. Symptoms may last hours to days, until the reflex arcs below the level of injury begin to regain function. This is a result of damage to the spinal cord, and obvious manifestations include pale, cold skin above the site of injury, and warm, pink skin below the site of injury. Anhidrosis (absence of sweating) may be present. Heart rate may be slow, requiring intervention.

Secondary injury may occur from impaired vasomotor tone, ischaemia, thrombosis, increased permeability, inflammatory and cellular dysfunction. Spinal cord oedema occurs 3–6 days after injury and may lead to a shocked state.[161]

Patient management

The extent of injury, whether complete (no sensory or motor function) or incomplete (some sensory or motor function), determines clinical medical management. Priority focuses on airway, breathing and circulation. The most risky time is the first 7–10 days after injury.[162]

Haemodynamic support is required and is usually provided in an escalating manner with fluid first followed by pharmacological agents to maintain targets. Mean arterial pressure augmentation may be required but is the subject of ongoing debate.[162]

Initial stabilisation and neck immobilisation

After neck and torso stabilisation, the patient with confirmed or suspected spinal cord injury is placed in a position that supports spinal precautions (neutral neck positioning with immobilisation) with spinal boards removed within 20 minutes if possible. Immobilisation may be achieved with sandbags either side of the head, the use of collars and log rolling.[161] Caution for spinal instability remains despite medical imaging clearance, due to the potential for spinal ligament damage. The patient is positioned supine, with their legs in alignment with the torso.

Elevation of the head may cause pooling of blood in the lower limbs, exacerbating hypotension,[163] and makes the patient sensitive to sudden position changes. It is important to note that while this is a standard practice it also may cause additional unintended issues for the patient such as discomfort, occipital pressure areas and impaired respiratory function. These precautions also inhibit airway interventions and increase risk of aspiration and raised intracranial pressure.[161]

Fluid therapy

Loss of sympathetic outflow requires close cardiac and haemodynamic monitoring for bradycardia and hypotension. Symptomatic bradycardia is treated and may require cardiac pacing if unresponsive to atropine. Therapies include fluid resuscitation with the addition of inotropes, if necessary, to improve vasomotor function. This increases preload and maintains a mean arterial pressure >80–85 mmHg[160,162] to restore spinal cord perfusion and to prevent secondary neuronal hypoperfusion.[164] This higher (supranormal) mean arterial pressure may be targeted to improve recovery and prevent secondary injuries.[164] Volume expansion with colloids and crystalloids or blood products will vary depending on patient situation; however, subgroup analysis in the SAFE trial indicated that colloids and hypotonic solutions may not be the best options.[49]

Respiratory support

Respiratory insufficiency is common[162] and, as such, respiratory function is closely monitored to prevent or minimise atelectasis, pneumonia[164] and secretion retention. The level of injury is indicative of the potential for respiratory muscle weakness (see Table 21.10). The diaphragm is innervated by the phrenic nerve (originating at C3–C5); any injury above C3 leads to complete respiratory muscle paralysis and patients will require ventilatory support.[164] Incomplete injuries between C3 and C5 may also require ventilation initially but subsequently recover some respiratory function. Intubation is complicated by any spinal cord injury as airway interventions cause some level of spinal movement and respiratory failure is an independent predictor of mortality in spinal cord injury.[161] Coughing, and therefore secretion clearance, is reliant on 'expiratory muscles' and, for patients with injuries that interfere with abdominal and intercostal muscle function, careful monitoring of the work of breathing and secretion clearance should be initiated. There will be varying levels of decreased respiratory function with substantially reduced lung volumes.

TABLE 21.10

Respiratory muscle innervation by cord level

CORD LEVEL INNERVATION	ACCESSORY MUSCLE
C3–C5 (mostly C4)	Diaphragm
C6	Serratus anterior
	Latissimus dorsi
	Pectoralis
T1–11	Intercostals
T6–L1	Abdominals

Adjunctive support

Hypothermia may be present, resulting from dilated peripheral blood vessels allowing radiant loss of heat. A patient is monitored for core temperature changes, and external warming devices may be required.

Paralytic ileus is a concern in the acute phase of injuries above T5, where disruption of integrative innervation pathways leads to unmodulated colonic functioning[165] and peristaltic hypomotility. Ileus may lead to respiratory compromise and should be managed. The patient should remain 'nil by mouth' and treatment includes gastric decompression, adequate intravenous hydration and electrolyte balance. Drug therapy with prokinetics, probiotics, aperients and intravenous neostigmine or lignocaine has been reported to be useful.

Pressure care is attended every second hour and, where Jordan frames are used, slats should be removed between use. The patient is susceptible to deep venous thrombosis particularly high risk when spinal cord injury is involved, so sequential calf compression devices and other prophylaxis such as anticoagulants are initiated early with D-dimers monitored regularly.

Resuscitation end points

End points of resuscitation in shock states are similar but will differ depending on the cause. Table 21.11 outlines some of the discussed targets.

TABLE 21.11

Resuscitation endpoints

PARAMETER	TARGETS/RECOMMENDATIONS	PRECAUTIONS
Blood pressure	Target diastolic blood pressure ≥65 mmHg Target systolic blood pressure >90 mmHg as soon as possible	This target may be higher depending on pre-morbid state and specific organ requirements such as closed head injury
Urine output	Target ≥0.5 mL/hour	
Serum lactate levels	There is evidence that serum lactate is a clear marker for outcome in patients[17,166] There have been suggestions that any patient with a lactate >4 should be managed in a critical care environment Improving lactate levels to 'normal' is associated with improved survival	For patients presenting to emergency with a suspicion of sepsis it should be measured and assessed in the first hour

TABLE 21.11 *continued*

PARAMETER	TARGETS/RECOMMENDATIONS	PRECAUTIONS
Arterial base deficit	In combination with lactate base deficit in shock is related to oxygen transport imbalance at the cellular level and it is a good marker with lactate level for adequacy of resuscitation[167]	A high base deficit (≥4) is indicative of abnormal oxygen utilisation and patients have a higher mortality
Oxygen monitoring	Monitoring of oxygen saturation is readily available and required when any shock state is suspected It is important to assess oxygen requirements even in the setting of acceptable oxygen saturation as increasing requirement is indicative of deterioration P/F ratio (partial pressure of oxygen-to-fraction of inspired oxygen ratio) may be used as a guide to assess the level of dysfunction given that the normal result is approximately 500 (100/0.21) Oxygenation should also be assessed through arterial blood gas sampling and utilisation assumptions may be made by comparing with a venous sample	A P/F ratio <250 in the presence of high supplemental oxygen should be regarded as indicative of serious respiratory dysfunction Any patient requiring maximum oxygen support should be investigated
Mixed venous oxygen saturation	Normal mixed venous oxygen saturation levels are between 60% and 80% It may be used to guide resuscitation but is an invasive method of monitoring Haemoglobin should be measured in conjunction with this variable	A reduced mixed venous saturation indicates increasing extraction and worsening shock state High levels may be seen that may be indicative of cellular dysfunction in relation to oxygen extraction
End-tidal carbon dioxide	End-tidal carbon dioxide monitors usually provide both numeric and graphic waveform displays of the concentration using non-invasive measurement of exhaled carbon dioxide[168] End-tidal carbon dioxide is an estimate of the patient's alveolar ventilation status 'Stat cap' devices are standard on resuscitation trolleys for supporting confirmation of endotracheal tube placement by quickly establishing if carbon dioxide is exhaled	End-tidal carbon dioxide monitoring is unreliable in the setting of increased ventilation perfusion (V/Q) mismatch with worsening arterial carbon dioxide retention and increased peripheral carbon dioxide production[20]
Preload	Preload should be maximised without overstretching Usually this is achieved using fluid bolus in shock states (refer to the relevant sections)	Where preload is leading to congestion and cardiac failure, pharmacotherapy and ventilator support may be required
Right ventricular end-diastolic volume index	Provides a clinical estimate of right ventricular preload and has a normal adult parameter of 60–100 mL/m^2 Observing for changes with fluid challenge may support resuscitation by providing information about volume responsiveness[169]	
Afterload	Afterload reduction strategies are employed in many shocked states to improve cardiac output as increased afterload increases the work of the myocardium Afterload is affected by vascular resistance Calculations for systemic vascular resistance (SVR) are used to measure afterload	During shock states, resistance is increased through constriction and oxygen and energy are required for function
Contractility	Contractility is not easily measured clinically but the improvement would be observed usually by increased cardiac output or other surrogate measures with the addition of inotropes	

P/F ratio = PaO$_2$/FiO$_2$

Summary

Shock is a generic term describing a syndrome and pervasive set of potentially life-threatening symptoms. The patho-physiological changes associated with shock feature a complex interaction of generic compensatory mechanisms that attempt to sustain perfusion and particularly oxygen delivery to the vital organ systems of the body. These protective responses are particularly strong in supporting cerebral perfusion and combine responses from the sympathetic nervous, endocrine and adrenal/renal systems. As shock develops cellular dysfunction occurs in response to the release of a large collection of systemic and local inflammatory mediators, which inevitably overwhelm cell function and lead to diffuse organ injury if shock continues unabated. The classification system described here differentiates shock into categories including hypovolaemic, cardiogenic and distributive; classification is dependent on aetiology. Distributive shock states result in impaired oxygen and nutrient delivery to the tissues as a result of failure of the vascular system (the blood distri-bution system). While there may be additional factors (e.g. infection) beyond simple failure to provide sufficient perfusion to the capillary bed due to widespread vascular dilation, the common factor for all underlying causes of distributive shock is widespread failure of the vasculature. The most common categories of distributive shock are associated with systemic inflammatory response syndrome, anaphylaxis and neurogenic shock.

Clear assessment is required to distinguish the type of shock aids in appropriate treatment decisions, targeting the cause and managing associated symptoms. Critical care nurses are in a position to provide clear assessment and first-line emergency management of the various shock states. Collaborative integrated care is important to provide the patient with the best possible outcome.

Case study

An independent 70-year-old man, Matthew, presented to the emergency department at 1630 hours with abdominal cramping, nausea and vomiting for the past day. Matthew had a history of end-stage renal failure, type 2 diabetes and hypertension. Previous hospital admission noted he was positive for MRSA. He attends the dialysis unit three times a week and is dialysed through a tunnelled catheter that had been in situ for 3 months with no complications. His initial observations in the emergency department included a blood pressure of 143/75 mmHg, heart rate of 93 beats per minute, temperature of 37.5°C and respiratory rate of 18 breaths per minute, with an oxygen saturation of 95%. Routine blood tests were ordered and 1000 mL of intravenous 0.9% sodium chloride was given as a 'bolus', with a second litre commenced and prescribed to be administered over the next 8 hours. Intravenous metaclopramide 10 mg was administered and blood cultures were taken after Matthew had been in the department for approximately 4 hours.

The next set of observations included a temperature of 38.5°C. Matthew was also noted to be drowsy with a GCS of 14. He was then transferred to the medical assessment unit pending admission to the renal ward. Blood cultures were taken prior to him being transferred for ongoing care.

The next morning Matthew was reviewed on the ward round and he continued to be drowsy with some abdominal pain. His observations included an increased temperature of 38.2°C, blood pressure of 160/80 mmHg and oxygen saturation of 94% on room air. His ongoing diagnosis was gastroenteritis although other types of infection were considered given his long-term medical issues. A stool culture was ordered and intravenous metronidazole and vancomycin prescribed. A note was made in the patient's medical record to administer the antibiotics after his dialysis treatment and following checking of blood culture results. An abdominal computerised tomography scan was ordered, which delayed dialysis. Just after Matthew left for the dialysis unit, the hospital microbiology department contacted the ward to report a preliminary positive blood culture for gram-positive cocci – this was not communicated to the staff in the dialysis unit. About 3 hours later, a medical officer was called to review him in the dialysis unit as he was looking unwell and, during dialysis, had rigors increasing abdominal discomfort with the following observations: temperature 38.6°C, heart rate 90 beats per minute, blood pressure 140/90 mmHg, respiratory rate 20 breaths per minute. The medical officer took additional blood cultures, ordered a stat dose of vancomycin after reviewing current blood pathology, noting the positive culture and increased white cell count of 24 × 10⁹/L.

When dialysis was concluded Matthew returned to the renal unit. There was no handover provided. An hour after his return to the ward his observations included a temp of 39.2°C, respiratory rate of 22 breaths per minute, SpO$_2$ 88% on room air and HR of 115 beats per minute with a decreased level of consciousness. These observations automatically triggered an immediate clinical emergency response call.

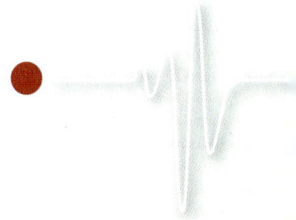

Matthew was assessed by the medical emergency team and transferred to ICU for ongoing care. He required intubation and ventilation to support respiratory function and noradrenaline to support blood pressure and continuous renal replacement therapy commenced. Matthew was persistently febrile over the next few days even with vancomycin in a therapeutic range. Matthew also had a fluctuating GCS and repeat CT scans indicated changes consistent with multiple cerebral infarcts.

Matthews's poor prognosis was considered by the medical team and discussed with his family. There was a decision made not to escalate interventions and to ensure Matthew's comfort by instituting palliative measures. Matthew died 12 days after admission.

This case study is a good example of care provided with confirmation bias towards gastroenteritis that probably led to less importance placed on providing antibiotic therapy. The delay to treatment may have been implicated in Matthew's decline and, given his pre-admission status, every effort should have been made to prevent this. Hospital processes and transfers between services are risky times where handover may be limited or incomplete. It is important in these cases to consider the checking procedures to ensure all interventions have been performed.

CASE STUDY QUESTIONS

1　Identify what the possible sources of infection are for Matthew.

2　What early clinical indications are there that Matthew is seriously unwell?

3　What opportunities existed during Matthew's time in the emergency department to optimise his 'sepsis path'?

RESEARCH VIGNETTE

Corfield AR, Lees F, Zealley I, Houston G, Dickie S, Ward K et al, on behalf of the Scottish Trauma Audit Group Sepsis Steering Group, 2013. Utility of a single early warning score in patients with sepsis in the emergency department, Emerg Med J 2014;31(6):482–7. doi:10.1136/emermed-2012-202186

Abstract

Background: An important element in improving the care of patients with sepsis is early identification and early intervention. Early warning score (EWS) systems allow earlier identification of physiological deterioration. A standardised national EWS (NEWS) has been proposed for use across the National Health Service in the UK.[170]

Aim: To determine whether a single NEWS on emergency department (ED) arrival is a predictor of outcome, either in-hospital death within 30 days or intensive care unit (ICU) admission within 2 days, in patients with sepsis.

Methods: Data were collected over a 3-month period as part of a national audit in 20 EDs in Scotland. All adult patients who were admitted for at least 2 days or who died within 2 days were screened for sepsis criteria. Patients with systemic inflammatory response syndrome criteria were included. An EWS was calculated based on initial physiological observations made in the ED using the NEWS.

Results: Complete data were available for 2003 patients. Each rise in NEWS category was associated with an increased risk of mortality when compared to the lowest category (5–6: OR 1.95, 95% CI 1.21 to 3.14), (7–8: OR 2.26, 95% CI 1.42 to 3.61), (9–20: OR 5.64, 95% CI 3.70 to 8.60). This was also the case for the combined outcome (ICU and/or mortality).

Conclusions: An increased NEWS on arrival at ED is associated with higher odds of adverse outcome among patients with sepsis. The use of NEWS could facilitate patient pathways to ensure triage to a high acuity area of the ED and senior clinician involvement at an early stage.

Critique

Vital signs falling outside of 'normal ranges' are associated with adverse events for patients. There are many reports that demonstrate systematic hospital challenges for inpatients who develop shock. Identified issues include failure to recognise or respond to deteriorating patients, inadequate or delayed treatment, unstable patient transfers and a lack of clinical supervision at the point of care. This has led to the implementation of track and trigger systems and development of various standards and performance indicators aimed at improving patient care.

This recently published multicenter prospective study in 20 Scottish emergency departments assessed a 'track and trigger' system for identifying sepsis patients at risk using the NHS Early Warning Score (NEWS). End points for the study included ICU admission within 2 days of attendance and 30-day in-hospital mortality.

Case note review was performed on more than 27,000 patients to determine if sepsis criteria were present. The sample was reduced to approximately 2000 with exclusion criteria applied. The NEWS is based on medical emergency team research and assigns a score to physiological derangements for six physiological parameters and the use of supplemental oxygen. The maximum score is 20 with higher scores indicating worsening patient state. The parameters appear in Table 21.12.

TABLE 21.12

NHS early warning score (NEWS)

	NHS EARLY WARNING SCORE						
	3	2	1	0	1	2	3
Respiration rate	≤8		9–11	12–20		21–24	≥25
Oxygen saturation	≤91	92–93	94–95	≥96			
Supplemental oxygen		Yes		No			
Temperature	≤35°		35.1–36°	36.1–38°	38.1–39°	≥39.1°	
Systolic blood pressure	≤90	91–100	101–110	111–219			≥220
Pulse	≤40		41–50	51–90	91–110	111–130	≥131
Conscious level				A			V, P, U

A = alert; V = voice; P = pain; U = unresponsive.

Adapted from Corfield AR, Lees F, Zealley I, Houston G, Dickie S, Ward K et al. Utility of a single early warning score in patients with sepsis in the emergency department. Emerg Med J 2014;31(6):482–7, with permission.

It is not surprising that patients admitted to ICU had a higher median NEWS score – it was more surprising that the ICU group was significantly younger. Increased age was associated with 30-day mortality. A score of ≥7 put patients at increased risk of ICU admission or death. There were a number of limitations acknowledged. At least 5% of the potential sample was excluded because of missing physiological observations so that scoring was incomplete. Poor compliance with scoring is not unusual and has been reported in other ED studies that have adopted scoring of physiological parameters.[171] This is an acknowledged problem for all track and trigger systems as more than one observation is required to complete the assessment.

Patients who were discharged within 2 days were also not included although the authors note that they may have had less incidence of significant illness. Patients that may have required ICU after 2 days were also excluded and this would potentially include patients where early deterioration may have been missed. Patients were also not followed up after discharge so outcomes are not known beyond the hospital stay.

The study continues to support the value of close, frequent clinical observation and the linking of signs and symptoms within the patient's overall physiological condition that provides the astute clinician with numerous indicators of the health or otherwise of the cardiovascular system and the impending shock syndrome. This study was a retrospective case note audit and, as such, it is not representative of the outcomes that may have been evident if the system was implemented within the jurisdiction and scoring was routine.

The criteria for scoring are based on reasonable data and are similar to other track and trigger observations. These scoring systems are of benefit in the setting of access to appropriate scoring tools such as standard observation charts with embedded scoring. They have the additional and often-cited benefit of supporting less-experienced clinicians in seeking help to interpret the patient's clinical state and gaining support to avoid deterioration such that late signs become an all-too-obvious message of imminent patient mortality. This is only the case when scoring is related to standards for escalation and the escalation response such as medical emergency teams or outreach services.

The scoring of NEWS is easy to apply and has been supported in the UK as a mechanism for early warning of deterioration but without supporting implementation strategies. A standard bedside observation chart could be used across jurisdictions and highlight appropriate calling criteria and escalation procedures. This has been demonstrated in the 'Between the Flags' program in New South Wales, Australia.[172] Standardisation in this way supports organisations to provide equitable service to patients. This jurisdiction-wide program includes a colour-coded chart, escalation procedure and in-depth online training modules. This program enables clinicians to respond appropriately and communicate effectively when patients deteriorate. Regardless of the method, these are important initiatives to combat avoidable in-hospital complications and deaths.

Learning activities

1 What are the implications for dosing patients receiving renal replacement therapies?

2 What assessments are important to obtain appropriate information for a patient presenting with signs of hypoperfusion?

3 What are key monitoring strategies to assess end-organ perfusion?

4 What are the common management strategies for all shock types?

Online resources

American Heart Association, www.heart.org/HEARTORG

Australian and New Zealand Anaesthetic Allergy Group, www.anzaag.com/Default.aspx

Australian and New Zealand Anaesthetic Allergy Group Anaphylaxis Management Guidelines, www.anzaag.com/Docs/PDF/Management%20Guidelines/Mx%20Guidelines%20Intro%20v1.1Jun13.pdf

Australian Commission on Safety and Quality in Healthcare, www.safetyandquality.gov.au/internet/safety/publishing.nsf/Content/home

Clinical Excellence Commission: Between the flags, www.cec.health.nsw.gov.au/programs/between-the-flags

National Blood Authority Australia, www.nba.gov.au

Patient Blood Management guidelines App: for iPad, www.blood.gov.au/pbm-ipad

Sepsis, www.ihi.org/Topics/Sepsis/Pages/default.aspx

Spinal cord injury network, https://spinalnetwork.org.au/

Surviving Sepsis, www.survivingsepsis.org/

TRANSFUSE, http://clinicaltrials.gov/show/NCT01638416 and http://clinicaltrials.gov/show/NCT00975793

World Allergy Organization, www.worldallergy.org/index.php

Further reading

Aitken LM, Williams G, Harvey M, Blot S, Kleinpell R, Labeau S et al. Nursing considerations to complement the Surviving Sepsis Campaign guidelines. Crit Care Med 2011;39(7):1800–18.

Australian Commission on Safety and Quality in Healthcare. Recognising and responding to clinical deterioration: background paper, <http://www.safetyandquality.gov.au/internet/safety/publishing.nsf/Content/AB9325A491E10CF1CA257483000C9AC4/$File/BackgroundPaper-2009.pdf>; June 2008.

Dellinger RP, Levy MM, Rhodes A, Annane D, Gerlach H, Opal SM et al. International guidelines for management of severe sepsis and septic shock, <http://www.survivingsepsis.org/Pages/default.aspx>; 2012.

Manji RA, Wood KE, Kumar A. The history and evolution of circulatory shock. Crit Care Clin 2009;25(1):1–29.

References

1 Adams F. The book of prognostics, by Hippocrates. In: eBooks@Adelaide University of Adelaide Library; 2007.

2 Bridges E, Dukes S. Cardiovascular aspects of septic shock: pathophysiology, monitoring, and treatment. Crit Care Nurs 2005;25:14-24.

3 Manji RA, Wood KE, Kumar A. The history and evolution of circulatory shock. Crit Care Clin 2009;25:1-29.

4 Barbee R, Reynolds P, Ward K. Assessing shock resuscitation strategies by oxygen debt repayment. Shock 2010;33:113-22.

5 Bangash MN, Kong ML, Pearse RM. Use of inotropes and vasopressor agents in critically ill patients. Br J Pharmacol 2012;165:2015-33.

6 Strehlow MC. Early identification of shock in critically ill patients. Emerg Med Clin North Am 2010;28:57-66.

7 Carlson KK, ed. AACN Advanced critical care nursing. St. Louis: Mosby; 2008.

8 Kolecki P. Hypovolemic shock, <http://emedicine.medscape.com/article/760145-overview>; 2014 [accessed 29.03.15].

9 Vincent J-L, De Backer D. Circulatory shock. N Engl J Med 2013;369:1726-34.

10 Vallet B, Wiel E, Lebuffe G. Resuscitation from circulatory shock: an approach based on oxygen-derived parameters. Berlin: Springer-Verlag; 2005.

11 Rosen IM. Oxygen delivery and consumption. Up-to-Date 2013; 2013.

12 Wilson WC, Grande CM. Trauma: critical care. Boca Raton, Florida: C R C Press LLC; 2007.

13 Galley HF. Oxidative stress and mitochondrial dysfunction in sepsis. Br J Anaesth 2011;107:57-64.

14 Fortin C, McDonald P, Fulop T, Lesur O. Sepsis, leukocytes, and nitric oxide (NO): an intricate affair. Shock 2010;33:344-52.

15 Wagner F, Baumgart K, Simkova V, Georgieff M, Radermacher P, Calzia E. Year in review 2007: Critical care – shock. Crit Care (London, England) 2008;12:227.

16 Mikkelsen ME, Miltiades AN, Gaieski DF, Goyal M, Fuchs BD, Shah CV et al. Serum lactate is associated with mortality in severe sepsis independent of organ failure and shock. Crit Care Med 2009;37:1670-7.

17 Phypers B, Pierce JT. Lactate physiology in health and disease. Continuing Education in Anaesthesia, Critical Care & Pain 2006;6:128-32.

18 Zhang Z, Xu X. Lactate clearance is a useful biomarker for the prediction of all-cause mortality in critically ill patients: a systematic review and meta-analysis. Crit Care Med 2014;42:2118-25.

19 Dutta TK, Sahoo R, Karthikeyan B. Capillary leak syndrome: desk to bedside. The Association of Physicians of India, <http://www.apiindia.org/pdf/pg_med_2007/Chapter-4.pdf>; 2013 [accessed 29.03.15].

20 Sherwood E, Toliver-Kinsky T. Mechanisms of the inflammatory response. Best Pract Res Clin Anaesth 2004;18: 385–405.

21 Caille V, Squara P. Oxygen uptake-to-delivery relationship: a way to assess adequate flow. Crit Care 2006;10 Suppl 3:S4.

22 Adams KL. Hemodynamic assessment: the physiologic basis for turning data into clinical information. AACN Clin Issues 2004;15:534-46.

23 Casserly B, Read R, Levy M. Hemodynamic monitoring in sepsis. Crit Care Clin 2009;25:803-23.

24 Moshkovitz Y, Kaluski E, Milo O, Vered Z, Cotter G. Recent developments in cardiac output determination by bioimpedance: comparison with invasive cardiac output and potential cardiovascular applications. Curr Opin Cardiol 2004;19:229-37.

25 Levin PD, Sprung CL. Another point of view: no swan song for the pulmonary artery catheter. Crit Care Med 2005;33:1123-4.

26 Böettger S, Pavlovic D, Gründling M, Wendt M, Hung O, Henzler D et al. Comparison of arterial pressure cardiac output monitoring with transpulmonary thermodilution in septic patients. Med Sci Monit 2010;16:PR1-7.

27 Weil M. Personal commentary on the diagnosis and treatment of circulatory shock states. Curr Opin Crit Care 2004;10:246–9.

28 Treacher D, Harvey C, Bradley R. Can cardiac output be assessed clinically with sufficient accuracy to be of value in patient management? Comparison with thermo-dilution in Intensive Care Unit patients. In: The Intensive Care Unit, UMDS, St Thomas' Hospital, London, UK; 2006.

29 Boyle M, Steel L, Flynn GM, Murgo M, Nicholson L, O'Brien M et al. Assessment of the clinical utility of an ultrasonic monitor of cardiac output (the USCOM) and agreement with thermodilution measurement. Crit Care Resusc 2009;11:198-203.

30 Dipti A, Soucy Z, Surana A, Chandra S. Role of inferior vena cava diameter in assessment of volume status: a meta-analysis. Am J Emerg Med 2012;30:1414-9.e1.

31 Pittman J, Bar-Yosef S, SumPing J, Sherwood M, Mark J. Continuous cardiac output monitoring with pulse contour analysis: a comparison with lithium indicator dilution cardiac output measurement. Crit Care Med 2005;33:2015-21.

32 Shah MR, Hasselblad V, Stevenson LW, Binanay C, O'Connor CM, Sopko G et al. Impact of the pulmonary artery catheter in critically ill patients: meta-analysis of randomized clinical trials. JAMA 2005;294:1664-70.

33 Harvey SE, Welch CA, Harrison DA, Rowan KM, Singer M. Post hoc insights from PAC-Man – the U.K. pulmonary artery catheter trial. Crit Care Med 2008;36:1714-21.

34 Rivers E, Nguyen B, Havstad S, Ressler J, Muzzin A, Knoblich B et al. Early goal-directed therapy in the treatment of severe sepsis and septic shock. N Engl J Med 2001;345:1368-77.

35 Ho BC, Bellomo R, McGain F, Jones D, Naka T, Wan L et al. The incidence and outcome of septic shock patients in the absence of early-goal directed therapy. Crit Care 2006;10:R80.

36 The ProCESS Investigators. A randomized trial of protocol-based care for early septic shock. N Engl J Med 2014;370(18):1683-93.

37 ARISE Investigators; ANZICS Clinical Trials Group, Peake SL, Delaney A, Bailey M, Bellomo R, Cameron PA, Cooper DJ et al. Goal-directed resuscitation for patients with early septic shock. N Engl J Med 2014;371(16):1496-506.

38 Vincent J-L. Give your patient a fast hug (at least) once a day. Crit Care Med 2005;33:1225–9.

39 Stennett A, Gainer J. TSC for hemorrhagic shock: effects on cytokines and blood pressure. Shock 2004;22 569–74.

40 Santry HP, Alam HB. Fluid resuscitation: past, present, and the future. Shock 2010;33:229-41.

41 Gutierrez G, Reines HD, Wulf-Gutierrez ME. Clinical review: hemorrhagic shock. Crit Care 2004;8:373-81.

42 Beekley A. Damage control resuscitation: a sensible approach to the exsanguinating surgical patient. Crit Care Med 2008;36:S267-74.

43 National Blood Authority. This work is based on/includes The National Blood Authority's Patient Blood Management Guideline: Module 1- Critical Bleeding/Massive Transfusion which is licensed under the Creative Commons Attribution-NonCommercial-ShareAlike 3.0 Australia licence. 2011.

44 Myburgh JA, Mythen MG. Resuscitation fluids. N Engl J Med 2013;369:1243-51.

45 Guidry C, Gleeson E, Simms ER, Stuke L, Meade P, McSwain NE Jr et al. Initial assessment on the impact of crystalloids versus colloids during damage control resuscitation. J Surg Res 2013;185:294-9.

46 Ball CG. Damage control resuscitation: history, theory and technique. Can J Surg 2014;57:55-60.

47 Duke MD, Guidry C, Guice J, Stuke L, Marr AB, Hunt JP et al. Restrictive fluid resuscitation in combination with damage control resuscitation: time for adaptation. J Trauma Acute Care Surg 2012;73:674-8.

48 Annane D, Siami S, Jaber S, Martin C, Elatrous S, Declère AD et al. Effects of fluid resuscitation with colloids vs crystalloids on mortality in critically ill patients presenting with hypovolemic shock: the CRISTAL randomized trial. JAMA 2013;310:1809-17.

49 Finfer S, Bellomo R, Boyce N, French J, Myburgh J, Norton R. A comparison of albumin and saline for fluid resuscitation in the intensive care unit. New Engl J Med 2004;350:2247-56.

50 Alderson P, Bunn F, Lefebvre C, Li WP, Li L, Roberts I at al. Human albumin solution for resuscitation and volume expansion in critically ill patients. Cochrane Database Syst Rev 2004;4 CD001208.

51 Lighthall G, Pearl R. Volume resuscitation in the critically ill: choosing the best solution: how do crystalloid solutions compare with colloids? J Crit Illness 2003;18:252–60.

52 Lopez-Plaza I. Massive blood transfusion. In: Transfusion medicine update, <http://www.itxm.org/tmu/ tmu1998/tmu4-98.htm>; 1998.

53 Criddle L, Eldredge D, Walker J. Variables predicting trauma patient survival following massive transfusion. J Emerg Nurs 2005;31:236–42.

54 Rappold JF, Pusateri AE. Tranexamic acid in remote damage control resuscitation. Transfusion 2013;53 Suppl 1:96S-9S.

55 Roberts I, Shakur H, Coats T, Hunt B, Balogun E, Barnetson L et al. The CRASH-2 trial: a randomised controlled trial and economic evaluation of the effects of tranexamic acid on death, vascular occlusive events and transfusion requirement in bleeding trauma patients. Health Technology Assessment 2013;17:1-79.

56 Gruen RL, Jacobs IG, Reade MC. Trauma and tranexamic acid. Med J Aust 2013;199:310-1.

57 Lim N, Dubois M, De Backer D, Vincent J-L. Do all nonsurvivors of cardiogenic shock die with a low cardiac index? Chest 2003;124:1885–91.

58 Ahrens TS, Prentice D, Kleinpell RM. Shock states. Critical care nursing certification: Preparation, review, and practice exams. 6th ed. New York: McGraw-Hill; 2010.

59 Hofer C, Furrer L, Matter-Ensner S, Maloigne M, Klaghofer R, Genoni M et al. Volumetric preload measurement by thermodilution: a comparison with transoesophageal echocardiography. Br J Anaes 2005; 94:748–55.

60 Agricola E, Bove T, Oppizzi M, Marino G, Zangrillo A, Margonato A et al. Ultrasound comet-tail images – a marker of pulmonary edema: a comparative study with wedge pressure and extravascular lung water. Chest 2005;127:1690–5.

61 Worthley L. Shock: a review of pathophysiology and management, Part 1. Crit Care Resusc 2000;2:55–65.

62 Di Marco J, Gersh B, Opie L. Antiarrhythmic drugs and strategies. In: Opie L, Gersh B, eds. Drugs for the Heart. 6th ed. Philadelphia: Elsevier; 2005.

63 Dubey L, Sharma S, Gautam M, Gautam S, Guruprasad S, Subramanyam G. Cardiogenic shock complicating acute myocardial infarction – a review. Acta Cardiologica 2011;66:691-9.

64 Blanton C, Thompson P. Cardiogenic shock and myocardial infarction in 19 Australian teaching hospitals. In: Cardiac Society of Australia and New Zealand, 49th ASM; 2001.

65 Carnendran L, Abboud R, Sleeper L, Gurunathan R, Webb J, Menon V et al. Trends in cardiogenic shock: report from the SHOCK Study. The SHould we emergently revascularize Occluded Coronaries for cardiogenic shocK? Eur Heart J 2001;22:472–8.

66 Menees DS, Peterson ED, Wang Y, Curtis JP, Messenger JC, Rumsfeld JS et al. Door-to-balloon time and mortality among patients undergoing primary PCI. N Engl J Med 2013;369:901-9.

67 Herget-Rosenthal S, Saner F, Chawla LS. Approach to hemodynamic shock and vasopressors. CJASN 2008;3:546-53.

68 Bodson L, Bouferrache K, Vieillard-Baron A. Cardiac tamponade. Curr Opin Crit Care 2011;17:416-24.

69 Menon V, White H, LeJemtel T, Webb J, Sleeper L, Hochman J. The clinical profile of patients with suspected cardiogenic shock due to predominant left ventricular failure: a report from the SHOCK Trial Registry. SHould we emergently revascularize Occluded Coronaries in cardiogenic shocK? J Am Coll Cardiol 2000;36:1071–6.

70 Topalian S, Ginsberg F, Parrillo JE. Cardiogenic shock. Crit Care Med 2008;36:S66-74.

71 Rahimtoola S. Acute rheumatic fever. In: Fuster V AR, O'Rourke RA, eds. Hurst's the Heart. New York: McGraw-Hill; 2004.

72 Leach RM, Treacher DF. The pulmonary physician in critical care 2: oxygen delivery and consumption in the critically ill. Thorax 2002;57:170-7.

73 Shoemaker W, Appel P, Kram H, Waxman K, Lee TS. Prospective trial of supranormal values of survivors as therapeutic goals in high-risk surgical patients. Chest 1988;94:1176–86.

74 Lesage A, Ramakers M, Daubin C, Verrier V, Beynier D, Charbonneau P et al. Complicated acute myocardial infarction requiring mechanical ventilation in the intensive care unit: prognostic factors of clinical outcome in a series of 157 patients. Crit Care Med 2004;32:100–5.

75 Park M, Sangean M, Volpe Mde S, Feltrim M, Nozawa F, Leite PF et al. Randomized, prospective trial of oxygen, continuous positive airway pressure, and bilevel positive airway pressure by face mask in acute cardiogenic pulmonary edema. Crit Care Med 2004;32:2507–15.

76 Management of complications following myocardial infarction (revised Feb 2012). In: eTG complete [Internet]. Melbourne: Therapeutic Guidelines Limited; 2014.

77 Poole-Wilson P, Opie L. Digitalis, acute inotropes and inotropic dilators: acute and chronic heart failure. In: Opie L, Gersh B, eds. Drugs for the heart. 6th ed. Philadelphia: Elsevier; 2005.

78 Lampard JG, Lang E. Vasopressors for hypotensive shock. Ann Emerg Med 2013;61:351-2.

79 Magder SA. The highs and lows of blood pressure: toward meaningful clinical targets in patients with shock. Crit Care Med 2014;42:1241-51.

80 Pirracchio R, Parenica J, Resche Rigon M, Chevret S, Spinar J, Jarkovsky J et al. The effectiveness of inodilators in reducing short term mortality among patient with severe cardiogenic shock: a propensity-based analysis. PLoS ONE 2013;8:e71659.

81 Follath F, Cleland J, Just H, Papp J, Scholz H, Peuhkurinen K et al. Efficacy and safety of intravenous levosimendan compared with dobutamine in severe low-output heart failure (the LIDO study): a randomised double-blind trial. Lancet 2002;360:196–202.

82 Mebazaam A, Barraud D, Welschbillig S. Randomized clinical trials with levosimendan. Am J Cardiol 2005;96:G74.

83 Moiseyev V, Poder P, Andrejevs N, Ruda M, Golikov A. Safety and efficacy of a novel calcium sensitizer, levosimendan, in patients with left ventricular failure due to an acute myocardial infarction: a randomized, placebo-controlled, double-blind study (RUSSLAN). Eur Heart J 2002;23:1422–32.

84 O'Connor C, Gattis W, Uretsky B, Adams KJ, McNutty SE, Grossman SH et al. Continuous intravenous dobutamine is associated with an increased risk of death in patients with advanced heart failure: insights from the Flolan International Randomized Survival Trial (FIRST). Am Heart J 1999;138:78–86.

85 Gersh B, Opie L. Which therapy for which condition? In: Opie L, Gersh B, eds. Drugs for the heart. 6th ed. Philadelphia: Elsevier; 2005.

86 Annane D, Bellissant E, Pussard E, Asmar R, Lacombe F, Lanata E et al. Placebo-controlled, randomized, double-blind study of intravenous enalaprilat efficacy and safety in acute cardiogenic pulmonary edema. Circulation 1996;94:1316–24.

87 The Acute Infarction Ramipril Efficacy (AIRE) Study Investigators. Effect of ramipril on mortality and morbidity of survivors of acute myocardial infarction with clinical evidence of heart failure: the Acute Infarction Ramipril Efficacy (AIRE) Study. Lancet 1993;342:821–8.

88 Thiele H, Zeymer U, Neumann FJ, Ferenc M, Olbrich HG, Hausleiter J et al. Intra-aortic balloon counterpulsation in acute myocardial infarction complicated by cardiogenic shock (IABP-SHOCK II): final 12 month results of a randomised, open-label trial. Lancet 2013; 382:1638-45.

89 Extracorporeal Life Support Organisation. ELSO guidelines for adult cardiac failure, <https://www.elso.org/Portals/0/IGD/Archive/FileManager/ e76ef78eabcusersshyerdocumentselsoguidelinesforadultcardiacfailure1.3.pdf>; 2013.

90 Extracorporeal Life Support Organisation. ELSO guidelines for ECMO centres, <https://www.elso.org/Portals/0/IGD/Archive/FileManager/ faf3f6a3c7cusersshyerdocumentselsoguidelinesecmocentersv1.8.pdf>; 2014.

91 Murray S. Bi-level positive airway pressure (BiPAP) and acute cardiogenic pulmonary oedema (ACPO) in the emergency department. Aust Crit Care 2002;15:51–63.

92 Agarwal R, Aggarwal AN, Gupta D, Jindal SK. Non-invasive ventilation in acute cardiogenic pulmonary oedema. Postgrad Med J 2005;81: 637–43.

93 Park M, Sangean M, Volpe Mde S, Feltrim M, Nozawa F, Leite PF et al. Randomized, prospective trial of oxygen, continuous positive airway pressure, and bilevel positive airway pressure by face mask in acute cardiogenic pulmonary edema. Crit Care Med 2004;32:2546–8.

94 Tallman T, Peacock W, Emerman C, Lopatin M, Blicker JZ, Weber J et al. Noninvasive ventilation outcomes in 2,430 acute decompensated heart failure patients: an ADHERE Registry Analysis. Acad Emerg Med 2008;15:355-62.

95 Bone RC, Balk RA, Cerra FB, Dellinger RP, Fein AM, Knaus WA et al. Definitions for sepsis and organ failure and guidelines for the use of innovative therapies in sepsis. ACCP/SCCM Consensus Conference Committee American College of Chest Physicians/Society of Critical Care Medicine. Chest 1992;101:1644–55.

96 Daniels R. Surviving the first hours in sepsis: getting the basics right (an intensivist's perspective). J Antimicrob Chemother 2011;66:ii11-ii23.

97 Finfer S, Bellomo R, Lipman J, French C, Dobb G, Myburgh J. Adult-population incidence of severe sepsis in Australian and New Zealand intensive care units. [Erratum appears in Intensive Care Med. 2004 Jun;30(6):1252]. Intens Care Med 2004;30:589-96.

98 Hicks P, Cooper DJ, Webb S, et al. The Surviving Sepsis Campaign: International guidelines for management of severe sepsis and septic shock: 2008. An assessment by the Australian and New Zealand Intensive Care Society. Anaes Inten Care 2008;36:149-51.

99 Kaukonen K, Bailey M, Suzuki S, Pilcher D, Bellomo R. Mortality related to severe sepsis and septic shock among critically ill patients in Australia and New Zealand, 2000–2012. JAMA 2014;311:1308-16.

100 Dellinger RP, Levy MM, Carlet JM, Bion J, Parker MM, Jaeschke R et al. Surviving Sepsis Campaign: international guidelines for management of severe sepsis and septic shock: 2008. Crit Care Med 2008;36:296-327.

101 Dellinger RP, Levy MM, Rhodes A, Annane D, Gerlach H, Opal SM et al. Surviving Sepsis Campaign: international guidelines for management of severe sepsis and septic shock: 2012. Crit Care Med 2012;41:580-637.

102 Dellinger R, Carlet J, Masur H, Gerlach H, Calandra T, Cohen J et al. Surviving Sepsis Campaign guidelines for management of severe sepsis and septic shock. Crit Care Med 2004;32:858–73.

103 Organizations JCoAoH. Raising the bar with bundles treating patients with an all-or-nothing standard. Jt Comm Pers Patient Saf 2006;6:5-6.

104 Finfer S. The Surviving Sepsis Campaign: robust evaluation and high-quality primary research is still needed. Intens Care Med 2010; 36:187-9.

105 Chamberlain DJ, Willis EM, Bersten AB. The severe sepsis bundles as processes of care: a meta-analysis. Aust Crit Care 2011;24:229-43.

106 Barochia A, Cui X, Vitberg D, Suffredini AF, O'Grady NP, Banks SM et al. Bundled care for septic shock: an analysis of clinical trials. Crit Care Med 2010;38:668-78.

107 Van den Berghe G, Schetz M, Vlasselaers D, Hermans G, Wilmer A, Bouillon R et al. Clinical review: intensive insulin therapy in critically ill patients: NICE-SUGAR or Leuven blood glucose target? J Clin Endocrinol Metab 2009;94:3163-70.

108 van den Berghe G, Wouters P, Weekers F, Verwaest C. Bruyninckx F, Schetz M et al. Intensive insulin therapy in the critically ill patients. N Engl J Med 2001;345:1359-67.

109 NICE-SUGAR Study Investigators, Finfer S, Chittock D, Su SY, Blair D, Foster D, Dhingra V et al. Intensive versus conventional glucose control in critically ill patients. N Engl J Med 2009;360:1283-97.

110 Griesdale DE, de Souza RJ, van Dam RM, Heyland DK, Cook DJ, Malhotra A et al. Intensive insulin therapy and mortality among critically ill patients: a meta-analysis including NICE-SUGAR study data. CMAJ 2009;180:821-7.

111 Schrier R, Wang W. Acute renal failure and sepsis. New Engl J Med 2004;351:159–69.

112 Ranzani OT, Monteiro MB, Ferreira EM, Santos SR, Machado FR, Noritomi DT. Reclassifying the spectrum of septic patients using lactate: severe sepsis, cryptic shock, vasoplegic shock and dysoxic shock. Revista Brasileira de Terapia Intensiva 2013;25:270-8.

113 Puskarich MA, Trzeciak S, Shapiro NI, Heffner AC, Kline JA, Jones AE. Outcomes of patients undergoing early sepsis resuscitation for cryptic shock compared with overt shock. Resuscitation 2011;82:1289-93.

114 Ranzani O, Monteiro M, Ferreira E, Santos SR, Machado FR, Noritomi DT et al. Stratifying septic patients using lactate: severe sepsis and cryptic, vasoplegic and dysoxic shock profile. Crit Care 2013;17:P37.

115 Bauer M. Multiple organ failure: update on pathophysiology and treatment strategies. In: Euroanesthesia: European Society of Anaesthesiology, 2005. Vienna, Austria; 2005, pp 203–6.

116 Marik PE, Varon J. Early goal-directed therapy: on terminal life support? Am J Emerg Med 2010;28:243-5.

117 Puskarich MA, Marchick MR, Kline JA, Steuerwald MT, Jones AE. One year mortality of patients treated with an emergency department based early goal directed therapy protocol for severe sepsis and septic shock: a before and after study. Crit Care 2009;13:R167.

118 Focht A, Jones AE, Lowe TJ. Early goal-directed therapy: improving mortality and morbidity of sepsis in the emergency department. Jt Comm J Qual Patient Saf 2009;35:186-91.

119 Rivers EP, Coba V, Whitmill M. Early goal-directed therapy in severe sepsis and septic shock: a contemporary review of the literature. Curr Opin Anaesthesiol 2008;21:128-40.

120 Mouncey PR, Osborn TM, Power GS, Harrison DA, Sadique MZ, Grieve RD et al for the ProMISe Trial Investigators. Trial of early, goal-directed resuscitation for septic shock. N Engl J Med 2015;372:1301-11. doi: 10.1056/NEJMoa1500896.

121 Padkin A, Goldfrad C, Brady AR, Young D, Black N, Rowan K. Epidemiology of severe sepsis occurring in the first 24 hrs in intensive care units in England, Wales, and Northern Ireland. Crit Care Med 2003;31:2332-8.

122 Brun-Buisson C, Meshaka P, Pinton P, Vallet B, Episepsis Study Group. EPISEPSIS: a reappraisal of the epidemiology and outcome of severe sepsis in French intensive care units. Intensive Care Med 2004;30:580-8.

123 Kumar A. Optimizing antimicrobial therapy in sepsis and septic shock. Crit Care Clin 2009;25:733-51.

124 Kumar A, Roberts D, Wood KE, Light B, Parrillo Je, Sharma S et al. Duration of hypotension before initiation of effective antimicrobial therapy is the critical determinant of survival in human septic shock. Crit Care Med 2006;34:1589-96.

125 Taccone FS, Laterre P-F, Dugernier T, Spapen H, Delattre I, Wittebole X et al. Insufficient beta-lactam concentrations in the early phase of severe sepsis and septic shock. Crit Care 2010:R126.

126 Dulhunty JM, Roberts JA, Davis JS, Webb SA, Bellomo R, Gomersall C et al. A protocol for a multicentre randomised controlled trial of continuous beta-lactam infusion compared with intermittent beta-lactam dosing in critically ill patients with severe sepsis: the BLING II study. Crit Care Resusc 2013;15:179-85.

127 Lipman J, Boots R. A new paradigm for treating infections: "go hard and go home". Crit Care Resusc 2009;11:276-81.

128 Finfer S, McEvoy S, Bellomo R, McArthur C, Myburgh J, Norton R. Impact of albumin compared to saline on organ function and mortality of patients with severe sepsis. Intensive Care Med 2011;37:86-96.

129 Myburgh JA, Finfer S, Bellomo R, Billot L, Cass A, Gattas D et al. Hydroxyethyl starch or saline for fluid resuscitation in intensive care. N Engl J Med 2012;367:1901-11.

130 Bagshaw SM, Chawla LS. Hydroxyethyl starch for fluid resuscitation in critically ill patients. Can J Anaesth 2013;60:709-13.

131 Myburgh J. CHEST and the impact of fraud in fluid resuscitation research. Crit Care Resusc 2011;13:69-70.

132 Perel P, Roberts I, Ker K. Colloids versus crystalloids for fluid resuscitation in critically ill patients. Cochrane Database Syst Rev 2013;2:CD000567.

133 Obritsch MD, Bestul DJ, Jung R, Fish DN, MacLaren R. The role of vasopressin in vasodilatory septic shock. Pharmacotherapy 2004;24:1050-63.

134 Lipiner-Friedman D, Sprung CL, Laterre PF, Weiss Y, Goodman SV, Vogeser M et al. Adrenal function in sepsis: the retrospective Corticus cohort study. Crit Care Med 2007;35:1012-8.

135 Magnotti L, Deitch E. Burns, bacterial translocation, gut barrier function, and failure. J Burn Care Rehab 2005;26:383-91.

136 Maragakis L. Recognition and prevention of multidrug-resistant Gram-negative bacteria in the intensive care unit. Crit Care Med 2010;38:S345-51.

137 Aitken LM, Williams G, Harvey M, Blot S, Kleinpell R, Labeau S et al. Nursing considerations to complement the Surviving Sepsis Campaign guidelines. Crit Care Med 2011;39:1800-18.

138 Young PJ, Weatherall M, Saxena MK, Bellomo R, Freebairn RC, Hammond NE et al. Statistical analysis plan for the HEAT trial: a multicentre randomised placebo-controlled trial of intravenous paracetamol in intensive care unit patients with fever and infection. Crit Care Resusc 2013;15:279-86.

139 Ellis A, Day J. Diagnosis and management of anaphylaxis. CMAJ 2003;169:307–11.

140 McLean-Tooke A, Bethune C, Fay A, Spickett G. Adrenaline in the treatment of anaphylaxis: what is the evidence? Br Med J 2003;327:1332–5.

141 Gold M. EpiPen epidemic or good clinical practice? J Paediatr Child Health 2003;39:376–7.

142 Nurmatov UB, Rhatigan E, Simons FER, Sheikh A. H_2-antihistamines for the treatment of anaphylaxis with and without shock: a systematic review. Ann Allergy Asthma Immunol 2014;112:126-31.

143 Dhami S, Panesar SS, Roberts G, Muraro A, Worm M, Bilo MB et al. Management of anaphylaxis: a systematic review. Allergy 2014;69:168-75.

144 Kanji S, Chant C. Allergic and hypersensitivity reactions in the intensive care unit. Crit Care Med 2010;38:S162-8.

145 Sampson HA, Munoz-Furlong A, Campbell RL, Adkinson NF Jr, Bock SA, Branum A et al. Second symposium on the definition and management of anaphylaxis: summary report – Second National Institute of Allergy and Infectious Disease/Food Allergy and Anaphylaxis Network symposium. [Reprint in Ann Emerg Med. 2006 Apr;47(4):373-80; PMID: 16546624]. J Allergy Clin Immunol 2006;117:391-7.

146 Berin MC, Sampson HA. Mucosal immunology of food allergy. Curr Biol 2013;23:R389-400.

147 Burks AW, Tang M, Sicherer S, Muraro A, Eigenmann PA, Ebisawa M et al. ICON: Food allergy. J Allergy Clin Immunol 2012;129:906-20.

148 Sicherer SH, Sampson HA. Food allergy. J Allergy Clin Immunol 2010;125:S116-25.

149 Boros C, Kay D, Gold M. Parent reported allergy and anaphylaxis in 4173 South Australian children. J Paediatr Child Health 2000;36:36–40.

150 Wood RA, Camargo CA Jr, Lieberman P, Sampson HA, Schwartz LB, Zitt M et al. Anaphylaxis in America: the prevalence and characteristics of anaphylaxis in the United States. J Allergy Clin Immunol 2014;133:461-7.

151 Simons FE, Frew AJ, Ansotegui IJ, Bochner BS, Golden DB, Finkelman FD et al. Practical allergy (PRACTALL) report: risk assessment in anaphylaxis. Allergy 2008;63:35-7.

152 Brown S. Clinical features and severity grading of anaphylaxis. J Allergy Clin Immunol 2004;114:371–6.

153 Pumphrey R. Anaphylaxis: can we tell who is at risk of a fatal reaction? Curr Opin Allergy Clin Immunol 2004;4:285–90.

154 Australian and New Zealand Anaesthetic Allergy Group–Australian and New Zealand College of Anaesthetists. Anaphylaxis management guidelines: Introduction, <http://www.anzaag.com/Docs/PDF/Management%20Guidelines/Mx%20Guidelines%20Intro%20v1.1Jun13.pdf>; 2013 [accessed 29.03.15].

155 Australasian Society of Clinical Immunology and Allergy Inc. Acute management of anaphylaxis guidelines, <http://www.allergy.org.au/health-professionals/papers/acute-management-of-anaphylaxis-guidelines>; 2013 [accessed 29.03.15].

156 Tang A. A practical guide to anaphylaxis. Am Fam Physician 2003;68:1325–32.

157 Wang J, Sampson HA. Treatments for food allergy: how close are we? Immunologic Res 2012;54:83-94.

158 Guly HR, Bouamra O, Lecky FE, Trauma Audit and Research Network. The incidence of neurogenic shock in patients with isolated spinal cord injury in the emergency department. Resuscitation 2008;76:57-62.

159 Summers RL, Baker SD, Sterling SA, Porter JM, Jones AE. Characterization of the spectrum of hemodynamic profiles in trauma patients with acute neurogenic shock. J Crit Care 2013;28:531 e1-5.

160 Dawodu S. Spinal cord injury: definition, epidemiology, pathophysiology. Medscape 2005.

161 Stevens RD, Bhardwaj A, Kirsch JR, Mirski MA. Critical care and perioperative management in traumatic spinal cord injury. J Neurosurg Anesthesiol 2003;15:215-29.

162 Ryken TC, Hurlbert RJ, Hadley MN, Aarabi B,Dhall SS, Gelb DE et al. The acute cardiopulmonary management of patients with cervical spinal cord injuries. Neurosurgery 2013;72 Suppl 2:84-92.

163 Jasmin L. Spinal cord trauma. In: MedlinePlus; 2013.

164 Miko I, Gould R, Wolf S, Afifi S. Acute spinal cord injury. Int Anesthesiol Clin 2009;47:37-54

165 Baumann A, Audibert G, Klein O, Mertes P. Continuous intravenous lidocaine in the treatment of paralytic ileus due to severe spinal cord injury. Acta Anaesthesiol Scand 2009;53:128-30.

166 Nguyen HB, Rivers EP, Knoblich BP, Jacobsen G, Muzzin A, Ressler JA et al. Early lactate clearance is associated with improved outcome in severe sepsis and septic shock. Crit Care Med 2004;32:1637-42.

167 Kincaid EH, Miller PR, Meredith JW, Rahman N, Chang MC. Elevated arterial base deficit in trauma patients: a marker of impaired oxygen utilization. J Am Coll Surg 1998;187:384-92.

168 St John RE. End-tidal carbon dioxide monitoring. Crit Care Nurs 2003;23:83-8.

169 Cheatham ML, Nelson LD, Chang MC, Safcsak K. Right ventricular end-diastolic volume index as a predictor of preload status in patients on positive end-expiratory pressure. Crit Care Med 1998;26:1801-6.

170 Corfield AR, Lees F, Zealley I, Houston G, Dickie S, Ward K et al, on behalf of the Scottish Trauma Audit Group Sepsis Steering Group. Utility of a single early warning score in patients with sepsis in the emergency department. Emerg Med J 2014;31(6):482–7.

171 Wilson SJ, Wong D, Clifton D, Fleming S, Way R, Pullinger R et al. Track and trigger in an emergency department: an observational evaluation study. Emerg Med J 2013;30:186-91.

172 Hughes C, Pain C, Braithwaite J, Hillman K. 'Between the flags': implementing a rapid response system at scale. BMJ Qual Saf 2014;23(9)714-7.

Chapter 22

Multiple organ dysfunction syndrome

Melanie Greenwood, Alison Juers

Learning objectives

After reading this chapter, you should be able to:

- define the common terminology related to multiple organ dysfunction syndrome
- describe the related pathophysiology of multiple organ dysfunction syndrome
- identify the clinical manifestations of multiple organ dysfunction syndrome
- identify patients at risk of developing multiple organ dysfunction, including predictors of mortality
- initiate appropriate monitoring, care planning and evaluation strategies for the patient with multiple organ dysfunction in relation to the current evidence base
- discuss treatment strategies that promote homeostasis in the patient with multiple organ dysfunction syndrome.

Introduction

The term multiple organ dysfunction syndrome (MODS) was established by an expert consensus conference in 1992 to describe a continuum of physiological derangements and subsequent dynamic alterations in organ function that may occur during a critical illness.[1,2] Previous terminologies in the literature were confusing. For example, multiple organ failure was a term commonly used, but somewhat misleading as normal physiological function can, in most cases, be restored in survivors of a critical illness who have temporary organ dysfunction.[3,4] Although the syndrome affects many organs, it also affects physiological systems such as the haematological, immune and endocrine systems. MODS therefore more accurately describes altered organ function in a critically ill patient who requires medical and nursing interventions to achieve homeostasis.[4]

MODS is associated with widespread endothelial and parenchymal cell injury because of hypoxic hypoxia, direct cytotoxicity, apoptosis, immuno-suppression and coagulopathy.[4] Four clinical stages describe a patient with developing MODS:[5]

1 increasing volume requirements and mild respiratory alkalosis, accompanied by oliguria, hyperglycaemia and increased insulin requirements

2 tachypnoea, hypocapnia and hypoxaemia, with moderate liver dysfunction and possible haematological abnormalities

3 developing shock with azotaemia, acid–base disturbances and significant coagulation abnormalities

4 vasopressor dependence with oliguria or anuria, ischaemic colitis and lactic acidosis.

Cellular damage in various organs in patients who develop MODS begins with the onset of local injury that is then compounded by activation of the innate immune system. This includes a combination of pattern recognition, receptor activation and release of mediators at the microcellular level, leading to episodes of hypotension or hypoxaemia and secondary infections.[4,5] The primary therapeutic goal for nursing and medical staff is prompt, definitive control of the source of infection or pro-inflammation[6] and early recognition of pre-existing factors that may lead to subsequent organ damage away from the initial site of injury. This pre-emptive therapy is instituted to maintain adequate tissue perfusion and prevent the onset of MODS. Recognition and response to early signs of clinical deterioration are therefore important to minimise further organ dysfunction.

In this chapter the pathophysiology of inflammatory and infective conditions that may lead to multiple organ dysfunction is described. System responses and specific organ dysfunction are discussed, expanding on dialogue in previous chapters, particularly Chapter 20. Assessment of the severity of MODS and nursing considerations in the treatment of the MODS patient are presented.

Pathophysiology

The syndrome of multiple organ dysfunction is most closely related to an outcome of sepsis, which is described in Chapter 21. MODS is a state characterised by aberrant cellular responses involving multiple organ systems and sequential processes. The pathogenesis of MODS is complex, simultaneously involving every cell type, neuro-hormonal axis and organ system.[7]

In brief, hypoxic hypoxia results from altered metabolic regulation of tissue oxygen delivery, which contributes to further organ dysfunction. Microcirculatory injury as a result of lytic enzymes, and vasoactive substances (nitric oxide, endothelial growth factor), is compounded by the inability of erythrocytes to navigate the septic microcirculation. Mitochondrial electron transport is affected by endotoxins in sepsis, nitric oxide and tumour necrosis factor alpha (TNF-α), leading to disordered energy metabolism (see Figure 22.1). This causes cytopathic or histotoxic anoxia.[8] This context of impaired oxygen utilisation where oxygen delivery is normal[7,8] results from diminished mitochondrial production of cellular energy – adenosine

FIGURE 22.1 Pathophysiology of cellular dysfunction.

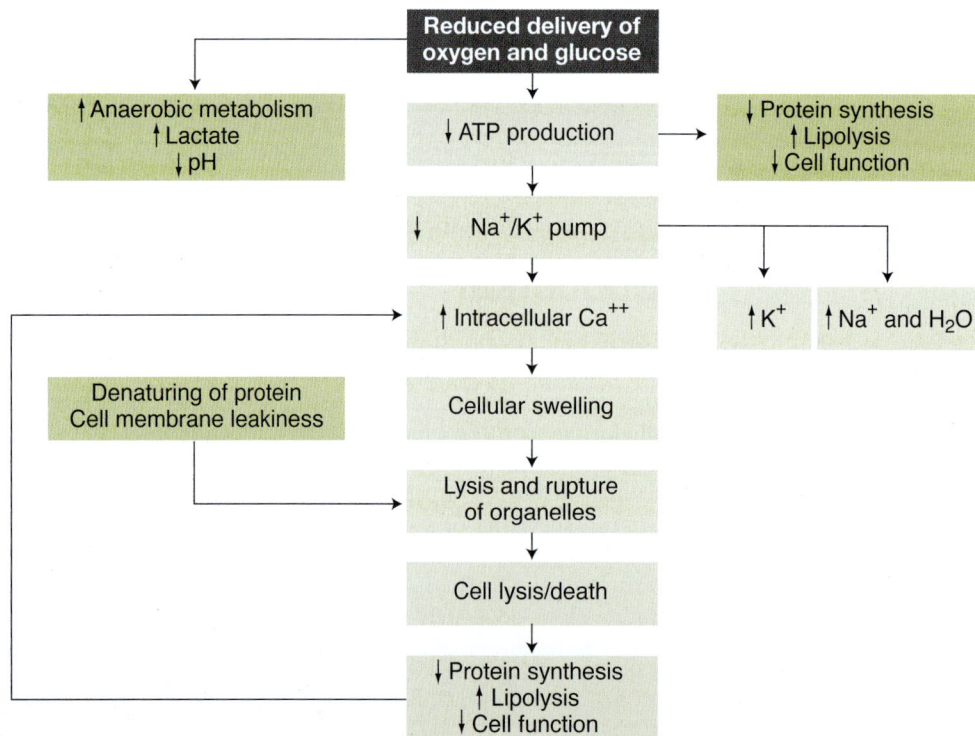

Adapted from Australian College of Critical Care Nurses. National Advanced Life Support Education Package: Pathophysiology of cellular dysfunction. Melbourne: Cambridge Press; 2004, with permission.

triphosphate (ATP) – despite normal or even supranormal intracellular oxygen levels.[9] Cellular hypoxia increases free radicals further compounding oxidative stress, which results in calcium entering the endoplasmic reticulum and mitochondria leading to cell death.[10] Cytopathic hypoxia appears resistant to resuscitation measures, and may ultimately worsen already-existing organ dysfunction. During sepsis or ischaemia, mitochondria respond by facilitating cell death rather than the restoration of homeostasis.[7]

Apoptosis is normal physiological programmed cell death and is the main mechanism to eliminate dysfunctional cells.[11] Apoptosis involves chromatin condensation, membrane blebbing, cell shrinkage and subsequent breakdown of cellular components into apoptotic bodies. This normally orderly process is deranged in critical illness, leading to tissue or organ bed injury and MODS. Pro-inflammatory cytokines released in sepsis may delay apoptosis in activated macrophages and neutrophils, but in other tissues, such as gut endothelium, accelerated apoptosis occurs.[8]

In contrast, necrosis is a form of cell death characterised by cellular swelling and loss of membrane integrity as a result of hypoxia or trauma. Necrosis has been termed 'cellular energy crisis',[11] and is unregulated resulting in loss of membrane sodium/potassium/ATP-ase pumps. This loss leads to cell swelling, rupture and spillage of intracellular contents into surrounding regions creating collateral damage.[11] Necrosis therefore can involve significant amounts of tissue and organ bed damage. Apoptosis differs from necrosis in that it does not seem to involve the recruitment of inflammatory cells or mediators to complete its task. Activation of an enzyme cascade systematically cleaves proteins and degrades the cell's nuclear deoxyribonucleic acid (DNA) with the end result being death of the cell. This requires energy from mitochondria and, if not available, necrosis of the cell occurs. Apoptosis and necrosis are processes important to understand in relation to future MODS research.

Increased concentrations of cell-free plasma DNA are present in various clinical conditions such as stroke, myocardial infarction and trauma, a likely result of accelerated cell death. Maximum plasma DNA concentrations correlated significantly with Acute Physiology and Chronic Health Evaluation (APACHE) II scores and maximum Sequential Organ Failure Assessment (SOFA) scores (described later in this chapter), with cell-free plasma DNA concentrations higher in hospital non-survivors than in survivors. Using regression analysis, maximum plasma DNA was an independent predictor of hospital mortality.[12]

Other cellular organelles may also exhibit pathological reactions in MODS. In ischaemia/reperfusion, endoplasmic reticulum loses its ability to process proteins, which induces the expression of heat shock proteins,[7] affecting transcription of proteins necessary for organ-specific functions. For example, liver cell metabolism, renal cell function or cardiac cell contractility may be affected.[7] This has led to the concept of a mode of hibernation[10,13] of cells at the expense of survival of the whole organism.[7]

Cellular communication is also altered in MODS. Cells normally communicate through highly interactive bidirectional neural networks.[14] The endothelium acts as a communication interface between cells, organs and systems and is involved in orchestration of systemic responses, including haemodynamic regulation, inflammation and coagulation; oxygen and nutrient delivery; oxidative stress; and sensing of psychological stress and neuroendocrine alterations.[7] In critical illness, endothelia release molecules that trigger the immune and neuroendocrine systems to produce a generalised inflammatory response.[7] The combination of the pathophysiological processes involved with the development of MODS, compensatory mechanisms and the effect on target organs and systems is now discussed.

Systemic response

After an overwhelming incident such as trauma, sepsis or non-infectious inflammation, a complex range of interrelated reactions occurs that result in a cascade of responses. The complex host-response generated involves the inflammatory immune systems, hormonal activation and metabolic derangements, resulting in multiple organ system involvement.[15,16] These host-responses are initially adaptive to maintain nutrient perfusion to the tissues; however, eventually organ systems become dysfunctional and fail, and the body is no longer able to maintain homeostasis[17] (see Figure 22.2).

Initially, pro-inflammatory mediators are released locally to fight foreign antigens and promote wound healing. Anti-inflammatory mediators are also released to downregulate the initial response to the insult.[18] If the local defence system is overwhelmed, inflammatory mediators appear in the systemic circulation and recruit additional leucocytes to the area of damage. A whole-body stress response ensues, further compounding the situation. If the pro-inflammatory mediators and the anti-inflammatory response are imbalanced, the patient may develop systemic inflammatory response syndrome (SIRS) and subsequent immunological dissonance[18] of organ dysfunction.[2,17,19]

Regardless of the trigger event, lymphocytes (T cells, B cells, natural killer cells) and macrophages are activated by cytokines (cellular signaling agents) to commence the inflammatory or anti-inflammatory response. A number of interleukins (IL) have been identified as key cytokines in pro-inflammatory (e.g. IL-1, IL-6; and similar to TNF-α actions) or anti-inflammatory (e.g. IL-10, IL-6, IL-4) responses. The inflammatory response results in clinical signs of hypoperfusion, culminating in shock.

Intracellular transcription factors, in particular nuclear factor kappa B (NF-κB), are important in innate and adaptive immunity,[20,21] as they regulate the transcription of genes involved in the inflammatory and acute stress response, leading to expression of TNF-α, interleukins and tissue factor.[21,22] NF-κB therefore plays an important role in response pathways in critical states including hypoxia, ischaemia, haemorrhage, sepsis, shock and MODS.[21,23,24]

The inflammatory cascade activates a number of prostaglandins and leucotrienes that also have pro- and anti-inflammatory effects. Thromboxane A_2 plays a role in the acute phase, in part due to stimulation of platelet

FIGURE 22.2   Tissue factor pathway.

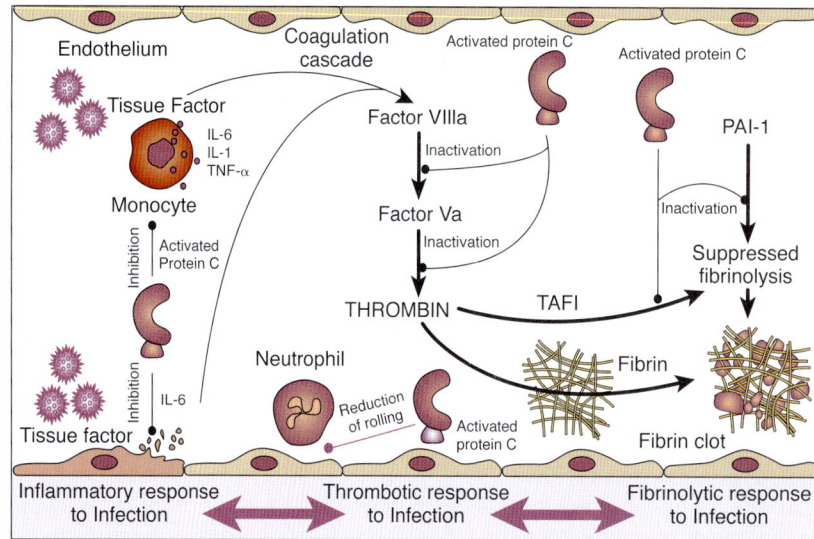

Courtesy of Bernard CR et al, (2001). Efficacy and safety of recombinant human activiated protein C for severe sepsis. N Eng J Med 344, 699-709.

aggregation, leading to microvascular thrombosis and tissue injury;[17] it may also play a role in pulmonary broncho-constriction and myocardial depression.

The specific pathophysiological concepts of inflammation, oedema and infection are discussed below.

Inflammation

Inflammation is part of innate immunity, a generic response to injury, and is normally an excellent mechanism to localise injury and promote healing.[25,26] The basis of this immune response is recognition of and an immediate response to an invading pathogen without necessarily having previous exposure to that pathogen.[27] Neutrophils, macrophages, natural killer cells, dendrites, coagulation and complement are the principal active components of the innate host response.[26]

The classic signs of inflammation are:

- pain
- oedema
- erythema and heat (from vasodilation)
- leucocyte accumulation and capillary leak.[25,26]

Nitric oxide and prostaglandins (e.g. prostacyclin) are the primary mediators of vasodilation and inflammation at the injury site.[26] Injured endothelium produces molecules that attract leucocytes and facilitate movement to the tissues. White blood cells accumulate by margination (adhesion to endothelium during the early stages of inflammation) and neutrophils accumulate at the injury site, where rolling and adherence to binding molecules on the endothelium occurs with eventual movement across the endothelium into the tissues.[26] Different blood components therefore escape the intravascular space and occupy the interstitial

space where they play the main role in successive phases of the inflammatory response. The endothelium thus plays a bidirectional mediating role between blood flow and the interstitial space where inflammation mainly takes place.[28] Macrophages, neutrophils and monocytes are responsible for phagocytosis and the production of toxic free radicals to kill invading pathogens.[27] The complement system, a collection of 30 proteins circulating in the blood, is also activated, with plasma and membrane proteins acting as adjuncts to inflammatory and immune processes.[27] When activated by inflammation and microbial invasion, these processes facilitate lysis (cellular destruction) and phago-cytosis (ingestion) of foreign material.[26,29]

Dysfunction of organ systems often persists after the initial inflammatory response diminishes; this is largely unexplained, although dysoxia (abnormal tissue oxygen metabolism and utilisation) has been implicated.[25,30] Hypoxia induces release of IL-6, the main cytokine that initiates the acute phase response. After reperfusion of ischaemic tissues, tissue and neutrophil activation forms reactive oxygen species (e.g. hydrogen peroxide) as a byproduct. These strong oxidants damage other molecules and cell structures that they come into contact with,[13,26] resulting in water and sodium infiltrate and cellular oedema.

Oedema

Oedema occurs as a consequence of alterations to tissue endothelium, with increased microvascular permeability or 'capillary leak'. As noted earlier, many mediators, including circulating cytokines, oxygen free radicals and activated neutrophils, alter the structure of endo-thelial cells, enabling larger molecules such as proteins and water to cross into the extravascular space.[26,31]

This response mechanism improves supply of nutrient-rich fluid to the site of injury but, if this becomes systemic, fluid shifts can lead to hypovolaemia or third-spacing (interstitial oedema) or affect other organs (e.g. acute lung injury, acute kidney injury).[26]

Infection and immune responses

Infection exists when there is one of the following: positive culture, serology,[32] presence of polymorphonuclear leucocytes in a normally sterile body fluid except blood or clinical focus of infection such as perforated viscus or pneumonia.[33]

The immune response to infection has both non-specific and specific actions, with inflammation and coagulation responses intricately linked in sepsis pathophysiology.[26,27,34,35] Tissue injury and the production of inflammatory mediators lead to:

- coagulation via the expression of tissue factor and factor VIIa complex (tissue factor pathway)[31,34–36]
- coagulation amplification via factors Xa and Va, leading to massive thrombin formation and fibrin clots (common coagulation pathway).[31,34]

Note that blood cell injury or platelet contact with endothelial collagen initiates the contact activation pathway.[34]

Procoagulation

Tissue factor is a procoagulant glycoprotein-signaling receptor,[37] expressed when tissue is damaged or cytokines are released from macrophages or the endothelium (see Figure 22.3). Prothrombin is formed, leading to thrombin and fibrin generation from activated platelets. Resulting clots are stabilised by factor XIII and thrombin-activatable fibrinolysis inhibitor.[34,37] Fibrinolysis is a homeostatic process that dissolves clots via the plasminogen–tissue plasminogen activator–plasmin pathway (involving antithrombin, activated protein C [APC] and tissue factor pathway inhibitor). APC:[38]

- reduces inflammation by decreasing TNF and NF-κB production
- reduces thrombin production when activated via thrombin–thrombomodulin complexes (anticoagulant action)
- inhibits thrombin-activatable fibrinolysis inhibitor and plasminogen activator inhibitor-1 (profibrinolytic action).[34,35]

APC is consumed in severe sepsis, and thrombomodulin is unable to activate protein C,[34,35,38] promoting a proinflammatory, prothrombotic state.[35]

Endocrine response

Physiological changes are triggered as a normal response to a stressor. In a critically ill patient, however, chronic activation of the stress response, including the hypothalamic–pituitary–adrenal (HPA) axis and the sympathetic–adrenal–medullary axis, results in ongoing production of glucocorticoid hormones and catecholamines.[20] This response interferes with the regulation of cytokine-producing immune cells, leading to immune dysfunction. Other compensatory mechanisms are instigated in an attempt to maintain supply and perfusion to organs.[18]

These homeostatic mechanisms are activated through positive or negative feedback systems to counteract stress. When stress is extreme or prolonged, these normal homeostatic mechanisms may be insufficient and a patient may respond through a sequence of physiological changes called the stress response. The stress response occurs in three stages: the alarm reaction, the resistance reaction and exhaustion (see Figure 22.4).[39]

FIGURE 22.3 Progression of SIRS–sepsis–shock–MODS.

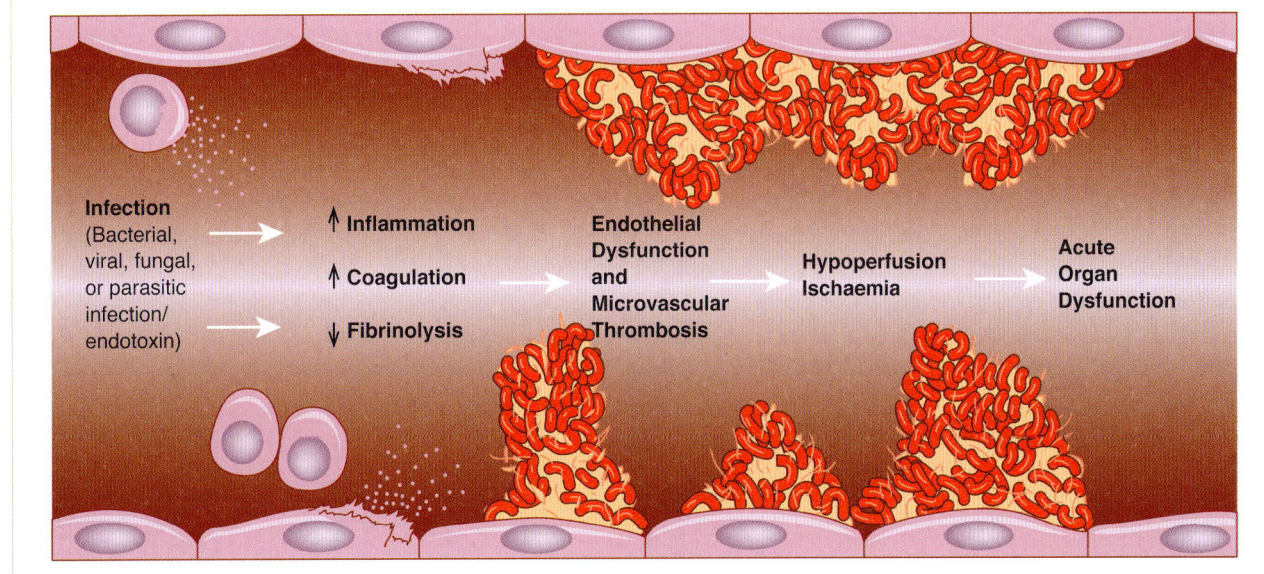

Infection (Bacterial, viral, fungal, or parasitic infection/endotoxin) → ↑ Inflammation ↑ Coagulation ↓ Fibrinolysis → Endothelial Dysfunction and Microvascular Thrombosis → Hypoperfusion Ischaemia → Acute Organ Dysfunction

FIGURE 22.4 Actions of the stress response.[39]

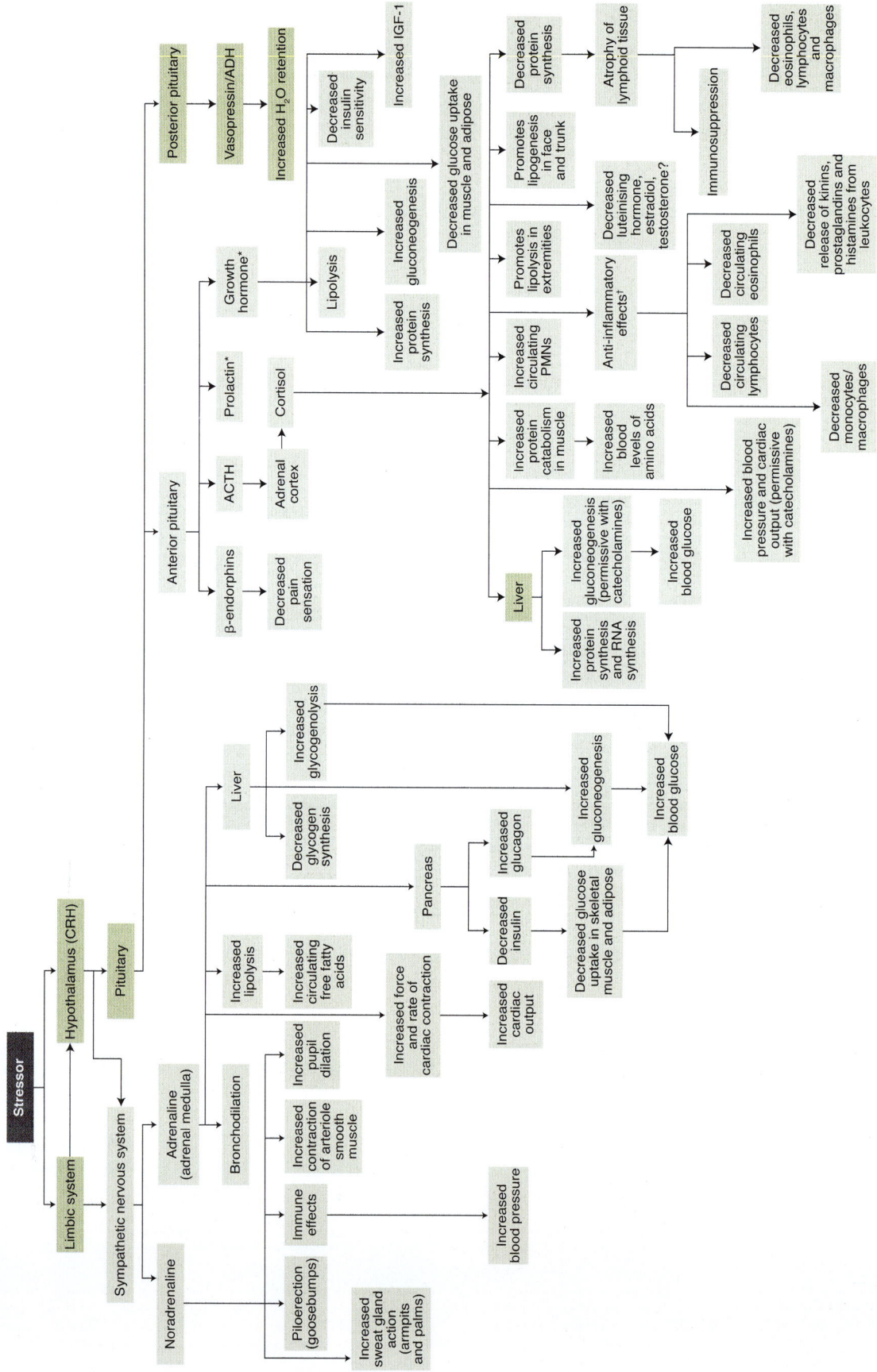

Adapted from McCance KL, Heuther SE, Brashers VL, Rote NS. Pathophysiology: The biological basis for disease in adults and children. 6th ed. Mosby Elsevier: St Louis; 2010, with permission.

The alarm reaction (flight-or-fight response)[39] is initiated when stress is detected, increasing the amount of glucose and oxygen available to the brain, skeletal muscle and heart. Two-thirds of total blood volume is also redistributed to support central circulation.[39] A rise in glucose production and the breakdown of glycogen in skeletal muscle increases circulating glucose levels, providing an immediate energy source. The long-lasting second stage is a resistance reaction, involving hypothalamic, pituitary and adrenal hormone release.[39] Response exhaustion occurs when these physiological changes can no longer maintain homeostasis.

Compensatory mechanisms

Internal equilibrium (homeostasis) is maintained by the nervous and endocrine systems, and these work symbiotically with other compensatory mechanisms, such as endothelial cells, to maintain cellular perfusion. The nervous system responds rapidly to maintain homeostasis by sending impulses to organs to activate neurohormonal responses (see Chapters 16 and 21). Autonomic dysfunction reflects 'uncoupling' of neurally mediated organ interactions in MODS[14] characterised by heart rate, baroreflex and chemoreflex variability. Endothelins (ET-1, ET-2, ET-3) are potent vasoconstrictors produced by endothelial cells that regulate arterial pressure.[23] The endocrine system works in a slow and sustained manner by secreting hormones, which travel via the blood to end-organs.

An initial acute-adaptive response is activated when an insult or stress occurs. For example, the body senses a disruption of blood flow through baroreceptor and chemoreceptor reflex actions: baroreceptors located in the carotid sinus detect changes in arterial pressure;[16] chemoreceptors co-located with the baroreceptors detect oxygen, carbon dioxide and hydrogen ion concentration. When alterations are sensed, the cardiovascular centre in the brain adjusts autonomic outflow accordingly.[39] In a patient with decreased tissue perfusion, there is increased peripheral vasoconstriction, contractility and heart rate. Blood flow is shunted to the vital organs (brain, heart, lungs), and away from less vital areas such as the gastrointestinal system, skin and reproductive organs.[40] Important hormonal regulators of blood flow are also activated from decreased blood flow to the kidneys, including adrenocorticotrophic hormone and the renin–angiotensin–aldosterone system (see Chapter 18). Adrenal medullary hormones, adrenaline and noradrenaline, vasopressin (antidiuretic hormone) and atrial natriuretic peptide also regulate blood flow to maintain adequate circulation and tissue oxygenation.[15,39,40]

Arterial pressure is a major determinant of tissue perfusion as it forces blood through the regional vasculature.[23] Hypotension (systolic blood pressure <90 mmHg or mean arterial pressure [MAP] <70 mmHg) results from either low systemic vascular resistance or a low cardiac output.[23] Glomerular filtration falls, leading to reduced urine output; low cerebral blood flow results in an altered level of consciousness; and other manifestations reflect low-flow states in other organ systems. To maintain oxygen supply, respirations and heart rate increase to meet organ oxygenation demands.[41] Heart rate variability is suggested as a strong predictor of mortality in MODS.[15] Organ dysfunction ensues if balance is not sufficiently restabilised (see Table 22.1).

Organ dysfunction

Organ dysfunction is a common clinical presentation in ICU. Patients with dysfunction in the respiratory, cardiovascular, hepatic or metabolic systems are 50% more likely to require ICU treatment and have a higher mortality than patients not requiring intensive care.[42] Timely identification of organ dysfunction is therefore critical, as early intervention reduces damage and improves recovery in organ systems. As each organ fails, the average risk of death rises by 11–23%.[43] The organ system that most commonly fails is the pulmonary system, followed by the cardiovascular, renal and haematological systems.[44] Organ and system

TABLE 22.1
Acute organ dysfunction[49,110]

ORGAN SYSTEM	CLINICAL PARAMETERS
Cardiovascular	Patient requires vasopressor support for systolic BP <90 mmHg or MAP <70 mmHg for 1 hour despite fluid bolus
Respiratory	Patient requires mechanical ventilation: PF ratio <250, PEEP >7.5 cmH$_2$O
Renal	Low urine output <0.5 mL/kg/h; raised creatinine >50% from baseline or requiring acute dialysis
Haematological	Low platelet count (<1,000,000/mm³) or APTT/PTT >upper limit of normal
Metabolic	Low pH with increased lactate (pH <7.3 and plasma lactate >upper limit of normal)
Hepatic	Liver enzymes >2 × upper limit of normal
Central nervous	Altered level of consciousness/reduced Glasgow Coma Scale score
Gastrointestinal	Translocation of bacteria, possible elevated pancreatic enzymes and cholecystitis

APTT = activated partial thromboplastin time; BP = blood pressure; MAP = mean arterial pressure; PEEP = peak end-expiratory pressure; PF = PaO$_2$/FiO$_2$ = partial pressure of arterial oxygen/fraction of inspired oxygen; PTT = partial thromboplastin time.

dysfunctions are a result of hypoperfusion, inflammation, cellular dysfunction and oedema. Dysfunctions of the cardiovascular (Chapters 10 and 12), respiratory (Chapters 14 and 15), renal (Chapter 18) and hepatic and gastrointestinal systems (Chapter 20) have been previously addressed. The next sections address the haematological, endocrine and metabolic systems. Neurological dysfunction is also common in the patient with MODS and complements previous discussions in Chapter 17.

Haematological dysfunction

SIRS and disseminated intravascular coagulation (DIC) have pivotal and synergistic roles in the development of MODS.[42] The coagulopathy present in MODS results from deficiencies of coagulation system proteins such as protein C, antithrombin III and tissue factor inhibitors.[8] Inflammatory mediators initiate direct injury to the vascular endothelium, releasing tissue factor, triggering the tissue factor pathway (extrinsic coagulation cascade) and accelerating thrombin production.[8] Coagulation factors are activated as a result of endothelial damage with binding of factor XII to the subendothelial surface and activation of factors VIII, X, XI, XII, calcium and phospholipid.[8] The final pathway is production of thrombin, which converts soluble fibrinogen to fibrin. Fibrin and aggregated platelets form intravascular clots.

Inflammatory cytokines also initiate coagulation through activation of tissue factor, a principal activator of coagulation. Endotoxins increase the activity of inhibitors of clot breakdown (fibrinolysis). Levels of protein C and endogenous activated protein C are decreased in sepsis; this inhibits coagulation cofactors Va and VIIa and acts as an antithrombotic in the microvasculature.[8]

Microvascular thrombosis that leads to MODS results from two major syndromes: thrombotic microangiopathy and DIC. Thrombotic microangiopathy is characterised by formation of microvascular platelet aggregates and occasionally fibrin formation. Typically, there is history of injury to the microvascular endothelium (e.g. thrombotic thrombocytopenic purpura, haemolytic uraemic syndrome, haemolytic anaemia, elevated liver enzymes and low platelet syndromes of pregnancy or antiphospholipid antibody syndrome).[42] Thrombotic microangiopathy usually presents with normal coagulation profiles such as prothrombin times and partial thromboplastin time.[45]

DIC results from widespread activation of tissue factor-dependent coagulation, insufficient control of coagulation and plasminogen-mediated attenuation of fibrinolysis.[45] This leads to formation of fibrin clots, consumption of platelets and coagulation proteins, occlusion of the microvasculature and resultant reductions in cellular tissue oxygen delivery.[45] DIC is most commonly a result of trauma or sepsis and is an exaggerated response to normal coagulation aimed at limiting infection and exsanguination and promoting wound healing.[45]

Thrombocytopenia (a platelet count of <80,000/mm^3 or a decrease of ≥50% over the preceding 3 days) signifies haematological failure,[46] with leucocytopenia/cytosis,

markers of coagulation and DIC also present.[47] Treatment is supportive and aimed at removing the triggering insults. Clinical biomarkers include a simultaneous rise in prothrombin time, activated partial thromboplastin time (aPTT) and thrombocytopenia.[35] A patient may exhibit bleeding from puncture sites (e.g. invasive vascular access), mucous membranes including bowel or upper gastrointestinal tract. Bruising or other subcutaneous petechiae may be evident. The skin should be protected from trauma.

Primary therapy is directed at the cause of the insult, with SIRS, ischaemia, uraemia, hepatotoxins and sources of infection, injury or necrosis managed concurrently. Aggressive resuscitation includes crystalloid or colloid administration and replacement of blood components and clotting factors using packed cells, platelets, cryoprecipitate and fresh frozen plasma. End points for haemoglobin, platelets and coagulation levels have not been agreed upon and replacement is therefore individualised.[48]

The role of heparin or fractionated heparin is controversial in the presence of sepsis, particularly in those with overt thromboembolism or extensive fibrin deposition, such as in purpura fulminans or ischaemia in the extremities.[49] Administration of APC in its role as inhibitor of the coagulation cascade is controversial. A Cochrane review of four studies involving 4911 participants (4434 adults and 477 paediatric patients) identified no reduction in risk of death (28-day mortality) in adult participants with severe sepsis, but was associated with a higher risk of bleeding. Effectiveness was not associated with the degree of severity of sepsis[52] and, therefore, APC is no longer commercially available.

Endocrine dysfunctions

Numerous endocrine derangements are noted in critically ill patients, including abnormalities in thyroid, adrenocortical, pancreas, growth and sex hormones. A high thyrotropin level is a significant independent predictor of non-survival in critically ill patients,[51] while subclinical hypothyroidism has significant negative effects on cardiac function and haemodynamic instability.[51,52]

Adrenal insufficiency

Adrenal insufficiency is present in approximately 30% of patients with sepsis or septic shock,[44,53,54,55] and is associated with chronic adrenal insufficiency and recent physiological stress, or in new-onset adrenal insufficiency.[51] This adrenal insufficiency can be caused by sepsis, surgery, bleeding and head trauma. Adrenal insufficiency as a cause of shock should be considered in any patient with hypotension with no signs of infection, cardiovascular disease or hypovolaemia. Incidence ranges from 0–95%,[56] partly because there is no standard definition for adrenal insufficiency.

Eosinophilia (>3% of total white blood cell count) is reported as a marker of adrenal insufficiency. Methods to diagnose acute adrenal insufficiency include: 1) a single random cortisol level check, or a change in cortisol level after endogenous adrenocorticotrophic hormone (ACTH) is administered; or 2) a short corticotrophin stimulation test with administration of high-dose ACTH. A change in cortisol level (≤9 mcg/dL) is considered relative adrenal insufficiency. It is, however, argued that patients with severe sepsis may have appropriate cortisol levels, but not the reserve function to respond to the stimulation test.[34]

Hypocalcaemia

Hypocalcaemia is common in patients with SIRS[58] and affects myocardial contractility and neuromuscular functions. The link between neuromuscular changes such as polyneuropathy or polymyopathy and critical illness has not been established beyond early investigations into corticosteroid use, neuromuscular blocking medication administration and prolonged mechanical ventilation.[58]

Neurological dysfunction

Evidence has highlighted that multiple organ dysfunction can result from severe traumatic brain injury or subarachnoid haemorrhage (see Chapter 17). Cardiovascular and respiratory dysfunction contribute to mortality in approximately two-thirds of all deaths following severe traumatic brain injury.[59] In non-traumatic subarachnoid haemorrhage the incidence and importance of life-threatening conditions from non-neurological physiology has been identified, including lethal arrhythmias, myocardial ischaemia and dysfunction and neurogenic pulmonary oedema.[59] The cause of cardiovascular and respiratory organ dysfunction following these acute, severe neurological events is associated with dysfunction of the sympathetic nervous system. Beta-blockers may modulate the sympathetic storm resulting from severe neurological injury.[59]

Critically ill patients may develop a syndrome of neuromuscular dysfunction characterised by generalised muscle weakness and an inability to wean successfully from mechanical ventilation. ICU-acquired weakness, including critical illness neuromyopathy syndromes, has been associated with risk factors including hypergylcaemia, SIRS, sepsis, MODS, renal replacement therapy, glucocorticoids, neuromuscular blocking agents and catecholamine administration.[60] The risk of ICU-acquired weakness is nearly 50% in patients with sepsis, MODS or protracted ventilation,[58] with short-term survival uncertain. Glycaemic control may be a potential strategy for decreasing ICU-acquired weakness.[60]

Survivors of sepsis-induced multiple organ dysfunction may also suffer long-term cognitive impairment, including alterations in memory, attention, concentration and/or global loss of cognitive function.[61] The participation of the brain during sepsis is poorly understood; septic encephalopathy is the more common neurological dysfunction, accounting for up to 70% of brain dysfunctions.[61] In Chapter 4 the physical, psychological and cognitive sequelae for survivors of a critical illness during their recovery are described.

Multiorgan dysfunction

MODS contributes to significant morbidity and use of intensive care resources worldwide. Patients with MODS have an increased ICU length of stay when compared to high-risk patients without multiple organ involvement[63,63] and very high 5-year mortality.[64] The epidemiology of MODS varies with North American and Australian studies in post-injury organ failure indicating a reduction in incidence,[62,63] versus increasing incidence reported in a recent German study.[65] These contrasting findings are in part due to different inclusion/exclusion criteria and MODS scoring systems used. Internationally, a reduction or stabilisation of MODS-related mortality is reported;[62,63,65] however, data from the developing world are scant. Mortality 15 years ago was estimated at 40–60%, rising with subsequent organ dysfunction.[43,66,67] More recent data in post-injury MODS indicate mortality rates between 11% and 27%.[62,63,68] This overall decrease in mortality is occurring despite increasing patient acuity and may reflect improvements in the delivery of critical care.[6]

Scoring systems

Organ dysfunction can be a consequence of a primary insult or a secondary insult due to circulating mediators (e.g. the patient with acute lung injury from pneumonia that also has renal dysfunction or failure as a consequence). This is sometimes quantified by scoring systems, traditionally used for predicting mortality but increasingly being explored as clinical management tools.[69–71,72] These systems are continually being tested and modified, to assess organ dysfunction severity and prognosis in an effort to identify patients who will benefit most from timely clinical intervention.[71] Scoring systems such as APACHE, simplified acute physiology score and mortality probability models account for information relating to a 24-hour cycle of patient data (commonly in the first 24 hours of admission), but do not account for the dynamic nature of many of the factors that affect clinical outcomes, thus potentially limiting their use for early MODS diagnosis and intervention.

Specific instruments designed to assess organ dysfunction or failure include the sepsis-related/SOFA score, the more trauma-specific Denver multiple-organ failure score, the multiple organ dysfunction score and the logistic organ dysfunction system.[63,70,72–75] Traditionally, SOFA uses the worst values for six commonly measured clinical parameters within a 24-hour period: PaO_2/FiO_2 (PF ratio), an index that may be used to characterise acute respiratory distress syndrome;[75] platelet count; bilirubin level; blood pressure; Glasgow Coma Scale score; and urine output or creatinine concentration. As the number of dysfunctional organ systems increases, there is a rise in mortality as measured by SOFA scores (see Table 22.2). Many variations of SOFA-based models have emerged in the literature, such as single SOFA scores calculated at admission or at a set time after admission, sequential SOFA scores (mean SOFA score), dynamic SOFA scores and scores of separate SOFA components.[69,70] SOFA scores at admission are comparable with severity of illness models such as APACHE or the simplified acute physiology score for predicting mortality.[70] SOFA scoring has the advantage of ease of use, as the clinical and laboratory data required are routinely available. As such, the use of dynamic SOFA scoring as a means of monitoring patient response to treatments is being explored.[69,71] Other scoring systems that allow pre-hospital identification of trauma patients predisposed to MODS are also being developed.[72] Overall, there is no one universally accepted gold standard scoring system with different systems used in MODS research.[76,77]

Other factors

Biomarkers such as lactate, base deficit and platelet count are also being studied as indicators of occult hypoperfusion and severity of organ dysfunction.[78–81] Blood lactate levels are routinely collected in the early stage of ICU admission, supporting early resuscitation as a management strategy to prevent organ dysfunction. Serial lactate scores may therefore be appropriate to guide optimal oxygen delivery in early resuscitation, with hyperlactataemia a sign of impending organ dysfunction. With the production of point-of-care lactate analysers, pre-hospital lactate levels may also identify patients predisposed to MODS and influence care delivery.[82] Prospective, well-controlled studies are, however, needed to confirm the role of lactate and other biomarkers in MODS management.[79–82]

Variations in the human DNA sequences can affect the way a person responds to disease. Researchers have studied the gene code for plasminogen activator inhibitor 1 (PAI-1), which is a key element in the inhibition of fibrinolysis and is active during acute inflammation[84] (the gene most studied is found at the 4G/5G insertion/deletion loci), and have found that different aspects bind as either a repressor (5G) or activator (4G) protein. For example, the 4G allele (position on the gene) of the 4G/5G gene sequence variation has been associated with increased susceptibility to community-acquired pneumonia and increased mortality in cases of severe pneumonia. It has also been reported to affect the risk of developing severe outcomes and higher mortality in meningococcal sepsis and trauma.[84] Among critically ill patients with severe sepsis due to pneumonia, carriers of the PAI-1 4G/5G genotypes have higher risk for MODS and septic shock.[84] In future, identification of genetic factors may assist selection of appropriate therapy for the patient at risk. Experimental BRCA1 gene therapy research is showing early promising results on key cellular processes involved in stimulating DNA repair and cellular defense.[84]

Patient management

Improvement in patient survival with MODS is thought to be due to improved identification of patients predisposed to MODS, improved shock and critical care management, awareness of secondary insults and a better understanding of the risk factors associated with MODS. Current prevention and management strategies therefore focus on identifying at-risk patients via scoring systems or biomarkers, efficient shock resuscitation, timely treatment of infection, exclusion of secondary inflammatory insults and organ support.[61,76,81]

TABLE 22.2
Sequential organ failure assessment (SOFA) score[69,110]

SOFA SCORE	0	1	2	3	4
Respiration PaO$_2$/FiO$_2$	>400	≤400	≤300	≤200[a]	≤100[a]
Coagulation platelets × 10³/mm³	>150	≤150	≤100	≤50	≤20
Liver bilirubin	<1.2 mg/dL >32 micromol/L	1.2–1.9 20–32	2.0–5.9 33–101	6.0–11.9 102–204	>12.0 >204
Cardiovascular hypotension	MAP >70 mmHg	MAP <70 mmHg	Dopamine ≤5 or Dobutamine (any dose)[b]	Dopamine >5 or adrenaline ≤0.1 or noradrenaline ≤0.1[b]	Dopamine >15 or adrenaline >0.1 or noradrenaline >0.1[b]
CNS Glasgow Coma Scale	15	13–14	10–12	6–9	<6
Renal creatinine or urine output	<1.2 mg/dL <110 micromol/L	1.2–1.9 110–170	2–3.4 171–299	3.5–4.9 300–440 or <500 mL/day	>5.0 >440 or <200 mL/day

[a]With respiratory support.

[b]Adrenergic agents administered for at least 1 hour (doses in *mcg*/kg per min).

FiO$_2$ = fraction of inspired oxygen; MAP = mean arterial pressure; PaO$_2$ = partial pressure of arterial oxygen.

Effective shock resuscitation

A number of interventions have been recommended to reduce mortality for patients with MODS due to sepsis. The Surviving Sepsis guidelines are based on clinical evidence graded according to the quality of evidence available.[81] The third version of the guidelines released in 2012 emphasises the importance of early recognition of sepsis-induced hypoperfusion and details resuscitation goals to be achieved within the first 6 hours of resuscitation. This treatment, known as early goal directed therapy (EGDT), created some controversy and dissent when released in the 2008 version of the guidelines (see Table 22.3) (see Chapter 21 for further discussion).

The multicentre, prospective, observational ARISE study (Australasian Resuscitation In Sepsis Evaluation) assessed the resuscitation practices and outcomes in patients presenting to emergency departments with sepsis with hypoperfusion or septic shock. Overall in-hospital mortality of 23% was comparable to in-hospital mortality reported in studies of early EGDT.[85] The study confirmed that protocolised central venous oxygenation saturation-directed EGDT was not routinely practised in Australia or New Zealand, and recommended that EGDT not be adopted in Australia and New Zealand without further multicentre randomised controlled trials.[85] While evidence of the benefits of EGDT from a quality improvement perspective is emerging,[81,86,87] these benefits may be due to increased awareness of sepsis management rather than EGDT.[88] In addition, the complex invasive technologies that underpin EGDT are not practical in resource-limited low- and middle-income countries.[88] Early resuscitation in severe sepsis does appear to improve patient outcomes;[89] however, evidence in relation to which components of EGDT are effective is lacking. One study has reported no

BOX 22.1

Surviving Sepsis campaign

The Surviving Sepsis campaign is an international collaborative formed in 2003 to reduce the mortality of sepsis. Guidelines for the management of severe sepsis and shock were updated in 2008 and 2012 and offer a comprehensive list of graded recommendations to care for these patients.[81] Many of the recommendations for practice have implications for critical care nurses and the multidisciplinary team (see *Online resources*).

Adapted from Dellinger R, Levy M, Rhodes A, Annane D, Gerlach H, Opal SM et al. Surviving Sepsis Campaign: international guidelines for management of severe sepsis and septic shock: 2012. Crit Care Med 2013;41(2):580–637, with permission.

mortality benefit for patients with severe sepsis/septic shock resuscitated with the protocol using continuous central venous oxygen saturation versus lactate clearance as a measure of adequate tissue oxygen delivery.[90] Large prospective clinical trials of EGDT include the US-based ProCESS (Protocolized Care for Early Septic Shock) trial, the Australian ARISE (Australasian Resuscitation in Sepsis Evaluation) trial and the UK ProMISe (Protocolised Management In Sepsis) trial.[91] The ProCESS trial showed no improvement in outcomes for patients with septic shock who received protocol-based resuscitation in the emergency department.[92] Similarly, the ARISE and ProMISe studies also did not detect a significant decrease in sepsis mortality with the use of EGDT. See Chapter 21 for further discussion of resuscitation in shock.

Early treatment of infection

Timely treatment of infection appears important in the prevention and management of MODS, with early antimicrobial therapy in septic shock recommended in the Surviving Sepsis guidelines. The Cooperative Antimicrobial Therapy of Septic Shock Database Research Group identified that:

- inappropriate initial antimicrobial therapy was associated with a five-fold decrease in survival to hospital discharge[94]
- the incidence of early acute kidney injury increased with delays in antimicrobial therapy from the onset of hypotension.[94]

Other studies support the Surviving Sepsis guidelines recommendation of antimicrobial therapy within the first hour of diagnosing severe sepsis.[95–97] As early antimicrobial administration may be difficult to achieve given competing patient management priorities (e.g. airway management, volume resuscitation, vasopressor administration), systems must be developed to promote early administration.[96] Nurses are in a pivotal position to ensure these guidelines or processes are developed, implemented and evaluated.

TABLE 22.3

EGDT in severe sepsis: initial targets[82]

ITEM	TARGET
CVP	8–12 mmHg 12–15 mmHg in mechanically ventilated patient or patient with decreased ventricular compliance
MAP	≥65 mmHg
Urine output	≥0.5 mL/kg/h
ScvO$_2$/ SvO$_2$	≥70%/≥65%

CVP = central venous pressure; MAP = mean arterial pressure; ScvO$_2$ = central venous oxygen saturation; SvO$_2$ = mixed venous oxygen saturation.

Adapted from Dellinger R, Levy M, Rhodes A, Annane D, Gerlach H, Opal SM et al. Surviving Sepsis Campaign: international guidelines for management of severe sepsis and septic shock: 2012. Crit Care Med 2013;41(2):580–637, with permission.

Practice tip

Tips for promoting early antimicrobial administration in severe sepsis/septic shock:[82,96,97]

- Ensure high priority in severe sepsis/septic shock algorithms.
- Do not delay antimicrobial administration if difficulty sampling blood cultures (cultures need to be collected within 45 minutes of diagnosis of severe sepsis or septic shock).
- Ensure adequate supply of antimicrobials in the emergency department and ICU that fit local colonisation patterns.
- Utilise appropriate antibiotics that can be given via intravenous push vs longer infusion.
- Emphasise education of staff on the significance of early administration of initial antimicrobial.
- Consider other potential barriers to early antimicrobial administration in your facility.

Combination antibiotic therapy may offer a survival benefit in septic shock, but may be deleterious to patients with a low mortality risk.[97] Certainly, antibiotic overuse and misuse is of concern given the emergence of antibiotic resistance.[98] Other factors that can lead to antibiotic failure in the critically ill include increased volume of distribution secondary to expanded extracellular volume, transient increased drug clearance due to elevated cardiac output (early sepsis) and increased free-drug levels secondary to reduced serum albumin. Maximum antibiotic dosage levels on day 1 of therapy, guided by predicted volume of distribution, are therefore recommended in life-threatening infections, as inadequate antibiotic penetration can occur due to impaired vascularity of infected tissue (inhibits delivery of antibiotic), antibiotic antagonism (uncommon but possible with combination therapy) and coexisting unrecognised bacterial infection.[81,97,99] Subsequent antibiotic dosing must be guided by drug clearance. This will be influenced by the associated organ dysfunction.[100] Nursing assessment of patient response to antibiotic therapy (resolution or exacerbation of signs of sepsis) and surveillance for sites of unrecognised infection are also important.

Source control (e.g. abscess drainage, removal of infected necrotic tissue or potentially infected device) is also an essential aspect of infection control and should be implemented within the first 12 hours of diagnosing severe sepsis or septic shock. The method of source control chosen should always involve a risk/benefit analysis as source control interventions can exacerbate complications.[81]

Steroid therapy

As septic shock is a major complication of infectious processes, the relationship between the immune, coagulation and neuroendocrine systems has been explored.[101] The role of corticosteroids in the treatment of septic shock

has led to a number of trials that suggested some survival benefit for low-dose corticosteroid therapy. More research is required, however, because of conflicting findings from individual studies.

Therapy with corticosteroids at a physiological dose, rather than a high dose, followed observations that patients with septic shock who had a reduced response to corticotropin were more likely to have increased mortality, and that pressor response to noradrenaline may be improved by the administration of hydrocortisone.[102] A trial exploring steroid use in sepsis demonstrated reduced vasopressor requirements and early lower mortality, but no difference in 1-year survival.[55] A multicentre trial demonstrated that hydrocortisone administration did not improve survival in patients with septic shock. Shock reversal was shorter in patients who received hydrocortisone, but there were more episodes of infection including new sepsis and septic shock.[102] Although the largest trial of corticosteroids in patients with septic shock, the study was not adequately powered to detect a clinically important treatment and so findings are to be interpreted with caution.[103] It is therefore appropriate to reserve corticosteroids for patients with septic shock whose blood pressure is poorly responsive to fluid resuscitation and high-dose vasopressor therapy.[103] Long-term treatment with corticosteroids may result in an inadequate response of the adrenal axis to subsequent stress such as infection, surgery or trauma, with resulting onset or worsening of shock. Other studies using corticosteroids for adrenal insufficiency in critically ill patients demonstrated lower mortality.[8]

Corticosteroid administration is associated with hyperglycaemia and may affect patient outcomes, necessitating insulin therapy to normalise blood glucose levels. A multicentre trial (Corticosteroids and Intensive Insulin Therapy for Septic Shock [COIITS])[104] demonstrated that intensive insulin therapy did not improve in-hospital mortality for patients treated with hydrocortisone and oral fludrocortisones for septic shock.

Glycaemia control

Hyperglycaemia is common in critically ill patients as a result of stress-induced insulin resistance and accelerated glucose production, and excessive circulating levels of glucagon, growth hormone, sympathomimetics and glucocorticoids (see Chapter 19). An increased caloric intake from parenteral or enteral nutrition will also increase glucose levels. Hyperglycaemia has undesirable effects such as fluid imbalance, immune dysfunction, promoting inflammation, abnormalities in granulocyte adherence, chemotaxis, phagocytosis and intracellular killing.[34] Resulting associations between hyperglycaemia and adverse clinical outcomes have been reported in many observational studies.[34,105] Potential benefits of exogenous insulin administration include normalising immune function, improving oxygen delivery to ischaemic areas of myocardium, tissue repair and preventing transfusion, dialysis and critical illness polyneuropathy.[34] Intensive insulin therapy has also been suggested to improve morbidity, reducing the risk of sepsis, excessive inflammation and multiple organ failure, transfusion requirements and dependence on mechanical ventilation.[106]

The Normoglycaemia in Intensive Care Evaluation and Survival Using Glucose Algorithm Regulation study (NICE-SUGAR) examined tight glycaemic control with insulin during critical illness.[106] Maintaining blood glucose at less than 10 mmol/L resulted in 10% reduction in 90-day mortality compared to a tighter glycaemic control target (4.5–6.0 mmol/L).[105] Lower target blood sugar levels are therefore not recommended for managing glycaemia in critically ill patients.

Exclusion of secondary insults and organ support

Prevention of secondary inflammatory insults and organ support include a broad range of interventions including use of massive transfusion protocols,[107] recognition of abdominal compartment syndrome via urine catheter manometry,[108] lung protective ventilation,[82] early nutritional support,[108,109] glycaemic control,[106] haemodynamic support using vasopressors and intropes[82] and renal replacement therapy.[81] Routine evidence-based measures are also essential, including hygiene; bowel management; pressure area, mouth and eye care; and other processes of care (e.g. FASTHUG; see Chapter 21).

Awareness of the latest evidence that underpins management of these complex patients is important.

Contemporary research is focusing on homogeneous subgroups of critically ill patients in an effort to refine MODS treatment, as opposed to heterogeneous groups where treatment impacts may be hidden by patient diversity.[76] There is a surprising dearth of literature specifically addressing the complex nursing care required by a MODS patient. These patients require highly skilled nurses who are able to balance competing priorities via ongoing patient assessment, care planning, monitoring and evaluation. The complex care required to nurse the MODS patient is highlighted in the clinical case study.

> **Practice tip**
>
> Tips for detecting haematological dysfunction in the patient with MODS:[48,56]
> - Monitor the skin for significant bruising or petechiae.
> - Check the sites of invasive devices such as arterial, central venous access or urinary catheters for bleeding.
> - Test urine or faeces for occult blood.
> - Note oral bleeding during mouth care or from the nose when nasal cleansing.
> - Detect progressive changes in coagulation or platelet profiles.

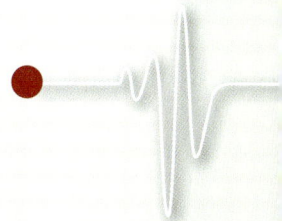

Summary

Multiple organ dysfunction is a common presentation to critical care units across the world. Critical care nurses require high-level knowledge of pathophysiology and early recognition of failure of individual organs and the antecedents to the development of organ failure. The pathophysiological consequence of systemic inflammatory response and sepsis requires understanding of individual organ function and responses to stressors so that pre-emptive strategies can be initiated to prevent further organ failure and support individual organs. Patients with MODS are complex patients to manage, requiring highly skilled nursing care that involves vigilant assessment, planning of intervention priorities, monitoring and ongoing treatment evaluation. Well-developed time management skills are required to include all routine cares and required treatment. Balancing care priorities begins on patient presentation as highlighted by the importance of initial resuscitation and early antimicrobial therapy.

Case study

Mrs Crisp, aged 30, presented to the maternity ward in the early stages of labour. Despite an elevated blood pressure (160/105 mmHg) on arrival, Mrs Crisp progressed to a normal vaginal delivery of a healthy baby boy. Mrs Crisp was moved from the delivery suite to spend time bonding with her baby following the birth. Approximately 6 hours later she began to complain of abdominal pain in the upper right quadrant. Paracetamol was provided; however, the pain continued, radiating to the epigastrium and shoulder. Mrs Crisp was nauseated and felt faint. Her blood pressure was noted to be 90/60 mmHg with a heart rate of 125 beats per minute. Nursing staff called the medical officer who, in collaboration with critical care medical staff, ordered a series of investigations. The blood results showed haemoglobin of 75 g/L, platelets of 57,000 × 10⁹, INR 1.6, fibrinogen of 1.4 g/L with deranged liver function tests. Chest computed tomography revealed no evidence of pulmonary emboli.

Chest auscultation revealed a decreased air entry to the right lower base; she appeared cool to the touch with respirations of 26 per minute. Abdominal assessment revealed tenderness in the right hypochondria and a relatively rigid abdomen. The uterus was contracting normally at this point in her postpartum period. Mrs Crisp had not passed urine at this stage. A cannula was inserted, and fluid and oxygen therapy commenced. Arrangements were made for urgent transfer to critical care for ongoing support. In critical care Mrs Crisp was intubated, ventilated and continued to display signs of shock with low blood pressure, reduced urine output and abdominal pain. She received an urgent surgical review as the CT abdomen revealed a rupture of the liver with bleeding in the subcapsular region. Mrs Crisp was transferred to the operating theatre for surgical repair.

On return from theatre Mrs Crisp remained intubated and ventilated with a controlled ventilation rate of 12 breaths per minute, tidal volumes of 8 mL/kg, positive end-expiratory pressure of 5 cmH$_2$O and fraction of inspired oxygen (FiO$_2$) of 0.5. Her respiratory status became unstable with increasing oxygen requirements (FiO$_2$ 0.8) and her oxygen saturation decreased to 90%. Blood gas results revealed pH 7.30, PaCO$_2$ 60 mmHg. Her inspiratory airway and plateau pressures increased and a diagnosis of acute respiratory distress syndrome was made based on a PaO$_2$/FiO$_2$ ratio of less than 200 and infiltrates on her chest X-ray.

Despite therapeutic interventions Mrs Crisp continued to be haemodynamically unstable. Her blood pressure remained low and a noradrenaline infusion of 15 mcg/min was commenced aiming to achieve a mean arterial pressure of 65–70 mmHg. Urine output decreased on day 2 to 15 mL/h. Central venous pressure was recorded as 14 cmH$_2$O and fluid filling did not increase her urine output. Diuretic therapy in the form of frusemide was trialled as a continuous infusion with some increase in her urine output. A diagnosis of acute renal failure was made (creatinine 141 micromol/L) and continuous venovenous haemodiafiltration renal replacement therapy commenced. Mrs Crisp had marked coagulopathy that resulted in DIC requiring administration of blood products (platelets and fresh frozen plasma) to replace consumed clotting factors.

Enteral feeds and a prokinetic were commenced early in the course of her admission to support nutritional status; this was tolerated with low residual gastric volume. Over the following few days the condition of Mrs Crisp slowly improved with lung mechanics and renal function returning to baseline levels and weaning of therapy commenced. On day 8 Mrs Crisp was extubated and discharged to the ward to continue her recovery and rehabilitation.

DISCUSSION

The period of time where Mrs Crisp was most at risk of multiple organ dysfunction was during the episode of hypotension. The loss of blood from the liver tear was physiologically compensated for initially through centralisation of cardiac output as a result of a vasomotor response resulting in vasoconstriction and tachycardia. The respiratory system increased oxygenation uptake through augmenting respirations; however, the reduced haemoglobin level lowered the oxygen-carrying capacity. As blood loss continued other compensatory mechanisms came into play. The stress response triggered a cascade of neuroendocrine and other hormonal events. Coagulation factors were consumed due to activation of tissue factor pathway activation leading to disseminated intravascular coagulation with resulting loss of platelets and fibrinogen levels. Microcirculatory failure and the continued vasoconstriction with altered vascular filling resulted in renal and liver dysfunction. This was reflected by her reduced urine output, elevated creatinine levels and deranged liver function test results.

Fortunately for Mrs Crisp, early intervention through the administration of fluids and blood products, invasive respiratory support and surgical repair of the liver tear resulted in a short course of multiple organ dysfunction. The critical care she received prevented many adverse effects of critical illness and psychological care resulted in minimal disruption to the mother and baby bonding.

The case highlights the significant part that early identification of patient deterioration with appropriate and timely management plays in averting longer periods of multiple organ dysfunction.

CASE STUDY QUESTIONS

1 Identify the organs and body systems that failed in the case of Mrs Crisp. Include in your answer the clinical signs that indicated MODS.

2 Develop a care plan for Mrs Crisp for her stay in critical care. Ensure that you include routine cares as well as care specifically targeted at organ support. Discuss your plan with an experienced colleague.

3 List some of the important assessment findings that influenced the care of Mrs Crisp during her stay in critical care.

RESEARCH VIGNETTE

Andruszkow H, Veh J, Mommsen P, Zeckey C, Hildebrand F, Frink M. Impact of the body mass on complications and outcome in multiple trauma patients: what does the weight weigh? Mediators Inflamm 2013; doi: 10.1155/2013/345702. Epub 2013 Aug 19

Abstract

Obesity is known as an independent risk factor for various morbidities. The influence of an increased body mass index (BMI) on morbidity and mortality in critically injured patients has been investigated with conflicting results. To verify the impact of weight disorders in multiple traumatized patients, 586 patients with an injury severity score >16 points treated at a level I trauma center between 2005 and 2011 were differentiated according to the BMI and analyzed regarding morbidity and outcome. Plasma levels of interleukin- (IL-) 6 and C-reactive protein (CRP) were measured during clinical course to evaluate the inflammatory response to the "double hit" of weight disorders and multiple trauma. In brief, obesity was the highest risk factor for development of a multiple organ dysfunction syndrome (MODS) (OR 4.209, 95% CI 1.515–11.692) besides injury severity (OR 1.054, 95% CI 1.020–1.089) and APACHE II score (OR 1.059, 95% CI 1.001–1.121). In obese patients as compared to those with overweight, normal weight, and underweight, the highest levels of CRP were continuously present while increased systemic IL-6 levels were found until day 4. In conclusion, an altered posttraumatic inflammatory response in obese patients seems to determine the risk for multiple organ failure after severe trauma.

Critique

The researchers set the background to the work by drawing attention to the conflicting results of previous research studies into the influence increased body mass of critically injured patients has on morbidity and mortality. The researchers questioned the role that inflammation had on the posttraumatic systemic immune response in critically injured obese and normal or underweight participants in the study population. The results from the study revealed obesity as the highest risk factor for the development of MODS though it had little impact on mortality. Obese patients were admitted with increased interleukin-6 levels for the first 4 days and showed sustained elevation in CRP levels for the study period. Increased interleukin-6 levels were positively correlated with the incidence of MODS during the whole study period while elevated CRP levels were positively correlated with MODS after day 3.

The authors suggest that increased adipose tissue content results in elevated pro-inflammatory adipokines, which have a number of effects on the critically ill multiple trauma patient. These effects resulted in an increased incidence of MODS in the obese study population. Study limitations are noted in that a substantial number of patients were excluded due to missing weight and height data, which was noted to be comparable to other studies. BMI was also questioned as presenting an accurate tool to determine weight disorders though this was felt by the authors to be a safe measurement as it represented the most widely accepted parameter in the literature quoted in the study.

The final summation by the study authors advised that obesity was revealed as an independent risk factor for the development of MODS in severely traumatised patients. The role that nutrition status plays in the post-traumatic clinical course was put forward for consideration as important in therapeutic strategies for patients suffering from major trauma.

The study was well designed and it is a significant study in relation to the growing incidence of obesity amongst the critically ill traumatised patients who are admitted to critical care. The relationship of obesity to MODS and mortality outcomes for patients with trauma should encourage future prospective trials that may translate into improved healthcare outcomes for critically ill patients.

Learning activities

1 Identify five key elements essential in managing the patient with emergent MODS.

2 Outline four strategies that promote early antimicrobial administration and therefore the prevention and management of MODS, in the patient with severe sepsis and septic shock.

3 Identify eight strategies that aim to minimise secondary insult and provide organ support for the MODS patient.

Online resources

The Institute for Healthcare Improvement (IHI) is a non-profit organisation for advancing the quality and value of health care. Search the site for sepsis-related information about improving care and severe sepsis bundles, www.ihi.org

The Surviving Sepsis guidelines webpage provides access to full text documents, references, presentations, updated position statements and tools related to the guidelines, www.survivingsepsis.org

The US National Institutes of Health clinical trials registry. Search the site for current trials in MODS, www.clinicaltrials.gov

Further reading

Dellinger R, Mitchell M, Rhodes A, Annane D, Gerlach H, Opal SM et al. Surviving Sepsis campaign: international guidelines for management of severe sepsis and septic shock: 2012. Crit Care Med 2013;41(2):580–637.

Fröhlich M, Lefering R, Probst C, Paffrath T, Schneider MM, Maegele M et al. Epidemiology and risk factors of multiple-organ failure after multiple trauma: an analysis of 31,154 patients from the TraumaRegister DGU. J Trauma Acute Care Surg 2014;76(4):921–8.

Lone N, Walsh T. Impact of intensive care unit organ failures on mortality during five years after a critical illness. Am J Respir Crit Care Med 2012;186(7):640–7.

Moore FA, Moore EE. The evolving rationale for early enteral nutrition based on paradigms of multiple organ failure: a personal journey. Nutr Clin Practice 2009;24(3):297–304.

Nydam TL, Kashuk JL, Moore ED, Johnson JL, Burlew CC, Biffl WL et al. Refractory postinjury thrombocytopenia is associated with multiple organ failure and adverse outcomes. J Trauma 2011;70(2):401–7.

Sauaia A, Moore E, Johnson J, Chin T, Banerjee A, Sperry JL et al. Temporal trends of postinjury multiple-organ failure: still resource intensive, morbid, and lethal. J Trauma Acute Care Surg 2014;76(3):582–93.

Ulldemolins M, Roberts J, Lipman J, Rello J. Antibiotic dosing in multiple organ dysfunction syndrome. Chest 2011; 139(5):1210–20.

References

1 Jackson W, Gallagher C, Myhand R, Waselenko J. Medical management of patients with multiple organ dysfunction arising from acute radiation syndrome. Brit J Radiol 2005;27: 161–8.

2 Bone R, Balk R, Cerra F, Dellinger R, Fein A, Knaus WA et al. Definitions for sepsis and organ failure and guidelines for the use of innovative therapies in sepsis. The ACCP/SCCM Consensus Conference Committee. American College of Chest Physicians/Society of Critical Care Medicine. Chest 1992;101(6):1644–55.

3 Al-Khafaji A, Sharma S. Multisystem organ failure of sepsis. eMedicine Critical Care, <http://emedicine.medscape.com/article/169640-overview>; 2010.

4 Marshall JC. The multiple organ dysfunction syndrome. Surgical treatment: evidence based and problem oriented, <http://www.ncbi.nlm.nih.gov/bookshelf/br.fcgi?book=surg&part=A5364>; 2001.

5 Deitch E. Multiple organ failure: pathophysiology and potential future therapy. Ann Surg 1992;216(2):117–34.

6 Barie P, Hydo L, Shou J, Eachempati S. Decreasing magnitude of multiple organ dysfunction syndrome despite increasingly severe critical surgical illness: a 17-year longitudinal study. Trauma 2008;65(6):1227–35.

7 Papathanassoglou E, Bozas E, Giannakopoloulou M. Multiple organ dysfunction syndrome pathogenesis and care: a complex systems' theory perspective. British Association of Critical Care Nurses. Nurs Critical Care 2008;13(5):249–59.

8 Pinsky M, Al Faresi F, Brenner B, Dire D, Filbin M, Flowers F et al. Septic shock. eMedicine Critical Care, <http://emedicine.medscape.com/article/168402-overview>; 2011.

9 Fink M. Cytopathic hypoxia in sepsis. Acta Anaesthesiol Scand 1997;110 (Suppl):87–95.

10 Duran-Bedolla J, Montes de Oca-Sandoval M, Saldana-Navor V, Villalobos J, Rodriguez M, Rivas-Aranchibia S. Sepsis, mitochondrial failure and multiple organ dysfunction. ClinInvest Med 2014;37(2):E58-E69.

11 Henke K, Eigisti J. Self-annihilation: a cell's story of suicide. Dimens Crit Care Nurs 2005;24(3):117–19.

12 Saukkonen K, Lakkisto P, Varpula M, Varpula T, Voipio-Pulkki L-M, Pettilä V et al. Association of cell-free plasma DNA with hospital mortality and organ dysfunction in intensive care unit patients. Intensive Care Med 2007;33(9):1624–7.

13 Singer M. The role of mitochondrial dysfunction in sepsis induced multi-organ failure. Virulence 2014;5(1):66-72.

14 Schmidt H, Lotze U, Ghanem A, Anker SD, Said SM, Braun-Dullaeus R et al. Relation of impaired interorgan communication and parasympathetic activity in chronic heart failure and multiple-organ dysfunction syndrome. J Crit Care 2014;29(3):367-73.

15 Mizock BA. Metabolic derangements in sepsis and septic shock. Crit Care Clinics 2000;16(2):319–36.

16 Singer M, De Santis V, Vitale D, Jeffcoate W. Multiorgan failure is an adaptive, endocrine-mediated, metabolic response to overwhelming systemic inflammation. Lancet 2004;364(9433):545–8.

17 Bone RC. Immunologic dissonance: a continuing evolution in our understanding of the systemic inflammatory response syndrome (SIRS) and the multiple organ dysfunction syndrome (MODS). Ann Internl Med 1996;125(8):680–87.

18 Jastrow K, Gonzalez E, McGuire M, Suliburk J, Kozar R, Iyengar S et al. Early cytokine production risk stratifies trauma patients for multiple organ failure. J Am Coll Surg 2009;3(209):320–31.

19 Bridges EJ, Dukes S. Cardiovascular aspects of septic shock: pathophysiology, monitoring, and treatment. Crit Care Nurs 2005;25(2):14–40.

20 Padgett DA, Glaser R. How stress influences the immune response. Trends Immunol 2003;24(8):444–8.

21 Hubbard WJ, Bland KI, Chaudry IH. The role of the mitochondrion in trauma and shock. Shock 2004;22(5):395–402.

22 Adrie C, Pinsky MR. The inflammatory balance in human sepsis. Intensive Care Med 2000;26(4):364–75.

23 Magder S, Cernacek P. Role of endothelins in septic, cardiogenic, and hemorrhagic shock. Can J Physiol Pharmacol 2003;81(6):635–43.

24 Zingarelli B, Sheehan M, Wong HR. Nuclear factor-kappaB as a therapeutic target in critical care medicine. Crit Care Med 2003;31(Supp):S105–11.

25 Brealey D, Brand M, Hargreaves I, Heales S, Land J, Smolenski R et al. Association between mitochondrial dysfunction and severity and outcome of septic shock. Lancet 2002;360(9328):219–23.

26 Sherwood E, Toliver-Kinsky T. Mechanisms of the inflammatory response. Best Prac Res Clin Anaesthesiol 2004;18(3):385–405.

27 Weigand M, Horner C. The systemic inflammatory response syndrome. Best Prac Res Clin Anaesthesiol 2004;18(3):455–75.

28 Arias J-I, Aller M-A, Arias J. Surgical inflammation: a pathophysiological rainbow. J Translation Med 2009;7(19), < http://www.translational-medicine.com/content/pdf/1479-5876-7-19.pdf>.

29 Kirschfink M. Controlling the complement system in inflammation. Immunopharmacol 1997;38(1–2):51–62.

30 Dishart MK, Schlichtig R, Tonnessen TI, Rozenfeld RA, Simplaceanu E, Williams D et al. Mitochondrial redox state as a potential detector of liver dysoxia in vivo. J Applied Physiol 1998;84(3):791–7.

31 Fishel RS, Are C, Barbul A. Vessel injury and capillary leak. Crit Care Med 2003;31(8):S502–11.

32 Calandra T, Cohen J. The international sepsis forum consensus conference on definitions of infection in the intensive care unit. Crit Care Med 2005;33(7):1538–48.

33 Micek ST, Shah RA, Kollef MH. Management of severe sepsis: integration of multiple pharmacologic interventions. Pharmacotherapy 2003;23(11):1486–96.

34 Amaral A, Opal SM, Vincent JL. Coagulation in sepsis. Intensive Care Med 2004;30(6):1032–40.

35 Rice TW, Bernard GR. Drotrecogin alfa (activated) for the treatment of severe sepsis and septic shock. Am J Med Sci 2004;328(4):205–14.

36 Sharma S, Eschun G. Multisystem organ failure of sepsis. eMedicine Critical Care, <http://www.emedicine.com/med/topic3372.htm>; 2004.

37 Doshi SN, Marmur JD. Evolving role of tissue factor and its pathway inhibitor. Crit Care Med 2002; 30(Suppl):S241–50.

38 Liaw P. Endogenous protein C activation in patients with severe sepsis. Crit Care Med 2004;32(5):S214–18.

39 McCance KL, Heuther SE, Brashers VL, Rote NS. Pathophysiology: The biological basis for disease in adults and children. 6th ed. Mosby Elsevier: St Louis; 2010.

40 Hameed SM, Aird WC, Cohn SM. Oxygen delivery. Crit Care Med 2003;31(12Suppl):S658–67.

41 Trager T, DeBacker D, Radermacher P. Metabolic alterations in sepsis and vasoactive drug-related metabolic effects. Curr Opin Crit Care 2003;9(4):271–8.

42 Sundararajan V, Macisaac C, Presneill J, Cade J, Visvanathan K. Epidemiology of sepsis in Victoria, Australia. Crit Care Med 2005;33(1):71–80.

43 Ferreira FL, Bota DP, Bross A, Melot C, Vincent JL. Serial evaluation of the SOFA score to predict outcome in critically ill patients. JAMA 2001;286(14):1754–8.

44 Micek ST, Isakow W, Shannon W, Kollef MH. Predictors of hospital mortality for patients with severe sepsis treated with drotrecogin alfa (activated). Pharmacotherapy 2005;25(1):26–34.

45 Gando S. Microvascular thrombosis and multiple organ dysfunction syndrome. Crit Care Med 2010;38(2Suppl):S35–42.

46 Department of Health and Ageing. Schedule of pharmaceutical benefits [database on the Internet]. Canberra: Department of Health and Ageing, <http://www.health.gov.au/pbschedule>.

47 Ely EW, Kleinpell RM, Goyette RE. Advances in the understanding of clinical manifestations and therapy of severe sepsis: an update for critical care nurses. Am J Crit Care 2003;12(2):120–33.

48 Bougle A, Harrois A, Duranteau J. Resuscitative strategies in traumatic haemorrhagic shock. Ann Intensive Care 2013;3(1):1-9, <http://www.annalsofintensivecare.com/content/3/1/1>.

49 Bauer M, ed. Multiple organ failure – update on pathophysiology and treatment strategies. Euroanesthesia Conference Proceedings; Vienna, Austria May 28–31: European Society of Anaesthesiology; 2005.

50 Martí-Carvajal A, Salanti G, Cardona-Zorrilla A. Human recombinant activated protein C for severe sepsis. Cochrane Reviews, <http://www2.cochrane.org/reviews/en/ab004388.html>; 2007.

51 Ho H, Chapital AD, Yu M. Hypothyroidism and adrenal insufficiency in sepsis and hemorrhagic shock. Arch Surg 2004;139(11):1199–203.

52 Annane D, Bellissant E, Bollaert P, Briegel J, Keh D, Kupfer Y. Corticosteroids for treating severe sepsis and septic shock (review). Cochrane Reviews, <http://www2.cochrane.org/reviews/en/ab002243.html>; 2004.

53 Annane D, Bellissant E, Cavaillon JM. Septic shock. Lancet 2005;365(9453):63–78.

54 Annane D, Sebille V, Charpentier C, Bollaert PE, Francois B, Korach JM et al. Effect of treatment with low doses of hydrocortisone and fludrocortisone on mortality in patients with septic shock. JAMA 2002;288(7):862–71.

55 Zaloga G, Marik P. Hypothalamic–pituitary–adrenal insufficiency. Crit Care Clin 2001;17(1):25–41.

56 Kinney M, Dunbar S, Brooks-Brunn J, Molter N, Vitello-Cicciu JM. AACN's Clinical reference for critical care nursing. St Louis: Mosby; 1998.

57 Hermans G, De Jonghe B, Bruyninckx F, Van den Berghe G. Clinical review: critical illness polyneuropathy and myopathy. Crit Care 2008;12(6):238–47.

58 Kemp CM, Johnson C, Riordan W, Cotton B. How we die: the impact of non neurologic organ dysfunction after severe traumatic brain injury. Am Surg 2008;74(9):866–72.

59 Stevens R, Dowdy D, Michaels R, Mendez-Tellez P, Pronovost P, Needham D. Neuromuscular dysfunction acquired in critical illness: a systematic review. Intensive Care Med 2007;33(11):1876.

60 Streck E, Commin C, Barichello T, Quevedo J. The septic brain. Neurochem Res 2008;33:2171–7.

61 Dewar D, Tarrant S, King K, Balogh Z. Changes in the epidemiology and prediction of multiple organ failure after injury. J Trauma Acute Care Surg 2013;74(3):774-9.

62 Sauaia A, Moore E, Johnson J, Chin T, Banerjee A, Sperry JL et al. Temporal trends of post-injury multiple-organ failure: still resource intensive, morbid, and lethal. J Trauma Acute Care Surg 2014;76(3):582-93.

63 Lone N, Walsh T. Impact of intensive care unit organ failures on mortality during five years after a critical illness. Am J Respir Crit Care Med 2012;186(7):640-47.

64 Fröhlich M, Lefering R, Probst C, Paffrath T, Schneider MM, Maegele M et al. Epidemiology and risk factors of multiple-organ failure after multiple trauma: an analysis of 31,154 patients from the TraumaRegister DGU. J Trauma Acute Care Surg 2014;76(4):921-928.

65 Angus DC, Linde-Zwirble WT, Lidicker J, Clermont G, Carcillo J, Pinsky MR. Epidemiology of severe sepsis in the United States: analysis of incidence, outcome, and associated costs of care. Crit Care Med 2001;29(7):1303–10.

66 Peres Bota D, Melot C, Lopes Ferreira F, Nguyen BV, Vincent J-L. The multiple organ dysfunction score (MODS) versus the sequential organ failure assessment (SOFA) score in outcome prediction. Intensive Care Med 2002;28(11):1619–24.

67 Minei JP, Cuschieri J, Sperry J, Moore EE, West MA, Harbrecht BG et al. The changing pattern and implication of multiple organ failure after blunt injury with hemorrhagic shock. Crit Care Med 2012;40(4):1129-35.

68 Anami EH, Grion CM, Cardoso LT, Kauss IA, Thomazini MC, Zampa HB et al. Serial evaluation of SOFA score in a Brazilian teaching hospital. Intensive Crit Care Nurs 2010;26:75–82.

69 Minne L, Abu-Hanna A, de Jonge E. Evaluation of SOFA-based models for predicting mortality in the ICU: a systematic review. Crit Care 2008;12(6):R161.

70 Jones A, Trzeciak S, Kline J. The sequential organ failure assessment score for predicting outcome in patients with severe sepsis and evidence of hypoperfusion at the time of emergency department presentation. Crit Care Med 2009;35(5):1649–54.

71 Vogel JA, Liao MM, Hopkins E, Seleno N, Byyny RL, Moore EE et al. Prediction of postinjury multiple-organ failure in the emergency department: development of the Denver Emergency Department Trauma Organ Failure Score. J Trauma Acute Care Surg 2013;76(1):140-5.

72 Khwannimit B. A comparison of three organ dysfunction scores: MODS, SOFA and LOD for predicting ICU mortality in critically ill patients. J Med Assoc Thai 2007;90(6):1074–81.

73 Heldwein M, Badreldin A, Doerr F, Lehmann T, Bayer O, Doenst T et al. Logistic Organ Dysfunction Score (LODS): a reliable postoperative risk management score also in cardiac surgical patients? J Cardiothorac Surg 2011;6:110.

74 Sauaia A, Moore, E, Johnson J, Ciesla D, Biffl W, Banerjee A. Validation of post-injury multiple organ failure scores. Shock 2009;31(4):438-47.

75 Rice TW, Wheeler AP, Bernard GR, Hayden DL, Schoenfeld DA, Ware LB. Comparison of the SpO_2/FiO_2 ratio and the PaO_2/FiO_2 ratio in patients with acute lung injury or ARDS. Chest 2007;4(2):410-7.

76 McConnell K, Coopersmith C. Organ failure avoidance and mitigation strategies in surgery. Surg Clin N Am 2012;92:307-19.

77 Nydam TL, Kashuk JL, Moore EE, Johnson JL, Burlew CC, Biffl WL et al. Refractory postinjury thrombocytopenia is associated with multiple organ failure and adverse outcomes. J Trauma 2011;70(2):401-6.

78 Jansen TC, van Bommel J, Mulder PG, Lima AP, van der Hoven B, Rommes JH et al. Prognostic value of blood lactate levels: does the clinical diagnosis at admission matter? J Trauma 2009;66:377-85.

79 Honore P, Joannes-Boyau O, Boer W, Collins V. Regional occult hypoperfusion detected by lactate and sequential organ failure assessment subscores: old tools for new tricks? Crit Care Med 2009;37(8):2477–8.

80 Jansen T, van Bommel J, Woodward R, Mulder P, Bakker J. Association between blood lactate levels, sequential organ failure assessment subscores, and 28-day mortality during early and late intensive care unit stay: a retrospective observational study. Crit Care Med 2009;37(8):2369–74.

81 Dellinger R, Levy M, Rhodes A, Annane D, Gerlach H, Opal SM et al. Surviving Sepsis Campaign: international guidelines for management of severe sepsis and septic shock: 2012. Crit Care Med 2013;41(2):580-637.

82 Guyette F, Suffoletto B, Castillo J, Quintero J, Callaway C, Puyana JC. Prehospital serum lactate as a predictor of outcomes in trauma patients: a retrospective observational study. J Trauma 2011;70(4):782-6.

83 Madách K, Aladzsity I, Szilágyi Á, Fust G, Gál J, Pénzes I et al. 4G/5G polymorphism of PAI-1 gene is associated with multiple organ dysfunction and septic shock in pneumonia induced severe sepsis: prospective, observational, genetic study. Crit Care 2010;14(2):R79.

84 Teoh H, Quan A, Creighton AK, Bang KW, Singh KK, Shukla PC et al. BRCA1 gene therapy reduces systemic inflammatory response and multiple organ failure and improves survival in experimental sepsis. Gene Ther 2013;20:51-61.

85 Peake S, Bailey M, Bellomo R, Cameron P, Cross A, Delaney A et al. Australasian resuscitation of sepsis evaluation (ARISE): a multi-centre, prospective, inception cohort study. Resuscitation 2009;80:811–18.

86 Levy M, Dellinger R, Townsend S, Linde-Zwirble W, Marshall J, Bion J et al. The Surviving Sepsis Campaign: results of an international guideline-based performance improvement program targeting severe sepsis. Crit Care Med 2010;38(2):367–74.

87 Finfer S. The Surviving Sepsis Campaign: robust evaluation and high-quality primary research is still needed. Crit Care Med 2010;38(2):683–4.

88 Becker JU, Theodosis C, Jacob ST, Wira CR, Groce NE. Surviving sepsis in low-income and middle-income countries: new directions for care and research. Lancet Infect Dis 2009;9(9):577–82.

89 Rivers E. Management of sepsis: early resuscitation. Clin Chest Med 2008;29:689–704.

90 Jones A, Shapiro N, Trzeciak S, Arnold R, Claremont H, Kline J et al. Lactate clearance vs central venous oxygen saturation as goals of early sepsis therapy – a randomized clinical trial. JAMA 2010;303(8):739-46.

91 The ProCESS/ARISE/ProMISe Methodology Writing Committee. Harmonizing international trials of early goal-directed resuscitation for severe sepsis and septic shock: methodology of ProCESS, ARISE, and ProMISe. Intensive Care Med 2013;39:1760-75.

92 The ProCESS Investigators. A randomized trial of protocol-based care for early septic shock. N Eng J Med 2014;370(18):1683-93.

93 Kumar A, Ellis P, Arabi Y, Roberts D, Light B, Parrillo JE et al. Initiation of inappropriate antimicrobial therapy results in a fivefold reduction of survival in human septic shock. Chest 2009;136(5):1237–48.

94 Bagshaw S, Lapinsky S, Dial S, Arabi Y, Dodek P, Wood G et al. Acute kidney injury in septic shock: clinical outcomes and impact of duration of hypotension prior to initiation of antimicrobial therapy. Intensive Care Med 2009;35:871–81.

95 Gaieski D, Mikkelsen M, Band R, Pines J, Massone R, Furia FF et al. Impact of time to antibiotics on survival in patients with severe sepsis or septic shock in whom early goal-directed therapy was initiated in the emergency department. Crit Care Med 2010;38(4):1045–53.

96 Lily C. The ProCESS trial – a new era of sepsis management. N Eng J Med 2014;370(18):1750-1.

97 Sharma S, Kumar A. Antimicrobial management of sepsis and septic shock. Clin Chest Med 2008;29:677–87.

98 Kumar A, Safdar N, Kethireddy S, Chateau D. A survival benefit of combination antibiotic therapy for serious infections associated with sepsis and septic shock is contingent only on the risk of death: a meta-analytic/meta-regression study. Crit Care Med 2010;38(8):1651–64.

99 Pines J. Timing of antibiotics for acute, severe infections. Emerg Med Clin N Am 2008;26:245–57.

100 Ulldemolins M, Roberts J, Lipman J, Rello J. Antibiotic dosing in multiple organ dysfunction syndrome. Chest 2011;139(5):1210-20.

101 Finfer S. Corticosteroids in septic shock. N Engl J Med 2008;358(2):188–90.

102 Sprung C, Annane D, Keh D, Moreno R, Singer M, Freivogel K et al. Hydrocortisone therapy for patients with septic shock. N Engl J Med 2008;358(2):111–24.

103 Mason P, Al-Khafaji A, Milbrandt E, Suffoletto B, Huang D. CORTICUS: the end of unconditional love for steroid use? Crit Care 2009;13(4):309.

104 Investigators TCS. Corticosteroid treatment and intensive insulin therapy for septic shock in adults: a randomised controlled trial. JAMA 2010;303(17):1694–8.

105 Vanhorebeek I, De Vos R, Mesotten D, Wouters P, De Wolf-Peeters C, Van den Berghe G. Protection of hepatocyte mitochondrial ultrastructure and function by strict blood glucose control with insulin in critically ill patients. Lancet 2005;365(9453):53–9.

106 Finfer S, Chittock D, Yu-Shhuo S, Blair D, Foster D, Dhingra V et al. Intensive versus conventional glucose control in critically ill patients. N Engl J Med 2009;360(13):1283–97.

107 Vincent J. Metabolic support in sepsis and multiple organ failure: more questions than answers. Crit Care Med 2007;35(9Suppl):S436–40.

108 Moore F, Moore E. The evolving rationale for early enteral nutrition based on paradigms of multiple organ failure: a personal journey. Nutrition Clin Prac 2009;24(3):297–304.

109 Australian College of Critical Care Nurses. National Advanced Life Support Education Package: Pathophysiology of cellular dysfunction. Melbourne: Cambridge Press; 2004.

110 Vincent J, Moreno R, Takala J, Willats S, De Mendonca A, Bruining H et al. The SOFA (sepsis related organ failure assessment) score to describe organ dysfunction/failure. Intensive Care Med 1996;22:707–10.

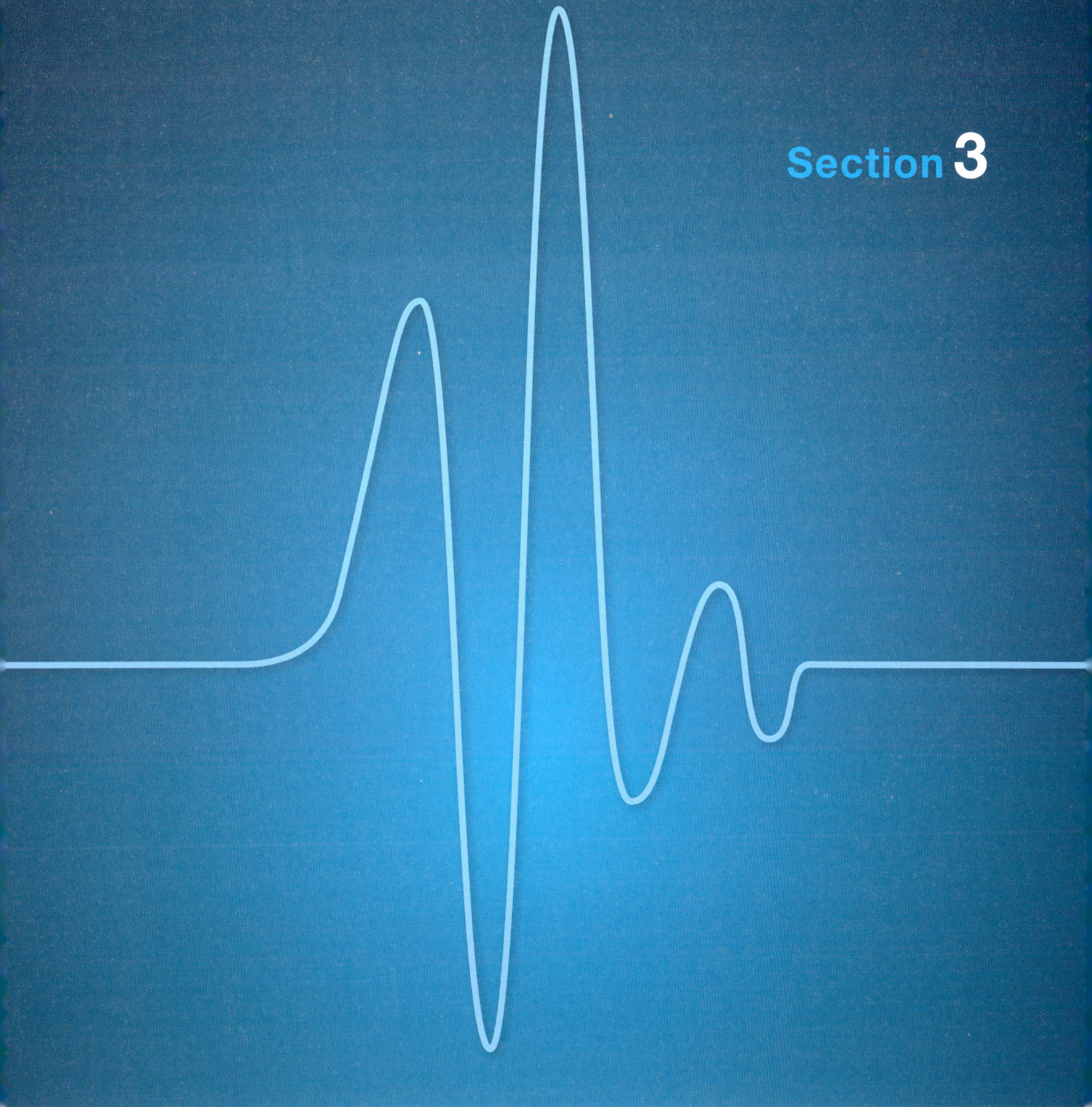

Specialty practice

Chapter 23

Emergency presentations

David Johnson, Julia Crilly

Learning objectives

After reading this chapter, you should be able to:

- describe the uniqueness of the emergency care environment
- describe the different international triage models and outline the development of Australasian triage models
- discuss the process of initial patient assessment and triage nursing practice
- integrate emergency nursing principles and practice in initial patient care
- describe the various roles of extended nursing practice in the emergency setting
- describe the principles and practice of patient preparation for retrievals or transfers
- discuss the principles for the management of disaster victims in the emergency department
- discuss the initial nursing management of common presentations to the ED, including respiratory or neurological dysfunction, chest pain, abdominal pain, poisoning, envenomation, submersion and heat illness.

Introduction

Emergency nursing practice covers an enormous range of clinical presentations. The focus of this book is critical care, and this chapter discusses conditions of clinical presentations at the critical end of the practice spectrum. Please read in conjunction with Chapters 24 and 25, which describe the management of additional common presentations to the emergency department (ED): trauma and resuscitation emergencies, respectively. Chapter 1 contains information on extended nursing roles relevant to emergency nursing.

In this chapter the organisational systems and processes of care in an ED environment, including triage, specifics of ED extended practice nursing roles, multiple casualties/disaster management and transport/retrieval of critically ill patients, are described. Details of a select group of the most common emergency presentations and conditions related to critical care practice are then described. The initial clinical assessment and incidences of these common presentations are discussed, and the likely diagnoses associated with these presentations and their initial management in the ED are identified. Ongoing management of these selected conditions is covered in Section 2 of this text.

Emergency nursing practice is the holistic care of individuals of all ages who present with perceived or actual physical and/or emotional alterations. These presentations are often undiagnosed and require a range of prompt symptomatic and definitive interventions. Emergency clinical practice is usually unscheduled, episodic and acute in its nature, and is therefore unlike any other type of nursing in the demands it places on nursing staff.[1,2] In many instances the emergency nurse is the first healthcare professional to be in contact with an acutely ill or injured patient. Patient presentations include a full range of acuity across the spectrum of possible illnesses, injuries and ages.

Background

Emergency nursing is unique, in that it involves the care of patients with health problems that are often undiagnosed on presentation but perceived as sufficiently acute by the individual to warrant seeking emergency care in the hospital setting. As patients present with signs and symptoms rather than medical diagnoses, refined assessment skills are paramount. Many skills required by emergency nurses are based on a broad foundation of knowledge that serves as a guide in collecting information, making observations and evaluating data, and sorting and analysing relevant information.[3–7] This foundation enables an emergency nurse to communicate appropriately with other members of the healthcare team, and to implement appropriate independent and collaborative nursing interventions.

Emergency nurses are specialists in acute episodic nursing care, and their knowledge, skills and expertise encompass almost all other nursing specialty areas. Emergency nurses therefore possess a unique body of knowledge and skill sets to manage a wide variety of presentations across all age groups; this includes familiarity with general physical and emotional requirements of each age group as these relate to their presenting health needs.[2–4,7] ED nurses work collaboratively with pre-hospital emergency personnel, doctors and other healthcare providers and community agencies to provide patient care.[2,3,5] Roles in the ED include triage, direct patient care, patient flow, implementing medical orders, providing emotional support during crises, documenting and arranging ongoing care, admission to the hospital, transfer to another healthcare facility or discharge into the community.[5,6]

Triage

Central to the unique functions of an ED nurse is the role of triage, perhaps the one clinical skill that distinguishes an emergency nurse from other specialist nurses. Triage literally means 'to sieve or sort', and it is the first step in any patient's management on presentation to an ED.[1–3,7]

History of triage

Triage was first described in 1797 during the Napoleonic wars by Surgeon Marshall Larrey, Napoleon's chief medical officer,[8] who introduced a system of sorting casualties that presented to the field dressing stations. His aims were military rather than medical, however, so the highest priority was given to soldiers who had minor wounds and could be returned quickly to the battle lines with minimal treatment.[1,8]

The documented use of triage was limited until World War I, when the term was used to describe a physical area where sorting of casualties was conducted, rather than a description of the sorting or triage process itself.[9] Triage continued to develop into a formalised assessment process, with subsequent adoption of initial categorising of patient urgency and acuity within most civilian EDs.[1,8–10]

International approaches to triage

The triage process has evolved internationally, particularly over the past two decades. Four main triage scales are available and, although used in the country in which they were developed, they have also been implemented or adapted in other health services. The Canadian Emergency Department Triage and Acuity Scales (CTAS)[11], the Manchester Triage Scale (MTS)[3] and the Australasian Triage Scale (ATS)[12,13] are the most common five-level triage scales used with the ATS being reported as the most reliable.[14] In the USA, three-level triage scales have historically been used; however the Emergency Severity Index (ESI),[15] a five-level triage scale, was developed in the late 1990s and has been implemented in a small number of hospitals.[7] Three-level triage scales do not fare as well as the five-level scales in terms of measures such as agreement, discrimination, sensitivity, specificity and accuracy.[16] Newer triage systems have been developed, e.g. the four-level Taiwan Triage System[17] and the Soterion Rapid Triage System.[18] These newer systems are not widely reported or implemented and require further testing.[19]

Characteristics of the ATS, CTAS, MTS and ESI five-level triage scales are presented in Table 23.1.[7] Although somewhat similar, there are variations in some aspects such as timeframes for which a person should wait to see a doctor. For example, the ESI does not define expected time intervals to doctor evaluation, and not all scales are adapted to specific populations, such as paediatrics, or settings, such as rural environments. The Manchester Triage System differs to the ATS, CTAS and ESI in that it uses an algorithm approach with 52 presenting complaints to derive a triage score. The other systems use a slightly different approach where a combination of observation, history taking and physical examination facilitates the nurse's judgement to apply a triage score. Updates to and computerisation of previous guidelines have been undertaken over the years.[20] Educational materials to support each of the scales are available. An International Triage Scale has been proposed but requires development and testing.[20]

TABLE 23.1

Comparison of characteristics of the ATS, CTAS, MTS and ESI 5-level triage scales

CRITERION	CTAS	ATS	ESI	MTS
Time to triage assessment	10 min	NS	NS	NS
Time to nurse assessment	Based on initial triage	NS	NS	NS
Time to doctor assessment	Immediate/15/ 30/60/120 min	Immediate/10/ 30/60/120 min	NS	Immediate/10/60/ 120/240 min
Fractile response time (CTAS)/performance threshold (NTS)	I-98, II-95, III-90,IV-85, V-80	I-97.5, II-95, III-90, IV-90, V-85	NS	NS
Pain scale	10-point scale	NS	>7/10 *consider* up-triage to ESI level 2	A major factor considered for each chief complaint
Paediatrics	Used in CTAS	NS but generally recognised	Paediatric VS criteria included to help determine ESI level 2 vs 3; fever criteria for <24 months included	Not addressed in the algorithm
Sentinel diagnoses	Yes	Yes	Not used	52 chief complaints vs sentinel diagnosis
Expected admission rates	Specified	Defined using actual data from multiple sites	Benchmarking data available	NS
Education implementation material	Web-based training available for a fee	Training video; Website: http://www. acem.org.au/open/ documents/triage.htm	Available for purchase from ENA (www.ena.org)	Published manual: Manchester Triage Group. Emergency triage. Plymouth: BMJ Publishing Group; 1997
Rural setting	Yes	NS	NS	NS
Additional comments			Uses acuity to identify level 1 and 2 patients, and resources to identify levels 3–5	Algorithmic approach that uses 52 chief complaint-based flow charts; the triage nurse then continues an algorithmic approach and assesses life threat, pain, haemorrhage, consciousness level, temperature and acuteness for each chief complaint

Note: the ATS performance thresholds have since been revised to: 100%, 80%, 75%, 70%, 70%.[26]

NS = not specified; VS = vital sign; MTS = Manchester Triage Scale.

Adapted from Fernandes CM, Tanabe P, Gilboy N, Johnson LA, McNair RS, Rosenau AM et al. Five-level triage: a report from the ACEP/ENA Five-level Triage Task Force. J Emerg Nurs 2005;31(1):39-50; quiz 118, with permission.

Development of triage processes: Focus on Australia and New Zealand

Australia is a world leader in the development of emergency triage and patient classification systems. Because other triage systems (CTAS, MTS, ESI) have primarily been adapted from the Australian system,[20] the focus here is on the development of the Australian and New Zealand ATS. In the late 1960s patients presenting to 'casualty' departments in Australia were not always triaged,[1,2,4] with many EDs using random models of care; ambulance presentations were given priority and the 'walking wounded' seen in order of arrival. In the mid-1970s, staff at Box Hill Hospital in Melbourne developed a five-tiered system that included a time-based scale and different colours on the medical record to indicate priority.[1,9,21] Subsequent modification and refinement led to the Ipswich Scale in the 1970s–80s.[1,2,4,5,21] These early triage systems reinforced the concepts developed by Larrey, and established a process for patient presentations to be seen in order of clinical priority rather than time of attendance. In the 1990s the impacts of community expectations and national health policy led to further enhancements of triage systems in Australia, and the Ipswich triage scale was adapted into the national triage scale. The National Triage Scale was subsequently tested and demonstrated to have the essential characteristics of utility, reliability and validity.[1,2,4,5,12,13,20,21] In 1993, the NTS was adopted by the Australasian College for Emergency Medicine in its triage policy,[21] and subsequently renamed the ATS as it was implemented in most EDs in Australia and New Zealand (see Table 23.2).[4]

TABLE 23.2
ATS category characteristics[5,13,22]

ATS CODE	TYPICAL DESCRIPTION
1	**Immediately life-threatening** (or imminent risk of deterioration) Patients are critically ill, and require immediate transfer to a resuscitation area for initial resuscitation, with no delay at triage. The majority will arrive by ambulance, and will be suffering: • multi-trauma • shock • unconsciousness • convulsions • extreme dyspnoea • cardiorespiratory arrest
2	**Imminently life-threatening** Patients 'at high risk' of critical deterioration or have very severe pain from any cause. Assessment and treatment needs to commence within 10 minutes for: • chest pain or other symptoms suggestive of myocardial ischaemia, pulmonary embolism or aortic dissection • important time-critical treatment (e.g. thrombolysis, antidote) • severe abdominal pain or other symptoms suggestive of ruptured aortic aneurysm • severe dyspnoea from any cause • altered levels of consciousness • acute hemiparesis/dysphasia • fever, rash, headache, suggestive of sepsis or meningitis • severe skeletal trauma such as femoral fractures or limb dislocations • very severe pain from any cause (practice mandates the relief of pain or distress within 10 minutes)
3	**Potentially life-threatening or situational urgency** Patients have significant illness or injury and should have assessment and treatment commenced within 30 minutes of presentation. Typical patients include those with: • moderately severe pain from any cause (e.g. abdominal pain, acute headache, renal colic), but not suggestive of critical illness; practice mandates relief of severe discomfort or distress within 30 minutes • symptoms of significant infections (e.g. lung, renal) • moderate injury (e.g. Colles' fracture, severe laceration without active haemorrhage) • head injury, with transient loss of consciousness • persistent vomiting/dehydration
4	**Potentially serious** The patient's condition may deteriorate, or adverse outcome may result, if assessment and treatment is not commenced within 1 hour of arrival. Patients have moderate symptoms, symptoms of prolonged duration or acute symptoms of low-risk pre-existing conditions, including: • minor acute trauma (e.g. sprained ankle) • minor head injury, no loss of consciousness • mild haemorrhage • earache or other mildly painful conditions • practice mandates relief of discomfort or distress within 1 hour • there is a potential for adverse outcome if time-critical treatment is not commenced within 1 hour • likely to require complex work-up and consultation and/or inpatient management
5	**Less urgent** The patient's condition is minor or chronic; acute symptoms of minor illness, symptoms of chronic disease or with a duration of greater than 1 week. Symptoms or clinical outcome will not be significantly affected if assessment and treatment are delayed up to 2 hours from arrival. Examples include: • chronic lower back pain with mild symptoms • minor wounds: small abrasion/minor lacerations • most skin conditions • clinical administrative presentations (e.g. results review, medical certificates, repeat prescriptions)

The process of triage

All patients presenting to an ED should be triaged on arrival by a suitably experienced and trained registered nurse.[2,12,15,22,23] This assessment represents the first clinical contact and the commencement of care in the department. The ideal features of a triage area are: a well-signposted location close to the patient entrance; ability to conduct examination and primary treatment of patients in privacy; close proximity to the acute treatment and resuscitation areas; and appropriate resources including an examination table, thermometer, a sphygmomanometer, stethoscope, glucometer and pulse oximetry.[2,4,12] Access to emergency equipment, communication devices (such as telephone, emergency buzzer), standard precaution equipment (such as gloves and hand-wash) and paper/electronic recording facilities are also important.[24]

As the first clinician in the ED to interview the patient, the triage nurse gathers and documents information from the patient, family and friends, or pre-hospital emergency personnel. Professional maturity is required to manage the stress inherent in dealing with an acutely ill patient and family members (under significant stress themselves), while rapidly making informed judgement on priorities of care for a wide range of clinical problems.[7,12]

The triage nurse receives and records information about the patient's reason for presentation to the ED, beginning with a clear statement of the complaint, followed by historical information and related relevant details, such as time of onset, duration of symptom/s and what aggravates or relieves the symptom/s. A brief, focused physical assessment including vital signs may be undertaken to identify the urgency and severity of the condition, and may be collected as part of the triage process to inform decision making.[5,12,13] Triage assessment generally should be no longer than 2–5 minutes, balancing between speed and thoroughness.[13] From the information collected, the triage nurse determines the need for immediate or delayed care,[1–3,7] and assigns the patient a 1–5 ATS category in response to the statement: *This patient should wait for medical assessment and treatment no longer than ….*[13]

Patients with acute conditions that threaten life or limb receive the highest priority while those with minor illness or injury are assigned a lower priority. It may not be possible to categorise the patient correctly in all instances, and it is better to conservatively allocate priority to ensure the patient is seen sooner, if the triage category is unclear.[3,8,12,13] Importantly, a triage allocation is flexible and can be altered at any time.[5–8,13] If a patient's condition changes while awaiting medical assessment/treatment, or if additional relevant information becomes available that impacts on the patient's urgency, the patient should be re-triaged to a category that reflects the determined urgency.[13,25] Frequent, ongoing observation and assessment of patients is therefore routine practice following the initial triage assessment.

> **Practice tip**
>
> Triage decisions must be accurate, ensure the patient's safety and be reproducible across clinicians and departments. The decision regarding triage urgency should not be clouded by factors other than the patient's clinical condition.[7,22] If it is unclear what triage category should be assigned, the patient should be allocated a higher category.

The premise for a triage decision is that utilisation of valuable healthcare resources should provide the greatest benefit for those most in need, and that persons in need of urgent attention always receive that care.[13,25] Triage encompasses the entire body of emergency nursing practice, and nurses complete a comprehensive triage education program prior to commencing this role. Formal triage training resources have been developed that provide the essential education components to promote consistency in application of the triage score, depending on the scales used.[7,13,15,25]

Triage categories

After triage assessment is undertaken on arrival, patients are allocated one of five triage categories depending on the triage scale used (see Tables 23.1 and 23.2). Prompt assessment of airway, breathing, circulation and disability remains the cornerstone of patient assessment in any clinical context, including triage.

Triage assessment

Patient assessment at triage has three major components: quick, systematic and dynamic. Speed of assessment is required in life-threatening situations, with the focus on airway, breathing, circulation and disability, and a quick decision on what level of intervention is required. A systematic approach to assessment is used for all patients in all circumstances, to ensure reproducibility. Finally, the triage assessment must be dynamic, in that several aspects can be undertaken at once, and acknowledges that a patient's condition can change rapidly after initial assessment. Various assessment models are available, but fundamentally they all include components of observation, history taking, primary survey and secondary survey.[1–4,6,13,15,25]

Patient history/interview

The triage interview provides the basis for data gathering and clinical decision making regarding patient acuity. After an introduction, the triage nurse asks person-specific, open-ended questions. Use of close-ended questions or summative statements enables clarification and confirmation of information received, and a means of checking understanding by the patient.[26] Privacy is important to ensure that the patient is comfortable in answering questions of a personal nature. Most EDs need to balance providing an area that is private and accessible, yet safe for staff to work in relative isolation.

A large component of the triage assessment may be based on subjective data, which are then compared and combined with objective data obtained through the senses of smell, sight, hearing and touch to determine a triage category. If time permits, vital signs such as pulse, blood pressure, respiratory rate, oxygen saturation, temperature and blood glucose level can be measured to assist in estimating urgency.[24] One aspect of the history that is difficult to quantify is intuition. This is that 'sixth sense or gut feeling' that tells us that something not yet detectable is wrong with the patient. This unexplained sense is difficult to outline or apply scientific research models to, but has a role to play in patient assessment and should be acknowledged when something 'doesn't feel right'.[6,13,25]

Primary survey

While taking a patient history, the triage nurse also simultaneously conducts a primary survey. As noted earlier, airway, breathing, circulation and neurological function are observed. If any major problem is observed (or a patient is identified as ATS Category 1 or 2), the interview is ceased and the patient is transferred immediately to the acute treatment or resuscitation area.[8,24]

Secondary survey and physical examination

A secondary survey, involving a concise, systematic physical examination, is conducted after the patient history and primary survey have been completed. The equipment used includes a thermometer, stethoscope, oxygen saturation monitor and sphygmomanometer, in combination with clinical skills. This examination is not comprehensive but focuses on the presenting complaint while avoiding tunnel vision and wrong conclusions.[3,26] Remember that the patient may not be able to lie down or be exposed for an examination in the triage area, and may be distressed. The triage process should reflect a system of rapid assessment that is reproducible and adaptable to a variety of presentations. The secondary survey may be performed by the triage nurse if time permits or by another registered nurse who may be able to initiate appropriate investigations (such as X-rays) or initial management (such as analgesia), according to hospital protocols.[24] Further information regarding advanced practice roles such as the clinical initiatives nurse is presented in Chapter 1.

Practice tip

The triage physical assessment should be quick, accurate and concise, focusing on the presenting complaint.

Approaches to triage assessment

A range of approaches to nursing assessment is applicable to triage assessments (see Table 23.3).[8] Body systems approach enables systematic examination of each body system to discover abnormalities (i.e. central nervous

TABLE 23.3
Aids to triage assessment[8]

MNEMONIC	COMPONENTS
SOAPIE	**S**ubjective data **O**bjective data **A**ssessment (to enable formulation of a …) **P**lan (that is …) **I**mplemented (and …) **E**valuated (as to its success)
AMPLE	**A**llergies **M**edications **P**ast medical history **L**ast food and fluids ingested **E**nvironmental factors and **E**vents leading to presentation
PQRST	**P**rovoking or **P**recipitating factors **Q**uality and **Q**uantity (severity) of the symptom **R**egion/**R**adiation **S**ymptoms associated **T**ime of onset and duration of episode, and **T**reatment

system, cardiovascular system, respiratory system, gastrointestinal system etc).[6,13,15] Detailed descriptions of systems assessment are available elsewhere in the text.

Triage assessment of specific patient groups

While triage assessment is a complex process for a range of patient presentations, some specific groups are more demanding, such as mental health, paediatric, older and mass casualty patients.

Mental health presentations

Patients with psychiatric problems presenting to an ED should be triaged, assessed and treated as for other presenting patients, with particular attention to appropriate initial medical assessment and management.[6,13,22,26,27]

Resources outlining specific mental health triage category descriptors are readily available and relate specific aspects of mental health presentation with clinical urgency and triage categories (see Table 23.4),[27] including an outline of suggested responses, such as patient placement requirements based on the level of risk and urgency.[6,13,22,25–30] Although the triage process has the same underlying principles, factors associated with mental health presentations may vary between geographical settings and countries where there are differences in health system structure, financing and sociocultural contexts.[27,31,32]

Paediatric presentations

Children presenting to the ED are assessed and assigned a triage category as for adults, although vital differences in paediatric anatomy, physiology and clinical

TABLE 23.4

Examples of a mental health triage tool[26]

ATS	OBSERVATION	ACTION
1 Immediate	Severe behavioural disorder with immediate threat of dangerous violence to self or others	• Provide continuous visual observation in safe environment • Ensure adequate personnel to provide restraint/detention
2 Emergency	Severe behavioural disturbance with probable risk of danger to self and others	• Provide continuous visual observation in safe environment • Use defusing techniques • Ensure adequate personnel to provide restraint/detention
3 Urgent	Moderate behavioural disturbance or severe distress with possible danger to self and others	• Provide safe environment, frequent visual observations every 10 minutes
4 Semi-urgent	Semi-urgent mental health problem with no immediate risk to self or others	• Regular visual observations at a maximum of every 30 minutes
5 Non-urgent	No behavioural disturbance or acute distress with no danger to self or others	• Regular visual sighting at a maximum of 1-hour intervals

presentations should be considered (see Chapter 27). The reliance on information from parents or primary carers and their capacity to identify deviations from normal are important, particularly in supporting recognition of often subtle indicators of serious illness in infants and young children. Paediatric triage resources are available to assist in identifying physiological alterations and applying a triage category based upon identified physiological discriminators.[3,15,26,33] Other important points to consider include the following:

• Children may suffer rapid decompensation due to limited physiological reserves.[13,22,34]
• Children are less able to tolerate pain in either physical or psychological terms.[13,22,34]
• It is difficult to rationalise long waiting periods with a child or parent of a sick child. The longer they wait, the more difficult an examination becomes.[13,22,34]
• Parents are much less tolerant of waiting times for their sick child than they would be for themselves.[13,22,34]
• The spectrum of childhood illnesses presenting to EDs varies between countries that are developing and those that have more established health systems.[33,34]

Practice tip

A short time is a long time in the life of a child; they may develop serious illness in a much shorter time than for an adult.

Adapted from Durojalve L, O'Meara M. A study of triage in paediatric patients in Australia. Emerg Med 2002;4: 67-76, with permission.

Older persons

With the ageing population globally, there is a trend towards an increase in the use of emergency services by older persons. While older persons should be triaged according to their presenting complaint, this can be complicated by a number of factors.[35] It is therefore important to consider additional comorbidities, place of residence, medications and cognitive function when triaging older adults.[36] Evidence-based recommendations[37–39] and policy guidelines[40] for the management of older persons in the ED are available with additional recommendations provided by key organisations.[36,37] Important points to remember when triaging the elderly are the following:

• Older persons have an increased medical complexity and nursing dependency.[39]
• Be attuned to the potential signs of elder abuse,[39] and the presence of pressure sores.
• Note the use of aids such as hearing aids, glasses and walking sticks that assist with activities of daily living.
• The older person (particularly if from an aged care facility) may have an advanced medical directive that should be used to ensure their wishes are respected in the event of a life-threatening illness.[39]

Practice tip

When triaging older people important considerations include other illnesses they may have, where they live, medications they are on and changes in their cognitive function.

Chemical, biological and radiological events

Since the Japanese doomsday cult Aum Shinrikyo released sarin nerve gas on the Tokyo subway in March 1995, killing 12 people, terrorist incidents and hoaxes involving toxic or infectious agents have been on the rise. The ease of obtaining non-nuclear radioactive material may mean that 'dirty bombs'[41,42] are more likely to be used as an explosive device. The availability and the impact of chemical and biological threat materials are both relatively high, with potentially devastating impact.[43–46] Because biological and chemical agents are so dissimilar, each category will be dealt with separately but there are common elements or characteristics.

Chemical agents

Chemical agents are supertoxic chemicals used for the purpose of poisoning victims. They are similar to hazardous industrial chemicals, but hundreds of times more toxic.[44] For example, the 1995 sarin attack in Tokyo caused 1039 injuries and at least 4000 people with psychogenic symptoms.[44] Sarin is approximately 60 times more toxic than methylisocyanate. To put this in perspective, a leak of methylisocyanate from a factory in Bhopal, India, in 1984 caused 200,000 people to be effected, 10,000 severely affected and 3300 deaths.[47] Relatively small quantities of a military grade chemical agent could have the same capability to produce large numbers of casualties (symptomatic and psychological).[44,45]

Table 23.5 provides a summary of the more common chemical agents, their effects, clinical presentations and treatments. It needs to be stressed that specialised personal protective equipment (PPE) and specialist training are required to manage these situations.[48]

Biological agents

The use of biological weapons is not a recent concept.[44,45] Biological agents have the longest history of use, dating back to the 14th century.[45] Biological agents are living organisms or toxins that have the capacity to cause disease in people, animals or crops. Toxins are a special type of poisonous chemical categorised as biological agents because they were created by living organisms. They generally behave like chemical agents and serve the same function: to poison people.

Biological agents are relatively inexpensive to produce and have the potential to be devastating in their effects. Organisms such as anthrax, plague and smallpox have been the agents of greatest concern from a potential terrorist use perspective.[43] Table 23.6 presents an outline of biological agents, clinical presentations and treatments.

Radiological agents

Radiological materials can pose both an acute and long-term hazard to humans. In many ways, they behave like some of the chemical agents in that they cause cellular damage. A major difference is that radiological agents do not necessarily have to be inhaled or come in contact with the skin to do damage.[41]

The deployment of a nuclear weapon would be catastrophic, as evidenced by events such as Hiroshima or industrial accidents as occurred at Chernobyl. While very different, both events produced immediate injury and had long-term effects of ionising radiation on large populations.[43] The event of highest risk is likely to be a 'dirty bomb' that combines conventional explosives with any available radioactive source.[43]

Psychological effects

A chemical, biological or radiological terrorism incident may or may not result in mass casualties and fatalities as intended. However, large numbers of psychological casualties are very likely and, therefore, regardless of the effectiveness of the attack and number of people actually exposed to the agent, there will most likely be a mass casualty situation.[43] The psychological implications of chemical and biological weapons may be worse

---

TABLE 23.5

Summary of common chemical agents, effects, clinical presentations and treatments[42–45]

TYPE OF CHEMICAL	EFFECT	EXAMPLE	CLINICAL PRESENTATION	ANTIDOTES/TREATMENT
Nerve agent	Inhibits the activation of acetylcholinesterase	Sarin VX Soman Tabun	Muscarinic and nicotinic signs	Atropine 2-Pyridine aldoxime methyl chloride Benzodiazepines
Blood agents	Binds with cytochrome oxidase, causing hypoxia	Cyanide	Hypoxia	Cyanide kit Sodium nitrite Sodium thiosulfate
Vesicants	Chemical burns	Mustard gas Lewisite	Burns and blisters	Decontamination with soap and water
Pulmonary agents	Irritation to the respiratory tract	Chlorine phosgene	Respiratory distress Pulmonary oedema	Oxygen

TABLE 23.6

Summary of biological agents, clinical presentations and treatments[43,44,46,47]

BIOLOGICAL GROUP	EXAMPLE	CLINICAL PRESENTATION	TREATMENT
Virus	Smallpox (variola)		Supportive care
Bacteria	Anthrax (*Bacillus anthracis*)	Inhalational • Respiratory failure • Widened mediastinum • Severe sepsis	Antibiotics
	Plague (*Yersinia pestis*)	Pneumonic plague • Respiratory failure • Haemoptysis • Painful lymph nodes	Antibiotics
Toxin	Botulism (*Clostridium botulinum*)		Supportive care Botulism immune globulin

than the physical ones. Chemical and biological weapons are weapons of terror; part of their purpose is to wreak destruction via psychological means by inducing fear, confusion and uncertainty in everyday life.[49]

The long-term social and psychological effects of an episode of chemical or biological attack, real or suspected, would be as damaging as the acute ones, if not more so.[50]

Major challenges for chemical, biological or radiological responders

A well-delivered chemical or biological event would be catastrophic and exposure for emergency workers likely, as occurred previously when 110 staff developed signs and symptoms of exposure following the 1995 sarin attack in Tokyo.[51]

To protect staff, there must be clear procedures for dealing with potentially exposed or contaminated patients. This begins with proper assessment of a patient in need of isolation or decontamination and includes understanding of what PPE is appropriate and the capability of staff to effectively use the PPE. Emergency personnel must also have immediate access to the PPE that they need to limit their risk of exposure. However, the issue is complex: advanced levels of PPE require advanced training and special skills to be used safely. Decontamination of patients with chemical exposure is a high-risk activity for untrained staff.[51,52]

Advanced clinical skills

Within the ED, there has been an evolution of advancing the clinical roles and skill set for nurses. This has come about largely in response to an increasing number of emergency presentations, and to improve performance in patient flow, waiting times, length of stay and patient satisfaction.[51–53] Within the ED, advanced clinical roles, as discussed in more detail in Chapter 1, mean that registered nurses with advanced clinical skills can progress patient assessment and management through nurse-initiated radiology and nurse-initiated analgesia.

Nurse-initiated radiology

Nurse-initiated radiology ordering enables radiological investigations of extremities,[54] joints such as hips and shoulders, the chest and abdomen according to clinical protocols that list inclusion and exclusion criteria[55] based on findings from the patient's history and clinical examination. The inclusion criteria reflect well-established clinical indicators. While nurse-initiated radiology ordering is often undertaken as an extended triage nurse function, it can be performed by any accredited nurse. The use of nurse-initiated radiology, especially in association with extremity injuries, is safe and accurate, reducing both waiting time and department transit time and improving both patient and staff satisfaction.[53–57]

Nurse-initiated analgesia

Although pain is a common complaint in the majority of patients presenting to the ED,[58,59] timeliness, adequacy and appropriateness of analgesia administration have been suboptimal[58,59] and contribute to poor patient satisfaction.[58] Consequently, many EDs have developed nurse-initiated analgesia protocols, standing orders or pathways to enable designated emergency nurses to implement analgesia regimens before medical assessment. These protocols are locally derived and note patient inclusion and exclusion criteria for managing mild, moderate or severe pain in both adult and paediatric patients, and often include administration of an antiemetic.[58,59] A numerical pain rating scale or a visual analogue scale is used to direct the type and route of analgesia administration. Severe pain protocols outline intravenous (IV) narcotic administration, including incremental and total maximum administration dosages. After administration of the initial dose, the administering nurse gives subsequent doses in response to patient assessment of pain score and vital signs (pulse, blood pressure and respiratory rate). Protocols directed towards moderate and minor pain may include either single or incremental IV or oral analgesia. Nurse-initiated analgesia protocols are safe and effective, shortening the time ED patients wait for analgesia,[59–61] which should assist in improving patient outcomes and satisfaction.

Retrievals and transport of critically ill patients

The care of an acutely ill patient often includes transport, either within a hospital to undergo tests and procedures or between hospitals to receive a higher level of care or to access a hospital bed. The movement of critically ill patients places the patient at a higher risk of complications during the transport period[62–65] because of condition changes, inadequate availability of equipment or support from other clinicians or the physical environment in the transport vehicle. For this reason the standard of care during any transport must be equivalent to, or better than, that at the referring clinical area.[62,66,67] Safe transport of patients requires planning and stabilisation by staff with appropriate skills and experience. This section focuses on the movement of critically ill patients between hospitals.

Retrievals

Although there are a variety of retrieval or transport models, most retrieval teams comprise doctors, nurses and paramedics with specialised training in critical care. The skills of the escort personnel need to match the acuity of the patient, so that they can respond to most clinical problems.[68,69] Thus, retrieval team staff need to deliver high-level critical care equal to the standard of the receiving centre, but need to be familiar with the challenges associated with working outside the hospital environment. Standards and guidelines for the transport of critically ill patients have been established by the College of Critical Care Medicine and the Australasian College for Emergency Medicine,[62] the Intensive Care Society,[69] American College of Critical Care Medicine[68] and the Association of Anaesthetists of Great Britain and Ireland.[70]

When transporting an unstable patient it is essential that a minimum of two people focusing solely on the clinical care aspects of the patient are present, in addition to other staff transporting the patient and equipment. The transport team leader is usually a medical officer with advanced training in critical care medicine or, for the transport of critical but stable patients, a registered nurse with critical care experience. The precise composition of the transport team can depend on the clinical circumstances in each case. The skill set includes advanced cardiac life support, arrhythmia interpretation and treatment and emergency airway management.[68]

Preparing a patient for inter-hospital transport

Adequate and considered preparation for the transport of a critically ill patient from one hospital area to another should be appropriately planned and not compromised by undue haste. Appropriate evaluation and stabilisation are required to ensure patient safety during transport,

including assessment of airway, breathing, circulation and suitable IV access.[62,68,70]

If potential airway compromise is suspected, careful consideration should be given to an elective intubation prior to transport rather than an emergency airway intervention in a moving vehicle or a radiology department. A laryngeal mask airway is not an acceptable method of airway management for critically ill patients undergoing transport because of the problems associated with movement.[68] A nasogastric or orogastric tube is inserted in all patients requiring mechanical ventilation.

Fluid resuscitation and inotropic support are initiated prior to transporting the patient. Planning for the trip needs to include adequate reserves of blood or other IV fluid for use during transport. If the patient is combative or uncooperative, the use of sedative and/or neuromuscular blocking agents and analgesia may be indicated.[68] A syringe pump with battery power is the most appropriate method for delivering medications for sedation and pain relief. A urinary catheter is inserted for transports of extended duration and all unconscious patients.[68,69]

Equipment essential for transport includes:

- equipment for airway management, sized appropriately and transported with each patient (check for operation before transport)
- portable oxygen source of adequate volume to provide for the projected timeframe, with a 30-minute reserve
- a self-inflating bag and mask of appropriate size
- handheld spirometer for tidal volume measurement
- available high-pressure suction
- basic resuscitation drugs, and supplemental medications, such as sedatives and narcotic analgesics (considered in each specific case)
- a transport monitor, displaying electrocardiogram (ECG) and heart rate, oxygen saturation, end-tidal CO_2 and as many invasive channels as required for pressure measurements.

The patient's identification bracelet should be checked and verified, medical records and relevant information such as laboratory and radiology findings are copied for the receiving facility, and other documentation includes initial medical evaluation and medical officer to medical officer communication, with the names of the accepting doctors and the receiving hospital.[67–69]

Patient monitoring during transport

Critically ill patients undergoing transport receive the same level of monitoring as they would have in a critical care unit. Monitoring equipment should be selected for its reliable operation under transport conditions, as monitoring can be difficult during transport; the effects of motion, noise and vibration can make even simple clinical observations (e.g. chest auscultation or palpation) difficult, if not impossible.[71] The monitor should have a capacity for storing and reproducing patient bedside data and printouts during transport.[62,68,71] As transport of mechanically ventilated patients is associated with risk,[62,68,71,72] consistent ventilation and oxygenation should be a goal; transport ventilators provide more constant ventilation than manual ventilation. An appropriate transport ventilator provides full ventilatory support, monitors airway pressure with a disconnect alarm and should have adequate battery and gas supply for the duration of transport.[62]

Adverse events during transport of critically ill patients fall into two categories:[62,72,73] 1) equipment dysfunction, such as ECG lead disconnection, loss of battery power, loss of IV access, accidental extubation, occlusion of the endotracheal tube or exhaustion of oxygen supply (at least one team member should be proficient in operating and troubleshooting all equipment), and 2) physiological deteriorations related to the critical illness. Mechanisms for audit, quality improvement and teaching purposes should be in situ to allow for feedback, performance review and service improvements.[62,68–71]

Multiple patient triage/disaster

Disaster triage is a process designed to provide the greatest benefit to multiple patients when treatment resources and facilities are limited. Disaster triage systems differ from the routine triage system used within the ED (e.g. the ATS, MTS): system care is focused on those victims who may survive with proper therapy, rather than on those who have no chance of survival or who will live without treatment. The system was first devised during war as a method of managing large numbers of battlefield casualties. Today it is applicable for treating multiple victims of illness or injury outside and within the hospital setting. Variations exist between states and countries regarding disaster victim triage classifications. It is therefore important to be familiar with local plans and policy.[13,22,74]

Triage of mass victims may be necessary in common situations, such as vehicle collisions with multiple occupants, as well as other large-scale disasters, such as earthquakes, floods, bushfires, damaging storms, public transport incidents or explosions. The principles of triage vary little, though the methods used to communicate triage information and to match victims with available resources may differ. Triage at the scene of a major incident or disaster is commenced by the first qualified person to arrive (i.e. the one with the most medical training). This person is initially responsible for performing immediate primary surveys on all victims and for determining and communicating the numbers and types of resources needed to provide initial care and transport.[8]

In Australia, New Zealand, the United Kingdom and the United States of America disaster systems have up to five triage categories (depending on jurisdictional and local protocols), usually with corresponding colours. Despite slight variation, the aim is similar: to provide the best level of care and ensure the highest number of survivors. Those who are mortally injured but alive may

be given a low treatment priority, though this will almost certainly ensure their death. These decisions are therefore best made by an experienced doctor. In a situation with a large number of casualties, one or more doctors should be present at the site to lead the triage effort. Further, it is not within the scope of practice of non-physician emergency personnel to pronounce a patient dead, but properly trained ambulance or rescue personnel can recognise the signs of death for the purposes of triage until doctors can formally declare death.[63,64]

Emergency department response to an external disaster: receiving patients

Disasters may produce mass victims on a scale that means routine processes and practices in the ED and hospital will be overwhelmed. The ED response to an external disaster forms part of the overall hospital response, outlined in a hospital disaster plan. The ED response plans also sit within the larger context of other health disciplines where there is a consideration of the prevention of, preparedness for, response to and recovery from the health problems arising from a disaster.[64] These plans are reviewed regularly for currency, and practised for preparedness. The following aspects form part of ED planning and response to receiving patients from an external disaster.[64,65,74]

Department preparation

If the disaster site is close to the hospital, a significant number of disaster victims will self-evacuate from the site and arrive at the hospital without any prehospital triage, treatment or decontamination before any formal notification has been received. In this instance the ED will need to declare the incident and commence the notification process required.[64] The ED may be quickly overwhelmed with arriving patients; the closest local medical facility may receive up to 50–80% of the disaster victims within 90 minutes of the incident.[65] On notification of a disaster response a number of key positions should be allocated (medical coordinator, nursing coordinator, triage nurse, medical triage officer). These personnel are senior staff with specific disaster training and knowledge of the hospital's disaster plan.[63,64,74] Nursing and medical coordinators are responsible for allocating staff to specific duties; all designated roles are outlined on action cards available for staff to read prior to commencing their roles.[65]

The capacity of the ED to accommodate a large influx of patients needs to be maximised. Patients currently in the department are reviewed for a decision to admit. Patients requiring admission are transferred out of the department to a suitable location in the hospital. Patients suitable for discharge or referral to their local medical officer, including patients with minor complaints currently waiting, should be discharged or referred to community resources. A small number of patients may need to remain in the ED, and their care will need to be prioritised in conjunction with arriving disaster victims.[62–65]

Areas of the department are designated to accommodate the expected severity of the victims (e.g. resuscitation room for priority 1 patients, observation areas for priority 2). Walking wounded casualties with relatively minor injuries and who are unlikely to require admission to hospital are best accommodated in a treatment area outside the ED, as this reduces congestion and increases the capacity for more significantly-injured victims to be managed.[64]

Additional staff members are notified from the current staff lists to participate in the disaster management. Staff members are allocated to teams to manage bed spaces within designated treatment areas. Additional staff from outside the ED may be deployed to assist; these staff should be teamed with routine ED staff because of their familiarity with the layout and location of equipment and other resources. It is important to recognise the need to replace staff to avoid fatigue, especially in incidents of a protracted nature. Therefore, not all staff should be called in initially. Where possible, staff who usually work together on a daily basis should work in teams during the disaster period.[64,65,74]

Triage and reception

Routine, day-to-day triage and reception processes will be ineffective when receiving large numbers of disaster victims. A registration process for disaster victims generally involves collecting minimal personal information from the patients, where possible, and the allocation of a prepared disaster hospital number used for identification and ordering investigations.[8,74] Triage assessments will often be undertaken by both a medical officer and a nurse, and the process will be brief and focused. Most victims will have been allocated a triage tag in the field, but are reevaluated for any changes, as their condition may have deteriorated. Triage assessment is based on observations of the nature and extent of the victims' injuries. Patients present in the ED prior to disaster notification are considered part of the disaster event and triaged in the same manner.[4,8,65]

Treatment

Treatment provided during a disaster will not reflect routine practices; priorities focus on resuscitation, identification of serious injuries, identification of patients requiring urgent surgery and stabilisation of patients for transfer out of the ED. The best overall outcomes during a disaster are achieved when the routine principles of resuscitation and management are adapted to reflect the resources available.[64,65]

Transfer from the ED

Patients are triaged, stabilised and transferred out to the operating theatre or other clinical areas as soon as possible using designated transfer staff and a coordinated process outlined in the hospital plan. This will maintain the effectiveness and efficiency of the department as victims continue to arrive. During and after the incident, opportunity for staff to debrief is an important aspect to manage staff psychosocial wellbeing.[8,74]

Respiratory presentations

Patients with respiratory dysfunction are common presentations to the ED and are seen across all age groups. Respiratory symptoms can be associated with a broad range of underlying pathologies. This section will discuss the initial assessment and treatment of several common respiratory diseases seen in the ED. Chapter 14 provides more detailed information regarding respiratory diseases.

Presenting symptoms and incidence

Patients presenting with respiratory complaints may display a range of symptoms. These symptoms will vary based upon the age of the patient, the underlying cause of the symptoms and the severity of the underlying condition. A list of frequently encountered respiratory signs and symptoms can be found in Box 23.1.[75–77]

BOX 23.1

Signs and symptoms commonly associated with respiratory presentations[75,76]

- Shortness of breath
- Dyspnoea (painful or difficulty breathing)
- Decreased SaO_2
- Cyanosis
- Alteration in respiratory rate – tachypnoea/bradypnoea
- Alterations in respiratory depth or pattern
- Use of accessory muscles
- Intercostal and/or subcostal recession
- Inability to speak in full sentences
- Wheeze
- Stridor (upper airway respiratory disorders)
- Alterations in level of consciousness
- Anxiety/feeling of impending doom

Shortness of breath or dyspnoea is a frequent symptom or complaint on presentation to the ED. Respiratory presentations are not isolated to any one specific patient population or age group and are frequently encountered in patients across the lifespan. Dyspnoea, while commonly associated with respiratory conditions such as asthma, pneumonia, chronic obstructive pulmonary disease and cardiac conditions, has multiple aetiologies and can be caused by disease in almost any organ system. Shortness of breath is a significant symptom and is commonly associated with the need for hospital admission.[77–79]

Assessment, monitoring and diagnostics

On arrival, patients with respiratory complaints should be quickly assessed utilising a systematic approach to determine whether there is any potentially life-threatening disturbance to the airway, breathing or circulation that requires immediate medical assessment and/or resuscitative intervention.

Initial assessment should include a thorough history focused on the presenting complaint/s. A detailed history may often identify the underlying process; however, the emergency clinician should maintain a high index of suspicion of other potential causes during the initial assessment.[77,78] The history should focus on the nature of symptoms, the timing of the onset of symptoms, associated features, the possibility of trauma or aspiration and past medical history, especially the presence of chronic respiratory conditions. After obtaining a history, a physical assessment of the respiratory system should be undertaken (see Chapter 13 for a detailed description of respiratory physical assessment).

Patients with significant respiratory symptoms are best managed in an acute monitored bed or resuscitation area of the emergency department. A set of observations including heart rate, respiratory rate, blood pressure, temperature and oxygen saturation should be completed and the patient's heart rate and oxygen saturation can be continuously monitored. Pulse oximetry plays an important role in the monitoring of the patient with a respiratory complaint. The recognition of hypoxaemia is significantly improved with the use of pulse oximetry.[80]

IV access should be obtained and venous blood samples may be collected for full blood count, urea, electrolytes and creatinine where clinically indicated. A chest X-ray (CXR) should be ordered in most instances. The CXR is one of the most useful investigations in the patient with a respiratory presentation. Interpretation of the CXR does not provide 100% accuracy in distinguishing between possible underlying pathologies, and may appear normal in some instances. Therefore, interpretation of the CXR should always be performed in light of the clinical history and other examination findings.[79] An arterial blood gas is often indicated in patients with a significant respiratory presentation. The arterial blood gas will provide useful information that assists in identifying alterations to oxygenation, ventilation and acid–base status.[79] Spirometry or peak flow measurements may also be utilised in the assessment of the patient. Peak expiratory flow rate, forced vital capacity and forced expiratory volume in 1 second are useful in determining the nature of the underlying respiratory condition and, when the values are compared to predicted normal values, are useful in determining severity. These tests are, however, effort- and technique-dependent and may not be able to be performed by the patient who is acutely short of breath.[79]

Oxygen therapy should be commenced early in patients presenting with signs of acute respiratory compromise, including patients known to have chronic obstructive pulmonary disease. Patients with acute hypoxia require oxygen. The often mentioned complications associated with oxygen, especially in the patient with known chronic obstructive pulmonary disease, are uncommon. Such complications are concentration- and

time-dependent having a slow onset, which allows time for monitoring with pulse oximetry, arterial blood gas analysis and clinical review.[79]

Patient diagnoses and management

The common diagnoses related to patients who present with shortness of breath are asthma, respiratory failure and pneumonia.[78]

Asthma

Asthma is a very common reason for patients presenting to Australasian emergency departments. Over 2.2 million Australians have asthma: up to 16% of children and 12% of adults are affected by the condition.[81–85] In other developed countries like the USA asthma is the most common respiratory disease affecting between 4% and 5% of the population.[85] Asthma is a chronic inflammatory disease of the airways in which many cells and cellular elements play a role, including mast cells, eosinophils, T lymphocytes, macrophages, neutrophils and epithelial cells. The inflammatory changes cause recurrent episodes of wheezing, breathlessness, chest tightness and coughing associated with widespread reversible airflow obstruction of the airways. This airflow obstruction or excessive narrowing is a result of airway smooth muscle contraction and swelling of the airway wall due to smooth muscle hypertrophy, inflammatory changes, oedema, goblet cell and mucous gland hyperplasia and mucus hypersecretion.[84,85]

Normally, airways widen during inspiration and narrow in expiration. In asthma, the above responses combine to severely narrow or close the lumen of the bronchial passages during expiration, with altered ventilation and air trapping.[84,85] The causes of asthma are related to many factors, including allergy,[81] infection (increased reaction to bronchoconstrictors such as histamine),[81–85] irritants (e.g. noxious gases, fumes, dusts, dust mites, powders) or heredity, although the exact role or importance of any hereditary tendency is difficult to assess.[85]

A patient usually has a history of previous asthma attacks. Often, an acute episode follows a period of exercise or exposure to a noxious substance, or a known allergen. The onset of the asthma may be characterised by vague sensations in the neck or pharynx, tightness in the chest with breathlessness, loose but non-productive cough with difficulty in raising sputum, difficulty breathing, particularly on expiration, with increasing severity as the episode continues; apprehension and tachypnoea may follow as the patient becomes hypoxic, with audible wheezing.[84,85]

The characteristics and initial assessment of acute mild, moderate and severe/life-threatening asthma in adults are outlined in Table 23.7. The associated clinical management guidelines for acute asthma are outlined in Table 23.8. Be alert to the high-risk patient whose ability to ventilate is impaired: this is a life-threatening condition. Such patients will exhibit an inability to talk, central cyanosis, tachycardia, use of respiratory accessory muscles, a silent chest on auscultation and a history of previous intubation for asthma.[81–88]

TABLE 23.7

Initial assessment and characteristics of acute asthma[84,85]

	SEVERITY OF ATTACK		
SYMPTOMS	MILD	MODERATE	SEVERE OR LIFE-THREATENING
Able to talk in	Sentences	Phrases	Words
Physical exhaustion	No	No	Yes, may have paradoxical chest wall movement
Pulse oximetry (room air)	>94%	90–94%	<90%; cyanosis may be present
Pulse rate	<100/min	100–120/min	>120/min; below 60/min
Level of consciousness	Normal	May be agitated	Confused, drowsy or agitated
Wheeze intensity	Variable	Moderate–loud	Often quiet
Central cyanosis	Absent	May be present	Likely to be present
Peak expiratory flow (% predicted)	>75%	50–75%	<50% or an inability to perform the test
Arterial blood gases	Test not necessary	If initial response is poor	Yes

TABLE 23.8

Initial clinical management in acute asthma[84,88]

	MILD	MODERATE	SEVERE OR LIFE-THREATENING
Hospital admission necessary	Probably not	Likely to be required	Yes, consider ICU
Oxygen	High flow of at least 8 L/min, titrated to maintain SaO_2 >90%, preferably >94%. Monitor effect by oximetry. Frequent measurement of arterial blood gases in severe asthma if not responding		
Beta-2-agonist via a metered-dose inhaler and spacer *or* nebulised solution with 8 L/min O_2	Salbutamol 8–12 puffs *or* Salbutamol 5 mg	Salbutamol 8–12 puffs *or* Salbutamol 5–10 mg every 1–4 hours	Salbutamol 8–12 puffs every 15–30 min *or* Salbutamol 5–10 mg every 15–30 min If no response to aerosol give salbutamol 250 mcg IV bolus and then 5–10 mcg/kg/h
Ipratropium bromide metered dose inhaler or spacer *or* nebulised solution	Not necessary Not necessary	Optional Optional	6 puffs (20 mcg/puff) with salbutamol every 2 hours 2 mL 0.05% (500 mcg) ipratropium bromide with salbutamol 2-hourly
Steroids	Yes (consider oral)	Yes, oral 0.5–1.0 mg/kg	IV hydrocortisone 250mg 6-hourly
Other agents	Not indicated	Not indicated	For life-threatening and no response, magnesium sulfate 2 g IV over 10 min may help
CXR (and other investigations	Not usually necessary	Not necessary unless focal signs present, or no improvement with therapy	Necessary if no response to initial therapy or suspect pneumothorax/infection Check for hypokalaemia
Observations	Regular	Continuous	Continuous

Acute respiratory failure

Acute respiratory failure exists when the lungs do not provide sufficient gas exchange to meet the body's need for oxygen consumption, carbon dioxide elimination or both. Acute respiratory failure results from a number of causes.[89] When alveolar ventilation decreases, arterial oxygen tension falls and carbon dioxide rises. The rise in arterial carbon dioxide produces increased serum carbonic acid and pH falls, resulting in respiratory acidosis.[90] If uncorrected, low arterial oxygen combines with low cardiac output to produce diminished tissue perfusion and tissue hypoxia. Anaerobic metabolism results in increased lactic acid, aggravating the acidosis caused by carbon dioxide retention. In the process, a wide range of symptoms develop, involving the central nervous and cardiovascular systems.[84] Arterial blood gases confirm the diagnosis, with hypercarbia and a partial pressure of carbon dioxide in the arterial blood >45 mmHg and hypoxaemia evidenced by a partial pressure of oxygen in the arterial blood <80 mmHg, and a low pH evident. A CXR identifies the specific lung disease.[89]

Clinical management focuses on correction of hypercapnia, treatment of hypoxaemia, correction of acidosis and identification and correction of the specific cause[89] (see Chapter 14). For a spontaneously breathing patient, administer oxygen by Venturi mask (24%) or nasal cannula. Adjust oxygen therapy, according to arterial blood gas findings at 15–20-minute intervals, to achieve a partial pressure of oxygen in the arterial blood of 85–90 mmHg. For a patient with inadequate respiratory effort, non-invasive ventilation may be instituted (see Chapter 15). In an apnoeic situation, initiate ventilatory assistance with bag–mask ventilation (see Chapter 15) prior to endotracheal intubation, and then commence mechanical ventilation.

Pneumonia

Pneumonia is an acute inflammatory condition of lung tissue caused by a variety of viral and bacterial organisms, fungi and parasites.[76,87,91] These organisms cause an inflammatory response from the cells involved in the affected segment of lung tissue. Pneumonia may occur in previously healthy patients, but more often it is associated with conditions that impair the body's defence mechanisms[76,87,91] (see Chapter 14). The predominant symptoms associated with pneumonia are a combination of cough, chest pain (usually pleuritic), dyspnoea, fever (with or without chills) and mucoid, purulent or bloody sputum, with an abrupt or gradual onset.[87,91] A physical examination demonstrates tachypnoea, fever, tachycardia, possible cyanosis, diminished respiratory excursion due to pleuritic pain, end-respiratory crackles or rales on auscultation with bronchial breathing over areas of consolidation[76,87,91] (see Chapter 14).

Investigations include a CXR, which may reveal varying infiltrates – interstitial, segmental or lobar. The CXR, however, may initially be clear until later in the illness and following adequate rehydration.[79] Venous blood samples will be analysed to identify a raised white cell count (i.e. leucocytosis). Blood cultures and sputum cultures will also be acquired to assist in identifying the causative organism. Arterial blood gases will assist in determining the degree of impaired gas exchange. Hypoxaemia and often hypocarbia may be present.[76]

Initial treatment involves administration of oxygen therapy via face mask. Oxygen therapy should be evaluated frequently in response to arterial blood gas results and pulse oximetry. Treatment will routinely require IV fluid therapy to ensure adequate hydration, and administration of antibiotics orally or parentally in accordance with existing antibiotic guidelines or suspected infective agent (see Chapter 14). Ventilatory support may be required in some cases; in spontaneously breathing patients non-invasive ventilation via a face mask should be utilised before invasive ventilation. Mechanical ventilation is not normally required unless there is some underlying cardiopulmonary disease.[76,87]

Chest pain presentations

Chest pain or chest discomfort is a common presenting complaint to the ED and can be associated with a number of different clinical conditions, several of which are associated with life-threatening pathology.[92] The identification of cardiac-related chest pain is important. During an initial assessment it may be difficult to differentiate between non-cardiac and cardiac causes of chest discomfort based on pain characteristics such as intensity, location, radiation and other associated symptoms.[92,93] Therefore, it is important to consider any presentation in which chest pain is a feature as cardiac in origin until a cardiac cause has been ruled out or another cause has been confirmed.

Description of presenting symptoms and incidence

The incidence of acute chest pain presentations appears to be increasing as patients are more aware of the importance of early treatment for myocardial infarction due to public awareness campaigns.[92,94] In American EDs up to 7% of all presentations are for complaints of chest pain.[95] The pain or discomfort associated with chest pain presentations is often described in a variety of ways in terms of onset, intensity, duration and radiation (see Table 23.9).

Up to 9% of patients who will go on to be diagnosed with an acute coronary syndrome (ACS) may present with a number of these associated symptoms but without chest pain. These patients tend to be elderly, female, diabetic and non-white minorities.[96–98] Therefore, it is important to consider the possibility of a cardiac presentation in patients presenting with these associated symptoms even in the absence of chest pain.[9]

Assessment, monitoring and diagnostics

Any patient presenting with a complaint of chest pain requires urgent assessment, generally within 10 minutes of

TABLE 23.9

Features of chest pain[92,94–97]

CHEST PAIN FEATURE	DESCRIPTION
Description	Typical: pressure, a weight on the chest, tightness, constriction about the throat, an aching feeling Less typical: epigastric, indigestion, stabbing, pleuritic, sharp
Onset	Unprovoked or gradual With physical exertion or emotional stress
Intensity	Mild to severe
Radiation	To one or both arms, neck, jaw or back
Associated symptoms	Shortness of breath, nausea, vomiting, weakness, dizziness, anxiety, feeling of impending doom, palpitations, diaphoresis

arrival to the ED. Any patient with evidence of a disturbance to airway, breathing or circulation requires close monitoring, immediate medical assessment and resuscitative interventions. The initial assessment should include a 12-lead ECG and a history of the presenting complaint including an evaluation of the pain utilising a systematic approach. The ECG should be rapidly evaluated for the presence of ST-segment elevation or a new left bundle branch block suggestive of an acute myocardial infarction (AMI) so that time-critical treatment can be initiated. If the initial ECG is non-diagnostic and symptoms continue, repeat ECGs should be performed at 15-minute intervals.[92,95,96]

The patient should have cardiac monitoring commenced in order to identify any life-threatening arrhythmias. Supplemental oxygen should also be commenced if indicated to potentially improve PaO_2 and increase oxygen availability, especially in the presence of myocardial ischaemia;[99] however this is a routine intervention currently being reviewed. An IV cannula should be inserted and routine venous blood samples collected for troponin T or troponin I, cardiac enzymes that, when elevated, suggest myocardial injury. Cardiac enzymes are usually repeated within 6–8 hours of ED presentation.[99] A physical examination should also be performed. The physical examination may be of limited value in identifying cardiac causes of the pain but will be beneficial in identifying non-cardiac causes of the pain or complications associated with cardiac-related conditions.[92,94,96] The examination should also include assessment of the abdomen as a number of significant abdominal complaints may also present with chest pain as a feature.[92–94] A CXR should also be performed in order to identify any potential causes for the patient's pain.

Patient diagnoses and management

Acute coronary syndromes

Chest pain of cardiac origin results from reduced or obstructed coronary blood flow, commonly due to atherosclerosis, although coronary artery spasm or an embolism may also be involved.[92–94] Angina, whether stable or unstable, is a temporary condition in which there is no damage to the myocardial cells. A time-critical obstruction results in death or necrosis of a segment of myocardial cells resulting in an AMI.[93]

ACS collectively describes unstable angina and AMI. Coronary heart disease is the largest single cause of death and the commonest cause of sudden death in Australia and New Zealand.[100] It is the leading cause of premature death and disability in both countries, although death rates have fallen since the 1960s. Over half of all coronary heart disease deaths were from AMI.[101] ACS is the most common life-threatening condition seen in the ED and therefore represents an important area of clinical practice in the ED.[101,102] Chapters 10 and 11 provide additional information about presentations of cardiac dysfunction, including pathophysiology, clinical manifestations and treatment of cardiac conditions. This section summarises clinical management processes in the ED.[93]

The initial management in the ED is focused on rapid identification of patients with AMI and their suitability for reperfusion therapy. Reperfusion therapy consists of the administration of thrombolytic drugs with or without percutaneous coronary intervention (angioplasty ± stent). Percutaneous coronary intervention is generally only available to patients in larger centres where there is access to such resources. If percutaneous coronary intervention is not available, suitable patients should be managed with thrombolysis.[93]

The ongoing management in the ED for patients with ACS includes oxygen therapy, administration of aspirin 300 mg – if not already administered by pre-hospital personnel – and pain relief. Pain relief management generally includes the administration of IV morphine in small incremental doses. Pain relief may also include the administration of nitrates initially via the sublingual route; however, if pain persists despite IV morphine, the administration of IV nitrates may be indicated.[102] The patient and their family should also be provided reassurance, information and emotional support.

Patients without initial evidence of AMI are subsequently stratified into high-, intermediate- and low-risk groups based upon the presence of a number of clinical features associated with the presentation including the significance and duration of pain, ECG findings, past history, cardiovascular disease risk factors and cardiac enzyme results.[99] Specific ongoing treatment and management is then guided by the associated risk pathway.[93,99]

Thoracic aortic dissection

Thoracic aortic dissection (TAD) occurs when there is a tear in the intimal layer of the vessel wall. Blood passes through the tear, separates the intima from the vessel media or adventitia and results in a false channel. Shear forces lead to dissection propagation as blood flows through the false channel.[96,103] The incidence of TAD is quite low; ACS is 80 times more common. Identification of this life-threatening condition in the patient presenting with chest pain is important as patients often require immediate surgery. TAD is most commonly seen in men aged 50 to 70 years who have a history of hypertension. Other risk factors include Marfan's disease and other connective tissue disorders, cocaine or ecstasy use, pregnancy and aortic valve replacement.[98] TAD is associated with an acute and sudden onset of severe pain that is maximal at symptom onset. Pain is usually located in the midline and may be present in the back and rarely radiates. The pain is often described as sharp, tearing or ripping in nature.[98] Patients may also have pulse deficits or blood pressure differences (>20 mmHg) between the upper arms. CXR will be abnormal in 80–90% of cases with a widened mediastinum seen in approximately 50% of cases.[103,104] Patients will most commonly have the diagnosis confirmed using contrast computed tomography. The management of TAD is aimed at aggressive control of blood pressure and pulse with sodium nitroprusside and beta-blockers, relief of pain with narcotic analgesia and referral and/or transport to cardio-thoracic services for definitive surgical intervention.[103,104]

Abdominal symptom presentations

Acute abdominal pain is a common complaint, accounting for 5–10% of all presentations to the ED.[105–107] Specific cause for the presenting abdominal pain will not be found in 30–40% of patients of all ages;[105] for children, a diagnosis of non-specific abdominal pain accounts for up to 60% of cases.[108] About 20% of adult patients presenting will require surgical intervention and/or hospital admission.[108,109]

Common causes in the elderly include biliary tract disease (25%), diverticular disease (10%), bowel obstruction (10%) or malignancy (13%).[110] Elderly patients are more likely to have catastrophic illnesses rarely seen in younger patients, including mesenteric ischaemia, leaking or ruptured abdominal aortic aneurysm and myocardial infarction.[105,106,109] Up to a third require surgical intervention,[108] while 15% will not have a cause for their abdominal pain found.[110] Presentations by elderly patients are often complicated by delays in seeking medical attention, atypical presentations, associated medical conditions and comorbidities, medications and cognitive function.

Assessment, monitoring and diagnostics

Patients presenting with abdominal pain are assessed quickly for any disturbance to airway, breathing or circulation requiring close monitoring, immediate medical assessment and/or resuscitative interventions. Abnormal vital signs are suggestive of clinically significant abdominal pain.[109] A thorough history includes location and timing of onset; quantity, quality and radiation of pain; associated symptoms, previous history and general state of health. A complaint-specific history and physical examination is performed for a differential diagnosis.[105,106,109] Physical assessment includes visual inspection of the abdomen with the patient in a supine position, followed by auscultation, then gentle palpation and percussion of all four quadrants of the abdomen, working towards the area of reported pain.[110,111] While location of the pain is important, it can be misleading, as various pathological processes can localise to different areas of the abdomen (see Figure 23.1).[112] An ECG is considered to rule out myocardial ischaemia or infarction, as some cardiac patients may present with upper abdominal pain as the predominant symptom. Myocardial ischaemia may also be caused by the physiological stress of the intra-abdominal pathology.[105]

Administration of narcotic analgesia in acute abdominal pain does not hinder assessment or obscure abdominal findings, nor cause increased morbidity or mortality, and may allow for a better abdominal examination.[113,114] Incremental doses of a narcotic can minimise pain but not palpation tenderness. Analgesics enable relaxation of the patient's abdominal muscles and decrease anxiety, potentially improving information obtained from the physical examination.[61,113]

Venous blood samples are collected for full blood count, urea, electrolytes, creatinine and amylase and lipase.[111] A dipstick urinalysis can suggest specific disease. For example, leucocytes and/or blood in the urine can suggest a urinary tract infection and haematuria can suggest renal colic, but should be considered in the context of other clinical findings and formal microscopy.[111] Women of child-bearing age with abdominal pain provide the challenge of a broader range of potential causative pathologies, although history and physical examination are unreliable in determining pregnancy.[111] If pregnancy or a pregnancy-related disorder is possible, a urine beta-human chorionic gonadotrophin test is performed. Test sensitivity is extremely high; a positive finding occurs within a few days of conception, and accuracy is comparable to blood sampling. An ectopic pregnancy may be missed if pregnancy is not considered; an ectopic pregnancy is extremely unlikely if the beta-human chorionic gonadotrophin result is negative.[111]

Patient diagnoses and management

Common abdominal diagnoses for acute abdominal pain are abdominal aortic aneurysm, appendicitis and bowel obstruction.

FIGURE 23.1 An algorithm for triaging commonly missed causes of acute abdominal pain.

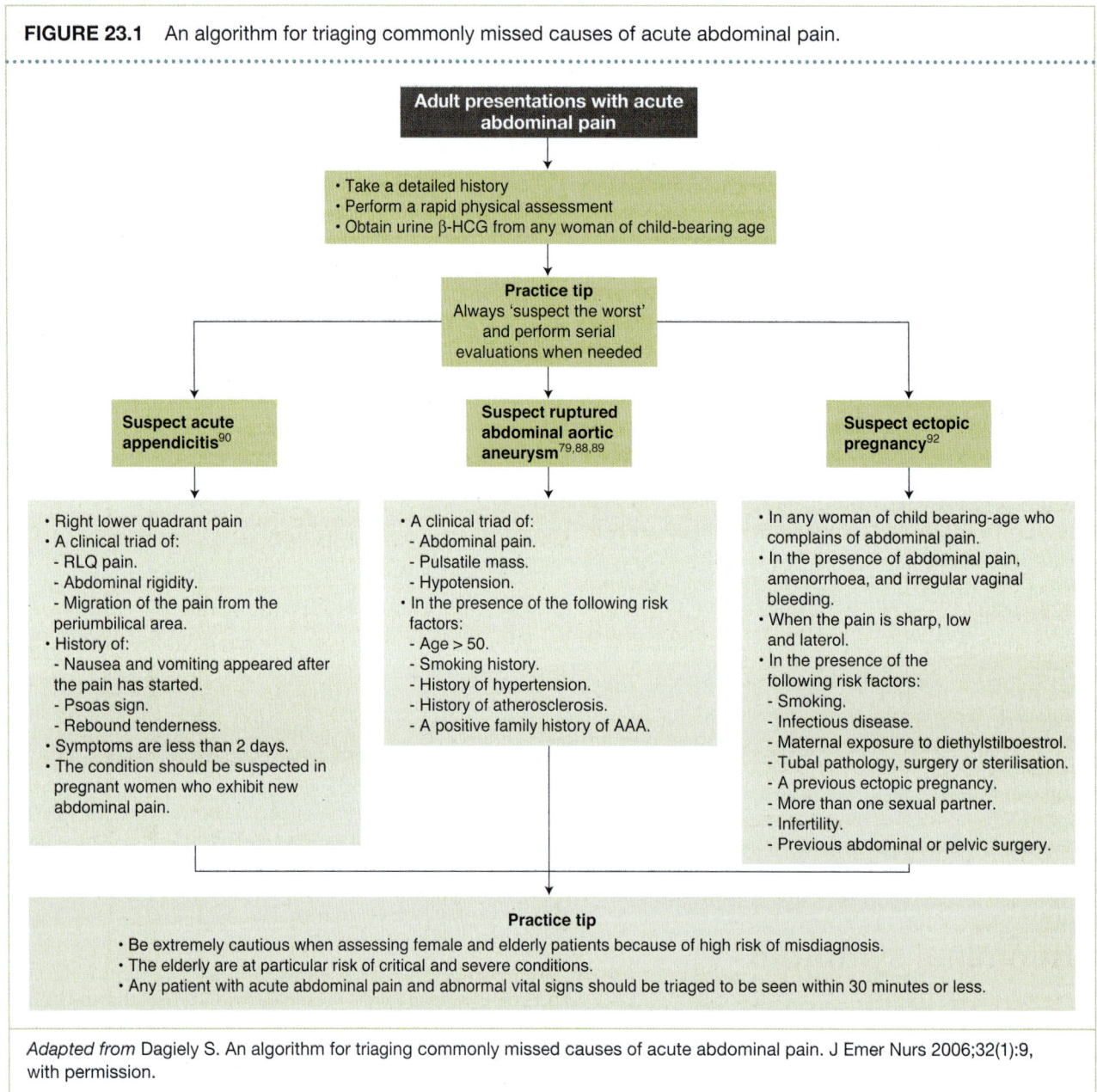

Adapted from Dagiely S. An algorithm for triaging commonly missed causes of acute abdominal pain. J Emer Nurs 2006;32(1):9, with permission.

Abdominal aortic aneurysm

Abdominal aortic aneurysm is more likely to develop in men than women,[115] is a common cause of death in all patients over the age of 65 years and is responsible for 0.8% of all deaths.[108,116] The traditional presentation is acute pain in the back, flank or abdomen, with hypotension and a palpable abdominal mass in the older patient.[116] Missed diagnoses primarily occur because physical examination is frequently unreliable.[116] Many patients with dissecting abdominal aortic aneurysm are misdiagnosed with renal colic because of haematuria present, no palpable pulsatile mass and flank pain.[116] Other common misdiagnoses include diverticulitis, gastrointestinal haemorrhage, AMI and musculoskeletal back pain.[116] Abdominal aortic

aneurysms are surgically repaired more than any other type of aneurysm. Unless a patient receives immediate resuscitation and surgical intervention, a ruptured abdominal aortic aneurysm is fatal.[116]

Appendicitis

Appendicitis is the most common acute abdominal pain presentation worldwide that requires a surgical intervention. About 8% of people in Western countries will have appendicitis during their lifetime.[117] Along with pain (usually in the right lower quadrant), other presenting symptoms may include nausea and vomiting.[117] Diagnosis is based on clinical assessment as there is no specific test available to confirm diagnosis.[118] Appendicitis can mimic almost all acute abdominal pain presentations, and is frequently misdiagnosed as gastroenteritis during the initial ED visit, pelvic inflammatory disease or urinary tract infection.[111] Although it is a well-studied disease, appendicitis continues to be difficult to diagnose in ED because of its varied presentations. Elderly patients require careful consideration due to associated comorbidities[117] and women of childbearing age are commonly misdiagnosed due to anatomical changes associated with pregnancy. Treatment includes management of pain-related symptoms and provision of IV hydration.[118] Definitive treatment is surgical removal of the appendix.[118]

> ### Practice tip
>
> Elderly patients require careful consideration due to associated comorbidities and age-related changes to their response to illness.

Bowel obstruction

A bowel obstruction commonly results from impaired peristaltic movement, hernias, adhesions and neoplasms.[119,120] Presentation includes poorly localised colicky pain that increases in intensity and location, with subsequent abdominal swelling and vomiting of faecal fluid.[119,120] Management includes both conservative options (management of symptoms, placement of a nasogastric tube and replacement of IV fluids) and surgical therapy for neoplasms or hernias.[119,120]

Ectopic pregnancy

An ectopic pregnancy is implantation outside the uterus, most commonly in the fallopian tubes. Ectopic pregnancies in the developed world occur at a rate of about 11:1000 diagnosed pregnancies.[121] The incidence is thought to be higher in developing countries but specific numbers are unknown.[122] Presenting symptoms can include lower abdominal pain that can become severe, feeling faint, bleeding or shoulder tip pain. Management is guided by the patient's haemodynamic state. Stable patients with no tubular ectopic may be managed with observation and drugs such as methotrexate; haemodynamically unstable patients will require resuscitation and surgical intervention.[122]

Acute stroke

Cerebrovascular disease is highly prevalent in developed countries. In some countries that have seen continuing industrialisation (such as Asia and Africa) the increasingly unhealthy lifestyle is being reflected in diseases including cerebrovascular disease.[123] In China, different epidemiological changes, such as an ageing population, high prevalence of smoking and hypertension, are expected to result in an increase in stroke rates.[123] In Australia, cerebrovascular disease is the third-largest cause of death.[124] Around 60,000 acute cerebrovascular accidents or recurrent strokes are reported each year with around half occurring

in persons aged over 75 years.[125] The two general stroke classifications are:

- Ischaemic strokes are precipitated by disrupted blood flow to an area of the brain as a result of arterial occlusion. Acute ischaemic stroke presentations are now referred to as a 'brain attack', to promote early presentation for access to time-critical treatments[126–128] and because the pathophysiology and current treatment of acute ischaemic stroke mimics that of AMI. From an ED perspective, serious long-term disability can be minimised if ischaemic stroke is recognised and treated promptly; that is, within 3 hours of symptom onset.[127,129]

- Haemorrhagic strokes are caused by rupture of a blood vessel, which produces bleeding into the brain parenchyma. (Chapter 17 details the pathophysiological processes.)

For patients diagnosed with an ischemic stroke, 13–25% will die within the first 30 days and 60% within 10 years.[130–132] Permanent disability requiring care in a nursing home or other long-term facility is required for around 10%.[125,130]

Assessment, monitoring and diagnostics

Symptoms of stroke are common amongst patients presenting to the ED; presenting signs vary from profound alterations in level of consciousness and limb hemiplegia to mild symptoms affecting speech, cognition or coordination. Symptoms may include confusion, dizziness, ataxia, visual disturbances, dysphasia or receptive and expressive aphasia, dysphagia, weakness and numbness or tingling of the face, arm or leg, which is usually unilateral.[125,129,131] Many disorders resemble a stroke presentation so emergency clinicians must quickly determine if another condition is responsible for the patient's neurological deficits. Other conditions include post-ictal phase following seizures, migraine with neurological deficits, hypoglycaemia or hyperglycaemia, systemic infections, brain tumours, hyponatraemia and hepatic encephalopathy.[124,129]

The focus of initial assessment is airway, breathing, circulation and disability. Of note, for airway assessment, stroke symptoms include altered muscle function, affecting swallowing and speech functions. A patient with a Glasgow Coma Scale (GCS) score of 9 or less may require intubation to protect and secure the airway.[123] The patient's breathing pattern should be assessed and continually monitored. Hypertension is common, with the increase improving any cerebral ischaemia so this should not be lowered unless dangerously high or contraindicated.[126] Hypotension or dehydration decreases cerebral blood flow and perfusion and should be corrected, although fluid replacement is instituted with caution.[131] Vital signs are documented every 15 minutes during drug therapy to identify changes suggestive of internal bleeding. Maintaining blood pressure less than 185/110 mmHg during fibrinolytic infusion decreases the risk of intracerebral haemorrhage.[128]

A thorough assessment of neurological disability should be undertaken, including a GCS (see Chapter 16). An ECG is recorded to detect any abnormal rhythm such as atrial fibrillation, which may be associated with stroke presentation.[123] IV access is obtained to administer medications, and collect blood for electrolytes, haematology and coagulation studies. Assessment of blood glucose will rule out hypoglycaemia or hyperglycaemia as a cause of the presenting symptoms. Abnormal glucose levels adversely affect cerebral metabolism.[126] After obvious alternative diagnoses are excluded, a brain computed tomography scan determines whether a stroke is haemorrhagic or ischaemic in origin. While a new-onset ischaemic stroke may not be evident for up to 24 hours, blood in the cranial cavity will be apparent immediately. Patients with any sign of haemorrhage are excluded for fibrinolytic therapy.[127]

Management

Acute ischaemic stroke management includes timely administration of a fibrinolytic agent in appropriately selected patients (see Box 23.2), which facilitates reperfusion, minimises tissue damage and reduces long-term stroke sequelae. Longer times between symptom onset and fibrinolytic infusion are associated with higher rates of morbidity and mortality.[125] Early presentation is therefore essential to instigate appropriate assessments and investigations, including computed tomography scanning, and then thrombolytic administration and still fall within the narrow treatment window. Acute stroke unit care, with specialised teams dedicated to the rapid assessment and management of presentations, can significantly reduce death and disability[125] (see Chapter 17).

Overdose and poisoning

Poisoning is a common clinical presentation throughout the world. Worldwide up to 9% of deaths are related to drug and alcohol misuse in the age group between 15 and 29.[133–138] In developed counties up to 25% of successful suicides are due to poisoning.[135] In Australia and New Zealand, poisoning accounts for 1–5% of admissions to public hospitals.[133–135,137]

Current clinical management with supportive and/or symptomatic control has resulted in death rates as low as 0.5% for overdose admissions to hospitals in developed countries.[135]

The usual types of poisoning encountered as ED presentations include self-poisoning with prescribed drugs, ingestion of illicit drugs and common dangerous substances (e.g. detergents, cleansers; psychotropic agents; analgesics; insecticides; paracetamol, aspirin).[139] A range of artificial and naturally occurring substances can produce acute poisonings. The toxicity of a substance depends on numerous factors, such as dose, route of exposure and the victim's pre-existing conditions. Poisoning, whether intentional or unintentional, can occur at any time, and may involve single or multiple substances.[133–137]

The vast amount of knowledge required concerning all poisons prompted the development of poison control information centres to provide specific information and guidance for healthcare providers and the general public on the management of a poisoned patient; to collect statistics on toxic substances; and to educate the public on the prevention or recognition of toxic exposures.[136] Other initiatives to limit the incidence and severity of acute poisoning include the control of drugs, specific information on labels, the introduction of blister packs and enforced safety standards such as childproof caps.[136,140,141]

Assessment, monitoring and diagnostics

The poisoned patient may present with a wide range of clinical features from no symptoms through to a

---

BOX 23.2

Criteria for administering fibrinolytic therapy in ischaemic stroke[127]

Inclusion criteria (all must be positive):
- Age ≥18 years
- Clinical diagnosis of ischaemic stroke with measurable neurological deficit
- Time of symptom onset <180 min and well established

Exclusion criteria (all must be negative):
- Evidence of intracranial haemorrhage on non-contrast head computed tomography
- Only minor or rapidly improving stroke symptoms
- High suspicion of subarachnoid haemorrhage, even with normal computed tomography
- Active internal bleeding
- Known bleeding condition, including but not limited to platelets <100,000/mm^3

- Patient received heparin within 48 h and had an elevated activated partial thromboplastin time (PTT)
- Current use of oral anticoagulants (e.g. warfarin)
- Recent use of anticoagulant and elevated international normalised ratio (INR) or prothrombin time (>15 s) or
- Intracranial surgery or serious head trauma, or previous stroke within 3 months
- Major surgery or serious trauma within 14 days
- History of intracranial haemorrhage, arteriovenous malformation, or aneurysm
- Witnessed seizure at stroke onset
- Recent acute myocardial infarction
- Systolic blood pressure >185 mmHg or diastolic blood pressure >110 mmHg at time of treatment

life-threatening condition or the potential to deteriorate rapidly, and should always be assessed immediately. Triage decisions should be based on the potential for rapid deterioration and the need for urgent intervention. Resuscitation may be necessary before any further definitive care can be commenced. The priorities of care for all patients include the assessment and maintenance of an airway, adequate ventilation and circulation.[134,136] Successful resuscitation may require removal of the toxin, counteraction of the poisoning by an antidote if available, and the treatment or support of symptoms.[133–137] It is extremely important to note that many drugs such as paracetamol may have limited initial effects but serious, potentially fatal consequences if not treated in a timely manner.[134,141]

An accurate history is often the most significant aid in directing care. If a history is unobtainable or uncertain, there are several general guidelines that may prove helpful for dealing with the patient who has an altered mental state or conscious level[133–137] (see Table 23.10).

Poisoning should always be considered when dealing with a patient who has a sudden-onset, acute illness. If there is a strong suspicion of poisoning, a clinician should attempt to compare the patient's presentation with symptoms caused by the suspected toxin and the likelihood of exposure.

Accidental poisonings are the commonest cause of medical emergencies in the paediatric patient population. Childhood ingestions tend to be accidental and to involve a single substance. Intentional poisonings occur more often with adults, and are more likely to involve multiple substances.[135,137,139] Poisonings in the aged population

are often complicated by coexisting medical conditions, which may exaggerate the effects or impair the excretion of the substances involved. Boys are more likely to be the victims of poisoning than girls. Adult women attempt suicide with poisons more often than men, but men's suicide intentions are associated with a higher mortality rate.[135,137,139]

> ### Practice tip
>
> Poisonings in the aged population are often complicated by coexisting medical conditions, which may exaggerate the effects or impair excretion of the substances involved.

Previous history

Patients with existing medical conditions often have multiple medications that could be either intentionally or unintentionally ingested. The use of multiple drugs may cause untoward reactions. A patient with a history of depression may attempt suicide with psychotropic drugs.[133–137] A quick onset and acute illness or condition should raise the level of suspicion of a poisoning, especially if there is no history of previous signs or symptoms that suggest another cause.

Suspected toxin

Rescue personnel, family or friends should bring any container, plant product or suspected toxin with the patient to the hospital, as long as the substance presents no risk of contamination to the person retrieving it. A child's play area should be inspected for possible sources of toxins.[133–137]

Time of poisoning

History should include time of exposure, onset of symptoms and time since treatment began. Alcohol is the commonest drug taken with other intentional self-poisonings, and can potentiate a range of medication effects and increase the incidence of vomiting and potential aspiration.[134,136] Poisonings in children tend to occur most often just prior to mealtimes, when they are hungry. Adults may take substances late in the evening, fall asleep and be found several hours later.[134]

A thorough assessment may provide clues about an unconscious, uncooperative or suspicious presentation. Assess for respiratory effort, skin colour, pupil size and reactivity, reflexes and general status. Auscultation of the lung fields, the apical pulse and presence of active bowel sounds provide a baseline for further assessment and clues about current problems. Check blood pressure as often as necessary to determine cardiovascular stability. Percuss the thorax and abdomen to detect accumulations of fluid or air.[134,136] Needle marks, pill fragments, uneaten leaves or berries or drug paraphernalia assist in a diagnosis.[134,136] The presence of pressure areas on the skin may indicate how long the patient has been unresponsive. Any odours are important to note. An oily-garlicky smell may be due

TABLE 23.10

Acronyms outlining potential causes of altered levels of consciousness[133–136]

ACRONYM	CAUSE	ACRONYM	CAUSE
T	**T**rauma	A	**A**lcohol and other toxins
I	**I**nfection	E	**E**ndocrine
			Encephalopathy
P	**P**sychogenic		**E**lectrolyte abnormality
	Porphyria		
		I	**I**nsulin/diabetes
S	**S**eizure		
	Syncope	O	**O**xygen: hypoxia of any cause
	Space-occupying lesion		**O**piates
		U	**U**raemia

to pesticides. Other odours may indicate chronic medical disorders (e.g. fruity odour with diabetic ketoacidosis) or neglect of personal hygiene.[142,143]

Practice tip

Odours are important to note, as they may reflect not only poisoning but other medical disorders, for example a fruity odour may reflect diabetic ketoacidosis.

Toxicology screens include an analysis of serum and urine to determine the presence and amount of a substance. Laboratory levels are helpful but must be considered according to the nature of the substance and its rate of metabolism. Certain substances are sequestered in fatty tissues or are bound to serum proteins, and may be present with a misleadingly low serum level.[133,136] Serum electrolytes, non-electrolytes, osmolality, arterial blood gases and urine electrolytes are used to determine the patient's overall status or response to therapy. Continuous cardiac monitoring supplemented with a 12-lead ECG or invasive monitoring devices may be required to help provide symptomatic care.[134,136]

Initial and ongoing care of the victim follows three principles:[134,136]

1 preventing further absorption of the toxin
2 enhancing elimination of absorbed toxin from the body
3 preventing complications by providing symptomatic or specific treatments, including psychiatric management.

Management: Preventing toxin absorption

Ingested poisons are best removed while still in the upper gastrointestinal tract when possible. Emesis and gastric lavage were utilised in the past to empty the stomach, although a significant body of evidence now suggests that these are relatively ineffective and effectiveness decreases rapidly after 1 hour.[134,136] Both the patient and substance should be evaluated for appropriateness of gastric emptying.[134,136]

The patient's consciousness level, gag reflex and ability to vomit while protecting the airway from aspiration should be considered. Any central nervous system depressants are capable of obtunding the protective gag or cough reflex. If the ingested substance has a rapid onset of action, such as with benzodiazepines, it is safer to avoid emetics because of the risk of a sudden fall in the level of consciousness.[134,136]

Ingested poisons

Evaluate the substance ingested to determine whether gastric emptying is appropriate. The physical properties of a drug may make it more responsive to a particular type of gastric emptying. For example, the antimuscarinic effect of tricyclic antidepressants on gut motility can prolong gastrointestinal absorption, increasing plasma levels.[144] Also, consider the effects of substances on tissue. Corrosives, such as acids, alkalis and iron supplements, produce irritation and tissue breakdown when in contact with the skin or mucous membranes. Recognition is important, as therapy may cause further injury. Emesis could be contraindicated, and a lavage tube may further traumatise injured tissue.[145] Ipecac syrup and vomiting are generally ineffective against a substance with an antiemetic property, such as phenothiazines.[134,136] Waiting for emesis also causes further delay in definitive treatment. Other substances have natural emetic qualities if taken in sufficient doses (e.g. hand soaps and liquid soap detergents).[136]

Evaluate other substances on an individual basis. Most petroleum distillates, such as furniture polish or cleaning fluids, present a greater hazard for chemical pneumonitis than a systemic intoxication.[133] Even very small amounts can quickly disperse over the lung surface if accidentally introduced into the trachea. Avoid emesis or lavage when the chance of aspiration is high.[133] There are situations, however, when the amount, character or additional chemicals present make it necessary to remove the ingested substance from the stomach. Occasionally, therapy is based on the reported amount taken or time since ingestion. Time since ingestion is important in order to rule out the benefit of therapy. The stomach tends to empty its contents after 1 hour, unless a substance that slows gastric motility has been ingested. For example, narcotics can slow peristalsis and may be found in the stomach several hours after ingestion.[134,136] A patient may also underreport the dosage to avoid an obviously unpleasant experience. Although conservative management with observation is appropriate in certain situations, the risk of not treating might be greater in others.[134,136,146] If a large number of tablets or pills are consumed at one time, they may clump together in the stomach and form a mass that is too large to pass out of the pylorus (e.g. aspirin).[146]

Once a substance enters the lower gastrointestinal tract, it can be absorbed into the mesenteric circulation. As absorption can vary according to substance, slow-release characteristics, rate of peristalsis and the presence of other substances, it is possible for a poison to be present in the bowel for an extended period of time. If intestinal motility can be stimulated or the toxin permanently bound until excretion, then further absorption is reduced.[134,136] Activated charcoal is a refined product with an enormous surface area that binds to a large range of substances to enhance elimination, and is the most effective decontaminating agent currently available.[134,136]

A solution of either water or sorbitol is mixed with approximately 15–30 g of activated charcoal to form a thick, liquid slurry that can be given to a compliant patient orally or through a nasogastric tube. It may be mixed with a cathartic, which reduces the time the substance or the charcoal is in contact with the bowel wall, although there is no evidence that this improves clinical outcome.[134,136] However, there is no clinical evidence that adding cathartic agents such as sorbitol improves the clinical outcome.[134]

It has been suggested that effectiveness can be improved through repeated administration of activated charcoal, by ensuring that the entire drug is absorbed, as well as by interrupting the reabsorption of any drug in the enterohepatic circulation.[134] Cathartic agents such a sorbitol and polyethylene glycol reduce gastric transit time, reducing the time a drug spends in the gastrointestinal tract, in theory limiting the time available for drug absorption; however, this has not been demonstrated to significantly improve outcomes.[134,136] Unfortunately, not all poisons ingested can be bound by charcoal, such as alcohol and heavy metals.[134,136]

Inhaled poisons

A patient poisoned by inhalation of toxic gases or powders should be removed from the source as soon as it is safe to do so. Attempts to remove the substance, which is usually a vapour, gas or fine particulate matter, from the lung are not normally useful.[134,136] The history of a patient suspected of an inhaled poison should include time of exposure, the duration of exposure, the onset of symptoms, suspected inhalant and time since treatment began.

Staff involved in direct care of the patient should take precautions to avoid unprotected contact to reduce the risk of self-contamination with unknown substances. For many inhaled poisons clothing may contain significant amounts of the poison and serve as a continuous source of the toxin. Contaminated linen and clothes should be removed carefully, sealed in a bag and destroyed.[134,136]

Contact poisons

Contact poisons are dangerous because of their ability to enter the body via the skin or mucous membranes. All clothing and all of the toxic substance should be carefully removed, preferably with an irrigating and neutralising solution. Precautions to avoid direct skin contact and reduce the risk of self-contamination should be used. Clothing may contain significant residual amounts of the poison and serve as a continuous source of the toxin. Contaminated linen and clothes should be sealed in a bag and destroyed.[134,136]

Management: Enhancing elimination of the toxin from blood

After a substance has entered the bloodstream, it is normally excreted from the body either in an unchanged form or after liver metabolism and detoxification. Various metabolic byproducts are eliminated in the bile and faeces or urine. Urinary excretion of substances can be enhanced by increasing the filtration process by forcing diuresis and the administration of large volumes of IV solutions and/or diuretics. Enhanced secretion can also occur by inhibiting absorption in the renal tubules or by stimulating the secretion of substances into the urine.[134,136,146]

Alkalinisation of urine

Manipulation of the absorption or secretion process of a drug can be assisted by chemically altering the structure of some substances. All substances break down into ions at a specific pH for that substance. Altering the pH of urine with acidifying or alkalising drugs allows the poison to be forced into an ionic state and then excreted in the urine. This ion trapping process is effective only for substances that are primarily eliminated by the kidneys,[134,136] for example salicylates and tricyclic antidepressants.[134]

Haemodialysis or haemoperfusion

If a dangerous amount of a poison is present or if renal failure is evident, haemodialysis or haemoperfusion may be used to enhance excretion. Dialysis is effective in removing substances that are reversibly bound to serum proteins, or not stored in body fat, only. This is a highly invasive approach and is normally reserved for life-threatening cases (see Chapter 18 for further discussion).[133,136]

Management: Preventing complications and specific symptomatic care

Supportive care is the key element in managing an acutely poisoned patient. Once a patient has either ingested or been exposed to many poisons, there are limited options other than to treat the symptoms as they appear or become clinically significant (see Table 23.11).

TABLE 23.11
Summary of the management of poisoning victims[133–136]

AIM	ACTION
Prevent absorption of toxin	• Ingested toxins: activated charcoal is the most effective method of reducing adsorption • Inhaled toxins: remove victim from source of contamination and administer oxygen or provide fresh air • Contact toxins: remove any substances from the body surface, preferably with copious amounts of irrigating fluid. Remove clothing and place in a sealed bag to reduce vapour hazards. Use special caution with corrosive materials and pesticides
Enhance elimination of the toxin from the blood	Ingested or injected toxins: administer an antidote or antagonist if available (e.g. naloxone for opiates; flumazenil for benzodiazepines). Employ forced diuresis, for acidification or alkalinisation of the urine; and haemodialysis
Prevent complications by providing symptomatic or specific treatment	Carefully monitor all vital systems. Continually reassess patient for changes or response to therapy. Administer antidotes as prescribed. Provide symptomatic care as needed for: cardiac arrhythmias, CNS depression or stimulation, fluid and electrolyte imbalances, acid–base disturbances, renal function, effects of immobility

TABLE 23.12

Common emergency antidotes[133–136]

POISONING	ANTIDOTE
Benzodiazepines	Flumazenil
Opioids	Naloxone
Paracetamol	N-Acetylcysteine
Organophosphates	Atropine and pralidoxime
Tricyclic antidepressants	Sodium bicarbonate
Carbon monoxide	Oxygen
Insulin	Dextrose

Antidotes act to antagonise, compete with or override the effects of the poison, although few specific antidotes exist for toxins (see Table 23.12). In some cases, an absorbed toxin can be rendered benign by the use of an antidote (e.g. the interaction between naloxone and opiates). For chelating agents, such as desferrioxamine for iron poisoning, a non-toxic compound is formed that is then safely eliminated from the body.[133–136] The effect of an antidote may be only temporary if the antidote has a shorter half-life than the poison. Most antidotes are given either in a specific dose or at a response to dose rate.[133–136] For many poisonings, symptomatic care involves support and protection of vital organ systems. Routine and frequent physical assessment of respiratory, cardiovascular and renal function enables identification of potential problems. If large volumes of fluids or drugs that alter serum pH are administered, the patient's electrolyte and acid–base balance are also monitored.

A poisoning may be the physical manifestation of an emergency or crisis that requires emotional support. A patient may have underlying emotional conflict/s or mental health problems, regardless of whether the poisoning was intentional or accidental. Psychological care is, therefore, an important component for all patients presenting with poisoning.[133–136] Many facilities offer the services of a mental health worker while the patient is still in the ED. If the patient's condition is stable and the poisoning has not altered their mental state, early intervention is appropriate.

For adult patients, the desire for treatment is not as important as the manner in which treatment is received. Even though patients may initially refuse care, if approached in a non-threatening way and given some form of control, they will usually comply. If threatened with force or restraints, they are placed in the position of either submitting to coercion or resisting therapy in order to 'protect' themselves. A paediatric patient may be too young either to fully understand or to effectively cooperate with staff.

Central nervous system depressants

A large number of common medications are capable of depressing levels of consciousness, thought processes or important regulatory centres located within the central nervous system (CNS). The clinical findings associated with CNS alteration can vary a great deal from drug class to class or within the same drug family, as physical effects are dependent on the chemical structure of the drug, the dose, the route of exposure, any other co-ingested drugs and the rate of drug metabolism. In addition, the chemical structure and/or purity of illicit drugs may be affected by variations or deliberate aberrations in the manufacturing process.[147–149] Drugs in this section include sedatives, hypnotics, tranquillisers and narcotics.

Assessment

The predominant observed effect is an altered level of CNS function.[147–149] A spectrum of physical findings is possible with the selective action of the specific drug on inhibitory or excitatory centres of the brain: effects can vary from mild euphoria to convulsions, or mild sedation to coma, dependence, addiction and tolerance. Narcotics constrict the pupil, and some patients experience nausea and vomiting due to a stimulation of the chemoreceptor trigger zone in the medulla.[142,147–149]

A narcotic overdose is distinctive, with a set of readily identifiable features. These features include a decreased respiratory rate and tidal volume, constriction of the pupil, hypotension and an altered level of consciousness.[147–149] Other factors may, however, affect these findings as outlined in Box 23.3.

Patients with an altered level of consciousness are subject to injury from decreased sensory ability or prolonged immobilisation. Reddened areas over bony prominences or pressure points appear within a short

BOX 23.3

Factors confounding diagnosis of narcotic overdose[142,147–149]

- A decreased respiratory effort may produce hypercarbia, which in turn may cause pupil dilation.
- Chronic narcotic users tend to have multiple problems associated with their drug use or lifestyle, which may modify findings.
- CNS depressants in sufficiently high dose cause depression of vital regulatory centres in the brain.
- Altered respirations cause hypoventilation, stasis of secretions and atelectasis. The resultant hypoxia serves to further aggravate the sensorium and cerebral functioning.[149]
- Narcotics may produce idiopathic pulmonary oedema.[142,147–149]
- CNS depressants often possess the ability to cause peripheral vasodilation, with a resultant hypotension and tachycardia.
- Arrhythmias may occur because of cardiac conduction effects or tissue hypoxia.[142,147–149]

time. Skin blisters indicate altered blood flow, usually due to excessive pressure. Actual skin breakdown can occur within 3 hours. If external pressure or altered circulation to an extremity is allowed to continue for over 4 hours, compartment syndrome may develop.[147–149]

Effects of multiple drug use

A patient who ingests a combination of drugs may experience toxicity because of additive or synergistic effects.[147–149] Illicitly produced drugs will most likely have had substances added (e.g. glucose powders, icing sugar, talcum powder) to dilute or 'cut' them, to increase the volume of their supply and thus profit to the supplier.[147–149] Users may also intentionally inject other drugs (e.g. antihistamines, amphetamines, benzodiazepines) to modify or potentiate the effects of narcotics.[147–149]

Potential for acute or active infections

The use of non-sterile solutions and equipment and the sharing of injection equipment significantly increase the likelihood of acute or active infections. Frequent exposure and a depressed immune response also predispose a patient to severe infections, such as hepatitis, osteomyelitis, infective bacterial endocarditis and encephalitis/meningitis.[147–149]

Management

General principles for the management of a patient with ingestion of a toxic substance with a reduced level of consciousness apply. Prevent continued absorption by administering activated charcoal for oral ingestions, and provide symptomatic care (see Table 23.13).[147–149]

Central nervous system stimulants

CNS stimulants increase the activity of the reticular activating system, promoting a state of alertness and affecting the medullary control centres for respiratory and cardiovascular function. Many illegal stimulants are poorly manufactured, with no guarantee of purity or consistency in dosage. The possibility of overdose is therefore always present, producing profound CNS excitation.[147–149] Commonly used stimulants include amphetamines, dextroamphetamine, methylphenidate, lysergic acid diethylamide (LSD), phencyclidine (PCP), caffeine, cocaine and methamphetamines[147,150] (see Table 23.13).

Assessment

Both psychological and physical symptoms are produced. A patient may demonstrate repetitive, non-purposeful movements, grind their teeth and appear suspicious of or paranoid about others. Physiological stimulation causes an increase in metabolism, with flushing, diaphoresis, hyperpyrexia, pupillary dilation and vomiting evident. Dizziness, loss of coordination, chest pains, palpitations or abdominal cramps may also occur. During the acute phase of poisoning, severe intoxication and loss of rational mental functioning may lead individuals to behave irrationally and even attempt suicide. Anxiousness and a general state of tension may also lead the affected person to attempt to harm others.[147,150] Death is possible from cardiovascular collapse or as a sequela to convulsions and acute drug toxicity.[147,150]

Management

If a patient has ingested the drug, emesis or lavage is of little value, and an individual risk–benefit assessment is

---

TABLE 23.13

Assessment and management of specific drug overdoses[147–149,153–155]

TYPE OF POISONING	GENERAL MANAGEMENT	ANTIDOTE	CLINICAL CONSIDERATIONS
CNS depressants (morphine, heroin, methadone, oxycodone)	Supportive care of airway, breathing, circulation	Naloxone hydrochloride (Narcan); specific reversal agent	Action of naloxone may be much shorter than the duration of effect of the drug; the patient may need to be observed for return of unconsciousness
CNS stimulants	Supportive care of airway, breathing, circulation	Benzodiazepines may be used to reduce symptoms	Reduce stimulation in the surrounding environment; monitor cardiovascular status and temperature
Salicylate	Observe for hyperventilation and acid–base disturbances	Nil; charcoal may be used	Monitor electrolyte changes and increases in fever
Paracetamol	Careful history required to determine time and amount taken; initially vague symptoms	N-Acetylcysteine	Antidote must be given within the specified time range; consider the effects of other drugs (i.e. paracetamol and codeine combinations); monitor for signs of hepatotoxicity
Carbon monoxide	Supportive care of airway, breathing, circulation	High concentrations of oxygen therapy	Hyperbaric oxygen may be required; monitor carboxyhaemoglobin; oxygen saturation monitors will give erroneously high readings
Organophosphates	Decontamination; supportive care of airway, breathing, circulation	Pralidoxime chloride; benzodiazepines	Maintain careful decontamination and personal safety considerations

required. Gastric emptying may precipitate more severe agitation with a concomitant rise in blood pressure, pulse rate and metabolism.[147,150] Activated charcoal and cathartics may be administered to promote elimination. Ongoing emergency management includes:

- support of vital functions[147,150]
- reduction of external stimulation by placing the patient in a quiet, non-threatening environment where a supportive person can attempt to calm and 'talk the person down' while observing for untoward reactions
- sedating when necessary, although it is not desirable to give more medications in a precarious situation; sedation may be needed to control seizures or keep the patient from self-harm.[147,150]

> **Practice tip**
>
> Note that there are no specific antidotes for CNS stimulants.

Amphetamines and designer drugs

Amphetamines and designer drugs have been drugs of abuse for a number of years. Originally, many of them were designed and introduced as anaesthetic agents, decongestants or for other legitimate purposes. Amphetamines are chemically related to the anaesthetic ketamine, with a similar CNS response.[147,150] Most drugs in this group were discontinued or controlled because of the delirium and agitation experienced by the patients who had received them; paradoxically, these effects led to their popularity as recreational drugs.[147,150] Amphetamines are synthetic sympathomimetic drugs; they are available in oral, intranasal or IV forms; crystalline rock forms such as 'ice' are smoked. Death may occur from overdose, self-mutilation or dangerous activities such as diving or walking on roads.[147,150,151]

Assessment

Depending on the dose, route and time since exposure, a person exhibits characteristic behavioural and physical changes. With high-dose intoxication, the patient has pronounced CNS involvement – altered levels of consciousness, seizure activity or a loss of protective gag, corneal and swallow reflexes. Nystagmus is a classic sign, along with hypertension and an elevated body temperature. A significant rise in arterial pressure presents a risk for intracerebral haemorrhage. One of the distinguishing features of amphetamines is their ability to produce coma without affecting respirations.[147,150] The patient may risk dehydration and renal failure if muscle breakdown has occurred. A high urine output should be maintained and serum urea and creatinine levels monitored to detect a decrease in renal function.[147,150]

Lower dose intoxications do not produce unconsciousness but typically cause behavioural patterns that reflect depersonalisation and distorted perceptions

of events or other people. The patient's physical and mental responses may be dulled and slow, or abusive and delusional. Intoxication is marked by paranoid thoughts, with the patient responding to therapeutic or friendly gestures with behaviours ranging from apprehension to aggressive hostility. To avoid stimulating the patient and thereby intensifying the behaviour, a quiet environment should be provided for initial assessment and treatment, although this is often difficult in the ED.[147,150]

> **Practice tip**
>
> Noxious environmental stimulation such as bright lighting, loud noises and activity can provoke these patients to become anxious and uncooperative.

Management

Gastric emptying is normally ineffective due to delays in seeking treatment. If a patient presents early, activated charcoal and cathartics are useful in preventing further absorption. Noises, sights and sounds provoke paranoid ideation and may present a risk to staff and other patients. 'Talking down' is usually not successful and probably only serves to exacerbate the situation. If the patient is demonstrating hostile or self-abusive forms of behaviour, restraints may be needed to protect him/her and any others present. The use of physical restraints is not without danger, and they should never be used as a substitute for a more desirable environment. If the threat of danger or psychosis is significant, sedatives such as diazepam or haloperidol may be necessary to control the patient's behaviour. IV diazepam is also used to control frequent seizure activity.[147,150]

Salicylate poisoning

Aspirin is the commonest form of salicylate in the home and is found in many over-the-counter medications, such as combination analgesic and topical ointments.[152] Aspirin may be ingested orally, absorbed through the rectal mucosa, or applied to the skin in topical preparations. Under normal circumstances, the kidneys serve as the principal organ of excretion. At one time, aspirin was the commonest form of poisoning in children.[140,152,153] In response to the problem, legislation has been implemented to limit the number of tablets per pack and to introduce packaging with childproof caps. In Australia salicylate poisoning is now relatively uncommon, accounting for about 0.3% of calls to poison information centres.[154] The three common types of aspirin overdose are: accidental ingestion (more common in young children); intentional ingestion (more common in adults); and chronic toxicity (occurs in any age group).[146,154]

Assessment, monitoring and diagnostics

Intentional or accidental ingestion is straightforward, with a clear history of poisoning. Chronic toxicity is, however, often unrecognised. Many individuals are not aware of correct dosages, may combine multiple drugs, each of which contains aspirin, or may have impaired excretion due to dehydration. The symptoms of chronic aspirin overdose include dehydration, lethargy and fever and resemble the original problem being treated, and some people will continue treating themselves with aspirin for these symptoms. Chronic toxicity has a higher mortality than acute ingestion.[146,154]

Toxicity may result if aspirin is ingested in amounts greater than 150 mg/kg. Aspirin toxicity can result in tachypnoea, fever, tinnitus, disorientation, coma and convulsions.[146,154] Acid–base disturbances arise from a direct stimulatory effect on the respiratory centre in the CNS. An increased rate and depth of respirations causes hypocarbia and respiratory alkalosis, with renal compensation by bicarbonate elimination. However, salicylates also alter metabolic processes, resulting in metabolic acidosis. Blood gases can therefore reflect acidosis, alkalosis or a combination of the two. Tinnitus is a symptom of the effect of aspirin on the 8th cranial nerve.[146,154]

Aspirin interferes with cellular glucose uptake, causing initial hyperglycaemia. Cellular levels of glucose become depleted and the patient then demonstrates hypoglycaemic effects, particularly those related to the central nervous system. Later, serum levels may be either normal or hypoglycaemic.[146,154] Patients may be nauseated and vomit after ingestion, causing fluid and electrolyte imbalance.[146,154] Aspirin use is also associated with local tissue irritation and gastrointestinal bleeding. Normal platelet function is altered by aspirin, with an increased tendency for bleeding. Concomitant use of anticoagulants increases the risk of haemorrhage.[146,154]

Management

Absorption can be reduced with activated charcoal. Repeat doses should be given for patients with signs of ongoing absorption.[146,153,154] Urine alkalisation and forced diuresis can significantly increase elimination, as salicylates are weak acids excreted by the kidneys.[146,153,154] Haemodialysis is reserved for extreme cases with profound acidosis, high blood levels, persistent CNS symptoms or renal failure.[146,154]

As salicylates have no known specific antidote,[146,153,154] supportive therapy includes prevention of dehydration by carefully monitoring fluid output and providing adequate fluid replacement and monitoring serum electrolytes for imbalance and replacing as needed. Evaluate arterial blood gases to determine whether the patient continues to have an effect from aspirin toxicity or is not responding to therapy. Temperature elevations should be controlled with external cooling methods if fever develops.

Paracetamol poisoning

The incidence of paracetamol, also known as acetaminophen, toxicity is associated with approximately half of all Australasian toxic ingestions, due in part to its common availability as an analgesic/antipyretic agent.[140,152] The drug is absorbed in the stomach and small bowel, with 98% metabolised by the liver using one of two mechanisms: most is via a pathway that breaks down into non-toxic byproducts; the second hepatic pathway usually metabolises about 4% of the drug, but the process has a toxic byproduct. The liver is capable of detoxifying the toxic byproduct by combining it with a naturally occurring substance, glutathione. In an overdose or when the minor pathway has already been stimulated (e.g. concomitant barbiturate use), more paracetamol is metabolised by the secondary pathway and the toxic byproduct accumulates, quickly consuming the available glutathione, resulting in liver tissue destruction.[140,152,155]

Assessment, monitoring and diagnostics

The amount of paracetamol ingested is best determined from the patient history, as serum levels, although helpful, can be easily distorted. A nomogram is used to plot measured levels against time post-ingestion as a relative indicator of toxicity. A relatively small dose of 200 mg/kg paracetamol is considered to be toxic, although hepatotoxicity occurs after an ingestion of 140 mg/kg or 10 g in a single dose.[152,155–157]

Liver function studies are helpful to recognise the development of hepatic dysfunction or damage. These include liver enzymes, serum bilirubin, protein, prothrombin time, partial thromboplastin time and platelets.[140,152,155] Three phases of toxic damage resulting from excess paracetamol are presented in Table 23.14.[140,152,155–157]

TABLE 23.14

Phases of toxic damage resulting from an excess of paracetamol[140,152,155–157]

PHASE	TIMEFRAME	SYMPTOMS
Phase 1	First 24 hours	Vague symptoms of nausea, vomiting and malaise
Phase 2	24–48 hours	Vague symptoms subside; onset of right upper quadrant pain due to hepatic injury; urine output may decrease as paracetamol potentiates the effect of antidiuretic hormone; liver enzymes, bilirubin, proteins and clotting studies may be abnormal
Phase 3	60–72 hours	Liver impairment becomes more obvious, with jaundice, coagulation defects, hypoglycaemia and hepatic encephalopathy; renal failure or cardiomyopathy may also occur; death from hepatic failure occurs in approximately 10% of severe overdose

Management

Absorption can be reduced with activated charcoal when the patient presents to hospital early; however, following periods of 2 hours or greater since ingestion activated charcoal is unlikely to be very effective. Haemodialysis with a charcoal dialysate has been used in an attempt to remove unchanged paracetamol from the liver, but this does not remove the toxic byproduct. Forced diuresis is also not effective, because little paracetamol (about 2%) is removed by the kidneys.[140,152,155]

The specific therapy for paracetamol poisoning is administration of the antidote, N-acetylcysteine, which is structurally similar to glutathione and binds to the toxic byproduct. When given within 24 hours of an acute ingestion, N-acetylcysteine is effective in preventing hepatic damage. [140,152,155]

Carbon monoxide poisoning

Carbon monoxide is a gaseous byproduct of incomplete fuel combustion, and is present where there is a flame in a confined space with improper ventilation or air exchange. Levels of carbon monoxide can accumulate rapidly, and the gas is dangerous as it is colourless, odourless, tasteless and non-irritating[156,158,159] Common sources of carbon monoxide are faulty radiant heaters, kerosene lamps, cooking stoves, engine exhausts and fireplaces. Acute carbon monoxide poisoning is the commonest form of successful poisoning in three of the world's most developed countries.[156,158,159]

Assessment, monitoring and diagnostics

Haemoglobin has a 210–240-fold greater affinity for carbon monoxide than for oxygen, and shifts the oxygen–haemoglobin curve to the left (see Chapter 13). As carbon monoxide displaces oxygen from red blood cells, the patient experiences hypoxaemia and hypoxia.[156,158,159] Headache, nausea and vague pains are often experienced at onset of poisoning, and the patient may feel increasingly tired and sleepy, have difficulty concentrating and fail to recognise the onset of poisoning. With higher levels of inhalation, the patient may be tachypnoeic, tachycardic and experience loss of consciousness. A characteristic red colour presents in the lips with skin flushing.[156,158,159] The most important factors in determining carbon monoxide poisoning are a history of exposure with an elevated blood carboxyhaemoglobin level.[156,158,159]

Management

As CO is an inhaled toxin, the patient should be removed from the contaminated environment to prevent further absorption and allowed to breathe fresh air until 100% oxygen can be administered, although this may be ineffective because of the bond between carbon monoxide and haemoglobin. High flow high concentration oxygen administration will, however, substantially reduce the half-life of carbon monoxide.[159] Hyperbaric oxygenation is used to treat severe cases of carbon monoxide poisoning, as pressurised oxygen reduces the half-life of the carboxyhaemoglobin molecule and shortens the duration of its effects.

Mild-to-moderate poisoning can be managed without the use of hyperbaric oxygen, as hyperbaric oxygenation is not available at every facility. Treatment depends on carboxyhaemoglobin serum levels, time since exposure, transport time to the hyperbaric chamber and the clinical symptoms of the patient.[156,158,159] Patients should be monitored for adverse effects of hypoxia, as they may have convulsions, cardiac arrhythmias and acid–base disturbances.

Corrosive acids

A number of substances are discussed here due to their similar ability to cause local tissue injury. Some common acids involved in toxic emergencies are acetic acid (vinegar), carbolic acid (phenol disinfectants), chlorine (swimming pools, sanitising agents), hydrochloric acid (pools, cleaning agents), hydrofluoric oxalic (laundry agents), sodium bisulfate (toilet cleaning agents that become acidic when added to water) and sulfuric acid (car battery acid).

Ingested corrosives can produce immediate or late life-threatening complications. In general, acids dissolve tissue and destroy haemoglobin.[160] Swallowing a strong acid can produce ulceration and perforation of oral and oesophageal mucosa, presenting a danger for haemorrhage and mediastinitis, and cardiac arrest as a result.[160,161] The late sequelae of swallowing a corrosive substance involve mucosal scarring with constriction and mechanical obstruction of the oesophagus.

Assessment

Physical findings are site-specific and relate to the type of exposure – ingestion, inhalation or contact (see Table 23.15). Ingested acids present as burns to the mouth and pharynx. Patients able to vocalise complain of pain, gastric irritation with vomiting and haematemesis. Fumes

---

TABLE 23.15

Summary of assessment and management of acid and alkali exposure[160–162]

	CORROSIVE ACIDS OR CORROSIVE ALKALIS
Assessment	• Burns to skin, mouth, pharynx or oesophagus • Gastric irritation with nausea and vomiting
Management	• Airway • Breathing • Circulation • Decontamination
Prevent absorption	• Do not induce vomiting • Remove contaminated clothing • Flush the skin with copious amounts of water
Enhance elimination	• Administer chelating agents if they exist, such as calcium gluconate for hydrofluoric acid
Symptomatic management	• Protect burnt skin with sterile dressings • Monitor respiratory status

from an ingested substance may cause pneumonitis. Contact with skin or eyes is similar to other types of burns, with a sharply defined blister or wound, inflammation, pain and ulceration. Hypotension and cardiovascular collapse are also possible when damage occurs to underlying vital structures.[160,162]

Inhalation irritates respiratory tissues, producing direct damage, oedema and alterations in ventilation. Patients may initially experience coughing, choking, gasping for air and increased respiratory secretions. Clinicians should assess and monitor any obvious tissue injury, impaired respiratory function and subsequent effects of hypoxia and pulmonary oedema, which may occur up to 6–8 hours later.[145,160,162] Arterial blood gases, ventilation studies, serial chest X-rays and frequent physical assessments are used to monitor for changes.

Management

Contaminated clothing should be removed to prevent recontamination. Patients with external contamination should be washed thoroughly to remove any remaining surface material that may come into contact with treating staff. For acid contact with skin or eyes, begin immediate flushing with a non-reactive liquid and continue to do so for at least 15 minutes to guarantee complete removal. In most cases water will be the safest and best available liquid. Provide skin or eye protection with a sterile dressing.[145]

For ingested acids, emesis or lavage should not be attempted, as the substance will cause additional damage when ejected from the stomach. A gastric tube may also cause structural damage by penetrating or irritating friable tissues.[145,160] Do not attempt to neutralise the acid, as this may result in a chemical reaction and generate heat as a byproduct, with potential further burning and damage to the patient.[145,160] Suctioning of oral secretions should be done carefully and with as much visualisation of tissues as possible. A patient may be given water or milk to irrigate the upper gastrointestinal tract, although extreme care is required to ensure that the airway is adequately protected because there is a risk of aspiration.[160]

Corrosive alkalis

Alkalis produce tissue destruction on contact by interacting with tissue component fats and proteins and producing necrotic tissue. Erosion of the oesophagus and stomach occurs if ingested orally, and peritonitis or mediastinitis may develop as sequelae. Late effects are similar to those produced by acids. Oesophageal strictures due to scarring are common post-ingestion. About 25% of patients who ingest a strong alkali will die from the initial insult.[160]

Skin contact and ingestion are the commonest types of injury from an alkali; however, ingestion is the most immediately life-threatening form of contact. Alkalis involved in toxic emergencies include many substances found around the house, such as detergents and cleaning agents that contain ammonia; cement and builder's lime; low-phosphate detergents; dishwasher detergents that contain sodium carbonate; and laundry bleaches that contain sodium hypochlorite.[160]

Assessment

The immediate response to ingestion is increased secretions, pain, vomiting or haemoptysis. Signs of perforation include fever, respiratory difficulty or peritonitis. Approximately 98% of patients develop strictures.[145,160,161] Alkalis and skin contact produce a soap-like substance because of the interaction with tissue fats, giving a slimy, soapy feeling.[145,160,161]

Management

Induced vomiting or gastric lavage should not be attempted for ingested alkalis, as these will be neutralised by stomach acid. Lavage tubes may cause further tissue damage.[145,160,161] External contact with alkalis necessitates copious irrigation of the point of contact. Continue irrigation for at least 15 minutes; in the case of the eye, irrigation may be necessary for up to 30 minutes. Cover all wounds after irrigation with sterile dressings to reduce the risk of infection.

A patient should be nil by mouth until an inspection of the mouth and throat is conducted to determine the amount and extent of burns. An oesophagoscopy will identify the degree of injury and enable direct irrigation of any affected areas of mucosa.[145] Alkalis that contain phosphates may produce a systemic hypocalcaemia, and IV calcium gluconate may be required. Continue to monitor for systemic effects of perforation or tissue injury.[145]

Petroleum distillates

Petroleum distillates are common substances, and account for 7% of all poisonings.[163] Typical petroleum products are benzene, fuel oils, petrol, kerosene, lacquer diluents, lubricating oil, mineral oil, naphthalene, paint thinners and petroleum spirits. Toxicity depends on: route of exposure (ingestion or aspiration); volatility (ease with which the substance evaporates); viscosity (density or thickness); amount ingested; and presence of other toxins.[163]

Products with a low viscosity are more likely to be aspirated and can quickly spread over the lung surface. Substances with low viscosity and high volatility, for example benzene, kerosene, and turpentine, are toxic in doses as low as 1 mL/kg, with death from doses of 10–250 mL. Mortality is increased if an additional toxic substance is present, or if accidental aspiration occurs.[163]

Assessment

Aspiration causes pneumonitis with low-grade fever, tachypnoea, coughing, choking, gagging and pulmonary oedema as a late effect.[163,164] As petroleum distillates are fat solvents and rapidly cross the lipid-rich cell membrane, nerve tissue is especially sensitive to injury. A patient may exhibit local effects, such as depressed nerve conduction, or varied central effects, such as feelings of wellbeing, headache, tinnitus, dizziness, visual disturbances, through to respiratory depression, altered levels of consciousness, convulsions and coma.[164]

Management

In the awake and alert patient, the decision to treat is based on the physical properties of the substance, the likelihood of aspiration or other complications and the amount consumed.[163,164] When preventing absorption, careful consideration needs to be given to gastric emptying, as neither induced vomiting nor gastric lavage is recommended.

The patient's respiratory status should be immediately assessed for possible aspiration. A patient that is coughing, has cyanosis or appears hypoxic may have aspirated or developed chemical pneumonitis.[145] If the patient is lethargic or unconscious, an endotracheal tube must be placed for adequate airway protection,[145,163,164] although this heightens the risk of aspiration as hydrocarbons adhere to the tube and increase the risk of chemical pneumonitis.[145,163,164]

Organophosphates

Organophosphates are a large and diverse group of chemicals used in domestic, industrial and agricultural settings (e.g. insecticides, herbicides).[133,143] The primary effect of organophosphates is binding and inactivation of acetylcholinesterase, a neurotransmitter that metabolises acetylcholine.[133,143]

Organophosphates can be absorbed through the skin, ingested or inhaled. Although most patients become symptomatic soon after ingestional exposure, the onset and duration of action depend on the nature and type of compound, the degree and route of exposure, the mode of action of the compound, its lipid solubility and rate of metabolic degradation.[133,143,165]

Mortality rates range from 3% to 25%, with organophosphate poisonings the commonest mode of suicide in some developing countries, including Sri Lanka and Fiji.[166] In one Australian study, 36% of patients had suicidal intentions, compared with 65–75% in developing countries.[166] Men aged 30–50 years were more likely to attempt suicide with organophosphates. Common complications include respiratory distress, seizures and aspiration pneumonia, with respiratory failure the commonest cause of death.[166]

Assessment, monitoring and diagnostics

The clinical findings of organophosphate poisoning can be divided into three broad categories: muscarinic effects, nicotinic effects and effects on the central nervous system. Common muscarinic manifestations are summarised by the mnemonic SLUDGE: **S**alivation, **L**acrimation, **U**rination, **D**efecation, **G**I upset, **E**mesis.[133,143,165] Other symptoms include bradycardia, hypotension, bronchospasm, cough, abdominal pain, blurred vision, miosis and sweating. Nicotinic effects include muscle fasciculations, cramping, weakness and diaphragmatic failure. Autonomic effects include hypertension, tachycardia, pupillary dilation and pallor.

CNS effects include anxiety, restlessness, confusion, ataxia, seizures, insomnia, dysarthria, tremors, coma and paralysis. The three types of paralysis that may result from organophosphate poisoning are described in Table 23.16.[133,143,165,166]

Laboratory diagnosis is based on the measurement of cholinesterase activity using either erythrocyte or plasma levels; erythrocyte cholinesterase is more accurate, but plasma cholinesterase is easier to test and is more widely available. Erythrocyte acetylcholinesterase is found in the grey matter of the central nervous system, red blood cells, peripheral nerve and muscle. Plasma cholinesterase circulates in plasma and is found in white matter of the central nervous system, pancreas and heart.[133,143,165,166] Mild poisoning is when the cholinesterase activity is reduced to 20–50% of normal; moderate poisoning occurs when activity is 10–20% of normal; and severe poisoning occurs at less than 10% of normal cholinesterase enzyme activity. Levels do not, however, always correlate with clinical illness.[143]

Management

Initial priorities in managing organophosphate poisoning are airway, breathing and circulation, incorporating D for danger, as organophosphates also present considerable risk to staff caring for the patient, especially during the initial phases of management. All of the patient's clothing should be removed and considered as hazardous waste. The patient's

---

TABLE 23.16

Types of paralysis that may result from organophosphate poisoning[133,143,165,166]

TYPE	ONSET	PRESENTATION	DURATION OF SYMPTOMS
Type 1	Occurs shortly after exposure	Acute paralysis secondary to persistent depolarisation at the neuromuscular junction	
Type 2	24–96 hours after resolution of acute cholinergic poisoning	Paralysis and respiratory distress. Proximal muscle groups are involved, with relative sparing of distal muscle groups	Up to 3 weeks
Type 3	2–3 weeks after exposure to large doses of certain organophosphates	Distal muscle weakness with relative sparing of the neck muscles, cranial nerves and proximal muscle groups	Up to 12 months

decontamination with soap and water is a priority, as soap with a high pH breaks down organophosphates.[143,165] Staff must use personal protective equipment, such as neoprene or nitrile gloves, and gowns are worn when decontaminating patients. Charcoal cartridge masks for respiratory protection are useful, although recent evidence suggests that the nosocomial risk to staff may not be as significant as was once thought.[165] Intubation is commonly required after significant exposure, due to respiratory distress from laryngospasm, bronchospasm or severe bronchorrhoea. Continuous cardiac monitoring and an ECG are used to check for bradycardias. Activated charcoal is used for gastric decontamination for those patients who have ingested organophosphate. The mainstay of treatment is atropine and pralidoxime, with a benzodiazepine used for seizure control.[165,166] Atropine blocks acetylcholine receptors and halts the cholinergic stimulation. Very large doses of atropine are usually required, 1–2 g IV, and repeated if muscle weakness is not relieved or the signs of poisoning recur. Clearing of bronchial secretions is the end point of atropine administration, not pupil size or the absolute dose.[133,165,166] Pralidoxime hydrochloride reactivates acetylcholinesterase and is effective at restoring skeletal muscle function, but is less effective at reversing muscarinic signs. Over time, the bond between organophosphate and cholinesterase becomes permanent and the effectiveness of pralidoxime diminishes[165,166] The current recommendation is administration within 48 hours of organophosphate poisoning.[166] Benzodiazepines are clinically indicated through their binding to specific receptor sites, potentiating the effects of gamma-aminobutyrate and facilitating inhibitory transmitters for management of seizures.[133,143,165,166]

Envenomation

Venomous animals can be land-based or marine-based, and their distribution ranges from broad to very specific locations. Exposure of humans to venom produces a large and varied range of symptomatology, which often results in an emergency presentation. It is therefore important for critical care nurses to be familiar with the types of potentially venomous animals inhabiting the catchment area of their health setting. From a first aid perspective it is vital nurses are familiar with the presentation and management of specific life-threatening or injury causing envenomations, including the use of antivenom when one exists. Most countries have local poison information centres for advice from expert toxicologists (see *Online resources*). Common envenomations across Australia and New Zealand are described below.

Redback/katipo spider bite

Description and incidence

The redback spider (*Latrodectus hasseltii*) is found throughout Australia but more commonly in temperate regions. Tasmania has the lowest frequency of reported bites, while areas around Alice Springs, Perth and Brisbane are especially infested.[167] The redback spider is easily identifiable by the presence of a red, orange or brownish stripe on its characteristic black, globular abdomen. The female is much larger than the male; generally only the female is considered dangerous. Juveniles are smaller, more variably coloured and may lack any spots or stripes. Bites from both male and juvenile spiders may result in symptoms, although these tend to be less significant than bites from females.[168]

The redback spider has also become established outside Australia, including in New Zealand, Japan and South America.[168,169] Although bites are rare, small populations of redback spiders have been reported in Central Otago (South Island) and New Plymouth (North Island) since the early 1980s.[168,169] The only other venomous spider in New Zealand is the katipo (*Latrodectus katipo*) from the same genus as the redback. The katipo has a black, rounded body, slender legs and a red stripe on the abdomen. Adult males and juveniles are black and white and are smaller than females.[170] Symptoms of katipo spider bite are similar to those of the redback spider and, where indicated, redback antivenom is used to treat bites.

A redback spider bite is a frequent cause for ED presentations and the most clinically significant spider bite in Australia.[168,171] Most bites are minor, with either minimal or no symptoms and requiring no antivenom. In approximately 20% of cases, significant envenomation occurs and antivenom administration is generally indicated, although death is extremely unlikely in untreated cases.[172] Redback antivenom is the most commonly administered antivenom in Australia.[168]

Clinical manifestations

Envenomation by a redback spider is known as latrodectism; the venom contains excitatory neurotoxins that stimulate release of catecholamines from sympathetic nerves and acetylcholine from motor nerve endings.[168,172] Signs and symptoms associated with a significant envenomation are distinctive, and diagnosis is by clinical findings. Initially, there is a minor sting at the bite site, where the spider may or may not have been seen. Over the first hour the bite becomes progressively painful to severe, spreading proximally with and involving swollen and tender local lymph nodes. Localised sweating at the bite site or limb or generalised sweating may appear, associated with hypertension and malaise. Pain eventually becomes generalised and may be expressed as chest, abdominal, head or neck pain suggestive of other acute conditions such as myocardial infarction.[171]

Progression of symptoms generally occurs in less than 6 hours but may take up to 24 hours. People with minor untreated bites may experience symptoms for several weeks.[168,172] Other less common signs and symptoms include local piloerection, nausea, vomiting, headache, fever, restlessness/insomnia, tachycardia and neurological symptoms such as muscle weakness or twitching.[168,172,173]

Assessment

Patients presenting with pain from a bite who have the offending spider with them are straightforward in terms of initial assessment. Identification of the spider is confirmed and a history of the event obtained, including the time of the bite and any first aid initiated. A brief assessment of the bite site and the involved limb is undertaken, including the extent of pain, presence of sweating and painful tender lymph nodes, and a baseline set of vital signs. Patients are then placed in a suitable area for medical assessment and ongoing observation.[173]

Adult patients presenting with vague limb pain, or preverbal children who are 'distressed' and 'cannot be settled', may be unaware that they have been bitten by a redback. The pain may not have been felt at the time of the bite and no spider may have been seen. Thorough history taking, physical assessment and knowledge of the effects of latrodectism enable detection of a suspected spider bite.[173]

Management

There is no recommended definitive first aid for a redback spider bite. Application of cold packs to the bite site and administration of simple analgesia, such as paracetamol, may assist with local pain relief. The use of a pressure immobilisation bandage is not necessary, as symptom progression is slow and not life-threatening,[168,172–174] and will cause further pain only in the affected limb. Remove any pressure bandage that was applied during first aid after identification of the spider is confirmed.[168]

Presence of the above symptoms (pain, swelling, localised sweating at the site) indicates systemic envenomation requiring administration of redback spider antivenom.[168,172] Prior to administration, the patient should be placed in a clinical area with readily available resuscitation equipment to treat any anaphylactic reaction, although this is rare. An IV cannula is inserted and adrenaline 1:1000 is prepared for the possibility of anaphylaxis.

The initial dose of Redback Spider Antivenom is 2 ampoules administered intramuscularly (IM) (500 units; approximately 1.5 mL each ampoule), and symptoms should subside over the next 30–60 minutes. Complete resolution of symptoms requires no specific further treatment. If there has not been complete resolution of symptoms after 2 hours a further 2 doses of antivenom are given. If after a further 2 hours there is incomplete resolution of symptoms or no discernable response after 4 ampoules of antivenom, expert advice should be sought via the local poison information centre. Patients who are symptom-free after 6 hours of observation or the admin-istration of antivenom can be discharged home with instructions to re-present should any symptoms return. Antivenom may be effective days after the bite, and possibly longer; however, a larger amount of antivenom is usually required.[168,172] IV administration has been advocated in severe cases or where there is poor response to IM administration.[168,172] The manufacturer recommends that, for life-threatening envenomation, the IV route may be used after first diluting the antivenom to 1:10 with Hartmann's solution and the antivenom administered over 20 minutes.[172,175] IV administration is safe with reactions uncommon (less than 5%).[176] No significant benefit of IV

administration over IM administration was demonstrated in a randomised controlled trial, so there is little evidence to justify one route of administration over another.[176] Redback spider antivenom administration in various stages of pregnancy has not been associated with direct or indirect harmful effects to the fetus.[168,172]

> **Practice tip**
>
> Observations for the development or progression of symptoms of a redback envenomation focus on development of local pain that spreads proximally and increases in intensity, development of sweating (either local or generalised) and hypertension.

Funnel-web spider bite

Description and incidence

Funnel-web spiders are the most venomous spiders to humans worldwide,[173,177] and Australian funnel-web spiders (*Atrax* or *Hadronyche* genera) are found primarily along the east coast. The Sydney funnel-web spider (*Atrax robustus*) is found mainly around Sydney, while other species are found in eastern New South Wales and central and southern Queensland. The spider is large, black or dark brown and approximately 3 cm long in the body. Male spiders have smaller bodies and are significantly more toxic than females.[177]

Clinical manifestations

Funnel-web spider bites are potentially rapidly lethal; however, only 10–20% of bites result in systemic enven-omation, with the majority being minor and not requiring antivenom. The bite is extremely painful, and fang marks may be seen. Signs and symptoms of systemic enven-omation may appear within 10 minutes, and include perioral tingling and tongue fasciculation, increased salivation, lacrimation, piloerection, sweating; nausea, vomiting, headache; hypertension, tachycardia; dyspnoea, pulmonary oedema; irritability, decreased consciousness and coma.[172,178] Regardless of the presence of symptoms, all possible funnel-web spider bites are managed as a medical emergency.[172]

Assessment

Patients with suspected funnel-web spider bites are rapidly assessed for the presence of any signs and symptoms of envenomation and allocated an ATS triage category of 1–3, based on presenting symptoms. A pressure immobili-sation bandage is applied if this was not done during initial first aid. Patients with signs of envenomation are moved to a resuscitation area for immediate treatment, including urgent antivenom administration and management of the clinical effects of envenomation. Monitoring and assessment for potentially serious manifestations focus on:

- airway compromise due to decreased level of consciousness, requiring airway protection with an airway adjunct or endotracheal intubation

- breathing for respiratory compromise due to pulmonary oedema, requiring continuous positive airway pressure or intubation/ventilation with positive end-expiratory pressure (see Chapter 15)
- circulatory compromise due to profound hypotension, although a late sign with hypertension more commonly seen, requires IV access and volume replacement. Circulatory compromise/failure may lead to cardiac arrest requiring cardiopulmonary resuscitation (see Chapter 25).

All patients require full monitoring with constant nursing observation. A patient with no signs of envenomation on arrival has a detailed history taken regarding the circumstances of the bite, the time of bite, a description of the spider and any first aid undertaken. The patient is then regularly assessed for any symptoms suggesting systemic envenomation. After thorough medical assessment, if there are no signs of systemic envenomation, any first aid such as a pressure immobilisation bandage is removed and the patient observed for 6 hours.[172] With no diagnostic test for funnel-web spider envenomation and no venom detection procedure available,[172] clinical diagnosis is based on the history and symptoms.

Management

For signs of systemic envenomation, 2 ampoules of funnel-web spider antivenom are administered slowly IV over 15–20 minutes;[177,178] premedication is not required,[172] although the patient is observed closely for anaphylaxis. In severe envenomation associated with dyspnoea, pulmonary oedema or decreased level of consciousness, the initial antivenom dose should be doubled to 4 ampoules.[177,178] More antivenom may be required until all major symptoms have resolved (severe bites often require 8 ampoules).[172,177,178] The antivenom dose for children is the same as the adult dose.[172,177,178] First aid measures such as a pressure immobilisation bandage can be removed after antivenom administration and the symptoms have stabilised; this may take several hours.[172]

Snake bites

Worldwide there are a variety of snakes that have the capacity to envenomate humans and cause life-threatening clinical features; broadly these snakes fall into three groups, elapids, pit vipers and cobras. Elapids are mostly encountered throughout Australasia, pit vipers in the Americas and cobras in Africa and south Asia.[167,179,180]

The focus of this section will be on the life-threatening Australasian elapid species.

Description and incidence

Australasia is inhabited by a large number of snakes (over 140 recognised snakes from 30 different species; 25% of all known venomous snakes, and 40% of all dangerous front-fanged snakes or elapids).[167,179,180] New Zealand has no known venomous terrestrial snakes.[167] Australian venomous snakes are found in both rural areas and residential and metropolitan areas, especially when in close proximity to bush land and in periods of drought. The incidence of snakebite is estimated at 500–3000 each year, with approximately 200–500 cases requiring treatment with antivenom.[180] There are on average 1–3 deaths per year, although this may be higher due to unrecognised snake bites.[180]

Clinical manifestations

The majority of snake bites do not result in significant envenomation.[181] Bites are generally recognised by the patient at the time because of associated pain, although some bites are unrecognised. The bite site may show minimal to obvious signs of punctures or scratches, with accompanying swelling and bruising. Multiple bites are possible and are generally associated with major envenomation.[172,181] Australian snake venoms contain various toxins that are responsible for the systemic effects[172,181,182] (see Table 23.17). Renal damage may occur as a consequence of myoglobinuria from severe rhabdomyolysis or haemoglobinuria associated with coagulopathies,[181] leading to acute renal failure (see Chapter 18).[180]

Assessment

Patients presenting with snake bite(s) are allocated a high priority for assessment and treatment even if they appear well on arrival. Patients who present without effective first aid measures (the application of a pressure immobilisation bandage and splint) have these applied immediately.[181] The pressure immobilisation bandage is applied with a broad (15-cm) bandage, commencing over the bite site with the same pressure that would be used for a sprained ankle. The bandage is then extended to cover the whole limb, including fingers/toes, and the limb is splinted and immobilised.[183] Correct application of the pressure bandage is important, as any benefit is lost with bandages that are too loose, not applied to the whole limb or with no splinting or immobilisation.[183] Elasticised bandages are superior to crepe bandages in obtaining and maintaining adequate pressure.[184] Do not wash the wound prior to applying the pressure immobilisation bandage, as swabbing of the bite site is used when performing venom detection. The patient should not mobilise to minimise distribution of any injected venom. Once applied, the pressure immobilisation bandage is not removed until the patient is in a healthcare location that is stocked with antivenom.[180]

> **Practice tip**
>
> Pressure immobilisation may be contraindicated or ineffective in bites from exotic snake species. Many of these non-Australasian species of snake have venoms that cause local tissue destruction. For example, pit vipers and cobras can both cause extensive localised tissue damage. Immobilisation is the mainstay of first aid.[180,181]

TABLE 23.17

Characteristics and clinical manifestations of snake venom[172,181,182]

TOXIN	EFFECTS	SIGNS AND SYMPTOMS
Neurotoxin	Blocks transmission at the neuromuscular junctions, causing skeletal and respiratory muscle flaccid paralysis, presynaptic and/or postsynaptic	• Ptosis (drooping of upper eyelids) • Diplopia (double vision) • Ophthalmoplegia (partial or complete paralysis of eye movements) • Fixed, dilated pupils • Muscle weakness • Respiratory weakness, paralysis
Haemotoxin	Causes coagulopathies, resulting in either: • defibrination with low-fibrinogen, unclottable blood, but usually with a normal platelet count or • direct anticoagulation with normal fibrinogen and platelet count Both cause an elevated prothrombin ratio and international normalised ratio	• Bleeding from bite wounds • Bleeding at venipuncture sites • Haematuria
Myotoxin	Causes myolysis, resulting in generalised destruction of skeletal muscles with high serum creatine kinase and leading to myoglobinuria and occasionally severe hyperkalaemia	• Muscle weakness • Muscle pain on movement • Red or brown urine, which tests positively to blood

A brief and focused history explores the time and circumstances of the bite, a description of the snake (colour, length), geographical location and the application of any first aid. The patient is assessed for general symptoms including headache, nausea, vomiting, abdominal pain, collapse, convulsions and anxiety, although these alone do not indicate envenomation.[180,181] Additional signs and symptoms include blurred or double vision, slurred speech, muscle weakness, respiratory distress, bleeding from the bite site or elsewhere and pain and swelling at the bite site and associated lymph nodes.

Patients with suspected snake bite are located in an acute area with full monitoring available, with symptomatic patients placed in a resuscitation area. The patient requires insertion of IV access devices and collection of blood for pathology tests including full blood count, urea, electrolytes, creatine, creatinine kinase and full coagulation studies. Unnecessary venipunctures should be avoided, including sites where it may be difficult to control bleeding should it occur. Healthcare settings without ready access to pathology services may need to perform whole blood clotting time testing at the bedside to assess for any coagulopathy.

All probable snake bites require observation for at least 12 hours, as some serious symptoms may be delayed.[180,181] Patients should be assessed for tachycardia, hypotension or hypertension, and falling oxygen saturation, altered respiratory rate, forced vital capacity or peak expiratory flow rate, indicating respiratory muscle paralysis.[181] Frequent neurological observations focus on identification of muscle weakness and paralysis; clinicians should note any ptosis, diplopia, dysphagia, slurred speech, limb weakness or altered levels of consciousness. An indwelling catheter should be inserted for close monitoring of urine output and presence of any myoglobin in urine.

To identify the likely snake involved and thus the correct antivenom required, a bedside snake venom detection kit is used at the bite site or with a urine sample. A swab of the washings from the bite area is collected by leaving the pressure immobilisation bandage on and creating a window over the bite site to expose the bitten area. Testing takes about 25 minutes. If there are signs of systemic envenomation, urine can be used to perform the test; blood should be avoided, as it is unreliable. A positive result indicates that venom from a particular snake is present, but does not mean that systemic envenomation has occurred, while a negative result does not exclude systematic envenomation.[179,181]

> **Practice tip**
>
> Whole blood clotting time is performed by drawing 10 mL venous blood and placing in a glass test tube. If the blood has not clotted within 10 minutes, a coagulopathy is likely to exist, suggesting envenomation.[182]

In patients with known snake bite and systemic envenomation, antivenom administration is required if there is any degree of paralysis, significant coagulopathy, any myolysis (myoglobinuria or creatinine kinase >500 micrograms per litre), unconsciousness and/or convulsions. In an asymptomatic patient with normal pathology and a negative or positive snake venom detection result, it is likely that envenomation has not occurred. In this case, the pressure immobilisation bandage can be removed under close observation in a resuscitation area. The patient is fully reevaluated including repeat blood tests, assessing coagulation parameters, within 1–2 hours after removal of the pressure bandage. If the patient's condition remains unchanged, further observation and repeat blood tests at 6 and 12 hours are required. Patients with no evidence of envenomation after 12 hours may be discharged.[179,181]

Management

A patient with evidence of systemic envenomation requires antivenom administration; monovalent antivenom is used in preference to polyvalent antivenom when identity of the snake species is known. Polyvalent antivenom is a mixture of all monovalent antivenoms, and is therefore used for severe envenomation where the identity of the snake is unknown and the patient's condition does not allow time for a snake venom detection kit result, or where there is insufficient monovalent antivenom available.[179,181] Expert advice from a poison information centre may assist in identifying the snake, based on known habitats and distribution as well as presenting symptoms. Antivenom is always administered IV in a diluted strength of 1:10 (or less if volume is a concern) via an infusion. Administration is commenced slowly while observing for signs of any adverse reaction. The infusion rate can be increased if no reaction occurs, with the whole initial dose administered over 15–20 minutes. The dose will vary depending on the type of antivenom, type of snake and number of bites; the use of 4–6 ampoules is not uncommon in severe envenomation.[172,181] Use of premedication before antivenom administration is controversial; at present the antivenom manufacturer does not recommend any premedication to reduce the chance of anaphylaxis. Regardless of whether a premedication is used, prepare to treat anaphylaxis.[179,181,185]

When the patient's condition has stabilised after the initial dose of antivenom, the pressure immobilisation bandage is removed, with continuous close observation for any clinical deterioration caused by the release of venom contained by the pressure bandage. If deterioration is evident, further antivenom and reapplication of the pressure immobilisation bandage may be required.[182] Patients without signs of deterioration still require ongoing observation in a high dependency unit/intensive care unit and repeat testing of coagulation at 3 and 6 hours post-antivenom administration should be done. Ongoing observation and pathology studies will occur for at least 24 hours.[181]

In children, management for snake bite is similar, with antivenom dosages the same as for an adult. Dilution volume can be reduced (from 1:10 to 1:5) for children.[180]

Box jellyfish envenomation

Chironex fleckeri (box jellyfish) is one of the world's most dangerous venomous animals.[167] The jellyfish is a cubic (box-shaped) bell measuring 20–30 cm across and weighing up to 6 kg. Four groups of tentacles, with up to 15 tentacles in each group, can stretch up to 2 m and total length can exceed 60 m. Importantly, the animal is transparent in water and is therefore difficult to identify.[186,187]

The tentacles are covered with millions of stinging nematocysts, each a spring-loaded capsule that contains a penetrating thread that discharges venom. Threads are 1 mm in length and capable of penetrating the dermis of adult skin. The tentacles also produce a sticky substance that promotes adherence to a victim's skin, causing some tentacles to be torn off and remain attached to the person, where the nematocysts remain active.[167]

Description and incidence

Most stings occur during the summer months (December, January) in the tropical waters of northern Australia, from Gladstone in Queensland around to Broome in Western Australia, on hot, calm and overcast days when the jellyfish moves from the open sea to chase prey in shallow water.[167,186,187] The exact incidence of stings is difficult to determine, but they are common in children. One ED reported 23 confirmed *C. fleckeri* stings in a 12-month period.[188] There have been at least 63 confirmed deaths from envenomation by *Chironex fleckeri* in the Indo-Pacific region.

Clinical manifestations

Most stings are minor, with clinically significant stings occurring from larger jellyfish. Stings generally occur on the lower half of the body, and are characterised by immediate and severe pain. Pain increases in severity and may cause victims, especially children, to become incoherent. While mechanisms of toxicity remain poorly understood, death is thought to occur from central respiratory failure, or cardiotoxicity leading to atrioventricular conduction disturbances or paralysis of cardiac muscle. Victims may become unconscious before they can leave the water following envenomation, and death can occur within 5 minutes.[167,186,187]

Multiple linear lesions, purple or brown in colour, are seen on the area where tentacle contact occurs. A pattern of transverse bars is usually seen along the lesions, along with an intense acute inflammatory response, initially as a prompt and massive appearance of wheals, followed by oedema, erythema and vesicle formation, which can lead to partial- or full-thickness skin death.[167,189]

Assessment

Patients presenting to ED after potential box jellyfish sting are easily diagnosed based on the history, the presence of pain and their skin lesions as outlined above. Generally, some form of pre-hospital management or first aid will have been instituted. On arrival, patients with signs of clinically significant stings, alteration in consciousness, cardiovascular or respiratory function, or those with severe pain are seen immediately.

Management

Treatment focuses on appropriate first aid, administration of adequate pain relief, symptomatic management of cardiovascular and respiratory effects and the administration of box jellyfish antivenom when indicated. First aid measures include liberal application of vinegar to the sting area for 30–60 seconds. Vinegar inactivates the undischarged nematocysts, so removal of any remaining tentacles should occur simultaneously to prevent further envenomation.[167,189,190] Mild stings respond to the application of ice packs and simple oral analgesia, after the application of vinegar.[167,188] Patients with moderate-to-severe pain require IV narcotic analgesia. For patients with continuing severe pain, antivenom is administered along with continued parenteral analgesia.[187]

Patients are observed for the development of cardio-respiratory symptoms, including arrhythmias. Management focuses on specific clinical effects, ranging from oxygen administration and IV fluid resuscitation through to intubation/mechanical ventilation or cardiopulmonary resuscitation.[167,189] Antivenom is indicated in patients with cardiorespiratory instability, cardiac arrest or severe pain unrelieved by narcotic analgesia.[187] Antivenom is carried by prehospital personnel, and administration may occur prior to ED presentation. A 20,000-unit ampoule of box jellyfish antivenom is diluted in 10 mL isotonic saline and administered IV over 5–10 minutes.[188] The number of ampoules used varies with clinical status: at least one for cardiorespiratory instability; up to three for life-threatening situations with an inadequate response; and at least six for a cardiac arrest.[167,189]

While the application of a pressure immobilisation bandage to affected limbs after vinegar application was previously recommended as a first aid intervention, there is little current evidence supporting this in box jellyfish stings, and its application may promote additional venom release and therefore be potentially dangerous.[187,191] Some animal research has suggested a role for magnesium sulfate in management for patients not responding to antivenom.[192]

Practice tip

The Australian Resuscitation Council currently recommends that a pressure immobilisation bandage not be used in the management of jellyfish stings.

Adapted, with permission, from Australian Resuscitation Council. Guideline 8.9.6. Envenomation – jellyfish stings, <http://resus.org.au/download/9_4_envenomation/guideline-9-4-5july10.pdf>; 2005 (updated July 2010) [accessed 12.14].

Irukandji envenomation

The Irukandji is a small marine jellyfish, with stinging tentacles capable of causing intense pain and catechol-amine release.[194]

Description and incidence

Irukandji syndrome is a poorly-understood marine enven-omation encountered in far northern and northwestern areas of Australia. Death is uncommon and attributed to cerebral haemorrhage and is associated with other comorbid conditions.[195]

Assessment

People stung by an Irukandji may have no symptoms initially, but may develop symptoms up to 1 hour after being stung. Irukandji syndrome produces clinical features of severe lower back pain, muscle cramps; raised blood pressure, pulse; and respiratory compromise, vomiting and anxiety.[194] A patient with suspected Irukandji enven-omation is placed in an acute area with full monitoring available.

Management

The mainstays of patient management are pain control and symptom management. Application of vinegar has been part of first aid treatment but, due to delay in the presentation of symptoms following a sting, this may be of limited value.[190] Evidence is emerging indicating that washing the area with either fresh or salt water may also be effective. Pain is severe, and opioid analgesia may be required; if requirements for opioids are very high, fentanyl is considered.[194] There is anecdotal evidence that magnesium sulfate may have a role in the management of Irukandji syndrome not responsive to the above treatments, but this remains unproven.[190]

Ciguatera

Ciguatera is a type of seafood poisoning caused by the consumption of fish, especially certain tropical reef fish, which contain one or more naturally-occurring neuro-toxins from the family of ciguatoxins. Ciguatera is reported as the most common form of seafood poisoning in the world,[196] and is considered a mild non-fatal disease, with a worldwide mortality rate ranging from 0.1–20%.[197] Ciguatera as a tropical disease confined to latitudes 35°North–35°South is no longer tenable, as tropical fish are now marketed throughout the world and some species, such as tuna, mackerel and dolphin fish, also migrate considerable distances. In Australia, there have been numerous outbreaks of ciguatera poisoning in Sydney and as far south as Melbourne.[197,198]

Ciguatera toxins (ciguatoxins) are among the deadliest poisons known, reportedly 1000 times more potent than arsenic.[199] These heat-stable toxins originate from a microorganism that attaches to certain species of algae in tropical areas around the world; these toxins become altered after ingestion by progressively larger fish up the food chain.[191,197]

Clinical manifestations and diagnosis

Ciguatera poisoning typically presents as an acute gastro-intestinal illness, followed by a neurological illness with classical symptoms of heat and cold reversal of sensation that may last for a few days after consumption of contam-inated fish[191] (see Table 23.18).

A patient may become sensitive to repeated exposure to ciguatoxins;[191,197] additional exposure to poisoning from ciguatera may be more severe than the first episode. Importantly, patients exposed to ciguatera suffer recur-rences following the consumption of seemingly innocuous

TABLE 23.18
Symptoms of ciguatera[191,197]

GASTROINTESTINAL	NEUROLOGICAL	CARDIOVASCULAR	OTHER SYMPTOMS
Abdominal pain	Paraesthesias in extremities and around	Bradycardia	Dermatitis
Nausea	the mouth, tingling, burning and pain	Tachycardia	Rash
Vomiting	Painful extremities	Hypotension	Arthralgia and myalgia
Diarrhoea	Paradoxical temperature reversal where	Hypertension	General weakness
	hot feels cold and cold feels hot	Arrhythmia	Salivation
	Temperature sensitivity		Dyspnoea
	Vertigo		Neck stiffness
	Dental pain where teeth feel loose		Headache
	Blurred vision		Ataxia
	Tremor		Sweating
			Metallic taste in the mouth

foods (e.g. nuts, nut oils, caffeine, alcohol or animal protein foods),[197,199] with relapses months or years after the initial poisoning.[199]

Diagnosis is made on a patient's history and clinical features: consumption of fish followed by an acute gastrointestinal and neurological illness. There is no conclusive diagnostic test for the presence of ciguatoxins.[197,199]

Management

Treatment of ciguatera poisoning is supportive care and symptom management. Mannitol has been recommended, although this is only effective if used in the first 48–72 hours of the illness.[191,197]

Scombroid fish poisoning

Scombroid poisoning is a form of food poisoning caused by the combination of inadequately cooled fish and the bacterial decomposition of the fish flesh resulting in a release of histamine. The active component of scombrotoxin is histamine. The main groups of fish associated with this type of poisoning are the *Scombridae*, that is tuna and mackerels; however, other fish such as mahi-mahi have also been known to have illness-causing potential.[200] Scombrotoxin is not inactivated by the cooking process.

Clinical manifestations and diagnosis

People normally start feeling unwell in about 30 minutes after eating fish affected with scombrotoxin, with flushing, development of a rash and urticaria. This may be followed by more profound symptoms such as tachycardia, pounding headaches, difficulty breathing and collapse due to hypotension.[200] Deaths have been recorded from this; recently, two Australian tourists died from the same meal while travelling in Bali.

Management

The mainstays of treatment are controlling the histamine reaction with antihistamines and supportive nursing care for symptoms. Histamine-2 receptor blockers have been shown to be useful for up to 24 hours following the development of symptoms. This prolonged treatment allows the scombrotoxin to be eliminated from the patient's system. Importantly, while this may appear to have the clinical features of an allergic reaction, drugs such as adrenaline and corticosteroids do not play a role in management.

Near-drowning
Description and incidence

Submersion incidents are often preventable events associated with significant mortality and morbidity in both adults and children, usually necessitating an ED presentation and subsequent hospital admission. Worldwide, there are an estimated 359,000 drowning deaths annually with children, males and those with increased access to water most at risk.[201] The location of drowning varies from country to country. In the USA, artificial pools and natural bodies of freshwater were common drowning locations, particularly for children.[202] In Australia, drowning often occurred in non-tidal lagoons, lakes and surf beaches.[203] In Uganda, lakes and rivers were common sites particularly for young males.[204] A bimodal distribution of deaths is seen in children, with a peak in the toddler age group (0–4 years) and a second peak in young adolescent males (15–19 years).[201,205–207]

It is estimated that, for every drowning death, there are 4–5 near-drowning hospital admissions and 14 ED presentations.[205,206,208] Near-drowning is also associated with high-impact injuries, especially boating or personal watercraft incidents and shallow-diving-related injuries. Associated cervical spine injury is seen in 0.5% of near-drowning cases.[205]

Clinical manifestations

The sequence of events in drowning has been identified primarily by animal studies, highlighting an initial phase of panic struggling, some swimming movements and sometimes a surprise inhalation. There may be aspiration of small amounts of water at this time that produces laryngospasm for a short period. Apnoea and breath-holding occur during submersion and are often followed by swallowing large amounts of water with subsequent vomiting, gasping and fluid aspiration. This leads to severe hypoxia, loss of consciousness and disappearance of airway reflexes, resulting in further water moving into the lungs prior to death.[205,209,210]

Approximately 80–90% of submersion victims suffer 'wet drowning' as described above, with aspiration of water into the lungs resulting from loss of airway reflexes and laryngospasm. Approximately 10–15% of victims have sustained laryngospasm, and no detectable amount of water will be aspirated (known as 'dry drowning'), with the resulting injury secondary to anoxia.[205,206] Pre-existing medical conditions predispose a person to drowning and should be considered during management, including seizures, arrhythmia (especially torsades de pointes associated with long Q-T interval), coronary artery disease, depression, cardiomyopathy (dilated or hypertrophic obstructive), hypoglycaemia, hypothermia, intoxication or trauma.[209]

Pulmonary manifestations after aspiration of fresh or salt water differ, as fresh water is hypotonic and when aspirated moves quickly into the microcirculation across the alveolar–capillary membrane. With fresh water aspiration, surfactant is destroyed, producing alveolar instability, atelectasis and decreased lung compliance and resulting in marked ventilation/perfusion mismatching.[205,206,208,209] In contrast, salt water has 3–4 times the osmolality of blood and, when aspirated, draws damaging protein-rich fluid from the plasma into the alveoli, resulting in both interstitial and alveoli oedema, with associated bronchospasm and subsequent shunting and ventilation/perfusion mismatch.[205,208,209]

Despite these different physiological effects from aspirated fresh and salt water, the resulting clinical manifestation is the same: profound hypoxaemia secondary to ventilation/perfusion mismatch with intrapulmonary shunting (see Figure 23.2).[205,208,209] Patients with evidence

of fluid aspiration often progress to develop severe acute respiratory distress syndrome within a very short time.[205] No significant effects on electrolytes are noted in humans, as rarely more than 10 mL/kg and commonly no more than 4 mL/kg of water is aspirated, while clinically significant electrolyte disturbances occur when over 22 mL/kg has been aspirated.[205,208,209]

Cardiovascular effects are influenced by the extent and duration of hypoxia, derangement of acid–base status, the magnitude of the stress response and hypothermia.[205] Ventricular arrhythmias and asystole may result from hypoxaemia and metabolic acidosis. Acute hypoxia results in release of pulmonary inflammatory mediators, which increase right ventricular afterload and decrease contractility.[205,208,209] Hypotension is commonly seen due to volume depletion secondary to pulmonary oedema, intracompartmental fluid shifts and myocardial dysfunction.[205]

Severe hypoxic and ischaemic injury is the most important factor related to outcome and subsequent quality of life. Other factors influencing the extent of injury include water temperature and submersion time, stress during submersion and coexisting cardiovascular and neurological disease.[205,208,209,211,212] Prediction of death or persistent vegetative state in the immediate period after near-drowning is difficult. Patients awake or with only blunted consciousness on presentation usually survive without neurological sequelae. A third of patients admitted in coma or after cardiopulmonary resuscitation will survive neurologically intact or with only minor deficits, while the remaining two-thirds of patients will either die or remain in a vegetative state.[205]

Hypothermia is a well-documented feature in submersion victims.[205,208,209,212] Incidents of submersion times of greater than 15 minutes where victims recovered with a good neurological outcome all occurred in very cold water (<10°C). While the exact mechanisms in these outcomes are unclear, acute cold submersion hypothermia may be protective against cerebral insult by: very rapid cooling in victims with low levels of subcutaneous fat who have aspirated a large amount of very cold water; induced muscle paralysis leading to minimal struggling and very little oxygen depletion; and the heart gradually slowing to asystole in the presence of profound hypothermia.[205,208,209,212] In these cases prolonged resuscitative efforts may be warranted, including active and aggressive re-warming interventions, that should not be abandoned until the patient has been re-warmed to at least 30°C.[208]

Assessment

Continuously monitor heart rate, blood pressure and oxygen saturation, and assess neurological status, including any seizure activity. Deterioration is evident with a falling level of consciousness, a high alveolar–arterial gradient, respiratory failure evidenced by a partial pressure of carbon dioxide in the arterial blood >45 mmHg or worsening blood gas results.[208] Caution should be taken to avoid activities that may cause a rise in intracranial pressure.

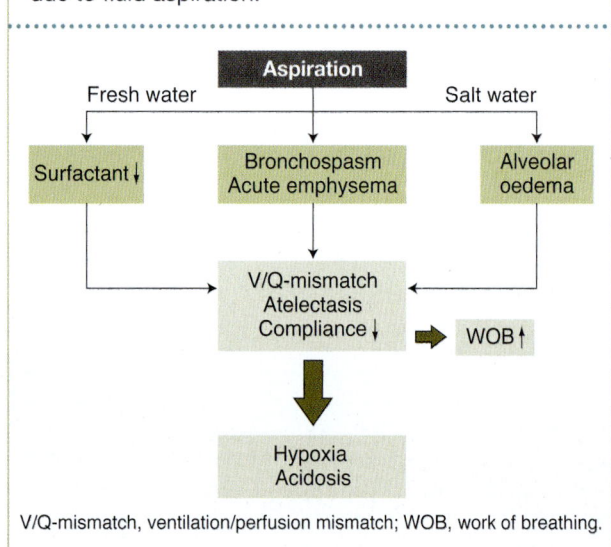

FIGURE 23.2 Pathophysiology of respiratory failure due to fluid aspiration.[205,206,208,209]

V/Q-mismatch, ventilation/perfusion mismatch; WOB, work of breathing.

A 12-lead ECG identifies any arrhythmias that result from acidosis and hypoxia rather than electrolyte abnormalities. The patient should be managed conventionally (see Chapter 11).[208] All patients require serial CXR, as lung fields often worsen in the first few hours. In clinically significant submersions, the CXR will typically show bilateral infiltrates undifferentiated from other causes of pulmonary oedema.

Management

The condition of the patient, the environment and the skill of the attending rescue personnel will influence prehospital management of the post-submersion patient, and the adequacy of initial basic life support at the scene is the most important determinant of outcome.[213] The Heimlich manoeuvre should not be performed in an attempt to remove aspirated water, as it is ineffective and likely to promote aspiration of gastric contents. Supplemental oxygen 100% is administered as soon as possible.[211–213]

For patients presenting to the ED in cardiac arrest, active resuscitation measures continue (see Chapter 25), although the need for continued cardiopulmonary resuscitation is generally associated with a poor neurological outcome; however, patients experiencing submersions in very cold water may have a better outcome.[213] The focus of management for patients with spontaneous circulation includes respiratory support and the correction of hypoxia, neurological assessment and maintenance of optimal cerebral perfusion, cardiovascular support and maintenance of haemodynamic stability, correction of hypothermia and management of other associated injuries.

All patients require 100% supplemental oxygen via a non-rebreathing mask initially, unless mechanical ventilation is required. Patients without any respiratory symptoms should be observed for 6–12 hours, until there is a GCS greater than 13, normal CXR, no signs of respiratory distress and normal oxygen saturation on room air.[205,208,212,213] Alert patients unable to maintain adequate oxygenation should be considered for continuous positive airway pressure or bi-level positive airway pressure prior to intubation provided they are able to maintain their own airway, with its effect on circulation monitored closely (see Chapter 15).

While cerebral oedema and intracranial hypertension is often seen in hypoxic neuronal injury, only general supportive measures are recommended as there is insufficient evidence to indicate that invasive intracranial pressure monitoring and related management improve outcomes.[205,208,212,213] Any seizures should be promptly treated with appropriate measures (see Chapter 17). Acute respiratory distress syndrome should be managed with non-invasive ventilation if possible.[209] Barbiturate-induced coma or corticosteroids are not recommended as there is no evidence of improvement in outcome.[209,211]

Cardiovascular support may require a multifaceted approach, initially by improving hypoxia and correcting circulating volume. Hypotensive patients require rapid volume expansion (crystalloid or colloid) and an indwelling catheter for hourly urine measurement. Patients with persistent cardiovascular compromise may require inotropic support in conjunction with invasive haemodynamic monitoring.[205,208,212,213]

Patients presenting with associated high-impact or shallow-diving mechanisms should have cervical spine immobilisation instituted with the application of a rigid cervical collar, especially for complaints of neck pain or an altered level of consciousness (see Chapter 17). The management of hypothermia and re-warming methods outlined below are appropriate for the management of near-drowning.

Hypothermia
Description and incidence

Hypothermia is a core body temperature that is lower than 35°C (measured centrally by oesophageal or rectal probe) and occurs with exposure to low ambient temperatures that are influenced by low environmental temperatures, humidity, wind velocity, extended exposure time or cold water immersion.[214–216] Cold injury is a common occurrence in those climates with cooler ambient conditions; however, when body heat is lower than the surrounding environmental conditions, it can easily develop so it is not an uncommon problem in Australia and New Zealand, despite the relatively warm weather zones in the former. The very young and very old are most susceptible to injury.[214,217] A normal core temperature of 37°C has a variation of 1–2°C. Temperature maintenance is essential for normal homeostatic functioning, and normal adaptive mechanisms can respond to reductions in ambient temperature.

Clinical manifestations

When skin temperature is reduced after exposure to the cold, sympathetic stimulation occurs causing peripheral vasoconstriction, decreased skin circulation and shunting of blood centrally to vital organs. Blood pressure, heart rate and respiratory rate rise, and shivering (involuntary clonic movements of skeletal muscle) stimulates metabolic activity to produce heat and blood flow to striated muscles[214] to maintain a normal core temperature. If continued exposure to cold occurs these compensatory functions fail, and hypothermia results.[214,216]

Ambient temperatures need not be particularly low, as other contributing factors such as wind or a person having wet clothing may be significant. A patient with a decreased level of consciousness may present with hypothermia after lying on a cool surface.[214] As a person's core temperature drops, progressive cardiac abnormalities occur; normal sinus rhythm may progress to sinus bradycardia, T-wave inversion, prolonged P–R and Q–T intervals, atrial fibrillation and ventricular fibrillation.[214] A QRS abnormality, the Osborn wave, represented by a positive deflection at the junction of the QRS and ST segments, is frequently described as being characteristic of cold injury.[218]

TABLE 23.19

Physiological effects of hypothermia[214–216,218–221]

PHYSIOLOGICAL EFFECTS	DEGREE OF HYPOTHERMIA		
	MILD (32–35°C)	MODERATE (28–32°C)	SEVERE (<28°C)
General metabolic	Shivering Raised oxygen consumption Hyperkalaemia	Raised oxygen consumption Acidosis	Normal metabolic functions fail
Cardiac	Vasoconstriction Tachycardia Increased cardiac output	Atrial arrhythmias Bradycardia	Ventricular arrhythmias Decreased cardiac output
Respiratory	Tachypnoea Bronchospasm	Decreased respiratory drive	Apnoea
Neurological	Confusion Hyperreflexia	Lowered level of consciousness Hyporeflexia	Coma Absent reflexes
Coagulation	Platelet dysfunction Impaired clotting enzyme function Increased blood viscosity	Increased haematocrit	Lower bleeding times due to failure of clotting systems

Metabolic acidosis and blood-clotting abnormalities are common, as well as hypoglycaemia, which occurs because of depletion of glycogen stores caused by excessive shivering. Hyperglycaemia can be present because of inhibition of insulin action due to the lowered temperature.[214–216,218–221] The physiological alterations that accompany lowering of core temperature to below 30°C are summarised in Table 23.19.[214–216,218–221]

Management

A patient with severe hypothermia may appear dead: cold, pale, stiff, with no response to external stimulation. Successful resuscitation of patients has occurred at temperatures as low as 17°C, due to the low body temperature protecting vital organs from hypoxic injury.[215,216,218,219] This is reflected in the anecdotal phrase, 'patients are not dead until they are warm and dead'.[215] In most cases, therefore, resuscitation should continue until the patient's core temperature reaches 30°C.[215,216,218,219]

> **Practice tip**
>
> Removing wet clothing and drying the patient is an extremely important first aid measure for a cold wet to prevent further cooling.

If a patient's core temperature is below 32°C, 'core rewarming' is indicated. This approach is favoured, as experimental evidence indicates that return to normal cardiovascular function is more rapid with temperature rises of up to 7.5°C per hour.[214,216] A number of invasive internal warming options are available, including peritoneal lavage, although the most effective of all internal methods is cardiopulmonary bypass, as it transfers heat at a rate several times faster than any other methods available,

that being approximately 7.5°C per hour.[217,219] While the technique is efficient, it is obviously more invasive and carries associated risks, and so is reserved for profoundly hypothermic patients.[214]

External warming is indicated only if the core temperature is above 32°C, as this may cause vasodilation and hypovolaemic shock. Shunting of cold peripheral blood to the core may also lead to further chilling of the myocardium and ventricular fibrillation.[214,216] External warming using warm blankets, forced warm air blankets and heat packs in contact with the patient's body should raise body temperature by approximately 2.5°C per hour.[214,216] Inhalation rewarming with oxygen warmed to 42–46°C is also effective, as around 10% of metabolic heat is lost through the respiratory tract.[219]

> **Practice tip**
>
> Always measure the blood glucose of hypothermic patients to exclude hypoglycaemia as a reason for an altered conscious state.

Recovery of patients with temperatures as low as 13.7°C has occurred, so death in hypothermia is defined as failure to revive with rewarming. Hence unless there are other factors preventing survival, resuscitation should continue until the patient's temperature reaches at least 30°C–32°C.[216]

Hyperthermia and heat illness
Description and incidence

Potentially one of the more significant environmental fears expressed by many scientists is the issue of climate change and the consequence of heat-related illness worldwide.

Global warming and events such as recurrent prolonged hot weather days have recently caused numerous deaths through Europe, the USA and Australia and scientists are predicting the events will become more common.[217,222] Heat-related illness is common in Australia and represents a significant public health risk, although there are only limited deaths compared to what has happened in the USA and Europe.[217,222]

Heat-related illness can affect any age group; however it is the very young, because of their larger surface area, reduced sweating capacity and inability to access their own fluids, and the older person, who may have fluid restrictions because of other health reasons or taking medications that affect their capacity to sweat and a tendency to layer clothing, who are at the highest risk.[217,222] The other vulnerable group is those in the younger age groups undertaking physical activity during hot weather periods whether because of work or sports.

Alterations in thermoregulatory function cause varying degrees of heat illness, categorised as three types: heat cramps, heat exhaustion and heat stroke.[217,222] Excessive exposure to heat substantially increases fluid and electrolyte losses from the body.[217,222] The loss of both fluids and electrolytes in addition to impaired organ function leads to the complications of heat illnesses. Factors contributing to heat illness include elevated ambient temperature, increased heat production due to exercise, infection and drugs such as amphetamines, phenothiazines or other stimulants.[217]

Clinical manifestations

Environmental heat illness is more likely to develop when the ambient temperature exceeds 32–35°C and the humidity is greater than 70%.[217,222] Assessment of the patient's physical state and vital signs including GCS score provides some evidence of hypovolaemia and potential or impending shock.

Heat exhaustion is a more severe form of heat illness and is associated with severe water or salt depletion due to excessive sweating; the patient's temperature may range between normal and below 40°C.[217,222] Combined water and salt losses cause muscle cramps, nausea and vomiting, headache, dizziness, weakness, fainting, thirst, tachycardia, hypotension and profuse sweating, but with normal neurological function.[217]

Heat stroke is the most severe and serious form of heat-related illness, with temperatures above 41°C and impaired neurological function. Heat stroke is a profound disturbance of the body's heat-regulating ability, and is often referred to as 'sunstroke', although it relates to the body's inability to dissipate heat, loss of sweat function and severe dehydration, rather than actual sun exposure.[217,222,223]

Management

Initial management of the hyperthermic patient focuses on airway, breathing and circulation,[217,222,224] correction of urgent physiological states such as hypoxia, severe potassium imbalances and acidosis. A heat-stressed patient can have large fluid losses and require prompt fluid resuscitation, preferably isotonic sodium chloride solution.[217,222] Total water deficit should be corrected slowly; half of the deficit is administered in the first 3–6 hours, with the remainder over the next 6–9 hours.[222]

Rapid cooling is the second priority: lowering core temperature to less than 38.9°C within 30 minutes improves survival and minimises end-organ damage.[222] The ideal goal is to reduce the core temperature by 0.2°C/min.[222] Non-invasive external methods of cooling include removal of clothing and covering the patient with a wet, tepid sheet. Ice packs can be placed next to the patient's axillae, neck and groin. Invasive cooling measures such as iced gastric lavage and cardiopulmonary bypass are reserved for the patient who fails to respond to conventional cooling methods.[217,222] Core body temperature should be monitored using a continuous rectal or tympanic probe. No randomised clinical trials have compared the effectiveness of different cooling methods.[222]

Summary

This chapter has provided an overview of important emergency systems and processes, outlining the practice of initial assessment and prioritisation of patients presenting to the ED through the unique nursing process of triage. The role of the emergency nurse in the initial assessment, intervention and management of the patient has been described. The initial ED management of common emergency presentations was outlined, reflecting current practice and based on the latest available evidence.

The emergency environment is dynamic, and it was beyond the scope of this chapter to describe the full extent of emergency nursing practice and the clinical entities that are frequently managed. It is therefore important for a critical care nurse to be familiar with the content provided in the other chapters in this text, as well as other resources. As noted at the beginning of this chapter, other common presentations to the ED, such as trauma and cardiorespiratory arrest, are described in Chapters 24 and 25.

Emergency nursing is a demanding specialty area of practice, as are all areas of specialty practice. The challenges with emergency nursing come with the volumes of predicable patient groups, changing demographics in our community and the unpredictable or unusual presentations. Emergency nurses need to prepare themselves with a broad knowledge base, adaptability to change and resilience to meet these demands.

Case study

0750 h: Maria Baxter, a 42-year-old woman, presented to the ambulance bay of the ED in a private car and accompanied by her family for evaluation after a suspected overdose of insecticide. Maria's partner and sister approached the triage area stating that the patient had taken 'another overdose and was vomiting'. The triage nurse questioned Maria's sister who revealed that she had deliberately drunk approximately one cup of 'insect killer'.

The triage nurse protected herself with a pair of gloves and a patient gown, then went to assess Maria, who was sitting in the backseat of the car. On initial triage assessment, Maria was alert and able to talk, stating that she 'felt unwell'. The triage nurse noted that she had vomited and that there was a strong smell of a garlicky oily-type substance coming from the car. The triage nurse immediately removed herself from the area and contacted the shift coordinator of the ED to inform her of the incident, the need for assistance and that staff should adopt a standard approach to a chemically contaminated patient.

Maria remained in the car while staff prepared a treatment area that was isolated from the department (a single room with negative-pressure air flow and high-volume air extraction). Staff also applied personal protective equipment to guard themselves from contamination. Three suitably-clothed nursing staff helped Maria from the car. After minimal assessment, she was taken to an external shower, where she had her clothing removed and placed in a sealed contaminated-waste bag. The patient was then given a shower using warm, soapy water. It was noted at this point that an oily substance on and around her mouth and hands turned white when water was applied. This was thoroughly removed and Maria was placed in the isolation room of the ED.

0803 h: Maria was formally triaged with an ATS of 2, meaning she should be seen by a doctor within 10 minutes, based on her exposure to the chemical and the level of response required. Her initial observations were: alert with pink, warm and dry skin; pulse 72 beats per minute; blood pressure 117/71 mmHg; oxygen saturation 100%. Cardiac monitoring and supplemental oxygen therapy (6 L/min via Hudson mask) were commenced. An IV cannula was inserted by an ED nurse and venous blood samples were collected.

0810 h: Initial medical assessment noted the following additional history:

- Maria vomited twice, once in the car and once in the ED; this was followed by an episode of diarrhoea.
- Maria had taken an intentional ingestion of chlorpyrifos, estimated to be approximately half a cup at 0630–0645 h. Maria stated that she wanted to kill herself.
- The family members who had accompanied her appeared asymptomatic: that is, they had no physical signs of organophosphate adsorption at this time; however, they were complaining of headaches and feeling ill from the smell.
- On the container supplied by the family, the information label read 'Super Buffalo Fly Insecticide, 20% chlorpyrifos, 65% liquid hydrocarbon'.

0815 h: The Poisons Information Hotline was contacted for advice, with the following information provided:

- Symptoms may have a delayed onset.
- The solution contains active metabolites.
- A serum cholinesterase level should be collected.
- An oral dose of activated charcoal should be administered.
- A dose of atropine may be given as a heart rate response test.
- Administration of pralidoxime was suggested if there was no response to atropine or an exacerbation of symptoms was seen.

0825 h: Maria's pulse rate was noted to be 110 beats per min. A dose of atropine 0.5 mg IV was administered and her pulse rate rose to 125 beats per min. A CXR was also ordered.

0830 h: Maria developed mild sweating of the face and forehead. There was no increase in salivation but a large amount of clear saliva was noted on the tongue. No muscle fasciculations were evident, and Maria's pupils fluctuated from 4 mm to 1 mm in size. On auscultation her chest was clear, and good power was evident in all limbs. At this time, staff discussed Maria's progress with her concerned family, including the potentially serious nature of the ingestion, and offered emotional support.

0845 h: Maria developed widespread muscle tremors but retained good muscle strength, including the ability to cough and maintain adequate respiratory function. Her pulse rate rose to 144 beats per minute with a blood pressure of 140/90 mmHg. A pralidoxime loading dose was ordered (1 g in 100 mL isotonic saline) and commenced over 30 minutes, followed by a pralidoxime infusion (at 400 mg/h).

0850 h: An ICU review was requested and Maria was seen by the intensive care consultant. The consultant agreed with the current management plan and accepted Maria as a suitable admission to the ICU. At that time a bed was available and ready. The earlier CXR was reviewed and noted to be clear. The ICU consultant also noted that the ECG showed a sinus tachycardia with no rhythm disturbances. At this time, emergency staff caring for Maria began complaining of nausea and headaches. A rotation of the staff caring for Maria was commenced.

0900 h: Maria had an increase in sweating, further diarrhoea, had developed a cough and increased salivation, which required suctioning. But Maria was still able to talk, and her GCS remained at 15. Other observations were: heart rate 130 beats per min, respiratory rate 24 breaths per min, blood pressure 140/95 mmHg and oxygen saturation 99%.

0910 h: With an ICU bed available, a transfer to the ICU was undertaken. Maria was transferred with full monitoring and resuscitation equipment and with the ICU consultant, emergency doctor and an emergency nurse escort.

0915 h: Maria's condition suddenly deteriorated during transport to the ICU. Her level of consciousness decreased, along with her respiratory effort. She was noted to be profoundly weak, with widespread piloerection and muscle tremors. Assisted ventilation with bag–valve–mask resuscitator commenced.

0920 h: On arrival in the ICU Maria was unable to protect her airway due to profound weakness and a reduced GCS. She was intubated with midazolam 3 mg and vecuronium 10 mg given for induction.

Summary of ICU admission: Maria required 3 days of ventilation. A pralidoxime infusion was required for 2 days due to depleted cholinesterase levels. On extubation, Maria complained of a headache and generalised weakness, but was able to eat, drink and mobilise. She spent a total of 5 days in the ICU before being discharged to the mental health service.

Mental health admission summary: Maria was diagnosed as having a maladaptive situational response and moderate depression with ongoing suicidal thoughts. She stated to staff that she would not use insect killer again and had no other formal plan of how she might harm herself. The mental health admission was for a total of 5 days. At hospital discharge Maria had no suicidal ideation. A community mental health team follow-up was arranged.

CASE STUDY QUESTIONS

1 Why did Maria have her clothing removed and then her body washed with soapy water before entering the ED?

2 Outline the physiological effects of atropine administration in the context of this poisoning. What are the clinical end points for atropine therapy and how should this be monitored?

3 Pralidoxime is one pharmacological agent available to treat patients with symptomatic organophosphate exposure. How does this drug work?

4 Maria's family members requested to visit her during the initial management phase in the ED. How would you handle this request?

Please consider the following issues:

a the current clinical safety for the patient

b management of family exposure to this substance/poisoning

c containment of the potential distribution of the substance within the ED.

RESEARCH VIGNETTE

Muntlin A, Carlsson M, Safwenberg U, Gunningberg L. Outcomes of a nurse initiated IV analgesic protocol for abdominal pain in an emergency department: a quasi-experimental study. Int J Nurs Stud 2011;48(1):13–23

Background: Abdominal pain is one of the most frequent reasons for seeking care in an emergency department. Surveys have shown that patients are not satisfied with the pain management they receive. Reasons for giving inadequate pain management may include poor knowledge about pain assessment, myths concerning pain, lack of communication between the patient and healthcare professional and organizational limitations.

Objectives: The aim of the study was to investigate the outcome of nursing assessment, pain assessment and nurse-initiated IV opioid analgesic compared to standard procedure for patients seeking emergency care for abdominal pain. Outcome measures were: (a) pain intensity, (b) frequency of received analgesic, (c) time to analgesic, (d) transit time, and (e) patients' perceptions of the quality of care in pain management.

Design: A quasi-experimental (before–during–after) design was used.

Setting: The study was conducted in an emergency department at a Swedish university hospital.

Participants: Patients with abdominal pain seeking care in the emergency department were invited to participate. A total of 50, 100 and 50 patients, respectively, were included for the three phases of the study. The inclusion criteria were: ongoing abdominal pain not lasting for more than 2 days, ≥18 years of age and oriented to person, place and time. Exclusion criteria were: abdominal pain due to trauma, in need of immediate care and pain intensity scored as 9–10.

Methods: The patients' perceptions of the quality of care in pain management in the emergency department were evaluated by means of a patient questionnaire carried out in the three study phases. The intervention phase included education, nursing assessment protocol and a range order for analgesic.

Results: The nursing assessment and the nurse-initiated IV opioid analgesic resulted in significant improvement in frequency of receiving analgesic and a reduction in time to analgesic. Patients perceived lower pain intensity and improved quality of care in pain management.

Conclusions: The intervention improved the pain management in the emergency department. A structured nursing assessment could also affect the patients' perceptions of the quality of care in pain management in the emergency department.

Critique

This paper described the effect of introducing a nurse-led analgesia protocol for patients who presented to an ED in Sweden with abdominal pain. Pain management in the ED in this and other groups is often poorly done everywhere. In order to improve care delivery for this group of patients, a strategy that focused on nurse assessment, pain assessment and nurse-initiated IV opioid analgesia was introduced. Educational sessions were delivered over a one-month period prior to the introduction of the intervention. Most (n = 47) of the 50 registered nurses participated in this requirement to use the analgesic order that was developed based on the literature and clinical experience. It was also validated by the head of the ED, specialists in general surgery and registered nurses working in the ED for relevance and clinical applicability. The order was based on a pain score range, following assessment of the patient, and considered inclusion and exclusion criteria (e.g. allergy to morphine, pregnant, pain intensity >8, circulation or respiratory condition) to assure patient safety and prevent adverse events (of which there were none).

Outcomes measures included: pain intensity, frequency of received analgesic, time to analgesia, transit time in the ED and patients' perceptions of the quality of care in pain management. These outcomes were measured before (phase A1), during (phase B) and after (phase A2) the introduction of the intervention. This was a strong design given the inability to undertake a randomised controlled trial (the optimal design choice to study the effect of an intervention) due to practical and financial reasons. The authors provide justification for their sample size requirements (n = 50 in A1, 100 in B, 50 in A2) that was based on a power calculation and previously documented evidence of clinical significance. The tools and outcomes used in the study were based on previous research and, where indicated, have been validated with minor adaption made in this study to suit the ED setting. The analysis, consisting of descriptive and inferential statistics, was clear, thorough and considered, including Bonferroni correction to avoid reporting mass significance when using the one-way analysis of variance test. Recognising potential areas where bias may occur, the authors present important information such as: dropouts were not different in terms of age and gender to the group that was included and there were no significant differences between patients in the three phases with respect to background information.

Results from the study indicate that a structured nurse assessment protocol and nurse initiated IV opioid analgesic can increase the frequency of pain assessment and received analgesia while also reducing the patient's waiting time for analgesia in the ED (median times: A1, 1.8 h; B, 1.0 h; A2, 1.7 h). Although there were some limitations to this study, such as some external dropouts and incompleteness of questionnaires, there is some degree of generalisability of the results to other settings with similar findings noted elsewhere.

Overall, this is a good example of a well-conducted study demonstrating how an evidence-based approach to changes in nursing care can result in positive patient and service outcomes at a relatively low cost.

Learning activities

These learning activities will require you to investigate plans that exist in your clinical areas, and demonstrate an understanding of an approach to a chemically contaminated patient, important emergency interventions and aspects of personal protection for the responder and the clinical unit where the patient has presented.

1   Review your department's plan for the management of a potentially chemical-contaminated patient.

2   Outline what PPE your department has available for staff use.

3   Describe the routes by which organophosphates can be absorbed and how inadvertent staff exposure can be minimised.

Online resources

American Emergency Nurses Association, www.ena.org

Australasian College for Emergency Medicine, www.acem.org.au

Australian College of Emergency Nursing, https://acen.com.au

Australian Institute of Health and Welfare, www.aihw.gov.au

Australian Venom Research Unit, www.avru.org

Best Bets, www.bestbets.org

Clinical Toxinology Resources, Women's and Children's Hospital, Adelaide, www.toxinology.com

College of Emergency Nursing Australasia, www.cena.org.au

College of Emergency Nursing New Zealand, www.nzno.org.nz/groups/colleges/college_of_emergency_nurses

Commonwealth Serum Laboratories Antivenom Handbook eMedicine, www.emedicine.com

Emergency Nursing World, http://enw.org

National Asthma Council of Australia, www.nationalasthma.org.au

National Institute of Clinical Studies, Emergency Care Community of Practice Project, www.nicsl.com.au

New Zealand Health Information Service, www.nzhis.govt.nz

New Zealand Ministry of Health, www.moh.govt.nz

Poisons Information Australia, telephone: 131126

Poisons Information New Zealand, phone: 0800 POISON or 0800 764766

The Cochrane Centre, http://acc.cochrane.org

Further reading

White J. A clinician's guide to Australian venomous bites and stings: Incorporating the updated CSL Antivenom Handbook. CSL Ltd, <http://www.toxinology.com/fusebox.cfm?staticaction=generic_static_files/cgavbs_avh.html>; 2013.

References

1 Pink N. Triage in the accident and emergency department. Aust Nurs J 1977;6(9):35–6.

2 Australasian College for Emergency Medicine. National Triage Scale. Emerg Med 1994;6(2):245-6.

3 Manchester Triage Group. Emergency triage. 1st ed. London: BMJ Publishing; 1997.

4 Australasian College for Emergency Medicine. Australasian triage scale. Emerg Med 2002;14:335-6.

5 Whitby S, Ieraci S, Johnson D, Mohsin M. Analysis of the process of triage: The use and outcome of the National Triage Scale. Canberra: Commonwealth Department of Family Services; 1997.

6 Kelly A, Richardson D. Training for the role of triage in Australasia. Emerg Med 2001;113:230-2.

7 Fernandes CM, Tanabe P, Gilboy N, Johnson LA, McNair RS, Rosenau AM et al. Five-level triage: a report from the ACEP/ENA Five-level Triage Task Force. J Emerg Nurs 2005;31(1):39-50; quiz 118.

8 Kitt S. Emergency nursing: A physiological and clinical perspective. 2nd ed. Philadelphia: WB Saunders; 1995.

9 McMahon M. ED triage: Is a five level triage system the best? Am J Nurs 2003;103(3):61-3.

10 Robertson-Steel I. Evolution of triage systems. Emerg Med J 2006;23(2):154-5.

11 Canadian Association of Emergency Physicians. Implementation guidelines for the Canadian emergency department Triage and Acuity Scale (CTAS), <http://caep.ca/resources/ctas/implementation-guidelines> [accessed 12.14].

12.College of Emergency Nursing Australasia. Position Statement Triage Nurse, <http://www.cena.org.au/>; 2009 [accessed 12.14].

13 Australian College for Emergency Medicine. Guidelines for implementation of the Australasian Triage Scale in Emergency Departments, <https://www.acem.org.au/getattachment/d19d5ad3-e1f4-4e4f-bf83-7e09cae27d76/G24-Implementation-of-the-Australasian-Triage-Scal.aspx>; 2005 [accessed 12.14].

14 van der Wulp I, van Stel HF. Calculating kappas from adjusted data improved the comparability of the reliability of triage systems: a comparative study. J Clin Epidemiol 2010;63(11):1256-63.

15 Gilboy N, Tanabe P, Travers DA, Rosenau A. The Emergency Severity Index (ESI): A triage tool for emergency department. Version 4, <http://www.ahrq.gov/professionals/systems/hospital/esi/esi1.html>; 2012 [accessed 12.14].

16 Travers DA, Waller AE, Bowling JM, Flowers D, Tintinalli J. Five-level triage system more effective than three-level in tertiary emergency department. J Emerg Nurs 2002;28(5):395-400.

17 Ng CJ, Hsu KH, Kuan JT, Chiu TF, Chen WK, Lin HJ et al. Comparison between Canadian Triage and Acuity Scale and Taiwan Triage System in emergency departments. J Formos Med Assoc 2010;109(11):828-37.

18 Maningas PA, Hime DA, Parker DE, McMurry TA. The Soterion Rapid Triage System: evaluation of inter-rater reliability and validity. J Emerg Med 2006;30(4):461-9.

19 Farrohknia N, Castren M, Ehrenberg A, Lind L, Oredsson S, Jonsson H et al. Emergency department triage scales and their components: a systematic review of the scientific evidence. Scand J Trauma Resusc Emerg Med 2011;19:42.

20 FitzGerald G, Jelinek GA, Scott D, Gerdtz MF. Emergency department triage revisited. Emerg Med J 2010;27(2):86-92.

21 Commonwealth Department of Health and Family Services and the Australian College of Emergency Medicine. Australian national triage scale: a user's manual. Pardy M, ed. Canberra: CDHFS; 1997.

22 College of Emergency Nursing Australasia. Position Statement Triage and the Australasian Triage Scale, <http://cena.org.au/wp-content/uploads/2014/10/2012_06_14_CENA_-_Position_Statement_Triage.pdf>; 2012 [accessed 12.14].

23 Jelinek C, Little M. Inter-rater reliability of the national triage scale over 11,500 simulated occasions of triage. Emerg Med 1996;8:226-30.

24 Western Australian Centre for Evidence Informed Healthcare Practice. Triage in the Emergency Department. Western Australia: Curtin University, <http://www.bhi.nsw.gov.au/__data/assets/pdf_file/0016/170620/Examples_of_triage_conditions.pdf>; 2011 [accessed 12.14].

25 Tanabe P, Gilboy N, Travers DA. Emergency Severity Index version 4: clarifying common questions. J Emerg Nurs 2007;33(2):182-5.

26 Department of Health and Ageing. Emergency triage education kit. http://www.health.gov.au/: Australian Government, <http://www.health.gov.au/internet/main/publishing.nsf/Content/casemix-ED-Triage+Review+Fact+Sheet+Documents>; 2007 [accessed 12.14].

27 Mental Health and Drug and Alcohol Office. Mental Health Triage Policy. Sydney: NSW Government, <http://www.health.nsw.gov.au/>; 2012 [accessed 12.14].

28 Mental Health and Drug and Alcohol Office. Mental Health for Emergency Department – A reference guide. Sydney: NSW Department of Health; 2009.

29 Broadbent M, Jarman, Berk M. Emergency department mental health triage scales improve outcomes. J Eval Clin Pract 2004;10(1):57-62.

30 Department of Human Services. Mental health care: Framework for emergency department services. Melbourne: Victorian Government Department of Human Services, <http://www.health.vic.gov.au/mentalhealth/emergency/framework.htm>; 2007 (updated May 2014) [accessed 12.14].

31 Larkin GL, Claassen CA, Emond JA, Pelletier AJ, Camargo CA. Trends in U.S. emergency department visits for mental health conditions, 1992 to 2001. Psychiatr Serv 2005;56(6):671-7.

32 Adeosun I, Adegbohun AA, Jeje OO, Oyekunle OO, Omoniyi MO. Urgent and nonurgent presentations to a psychiatric emergency service in Nigeria: pattern and correlates. Emerg Med Int 2014;2014:479081.

33 Buys H, Muloiwa R, Westwood C, Richardson D, Cheema B, Westwood A. An adapted triage tool (ETAT) at Red Cross War Memorial Children's Hospital Medical Emergency Unit, Cape Town: an evaluation. S Afr Med J 2013;103(3):161-5.

34 Durojalve L, O'Meara M. A study of triage in paediatric patients in Australia. Emerg Med 2002;4: 67-76.

35 Bertolote JM, Fleischmann A, Butchart A, Besbelli N. Suicide, suicide attempts and pesticides: a major hidden public health problem, Editorial. Bull WHO 2006;84(4):260-1.

36 Australian and New Zealand Society of Geriatric Medicine. The management of older patients in the emergency department, <http://www.anzsgm.org/managementofolderpatientsintheemergencydepartment.pdf>; 2008 [accessed 12.14].

37 Carpenter CR, Bromley M, Caterino JM, Chun A, Gerson LW, Greenspan J et al. Optimal older adult emergency care: introducing multidisciplinary geriatric emergency department guidelines from the American College of Emergency Physicians, American Geriatrics Society, Emergency Nurses Association, and Society for Academic Emergency Medicine. J Am Geriatr Soc 2014;62(7):1360-3.

38 Carpenter CR, Platts-Mills TF. Evolving prehospital, emergency department, and "inpatient" management models for geriatric emergencies. Clin Geriatr Med 2013;29(1):31-47.

39 Arendts G, Lowthian J. Demography is destiny: an agenda for geriatric medicine in Australasia. Emerg Med Australas 2013;25(3):271-8.

40 Australasian College of Emergency Medicine. Policy on the care of elderly patients in the emergency department, <https://www.acem.org.au/getattachment/1b47b3b9-0643-4860-b3c9-52435d8cf8d0/Policy-on-the-Care-of-Elderly-Patients-in-the-Emer.aspx>; 2013 [accessed 12.14].

41 Karam A. Radiological incidents and emergencies. In: Veenema TG. Disaster nursing and emergency preparedness for chemical, biological and radiological terrorism and other hazards. 2nd ed. New York: Springer Publishing Company; 2007, pp 521–45.

42 Colella M, Thompson S, McIntosh S, Logan M. An introduction to radiological terrorism. J Emer Manag 2005;20(2):9-17.

43 Thornton R, Court B, Meara J, Murray V, Palmer I, Scott R et al. Chemical, biological, radiological and nuclear terrorism: an introduction for occupational physicians. Occup Med (Lond) 2004;54(2):101-9.

44 Veenema TG, Benitez J, Benware S. Chemical agents of concern. In: Veenema TG (ed). Disaster nursing and emergency preparedness for chemical, biological and radiological terrorism and other hazards. 2nd ed. New York: Springer Publishing Company; 2007, pp 483–505.

45 Croddy E, Ackerman G. Biological and chemical terrorism: a unique threat. In: Veenema TG (ed). Disaster nursing and emergency preparedness for chemical, biological and radiological terrorism and other hazards. 2nd ed. New York: Springer Publishing Company; 2007, pp 365–89.

46 Pigott D, Kazzi Z. Biological agents of concern. In: Veenema TG (ed). Disaster nursing and emergency preparedness for chemical, biological and radiological terrorism and other hazards. 2nd ed. New York: Springer Publishing Company; 2007, pp 403-23.

47 Varma. D, Guest. I. The Bhopal accident and methyl isocyanate toxicity. J Toxicol Environ Health 1993;40(4):513-29.

48 Kumar V, Goel R, Chawla R, Silambarasan M, Sharma RK. Chemical, biological, radiological, and nuclear decontamination: recent trends and future perspective. J Pharm Bioallied Sci 2010;2(3):220-38.

49 Ollerton JE. Emergency department response to the deliberate release of biological agents. Emerg Med J 2004;21(1):5-8.

50 Wessely S, Hyams KC. Editorials: Psychological implications of chemical and biological weapons. Long term social and psychological effects may be worse than acute ones. BMJ 2001;323:878.

51 Okumura T, Hisaoka T, Yamada A, Naito T, Isonuma H, Okumura S et al. The Tokyo subway sarin attack – lessons learned. Toxicol Appl Pharmacol 2005;207(2 Suppl):471-6.

52 Morris J, Ieraci S, Bauman A, Mohsin M. Emergency department work practices review project: introduction of work practice model and development of clinical documentation system specifications. Sydney: NSW Department of Health; 2001.

53 Fry M, Borg A, Jackson S, McAlpine A. The advanced clinical nurse a new model of practice: meeting the challenge of peak activity periods. Aust Emerg Nurs J 1999;2(3):26-8.

54 Patel H, Celenza A, Watters T. Effect of nurse initiated X-rays of the lower limb on patient transit time through the emergency department. Australas Emerg Nurs J 2012;15(4):229-34.

55 Fry M. Triage nurses order x-rays for patients with isolated distal limb injuries: a 12-month ED study. J Emerg Nurs 2001;27(1):17-22.

56 Lindley-Jones M, Finlayson B. Triage nurse requested x rays – are they worthwhile? J Accid Emerg Med 2000;17(2):103-7.

57 Fry M. Expanding the triage nurses role in the emergency department: how will this influence practice? Aust Emerg Nurs J 2002;5(1):32-6.

58 McCallum T. Pain management in Australian emergency departments: a critical appraisal of evidence based practice. Aust Emerg Nurs J 2004; 6(2):9 13.

59 Fry M, Holdgate A. Nurse-initiated intravenous morphine in the emergency department: efficacy, rate of adverse events and impact on time to analgesia. Emerg Med 2002;14:246-54.

60 Coman M, Kelly A. Safety of a nurse-managed, titrated analgesia protocol for the management of severe pain in the emergency department. Emerg Med 1999;11:128-32.

61 Muntlin A, Carlsson M, Safwenberg U, Gunningberg L. Outcomes of a nurse-initiated intravenous analgesic protocol for abdominal pain in an emergency department: a quasi-experimental study. Int J Nurs Stud 2011;48(1):13-23.

62 Australasian College for Emergency Medicine Australian and New Zealand College of Anaesthetists Joint Faculty of Intensive Care Medicine. Minimum standards for transport of critically ill patients, <http://www.anzca.edu.au/resources/professional-documents/pdfs/ps52-2013-guidelines-for-transport-of-critically-ill-patients.pdf>; 2003 (updated Nov 2013) [accessed 12.14].

63 Advanced Life Support Group. Major incident medical management and support: the practical approach. 2nd ed. London: BMJ Books; 2002.

64 Emergency Management Australia. Australian emergency manuals series Part 3. Emergency management practice, Vol. 1, Service provision; manual 2. Disaster medicine. Australian Government. 2nd ed. Australian Emergency Management Institute, <https://ema.infoservices.com.au/collections/handbook>; 2010.

65 Brennan R, Bradt D, Abrahams J. Medical issues in disasters. In: Cameron P, Jelinek G, Kelly A-M, Murray L, Brown A, eds. Textbook of adult emergency medicine. 3rd ed. Edinburgh: Churchill Livingstone Elsevier; 2009, pp 785-93.

66 Wallen E, Venkataraman S, Grosso M, Kiene K, Orr RA. Intrahospital transport of critically ill paediatric patients. Crit Care Med 1995;23:1588-95.

67 Waddell G. Movement of critically ill patients within hospital. BMJ 1975;2(5968):417-19.

68 Warren J, Fromm R, Orr R, Rotello L, Horst H. Guidelines for the inter- and intrahospital transport of critically ill patients. Crit Care Med 2004;32(1):256-62.

69 Whiteley S, Gray A, McHugh P, O'Riordan B. Guidelines for the transport of the critically ill adult: standards and guidelines:, <http://critical caremedicine.pbworks.com/f/Transport+of+Critically+Ill+Patient~ICS.PDF>; 2002 [accessed 12.14].

70 Goldhill D, Gemmell L, Lutman D, McDevitt S, Parris M, Waldmann C et al. Interhospital transfer. <http://www.aagbi.org/sites/default/files/interhospital09.pdf>; 2009 [accessed 12.14].

71 Ehrenwerth J, Sorbo S, Hackel A. Transport of critically ill adults. Crit Care Med 1986;14(6): 543-7.

72 Braman S, Dunn S, Amico C, Millman R. Complications of intrahospital transport in critically ill patients. Ann Intern Med 1987;107(4):469-73.

73 Duke G, Green J. Outcome of critically ill patients undergoing interhospital transfer. Med J Aust 2001;174:122-5.

74 American College of Emergency Physicians. Hospital Disaster Preparedness Self-Assessment Tool, <http://www.acep.org/content.aspx?id=912052002> [accessed 12.14].

75 Tallman T. Acute bronchitis and upper airways. In: Tintinalli J, Stapczynski J, Ma J, Cline D, Cydulka R, Meckler G, eds. Emergency medicine; A comprehensive study guide. American College of Emergency Physicians. 7th ed. New York: McGraw-Hill; 2011, pp 445-58.

76 Emerman C, Anderson E, Cline D. Community acquired pneumonia, aspiration pneumonia. In: Tintinalli J, Stapczynski J, Ma J, Cline D, Cydulka R, Meckler G, eds. Emergency medicine; A comprehensive study guide. American College of Emergency Physicians. 7th ed. New York: McGraw-Hill; 2011, pp 479-91.

77 Wills CP, Young M, White DW. Pitfalls in the evaluation of shortness of breath. Emerg Med Clinics N Am 2010;28:163-81.

78 Sarko J, Stapczynski J. Respiratory distress. In: Tintinalli J, Stapczynski J, Ma J, Cline D, Cydulka R, Meckler G, eds. Emergency medicine; A comprehensive study guide. American College of Emergency Physicians. 7th ed. New York: McGraw-Hill; 2011, pp 465-73.

79 Hore C, Roberts J. Respiratory emergencies: the acutely breathless patient. In: Fulde G, ed. Emergency medicine: The principles of practice. Sydney: Elsevier; 2009, pp 122-39.

80 Callahan JM. Pulse oximetry in emergency medicine. Emerg Med Clin N Am 2008;26:896-79.

81 Kelly A. Asthma. In: Cameron P, Jelinek G, Kelly A-M, Murray L, Brown A, eds. Textbook of adult emergency medicine. 3rd ed. Edinburgh: Churchill Livingstone Elsevier; 2009, pp 279-82.

82 Australian Centre for Asthma Monitoring. Asthma in Australia, <http://www.aihw.gov.au/publication-detail/?id=10737420159>; 2011 [accessed 12.14].

83 Powell C, Kelly A, Kerr D. Lack of agreement in classification of the severity of acute asthma between emergency physician assessment and classification using the National Asthma Council Australia guidelines. Emerg Med 2003;15(1):49-53.

84 National Asthma Council Australia. Asthma management handbook, <http:www.nationalasthma.org.au/cms/index.php>; 2014 [accessed 05.14].

85 Cyudlka R. Acute asthma in adults. In: Tintinalli J, Stapczynski J, Ma J, Cline D, Cydulka R, Meckler G, eds. Emergency medicine; A comprehensive study guide. American College of Emergency Physicians. 7th ed. New York: McGraw-Hill; 2011, pp 468-75.

86 Hillman K, Bishop G. Specific respiratory problems. Clinical intensive care and acute medicine. 2nd ed. Cambridge: Cambridge University Press; 2004, pp 325-73.

87 Putland M. Community acquired pneumonia. In: Cameron P, Jelinek G, Kelly A-M, Murray L, Brown A, eds. Textbook of adult emergency medicine. 3rd ed. Edinburgh: Churchill Livingstone; 2009. p. 283-93.

88 Lazarus SC. Clinical practice. Emergency treatment of asthma. N Engl J Med 2010;363(8):755-64.

89 Bates C, Cydulka R. Chronic obstructive pulmonary disease. In: Tintinalli J, Stapczynski J, Ma J, Cline D, Cydulka R, Meckler G, eds. Emergency medicine; A comprehensive study guide. American College of Emergency Physicians. 7th ed. New York: McGraw-Hill; 2011, pp 511-9.

90 Naughton M, Tuxen D. Acute respiratory failure in chronic obstructive pulmonary disease. In: Bersten A, Soni N, Oh T, eds. Oh's intensive care manual. 5th ed. Oxford: Butterworth-Heinemann; 2003, pp 297-308.

91 Murrie J, Wu L. Factors influencing in-hospital mortality in community-acquired pneumonia: a prospective study of patients not initially admitted to the ICU. Chest 2005;127:1260-70.

92 Green G, Hill P. Approaches to chest pain. In: Tintinalli J, Stapczynski J, Ma J, Cline D, Cydulka R, Meckler G, eds. Emergency medicine; A comprehensive study guide. American College of Emergency Physicians. 7th ed. New York: McGraw-Hill; 2011, pp 333-43.

93 Hollander J. Acute coronary syndromes: acute myocardial infarction and unstable angina. In: Tintinalli J, Stapczynski J, Ma J, Cline D, Cydulka R, Meckler G, eds. Emergency medicine; A comprehensive study guide. American College of Emergency Physicians. 7th ed. New York: McGraw-Hill; 2011, pp 343-59.

94 Goodacre S. Chest pain. In: Cameron P, Jelinek G, Kelly A-M, Murray L, Brown A, eds. Textbook of adult emergency medicine. 3rd ed. Edinburgh: Churchill Livingstone Elsevier; 2009, pp 205-7.

95 Whelan P, Whelan A. The approach to the patient with chest pain, dyspnoea or haemoptysis. In: Fulde G, ed. Emergency medicine: The principles of practice. Sydney: Elsevier; 2009, pp 96-107.

96 Parsonage WA, Cullen L, Younger JF. The approach to patients with possible cardiac chest pain. Med J Aust 2013;199(1):30-4.

97 Jones ID, Slovis CM. Pitfalls in evaluating the low risk chest pain patient. Emerg Med Clinic N Am 2010;28:183-201.

98 Woo KC, Schnieder JI. High risk chief complaints 1: chest pain – the big three. Emerg Med Clinics N Am 2009;27:685-712.

99 Queensland Government. Cardiac chest pain risk stratification pathway, <http:www.health.qld.gov.au/caru/pathways/docs/pathway_chstpain.pdf>; 2012 [accessed 12.14].

100 Edwards N, Varma M, Pitcher D. Changing names, changing times, changing treatment: an overview of acute coronary syndromes. Br J Resusc 2005;4:6-10.

101 National Centre for Monitoring Cardiovascular Disease. Heart, stroke and vascular diseases, <http://www.aihw.gov.au/publication-detail/?id=6442467236>; 2001 [accessed 2014 Dec].

102 Goodacre S, Kelly AM. Acute coronary syndromes. In: Cameron P, Jelinek G, Kelly A-M, Murray L, Brown A, eds. Textbook of adult emergency medicine. 3rd ed. Edinburgh: Churchill Livingston; 2009, pp 208-14.

103 Prince L, Johnson G. Aortic dissection and aneurysms. In: Tintinalli J, Stapczynski J, Ma J, Cline D, Cydulka R, Meckler G, eds. Emergency medicine; A comprehensive study guide. American College of Emergency Physicians. 7th ed. New York: McGraw-Hill; 2011, pp 404-9.

104 Drake TR. Aortic aneurysms and aortic dissection. In: Markovchick VJ, Pons PT, eds. Emergency medicine secrets. 3rd ed. Philadelphia: Hanley & Belfus; 2003, pp 154-7.

105 Gallagher EJ, Lukens TW, Colucciello SV, Morgan DL. Clinical policy: critical issues for the initial evaluation and management of patients presenting with a chief complaint of non traumatic abdominal pain. Annal Emerg Med 2000;36(4):406-15.

106 Graff L, Robinson D. Abdominal pain and emergency department evaluation. Emerg Med Clin N Am 2001;19(1):123-35.

107 Lameris W, van Randen A, Dijkgraaf MG, Bossuyt PM, Stoker J, Boermeester MA. Optimization of diagnostic imaging use in patients with acute abdominal pain (OPTIMA): design and rationale. BMC Emerg Med 2007;7:9.

108 Kamin RA, Nowicki TA, Courtney DS, Powers RD. Pearls and pitfalls in the emergency department evaluation of abdominal pain. Emerg Med Clin N Am 2003;21(1):61-72.

109 O'Toole J. Abdominal pain: pathophysiology, etiology, diagnosis, and therapy (pain management in the ED). Top Emerg Med 2002;24(1):46-51.

110 Trott A, Lucas R. Acute abdominal pain. In: Rosen P, ed. Emergency medicine: Concepts and clinical practice. 4th ed. St Louis: Mosby; 1998, pp 1888-903.

111 Chan K, Seow E. Approaches to abdominal pain. In: Cameron P, Jelinek G, Kelly A-M, Murray L, Brown A, eds. Textbook of adult emergency medicine. 3rd ed. Edinburgh: Churchill Livingstone Elsevier; 2009, pp 316-25.

112 Dagiely S. An algorithm for triaging commonly missed causes of acute abdominal pain. J Emer Nurs 2006;32(1):9.

113 Paseo C. Pain in the emergency department: withholding pain medication is not justified. Am J Nurs 2003;103(7):73-4.

114 National Institute of Clinical Studies. Pain medication for acute abdominal pain, <http://www.nhmrc.gov.au/_files_nhmrc/file/nics/material_resources/pain_medication_aute_abdominal_pain.pdf>; 2008 [accessed 12.14].

115 Tillman K, Lee OD, Whitty K. Abdominal aortic aneurysm: an often asymptomatic and fatal men's health issue. Am J Mens Health 2013;7(2):163-8.

116 Chung CH. Aneurysms. In: Cameron P, Jelinek G, Kelly A-M, Murray L, Brown A, eds. Textbook of adult emergency medicine. 3rd ed. Edinburgh: Churchill Livingstone; 2009, pp 269-72.

117 Nshuti R, Kruger D, Luvhengo TE. Clinical presentation of acute appendicitis in adults at the Chris Hani Baragwanath Academic Hospital. Int J Emerg Med 2014;7(1):12.

118 Banerjee A. Acute appendicitis. In: Cameron P, Jelinek G, Kelly A-M, Murray L, Brown A, eds. Textbook of adult emergency medicine. 3rd ed. Edinburgh: Churchill Livingstone; 2009, pp 350-3.

119 Yates K. Bowel obstruction. In: Cameron P, Jelinek G, Kelly A-M, Murray L, Brown A, eds. Textbook of adult emergency medicine. Edinburgh: Churchill Livingstone; 2009, pp 325-7.

120 Vallicelli C, Coccolini F, Catena F, Ansaloni L, Montori G, Di Saverio S et al. Small bowel emergency surgery: literature's review. World J Emerg Surg 2011;6(1):1.

121 Bryan S. Ectopic pregnancy and bleeding in early pregnancy. In: Cameron P, Jelinek G, Kelly A-M, Murray L, Brown A, eds. Textbook of adult emergency medicine. Edinburgh: Churchill Livingstone; 2009, pp 592-4.

122 Sivalingam VN, Duncan WC, Kirk E, Shephard LA, Horne AW. Diagnosis and management of ectopic pregnancy. J Fam Plann Reprod Health Care 2011;37(4):231-40.

123 Kinlay S. Changes in stroke epidemiology, prevention, and treatment. Circulation 2011;124(19):e494-6.

124 Brain Foundation. Stroke 2014. <http://brainfoundation.org.au/component/content/article/3-stroke/64-does-stroke-affect-many-australians>; 2014 [accessed 12.14].

125 Stroke Foundation. Clinical guidelines for acute stroke management, <http://brainfoundation.org.au/component/content/article/3-stroke/64-does-stroke-affect-many-australians>; 2010 [accessed 12.14].

126 Somes J, Bergman DL. ABCDs of acute stroke intervention. J Emerg Nurs 2007;33(3):228-34.

127 Goldstein LB, Adams R, Alberts MJ, Appel LJ, Brass LM, Bushnell CD et al. Primary prevention of ischemic stroke: a guideline from the American Heart Association/American Stroke Association Stroke Council (co-sponsored by the Atherosclerotic Peripheral Vascular Disease Interdisciplinary Working Group; Cardiovascular Nursing Council; Clinical Cardiology Council; Nutrition, Physical Activity, and Metabolism Council; the Quality of Care and Outcomes Research Interdisciplinary Working Group). Stroke 2006;37:1583-633.

128 Krock AB, Massaro L. Facilitating ED evaluation of patients with acute ischemic stroke. J Emerg Nurs 2008;34(6):519-22.

129 Adams HP, Adams RJ, Brott M, del Zoppo G, Furlan A, Goldstein LB et al. Guidelines for the early management of patients with ischemic stroke. Stroke 2003;34:1056-83.

130 Nedeltchev K, Renz N, Karameshev A, Haefeli T, Brekenfeld C, Meier N et al. Predictors of early mortality after acute ischaemic stroke. Swiss Med Wkly 2010;140(17-18):254-9.

131 Schretzman D. Acute ischemic stroke. Dimens Crit Care Nurs 2001;20(2):14-7.

132 van Wijk I, Kappelle LJ, van Gijn J, Koudstaal PJ, Franke CL, Vermeulen M et al. Long-term survival and vascular event risk after transient ischaemic attack or minor ischaemic stroke: a cohort study. Lancet 2005;365(9477):2098-104.

133 Murray L, Daly F, Little M, Cadogan M, eds. Toxicology handbook. Sydney: Elsevier; 2007.

134 Murray L. Approaches to the poisoned patient. In: Cameron P, Jelinek G, Kelly A-M, Murray L, Brown A, eds. Textbook of adult emergency medicine. Edinburgh: Churchill Livingstone; 2009, pp 893-9.

135 Gunnell D, Ho D, Murray V. Medical management of deliberate drug overdose: a neglected area for suicide prevention. Emerg Med J 2004;21:35-8.

136 Hack J, Hoffman R. General management of poisoned patients. In: Tintinalli J, Kelen G, Stapczynski J, eds. Emergency medicine: A comprehensive study guide. 6th ed. New York: McGraw-Hill; 2004, pp 1015-22.

137 Yates K. Accidental poisoning in New Zealand. Emerg Med 2003;15(3):244-9.

138 World Health Organization. Management of substance abuse, <http://www.who.int/substance_abuse/en/>; 2012 [accessed 12.14].

139 Miller M, Draper G. Statistics on drug use in Australia 2000. Canberra: Australian Institute of Health and Welfare; 2001.

140 Wazaify M, Kennedy S, Hughes CM, McElnay JC. Prevalence of over-the-counter drug-related overdoses at accident and emergency departments in Northern Ireland – a retrospective evaluation. J Clin Pharm Ther 2005;30(1):39-44.

141 Hawton K, Simkin S, Deekes J, Cooper J, Johnston A, Waters K et al. UK legislation on analgesic packs: before and after study of long term effects on poisonings. Br Med J 2004;329:1076-84.

142 Braitberg G, Kerr F. Central nervous system drugs. In: Cameron P, Jelinek G, Kelly A-M, Murray L, Brown A, eds. Textbook of adult emergency medicine. Edinburgh: Churchill Livingstone; 2009, pp 906-17.

143 Roberts DM. Pesticides. In: Cameron P, Jelinek G, Kelly A-M, Murray L, Brown A, eds. Textbook of adult emergency medicine. Edinburgh: Churchill Livingstone; 2009, pp 966-73.

144 Mills K. Tricyclic antidepressants and serotonin syndromes. In: Tintinalli J, Kelen G, Stapczynski J, eds. Emergency medicine: A comprehensive study guide. 6th ed. New York: McGraw-Hill; 2004, pp 1025.

145 Dowsett R. Corrosive ingestion. In: Cameron P, Jelinek G, Kelly A-M, Murray L, Brown A, eds. Textbook of adult emergency medicine. Edinburgh: Churchill Livingstone; 2009, pp 958-61.

146 Yip L. Aspirin and salicylates. In: Tintinalli J, Stapczynski J, Ma J, Cline D, Cydulka R, Meckler G, eds. Emergency medicine; A comprehensive study guide. American College of Emergency Physicians. 7th ed. New York: McGraw-Hill; 2011, pp 1243-6.

147 Daly F. Drugs of abuse. In: Cameron P, Jelinek G, Kelly A-M, Murray L, Brown A, eds. Textbook of adult emergency medicine. Edinburgh: Churchill Livingstone; 2009, pp 943-52.

148 Quan D. Benzodiapines. In: Tintinalli J, Stapczynski J, Ma J, Cline D, Cydulka R, Meckler G, eds. Emergency medicine; A comprehensive study guide. American College of Emergency Physicians. 7th ed. New York: McGraw-Hill; 2011, pp 1216-9.

149 Doyon S. Opiods. In: Tintinalli J, Stapczynski J, Ma J, Cline D, Cydulka R, Meckler G, eds. Emergency medicine; A comprehensive study guide. American College of Emergency Physicians. 7th ed. New York: McGraw-Hill; 2011, pp 1230-4.

150 Prosser J, Perrone J. Cocaine, methamphetamines, other amphetamines. In: Tintinalli J, Stapczynski J, Ma J, Cline D, Cydulka R, Meckler G, eds. Emergency medicine; A comprehensive study guide. American College of Emergency Physicians. 7th ed. New York: McGraw-Hill; 2011, pp 1234-8.

151 Prybys K, Hansen K. Hallucinogens. In: Tintinalli J, Stapczynski J, Ma J, Cline D, Cydulka R, Meckler G, eds. Emergency medicine; A comprehensive study guide. American College of Emergency Physicians. 7th ed. New York: McGraw-Hill; 2011, pp 1079-84.

152 Graudins A. Paracetamol. In: Cameron P, Jelinek G, Kelly A-M, Murray L, Brown A, eds. Textbook of adult emergency medicine. 3rd ed. Edinburgh: Churchill Livingstone; 2009, pp 928-30.

153 Clinical practice guidelines. Salicylate poisoning, <http://www.rch.org.au/clinicalguide/guideline_index/Salicylates_Posioning/>; 2014 [accessed 12.14].

154 Graudins A. Salicylate. In: Cameron P, Jelinek G, Kelly A-M, Murray L, Brown A, eds. Textbook of adult emergency medicine. 3rd ed. Edinburgh: Churchill Livingstone; 2009.

155 Daly FS, Fountain JS, Murray L, Graudins, Buckley NA. Consensus Statement. Guidelines for the Management of Paracetamol Poisoning in Australia and New Zealand; Explanation and Elaboration. Med J Aust 2008;188(5):296-302.

156 Wolf SJ, Heard K, Sloan EP, Jagoda AS. Clinical Policy: Critical Issues in the Management of Patients Presenting to the Emergency Department with Acetaminohen Overdose. J Emerg Nurs 2008;34(2):292-313.

157 Guidelines CP. Paracetamol poisoning, <http://www.rch.org.au/clinicalguide/cgp.cfm?doc_id=5436>; 2014.

158 Buckley N. Carbon monoxide. In: Cameron P, Jelinek G, Kelly A-M, Murray L, Brown A, eds. Textbook of adult emergency medicine. Edinburgh: Churchill Livingstone; 2009.

159 Goldstein M. Carbon monoxide poisoning. J Emerg Nurs 2008;34(6):538-42.

160 Bouchard N, Wallace A. Caustics. In: Tintinalli J, Stapczynski J, Ma J, Cline D, Cydulka R, Meckler G, eds. Emergency medicine; A comprehensive study guide. American College of Emergency Physicians. 7th ed. New York: McGraw-Hill; 2011, pp 2992-1297.

161 Javed A, Pal S, Krishnan EK, Sahni P, Chattopadhyay TK. Surgical management and outcomes of severe gastrointestinal injuries due to corrosive ingestion. World J Gastrointest Surg 2012;4(5):121-5.

162 Bruno R, Wallace A. Caustics. In: Tintinalli J, Kelen G, Stapczynski J, eds. Emergency medicine: A comprehensive study guide. 6th ed. New York: McGraw-Hill; 2004, pp 1130-4.

163 Wax P, Wong S. Hydrocarbons and volatile substances. In: Tintinalli J, Stapczynski J, Ma J, Cline D, Cydulka R, Meckler G, eds. Emergency medicine; A comprehensive study guide. American College of Emergency Physicians. 7th ed. New York: McGraw-Hill; 2011, pp 1287-92.

164 Lifshitz M, Sofer S, Gorodischer R. Hydrocarbon poisoning in children: a 5-year retrospective study. Wildern Environ Med 2003;14(2):78-82.

165 Little M, Murray L. Consensus statement: risk of nosocomial organophosphate poisoning in emergency departments. Emerg Med Australas 2004;16:456-8.

166 Robey W, Meggs W. Insecticides, herbicides, rodenticides. In: Tintinalli J, Stapczynski J, Ma J, Cline D, Cydulka R, Meckler G, eds. Emergency medicine, A comprehensive study guide. American College of Emergency Physicians. New York: McGraw-Hill; 2011, pp 1134-43.

167 Sutherland S, Tibbals J. Australian animal toxins: the creatures, their toxins and care of the poisoned patient. 2nd ed. Melbourne: Oxford University Press; 2001.

168 Nimorakiotakis B, Winkel KD. Spider bite – the redback spider and its relatives. Aust Family Phys. 2004;33(3):153-7.

169 Health NZMo, ed. Spiders in New Zealand: what to look out for and keeping yourself safe. Wellington, NZ: New Zealand Ministry of Health; 2003.

170 Slaughter RJ, Beasley DM, Lambie BS, Schep LJ. New Zealand's venomous creatures. NZ Med J 2009;122(1290):83-97.

171 Isbister G, Gray M. Latrodectism: a prospective cohort study of bites by formally identified redback spiders. Med J Aust 2003;179:88-91.

172 New South Wales Health Statewide Services Branch. Snakebite and spiderbite clinical management guidelines, <http://www0.health.nsw.gov.au/policies/gl/2014/pdf/GL2014_005.pdf>; 2013 [accessed 12.14].

173 Isbister GK. Spider bite: a current approach to management. Aust Prescrib 2006;156-158(29):6.

174 Isbister GK. Safety of I.V. administration of redback spider antivenom. Int Med J 2007;37:820-2.

175 Commonwealth Serum Laboratories. Red back spider antivenom: product information, <http://www.csl.com.au/docs/1002/757/Red-Back-Spider-AV_PI_V5_Clean_TGA-Approved_8-January-2014.pdf#search=Red back spider antivenom Product information>; 2014.

176 Isbister GK, Brown SGA, Miller M, Tankel A, MacDonald E, Sokes B et al. A randomised controlled trial of intramuscular vs. intravenous antivenom for latrodectism – the RAVE study. QJM 2008;101:557-65.

177 Isbister G, Graudins A, White J, Warrell D. Antivenom treatment in arachnidism. J Toxicol 2003;41(3):291-300.

178 Commonwealth Serum Laboratories. Funnel web spider antivenom: product information 2013. Commonwealth Serum Laboratories, 2014 #113.

179 Stewart C. Snake bite in Australia: First aid and envenomation management. Accid Emerg Nurs 2003;11:106-11.

180 Australian Venom Research Unit. Snakebite in Australia. University of Melbourne, <http://www.avru.org/health/health_snakes.html>; 2011.

181 Isbister GK. Snake bite: a current approach to management. Aust Prescrib 2008;28(5):125-9.

182 White J. Snakebite and spiderbite: management guidelines for New South Wales Health Department, <http://www0.health.nsw.gov.au/policies/gl/2014/pdf/GL2014_005.pdf>; 2013 [accessed 12.14].

183 Currie BJ, Canale E, Isbister GK. Effectiveness of pressure-immobilization first aid for snakebite requires further study. Emerg Med Australas 2008;20:267-70.

184 Canale E, Isbister GK, Currie BJ. Investigating pressure bandaging for snakebite in a simulated setting: bandage type, training and the effect of transport. Emerg Med Australas 2008;21:184-90.

185 Currie B. Clinical toxicology: a tropical Australian perspective. Ther Drug Monit 2000;22(1):73-8.

186 Australian Venom Research Unit. Box jellyfish, <http://www.avru.org/general/general_boxjelly.html>; 2011 [accessed 12.14].

187 Bailey P, Little M, Jelinek G, Wilce J. Jellyfish envenoming syndromes: unknown toxic mechanisms and proven therapies. Med J Aust 2003;178:34-7.

188 O'Reilly G, Isbister G, Lawrie P, Treston G, Currie B. Prospective study of jellyfish stings from tropical Australia, including the major box jellyfish *Chironcx fleckeri*. Med J Aust 2001;175:652-5.

189 Burnett J, Currie B, Fenner P, Rifkin J, Williamson J. Cubozoans ('box jellyfish'). In: Williamson J, Fenner P, Burnett J, eds. Venomous and poisonous marine animals: Medical and biological handbook. Sydney: University of New South Wales Press; 1996, pp 236-83.

190 Li L, McGee RG, Isbister G, Webster AC. Interventions for the symptoms and signs resulting from jellyfish stings. Cochrane Database Syst Rev 2013;12:CD009688.

191 Little M. Marine envenomation and poisoning. In: Cameron P, Jelinek G, Kelly A-M, Murray L, Brown A, eds. Textbook of adult emergency medicine. Edinburgh: Churchill Livingstone; 2009, pp 993-7.

192 Ramsasamy S, Isbister GK, Seymour JE, Hodgson W. The in vivo cardiovascular effects of box jellyfish *Chironex fleckeri* venom in rats: efficacy of pre treatment with antivenom, verapamil and magnesium sulfate. Toxicon 2004;43(6):685-90.

193 Australian Resuscitation Council. Guideline 8.9.6. Envenomation – jellyfish stings, <http://resus.org.au/download/9_4_envenomation/guideline-9-4-5july10.pdf>; 2005 [accessed 12.14].

194 Little M, Pereria P, Mulchay R, Cullen P. Marine envenomation. Emerg Med Aust 2001;13(3):390-2.

195 Fenner P, Hadock J. Fatal envenomation by jellyfish causing Irukanji syndrome. Med J Aust 2002;177:362-3.

196 Lewis R. Australian perspectives on a global problem. Toxicon 2006;48(7):799-809.

197 Arnold T. Ciguatera, <http://emedicine.medscape.com/article/813869-overview>; 2010 [accessed 12.14].

198 Dickey RW, Plakas SM. Ciguatera: a public health perspective. Toxins in Seafood 2010;56(2):123-36.

199 Sobel J, Painter J. Illnesses caused by marine biotoxins. Clinic Infect Dis 2005;41(9):1290-6.

200 McGauly P, Mahler S. Food and waterbourne disease. In: Tintinalli J, Stapczynski J, Ma J, Cline D, Cydulka R, Meckler G, eds. Emergency medicine; A comprehensive study guide. American College of Emergency Physicians. 7th ed. New York: McGraw-Hill; 2011, pp 1062-70.

201 World Health Organization. Drowning, Fact sheet No. 347, <http://www.who.int/mediacentre/factsheets/fs347/en/>; 2014 [accessed 12.14].

202 Brenner RA, Trumble AC, Smith GS, Kessler EP, Overpeck MD. Where children drown, United States, 1995. Pediatrics 2001;108(1):85-9.

203 Mackie IJ. Patterns of drowning in Australia, 1992–1997. Med J Aust 1999;171(11-12):587-90.

204 Kobusingye O. The global burden of drowning: Africa. In: Bierens J, ed. Handbook on drowning: Prevention, rescue and treatment. Netherlands: Springer; 2003.

205 Hasibeder W. Drowning. Curr Opin Anaesth 2003;16(2):139-45.

206 Martinez FE, Hooper AJ. Drowning and immersion injury. Anaesth Intens Care Med 2014;15(9):420-3.

207 Bernocchi P, Scalvini S, Tridico C, Borghi G, Masella C. Healthcare continuity from hospital to territory in Lombardy: TELEMACO project. Am J Manag Care 2012;18(3):e101-e8.

208 Shepherd S. Submersion injury, near drowning, <http://www.patient.co.uk/doctor/Drowning-and-near-drowning.htm>; 2010 [accessed 12.14].

209 Moon R, Long R. Drowning and near-drowning. Emerg Med 2002;14(4):377-86.

210 World Health Organization. Guidelines for safe recreational water environments: Drowning and injury prevention, <http://www.who.int/water_sanitation_health/bathing/srwe1/en/> [accessed 05.14].

211 Ibsen L. Submersion and asphyxial injury. Crit Care Med 2002;30(11 Suppl):402-8.

212 Handley AJ. Drowning. BMJ 2014;348:g1734.

213 Fiore M. Near drowning, <http://www.emedicine.com/ped/topic2570.htm>; 2009 [accessed 12.14].

214 Rodgers I. Hypothermia. In: Cameron P, Jelinek G, Kelly A, Murray L, Heyworth J, eds. Textbook of adult emergency medicine. Edinburgh: Churchill Livingstone; 2009, pp 852-4.

215 Ko C, Alex J, Jefferies S, Parmar J. Dead? Or just cold?: profound hypothermia with no signs of life. Emerg Med J 2002;19:478-9.

216 Bressen H, Ngo B. Hypothermia. In: Tintinalli J, Stapczynski J, Ma J, Cline D, Cydulka R, Meckler G, eds. Emergency medicine; A comprehensive study guide. American College of Emergency Physicians. 7th ed. New York: McGraw-Hill; 2011, pp 1335-9.

217 Rodgers I, Williams A. Heat related illness. In: Cameron P, Jelinek G, Kelly A, Murray L, Heyworth J, eds. Textbook of adult emergency medicine. Edinburgh: Churchill Livingstone; 2009, pp 848-51.

218 Krantz M, Lowery C. Giant Osborne waves in hypothermia. N Engl J Med 2005;352(2):184.

219 Tsuei B, Kearney P. Hypothermia in the trauma patient. Injury 2005;35(1):7-15.

220 Sessler D. Complications and treatment of mild hypothermia. Anesthesiology 2001;95(2):531-43.

221 Hildebrand F, Giannoudis P, van Grievensen M, Chawda M, Pape H-S. Pathophysiologic changes and effects of hypothermia on outcome in elective surgery and trauma patients. Am J Surg 2004;187(3):363-71.

222 Waters T, Al-Salamah M. Heat emergencies. In: Tintinalli J, Stapczynski J, Ma J, Cline D, Cydulka R, Meckler G, eds. Emergency medicine; A comprehensive study guide. American College of Emergency Physicians. 7th ed. New York: McGraw-Hill; 2011, pp 1339-44.

223 Physicians for Social Responsibility. The medical and public health impacts of global warming, <http://www.psr.org/resources/the-medical-and-public-health-impacts-of-global-warming.pdf> [accessed 12.14].

224 Yeo T. Heat stroke: a comprehensive review. AACN Clin Issues 2004;15(2):280-93.

Chapter 24

Trauma management

Catherine Bell, Kerstin Prignitz Sluys

Learning objectives

After reading this chapter, you should be able to:

- identify the benefits and limitations of an organised trauma system
- describe the rationale for a systematic approach to the patient who has sustained injuries
- discuss the benefits of appropriate management of the patient with serious injury and/or multitrauma
- describe the acute management of the patient with multiple serious fractures
- describe the acute management of patients with burn injuries, abdominal injuries and chest trauma
- describe the nurse's role in managing the trauma patient undergoing interim damage-control surgery.

Introduction

Trauma is one of the leading public health problems and the most common avoidable cause of death among children and adults under 45 years of age throughout the world.[1-5] The World Health Organization (WHO) reports that almost 6 million people die every year and 100 million are admitted to hospital after traumatic injury, accounting for 16% of the world's disease burden.[2,4] Survivors incur temporary or permanent impairments and disabilities resulting in human suffering, major social consequences and economic cost for the individual, families and society. The most common cause of death from trauma worldwide is traffic accidents, and more than 90% of the deaths occur in low and middle income countries.[6]

The injury epidemiology for trauma differs with severity. The majority of trauma patients requiring admission to an ICU are those with more serious injuries that are associated with motor vehicles, motorbikes and pedestrian collisions. Falls, self-inflicted injuries and assaults are less common, but still frequent, causes of trauma requiring critical care admission. A significant proportion of injured patients admitted to critical care have experienced neurotrauma (see Chapter 17), while other common injuries include multiple fractures and injury to internal organs in the thorax and abdomen.

The systematic organisation of trauma systems, major changes in practice and delivery of time-critical interventions have made the traditional boundaries more seamless between pre-hospital emergency medical service and hospital-based emergency, surgery, radiology and intensive care services, improving the survival of trauma patients in recent years. Consequently, a greater number of patients with severe multiple injuries are now admitted to critical care units. These patients generally require complex nursing care, often for lengthy periods, both within the critical care unit and beyond. The common traumatic injuries that result in admission to critical care and the principles of management are outlined in this chapter.

Trauma systems and processes

A trauma system can be defined as:

an assembly of health care processes intended to improve survival among injured patients by reducing the time interval between injury and definitive treatment, and by assuring that appropriate resources and personnel are immediately available when a patient presents to a hospital'.[7]

Trauma systems should be 'designed to provide citizens with prompt, safe and effective access to the health-care system in times of urgent need. Each system must be defined by local needs and assessments of capacity and developed with due regard for local culture, legislation, infrastructure, health-system capacity, economic considerations and administrative resources'.[8 p 13]

Over the last 30 years there has been significant evolution of trauma systems and planning for how major trauma is managed.[9] The World Health Organization (WHO) suggest that pre-hospital trauma care systems cannot function in isolation and must be fully integrated into existing public health and healthcare infrastructure to be effective.[8,10]

Trauma systems are inclusive of all areas of health care that are involved in the management of the trauma patient from injury through to discharge or death, to enable the scope of improvement to be targeted at any area across the continuum of care.[11,12] Although many studies have found that regionalisation of trauma care has been associated with reduced mortality,[13] the impact on the quality of survival of trauma patients has not been systematically explored.[14] One possible explanation for improved outcome in those patients who are admitted to a major trauma service is the expertise and experience of all staff caring for this cohort and the greater access to rehabilitation services, which may contribute to improved functional outcome.[14,15]

Despite the lack of empirical evidence supporting the benefits of implementing trauma systems,[16] internationally it is suggested that the mortality rate is reduced by 15–40% when a trauma system is implemented.[9] In developed countries where trauma systems have been established the likelihood of continued improvement in mortality is seen to be small in comparison to the initial reduction observed when a trauma system is first implemented.[9]

Pre-hospital care

There are multiple purposes of pre-hospital care, including:

- providing appropriate care at the scene
- transporting the patient to the most appropriate healthcare facility for further management
- reducing the occurrence of preventable death and disability associated with trauma.

The optimal pre-hospital trauma care model is in doubt with the debate of whether pre-hospital time or initial treatment occurring in a hospital is the more relevant to decreasing mortality in the trauma population.[17] The focus of treatment should be on:

- rapid primary assessment
- maintaining a patent airway
- immediate control of external haemorrhage
- immobilisation of the patient
- rapid transfer to an appropriate trauma centre.[18]

The principle of the 'golden hour' is commonly referred to in trauma literature, with the belief that trauma patients have better outcomes if they are provided definitive care within 60 minutes of injury. This is the basis for concepts such as 'scoop and run', aeromedical transport and trauma centre designation with trauma teams in place that are seen to have an impact on the management of the injured patient.[19] In the USA a reduction in mortality in those patients transported by air rather than traditional methods has been seen,[20] whereas others have suggested that the timely triage of the injured to the closest most appropriate facility is essential.[21]

In countries with large distances to designated trauma centres this can pose a problem; however, it has been shown that the disadvantage of spending more time at the scene is possibly diluted by the delivery of high standards of care using the principles of Advanced Life Support (ALS). There is controversy about whether treating life-threatening events at the scene or first hospital rather than at a trauma centre reduces mortality or not.[17,20,22] Treatment at the scene may be delivered by personnel with differing levels of expertise worldwide, with some countries in Europe having doctors at the scene while countries such as Australia, the USA and UK have highly trained paramedics.[21] Other countries may rely on first responders who may only have the capacity to administer Basic Life Support (BLS).[10]

In areas where trauma systems have been implemented processes are in place to facilitate advance notice being given to the trauma centre to enable the assembly of a multidisciplinary group of health professionals who can provide immediate assessment, resuscitation and treatment of the injured patient.[23–25] Such trauma teams have been shown to provide benefit in the early management of trauma patients, and are reviewed later in this chapter.[25,26]

Transport of the critically ill trauma patient

Transporting severely injured patients directly from the scene of injury to a designated trauma centre is considered optimal;[12,27] however, there are risks involved in any transfer and the goal should be to provide the best care possible while reducing those risks to the patient.[21,23] In general, with any patient transfer the level of health care available should be maintained or increased at each stage.[13]

Transport of critically injured patients occurs at two stages in the patient's care. Primary transport occurs from the scene of injury to the first healthcare facility that provides care to the patient; this is sometimes referred to as pre-hospital transport. Secondary transport occurs between healthcare facilities; this is sometimes referred to as inter-hospital transport. This chapter concentrates on secondary transport, although many of the principles are similar for both stages of transport. Secondary transport principles are also relevant for critically injured patients being transferred within departments in a healthcare facility (see Chapter 6). Transport of a patient between healthcare facilities may occur for clinical reasons, such as specialist or higher levels of care being required, or for non-clinical reasons, such as bed availability. It is preferable for patient transfer to be for clinical reasons only.

Secondary transport of critically injured patients may occur via ground or air (by fixed-wing aircraft or helicopter).[28] The decision as to what form of transport to use will depend on:

- the condition of the patient
- the potential impact of the transport medium on the patient
- the distance to be covered
- the urgency of the transport
- the environmental conditions
- the resources available
- the expertise of the respective transport teams.

Amenities such as landing sites, particularly for helicopters, being in close proximity to healthcare facilities must also be considered. Different jurisdictions activate air retrieval using helicopters when the distance for the transport is beyond a certain point, with the minimum distance ranging from 16 to 80 km.[11,27,29,30]

It is essential that the standard of care is not compromised during transport of critically injured patients. Minimum standards exist that outline the requirements for transport of critically injured patients, and these should be referred to for full details.[27,31,32] Consideration should be given to both the conscious patient and the restless, anxious or combative patient in ensuring adequate preparation prior to transfer. These preparations might include anti-emetics and sedation to ensure the safety of both the patient and the personnel involved in the transport.[21]

The following principles apply during such phases of care:

- There must be adequate preparation of the patient and equipment.
- Transport must occur by personnel with appropriate levels of expertise.
- Necessary equipment, including batteries and pumps, should be secured.
- Patients should be stabilised prior to transport (while balancing the need for timely transport).
- Monitoring of relevant aspects of the patient's care is essential.
- Adequate vascular access and airway control must be secured prior to commencing transport.
- Effective communication is mandatory between referring, transporting and receiving personnel.
- Documentation, including X-rays and scans, should accompany the patient and should cover the patient's status, assessment and treatment before, during and on completion of the transport.
- Relatives should be informed of the transfer, including destination, and provided with assistance for their own travel arrangements.[32] Checklists itemising many of these principles, sometimes attached to an envelope containing all transfer documentation, are often used to ensure that all necessary actions are undertaken.[30]

Trauma reception

Reception of the trauma patient at the emergency department of the hospital is generally performed by the triage nurse, with patients managed in a designated resuscitation area and received by a trauma team.[13] In the severely injured patient it is usual for a multidisciplinary team to receive the patient and commence assessment and treatment concurrently. In the setting of a mass-casualty incident, triage may be performed in the field. Despite documented benefits, such as shorter emergency department (ED) time, ED to computed tomographic imaging time, ED to operating room time and improved survival, having a trauma team is not universal, even within advanced trauma systems.[33] For example, only 20% of UK hospitals have a trauma team available.[13]

In the ED, the trauma team receives the patient after a comprehensive, clear handover that is heard by the entire team. The importance of a handover from the paramedics cannot be overestimated.[34]

The formal process of triage provides a means of categorising patients based on threat to life. Although there are many different triage systems in use the most commonly used ones are the MTS, the Canadian Triage Assessment Scale and the Australasian Triage Score (ATS). The Canadian Triage Assessment Scale and the ATS are similar as they both use a time-to-treatment objective scale, while the MTS is an algorithm-based approach to decision making involving the selection of one of 52 algorithms.[35,36] See Chapter 23 for further description of the ATS.

Primary survey

Priorities of care are similar to those in all health settings, with airway, breathing and circulation taking precedence during the primary survey (see Chapter 23). Disability and exposure/environment are essential elements that should follow.[37] These components of care will often occur simultaneously rather than sequentially and are designed to identify immediately life-threatening injuries.[37]

Compromise to airway and breathing may result from direct injury, for example to the trachea, or indirectly through decreased level of consciousness. Compromise to circulation is usually as a result of significant blood loss although it may occur as a result of injuries, such as cardiac contusions in chest trauma, or the patient's pre-existing disease. The evaluation of patients after trauma must be rapid, systematic and organised, and include:

- airway with cervical spine precautions
- breathing
- circulation with control of external haemorrhage
- disability, including brief neurological assessment
- exposure/environment, including prevention of hypothermia when removing clothing[37]
- prevention of complications or further compromise.

Secondary survey

Following stabilisation of the life-threatening problems identified during the primary survey, patients should undergo a secondary survey (see Chapter 23). This is a systematic examination of the body regions to identify injuries that have not yet been recognised. It is essential that both the front and the back of the patient, as well as areas covered by clothing, are examined during this process.

Tertiary survey

A tertiary survey should be conducted upon the arrival of trauma patients in the ICU, or soon after. The purpose of this third survey is to identify injuries that have not yet been detected, assess initial response to treatment and plan assessment and management strategies for future care.

The tertiary survey consists of another head-to-toe physical examination, assessment of the patient's condition in the context of his/her earlier condition and the treatment that has been administered, a full review of all diagnostic information gained so far and acquisition of the patient's past health history if family members or friends are available. A systematic approach will minimise the number of injuries that are not identified during the first 24 hours of care. It is also important to repeat the tertiary survey after the patient regains consciousness and begins to mobilise. Joint injuries may only become apparent during weight-bearing movements.

Radiological and other investigations

Initial radiological investigations will usually be performed in the emergency department using portable equipment. A radiographer is often a member of the trauma team that is activated on notification of the imminent arrival of a severely injured trauma patient. Radiological investigation is dependent on the type of injury sustained, but will generally consist of a portable X-ray of the injured area/s if these include the chest, cervical spine or pelvis. Other X-rays at this stage are rarely beneficial, or rarely change the course of treatment.

If the patient is sufficiently stable after the secondary survey, more extensive investigation in the radiology department should be undertaken. This will include CT scans. It is essential that clinicians consider investigations carefully, to ensure that all necessary imaging is undertaken; for example, where a CT scan of the brain is required it is often prudent to also undertake a CT scan of the cervical spine. However, care should be taken to avoid investigations that will not change the planned treatment but may delay urgent interventions such as surgery. Current controversies in radiation exposure and lifetime-associated cancer risks need to also be considered.[21]

Furthermore, there are not insignificant implications of moving the patient on and off imaging tables for repeated imaging. The patient should be accompanied and monitored by a competent nurse during all transfers for investigation. Where the patient is requiring ongoing advanced life support such as fluid resuscitation or airway monitoring, it may also be appropriate for a medical officer to accompany the patient.

Further radiological investigation may be required as part of the tertiary survey. This will depend on the radiological examinations that have been undertaken as part of the secondary survey, the treatment that has already been administered and the current condition of the patient.

Focused assessment with sonography for trauma

Where abdominal trauma is suspected, a focused assessment with sonography for trauma (FAST) examination[22,23] is likely to be used as part of the secondary survey to determine whether free fluid is present in the abdominal cavity. The abdomen is scanned in four zones – pericardial, Morison's pouch (right upper quadrant), splenorenal (left upper quadrant) and pelvis (Douglas' pouch). This generally takes 1–2 minutes when performed by an experienced, credentialled clinician. Findings are regarded as positive (fluid [blood] observed), negative or equivocal. Technical difficulties can be experienced with obese patients. While a positive FAST is useful in identifying if a patient should receive urgent surgical intervention, a negative FAST does not rule out significant abdominal trauma, and the low sensitivity of FAST remains a concern for trauma clinicians.[22] Where a patient is undergoing a prolonged trauma resuscitation phase, there may be an indication to repeat the FAST after 20 minutes. The use of FAST examination outside the trauma resuscitation and reception phase is occurring more often and can be undertaken in any clinical setting where there is a suspicion of internal haemorrhage or pneumothorax.[24]

Trauma teams

There are a number of different ways to organise the early care of trauma patients. The most common method used is through the establishment of multidisciplinary trauma teams that can provide immediate, expert assessment, resuscitation and treatment of traumatised patients, especially those with multiple injuries.[38] The purpose of the trauma team is to provide a coordinated and collaborative approach by relevant specialists to the injured trauma patient in a designated resuscitation area[10,38,39] with the performance of the team being greater than the sum of the individuals.

Many hospitals that receive trauma patients operate trauma teams that are either activated or placed on standby, via pagers or telephone, based on communications from paramedic personnel in the pre-hospital setting.[40] This activation is based on a combination of physiological and injury criteria (Table 24.1). Age is sometimes added to the patient criteria, with those under 5 years or over 65 years receiving particular attention. A number of hospitals have two levels of trauma team activation, with patients with more severe injuries activating the full trauma team and those with less severe injuries activating a partial team. The use of two-tiered trauma team activation has not been shown to affect patient outcomes.[25]

TABLE 24.1

Criteria for activation of trauma teams[131,130]

PHYSIOLOGICAL CRITERIA	INJURY CRITERIA
Heart rate <50 or >120 beats/min	Penetrating injury to head, neck or torso
Respiratory rate <10 or >29 breaths/min	Burn to ≥20% body surface area
Systolic blood pressure <90 mmHg	Fall ≥5 metres
Glasgow Coma Scale score <10	Multiple trauma
Skin pale, cool or moist	Crush or degloving injury to extremity
Paralysis	Amputation proximal to the wrist or ankle
Trauma arrest	Motor vehicle crash with ejection

Adapted with permission from:

Richards CE, Mayberry JC. Inital management of the trauma patient. Crit Care Clin 2004;20(1):1–11.

Kohn MA, Hammel JM, Bretz SW, Stangby A. Trauma team activation criteria as predictors of patient disposition from the emergency department. Acad Emerg Med 2004;11(1):1–9.

Common clinical presentations

Trauma generally occurs to a specific area of the body (e.g. the chest or the head) or consists of an injury caused by a specific external cause (e.g. burns). This section has been arranged according to these specific types of injury, including skeletal, chest, abdominal and from burns. Specific considerations relating to penetrating injuries have been covered separately, although the majority of care for patients with penetrating injuries will follow the principles of the area of injury. For example, a patient with a penetrating injury of the abdomen will generally be cared for in the same way as all patients with abdominal trauma.

Patients with multi/poly-trauma will also be cared for according to the principles of care for each specific injury, although consideration of priorities is essential. Care should follow the common principles of airway, breathing and circulation as developed by the American College of Surgeons over 30 years ago,[23] hence concentrating on respiratory and circulatory compromise first, before moving on to the treatment of other injuries. The relative importance of other injuries, for example neurological trauma or skeletal trauma, will vary for each individual patient and will be dependent on the physiological impact of the injuries. Neurological and spinal cord injury are reviewed in Chapter 17.

Mechanism of injury

Trauma refers to the physical injury that is caused by a mechanism of injury or kinetic injury. The principles of kinetic energy associated with blunt trauma are generally those of acceleration and deceleration forces that can lead to shearing or compression injuries, while penetrating injury is proportional to the velocity of the object striking tissue and the associated energy dissipation leading to either permanent or temporary cavitation.[37]

The most common mechanisms of injury are either blunt or penetrating injury. The third, less common mechanism of injury is blast injury, usually as a result of explosions that can be related to industrial or recreational accidents or terrorist acts. The mechanisms of blast injuries include:

- primary blast injury – blast overpressure reaches the person and transmitted forces exert their effects on the body, causing direct tissue damage
- secondary blast injury – created by debris that is physically displaced by the blast overpressure
- tertiary blast injury – caused when the person is physically displaced by the force of the peak overpressure and blast winds leading to blunt traumatic injuries being sustained
- quaternary blast injury – miscellaneous blast injuries caused directly by the explosion including injuries such as burns, toxic substance exposure
- quinary blast injury – a hyperinflammatory state manifested by hyperpyrexia, diaphoresis, low CVP and positive fluid balance.[41]

In 2008 traumatic injury was ranked as the ninth leading cause of unintentional injury, and by 2030 it is predicted to be the fifth leading cause of injury.[6] Leading causes of injury include road traffic crashes, drowning, burns, poisoning and falls.[42] The mechanism of injury is recognised as affecting both survival and requirements for admission to ICU. The largest proportion of serious injuries is related road crashes and makes up approximately 33% of unintentional injury deaths.[42,43] Patients who are injured in a road traffic crash experience a similar mortality to those injured through falls (approximately 3% in all patients and 10–17% in major injury patients), with both groups having a higher mortality than patients injured in assaults and collisions with objects (<1% in all patients and 12% in major injury patients).[41,42] While motor vehicle related deaths in Australia and many developed countries have fallen, the numbers of pedal cyclist deaths and drownings have increased over the same period.[42] Falls account for one-third of injuries in the over-65-years age group or approximately 11% of unintentional injury deaths,[40] with approximately 20% requiring healthcare attention.

Injuries sustained in road traffic crashes tend to be more severe given the high velocity of the trauma and account for the greatest number of major injuries, including those injuries that require admission to a critical care unit.[43] In addition, they are associated with a higher proportion of disability life-years lost annually with road traffic injuries accounting for approximately 17.5% in comparison to 12.2% for falls as reported by the World Health Organization.[42]

The older age group, with associated comorbidities, is likely to account for many of the deaths in the group injured through falls. In addition, patients injured in road traffic crashes tend to spend longer in the intensive care unit than patients injured through falls or assaults and collisions, and experience a greater number of injuries.[43]

Generic principles of management of the injured patient

Nursing care of trauma patients is characterised by the need to integrate practices directed towards limiting the impact of the injury and healing injuries to multiple body areas in a complex process. The delivery of critical care services must be systematic and must cross both team and departmental barriers to achieve a coordinated approach. This section outlines the principles of care relevant to all trauma patients, including positioning, mobilisation and prevention or minimisation of the trauma triad components of hypothermia, acidosis and coagulopathy.

Positioning and mobilisation

Appropriate positioning and mobilisation can be a significant challenge, especially in those patients with multiple injuries that create competing needs. Positioning refers to the alignment and distribution of the patient in the bed, for example supine, Fowler, semirecumbent or prone. In addition to these fundamental nursing postures, there is positioning of the limbs (i.e. elevated arms and legs). Mobilisation refers to the movement of joints by the patient, to shift from one place to another. This movement may be restricted to rolling within the bed, or moving out of the bed.

The principles of positioning and mobilisation are generally not different from those in other critically ill patients, and should incorporate the need to:

- promote the patient's comfort
- maintain the patient's and staff members' safety
- prevent complications
- facilitate delivery of care.

Difficulty in positioning and mobilisation is often experienced when there is concern for the stability of the patient's spine, in particular the cervical spine in the unconscious patient. Specific protocols such as the NEXUS criteria and the Canadian C-Spine Rule[21] are used for confirming the absence of injury to the cervical spine. Patients are considered to be at extremely low risk of cervical spine injury if the following criteria are met:

- no midline cervical spine tenderness
- no focal neurological deficit
- no evidence of intoxication
- no painful distracting injuries
- no altered mental status.[44]

For those patients who exhibit any of the above criteria a clinical examination is unreliable and radiographic assessment is advised. The debate continues as to whether these protocols should be used in any patient who is unconscious, intoxicated or complaining of cervical soreness or abnormal neurology. The following principles should be incorporated into confirming the presence or absence of injury:[21,44]

- Obtain a detailed history of the injury wherever possible, including specific investigation of mechanisms of injury that might exert force on the cervical spine. A high index of suspicion should remain, particularly in the setting of injuries often associated with cervical spine injury, including craniofacial trauma, rib fractures, pneumothoraces and damage to the great vessels and/or trachea.
- Undertake plain X-rays of the full length of the spine, interpreted by a radiologist.
- Where any abnormality exists in clinical or radiological assessment, or the patient remains unconscious, a CT or MRI may be undertaken, and this must be reported on by a radiologist.
- A correctly fitted hard collar should remain in place only until the patient is appropriately reviewed and the chance of a cervical spine injury is eliminated. If a collar is required for more than 4 hours, a long-term collar (e.g. Philadelphia, Aspen or Miami J) should be used.
- Maintain appropriate pressure area care to areas under the hard collar as well as the usual pressure points until cervical clearance is gained.[45]

The practice of maintaining a patient in a hard collar for days without active attempts to gain cervical clearance should be avoided at all costs.

The two methods available for moving the trauma patient are staff manual handling and lifting hoists.

Generally, trauma patients can be log-rolled (see Figure 24.1 for initial care) as frequently as required for nursing care. Any restrictions to patient positioning and weight bearing due to injuries or physiological status must be considered through this process; it is essential that care be taken to prevent any worsening of injuries due to handling of the patient. Although the benefits of immobilisation of the cervical spine have not been demonstrated through research, it is a practice that is supported by years of cumulative trauma and triage clinical experience[45] and should be used to prevent worsening of injuries.

Knowledge of the position restrictions for each limb, including all weight-bearing joints and the vertebrae, is imperative to avoid secondary iatrogenic injury. Certain injuries will impose position and mobility restrictions (see Table 24.2).

Practice tip

When planning positioning and mobilisation of the trauma patient, ascertain the weight-bearing status of each injured limb/body region, then determine positions or methods of mobilisation that are appropriate. Consultation with allied health professionals such as physiotherapists may aid in planning.

Practice tip

The NEXUS low-risk criteria have been widely accepted as identifying patients in whom further examination is unnecessary and cervical spine injury can be excluded on the basis of clinical examination.[44]

Adapted with permission from Ackland H. Spinal clearance management protocol. Melbourne: Alfred Health, <http://www.alfred.org.au/Assets/Files/SpinalClearanceManagement Protocol_External.pdf>; updated 24.11.09.

The 'trauma triad'

The critically injured patient can experience the 'trauma triad' of hypothermia, acidosis and coagulopathy. These pathophysiological conditions can occur individually; however, they often occur simultaneously. Hypothermia is a known contributor to the development of acidosis and coagulopathy. This relationship between the three conditions can contribute to a mortality rate of 35–90% in severe trauma patients.[46,47]

Acidosis has been discussed in earlier chapters so is reviewed here only as it interacts with hypothermia and coagulopathy in the trauma setting. Low cardiac output, hypotension, hypoxia, hypothermia and rhabdomyolysis

---

FIGURE 24.1 Spine movement precautions.[123]

Cervical Spine Immobilisation Procedure

Cervical spine stabilization should be performed as a team, generally four people working together.
Note: some patients (such as those with a compromised airway, neck deformities, or penetrating injuries) may not be able to tolerate lying flat.

1   The lead clinician is positioned at the head of the patient with hands on either side of the patient's head. Manual inline stabilization is maintained throughout the entire procedure by placing the hands on the patient with fingers along the mandible

2   Assess the patient's motor and sensory level by asking the patient (if applicable) to wiggle his or her toes and fingers. Touch the patient's arms and legs to determine sensory response

3   One assistant is to apply and secure an appropriately fitting cervical collar. Follow the directions for sizing that comes with each collar. An ill-fitting collar can cause pain, occlude the patient's airway, or fail to give appropriate immobilization

4   Straighten the patient's arms and legs, and position team members so that they are both on the same side of the patient at the shoulders and hips

5   On the lead clinician's count, the patient is rolled on the backboard as a unit

6   Straps should be placed so that the patient is secured to the backboard at the shoulders, hips and proximal to the knees

7   The patient's head should be further immobilized with head blocks or towel rolls. Tape or straps should not be placed across the chin

8   Manual in-line stabilization is maintained until the head and neck are immobilized

9   The patient's motor and sensory function should be reassessed after the patient is immobilized.

Modified from Howard PK, Steinmann RA, Sheehy SB. Sheehy's emergency nursing: Principles and practice. St Louis: Mosby Elsevier; 2010, with permission.

TABLE 24.2

Position and mobility restrictions in trauma patients

TYPE OF INJURY	RESTRICTIONS
Traumatic brain injury	• Nurse head up 15–30° • Side-lying as tolerated • Full tilt on bed if cervical spine not yet cleared of injury • Occasionally nursed flat if ICP problematic
Facial trauma	• Generally nurse in head-elevated position to reduce swelling, using either full bed tilt or back rest elevation
Chest trauma	• Nurse in varying positions from semi-Fowler to side-lying • Postural drainage (head down) usually beneficial if not contraindicated by other injuries (e.g. head or facial)
Abdominal trauma	• Nurse in varying positions from semi-Fowler to side-lying • Preferable to have some degree of hip flexion when lying supine to reduce abdominal suture line tension
Pelvic trauma	• Position restrictions are dependent on severity of fracture(s), use of external fixateurs and degree of stabilisation • Some patients may sit out of bed and ambulate with external pelvis fixateur in situ • Position restrictions require regular review, as changed or loss of fixation may affect recovery
Extremity trauma	• Significant position restrictions may include limb elevation, avoidance of side-lying or limited movement

ICP = intracranial pressure.

are common causes of acidosis in the trauma setting. The increased recognition of the importance of this triad in the trauma setting has led to the development of damage-control surgery.[48] The principle of this surgery is reviewed below.

Hypothermia

Hypothermia is defined as a core temperature <35°C[46,49] and is associated with high morbidity and mortality. Even in subtropical environments, hypothermia is identified in approximately 10% of major trauma cases during the pre-hospital or in-hospital phase of care.[50,51]

Uncontrolled causes of hypothermia can be endogenous or accidental.[51–54] Endogenous causes include metabolic dysfunction with decreased heat production or central nervous system dysfunction with insufficient thermoregulation such as in neurological trauma. Dermal dysfunction, such as a burn, is another endogenous cause of hypothermia.

Accidental hypothermia can occur without thermoregulatory dysfunction, and generally occurs in the trauma patient as a result of environmental exposure either at the injury site or during transport to, or between, healthcare facilities, as a result of large-volume fluid resuscitation[46] or during prolonged surgical procedures. The pathophysiological changes associated with hypothermia vary depending on the severity, and are outlined in Chapter 23. Of particular relevance, shivering leads to increased oxygen consumption and acidosis; platelet dysfunction leads to impaired clotting,[50,52,54] while haemorrhage reduces the circulating volume, which in turn may lead to a reduction in core body temperature and hypoperfusion of tissues. Hypoperfusion may cause hypoxia and subsequent production of lactic acid, which in turn slows the clotting cascade allowing haemorrhage to continue.[46]

Measures to reduce the incidence of hypothermia – or to correct it when it is present – in the trauma setting include:

• ensuring the patient is adequately covered during transport and hospital care
• warm intravenous fluids
• using warm blankets or electrical warming blankets
• adjusting the temperature in the operating room where feasible.[53]

In extreme cases of hypothermia methods of rewarming, such as cardiopulmonary bypass and peritoneal dialysis or lavage, might be used.

Coagulopathy

Coagulopathy is a term used for a group of conditions in which there is a problem with the process of blood clotting.[46] These are widespread in the trauma setting, ranging from mild defects in coagulation function to life-threatening coagulopathy. Defects in coagulation may be caused by dilution, hypothermia, acidosis, tissue damage or the effects of the underlying disease.[46,53,55]

Dilution results from the transfusion of either crystalloid or colloid fluids, and occurs as the concentration of coagulation factors in the patient's blood is diluted with the transfused fluid. It should be remembered that transfusion of red blood cells has the same effect, as whole blood or packed cells have undergone some dilution and have reduced viability of platelets.[56]

Preventing or intervening early in acute traumatic coagulopathy is an important goal for all major traumas, but may be even more important in the elderly or chronic disease population who are on anticoagulants and antiplatelet agents.[47,57]

> **Practice tip**
>
> Check whether trauma patients are on anticoagulant or antiplatelet agents, particularly those patients who have chronic disease or are elderly. If patients are taking these medications, be on the alert for complications associated with coagulopathy.

Hypothermia causes coagulopathy because many of the enzymatic reactions in coagulation are temperature-dependent.[53] Platelet and thromboplastin function both decline with even moderate (34°C) hypothermia, while hypothermia stimulates fibrinolysis.[46,53]

Acidosis reduces the activity of both extrinsic and intrinsic coagulation pathways, as well as platelet function. This is particularly pronounced with a pH below 6.8.[53] Tissue damage causes endothelial disruption and defibrination, which promote the systemic activation of coagulation; this is particularly profound in patients with brain injury due to the high level of thromboplastin in brain tissue.[51,53,58]

The final cause of coagulopathy in trauma is the underlying disease present in many patients. Patients may have a coagulation defect, such as haemophilia or von Willebrand's disease, or liver disease with resultant compromise to coagulation on an ongoing basis. Alternatively, patients may be taking anticoagulants, such as aspirin or warfarin, as treatment for other health conditions.[51,59]

Treatment of coagulopathy should focus first on prevention of coagulopathy and then on amelioration as required. Prevention strategies include:[56]

- maintaining normothermia in critically injured patients through the use of blankets and warming devices and minimisation of exposure and theatre time
- administering as little resuscitation fluid as is necessary to maintain adequate circulation
- achieving control of haemorrhage as soon as possible, through techniques such as low-pressure resuscitation and damage-control surgery.

Traumatic injury often necessitates large volume replacement of blood volume to increase perfusion. Even protocols such as Advanced Trauma Life Support do not provide clear guidance on the administration of pro-coagulation products to optimally resuscitate patients while also maintaining the ability to form clots.[60] There is a strong need to ensure that patients are not overtransfused, and regular monitoring of coagulation factors including haematocrit, platelet count, prothrombin time (PT), activated partial thromboplastin time (APTT), thrombin time (TT) and fibrinogen levels will assist in achieving this aim. The international normalised ratio (INR) should be measured at the beginning of the process and repeated if abnormal.

Treatment includes transfusion of platelets, fresh frozen plasma (FFP) and cryoprecipitate, as well as the plasma derivatives showing promise in this area of treatment.[60] While transfusion of platelets is specifically directed towards increasing the circulating concentration of platelets, administration of FFP is directed at increasing the levels of fibrinogen and other coagulation factors. Cryoprecipitate is made by freezing and thawing individual units of FFP and collecting the precipitate, a process that concentrates fibrinogen, von Willebrand factor, factor VIII and factor XIII.

Damage-control surgery

The goals of controlling haemorrhage and prevention of contamination while limiting the stress of surgery to the patient are the underlying principles of damage-control surgery (DCS).[55] Initially, DCS was used for injuries sustained in the abdomen but this has now expanded to include thoracic, skeletal and vascular injuries.[61]

DCS can be seen as encompassing up to five stages including: 1) the early recognition of relevant patients, 2) repair of structures to achieve haemostasis and restore distal vascularity, 3) correction of physiological insult from the initial trauma and subsequent surgery, 4) secondary return to theatre for definitive surgical procedures and 5) final closure of injury once the visceral oedema has subsided in those patients where it is required.[55,62] This approach to surgical correction of traumatic injuries gained favour through the latter part of the 1990s and is intended to reduce the development of the triad of complications of hypothermia, acidosis and coagulopathy.[55,61] Mortality among patients in the 1990s who received traditional definitive surgery versus the newer concept of DCS was similar, although a subset of patients with multiple visceral injuries and a vascular injury showed improved survival with DCS (77% vs 11%).[61]

Other adjuncts to DCS and damage-control resuscitation include topical haemostatic agents and now tranexamic acid after the results of the CRASH-2 (Clinical Randomisation of an Antifibrinolytic in Significant Haemorrhage 2) trial demonstrated benefit.[32,48] Other pharmacological agents may emerge as future therapies; however, the utilisation of interventional radiology for endovascular management of bleeding is proving useful in the massively injured patient.[55,61]

Nursing a patient who undergoes damage-control surgery requires recognition of the principles and aims of the surgery, as well as flexibility in the care of the patient after the initial surgery but before definitive surgery. In the emergency department setting there is a need to undertake a rapid, systematic evaluation of the patient and prepare him or her for rapid transfer to the operating room. It is essential to implement all measures possible to preclude the components of the trauma triad, while avoiding any delays to surgery. When the patient is admitted to the ICU postoperatively, the standard mechanisms for the treatment of hypothermia, acidosis and coagulopathy, as discussed above, should be implemented. After damage-control surgery, patients may also have an open abdomen with temporary dressings or skeletal fractures with external fixateurs in situ and may require multiple return trips to theatre to achieve final closure.

Skeletal trauma

Skeletal trauma involves injury to the bony structure of the body. Although skeletal injuries alone rarely result in the patient being admitted to critical care, damage to surrounding blood vessels and nerves, as well as potential complications such as fat embolism syndrome[63] and rhabdomyolysis, may cause the patient to become seriously ill. Patients with skeletal trauma who require admission to ICU include those with multiple injuries, severe pelvic fractures (often associated with significant blood loss), long bone fractures (often associated with fat embolism syndrome [FES]) and thoracic injuries such as flail segment. A small number of people with crush injuries that cause significant damage to muscles, often resulting in rhabdomyolysis, also require admission to the ICU.[64,65]

Skeletal trauma is the form of trauma that causes the highest number of patients to be admitted to hospital for 24 hours or more, with approximately 50% of patients experiencing a fracture as their main injury.[66] More than 70% of all patients with major trauma need at least one surgical procedure, with survivors experiencing poor functional outcome or quality of life, especially those with lower limb injury.[64]

Pathophysiology

Bone is composed of an organic matrix as well as bone salts. The majority of the organic matrix is collagen fibres and the remainder is ground substance, a homogeneous gelatinous medium composed of extracellular fluid plus proteoglycans.[67,68] Calcium and phosphate are the primary ions in bone salts, although there are smaller amounts of magnesium, sodium, potassium and carbonate ions. These ions combine to form a crystal known as hydroxyapatite.

A fracture is simply defined as a break in the continuity of a bone. Fractures generally occur when there is force applied that exceeds the tensile or compressive strength of the bone. In patients sustaining a major injury (injury severity score ≥16 [1998 version] or ≥12 [2008 version]),[69] fractures are the primary injury in more than 15% of cases, although many patients experience a fracture in addition to other serious injury resulting in ICU admission.[66]

Fractures are classified as either complete or incomplete. A complete fracture is where the bone is broken all the way through, while incomplete fractures only involve part of the bone. Fractures are also classified according to the direction of the fracture line, and include linear, oblique, spiral and transverse fractures. Finally, fractures are classified as either open or closed, with those patients who sustain an open fracture having a higher risk of delayed healing or non-union compared with closed fractures. Loss of the haematoma that initiates the inflammatory phase of fracture healing and contamination leading to infection are causative influences behind delayed healing or non-union.[70]

A fracture causes disruption to the periosteum, blood vessels, marrow and surrounding soft tissue, resulting in a loss of mechanical integrity of the bone. When a fracture occurs, there is initial bleeding and soft tissue damage around the site, with haematoma formation within the medullary canal.[70] The healing sequence that follows a fracture depends on the type of fracture fixation that is used. When a fracture is fixed using a method that eliminates the interfragmentary gap and provides stability

to the site, such as in screwing or wiring, primary healing takes place.[71] When a fracture is fixed in a manner that reduces but does not eliminate movement around the fracture site, secondary healing takes place.[71]

In primary healing, also referred to as direct union, the haematoma that initially formed is eliminated by the apposition of fracture ends during reduction. Once the bone ends are intact, osteoclasts form cutting cones that, in turn, form new haversian canals across the fracture gap.[68] These contain blood vessels that are essential to primary bone healing. By 5–6 weeks after the fracture, osteoblasts will fill the canals with osteons, which are the basic structure of the new bone. Although the bone is now formed, the strength and shape continues to develop over coming weeks. Clinical evaluation of whether a fracture has healed is based on both radiographic and clinical findings; however, associated injuries may confound the ability to use clinical criteria.[64,71]

In contrast to primary healing, secondary healing is characterised by an intermediate phase, where a callus of connective tissue is first formed and then replaced by bone.[68] The secondary healing phase begins with an inflammatory phase in which the haematoma clots and provides initial support, then inflammatory cells invade the haematoma to remove necrosed bone and debris. The reparative phase begins 1–2 weeks after the fracture and consists of immature woven bone being laid down and strengthened through a process known as mineralisation. The final remodelling stage consists of replacement of the woven bone by lamellar bone, through osteoblasts secreting osteoid that is mineralised and forms interstitial lamellae.[68] The remodelling of these structures occurs in response to appropriate levels of mechanical loading during this phase.[64]

Fat embolism

Fat embolism syndrome[63] may occur in patients who have experienced a fracture of a long bone, particularly if multiple fractures or fractures to the middle or proximal parts of the femur are experienced. Fractures to the pelvis can also lead to a fat embolism. Incidence of FES is low (<1%). FES consists of fat in the blood circulation associated with an identifiable pattern of clinical signs and symptoms that include hypoxaemia, neurological symptoms and a petechial rash.[65] Patients generally present 12–72 hours after they have experienced a relevant fracture and often require admission to a critical care unit for assessment and treatment, including mechanical ventilation.[72]

Internationally, there continues to be disagreement regarding the pathophysiological changes associated with FES, although there is general consensus on the following principles. It has been accepted that there is a mechanical component to the changes that take place in FES, where fat is physically forced into the venous system and causes physical obstruction of the vasculature.[72] Although marrow pressure is normally 30–50 mmHg, it can be increased up to 800 mmHg during intramedullary reaming (the process where the medullary cavity of the bone is surgically enlarged to fit a surgical implant such as a tibial nail), consequently reaching a pressure significantly above pressures throughout the vasculature.[72]

A second theory, associated with the biochemical changes that occur during trauma, proposes that trauma is associated with a higher level of circulating free fatty acids, which cause destabilisation of circulating fats and/or direct toxicity to specific tissues, including pulmonary and vascular endothelium.[72]

Rhabdomyolysis

Rhabdomyolysis is a potentially life-threatening condition and is caused by either acquired or inherited factors. Nine percent of cases occur as a result of trauma, 34% are due to substance abuse and 11% from medications.[73] Rhabdomyolysis is the breakdown of muscle fibres resulting in the distribution of the cellular contents of the affected muscle throughout the circulation, and occurs during the reperfusion of injured muscle. There are two phases of injury that are essential for the development of rhabdomyolysis: the first is when muscle ischaemia occurs and the second is with reperfusion of the injured muscle. The length of time that muscle is ischaemic affects the development of rhabdomyolysis, with periods of less than 2 hours generally not producing permanent damage whereas periods longer than 2 hours can result in irreversible anatomical and functional changes.[74] Presentation varies widely across patient groups and ranges from asymptomatic elevated creatinine kinase (CK) to life-threatening conditions with electrolyte disturbances, cardiac arrhythmias, acute renal failure and disseminated intravascular coagulation (DIC).[73]

Clinical manifestations

Common forms of skeletal trauma include the following:

- Long bone fractures – the long bones are the humerus, radius, ulna, femur, tibia and fibula. Fractures of these bones are serious and can carry a high level of morbidity, especially if they involve a joint such as a trimalleolar fracture of the ankle (distal tibia and fibula). In many cases definitive surgical management is required, with internal fixation.

- Dislocations – all joints are at risk of traumatic dislocation, depending on the mechanism of injury. Dislocations can be limb-threatening if they cause neurovascular compromise. Reduction of traumatic dislocation is a medical emergency.

- Open fractures (compound) – any break in the skin that communicates directly with the fracture is classified as an open fracture. Open fractures carry a higher infection risk and require surgical treatment within 8 hours.[70,75]

- Traumatic amputation – amputation refers to an avulsion in which the affected limb or body appendage is completely separated from the body. This can occur when a digit or extremity is sheared off by either mechanical or severing forces, for

example amputation of a thumb by a bandsaw. Traumatic amputations vary in severity and ongoing compromise, with a clean-cut amputation more likely to be successfully reattached than a crushed extremity. Criteria that inform the surgical decision-making process include: the amount of tissue loss; location on the body at the connection site; damage to underlying and surrounding tissues, bones, nerves, tendons/muscles and vessels; and condition of the amputated part.

- Fractures of the pelvis – the pelvis is the largest combined bony structure in the body and serves to provide an essential supporting framework for ambulation and protection of pelvic organs. Major blood vessels and nerves traverse the pelvic bones, supplying the lower limbs and pelvic organs. Therefore, injury to any part of the pelvis is serious. The three bones that comprise the pelvic ring are the two innominate bones (ilium and pubic rami) and the sacrum. Due to its reinforced structure, the amount of force required to fracture the pelvis is substantial. Fractures of the pelvis can affect one or both sides of the pelvis, and be stable or unstable. A variety of classification systems exist to describe the severity of pelvic fractures, the most common being the Tile classification (see Figure 24.2).

- Fractures of the spinal column (see also Chapter 17) – the spinal column includes all of the bony components in the cervical, thoracic and lumbar vertebral regions. Fractures of the vertebra are common in trauma patients, but the actual incidence of fracture without spinal cord injury in multitrauma patients is not well described. Not all fractures cause vertebral column instability with the subsequent risk of spinal cord damage. A spinal column fracture will be diagnosed as mechanically stable or unstable and this will affect the positioning and possible activity of the patient.

- Discoligamentous injuries of the spinal column (see also Chapter 17) – the soft tissue components of the spinal column include the spinal cord, the intervertebral discs and the spinal ligaments. An injury to the spinal column can disrupt one or more of these structures with or without fracture. These injuries can be highly unstable and the nurse must be vigilant with spinal precautions and the fitting and management of the patient requiring a spine orthosis (see Figure 24.1).

Patient management

There are several major considerations for the nurse managing the critically ill patient with skeletal trauma. These include appropriate assessment as well as application of traction, management of any amputated parts and stabilisation of pelvic fractures and spine precautions. These latter aspects of care will be conducted in collaboration with medical and allied health colleagues.

FIGURE 24.2 Tile classification for pelvic fractures.[124]

Tile A

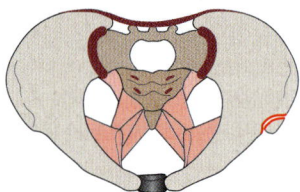

A1
Avulsion injury
Not involving the ring

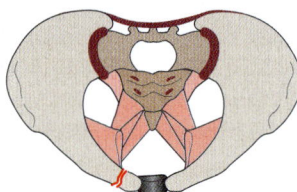

A2
Stable
Minimal displacement

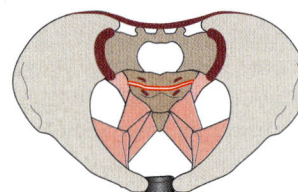

A3
Transverse fractures of
sacrum or coccyx

Tile B

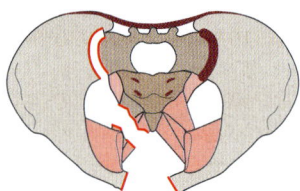

B1
Unilateral

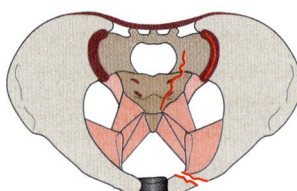

B2
Lateral compression injury
Internal rotation instability

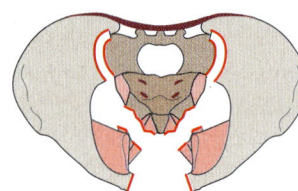

B3
Bilaterally rotational instability

Tile C

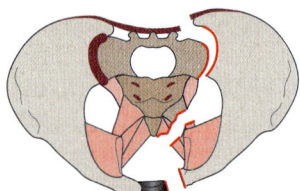

C1
Unilateral

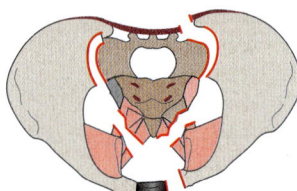

C2
Bilateral
One side rotationally unstable
One side vertically unstable

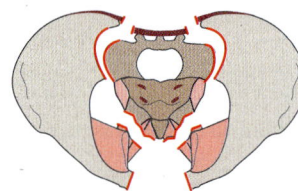

C3
Bilaterally vertically unstable

Reproduced from Kobziff L. Traumatic pelvic fractures. Orthopaed Nurs 2006;25(4):235–41; quiz 42-3, with permission.

Bones are very vascular structures and can be the cause of substantial blood loss in the trauma patient. The critical care nurse should therefore be cognisant of the potential for extensive blood loss in common fractures (Table 24.3).

Given the potential for extensive blood loss, as well as the frequent close proximity of nerves and blood vessels to bones, neurovascular assessment of the patient with skeletal trauma is essential (Table 24.4).

Splinting

One of the major emergent management strategies for haemorrhage control in the patient with skeletal trauma is splinting. Splinting is a potentially life-saving intervention and is generally undertaken by nursing staff. The purpose of splinting is to align and immobilise the

TABLE 24.3

Potential blood loss caused by fractures[37]

FRACTURE	BLOOD LOSS (ML)
Humerus	500–1500
Elbow	250–750
Radius/ulna	250–500
Pelvis	500–3000
Femur	500–3000
Tibia/fibula	250–2000
Ankle	250–1000

Adapted with permission from McQuillan KA, Makic MBF, Whalen E. Trauma nursing: from resuscitation through rehabilitation. St Louis, Mo: Saunders/Elsevier; 2009.

TABLE 24.4

Neurovascular observations of the skeletal trauma patient

Note: should be undertaken on all injured limbs both pre- and postoperatively as required.

OBSERVATION	PROCESS	COMMENTS
Skin colour	State the skin colour of the area inspected as it compares with the unaffected part NB: distal limb pulses may be difficult to palpate in the injured limb; a warm pink limb is a perfused limb	Pink: normal perfusion Pale: reduced perfusion Dusky, purple or cyanotic discolouration: usually indicating significantly reduced perfusion Demarcated: a distinct line where the skin colour changes to dusky (usually follows the vessel path)
Skin temperature to touch	State the ambient temperature of the skin to touch as it compares with normally perfused skin at room temperature	Normal: not discernibly cold to touch Reduced skin temperature indicates reduced perfusion
Voluntary movement	The patient should be able to move the non-immobilised distal part of any injured limb (i.e. fingers and toes of a plastered limb)	It is important to assess range of motion where that is possible, provided this will not aggravate the injury. Reduced movement may indicate compromise to either the nerve or blood supply to the limb
Sensation	The patient should be able to report normal sensation to touch	Sensation should be assessed in nerve distributions (i.e. all fingers and toes). Reduced sensation may indicate compromise to either the nerve or blood supply to the limb

bone, which alone has remarkable haemorrhage control properties. Every fractured bone that has not undergone definitive orthopaedic management requires splinting. Examples of intermediate stabilisation of fractures include:

- Positioning of injured limbs – all patients who have any form of splint in situ may need to have it elevated to promote venous return and minimise tissue oedema. In the ICU the trauma patient will often be nursed flat, with the bed on tilt for a head-elevation position. In these circumstances, the injured dependent limb must be elevated on pillows. Care must be taken to ensure that elevation does not place pressure on any part of the limb: for example, a hand sack made from a pillowcase tied to an IV pole should not be used, as it places direct pressure on the path of the median nerve and can cause an iatrogenic neurapraxia.
- Wooden/air splints – are padded appliances that are strapped to the injured limb. Ideally, no patient should remain in wooden splints for longer than 4 hours, as pressure may build up on pressure points.
- Plaster backslab – limbs with fractures will often swell as a physiological response to injury; a plaster backslab composed of layered plaster of Paris is the preferred treatment, as it accommodates swelling and can easily be loosened by nursing staff at any time of day. It is imperative that this be adequately padded within the limitations of providing structural support to the limb. Poorly made or ill-fitting backslabs can cause major

complications, such as pressure sores or displacement of fractures.

- Traction – may be required as part of fracture management, and involves the application of a pulling force to fractured or dislocated bones. There are three types of traction:
  - skeletal, where traction pins are anchored into the bone (i.e. Steinmann pin)
  - skin, where the body is gripped, as in the use of slings and bandages
  - manual, applied by a clinician pulling on a body part, such as in the reduction of dislocation. It may also be applied to maintain the traction during such nursing care manoeuvres as log-rolling or repositioning of the traction.

The principles of traction are to achieve the goal of alignment of bones while preventing complications. Remember that incorrectly applied traction is painful and can exacerbate the injury. The following should guide management of the patient with traction:

1 The grip or hold on the body must be adequate and secure.
2 Provision for counter-traction must be made.
3 Minimise friction.
4 Maintain the line and magnitude of the pull, once correctly established.
5 Frequently check the apparatus and the patient to ensure that: 1) the traction set-up is functioning as planned and 2) the patient is not suffering any injury as a result of the traction treatment.

> **Practice tip**
>
> No patient should remain in a wooden splint longer than 4 hours. Wooden splints must be changed to a resting backslab if prolonged immobilisation is required; this will maintain the injured limb in anatomical fracture alignment.

Traumatic amputations

Traumatic amputation is the separation of a limb or appendage from the body. During the pre-hospital phase any amputated body part should be wrapped in a clean or sterile (if available) cloth and placed in a plastic, waterproof bag inside an insulated cooler with ice. It is important that the ice does not come into direct contact with the amputated part. When managed using these principles, the amputated part may be viable for up to 6–12 hours before reattachment. Depending on any additional injuries, and the cardiovascular status of the patient, surgery for limb salvage will be scheduled as soon as possible.

Postoperative management will be guided by the type of surgery that was performed, specifically whether or not amputation occurred. Principles of postoperative care include:

- appropriate positioning of the affected limb, usually based on surgical orders
- frequent neurovascular observations, particularly observing for reperfusion injury, which manifests as an acute compartment syndrome or vascular trashing of distal vessels from a clot
- implementing changes in treatment initiated in response to altered perfusion in a timely manner
- psychological support to assist the patient in dealing with the injury.

> **Practice tip**
>
> Where there are any signs of deterioration of the re-implanted part, communication should occur directly between the nursing staff and the surgical consultant to ensure timely implementation of changes to optimise salvage of the amputated part.

> **Practice tip**
>
> For patients with amputations, on arrival in the emergency department:
>
> 1 Inspect the amputated part.
> 2 Clean with 0.9% saline solution and return to a clean plastic bag wrapped in 0.9% saline-soaked gauze. Surround with ice in a thermal cooler.

Pelvic stabilisation

Pelvic fractures can occur in 5–16% of patients with blunt trauma and can be uncomplicated and require no

surgical intervention, or they can be serious enough to be the primary cause of death from exsanguination.[76] The mortality rate from pelvic fracture ranges from 18% to 40% with death usually occurring within 24 hours of injury, frequently as a result of haemorrhage.[76,77] Appropriate assessment and management of pelvic fractures is essential and should encompass diagnostic evaluation, non-invasive pelvis stabilisation, abdominal evaluation, the requirement for surgical intervention and angiography.[78]

The initial management of the patient with a fractured pelvis involves assessment and splinting. Assessment should encompass the following two aspects:[77]

1 haemodynamic status – to identify signs of ongoing blood loss and determine fluid resuscitation requirements
2 stability of the pelvic ring – assessed with the aid of clinical examination and diagnostic imaging. Palpation and inspection of the anterior and posterior pelvis for signs of trauma, including tenderness in the conscious patient, is generally adequate.[77]

The orthopaedic surgeon may elect to undertake further clinical assessments incorporating 'springing' of the pelvis, although it should be noted that this may aggravate the injury and cause additional bleeding.[77] Nursing staff would not normally conduct such assessment, unless under appropriate specialist guidance in a setting such as remote area trauma nursing or tele-health consultation.

Non-invasive pelvic binding, in the form of either a bedsheet or a proprietary pelvic binder, may make a significant impact on patient morbidity and mortality.[76,78] Such a manoeuvre will stabilise the pelvis and assist in approximating bleeding vessels, thereby assisting in haemostasis (see Figure 24.3).

Pelvic binders are temporary devices,[76–78] and ideally will not be left in situ for longer than 4 hours. If a patient

FIGURE 24.3 Application of a pelvic binder.

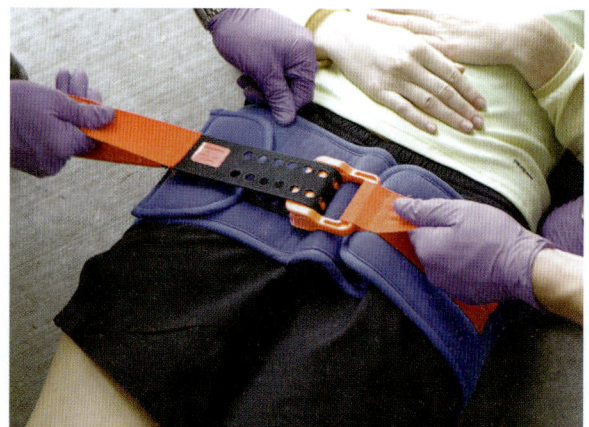

Courtesy Ferno Australia

is to remain in the binder longer than 4 hours, nursing staff must take care to minimise pressure. Conscious patients should be advised to report signs of increasing pressure, such as positional paraesthesia. Increasing abdominal swelling may indicate a need to reposition the binder. Position restrictions should be clarified by all members of the healthcare team, especially if the patient will be in the binder for a lengthy period. The patient may be able to be log-rolled and side-lain with a pelvic binder in situ. Release of a pelvic binder should by undertaken only with caution and as part of definitive care (e.g. within the operating theatre), with all relevant members (particularly the orthopaedic or trauma surgeon) of the healthcare team present.[77]

Invasive pelvic fixation uses an external fixateur (Figure 24.4) to achieve pelvic stabilisation.[77,78] The application of an external bridging frame (either anterior or posterior) to stabilise the pelvis may be an interim or definitive treatment measure that may be in situ for days or weeks. Patients in external fixation may be permitted to mobilise, although the extent of mobilisation will depend on the stability of the fracture. While the external fixateur is in place, the following nursing care is required:

- pin site care – usually cleaned with isotonic saline and left open unless there is a large amount of exudate, in which case the pin sites may be covered with dry absorbent dressing; care should be taken to identify gaping or stretched skin around the site, as this may require surgical intervention

- analgesia – based on patient reports of pain and taking into account planned activities such as mobilisation and physiotherapy

- mobilisation – based on stability of the pelvis, and in consultation with the surgeon

- patient education – particularly regarding the safety of the procedure and mobilisation and rehabilitation plans.

Pelvic embolisation involves interventional radiology to control haemorrhage in patients with pelvic fractures. Because of the large arteries that traverse the pelvis, arterial bleeding can be the cause of substantial blood loss in 10–20% of cases. The timing of embolisation, particularly in relation to stabilisation, remains controversial, and is dependent on the availability of appropriately trained staff and resources.[78]

Spine orthoses

The cervical collar or orthosis is the most commonly used splint to immobilise the cervical spine. It commonly remains in situ for >24 hours in an ICU setting. This particular type of splinting is associated with an increased risk of pressure ulceration in immobile patients due to unrelieved pressure, shearing forces, moisture or foreign bodies beneath the collar. Collar care is an essential component of critical care practice. Any dirt, grit, glass and road grime must be removed from under the collar, particularly in the occipital regions. The patient should side-lie as much as possible and the collar should be

FIGURE 24.4 External fixateur: pelvis.[128]

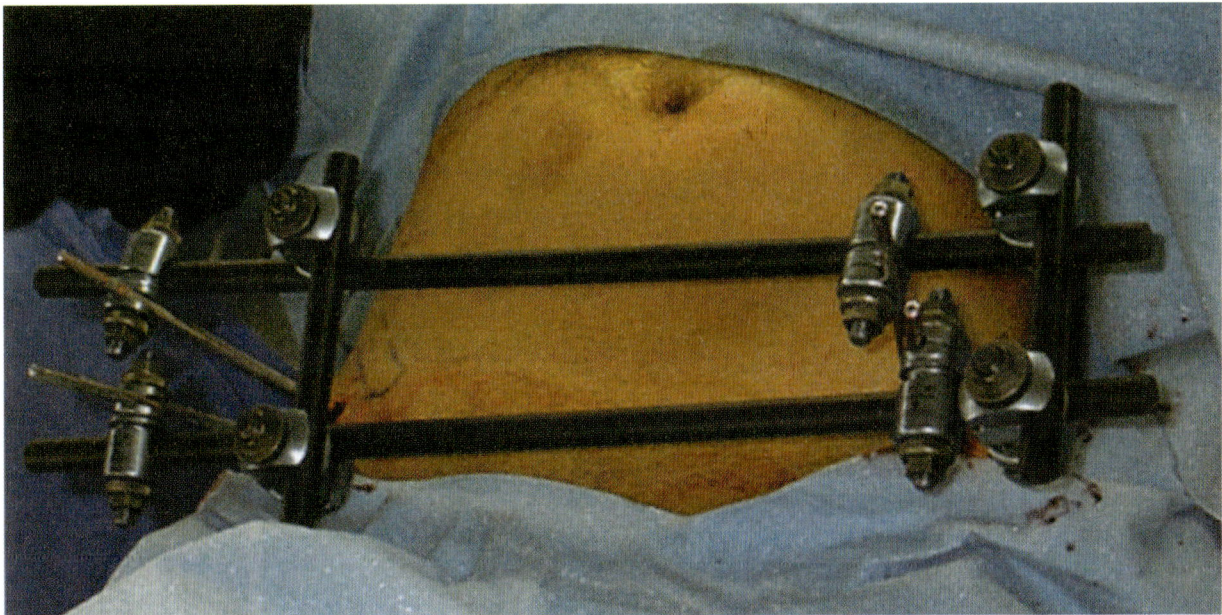

Reproduced from Wiss DA, Ovid Technologies I. Fractures. Philadelphia: Lippincott Williams & Wilkins; 2006: Figure 37.21, p 634, with permission.

TABLE 24.5
Spinal precautions[44]

ACTION	RATIONALE	AIM	METHOD
Head hold	To maintain the cervical spine in a neutral position during any position change	To prevent flexion, extension and lateral head tilting during any movement	1 Nurse holds head from head of bed – the head is held firmly by placing one hand around the patient's jaw with fingers spread to cup the jaw and hold the endotracheal tube as necessary. The forearm is used to support the side of the head 2 Nurse holds head from side of bed – nurse stands on side of bed that the patient will be rolled towards. One hand is placed firmly under the patient's occiput. Ensure nurse is in a position to support the weight of the head. The other hand holds the jaw and endotracheal tube as necessary. The patient is rolled onto the forearm of the nurse holding the head, which completes the biomechanical support for the head thus immobilising the cervical spine during the rolling
Log roll	To maintain the entire spine in anatomical alignment position during any position change	To prevent rotational torsion on the spinal column by minimising twisting of the craniocervical, cervicothoracic and thoracolumbar junctions of the spinal column	The patient is rolled in one smooth motion with assistants supporting the shoulder and pelvic girdles. Another assistant supports the legs so the patient moves in one plane The patient is rolled in one smooth motion with the nurse holding the head issuing the command to start and stop the manoeuvre

removed while maintaining spinal precautions (see Table 24.5) and the underlying skin integrity assessed at least every 4 hours. Other examples of spine orthoses include a halothoracic brace and thoracolumbar/truncal anti-flexion bracing.

Chest trauma

Chest trauma is recognised as a severe, potentially life-threatening form of injury that may require admission to critical care. Chest trauma may be blunt in nature, often being experienced during road traffic crashes, and can be associated with injuries to other areas of the body or penetrating in nature. Penetrating injuries are often experienced during gunshot or stabbing injuries.[79]

Chest trauma represents approximately 10% of injuries that require admission to hospital for more than 24 hours, although this proportion grows to over 15% when only patients with major injury (injury severity score >15) are considered. Chest trauma represents approximately 15% of the injured patients requiring admission to the ICU. The incidence of chest trauma varies, depending on the external cause of the injury, with approximately 20–30% of road traffic crash injuries occurring to the chest,[80] 30% of stabbing injuries occurring to the chest and 10–15% of assault and fall injuries resulting in injuries to the chest. Associated mortality ranges from 20% to 25% with reported mortality rates up to 60% in America and Europe.[79,81–83]

Pathophysiology

The chest consists of the thoracic cavity and the organs contained within. The thoracic cavity is made up of two structures, including a bony cavity consisting of the ribs, sternum, scapulae and clavicles, and the second muscular structure of the respiratory muscles and diaphragm. The organs contained in the chest include the lungs, airways, heart, blood and lymph vessels and oesophagus.

As in all trauma, chest trauma can be penetrating or blunt in nature. Penetrating trauma is generally caused by blades or bullets and results in damage to the structures and organs in the chest, as well as disruption of the normal negative intrapleural pressure leading to a pneumothorax. Blunt chest trauma generally occurs as a result of road traffic crashes, falls and assaults or collisions.

Chest trauma can be separated into injury to the thoracic structure, including the ribs and diaphragm; injury to the lung, airways and associated tissue; injury to the heart and associated tissue; or injury to the vascular or digestive system located in the chest.

Chest trauma covers a broad array of injuries and severity, and ranges from relatively minor injuries (e.g. abrasions and fracture of a single rib) to major, immediately life-threatening injuries (e.g. cardiac rupture or tension pneumothorax). In 70–90% of patients who sustain a severe chest injury there are associated injuries to other regions of the body, including the head, neck, spine, abdomen and limbs.[83,84]

Chest trauma includes the following:

- Rib fractures – a very common form of chest trauma, often a source of severe pain and often associated with other injuries such as haemothorax, pneumothorax and pulmonary contusion.[83]

- Flail chest – fractures to two or more ribs, in two or more places, resulting in a freely-moving section of the rib cage. The production of a flail segment is dependent on a number of factors, including the extent of adjacent soft tissue support.[80] Usually such fractures occur in the anterior or lateral sections of the rib cage, where there is less muscle protection. The significant impact of this injury is paradoxical movement of the flail segment during spontaneous ventilation, so that when a patient inspires, the flail segment moves inwards with the negative intrapleural pressure instead of expanding with the rib cage. Compromised respiratory function is caused by the increased work of breathing that this ineffective flail segment creates as well as the contused lung that normally occurs underneath the flail segment.[80]

- Diaphragmatic injuries – generally consist of diaphragmatic rupture when there has been a significant rise in intra-abdominal pressure, usually with compression injuries.[85] When the rupture is sufficiently large, protrusion of the abdominal contents into the thoracic space, resulting in respiratory compromise, is likely. Bilateral diaphragmatic injury is uncommon, with the majority involving the left hemidiaphragm, with 75% of injuries caused by blunt trauma.[86]

- Pulmonary contusion – consists of bruising to the lung tissue, usually as a result of mechanical force. This bruising is followed by diffuse haemorrhage and interstitial and alveolar oedema, resulting in impaired gas exchange due to shunting and leading to hypoxia and increased oxygen requirements.[85] This injury represents the most common internal injury after blunt thoracic trauma and has been estimated to affect 30–70% of injured patients.[80,84]

- Pneumothorax – the accumulation of air in the pleural space.[84] A pneumothorax may be closed (no contact with the external atmosphere) or open (a communicating channel with the atmosphere).[87] Closed pneumothoraces are generally caused by blunt chest trauma and result from a fractured rib puncturing the lung parenchyma. Open pneumothoraces generally occur in the setting of penetrating trauma, where air is able to move from the external atmosphere to the pleural space during inspiration. If not all of the inspired air is able to escape during expiration, due to a tissue flap or similar obstruction covering the opening, the volume of the pneumothorax will gradually expand and cause collapse of the adjacent lung, with resultant hypoxaemia. Where air is not able to escape at all from the pleural space, this is referred to as a tension pneumothorax, and rapidly becomes a life-threatening event due to the increasing pressure on the lungs, heart and trachea.[79,87] With the use of imaging modalities such as CT scan the phenomenon

of occult pneumothorax (pneumothorax detected on CT scan that was not diagnosed on X-ray) has appeared, with a reported incidence of 2–7%. Up to 76% of pneumothoraces have been identified as occult when the CXR was read in the acute resuscitation setting by the trauma team.[83]

- Haemothorax – the accumulation of blood in the pleural space. Blood may collect from the chest wall, the lung parenchyma or major thoracic vessels.[88] Breath sounds are usually reduced on the side of the haemothorax and percussion is noted to be dull rather than hyper-resonant.[79] Small haemothoraces (<200 mL blood) may not be apparent on clinical or radiological investigation, although respiratory compromise is likely to be present. Initial management of a haemothorax is the insertion of a chest tube to allow for drainage of the accumulated blood. Optimal evacuation of residual clots and breakdown of adhesions and loculated effusions is important to prevent complications such as empyema or fibrothorax and can be achieved using a surgical approach in the later phase of care.[88]

- Cardiac trauma – encompasses a number of different injuries, ranging from relatively mild bruising of the heart muscle to rupture of the heart wall, septum or valves or damage to the coronary arteries.[89] The right side of the heart is most commonly injured,[83] probably as a result of the anterior placement of this side of the heart in the thorax.

- Aortic injuries – generally, injuries to the brachiocephalic, left subclavian or right subclavian branches of the aorta are associated with high mortality at the scene. Aortic injury is divided into minor and significant injuries. Minor injuries usually involve a small intimal tear with small peri-aortic haematoma, while significant injuries include the intima and full thickness of media with associated high risk of rupture.[79] Aortic transection and rupture is associated with >80% mortality within the first 30 minutes of injury;[89] those who do survive to hospital frequently have a significant injury.[79]

- Tracheobronchial injuries – tend to occur as a result of direct blunt trauma and in close proximity to the carina, but are relatively rare.[83] Larger defects result in dyspnoea (with or without respiratory distress) while smaller injuries may initially go unnoticed. Many subtle presentations will manifest as mediastinal air on CT scan.[83]

Clinical manifestations

Injuries to the thoracic cavity can manifest according to the structures and systems involved (see Table 24.6). When multiple organs and systems are involved, the combined injuries pose an increased threat to life.

TABLE 24.6

Clinical manifestations of chest trauma

SYSTEM	MANIFESTATION	CLINICAL SIGNS AND SYMPTOMS
Respiratory • Airways • Lungs • Diaphragm	Any sign of respiratory compromise, noting that serial observations are an important indicator of imminent decompensation	Abnormal respiratory rate (<12 or >20 breaths/min) Abnormal chest wall movement, including asymmetrical chest wall expansion Reduced breath sounds Obstructed airway Hypoxia (<94%) Hypercarbia Apnoea Dyspnoea Orthopnoea Crepitus/surgical emphysema
Cardiovascular • Heart • Great vessels	Circulatory insufficiency resulting in decreased tissue perfusion	Abnormal heart rate (<60 or >100 beats/min) Arrhythmia In severe cases, pulseless electrical activity (see Chapter 9) Pulsus alternans Decreased cardiac output Lowered blood pressure (systolic <100 mmHg) Reduced peripheral perfusion Confusion and reduced consciousness level
Gastrointestinal • Oesophageal rupture	Perforation and contamination of mediastinum	Crepitus Haemopneumothorax Pain Cough Stridor Bleeding Sepsis (late)
Systemic • Air embolism	May occur in response to injury of a vessel that traverses an air space; manifestations will vary depending on location and associated injuries	Varied depending on location, but may include: • Focal neurological sign • Cardiac deterioration

Patient management

Given the underlying structures of heart, lungs and great vessels, chest trauma can cause rapid deterioration in the patient. Ongoing and thorough assessment, particularly in relation to the signs and symptoms outlined in Table 24.6, is essential. Other essential aspects of care include patient positioning and management of pain relief.

Assessment

Initial assessment in the emergency department should be conducted on an ongoing basis, with formal documentation of these findings occurring every few minutes until stabilisation. The frequency of ongoing assessment will then be based on the patient's condition, but is likely to be needed every 15 minutes initially, reducing to hourly with transfer to the critical care unit. Signs of chest trauma that represent life-threatening emergencies include the following.

• Cardiac tamponade – as blood collects in the pericardium, the venous return to the heart is impeded, resulting in reduced cardiac output. Signs of cardiac tamponade include:

◦ elevated heart rate
◦ reducing pulse pressure, with falling systolic BP and rising diastolic BP
◦ increased preload (CVP and/or PCWP)
◦ distended neck veins
◦ signs of reduced cardiac output, including lower level of consciousness, poor peripheral perfusion and reduced urine output.

• Tension pneumothorax – the lung or lungs collapse as the pleural space fills with air that cannot escape (see Figure 24.5). As the volume of air grows with each breath, the thoracic cavity contents are compressed or pushed against the opposite side of the chest. Signs of tension pneumothorax include:
◦ elevated heart rate
◦ increased respiratory rate
◦ decreased air entry, particularly over the affected lung
◦ tracheal deviation
◦ distended neck veins
◦ surgical emphysema.

FIGURE 24.5 Right tension pneumothorax.

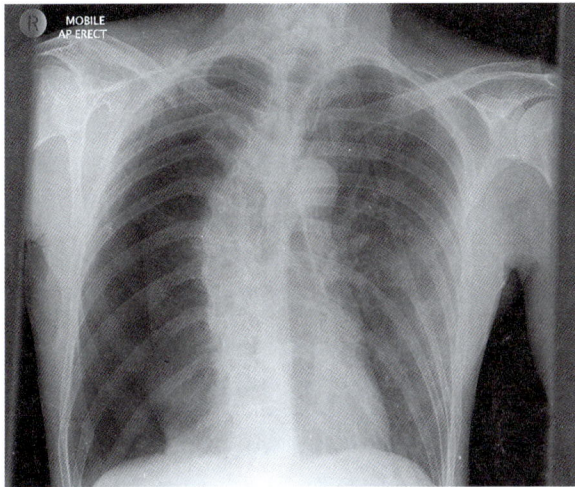

Courtesy The Alfred, Melbourne.

Practice tip

Unexplained hypotension in a patient with chest trauma may indicate a tension pneumothorax; an urgent chest X-ray is required for diagnosis.

Positioning

Early mobilisation of the patient with chest trauma is vital to prevent the complications of prolonged bed rest and immobility. Patients should be nursed side-to-side and in a variety of positions, including sitting upright. The extent to which the patient can be mobilised is dependent on other injuries. Patients should be mobilised to sit out of bed as soon as they are conscious and their injuries permit.

Care must be taken to accommodate the increased work of breathing that is associated with injuries to the lungs. Appropriate use of supplemental oxygen will assist the patient's exercise tolerance. Further, if the patient is mechanically ventilated, additional mechanical support (i.e. transient increase in pressure support) may be applied to assist the patient's exercise tolerance. Being unable to catch their breath is a terrifying experience that is likely to result in increased levels of anxiety for patients, and should be avoided wherever possible.

Pain relief

The principles of managing pain in chest trauma patients are similar to those for other patients, although the potential severity of pain, particularly as a result of fractured ribs, should not be underestimated. Effective pain management in the chest trauma patient is a major determinant of maintaining adequate spontaneous breathing. Avoiding mechanical ventilation is a major goal in the less-severe group of chest trauma patients, so effective deep-breathing and coughing must be promoted.

Pain relief will normally include IV opioids, but may also include intercostal or epidural analgesia and non-steroidal anti-inflammatory agents in selected patients (see Chapter 7). Non-pharmacological means such as the use of supplemental oxygen, use of cold packs early and heat packs late in the treatment course, massage, relaxation and diversion techniques should also be considered. Providing and maintaining a comfortable posture for the patient that includes the elevation and support of injured limbs has remarkable analgesic properties. A confident, competent and efficient nurse who engenders trust from both the patient and family is very comforting.

Surgical management of injury

Surgical intervention in the chest trauma patient is generally limited to repair of tears and lacerations, for example repair of vessel injuries including rupture, lung lacerations, heart injuries including lacerations and valvular injury. A ruptured diaphragm or oesophageal perforation will also be repaired surgically.

The emergency thoracotomy has proven beneficial in a select group of patients with penetrating trauma and less than 15 minutes of cardiopulmonary resuscitation; however, it is generally recognised as not providing benefit in patients with blunt chest trauma. While different techniques are used in different settings, the main access to the thoracic cavity is via a left thoracotomy, a midline sternotomy or a 'clam shell' incision. Initial assessment of the patient is used to determine the need for a thoracotomy in either the emergency department or the operating room. Nurses working in a trauma reception facility that has the capacity for emergency thoracotomy should be familiar with the equipment and process for this procedure. Postoperative nursing care of these patients should follow the same principles as for patients who have undergone routine cardiothoracic surgery.

Chest drainage

When injury to the pleura occurs, air or blood collects between the two layers of the pleura, causing collapse of the underlying area of lung and loss of the negative intrapleural pressure. Insertion of an intercostal catheter drains the air and/or blood from between the pleura, resulting in reinstatement of the negative intrapleural pressure and reinflation of the underlying lung.

A central principle in the treatment of chest trauma is the use of the intercostal catheter (ICC) for chest drainage purposes. The principles of chest drainage include the following:

- The lungs are encased in a potential space. The visceral pleura attaches to the parietal pleura via surface tension, creating a negative intrapleural pressure and attaching the lung to the chest wall. During inspiration the rib cage moves out and the diaphragm contracts and moves down, increasing the size of the intrathoracic space. Air moves from an area of higher pressure in the environment to an area of lower pressure within the lungs along a pressure gradient.

- An intercostal catheter is inserted into the pleural space, passing between the ribs. The ICC is designed to drain both air and fluid as required.

- The drainage system and seal provides an ongoing means of removing air and/or fluid from the pleural space, while preventing air from the atmosphere entering via the ICC. If the traditional glass bottle system is being used, the seal is provided by placing the distal end of the ICC under water (usually 2 cm). The catheter should not be placed under excessive levels of water, as this creates resistance and will limit air and fluid escaping from the pleural space.

- Suction is often added to the drainage system to promote drainage of fluid.

Care of the chest trauma patient with intercostal drainage is directed towards ensuring sterility and patency of the system and assessing the amount and type of drainage, as well as the impact on the patient (Table 24.7). Additional considerations include the following:

- ICC may be positional, or alternatively haemo/pneumothoraces may be loculated. Repositioning of either the patient or the catheter may be necessary.

- Side-lying or lifting the patient, especially with a frame, may kink or disconnect the ICC.

- Surgical emphysema around the site of the ICC may dislodge the tip of the catheter out of the pleural cavity as the emphysema swells. Ongoing assessment, including a chest X-ray, is required to confirm the position of the ICC.

- Movement of the patient, including sitting upright, will assist with fluid drainage; the volume of drainage should be assessed after moving the patient.

- Monitoring of respiratory function should continue after removal of the ICC to detect recollection of air or fluid.

Practice tip

Fresh, brightly-coloured blood drained from the ICC indicates continued active bleeding, while dark blood usually indicates older blood that has been resting in the pleural space for some time.

Ventilatory support

Ventilatory support is often required for patients with chest trauma (see Chapter 15 for general principles). The following specific considerations apply:

- Non-invasive ventilation – care should be taken based on associated injuries, with contraindications including fractured base of skull or facial fractures.

- Intubation – haemoptysis is relatively common in patients with lung injury, and care must be taken to ensure removal of blood clots from the endotracheal tube (ETT). Heated, humidified air and regular suctioning will assist with maintaining ETT patency.

TABLE 24.7
Assessment of chest drainage

CHARACTERISTIC	DESCRIPTION
Water seal	Ensure there is sufficient water in the water seal chamber
Bubbling	Continued bubbling indicates an air leak
Drainage	Observe the nature and volume of fluid exudate (NB: >1500 mL stat or 200/mL/h for 2–4 hours; surgical exploration may be required)
Patency	Ensure the intercostal catheter is not blocked, remove any blood clots
Swinging	Oscillation of fluid in the ICC confirms patency, as this reflects the changes in intrapleural pressure with respiration; such oscillation should continue even when the lung has re-expanded
Suction	If suction is ordered, check the appropriate level is being delivered

---

- Airway injury – initiation of positive pressure ventilation in the chest trauma patient may identify damage to a small airway that previously went unnoticed (damage to a large airway will usually have been detected early in the assessment phase). Treatment will depend on the severity and location of the rupture, but usually requires decompression of the pleura with an ICC, possibly surgical intervention and advanced respiratory support such as independent lung ventilation.

- Use of tracheostomy – this may be required for patients with injury to the trachea and is managed using the same principles as with any patient with a tracheostomy.

Allied health interventions

Physiotherapy is generally required for chest trauma patients. The primary aspects of care include chest physiotherapy, given the often extended episodes of mechanical ventilation and bed rest that are required, as well as mobility exercises. Occupational therapy particularly offers benefits to the long-term ventilated patient in terms of diversion activity, while social work is often beneficial for patients with ongoing disability and financial and social problems. Early referral of selected patients to allied health professionals has the potential to significantly influence patient outcome.

Abdominal trauma

Any organ or structure in the abdominal cavity can be injured. Abdominal trauma presents unique challenges to clinicians due to the abdominal cavity's high diversity of organs and structures. Approximately 10–15% of blunt trauma patients experience intra-abdominal injury[63,90] with high associated morbidity and mortality;[63,91] hence the need for early, accurate diagnosis and treatment is paramount.

Recent advances in diagnostic and treatment techniques for abdominal trauma have seen an increased emphasis on non-operative management for solid organ injury, with more recent increases in the use of angioembolisation. These two clinical treatment innovations place an emphasis on excellent patient monitoring and, in some instances, higher ICU utilisation for selected cases.[92]

Pathophysiology

The abdominal cavity consists of a range of tissues and organ structures, including musculoskeletal, solid and hollow organs, vessels and nerves. Musculoskeletal structures include the major abdominal muscle groups forming the abdominal wall, as well as the lumbar vertebrae and pelvis. Solid organs include the liver, spleen, pancreas, kidneys and adrenal glands (and ovaries in women). Hollow organs include the stomach, small and large intestines, gallbladder and bladder (and uterus in women). Finally, the vessels and nerves include a complex array of all abdominal blood vessels (arterial and venous), lymphatics and nerves including neural plexuses and the spinal cord. Traumatic abdominal injuries are classified as being extraperitoneal, intraperitoneal and/or retroperitoneal. Importantly, a patient can have any mix or multiples of these. The classification of injury guides clinical decision making.

The pathophysiology of abdominal trauma is largely related to the structure(s) injured. Careful serial assessments are essential to identify changing clinical manifestations. The most common clinical manifestation of abdominal trauma is haemorrhage and/or signs of an acute abdomen, such as pain, tenderness, rigidity and bruising. Importantly, these are life-threatening signs and require immediate surgical intervention.

The most significant sign of abdominal trauma in the conscious patient is thought to be pain, although in a recent systematic review abdominal pain along with abdominal tenderness with palpation were less predictive in identifying intra-abdominal injuries than other investigations.[90] Where hollow viscus perforation has occurred, such as bruising across the area of the abdominal seatbelt, small bowel perforation may be present. These patients are characterised by pain out of proportion to that expected with superficial abdominal wall contusions. Other signs of abdominal trauma can be related to the structure that has been injured. For example, haematuria demonstrates trauma to some part of the urinary tract, including the kidneys.

The abdomen is susceptible to injury from a variety of external causes, both blunt and penetrating (see discussion of penetrating injuries below). A key aspect to remember with any abdominal injury is that the superficial injury does not always reflect what lies below. For example, it is not possible to be certain of the trajectory that a bullet took after it passed through the skin.

Contusion/laceration

Sudden deceleration of moving body tissues can result in laceration or haemorrhage into the tissues (contusion). This is related to the tearing of the tissues that occurs due to inertia, or the tendency of tissues to resist changes in speed or direction (e.g. to keep moving forwards when the body has stopped moving, resulting in a tearing action to the tissues). Any structure in the abdomen is susceptible to this type of injury. Commonly, the liver and spleen are the worst-affected organs, largely related to a seatbelt injury in motor vehicle collisions. Laceration of a solid organ can be a minor injury that is appropriately monitored and managed conservatively; alternatively, a similar injury can lead to exsanguination (e.g. a liver laceration into the hilum that involves the inferior vena cava). Hollow viscus can be contused, as can the mesentery and peritoneum.

Perforation

Full-thickness injury, or perforation, to a hollow viscus organ is life-threatening. Perforation of the intestine can result in peritoneal soiling and ischaemic bowel. Small bowel injuries are particularly difficult to diagnose;[92] if diagnosis is delayed, morbidity can be severe. The abdominal seatbelt sign – in other words, bruising across the anterior abdominal wall that follows the path of the lap and sash of the seatbelt – is a sentinel sign for hollow viscus perforation.[93,94] A high index of suspicion should be given to passengers of motor vehicle crashes who present with a seat belt sign as it has been shown that they have twice the odds of sustaining an abdominal injury. One thought behind this finding is that adult passengers tend to sit further back from the instrument panel where the frontal airbag deploys, and may have different safety belt force loading characteristics.[95] Importantly, patients with this type of abdominal trauma can present late (by days). If presenting late, the usual clinical manifestations are pain, peritonitis and sepsis.[93,94]

Secondary injury: Abdominal compartment syndrome

The abdominal viscera are highly vascular and subject to vascular engorgement during massive fluid resuscitation. Where this occurs, there is an acute rise in intra-abdominal pressure (IAP). In severe cases, the IAP will rise to the point where cardiorespiratory function is compromised. This is a surgical emergency and the abdominal cavity requires decompression immediately. The incidence of abdominal compartment syndrome is difficult to determine because of the different assessment and measurement techniques used, but has been reported to be 6–14% in trauma patients.[96]

A high level of suspicion for abdominal compartment syndrome should be retained for all patients with abdominal trauma as well as those who have had abdominal surgery for other reasons. Clinical examination, looking for a distended and firm abdomen, is insensitive in the early stages of abdominal compartment syndrome with detection in only 40–60% of cases;[96] however, these signs should be identified if abdominal compartment syndrome progresses to a late state. Proactive detection of abdominal compartment syndrome is more effectively carried out through the use of routine IAP measurements in patients with the potential to develop abdominal compartment syndrome. While agreement regarding the level of IAP that indicates abdominal compartment syndrome does not exist, values above 20 mmHg generally require investigation; and pressures above 25 mmHg, in association with other clinically relevant findings such as firm or distended abdomen and the systemic effects outlined above, often indicate a need for urgent surgery.[97] It may also be appropriate to monitor the abdominal perfusion pressure,[98] which is the mean arterial pressure minus the IAP. Although not validated it is recommended to maintain an arterial perfusion pressure between 50 and 60 mmHg or higher if possible.[96] See Chapter 20 for a detailed review of abdominal compartment syndrome including IAP monitoring and subsequent management.

Patient management

Recent trends have seen an increasing use of non-operative care of patients with abdominal injury. In these patients, monitoring for deterioration is essential, as is the ability to activate surgery and care for patients accordingly. Care of patients after abdominal trauma also includes effective diagnosis, surgical or radiological interventions, and associated care. Damage-control surgery is now a mainstay in management.

With the high use of non-operative management techniques for solid organ injury, the role of monitoring of patients with abdominal trauma is pivotal. Nurses must be cognisant of the clinical signs of abdominal injury, especially haemorrhage, and act on these immediately (see Table 24.8). Specific aspects of nursing care for patients after abdominal trauma include pain management, monitoring and postoperative care. Patients often experience severe pain as a result of both the primary trauma and any surgical intervention for repair (see Chapter 7).

Vital sign monitoring is a mainstay of nursing management in patients with abdominal trauma, and all patients should have appropriate monitoring (as outlined in trauma reception). It is also essential that patients receive a urinalysis after incurring abdominal trauma in order to identify trauma to the urinary system.

Where the patient has undergone a trauma laparotomy, postoperative care is standard as for any patient who has undergone an abdominal surgical procedure. The specific nursing care elements will depend on what organ has been injured and the surgical procedure undertaken. Careful attention must be paid to general nursing care elements for all patients (see Chapter 6).

Postoperative feeding and bowel care should be discussed with the healthcare team and plans made early to avoid delays and adverse events such as constipation (see Chapter 19 for principles of feeding). A paralytic ileus is a common manifestation of the critically-ill abdominal trauma patient. Ensuring that the gut is decompressed, with a functional enterogastric tube that is correctly positioned, is essential. Because constipation is a common problem, early intervention and implementation of a bowel care protocol for trauma should be considered (see Chapter 6).

Diagnosis in the trauma setting consists of a thorough clinical assessment, the potential use of FAST, diagnostic peritoneal lavage (DPL), abdominal computed tomography (CT)[68] and laparotomy or laparoscopy. Clinical assessment may reveal clinical signs such as skin bruising, lacerations, signs of abdominal rigidity and guarding. The various locations of clinical signs are clues to potential abdominal injury. The results of this phase of the investigation will determine what additional diagnostic tests are undertaken. FAST is rapidly becoming an extension of the clinical assessment in abdominal trauma patients.

Diagnostic peritoneal lavage

Diagnostic peritoneal lavage (DPL) is a procedure that can be undertaken rapidly to assess for intra-abdominal bleeding, although it is frequently only used where FAST or CT is not available.[99] DPL may be performed on a patient with unexplained persistent signs of shock (hypotension ± tachycardia); where the abdominal clinical examination and FAST is inconclusive; or where there is a high index of suspicion of intra-abdominal injury. DPL can identify the presence of haemorrhage but gives no indication of its source.[92,100] Disadvantages of DPL include:

- high level of invasiveness and associated complications
- inability to detect retroperitoneal injuries
- potential interference with the interpretation of subsequent CT scans.[92]

TABLE 24.8
Common signs of abdominal injury[133]

SIGN	DESCRIPTION	SUSPECTED INJURY
Grey Turner's sign	Blueish discolouration of the lower abdomen and flanks 6–24 hours after onset of bleeding	Retroperitoneal haemorrhage
Kehr's sign	Left shoulder tip pain caused by diaphragmatic irritation	Splenic injury, although can be associated with any intra-abdominal bleeding
Cullen's sign	Bluish discolouration around the umbilicus	Pancreatic injury, although can be associated with any peritoneal bleeding
Coopernail's sign	Ecchymosis of scrotum or labia	Pelvic fracture or pelvic organ injury

Adapted with permission from Eckert KL. Penetrating and blunt abdominal trauma. Crit Care Nurs Q 2005;28(1):41–59.

Abdominal computed tomography

Abdominal computed tomography[68] is recognised as having high sensitivity and specificity in the setting of abdominal trauma and is therefore accepted as a diagnostic mainstay in this group of patients, particularly for patients with blunt trauma who are haemodynamically stable.[90,92] The main exception to this is where the results of a FAST examination are positive and the patient is taken to surgery urgently. The use of abdominal CT in patients with a penetrating injury has an accuracy rate >90% when combined with the administration of oral, rectal and intravenous contrast with some evidence suggesting that triple contrast CT may reduce the need for operative investigation of these injuries.[101] An important pitfall for CT imaging in abdominal trauma occurs when the patient has arrived at the scanner so quickly after the injury that major blood loss is not apparent and the extent of the injury is missed or underevaluated. A high index of suspicion in the setting of a negative CT and extensive abdominal trauma should remain, particularly if signs of shock develop.

Debate currently exists as to the role of oral contrast in the trauma patient who must remain supine and immobilised in a cervical collar. It is essential that nursing assessment for the risk of aspiration be conducted, and to be prepared to manage the vomiting patient. Any supine patient given radiographic contrast should not be left unattended, and there should be sufficient staff available at short notice to roll the patient onto their side if he/she vomits. The healthcare team should discuss the risk of vomiting prior to ordering the test so that an informed decision can be made regarding the risk–benefit ratio on an individual case basis. Oral contrast has been demonstrated to be highly effective in revealing hollow viscus injury, and therefore has a place in the diagnostic evaluation of abdominal trauma.

Laparotomy/laparoscopy

The role of diagnostic operations such as laparotomy/laparoscopy is well described in the literature,[102] and is essential to aid diagnosis (laparoscopy) and provide appropriate treatment to control haemorrhage and repair organ injury (laparotomy). When this procedure is considered appropriate, rapid transit to the operating room should be undertaken. As the consequences of missed or delayed diagnosis of abdominal injury can be catastrophic for the patient, opening the peritoneal cavity to exclude injury in selected cases is a necessity. In an analysis of 51 studies the conversion rate from laparoscopy to laparotomy was 33.8%, of which 16% were non-therapeutic and 11.5% were negative.[102]

Embolisation

Interventional radiology is an option in the management of abdominal trauma. Via an arterial approach, the interventional radiologist can insert cannulae to identify arterial blushes (bleeders). Once identified, the vessel can be ligated via mechanical coiling or blocked chemically. Embolisation aims to achieve haemostasis and salvage organs without the need for surgery, which in turn may reduce the resuscitation period and requirements for transfusion.[103] In patients with vascular injuries within the abdominal cavity the treatment of choice is percutaneous selective embolization, which is directed to the injury site by the previously performed CT examination.[103] The patient undergoing embolisation for the control of haemorrhage requires meticulous monitoring and an ability to respond immediately to hypovolaemic shock should the bleeding worsen.

Management of the patient with an open abdomen

In cases of severe abdominal trauma, the abdominal trauma patient may be returned to the ICU with an open abdomen, or laparotomy, covered with a temporary wound-closure system. There are various types of open abdominal dressings with negative pressure therapy techniques becoming the most extensively used. The principal aim of the dressing is to provide coverage for the contents of the peritoneum if these are too swollen to fit beneath the closed skin or where there is a need for repeated opening of the abdomen.[104] Ultimately, the aim is to close the skin as soon as possible, when the patient's physiological status normalises. It is possible for these abdominal dressings to cause a secondary abdominal compartment syndrome if they are too restrictive. Another challenge for the patient with the open abdomen is the potential for the development of enteroatmospheric fistulas.[104,105]

The primary aims of managing a patient with an open abdomen include minimising complications of prolonged immobility, observing for signs of ongoing abdominal compartment syndrome, restoring the patient's physiology to normal and supporting the patient and family through a psychologically distressing time. Understandably, both the patient and their family can be distressed by the appearance of an open abdomen. There are no specific position restrictions for a patient with an open abdomen, but haemodynamic status is often labile so that care must be taken with side-lying and hygiene care.

Splenic injuries

The spleen is the solid organ most commonly injured in blunt trauma.[92,103] Its location (under the ribs) also makes it vulnerable to secondary injury from fractured ribs. Splenic injury should always be suspected in those patients who have sustained a direct blow to the abdomen, as it is a large organ. The most common sign of splenic injury is pain over the left upper quadrant. There may be no changes to vital sign parameters until the patient has incurred significant circulating blood loss. Splenic injury is categorised in a scale consisting of five levels; this scale is designed to aid classification for management and research purposes[105] (see Table 24.9).

The spleen has an immunological function that is not well understood. After splenectomy, patients are at increased risk of infection and therefore require careful education regarding lifelong risks. The role of immunisation after splenectomy is very important, and the patient must be counselled regarding the necessity for follow-up on immunisations.[106] Prior to discharge from the hospital, the patient should be administered the first round of immunisations. The current recommendation for predischarge immunisations includes:

- pneumococcal vaccine
- meningococcal vaccines
- influenza vaccine.[107]

The patient will also be commenced on antibiotic prophylaxis and should be advised to wear a medi-alert disk or card and consult specialist travel advice when travelling.[107]

Liver injuries

The liver is a vital organ, with liver failure being a fatal condition unless reversible. After the spleen, the liver is the next most common solid organ injured.[103] Any injury to this highly vascular organ is serious and requires surgical review. As the largest abdominal solid organ traversing the midline, the liver is susceptible to injury from any external forces applied to the abdomen, for example seatbelt injuries and abdominal blows from an assault. Liver injuries are graded using the six-level liver injury scale[105] (see Table 24.10). The treatment of liver injuries is largely dependent on the nature of the injury or injuries to the liver itself, presence of concomitant injuries, premorbid status and overall injury severity. The treatment options may also be guided by the services and expertise that your health agency can offer the patient.

The overwhelming aim of the management of liver injuries is to preserve liver function. This is achieved by controlling haemorrhage, resting the patient and close monitoring. Most liver injuries can be managed non-operatively. In these cases it is imperative that the patient be closely monitored for signs of haemorrhage and that the capacity for laparotomy is available at short notice if required. In some cases, embolisation may be considered for arterial haemorrhage.[92] Late complications of liver injury include infection, haematoma, bile leak and late haemorrhage.

Penetrating injuries

Trauma is broadly categorised according to whether the external cause of injury was blunt or penetrating. Penetrating trauma refers to a mechanism of injury where the skin has been cut through the insertion of a foreign object. The most common examples include knife and gunshot wounds, although solid objects such as fences, signposts and tools can cause penetrating trauma. Penetrating trauma is significantly different from blunt trauma in that the injury is largely localised to a single body region. Exceptions to this may occur: for example, with firearm wounds if there are multiple bullet-entry wounds or multiple knife-stab sites.

Care must be taken when caring for patients with penetrating injury to prevent injury to staff. This is particularly important when the patient presents with a knife in situ or a large, protruding foreign object in their body. It should also be noted that some penetrating trauma occurs as a result of a criminal act, and it is essential to observe rules governing forensic evidence. Police should be notified by the senior clinician involved in providing care.

TABLE 24.9

Spleen injury scale[134]

GRADE[a]	INJURY TYPE	DESCRIPTION OF INJURY
I	Haematoma	Subcapsular, <10% surface area
	Laceration	Capsular tear, <1 cm parenchymal depth
II	Haematoma	Subcapsular, 10–50% surface area
		Intraparenchymal, <5 cm in diameter
	Laceration	Parenchymal depth 1–3 cm not involving a trabecular vessel
III	Haematoma	Subcapsular, >50% surface area or expanding
		Ruptured subcapsular or parenchymal haematoma
		Intraparenchymal haematoma >5 cm or expanding
	Laceration	Parenchymal depth >3 cm or involving trabecular vessels
IV	Laceration	Laceration involving segmental or hilar vessels producing major devascularisation (>25% of spleen)
V	Laceration	Completely shattered spleen
	Vascular	Hilar vascular injury that devascularises spleen

[a]Advance one grade for multiple injuries, up to grade III.

Adapted with permission from Olthof DC, van der Vlies CH, Scheerder MJ, de Haan RJ, Breenen LFM, Goslings JC, van Delden OM. Reliability of injury grading systems for patients with blunt splenic trauma. Injury 2014;45(1):146–50.

TABLE 24.10

Liver injury scale[37]

	GRADE[a]	INJURY DESCRIPTION
I	Haematoma	Subcapsular, <10% surface area
	Laceration	Capsular tear, <1 cm parenchymal depth
II	Haematoma	Subcapsular, 10–50% surface area
		Intraparenchymal, <10 cm in diameter
	Laceration	Parenchymal depth 1–3 cm, <10 cm in length
III	Haematoma	Subcapsular, >50% surface area or expanding
		Ruptured subcapsular or parenchymal haematoma
	Laceration	Parenchymal depth >3 cm
IV	Laceration	Parenchymal disruption involving 25–75% of hepatic lobe or 1–3 Couinaud's segments within a single lobe
V	Laceration	Parenchymal disruption involving >75% of hepatic lobe or >3 Couinaud's segments within a single lobe
	Vascular	Juxtahepatic venous injuries; i.e. retrohepatic vena cava/central major hepatic veins
VI	Vascular	Hepatic avulsion

[a]Advance one grade for multiple injuries, up to grade III.

Adapted with permission from McQuillan KA, Makic MBF, Whalen E. Trauma nursing: from resuscitation through rehabilitation. St Louis, Mo: Saunders/Elsevier; 2009.

Clinical manifestations

The clinical manifestations of penetrating injuries are dependent on where in the body the penetrating injury has occurred, the underlying organs and the amount of force and dispersion caused by the injury. For example, a high-velocity bullet will cause substantial tissue damage in a wider area than just the bullet's track. The clinical manifestations of penetrating trauma can be divided into two broad types:

1 conspicuous – where the penetrating article is grossly visible (e.g. a shard of glass, a branch or a knife); care must be taken not to focus solely on the visible cause of injury but to continue to undertake a systematic trauma assessment

2 inconspicuous – where the penetrating article is not immediately visible and may become apparent only during the systematic trauma assessment of the patient (e.g. with gunshot wounds and projectiles); in these injuries the visual signs on the external skin may not reflect the catastrophic injury underlying it (e.g. ventricle lacerations or serious vascular injury).

Patient management

Patients with penetrating injury will be cared for based on the severity and area of injury they have sustained. Surgical intervention is usually more urgent than that seen with blunt injury, as bleeding may be occurring from a ruptured organ or vessel either into a body cavity or externally. For this reason, the incidence of procedures such as laparotomy and thoracotomy is high in patients with a penetrating injury.

In the emergency setting the following considerations are generally unique to the patient with a penetrating injury:

- Stabilise the foreign object. This may require padding and/or taping an object, for example a knife, to ensure minimal movement and prevent further damage until definitive care to remove the object.

- Care for the patient in a non-standard position. This will be dependent on how and where any foreign object is protruding from the body. For example, it may be necessary to care for a patient in the side-lying or prone position until the object is removed.

- Use minimal volume resuscitation. This describes the practice of only resuscitating a patient sufficiently to maintain adequate perfusion to essential organs until definitive repair of the wound can be undertaken.[108]

- Provide psychosocial care of the patient and family. It is possible that patients with penetrating injury will need specific psychosocial care, particularly when the injury has occurred as a result of assault.

Burns

Recent improvements in both shock and sepsis management have resulted in patients with severe and extensive burn injuries spending long periods of time in the critical care environment. Burn injuries occur as a result of thermal, electrical or chemical injury and cause both local and systemic changes to a patient. An understanding of these changes will assist with planning appropriate care for this group of patients.

In recent years, improved survival, reduced hospital length of stay and a decrease in morbidity and mortality has been seen in burns patients. This is primarily due to a better understanding of burns pathophysiology and advancements in care that include improvements in resuscitation protocols, improved respiratory support, management of the hypermetabolic response, rigid infection control monitoring, early excision and burn wound closure, use of skin substitutes and early nutritional support.

Burn injuries are highly variable and individual injuries that affect all ages and social groups. In general terms, assessment is based on the size, depth and anatomical site of the injury, mechanism of injury and the presence of coexisting conditions. The World Health Organization estimates that more than 300,000 deaths are fire-related every year, the majority occurring in developing countries.[109] Due to improvements in both surgical treatment and intensive care management strategies the outcomes of burn patients have continued to improve; however, they still require complex interdisciplinary therapeutic approaches to optimise management.[110]

All patients with a serious burn injury should be referred to a specialised burns unit that is staffed and equipped appropriately to manage burns. The Australian and New Zealand Burns Association (ANZBA) criteria outline which burns patients require treatment in a specialised burns unit (see Box 24.1).

BOX 24.1

Criteria for treatment in a specialised burn centre[113]

- Burns greater than 10% of total body surface area (TBSA)
- Burns to special areas: face, hands, feet, genitalia, perineum, major joints
- Full-thickness burns greater than 5% of TBSA
- Electrical burns
- Chemical burns
- Burns with an associated inhalation injury
- Circumferential burns of the limbs or chest
- Burns in the very young or very old
- Burns in people with pre-existing medical disorders that could complicate management, prolong recovery or increase mortality
- Burns with associated trauma
- The possibility of non-accidental injury in children

Adapted with permission from Australian and New Zealand Burns Association. Early management of severe burns (EMSB). Albany Creek: Australian and New Zealand Burns Association; 2013.

Pathophysiology

The skin is the largest organ in the human body and accounts for 15% of its weight. The skin has multiple purposes, including protection from infection, regulation of body heat and function as a vapour barrier.

The skin consists of three layers: the epidermis, the dermis and subcutaneous tissue.[39] The epidermis is the outer layer, and is composed of stratified epithelial cells that protect against infection and conserve moisture. This layer is characterised by having regenerative ability. The dermis, as the middle layer, is between 1 and 4 mm thick, although thinner in the elderly and the very young. It is composed of an outer papillary dermis and an inner reticular dermis, and supplies nutrients to the epidermis. The dermis contains all the accessory structures including blood vessels, nerve endings, the sweat and sebaceous glands and the hair follicles. The dermis itself does not have regenerative ability, but because the glands, vessels and follicles are lined with epidermis, burns that involve this layer may still regenerate. The innermost layer, the subcutaneous tissue, consists of adipose and connective tissue. This layer has no regenerative ability.

Local changes

Local changes include the zones of coagulation, stasis and hyperaemia (see Figure 24.6) and the specific changes are outlined below.[21,39,111]

- Zone of coagulation: occurs at the point of maximum damage. Irreversible tissue loss occurs in this zone due to coagulation of the constituent proteins.

- Zone of stasis: surrounds the zone of coagulation and is an area of decreased tissue perfusion. Changes that contribute to this stasis include microthrombus formation, neutrophil adherence, fibrin deposition and endothelial swelling. Tissue in this zone is potentially salvageable if sufficient resuscitation is achieved to increase tissue perfusion. If insufficient resuscitation occurs, or if there are additional insults of hypotension, infection or oedema, tissue within this zone may convert to the zone of coagulation.

- Zone of hyperaemia: is the outermost zone. It experiences increased tissue perfusion as a result of local inflammatory response, which results in local vasodilation and an increase in vascular permeability. Tissue in this zone will usually recover, unless there are prolonged or severe periods of hypotension, infection or oedema.

Systemic changes

With a burn injury of >30% total burn surface area (TBSA), microcirculation vessel wall integrity is altered resulting in fluid and protein loss into the interstitium. The protein loss results in a reduction in osmotic pressure that further insults circulating volume. Changes to the cardiovascular, respiratory, metabolic and immunological systems occur as a result of the release of cytokines and other inflammatory mediators in response to the injury (see Table 24.11).

FIGURE 24.6 Zones of burn damage.[127]

FIGURE 24.6 Zones of burn damage.[127]

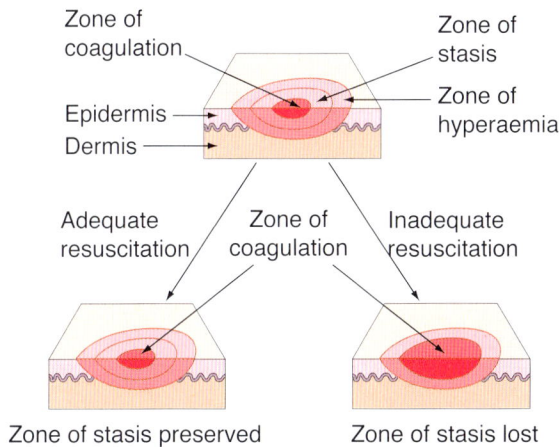

Reproduced from Stehan H, Peter D. ABC of burns. Br Med J 2004;328(7452):1366, with permission.

TABLE 24.11

Systemic changes that occur with burn injuries[135]

SYSTEM AFFECTED	PATHOPHYSIOLOGICAL CHANGE
Cardiovascular system	• Increased capillary permeability leading to capillary leak of intravascular proteins and fluids to interstitial compartment • Peripheral and splanchnic vasoconstriction • Reduced myocardial contractility • Systemic hypovolaemia due to above, plus fluid loss from burn
Respiratory system	• Bronchoconstriction • Adult respiratory distress syndrome
Metabolic system	• Increased basal metabolic rate (up to 3 times normal) • Above, plus splanchnic vasoconstriction, will lead to catabolism if patient not fed early and aggressively
Immunological system	• Downregulation of immune response

Adapted with permission from Grunwald TB, Garner WL. Acute burns. Plast Reconstr Surg 2008;121(5): 311e-319e.

Inhalation injury

The presence of an inhalation injury will increase mortality and morbidity in people with a dermal burn injury.[112] Inhalation injury consists of three components that may occur independently but often occur simultaneously, and include heat injury to the upper airways, effects of smoke on the respiratory system and inhalation of toxic gases.[112] This type of burn injury results in airway inflammation,

pulmonary shunting, augmented microvascular pressure gradient and severe hypoxaemic respiratory failure. Other than traditional ventilation strategies extracorporeal life support could be considered as a respiratory support option although the evidence clarifying benefits and limitations is limited (extracorporeal life support is discussed further in Chapter 15).[113] Diagnosis of an inhalation burn injury remains problematic, but it should be suspected if the injury was sustained in a closed spaced as well as if there are facial burns, singed nasal hairs or carbonaceous debris in the mouth or pharynx or in the sputum.[39,112] The specific changes are dependent on the types of substances inhaled at the time of injury. In addition, the size of the smoke particles that are inhaled will affect the location of any injury. If coarse smoke particles are inhaled, these will primarily be deposited in the upper tracheobronchial tree, while fine smoke particles will usually be lodged in the alveoli. Patients with inhalation burn injury will usually experience upper airway oedema and bronchospasm in the early stages, with the airway disease progressing to the small airways in subsequent days.[112,114] Bronchoscopy is useful to reveal injury to the large bronchi and therefore is recommended in the early evaluation of upper airway burn.[112,115]

Clinical manifestations

The most prominent clinical manifestations of burn injury are the dermal signs of injury. ANZBA uses the principles of the Early Management of Severe Burns (EMSB) course, which has been adopted internationally and categorises burns:[111,116]

1 Epidermal burns are limited to injury to the epidermis and tend to be very painful, with a common example being sunburn. The skin is pink to red in colour and remains intact. The surrounding tissues may be oedematous and there is no blistering. This burn injury will usually heal within 7 days.

2 Superficial partial-thickness burn injury involves the epidermal and superficial dermal layers and is generally red or mottled in appearance and the underlying skin will blanch with pressure, demonstrating that perfusion is intact; blisters are a hallmark symptom. This degree of burn injury is very painful and healing may take up to 14 days. There is usually a lot of wound exudate in the first 72 hours where the skin is broken.

3 Mid-dermal partial-thickness injuries extend a part way into the dermis. They have a large zone of damaged non-viable tissue extending into the dermis, with damaged but viable tissue at the base. Preservation of the damaged but viable tissue (particularly in the initial period following injury) is pivotal to preventing burn wound progression. As some of the nerve endings remain viable, pain is present but is less severe when compared to superficial burns. Similarly, as some of the capillaries remain viable, capillary return is present, albeit delayed. Blisters may be present and the underlying dermis is a variable colour (pale to dark pink).

4 Deep partial-thickness burns extend into the deep dermal layer. The tissue is a characteristic pink to pale ivory in appearance. It can also have a blotchy red base due to extravasation of red blood cells. The underlying tissue does not blanch and the hair is easily removed; sensation is reduced. These burns usually take in excess of 3 weeks to heal and are managed with surgical excision and closure.

5 Full-thickness burns destroy both layers of skin (epidermis and dermis) and may penetrate more deeply into underlying structures. These burns have a dense white, waxy or even charred appearance. The sensory nerves in the dermis are destroyed in a full thickness burn, and so sensation to pinprick is lost. The coagulated dead skin of a full thickness burn, which has a leathery appearance, is called eschar.

Assessment of the total body surface area (TBSA) of burns

The extent of injury is best described using the percentage of the total body surface area that sustained burns. The measurement of burn surface area is important during the initial management of people with burns for estimating fluid requirements and determining the need for transfer to a burns service. Erythema should not be included when calculating burn area.

There are several methods that provide a reproducible estimation of the area of surface area burns. These are:

- Rule of nines – for the adult population, the most widely known and easily applied method of estimating TBSA is the 'rule of nines' (see Figure 24.7). The principle of this assessment method is that most areas of the body constitute 9% (or multiples of 9%) of the TBSA.

- Palmar surface – the surface area of a patient's palm (including fingers) is about 1% total body surface area. This method of estimating TBSA is commonly taught but is yet to be validated. The palmar surface method can be used to estimate relatively small burns (<15% of total surface area) or very large burns (>85%, when unburnt skin is counted), but is inaccurate for medium-sized burns.

Patient management

Care can be considered in two phases. The first is the immediate priorities of care (outlined below) and including emergency principles, assessment and management of airway, breathing and circulation, and minimisation of hypothermia and hyperkalaemia. The second phase of care is that provided throughout the first 24 hours (see Table 24.12). Care of the burn patient beyond that time will follow the general principles for critically ill patients, with additional considerations relating to wound care.

Emergency principles of care

The patient should be removed from danger and the burning process should be stopped. The wound should

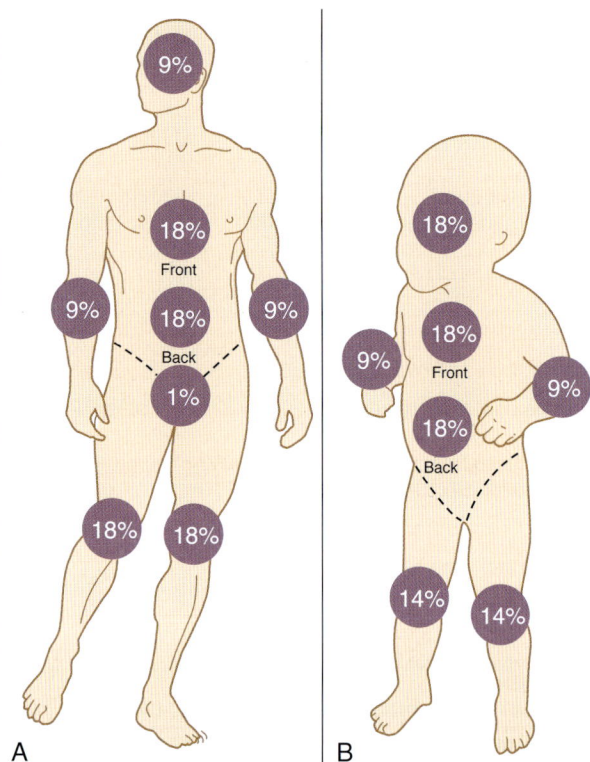

FIGURE 24.7 Diagram of the 'rule of nines': **A**, adult; **B**, child.[128]

Reproduced from Sheehy SB, Newberry L. Sheehy's emergency nursing: Principles and practice. St Louis: Mosby; 2003, with permission.

then be cooled to minimise the burden of injury. ANZBA recommends the application of cool running water for 20 minutes.[111] This is most useful immediately after injury but can be instigated up to 3 hours post-injury. The wound and the patient should then be covered to reduce risk of hypothermia. Adequate analgesia must be provided early in patient care.

Airway

All patients with burn injury require supplemental oxygen. Facial burns or carbonaceous sputum (sputum with signs of smoke or charcoal) may indicate a burn injury to the airway. A carboxyhaemoglobin of >10% within the first hour post-injury is strongly indicative of inhalation injury. Classic signs of obstruction including stridor, dyspnoea and hoarse voice warrant immediate intubation and should be considered early as worsening oedema can make intubation difficult. Airway stability is mandatory for safe transfer.[111]

Breathing

Carbonaceous pulmonary secretions are a hallmark of airway injury. Dyspnoea and tachypnoea are signs of respiratory distress, while pulmonary oedema will often ensue with airway burns.

TABLE 24.12

Acute nursing care after burn injury (first 24 hours)

ELEMENT OF CARE	MINOR BURN INJURY (<10%)	MAJOR BURN INJURY	CRITICALLY ILL
Fluid replacement	Generally not fluid loaded	Fluid replacement as per relevant formula	Major fluid replacement
Need for intubation and mechanical ventilation	Supplemental oxygen therapy. Only if airway burns are suspected or comorbidities require it	Supplemental oxygen therapy. Intubation and mechanical ventilation may be required with analgesia and in burns shock. Any airway burn in this group requires intubation	Mandatory
Respiratory and cardiovascular observations	Hourly TPR, BP, SpO$_2$ adapted according to patient status	Continuous ECG, SpO$_2$, temperature, urine output (hourly observations if not continuously monitored)	Continuous invasive haemodynamic, respiratory and urine output monitoring, including core temperature
Neurovascular observations	Assess neurovascular status of circumferential burns to chest and limbs (including fingers and toes)	Assess neurovascular status of circumferential burns to chest and limbs (including fingers and toes)	Assess neurovascular status of circumferential burns to chest and limbs (including fingers and toes)
Analgesia	Continuous, intermittent or patient-controlled (if patient capable) analgesia ± conscious sedation for dressings	Continuous intravenous analgesia ± conscious sedation for dressings	Continuous intravenous analgesia + sedation
Arterial blood gas, serum potassium; chloride and haemoglobin	Baseline and as indicated by patient's condition	Baseline and as indicated by patient's condition	Baseline and minimum 4-hourly depending on patient's condition, including temperature and ventilatory requirements
Haematology	Baseline and as indicated by patient's condition	Baseline and as indicated by patient's condition, noting that more frequent assessment will be needed if coagulopathy is present	Baseline and as indicated by patient's condition, noting that more frequent assessment will be needed if coagulopathy is present
Feeding	Oral intake should be monitored and encouraged	Enteral or oral intake should commence within 24 hours of injury (NB: burns of >20% TBSA require enteral feeding)	Enteral feeding should commence within 24 hours of injury
General burn dressings	Primary debridement undertaken by nursing staff with theatre debridement if indicated due to burn depth Burn escharotomy as indicated (unlikely unless circumferential injury)	Primary debridement undertaken by nursing staff with theatre debridement if indicated due to burn depth Burns escharotomy as indicated (likely with circumferential injury)	Primary debridement undertaken by nursing staff with theatre debridement if indicated due to burn depth Burns escharotomy as indicated (highly likely)

BP = blood pressure; ECG = electrocardiogram; SpO$_2$ = peripheral oxygen saturation; TBSA = total body surface area; TPR = temperature, pulse respiration.

Circulation

The massive interstitial and intracellular fluid shifts associated with acute burn injury will deplete circulating volume and result in shock if it remains uncorrected. Fluid resuscitation aims to anticipate and prevent rather than treat shock. ANZBA and EMSB guidelines recommend IV resuscitation in adults with burns >15% TBSA and children with burns >10% TBSA, although due to a lack of evidence there is still considerable variability in resuscitation protocols.[110]

Early intravenous cannulation (with two wide-bore cannulae) and the administration of high-volume fluids must begin immediately. ANZBA recommends crystalloid solution in the first 24 hours, with fluid administration titrated to patient response. One of the most widely accepted resuscitation formulas is the Modified Parkland formula, which recommends delivery of Hartmann's solution at the rate of 3–4 mL/kg/% TBSA over the first 24 hours commencing at the time of burn injury, with half the fluid administered within the first 8 hours and the remainder over the next 16 hours. Time delays for implementation of fluid resuscitation should be corrected by increasing infusion rates to reach targets. Fluid resuscitation should be guided by predetermined end points in combination with fluid volumes dictated by the formula. Precise end points for burns resuscitation remain debatable; at present ANZBA recommends urine output of 0.5–1 mL/kg/h in adults and 0.5–2 mL/kg/h in children. The evolution of 'fluid creep' has been reported due to over-resuscitation in the early phases of shock, which can result in complications such as acute lung injury, abdominal and extremity compartment syndrome, multi-organ failure and death.[109,110]

Patients with circumferential full thickness burn injury may require escharotomies due to the extensive oedema formation and the inelasticity of burn eschar. Delayed capillary return, a cool limb and increased pain manifest earlier than loss of palpable pulse.

The use of invasive monitoring in the burns patient is controversial, as the relevant catheters often require insertion through a burn and therefore provide a portal of entry for infection. However, all serious burns patients require an indwelling catheter for monitoring. Relevance of other monitoring capability will be determined on an individual patient basis based on cardiovascular status, need for inotropic support, extent of the burn and potential for infection.

Minimising hypothermia

Skin is an essential component of the body's natural thermoregulation mechanism, so loss of skin integrity, coupled with such treatment strategies as cooling the burn and administering high-volume fluid replacement, exposure of wounds following injury and during dressing changes, places the patient at high risk of hypothermia. Continuous temperature monitoring is essential, and strategies to maintain normothermia should be implemented immediately and continuously. Strategies include minimising exposure, warming fluids and warming the patient's environment. Warm blankets and heated humidified supplemental oxygen are also valuable adjuncts.

Hyperkalaemia

Cell destruction from the burn injury can result in high serum potassium levels, which should be monitored closely. Metabolic acidosis will exacerbate the hyperkalaemia, as intracellular exchange of hydrogen ions with potassium ions takes place.

Nutrition

Supplemental feeding is mandatory and should commence as soon as possible following severe burn injuries due to the hypermetabolism.[39] Patients with >20% TBSA are unable to meet their nutritional requirements orally. ANZBA and EMSB recommend enteric feeding in adults with burn injury >20% and >10% TBSA in children.

The multitrauma burns patient

The combination of traumatic injury and burn injury is not common, with an incidence of 5–7%, however the mortality and morbidity is significantly higher than in those patients who sustain an isolated traumatic or burn injury.[117] It is essential to combine the principles of care of the burns patient with those of the relevant injury as outlined below:

- Spinal injury – if the patient has potential spinal injuries in addition to the burn, spinal precautions must be maintained; however, cervical collars should not be used over a burnt neck or upper chest due to the potential for swelling and subsequent restriction. If a collar is used, changing to an appropriate size as the swelling worsens or goes down is essential.
- Skeletal injury – skin traction cannot be used in a patient with burn injury over a limb that also has a skeletal fracture; this will necessitate early internal fixation or the use of an external fixateur.
- Electrocution injuries – electrocution burns are largely internal burns that potentially cause devastating multiple internal injuries. The electrical current causes a burn at both the entry and exit sites. Where electrocution is confirmed or suspected the body must be inspected to identify all injuries. These may be in obscure places such as the hands and feet or even the back and scalp. Close monitoring for cardiac damage and rhabdomyolysis is essential.

Burn dressings

Mitigating infection is the primary aim of good burns nursing.[116] The greatest challenge is minimising the risk for cross-contamination, and patients should be nursed in a single room where possible. Burn dressings present a physical challenge, particularly when large areas of the body are affected.

The traditional burn dressing in the ICU is undertaken as a surgically clean technique. As part of the management of the burn injury, there are a number of specific issues that require attention. The following is a guide to specific aspects of burn management:

- Debridement – this refers to the excision of dead skin. Gentle scrubbing is generally used to remove loose tissue and burst blisters. Forceps and scissors may be required to lift and remove smaller areas of tissue. Extensive areas of debridement will usually be undertaken in the operating room.
- Blisters – small blisters should be left intact whereas large blisters may be aspirated or deroofed during debridement, although it should be noted that evidence regarding blister management is poor. Blisters over joints that are restricting movement should also be debrided.
- Escharotomy – an escharotomy is undertaken to a limb or side of the trunk for circumferential burns that are contracting and creating vascular compromise

to the underlying and distal tissues. The escharotomy is an incision through the eschar, and does not involve opening muscle fascia. The escharotomy immediately relieves the compression and is a limb-/life-saving surgical manoeuvre. The escharotomy is dressed as a burn to prevent infection.

- Skin grafts – these are required to cover the skin defect. They may be full-thickness or partial-thickness grafts, and may be harvested from the patient or, in some cases, obtained from a cadaver donor. Regardless of the type of skin graft, nursing care remains the same, with the aim being to maximise adherence. Specific nursing care of the graft site includes leaving the site intact and immobilising the graft site, applying the appropriate wound care regimen, preventing shearing injury to the graft site and minimising the risk for infection. With autografts, wound care will also be required for the donor site.[109]

- Skin substitutes – some products are available to cover partial-thickness wounds that provide a moist environment that stimulates epithelialisation. These are best reserved for 'clean' wounds. Some products are able to act as full-thickness substitutes that provide wound closure, protection from mechanical trauma and bacteria and a vapour barrier. Once the new dermis is created the substitute is removed.[109]

Summary

Care of the trauma patient presents the critical care nurse with multiple challenges. With the introduction of trauma systems the outcome and survival of injured patients has improved dramatically. The severity of injury and patient outcome are dependent on effective pre-hospital care, resuscitation and definitive surgical management on arrival at the hospital. Principles of resuscitation of the trauma patient are the same as for all patients, with a primary, secondary and tertiary survey being undertaken, and maintenance or correction of airway, breathing and circulation taking precedence. Prevention of the 'trauma triad' of hypothermia, acidosis and coagulopathy has the potential to significantly influence patient outcome. Consideration of the specific injury, with its resultant pathophysiological changes, is necessary to care effectively for patients with abdominal, chest, multiple or burn injuries. It is challenging work as trauma patients are largely a young and healthy population prior to injury and may experience significant ongoing compromise.

Case study

Helen is a 45-year-old, 70-kg woman from Hong Kong who has been working in Australia for several months. Her husband and son both reside in Hong Kong. Helen was a pedestrian walking with her headphones on and had stopped at an intersection where she was struck by a concrete mixer and dragged 200 metres. Glasgow Coma Score (GCS) was initially 3; however, it improved to 9 pre-hospital.

Helen met the major trauma triage criteria and was transferred via road to a major trauma hospital. Trauma team activation occurred prior to Helen's arrival. When Helen arrived in the emergency department (ED), a full team was present to assess and treat her. This team included a trauma surgeon, trauma nurse leader, emergency doctor, orthopaedic surgeon, anaesthetist, specialist nurses and support staff.

On arrival of the ambulance personnel Helen's vital signs were as follows:

- HR was 140 (sinus tachycardia), BP unrecordable, respiratory rate (RR) not recorded, unconscious GCS 3, SpO_2 92% on room air.
- IV cannula was inserted with 1 L normal saline administered during transport. Helen received O_2 and morphine for pain; her spine and left leg were both immobilised.
- First ABGs were: pH 7.03, pCO_2 56 mmHg, pO_2 447 mmHg, HCO_3^- 15 mEq/L, SpO_2 99%, Na 138 mmol/L, K 6.8 mmol/L. Cl⁻109 mmol/L, glucose 17.0 mmol/L; lactate was unavailable.
- Duration at scene was 8 minutes.

Ongoing assessment and treatment in the ED consisted of the following:

- HR was 76, SBP 60–70, RR not recorded, GCS fluctuating from 9 to 3, SpO_2 97% decreased to 79%.
- Primary survey was conducted.
- Initial resuscitation with 1 L normal saline, FAST negative, massive transfusion protocol activation, right subclavian CVC inserted, 7 units RBC administered, intubation, left lower leg splint, left thigh pressure bandage, pelvic binder applied.
- Duration in ED was 28 minutes.

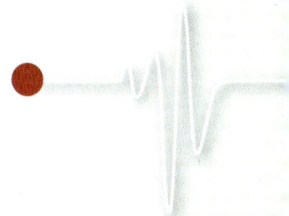

Observations and treatment in the operating theatre included:

- SBP was <100, HR >100, initial temp 33°C, increased to 37°C.

- Operations were trauma laparotomy and vacuum dressing, external fixateur and C-clamp to pelvis, external fixateur to left knee and right femur, left thigh exploration and repair left iliac artery, laparotomy and control iliac vein bleeding (avulsion injury), left lower eyelid canthotomy, repair facial and lip laceration, repair left hand laceration, left leg wound repair and vacuum dressing, left illiofemoral bypass, fasciotomy and haemostasis; indwelling catheter (IDC) insertion

- Duration in theatre was 11 h.

Injuries included: right tentorial subdural haemorrhage; left orbital fracture (#); left ribs # 3–12th; bilateral sacroiliac joint diastasis and left sacral alar #; left superior pubic rami #; left inferior ischial rami #; right femur #; dislocated left knee, pancreatic, duodenal and jejunal oedema and mesenteric haematoma; left subcostal artery injury; left inferior gluteal and left external iliac artery injury; left hand laceration; full thickness graze to mid back and sacral area; scalp haematoma.

On arrival in intensive care Helen had already received a total of 54 units red blood cells (RBC), 40 units fresh frozen plasma (FFP), 7 pooled units platelets, 750 mL cryoprecipitate, Novo 7 (noted in anaesthetics documentation, with dose not recorded), and cell saver had been used in theatre.

In ICU Helen was initially reported as being able to roll for pressure care; however, subsequently this was changed by the orthopaedic team to Jordan frame lift only due to pelvic fracture instability. Post fixation of her pelvic fracture and removal of external fixateurs this changed and Helen was only allowed to log roll to the left side with no side lying at all.

During day 1 Helen had rising creatine kinase (CK) levels (<30,000) and decreasing urinary output resulting in commencement of dialysis post insertion of a right internal jugular vascular catheter. She had high inotropic requirements (both noradrenaline and adrenaline) to maintain her mean arterial pressure >70 mmHg. An echocardiogram showed normal cardiac function. A warming blanket was used as Helen had hypothermia (temp 35°C) on arrival in ICU, no doubt as a result of the prolonged theatre time.

Consultation with trauma, orthopaedics and vascular teams occurred on day 1 regarding the viability of Helen's left leg. Discussion then occurred with Helen's family – her son was present, but other family members including Helen's husband were in Hong Kong. A decision was made to return Helen to theatre for a left hindquarter amputation.

A social worker worked with Helen's son to support him and to make travel arrangements for Helen's husband to come to Australia from Hong Kong; the social worker and nursing team continued to support the family throughout Helen's ICU stay.

Within ICU members of the multidisciplinary team who contributed to Helen's care included nursing and medical staff who provided patient and family care and support; physiotherapists delivering ongoing respiratory assessment, passive limb movements and assessment for increasing tone in all limbs; and the dietitian to assess nutritional requirements and provide total parenteral nutrition and enteral nutrition.

Other teams who contributed to Helen's care included:

- trauma team, which undertook the FAST in the ED and performed some of the surgical procedures initially and on an ongoing basis

- orthopaedic team, which undertook the orthopaedic surgical procedures and provided ongoing management in this area of her care

- vascular team, who were involved in the management of all arterial injuries including her amputation

- haematology team, who were involved in the management of her coagulopathy

- plastics team, which contributed expertise related to the management of full thickness graze and burn injuries

- faciomaxillary team, which completed an open reduction and internal fixation of her left orbit # on day 16 of admission

- renal team, who were involved with management of intermittent dialysis via a perma-cath

- speech therapy, who assessed Helen's swallow post extubation to ensure that she was safe to commence oral intake

- occupational therapy, who assessed Helen for post traumatic amnesia and contributed to her discharge planning, including the possibility of musculoskeletal and acquired brain injury rehabilitation.

Commencing on day 12 Helen was gradually woken. She had slow improvements in her conscious state and was able to tolerate a slow wean of her mechanical ventilation support. She was successfully extubated on day 13 of her admission.

Helen was initially confused and not speaking English, although she did recognise her husband and son when they visited and was often more settled during these times. Helen required frequent orientation to time and place and what had happened to her. Fortunately, she was able to speak and understand English, although this was not her native language, which was difficult for her. Helen was assessed for delirium and was treated for this during the days leading to her discharge to the ward; she also experienced depression in response to the injury and subsequent loss of independence. A plan was instituted for the ongoing assessment and management of this while in ICU and post discharge to the ward.

The social worker supported Helen and her family to assist with the many adjustments required as a result of her injury and subsequent loss of independence and changes to living arrangements as Helen previously lived in a first floor apartment with stair access only.

CASE STUDY QUESTIONS

1 Discuss the components of the 'trauma triad' and outline the practices that would prevent or ameliorate the triad.

2 Identify the likely causes of Helen's renal failure and discuss the preventative and treatment approaches that are available.

3 Discuss the management of massive blood transfusion and the treatment approaches that are available.

4 What is 'damage-control surgery' and why is this so important to survival in trauma patients? Describe the implications of the type of accident experienced by Helen and her likely injuries and treatment in relation to DCS.

5 Describe the practices that could be incorporated into Helen's care to reduce her psychological distress both during the initial weeks post injury and in the rehabilitation/discharge phase of her recovery.

RESEARCH VIGNETTE

Hyllienmark P, Brattstrom O, Larsson E, Martling CR, Petersson J, Olner A. High incidence of post-injury pneumonia in intensive care-treated trauma patients. Acta Anaesthesiol Scand 2013;57:848–54

Abstract

Introduction: Trauma patients are susceptible to post-injury infections. We investigated the incidence, as well as risk factors for development of pneumonia in intensive care unit (ICU)-treated trauma patients. In addition, we report pathogens identified in patients that developed pneumonia.

Methods: The study cohort consisted of 322 trauma patients admitted to the ICU at a level-one trauma centre following initial resuscitation. Patients 15 years or older with an ICU stay of more than 24 h were included. We investigated pre-hospital and hospital parameters during the first 24 h after admission and their possible association with pneumonia within 10 days of ICU admission.

Results: Majority of the patients were male (78%) and the median age was 41 years. The overall degree of injury was high with a median Injury Severity Score of 24. Overall 30-day mortality was 9%. Eighty-five (26%) patients developed pneumonia during their first 10 days in the ICU. Univariate logistic regression revealed that intubation in the field, shock, Glasgow Coma Scale (GCS) 3–8, major surgery within 24 h after admission, massive transfusion and injury severity score >24 were all risk factors for subsequent development of pneumonia. In the multivariable model, only GCS 3–8 was identified as an independent risk factor. In 42 out of the 85 cases of pneumonia, the diagnosis was defined by significant growth of at least one pathogen where *Enterobacteriaceae* and *Staphylococcus aureus* were the most common.

Conclusion: Pneumonia is a common complication among ICU-treated trauma patients. Reduced consciousness is an independent risk factor for development of pneumonia after severe injury.

Critique

This investigation was a single site study with an exploratory research design. The setting for the study was a mixed 13-bed ICU in a designated level 1 trauma centre in a university hospital in Stockholm, Sweden. The trauma centre served as the only referral centre for severe trauma cases in a region with a population of approximately 2 million inhabitants. This makes this study cohort a representative sample of severe trauma across urban and rural settings in this country. However, patients were excluded if they were admitted to the ICU from other receiving units, and it is not clear why the transferred patients were excluded; this may limit the generalisability of the results.

The study has several strengths. One is that all clinical data were entered prospectively into the databases, which likely minimised missed values and increased the accuracy and validity of the data. Another strength was that pneumonia was clearly and thoroughly defined based on radiographic criteria together with clinical or microbiological criteria as established by the Swedish intensive care registry (SIR); these are the same criteria developed by the CDC National Health and Safety Network with the exception that microbiological criteria are optional.[119] Pneumonia occurring after more than 48 hours of invasive mechanical ventilation was classified as ventilator-associated pneumonia (VAP). Other assessment requirements and interventions were also clearly described, e.g. massive transfusion was defined as more than 10 units of blood during the first 24 hours after admission.

The study included 322 patients for analysis. The characteristics of the cohort, with relatively low median age, male dominance and limited number of penetrating injuries, was representative of other European trauma ICU cohorts.[120,121] One-quarter of the patients developed pneumonia during their first 10 days post-injury, which is consistent with other studies. The key finding in this study was that reduced level of consciousness (GCS 3–8) was the single greatest independent risk factor for the development of post-injury pneumonia. Although the risk factors of intubation in the field, shock, major surgery, massive transfusion and severe injury had a univariate relationship with the outcome of pneumonia, they did not retain significance in the multivariable model. The investigators suggest that factors other than decreased consciousness, for example immobilisation, may contribute to the development of post-injury pneumonia.

This study was generally well designed. Further prospective, multicentre research is needed to address the complexity in the pathophysiology of multiple injuries and the association with pneumonia and VAP in trauma patients. The implications for clinical nursing are significant, as 25% of severe trauma patients have the potential of developing pneumonia and VAP in the first 10 days after a major trauma event. Trauma management includes the use of VAP bundle strategies containing different components such as body position, oral care, daily interruption in sedation and assessment of readiness for extubation, and use of specialised endotracheal tubes.[122] The efficacy and validity behind the components in the VAP bundle need to be investigated as there is a lack of evidence. Nurses, using their clinical expertise, can identify at-risk patients for developing VAP and play a vital role in the innovation and critical evaluation of the evidence behind interventions and contribute to improving trauma patients' safety and outcome.

Learning activities

1   Briefly describe why the mechanism of injury is important information in diagnosing injuries.
2   Describe the implications of the type of accident experienced by Helen and her likely injuries and treatment.

Online resources

American College of Surgeons, www.facs.org

Australasian College for Emergency Medicine, www.acem.org.au

Australasian Trauma Society, www.traumasociety.com.au

Australian and New Zealand Burn Association, www.anzba.org.au

Eastern Association for the Surgery of Trauma, www.east.org

European Society for Trauma and Emergency Surgery, www.estesonline.org

NSW Trauma Management Guidelines, www.itim.nsw.gov.au/go/itim-trauma-guidelines

NSW Trauma System, www.itim.nsw.gov.au/index.cfm

Royal Australasian College of Surgeons, www.surgeons.org

Society of Trauma Nurses, www.traumanurses.org

Trauma.org, an independent, non-profit organisation providing global education, information and communication resources for professionals in trauma and critical care, www.trauma.org

Victorian State Trauma System, www.health.vic.gov.au/trauma

World Health Organization, www.who.int/topics/injuries/en/

Further reading

McQuillan K, Whalen E, Flynn-Makick M. Trauma nursing: From resuscitation through rehabilitation. 4th ed. Philadelphia: Saunders, 2008.

Moloney-Harmon PA, Czerwinski SJ. Nursing care of the paediatric trauma patient. Cambridge: Elsevier, 2003.

Skinner DV, Driscoll PA. ABC of major trauma. 4th ed. West Sussex: Wiley, 2013.

Spahn DR, Bouillon B, Cemy V, Coast TJ, Duranteau J, Fernandez-Mondejar E et al. Management of bleeding and coagulopathy following major trauma: an updated European guideline. Crit Care 2013;17:R76. <http://ccforum.com/content/17/2/R76>.

Wolf SJ, Bebarta VS, Bonnett CJ, Pons PT, Cantrill SV. Blast injuries. Lancet 2009;374(9687):405–15.

References

1 Service NZHI. Selected morbitity data for publicly funded hospitals 2000/01. Wellington: Ministry of Health; 2004.

2 World Health Organization. Global burden of disease [Internet]. <http://www.who.int/healthinfo/global_burden_disease/GBD_report_2004 update_full>; 2004.

3 (AIHW) AIoHaW. Australia's health, 2010. Canberra: Australian Institute of Health and Welfare; 2010.

4 Begg S VT, Baker B, Stevenson C, Stanley L, Lopes AD. The burden of disease and injury in Australia 2003. Canberra: Australian Institute of Health and Welfare; 2007.

5 Bauer R, Steiner M. Injuries in the European Union, statistics summary 2005–2009. Vienna: European Commission; 2009.

6 World Health Organization. Global status on road safety: Time for action. Geneva: WHO, <http://whqlibdoc.who.int/publications/2009/9789241563840_eng.pdf>; 2009 [accessed 04.15].

7 Clay Mann N, Mullins RJ, Hedges JR, Rowland D, Arthur M, Zechnich AD. Mortality among seriously injured patients treated in remote rural trauma centers before and after implementation of a statewide trauma system. Med Care 2001;39(7):643–53.

8 World Health Organization. Prehospital trauma care systems. France: WHO, 2005.

9 Lendrum RA, Lockey DJ. Trauma system development. Anaesthesia 2013;68(Suppl 1):30-9.

10 World Health Organization. Guidelines for essential trauma care. Geneva: WHO, <http://www.who.int/violence_injury_prevention/publications/services/en/guidelines_traumacare.pdf>; 2004 [accessed 04.15].

11 Larsen KT, Uleberg O, Skogvoll E. Differences in trauma team activation criteria among Norwegian hospitals. Scand J Trauma Resusc Emerg Med 2010;18:21.

12 Davis MJ, Parr MJ. Trauma systems. Curr Opin Anesthesiol 2001;14(2):185-9.

13 Cameron PA, Gabbe BJ, Smith K, Mitra B. Triaging the right patient to the right place in the shortest time. Br J Anaesth 2014;113(2):226-33.

14 Gabbe BJ, Biostat GD, Simpson PM, Sutherland AM, Dip G, Wolfe R et al. Improved functional outcomes for major trauma patients in a regionalized, inclusive trauma system. Ann Surg 2012;255(6):1009-15 10.97/SLA.0b013e31824c4b91.

15 Joseph A, Pearce A. The future of trauma care. Injury 2012;43(5):539-41.

16 Henry JA, Reingold AL. Prehospital trauma systems reduce mortality in developing countries: a systematic review and meta-analysis. J Trauma Acute Care Surg 2012;73(1):261-8.

17 Gomes E, Araújo R, Carneiro A, Dias C, Costa-Pereira A, Lecky FE. The importance of pre-trauma centre treatment of life-threatening events on the mortality of patients transferred with severe trauma. Resusc 2010;81(4):440-5.

18 Duncan NS, Moran C. (i) Initial resuscitation of the trauma victim. Orthopaed Trauma 2010;24(1):1-8.

19 Lerner EB, Moscati RM. The golden hour: scientific fact or medical "urban legend"? Acad Emerg Med 2001;8(7):758-60.

20 Deakin CD, Søreide E. Pre-hospital trauma care. Curr Opin Anesthesiol 2001;14(2):191-5.

21 Cameron P. Textbook of adult emergency medicine. New York: Churchill Livingstone Elsevier; 2009.

22 Newgard CD, Schmicker RH, Hedges JR, Trickett JP, Davis DP, Bulger EM et al. Emergency medical services intervals and survival in trauma: assessment of the "golden hour" in a North American prospective cohort. Ann Emerg Med 2010;55(3):235-46.e4.

23 American College of Surgeons Committee on Trauma. Advanced trauma life support for doctors (ATLS). 8th ed. Chicago: American College of Surgeons Committee on Trauma; 2008.

24 Cherry RA, King TS, Carney DE, Bryant P, Cooney RN. Trauma team activation and the impact on mortality. J Trauma Acute Care Surg 2007;63(2):326-30 10.1097/TA.0b013e31811eaad1.

25 Kouzminova N SC, Palm E, McCullough M, Serck J. The efficacy of a two-tiered trauma activation system at a level 1 trauma center. J Trauma Acute Care Surg 2009;67(4):829-33.

26 Cameron PA, Gabbe BJ, Cooper DJ, Walker T, Judson R, McNeil J. A statewide system of trauma care in Victoria: effect on patient survival. Med J Aust 2008;189(10):546-50.

27 Garwe T, Cowan LD, Neas BR, Sacra JC, Albrecht RM. Directness of transport of major trauma patients to a lLevel I trauma center: a propensity-adjusted survival analysis of the impact on short-term mortality. J Trauma Acute Care Surg 2011;70(5):1118-27 10.097/TA.0b013e3181e243b8.

28 Cameron PA, Gabbe BJ, Smith K, Mitra B. Triaging the right patient to the right place in the shortest time. Br J Anaesth 2014;113(2):226-33.

29 Brown JB, Stassen NA, Bankey PE, Sangosanya AT, Cheng JD, Gestring ML. Helicopters and the civilian trauma system: national utilization patterns demonstrate improved outcomes after traumatic injury. J Trauma Acute Care Surg 2010;69(5):1030-6. doi: 10.97/TA.0b013e3181f6f450.

30 Nocera N SP. N.E.W.S Checklist (Abstract). Aust Emerg Nurs J 2001;4(1):31.

31 Nirula R, Maier R, Moore E, Sperry J, Gentilello L. Scoop and run to the trauma center or stay and play at the local hospital: hospital transfer's effect on mortality. J Trauma Acute Care Surg 2010;69(3):595-601. doi: 10.1097/TA.0b013e3181ee6e32.

32 Zalstein S, Danne P, Taylor D, Cameron P, McLellan S, Fitzgerald M et al. The Victorian major trauma transfer study. Injury 2010;41(1):102-9.

33 Tiel Groenestege-Kreb D, van Maarseveen O, Leenen L. Trauma team. Br J Anaesth 2014;113(2):258-65.

34 McCullough AL, Haycock JC, Forward DP, Moran CG. Early management of the severely injured major trauma patient. Br J Anaesth 2014; 113(2):234-41.

35 Department of Health and Ageing. Emergency triage education kit. In: Department of Health and Ageing, editor. Canberra: Australian Government; 2009.

36 Robertson-Steel I. Evolution of triage systems. J Emerg Med 2006;23:154-5.

37 McQuillan KA, Makic MBF, Whalen E. Trauma nursing: from resuscitation through rehabilitation. St Louis, Mo: Saunders/Elsevier; 2009.

38 Georgiou A, Lockey DJ. The performance and assessment of hospital trauma teams. Scand J Trauma Resusc Emerg Med 2010;18(1):66.

39 Shepherd MV, Trethewy CE, Kennedy J, Davis L. Helicopter use in rural trauma. Emerg Med Australas 2008;20(6):494-9.

40 Delprado AM. Trauma systems in Australia. Jf Trauma Nurs 2007;14(2):93-7. doi: 10.1097/01.JTN.0000278795.74277.cf.

41 Wolf SJ, Bebarta VS, Bonnett CJ, Pons PT, Cantrill SV. Blast injuries. Lancet 2009;374(9687):405-15.

42 Chandran A, Hyder AA, Peek-Asa C. The global burden of unintentional injuries and an agenda for progress. Epidemiol Rev 2010;32(1):110-20.

43 Ruseckaite R, Gabbe B, Vogel AP, Collie A. Health care utilisation following hospitalisation for transport-related injury. Injury 2012;43(9):1600-5.

44 Ackland H. Spinal clearance management protocol. Melbourne: Alfred Health, <http://www.alfred.org.au/Assets/Files/SpinalClearanceManagementProtocol_External.pdf>; updated 24.11.09 [accessed 04.15].

45 Theodore N, Hadley MN, Arabi B, Dhall SS, Gelb DE, Hurlbert RJ et al. Prehospital cervical spinal immobilization after trauma In: Guideline for the management of acute cervical spine and spinal cord injuries. Neurosurg 2013;72(Suppl 2):22-34.

46 Moffatt SE. Hypothermia in trauma. Emerg Med J 2013;30(12):989-96.

47 Mitra B, Tullio F, Cameron PA, Fitzgerald M. Trauma patients with the 'triad of death'. Emerg Med J 2012;29(8):622-5.

48 Thorsen K, Ringdal KG, Strand K, Søreide E, Hagemo J, Søreide K. Clinical and cellular effects of hypothermia, acidosis and coagulopathy in major injury. Br J Surg 2011;98(7):894-907.

49 Mylankal KJ, Wyatt MG. Control of major haemorrhage. Surgery (Oxford) 2010;28(11):556-62.

50 Langhelle A LD, Harris T, Davies G. Body temperature of trauma patients on admission to hospital: a comparison of anaesthetized and non-anaesthetised patients. Emerg Med J 2010;29(3):239-42.

51 Frith D, Brohi K. The acute coagulopathy of trauma shock: clinical relevance. Surgeon 2010;8(3):159-63.

52 Kheirbek T, Kochanek AR, Alam HB. Hypothermia in bleeding trauma: a friend or a foe? Scand J Trauma Resusc Emerg Med 2009;17(1):65.

53 Hess JR, Brohi K, Dutton RP, Hauser CJ, Holcomb JB, Kluger Y, et al. The coagulopathy of trauma: a review of mechanisms. J Trauma Acute Care Surg 2008;65(4):748-54. doi: 10.1097/TA.0b013e3181877a9c.

54 Ireland S, Endacott R, Cameron P, Fitzgerald M, Paul E. The incidence and significance of accidental hypothermia in major trauma: a prospective observational study. Resusc 2011;82(3):300-6.

55 Mylankal KJ, Wyatt MG. Control of major haemorrhage and damage control surgery. Surgery (Oxford) 2013;31(11):574-81.

56 Larson CR, White CE, Spinella PC, Jones JA, Holcomb JB, Blackbourne LH et al. Association of shock, coagulopathy, and initial vital signs with massive transfusion in combat casualties. J Trauma Acute Care Surg 2010;69(1):S26-S32. doi: 10.1097/TA.0b013e3181e423f4.

57 Mitra B, Cameron PA. Optimising management of the elderly trauma patient. Injury 2012;43(7):973-5.

58 Clement ND, Tennant C, Muwanga C. Polytrauma in the elderly: predictors of the cause and time of death. Scand J Trauma Resusc Emerg Med 2010;18:26.

59 Ganter MT, Pittet J-F. New insights into acute coagulopathy in trauma patients. Best Prac Res Clin Anaesthesiol 2010;24(1):15-25.

60 D'Angelo MR. Management of trauma-induced coagulopathy: trends and practices. AANA 2010;78:35-40.

61 Chovanes J, Cannon JW, Nunez TC. The evolution of damage control surgery. Surg Clin N Am 2012;92(4):859-75.

62 Godat L KL, Costantini T, Coimbra R. Abdominal damage control surgery and reconstruction: World Society of Emergency Surgery position paper. World J Emerg Surg 2013;8.

63 Diercks DB MA, Nazarian DJ, Promes SB, Decker WW, Fesmire FM. Clinical policy: critical issues in the evaluation of adult patients presenting to the emergency department with acute blunt abdominal trauma. Ann Emerg Med 2011;57(4):387-404.

64 Balogh ZJ, Reumann MK, Gruen RL, Mayer-Kuckuk P, Schuetz MA, Harris IA et al. Advances and future directions for management of trauma patients with musculoskeletal injuries. Lancet 2012;380(9847):1109-19.

65 Panteli M, Lampropoulos A, Giannoudis PV. Fat embolism following pelvic injuries: a subclinical event or an increased risk of mortality? Injury 2014;45(4):645.

66 Aitken LM LJ, Bellamy N. Queensland Trauma Registry: description of serious injury throughout Queensland, 2003. Herston: Centre of National Research on Disability and Rehabilitation Medicine; 2004.

67 Guyton AC, Hall JE. Textbook of medical physiology. Philadelphia: Elsevier Saunders; 2006.

68 Little N, Rogers B, Flannery M. Bone formation, remodelling and healing. Surgery (Oxford) 2011;29(4):141-5.

69 Association for the Advancement of Automotive Medicine. Abbreviated Injury Scale 2005: update 2008. Barrington: Association for the Advancement of Automotive Medicine; 2008.

70 Copuroglu C, Calori GM, Giannoudis PV. Fracture non-union: who is at risk? Injury 2013;44(11):1379.

71 Hak DJ, Fitzpatrick D, Bishop JA, Marsh JL, Tilp S, Schnettler R et al. Delayed union and nonunions: epidemiology, clinical issues, and financial aspects. Injury 2014;45(Suppl 2):S3-S7.

72 Sinha P, Bunker N, Soni N. Fat embolism – an update. Curr Anaesth Crit Care 2010;21(5):277-81.

73 Zutt R, van der Kooi AJ, Linthorst GE, Wanders RJA, de Visser M. Rhabdomyolysis: review of the literature. Neuromusc Disord 2014;24(8):651.

74 Bosch X, Poch E, Grau JM. Rhabdomyolysis and acute kidney injury. N Engl J Med 2009;361(1):62-72.

75 Lenarz CJ, Watson JT, Moed BR, Israel H, Mullen JD, Macdonald JB. Timing of wound closure in open fractures based on cultures obtained after debridement. J Bone Joint Surg 2010;92(10):1921-6.

76 Chesser TJS, Cross AM, Ward AJ. The use of pelvic binders in the emergent management of potential pelvic trauma. Injury 2012;43(6):667.

77 Walker J. Pelvic fractures: classification and nursing management. Nurs Stand (Royal College of Nursing (Great Britain): 1987) 2011;26(10):49.

78 Eckroth-Bernard K, Davis JW. Management of pelvic fractures. Curr Opin Crit Care 2010;16(6):582-6. doi: 10.1097/MCC.0b013e3283402869.

79 Roodenburg O, Roodenburg B. Chest trauma. Anaesth Intensive Care Med 2011;12(9):390-2.

80 Kiraly L, Schreiber M. Management of the crushed chest. Crit Care Med 2010;38(9 Suppl):S469-77.

81 Ahmad M, Sante ED, Giannoudis P. Assessment of severity of chest trauma: is there an ideal scoring system? Injury 2010;41(10):981-3.

82 Martínez RJA, Fernández CM, Alarza FH, Serna IM, de Alba AM, Bedoya MZ et al. Evolution and complications of chest trauma. Arch Bronchol (Archivos de Bronconeumología, English Edition). 2013;49(5):177-80.

83 Bernardin B, Troquet JM. Initial management and resuscitation of severe chest trauma. Emerg Med Clin North Am 2012;30(2):377-400.

84 Turkalj I, Stojanović S, Petrović D, Brakus A, Ristić J. Blunt chest trauma: an audit of injuries diagnosed by the MDCT examination. Vojnosanit Pregl 2014;71(2):161-6.

85 Burnside N. Blunt thoracic trauma. Surg 2014;32(5):254-60.

86 Dwivedi S, Gharde P, Bhatt M, Johrapurkar SR. Treating traumatic injuries of the diaphragm. J Emerg Trauma Shock 2010;3(2):173-6.

87 Fontaine EJ. Pneumothorax and insertion of a chest drain. Complications of chest drains. Surgery 2011;29(5):244-6.

88 Boersma WG SJ, Smit HJM. Treatment of haemothorax. Respir Med 2010;104(11):1583-7.

89 Bock JS BR. Blunt cardiac injury. Cardiol Clin 2012;30(4):545-55.

90 Nishijima DK, Simel DL, Wisner DH, Holmes JF. Does this adult patient have a blunt intra-abdominal injury? JAMA 2012;307(14):1517-27.

91 Groven S, Eken T, Skaga NO, Roise O, Naess PA, Gaarder C. Abdominal injuries in a major Scandinavian trauma center: performance assessment over an 8 year period. J Trauma Manag Outcomes 2014;8:9.

92 Prachalias AA. Isolated abdominal trauma: diagnosis and clinical management considerations. Curr Opin Crit Care 2014;20(2):218-25.

93 O'Dowd V, Lowery A, Khan W, Barry K. Seatbelt injury causing small bowel devascularization: case series and review of the literature. Emerg Med Int 2011;2011:675341.

94 Alsayali M, Winnett J, Rahi R, Niggemeyer LE, Kossmann T. Management of blunt bowel and mesenteric injuries: experience at the Alfred Hospital. Eur J Trauma Emerg Surg 2009;35(5):482-8.

95 Bansal V, Tominaga G, Coimbra R. The utility of seat belt signs to predict intra-abdominal injury following motor vehicle crashes. Traffic Injury Prevent 2009;10(6):567-72.

96 American College of Surgeons. Abdominal compartment syndrome: a decade of progress. J Am Coll Surg 2013;216(1):135-46.

97 Kirkpatrick AW, De Waele J, Jaeschke R, Malbrain ML, De Keulenaer B, Duchesne J et al. Intra-abdominal hypertension and the abdominal compartment syndrome: updated consensus definitions and clinical practice guidelines from the World Society of the Abdominal Compartment Syndrome. Intensive Care Med 2013;39:1190-206.

98 Gabbe BJ, Simpson PM, Sutherland AM, Wolfe R, Fitzgerald MC, Judson R et al. Improved functional outcomes for major trauma patients in a regionalized, inclusive trauma system. Ann Surg 2012;255(6):1009-15.

99 Rhodes CM, Smith HL, Sidwell RA. Utility and relevance of diagnostic peritoneal lavage in trauma education. J Surg Educ 2011;68(4):313-7.

100 Whitehouse JS, Weigelt JA. Diagnostic peritoneal lavage: a review of indications, technique, and interpretation. Scand J Trauma Resusc Emerg Med 2009;17:13.

101 Castrillon GA, Soto JA. Multidetector computed tomography of penetrating abdominal trauma. Sem Roentgenol 2012;47(4):371-6.

102 O'Malley E, O'Callaghan A, Coffey JC, Walsh SR. Role of laparoscopy in penetrating abdominal trauma: a systematic review. World J Surg 2012;37(1):113-22.

103 Wallis A, Kelly MD, Jones L. Angiography and embolisation for solid abdominal organ injury in adults: a current perspective. World J Emerg Surg 2010;5:18.

104 Demetriades D. Total management of the open abdomen. Int Wound J 2012;9(Supp 1):17-24.

105 Burlew CC. The open abdomen: practical implications for the practicing surgeon. Am J Surg 2012;204(6):826-35.

106 Langley JM, Dodds L, Fell D, Langley GR. Pneumococcal and influenza immunization in asplenic persons: a retrospective population based cohort study 1990–2002. BMC Infect Dis 2010;10:219.

107 Pasternack MS. Patient information: preventing severe infection after splenectomy (Beyond the Basics), < http://www.uptodate.com/contents/preventing-severe-infection-after-splenectomy-beyond-the-basics>; 2014.

108 Duchesne JC, Kimonis K, Marr AB, Rennie KV, Wahl G et al. Damage control resuscitation in combination with damage control laparotomy: a survival advantage. J Trauma 2010;69(1):46-52.

109 Bezuhly M, Fish JS. Acute burn care. Plast Reconstr Surg 2012;130(2):349e-58e. doi: 10.1097/PRS.0b013e318258d530.

110 Rex S. Burn injuries. Curr Opin Crit Care 2012;18(6):671-6. doi: 10.1097/MCC.0b013e328359fd6e.

111 Australian and New Zealand Burns Association. Early management of severe burns (EMSB). Albany Creek: Australian and New Zealand Burns Association; 2013.

112 Singh S, Handy J. The respiratory insult in burns injury. Curr Anaesth Crit Care 2008;19(5–6):264-8.

113 Asmussen S, Maybauer DM, Fraser JF, Jennings K, George S, Keiralla A et al. Extracorporeal membrane oxygenation in burn and smoke inhalation injury. Burns 2013;39(3):429-35.

114 Cancio LC. Airway management and smoke inhalation injury in the burn patient. Clin Plast Surg 2009;36(4):555-67.

115 Hassan Z, Wong JK, Bush J, Bayat A, Dunn KW. Assessing the severity of inhalation injuries in adults. Burns 2010;36(2):212-6.

116 Edgar D (ed). Burn survivor rehabilitation: principles and guidelines for the allied health professional. Australian and New Zealand Burn Association, <http://www.aci.health.nsw.gov.au/__data/assets/pdf_file/0003/154083/anzba_ahp_guidelines_october_2007.pdf>; 2007 [accessed 04.15].

117 Hawkins A, MacLennan PAP, McGwin GJ, Cross JM, Rue L. The impact of combined trauma and burns on patient mortality. J Trauma-Injury Infect Crit Care 2005;58(2):284-8.

118 Hyllienmark P, Brattstr ÖM, Larsson E, Martling CR, Petersson J, Oldner A. High incidence of post-injury pneumonia in intensive care-treated trauma patients. Acta Anaesthes Scand 2013;57(7):848-54.

119 Yokoe DS, Mermel LA, Anderson DJ, Arias KM, Burstin H, Calfee DP et al. Compendium of strategies to prevent healthcare associated infections. Infect Control Epidemio. 2008;29(Suppl 1):S12-21.

120 Michelet P, Brégeon F, Perrin G, D'Journo XB, Pequignot V, Vig V et al. Early onset pneumonia in severe chest trauma: a risk factor analysis. J Trauma 2010;68(2):395-400.

121 Cavalcanti M, Ferrer R, Morforte R, Garnacho A, Torres A. Risk and prognostic factors of ventilator-associated pneumonia in trauma patients. Crit Care Med 2006;34:4.

122 Munro N, Ruggiero M. Ventilator-associated pneumonia bundle: reconstruction of best care. AACN Adv Crit Care 2014;25(2):163-75.

123 Howard PK, Steinmann RA, Sheehy SB. Sheehy's emergency nursing: Principles and practice. St Louis: Mosby Elsevier; 2010.

124 Kobziff L. Traumatic pelvic fractures. Orthopaed Nurs 2006;25(4):235-41; quiz 42-3.

125 SAM Medical Products. Pelvic Sling II, <http://www.sammedical.com/products/sam-pelvic-sling-ii> [accessed 04.15].

126 Wiss DA, Ovid Technologies I. Fractures. Philadelphia: Lippincott Williams & Wilkins; 2006.

127 Stehan H, Peter D. ABC of burns. Br Med J 2004;328(7452):1366.

128 Sheehy SB, Newberry L. Sheehy's emergency nursing: Principles and practice. St Louis: Mosby; 2003.

129 Richards CE, Mayberry JC. Inital management of the trauma patient. Crit Care Clin 2004;20(1):1-11.

130 Kohn MA, Hammel JM, Bretz SW, Stangby A. Trauma team activation criteria as predictors of patient disposition from the emergency department. Acad Emerg Med 2004;11(1):1-9.

131 Eckert KL. Penetrating and blunt abdominal trauma. Crit Care Nurs Q 2005;28(1):41-59.

132 Olthof DC, van der Vlies CH, Scheerder MJ, de Haan RJ, Breenen LFM, Goslings JC, van Delden OM. Reliability of injury grading systems for patients with blunt splenic trauma. Injury 2014;45(1):146-50.

133 Grunwald TB, Garner WL. Acute burns. Plast Reconstr Surg 2008;121(5): 311e-319e.

Chapter 25

Resuscitation

Trudy Dwyer, Jennifer Dennett, Ian Jacobs

Learning objectives

After reading this chapter, you should be able to:

- identify the benefits of an international approach to resuscitation systems
- discuss the importance of basic life support in the context of advanced life support
- describe the safety precautions of defibrillation
- discuss the principles of therapeutic hypothermia
- discuss indications, actions and routes of administration of medications used in advanced life support
- outline the treatment algorithm for both shockable and non-shockable rhythms
- outline the nurse's role in facilitating family presence during an arrest.

Introduction

The continuum of critical illness for an individual can span the period before and beyond hospital admission. Resuscitation is often required outside the critical care environment. The 'cardiac arrest' team has evolved to use a more proactive, early intervention approach, utilising a range of rapid response systems and instruments to detect deterioration in patients' clinical status (see Chapter 3). It is well recognised that improved outcomes from cardiac arrest are dependent on early recognition and initiation of the 'chain of survival'.[1] This chapter introduces the resuscitation systems and processes in both the pre-hospital and the in-hospital settings. The chain of survival provides a framework for the management of the person experiencing cardiac arrest and resuscitation in specific circumstances. The chapter expands on the final link in the chain, advanced life support, to outline advanced airway management, rhythm recognition, administration of medications and post-resuscitation care. Resuscitation involves many moral and ethical issues, such as family presence during resuscitation, deciding when to cease or initiate resuscitation and near-death experiences (see Chapter 5).

Cardiac arrest

Coronary heart disease (CHD) is the leading cause of death in most industrialised countries, with over half of these being due to sudden cardiac arrest (SCA).[2,3] Despite advances in CHD management, survival outcome figures from SCA remain poor with the survival rate reported to be between 1% and 31% annually.[4] Survival after SCA is dependent on the presenting rhythm, early defibrillation, effective cardiopulmonary resuscitation, early advanced life support and post-resuscitation care.[5,6] Because the presenting rhythm with the majority of witnessed SCAs is ventricular fibrillation (VF), bystander cardiopulmonary resuscitation and early defibrillation are the major interventions influencing outcome after SCA.[2,6,7] The percentage of patients in out-of-hospital cardiac arrest (OHCA) presenting with VF is decreasing with time, possibly secondary to the use of beta-blockers or increased presence of implantable cardioverter-defibrillators.[8]

Incidence/aetiology of cardiac arrests

The prevalence of CHD varies worldwide; thus estimates of the incidence of SCA are difficult to obtain.[9] In Australia, CHD is the leading cause of disease burden (9%) and accounts for 16.5% of all deaths.[10] There are many factors that contribute to cardiac arrest. In adults, the most common cause of cardiac arrest is a primary cardiac event,[11] with coronary artery disease accounting for up to 90% of all victims.[12,13] CHD is the most likely cause of death in those over 35 years of age, compared to non-cardiac causes such as drowning, acute airway obstruction or trauma for people less than 35 years of age.[13]

While causes of cardiac arrest are numerous, most often it is associated with ventricular fibrillation triggered by an acutely ischaemic or infarcted myocardium or primary electrical disturbance.[3] Causes of cardiac arrest may be separated into two categories, primary and secondary, as displayed in Table 25.1.

TABLE 25.1
Causes of cardiac arrest

PRIMARY CAUSES	SECONDARY CAUSES
Acute myocardial infarction	Cessation of breathing
Cardiomyopathy	Airway obstruction
Electrical shock (low- and high-voltage)	Severe bleeding
	Hypothermia
Congenital heart disease (e.g. prolonged Q-T)	Hypoglycemia
	Drug-induced proarrhythmia
Drugs	Metabolic disturbance
	Electrical disturbance
	Trauma
	Neuromuscular disease

Adapted with permission from Konstantopoulou A, Tsikrikas S, Asvestas D, Korantzopoulos P, Letsas KP. Mechanisms of drug-induced proarrhythmia in clinical practice. World J Cardiol 2013;5(6):175.

Acute myocardial infarction is the most common precursor to cardiac arrest. In victims of trauma, drug overdose and drowning, the predominant cause of cardiac arrest is asphyxia. Cardiac arrest in children is less common and even more rarely sudden,[14,15] with the common causes being trauma, congenital heart disease, long QT syndrome, drug overdose, hypoxia and hypothermia. The most common arrhythmia in infants is bradycardia, and the prognosis is especially poor if asystole is present.[14,16] Chest compression should be started if the pulse is less than 60/minute with poor perfusion.[16]

Pathophysiology

In sudden cardiac arrest with cardiac origin, it is believed that myocardial ischaemia leads to ventricular irritability and the progression from ventricular tachycardia (VT) to VF and ultimately asystole.[17] After the onset of VF (in animal studies), carotid arterial blood flow continues for approximately 4 minutes even in the absence of cardiac compressions, as coronary perfusion pressure (the pressure gradient between the aorta and the right atrium) falls over this period.[17] This initial phase is characterised by minimal ischaemic injury, and it is during this time that defibrillation is most likely to result in the restoration of a perfusing rhythm, while initiation of effective cardiac compressions will increase the coronary perfusion pressure.[17]

Progression of the cardiac arrest beyond 4 minutes results in accumulation of toxic metabolites, depletion of high-energy phosphate stores and the initiation of ischaemic cascades.[17] Increasing probability of irreversible cellular injury exists where a cardiac arrest extends for longer than 10 minutes, and the return of a spontaneous circulation during this period may initiate a reperfusion injury[17] (see Chapter 11 for further discussion).

Resuscitation systems and processes

Since the rediscovery of the effectiveness of closed-chest cardiopulmonary resuscitation (CPR) in 1960 and its subsequent widespread adoption, CPR has saved the lives of many, potentially ensuring years of productive life.[18] As CPR quickly became one of the most widely-used and researched procedures, voluntary coordinating bodies developed throughout the world.[13] Organisations such as the European Resuscitation Council (ERC), the American Heart Association (AHA), the New Zealand Resuscitation Council (NZRC), the Heart and Stroke Foundation of Canada, the Resuscitation Council of Southern Africa and the Australian Resuscitation Council (ARC) established practice guidelines to improve standards in resuscitation, and coordinated resuscitation activities on a national basis.[19] However, as standardised recording of outcome data did not exist, resuscitation endeavours could not be compared meaningfully between countries.[19] Consequently, the International Liaison Committee on Resuscitation (ILCOR) was formed in 1992 to promote global discussion and consistency of guidelines between these international resuscitation councils.[19] The AHA, ARC, NZRC, ERC and ILCOR guidelines are subject to constant review and modification based on emerging scientific data. Guidelines and recommendations are classified according to scientific evidence. The most recent substantive guidelines from ILCOR were published in October 2010[20] and further revision will be published in 2015 but were not available at the time of publication.

Survival of arrests

Despite recent advances in resuscitation and technology, the survival rate for OHCA to hospital discharge remains low at about 6.7–8.4%.[2,3] Factors associated with higher rates of mortality for adults are: age over 80 years, unwitnessed arrest, delays before commencing CPR, delayed defibrillation (pre-shock pauses) and delays prior to resumption of CPR (post-shock pauses) and non-ventricular tachycardia/fibrillation rhythm.[21] The outcome statistics for children after OHCA are similarly poor.[14] Marked differences in the inclusion criteria and outcome definitions may, however, also explain the wide variations in survival rates from cardiac arrests. In recognition of these variations, the Utstein guidelines were developed and implemented to consistently document, monitor and compare out-of-hospital cardiac arrests. These guidelines:

- establish uniform terms and definitions for out-of-hospital resuscitation
- establish a reporting template for resuscitation studies to ensure comparability
- define time points and time intervals relating to cardiac resuscitation
- define clinical items and outcomes that emergency medical systems should gather
- develop methods for describing resuscitation systems.

In-hospital resuscitation has survival to hospital discharge rates of around 18–25%.[22–24] The majority of cardiac arrests occur on the general wards where patients are not monitored and the predominant presenting rhythms are VF/VT (16.9%) and asystole/pulseless electrical activity (PEA) (72.3%).[23] Many factors such as age, time of day, presence or absence of morbidity before or during the hospital admission, absence of 'not-for-resuscitation' orders, quality of the CPR, asystole and non-ICU location contribute to the low in-hospital survival rates.[25,26]

Chain of survival

To optimise a person's chance of survival, the 'chain of survival' strategy has been developed,[27] which represents a sequence of four events that must occur as quickly as possible: early recognition, early CPR, early defibrillation and post-resuscitation care (see Figure 25.1). These time-sensitive, sequential actions must occur to optimise a cardiac arrest victim's chances of survival. Communities with integrated links along this chain have demonstrated higher survival rates after OHCA than those with deficiencies in these links.[2,26]

Early recognition of cardiac arrest

The chain of survival begins with early recognition of a medical emergency and the activation of a rapid response system.[2,28] However, the chain of survival has not always been adequate when a cardiac arrest occurs in the hospital, from the point of view of early recognition, timeliness or availability of equipment or staff.[25,29] Two-thirds of in-hospital cardiac arrests are potentially avoidable, with up to 84% of all in-hospital cardiac arrests demonstrating evidence of deterioration in the 6–8 hours preceding the arrest.[30,31] In recent years early warning systems, based on abnormal vital signs, have been implemented to facilitate the early recognition of the deteriorating patient (see Table 25.2)[32–36] (see Chapter 3 for further discussion). While the best early warning scoring system continues to be debated, in the United Kingdom the National Early Warning Score (NEWS) shows promise with the early identification of patients at risk of unexpected ICU admission or cardiac arrest.[37] To further facilitate

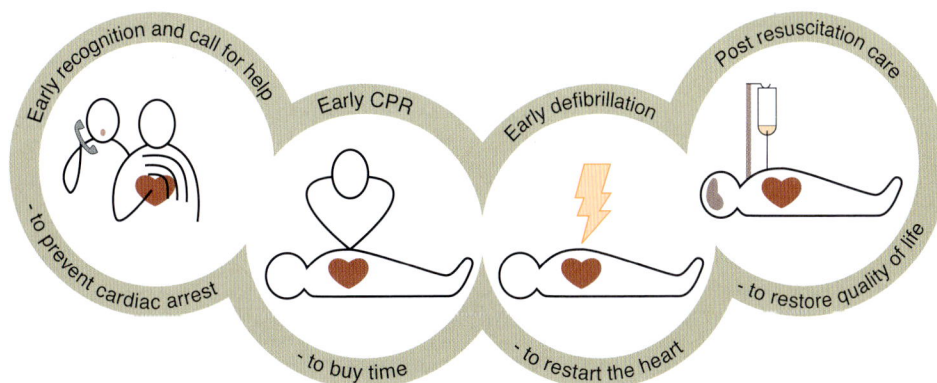

FIGURE 25.1 Chain of survival.

Courtesy of Laerdal.

TABLE 25.2

Early calling criteria

AREA	ADULTS	CHILDREN	
		0–12 MONTHS	**1–8 YEARS**
Airway	Threatened	Threatened	Threatened
Breathing	All respiratory arrests RR <8 RR >27 SpO$_2$ <90%	All respiratory arrests RR <20 RR >50 Grunting respirations SpO$_2$ <90%	All respiratory arrests RR <15 RR >35 SpO$_2$ <90%
Circulation	All cardiac arrests PR <50 PR >130 Systolic BP <90	All cardiac arrests PR <100 PR >180 Systolic BP <50 Capillary return >4 seconds Marked pallor	All cardiac arrests PR <90 PR >160 Systolic BP <80
Neurology	Sudden fall in the level of consciousness (fall in the Glasgow Coma Scale score of ≥2 points) Repeated or prolonged seizures	Floppy Unresponsive Depressed conscious level Prolonged seizures	Floppy Unresponsive Depressed conscious level Prolonged seizures
Other	Any patient you are seriously worried about who does not fit the above criteria		

Note: these values are a guide and vary with different organisations.

BP = blood pressure; PR = pulse rate; RR = respiratory rate.

Adapted from:

Prytherch DR, Smith GB, Schmidt PE, Featherstone PI. ViEWS – Towards a national early warning score for detecting adult inpatient deterioration. Resuscitation 2010;81(8):932–7

Smith GB, Prytherch DR, Meredith P, Schmidt PE, Featherstone PI. The ability of the National Early Warning Score (NEWS) to discriminate patients at risk of early cardiac arrest, unanticipated intensive care unit admission, and death. Resuscitation 2013;84(4):465–70.

earlier activation of the rapid response teams, family and patients have been provided with a means to activate the team on a patient's behalf.[38]

Basic life support

When a patient is identified as in potential or actual arrest, a primary and secondary survey should be conducted in the DRSABCD sequence:[39]

- **D**anger – check for danger (hazards or risks to safety).
- **R**esponsive – check for response (if responsive/ unconscious).
- **S**end – send for help.
- **A**irway – open the airway. Airway assessment is undertaken to establish a patent airway while maintaining cervical spine support (if injury is suspected).
- **B**reathing – check breathing. Breathing includes the assessment and establishment of breathing, noting rate, pattern, chest movement and tissue oxygenation.
- **C**PR – start CPR. Give 30 chest compressions (almost 2 compressions/second) followed by 2 breaths.
- **D**efibrillation – attach an automated external defibrillator as soon as available and follow its prompts.

Continue CPR until responsiveness and normal breathing return. Ideally, these interventions are performed simultaneously or in rapid sequence and will take no longer than 60–90 seconds to complete. This systematic approach correlates closely with the principles of basic life support (BLS) in that, where a life-threatening abnormality is detected, immediate intervention is required before further assessment (see Figure 25.2).

Airway

Recognition of airway obstruction includes listening for inspiratory (stridor), expiratory or grunting noises. The work of breathing can be assessed by the respiratory rate, intercostals, subcostal or sternal recession, use of accessory muscles, tracheal tug or flaring of the alae nasi. Nasal flaring is especially evident in infants with respiratory distress. Noisy breathing is obstructed breathing, but the volume of the noise is not an indicator of the severity of respiratory failure. Should obstruction to air flow be detected, then the airway should be opened using three manoeuvres: the head-tilt, chin-lift and jaw thrust. Assess a person's airway without turning them onto the side unless the airway is obstructed with fluid (vomit or blood) or submersion injuries.[39]

FIGURE 25.2   Basic life support flow chart.[1]

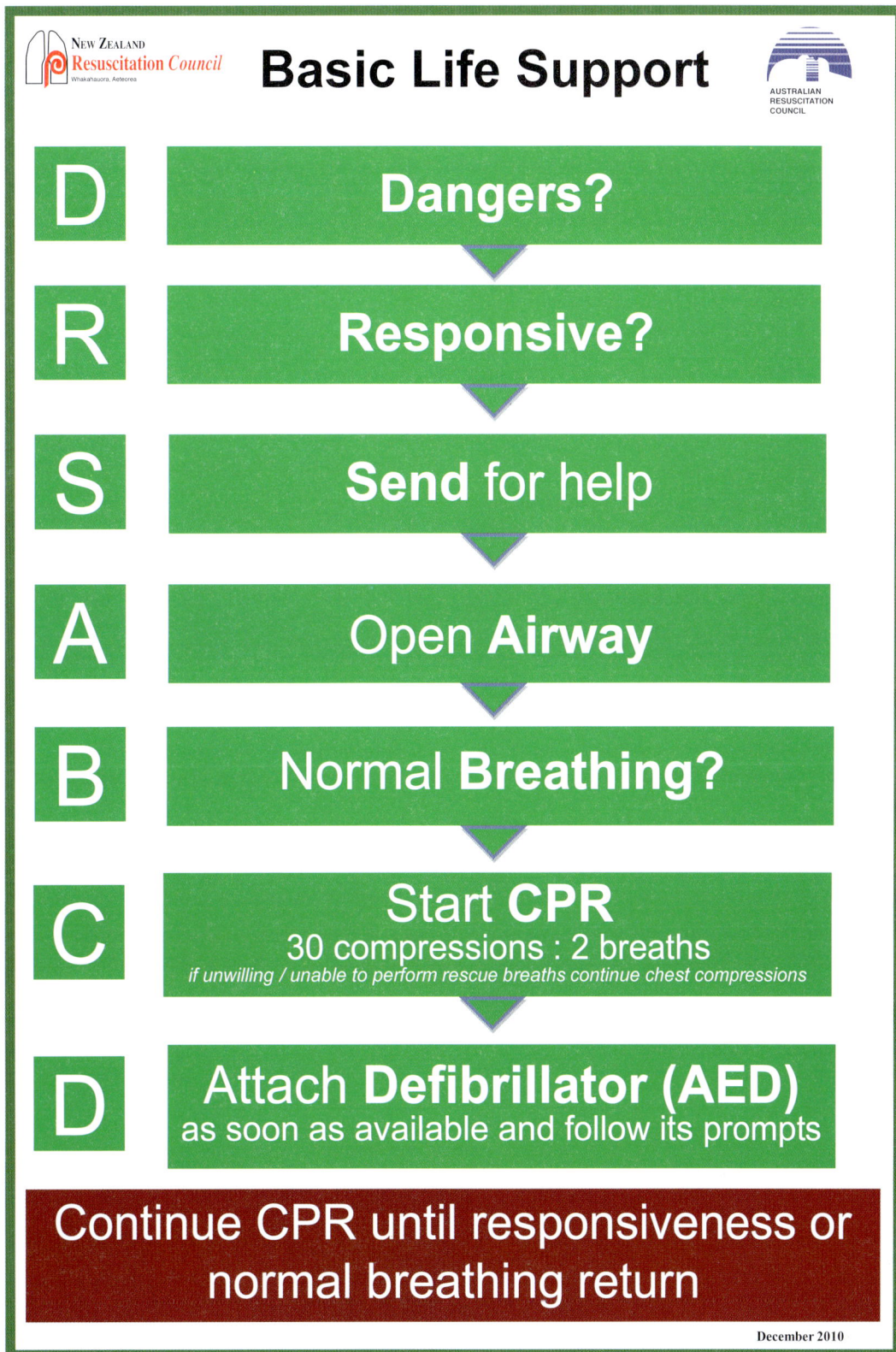

Australian resuscitation flow chart reproduced with permission.

The airway of the infant differs from that of the older child or adult in that the infant has a large head and tongue and small mouth, and the larynx is narrower, shorter, more anterior and acutely angled.[17] The airway of an infant is also more cartilaginous and can be easily occluded when the neck is hyperextended; in addition, the large tongue can easily fall back to obstruct the pharynx.[40] Hence, the head of an infant should be maintained in the neutral position, whereas a child aged 1–8 years will require the 'sniffing position', with varying degrees according to age. The chin-lift and head-tilt manoeuvres may be used in children to obtain the appropriate positioning for age. Jaw thrust may be used if head-tilt/chin-lift is contra-indicated.[40] Do not use the finger sweep to clear the airway of an infant, as this may result in damage to the delicate palatal tissues and cause bleeding, which can worsen the situation. Use of finger sweep can force foreign bodies further down into the airway.[40] Suction is more useful for removing vomitus and secretions.

Practice tip

An infant will only require 5 to 8 cc/kg with each ventilation.[126]

Reproduced with permission from Yost CC, Bloom R. Neonatal resuscitation. Crit Care Obstetr 2010:108.

Breathing

To assess for the presence of breathing, look, listen and feel for breath sounds for no more than 10 seconds. If the person is unresponsive with absent or abnormal breathing, call for help and compressions should be commenced immediately. Agonal gasps are not to be considered as normal breathing. Typically, the arterial blood will remain saturated with oxygen for several minutes following the cardiac arrest and, as cerebral and myocardial cell oxygenation is limited more by the absence of cardiac output as opposed to the reduced PaO_2, effective compressions are more important than rescue breaths.[27]

Cardiopulmonary resuscitation

Individuals should commence cardiac compressions if the victim is unconscious, unresponsive, not moving and not breathing normally. Where possible, change the person delivering the compressions every 2 minutes. Pulse check by lay rescuers and health professionals in BLS is not recommended. Assessment of effective chest compression by healthcare professionals may be made by continuous end tidal CO_2 ($ETCO_2$) monitoring. For CPR to be effective the patient should be flat, supine and on a firm surface. The chest should be compressed in the midline over the lower half of the sternum, which equates to the 'centre of the chest', at a depth of 5–6 cm (in adults) and at a rate of 100–120 compressions per minute for adults, infants and children, with the rate rising to 120/min for the newborn.[27] CPR should be initiated when the heart rate is 60 beats/min for the neonate, infant and the small child and 40 beats/min for the large child. Performed correctly, external cardiac compressions (ECC) can produce a systolic blood pressure peak of 60–80 mmHg (in adults) and a cardiac output of 20–30% of normal.[27,41] With external chest compressions it takes time to reach optimal levels of coronary perfusion pressure and, ultimately, blood flow. Any interruption to chest compressions therefore decreases the coronary perfusion pressure and resultant blood flow, ultimately reducing survival.[42] After 30 compressions open the airway and give two breaths.[43]

Survival potentially improves when an individual receives a higher number of chest compressions during CPR, even if the person receives fewer ventilations. Because of this, it is recommended that a 30:2 compression-to-ventilation ratio is used in adults, children and infants regardless of the number of rescuers, and 3:1 for neonates. Having noted this, in the advanced life support paediatric setting, the compression ratio changes to 15:2 and a ratio of 3:1 for the newborn with any number of rescuers (see Table 25.3). The average person may not only be reluctant to initiate mouth-to-mouth resuscitation,[44] but will also take 8 seconds to deliver one

---

TABLE 25.3

CPR for adults, children and infants

AGE	AIRWAY	COMPRESSION (CPR)	1 OR 2 PERSON
Infants <1 year	Jaw support or chin-lift (no head-tilt)	Two fingers or two overlying thumbs on the lower end of the sternum with hands encircling the chest (preferred), 100 beats/min	30:2 PALS 15:2 (2 rescuers)
Younger child: 1–8 years	Head-tilt more than infants but less than adults	Heel of one hand, 100 beats/min	30:2 PALS 15:2 (2 rescuers)
Older child: 9–14 years	Head-tilt	Two hands, 100 beats/min	30:2 PALS 15:2 (2 rescuers)
Adult	Head-tilt	Two hands, 100–120 beats/min	30:2

PALS = paediatric advanced life support.

Adapted with permission from Australian Resuscitation Council and New Zealand Resuscitation Council (ARC and NZRC). Australian Resuscitation Council Guidelines. Victoria, Australia: Australian Resuscitation Council, <http://www.resus.org.au>; 2014.

breath.[45] When a rescuer is reluctant to perform rescue breaths, external cardiac compression (ECC) without expired air resuscitation (EAR) should be encouraged, as the generally held belief is that ECC alone is better than no CPR at all.[46,47]

Evaluation during resuscitation

Maintenance of an effective cardiac output during CPR is evaluated by palpating the carotid or femoral pulse in adults (brachial in children); this was once the 'gold standard' for assessing circulation. However, neither lay-persons nor professionals can rapidly (in less than 10 s) and accurately perform this step. Pulse checks are not recommended for evaluation after defibrillation until 2 minutes of CPR have been performed, regardless of the rhythm post defibrillation.

The use of capnometry as a non-invasive technique for monitoring the effectiveness of CPR is recommended.[12] As the partial pressure of the $ETCO_2$ concentration correlates with pulmonary blood flow during CPR, the adequacy of resuscitation efforts is evaluated by measuring this parameter. $ETCO_2$ also correlates with cardiac output, return of spontaneous circulation (ROSC) and outcomes in cardiac arrest.[48,49] A mean $ETCO_2$ of 20 mmHg or above has been associated with survival from cardiac arrest, while a mean $ETCO_2$ <10 mmHg is associated with poor outcomes.[49] A rise in $ETCO_2$ during CPR may indicate the return of spontaneous circulation.[50] Having noted this, hyperventilation during CPR is not recommended and may be harmful. Near infrared spectroscopy can be used to measure regional cerebral oxygen saturation. A higher mean somatic tissue oxygenation (sSO_2) is associated with higher ROSC.[49] Similarly, animal studies indicate that hyperventilation is associated with raised thoracic pressure, decreased coronary and cerebral perfusion and reduced return of spontaneous circulation. Clinical studies show that rescuers consistently hyperventilate patients during a cardiac arrest.[51]

Devices to augment compression

As external cardiac compression supplies only 30% of normal cardiac output[52] and 15% of normal cerebral blood flow, there is a great need to find ways to improve cardiac compression. While no circulatory adjunct is currently recommended, several are being routinely used in the pre- and in-hospital settings.[53] A few of the devices are outlined in Table 25.4.

Given the limited available information on the outcomes associated with use of any of these devices and the absence of evidence to demonstrate these devices are superior to conventional manual CPR, no device is currently recommended as a routine substitute for manual CPR.[20,54,55] There is, however, a growing incidence of the use of some of these devices in the pre-hospital environment and in situations where it is difficult to provide high-quality compressions such as during transport, prolonged cardiac arrests and cardiac catheter laborites.[55] These devices should be used in a properly supervised program and the users should be well trained.[39,53]

Practice tip

CPR should commence if the patient is unconscious, unresponsive, not moving and not breathing, even if the patient is taking the occasional gasp.

Reproduced with permission from Australian Resuscitation Council and New Zealand Resuscitation Council (ARC and NZRC). Australian Resuscitation Council Guidelines. Victoria, Australia: Australian Resuscitation Council; 2014. Available from: http://www.resus.org.au/.

Defibrillation

While CPR has been associated with improved survival to discharge from hospital, it cannot be substituted for the definitive treatment of early defibrillation. It is thought that CPR will supply sufficient oxygen to the brain and heart until defibrillation is available. Ultimately, despite

---

TABLE 25.4
Augment compression devices[54,127,128]

DEVICE	DESCRIPTION
Active compression–decompression (ACD-CPR)	• Utilises a small portable device to compress and decompress the chest ('plunger method') • Enhances ventilation and venous return by raising the negative intrathoracic pressure, which facilitates venous return, thus priming the heart for subsequent compressions[127]
Interposed abdominal compression (IAC) combined with CPR (IAC-CPR)	• Least technical device • The abdomen is compressed (midway between the xiphisternum and the umbilicus) alternately with the rhythm of chest compression • Rarely utilised method • Results in increased resistance in the descending aorta, thus raising the coronary perfusion pressure[128]
Non-invasive automated chest compression device (e.g. AutoPulse)	• Utilises a load-distributing band (LDB) to compress the anterior chest • The device is built around a backboard that contains a motor[54] • The motor tightens or loosens LDB around the patient's chest

the most effective CPR, the single-most important cause of decreased prognosis in pulseless VT/VF cardiac arrests is a delay in electrical defibrillation.[3]

Precordial thump

A precordial thump is a single, sharp blow delivered with a clenched fist to the mid-sternum of a victim's chest from a height of 25–30 cm above the sternum.[7] The mechanical energy generated by the precordial thump may generate a few joules, and therefore is applied within the first few seconds of onset of a shockable rhythm, but it has a very low success rate at converting VF/VT to a perfusing rhythm.[56,57] Because of the very low success rate and the brief period for application, delivery of the thump must not delay accessing help or a defibrillator. Only in situations where the VF arrest is witnessed and monitored and a defibrillator is not immediately on hand (i.e. critical care environments) would the delivery of the precordial thump be appropriate.[20]

Electrical defibrillation

Defibrillation is the passage of a current of electricity through a fibrillating heart to simultaneously depolarise the mass of myocardial cells and allow them to repolarise uniformly to an organised electrical activity.[12]

Practice tip

Effective BLS can slow the loss of amplitude and waveform of VF. Interruptions to effective CPR should be kept to a minimum.

Reproduced with permission from Deakin CD, Nolan JP, Soar J, Sunde K, Koster RW, Smith GB et al. European Resuscitation Council Guidelines for Resuscitation 2010 Section 4. Adult advanced life support. Resuscitation 2010;81(10):1305–52.

There are two types of external defibrillators: the manual external defibrillator and the automatic external defibrillator (AED). The AED can be either fully automatic or semiautomatic. The manual defibrillator requires the user to be able to immediately and accurately recognise arrhythmias and make the decision whether to initiate defibrillation or not. In comparison, the AED automatically detects and interprets the rhythm without relying on the user's recognition of arrhythmias. AEDs can be operated in both manual and semiautomatic mode. When using an AED, the user determines whether the person is unresponsive, not breathing and pulseless.[58] After checking for a pulse, the AED requires only four steps to operate: 1) turn power on; 2) place self-adhesive electrodes on a victim's chest; 3) rhythm analysis follows (hands-off period); 4) then (if advised by the machine) press the shock button. The AED will automatically interpret the cardiac rhythm and, if VF/VT is present, will advise the operator to provide a shock. This 'hands-off' period using the AED may result in significant interruptions to chest compressions and adversely impact patient survival. Health professionals with expertise in rhythm

recognition may reduce the 'hands-off' period using a manual defibrillator.[59,60] The combined pre-shock and the post-shock pause ideally should be less than 5 seconds.[12] This can be achieved by continuing compressions while the defibrillator is charging and resuming chest compressions immediately after the delivery of the shock. Fully automatic defibrillators are programmed to assess the rhythm, charge the defibrillator and deliver shocks without user intervention.

To facilitate early defibrillation, ILCOR endorses the concept of non-medical individuals being authorised, educated and encouraged to use defibrillators.[12] This public access to early defibrillation has seen the placement of defibrillators on aircraft, in casinos and cricket grounds, with non-medical personnel such as police, flight attendants, security guards, family members and even children successfully initiating early defibrillation.[60] The effectiveness of training non-traditional out-of-hospital first responders to use the AED has improved survival to discharge rates.[20] Similarly, in-hospital cardiac arrests also occur in any area, and all healthcare workers should be capable of initiating early defibrillation.[12] The ARC notes that, while BLS does not have to include the use of adjunctive equipment, the use of AEDs by persons with education in their use is supported and should be taught. Figure 25.3 outlines the integration of defibrillation with BLS.

Practice tip

When using the defibrillator in manual mode, limiting the pre-shock analysis pause to 5 seconds should improve survival.

For 90% of people in VF, return of a perfusing rhythm will occur after a single shock.

However, it is rare that a pulse will be palpable with the perfusing rhythm; hence the immediate resumption of chest compressions in the post-shock period is supported.[12] Failure to successfully convert VF after the single-shock strategy may indicate the need for a period of effective CPR (30:2) for 2 minutes and rhythm re-analysis, followed by shock if indicated.[12] A single-shock strategy is now recommended for all patients in cardiac arrest requiring defibrillation for VF or pulseless VT.[39] Not all of the electrical energy delivered during defibrillation will traverse the myocardium. Table 25.5 outlines some of the common factors contributing to the success or failure of defibrillation. Studies have demonstrated that lower-energy biphasic defibrillators are associated with greater first-shock efficacy, require lower joules, cause less myocardial dysfunction and increase return of spontaneous circulation when compared with the monophasic defibrillator.[61,62] The optimum defibrillation energy level is that which sufficiently abolishes the arrhythmia to enable the return of an organised rhythm, with minimal myocardial damage.[12,61] Other biphasic energy levels may be used providing there is relevant clinical data for

FIGURE 25.3 Advanced life support flow chart.[1]

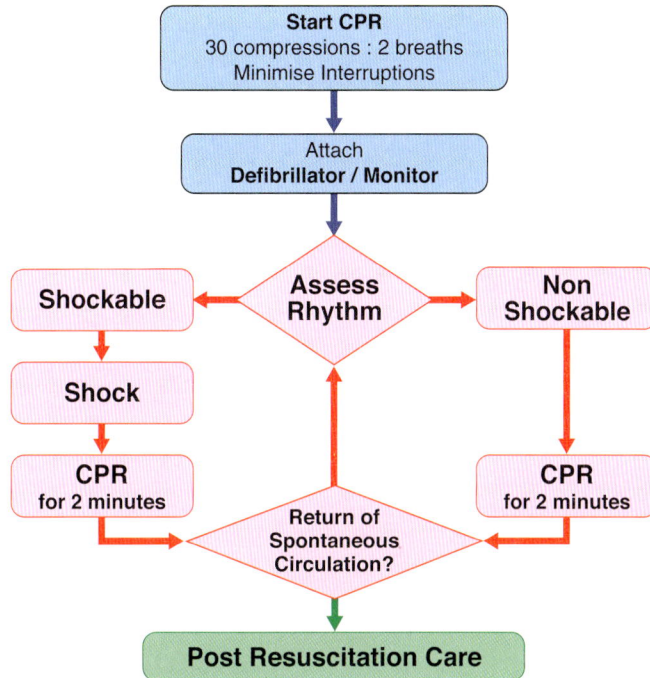

Australian resuscitation flow chart reproduced with permission.

TABLE 25.5

Factors contributing to the success or failure of defibrillation[129-132]

SUCCESS	FAILURE	PRECAUTIONS
• VF duration • Early defibrillation (if VF <3 min) • Initial CPR (if VF >3 min) • Presenting rhythm (VT/VF) • Paddle/pad size and placement • Use of self-adhesive pads	• Inadequate contact with the chest (excessive chest hair) • Faulty positioning of the paddles • Synchronise button in the 'on' position, flat battery or fractured lead • Positioning over bone/fat or breast tissue, chest size • Drying out of gel conduction pads • Patient factors: acidosis, hypoxia, electrolyte imbalance, drug toxicity, hypothermia • Time of respiration (best delivered at end-expiration) • PEEP and auto-PEEP (air-trapping) should be minimised • Paddles/electrodes too small (8–12 cm electrodes for adults)	• Place defibrillation electrodes at least 8 cm away from ECG electrodes, or implantable medical devices, pacemakers, vascular access devices • Remove medication patches, wipe the area before applying defibrillation electrodes • Do not defibrillate unless all clear of the bed/patient • Do not charge/discharge paddles in the air • Do not have the patient in contact with metal • Do not allow oxygen to flow onto the patient during delivery of the shock (at least 1 m from the patient) • Ensure the chest is dry • Do not use electrode gels and pastes as these can spread between the paddles and potentially spark

ECG = electrocardiogram; PEEP = peak end-expiratory pressure; VF = ventricular fibrillation; VT = ventricular tachycardia.

Developed from:

Ristagno G, Li Y, Gullo A, Bisera J. Amplitude spectrum area as a predictor of successful defibrillation. In: Anaesthesia and Pharmacology of Intensive Care Emergency Medicine APICE: Springer; 2011, pp 141–60

Monteleone PP, Borek HA, Althoff SO. Electrical therapies in cardiac arrest. Emerg Med Clin North Am 2012;30(1):51–63

Link MS, Atkins DL, Passman RS, Halperin HR, Samson RA, White RD et al. Part 6: Electrical therapies automated external defibrillators, defibrillation, cardioversion, and pacing: 2010 American Heart Association Guidelines for Cardiopulmonary Resuscitation and Emergency Cardiovascular Care. Circulation 2010;122(18 suppl 3):S706–19

Morley P. Cardiopulmonary resuscitation. In: Harley I, Hore P, eds. Anaesthesia: An introduction. 5th ed. East Hawthorn, Victoria: IP Communications; 2012, pp 174–89.

a specific defibrillator that suggests that an alternative energy level provides adequate shock success.[1,63] If the initial shock is unsuccessful, subsequent shocks should be delivered at the initial dose or higher energy levels may be selected.[12,62] In children, it is recommended 4 J/kg for the initial and subsequent shocks for both biphasic and monophasic defibrillators.[12] Standard adult AEDs and pads are suitable for use in children older than 8 years. Ideally, for children between 1 and 8 years, paediatric pads and an AED with paediatric capability should be used.[1,64] These pads are placed as per the adult methodology. If the AED does not have a paediatric mode or paediatric pads, the standard adult AED and pads can be used.[25] Defibrillation of infants less than 1 year of age is not recommended.[12]

The importance of early, uninterrupted chest compressions and early defibrillation are well promulgated in the ILCOR guidelines.[12] As the length of time from collapse is difficult to accurately estimate, it is imperative rescuers perform chest compressions until the defibrillator is both available and charged.[65,66]

Advanced life support

Basic life support provides about 20–30% of normal cardiac output and a fraction of inspired oxygen (FiO_2) of 0.1–0.16. Consequently, a significant number of patients rely on the provision of advanced life support (ALS) for survival. ALS extends BLS to provide the knowledge and skills essential for the initiation of early treatment and stabilisation of people post-cardiac arrest. Advanced skills traditionally include defibrillation, advanced airway management and the administration of resuscitation drugs. While BLS is generally initiated prior to ALS, where a defibrillator and a person trained in its use are available, defibrillation takes precedence over BLS and ALS. The ARC and NZRC algorithm for management of cardio-pulmonary arrest (see Figures 25.3 and 25.4) outlines the two decision paths of therapy in ALS: 1) defibrillation and CPR for pulseless VT/VF (shockable) and 2) identifying and treating the underlying cause for non-VT/VF (non-shockable).

Advanced airway management

A person with signs of acute respiratory distress should be administered oxygen at the highest possible concentration, including initially during CPR.[43] Oxygen should never be withheld for fear of adverse effects, as rescue breaths provide an inspired oxygen concentration of only 15–18%. The administration of oxygen alone does

FIGURE 25.4   Advanced life support for infants and children flow chart.[1]

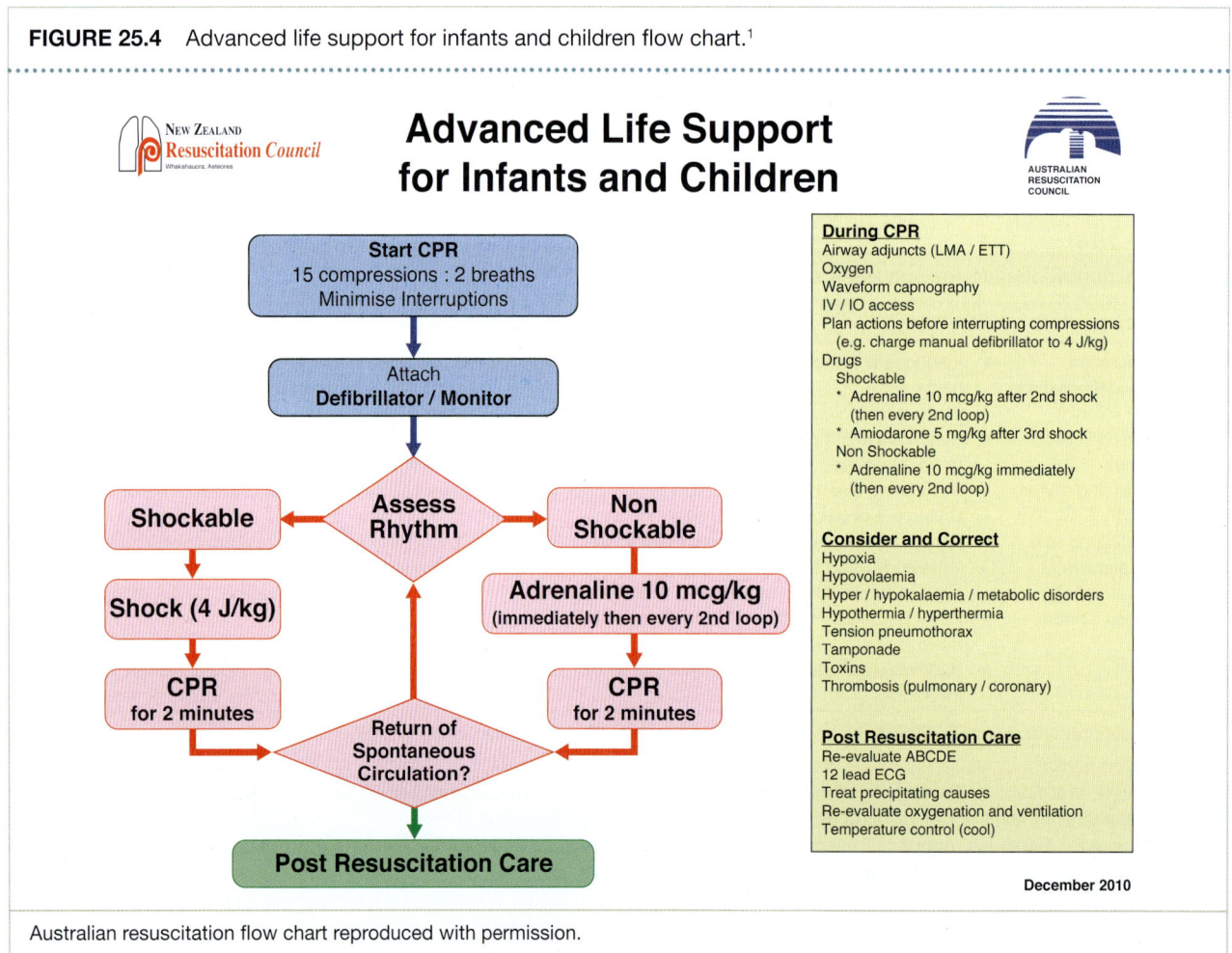

Australian resuscitation flow chart reproduced with permission.

not result in adequate ventilation and, as such, the establishment of an effective airway is paramount. Airway management is essential in the performance of CPR, and may be administered using a variety of techniques. These may include: compression-only CPR with high-flow oxygen by face-mask, bag-mask ventilation, insertion of a supraglottic airway (SGA) device that does not require laryngoscopy or tracheal intubation.[67]

The choice of advanced airway adjunct is determined by the availability of equipment and experienced personnel[67] (see Table 25.6 and Chapter 15):

- oropharyngeal (Guedel's) airway
- nasopharyngeal airway
- laryngeal mask airway
- oesophageal–tracheal combitube laryngeal tube (King airway)
- endotracheal intubation
- tracheostomy.

While the endotracheal tube (ETT) is considered the 'gold standard' for airway management in a cardiac arrest, as it protects the airway, assists effective ventilation, ensures delivery of high concentrations of oxygen and eases suctioning, no studies have found that ETT use during a cardiac arrest increases survival. It is vital that CPR not be interrupted for more than 10 seconds during attempts

TABLE 25.6

Adjuncts used during resuscitation[1,12,133–135]

AIRWAY TYPE	DESCRIPTION	PRACTICE CONSIDERATIONS
Oropharyngeal (Guedel's) airway	Conforms to the curve of the palate, moving the tongue forward away from the posterior pharyngeal wall Sizes from 000–5	Incorrect size or placement may contribute to airway obstruction by pushing the tongue back into the pharynx. Unlike adult insertion, the insertion of the oropharyngeal airway in infants and young children is inserted right-way-up; a tongue depressor or laryngoscope should be used to aid insertion
Nasopharyngeal airway	Soft tube inserted into the nasopharynx	Use with caution in patients with head injuries With the exception of infant's head-tilt, jaw support or jaw thrust is still necessary when using either the oropharyngeal or the nasopharyngeal airway
Bag–valve–mask (BVM) systems	A self-inflating bag that may be connected to a face mask, laryngeal mask airway or endotracheal tube (ETT)	BVMs are often inappropriately used and offer no protection to the airway Two-person technique is preferable Single-person BVM ventilation may result in a poor seal around the patient's mouth and the delivery of less than optimal tidal volumes[12] When using a BVM it is best performed using two rescuers, although not always possible As the airway is not protected, smaller tidal volumes with supplementary oxygen can provide adequate oxygenation and reduce the risk of gastric inflation, regurgitation and aspiration The mask should be used right-way-up with children and upside-down with infants The soft circular mask is preferred for infants, as it provides an excellent seal with low dead space
Laryngeal mask airway (LMA)	Consists of a tube with an elliptical cuff fitted at the distal end that inflates in the hypopharynx around the posterior perimeter of the larynx The LMA is inserted orally using a blind technique so that the distal end of the mask abuts against the base of the hypopharynx, behind the cricoid cartilage, and the cuff is inflated to form an airtight seal around the larynx	The LMA is used as a first-line adjunct when endotracheal intubation is not available The LMA is easier to insert than a Combitube, more rapidly inserted and requires less equipment than the ETT When used as a first-line airway device, the LMA provides a clear airway with a significantly lower risk of gastric overinflation and regurgitation than the BVM[12] As with adults, the LMA can be used safely and effectively in infants[133] LMA: size 1 for <5 kg; size 1.5, 5–10 kg; size 2, 10–20 kg; size 2.5, 20–30 kg; size 4, 50–70 kg; size 5, 70–100 kg; size 6, >100 kg Use in newborns over 34 weeks gestation and weighing more than 2 kg[133] Complications of LMA include gastric aspiration, partial airway obstruction, coughing or gastric insufflation Contraindications include patients unable to open their mouths adequately; pharyngeal pathology; airway obstruction at or below level of the larynx; low pulmonary compliance or high airway resistance; or increased risk of aspiration

TABLE 25.6 *continued*

AIRWAY TYPE	DESCRIPTION	PRACTICE CONSIDERATIONS
Oesophageal–tracheal Combitube (ETC)	The ETC is a double-lumen airway with proximal and distal cuffs that is passed into the oesophagus	It is effective in maintaining an airway when performed by unskilled personnel and is a suitable alternative to tracheal intubation The ETC enables ventilation, whether it is positioned in the oesophagus or the trachea Only one size needed for most adults
Laryngeal tube (LT)	Airway tube with a small oesophageal cuff and a larger pharyngeal cuff. The distal tip is positioned in the upper oesophagus	Use is comparable to classic LMA and ProSeal LMA[134]
I-gel	The cuff of the I-gel is made of gel and does not require inflation	Very easy to insert with minimal training.[12] Enables continuous chest compression without interruption for ventilation[135]
Endotracheal tube (ETT)	During intubation, direct application of firm pressure to the cricoid cartilage is required to compress the oesophagus between the trachea and vertebral column and minimise/prevent regurgitation of gastric contents	Endotracheal intubation is a difficult skill to acquire and maintain In addition to routine clinical methods, ETT placement can be confirmed by either measurement of ETCO$_2$ or use of an oesophageal detector; the latter is more reliable in a non-perfusing rhythm (Class IIb) Immediate complications associated with intubation include oesophageal intubation; right main bronchi intubation; or ETT occlusion (kinking, sputum, cuff, blood)

Developed from:

Australian Resuscitation Council and New Zealand Resuscitation Council (ARC and NZRC). Australian Resuscitation Council Guidelines. Victoria, Australia: Australian Resuscitation Council, <http://www.resus.org.au>; 2014.

Deakin CD, Nolan JP, Soar J, Sunde K, Koster RW, Smith GB et al. European Resuscitation Council Guidelines for Resuscitation 2010 Section 4. Adult advanced life support. Resuscitation 2010;81(10):1305–52

Zhu X-Y, Lin B-C, Zhang Q-S, Ye H-M, Yu R-J. A prospective evaluation of the efficacy of the laryngeal mask airway during neonatal resuscitation. Resuscitation 2011;82(11):1405–9.

Yamaga S, Une K, Kyo M, Suzuki K, Kobayashi Y, Nakagawa I et al. Gas insufflation in the stomach during cardiopulmonary resuscitation using laryngeal tube ventilation in comparison with bag-valve-mask ventilation. Circulation 2012;126(21 Supplement):A295.

Soar J. Which airway for cardiac arrest? Do supraglottic airways devices have a role? Resuscitation 2013;84(9):1163–4.

at endotracheal intubation. Waveform capnography or an oesophageal detector device should be applied to confirm the ETT placement.[12,67]

ETCO$_2$ may also be used to monitor the quality of the CPR. Given the limitations noted in Table 25.6, a variety of adjunct airway/ventilation management devices are available, such as: bag–mask ventilation (BMV); supraglottic airways devices such as the laryngeal mask airway (LMA) and the classic laryngeal mask airway; the oesophageal-tracheal airway (Combitube); and the I-gel. The benefit of the supraglottic airways devices is that they are easily inserted without interruption to chest compressions. Currently, there is no evidence to support the routine use of any particular advanced adjunct airway devices.[67] Healthcare professionals trained to use supraglottic airway devices (e.g. LMA) may consider their use for airway management during cardiac arrest and as a backup or rescue airway in a difficult or failed tracheal intubation.

Once an airway has been established, continue chest compressions without interruption for ventilation. Ventilate the lungs at a rate of approximately 10 breaths a minute and an inspiratory time of 1 second with sufficient volume to produce a normal chest rise. Ventilation adjuncts may include:

- a simple face mask with filter and oxygen connector (pre-intubation)
- bag–valve–mask systems
- ventilators.

If available, automated ventilators can be used. These may be set to deliver a tidal volume of 6–7 mL/kg at a rate of 10 breaths/min. The automated ventilator may be used with either the face mask or other adjunct airway devices.[16] Having noted this, there is currently no evidence to suggest that the use of automated ventilators during cardiac arrest is more beneficial than bag–valve–mask devices.[16]

Rhythms

There is an association between the initial cardiac arrhythmias and survival to discharge after SCA. Cardiac arrest rhythms can be divided into two subsets:

1 ventricular fibrillation and pulseless ventricular tachycardia

2 non-VF/VT incorporating asystole and pulseless electrical activity.

The most common arrhythmias observed in SCA are pulseless VT and VF, with 60–85% of all patients initially presenting with these lethal arrhythmias.[6] In-hospital PEA occurs as the initial rhythm in approximately 30–37% of cases[68,69] and the overall neurologically intact survival rate is 10%.[68] Asystole is the most common arrest arrhythmia in children (40% versus 35% in adults)[68] because their hearts respond to prolonged severe hypoxia and acidosis by progressive bradycardia leading to asystole.[12]

Ventricular fibrillation and pulseless ventricular tachycardia

As previously noted, the only intervention shown to unequivocally improve long-term survival after a VF or pulseless VT arrest is prompt and effective BLS, uninterrupted chest compressions and early defibrillation.[12] VT and VF rhythms are displayed in Figures 25.5 and 25.6. Energy levels and subsequent shocks are equivalent for both VF and pulseless VT.

Non-VF/VT

Non-VF/VT arrhythmias include pulseless electrical activity and asystole. PEA or electromechanical dissociation (EMD) reflects dissociation between the heart's electrical and mechanical activities, and the two terms are used interchangeably. It is important to note that PEA/EMD may present as any rhythm normally compatible with a pulse (e.g. sinus rhythm, sinus tachycardia/bradycardia). PEA is characterised by a stroke volume insufficient to produce a palpable pulse, despite adequate electrical activity.[70] Management of PEA includes identifying and correcting reversible causes, summarised as the 4 Hs and 4 Ts in Table 25.7.

TABLE 25.7

Causes of pulseless electrical activity

THE FOUR Hs	THE FOUR Ts
• Hypoxia	• Tamponade
• Hypovolaemia	• Tension pneumothorax
• Hypo/hyperthermia	• Toxins/poisons/drugs
• Hypo/hyperkalaemia and metabolic disorders	• Thrombosis: pulmonary/ coronary

Adapted with permission from: Australian Resuscitation Council and New Zealand Resuscitation Council (ARC and NZRC). Australian Resuscitation Council Guidelines. Victoria, Australia: Australian Resuscitation Council, <http://www.resus.org.au>; 2014.

FIGURE 25.5   Ventricular tachycardia.

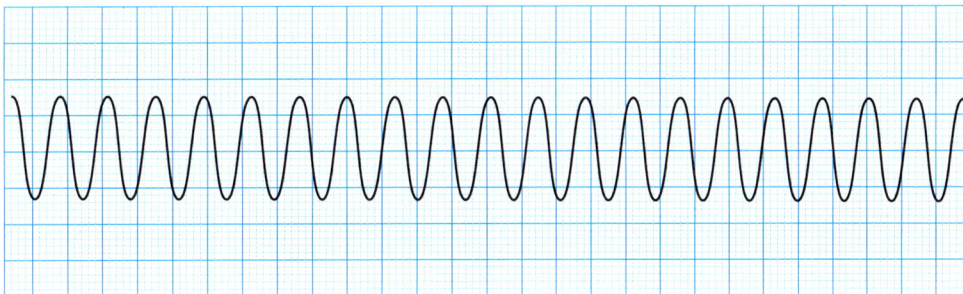

FIGURE 25.6   Ventricular fibrillation.

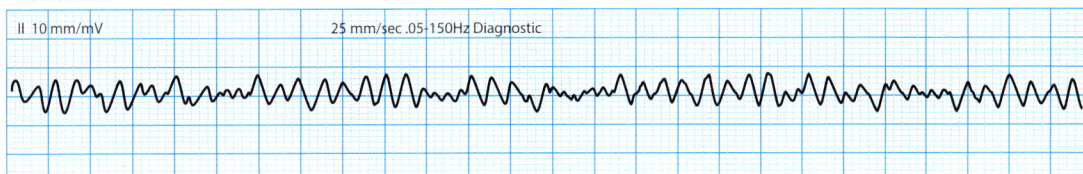

M3536A 26 Apr 2006 12 : 32 : 01: Delayed Alarms Paused Adult HR 133 bpm
Monitor Mode

II 10 mm/mV   25 mm/sec .05–150Hz Diagnostic

FIGURE 25.7 Asystole.

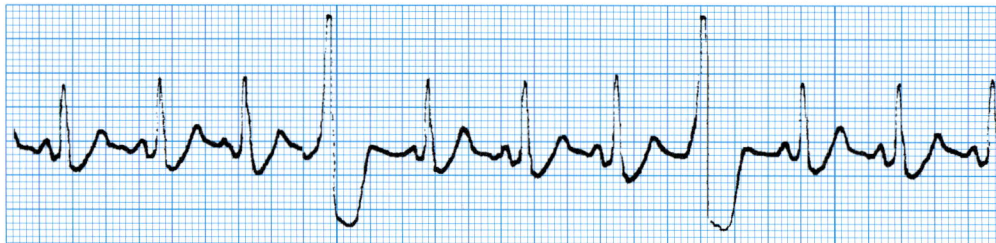

Careful confirmation of asystole (see Figure 25.7) on two leads and the absence of a palpable pulse are essential when making the decision to manage asystole. When an in-hospital arrest has an initial rhythm of asystole, survival to discharge has been reported as 10.66%.[68]

Medications administered during cardiac arrest

Resuscitation drugs can be administered during a cardiac arrest using a variety of routes including peripheral and central veins or intraosseously. Administration by the central venous route remains the optimal method, but the decision to access peripheral versus central cannulation will depend on the skill of the operator. Peripheral venous cannulation is the quickest and easiest method; however, the patient in cardiac arrest may have inaccessible peripheral veins.[23] Should a decision be made to insert a central line during a cardiac arrest, this must not take precedence over defibrillation attempts, CPR or airway maintenance. Medications inserted into a peripheral line should be flushed with at least 20 mL (adults) of an isotonic solution followed by at least 1 minute of continuous external cardiac compressions. Where there is difficulty accessing a peripheral vein, selected medications may be administered via an intraosseous route.[23] Tracheal administration of medication is no longer recommended as the dose delivered is unpredictable and the optimal dose is unknown.[23]

Intraosseous infusion involves the insertion of a metal needle with trocar (usually utilising a drill) into the bone marrow and provides a rapid, safe and reliable access to the circulation. The marrow sinusoids of long bones are a non-collapsible venous system in direct connection with the systemic circulation, allowing drugs to reach the central circulation as quickly as medications injected into central veins. Intraosseal access is safe and effective for use in patients of all age groups.[71] General blood specimens such as biochemistry values, blood cultures, haemoglobin and cross-match studies can also be taken from the marrow at cannulation.[17]

Practice tip

Attempts at peripheral cannulation in children should be aborted after 1 minute and an intraosseous needle inserted.

Vasopressors such as adrenaline and vasopressin have been used as adjuncts in cardiac arrests to improve the success of CPR. While there is no evidence that shows that the routine use of any vasopressor during a cardiac arrest will increase survival to discharge from hospital, adrenaline is still recommended.[12] A randomised controlled trial has shown that, although patients in cardiac arrest that receive adrenaline demonstrate significant improved likelihood of ROSC, significant improvement in their survival to discharge from hospital is not seen.[72]

The optimal dose of adrenaline in the pre-hospital and in-hospital settings remains unclear. Current recommendations propose that adrenaline 1 mg should be administered for VT/VF following the second shock and then every second loop thereafter. For asystole and EMD administer 1 mg of adrenaline in the initial loop, then every second loop (see Table 25.8).[1] Research on the use of vasopressin continues, with a meta-analysis reporting that using the drug during the resuscitation of cardiac arrest patients offers neither overall benefit nor disadvantage for the patient.[73] While there are reports that vasopressin produces no overall change in survival after cardiac arrest when compared with adrenaline, there is no evidence to support or refute the use of vasopressin as an alternative to or in combination with adrenaline.[74,75] The American Heart Association guidelines propose that vasopressin may replace the first or second dose of epinephrine during cardiopulmonary resuscitation.[76]

The optimal role and exact benefit of antiarrhythmic medications in cardiac resuscitation is yet to be fully elucidated, but they have very little, if any, role to play in the treatment of cardiac arrests.[12] The common antiarrhythmic drugs include amiodarone, magnesium, atropine and calcium (see Table 25.8). Lignocaine is no longer recommended as first-line management in cardiac arrest. Amiodarone is the leading antiarrhythmic medication because its safety and efficacy have been demonstrated.[77] If, after the third shock, the VT/VF has not reverted, a bolus injection of 300 mg of amiodarone is recommended and 150 mg for recurrent or refractory VT/VF. There is no evidence of improved survival with the use of atropine in a cardiac arrest with asystole or PEA.[23] Calcium chloride has little use in the management of arrhythmias unless caused by hyperkalaemia, hypocalcaemia or hypermagnesaemia, or an overdose of calcium

TABLE 25.8

Medications used during resuscitation

| ACTION | INDICATIONS | DOSE | | ADVERSE EVENTS |
		ADULTS	PAEDIATRIC	
Adrenaline is a catecholamine that increases aortic diastolic pressure and coronary artery perfusion by producing arteriolar vasoconstriction. It may facilitate defibrillation by improving myocardial blood flow during CPR. Traditionally the first-line medication for the treatment of VF and refractory VT, adrenaline has not demonstrated improved outcomes after cardiac arrest and has been associated with post-resuscitation myocardial dysfunction	VF and pulseless VT resistant to the three initial counter shocks PEA and asystole	VF and pulseless VT: 1 mg after the 2nd shock then after every second cycle PEA and asystole: 1 mg in the initial cycle, then every second cycle	VF and pulseless VT: 10 mcg/kg after the 2nd shock then after every second cycle PEA and asystole: 10 mcg/kg immediately, then every second cycle	Tachyarrhythmias; hypertension; coronary vasoconstriction; increased myocardial oxygen consumption
Amiodarone directly affects smooth muscle and blocks calcium channels and alpha-adrenergic receptors, resulting in coronary and peripheral arterial vasodilation and a reduction in afterload and systemic blood pressure	VT/VF refractory to three shocks Polymorphic VT and wide complex tachycardia of uncertain origin Control of haemodynamically stable VT when cardioversion unsuccessful (in the presence of LV dysfunction) Adjunct to electrical cardioversion of SVT Prophylaxis of recurrent VF/VT	Initial bolus dose: 300 mg in 20 mL dextrose. A further 150 mg could be considered for refractory cases *Periarrest:* An infusion of 15 mg/kg over 24 hours may be commenced	Initial dose: 5 mg/kg bolus over 2 minutes, which may be repeated to a maximum of 300 mg *Periarrest:* IV infusion 5–15 mcg/kg/min as continuous infusion (max of 1.2 g in 24 h)	Vasodilation and hypotension, bradycardia, heart block May have negative inotropic effects Use with caution in renal failure Avoid use in torsades de pointes and other causes of prolonged Q-T
Magnesium is a major intracellular cation resulting in smooth muscle relaxation and membrane stabilisation	Torsades de pointes with or without a pulse; cardiac arrest associated with digoxin toxicity Failure of defibrillation and adrenaline to reverse VF and pulseless VT Documented hypokalaemia or hypomagnesaemia	Bolus dose: 5 mmol *Periarrest:* May be followed by infusion of 20 mmol infused over 4 hours	IV or IO bolus: 0.1–0.2 mmol/kg May be followed by an infusion of 0.3 mmol/kg over 4 hours	Hypotension with rapid administration Use with caution if renal failure present Muscle weakness, paralysis and respiratory failure Tachycardia and excitement
Calcium is essential to nerve and muscle impulse formation and excitation	Hypocalcaemia, hyperkalaemia, overdose of calcium blockers	Bolus dose: 5–10 mL 10% calcium chloride (6.8 mmol)	0.2 mL/kg 10% calcium chloride, or 0.7 mL/kg 10% calcium gluconate via IV	Calcium is incompatible with a range of medications and may precipitate in IV lines Tissue necrosis with extravasation may occur

TABLE 25.8 continued

ACTION	INDICATIONS	DOSE		ADVERSE EVENTS
		ADULTS	PAEDIATRIC	
Sodium bicarbonate (NaHCO₃) is an alkaline agent that may be used to correct an acidosis. Routine administration of sodium bicarbonate for treatment of in-hospital and out-of-hospital cardiac arrest is not recommended	Correcting a metabolic acidosis (pH <7.1), or base deficit of ≤10 or after 15 min; pre-existing hyperkalaemia; tricyclic antidepressant overdose and urinary alkalinisation in overdose; or hypoxic lactic acidosis	Bolus dose: 1 mmol/kg administered over 2–3 min. As NaHCO₃ is incompatible with many medications, it should be administered by a separate line or flushed before and after administration	0.5–1 mmol/kg via IV or IO administered over 2–3 min	Should not be routinely administered Alkalosis, hypernatraemia, hyperosmolality, paradoxical cerebral acidosis, depressed cardiac contractility and metabolic acidosis
Potassium is an electrolyte essential for cell membrane stabilisation that is occasionally used in ALS	Persistent documented VF, suspected hypokalaemia or hypomagnesaemia, and cardiac arrest associated with digoxin toxicity	Slow bolus: 5 mmol	0.03–0.07 mmol/kg via slow administration IV or IO *Periarrest:* 0.2 mmol/kg/h as a continuous infusion; dilute with at least 50 times its volume and mix well, as can be fatal 0.2–0.5 mmol/kg/h to a max of 1 mmol/kg if hypokalaemia severe but not immediately life-threatening	Hyperkalaemia with bradycardia, hypotension with possible asystole and extravasation may lead to tissue necrosis

ECC = external cardiac compression; IO = intraosseous; LV = left ventricular; PEA = pulseless electrical activity; SI = sinoatrial; SVT = supraventricular tachycardia; VF = ventricular fibrillation; VT = ventricular tachycardia.

Adapted with permission from: Australian Resuscitation Council and New Zealand Resuscitation Council (ARC and NZRC). Australian Resuscitation Council Guidelines. Victoria, Australia: Australian Resuscitation Council, <http://www.resus.org.au>; 2014.

channel-blocking drugs. Sodium bicarbonate is no longer administered routinely,[76] as it may cause hypernatraemia, hyperosmolality and intracellular acidosis from the rapid ingress of CO_2 generated from its dissociation. However, it is recommended if the cardiac arrest is associated with hyperkalaemia or tricyclic antidepressant overdose.[12]

There are insufficient data to support the routine use of magnesium in cardiac arrests,[78] except if torsades de pointes is suspected.[12,76] Thrombolytics should not be routinely administered in a cardiac arrest, but they may be considered in adults with proven or suspected pulmonary embolism or acute thrombotic aetiology.[12] Effective CPR should be continued for at least 60–90 minutes following the administration of the fibrinolytic medication as there is evidence in these situations of good neurological outcome and survival following extended periods of CPR.[50]

During the arrest, strategies should be initiated to prevent the development of serious periarrest arrhythmias. Whenever possible, arterial blood gases, serum electrolytes and a 12-lead ECG should be obtained to assist with determining the precise rhythm and appropriate medical interventions.[16] The presence or absence of adverse signs and symptoms will dictate interventions. Adverse factors may include clinical evidence of:

- low cardiac output (unconscious, unresponsive, systolic BP <90 mmHg, increased sympathetic activity)
- reduced diastolic filling time (excessive tachycardia, e.g. heart rates of >150/min, wide complex tachycardia and supraventricular tachycardia)
- excessive bradycardia (heart rates of <40/min)
- raised end-diastolic filling pressure (presence of pulmonary oedema or raised jugular venous pressures)
- reduced coronary blood flow (chest pain).

Interventions can broadly be divided into three options for immediate treatment:

1 antiarrhythmics (refer to *periarrest* in Table 25.8)
2 electrical cardioversion
3 cardiac pacing.

Common periarrest arrhythmias and interventions are covered in Chapter 11. Antiarrhythmic interventions such as medications, physical manoeuvres and electrical therapies may be proarrhythmic.[16] These proarrhythmic interventions alter the cardiac depolarisation and/or repolarisation, lengthening or shortening the QT and predisposing to fatal arrhythmias.[79]

Fluid resuscitation

Fluid resuscitation may be considered if hypovolaemia is suspected as a possible cause of the cardiac arrest. Sodium chloride (0.9%) or Hartmann's solution are recommended as a rapid infusion in the initial stages of resuscitation (at least 20 mL/kg). There is no evidence to support the routine administration of fluids during a cardiac arrest in the absence of hypovolaemia.

Temporary cardiac pacing

During a cardiac arrest, temporary cardiac pacing may be required for sustained symptomatic bradycardia unresponsive to medical intervention. Two types of temporary cardiac pacing are utilised during a cardiac arrest: transvenous (invasive) and transcutaneous (external, non-invasive) pacemakers. As most current defibrillators have the capacity to pace, transcutaneous pacemakers are generally used in an arrest situation.

Ultrasound imaging

Ultrasound imaging has been shown to have some benefit in the detection and diagnosis of reversible causes of arrest including cardiac tamponade, pulmonary embolism, pneumothorax, aortic dissection or hypovolaemia. Placement of the probe at the sub-xiphoid position prior to stopping for planned rhythm assessment will facilitate views within 10 seconds and minimise chest compression interruptions.[20] While the use of imaging has not been shown to improve outcome, absence of heart motion on sonography during resuscitation is highly predictive of death.[20]

Special conditions

Although not common, there are some clinical presentations that require special considerations in a cardiac arrest scenario; these include pregnancy, electrical injuries and drowning. The principles of airway, breathing and circulation remain the same, but modifications must be made because of the physiological changes that occur.

Pregnancy

Researchers report that maternal mortality rates in the USA have either remained unchanged or increased in recent decades.[80] Precipitants included pulmonary embolism, trauma, peripartum haemorrhage, amniotic fluid embolism, eclamptic seizure, congenital and acquired cardiac disease, myocardial infarction, subarachnoid haemorrhage and cerebral aneurysm.[81] Regardless of the aetiology, resuscitation following cardiac arrest in late pregnancy is often unsuccessful. Hence, timely delivery by caesarean section in the setting of maternal cardiac arrest may save both infant and mother.

The principles of airway, breathing and circulation remain the same, but modifications must be made because of the physiological changes that occur with normal pregnancy.[82] A number of factors may need to be considered when resuscitating a pregnant woman. Any situation that affects haemodynamic status will be exacerbated in a supine position, as autocaval compression may result in a fall in cardiac output of up to 25%.[83] During CPR, the mother may be placed in the left lateral tilt (15–25°) or supine with a pillow under the right buttock, to displace the uterus from the inferior vena cava, facilitating venous return and cardiac output.[83–85] Often, the angle of the tilt is overestimated, potentially reducing the quality of the chest compressions.[84] The uterus may also be manually and gently displaced to the left to remove caval compression.[83–85] While ventilation-to-compression ratios remain the same for a pregnant woman, chest compression may be complicated by flaring of the ribs, raised diaphragm, obesity and breast hypertrophy.[82]

The superior displacement of stomach contents by the gravid uterus and a relaxed cardiac sphincter contribute to an increased risk of gastric aspiration in the pregnant woman.[82,86] Because of this increased risk, cricoid pressure should be applied until after the airway is protected by a cuffed tracheal tube.[85] Tracheal intubation should be attended to early, using a short-handled laryngoscope[86] or with a blade mounted at more than 90°,[85] as airway anatomy is altered with the larynx more anterior and superior, while the pharyngeal mucosa is slightly oedematous and friable.[85] A tracheal tube a size smaller than one normally chosen for a similar size non-pregnant woman may be used because of potential narrower airways secondary to oedema or swelling.[82] Defibrillation energy, drug doses and administration are in accordance with ALS guidelines.[85]

If maternal cardiac arrest occurs in the labour ward, operating room or emergency department and BLS and ALS measures are unsuccessful, the uterus should be emptied by surgical (scalpel) intervention within 4–5 minutes.[85] Maternal resuscitation may not be possible until the fetus is removed. Successful resuscitations have occurred after prompt surgical intervention.[85] Refer to Chapter 28 for additional information about critical illness and pregnancy.

Electrical injuries

Electrical burn injuries and lightning injuries are similar in that they occur infrequently, commonly cause widespread acute and delayed tissue damage and can arrest the heart and respiratory centre. Burn injuries are discussed in Chapter 24. This section focuses on the cardiac arrest situation. High-voltage electrocution is associated with a high incidence of cardiac abnormalities, including arrhythmias, prolongation of the QT interval, ST and T wave changes and myocardial infarction.[82] The most common cause of death with lightning injury is cardiac arrest due to VF or asystole or respiratory arrest.[87] Because of the potential for cardiac injuries, all patients should be admitted for cardiac monitoring.

A lightning strike may result in asystole followed by spontaneous return of circulation. If ventilation is initiated early and severe hypoxia does not ensue, a patient's chance of recovery should be better.[87] Initial response of BLS should always begin with D (danger), that is, avoidance of injury to the rescuer. Ensure that the environment is safe for rescuers by disconnecting the electrical supply, where possible, without touching the patient. Where high-voltage lines (power lines) are in contact with the person or the vehicle, no attempt should be made to extricate the person from the vehicle until the situation is deemed safe by an authorised electricity supply person. Once the environment is safe, commence BLS resuscitation. The neck and spine should be protected, as there may be trauma.

In lightning victims, emphasis is on the immediate resuscitation of those who appear unresponsive. Respiratory arrest may be prolonged due to paralysis of the medullary respiratory centre; if not corrected, cardiac arrest secondary to hypoxia ensues. Fixed, dilated pupils should not be used as a poor prognosis of outcome, as victims can benefit from prolonged resuscitation without major sequelae.[87]

Drowning

General issues in managing drowning presentations are discussed in Chapter 23. This section focuses on resuscitation of a cardiorespiratory arrest. Hypoxia and acute lung injury from drowning result in respiratory arrest that, if not corrected, may proceed to a cardiac arrest.[88] A patient's emotional state, associated diseases, previous hypoxia and water temperature all influence this progression.[82]

The primary goal of initial intervention is the relief of hypoxaemia[82] and restoration of cardiovascular stability.[88] Resuscitation of drowning victims follows BLS guidelines, with commencement as soon as practical. Rescue breathing may commence while the victim is still in the water, provided it is safe for the rescuer.[82] As drowning victims may have swallowed considerable amounts of water, vomiting and aspiration of gastric contents can be a major problem during resuscitation. To minimise the risks of inhalation, abdominal compression, the Heimlich manoeuvre and attempts to drain water from the lungs are not recommended. Instead, the victim should be placed on the side for the initial assessment of airway and breathing.[64] Cardiac arrest in these victims is secondary to hypoxia, so compression-only CPR is likely to be less effective and should be avoided.[82] Once experienced personnel arrive, ALS and administration of oxygen should be initiated. The principles of respiratory support and ventilation are discussed in Chapter 15, and treatment of the sequelae of a drowning victim is discussed in Chapter 23.

Resuscitation teams

Resuscitation teams should be organised to ensure that the individual skills of each member are used effectively and efficiently.[89] The exact composition of the resuscitation team will vary between organisations, but generally the team should possess the following skills:[89]

- advanced airway management and intubation skills
- intravenous access skills including central venous access
- defibrillation and external pacing abilities
- medication administration skills
- post-resuscitation skills.

As members of a resuscitation team in the hospital generally do not work together but come from all areas of the hospital, the team should have a designated leader. The team leader gives direction and guidance, assigns tasks and makes clinical decisions without directly performing specific procedures.[16,89] The leader should engender the team's trust. Where leaders initiate structure within the arrest team, members not only work together better, they also perform the tasks of resuscitation more quickly and more effectively.[89] The leader nominates the roles of arrest team members. Roles of team members include airway management, chest compression, medication administration (including IV access), documentation of events and care of family members. The team leader should be responsible for post-resuscitation transfer, documentation, communicating with family members and healthcare professionals and debriefing of the team.[89]

The resuscitation scenario is both complex and stressful for all participants. Often, participants express feelings that too many people are involved, with no one person in control. Unfortunately, the concept of the multi-disciplinary team, where all members' contributions are equally respected, is often not evident in the literature.[90] In addition, while nurses already present at a cardiac arrest in the hospital setting may be willing and competent to perform CPR, they may be prevented from doing so because of the arrival of the cardiac arrest team.[91,92]

Post-resuscitation phase

The aim of post-resuscitation care is the maintenance of cerebral and myocardial perfusion and the return of a patient to a state of best possible health. Resuscitation does not cease with the return of spontaneous circulation. However, ROSC after cardiac arrest does not always equate to a positive outcome for the patient. Mortality rates following in-hospital cardiac arrests vary between 67% and 71%.[93] This high mortality rate has been attributed to multiple organs that are involved with whole of body ischaemia during cardiac arrest. The reperfusion responses that occur following successful resuscitation are termed post-cardiac arrest syndrome.[93] Coordinated care and specific interventions initiated in the post-arrest phase can influence outcomes.[94] Control of body temperature, identification and treatment of acute coronary syndromes and optimisation of mechanical ventilation are a few of the targeted objectives of care (ARC and NZRC Guideline 11.8).[1]

Role of hypothermia in adults after cardiac arrest

During cardiac arrest, prolonged global ischaemia coupled with inadequate reperfusion during the immediate post-resuscitation period can lead to severe cerebral hypoxic injury.[95] Mild therapeutic hypothermia as part of the post-cardiac arrest management provides significant survival benefit as well as improved cardiac and neurological function.[95–97] Several cooling techniques are described in Box 25.1.

Therapeutic cooling consists of the induction, maintenance and rewarming phases.[98] ILCOR recommends that unconscious adult patients with spontaneous circulation after OHCA should be cooled to 32–34°C for 12–24 hours if the initial rhythm was VF. Optimal targeted temperature management continues to be examined with a recent randomised controlled trial reporting no statistically significant difference when comparing the survival and neurological outcomes of patients that were cooled to 33°C compared to those that were cooled to 36°C.[96] It is important to note that shivering post-hyperthermia fever must be avoided.[1] Persistent hyperglycaemia following cardiac arrest has been associated with poor neurological

---

BOX 25.1

Cooling techniques post-cardiac arrest

External:

- Cooling blankets/pads, ice packs, wet towels, fanning, tents and cooling helmets

Internal:

- Transnasal evaporating cooling
- IV administration of cold saline or Hartmann's solution (15–30 mL/kg at 4°C over 30 minutes to achieve a 1.5°C fall in core temperature)
- IV heat exchange device
- Peritoneal and pleural lavage (not generally used)

Adapted with permission from:

Nolan JP, Morley PT, Hoek TV, Hickey RW, Kloeck W, Billi J et al. Therapeutic hypothermia after cardiac arrest: an advisory statement by the Advanced Life Support Task Force of the International Liaison Committee on Resuscitation. Circulation 2003;108(1):118–21.

Nielsen N, Wetterslev J, Cronberg T, Erlinge D, Gasche Y, Hassager C et al. Targeted temperature management at 33 C versus 36 C after cardiac arrest. N Engl J Med 2013;369(23):2197–206.

Bernard SA, Gray TW, Buist MD, Jones BM, Silvester W, Gutteridge G et al. Treatment of comatose survivors of out-of-hospital cardiac arrest with induced hypothermia. N Engl J Med 2002;346(8):557–63.

Polderman KH, Herold I. Therapeutic hypothermia and controlled normothermia in the intensive care unit: practical considerations, side effects, and cooling methods. Crit Care Med 2009;37(3):1101–20.

---

outcome. Monitoring of blood sugar levels and treatment of hyperglycaemia (>10 mmol/L) with insulin is recommended in the post-cardiac arrest period.[1]

Near-death experiences

With the rise in survival rates after a critical illness, there are increasing numbers of documented near-death experiences and out-of-body experiences.[99,100] Near death has been described as unusual experiences during a close brush with death.[99,100] Experiences have typically included memories of bright tunnels of light, deceased relatives, out-of-body sensations, feelings of the presence of a deity and peace.[101,102] These experiences may vary between cultures: Euro-Americans may report a golden colour light whereas people from Tibet may report a clear light.[103] People report the experiences as pleasant, and they have resulted in positive life changes for the individual. After-effects of a near-death experience include absence of fear of death, a more spiritual view of life, less regard for material wealth and/or a heightened chemical sensitivity.[104] The incidence of near-death experiences after cardiac arrest is reported at 6–18%,[99] with the frequency generally being higher in people under 60 years of age.[104] Hence, an awareness of the incidence of near-death experiences and of the cultural differences and needs of the person with a reported near-death experience is essential post-cardiac arrest.[103] Chapter 8 provides more information about family and cultural care.

Special considerations

The chapter to this point primarily has focused on the physiological considerations of resuscitation to achieve the goal of preservation of cellular function. However, this outcome is only achieved in a minority of cases.[22–24] Decision making around the initiation of CPR and resuscitation interventions and the progression and termination of resuscitation involves a multitude of factors.

Family presence during an arrest

The practice of family members witnessing resuscitation has become more evident over time. This shift in practice has been attributed to increasing patient autonomy and the presence of family at a cardiac arrest in popular television shows. This has contributed to public support, and family members requesting – and expecting – to be present.[105,106] However, the issue of whether the family should be present during a cardiac arrest remains controversial. Proponents argue the importance of family being with loved ones during their last moments, as this shortens the period of grieving and provides closure. Indeed, professional resuscitation bodies recommend that family should be afforded the opportunity to be present. However, translating these recommendations into practice varies among healthcare personnel. Commonly cited is a concern that the family may interrupt the work of the resuscitation team, the ethical and medico-legal implications or concern about offending the family.[107,108] Contrary to these beliefs, there is limited evidence that family interfere with the performance of the resuscitation team.[107–109]

Conflicting evidence exists as to the psychological effects of such an event on the family. Effects have been documented as ranging from no adverse effects[108] through to expressions of distress, haunting consequences and trauma.[108] Indeed, families with experience recommend and support family presence as they believe it was beneficial for their loved one and helped them to adjust to the family member's death.[110] Where families are provided the option of being present, a staff member should be identified to have sole responsibility of supporting the family. Chapter 8 is dedicated to family and cultural care, providing additional information about family support.

Ceasing CPR

The decision to cease CPR is often difficult; continuing CPR beyond 30 minutes without ROSC is usually futile unless the arrest was compounded by hypothermia, submersion in cold water, lightning strike, drug overdose or other identified and treatable conditions such as intermittent VF/VT.[16] Prolonging resuscitation for more than 60 minutes may be beneficial for a severely hypothermic, child victim of near-drowning. Pupillary signs should not be used as a predictor of outcome in infants and children, as 11–33% of children with non-reactive pupils have survived long-term after CPR.[17] It is important to have eliminated all causes as far as possible.

Termination of resuscitation is a multifactorial process, influenced by provider comfort and experience, patient prognosis and the patient's desires, wishes and values. Organisational issues such as the local culture, protocols, resources and guidelines will all impact termination decisions. With scientific advances such as extracorporeal membrane oxygenation (ECMO) as a bridge for refractory ventricular fibrillation and evidence-based protocols becoming more widely implemented, current impressions of termination decisions will change over time.[111,112] It is appropriate to invite suggestions from team members, to ensure that all members are comfortable with a decision to stop the resuscitation attempt.[16] Ultimately, terminating CPR is equivalent to a determination of death, and must be made by a doctor. In some out-of-hospital circumstances it may be the paramedical staff who make this decision to stop CPR, essentially terminating resuscitation.[113] Because of this need, termination of resuscitation guidelines have been developed for use in the out-of-hospital setting. One prospectively validated termination of resuscitation guideline is the 'basic life support termination of resuscitation rule' which may be adopted to guide the termination of pre-hospital CPR in adults.[25] One such validated rule is described below.

In the pre-hospital setting stop CPR if:

- no return of spontaneous circulation
  and
- no shocks are administered
  and

- the arrest is not witnessed by emergency medical-services personnel.

Otherwise, the rule recommends transportation to the hospital, in accordance with routine practice.[114]

Legal and ethical considerations

Burgeoning technology in the 1960s enabled the support of oxygenation and circulation for people whose illnesses would have been lethal just a few years before. Enthusiasm for restoration of life led healthcare workers to routinely initiate CPR for all patients who died in hospital.[115] Unfortunately, this led to inappropriate resuscitation attempts and the realisation of the economic, medical and ethical burden to society when survivors had a resultant poor quality of life.[116,117] In the 1970s, growing concern about inappropriate application of CPR and patient's rights led authors to suggest means of forgoing resuscitation and involving patients in decision making.[118] Traditionally, the decision to initiate or withhold CPR was often made by the treating medical team in the absence of the patient or family.[119]

Hospitals responded by developing procedures for withholding CPR through the documentation of 'do not attempt to resuscitate' (DNAR) orders, doctor's orders for life-sustaining treatment, advance directives or living wills[119,120] (see Chapter 5). For patients or their surrogates to meaningfully participate in decision making about CPR and limitation-of-treatment orders, they must have some understanding of survival rates and adverse effects associated with such interventions.[117] Consequently, much debate has ensued over the right of a person to forgo treatment.

Research proposes that, while patients want to be involved in CPR decision making and want some form of advance directive, their knowledge is limited and often derived from television dramas.[119,121] Understanding of quality of life, morbidity and outcomes after CPR strongly influences their preferences.[122,123] Most patients, and indeed healthcare workers, commonly hold unrealistic expectations of CPR success,[121] and will often reverse their preference for commencing CPR once they are informed of the true probability of survival, functional status and quality of life after resuscitation.[124] When compared to the general public, survivors following cardiac arrest generally assess their quality of life as good 12 months post-arrest.[123] Regardless of this, healthcare workers continue to demonstrate a reluctance to discuss CPR options with patients.[125] Despite open discussion, variations in the timing of the orders, poor documentation and communication can result in CPR being inappropriately commenced.[120] Conversely, and contrary to medical and nursing opinions, some people choose CPR even when they have a terminal illness, coma or serious disability.[122]

Standardised orders for limitations on life-sustaining treatments (e.g. DNAR) should be considered to decrease the incidence of futile resuscitation attempts and to ensure that adult patients' wishes are honoured. These orders should be specific, detailed, transferable across healthcare settings and easily understood. Processes, protocols and systems should be developed that fit within local cultural norms and legal limitations to allow providers to honour patients' wishes about resuscitation efforts.[25] With the exception of a zero survival rate there remains no formal consensus on DNAR decision-making practices or the termination of resuscitation. While researchers have attempted to develop prognostic indicators for cardiac arrest outcome, moralists would argue that the use of such prognostic tools alone reflects utilitarianism, and that they should never be used in isolation of the input of the patient and healthcare team.

Summary

Outcomes for patients after in-hospital sudden cardiac arrest remain poor. Successful management of a patient following SCA depends largely on the timely implementation of the chain of survival. Nurses should understand the role of the chain of survival in the resuscitation of the person following cardiac arrest. The chain emphasises the importance of early recognition and intervention, continuous uninterrupted compressions and the early use of the defibrillator as a BLS skill. Understanding when to start, when to continue and when to stop are equally important and are influenced by multiple factors. Including the patient's wishes in decision making is of utmost importance to ensure futile resuscitation attempts are avoided. Despite the plethora of research on the topic of resuscitation, there is much we still do not know.

Case study

Matt, a fit, healthy 31-year-old, was playing football in a suburb of a major city on a Saturday afternoon when he suddenly collapsed on the field. Two other footballers on the scene knelt down to render aid. When Matt did not move they signalled for help, and an official first aid person at the scene ran onto the field to assess Matt. Matt was unconscious, unresponsive and not moving. Cardiopulmonary resuscitation was commenced by the first aid person utilising compression-only resuscitation at a rate of approximately 100 compressions per minute. The sports club at the field owned an AED; therefore another bystander ran into the club and brought the AED onto the field and attached the pads onto Matt's chest, while compressions continued. During this time the coach of Matt's team called triple zero (000).

The AED was turned on and instructed the first aid responders to 'stand clear'. The rhythm was analysed and a shock was advised and delivered as per the verbal cues, followed by immediate compressions. After one more minute of CPR the second first aid person took over compressions and gave the first responder a rest; after the second minute the AED once again advised a 'stand clear' message and analysed the rhythm, and a second shock was advised and delivered, with compressions again immediately recommenced.

An ambulance responded and arrived at the scene 14 minutes post-collapse. They assessed the situation and provided advanced life support measures as per the ARC guidelines. Compressions continued at a rate of 100 per minute and, on arrival of an intensive care paramedic, Matt was intubated with a size 8 endotracheal tube and ventilation via bag and valve with supplemental oxygen was continued. The ventilation rate was approximately 8–10 per minute. At 20 minutes after Matt collapsed, his cardiac rhythm was noted to be VF and he had been given four shocks from the AED and then a further two shocks by the paramedics. Matt had an intravenous cannula inserted and the first dose of adrenaline 1 mg was given, and then repeated every 3 minutes (after every second loop of the shockable side of the ALS flow chart). Amiodarone 300 mg IV was given after the third shock.

The ambulance was equipped with a mechanical automated chest compression device, which utilises a load distributing band that squeezes the entire chest and hence delivers high-quality cardiac compressions. Matt was rolled onto the device and the band was attached around his chest; the device was switched on and took over the compressions at a rate of 100 per minute.

A call was made to the closest tertiary hospital to alert the centre that the patient was in refractory ventricular fibrillation and request the possibility of rescue extracorporeal membrane oxygenation (ECMO). ECMO is indicated for potentially reversible, life-threatening forms of respiratory and/or cardiac failure that are unresponsive to conventional therapy. At no time during these procedures was there any sign of ROSC. Matt was transferred to the ambulance and transported to the major hospital with compressions and ventilations continuing.

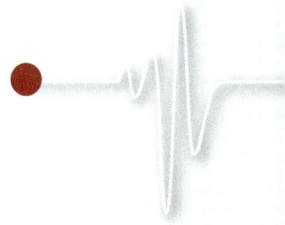

Upon arrival in the emergency department the ECMO response team was waiting and Matt's femoral vein and artery were percutaneously cannulated with size 15 and 17 French gauge catheters, respectively. He was connected to venous-arterial ECMO and cooled to 32–34°C with the intravenous administration of 2 litres of cold saline as per hospital protocol for therapeutic hypothermia. Once connected to ECMO the mechanical chest compression device was removed; however ventilation continued and Matt was taken to the cardiac interventional catheter laboratory for urgent percutaneous interventional therapy. At this time Matt had been in an arrested state for 1 hour and 20 minutes. During this time repeated shocks were given in an attempt to revert his refractory ventricular fibrillation.

Percutaneous interventional therapy demonstrated a 98% occlusion in the left anterior descending artery that was successfully stented. A further two shocks post-stent were given and Matt reverted to a sinus rhythm after the second shock. Matt was transferred to the intensive care unit and over the following 2 days was slowly weaned from ECMO. Post-resuscitation care included reducing the fraction of inspired oxygen as soon as possible with a targeted oxygen saturation of 90–95%, maintaining a normal $PaCO_2$, ensuring blood pressure was adequate (systolic pressure between 100 and 120 mmHg) and maintenance of therapeutic hypothermia for the first 24 hours. Matt was extubated on day 3 and was discharged home on day 8 with full neurological function to a very relieved family.

CASE STUDY QUESTIONS

1 Discuss the advantages and disadvantages of compression-only CPR.
2 What is the rationale for switching personnel during cardiac compressions?
3 Discuss the stage in the ALS flow chart that amiodarone is given.
4 Identify two common types of mechanical devices for cardiac compressions and how they augment blood flow.

RESEARCH VIGNETTE

Nielsen N, Wetterslev J, Cronberg T, Erlinge D, Gasche Y, Hassager C et al. Targeted temperature management at 33°C versus 36°C after cardiac arrest. N Engl J Med 2013;369(23):2197–206

Background: Unconscious survivors of out-of-hospital cardiac arrest have a high risk of death or poor neurologic function. Therapeutic hypothermia is recommended by international guidelines, but the supporting evidence is limited, and the target temperature associated with the best outcome is unknown. Our objective was to compare two target temperatures, both intended to prevent fever.

Methods: In an international trial, we randomly assigned 950 unconscious adults after out-of-hospital cardiac arrest of presumed cardiac cause to targeted temperature management at either 33 degrees C or 36 degrees C. The primary outcome was all-cause mortality through the end of the trial. Secondary outcomes included a composite of poor neurologic function or death at 180 days, as evaluated with the Cerebral Performance Category (CPC) scale and the modified Rankin scale.

Results: In total, 939 patients were included in the primary analysis. At the end of the trial, 50% of the patients in the 33 degrees C group (235 of 473 patients) had died, as compared with 48% of the patients in the 36 degrees C group (225 of 466 patients) (hazard ratio with a temperature of 33 degrees C, 1.06; 95% confidence interval [CI], 0.89 to 1.28; P=0.51). At the 180-day follow-up, 54% of the patients in the 33 degrees C group had died or had poor neurologic function according to the CPC, as compared with 52% of patients in the 36 degrees C group (risk ratio, 1.02; 95% CI, 0.88 to 1.16; P=0.78). In the analysis using the modified Rankin scale, the comparable rate was 52% in both groups (risk ratio, 1.01; 95% CI, 0.89 to 1.14; P=0.87). The results of analyses adjusted for known prognostic factors were similar.

Conclusions: In unconscious survivors of out-of-hospital cardiac arrest of presumed cardiac cause, hypothermia at a targeted temperature of 33 degrees C did not confer a benefit as compared with a targeted temperature of 36 degrees C. (Funded by the Swedish Heart-Lung Foundation and others; TTM ClinicalTrials.gov number, NCT01020916.)

CRITIQUE

In this study Nielsen aimed to determine whether cooling patients to 33°C provided any advantage compared to cooling patients to 36°C post cardiac arrest as part of a targeted temperature management strategy.[96] Randomisation of the 939 patients was undertaken using a computer generated sequence and permuted blocks of varying size were used to account for potential biases between study sites. Those who assessed patient outcomes were blinded to treatment allocation. In addition to the researchers who implemented a standardised protocol, a doctor who was blinded to treatment allocation performed a neurological evaluation 72 hours following completion of the trial interventions. The primary end point was survival at 180 days, with secondary outcomes being neurological outcome as assessed by the Cerebral Performance Category (CPC) and Modified Rankin scores. The study was powered to detect a 20% reduction in baseline mortality of 44% in the 33°C group compared with 55% in the 36°C group.

In assessing this study one should adopt a systematic approach of determining the study characteristics, understanding the results and assessing the applicability of the findings to the patients you manage. With regard to the study characteristics, Table 1 in the journal article provides the baseline characteristics of the patients and known prognostic factors (e.g. bystander CPR, age, sex, initial rhythm etc) in each of the treatment arms. Both groups appear to be very similar. It is interesting to note that both groups were initially quite hypothermic (35°C), time to commencement of basic life support was a median of 1 minute and approximately 80% of patients had an initial shockable rhythm. Figure 1 in the journal article demonstrates good temperature separation with each intervention reaching target temperature within 8 hours of randomisation and that temperature being maintained for the next 20 hours as per study protocol.

In understanding the findings of the study, the authors found no difference in either primary or secondary outcomes between the two interventions. Death at 180 days occurred in 48% and 47% of patients allocated to 33°C and 36°C, respectively (HR 1.01; 95% CI 0.87 to 1.15). Further, there was no difference observed in neurological outcome. The authors conclude that their study did not provide evidence that targeting a temperature of 33°C following out-of-hospital cardiac arrest offers any advantage over a target temperature of 36°C. The authors appropriately identified the limitations of their study.

So what does this mean for current practice? Firstly, it should be understood that this study was designed to detect a difference in outcome between the two treatment temperatures. It failed to detect any such difference. This is not the same as concluding the two temperatures were equivalent and the study was not designed as an equivalence trial. Equivalence trials are designed to test the hypothesis that the two interventions are not too different within predetermined values of what would be considered (often clinically) as equivalent. Secondly, as previously noted the proportion of patients with initial shockable rhythm and 50% of the study patients receiving basic life support within 1 minute are quite different to the mainstream population of out-of-hospital cardiac arrests. As such, the findings of this study may lack some generalisability in this regard. Further, it remains unknown if similar findings would be observed in patients presenting with pulseless electrical activity or asystole. Conversely, the implementation of a target temperature of 36°C may be logistically easier in the ICU and potential for complications related to therapeutic hypothermia.

This study does not provide any support to justify not initiating therapeutic hypothermia. The authors clearly state that the prevention of fever is important in this patient cohort and this is consistent with the current evidence. Accordingly, one should interpret the findings of this study as in support of a targeted temperature control strategy where a temperature range of 33°C to 36°C is maintained.

Learning activities

1   Does the study recommend a target body temperature of 33°C for unconscious patients admitted to hospital following out-of-hospital cardiac arrest?

2   What limitations did the commentary highlight in the above recommendation?

3   What, in research outcome terms, is the importance of the doctor who performed the neurological evaluations being blinded to treatment allocation?

4   What would be the practical advantage of a protocol change from therapeutic hypothermia to a targeted temperature of 36°C?

Online resources

American Heart Association (AHA), www.americanheart.org

Australian Resuscitation Council (ARC), www.resus.org.au

Center for Pediatric Emergency Medicine (CPEM), http://cpem.med.nyu.edu

European Resuscitation Council (ERC), www.erc.edu

International Liaison Committee on Resuscitation (ILCOR), www.ilcor.org/en/home

New Zealand Resuscitation Council (NZRC), www.nzrc.org.nz

The Regional Emergency Medical Services Council of New York City, www.nycremsco.org/default.asp

Further reading

Luo X, Zhang H, Chen G, Ding W, Huang L. Active compression–decompression cardiopulmonary resuscitation (CPR) versus standard CPR for cardiac arrest patients: a meta-analysis. World J Emerg Med 2013;4(4):266–72.

References

1 Australian Resuscitation Council and New Zealand Resuscitation Council (ARC and NZRC). Australian Resuscitation Council Guidelines. Victoria, Australia: Australian Resuscitation Council, <http://www.resus.org.au>; 2014 [accessed 07.14].

2 Gräsner J-T, Bossaert L. Epidemiology and management of cardiac arrest: what registries are revealing. Best Pract Res Clin Anaesthesiol 2013;27(3):293–306.

3 Sasson C, Rogers M, Dahl J, Kellermann A. Predictors of survival from out-of-hospital cardiac arrest a systematic review and meta-analysis. Circulation: Cardiovasc Q Outcomes 2010;3(2):63-81.

4 Gräsner J-T, Frey N. The best things to do – MTH and PCI after cardiac arrest? Resuscitation 2014;85(5):581-2.

5 Atwood C, Eisenberg M, Herlitz J. Incidence of EMS-treated out-of-hospital cardiac arrest in Europe. Resuscitation 2005;67:75-80.

6 Holmgren C, Bergfeldt L, Edvardsson N, Karlsson T, Lindqvist J, Silfverstolpe J et al. Analysis of initial rhythm, witnessed status and delay to treatment among survivors of out-of-hospital cardiac arrest in Sweden. Heart 2010;96:1826-30.

7 Rea TD, Pearce RM, Raghunathan TE, Lemaitre RN, Sotoodehnia N, Jouven X et al. Incidence of out-of-hospital cardiac arrest. Am J Cardiol 2004;93(12):1455-60.

8 Berdowski J, Berg RA, Tijssen JGP, Koster RW. Global incidences of out-of-hospital cardiac arrest and survival rates: systematic review of 67 prospective studies. Resuscitation 2010;81(11):1479-87.

9 Herlitz J, Engdahl J, Svensson L, Young M, Ängquist K-A, Holmberg S. Can we define patients with no chance of survival after out-of-hospital cardiac arrest? Heart 2004;90(10):1114-8.

10 Australian Institute of Health and Welfare (AIHW). Australia's health 2012. Australia's health series no. 12. Canberra: AIHW, <http://www.aihw.gov.au/publication-detail/?id=10737422172>; 2012.

11 Müller D, Agrawal R, Arntz H-R. How sudden is sudden cardiac death? Circulation 2006;114(11):1146-50.

12 Deakin CD, Nolan JP, Soar J, Sunde K, Koster RW, Smith GB et al. European Resuscitation Council Guidelines for Resuscitation 2010 Section 4. Adult advanced life support. Resuscitation 2010;81(10):1305-52.

13 Herlitz J, Svensson L, Engdahl J, Gelberg J, Silfverstolpe J, Wisten A et al. Characteristics of cardiac arrest and resuscitation by age group: an analysis from the Swedish Cardiac Arrest Registry. Am J Emerg Med 2007;25(9):1025-31.

14 Dickson EM, Anders NRK. Infant resuscitation. Curr Anaesth Crit Care 2004;15(1):53-60.

15 Atkins DL, Everson-Stewart S, Sears GK, Daya M, Osmond MH, Warden CR et al. Epidemiology and outcomes from out-of-hospital cardiac arrest in children: the Resuscitation Outcomes Consortium Epistry–Cardiac Arrest. Circulation 2009;119(11):1484-91.

16 Kleinman ME, de Caen AR, Chameides L, Atkins DL, Berg RA, Berg MD et al. Part 10: Pediatric basic and advanced life support: 2010 International Consensus on Cardiopulmonary Resuscitation and Emergency Cardiovascular Care Science with Treatment Recommendations. Circulation 2010;122(16 suppl 2):S466-S515.

17 Frenneaux M. Cardiopulmonary resuscitation – some physiological considerations. Resuscitation 2003;58(3):259-65.

18 Ballew K. Cardiopulmonary resuscitation: recent advances. BMJ 1997;314(7092):1462-6.

19 Cummins R, Chamberlain D, Hazinski M, Nadkarni V, Kloeck W, Kramer E. Recommended guidelines for reviewing, reporting, and conducting research on in-hospital resuscitation: the in-hospital 'Utstein style'. Circulation 1997;95(8):2213-39.

20 Nolan J, Soar J, Zideman D, Biarent D, Bossaert L, Deakin C et al. European Resuscitation Council guidelines for resuscitation 2010 Section 1. Executive summary. Resuscitation 2010;81(10):1219-76.

21 Cheskes S, Schmicker RH, Verbeek PR, Salcido DD, Brown SP, Brooks S et al. The impact of peri-shock pause on survival from out-of-hospital shockable cardiac arrest during the Resuscitation Outcomes Consortium PRIMED trial. Resuscitation 2014;85(3):336-42.

22 Kolte D, Khera S, Aronow W, Mujib M, Palaniswamy C, Jain D et al. Gender and racial/ethnic differences in survival after cardiopulmonary resuscitation for in-hospital cardiac arrest. J Am CollCardiol 2014;63(12_S).

23 Nolan JP, Soar J, Smith GB, Gwinnutt C, Parrott F, Power S et al. Incidence and outcome of in-hospital cardiac arrest in the United Kingdom National Cardiac Arrest Audit. Resuscitation 2014;85(8):987-92.

24 Girotra S, Nallamothu BK, Spertus JA, Li Y, Krumholz HM, Chan PS. Trends in survival after in-hospital cardiac arrest. N Engl J Med 2012;367(20):1912-20.

25 Soar J, Mancini M, Bhanji F, Billi J, Dennett J, Finn J et al. On behalf of the Education, Implementation, and Teams Chapter Collaborators. Part 12: Education, implementation, and teams: 2010 International Consensus on Cardiopulmonary Resuscitation and Emergency Cardiovascular Care Science with Treatment Recommendations. Resuscitation 2010;81:e288-e330.

26 Meaney P, Bobrow B, Mancini M, Christenson J, De Caen A, Bhanji F et al. Cardiopulmonary resuscitation quality: improving cardiac resuscitation outcomes both inside and outside the hospital: a consensus statement from the American Heart Association. Circulation 2013;128(4):417-35.

27 Koster R, Baubin M, Bossaert L, Caballero A, Cassan P, Castrén M et al. European Resuscitation Council Guidelines for Resuscitation 2010 Section 2. Adult basic life support and use of automated external defibrillators. Resuscitation 2010;81:1277-92

28 Brindley P, Simmonds M, Gibney R. Medical emergency teams: is there M.E.R.I.T? Can J Anesth 2007;54(5):389-91.

29 Smith GB. In-hospital cardiac arrest: is it time for an in-hospital 'chain of prevention'? Resuscitation 2010;81(9):1209-11.

30 Considine J, Botti M. Who, when and where? Identification of patients at risk of an in-hospital adverse event: implications for nursing practice. Int J Nurs Res 2004;10(1):21-31.

31 Kause J, Smith G, Prytherch D, Parr M, Flabouris A, Hillman K. A comparison of Antecedents to Cardiac Arrests, Deaths and EMergency Intensive care Admissions in Australia and New Zealand, and the United Kingdom – the ACADEMIA study. Resuscitation 2004;62(3):275-82.

32 DeVita M, Smith G, Adam S, Adams-Pizarro I, Buist M, Bellomo R et al. Identifying the hospitalised patient in crisis – a consensus conference on the afferent limb of Rapid Response Systems Resuscitation. 2010;81(4):375-82.

33 Laurens NH, Dwyer TA. The effect of medical emergency teams on patient outcome: a review of the literature. Int J Nurs Pract 2010;16(6): 533-44.

34 Prytherch DR, Smith GB, Schmidt PE, Featherstone PI. ViEWS – Towards a national early warning score for detecting adult inpatient deterioration. Resuscitation 2010;81(8):932-7.

35 McNeill G, Bryden D. Do either early warning systems or emergency response teams improve hospital patient survival? A systematic review. Resuscitation 2013;84(12):1652-67.

36 Chan P, Jain R, Nallmothu B, Berg R, Sasson C. Rapid response teams: a systematic review and meta-analysis. Arch Intern Med 2010;170(1):18-26.

37 Smith GB, Prytherch DR, Meredith P, Schmidt PE, Featherstone PI. The ability of the National Early Warning Score (NEWS) to discriminate patients at risk of early cardiac arrest, unanticipated intensive care unit admission, and death. Resuscitation 2013;84(4):465-70.

38 Ray EM, Smith R, Massie S, Erickson J, Hanson C, Harris B et al. Family alert: implementing direct family activation of a pediatric rapid response team. Joint Commission Journal on Quality & Patient Safety 2009 35(11):575-80.

39 Australian Resuscitation Council and New Zealand Resuscitation Council (ARC and NRZC). Australian Resuscitation Council, Airway: Guideline 4. Australian Resuscitation Council, <http://www.resus.org.au>; 2014.

40 Mackway-Jones K, Molyneux E, Phillips B, Wieteska K. Advanced paediatric life support: the practical approach. 4th ed. Oxford: Blackwell; 2005.

41 Wyllie J, Perlman J, Kattwinkel J, Atkins D, Chameides L, Goldsmith J et al. On behalf of the Neonatal Resuscitation Chapter Collaborators. Part 11: Neonatal resuscitation: 2010 International Consensus on Cardiopulmonary Resuscitation and Emergency Cardiovascular Care Science with Treatment Recommendations. Resuscitation 2010;81:e260-e87.

42 Berg R, Saunders A, Kern K, Hilwig R, Heidenreich J, Porter M. Adverse hemodynamic effects of interrupting chest compressions for rescue breathing during cardiopulmonary resuscitation for ventricular defibrillation cardiac arrest. Circulation 2001;104:2465-70.

43 Nolan J, Hazinski M, Billi J, Boettiger B, Bossaert L, de Caen A et al. Part 1: Executive summary: 2010 International Consensus on Cardiopulmonary Resuscitation and Emergency Cardiovascular Care Science With Treatment Recommendations Resuscitation. 2010;81 (1 Sup 1):e1-e25.

44 Dwyer T. Psychological factors inhibit family members' confidence to initiate CPR. Prehospital Emerg Care 2008;12(2):157-61.

45 Assar D, Chamberlain D, Colquhoun M, Donnelly P, Handley AJ, Leaves S et al. Randomised controlled trial of staged teaching for basic life support: skill acquisition at bronze stage. Resuscitation 2000;45:7-15.

46 Koster R, Sayre M, Botha M, Cave D, Cudnik M, Handley A et al. Part 5: Adult basic life support: 2010 International Consensus on Cardiopulmonary Resuscitation and Emergency Cardiovascular Care Science with Treatment Recommendations. Resuscitation 2010;81:e48-e70.

47 Bobrow B, Spaite D, Berg R, Stolz U, Sanders A, Kern K et al. Chest compression-only CPR by lay rescuers and survival from out-of-hospital cardiac arrest. JAMA 2010;304(3):1447-54.

48 Touma O, Davies M. The prognostic value of end tidal carbon dioxide during cardiac arrest: a systematic review. Resuscitation 2013;84(11):1470-9.

49 Nolan JP. High-quality cardiopulmonary resuscitation. Curr Opin Crit Care 2014;20(3):227-33.

50 Hartmann SM, Farris RW, Di Gennaro JL, Roberts JS. Systematic review and meta-analysis of end-tidal carbon dioxide values associated with return of spontaneous circulation during cardiopulmonary resuscitation. J Intensive Care Med 2014:0885066614530839.

51 Park SO, Shin DH, Baek KJ, Hong DY, Kim EJ, Kim SC et al. A clinical observational study analysing the factors associated with hyperventilation during actual cardiopulmonary resuscitation in the emergency department. Resuscitation 2013;84(3):298-303.

52 Delguercio L, Feins N, Cohn J, Coomaraswamy R, Wollman S, State D. Comparison of blood flow during external and internal cardiac massage in man. Circulation 1965;31(Suppl 1):171-80.

53 Wik L, Olsen J-A, Persse D, Sterz F, Lozano Jr M, Brouwer MA et al. Manual vs integrated automatic load-distributing band CPR with equal survival after out of hospital cardiac arrest. The randomized CIRC trial. Resuscitation 2014;85(6):741-8.

54 Brooks SC, Hassan N, Bigham BL, Morrison LJ. Mechanical versus manual chest compressions for cardiac arrest. Cochrane Database Syst Rev 2014;2:CD007260.

55 Soar J, Nolan JP. Manual chest compressions for cardiac arrest – with or without mechanical CPR? Resuscitation 2014;85(6):705-6.

56 Nehme Z, Andrew E, Bernard SA, Smith K. Treatment of monitored out-of-hospital ventricular fibrillation and pulseless ventricular tachycardia utilising the precordial thump. Resuscitation 2013;84(12):1691-6.

57 Pellis T, Kette F, Lovisa D, Franceschino E, Magagnin L, Mercante WP et.al. Utility of pre-cordial thump for treatment of out of hospital cardiac arrest: a prospective study. Resuscitation 2009;80:17-23.

58 Dwyer T, Mosel Williams L, Jacobs I. The benefits and use of shock advisory defibrillators in hospitals. Int J Nurs Pract 2004;10(2):86-92.

59 Tomkins WGO, Swain AH, Bailey M, Larsen PD. Beyond the pre-shock pause: the effect of prehospital defibrillation mode on CPR interruptions and return of spontaneous circulation. Resuscitation 2013;84(5):575-9.

60 Husain S, Eisenberg M. Police AED programs: a systematic review and meta-analysis. Resuscitation 2013;84(9):1184-91.

61 Morrison LJ, Henry RM, Ku V, Nolan JP, Morley P, Deakin CD. Single-shock defibrillation success in adult cardiac arrest: a systematic review. Resuscitation 2013;84(11):1480-6.

62 Hess EP, Atkinson EJ, White RD. Increased prevalence of sustained return of spontaneous circulation following transition to biphasic waveform defibrillation. Resuscitation 2008;77(1):39-45.

63 Wang C-H, Huang C-H, Chang W-T, Tsai M-S, Liu SS-H, Wu C-Y et al. Biphasic versus monophasic defibrillation in out-of-hospital cardiac arrest: a systematic review and meta-analysis. Am J Emerg Med 2013;31(10):1472-8.

64 de Caen AR, Kleinman ME, Chameides L, Atkins DL, Berg RA, Berg MD et al. Part 10: Paediatric basic and advanced life support. Resuscitation 2010;81(1 Supplement):e213-e59.

65 Chan PS, Krumholz HM, Spertus JA, Jones PG, Cram P, Berg RA et al. Automated external defibrillators and survival after in-hospital cardiac arrest. JAMA 2010;304(19):2129-36.

66 Christenson J, Andrusiek D, Everson-Stewart S, Kudenchuk P, Hostler D, Powell J et al. Chest compression fraction determines survival in patients with out-of-hospital ventricular fibrillation. Circulation 2009;120(13):1241-7.

67 Soar J, Nolan JP. Airway management in cardiopulmonary resuscitation. Curr Opin Crit Care 2013;19(3):181-7.

68 Morrison LJ, Neumar RW, Zimmerman JL, Link MS, Newby LK, McMullan PW et al. Strategies for improving survival after in-hospital cardiac arrest in the United States: 2013 consensus recommendations. A consensus statement from the American Heart Association. Circulation 2013;127(14):1538-63.

69 Hellevuo H, Sainio M, Olkkola KT, Tenhunen J, Hoppu S. Ventricular fibrillation/tachycardia, pulseless electrical activity and asystole are equally common initial rhythms in in-hospital cardiac arrest due to cardiac reasons. Resuscitation 2014;85:S34.

70 Rosborough JP, Deno DC. Electrical therapy for post defibrillatory pulseless electrical activity. Resuscitation 2004;63(1):65-72.

71 Leidel BA, Kirchhoff C, Braunstein V, Bogner V, Biberthaler P, Kanz K-G. Comparison of two intraosseous access devices in adult patients under resuscitation in the emergency department: a prospective, randomized study. Resuscitation 2010;81(8):994-9.

72 Jacobs IG, Finn JC, Jelinek GA, Oxer HF, Thompson PL. Effect of adrenaline on survival in out-of-hospital cardiac arrest: a randomised double-blind placebo-controlled trial. Resuscitation 2011;82(9):1138-43.

73 Mentzelopoulos SD, Zakynthinos SG, Siempos I, Malachias S, Ulmer H, Wenzel V. Vasopressin for cardiac arrest: meta-analysis of randomized controlled trials. Resuscitation 2012;83(1):32-9.

74 Wenzel V, Krismer AC, Arntz HR, Sitter H, Stadlbauer KH, Lindner KH. A comparison of vasopressin and epinephrine for out-of-hospital cardiopulmonary resuscitation. N Engl J Med 2004;350(2):105-13.

75 Layek A, Maitra S, Pal S, Bhattacharjee S, Baidya DK. Efficacy of vasopressin during cardio-pulmonary resuscitation in adult patients: a meta-analysis. Resuscitation 2014;85(7):855-63.

76 Neumar RW, Otto CW, Link MS, Kronick SL, Shuster M, Callaway CW et al. Part 8: Adult advanced cardiovascular life support: 2010 American Heart Association guidelines for cardiopulmonary resuscitation and cmergency cardiovascular care. Circulation 2010;122(18 suppl 3):S729-S67.

77 Lunxian T, Hu X, Qing H. Intravenous amiodarone for treatment of ventricular tachycardia and ventricular fibrillation [protocol]. Cochrane Database Syst Rev 2003(2).

78 Ong MEH, Pellis T, Link MS. The use of antiarrhythmic drugs for adult cardiac arrest: a systematic review. Resuscitation 2011;82(6):665-70.

79 Konstantopoulou A, Tsikrikas S, Asvestas D, Korantzopoulos P, Letsas KP. Mechanisms of drug-induced proarrhythmia in clinical practice. World J Cardiol 2013;5(6):175.

80 Clark SL, Christmas JT, Frye DR, Meyers JA, Perlin JB. Maternal mortality in the United States: predictability and the impact of protocols on fatal postcesarean pulmonary embolism and hypertension-related intracranial hemorrhage. Am J Obstet Gynecol 2014;211(1):32.e1-9.

81 Lewis G, ed. Saving mothers' lives: The continuing benefits for maternal health from the United Kingdom (UK) Confidential Enquires into Maternal Deaths. Seminars in Perinatology. Elsevier; 2012.

82 Soar J, Perkins GD, Abbas G, Alfonzo A, Barelli A, Bierens JJ et al. European Resuscitation Council guidelines for resuscitation 2010: Section 8. Cardiac arrest in special circumstances: electrolyte abnormalities, poisoning, drowning, accidental hypothermia, hyperthermia, asthma, anaphylaxis, cardiac surgery, trauma, pregnancy, electrocution. Resuscitation 2010;81(10):1400-33.

83 Lipman S, Cohen S, Einav S, Jeejeebhoy F, Mhyre JM, Morrison LJ et al. The Society for Obstetric Anesthesia and Perinatology consensus statement on the management of cardiac arrest in pregnancy. Anesth Analg. 2014;118(5):1003-16.

84 Jeejeebhoy FM, Zelop CM, Windrim R, Carvalho JC, Dorian P, Morrison LJ. Management of cardiac arrest in pregnancy: a systematic review. Resuscitation 2011;82(7):801-9.

85 Hoek TLV, Morrison LJ, Shuster M, Donnino M, Sinz E, Lavonas EJ et al. Part 12: Cardiac arrest in special situations 2010: American Heart Association guidelines for cardiopulmonary resuscitation and emergency cardiovascular eare. Circulation 2010;122(18 suppl 3):S829-S61.

86 Gupta S. Maternal cardiac arrest and resuscitation: some burning issues! J Obstet Anaesth Crit Care 2013;3(1):1.

87 Zafren K, Durrer B, Herry J-P, Brugger H. Lightning injuries: prevention and on-site treatment in mountains and remote areas: official guidelines of the International Commission for Mountain Emergency Medicine and the Medical Commission of the International Mountaineering and Climbing Federation (ICAR and UIAA MEDCOM). Resuscitation 2005;65(3):369-72.

88 Layon AJ, Modell JH. Drowning: update 2009. Anesthesiology 2009;110(6):1390-401.

89 Yeung JHY, Ong GJ, Davies RP, Gao F, Perkins GD. Factors affecting team leadership skills and their relationship with quality of cardiopulmonary resuscitation. Crit Care Med 2012;40(9):2617-21.

90 Hunziker S, Johansson AC, Tschan F, Semmer NK, Rock L, Howell MD et al. Teamwork and leadership in cardiopulmonary resuscitation. J Am CollCardiol 2011;57(24):2381-8.

91 Jones L, King L, Wilson C. A literature review: factors that impact on nurses' effective use of the medical rmergency yeam (MET). J Clin Nurs 2009;18(24):3379-90.

92 Dwyer T, Mosel Williams L, Mummery K. Defibrillation beliefs of rural nurses: focus group discussions guided by the theory of planned behaviour. Rural Remote Health 2005;5:322.

93 Nolan JP, Neumar RW, Adrie C, Aibiki M, Berg RA, Böttiger BW et al. Post-cardiac arrest syndrome: epidemiology, pathophysiology, treatment, and prognostication: a scientific statement from the International Liaison Committee on Resuscitation; the American Heart Association Emergency Cardiovascular Care Committee; the Council on Cardiovascular Surgery and Anesthesia; the Council on Cardiopulmonary, Perioperative, and Critical Care; the Council on Clinical Cardiology; the Council on Stroke. Resuscitation 2008;79(3):350-79.

94 Binks A, Nolan J. Post-cardiac arrest syndrome. Minerva Anestesiol 2010;76(5):362-8.

95 Nolan JP, Morley PT, Hoek TV, Hickey RW, Kloeck W, Billi J et al. Therapeutic hypothermia after cardiac arrest: an advisory statement by the Advanced Life Support Task Force of the International Liaison Committee on Resuscitation. Circulation 2003;108(1):118-21.

96 Nielsen N, Wetterslev J, Cronberg T, Erlinge D, Gasche Y, Hassager C et al. Targeted temperature management at 33 C versus 36 C after cardiac arrest. N Engl J Med 2013;369(23):2197-206.

97 Bernard SA, Gray TW, Buist MD, Jones BM, Silvester W, Gutteridge G et al. Treatment of comatose survivors of out-of-hospital cardiac arrest with induced hypothermia. N Engl J Med 2002;346(8):557-63.

98 Polderman KH, Herold I. Therapeutic hypothermia and controlled normothermia in the intensive care unit: practical considerations, side effects, and cooling methods. Crit Care Med 2009;37(3):1101-20.

99 Greyson B. Incidence and correlates of near-death experiences in a cardiac care unit. General Hospital Psychiatry 2003;25(4):269-76.

100 Greyson B. Getting comfortable with near death experiences. Missouri Med 2013;110(6):471.

101 James D. What emergency department staff need to know about near-death experiences. Adv Emerg Nurs J 2004;26(1):29-34.

102 Parnia S, Fenwick P. Near death experiences in cardiac arrest: visions of a dying brain or visions of a new science of consciousness. Resuscitation 2002;52(1):5-11.

103 Belanti J, Perera M, Jagadheesan K. Phenomenology of near-death experiences: a cross-cultural perspective. Transcultural Psychiatry 2008;45(1):121-33.

104 Cant R, Cooper S, Chung C, O'Connor M. The divided self: near death experiences of resuscitated patients – a review of literature. Int Emerg Nurs 2012;20(2):88-93.

105 Mazer MA, Cox LA, Capon JA. The public's attitude and perception concerning witnessed cardiopulmonary resuscitation. Crit Care Med 2006;34(12):2925-8.

106 Ong MEH, Chung WL, Mei JSE. Comparing attitudes of the public and medical staff towards witnessed resuscitation in an Asian population. Resuscitation 2007;73(1):103-8.

107 Hung MS, Pang S. Family presence preference when patients are receiving resuscitation in an accident and emergency department. J Adv Nurs 2011;67(1):56-67.

108 Jabre P, Belpomme V, Azoulay E, Jacob L, Bertrand L, Lapostolle F et al. Family presence during cardiopulmonary resuscitation. N Engl J Med 2013;368(11):1008-18.

109 Schmidt B. Review of three qualitative studies of family presence during resuscitation. The Qualitative Report 2010;15(3):731-6.

110 Dwyer TA. Predictors of public support for family presence during cardiopulmonary resuscitation: a population based study. Int J Nurs Stud 2015; in press, <http://dx.doi.org/10.1016/j.ijnurstu.2015.03.004>.

111 Stub D, Bernard S, Pellegrino V, Smith K, Walker T, Stephenson M et al. Issues in establishing the refractory out-of-hospital cardiac arrest treated with mechanical CPR, hypothermia, ECMO and early reperfusion (CHEER) study. Heart, Lung and Circulation 2012;21:S163.

112 Chen Y-S, Lin J-W, Yu H-Y, Ko W-J, Jerng J-S, Chang W-T et al. Cardiopulmonary resuscitation with assisted extracorporeal life-support versus conventional cardiopulmonary resuscitation in adults with in-hospital cardiac arrest: an observational study and propensity analysis. Lancet 2008;372(9638):554-61.

113 Adams BD, Benger J. Should we take patients to hospital in cardiac arrest? BMJ 2014;349:5659.

114 Morrison LJ, Eby D, Veigas PV, Zhan C, Kiss A, Arcieri V et al. Implementation trial of the basic life support termination of resuscitation rule: reducing the transport of futile out-of-hospital cardiac arrests. Resuscitation. 2014;85(4):486-91.

115 Lynn J, Gregory CO. Regulating hearts and minds: the mismatch of law, custom and resuscitation decisions. J Am Geriatr Soc 2003; 51(10):1502-3.

116 European Resuscitation Council. Part 2: ethical aspects of CPR and ECC. Resuscitation 2000;46:17-27.

117 Salins NS, Pai SG, Vidyasagar M, Sobhana M. Ethics and medico legal aspects of "not for resuscitation". Indian J Palliat Care 2010;16(2):66.

118 Rabkin M, Gillerman G, Rice N. Orders not to resuscitate. NEngl J Med 1976;295:364-72.

119 Kerridge I, Pearson S, Rolfe I, Lowe M. Decision making in CPR: attitudes of hospital patients and health care professionals. Med J Aust 1998;169:128-31.

120 Mockford C, Clarke B, Field R, Fritz Z, Grove A, Waugh N et al. A systematic review of do-not-attempt-cardiopulmonary-resuscitation (DNACPR) orders: summarising the evidence around decision making and implementation. Resuscitation 2014;85:S85.

121 Harris D, Willoughby H. Resuscitation on television: realistic or ridiculous? A quantitative observational analysis of the portrayal of cardiopulmonary resuscitation in television medical drama. Resuscitation 2009;80(11):1275-9.

122 Yuen JK, Reid MC, Fetters MD. Hospital do-not-resuscitate orders: why they have failed and how to fix them. J Gen Intern Med 2011;26(7):791-7.

123 Smith K, Andrew E, Lijovic M, Nehme Z, Bernard S. Quality of life and functional outcomes 12 months after out-of-hospital cardiac arrest. Circulation 2015;131(2):174-81.

124 Heyland D, Frank C, Groll D. Understanding cardiopulmonary resuscitation decision making: perspectives of seriously ill hospitalised patients and family members. Chest 2006;130:419-28.

125 Sharma RK, Jain N, Peswani N, Szmuilowicz E, Wayne DB, Cameron KA. Unpacking resident-led code status discussions: results from a mixed methods study. J Gen Int Med 2014;29(5):750-7.

126 Yost CC, Bloom R. Neonatal resuscitation. Crit Care Obstetr 2010:108.

127 Luo X, Zhang H, Chen G, Ding W, Huang L. Active compression-decompression cardiopulmonary resuscitation (CPR) versus standard CPR for cardiac arrest patients: a meta-analysis. World J Emerg Med 2013;4(4):266-72.

128 Babbs CF. The case for interposed abdominal compression CPR in hospital settings. Analg Resusc: Curr Res 2013;3:1. of. 2014;6:2.

129 Ristagno G, Li Y, Gullo A, Bisera J. Amplitude spectrum area as a predictor of successful defibrillation. In: Anaesthesia and Pharmacology of Intensive Care Emergency Medicine APICE: Springer; 2011, pp 141-60.

130 Monteleone PP, Borek HA, Althoff SO. Electrical therapies in cardiac arrest. Emerg Med Clin North Am 2012;30(1):51-63.

131 Link MS, Atkins DL, Passman RS, Halperin HR, Samson RA, White RD et al. Part 6: Electrical therapies automated external defibrillators, defibrillation, cardioversion, and pacing: 2010 American Heart Association Guidelines for Cardiopulmonary Resuscitation and Emergency Cardiovascular Care. Circulation 2010;122(18 suppl 3):S706-S19.

132 Morley P. Cardiopulmonary resuscitation. In: Harley I, Hore P, eds. Anaesthesia: An introduction. 5th ed. East Hawthorn, Victoria: IP Communications; 2012, pp 174–89.

133 Zhu X-Y, Lin B-C, Zhang Q-S, Ye H-M, Yu R-J. A prospective evaluation of the efficacy of the laryngeal mask airway during neonatal resuscitation. Resuscitation 2011;82(11):1405-9.

134 Yamaga S, Une K, Kyo M, Suzuki K, Kobayashi Y, Nakagawa I et al. Gas insufflation in the stomach during cardiopulmonary resuscitation using laryngeal tube ventilation in comparison with bag-valve-mask ventilation. Circulation 2012;126(21 Supplement):A295.

135 Soar J. Which airway for cardiac arrest? Do supraglottic airways devices have a role? Resuscitation 2013;84(9):1163-4.

Chapter 26

Postanaesthesia recovery

Paula Foran, Andrea Marshall

KEY WORDS

anaesthesia

neuromuscular
 blockade

postanaesthesia care

postoperative
 complications

Learning objectives

After reading this chapter, you should be able to:

- describe the principles of immediate postoperative care with regard to respiratory and cardiovascular management

- discuss the assessment and management of complications following surgery and general anaesthesia

- discuss the principles and possible complications of central neural blockade

- discuss the signs, symptoms and treatment for anaesthetic complications such as malignant hyperthermia, inadvertent hypothermia and awareness under anaesthesia.

Introduction

In 1751, realising that postoperative patients were vulnerable, the first Post Anaesthetic Care Unit was created.[1] By the 1940s the importance of recovering from anaesthesia was recognised. Areas close to the operating theatre were created allowing patients leaving the operating theatre to be closely monitored for signs of respiratory failure so that appropriate management could be instituted.[1] Today, perianaesthesia nursing is recognised as a specialty in its own right and postgraduate education opportunities exist to support nurses to develop expertise in this area.

While surgical techniques and anaesthetic medications have changed exponentially, the primary purpose of immediate postanaesthesia/postoperative care, whether provided in the postanaesthesia care unit (PACU) or intensive care unit (ICU), has altered little in the last 70 years. The focus remains on critical evaluation and stabilisation of patients after surgery, with an emphasis on anticipation and prevention of complications arising from either the anaesthetic or the surgical procedure.[2] While this chapter is titled 'Postanaesthesia recovery', it is worth noting that patients are also recovering from their own specific surgical procedure, which may require specific assessment and management.

Timely, appropriate surgery and high quality pre- and postoperative care may be key in preventing deaths in the first 48 hours after surgical procedures.[3] The Australian National Consensus Statement on essential elements for recognising and responding to clinical deterioration[4] reports that measurable physiological abnormalities occur prior to adverse events such as cardiac arrest and death and suggests that early recognition of changes in a patient's condition, followed by prompt and effective treatment, can minimise poor outcomes. Surgical complications are estimated to account for approximately 40% of all adverse events,[5] making surgical patients prime candidates for clinical deterioration. This increased risk might require some patients to be admitted to the intensive care unit following surgery, especially if they require ongoing high level assessment and management. Postoperative patients who are not critically ill may also be recovered in ICU after hours, and it is this group of patients to which this chapter is directed. In this chapter a brief overview of nursing the patient in the period following surgery and anaesthesia is provided with the focus being on the recovery of non-critically ill patients.

In this chapter we will review anaesthesia and commonly used anaesthetic agents, postanaesthesia nursing care and assessment and management of specific postoperative complications. We acknowledge that postanaesthesia care nursing is a specialty in its own right and that this chapter will provide an overview. We encourage readers to refer to the end of this chapter for further reading about this specialty.

Introduction to anaesthesia

There are five components to anaesthesia. These include hypnosis, analgesia, muscle relaxation, sympatholysis and amnesia. As a result of improvements in pharmacological agents used in anaesthesia we now see patients emerging from anaesthesia in minutes rather than hours and, consequently, patients can be discharged from perianaesthesia care more quickly. Critical care nurses, whether they specialise in postanaesthesia recovery or not, need a thorough understanding of the pharmacology related to anaesthesia as this underpins patient assessment and management.

Phases of anaesthesia

There are four stages to anaesthesia that a critical care nurse should recognise and consider when undertaking patient assessment. The initiation of analgesia through to the loss of consciousness constitutes stage I, or the stage of analgesia. This is the lightest level of anaesthesia and, although there is sensory and mental depression, patients can often obey commands, breathe normally and maintain protective reflexes.[6] Stage II begins with loss of consciousness and ends when a regular breathing pattern starts and the eyelid reflex is lost. Also called the stage of delirium, stage II is characterised by excitement. Responses such as vomiting and laryngospasm can also occur in this stage, although with newer anaesthetic agents most patients move through this stage quite quickly.

Stage III, the stage of surgical anaesthesia, lasts from the time of onset of regular breathing to breathing cessation. Patients in stage III anaesthesia will not respond when a surgical incision is made. In stage III patients will have sensory depression, loss of recall, depressed reflexes and some evidence of skeletal muscle relaxation. In stage III anaesthesia swallowing, retching and vomiting reflexes disappear sequentially during induction and reappear in the same order during emergence from anaesthesia.[6]

During recovery from anaesthesia, if the patient is breathing using diaphragmatic muscles but does not have intercostal muscle involvement, they are likely still in stage III of anaesthesia. Lack of muscle tone, particularly in the jaw and abdomen, also suggests that the patient is in stage III anaesthesia. As the anaesthesia lightens, respiration will have a normal rate and rhythm.

Stage IV of anaesthesia lasts from when respiration stops to failure of the circulatory system, hence is referred to as the stage of overdose. Determining the stage of anaesthesia cannot be done by assessing any single parameter. Rather, all clinical signs should be considered in relation to the patient's clinical condition and the particular anaesthetic agent used.

Anaesthetic agents

Once referred to as the 'art of anaesthesia', modern anaesthesia now rests firmly on scientific foundations; however, the practice still remains a mixture of science and art.[7] The aim of good anaesthesia is to provide the safest anaesthetic, in the lightest plane possible, which allows a given procedure to be performed while the patient is pain free. This is why other medications, such as muscle relaxants, will be given in conjunction with anaesthetic agents so that muscle relaxation can occur at a lighter stage of anaesthesia.

Non-opioid agents

Non-opioid intravenous agents include non-barbiturates, barbiturates and sedatives. Non-opioid drugs interact with gamma-aminobutyric acid (GABA), an inhibitory neurotransmitter in the brain, with the specific actions being drug dependent.

Non-barbiturates

Propofol is likely the most common non-barbiturate used clinically. Its unique pharmacological characteristics include quick onset, relatively short emergence time and minimal side effects, making propofol (2,6-diisopropylphenol) one of the most widely used short-acting intravenously administered anaesthetic/hypnotic drugs.[8] Propofol as a 1% solution is administered intravenously at a dose of 1.5 to 2.5 mg/kg for induction,[9] although lower doses are used for elderly patients and those with hypovolaemia or cardiac disease.[10] As a single agent propofol is usually administered quickly (over 15 seconds) with unconsciousness occurring in about 30 seconds. With a half-life of 2–9 minutes, emergence from this drug is rapid and there are usually few effects on the central nervous system. If continuous infusion of propofol has been used for more than 12 hours, a longer recovery period can be expected.[10]

When administered, propofol can decrease cerebral blood flow, cerebral perfusion pressure and intracranial pressure. Blood pressure and cardiac output are also reduced and this can be more pronounced in those patients with compromised left ventricular function and hypovolaemia. The depressant effect of propofol on the respiratory system may result in airway and ventilatory support being required for those patients who are not already intubated and ventilated. There is some suggestion in the literature that propofol may have some short-acting analgesic properties,[11] although this effect is not well established and conflicting results exist in the literature.[12]

Practice tip

Propofol administered to elderly patients can result in a significant drop in blood pressure. Therefore, this group of patients should be carefully monitored.

Etomidate is a short-acting hypnotic agent without any analgesic effects. Although not available in all countries, and not licensed for use in Australia, etomidate is used in many countries, especially for intubation of critically ill patients, mainly because of the minimal cardiovascular effects of the drug.[13] Etomidate causes only a slight increase in heart rate and slight decrease in blood pressure. Cardiac index and peripheral vascular resistance are not significantly influenced and the drug does not seem to be arrhythmogenic. Controversy does exist around the use of etomidate because it inhibits steroid synthesis with adrenal suppression lasing for 5–8 hours following a single dose.[14] Consequently etomidate should only be administered to select patients.

Barbiturates

Barbiturates as an intravenous anaesthetic agent have a long history, and thiopental sodium was used frequently until the 1990s but is used less frequently since the introduction of non-barbiturates such as propofol.[15] Previously, thiopental sodium was used in conjunction with other anaesthetics because it had poor analgesic properties. The disadvantages of thiopental sodium also include adverse effect on respiratory function, coughing, laryngospasm and bronchospasm. The highly alkaline pH of the drug could also contribute to tissue necrosis if extravenous administration occurred. Thiopental sodium also has antianalgesic properties at low doses, so patients recovering from surgery may have more pain and therefore be irritable and restless in the initial recovery phase.[10]

Practice tip

Obese patients administered thiopental sodium may have delayed wakening because the drug is highly fat soluble.

Inhalation anaesthesia

Assessing emergence from inhalation anaesthesia requires an understanding of the pharmacological effects of these agents, and an overview of their characteristics. A brief summary of these agents is provided in Table 26.1. These agents are essentially depressant drugs and some are more

TABLE 26.1

Common inhalation anaesthetic agents[6]

AGENT	CHARACTERISTICS
Isoflurane	• Reduces systemic arterial blood pressure and systemic vascular resistance • Heart rate increased during recovery • Produces respiratory depression • Produces skeletal muscle relaxation in a dose-related fashion • Does not sensitise the myocardium to catecholamines compared to halothane so fewer arrhythmias are observed • Patient awakens 15–30 minutes following termination of anaesthetic gas but may be longer if surgery exceeds 45–60 minutes
Sevoflurane	• Emergence from anaesthesia occurs in minutes • Decreases blood pressure and systemic vascular resistance • A respiratory depressant • Does not increase risk of arrhythmias • Can increase intracranial pressure in a dose-related manner
Desflurane	• Extremely rapid emergence • Dose-related decrease in blood pressure • Low rate of cardiac arrhythmias • Irritates respiratory tract and induces coughing • May induce laryngospasm • Almost totally eliminated by the respiratory system
Nitrous oxide	• No side effects unless hypoxia is present • Non-toxic and non-irritating • Can be administered alone or in combination with other agents • Diffusion hypoxia can occur when not enough nitrous oxide is removed from the lungs at the end of the surgical procedure

likely to affect myocardial and respiratory function than others. Because of respiratory depression, during recovery it is essential that patients are encouraged to continue taking deep breaths. The increased rate and depth of breathing can also assist with eliminating the agents into the atmosphere.

Practice tip

Encouraging deep breathing during the recovery period is essential to promote removal of inhalation gases.

Opioids

Opioids are an important agent in the anaesthetic process and the postoperative period, with their main purpose being to provide analgesia. Opioids also enhance the effectiveness of inhaled anaesthetics allowing lower doses to be provided. In the postoperative period, opioids are commonly administered to alleviate pain associated with the surgical process.

Opioids, whether they are natural or synthetic substances, bind to receptors producing a morphine-like or opioid agonist effect.[16] Opioid receptors include the mu (μ), delta (δ) and kappa (κ) receptors located in the central nervous system, mostly in the brain stem and spinal cord. The mu receptors, specifically the mu-1 receptors, are responsible for supraspinal analgesia effects when stimulated. When mu-2 receptors are stimulated hypoventilation, bradycardia, physical dependence, euphoria and ileus can occur.

The most common opioid drugs used for pain relief in the postoperative period include morphine and fentanyl (Table 26.2) with morphine the most widely used and the standard against which other pain-relieving agents are compared.[17] Pethidine is no longer commonly used for long-term pain relief due to the accumulation of normeperidine over time, which can result in central nervous system toxicity.[18]

Practice tip

Morphine is metabolised by the liver and the metabolites are excreted by the kidneys so the analgesic and sedating effects can be prolonged and potentially dangerous for patients with renal failure.

Practice tip

Pethidine (meperidine) is metabolised in the liver to normeperidine. Elderly patients have less tolerance to the central depressant effects of pethidine so this drug should be avoided or the dose limited to 25 mg.

Spinal and epidural opioid administration

Opioids can be administered as part of either spinal or epidural anaesthesia. In spinal anaesthesia, drugs are administered into the cerebral spinal fluid that surrounds

---

TABLE 26.2

Opioid analgesics used for postoperative pain relief[16]

DRUG	DOSE[a]	ADVANTAGES	DISADVANTAGES
Morphine	IV: 4–10 mg Peak analgesic effect within 20 minutes; duration 2 hours IM: 10 mg Onset of action approximately 20 minutes with peak effect in 45–90 minutes; duration of action 4 hours	Minimal effect on heart rate/rhythm and blood pressure	Depresses respiratory rate and tidal volume Can cause orthostatic hypotension and syncope Can cause nausea and vomiting Causes histamine release
Fentanyl	IV: 1–2 mcg/kg OR 25–100 mcg PRN for analgesia Onset of action 4–6 minutes; peak effect within 5–15 minutes; duration 20–40 minutes IM: Onset of action 7–15 minutes; duration 1 to 2 hours	Has little or no hypotensive effect Usually does not cause nausea and vomiting	Delayed onset respiratory depression because of a secondary peak in the concentration of the drug occurs 45 minutes after apparent recovery Rapid IV administration can provoke bronchial constriction
Pethidine hydrochloride (meperidine hydrochloride)	IV: 25–50 mg every 3–4 hours IM: 25–100 mg every 3–4 hours IM: Onset of action 10 minutes; duration of action 2 to 4 hours	Minimal cardiovascular effects although a transient increase in heart rate may occur with IV administration	May slow rate of respiration but this usually returns to normal within 15 minutes of IV injection Can cause histamine release Causes orthostatic hypotension

[a]Average recommended doses for adults.

IM = intramuscular; IV = intravenous.

the spinal cord, and puncture of the dura is required for this administration. In contrast with epidural administration, the drugs are delivered outside the dura.[19] Administration of morphine (0.1 to 0.2 mg) directly into the spinal fluid results in a maximal concentration within 5–10 minutes; the duration of action is 80–200 minutes. In contrast, a higher dose of morphine is required when administered into the epidural space (5 mg) with pain relief in effect within 30–60 minutes that can last up to 24 hours. Additional morphine can be administered via the epidural route if required to a maximum of 10 mg in 24 hours. Fentanyl and sufentanil can also be administered epidurally and are more suited for continuous infusion.

Opioid antagonists

Should opioid-induced respiratory depression occur in the postanaesthesia period an opioid antagonist might be needed. Naloxone is a pure opioid antagonist that reverses the depressant effects of the drug and is usually administered in a titrated fashion, assessing patient response. A dose of 0.1 mg to 0.2 mg is usually sufficient. The onset of action is quick and occurs within 1–2 minutes of administration; the half-life is 30–80 minutes.[20] After 3–5 minutes, if reversal is still not achieved, additional doses of naloxone can be administered.[21]

When intrathecal or epidural opioids are administered close observation of the patient, particularly respiratory and conscious state, is essential as there may be delayed respiratory depression. Caution should also be taken with additional opioid administration during the first 24 hours as the half-life of opioids administered via these routes is increased.

Benzodiazepines and benzodiazepine antagonists

Benzodiazepines are sedatives that depress the limbic system and may cause some cortical depression.[22] They interact with GABA, the inhibitory neurotransmitter, causing decreased orientation through a hypnotic effect, retrograde amnesia, anxiolysis and skeletal muscle relaxation.[10] The hypnotic action of benzodiazepines is enhanced by the effects of opiates and barbiturates.

Midazolam is the most popular benzodiazepine used in anaesthesia and critical care and has a wide variety of uses including procedural sedation and induction of anaesthesia. While routine premedications are no longer given, midazolam can be used for some patients to allay anxiety[23] and is also an intraoperative adjunct to both inhalation and regional anaesthesia. Midazolam affects the benzodiazepine receptors in the central nervous system causing reduced anxiety and profound anterograde amnesia. Midazolam has a rapid onset of action — less than 60 seconds – with a peak effect seen within 2–5 minutes.[24] The duration of action is between 1 and 3 hours. Cardiovascular effects of midazolam include decreased blood pressure, increased heart rate and reduced systemic vascular resistance; thus

it should be used with caution in patients with known myocardial ischaemia. In small doses midazolam is used as an anti-emetic.[25]

> ### Practice tip
>
> Midazolam does not affect intracranial pressure and, therefore, can safely be used in patients with intracranial pathology or who are undergoing neurosurgery.

Although not commonly used, diazepam and lorazepam are longer acting benzodiazepines that may be used for induction and as an adjunct to intravenous anaesthesia. Both diazepam and lorazepam have a longer half-life and delayed onset of effect compared to that of midazolam.[10] Diazepam has few cardiovascular depressant effects but is known to cause slight respiratory depression, an effect that is enhanced when it is administered at the same time as opiates.

If required, the pharmacological effects of benzodiazepines can be reversed. Flumazenil is a benzodiazepine agonist that should be administered intravenously in 0.1-mg increments to avoid rapid reawakening. The usual dose is 0.4 mg and the maximum amount administered should be no more than 1.0 mg.[10] The drug takes effect within 5 minutes of administration and has a duration of action between 1 and 2 hours.

> ### Practice tip
>
> Flumazenil has a shorter duration of action than most benzodiazepines so patients should be carefully assessed for resedation after the initial dose is administered. If signs of resedation are evident, additional flumazenil can be administered every 20 minutes to a maximum dose of 3.0 mg in a 1-hour period.

Non-specific effects of benzodiazepines can be reversed with the administration of physostigmine, an anticholinesterase that crosses the blood–brain barrier. Physostigmine inhibits acetylcholinesterase making increased amounts of acetylcholine available at the central nervous system receptors that are affected by benzodiazepines. Doses of 0.5 mg to 1.0 mg should be slowly administered in order to avoid cholinergic side effects.[10]

Butyrophenones

As sedative agents, butyrophenones such as haloperidol and droperidol produce a state of profound calm and immobility where the patient appears to be pain free and dissociated from their surroundings. Butyrophenone use in anaesthesia is, however, uncommon. Haloperidol is rarely used because of its long duration of action and high incidence of extrapyramidal side effects. Droperidol can be used on its own or in conjunction with fentanyl as part of a neurolept analgesic technique. Droperidol is also administered in small doses (0.625–1.25 mg intravenously) in the postoperative period to manage nausea and vomiting.[25]

Practice tip

Some patients who have received droperidol report feeling terrified and unable to express how they feel while also having an outward appearance of being very calm. It is important that in the postanaesthesia period support is provided to patients even if they appear calm.

In the postanaesthesia period, regular stimulation of the patient and encouragement of deep breathing is necessary as patients can drift back to sleep and have slow and/or shallow respirations. In some instances patients who have received droperidol have become apnoeic.[10]

Neuromuscular blocking agents

Since the 1940s neuromuscular blocking agents have been used as pharmacological agents in anaesthesia. Although not all patients will require neuromuscular blockade during anaesthesia, these agents may be given to facilitate endotracheal intubation. Muscle relaxation is also indicated to facilitate some surgical procedures such as abdominal surgery, in ophthalmic surgery to relax extraocular muscles and to facilitate mechanical ventilation. Nurses who are responsible for the assessment and management of the postoperative patient should understand the physiology of neuromuscular transmission and mechanism of action of the various neuromuscular blocking agents that may be used in anaesthesia.

The neuromuscular junction has three components: the motor nerve fibre, the synaptic cleft and the motor end-plate of striated muscle (see Figure 26.1).

Acetylcholine (ACh), a neurotransmitter that is deactivated by the cholinesterase family of enzymes, is stored and released from the presynaptic terminal and is the only neurotransmitter used in the somatic nervous system.[26] ACh receptors are located on the motor end-plate and, when bound to ACh, membrane channels open and this results in an influx of sodium ions causing depolarisation of the motor end-plate membrane. Potassium ions exit causing repolarisation, allowing the membrane potential to again become negative. These sequences allow muscle contraction to occur. ACh is broken down by acetylcholinesterase, which is present in the synaptic cleft, and is metabolised before the excited muscle returns to its resting state. The broken down ACh elements are then used for the manufacture of new ACh molecules in the nerve terminal ending.

Non-depolarising neuromuscular blocking agents

Non-depolarising neuromuscular blocking agents block the action of ACh at the postsynaptic receptor sites in the neuromuscular junction (Figure 26.2) by competing with ACh at these binding sites and blocking neuromuscular transmission.[28] There are many different types of non-depolarising neuromuscular blocking agents, and their availability and use varies internationally.[29] Although the end effect of these agents is similar, their pharmacological effects differ in relation to onset of action, duration of effect and excretion (Table 26.3).

Residual neuromuscular block is a complication that can occur following use of neuromuscular blockade[32] and can result in adverse respiratory complications.[33]

FIGURE 26.1 Neuromuscular junction.[27]

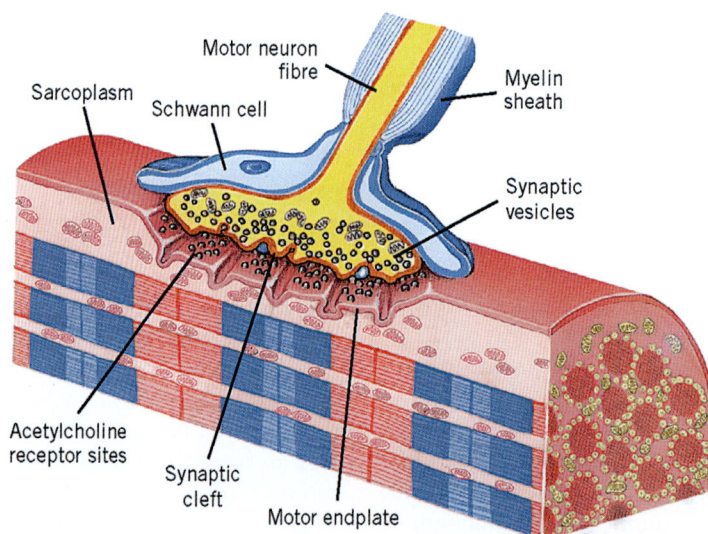

Adapted from Patton KT, Thibodeau GA. Anatomy and physiology. 7th ed. St Louis: Mosby; 2010, with permission.

TABLE 26.3

Pharmacological overview of commonly used non-depolarising neuromuscular blocking agents[30]

	PANCURONIUM	VECURONIUM BROMIDE	ATRACURIUM BESYLATE	CISATRACURIUM BESYLATE	ROCURONIUM BROMIDE
Dose for intubation (mg/kg)	0.06–0.1	0.08–0.1	0.4–0.5	0.1–0.2	0.1
Intubation to relaxation time (min)	4.0	2.5–3.0	2.0–2.5	2.8–3.4	1.0–2.0
Dose for muscle relaxation (mg/kg)	0.04–0.08	0.05–0.06	0.2–0.5	2.5	0.6–1.0
Recovery time (min)	84–114	30–60	30–45	55–75	30–90
Reversible	Yes	Yes	Yes	Yes	Yes
Time to reversal (after initial dose, in min)	40–60	25–80 (dose dependent)	20–35	10–15	5–10
Cumulative effects	Yes	Slight	No	No	No
Fasciculations and muscle soreness	No	None	No	No	No
Risk of histamine release	Slight to none	None	Minimal	No	No
Cardiovascular effects	Slight increase in pulse and increase in blood pressure	None	Few	None	None

Adapted with permission from Drain CB. Neuromuscular blocking agents. In: Odom-Forren J, ed. Perianesthesia nursing: A critical care approach. 6th ed. St Louis: Elsevier; 2013.

FIGURE 26.2   A, Normal muscle contraction. **B**, Neuromuscular blockade.[31]

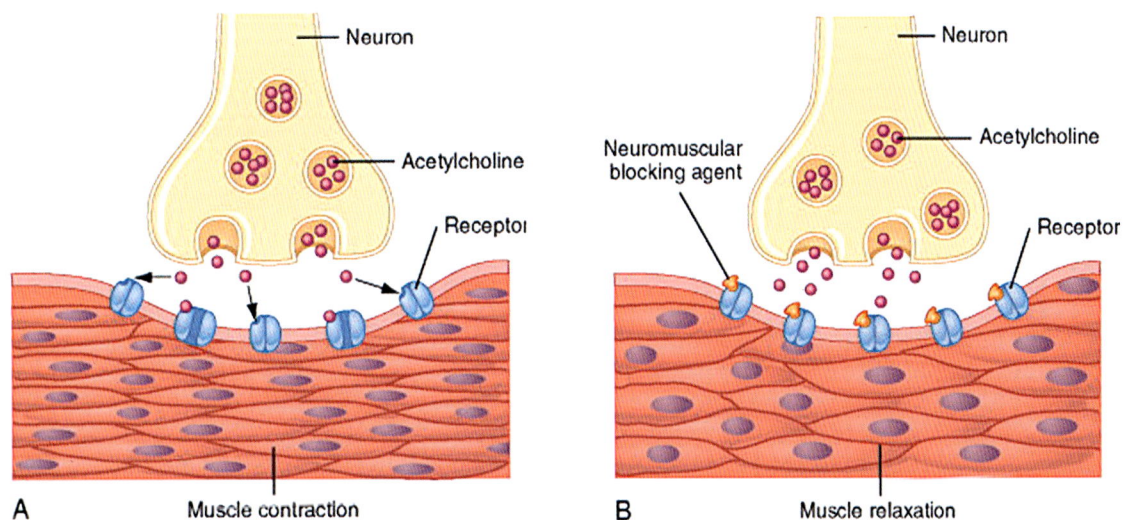

Adapted from Siedlecki SL. Pain and sedation. In: Carlson K, ed. Advanced critical care nursing. St Louis: Saunders; 2009, Figure 4-13, p 79, with permission.

Pharmacological reversal of neuromuscular block can be used when the effects of the neuromuscular blocking agent remain present at the end of the surgery. Conventional reversal of neuromuscular blockade involves administration of an anticholinesterase. Anticholinesterase inhibits the action of cholinesterases that inactivate ACh, thus potentiating the effects of the neurotransmitter ACh, and helps restore skeletal muscle activity.[30] To avoid residual neuromuscular blockade anticholinesterases should be administered at least 20 minutes prior to extubation to help facilitate complete recovery of neuromuscular function.[34] Anticholinesterases stimulate the muscarinic receptors and elicit side effects including bradycardia, arrhythmias, bronchospasm as well as nausea and vomiting. For this reason antimuscarinic agents such as atropine or glycopyrrolate must be administered at the same time as the reversal agent.[26]

Sugammadex is also used to reverse the effect of neuromuscular blockade, specifically when the agents rocuronium and vecuronium are used. Sugammadex is the first selective neuromuscular drug binding agent and reverses the effect of the neuromuscular blocking drugs through encapsulation. Hypersensitivity to sugammadex can occur within the first 5 minutes following administration and, as such, patients receiving this drug should be closely monitored for signs of drug-induced hypersensitivity.[35]

> **Practice tip**
>
> When patients return from surgery, review their anaesthetic record to see whether a neuromuscular blocking agent has been used and, if it was, whether a reversal agent was given.

> **Practice tip**
>
> When dyspnoea occurs there is sometimes initial confusion between narcosis and residual muscle relaxants. Patients with narcosis may have a normal tidal volume but the rate is slow; residual muscle relaxant patients breathe very poorly due to a mechanical problem with their muscles of respiration but their respiratory effort is not impaired.

Depolarising neuromuscular blocking agents

Suxamethonium, also known as succinylcholine, is the only depolarising neuromuscular blocking agent used in anaesthesia. Suxamethonium is most often used in rapid sequence induction for the purpose of endotracheal intubation. Suxamethonium works at the site of the acetylcholine receptor and causes persistent depolarisation at the motor end-plate.[30] Patients administered suxamethonium demonstrate muscle fasciculations because of the sudden increase in acetylcholine at the motor end-plate.

A typical dose of suxamethonium is 0.5–1.5 mg/kg administered intravenously. The onset of action is rapid, usually within 30–60 seconds of administration. The very rapid onset of paralysis when using suxamethonium remains its true advantage as a patient can be intubated almost immediately. Suxamethonium administration can induce hyperkalaemia so its use in patients with electrolyte disorders, such as those with severe burns or diabetic ketoacidosis, is not recommended.[36] The duration of action of suxamethonium is relatively short as the drug is hydrolysed rapidly by plasma pseudocholinesterase. Paralysis associated with administration of suxamethonium usually only lasts 5–10 minutes. Some patients may have reduced pseudocholinesterase activity. This can be an acquired deficiency that might be associated with liver disease, severe anaemia, malnutrition, prolonged pyrexia, pregnancy and renal dialysis. Congenital deficiencies in pseudocholinesterase are relatively uncommon.

> **Practice tip**
>
> Patients with either acquired or congenital pseudocholinesterase deficiency may remain paralysed for prolonged periods of time and may require mechanical ventilation for up to 48 hours.

Factors influencing neuromuscular blocking agents

There are a number of factors that can influence neuromuscular blocking agents. Many of these include drug interactions and alterations in electrolyte balance (Table 26.4). Dehydration can also increase the sensitivity to skeletal muscle relaxants because of increased neuromuscular excitability, slowed renal function and drug excretion and increased plasma concentration of the relaxant. Acid–base balance can also influence neuromuscular blockade where acidosis and increased carbon dioxide levels result in a stronger effect of the neuromuscular blocking agent pancuronium.[30] Hypothermia can antagonise the effect of neuromuscular blocking agents, as with pancuronium, or can potentiate the effect as seen with suxamethonium.

Non-steroidal anti-inflammatory drugs

Non-steroidal anti-inflammatory drugs such as ketorolac and indomethacin can be used as analgesics in the postoperative period, although indomethacin is used much less frequently. Ketorolac has analgesic, anti-inflammatory and anti-pyretic actions and works by inhibiting the cyclooxygenase enzyme system, thereby decreasing prostaglandin synthesis. Ketorolac is administered by intramuscular or intravenous injection or given orally. An intramuscular dose of 30 mg as a loading dose can be followed by a further 15 mg after 6 hours. Ketorolac can also be used in conjunction with opioids for effective postoperative pain relief. The peak effect of ketorolac occurs in approximately 45–60 minutes so it can be administered approximately 1 hour before the end of the surgical procedure so that maximal pain relief occurs at emergence from anaesthesia.

> **Practice tip**
>
> The recommended dose range of ketorolac is 15–60 mg. Lower doses of ketorolac should be administered to the elderly.

Dissociative anaesthetics

Ketamine is a dissociative drug that selectively blocks pain conduction and perception yet does not depress those parts of the central nervous system not involved in pain transmission and perception.[10] When patients are administered ketamine they experience profound analgesia and unconsciousness but respiratory function is usually unimpaired. Ketamine can induce bronchodilation and some published case reports suggest that this drug might be useful in asthma, although adequately powered randomised controlled trials are required before definitive recommendations can be made about this treatment.[37] Ketamine also causes increased cerebral blood flow so should be avoided in those patients at risk of developing increased intracranial pressure.

Of particular importance to the nurse managing a postoperative patient who has received ketamine is an understanding that psychic aberrations can occur on emergence from anaesthesia. Patients can experience vivid dreaming with or without psychomotor activity. They can appear confused, irrational and have hallucinations. These effects can be managed by avoiding early verbal or tactile stimulation. If the patient does have augmented psychomotor responses and irrational behavior, medications such as dexmedetomidine or a benzodiazepine can be administered.

> **Practice tip**
>
> Ketamine can be used as a sole anaesthetic agent for paediatric patients who appear to be less prone to psychic disturbances.

Drug interactions

Many patients undergoing anaesthesia will be taking medications in addition to those required for surgery and anaesthesia. Whenever two or more drugs are given to a patient there is a potential for drug interactions to occur. Such interactions can have a potentially negative effect on the patient and knowledge of these interactions will help guide nursing assessment. Table 26.4 provides a summary of common medications and how these can interact with pharmacological agents used in surgery and anaesthesia.[38]

> **Practice tip**
>
> Some antibiotics such as gentamycin can potentiate non-depolarising muscle relaxants and make reversal of these agents more difficult

---

> **BOX 26.1**
>
> **Monoamine oxidase inhibitors**
>
> The interaction of this class of drug with common anaesthetic agents is important to recognise. Although monoamine oxidase inhibitors (MAOI) are not as commonly used as in the past, many patients may still be prescribed these for management of depression. MAOIs inhibit N-demethylase and thus decrease the breakdown of pethidine/meperidine. A type I response to this drug interaction includes seizures, agitation, rigidity and hyperpyrexia. A Type II response includes hypotension, respiratory depression and coma.
>
> *Adapted from* Rasool F, Ghafoor R, Lambert DG. Antidepressants and antipsychotics: anaesthetic implications. Anaesth Intensive Care Med 2014;15(7):314–17.

Local and regional anaesthesia

Local anaesthesia works by blocking nerve conduction so that the patient does not feel painful stimuli. Local anaesthetics work by binding to sodium channels, keeping them open and inactive thus preventing depolarisation and transmission of the neuronal action potential. A second mechanism may also cause disruption of the ion channel when local anaesthetic molecules are incorporated into the cell membrane (Figure 26.3). The sensitivity to local anaesthetics depends on the nerve fibres, with sensitivity increased for the smaller nerve fibres. Myelinated fibres are also blocked before non-myelinated fibres, if they are of the same diameter.

> **Practice tip**
>
> Administration of local anaesthetics results in loss of nerve function, and consequently pain, temperature, touch and proprioception are affected. Skeletal muscle tone is the last to be affected. This explains why patients may be able to feel touch but not pain after receiving local anaesthesia.

Assessment and management of the patient receiving local or regional anaesthesia is provided later in this chapter.

Assessment and management in the postoperative period

When caring for a patient immediately after surgery, it is essential that the nurse has a full understanding of the possible complications of each individual procedure that has been performed. If a nurse is allocated a patient and they do not understand the surgical procedure they must ask, possibly at the time of anaesthetic handover, to gain an understanding of what complications might occur in their patient. It is beyond the scope of this text to discuss all possible procedural complications. However, some

TABLE 26.4
Drug–drug interactions[38]

DRUG	INTERACTION	RESULT	MECHANISM
ANTIHYPERTENSIVE DRUGS			
Propranolol	Inhalation anaesthetics	Bradycardia, hypotension	Additive effect
	Lignocaine	Enhanced negative inotropic effect	Propranolol reduces liver blood flow and lignocaine clearance
	Heparin	Myocardial depression	Heparin increases free fatty acids, which displace propranolol from plasma protein binding sites, leading to increased free propranolol
Lignocaine	Non-depolarising muscle relaxants	Increased duration of neuromuscular blockade	Synergistic effect
Digitalis	Suxamethonium /succinylcholine	Arrhythmias	Direct effect or caused by hyperkalaemia that can be induced by succinylcholine
	Thiazide diuretics	Increased potassium excreted by kidneys	Combined effect of two drugs on kidneys promotes potassium excretion
Quinidine	Digitalis	Can produce digitalis intoxication	Decreased digitalis clearance and increased concentration of digitalis
	Myasthenia gravis plus skeletal muscle relaxants	Postoperative respiratory depression	Blockade of acetylcholine receptors at neuromuscular postsynaptic membrane
ANTIBIOTICS			
Neomycin Streptomycin Dihydrostreptomycin Polymyxin A Polymxyin B Colistin Viomycin Paromomycin Kanamycin Lincomycin Gentamicin Tetracycline	Non-depolarising skeletal muscle relaxants	Potentiate non-depolarising muscle relaxants, respiratory depression	Neuromuscular blockade caused by reduction in amplitude of end-plate potential
OPIOIDS			
Morphine Fentanyl Sufentanil Remifentanil	Inhalation anaesthetics	Potentiation, respiratory and cardiovascular depression	Depressant effects of inhalation anaesthetics and opioids are additive
Pethidine/meperidine	Inhalation anaesthetics	Potentiation, respiratory and cardiovascular depression	Depressant effects of inhalation anaesthetics and opioids are additive
	Enovid Norinyl	Birth control pill potentiates pethidine/meperidine	Excess female sex hormones with oral contraceptive therapy, which may slow metabolism of pethidine/meperidine
	MAOI	MAOI interacts with pethidine/ meperidine metabolite	Type I: seizures Type II: hypotension

DRUG	INTERACTION	RESULT	MECHANISM
SYMPATHOMIMETIC AMINES			
Adrenaline	Inhalation anaesthetics	Cardiac arrhythmias	Anaesthetic agents may sensitise myocardium to endogenous and exogenous catecholamines
ELECTROLYTES			
Increased extracellular potassium	Skeletal muscle relaxants	Increased resistance to depolarisation and greater sensitivity to non-depolarising muscle relaxants	Acute increase in extracellular potassium increases end-plate transmembrane potential, thus causing hyperpolarisation
Decreased extracellular potassium	Skeletal muscle relaxants	Increased effects of depolarising muscle relaxants and increased resistance to non-depolarising muscle relaxants	Acute decrease in extracellular potassium lowers resting end-plate transmembrane potential
Increased calcium levels	Non-depolarising skeletal muscle relaxants	Decreased response	Calcium increases release of acetylcholine and enhances excitation–contraction coupling mechanism
Magnesium ions	Muscle relaxants	Potentiation	Magnesium ions cause partial muscle relaxation by blocking release of acetylcholine
Calcium chloride	Digitalis	Additive effect on heart	High concentrations of calcium inhibit positive inotropic actions of digitalis and potentiate digitalis toxicity
MISCELLANEOUS			
Furosemide Thiazide Ethacrynic acid	Non-depolarising skeletal muscle relaxants	Intensified neuromuscular block	Electrolyte imbalance (hypokalaemia)
Procaine Lignocaine	Non-depolarising and depolarising skeletal muscle relaxants	Enhanced neuromuscular blockade	Decreased end-plate potential
Lithium	Non-depolarising and depolarising skeletal muscle relaxants	Potentiated neuromuscular blockade	Lithium ions are substituted for sodium ions at presynaptic level
Chlorpromazine	Non-depolarising skeletal muscle relaxants	Enhanced neuromuscular blockade	Potentiation of neuromuscular blockade
All inhalation anaesthetics	Non-depolarising skeletal muscle relaxants	Augment block in dose-dependent manner	Central nervous system depression or presynaptic inhibition of acetylcholine
Insulin	Corticosteroids, oral contraceptives, loop and thiazide diuretics	Reduction in effects	Insulin antagonises effects
Hydrocortisone Dexamethasone Prednisone	Phenobarbital	Decreased effect of the steroids	Increased metabolism

Adapted from Nagelhout JJ. Basic principles of pharmacology. In: Odom-Forren J, ed. Perianesthesia nursing: A critical care approach. 6th ed. St Louis: Elsevier; 2013, with permission.

FIGURE 26.3 Mechanism of action for local anaesthesia.[39]

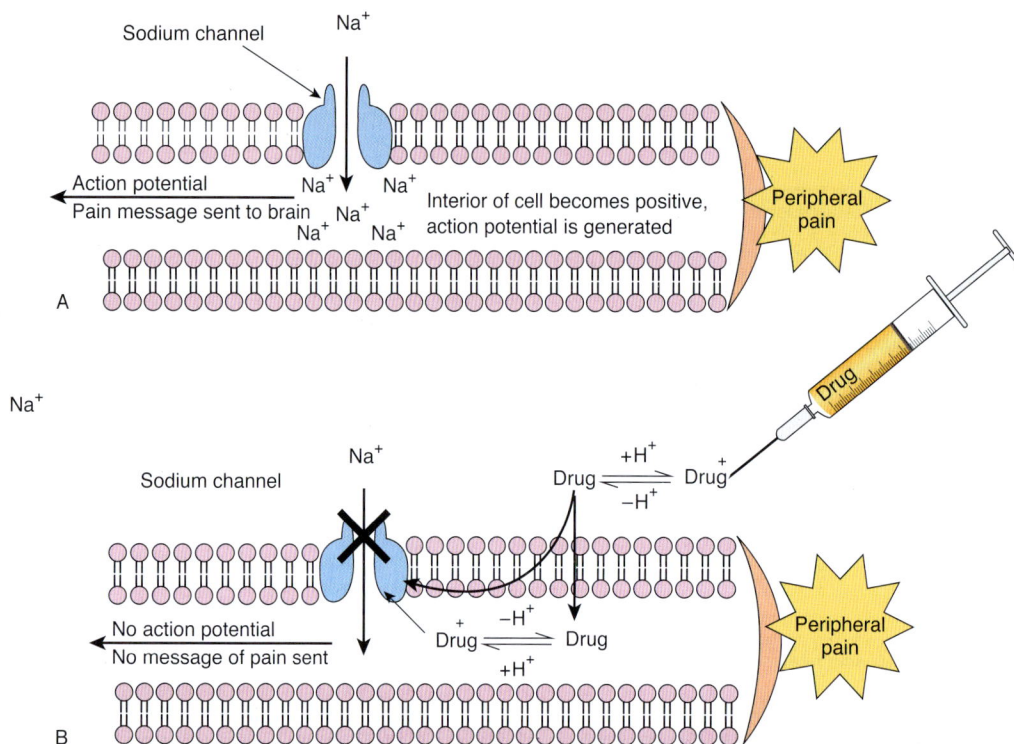

Adapted from Friel CJ, Eliadi C, Pesaturo KA. Local anesthetic use in perioperative areas. Perioperative Nurs Clin 2010;5:203–14, with permission.

examples of specific complications include: water intoxication and/or sodium depletion in surgery that flushes large amounts of saline solution or water under pressure (e.g. trans-urethral resection of the prostate [TURP], endometrial ablation); upper airway obstruction following surgery under the muscle layer of the neck (thyroidectomy, parotid cyst); postpartum haemorrhage (post lower uterine segment caesarean section) requiring assessment with fundal height measurements; specific vascular observations for patients following free flap surgery (deep inferior epigastric perforators [DIEP] or transverse rectus abdominis myocutaneous [TRAM]), not just observing for arterial vascularity but also venous engorgement; and cervical shock in gynaecological patients that causes both a fall in blood pressure and heart rate.

Anaesthetic handover

Handover is an important component that will help guide postoperative assessment and management. However, research suggests that postoperative patient handovers can be fraught with technical and communication errors and, if not done properly, may have potentially negative impacts for patient safety.[40] There is no standardised and agreed approach to handover; however, it is recognised that some form of standard process is required.[40] A formal handover will be provided by the treating anaesthetist to the nurse who will be caring for the patient at the time of transfer of care. The quality of the handover must be such that it allows the nurse to safely assume responsibility for the patient. It is important for nurses to understand this process, knowing what information needs to be gleaned from the handover as they accept responsibility for the patient's care. In some hospitals there is also a nursing handover from the perioperative nurse that may provide information about the surgical procedure, dressing, drain tubes and any notable intraoperative events. There are a variety of different handover tools available internationally, many of which incorporate similar elements. For example, the SBAR mnemonic is used to guide handover through discussion of the:

Situation

Background

Assessment

Recommendation.

The Australian and New Zealand College of Anaesthetists recommended the ISOBAR acronym, which represents:

Identification to ensure that the patient is correctly identified

Situation, including current clinical status and patient-centred care requirements

Observations – latest observations

Background and history

Assessment and **a**ctions to establish an agreed management plan

Responsibility and **r**isk management.[41]

Consistency in the handover method will help enhance its quality so it is important to know which approach is used in your hospital.

Respiratory assessment and management

Immediately after surgery patients are susceptible to events that can compromise adequacy of ventilation and oxygenation, thus airway and respiratory management skills are fundamental for nursing staff caring for this group.[42] What differentiates non-critically ill postoperative patients from other ICU patients is the residual effects of anaesthesia medications that may include, but are not limited to, narcotics, sedatives, hypnotics, inhalational gases, muscle relaxants, intravenous fluids and blood products.[42] These medications can cause decreased rate and depth of breathing, which contributes to alveolar hypoventilation and consequently results in increased levels of carbon dioxide and decreased levels of oxygen in the blood. Anaesthetic agents can also contribute to blunted responses to carbon dioxide and an overall decrease in minute ventilation.[43] It is important to have a detailed knowledge and understanding of the respiratory system and how to assess the respiratory function of postanaesthesia patients. For a detailed discussion of respiratory assessment and monitoring, please refer to Chapter 13.

Assessment and management of the airway

One of the most common complications seen in the immediate postanaesthesia period is airway obstruction.[44] The depressant effects of anaesthesia can mean that the postoperative patient is not able to protect or maintain a patent airway. Signs that the patient might have an airway obstruction include increased respiratory effort, respiratory muscle retraction, abnormal breath sounds and signs of altered gas exchange. In many cases opening the airway by tilting the head backward and extending the neck (if not contraindicated) can help restore airway patency. Artificial airways may be used to prevent obstruction that occurs when the patient's tongue and epiglottis fall back on the posterior pharyngeal wall.

All airway complications are serious as they all, in some way or another, obstruct the airway to varying degrees and put the patient at risk of decreased oxygenation and possible hypoxia. These complications can be from an upper airway obstruction such as laryngeal spasm, subglottic oedema or lower airway obstruction such as bronchospasm and non-cardiogenic pulmonary oedema. They may result from a simple problem, such as poor mandibular positioning where the tongue falls back obstructing the airway, to a complete laryngeal

spasm with no air entry.[44] Any of these problems can cause life-threatening hypoxia if not rectified immediately.

Some patients may leave the operating theatre with a laryngeal mask or endotracheal tube in situ that can be removed once they are awake and able to maintain their own airway. In an intubated patient a systematic approach to determining whether the patient is ready to be extubated can help avoid extubation failure.[45] This approach should include assessing whether the patient is awake, cooperative and able to follow commands. Reversal of non-depolarising muscle relaxants should be noted and the train-of-four assessed if there is concern about the patient's neuromuscular function. The patient should be normothermic and, if airway oedema is suspected, an endotracheal tube leak test should be performed where the cuff is deflated and breathing assessed prior to tube removal.

Assessment and management of ventilatory capacity and oxygenation

The altered respiratory rate and depth that may occur as a result of anaesthesia require focused assessment and understanding of the ways in which anaesthetic agents can influence both ventilator capacity and oxygenation in the postoperative period. For accurate assessment of respiratory rate, measurement will need to be taken by observing respirations over a 1-minute period; this process makes it the vital sign that is most often neglected in clinical practice.[46] Recent research suggests that respiratory rate is considered an inferior vital sign to blood pressure, heart rate and temperature measurement.[47] Inaccurate assessment of respiratory rate continues despite recognition that it is considered to be the single most important vital sign in detecting patient deterioration.[46] Assessment of respiratory rate in the period following general anaesthesia is of particular importance as patients may have received several pharmacological agents, including neuromuscular blockade, narcotics and sedative agents, that could directly influence respiratory function. Respiratory rate and depth directly influence minute ventilation and gas exchange. Capnography can be used to assess end-tidal carbon dioxide measurements[48] and pulse oximetry can be used to assess oxygen saturation. More accurate and detailed assessment of gas exchange requires arterial blood gas analysis. Depending on the nature of the surgical intervention, some patients may require a more detailed respiratory assessment that incorporates inspection, palpation, percussion and auscultation (see Chapter 13).

Practice tip

Following a pneumonectomy, the post-pneumonectomy space fills with air and on chest X-ray the trachea should be midline. A chest tube is inserted and specific orders on clamping and releasing the drain are given by the surgeon. Unexpectedly rapid accumulation of fluid in the post-pneumonectomy space might indicate haemorrhage.

Because respiratory effort can be compromised, almost all postoperative patients will receive supplemental oxygen, and with all patients the amount of oxygen received should be guided by the patient's clinical condition and assessment of arterial oxygen saturation. Oxygen therapy helps to wash out residual anaesthetic gases and provides a higher concentration of inspired oxygen for patients who may have residual effects of sedative and neuromuscular blocking agents causing hypoventilation. Patients who have had central neural blockade (epidural or spinal) or regional blocks will be assessed individually for oxygen requirements (see Chapter 13). Some patients may require respiratory support in the postoperative period and will remain intubated and ventilated for a period of time after surgery. If patients require ongoing mechanical ventilation they may require admission to ICU. For a detailed understanding of patients requiring mechanical ventilation and ongoing respiratory support please refer to Chapter 15.

Cardiovascular assessment and management

When making an assessment of cardiovascular function, it is worth remembering and evaluating the three vital components of the circulatory system: the heart as a pump, circulating blood volume and the arteriovenous system.[2] All these factors come together to ensure adequate tissue perfusion, which is reliant on a satisfactory cardiac output.[2] In the postanaesthesia period assessment of cardiovascular function will be frequently undertaken with monitoring of blood pressure and heart rate. Detailed description of cardiovascular assessment is provided in Chapter 9.

Postoperative patients are at risk of developing cardiovascular complications as they will have generally had some degree of blood loss, will have been administered anaesthetic medications or have temperature changes that may have altered vascularity. For example, central neural blockage will cause vascular vasodilation and interference to the body's sympathetic responses, which can lead to hypotension. Conversely, hypertension can be present when patients experience pain.

Hypotension can be transient or more sustained. Transient hypotension can occur in relation to drug administration. Conversely, more sustained hypotension and the development of shock can occur in relation to blood loss or from an altered distribution of flow that occurs secondary to sympathetic blockade and vasodilation that can occur in regional anaesthesia. Decreased cardiac output might be seen in some patients and could be related to decreased preload that occurs in hypovolaemia or decreased cardiac output secondary to myocardial injury contractility as a result of either myocardial injury or cardiac output and vasodilatory states.[49] Shock is characterised by a decrease in blood pressure (20–30% decrease from the patient's baseline) and an increase in heart rate, and is not an uncommon occurrence in postoperative patients.[44] Cardiovascular compromise that results from blood and fluid loss can lead to hypovolaemic shock.

Specific assessment and management strategies for the patient with shock are provided in Chapter 21.

Practice tip

Inadvertent hypothermia will cause vasoconstriction that may mask a low circulating blood volume.

Fluid and electrolyte balance

Postoperative patients are also particularly vulnerable to fluid and electrolyte imbalances due to the restrictions on fluid and electrolytes preoperatively, fluid loss during surgery, the patient's physical status and the associated stressors of surgery.[2] The normal bodily response to the stress of a surgical procedure is for the renal system to retain water and sodium.[2] For these reasons, the patient requires a full body assessment of their fluid and electrolyte status.[2] The primary goals of fluid management in the immediate postoperative phase are to maintain adequate intravascular volumes, left ventricular filling pressures, cardiac output, blood pressure and the delivery of oxygen to the tissues.[50] Normal concentrations of electrolytes and body fluids are vital to maintain the physiological function of all bodily systems.[50] The goals and strategies for volume replacement are patient dependent and should take into consideration the preoperative condition of the patient, cardiovascular status and intraoperative fluid losses.[51]

Pain assessment and management

Experiencing postoperative pain has been found to be the most common fear of surgical patients.[52] Effective pain management is considered to be both a right and an expectation of care for all patients following surgery.[53] Despite this, the practice of providing adequate postoperative pain relief continues to be inadequate.[52,54] Pain was once thought to be simply an unfortunate side effect of surgery with no detrimental effects; however, current research does not support this contention.[52]

Inadequate pain relief has been shown to alter the body's metabolic responses, which can delay recovery, extend hospital length of stay, increase morbidity rates and potentially lead to the development of a chronic pain state.[52] Conversely, effective pain control reduces postoperative complications, facilitates rehabilitation and provides a more rapid recovery from surgery.[52] For a detailed discussion on pain assessment and pain management please refer to Chapter 7. More information on pain medications is also provided in Chapter 7 and earlier in this chapter in the discussion on anaesthetic drugs. Specifically, a summary of opioid analgesics is provided in Table 26.2.

It is firmly believed that adequate pain relief requires more than one analgesic, and this approach is referred to as 'multimodal analgesia'.[55] Specific pain management techniques relevant to the postoperative period also include a mix of narcotic and non-narcotic analgesics, patient-controlled analgesia, central neural blockade and peripheral nerve blocks.

A number of randomised controlled trials have been conducted to examine the effectiveness of intravenous paracetamol (acetaminophen) in relieving postoperative pain and data suggest that it may be effective in a range of inpatient and ambulatory procedures such as total abdominal hysterectomy, tonsillectomy, caesarean section, joint replacement and laparoscopic cholecystectomy.[56] Intravenous paracetamol may also help reduce nausea in postoperative patients.[57]

Tramadol is also an effective agent for pain relief. Tramadol binds to mu-opioid receptor and also inhibits the reuptake of serotonin and noradrenaline.[58] Tramadol can be administered intravenously and is also available in oral and rectal preparations. The primary advantage of tramadol is the relative lack of respiratory depression, an important consideration in the immediate postoperative period.[55]

Two categories of non-steroidal anti-inflammatory drugs (NSAIDs) are available: non-selective, which inhibit both COX-1 and COX-2 pathways (ibuprofen, naproxen, ketorolac, diclofenac); and selective, which only inhibit COX-2 (celecoxib).[55] All of these analgesics add to the repertoire of multimodal pain relief.

Patient-controlled analgesia

Patient-controlled analgesia (PCA) can be effective for many patients requiring ongoing pain relief following surgery. The goal of PCA is to avoid the peaks and valleys of analgesia because the patient is able to control when pain relief is administered.[59] The patient is also able to anticipate activities such as rolling or coughing that are associated with increases in pain and is able to self-administer a narcotic bolus prior to the activity to manage any pain that might occur. Following a loading dose of analgesia the PCA pump is programmed based on the patient's needs and the pharmacokinetics of the drug being administered. The parameters programmed into the PCA pump include the bolus dose and a lockout interval. This allows the patient to attain immediate analgesia with the lockout interval preventing acute increases in the amount of drug delivered.[60] Occasionally, patients will require low-dose continuous administration through the PCA to maintain effective pain relief.[59]

Regional anaesthesia

Regional anaesthesia is a broad term to describe nerve blocks that block a region, for example arm blocks or femoral blocks. Regional anaesthesia involves injecting a local anaesthetic near major nerve bundles. To improve accuracy of drug delivery selected nerves can be located using ultrasound guidance or a nerve stimulator.[61]

Central neural blockade – epidural/ spinal

Central neural blockade or neuraxial anaesthesia is a generic term for epidural, spinal, epidural–spinal or caudal anaesthesia,[62] which blocks pain during a surgical procedure. Many of the medications used in epidural or spinal anaesthesia can continue to provide pain relief in the postoperative period, with local anaesthetic agents having differing durations of action. Local anaesthetic agents with adrenaline may be given if a longer duration of action is required.[62]

> **Practice tip**
>
> Patients who have received a spinal blockade will have a greater motor block than those with an epidural. This is because the local anaesthetic is injected into the subarachnoid space with the cerebrospinal fluid where the spinal nerves are not myelinated, providing a denser motor block.

Care of the patient following epidural or spinal anaesthesia requires an understanding of the possible complications associated with this type of anaesthesia. A wide range of complications can occur from minor irritations to possibly life-threatening conditions[63] and include high spinal block, hypotension, bradycardia, spinal and epidural haematoma, post-dural puncture headache, nausea and vomiting, urinary retention and transient neurological symptoms.[62] In addition to normal post-operative observations, continual assessment for possible complications should be maintained including: observation of the epidural catheter site for bleeding, catheter migration, swelling or redness; discussion with the patient regarding the onset of pain or tenderness at the catheter site; and protective care and observation of anaesthetised limbs.[62,63]

High spinal block

Assessing dermatomes after spinal and epidural anaesthesia is important to identify exaggerated dermatome spread that can occur (Figure 26.4).[64] Reduced doses of medications are necessary for select patients in whom a normal dose might be excessive. Some patients may also experience an unusual sensitivity or spread of local anaesthetic, which can lead to high spinal block.[64] Signs and symptoms may include dyspnoea, numbness or weakness in the upper extremities, nausea that often precedes hypotension and bradycardia.[64] Blocking of the cardiac sympathetic fibres from T1–T4 may cause loss of chronotropic and inotropic drive and a fall in cardiac output, which results in hypotension and bradycardia.

> **Practice tip**
>
> Elderly, pregnant, obese or very short patients may have excessive dermatome spread if administered normal doses of spinal or epidural anaesthesia.

Careful assessment of dermatome levels must be performed. Ice is often used to assess sensory block as hot and cold pass on the same pathway as pain. Central neural blockade not only blocks sensory fibres but also motor function and sympathetic outflow. The level of muscle block can be assessed using the Bromage score[66] (Table 26.5).

FIGURE 26.4 Dermatomes.[65]

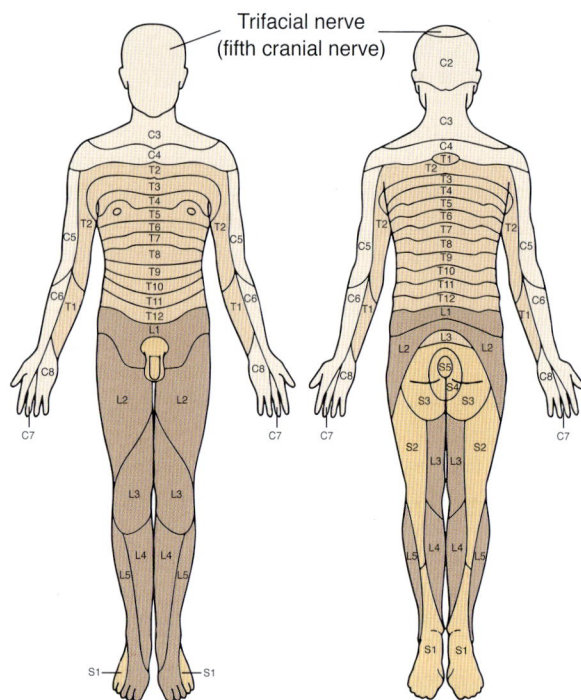

Trifacial nerve
(fifth cranial nerve)

Adapted from Nagelhout J, Plaus K. Nurse anesthesia.
4th ed. St Louis: Saunders; 2010, with permission.

TABLE 26.5

Modified Bromage score[66]

SCORE	CRITERIA
1	Complete block (unable to move feet or knees)
2	Almost complete block (able to move feet only)
3	Partial block (just able to move knees)
4	Detectable weakness of hip flexion while supine (full flexion of knees)
5	No detectable weakness of hip flexion while supine
6	Able to perform partial knee bend

Note: This modified Bromage score differs from the original score by including two additional criteria. The other substantial difference is that the original Bromage score[98] began with grade I, which was free movement of legs and feet, whereas in this modified Bromage scale score 1 is complete block.

Adapted from Breen TW, Shapiro T, Glass B, Foster-Payne D, Oriol NE. Epidural anesthesia for labor in an ambulatory patient. Anesth Analg 1993;77(5):919–24, with permission.

The level of differential blockade is judged by finding the level of sensory block with temperature sensitivity and recognising that the sympathetic block may be two or more segments higher. Motor blockade will be approximately two segments lower.[64] Sympathetic cardiac accelerator fibres arise from T1–T4 (at and above mid-nipple level). Close monitoring of heart rate and blood pressure should be initiated when the sensory block is sitting around T6 because of the potential for sympathetic outflow to be blocked.[64] A block at T1–T4 may produce profound bradycardia and hypotension from arterial dilation and venous pooling.[64] Consequently, a significant fall in cardiac output may occur without the body being able to compensate through the usual sympathetic responses. This change in patient condition should be treated as a medical emergency and treatment for shock implemented. Bradycardia can be treated with atropine and hypotension with fluid resuscitation therapy and/or vasopressors.[64] High spinal blocks can affect respiratory muscles so ongoing assessment of respiratory function should be initiated and airway support provided as required.

Urinary retention

A block at the level of S2–S4 root fibres decreases urinary bladder tone and may inhibit a patient's ability to void, and epidural opioids can also interfere with normal voiding.[64]

These effects seem to be more pronounced in men and urinary bladder catheterisation should be used for all but the shortest acting blocks.[64] If a patient with a central neural block does not have a catheter postoperatively, close observation for urinary retention will be necessary as persistent bladder dysfunction can also be a manifestation of serious neural injury.[64] The patient may not experience the sensation of a full bladder and, where suspected, performing a bladder scan would be indicated. If the bladder is full and the patient is unable to void, a catheter may need to be inserted until bladder muscle function returns.

Transient neurological symptoms

In administering a spinal or epidural anaesthetic a needle passes through the skin, subcutaneous tissues, muscle and ligaments. It is therefore not surprising that this procedure may cause varying degrees of tissue trauma such as bruising and localised inflammatory responses, with or without reflex muscle spasm. These muscle spasms may be responsible for postoperative backache,[64] which is usually mild and self-limiting. Backache can be treated with warm/cold packs or mild analgesics. Pain must be monitored carefully per the chance it may be an important clinical sign of more serious complications, such as epidural haematoma and abscess.[64]

Spinal or epidural haematoma

Spinal and epidural haematomas are rare but devastating complications that can occur following regional anaesthesia. The incidence of epidural haematoma associated with neuraxial anaesthesia is reported to be less than 1:150,000 and one in 2.2 million patients receiving spinal anaesthesia.[67] Both epidural and spinal haematomas are more likely to occur in patients who have abnormal coagulation levels, either disease-related or as a result of pharmacological therapies.[64] Consequently, coagulation studies must be performed prior to neuraxial anaesthesia being considered as changes in clotting profiles are an absolute contraindication to insertion of these blocks. Clotting status must also be performed prior to removal of the catheter and strict guidelines exist for removal in patients who are receiving prophylactic anticoagulants,[63] with recommendations specific to the anticoagulation medication used.

Epidural haematoma can lead to compression of the spinal nerves causing various degrees of irreversible damage. The symptoms of haematoma include sharp back and leg pain with a motor weakness and/or sphincter dysfunction.[64] Recognition of these symptoms can be delayed until after the effect of the anaesthesia has dissipated. In the event of such symptoms it is vital to call for immediate medical assistance. Rapid neurological imaging such as a computed tomography or magnetic resonance imaging scan should be performed to assess the location, size and extent of the haematoma as neurological outcomes are vastly improved if decompression occurs within 8–12 hours.[64]

Practice tip

Care must be taken when removing the epidural catheter as up to half of reported incidents of epidural haematoma are associated with catheter removal. Monitoring sensory observations after epidural removal is important to assess for complications, especially in those patients with abnormal clotting.

Post-dural puncture headache

Post-dural puncture headache is not an uncommon complication of interventional neuraxial blockade[68] and is the most common complication of spinal anaesthesia in the obstetric population.[69] If either a spinal or epidural needle accidentally tears the dura enough to cause cerebrospinal fluid to leak out, this may cause a post-dural puncture headache. Cerebrospinal fluid is regenerated about 3 to 5 times over each day at a rate of approximately 0.3 mL per minute.[68] Although the exact mechanism of the headache is theoretical, experts believe that there appears to be a definitive relationship between the loss of cerebrospinal fluid from the dural tear and the manifestation of symptoms and, put very simply, fluid loss disrupts the buoyancy of the brain.[68]

Conservative management of this condition includes assisting the patient with full bed rest, maintaining adequate hydration and assisting administering prescribed medications such as analgesics and caffeine. An epidural blood patch can be used to manage post-dural puncture headaches. This is done by taking approximately 10 mL of autologous blood and injecting it into the epidural space where the tear has occurred. The blood covers the area of dural puncture and prevents further leakage of cerebrospinal fluid.[69]

Management of nausea and vomiting

Postoperative nausea and vomiting (PONV) is a concern for patients and clinicians alike and affects as many as one-third of patients receiving anaesthesia. As the most undesirable postoperative complication, PONV also can contribute to complications such as wound dehiscence, aspiration, increased intracranial pressure and increased cardiovascular demand. For some patients deep breathing, a cool cloth on the forehead and reassurance can help assist with nausea; however, for most postoperative patients pharmacological interventions will be necessary. Common pharmacological agents for the management of nausea and vomiting are listed in Table 26.6.

Thermoregulation

The body has a highly sensitive system that provides a balance between heat production and heat loss. This consists of a complex feedback system that senses afferent messages, compares them to a central integrated set-point and sends reflex efferent messages to either cause vasoconstriction when the patient is cold or vasodilation when the patient is hot. Anaesthesia and the operating suite environment provide the perfect storm for the development of inadvertent hypothermia with the cold environment, exposure, opened body cavities, suppression of the thermoregulation centre and medications that cause vasodilation. Inadvertent or unplanned hypothermia is defined as a core temperature below 36°C[70] and is divided into three categories, mild (34–36°C), moderate (30–34°C) and severe (≤30°C).[71] Unlike the exposure hypothermia discussed in Chapter 23, inadvertent or unplanned hypothermia generally falls within the mild range but still has devastating consequences and is associated with increased mortality rates in postoperative patients.[72] Sequelae of this condition may include infection, impaired wound healing, adverse cardiac events, altered drug metabolism, impaired coagulation and increased postoperative discomfort.[44]

The pathophysiological effects of hypothermia include a left oxyhaemoglobin shift, increased oxygen requirements and the ability of vasoconstriction to mask a low circulating blood volume. Recognising these effects, nursing care should include rewarming the patient, providing supplemental oxygen and close monitoring of blood pressure during rewarming because of the potential for the patient to decrease their systolic blood pressure as vasoconstriction is reversed. Accurate temperature measurements reflecting the patient's core temperature are required and rewarming with external warming devices can be used (see Chapter 23).

Practice tip

During rewarming, patients with inadvertent hypothermia may initially decrease their body temperature before it starts to rise. This does not mean that the first temperature reading was inaccurate; rather, it is an indication of a phenomenon called 'after fall' that occurs when rewarming hypothermic patients.

TABLE 26.6

Pharmacological interventions for postoperative nausea and vomiting[44]

DRUG (RECEPTOR SITE AFFINITY)	DOSE[a]	DURATION OF ACTION	ADVERSE EFFECTS	COMMENTS AND RECOMMENDATIONS FOR USE
Droperidol (dopamine)	Adult: 0.625–1.25 mg IV Paediatric: 20–50 mcg/kg IV (children ≥2 years)	12–24 hours	Sedation, hypotension, EPS	Higher doses and doses that are repeated too soon can cause sedation, EPS and QT prolongation
Prochlorperazine (dopamine)	Adult: 5–10 mg IM or IV; 25 mg PR Paediatric:[b] 0.13 mg/kg IM; 0.2 mg/kg PO 2–3 times daily; 0.1 mg/kg 3–4 times daily PR	2–6 hours IV, IM, PO; 12 hours PR	Sedation, hypotension, EPS	Effective first-line agent
Promethazine (dopamine, histamine, acetylcholine)	Adult: 6.25–25 mg IM, IV or PR Paediatric (≥2 years of age): 0.25–0.5 mg/kg IV, IM, PR[c]	4 hours	Sedation, hypotension, EPS	Good for patients with motion sickness or undergoing surgery affecting vestibular apparatus
Diphenhydramine (histamine, acetylcholine)	Adult: 12.5–50 mg IM, IV Paediatric (≥2 years of age): 1 mg/kg IV or PO (maximum, 25 mg for <6 years of age)	4–6 hours	Sedation, dry mouth, blurred vision, urinary retention	Good for patients with motion sickness or undergoing surgery affecting vestibular apparatus
Metoclopramide (dopamine)	Adult: 10–20 mg IV Paediatric: 0.15–0.25 mg/kg	6–8 hours	Sedation, hypotension, EPS	Increases gastric motility; good if nausea or vomiting is from gastric stasis; reduce dose to 5 mg in renal impairment; consider diphenhydramine to prevent EPS in children
Ondansetron (serotonin)	Adult: 4 mg IV; 4, 8 mg ODT or wafer Paediatric: 0.05–0.1 mg/kg	Up to 24 hours	Headache, lightheadedness, constipation	Much more effective for vomiting than nausea; 2 mg may be sufficient to treat PONV in PACU
Granisetron (serotonin)	Adult: 1 mg IV over 30 seconds Paediatric: N/A	Up to 24 hours	Headache, lightheadedness	Much more effective for vomiting than nausea
Palonosetron (serotonin)	Adult: 0.075 mg IV	24 hours	Headache, constipation	Prolonged duration of action; given immediately before induction of anaesthesia
Scopolamine (acetylcholine)	Adult: 1.5 mg transdermal patch Paediatric: N/A	72 hours[d]	Sedation, dry mouth, visual disturbances, dysphoria, confusion, disorientation, hallucinations	Good for patients with motion sickness or undergoing surgery affecting vestibular apparatus; apply 4 hours before exposure
Dexamethasone	Adult: 4–10 mg IV Paediatric: 0.5–1 mg/kg	Up to 24 hours	Watch blood sugar in patients with diabetes; watch for fluid retention, especially in cardiac patients	Generally well tolerated in healthy patients; may take time (hours) to work – administer before induction of anaesthesia
Apretitant	Adult: 40 mg PO 1–3 hours before anaesthesia	Up to 24 hours	Generally well tolerated	Oral prophylaxis only; caution with patients taking warfarin; can reduce effectiveness of oral contraceptives

[a]Unless otherwise indicated, paediatric doses should not exceed the adult dose for each antiemetic agent.

[b]Children weighing more than 10 kg or older than 2 years of age only. Change from IM to PO as soon as possible. With administration PR, dosing interval varies from 8–24 hours depending on child's weight.

[c]Maximum of 12.5 mg in children younger than 12 years.

[d]Remove after 24 hours when used to prevent or treat PONV. Instruct patient to wash the patch site and hands thoroughly.

ECG = electrocardiogram; EPS = extrapyramidal symptoms, such as motor restlessness or acute dystonia; IM = intramuscular; IV = intravenous; ODT = orally disintegrating tablets; PACU = postanaesthesia care unit; PO = orally; PONV = postoperative nausea and vomiting; PR = per rectum.

Adapted from: O'Brien D. Postanesthesia care complications. In: Odom-Forren J, ed. Perianaesthesia nursing: A critical care approach. St Louis: Elsevier; 2013, with permission.

The postoperative bariatric patient

The prevalence of obesity is increasing[73] and therefore management of the bariatric or obese patient in the postoperative period warrants detailed discussion. Bariatric patients undergoing anaesthesia will have particular needs in the postanaesthesia period, irrespective of the surgical procedure. For example, the higher incidence of cardiovascular disease means that careful electrocardiographic monitoring should be implemented during recovery from anaesthesia. Assessment of haemodynamic status is important, as it is with any postoperative patient, and accurate measurement of blood pressure is contingent on the use of appropriately sized blood pressure cuffs.

Bariatric patients are also at increased risk for resedation because many anaesthetic drugs are lipophilic and metabolised more slowly by obese patients. Because of increased respiratory compromise, opioid should be used with caution and other pain management strategies, such as the use of non-steroidal anti-inflammatory agents, local anaesthesia or oral analgesia, should be considered.[74]

Specific assessment and management relative to the bariatric patient includes consideration for the prevention of venothromboembolism and pressure injuries. Proper fitting of compression stockings should be monitored so that a tourniquet effect of the stockings is avoided. Knowledge of the surgical procedure and intraoperative positioning will help guide assessment of the patient for signs of intraoperative pressure injury. Intravenous access should be monitored closely as initiating intravenous access can be challenging in this patient group.

The most important consideration in the postoperative period is the assessment of respiratory function. There is a direct correlation between the degree of obesity a patient suffers and the risk and rate of pulmonary complications.[75] Airway management may be difficult and hazardous due to anatomical features such as a large tongue and excessive pharyngeal and palatal soft tissue impairing vision and making mask ventilation awkward.

The dynamics of respiration are also altered in bariatric patients. There is a profound effect on the mechanics of the respiratory system with increased oxygen consumption and carbon dioxide production. Normocarbia is maintained by an increase in minute ventilation to expel increased carbon dioxide produced through metabolic activity of fat and the increased expenditure required for mobility and breathing.[76] Reduction in chest wall compliance also contributes to the increased work of breathing. Functional residual capacity may also decline particularly if the weight of the chest wall exceeds alveolar closing capacity, which results in small airway closure, ventilation perfusion mismatch and subsequent hypoxia.[76] Postoperatively, decreased lung function and capacity is expected for approximately 5 days and acute airway obstruction is more likely during this period.[76]

Provided cardiovascular stability is established it may be best to position obese patients sitting up. If the weight of the chest wall exceeds the closing capacity of the alveoli,

the alveoli will collapse and desaturation will occur. By sitting the patient up, the weight of the chest wall is lessened allowing greater tidal volume. If the patient is hypotensive, a discussion with medical staff would be required to assess which problem is worse; however, the 'banana' position (head up and feet up) may be required. It is essential to provide support for positioning to ensure upright sitting position is maintained. If edentulous replace the teeth as these will assist in upper airway support.

Assessment and management of specific postoperative complications

Laryngospasm

Laryngospasm is an involuntary forceful spasm of the laryngeal musculature that is caused by stimulation of the superior laryngeal nerve.[77] It is more common in young paediatric patients than in adults, and is most common in infants 1–3 months old.[77] Laryngeal spasm can result in an incomplete or complete airway obstruction,[78] with the latter being more uncommon. Prevention of this condition includes extubating patients either deeply asleep or fully awake (but not in between) and causes include fluid or secretions on the vocal cords.

Treatment of laryngospasm includes gentle positive-pressure ventilation, forward jaw thrust and intravenous lignocaine (1–1.5 mg/kg).[79] If hypoxia develops, paralysis with intravenous suxamethonium (0.5–1 mg/kg) or rocuronium (0.4 mg/kg) and controlled ventilation may be required.[77]

Signs and symptoms of laryngeal spasm include inspiratory stridor, dyspnoea, a distressed/sweating patient and on auscultation an upper airway noise can be heard. As postoperative patients generally have supplemental oxygen, these symptoms may or may not include a decrease in oxygen saturations in mild laryngeal spasm. Treatment of this condition will include sitting the patient up to facilitate ventilation, supplemental oxygen, gentle suctioning of the upper airway and providing airway support as required.[78] It is important to reassure the patient as anxiety can exacerbate the condition.

Non-cardiogenic pulmonary oedema

Pulmonary oedema may be defined simply as increased total lung water. Non-cardiogenic pulmonary oedema is where increased lung water occurs in the absence of a cardiac aetiology. In the post-anaesthesia period non-cardiogenic pulmonary oedema can occur because of upper airway obstruction such as laryngospasm,[80] bolus dosing with naloxone, reversal of neuromuscular blockade[81] or significant hypoxia.[44] In young athletic males, non-cardiogenic pulmonary oedema may occur in relation to the generation of negative intrathoracic pressure during an upper airway obstruction[82] as the diaphragm contracts against a closed or semi-closed glottis.[77] The severity of pulmonary oedema corresponds to the degree to which high negative inspiratory pressures are generated.[82] Symptoms usually occur within 1 hour of the upper airway obstruction, but may present as much as 6 hours later.[44] The patient may then develop sudden respiratory distress, tachypnoea, cough, shortness of breath, sudden decrease in oxygen saturation and the classic sign of pink frothy sputum.[44] Vital signs may or may not change.

Rapid diagnosis and treatment are essential to alleviate this respiratory complication. Treatment of this condition includes providing supplemental oxygenation. Continuous positive airway pressure can be used and, if the patient requires airway management, they may be intubated and mechanically ventilated with positive end-expiratory pressure.[44] For further information on oxygenation and caring for an intubated patient, please see Chapter 15.

Subglottic oedema/post-intubation croup

Subglottic oedema or post-intubation croup is a complication that occurs later than laryngospasm, but will almost always appear within 3 hours following extubation.[77] Although this condition can occur in adults, it is most commonly seen in the 1–4 year age group.[44] The risk of developing subglottic oedema can be lessened in children by allowing a slight gas leak around the endotracheal tube.[77]

Signs and symptoms of subglottic oedema include inspiratory stridor, retractions, hoarseness, crowing respiration and a croup-like cough and a patient who is apprehensive and restless. Humidified oxygen may help reduce airway swelling and nebulised racemic adrenaline can also help reduce subglottic oedema. If additional treatment is required, a helium–oxygen mixture can be used or dexamethasone administered.[44]

Bronchospasm

Bronchospasm is a lower airway obstruction, characterised by spasmodic smooth muscle contraction that causes narrowing of the bronchi and bronchioles.[44] Generally, bronchospasm will occur in patients with a pre-existing pulmonary illness such as asthma or chronic obstructive pulmonary disease, but it may also develop in healthy patients in the presence of allergy, anaphylaxis or pulmonary aspiration. For this reason, if a patient without pulmonary pathology develops bronchospasm, a high degree of suspicion should be employed by the nurse to ensure that the underlying cause is not allergic or due to pulmonary aspiration.

Signs and symptoms of bronchospasm include coughing, distinct wheeze upon auscultation, noisy shallow respiration, chest retractions, use of accessory muscles, prolonged expiratory phase of respiration, hypertension and tachycardia. The nurse should sit the patient up, provide assisted oxygen, call for medical assistance and reassure the patient.

Initial management of this patient will include removal of the identified cause if possible,[44] and treatment will depend on the cause, specific symptoms and severity of the bronchospasm. This may include humidified oxygen, administration of a beta-2-adrenergic agonist, intubation and intermittent positive pressure ventilation and perhaps antibiotics. Antihistamines and steroids may also be required.[44]

Aspiration pneumonitis

Mendelson syndrome, aspiration of gastric content that results in a severe pulmonary complication, was first reported in 1946.[83] Preoperative patient preparation, including fasting, is aimed at minimising the risk of aspiration. Pregnant women, those with gastro-oesophageal reflux disease, obese and non-fasting patients are all at increased risk of aspiration pneumonitis.[83]

Clinical progression after aspiration varies widely, from no and very mild symptoms to bronchopneumonia and possible development of acute respiratory distress syndrome.[83] The severity of progression is increased by several factors including the aspirate pH, quantity of aspirate and the presence of solid particles.[83] Symptoms include tachypnoea, tachycardia, cough and possible bronchospasm.[44] While this condition may be dramatic on onset it can also be insidious in nature. Bronchospasm that occurs in a healthy patient should be investigated further.

Awareness under anaesthesia

Awareness under anaesthesia results from an imbalance between anaesthetic need and delivery and is an uncommon complication of anaesthesia, affecting only 0.1–0.2% of all surgical patients. Patients who have experienced awareness under anaesthesia report a perception of paralysis, being aware of conversations and surgical manipulations alongside feelings of helplessness, fear and pain. Depth of anaesthesia is assessed through monitoring of vital signs; however, in some patients this is unreliable.[84] There is growing evidence suggesting the awareness can lead to the development of post-traumatic stress disorder,[85,86] so appropriate management of patients with this condition is essential.

If a patient awakes from anaesthesia and tells you that they have suffered awareness under anaesthesia, comfort and support should be provided to the patient. Explain that the operation is over and that they are safe. The treating anaesthetist should be contacted immediately. It is important not to dismiss the patient's comments or contradict them in any way. Their report should be taken seriously and documented accurately in the patient's notes and through established hospital incident reporting systems.

Emergence delirium

Emergence delirium is a well-known phenomenon that may occur in the postoperative period.[87] In its milder form an awake patient may exhibit restlessness, disorientation, irrational conversations and inappropriate behaviour, and this may be referred to as emergence excitement.[44] Emergence delirium can also include symptoms such as hallucinations, hypersensitivity to external stimuli and hyperactivity, with the patient often screaming and thrashing.[44,87] On assessment the patient's eyes can appear glazed and they do not respond to verbal dialogue. Raised voices tend to worsen the situation so calm, confident reassurance is advised.

Children have a higher incidence, along with adults who have suffered a recent tragedy or bereavement, severe preoperative anxiety, a history of drug dependency or psychiatric illness or who have had certain medications including ketamine, droperidol, opioids, benzodiazepines, scopolamine, atropine or large doses of metoclopramide.[44]

Clinical management of emergence delirium includes protecting the patient from self-injury, ensuring your own safety and calling for assistance. Patients should be assessed for hypoxia as a possible cause of the behaviour. If the cause of emergence delirium is known the cause should be treated. Sedation may be required.[44] Clinical evidence also suggests that emergence delirium is increasingly seen among military personnel who have seen active service.[88]

If you have prior knowledge that a patient is prone to emergence delirium, preparations can be made for their safe recovery by obtaining protective cot or bed sides to prevent injury, and ensuring appropriate human resources are available to help physically manage the patient if necessary.

> **Practice tip**
>
> Postoperative delirium often lasts about 20 minutes with the patient eventually falling back to sleep before waking with no recollections of the incident.

Delayed emergence

Time to emerge from anaesthesia is variable between patients, and may depend on a multitude of factors including the type of anaesthesia and length of surgery.[89] Occasionally, the time for a patient to awake may be slower than expected[44] and this could be due to a plethora of factors.[89]

Delayed emergence may occur in a patient who was recovering in the ICU, or may be the reason for an admission to ICU. The most common cause of delayed awakening is prolonged effect from anaesthesia and associated medications, but it could also be due to metabolic complications including hypoglycaemia, hyponatraemia, hypocalcaemia, hypomagnesaemia, hypercarbia, hypoxia, hypothermia, hypovolaemia or neurological injury.[44] The primary management is always in support of airway, breathing and circulation, while the cause is sought.[89]

Malignant hyperthermia

Malignant hyperthermia is a rare, catastrophic, often fatal syndrome that is triggered by volatile anaesthetic agents and suxamethonium.[90] It is an autosomal dominant disorder of the skeletal muscle that occurs only in genetically predisposed humans.[90] The incidence of this disorder is thought to be somewhere between 1:3000 and 1:50,000 anaesthetics.[91] Case fatality rate has fallen from 70% in the 1970s to less than 10% in 2006.[92] Although its pathogenesis is relatively well understood, there is wide variability

in the time of onset and the presentation of clinical signs and symptoms.[93]

Although most cases of malignant hyperthermia occur within 30 minutes of anaesthesia and therefore will be seen and treated in the operating suite, some patients may have delayed symptoms up to 12 hours postoperatively.[92] In some circumstances the delayed onset has hindered timely recognition and treatment.[93] Patients presenting with febrile illness after surgery should be assessed for malignant hyperthermia. This is a particularly important consideration for those patients who are discharged home after surgery but re-present to the hospital emergency department.[90]

In malignant hyperthermia an intracellular skeletal muscle biochemical defect and exposure to trigger agents results in excessive amounts of calcium in the myoplasm released by the sarcoplasmic reticulum. The resultant high level of calcium causes intense skeletal muscle contraction, which in turn causes heat production, increased oxygen consumption and increased carbon dioxide production.[91] Malignant hyperthermia is a cyclic process that liberates heat and produces lactic acid.[94] Cell membrane disruptions lead to potassium, phosphate, magnesium and myoglobin leakage into the extracellular fluid, which results in increased serum levels.[95] Early symptoms of malignant hyperthermia include tachycardia, tachypnoea, sweating, rise in end-tidal carbon dioxide levels, hyperthermia and possibly master muscle spasm.[96] Treatment of malignant hyperthermia is detailed in Box 26.2.

> **BOX 26.2**
>
> **Management of malignant hyperthermia**
> - Stop trigger agents immediately.
> - Administer 100% oxygen and hyperventilate.
> - Call for help – press emergency bell.
> - Contact the operating theatre to get specialised help from an anaesthetist.
> - Obtain sodium dantrolene, the treating agent, and administer 2.5 mg/kg up to 10 mg/kg.
> - Notify pharmacy department to replenish stores of sodium dantrolene.
> - Use aggressive cooling to prevent the patient reaching the thermal critical level of >40.6°C.
> - Assist in associated management of arrhythmias and electrolyte imbalance.
> - Assess cardiac function, urine output and colour (urinary catheterisation may be required).
>
> *Adapted with permission from:*
>
> Hooper VD. Care of the patient with thermal imbalance. In: Odom-Forren J, ed. Perianesthesia nursing: A critical care approach. 6th ed. St Louis: Elsevier; 2013
>
> Hirshey Dirksen S, Van Wicklin S, Ledrut Mashman D, Neiderer P, Merritt D. Developing effective drills in preparation for a malignant hyperthermia crisis. AORN 2013;97(3):330–52.

The treating medication, dantrolene sodium, is a skeletal muscle relaxant that decreases the amount of calcium released by the sarcoplasmic reticulum, thus reversing the pathophysiology of malignant hyperthermia. The dose of dantrolene sodium in malignant hyperthermia is 2.5 mg/kg given intravenously, regardless of age with no upper dose limit.[97] Dantrolene sodium when given intravenously has a half-life of 5 hours; some patients may require up to 30 mg/kg over 24 hours.[98] Because symptoms reoccur in 25% of patients subsequent doses of dantrolene sodium are required, usually as 1 mg/kg over 6 hours for the first 24–48 hours.[99, 100]

Practice tip

Sodium dantrolene must be reconstituted with sterile water because of compatibility issues. Reconstituted sodium dantrolene is very alkalotic (pH 9.5) so care must be taken to prevent extravasation. Patients receiving this drug should be monitored for thrombophlebitis.

Transferring care of the postoperative patient: discharge to an inpatient ward

Without question, the immediate postoperative period will require high quality, safe nursing care to detect and/or prevent serious complications.[101] Many factors affect the patient's response to anaesthesia and surgery, thus the length of stay for each patient will vary.[101]

For this reason most PACUs have discharge criteria that involve a thorough assessment of the patient's vital signs, pain, conscious state, nausea and vomiting and escalation of care plan prior to patient discharge from the PACU.[101] These criteria are used to determine when a patient is ready to be discharged to the ward and can be used in the ICU when non-critically ill patients are in ICU recovering from anaesthesia (Table 26.7). Critically ill postoperative patients will have their discharge managed by the ICU clinician team.

TABLE 26.7
Discharge criteria for the postoperative patient

Conscious state	• Conscious and able to respond appropriately to verbal stimuli
Respiratory function	• Able to protect his or her own airway • Has a cough reflex • Respiratory rate must be greater than 12 breaths per minute • Oxygen saturation should be >95% on room air and assessed at least 10 minutes after oxygen discontinued • Need for supplemental oxygen should be determined by medical team for those patients who do not have an oxygen saturation >95% on room air
Cardiovascular function	• Vital signs need to be within normal limits and considered in relation to the patient's preoperative vital signs. Heart rate and blood pressure should be within 20% of preoperative
Temperature	• Patient's core temperature should be between 36°C and 37°C
Pain	• The patient should be pain free or have pain at a manageable level
Nausea and vomiting	• The patient should be free from nausea and vomiting • Patients with persistent nausea may return to the ward after liaison with medical staff and appropriate ongoing management in place
Wound care	• Dressings should be dry and intact • Drains should be labelled with amount, date and time. Drainage should be assessed to ensure excessive drainage is not present • Women who have had a lower caesarean section will have their fundal height assessed. The fundal height should be equal to or less than the level of the umbilicus
Neurological and neurovascular observations	• Should be within normal limits
Documentation	• Nursing documentation completed legibly in ink • Ensure medical staff have written up appropriate notes and orders

Summary

In conclusion, patients who have received anaesthesia and undergone surgical procedures are vulnerable to a multitude of different complications. Although they may not be critically ill, patients who are transferred to the ICU immediately following surgery require close monitoring and observation. Respect for, and knowledge and understanding of, such complications will allow the nurse to provide a safer postoperative journey.

Case study

Mr Jones is a 62-year-old man who presented with a compound fracture of his left tibia and fibula following a workplace fall. He has had one past anaesthetic with no untoward events and no family history of anaesthetic complications. Due to his past history of unstable Prinzmetal angina and COPD he is sent to the intensive care unit postoperatively for specialised cardiac and respiratory monitoring and nursing care. Mr Jones received a full relaxant general anaesthetic. He was induced with propofol and anaesthesia was maintained with nitrous oxide and isoflurane. Mr Jones had an uneventful operative period and was safely transferred to the ICU at 1930 hours. He remained intubated and ventilated, with a plan for extubation the next morning if his condition was stable. He was in sinus rhythm with no ischaemic episodes.

At 1950 hours, Mr Jones developed tachycardia, became hypertensive and was noted to have an end-tidal CO_2 level rapidly rising from 36 mmHg to 59 mmHg. The nursing staff increased his ventilation rate and contacted medical staff, but the CO_2 levels continued to rise to 75 mmHg at 2005 hours. It was then noted by the nursing and medical staff that the patient was hot to touch and was also suffering from muscular-skeletal stiffness.

At this point a diagnosis of malignant hyperthermia was made. An oesophageal temperature probe was inserted revealing a temperature of 39.2°C.

Sodium dantrolene was administered at 2.5 mg/kg (180 mg) at 2015 hours with good effect. At 2025 hours, the patient's temperature began to decrease, CO_2 was 45 mmHg, HR and BP were lower and skeletal muscle stiffness ceased.

Three additional dantrolene doses (1 mg/kg) were given every 6 hours. The remainder of the patient's stay was uneventful.

DISCUSSION

Malignant hyperthermia is at the forefront of thinking while the patient is in the perioperative environment, but once they leave the operating suite, it may be more difficult to diagnose and less easily understood. This patient had routine normal blood gases throughout the operation revealing that, while the condition was triggered by the volatile anaesthetic agents during the operation, the condition did not present itself until after the operation was complete.

Malignant hyperthermia is most likely to occur in the operating room; however, it can also present in the PACU and possibly up to 12 hours postoperatively,[92] making this condition one that needs to be understood by intensive care nurses caring for postoperative patients.

CASE STUDY QUESTIONS

1 Describe the pathogenesis of malignant hyperthermia.
2 Discuss the risk factors for malignant hyperthermia in relation to the patient described in this case study.
3 What signs and symptoms did Mr Jones have that are consistent with malignant hyperthermia?

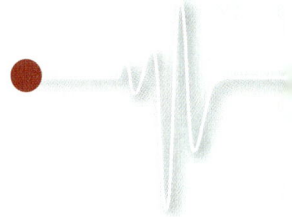

RESEARCH VIGNETTE

Karadag M, Iseri OP. Determining health personnel's application trends of new guidelines for perioperative fasting: findings from a survey. J Perianesthes Nurs 2014;29(3):175–84[102]

Introduction: For over a century, the discontinuation of oral food intake preoperatively after midnight has been routinely applied. Although routine fasting during the night before elective surgery has been abandoned by many modern centers, preoperative fasting after midnight continues as a routine practice.

Purpose: The purpose of this study was to determine trends in health personnel's application of new guidelines for preoperative fasting.

Materials and methods: The research sample of this descriptive study consisted of 73 nurses and physicians who were working in the surgical clinics during the time when the study was conducted and who agreed to participate in the study. The data of the study were collected using a questionnaire designed by the researchers.

Finding: Of the health personnel included in the study group, 43.8% routinely kept adult patients fasting after midnight, 34.2% discontinued solid food intake 8 hours preoperatively, 5.5% discontinued solid food intake 6 hours preoperatively, and 34.2% discontinued the intake of clear and particulate liquids 4 to 8 hours preoperatively. Compliance of the American Society of Anesthesiologists' "2-4-6-8 rule" by health staff was very low.

Conclusions: This study was carried out in a hospital and based on the statements of health staff. Therefore, the findings of the study are suggestive in nature and cannot be generalized. We recommend that the study should be conducted with larger sample groups and that actual preoperative fasting periods of the patients should be determined.

CRITIQUE

Fasting is a well-established practice that is thought to help prevent aspiration of gastric contents during the perioperative period. Perioperative fasting can, however, be distressing for the patient and can contribute to headache, unrest, dehydration, hypovolaemia and hypoglycaemia. It may also contribute to postoperative nausea.[103] There is a body of research now established that suggests all-night fasting may not be required and that patients can consume clear liquids (up to 150 mL) up to 2 hours preoperatively with no effect on the gastric contents or gastric pH.[104] New guidelines have been established for preoperative fasting based on the 2-4-6-8 hour rule where: 2 – the consumption of water up to 2 hours before anaesthetic induction; 4 – the consumption of mother's milk by infants and children up to at least 4 hours; 6 – the consumption of solid, light food, milk and beverages containing milk up to at least 7 hours; and 8 – the consumption of heavy foods, such as meat products, up to 8 hours are allowed. Despite these guidelines fasting from midnight continues to be common practice in many areas worldwide.

In this study, Karadag and Iseri[102] set out to describe trends in health personnel's application of new guidelines for preoperative fasting. They targeted the entire population of one hospital and 73 nurses and physicians working in surgical clinics agreed to participate; the majority (68.5%) of the respondents were nurses. Further detail about the setting (such as the size of the hospital, number of surgical beds) is not provided. The response rate for this study is also not provided so it is possible that this study reflects the views of only a few within this organisation. The researchers developed their own data collection instrument, which was pilot tested and modified before use.

Almost half (43.8%) of respondents fasted adult patients after midnight. Roughly one-third (34.2%) discontinued solid food 8 hours before surgery and only a few (5.5%) discontinued food 6 hours preoperatively. A more liberal approach was taken with children. There was no institutional approach to preoperative fasting with practice being guided by individual physicians.

This study supports existing literature that suggests conservative approaches continue to be used in healthcare settings worldwide.[105] What the authors highlight here is an ongoing gap between current evidence-based recommendations and clinical practice. The science behind this study is simplistic but clearly describes the issue in one institution, noting that their findings reflect those of others. What is surprising is that the authors did not take the opportunity to develop an understanding of what was driving this clinical practice either at an individual or organisational level. Presumably, the authors recognise preoperative fasting as an area for practice change but have not incorporated data collection in this study that would help them to identify targeted interventions for behaviour change. This is recently published work; incorporation of a knowledge translation or implementation science study to understand barriers and facilitators to this practice will help inform the development of a multifaceted intervention to change practice.

Learning activities

1 How might you recognise if a patient is experiencing emergence delirium?

2 Subglottic oedema occurs mainly in young children but can also be observed in adults. Subglottic oedema may be observed as long as 3 hours post-extubation. What signs and symptoms might you observe in the patient with subglottic oedema?

3 Bariatric patients undergoing surgery warrant special consideration. What specific assessment might you undertake for this specific patient group?

Online resources

American Society of Anesthesiologists, www.asahq.org

American Society of PeriAnesthesia Nurses, www.aspan.org

Association of Anaesthetists of Great Britain and Ireland, www.aagbi.org

Association of PeriOperative Registered Nurses, www.aorn.org

Australian College of Operating Room Nurses, www.acorn.org.au

Practice guidelines for postanesthetic care: an updated report by the American Society of Anesthesiologists Task Force of Postanesthetic Care, www.guideline.gov/content.aspx?id=43896

Operating Room Nurses Association of Canada, www.ornac.ca

Further reading

British Journal of Anaesthetic and Recovery Nursing

Journal of PeriAnesthesia Nursing

Odom-Forren J (ed). Drain's perianesthesia nursing: A critical care approach. 6th ed. St Louis: Elsevier; 2013.

Strunden MS, Heckel K, Goetz AE, Reuter DA. Perioperative fluid and volume management: physiological basis, tools and strategies. Ann Intensive Care 2011;1(1):2.

References

1 American Society of PeriAnesthesia Nurses. ASPAN's history timeline, <http://www.aspan.org/AboutUs/History/tabid/3146/Default. aspx#Beginning>; 2012.

2 Schick L. Assessment and monitoring of the perianesthesia patient. In: Odom-Forren J (ed). Perianaesthesia nursing: A critical care approach. 6th ed. St Louis: Elsevier; 2013.

3 Mullen R, Scollay J, Hecht G, McPhillips G, Thompson A. Death within 48h – adverse events after general surgical procedures. Surgeon 2012;10(1):1–5.

4 Australian Commission on Safety and Quality in Healthcare. National consensus statement: Essential elements for recognising and responding to clinical deterioration. Sydney: ACSQHC; 2010, pp 1-20.

5 de Vries EN, Ramrattan MA, Smorenburg SM, Gouma DJ, Boermeester MA. The incidence and nature of in-hospital adverse events: a systematic review. Qual Saf Health Care 2008;17(3):216-23.

6 Drain CB. Inhalation anesthesia. In: Odom-Forren J, ed. Perianesthesia nursing: A critical care approach. 6th ed. St Louis: Elsevier; 2013.

7 Butterworth J, Mckey D, Wasnick J. The practice of anesthesiology. In: Butterworth J, Mackey D, Wasnick J, eds. Morgan and Mikhail's clinical anesthesiology. 5th ed. New York: McGraw-Hill; 2013.

8 Loryan I, Lindqvist M, Johansson I, Hiratsuka M, van der Heiden I, van Schaik RH et al. Influence of sex on propofol metabolism, a pilot study: implications for propofol anesthesia. Eur J Clin Pharmacol 2012;68(4):397-406.

9 Smith S, Scarth E, Sasada M. Drugs in anaesthesia and intensive care. 4th ed. Oxford: Oxford University Press; 2011.

10 Drain CB. Nonopioid intravenous anesthetics. In: Odom-Forren J, ed. Perianesthesia nursing: A critical care approach. 6th ed. St Louis: Elsevier; 2013.

11 Bandschapp O, Filitz J, Ihmsen H, Berset A, Urwyler A, Koppert W et al. Analgesic and antihyperalgesic properties of propofol in a human pain model. Anesthesiology 2010;113(2):421-8.

12 Frolich MA, Price DD, Robinson ME, Shuster JJ, Theriaque DW, Heft MW. The effect of propofol on thermal pain perception. Anesth Analg 2005;100(2):481-6.

13 Cies J, Moront M, Parker J, Ostrowicki R, DaSilva S. Use of etomidate for rapid sequence intubation (RSI) in pediatric trauma patients: a national survey. Crit Care Med 2013; 12 (Suppl):A236.

14 Flynn G, Shehabi Y. Pro/con debate: is etomidate safe in hemodynamically unstable critically ill patients? Crit Care 2012;16(4):227.

15 Yang HS, Kim T-Y, Bang S, Yu G-Y, Oh C, Kim S-N et al. Comparison of the impact of the anesthesia induction using thiopental and propofol on cardiac function for non-cardiac surgery. J Cardiovascular Ultrasound 2014;22(2):58-64.

16 Drain CB. Opioid intravenous anesthetics. In: Odom-Forren J, ed. Perianesthesia nursing: A critical care approach. 6th ed. St Louis: Elsevier; 2013.

17 Gandhi K, Baratta JL, Heitz JW, Schwenk ES, Vaghari B, Viscusi ER. Acute pain management in the postanesthesia care unit. Anesthesiol Clin 2012;30(3):e1-15.

18 McKeen MJ, Quraishi SA. Clinical review of intravenous opioids in acute care. Journal of Anesthesiology & Clinical Science [Internet]. 2013; 2.

19 Bujedo BM, Santos SG, Azpiazu AU. A review of epidural and intrathecal opioids used in the management of postoperative pain. J Opioid Manag 2012;8(3):177-92.

20 Howlett C, Gonzalez R, Yerram P, Faley B. Use of naloxone for reversal of life-threatening opioid toxicity in cancer-related pain. J Oncol Pharm Pract 2014 Sep 16. pii: 1078155214551589.

21 Barone CP, Walthall B, Fenton M, Tinsley M, Fikes BD. Better pain relief in the PACU. OR Nurse 2010;4(1):21-6.

22 Simon MV. Intraoperative neurophysiology. New York: Demos Medical Publishing; 2010.

23 Banchs RJ, Lerman J. Preoperative anxiety management, emergence delirium, and postoperative behavior. Anesthesiol Clin 2014;32(1):1-23.

24 Lu F, Lin J, Benditt DG. Conscious sedation and anesthesia in the cardiac electrophysiology laboratory. J Cardiovasc Electrophysiol 2013;24(2):237-45.

25 Gan TJ, Diemunsch P, Habib AS, Kovac A, Kranke P, Meyer TA et al. Consensus guidelines for the management of postoperative nausea and vomiting. Anesth Analg 2014;118(1):85-113.

26 Farooq K, Hunter JM. Neuromuscular blocking agents and reversal agents. Anaesthesia and Intensive Care Medicine 2014;15(6):295-9.

27 Patton KT, Thibodeau GA. Anatomy and physiology. 7th ed. St Louis: Mosby; 2010.

28 Butterworth J, Mackey D, Wasnick J. Neuromuscular blocking agents. In: Butterworth J, Mackey D, Wasnick J, eds. Morgan and Mikhail's clinical anesthesiology. 5th ed. New York: McGraw-Hill Medical; 2013.

29 Naguib M, Kopman AF, Lien CA, Hunter JM, Lopez A, Brull SJ. A survey of current management of neuromuscular block in the United States and Europe. Anesth Analg 2010;111(1):110-9.

30 Drain CB. Neuromuscular blocking agents. In: Odom-Forren J, ed. Perianesthesia nursing: A critical care approach. 6th ed. St Louis: Elsevier; 2013.

31 Siedlecki SL. Pain and sedation. In: Carlson K, ed. Advanced critical care nursing. St Louis: Saunders; 2009.

32 Plaud B, Debaene B, Donati F, Marty J. Residual paralysis after emergence from anesthesia. Anesthesiology 2010;112(4):1013-22.

33 Murphy GS, Brull SJ. Residual neuromuscular block: lessons unlearned. Part I: definitions, incidence, and adverse physiologic effects of residual neuromuscular block. Anesth Analg 2010;111(1):120-8.

34 Brull SJ, Murphy GS. Residual neuromuscular block: lessons unlearned. Part II: methods to reduce the risk of residual weakness. Anesth Analg 2010;111(1):129-40.

35 Tsur A, Kalansky A. Hypersensitivity associated with sugammadex administration: a systematic review. Anaesthesia 2014;69(11):1251-7.

36 Ben Salem C, Badreddine A, Fathallah N, Slim R, Hmouda H. Drug-induced hyperkalemia. Drug Saf 2014;37(9):677-92.

37 Jat KR, Chawla D. Ketamine for management of acute exacerbations of asthma in children. Cochrane Database Syst Rev 2012;11:CD009293.

38 Nagelhout JJ. Basic principles of pharmacology. In: Odom-Forren J, ed. Perianesthesia nursing: A critical care approach. 6th ed. St Louis: Elsevier; 2013.

39 Friel CJ, Eliadi C, Pesaturo KA. Local anesthetic use in perioperative areas. Perioperative Nurs Clin 2010;5:203-14.

40 Segall N, Bonifacio A, Schroeder R, Barbeito A, Rogers D, Thornlow D et al. Can we make postoperative patient handovers safer? A systematic review of the literature. Anesth Analg 2012;115(1):102-15.

41 The Australian and New Zealand College of Anaesthetists. Statement on the handover responsibilities of the anaesthetist: bBackground paper. Melbourne: The Australian and New Zealand College of Anaesthetists, <http://www.anzca.edu.au/resources/professional-documents/pdfs/ps53bp-2013-statement-on-the-handover-responsibilities-of-the-anaesthetist-background-paper.pdf/view?searchterm=handover>; 2013 [accessed 25.04.14].

42 Wright S. Assessment and management of the airway, In: Odom-Forren J, ed. Perianaesthesia nursing: A critical care approach. 6th ed. St Louis: Elsevier; 2013.

43 Hedenstierna G. Oxygen and anesthesia: what lung do we deliver to the post-operative ward? Acta Anaesthesiol Scand 2012;56(6):675-85.

44 O'Brien D. Postanesthesia care complications. In: Odom-Forren J, ed. Perianesthesia nursing: A critical care approach. St Louis: Elsevier; 2013.

45 Howie WO, Dutton RP. Implementation of an evidence-based extubation checklist to reduce extubation failure in patients with trauma: a pilot study. AANA J 2012;80(3):179-84.

46 Subbe C. Failure to rescue: using rapid response systems to improve care of the deteriorating patient in hospital Clinical Risk 2013;19(1):6-11.

47 Cooper S, Cant R, Sparkes L. Respiratory rate records: the repeated rate. J Clin Nurs 2014;23(9–10):1236-8.

48 Kasuya Y, Akca O, Sessler DI, Ozaki M, Komatsu R. Accuracy of postoperative end-tidal PCO_2 measurements with mainstream and sidestream capnography in non-obese patients and in obese patients with and without obstructive sleep apnea. Anesthesiology 2009;111(3):609-15.

49 Anderson M, Watson G. Traumatic shock: the fifth shock. Journal of Trauma Nursing, <http://eds.a.ebscohost.com.ezproxy-m.deakin.edu.au/ehost/detail?vid=4&sid=1306eb51-af87-4e3d-b582-06ca07c14ae3%40sessionmgr4002&hid=4202&bdata=JnNpdGU9ZWhvc3QbGl2ZSZzY29wZT1zaXRl#db=ccm&AN=2012065447>; 2013 [accessed 16.07.14].

50 Malina P. Fluid and electrolytes. In: Odom-Forren J, ed. Drain's perianaesthesia nursing: A critical care approach. St Louis: Elsevier; 2013.

51 Strunden MS, Heckel K, Goetz AE, Reuter DA. Perioperative fluid and volume management: physiological basis, tools and strategies. Ann Intensive Care 2011;1(1):2.

52 Samaraee A, Rhind G, Saleh U, Bhattachacharya V. Factors contributing to poor post-operative abdominal pain management in adult patient: a review. The Surgeon 2010;8:151-8.

53 Bucknall T, Manias E, Botti M. Acute pain management: implications of scientific evidence for nursing practice in the postoperative context. Int J Nurs Pract 2001;7(4):266-73.

54 Hartog CS, Rothaug J, Goettermann A, Zimmer A, Meissner W. Room for improvement: nurses' and physicians' views of a post-operative pain management program. ACTA Anesthesiol Scand 2010;54(3):277-83.

55 Ulufer Sivrikaya G. Multimodal analgesia for postoperative pain management. In: Pain managment: Current issues and opinions. Rijeka, Croatia: InTech, <http://www.intechopen.com/books/pain-management-current-issues-and-opinions/multimodal-analgesia-for-postoperative-pain-management>; 2012.

56 Macario A, Royal MA. A literature review of randomized clinical trials of intravenous acetaminophen (paracetamol) for acute postoperative pain. Pain Pract 2011;11(3):290-6.

57 Apfel CC, Turan A, Souza K, Pergolizzi J, Hornuss C. Intravenous acetaminophen reduces postoperative nausea and vomiting: a systematic review and meta-analysis. Pain 2013;154(5):677-89.

58 Vickers MD, O'Flaherty D, Szekely SM, Read M, Yoshizumi J. Tramadol: pain relief by an opioid without depression of respiration. Anaesthesia and Intensive Care Medicine 1992;47(4):291-96.

59 Pasero C. Pain management. In: Odom-Forren J, ed. Perianaesthesia nursing: A critical care approach. 6th ed. St Louis: Elsevier; 2013.

60 Nikolajsen L, Haroutiunian S. Intravenous patient-controlled analgesia for acute postoperative pain. European Journal of Pain Supplements 2011;5(S2):453-56.

61 Australian and New Zealand College of Anaesthetists. Types of anaesthesia. Melbourne: Australian and New Zealand College of Anaesthetists, <http://www.anzca.edu.au/patients/types-of-anaesthestist> [accessed 22.08.14].

62 Moos D. Regional anaesthsia. In: Odom-Forren J, ed. Perianaesthesia nursing: A critical care approach. St Louis: Elsevier; 2013.

63 Weetman C, Allison W. Use of epidural analgesia in post-operative pain management. Nurs Stand 2006;20(44):54-64; quiz 6.

64 Butterworth J, Mackey D, Wasnick J. Spinal, epidural, and caudal blocks. In: Butterworth J, Mackey D, Wasnick J, eds. Morgan and Mikhail's clinical anesthesiology. 5th ed. New York: McGraw-Hill Medical; 2013.

65 Nagelhout J, Plaus K, eds. Nurse anesthesia. 4th ed. St Louis: Saunders; 2010.

66 Breen TW, Shapiro T, Glass B, Foster-Payne D, Oriol NE. Epidural anesthesia for labor in an ambulatory patient. Anesth Analg 1993;77(5):919-24.

67 Goswami D, Das J, Deuri A, Deka AK. Epidural haematoma: rare complication after spinal while intending epidural anaesthesia with long-term follow-up after conservative treatment. Indian J Anaesth 2011;55(1):71-3.

68 Shaparin N, Gritsenko K, Shapiro D, Kosharskyy B, Kaye D, Smith HS. Timing of neuraxial pain interventions following blood patch for post dural puncture headache. Pain Physician 2014;17(2):119-1125.

69 Karagucuchi M, Hashizume K, Watanabe K, Inoue S, Furuya H. Fluoroscopically guided epidural blood patch in patients with postdural headache after spinal and epidural anesthesia. J Anesth 2011;25(3):450-3.

70 Bernard H. Patient warming in surgery and the enhanced recover. Brit J Nurs 2013;22(6):319-25.

71 Mulry D, Mooney B. Prevention of perioperative hypothermia. WIN 2012;20(2):26-7.

72 Moola S, Lockwood C. Effectiveness of statagies for the management and/or prevention of hypothermia within the adult perioperative environment. Int J Evid Based Healthc 2011;9(4):337-45.

73 Mhyre J. Anaesthetic management for the morbidly obese pregnant woman. Int Anesthesiol Clin 2007;45(1):51-70.

74 Lloret-Linares C, Lopes A, Decleves X, Serrie A, Mouly S, Bergmann JF, et al. Challenges in the optimisation of post-operative pain management with opioids in obese patients: a literature review. Obes Surg 2013;23(9):1458-75.

75 Clifford T. Care of the obese patient undergoing bariatric surgery. In: Odom-Forren J, ed. Perianaesthesia nursing: A critical care approach. St Louis: Elsevier; 2013.

76 Mendon J, Pereiraa H, Xaráa D, Santosa A, Abelhaa F. Obese patients: respiratory complications in the post-anesthesia care unit. Rev Port Pneumol 2014;20(1):12-9.

77 Butterworth J, Mackey D, Wasnick J. Airway management. In: Butterworth J, Mackey D, Wasnick J, eds. Morgan and Mikhail's clinical anesthesiology. 5th ed. New York: McGraw-Hill Medical; 2013.

78 Drain CB. The respiratory system. In: Odom-Forren J, ed. Drain's perianaesthesia nursing: A critical care approach. 6th ed. St Louis: Elsevier; 2013.

79 Erb T, von Ungern-Sternberg B, Keller K, Frei F. The effect of intravenous lidocaine on laryngeal and respiratory reflex responses in anaesthetised children. Anaesthesia 2013;68:13-20.

80 Sharma S, Samplay M, Marshnay S. Pulmonary edema after thyroidectomy. Case report and review. Internet J Anesthesiol 2008;18:ISSN: 1092–406X.

81 Raiger LK, Naithani U, Vijay BS, Gupta P, Bhargava V. Non-cardiogenic pulmonary oedema after neostigmine given for reversal: a report of two cases. Indian J Anaesth 2010;54(4):338-41.

82 Tarrac S. Negative pressure pulmonary edema – a postanesthesia emergency. Journal of Peri-Anestheia Nursing 2003;18(5):317-23.

83 Wetsch WA, Spöhr FA, Hinkelbein J, Padosch SA. Emergency extracorporeal membrane oxygenation to treat massive aspiration during anaesthesia induction. A case report. Acta Anaesthesiol Scan 2012;56(6):797-800.

84 Russell IF. The ability of bispectral index to detect intra-operative wakefulness during isoflurane/air anaesthesia, compared with the isolated forearm technique. Anaesthesia 2013;68(10):1010-20.

85 Levinson C, Rodebaugh T, Bertelson A. Prolonged exposure therapy following awareness under anesthesia: a case study. Cognitive and Behavioral Practice 2013;20(1):74-80.

86 Leslie K, Chan MT, Myles PS, Forbes A, McCulloch TJ. Posttraumatic stress disorder in aware patients from the B-aware trial. Anesth Analg 2010;110(3):823-8.

87 Munk L, Hoist Andersen L, Gögenur I. Emergence delirium. J Periop Pract 2013;23(11):251-4.

88 McGuire J. The incidence of and risk factors for emergence delirium in U.S. military combat veterans. Journal of Peri-Anestheia Nursing 2012;27:236-45.

89 Saranagi S. Delayed awakening from anaesthesia. Internet J Anesthesiol, <http://eds.a.ebscohost.com.ezproxy-m.deakin.edu.au/ehost/detail?vid=15&sid=aec87267-0242-4080-b015-592069f17aac%40sessionmgr4003&hid=4103&bdata=JnNpdGU9ZWhvc3QtbGl2ZSZzY29wZT1zaXRl#db=ccm&AN=2010177084>; 2008 [accessed 6.07.14].

90 Cain C, Riess M, Gettrust L, Novalija J. Malignant hyperthermia crisis: optimizing patient outcomes through simulation and interdisciplinary collaboration. AORN 2014;99 (2):300-11.

91 Hirshey Dirksen SJ, Larach MG, Rosenberg H, Brandom BW, Parness J, Lang RS et al. Future directions in malignant hyperthermia research and patient care. Anesth Analg 2011;113(5):1108-18.

92 Hommertzheim R, Steinke E. Malignant hypertermia: the perioperative nurse's role. AORN J 2006;83(1):151-63.

93 Banek R, Weatherwax J, Spence D, Perry P, Muldoon S, Capacchione J. Delayed onset of suspected alignant hyperthermia during sevoflurane anesthesia in an Afghan trauma patient: a case report. AANA J 2013;81(6):441-5.

94 Hooper VD. Care of the patient with thermal imbalance. In: Odom-Forren J, ed. Perianesthesia nursing: A critical care approach. 6th ed. St Louis: Elsevier; 2013.

95 Hirshey Dirksen S, Van Wicklin S, Ledrut Mashman D, Neiderer P, Merritt D. Developing effective drills in preparation for a malignant hyperthermia crisis. AORN 2013;97(3):330-52.

96 Larach M, Gronert G, Allen G, Brandom B, Lehman E. Clinical manifestation, treatment and complications of malignant hyperthermia in North America from 1987 to 2006. Aneth Analg 2010;110 (2):498-507.

97 Bromage PR. Epidural analgesia. Philadelphia: WB Saunders; 1978. p 144.

98 Seifert PC, Wahr JA, Pace M, Cochrane AB, Bagnola AJ. Crisis management of malignant hyperthermia in the OR. AORN J 2014;100(2): 189-202 e1.

99 Carter-Templeton H. Awake to danger: temperature rising. Nursing Made Incredibally Easy 2006;4(4):10-1.

100 Mitchell-Brown F. Turn down the heat. Nursing 2012;42(5):39-44.

101 Clifford T. Length of stay – discharge criteria. J Perianesth Nurs 2014;29(2):159-60.

102 Karadag M, Pekin Iseri O. Determining health personnel's application trends of new guidelines for perioperative fasting: findings from a survey. J Perianesth Nurs 2014;29(3):175-84.

103 Murphy GS, Ault ML, Wong HY, Szokol JW. The effect of a new NPO policy on operating room utilization. J Clin Anesth 2000;12(1):48-51.

104 Ljungqvist O, Soreide E. Preoperative fasting. Br J Surg 2003;90(4):400-6.

105 Bulfone G, Juana M, Bresadola V. Differences between clinical practices and literature: recommendations in the preoperative fasting and skin preparation. Int Nurs Perspect 2008;8:13-20.

Chapter 27

Paediatric considerations in critical care

Tina Kendrick, Anne-Sylvie Ramelet

Learning objectives

After reading this chapter, you should be able to:

- consider and anticipate the specific needs of critically ill infants and children
- describe common conditions that lead to critical illness in infants and children
- discuss and apply age-appropriate assessment, monitoring and management of critically ill infants and children
- identify age-appropriate parameters and care required by critically ill infants and children who require ventilation
- discuss psychological and emotional care required by critically ill infants and children, and their families
- consider the child's family in all interactions.

Introduction

This chapter focuses on specific considerations for the care of critically ill infants and children experiencing, or at risk of experiencing, common life-threatening conditions. These include respiratory diseases common in the paediatric population, major trauma, shock and sepsis. It is aimed at the critical care nurse who encounters paediatric patients occasionally and, while not designed to meet all the needs of specialist paediatric critical care nurses, it provides a summary of the assessment, monitoring and care required by critically ill children. A systems approach has been used in this chapter for convenience, although paediatrics is a specialty defined by age rather than body systems.

Not only will children experience different patterns of illness and injury compared to adults, their behavioural and physiological responses to illness differ. It is important that the child's primary caregiver, who will usually be a parent (the term used throughout this chapter), be included in planning many aspects of care. While members of the critical care team are expert in management of critical illness, parents are generally the experts on their child, can provide the child's health history and know how best to settle the child in addition to knowing what their 'normal' behaviours are. For these reasons, parental concern should never be ignored or down-played, as this child-centred knowledge makes them valuable members of the team.

Over 11,000 children in Australia and New Zealand required admission to intensive care units (ICUs) in 2013.[1] Children account for almost 6% of all ICU admissions in Australia and New Zealand, representing a figure of 1.72 admissions per 100,000 children, a slightly higher figure than in the UK (1.53/100,000).[1] 50% of these children required mechanical ventilation[1] compared with around 39% of adults in intensive care,[2] indicating a 5% reduction in children requiring ventilation over the past 2 years. While almost 80% of critically ill children were admitted to specialist paediatric ICUs (PICUs), a significant number were managed in or retrieved from adult ICUs.[1] In many circumstances, children will respond effectively to initial resuscitation, particularly support of breathing and fluid resuscitation, and may not require transfer to a specialist PICU.

The age distribution of children in ICUs has remained the same for many years, with the figures from 2013 showing that children under the age of 5 years represent just under 67% of admissions, with 57% of this age group under 12 months of age and 24% under 4 weeks of age.[1] Boys make up almost 58% of children admitted to ICUs.[1] The overall ICU mortality rate is 9.2% for Australia and 10.3% for New Zealand;[2] however, the paediatric mortality rate is 2.6%.[1,2] Over the past 30 years, although length of stay and severity of illness in Australian PICUs have not essentially changed, mortality has halved while disability has increased.[3] Although other developed countries have not yet reported their own experiences, this trend is likely to be worldwide, reflecting the technological advances made generally in ICU care.

Anatomical and physiological considerations in children

Children require age- and developmentally-appropriate care. An appropriate range of paediatric equipment is required to assess, monitor and treat all ages and sizes of infants and children. General considerations based on differences between children and adults are described and then a systems approach is used to identify specific differences. The terms 'infants' and 'children' are used throughout the remainder of this chapter. 'Infants' includes children up to the age of 1 year and all other age groups are 'children'.

A number of general considerations, based on anatomical and physiological differences from adults, need to be considered for the critically ill child.

- Children have increased surface area-to-volume ratio compared with adults, which leads to increased heat loss and insensible fluid losses, placing infants and children at increased risk of developing hypothermia and dehydration. Providing an environment that maintains the infant and small child's body temperature is essential. Avoid exposing infants and children more than necessary; use warming blankets,

open care systems for all newborns and infants under 4 kg and overhead heaters when exposure is unavoidable. Temperature monitoring is required when using any heating devices to avoid iatrogenic thermal injury.

- Lower glycogen stores and increased metabolic rate predispose infants to hypoglycaemia. There are few standard doses in PICU; rather, medication doses and fluid requirements are calculated on age and kilograms of body weight. Weight of infants and children should therefore be estimated as accurately as possible. The Broselow tape measure is a colour-coded length-based method developed in North America to estimate weight for the use of resuscitation equipment sizes and drug doses. It is particularly accurate in children under 12 and up to 35 kg[4] and has been found to perform well across Asian and African countries.[5–7] Differences may occur in estimated weight of children of different origin and overweight children. The addition of body habitus in the newly developed paediatric advanced weight prediction in the emergency room (PAWPER) tape improves performance of length-based tapes.[8]

- Fluid requirements are based on body weight, and aim to ensure adequate hydration while preventing fluid overload. Maintenance intravenous (IV) fluids for infants and young children typically require the addition of glucose. Isotonic sodium chloride is recommended as the first choice fluid bolus in paediatric resuscitation.[9] Table 27.1 provides a guide for fluid maintenance requirements of children based on body weight.

- Excluding the newborn period, normal values for all blood gas and serum electrolyte levels are the same as adult levels. Creatinine and urea levels will vary with age.

Practice tip

To estimate weight, use the Broselow tape measure in the following way: 1) place the tape so the red arrow is positioned at the top of the child's head, 2) align the tape parallel to the side of the child who must be lying in a supine position, 3) extend the legs straight and 4) bend the ankle so the toes are pointing straight up. Look at the weight in the coloured areas directly under the bottom of the foot.

Practice tip

If paediatric oxygen masks are not available, an adult-sized mask, including a partial non-rebreather mask, can be used in an emergency. Place the nose section under the child or infant's chin in the 'upside-down' position.

TABLE 27.1
Guide to maintenance water in healthy children

For each of the first 10 kg body weight: 100 mL/kg/day or 4 mL/kg/hour
+ for each of the second 10 kg of body weight: 50 mL/kg/day or 2 mL/kg/hour
+ for every subsequent kg of body weight: 20 mL/kg/day or 1 mL/kg/hour

WEIGHT (KG)	ML/H	ML/KG/DAY
4	16	100
6	24	100
8	32	100
10	40	100
12	44	88
14	48	82
16	52	78
18	56	75
20	60	72
30	70	56
40	80	48
50	90	42
60	100	38
70	110	36

Adapted from Cavari Y, Pitfield AF, Kissoon N. Intravenous maintenance fluids revisited. Pediatr Emerg Care 2013; 29:1225–31.[243]

TABLE 27.2
Target cerebral perfusion pressure (CPP) by age

AGE	DESIRABLE MINIMUM CPP
Infants under 1 year	45–50 mmHg
Children 1–10 years	>55 mmHg
Children over 10 years	>65 mmHg

Adapted from Allen BB, Chiu Y, Gerber LM, Ghaja J, Greenfield JP. Age-specific cerebral perfusion pressure thresholds and survival in children and adolescents with severe traumatic brain injury. Pediatr Crit Care Med 2014;15:62–70.[12]

Central nervous system

Many central nervous system functions, such as locomotion and hand–eye coordination, will take from months to years to fully develop. Functions of the cerebral cortex are particularly underdeveloped, with myelination of all major nerve tracts continuing throughout infancy.[10] Consequently, assessment and management priorities will be dictated by the level of neurological maturity of the infant or child. The plasticity inherent in the brain of the infant may compensate for injury more readily than in older children and adults in some circumstances, with other areas of the infant's brain taking over function. Because the eight cranial bones are not yet fused, infants' skulls cope with both birth and ongoing growth, which is greatest in the first 2 years of life. In the first year, the cartilaginous sutures fuse at two points to form the posterolateral fontanelle. The larger anterior fontanelle closes during the second year as bone is laid down. By around 5 years of age, the sutures of the child's skull are completely fused.[11] However, the thinner skull will provide less protection to underlying tissues than the adult skull.

A common misconception is that the Monro-Kellie doctrine (see Chapter 16) does not apply to young children and infants with a more compliant skull. While slow rises in intracranial volume may be accommodated over time in children under 3 years of age, they will usually be accompanied by growing head circumference, making routine measurement of head circumference in children under 3 years of age an important assessment. However, the less rigid skull of the older child will not compensate for acute rises in intracranial volume, and the child will display symptoms of neurological compromise.[12] Normal ranges of intracranial pressure (ICP) and cerebral perfusion pressure (CPP) have not been formally studied in infants and children, but are presumed to be lower than in adults, reaching adult range by adolescence. Values that are commonly used to guide treatment are age-related and are displayed in Table 27.2.

Cardiovascular system

Infants produce both fetal and adult haemoglobin up to 6 months of age, when levels of fetal haemoglobin (approximately 60–70% to this point) fall rapidly and production of adult haemoglobin predominates.[10] Fetal haemoglobin allows greater amounts of oxygen to be carried for any given PaO_2 in utero and in infancy. Circulating blood volume per kilogram decreases with age; in the infant, circulating volume is approximately 85 mL/kg, with total body water accounting for 70% of body mass, adjusting to the adult values of 65 mL/kg and total body water of 60%.[10] The apex beat is heard at the fourth intercostal space, mid-clavicle and, by around 7 years of age, the left ventricle has grown and the apex beat can be heard at the fifth intercostal space, as in adults. An infant's cardiac output is approximately 500 mL/min, which, relative to body weight, is about twice that of an adult.[11] Heart rate is a major determinant of cardiac output in infants and young children, as there is limited ability to increase stroke volume. Tachycardia is an early sign of distress, but bradycardia is an ominous sign in infants and young children, as they are more dependent on a high heart rate to maintain cardiac output. In infants, bradycardia of 60/min and below requires resuscitation.

Arterial blood pressure should be appropriate for age, weight and clinical condition. Mean arterial pressure is generally used. Monitoring blood pressure using correct cuff sizes is important because incorrect cuff size is a

TABLE 27.3

Age-related ranges for mean blood pressure

AGE	MEAN BP (MMHG)
Term	40–60
3 months	45–75
6 months	50–90
1 year	50–90
3 years	50–90
7 years	60–90
10 years	60–90
12 years	65–95
14 years	65–95

Adapted from NSW Clinical Excellence Commission. Between the flags standard paediatric observation charts. 2nd ed. Sydney: NSW Health; 2013.[244]

common cause of inaccurate blood pressure readings in children. Diastolic blood pressure is recorded at Korotkoff sound 5 (K5); age-related parameters for mean blood pressure are displayed in Table 27.3.

Paediatric considerations for cardiovascular assessment

Cardiovascular assessment in children includes clinical parameters that are similar to those observed in adults. The normal values are, however, age and weight dependent. Indirect evidence of poor systemic perfusion in infants may include:[13]

- feeding difficulties
- abdominal distension
- fluid imbalances
- temperature instability
- hypoglycaemia
- hypocalcaemia
- apnoea.

Neurological changes with poor systemic perfusion in children are irritability, then disorientation or lethargy. Clinical signs of reduced cardiac output, typically seen in shock, are similar to adults.[14]

Respiratory system

The child's respiratory system, including airways, continues to mature until at least 8 years of age; therefore the paediatric airway is described and managed differently from the adult's. Structural and mechanical differences predispose infants and young children to respiratory compromise. Respiratory compromise leading to apnoeas and even respiratory arrest is a relatively common occurrence in the paediatric population, although specific incidences of occurrence have not been determined.

The newborn's larynx is just one-third of the diameter of the adult larynx.[11] Narrow nasal passages, in combination

with being obligatory nose-breathers up to 5–6 months of age, mean that infants may experience respiratory distress if nasal passages become oedematous or contain secretions such as mucus or blood. With the airway of an infant measuring around 6 mm in diameter at the level of the cricoid, obstruction is more likely. The paediatric airway is characterised and differentiated from an adult airway by the following features (see Figures 27.1 and 27.2):[11,15]

- short maxilla and mandible
- large tongue
- floppy epiglottis
- shorter trachea
- more acute angle of airway, particularly notable when attempting to visualise with a laryngoscope
- a more cephalad larynx that moves distally as the neck grows
- a cricoid ring that is the narrowest portion of the airway
- smaller lower airways, less developed with fewer alveoli
- true alveoli not present until 2 months, with full complement developed by around 8 years of age
- little smooth muscle present in airways
- little collateral ventilation in airways, as the pores of Kohn and canals of Lambert are not fully developed until around 3 to 4 years of age.

TABLE 27.4

Age-related heart and respiratory rates

AGE	RESPIRATORY RATE 10TH–90TH CENTILE	HEART RATE 10TH–90TH CENTILE
Birth–3 months	34–57	123–164
3–6 months	33–55	120–164
6–9 months	31–52	114–152
9–12 months	30–50	109–145
12–18 months	28–46	103–140
18–24 months	25–40	98–135
2–3 years	22–34	92–128
3–4 years	21–29	86–123
4–6 years	20–27	81–117
6–8 years	18–24	74–111
8–12 years	16–22	67–103
12–15 years	15–21	62–96
15–18 years	13–19	58–92

Adapted with permission from Fleming S, Thompson M, Stevens R, Heneghan C, Pluddermann A, Maconochie I et al. Supplement to: normal ranges of heart rate and respiratory rate in children from birth to 18 years of age: a systematic review of observational studies. Lancet [Internet]. 2011 [cited 17.09.14]; 377.[245]

FIGURE 27.1 Anatomy of the adult airway.

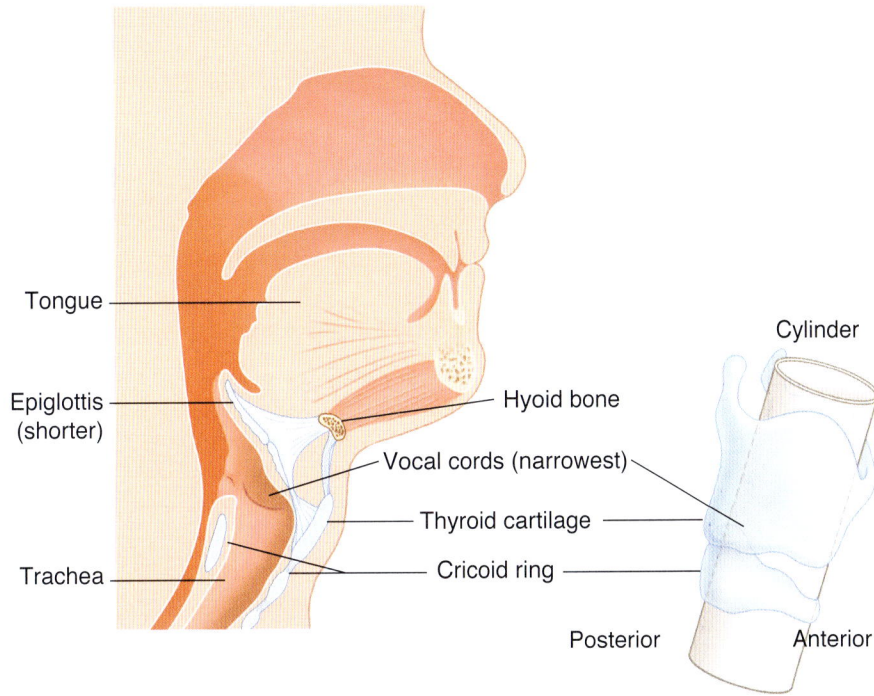

Courtesy Susan Gilbert.

FIGURE 27.2 Anatomy of the paediatric airway.

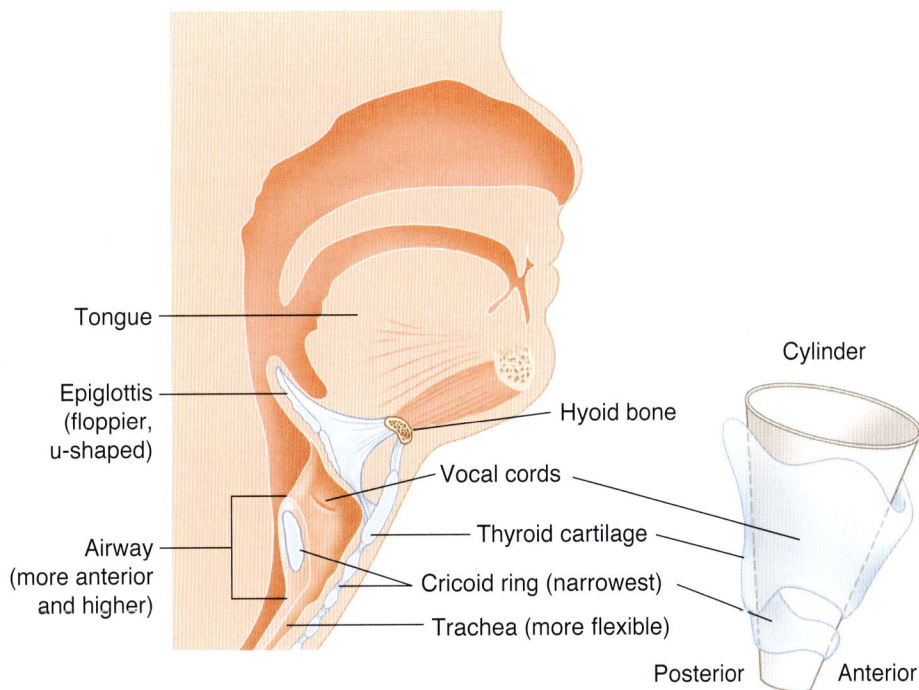

Courtesy Susan Gilbert.

Paediatric respiratory assessment

The thoracic cavity of infants and children is characterised by a thin chest wall that is highly compliant, with poorly developed intercostal and accessory muscles. The diaphragm is the most important muscle for infants and children in respiration, with abdominal muscles also used. The compliant chest wall prevents generation of high intrathoracic pressures, meaning that infants and young children are unable to significantly increase tidal volume; rather, they increase minute volume by breathing faster. This means that tachypnoea is a normal response to illness in infants and children, and a slowing respiratory rate in children may indicate impending collapse rather than clinical improvement.[16]

Assessing airway patency is important. Talking and crying indicate that the infant or child is maintaining their own airway. Adventitious airway noises in children include wheeze, stridor and grunting. In infants, grunting may be heard and is an attempt by the baby to produce positive end-expiratory pressure (PEEP). Infants and children who are grunting, gasping or unconscious need urgent assessment for possible endotracheal intubation.

Other observed signs of respiratory distress in infants and children up to about 8 years old include head bobbing in infants, nasal flaring and paradoxical chest movement observed in several locations on the chest and known as recessions. Recessions can be observed at the costal margin, or subcostal; between the ribs, or intercostal; at the sternum, or sternal; and at the trachea, called tracheal tug. Oral feeding is difficult for infants in moderate-to-severe respiratory distress due to limitations associated with sucking and breathing at the same time. In addition, tachypnoea greater than 60–80 breaths/min may lead to vomiting and aspiration.[17] For these reasons, initial enteral feeding might not be possible or desirable, so nutrients should be given as parenteral nutrition until enteral feeding is tolerated.[18]

Diagnosis of an upper or lower respiratory illness may be made, using the history of the symptoms from the parent or the child when age-appropriate, in conjunction with physical assessment of the child. Assessment of the rate, rhythm, effort and pattern of breathing according to age as well as colour and agitation should be undertaken. Similar to how heart rate is used to increase cardiac output, children compensate to maintain oxygenation for some time by breathing more rapidly until they become fatigued, when they are likely to become hypoxic and ultimately apnoeic.

Gastrointestinal tract

There are few differences between the child's and adult's gastrointestinal tract (GIT) outside the neonatal period, although a palpable liver below the costal margin is a normal finding. It will be up to 3 cm below the costal margin in normal infants, decreasing to 1 cm by 4–5 years of age, and should no longer be palpable in adolescents. In the neonate, a relative pancreatic amylase deficiency means utilisation of starches is less effective. Fats are also absorbed

less well, which is the reason why higher-fat milks such as cow's milk are not ideal for infants. Protein synthesis and storage is, however, enhanced in the neonate.[10]

As the infant liver is not completely mature at birth, gluconeogenesis is deficient, causing low and unstable blood sugar level in the first weeks of life. The infant is therefore reliant on fat stores until normal feeding is established.[11] Formation of plasma proteins and clotting factors are likely to be inadequate in the first weeks of life, thus all newborns in Australasia and many other areas of the world are given vitamin K shortly after birth to prevent bleeding. Blood glucose monitoring and provision of early nutrition are essential aspects of care, especially for infants. Children normally have increased metabolic demands to achieve growth but have fewer energy stores than adults.

Other systems and considerations

The following section presents the paediatric considerations of the genitourinary, musculoskeletal and integumentary systems.

Genitourinary system

The small developing pelvic bones of infants and young children cause adult pelvic organs, such as the bladder, to be located in the lower abdominal cavity. Urine output in children is calculated in mL/kg bodyweight/h. In infants with immature kidney function and limited ability to conserve water, urine output should be 1–2 mL/kg/h. In the first month of life, infants have limited capacity to concentrate urine to only 1.5 times their plasma osmolality, whereas adults concentrate their urine to 3–4 times plasma osmolality. The higher metabolic rate of infants produces twice the acid that an adult will, leading to a tendency to acidosis in critical illness.[10,19] By 6 months of age, normal urine output should be 1 mL/kg/h, and by adolescence 0.5–1 mL/kg/h is considered normal. Catheterisation is generally required in critically ill infants and children for accurate hourly measurement of urine output. Where this is not possible, particularly where small sizes of indwelling catheters are not readily available, weighing nappies will provide an interim estimate of urine output. Inserting feeding tubes in place of a urinary catheter is not recommended.

Practice tip

Where catheterisation is not possible, nappies can be weighed to estimate urine output. Use an indelible marker to record the dry weight of a disposable nappy on the nappy itself. This weight is then subtracted from the nappy's wet weight to give an estimate of volume, with 1 g equivalent to 1 mL.

Musculoskeletal system

Children have less developed musculature than adults, with less protection from external forces that collide with the child. Conversely, a child's skeleton is more cartilaginous than adults and therefore more pliable. As a result, rib fractures rarely accompany chest trauma in children whereas lung contusions are common.[19] The skeleton in children changes from less cartilaginous in nature at infancy to complete ossification and adult features during adolescence, so daily calcium requirements increase over childhood and adolescence.[10]

Integumentary system

Infants have a thinner epidermis, dermis and subcutaneous tissue that will continue to mature. This results in a greater susceptibility to absorption of chemicals, injury from adhesive tapes and any shearing force and loss of water and heat, particularly in the newborn period.[11] Critically ill children are more likely to develop pressure areas on the occiput, ear, sacrum, heel or thigh with pressure ulcers in children often associated with equipment pressing or rubbing on the skin. The Glamorgan paediatric pressure ulcer risk assessment scale is being used increasingly in paediatric settings, including PICUs.[20,21] The Glamorgan scale includes ten subscales: anaemia, equipment pressing, mobility, poor peripheral perfusion, pyrexia, serum albumin, surgery in last 4 weeks, weight <10th centile, continence and nutrition.[20]

Developmental considerations

Admission to ICU is very stressful for paediatric patients[22] and for their family.[23–25] The stressors, combined with the effects of critical illness, can lead to disturbances in normal child development and attachment. The psychological needs of children and families are not always met.[26] Factors that affect the psychosocial wellbeing of a critically ill child include loss of usual routines and self-control; family presence and role; family and friends visits, comfort; and the ICU environment.[22,27,28]

Knowledge and understanding of developmental psychology can help nurses assess and plan care for the critically ill child.[29,30] Identification of internal strengths, external supports and environmental modification can facilitate coping and reduce stress in these children.[31] Parental support is an important coping mechanism of infants and children during periods of stress. Strategies to facilitate coping in children of all ages include:

- facilitating parental presence at all times, including during invasive procedures and resuscitation[32,33]
- maintaining normal routines and rituals as much as possible, including story reading, bedtime routines and presence of favourite toys
- providing appropriate analgesia and sedation as well as non-pharmacological interventions
- providing opportunities for play and activities unrelated to treatment.

Erikson's psychosocial theory is helpful for understanding childhood development.[34] Erikson's theory asserts that people experience eight 'psychosocial crisis stages' that significantly affect their development and personality. The first five stages are presented below.

Infants (stage 1)

The first year of life is concerned with developing a sense of trust, laying a foundation for all future relationships.[29,34] The affective exchanges between infant and the primary caregiver provide a foundation for neurological development and lead to the creation of neural networks (particularly in the right hemisphere) that will influence the infant's personality and relationships with others throughout life.[35,36] Generally, up to the age of 6 months, infants are able to cope with limited separation from their mothers; however, changes to usual routine create anxiety and stress.[34] From about 6 to 18 months of age separation is the major fear, with changes to usual routine and environment resulting in anxiety.[34] Therefore, critically ill infants require parental presence and maintenance of normal routines, including breastfeeding, as much as is practicable.

Toddlers (stage 2)

The toddler period, between 1 and 3 years of age, is a time for establishing autonomy and independence. Control over bodily functions, increasing ability to communicate, ability to view the self as separate from others and being able to tolerate brief separation from the mother are all developmental characteristics during this period.[37] Toddlers tend to be egocentric in how they view the world, so illness, procedures and separation from parents may be perceived as punishment.[34] Their thinking processes include transduction, animism and ritual.[30] Transductive thinking allows a child to link unrelated objects or events, such as separation and endotracheal suction if suction occurs after the parent leaves the room. Animism attributes lifelike traits to inanimate objects, so the ventilator may become a hissing monster, or monitoring leads may be trying to trap them. Many toddlers have varying levels of ritual or sameness, including always eating off the same plate or a security toy or blanket. Regression, or loss of recently acquired skills such as toileting, may also occur during critical illness, creating further distress. When caring for critically ill toddlers, encourage parental presence and maintain as many of the usual rituals and routines as possible to facilitate coping.[38]

Preschool children (stage 3)

Children from 3 to 5 years of age fall into the preschool period of development. It is characterised by discovery, inventiveness, curiosity and the development of culturally and socially acceptable behaviour.[29,30,34] Preschoolers generally verbalise their needs reasonably well.[39] While thought processes become less ritualistic and negative, preschool children are still egocentric and magical thinking emerges, thus ideas about causality and linking events may be faulty. Fears, both real and imagined, are prevalent during this period.[30] For example, fears of monsters or being hurt may occur. They may also feel guilty as a result of illness.[34] There is, however, greater understanding of the passage of time, so parents can leave the preschooler for defined short periods. Hospitalisation remains difficult, but preschoolers respond to anticipatory preparation and concrete explanations.[29]

School-age children (stage 4)

Children from 5 to 11 years are usually referred to as being of school age. This period represents a widening of the sphere of influence from parents/family to include the school environment and peers.[30] A transition from egocentric thinking to concrete operations occurs,[29,30] with children becoming more independent and achievement-oriented for their sense of self-worth. They understand that an object may change its appearance but retains its qualities. For example, if some water is poured into a differently shaped glass, the volume remains the same, even though its appearance has changed. In the ICU, school-age children may have a distorted or fantasy-laden view, and will need concrete explanations. Sicker children are less able to cope with the ICU environment and are more likely to regress, which can have a significant impact on their sense of self-worth. Modesty and privacy are imperative at this age.[40] Preadolescence occurs between 10 and 11 years, and represents a time of turmoil and emotional upheaval.[30]

Adolescents (stage 5)

Adolescence is considered a time of transition from childhood to adulthood. It is typically represented by children aged 12–18 years, or teenagers. Internal changes relate to emotional upheaval, search for autonomy and transition of thought process from concrete to abstract, so they can imagine possible outcomes without actually experiencing them.[34] External changes relate to physical changes, such as the emergence of secondary sex characteristics, with a related preoccupation with bodily functions and image.[29]

A goal in adolescence is to develop an integrated sense of self, achieved through managing the conflicting demands of family and peers. Peer identity is essential to psychological growth and development, as is the gradual shift from family to peer orientation. Peer groups provide a way for adolescents to self-evaluate and to bolster self-esteem. Adolescents also target authority figures with retaliation and defiance. Conversely, adolescents will seek out non-parental adults, such as a teacher or relative, to obtain approval and acceptance.[41] Slote has described a process associated with adolescent illness.[41] The first phase is hopelessness and helplessness provoked by the equipment and environment. Adolescents often think they will not get better, and need to be given clear information about the expected course of the illness. They also need to be included as much as possible in decision making and encouraged to participate in their own care. Feeling helpless and defenceless is contrary to their normal feelings of invincibility and may result in antisocial behaviours. Adolescents must learn to accept the quest for autonomy has been temporarily interrupted. Acknowledging their feelings and setting clear behavioural limits can help an adolescent cope.[41] Adolescents may also experience fear and anxiety, which can be offset by clear explanations, and acknowledgement of feeling through articulation and reflection. Concern for body image is also paramount, particularly fear of mutilation and scarring. Physical appearance is important for acceptance into the peer group and for self-esteem.[41]

Family issues and consent

When children are admitted to an ICU, the whole family is affected by the hospitalisation. 'Family-centred care' (FCC) provides a framework for the care of children and their family in hospital[42] and is discussed in Chapter 8. FCC means that, during a hospital stay, nursing 'care is planned around the whole family, not just the individual child, and … all the family members are recognized as care recipients'.[42,p 1318] Parents should receive unbiased information at regular intervals, and be involved in the decision-making process and the care of their child. This parent–professional collaboration should be facilitated at all levels of health care.[42] As the developmental issues highlight, parents are essential to a child's coping with critical illness. Critically ill children are particularly vulnerable to short- and long-term emotional and psychological sequelae, but parental presence and participation in care can make a difference.[43]

Parents need to feel involved in their child's care, and this includes the need for information, communication, understanding the child's illness and being part of the decision-making process.[24,26,44,45] A partnership between staff and parents is the ideal situation, but parents often need to be reminded how to maintain the parental role and how they can effectively care for both their child's and their own psychological health.[46] Parents should be allowed to be present during potentially stressful situations such as endotracheal suction, cannulation and resuscitation if they choose to, providing adequate support from a nurse or another designated healthcare worker is given.[32] Being present at the end of their child's life may help parents through their grieving process.[33] Not allowing parents to be present during procedures is a form of paternalism that goes against the rights of the patient.[47] Parents should, however, be informed of their right to leave if they want to.

Consent and assent

Except for emergency treatment, parents or legal guardians need to consent to all aspects of medical care, including preventive, diagnostic or therapeutic measures for children. The legal age of consent differs between jurisdictions but is 18 years in major European countries and all Australian states, except New South Wales and South Australia, where the legal age for consent is 14 and 16 years, respectively.[48] Informed assent is described as providing permission for procedures when a child is not legally authorised or lacks sufficient understanding to provide informed consent but has the emotional maturity and intellectual capacity to agree to procedures.[49,50] To be considered competent, young people must be able to understand the nature of the decision as well as the consequences of making or not making the decision.[50] Whenever possible, it is recommended to obtain the child's assent for treatment or procedures. Children, even when deemed not competent, have the right to be informed and, when appropriate, to be asked for their permission. However, refusal of treatment by a child has no legal bearing when a parent has consented. Importantly, parents may also refuse to consent and, in that case, laws and legal mechanisms for resolving disputes may be used.[51]

Pain and sedation

Critically ill infants and children are particularly vulnerable to pain. If pain remains unrelieved it may cause short- and long-term physiological and psychological complications, such as increased risk of mortality and morbidity.[52] The assessment of pain in children is particularly challenging,[53] but the use of valid pain and sedation assessment tools has proved to be useful for the management of pain in critically ill children.[54–56] Prevention of procedural pain is important not only to avoid pain-related complications and emotional trauma, but also to facilitate the procedure.[57] Optimal level of sedation varies for each patient and will be dependent on the underlying diagnosis and severity of illness. Individualised sedation level targeted to the child's clinical status is therefore recommended to help maintain children in a comfortable state without compromising haemodynamic and respiratory status, while minimising other undesirable effects of analgesics and sedatives.

When the provision of analgesics and sedatives is necessary to keep children comfortable, there is a risk for withdrawal of these drugs when given over a prolonged period of time (>5 days).[58,59] Prevalence rates of withdrawal syndrome in PICU patients receiving benzodiazepines and/or opioids for 5 or more days was reported to be between 10% and 75%.[59,60]

Pain and sedation assessment

Recent advances in the assessment of pain and sedation show that pain and sedation remain problematic in paediatric critical care and highlight the need for routine assessment, documentation and effective communication of pain and sedation scores. Numerous pain assessment instruments have been developed, but few have been validated for the paediatric critical care population. Commonly used pain tools include the PICU Multidimensional Assessment Pain Scale (PICU-MAPS), the COMFORT scale, the COMFORT behaviour scale and the modified Faces Legs Activity Cry Consolability (FLACC) scale.

In combination with pain, assessment of sedation is paramount. The COMFORT behaviour scale and the State Behavioural Scale (SBS) are the tools that have the strongest psychometric properties and clinical utility to evaluate the level of sedation in infants and children in ICU.[61–63] The evaluation of withdrawal should be performed when opioids and/or benzodiazepines are administered for 5 days and longer, using valid tools, such as the Withdrawal Assessment Tool (WAT-1)[64] and the Sophia Observation Withdrawal Symptoms scale.[56]

Pain and sedation management

Painful procedures should be minimised when possible. Some non-pharmacological therapies have been shown to be beneficial alone in managing mild pain or in combination with drug therapy in infants and young children. These therapies include non-nutritive sucking (e.g. finger or pacifier) with or without sucrose (for infants up to 4 months)[65] or glucose,[66] swaddling, music therapy[67] and distraction with or without parental presence.[47]

Pharmacological treatment of pain and sedation in infants and children should be tailored to the child's need and condition. Continuous opioid (morphine) infusions are used at the lowest effective dose and minimum duration based on regular pain assessment. Fentanyl boluses are not recommended in neonates as they may cause glottic and chest wall rigidity.[68] Sedation management in children is similar to that in adults, except for the use of propofol, which should be used with caution in children. Although there is no strong evidence, propofol infusion in children has been associated with sudden myocardial failure and death[69] and prolonged infusion should be avoided.[70] More recent data show that propofol has an acceptable safety profile and could be used in children for short-term deep sedation under close monitoring of the airways.[71] Dexmedetomidine administered postoperatively in children demonstrated better analgesia and less shivering and agitation in PICU children than routine analgesia and sedation.[72] The most frequent adverse effects reported with dexmedetomidine have been hypotension and bradycardia, in 10% to 20% of children, respectively, but these effects can be resolved with dose reduction and careful monitoring,[73] Indications for the use of neuromuscular blocking agents in children, monitoring of the effects and management are similar to adult practice.[74]

Upper airway obstruction

Upper airway obstruction is common in infants and young children for two major reasons: the anatomical size of the airway and the frequency of respiratory infections experienced in early childhood. Congenital structural abnormalities and infections as well as foreign body aspiration are the three categories of causes of upper airway obstruction in children.

General description and clinical manifestations

General indicators of respiratory distress will be present in a child suffering from upper airway obstruction. Specific clinical signs of upper airway obstruction in children include:

- a longer inspiratory phase with unchanged expiratory phase
- stridor on inspiration

- chest wall recessions
- lower respiratory rate
- in infants, head bobbing and nasal flaring
- hoarseness
- drooling of saliva.[75]

The aim is to assess the child without causing further distress as a crying, agitated child can further increase the degree of obstruction and work of breathing, leading to respiratory collapse.[15] Observing and listening to the child's symptoms without disturbing them will provide important clues about the level and degree of obstruction the child is experiencing. The Paediatric Assessment Triangle (PAT) is a useful and widely used tool to facilitate rapid assessment of the child's appearance, work of breathing and skin circulation.[76] Stridor indicates obstruction in the upper airway, while wheeze is suggestive of lower airway disease. When stridor is also associated with a barking cough, it is likely to be croup. A softer stridor in a child who looks systemically unwell may indicate epiglottitis. When a previously well child presents with a sudden onset of stridor, it is likely to indicate foreign body aspiration, and eliciting the history of a sudden choking episode can clarify the diagnosis.[75]

Congenital airway abnormalities

Congenital structural abnormalities of the airway are present at birth; depending upon severity of obstruction, they may take hours to months to become apparent. These include laryngomalacia, laryngeal web, tracheomalacia and vascular rings. These infants and children require referral to a specialist paediatric centre for ongoing management and, if they develop respiratory infections, are likely to become compromised much more easily than children with normal airways.

Laryngomalacia is the most common cause of stridor in the newborn period. Stridor is produced by flaccid, soft laryngeal cartilage and aryepiglottic folds that collapse into the glottis on inspiration.[77] An inspiratory stridor, usually high-pitched, will be present. It may be intermittent, may decrease when the patient is placed prone with the neck extended, may increase with agitation and is usually present from birth or the first weeks of life. The infant's cry is usually normal. Feeding problems may be associated with increased respiratory distress. Laryngoscopy confirms the laryngomalacia diagnosis. Treatment is supportive, with only a small proportion of infants requiring airway reconstructive surgery. Where respiratory distress interferes with feeding and growth, a tracheostomy may be indicated.[78]

A laryngeal web is made of membrane that typically spreads between the vocal cords, with an inspiratory stridor present soon after birth. Diagnosis is confirmed by laryngoscopy. Treatment involves lysis in the case of thin membranous webs whereas a tracheostomy may be required for a thicker fibrotic web. Laryngeal webs can also develop after contracting illnesses such as diphtheria, and are occasionally reported in otherwise normal adults, typically at intubation for an operative procedure.[79]

Tracheomalacia and tracheobronchomalacia involve malformed cartilage rings, with lack of rigidity and an oval shape to the lumen. Secondary tracheomalacia is associated with prolonged intubation and prematurity and presents within the first year of life.[80] Malacias are characterised by wheezing and stridor on expiration, with collapse of the tracheal or bronchial lumen. Diagnosis is confirmed by fluoroscopy and bronchoscopy, which demonstrate tracheal collapse on expiration. As the infant grows, cartilaginous development improves the airway by about 2 years of age, but a number of children will require airway stenting or reconstructive surgery.[77,80]

Vascular rings result from congenital malformations of the intrathoracic great vessels, resulting in compression of the airways.[80] Infants present with stridor at birth or within the first few weeks of life. Other symptoms include wheezing, cough, cyanosis, recurrent bronchopulmonary infections and dysphagia. Diagnosis may be confirmed by CT scan, MRI scan or endoscopy, which reveals indentations secondary to the extrinsic pressure of the vasculature.[80] The anatomy of the vascular malformations is determined by angiography. Treatment is surgical correction of the vascular malformation.[80]

Monitoring and diagnostics

Initial monitoring and diagnostic studies for infants and children with upper airway obstruction are ideally of a non-invasive nature, to avoid distress.

Pulse oximetry is a non-invasive method of monitoring oxygenation. Arterial blood gases are performed only when absolutely necessary, as this may increase the child's distress and thus worsen the degree of obstruction. Continuous ECG monitoring is also indicated.

Lateral airway X-rays are unlikely to be helpful in the setting of croup and epiglottitis and, when they are likely to involve separating the child from a parent, are potentially harmful and not recommended.[15] When there is a less dramatic presentation of the infant or child, or when the diagnosis is not clear, as in the case of an inhaled foreign body, a chest X-ray may be diagnostic.

> **Practice tip**
>
> Close direct observation from a short distance away is an ideal nursing practice, accompanied by non-invasive monitoring. Ideally, the critical care nurse will be positioned to hear the child's stridor. Blood sampling, cannulation and other invasive procedures should be left until the airway has been secured, the child has been anaesthetised or airway obstruction is resolving.

Managing the paediatric airway

A child's airway may be managed in a number of ways. Simple positioning may be all that is required. Children will often assume an upright sitting position and may become more distressed if placed into the supine position; thus, when possible the best position for an infant or child with upper airway obstruction may be sitting on their parent's lap. Because of the anatomy and physiology of the respiratory tract, avoid extending the head of infants. Chin-lift and jaw-thrust are useful airway adjuncts in children to maintain an airway and to facilitate use of a bag–valve–mask. It may be necessary to use an oropharyngeal airway or nasopharyngeal airway, laryngeal masks and endotracheal intubation in an unconscious or sedated infant.[15,81]

Intubation

Intubation may be required to manage airway obstruction.[81] Uncuffed endotracheal tubes (ETT) have been traditionally favoured in paediatric practice over cuffed tubes. Inflating the cuff of a regular ETT can cause damage in prepubescent children, as the subglottic area is the narrowest portion of their airways. The recent availability of a paediatric-specific ETT with microcuff and markings to ensure correct placement below the glottis has facilitated ventilation when a leak is undesirable, including in the child with facial and airway burns,[82] for volume ventilation strategies, when using inhaled nitric oxide and for high frequency ventilatory strategies such as oscillation ventilation. Equipment necessary for paediatric intubation is shown in Figure 27.3. Figure 27.4 shows a range of sizes of uncuffed ETTs, 2.5 mm to 5.5 mm, that should be available in 0.5-mm increments, while cuffed ETTs are now available in sizes from 3 mm through to 9 mm. Selecting the correct ETT size includes having the recommended tube size plus tubes that are 0.5 mm larger and smaller than calculated. For children over 1 year of age, several formulae exist to calculate appropriate tube sizes, but the age-based

FIGURE 27.4 Range of ETT sizes.

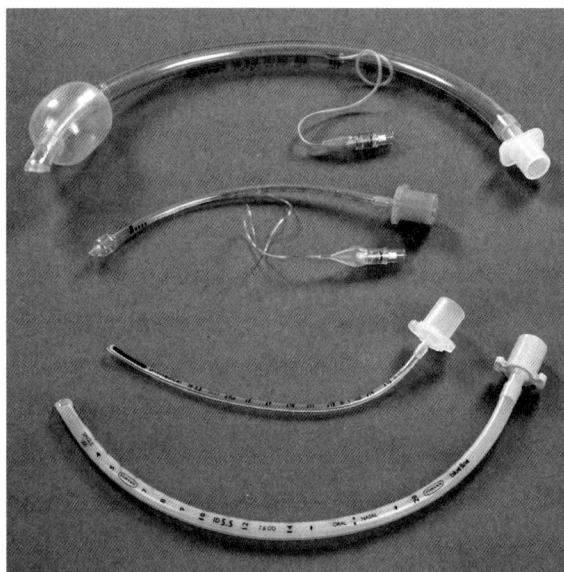

Courtesy Paul de Sensi.

and the fifth fingernail width-based predictions of ETT size remain the most commonly used. Recent research involving ultrasonography measurement may lead to a change in practice as bedside use of ultrasound increases.[83] Table 27.5 provides a guide for ETT sizes, suction catheter size and nasogastric tube size for infants and children.

FIGURE 27.3 Paediatric intubation equipment.

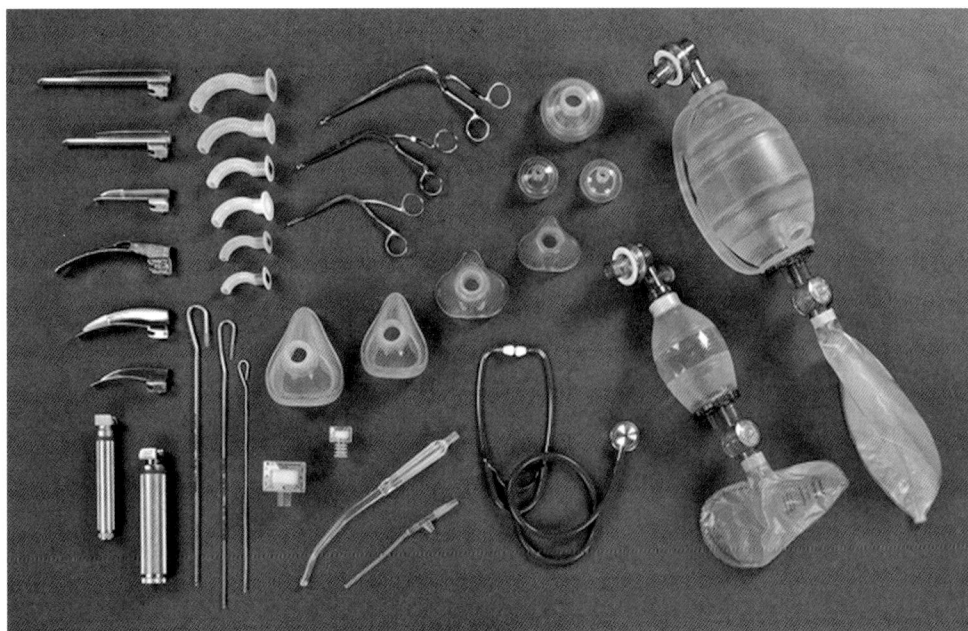

Courtesy Paul de Sensi.

TABLE 27.5
Endotracheal tube (ETT) and nasogastric tube (NG) sizes for infants and children

AGE	WEIGHT (KG)	ETT SIZE (MM ID)	AT GUM (CM)	AT NOSE (CM)	SUCTION CATHETER (FG)	NG TUBE (FG)
0	<3.0	2.5	6	7.5	5	8
0	3.0	3.0	8.5	10.5	6	8
0–3 months	3.5–5	3.5	9	11	6–8	10
3–12 months	6–9	3.5	10	12	6–8	10
1 year	10–12	4.0	11	14	8	10
2 years	13–14	4.5	12	15	8	12
3 years	14–15	4.5	13	16	8	12
4–5 years	16–19	5.0	14	17	8–10	12
6–7 years	20–23	5.5	15	19	10	14
8–9 years	24–29	6.0	16	20	10–12	14
10–11 years	30–37	6.5	17	21	12	14
12–13 years	38–49	7.0	18	22	12	16
14+ years	50–60	7.5	19	23	12	16
Adult	>60	8–9	20–21	24–25	12	16

FG = French gauge; ID = internal diameter.
Adapted from Shann F. Drug doses. 15th ed. Parkville, Victoria: Royal Children's Hospital; 2010.[247]

Practice tip

To calculate ETT tube size and length, use the following guides from the 2010 Australian and New Zealand Resuscitation Guidelines:[9]

- for term newborns ≥3 kg – size 3.0 mm or 3.5 mm (uncuffed tubes) or 3.0 mm (cuffed tubes)
- for infant up to 6 months – size 3.5 mm or 4.0 mm (uncuffed tubes) or 3.5 mm (cuffed tubes)
- for infant 7 to 12 months – size 4.0 mm (uncuffed tubes) or 3.5 mm (cuffed tubes)
- for children over 1 year – uncuffed tubes, size (mm) = age (years)/4 + 4; cuffed tubes, size (mm) = age (years)/4 + 3.5.

Adapted with permission from Australian Resuscitation Council. Techniques in paediatric advanced life support. Guideline 126. Melbourne, Australia: Australian Resuscitation Council; 2010.

The most common method used to intubate children is a modified rapid-sequence method. Rapid-sequence intubation is performed when the child may have a full stomach and is at risk of aspiration during intubation.[84] For children, the modification of technique involves bag–mask ventilation prior to intubation to prevent the occurrence of hypoxia.[85] It involves the practically simultaneous administration of sedative medication and a muscle relaxant immediately before intubation.[84,85] The main advantages of this method include avoidance of hypoxia, good airway visualisation with a relaxed jaw, open immobile vocal cords and the elimination of all movement, including gagging and coughing.[85] Careful consideration of appropriate induction agents is required for children with haemodynamic instability or a head injury/raised ICP as agents such as thiopentone, propofol and midazolam may not be appropriate or require dose modification.

Specific conditions affecting the upper airway

Bacterial and viral infections of the upper airway are common in children. Croup is the most common infection causing upper airway obstruction in children. Epiglottitis is now rarely seen since in countries where immunisation against *Haemophilus influenzae* type b (Hib) was introduced into the immunisation schedule. However, it is important to distinguish epiglottitis from croup in order to initiate appropriate management. Other less common infectious causes of upper airway obstruction seen in young children include bacterial tracheitis and retropharyngeal abscess. Diseases thought to have disappeared, such as Lemierre's syndrome and diphtheria, have not been completely eradicated with resurgences seen in recent years in both developed and developing countries.[86]

Infection of the lymphoid tissue around the nodes draining the nasopharynx, sinuses and eustachian tubes may cause pus to accumulate in the retropharyngeal space, leading to a retropharyngeal abscess. Presenting symptoms include history of upper respiratory tract infection (URTI), sore throat, fever, toxic appearance, meningismus, stridor, dysphagia and difficulty handling secretions.[87] Diagnosis is usually made on airway imaging or bronchoscopy.[88] Treatment involves surgical drainage and antibiotic administration. Short-term intubation may be required until swelling has resolved following surgery.

Croup

Croup (laryngotracheobronchitis) is the most common infective cause of upper airway obstruction in children aged 6 months to 6 years, with peak incidence at 2 years.[15,87,88] Croup is used to describe a set of symptoms caused by acute swelling causing obstruction in the upper airway (larynx, trachea and bronchi) from inflammation and oedema, caused mostly by the parainfluenza or influenza viruses, and is most commonly seen in winter months.[15] Recent advances in croup management have been responsible for a fall in the number of children requiring hospitalisation and intubation. Possible complications of croup include respiratory failure, respiratory arrest, hypoxic damage, secondary bacterial infection, acute pulmonary oedema, persistence or recurrence.[88]

Clinical manifestations

Croup is characterised by a barking or seal-like cough, inspiratory stridor and hoarse voice.[75] The severity of croup is assessed based on increased respiratory rate, increased heart rate, altered mental state, work of breathing and stridor. Stridor at rest is noted in moderate-to-severe croup and is often quite loud. If a child's stridor becomes softer but the work of breathing remains increased, it should be treated as an emergency as the obstruction may become more severe. The symptoms of croup are listed and compared with those of epiglottitis in Table 27.6. Diagnosis is made on physical assessment and the history of the illness.

Management

Management of croup depends on the severity of the upper airway obstruction. Children with moderate-to-severe croup should be given face-mask oxygen and allowed to adopt the position that they find most comfortable. Strategies such as positioning the child in a parent's lap and holding the face-mask close to their face may limit their distress and can have beneficial effects on oxygenation.[89]

Practice tip

If placement of a facemask to deliver oxygen causes increased agitation and worsens respiratory distress in young children, have the parent hold the mask near their child's face and increase the flow rate. 'Blow-over' oxygen will increase oxygen saturation and, as the child settles, mask or nasal cannulae can be reintroduced.

TABLE 27.6

Clinical features of croup and epiglottitis

	CROUP	EPIGLOTTITIS
Aetiology	Viral	Bacterial
Age	6 months–3 years	Infancy through adulthood
Onset	Subacute (over days)	Acute (over hours)
Fever	Mild (±38°C)	Severe (>38.5°C)
Cough	Present (often barking or seal-like)	Absent
Drooling	Absent	Present
Activity	Distressed	Lethargic
Colour	Pale/sick	Toxic
Obstruction	+++	+
Stridor	Inspiratory, high-pitched	Expiratory snore
Sore throat	Uncommon	Common
Position	Any	Tripod; sitting up
Course	Gradual worsening or improvement	Unpredictable; fatal if not treated
Season	Autumn–winter	Throughout the year

Adapted from Tibballs J, Watson T. Symptoms and signs differentiating croup and epiglottitis. J Paediatr Child Health 2010;47(3):77–82.[75]

The use of steroids in combination with nebulised adrenaline is responsible for significant improvement of symptoms in children within 12 hours of administration, abating the need for intubation in the vast majority of cases.[90] Nebulised adrenaline is efficacious in reducing airway inflammation, with effects seen within 5 minutes and lasting up to 2 hours. Although inhalations can be repeated, the benefits lessen with subsequent treatments. Adrenaline does not alter the course of croup.

Epiglottitis

Epiglottitis is inflammation of the epiglottis, frequently involving surrounding structures, with the classic description of a swollen, cherry-red, softened and floppy epiglottis, which tends to fall backwards, obstructing the airway.[88] Obstruction also occurs circumferentially, from the oedematous, inflamed aryepiglottic folds surrounding the larynx. It is typically caused by Hib and, since the introduction of childhood immunisation programs to protect against Hib infection in many countries, the incidence has dropped significantly, with one major Australian centre reporting no cases for the previous 3 years.[75] Hib infection can cause meningitis, septicaemia, septic arthritis and cellulitis as well as epiglottitis. The disease process and development of major symptoms progress rapidly over a few hours and an untreated child may become acutely obstructed. A child will make a full recovery without sequelae if diagnosis and treatment are appropriate and timely. Supraglottitis has emerged in recent times as a more accurate description of a similar range of symptoms as epiglottitis, and has been linked with the herpes virus and other organisms, requiring treatment with aciclovir and vancomycin.[88]

Clinical manifestations

The child with epiglottitis presents looking unwell with a fever and is unable to swallow secretions, drooling saliva and refusing to talk or swallow. The child may maintain an upright position, usually leaning with the head extended, supporting a sitting position with the arms stretched out behind in what is known as the tripod position. Hypoxaemia is usually present. Sudden respiratory arrest followed by cardiac arrest can occur unpredictably. Cardiac arrest is likely to be asystolic in rhythm due to either vagal stimulation or hypoxia secondary to airway obstruction.[88]

Management

The most important aspect in the management of epiglottitis is rapid diagnosis and minimal handling of the child until an airway is in place. Children with epiglottitis require urgent intubation because acute airway obstruction followed by cardiac arrest is a potential hazard. Thus, the aim of nursing management at this time is to keep the child as calm as possible until the airway is secured.[91] The child should be nursed propped up with pillows or on a parent's lap while arrangements are made for intubation. Procedures such as cannulation and examination of the throat should be avoided until the child's airway is secure.[91]

Prophylaxis with antibiotics is required for families and household contacts if there is an infant under 12 months of age and/or a child in the household under the age of 5 years who is not fully immunised. Where the infected child has attended childcare for more than 18 hours each week, staff and other children at the centre should receive antibiotic prophylaxis.[92]

Foreign body aspiration

Aspiration of a foreign body into the upper airway is another relatively common cause of obstruction in children. Infants tend to swallow food items such as nuts and seeds, while toddler-aged children tend to swallow coins, teeth etc.[93] An inhaled foreign body is likely to have a rapid onset with no previous symptoms. Sometimes the diagnosis is missed for days, weeks or even months, and the child's symptoms may be non-specific, such as a cough with or without blood-stained sputum.[93]

Clinical manifestations

Sudden onset of coughing, gagging and an audible stridor in a previously-well infant or child is suggestive of an inhaled foreign body.[15] However, an accurate history – such as a recent coughing or choking episode – is the most sensitive factor in making a diagnosis of inhaled foreign body.

Patient management

Management will depend on the location and level of the aspirated foreign body, as it may have lodged in the pharynx, oesophagus, larynx, trachea or bronchial tree. Coughing is encouraged for mild airway obstruction.[94] Up to five back blows may be successful in dislodging the foreign body, which may be followed by up to five chest thrusts and back blows. Direct laryngoscopy and removal of a foreign body using Magill forceps may be required for an acute episode when back blows and chest thrusts have been unsuccessful. When the foreign body has lodged below the carina, diagnosis and definitive treatment usually consist of removal of the foreign body via a bronchoscopy under general anaesthesia.[95]

The child experiencing lower airway disease

Lower airway disease in children is a common reason for admission to ICU. Infants under 12 months usually present with bronchiolitis or pneumonia. Asthma is more common in older children, but infants nearing 12 months of age may develop asthma and there is often confusion between bronchiolitis and asthma at this age.

Specific conditions affecting the lower airway

Bronchiolitis and asthma are commonly seen in children, and the management of each condition is discussed below. National and worldwide clinical guidelines for these conditions have been developed and are continually updated.[96,97]

Bronchiolitis

Viral bronchiolitis in infancy is characterised by obstruction of the small airways, resulting in air trapping and respiratory distress in infants less than 12 months of age. It is the commonest severe respiratory infection in infancy, although the course is usually mild to moderate and is self-limiting, usually requiring no treatment.[98] Severe infection represents less than 5% of all cases and is usually associated with prematurity, infants under 3 months of age or congenital heart disease. Respiratory syncytial virus (RSV) causes 90% of bronchiolitis cases.[99,100] Other causative agents are parainfluenza virus types 1, 2 and 3, influenza B, adenovirus types 1, 2 and 5 and *Mycoplasma*. RSV invades the epithelial cells of the bronchioles, spreading via the creation of syncytia, which are created when host cell membranes fuse with neighbouring cells. This results in destruction of the epithelium and patches of necrosis. The debris associated with epithelial shedding and mucus production lead to small airway blockage and the clinical features of bronchiolitis.

In temperate regions of Australia and New Zealand most cases of bronchiolitis occur between late autumn and early spring, with sporadic cases throughout the year. There is a paradoxical relationship between the incidence of RSV and other viral pathogens causing bronchiolitis. RSV epidemics occur when other respiratory pathogen epidemics are diminishing, and vice versa. The incidence rate of RSV infection varies between continents with rates as high as 225 per 1000 infants in the USA and 869/1000 infants in Australia.[101] The estimated RSV-related hospitalisation rates in Australia ranged from 2.2 to 4.5 per 1000/children less than 5 years of age to 8.7 to 17.4 per 1000/infants, with a total annual direct healthcare cost estimated to be up to 50 million dollars.[101] These figures are fairly similar to European figures, with 24/1000 infant admissions in the UK and 22 in Norway. There is also a higher incidence of bronchiolitis among Aboriginal people in Australia[103] and more severe illness when compared to non-indigenous people.[103] Younger children with one or more comorbidities are at higher risk of complications. RSV infection occurs throughout the year, with an annual peak during the winter months.

When bronchiolitis occurs, the highest risk for hospitalisation is infants under 6 months of age, those with exposure to tobacco smoke and underlying conditions such as congenital heart disease, prematurity and low socioeconomic group.[104,105] Severe disease, requiring admission to a PICU, is associated with prematurity, particularly in infants with chronic lung disease or a history of ventilation in the newborn period and congenital heart disease.

Clinical manifestations

Bronchiolitis is a clinical diagnosis, and non-isolation of a causative viral agent does not exclude the diagnosis. The clinical features of bronchiolitis are variable, and may include URTI symptoms such as rhinorrhoea (runny nose) and an irritating cough. Within 3 days the infant develops tachypnoea and respiratory distress, which may be mild, moderate or severe. An expiratory wheeze is often present with auscultation revealing fine to coarse crackles. Fever is present in approximately 50% of infants. In very young, premature or low-birth-weight infants, apnoea is often the presenting symptom, which then develops into severe respiratory distress.[106] The clinical course of bronchiolitis is usually 7–10 days; however, the effects of severe illness may last much longer. Indications for intensive care admission include: frequent and/or prolonged apnoeas; hypoxaemia despite administration of oxygen; haemodynamic instability; an obviously tiring infant; or decreased level of consciousness.[104]

Assessment and patient management

A thorough history and assessment are important to provide a foundation for management of bronchiolitis. The infant with acute bronchiolitis requires continuous cardiorespiratory monitoring and oxygen saturation monitoring. Management of infants presenting with bronchiolitis is largely supportive, as most pharmacological treatments are unproven. In general, management centres on supporting therapies, such as hydration and nutrition, oxygenation and maintaining vigilance for signs of deterioration that may require mechanical ventilation.[100] Prone

positioning and minimising the impact of procedures on the infant are also important, especially in infants less than 3 months. Recent innovations in less invasive respiratory support, such as increased use of non-invasive ventilation strategies as well as the use of humidified high flow oxygen therapy via nasal cannulae, can lead to reduced numbers of bronchiolitic infants requiring intubation and invasive ventilation.[107] Before high flow therapy can be recommended widely in severe bronchiolitis, issues of system monitoring and safety as well as staffing need to be established.

Asthma

Asthma is a lower respiratory tract disease characterised by mucosal and immune system dysfunction. There is a complex interaction between bronchial wall cells, inflammatory mediators and the nervous system. The chronic inflammatory process causes narrowing of bronchial airways, thus obstructing airflow. This leads to episodes of wheezing, breathlessness and chest tightening that are usually reversible. In an acute episode of asthma, wheeze is not always audible, but a prolonged expiratory phase is an early sign.[108]

Development of childhood asthma results from a combination of genetic, environmental and socioeconomic risk factors.[108–110] Increasing prevalence of asthma over the past 20–30 years may be linked to a higher incidence of genetic predisposition, independent of environmental factors. Some studies identify links between asthma and various regions of the human genome, but the linkages are not consistent. Certain racial groups, such as African Americans, when compared to Americans of European origin are also more likely to develop asthma and have complications, particularly those traditionally from tropical regions.[111] Once asthma has developed, there are triggers that may precipitate an attack. These include: viral illnesses, particularly respiratory viruses; tobacco smoke exposure; house dust mites; exercise; pet hair; food; and environmental allergens.

Asthma is one of the commonest paediatric presentations to emergency departments and its worldwide prevalence is growing with differences among various populations.[112,113] It is reported that as many as 20–30% of children in Western countries will develop wheeze or asthma symptoms;[114] the current disease rate is 9.6% in the USA,[115] 29.7% in the UK[117] and 31% in Australia.[117] Asthma prevalence is increasing,[114] is higher in boys and in urban areas,[113] but its mortality has declined over the past two decades, from 1–2/100,000 down to 0.8/100,000.[114]

Clinical manifestations

ICU admission is required when children present with respiratory failure due to an asthma exacerbation. These exacerbations can be due to viral infection and allergy, seasonal patterns, bacterial infections, environmental factors as well as psychological factors such as stress.[118,119] Other factors such as obesity and genetic predisposition may be important in reacting to beta-2 agonist therapy.[120]

These children exhibit clinical features associated with respiratory distress. Pulsus paradoxus, a phenomenon of palpable changes in blood pressure that occur with respirations, may also be present and can also be noted on plethysmography. Arterial blood gas analysis usually reveals a mild respiratory alkalosis and hypoxaemia initially; however, more severe asthma may show combined respiratory and metabolic acidosis and hypercapnia as the child tires and is unable to eliminate carbon dioxide.[121]

Patient assessment and management

Assessment of asthma severity is based on criteria such as the degree of respiratory failure as evidenced by cyanosis, length of sentences between breaths, retractions and hypoxia, as well as level of consciousness and degree of pulsus paradoxus. There are many scores available to assist in determining the severity of asthma, including the National Asthma Campaign guidelines, the Pulmonary Index Score, the Respiratory Failure Score and the Modified Dyspnoea Scale. Whatever method is used, assessments should be frequent and response to treatment recorded. Severe asthma that worsens and/or does not respond to treatment warrants admission to a PICU.[113]

The broad aims of management of severe asthma include maintaining oxygenation, rapid bronchodilation and treating any cardiovascular compromise.[122] In children with severe asthma, hypoxaemia results from ventilation/perfusion (V/Q) mismatch due to lower airway obstruction, in addition to hypoventilation, hypercarbia and pulmonary vasoconstriction related to acidosis. Hypoxaemia can result in further bronchoconstriction, hypotension, systemically-reduced oxygen availability, increased myocardial oxygen consumption and neurological symptoms such as agitation, confusion or decreased level of consciousness. Bronchodilators may worsen hypoxaemia through worsening V/Q mismatch or bronchoconstriction, due to the hyperosmolarity of the nebulised solution. In addition, rapid changes to the compliance of the airways together with hyperexpanded lungs may result in airway collapse.

Oxygen delivery is achieved by high-flow oxygen mask with a reservoir bag. All nebuliser therapy should be oxygen-driven. However, if hypoxaemia persists despite maximal bronchodilator therapy and oxygen administration, mask continuous positive airway pressure (CPAP) may be considered.

Beta-2-agonists, anticholinergics and steroids form the foundation of acute severe asthma management, but for children over 40 kg and those who have reached puberty it may be more appropriate to administer IV adrenaline. Beta-2-agonists act by relaxing bronchial smooth muscle, improving mucociliary transport and inhibiting mediator release. In severe to life-threatening asthma, inhaled short-acting beta-2-agonists combined with an anticholinergic is recommended as it improves lung function, decreases side effects such as nausea and tremor and decreases the risk for hospital admission if treated early.[123] Adverse effects of beta-2-agonist administration

include hypokalaemia, tachycardia, tremors, agitation and hyperglycaemia. Mild lactic acidosis may also occur. Intravenous salbutamol infusion should be considered when there is severe, life-threatening asthma refractory to inhaled treatment. Inhaled salbutamol may be discontinued once IV infusion has commenced, but should be re-established before ceasing the infusion. In acute severe episodes, salbutamol is usually given every 20 minutes; if there is little response, continuous nebuliser therapy may be required. In this instance, a feeding tube is inserted into the nebuliser and the chamber replenished as it empties. Anticholinergics, in combination with beta-2-agonists, improve lung function by augmenting the action of beta-2-agonists, blocking irritant receptors and bronchodilation of larger airways.[124]

Corticosteroids decrease airway inflammation, enhancing the effects of beta-2-agonists, and reduce mucus production. Oral and intravenous methods of administration are similarly efficacious. The effects of systemic steroids are apparent within 3–4 hours of administration, with maximal benefit achieved within 6–12 hours. There is little evidence to support giving inhaled steroids during an acute episode.

Magnesium sulfate promotes smooth muscle relaxation by inhibiting uptake of calcium. Intravenous magnesium sulfate has demonstrated efficacy in acute severe asthma and inhaled magnesium sulfate combined with a beta-2-agonist results in possible improved pulmonary function.[125]

Aminophylline has shown some benefit with regard to improved lung function in severe asthma that is unresponsive to inhaled bronchodilators and steroids. It is a bronchodilator, improving diaphragmatic contractility, and a central respiratory stimulant. However, the narrow therapeutic window and side effects of induced nausea and/or vomiting represent a non-negligible risk of complication; thus its use should be limited to managing asthma not responsive to other agents.[126]

Ventilation may be required when there is profound hypoxaemia, severe muscle fatigue or decreased level of consciousness.[108] However, as asthmatic children are at higher risk of complications such as barotrauma and air trapping, there is a higher risk of death associated with ventilation in this group of patients. Non-invasive positive pressure ventilation (NIV) is the first choice with some evidence that it rapidly corrects gas exchange abnormalities and assists with respiratory muscle fatigue.[127] The contraindications for NIV include: cardiac/respiratory arrest, severe encephalopathy, haemodynamic instability, facial surgery/deformity, high risk for aspiration, non-respiratory organ failure, severe upper gastrointestinal bleeding, unstable arrhythmia and upper airway obstruction.

Intubation may be necessary when signs of deterioration are present, such as elevated carbon dioxide levels, exhaustion, alteration of mental status, haemodynamic instability and refractory hypoxaemia.[128] Because of high airway pressures, a cuffed ETT should be used.

Children with acute asthma may have a raised metabolic rate and increased insensible losses, together with reduced oral intake. With increased intrathoracic pressure due to air trapping, even mild dehydration may compromise cardiac output. Therefore, adequate fluid replacement is necessary. In addition, pulmonary secretions will thicken and plug the airways if fluid intake is inadequate. IV fluids should be provided until the child's condition and oral intake improve.[129]

Nursing the ventilated child

Principals of mechanical ventilation were covered in Chapter 15. Issues such as gastric decompression, adequate analgesia and sedation and undertaking steps to prevent accidental extubation are similar to those for adults. Specific considerations for ventilating infants and children include:

- Most children are oxygenated before, during and after suctioning with 100% O_2.[130] The child's clinical status is monitored throughout the procedure.

- Heated humidification is preferred in children as they have limited respiratory reserve and are prone to airway blockage.[131,132]

- Endotracheal suctioning does not require normal saline instillation.[133,134]

- To prevent iatrogenic atelectasis, the suction catheter size should be less than or equal to two-thirds the internal diameter of the ETT. Suction pressure should be limited to −60 mmHg (−8 kPa) for infants, and up to −200 mmHg (−27 kPa) for adolescents. A suction regulator is useful to monitor the amount of applied negative pressure, as too much can result in atelectasis.

- Restraints may be required to limit the movement of the child, with the aim of preventing accidental extubation rather than maintaining the child in an immobile state. Restraints may be physical, such as arm boards or hand ties; or chemical, such as sedation.

Modes of ventilation

There are many modes of ventilation (see Chapter 15). This section includes information specifically related to paediatric ventilation. As with adults, arterial blood gases should be taken about 15–20 minutes after initiating mechanical ventilation.

Volume ventilation of children

Typically, volume ventilation is not used in infants under 5 kg due to the small tidal volumes, which risk being lost in the distensible tubing and leaking around the ETT. In addition, most volume ventilators do not have a constant fresh gas flow, so the infant has to work harder to trigger a breath. Some of the newer models of ventilator have attempted to overcome these problems. Steps in beginning volume ventilation for a child are as follows:[135,136]

1 Set a tidal volume of 5 to 8 mL/kg. This is a protective lung strategy approach and can be increased if needed to a maximum of 9 to 10 mL/kg.[136]

2 Set the rate at 20 breaths/min. This is lower than physiological for infants, but the slightly larger tidal volumes will compensate.

3 Set the FiO_2 at <0.6 and titrate according to oxygen saturation and blood gases.

4 Set the PEEP at 5 cmH$_2$O. This is slightly higher than physiological.

5 Set the trigger sensitive enough to allow the infant or child to trigger a breath without working too hard. If a continuous fresh gas flow is available, this is preferable. If autocycling occurs, decrease the trigger-setting sensitivity gradually until the autocycling stops.

Pressure ventilation of children

The pressure ventilation mode is most commonly used in infants weighing less than 5 kg or with children who have a large leak around an uncuffed ETT. Steps in beginning pressure ventilation for a child are as follows and should be based on arterial blood gases.[136,137]

1 Set the peak inspiratory pressure (PIP) at 18–20 cmH$_2$O.

2 Set the positive end expiratory pressure (PEEP) at 4–6 cmH$_2$O (rarely exceeds 7 cmH$_2$O).

3 Set the rate at 20 breaths/min.

4 Set the FiO_2 at <0.6 and titrate according to oxygen saturation and blood gases.

5 Set the trigger sensitivity to trigger a breath without autotriggering. Most pressure ventilators have a constant fresh gas flow, which allows the child to breathe spontaneously without increased effort.

Non-invasive ventilation

Non-invasive ventilation (NIV) refers to ventilatory support without an artificial airway in the trachea (see Chapter 15). In critically ill children with respiratory failure, NIV may be used to reduce the need for intubation. However, the evidence for its use in children is weak[139] and often extrapolated from adults.[139] Some studies showed that NIV decreases the rate of ventilator-associated pneumonia and reduces oxygen requirement in children with lower airway diseases when compared to conventional ventilation[141] and may be recommended as the first-line ventilation strategy as it may decrease the rate of intubation in mild-to-moderate ARDS and increase extubation success.[141]

High-frequency oscillatory ventilation

High-frequency oscillatory ventilation (HFOV) uses supra-physiological ventilatory rates and tidal volumes less than anatomical dead space to accomplish gas exchange. Typical ventilator rates are 3–15 Hz or 180–600 breaths/min (1 Hz = 60 breaths). HFOV is primarily used in managing infants and children with diffuse alveolar or interstitial disease requiring high peak distending pressures. Goals include maximising alveolar recruitment, minimising barotrauma and providing adequate alveolar gas exchange.

HFOV is delivered primarily by the use of a specialised ventilator that uses a diaphragm piston unit to actively move gas into and out of the lung, and a non-compliant breathing circuit. A major difference between HFOV and other forms of ventilation is that there is active expiration with oscillation versus passive expiration for conventional ventilation.[142] Unlike conventional ventilation, which uses bulk flow to deliver gas to the lungs, using smaller than dead space tidal volumes utilises the mechanisms of pendelluft, Taylor dispersion, asymmetrical velocity profiles, cardiogenic mixing and, to a very limited extent, bulk flow.[142] These are all terms used to describe the distribution of gas when rapid rates and tiny volumes are used.

Ventilation is dependent on amplitude (a determinant of tidal volume) much more than rate. With oscillation ventilation, lowering frequency (Hz) improves CO_2 removal. This is thought to occur because the oscillating diaphragm is able to move through a greater distance, thus increasing tidal volume by providing more inspiratory time and a longer expiratory time.[142]

The principal determinants of oxygenation are the same as those for conventional ventilation. Therefore, as with conventional ventilation, the alveoli must be opened and prevented from collapsing if hypoxaemia is to be corrected. HFOV theoretically achieves this through delivering a high mean airway pressure without imposing a large tidal volume, but there is insufficient evidence to promote its use over conventional ventilation.[142,143] It thus avoids over-distension and the risk of barotrauma.

Extracorporeal membrane oxygenation

Extracorporeal membrane oxygenation (ECMO) is an alternative method of providing ventilatory and/or cardiac support.[144,145] When used to support ventilation, ECMO allows the lungs to rest and heal. Ventilation settings are reduced to minimal to minimise the iatrogenic effects of positive pressure. There are two main methods of ECMO – venovenous and venoarterial. In venovenous ECMO large-bore cannulas are placed in large veins, such as the internal jugular or femoral.[146] The more common form of ECMO in paediatric patients, venoarterial, utilises the right internal jugular to drain blood and the right common carotid artery for blood return.[146,147] Alternative placement of cannulas for venoarterial ECMO after heart surgery is the right atrium and aorta. Venoarterial ECMO allows support of both circulation and ventilation. Essentially, blood is drained from the 'venous' line, pumped through a membrane to oxygenate the blood and remove CO_2, then returned through a filter via the 'arterial' cannula.[146,147]

Children are considered for ECMO if they have potentially reversible lung or cardiac injury, or shock that has not responded to conventional therapies.[148,149] Contraindications include irreversible brain or CNS injury, immunodeficiency or severe coagulopathy. Outcomes are generally positive, but ECMO centres need to maintain their competence by performing the procedure often.

The child experiencing shock

A detailed description of shock is given in Chapter 21, with specific paediatric considerations addressed here. Hypovolaemic, cardiogenic and septic shock (also termed distributive shock) are the most common types of shock in children. Cardiogenic shock is rare and is seen mainly after open-heart surgery and severe myocarditis or untreated shock. The infant with an undiagnosed congenital heart defect, in particular lesions that rely on the ductus arteriosus – known as duct-dependent lesions – can present in shock in the first weeks of life as the duct closes.[150] As infants and children presenting in hypovolaemic shock are likely to respond to fluid resuscitation alone, they may not require transfer to a specialist paediatric centre. However, children presenting with septic shock or cardiogenic shock will require transfer to a specialist paediatric centre for ongoing management, and contact should be made to initiate goal-directed therapy as soon as possible. Those children who do not respond to fluid volume alone will require invasive haemodynamic monitoring and possible pharmacological intervention. The development of shock in a hypovolaemic child is considered to indicate losses of at least 30 mL/kg.[14]

Sepsis is the leading cause of death in infants and children worldwide.[151] The mortality rate for septic shock in North American children is reported to be about 9%.[152] Septic shock is responsible for up to 30% of admissions in European PICUs, with a mortality rate of 10%.[153] In Australia and New Zealand, sepsis was responsible for about 8% of all deaths of children in PICU in 2013.[1] Causes of septic shock in infants and children are often different from those in adolescents and adults. The commonest infecting organisms are often age-related in children, and are listed in Table 27.7. Infants and children with either congenital or acquired immunocompromise

---

TABLE 27.7

Organisms causing sepsis in newborns, infants and children

AGE GROUP	COMMON ORGANISMS CAUSING SEPSIS
Newborns	Group B beta-haemolytic streptococci *Enterobacteriaceae* (such as *E. coli*) *Listeria monocytogenes* *Herpes simplex virus* *Staphylococcus aureus* *Neisseria meningitidis*
Infants	*Haemophilus influenzae* *Streptococcus pneumoniae* *Staphylococcus aureus* *Neisseria meningitidis*
Children	*Staphylococcus aureus* *Neisseria meningitidis* *Streptococcus pneumoniae* Enterobacteriaceae

Adapted from Maloney PM. Sepsis and septic shock. Emerg Med Clin North Am 2013;31:583–600.[13]

are at greater risk of developing septic shock.[14] Meningo-coccal sepsis remains the leading cause of septic shock in developed countries such as Australia and New Zealand.

Clinical manifestations

There are many similarities between children and adults in the clinical manifestations of shock (see Chapter 21). However, there are three major differences:[13,154]

1   Children with systemic inflammatory response syndrome have either abnormal temperature or elevated white cell count (or both) plus abnormal heart rate or elevated respiratory rate (or both).

2   In addition to the symptoms of cardiovascular dysfunction seen in adults, children may also present with a normal blood pressure with no inotrope requirements, but have two of the following: unexplained metabolic acidosis, increased lactate, oliguria, prolonged capillary refill time or core to peripheral temperature gap >3°C.

3   Systemic hypotension is not necessary to make the diagnosis of septic shock. Tachycardia in the absence of fever is a more reliable sign than hypotension, as up to 25% of the child's circulating volume may be lost before hypotension occurs. Hypotension is thus a late sign in children and may indicate late decompensated shock, particularly following fluid delivery.[13]

One other specific factor for children that is not relevant in the adult population is a higher risk of sepsis in preterm infants and in infants with cardiac defects or chronic lung disease.[13]

Patient assessment and diagnostics

Assessment of the child with shock is based on clinical assessment, with less reliance on biochemical testing than in adult shock.[14] Ideally, shock should be diagnosed before hypotension occurs. Hypothermia or hyperthermia and altered neurological status, which provides information about perfusion pressure, and peripheral vasodilation (warm shock) or vasoconstriction with capillary refill >2 seconds (cold shock) are clinical signs of shock in children.[14,155]

Careful respiratory and cardiovascular assessment is required, as described in this chapter and Chapters 13 and 11. Monitoring of children experiencing shock is the same as for adults (see Chapter 21). It consists of continuous monitoring of heart rate, SvO_2 saturation, quality of peripheral pulses, capillary refill, level of consciousness, peripheral skin temperature and urine output as indirect measures of cardiac output as well as serial blood gas, lactate and electrolyte analysis.[14] Diagnosis of septic shock can be difficult in children. When present, non-blanching rash is a specific sign of meningococcal septicaemia.[156]

> ## Practice tip
>
> As rash may be less visible in dark-skinned children, check soles of feet, palms of hands and conjunctivae in those children.

A certain proportion of children will present with non-specific symptoms or signs of infection, such as fever, vomiting, lethargy, irritability or headache and the conditions may be difficult to distinguish from other less serious infections.[13] Laboratory testing of samples of blood, urine, stool, sputum, cerebrospinal fluid and any obvious wounds or lesions is standard practice in adults and children.

Patient management

Early recognition of shock, institution of appropriate goal-directed therapy and targeting the causative agent remain the mainstays of managing septic shock in children as in adults. Goal-directed therapies such as oxygen therapy, fluid resuscitation, maintenance of acceptable blood pressure and institution of pharmacological treatment and other supportive treatments to achieve therapeutic goals are practised in managing shock in children, and are linked to better outcomes.[13,14,154]

Large amounts of fluid may be required by children despite peripheral oedema or absence of overt fluid loss.[154] The large African study – the FEAST trial[158] – demonstrated that fluid bolus of up to 40 mL/kg increased mortality in African children with sepsis; however, this study was conducted in a resource poor environment without access to inotropes, biochemical testing or mechanical ventilation. Where access to inotropes and mechanical ventilation is readily available, aggressive fluid resuscitation in the first hour before development of hypotension is linked to improved mortality in children with hypovolaemic and septic shock.[13,154,158] Intravascular access in children can be difficult and umbilical venous access in newborns and intraosseous access in children can be used before the placement of central lines.[159] The use of the EZ-IO® (Vidacare Corporations, Texas) paediatric intraosseous needle set and driver system has become common in practice.[9,154,160] Other kinds of manually inserted intraosseous needles are available and, regardless of type, intraosseous needles all allow rapid access to the intramedullary capillary network, facilitating delivery of fluids, drugs and blood products. The site of choice in infants and children is the proximal tibia, 2–3 cm below the tibial tuberosity.[9] Once sited, a syringe must be attached to aspirate and ascertain correct placement. Fluid boluses can then be given via syringe into the intramedullary space with the aim of restoring circulating volume, which will in turn facilitate venous access with improvement of peripheral perfusion.[154]

Similarly to adults, after appropriate volume resuscitation has been given and symptoms of shock are not resolving or hypotension is developing, inotropes and vasopressors are recommended.[154] Inotropic drugs that are recommended in children include noradrenaline, adrenaline and dopamine.[14,154,161] Vasodilators, including sodium nitroprusside or nitroglycerin, are used to recruit microcirculation; type III phosphodiesterase inhibitors are used to improve cardiac contractility. If shock persists and there is a risk for adrenal insufficiency, hydrocortisone therapy is recommended.[162] ECMO may also be considered for a child who appears to be developing irreversible shock.[163]

The child experiencing acute neurological dysfunction

There are many reasons why an infant or child can present with an acute episode of neurological dysfunction. Common presentations to an ICU include meningitis,[156,164] encephalitis,[165] seizures and encephalopathy[167,167] (see also Chapter 17). Assessment and recognition of the clinical features and management of the various causes of neurological dysfunction in children are the keys to achieving good outcomes.

Neurological assessment

To assess a child's level of consciousness, several different scales can be used. The Glasgow Coma Scale (GCS) is commonly used,[168] but the Glasgow Coma motor subscore is more appropriate for children.[169] Another reliable scale is the Full Outline of Unresponsiveness (FOUR) score; it includes four parameters (eye response, motor response, pupil reflexes and breathing) rated on a 0 to 4 scale, giving a possible score of between 0 (completely unresponsive) and 16.[170] The FOUR score and the GCS are both able to predict in-hospital morbidity and poor outcome at the end of hospitalisation.

Other neurological assessment parameters include:

- Pupils – assess size, reaction and symmetry.
- Posture – abnormal flexion posturing, often referred to as decorticate posturing, is a flexion response of the arms with either flexion or extension of the legs, while abnormal extension posturing, often referred to as decerebrate posturing, is an extension response of all limbs, where arms rotate externally. Both abnormal flexion and extension posturing in a previously normal child may indicate raised intracranial pressure.
- Meningism – this is indicated by neck stiffness in a child and full/bulging fontanelle in an infant.

Seizures

Seizures are covered in Chapter 17. The various aetiologies of seizures in children include febrile convulsions, CNS infection such as meningitis or encephalitis, metabolic imbalances, drugs, trauma or epilepsy. Seizures in children are common, with about 4–10% of children having an unprovoked seizure without recurrence.[171] Children between the ages of 6 months and 6 years are more likely to develop seizures.[172] Children, particularly those under 5 years, are at higher risk, as the developing brain has a lower threshold for seizures.[171] Febrile convulsions occur in 2–5% of children, commonly between the ages of 6 and 60 months.[173,174] Non-febrile seizures are typically more common in the neonatal period, with the incidence falling with age.[172]

Patient management

Management of the paediatric patient with seizures is similar to management of the adult (see Chapter 17), but there are some specific paediatric considerations.

The paediatric patient who is suffering seizures is more susceptible than an adult to hypoglycaemia. Hypoglycaemia may lead to secondary brain injury during and after seizures. Blood sugar levels should always be checked in children suffering from seizures and intravenous fluids containing glucose administered.[172,175]

The care of the seizing or post-ictal child is generally supportive, and includes monitoring for signs of ongoing seizures, administration of appropriate anticonvulsants and regular assessment of neurological function. In young infants, seizures may be difficult to determine and may include stiffening, staring and lip smacking rather than obvious clonic activity.[176]

Meningitis

Meningitis is an acute inflammation of the meninges that usually develops over 1–2 days. A fulminant form of meningitis caused by *Neisseria meningitidis* or meningococcal disease may develop over several hours. Organisms causing bacterial meningitis vary by age group. In infants under 3 months of age, group b *Streptococcus*, *E. coli*, *Streptococcus pneumoniae* and *Listeria* are the most likely agents. In children over 3 months of age meningococcus, *Haemophilus influenzae* type b and *Streptococcus pneumoniae* are more common.[156] The commonest causes of viral meningitis in infants and children include herpes simplex virus and the enteroviruses.[177] Tuberculous meningitis, while still rare, is becoming more common, particularly in immigrant families or those with recent travel to affected areas. Bacterial meningitis continues to have a poorer outcome than other forms of meningitis, despite advances in therapy.[178]

Incidence

Data on the incidence of meningitis are limited to the major bacterial types, particularly for infants and children over 2 months of age. Hib, meningococcal and pneumococcal infections are all notifiable.[179] Since the introduction of the Hib vaccine in Australia in 1993, Hib infection has fallen to 1.2/100,000 in 2005.[180] Of all reports of infection only 28% were meningitis, and the majority of infections were in children under 2 years of age.[180]

Meningococcus is the main cause of meningitis in children. Specific strains tend to be prevalent in different regions of the world, with serogroups A, B, C, Y, W and X the current strains responsible for almost all invasive disease.[181] In Europe, the Americas and Oceania serogroups B, C and Y have caused the majority of cases. Serogroup A has been associated with the highest incidence (up to 1000 per 100,000 cases), causing large outbreaks of meningococcal disease in sub-Saharan Africa and Asia while serogroups W-135 and X have emerged more recently and are responsible for major disease outbreaks in sub-Saharan Africa.[181] Available vaccines differ around the world based on the prevalent strains, so recent overseas travel and place of vaccination should be obtained in the history.

In Australia meningococcal disease occurs seasonally, with the main peak between June and October. Serogroups A, B and C account for 90% of cases in Australia, with serogroup B causing 66% of disease.[180] There are two main peaks of disease. The 0–4-years age group represents 31% of all cases and 17% occur in the 15–19-years age group.[179,180] The incidence of meningococcal disease in children aged 0–4 years is 10/100,000. Of children with invasive meningococcal disease, 47% have meningitis, with or without sepsis.[182,183] The mortality rate of meningococcal meningitis in children under 5 years of age is below 1%; with sepsis present the rate increases up to 10–15% in developed countries and up to 40% in developing countries.[181]

The incidence of invasive pneumococcal disease has significantly dropped in developed regions such as Europe, North America and Australia since the introduction of routine vaccination,[181] with a reported rate of 23.4 cases per 100,000 children aged less than 5 years in 2005.[184] The highest peak of pneumococcal disease is seen in children aged 1 year with a rate fluctuating between 26.5, 37 and 51/100,000 in Australia and in Europe, respectively.[185,186] The highest Australian incidence occurs in the Northern Territory, with Aboriginal children at highest risk.[187] Other risk factors include extreme prematurity, chronic lung disease, trisomy 21 (Down syndrome), diabetes and cystic fibrosis. Clinical manifestations or symptoms vary with the age of the child, duration of the illness and history of antibiotic use for the current illness.

Patient management

Initial management of the infant or child with meningitis includes assessment and management of the airway, breathing, circulation and disability. Rapid antibiotic therapy is recommended and likely to decrease case fatality.[179,188] Once the initial resuscitation has been completed, consideration should be given to correcting any biochemical abnormalities. In particular, blood sugar level should be checked and corrected in the early management phase. Once meningitis is suspected, a lumbar puncture (LP) is generally performed to confirm diagnosis, but if the child is haemodynamically unstable or has ongoing seizures, problems with ventilation or signs of raised intracranial pressure, the LP should be delayed and blood cultures obtained.[189]

Steroid use in meningitis has some benefit in reducing morbidity in adults,[190] but not in children.[191] However, steroids were shown to reduce the risk of severe hearing loss in children with bacterial meningitis.[191]

Infants and children with meningitis require intensive care management when there is a reduced level of consciousness, respiratory and/or circulatory compromise. The broad aims of management are to support ventilation and circulation, while preventing secondary brain injury. Regular assessment and monitoring of associated risks such as seizures, syndrome of inappropriate antidiuretic hormone secretion (SIADH) or cerebral salt wasting and sepsis is essential.

Encephalitis

The most common type of encephalitis in children is acute viral encephalitis, and the most common causative agent is herpes simplex virus (HSV).[192] Left untreated, HSV is almost uniformly fatal, with over half of survivors experiencing significant long-term morbidity. Other causes of encephalitis in children include:[192, p 155]

- enteroviruses (e.g. enterovirus 71, coxsackievirus, polio and echovirus)
- varicella zoster virus
- Epstein-Barr virus
- cytomegalovirus
- adenovirus
- rubella
- measles
- Murray Valley encephalitis (MVE) virus
- Kunjin virus.

Worldwide, the incidence of acute encephalitis ranges between 3.5 and 16 cases per 100,000 children.[192] Children under 1 year of age are at higher risk of developing encephalitis. Other risk factors include immune dysfunction and exposure to risk animals, or specific geographic location. For example, in Australia Murray Valley encephalitis and Kunjin viruses are endemic in the Kimberley region of the Northern Territory, and Japanese B virus has been reported on Cape York Peninsula and is endemic in Southeast Asia.[193]

Encephalitis symptoms are similar to meningitis, but often with a much slower onset. Progressively worsening headache, fever and decreased level of consciousness or behavioural changes characterise encephalitis. Focal neurological signs and seizures may indicate involvement of the meninges or spinal cord.[194]

Patient management

Prompt administration of acyclovir is warranted to all patients with clinical symptoms suggesting encephalitis due to high mortality and morbidity rates.[192] Other viruses are also treated with acyclovir. Ganciclovir is useful for resistant organisms, but is more toxic.[194,195] Intensive care management involves supporting ventilation and managing neurological complications such as seizures and cerebral oedema. If the child is unconscious on presentation, the disease course will be more severe.[194]

Gastrointestinal and renal considerations in children

Many critically ill infants and children are also at risk of developing complications involving the gastrointestinal tract (GIT). Although primary acute renal failure (ARF) is relatively rare in critically ill children, the incidence of renal impairment secondary to the underlying illness is recognised increasingly in children, although a paucity of prospective studies remains problematic. When new paediatric Risk, Injury, Failure, Loss and End-stage kidney disease (pRIFLE) criteria were applied, the total incidence of kidney injury in PICU ranged from 10% up to 50%.[196,197] Diagnoses associated with primary kidney injury in children are sepsis, haemolytic uraemic syndrome, oncological diagnoses and following congenital cardiac surgery.[153,196] Both primary and acquired kidney injury in children are associated with increased length of stay and increased mortality. Consequently, continuous renal replacement therapy (CRRT) should be considered earlier in management than has previously been the case and is discussed in Chapter 18. Critically ill children experiencing, or at risk of developing, acute renal failure will benefit from prompt transfer to a specialty PICU.

The child's GIT will need protection from developing ulceration and bleeding in critical illness. A potentially fatal complication, stress ulceration and bleeding has a current incidence of around 10% in critically ill children.[198] Clinically significant bleeding causing haemodynamic instability or requiring transfusion is reported in about 1.6% of children in PICU.[198] The same treatments can be used in both children and adults, with no one agent, dose or regimen standing out as better for minimising bleeding and ulceration or leading to fewer complications such as pneumonia.[198]

Nutritional considerations

The aims of nutrition in critically ill children are two-fold. First, children are at particular risk of malnutrition because they are growing and have greater energy requirements for their weight and less storage capacity than adults. Second, children are at particular risk of developing protein–calorie malnutrition, which can lead to immuno-dysfunction, increased risk of infections, morbidity and death in those children with organ dysfunction.[199,200]

Nutrition is also important in maintaining gut mucosa integrity, preventing the development of hypo- and hyperglycaemia, assisting with maintenance of immune function and in modulating the immune response as well as providing energy.[201] One barrier to achieving adequate nutrition for critically ill children is the fluid restrictions that are routine practice in the ICU, and both use of feeding protocol and liberalising fluids where possible to maximise enteral nutrition should be considered.[202]

When caring for critically ill infants and children, nutrition to support growth needs to be considered. Ideally, enteral feeding of critically ill children should commence within 12–24 hours of admission to ICU, but may not be achievable until the child is transferred to a specialist centre.[203] It may not be appropriate to commence feeds if the child requires transfer, surgery or intubation. A dietician should be consulted to advise on appropriate enteral feeding formulas for children, in addition to organising caloric supplementation of feeds.[204] The dietician can advise on handling of human milk while in hospital for breastfeeding mothers, who will need to express milk when the infant is not yet feeding orally or to provide milk for tube feeding. In addition, dieticians can assess the child's energy requirements and the amount of feed required to meet needs, as both under- and over-feeding have been identified as issues in PICU.[201,203,205]

Supplements and feeding

While promising work has been undertaken in adult critical care with the supplementation of feeds and total parenteral nutrition (TPN) with supplements including amino acids such as L-arginine, glutamine, taurine, nucleotides, omega-3 and omega-6 fatty acids, carnitine, antioxidants, prebiotics and probiotics, the same outcomes have not been reproduced in children to date.[18] The evidence for additives in enteral feeding is not clear-cut in children, and therefore routine supplementation for critically ill infants and children is not common practice.

Intravenous therapy for children

Until enteral feeding is established, critically ill infants and children will require maintenance IV fluids. Traditionally, hypotonic fluids – fluids containing a concentration of sodium lower than normal serum sodium – have been administered as maintenance fluids. These included the hypotonic formulation of 0.225% sodium chloride with 3.75% glucose. Over the past decade this formulation has largely been replaced with 0.45% sodium chloride and 2.5% glucose as iatrogenic hyponatraemia has been observed in otherwise-well children having surgery.[206,207] It has been common paediatric practice to use only 500-mL IV bags in children for safety reasons. In the modern era across Westernised countries, use of volumetric IV pumps and burettes has also been standard paediatric practice, although changes to larger volumes of IV formulations for children will need to be closely monitored.

The use of hypotonic fluids is under review in many countries, with increased level of monitoring of weight and serum electrolytes recommended. Hypotonic fluids are implicated in hospital-acquired hyponatraemia[207] and, for critically ill children, the capacity to excrete additional free water is often impaired. In addition, a number of common conditions seen in the ICU increase secretion of antidiuretic hormone (ADH), including pain, nausea and infections of the CNS, the GIT, the lung and post-surgery, thus promoting the retention of water.[208] The risk of developing cerebral oedema is increased in children, who also have increased body tissue water content, and studies indicate that there is an increased risk of developing acute hyponatraemia leading to seizures.

Infants and children generally require added glucose in IV fluids. In infants under 3 months, glucose concentration is increased to at least 5% and up to 10%. The addition of potassium chloride into maintenance fluids is common, particularly in fasting children, and requires serial monitoring of serum potassium. For fluid resuscitation in infants and children, the use of glucose-containing IV fluids is contraindicated, and 0.9% sodium chloride is the resuscitation fluid of choice across the life span, including in the delivery suite for newborn fluid resuscitation.[9]

Glucose control in children

Hyperglycaemia is associated with a worse outcome in infants and children requiring ICU admission.[209] But the predisposition to hypoglycaemia in children has meant that aggressive treatment of hyperglycaemia is not commonplace in critically ill children. The most recently published study demonstrated no difference in outcome, but an increase in hypoglycaemia in the tight glucose control arm.[210] Hypoglycaemia is documented to occur more frequently in two groups of non-diabetic children: those requiring mechanical ventilation and those requiring inotropic support.[211] Monitoring for hypoglycaemia continues to be an important assessment parameter, particularly in sicker children who require ventilatory support, inotropic support and where enteral feeding may be contraindicated. Hypoglycaemia may be an indicator of worsening organ function; therefore, further research needs to focus on the safety of insulin therapy in the non-diabetic critically ill child before aggressive routine management of hyperglycaemia can be recommended.[209–211]

Liver disease in children

Liver failure is relatively rare in children. It often arises as a primary problem in children from countries where viral hepatitis is endemic and is associated with paracetamol overdose and chronic liver disorders, toxins, autoimmune disease, malignancies, vascular and biliary tree malformations as well as unidentified causes.[212] Chapter 20 contains more detail on liver function and dysfunction. There are varying severities and forms of liver failure. Infants and children experiencing fulminant hepatic failure and hepatic encephalopathy, regardless of underlying cause, are critically ill, and require transfer to a specialist PICU for ongoing management and possible liver transplantation. Mortality rate is strongly linked with the development of cerebral oedema and intracranial hypertension, and is reported to be as high as 50% where cerebral oedema occurs.[212,213] Promising work with auxiliary liver transplant of partial livers and preservation of the native liver in predominantly older children with infections or toxic causes of their liver failure has demonstrated recovery of the native liver and subsequent withdrawal of immunosuppressive agents.[214] Many critically ill infants and children are at risk of developing some degree of liver dysfunction; therefore, liver function of all critically ill children requires careful monitoring and management. Clinical manifestations and management of infants and children with liver failure are similar to those of adults.

Paediatric trauma

Trauma is a leading cause of death in children and young adults in all developed countries; in the developing world it is second only to deaths from infections.[1,151] The approach to management of trauma in children is the same as in

adults. See Chapter 24 for details on trauma systems and trauma management. While there has been some evidence from North America that specialist paediatric trauma centres produce better outcomes for children suffering traumatic injuries, the largely spread-out and relatively small population distribution in Australia, New Zealand and many other countries means that children will often need to be treated initially in adult settings.[1]

Incidence and patterns of injury in children

Injury is a leading cause of death in all children over 1 year across the world and represents half of all deaths in children 10 years and older.[215] Road traffic injuries, burns and drowning kill many children, while falls represent the leading cause of presentation to emergency departments worldwide.[215] Children who live in regional and rural areas have increased rates of traumatic injuries and deaths from trauma, as do children from lower socioeconomic backgrounds with crowded living conditions.[215] The same pattern is reflected in Australian and New Zealand statistics.[216,217] Across Australia almost 68,000 children were hospitalised as the result of injury in 2009–2010, accounting for 12% of all paediatric admissions, with 34% of all children's deaths attributable to injury in 2008–2010.[217,218] In 2013, injury accounted for around 5% of admissions to Australian and New Zealand PICUs, with a 5.3% mortality rate, accounting for 11% of all deaths in PICUs in the 1–15-years age group.[1]

Injury patterns in children differ from adults, with traumatic brain injury, blunt trauma and more diffuse injuries more common in children. There is a bimodal injury pattern associated with age, with peak incidence occurring in children aged 1–4 years and a second peak during adolescence and young adulthood, reflecting the different activities associated with each group.[217,218] Infants and young children have a decreased sense of danger and reduced ability to protect themselves, while adolescents have increased exposure to higher risk activities in conjunction with exposure to alcohol, drugs and motor vehicles.[219] Time of day and seasonal factors play a role in childhood injury, with children more likely to be injured between 3 p.m. and 5 p.m., coinciding with the end of the school day, and during summer months, when the incidence of drowning increases.[217,220]

Injury-related deaths in children are highest in the transport deaths category, followed by drowning and assault.[218] Motor vehicle accidents involving children as passengers, pedestrians or cyclists are the commonest cause of injury in Australian children, with driveway injuries involving four-wheel drive or light commercial vehicles more likely to be fatal.[217] Trauma associated with the use of all-terrain vehicles such as quad bikes is becoming increasingly common, particularly in rural areas.[216] For children under 14, falling from one level to another, such as falling from a window, was the most common form of falls-related injury.[215,217]

Drowning is another leading cause of death in children, with more than 175,000 children drowning each year. In low and middle income countries across Southeast Asia and the Western Pacific, higher rates of drowning occur and are associated with playing, washing or collecting water from open bodies of water.[215] In wealthier countries such as Australia, drownings in this age group peak in the summer months and are more likely to be linked to recreational activities. Boys outnumber girls, with two-thirds being boys. Children under 5 years are more likely to drown by falling into backyard swimming pools while older children (5–14 years) drown during planned swimming or other recreational activities in pools and open waterways such as dams and rivers.[220]

In Europe drowning is associated with lower socioeconomic status, with a greater number of deaths by drowning in the poorer parts of eastern and southern Europe when compared to western Europe. In developing countries the incidence remains high, with deaths from drowning having the highest mortality rate for all injuries presenting in the emergency department.[221]

Risk factors

The kinetic forces involved in injury are associated with a more diffuse injury pattern and a greater incidence of multiple trauma in children, as more of the child's body is subjected to the traumatic forces.[219,222,223] Children generally have less subcutaneous fat and musculature, providing less protection to the liver, kidneys and spleen, leading to a higher incidence of lung contusions and abdominal trauma.[19,222] In addition, the relatively large head size of the infant, particularly, and the child leads to a high incidence of head injury.[219]

Primary survey and resuscitation

Initial stabilisation of children who have experienced a traumatic injury is likely to have occurred in the field. Once at the hospital, the primary survey is conducted to assess for, detect and stabilise the child with life-threatening injuries. Undertaking a primary survey and resuscitation uses the same structured approach in children and adults. Chapters 23 and 24 cover emergency presentations and trauma management; however, specific paediatric considerations are highlighted below.

Children sustaining trauma to the head, just as adults, are managed with cervical spine precautions including a collar, until the spine has been radiologically and clinically cleared.[223,224] A selection of paediatric hard collars should be available and the measuring guide used to ensure good fit. As the collar can cause neck flexion in infants and small children, the child's torso may need to be elevated with a folded blanket to maintain a neutral neck position. The head and neck are usually immobilised, with head blocks (e.g. rolled towels) placed either side of the head to maintain in-line stabilisation and tapes applied to the forehead and chin to prevent movement. The combative, uncooperative child will not tolerate this, and the actions are likely to increase the child's agitation and movement.

The critical care nurse can position themselves to maintain in-line stabilisation while talking and soothing the child or ideally, where parents are present, seek their assistance to console their child. Specific paediatric trauma boards are available that are designed to maintain the child's head in a neutral position.

Fluid resuscitation is a controversial area of practice in paediatric trauma, where therapies have been generally less well-studied than in adults. However, in a haemodynamically unstable child, including the child with a traumatic brain injury at risk of secondary brain injury from hypotension, fluid resuscitation of 20 mL/kg of 0.9% saline followed by reassessment is recommended.[225] If more than 20 mL/kg is required, immediate surgical assessment for bleeding is indicated.[223]

Exposure of the child, with temperature control, is necessary to assess the child completely for injuries. As hypothermia can develop quickly in children, overhead heating sources and blankets are ideally used to keep the child warm. Hypothermia in trauma patients is associated with increased risk for coagulopathy and mortality, as in adults, so providing warmth is essential paediatric trauma nursing care.[219] The child's right to privacy and dignity should also be considered and exposure minimised.

Secondary survey

Undertaking a secondary survey is similar in children and adults and is described in Chapter 24. Specific paediatric considerations are highlighted below.

In children, particularly those under 1 year of age, if injuries and the accompanying history do not seem to match, non-accidental injury should be considered and noted. History should be obtained from the child where possible, from any witnesses to the accident and from ambulance officers if they attended. Parents or caregivers will provide details of the child's past medical history, any medications and any known allergies.

Specific conditions

Specific injuries that are seen in children are discussed briefly under the headings of traumatic brain injury, chest trauma and abdominal trauma. Obtaining an accurate history of the accident or events leading up to an injury is useful in determining the type of injuries that children may have sustained. Regardless of aetiology, where a child has been involved in a motor vehicle accident (MVA) or sustained a fall, there are likely to be multiple injuries and the situation should be treated as such until other injuries have been considered and excluded.[219]

Traumatic brain injury

Traumatic brain injury (TBI) is a leading cause of deaths and injury worldwide in children. In developing regions such as Asia and Africa, traumatic brain injury is increasing as the population has increased access to motor vehicles.[226] In Australia and other developed economies, children experience the greatest number of head injuries of any age group.[227,228] TBI is often associated with MVA where the child is a vehicle occupant, a pedestrian or a cyclist, with falls and with near-drowning. TBI is described in detail in Chapter 17.

Around 8% of all children aged 1–15 years of age who died in Australasian ICUs had sustained a traumatic brain injury.[1] Age and gender are the most significant risk factors for TBI, with peak incidence in the 0–4-years group and in males.[1] Other factors to consider in children are the increased tendency of the immature brain of children to experience disruption of the blood–brain barrier and, unlike adults, for an increased cerebral blood volume to lead to cerebral oedema due to higher brain water content.[227]

In 2012, the Society of Critical Care Medicine published the second edition of their guidelines on the management of paediatric brain injury; however, the limitations of the paediatric research evidence that underpinned these has led to reliance on less rigorous studies and ongoing reliance on extrapolation from adult research evidence.[229] Since the clinical manifestations of TBI in children are very similar to those in adults, management is also very similar. The practice of hyperventilation should be avoided as it is associated with regional cerebral ischaemia.[229]

In terms of assessment, the GCS modified for children has previously been described in this text. Indications for ICP monitoring in children include all infants and children with a severe head injury, which equates to a GCS score of 8 or below that persists following adequate cardiopulmonary resuscitation, and those children who present with abnormal motor posturing and hypotension.[230] Combined with invasive haemodynamic monitoring, targeted therapy to manage both ICP and CPP remains an important part of treatment. While thresholds for treating intracranial hypertension in children have not been studied, it has been known since the 1980s that prolonged intracranial hypertension or high ICP levels will worsen outcome. An ICP of 20 mmHg is considered high in children, with 15 mmHg considered high in infants. ICPs of these values are the usual cut-off points and are likely to be treated with the aim of lowering ICP while maintaining an adequate CPP.[229]

Diagnosis

Diagnostic techniques and clinical management of children with TBI mirror those in adults[230] (see Chapter 17). The smaller size of children means that diagnostics such as mixed cerebral venous saturation and direct brain oxygen saturation are not yet common practice in paediatrics, with further work required in direct brain oxygen saturation to determine utility and parameters.[231] A high index of suspicion for spinal injuries in paediatric TBI should be maintained, as spinal cord injury without radiological abnormality on plain X-rays and CT is a feature of paediatric spinal injury.[224] While CT scans are available in more centres than MRI, they involve radiation exposure to the young spine and miss spinal cord injury without radiological abnormality. MRI has been more effective in determining spinal cord injury than CT and, as it involves no radiation exposure, is the investigation of choice to determine spinal injury in children.[224,232]

Treatment

Several of the therapies used in the treatment of the child with severe head injury are controversial, as they have lacked sufficient scientific rigour when the small number of studies were evaluated to make clear, high quality evidence recommendations.[229] Essentially, treatment of TBI in children is identical to adult management: minimising intracranial hypertension and maintaining optimal CPP while preventing secondary injury from hypoxia, hypercarbia and hypotension while reducing the risk of iatrogenesis from treatment. Hyperglycaemia that persists beyond 48 hours of the injury is associated with a worse outcome;[209] however, studies are yet to be undertaken to determine whether this is modifiable with the use of tight glycaemic control.

Hypothermia has not yet been shown to make a difference in outcome in children, as it has in newborns and adults with hypoxic-ischaemic brain injury. Moderate hypothermia (temperature maintained at 32–34°C) has been studied in children with disappointing results;[233] therefore, the current recommendation is to consider cooling for 48 hours for intractable intracranial hypertension within 8 hours of the injury, to avoid cooling for 24 hours or less and to avoid rewarming at a rate faster than 0.5°C per hour.[229]

The use of decompressive craniectomy for early indications of herniation, ongoing neurological deterioration or development of intractable intracranial hypertension that is refractory to treatment such as drainage of CSF, sedation and barbiturates has demonstrated good outcome for some children.[234,235] But the evidence for this is not strong.[229]

Outcomes from TBI in children are associated with the severity of the initial injury and the presence and control of secondary brain injury, as in adults. Hypotension and hypoxia prior to hospital admission are strongly linked to mortality and poor functional outcome, with some emerging evidence that hypertension and hyperglycaemia in the first 24 hours may also predict poor outcomes at one year post-injury.[209,229]

Chest trauma

Thoracic injuries in children rarely occur in isolation with traumatic injuries and are often accompanied by head and neck injuries. There is some evidence that thoracic injuries are indicative of a more severe injury; they have been associated with higher mortality.[223] Injury to the heart and great vessels, in particular, is associated with higher mortality. The combination of head injury and thoracic injury is also known to have higher mortality. Most chest injuries in children are sustained as a consequence of MVAs.[19] The pattern of injury in children is predominantly one of blunt trauma. Lung contusions are the commonest thoracic injury seen in children.[19,223] As the ribcage is much more compliant in children, ribs are rarely broken, but they can damage underlying structures such as the lungs, so pulmonary contusions, pneumothorax and haemothorax are often seen. The clinical manifestations, approach to assessment, monitoring and management of children sustaining thoracic trauma are similar to those in adults, and are discussed in Chapter 24. Children with thoracic injuries are generally managed in a specialist trauma centre equipped to manage children.[19]

Abdominal trauma

Abdominal trauma in children is a leading cause of death when combined with head injury.[236] Blunt trauma from MVAs is the most common mechanism of injury, but bicycle handlebars may also inflict a significant injury.[237] The liver and spleen are the most commonly injured organs in abdominal trauma and can usually be managed non-surgically.[238] The abdominal organs are relatively large in children, with less musculature and a more compliant ribcage, meaning that there can be injury to underlying organs with no apparent external injury.[239] Blunt trauma is common, while penetrating injury is less common, resulting from gunshot and stab wounds. These injuries are associated with older children and adolescents, though a thinner body wall may result in greater underlying organ damage, particularly if the flank is penetrated.[239]

During the primary survey, the child's abdomen should be exposed and may reveal signs such as bruising from bicycle handles, tyre marks, abrasions or contusions. Abdominal distension is a less reliable sign in children, as distension may be from air that is swallowed from pain and crying. However, as in adults, the primary survey may not include the abdomen if other immediately life-threatening injuries are present, such as thoracic and/or head injuries. These injuries will take precedence, so it may not be until the secondary survey can be undertaken that abdominal injuries are considered. The monitoring and management of children sustaining abdominal trauma is very similar to that of adults,[220] and is discussed in Chapter 24.

More judicious use of CT scanning in paediatric centres is practised in relation to increased concerns regarding radiation exposure to children.[240] Clinical indicators will determine the need for a CT scan of the abdomen, including children with multiple injuries, gross haematuria with a minor injury and children with haemodynamic instability with no obvious source of blood loss. Diagnostic peritoneal lavage has largely ceased with the increasing utility of and expertise with focused ultrasound in trauma (FAST) in emergency departments.[240] When FAST sonography is combined with elevated liver transaminases, the sensitivity and specificity of the screening increases to 88% and 98%, respectively.[241] Monitoring of blood in urine is a simple, useful technique to detect bladder and kidney injuries. Management of abdominal trauma generally requires only haemodynamic and laboratory monitoring in conjunction with supportive therapies such as fluid replacement, monitoring of urine output and pain management with the aim of detecting signs of haemorrhage.[219,242]

Summary

Critically ill infants and children have several anatomical and physiological differences that predispose them to different types of critical illness when compared to adults. Children's relative physiological and psychological immaturity means that their needs may be different from adults when critically ill. Family support is important and parental presence should be allowed at all times. Patterns of disease may be different from adults – for example, a high incidence of respiratory illness and a predisposition to sustaining multiple trauma – but children have a lower incidence of sepsis, heart failure, liver failure and renal failure than adults. The need for specialised nursing and medical care as well as adapted equipment means that many critically ill children will require transfer to a specialist paediatric centre.

Case study

John is a 10-year-old boy weighing 50 kg who felt unwell on waking. He had a mild fever, headache and felt generally unwell. His parents decided he should stay home from school. Mid-afternoon John was still unwell and had a rash developing on his legs and trunk that was not evident in the morning. John had drunk very little, had not eaten anything and vomited twice. Dad took John to their local hospital emergency department (ED) in the family car.

John arrived at the local hospital's ED at around 4 p.m. At triage John's temperature was 39.1°C, heart rate was 150 and respiratory rate 40. He seemed drowsy, but his GCS was 14/15. Capillary refill time was 3–4 seconds. His systolic blood pressure was 100 and staff could not determine his diastolic blood pressure via the electronic monitor. O_2 saturation in air was 99%. Widespread rash over his legs, trunk and back was noted. The emergency nursing staff assigned a triage category of 2. John had a peripheral cannula sited, bloods were taken, including a venous blood gas, blood cultures, full blood count and electrolytes. John received a litre of 0.9% NaCl. Venous blood gas showed pH 7.30, PvO_2 48, $PvCO_2$ 45, lactate 6.2 and base deficit 10. John also received 2 g of cefotaxime IV.

The emergency consultant examined John and found no symptoms consistent with meningism. The specialist paediatric retrieval service was contacted to transfer John to a specialist children's hospital. A second litre of 0.9% NaCl was administered as John's heart rate, blood pressure and capillary refill were unchanged following the first bolus. During the bolus John became combative and confused, so a decision was made to intubate him. As part of preoxygenation and preparation, the nurse assisting successfully inserted a nasopharyngeal airway to facilitate bag–mask ventilation.

John was intubated and then placed on the ED transport ventilator. The paediatric retrieval team arrived during intubation and undertook their assessment in preparation to move John to PICU in a children's hospital. Observations at this time showed: temperature of 39.7°C, heart rate 153, BP 135/82 (mean 95), capillary refill time 4 seconds, pupils equal and reactive (3 mm in size), ventilator rate 17 with end-tidal CO_2 ($ETCO_2$) 32 mmHg, good chest movement, mottled colour with widespread purpuric rash on face, trunk and limbs. John remained sedated and muscle relaxed from intubation. The retrieval team placed radial arterial and femoral central venous lines. A nasogastric tube and indwelling catheter (IDC) were already in situ. John had blood oozing around his nasopharyngeal airway, so he received 1 g of tranexamic acid and blood was sent for coagulation studies. The retrieval team conferenced with PICU prior to leaving ED and the paediatric intensivist recommended giving 3% NaCl 3 mL/kg before leaving for potential raised ICP. John had Hartmann's solution running at two-thirds of maintenance rate, was muscle relaxed for transfer and received fentanyl and midazolam for analgesia and sedation. Blood results prior to leaving showed: pH 7.29, $PaCO_2$ 38, PaO_2 240, base deficit 8, bicarbonate 18.7 and lactate 3.81, sodium 139, potassium 4.2, chloride 106, ionised calcium 1.23, haemoglobin 136, haematocrit 40%, urea 5.4 and creatinine 48. FiO_2 was weaned and the team departed. The one-hour transport was uneventful.

John was taken directly to PICU. He was placed on the ICU ventilator on pressure controlled SIMV mode, rate 14, peak pressure 22, PEEP 5, FiO_2 50%, pressure support 17, inspiratory time of 1 second. He was generating tidal volumes of 7–8 mL/kg, with good chest movement, equal air entry on auscultation, $ETCO_2$ 40 mmHg and SpO_2 100%. On ETT suction secretions were blood-stained and coffee ground aspirate was noted from the nasogastric tube. His urine output was 1–1.5 mL/kg/h. Blood was sent for full blood count; electrolytes including calcium, magnesium and phosphate; liver function tests; coagulation studies; and procalcitonin level. A cross-match was also requested. The procalcitonin result was telephoned through from pathology as it was >10. Coagulation studies showed an INR of 1.7 and APTT 50. John was ordered fresh frozen plasma IV. His nasopharyngeal airway was removed following this. He continued on IV cefotaxime.

Around 10 hours after PICU admission John experienced a hypotensive episode, with mean arterial pressure dropping to the 50s. He received a 5-mL/kg fluid bolus and commenced dopamine infusion at 10 mcg/kg/min. John's lactate result around this time was 3.3. Neurologically, John remained on morphine (20 mcg/kg/h) and midazolam infusions (2 mcg/kg/min) and was reacting purposefully to noxious stimuli such as suctioning. He remained on inotropic support, which was able to be weaned a little over the course of day 2. Ventilation was also able to be weaned slightly.

On day 3 John's tidal volumes dropped to 4 mL/kg, so his ventilation was increased. His blood pressure also dropped, with mean pressure in the 60s. Inotropic support was increased back to 10 mcg/kg/min. He was no longer responding to stimuli so morphine was reduced to 10 mcg/kg/h and midazolam reduced to 1 mcg/kg/min. Noradrenaline infusion commenced at 0.05 mcg/kg/min and dopamine was weaned off. Enteral feeds were commenced at 5 mL/h and planned to grade up over the next 8 hours as tolerated.

Over the next 24 hours, John began coughing spontaneously and on suction and began moving all limbs to painful/noxious stimuli and when pressure care and other essential nursing care was attended. His noradrenaline infusion maintained his mean blood pressure between 65 and 75 mmHg. INR on coagulation studies had returned to normal at 1.1 and lactate remained under 2.

Over the course of night 4, John became agitated at times, requiring sedation boluses. After 4 days in PICU, John's inotropes were able to be weaned off and he was maintaining normal blood pressure. He was tolerating feeds. The rash, though widespread, was beginning to heal and lessen in parts such as his face. His family was greatly relieved at these improvements. It was planned for John to be extubated the next morning (day 6). Inotropes had been off for almost 24 hours and his coagulopathy had resolved. Midazolam infusion was ceased at 0600 of day 6 in anticipation of extubation later that morning following a trial of CPAP. John was able to be extubated at 1230 following a normal blood gas result on CPAP. By mid-afternoon, John appeared awake, recognising and responding to his family. He had a hoarse voice when speaking. John had a settled afternoon and night, requiring low flow oxygen via face mask and had commenced drinking and eating a small amount. At 0700 he was examined by the intensivist who declared he could be transferred to a ward bed. John left PICU for the ward at 11 a.m. on day 7 of his PICU stay.

John continued to receive intravenous antibiotics. His rash continued to heal. He was able to get out of bed and walk for short distances and by day 10 he was walking around the bed and able to shower with minimal assistance. On day 12, John was able to be discharged home from hospital. After 6 days at home, John returned to school for a half day prior to the weekend.

CASE STUDY QUESTIONS

1 What is the most likely diagnosis for John, based on his presentation and illness trajectory?

2 Describe a preferred approach to intubation of a shocked child. Calculate the ETT size for John.

3 John has a communicable disease that requires notification to the department of health. Consider which of John's contacts will require treatment with prophylactic therapy. What is the guideline/ recommendation in your state and hospital?

4 John has been experiencing blood-stained ETT aspirates, blood-stained secretions from nasogastric aspiration and blood oozing from around the nasopharyngeal airway. Provide two rationales for this bleeding and consider nursing actions and their effects.

RESEARCH VIGNETTE

Colville GA, Pierce CM. Children's self-reported quality of life after intensive care treatment.
Pediatr Crit Care Med 2013;14:7e85–e92

Abstract

Objectives: Study was to establish children's own views of their outcome.

Design: Prospective cohort study: A number of studies have reported on parental/clinician reports of children's quality of life after intensive care treatment.

Setting: Twenty-one bed PICU in a tertiary Children's Hospital.

Patients: Ninety-seven children aged over 7 years, with no pre-existing learning difficulties, consecutively admitted to PICU over an 18 month period.

Interventions: Patients completed the Pediatric Quality of Life Inventory and a post-traumatic stress screener, at 3 months and again at 1 year (n = 72) after discharge from PICU.

Measurements and main results: At 3 months post-discharge, the mean total Pediatric Quality of Life Inventory score reported by the PICU group was lower than that reported in the literature for a non-clinical community sample (PICU mean = 79.1 vs community mean = 83.9, p = 0.003), but by 1 year, they were comparable (82.2, p = 0.388). The mean physical functioning subscale score remained lower (PICU mean = 81.6 vs community mean = 88.5, p = 0.01), but improved significantly from 73.4 at 3 months (p = 0.001).

Sub-group analyses revealed that the elective group reported higher emotional functioning than the community sample (91.0, p = 0.005 at 3 months and 88.2, p = 0.038 at 1 year vs community mean = 78.5), and made significant gains in social functioning between time points (79.1 to 91.4, p = 0.015).

Finally, although total PedsQL scores at 1 year were not associated with measures of severity of illness during admission, they were significantly negatively associated with concurrent post-traumatic stress symptom scores (r = −0.40, p = 0.001).

Conclusions: The self-report version of the Pediatric Quality of Life Inventory proved to be a feasible and sensitive tool for assessing health related quality of life in this group of PICU survivors.

Critique

This study addresses an innovative way of reporting HRQOL in a heterogeneous sample of PICU survivors. The authors highlighted the documented poor agreement between proxy measurement of HRQOL by parents and self-reported measures by children. Although not the focus of the study, it would have been interesting to have the parents' perception of their child's HRQOL to compare with self-reported measurements, especially as a parent-report version is available for children aged 2 to 18 years. The study was nested in another study, which means that the authors could benefit from the study structure and process put in place in the primary study to collect the HRQOL data in the same sample. The instrument choice was justified by using a well-validated instrument for children aged between 5 and 18 years, including three versions specifically tailored to developmental ages (5–7 years, 8–11 years and 12–18 years). To meet the objective of the study, HRQOL was measured at two time points with sufficient time in between for potential HRQOL improvement. Rigorous data analyses were demonstrated with subgroup analyses (e.g. elective versus non-elective PICU admission) and tests of associations with potential confounding factors, such as the pediatric index of mortality, length of stay and post-traumatic stress scores.

The findings were clearly stated in tabulated form. The findings demonstrate HRQOL of PICU survivors is similar to that of healthy children 1 year after PICU discharge. Although below the norm at 3 and 12 months post-discharge, improvement in physical functioning was clinically significant. This is noteworthy, considering the sample severity of illness and the type of life-threatening conditions (e.g. 27 of 72 had traumatic brain injury).

The inclusion of children who were able to self-report only limits the generalisability of results to older PICU survivors. In addition, children with learning disabilities or those unable to self-report (e.g. severe TBI) were excluded from the study. This could have potentially positively biased the results. Finally, the number of children lost to follow-up at 12 months was significant. This is an inherent problem of longitudinal design. Due to the importance of this type of follow-up, researchers should keep concentrating their efforts on this issue. This study's findings demonstrate possible follow-up of children after PICU discharge using self-reported HRQOL questionnaires.

Learning activities

The questions below relate to the following scenario.

An 18-month-old child has presented to your emergency department with upper airway symptoms. The child is on her mother's lap and looks distressed and has an audible stridor. This is the first time this child has attended an emergency department.

1 Consider your approach to assessing children in this age group and this particular child.
2 What are the important aspects of history to elicit that will aid in making a diagnosis?
3 If you are thinking of a diagnosis, what are the important aspects to consider in terms of anatomy and symptoms?

Online resources

International educational platform for paediatric intensive care, http://openpediatrics.org

Meningitis information, www.meningitis.com

NSW Clinical Excellence Commission Sepsis program resources, www.cec.health.nsw.gov.au/documents/programs/sepsis/july-2013/sepsis-toolkit-june-2013.pdf

Paediatric Sepsis Initiative, www.wfpiccs.org/projects/sepsis-initiative

Royal Children's Hospital, Melbourne, www.rch.org.au/rch

Further reading

Butler A, Copnell B, Willetts G. Family-centred care in the paediatric intensive care unit: an integrative review of the literature. J Clin Nurs 2014;23:2086-99.

Curley MA, Wypij D, Watson RS, Grant MJ, Asaro LA, Cheifetz IM et al. Protocolized sedation vs usual care in pediatric patients mechanically ventilated for acute respiratory failure: a randomized clinical trial. JAMA 2015;313(4):379–89.

Dixon M, Crawford D. Paediatric intensive care nursing. Chichester, West Sussex: Wiley-Blackwell; 2012.

McAlvin SS, Carew-Lyons A. Family presence during resuscitation and invasive procedures in pediatric critical care: a systematic review. Am J Crit Care 2014;23:477-84.

Milési C, Baleine J, Matecki S, Durand S, Combes C, Novais ARB et al. Is treatment with a high flow nasal cannula effective in acute viral bronchiolitis? A physiologic study. Int Care Med 2013;39:1088-94.

Rimensberger PC. Pediatric and neonatal mechanical ventilation. Berlin: Springer-Verlag; 2015.

Verger J. Nutrition in the pediatric population in the intensive care unit. Crit Care Nurs Clin North Am 2014;26:199-215.

References

1 Alexander J, Millar J, Slater A, Woosley J. Report of the Australian and New Zealand Paediatric Intensive Care Registry 2013. Melbourne, Australia: Australian and New Zealand Intensive Care Society; 2014.

2 Australian and New Zealand Intensive Care Society. ANZICS Centre for Outcome and Resource Evaluation Annual Report 2012-2013. Melbourne: ANZICS; 2014.

3 Namachivayam P, Shann F, Shekerdemian L, Taylor A, van Sloten I, Delzoppo C et al. Three decades of intensive care: who was admitted, what happened in intensive care, and what happened afterward. Pediatr Crit Care Med 2010;11:549-55.

4 Rosenberg M, Greenberger S, Rawal A, Latimer-Pierson J, Thundiyil J. Comparison of Broselow tape measurements versus physician estimations of pediatric weights. Am J Emerg Med 2011;29:482-8.

5 Trakulsrichai S, Boonsri C, Chatchaipun P, Chunharas A. Accuracy of three methods used for Thai children's body weight estimation. J Med Assoc Thai 2012;95:1194-99.

6 Geduld H, Hodkinson PW, Wallis LA. Validation of weight estimation by age and length based methods in the Western Cape, South Africa population. EMJ 2011;28:856-60.

7 House DR, Ngetich E, Vreeman RC, Rusyniak DE. Estimating the weight of children in Kenya: do the Broselow tape and age-based formulas measure up? Ann Emerg Med 2013;61(1):1-8.

8 Wells M, Coovadia A, Kramer E, Goldstein L. The PAWPER tape: a new concept tape-based device that increases the accuracy of weight estimation in children through the inclusion of a modifier based on body habitus. Resuscitation 2013;84:227-32.

9 Australian Resuscitation Council. Techniques in paediatric advanced life support. Guideline 126. Melbourne, Australia: Australian Resuscitation Council; 2010.

10 Guyton AC, Hall JE. Fetal and neonatal physiology. In: Hall JE. Guyton and Hall textbook of medical physiology. 12th ed. Philadelphia: Saunders; 2011, pp 1019-30.

11 Blackburn ST. Maternal, fetal and neonatal physiology: A clinical perspective. 4th ed. Missouri: Elsevier Saunders; 2013.

12 Allen BB, Chiu Y, Gerber LM, Ghaja J, Greenfield JP. Age-specific cerebral perfusion pressure thresholds and survival in children and adolescents with severe traumatic brain injury. Pediatr Crit Care Med 2014;15:62-70.

13 Maloney PM. Sepsis and septic shock. Emerg Med Clin North Am 2013;31:583-600.

14 Mtaweh H, Trakas EV, Su E, Carcillo JA, Aneja RK. Advances in monitoring and management of shock. Pediatr Clin North Am 2013;60:641-54.

15 Primhak R. Evaluation and management of upper airway obstruction. Paediatr Child Health 2012;23:301-6.

16 Hammer J. Acute respiratory failure in children. Paediatr Respir Rev 2013;14:64-9.

17 Oymar K, Skjerven HO, Mikalsen IB. Acute bronchiolitis in infants: a review. Scand J Trauma Resusc Emerg Med 2014;22:22-3.

18 Joffe A, Anton N, Lequier L, Vandermeer B, Tjosvold L, Larsen B et al. Nutritional support for critically ill children. Cochrane Database Syst Rev 2009;(2):CD005144.

19 Tovar JA, Vazquez JJ. Management of chest trauma in children. Paediatr Respir Rev 2013;14:86-91.

20 Anthony D, Willock J, Baharestani M. A comparison of Braden Q, Garvin and Glamorgan risk assessment scales in paediatrics. J Tissue Viability 2010;19(3):98-105.

21 Willock J. Interrater reliability of the Glamorgan scale: overt and covert data. Br J Nurs 2013;22(20):S4, S6, S8-9.

22 Rennick JE, Rashotte J. Psychological outcomes in children following pediatric intensive care unit hospitalization: a systematic review of the research. J Child Health Care 2009;13:128-49.

23 Colville G, Darkins J, Hesketh J, Bennett V, Alcock J, Noyes J. The impact on parents of a child's admission to intensive care: integration of qualitative findings from a cross-sectional study. Intensive Crit Care Nurs 2009;25(2):72-79.

24 Foster M, Whitehead L, Maybee P. Parents' and health professionals' perceptions of family centred care for children in hospital, in developed and developing countries: a review of the literature. Int J Nurs Stud 2010;47:1184-93.

25 Harrison TM. Family-centered pediatric nursing care: state of the science. J Pediatr Nurs 2010;25:335-43.

26 Sturdivant L, Warren NA. Perceived met and unmet needs of family members of patients in the pediatric intensive care unit. Crit Care Nurs Q 2009;32:149-58.

27 Colville G. The psychologic impact on children of admission to intensive care. Pediatr Clin North Am 2008;55:605-16.

28 Melnyk BM, Crean HF, Feinstein NF, Fairbanks E, Alpert-Gillis LJ. Testing the theoretical framework of the COPE program for mothers of critically ill children: an integrative model of young children's post-hospital adjustment behaviors. J Pediatr Psychol 2007;32(4):463-74.

29 Dunkel CS, Sefcek JA. Eriksonian lifespan theory and life history theory: sn integration using the example of identity formation. Rev Gen Psychol 2009;13(1):13-23.

30 Piaget J. The child's conception of the world: A 20th-century classic of child psychology. Baltimore: Rowman & Littlefield; 2007.

31 Roberts CA. Unaccompanied hospitalized children: a review of the literature and incidence study. J Pediatr Nurs 2010;25:470-76.

32 Dudley NC, Hansen KW, Furnival RA, Donaldson AE, Van Wagenen KL, Scaife ER. The effect of family presence on the efficiency of pediatric trauma resuscitations. Ann Emerg Med 2009;53:777-84 e3.

33 Tinsley C, Hill JB, Shah J, Zimmerman G, Wilson M, Freier K et al. Experience of families during cardiopulmonary resuscitation in a pediatric intensive care unit. Pediatrics 2008;122:e799-804.

34 Erikson EH. Identity and the life cycle. New York: Norton & Company; 1994.

35 Schore AN. Affect regulation and the origin of the self: The neurobiology of emotional development. Hillsdale, NJ: Lawrence Erlbaum Associates; 1994.

36 Schore JR, Schore AN. Modern attachment theory: the central role of affect regulation in development and treatment. Clinical Social Work Journal 2008;36:9-20.

37 Beilin H, Pufall PB. Piaget's theory prospects and possibilities. Hillsdale, NJ: Lawrence Erlbaum Associates; 1992.

38 Wheeler HJ. The importance of parental support when caring for the acutely ill child. Nurs Crit Care 2005;10(2):56-62.

39 Coyne I. Consultation with children in hospital: children, parents' and nurses' perspectives. J Clin Nurs 2006;15(1):61-71.

40 Hockenberry M, Wilson D. Wong's essentials of pediatric nursing. 9th ed. St Louis: Mosby Elsevier; 2013.

41 Slote RJ. Psychological aspects of caring for the adolescent undergoing spinal fusion for scoliosis. Orthop Nurs 2002;21(6):19-31.

42 Shields L, Pratt J, Hunter J. Family centred care: a review of qualitative studies. J Clin Nurs 2006;15:1317-23.

43 Davidson JE, Powers K, Hedayat KM, Tieszen M, Kon AA, Shepard E et al. Clinical practice guidelines for support of the family in the patient-centered intensive care unit: American College of Critical Care Medicine Task Force 2004–2005. Crit Care Med 2007;35:605-22.

44 Jackson C, Cheater FM, Reid I. A systematic review of decision support needs of parents making child health decisions. Health Expect 2008;11:232-51.

45 Lam LWC, A.M.; Morrissey J., Chang AM, Morrissey J. Parents' experiences of participation in the care of hospitalised children: a qualitative study. Int J Nurs Stud 2006;43:535-45.

46 Cleveland LM. Parenting in the neonatal intensive care unit. J Obst Gynecol Neonatal Nurs 2008;37:666-91.

47 Kuzin JK, Yborra JG, Taylor MD, Chang AC, Altman CA, Whitney GM et al. Family-member presence during interventions in the intensive care unit: perceptions of pediatric cardiac intensive care providers. Pediatrics 2007;120:e895-e901.

48 National Health and Medical Research Council. National Statement on Ethical Conduct in Human Research. Canberra, Australia: Australian Government, <http://www.ag.gov.au/cca>; 2007 [accessed 7.12.14].

49 De Lourdes Levy M, Larcher V, Kurz R; Ethics Working Group of the Confederation of European Specialists in Paediatrics. Informed consent/assent in children. Statement of the Ethics Working Group of the Confederation of European Specialists in Paediatrics (CESP). Eur J Pediatr 2003;162:629-33.

50 Roberson AJ. Adolescent informed consent: ethics, law, and theory to guide policy and nursing research. J Nurs Law 2007;11(4):191-6.

51 Munro ER, Ward H. Balancing parents' and very young children's rights in care proceedings: decision-making in the context of the *Human Rights Act 1998*. Child Family Social Work 2008;13:227-34.

52 Walker SM. Pain in children: recent advances and ongoing challenges. Br J Anaesth 2008;101(1):101-10.

53 Ramelet A-S, Abu-Saad HH, Rees N, McDonald S. The challenges of pain measurement in critically ill young children: a comprehensive review. Aust Crit Care 2004;17:33-45.

54 Thomas M, Dhanani S, Irwin D, Writer H, Doherty D. Development, dissemination and implementation of a sedation and analgesic guideline in a pediatric intensive care unit...it takes creativity and collaboration. Dynamics 2010;21(4):16-25.

55 O'Connor M, Bucknall T, Manias E. Sedation management in Australian and New Zealand intensive care units: doctors' and nurses' practices and opinions. Am J Crit Care 2010;19:285-95.

56 Byrd PJ, Gonzales I, Parsons V. Exploring barriers to pain management in newborn intensive care units: a pilot survey of NICU nurses. Adv Neonatal Care 2009;9:299-306.

57 Neuhauser C, Wagner B, Heckmann M, Weigand MA, Zimmer KP. Analgesia and sedation for painful interventions in children and adolescents. Deutsches Aerzteblatt International (German). 2010;107(14):241-47, I-II, I.

58 Anand KJS, Willson DF, Berger J, Harrison R, Meert KL, Zimmerman J et al. Tolerance and withdrawal from prolonged opioid use in critically ill children. Pediatrics 2010;125:e1208-25.

59 Birchley G. Opioid and benzodiazepine withdrawal syndromes in the paediatric intensive care unit: a review of recent literature. Nurs Crit Care 2009;14(1):26-37.

60 Fisher D, Grap MJ, Younger JB, Ameringer S, Elswick RK. Opioid withdrawal signs and symptoms in children: frequency and determinants. Heart Lung 2013;42:407-13.

61 Ista E, de Hoog M, Tibboel D, van Dijk M. Implementation of standard sedation management in paediatric intensive care: effective and feasible? J Clin Nurs 2009;18:2511-20.

62 Ista E, van Dijk M, Tibboel D, de Hoog M. Assessment of sedation levels in pediatric intensive care patients can be improved by using the COMFORT "behavior" scale. Pediatr Crit Care Med 2005;6:58-63.

63 Dingeman RS, Mitchell EA, Meyer EC, Curley MA. Parent presence during complex invasive procedures and cardiopulmonary resuscitation: a systematic review of the literature. Pediatrics 2007;120:842-54.

64 Franck LS, Oulton K, Bruce E. Parental involvement in neonatal pain management: an empirical and conceptual update. J Nurs Scholarsh 2012;44:45-54.

65 Harrison D, Yamada J, Adams-Webber T, Ohlsson A, Beyene J, Stevens B. Sweet tasting solutions for reduction of needle-related procedural pain in children aged one to 16 years. Cochrane Database Syst Rev, <http://www.mrw.interscience.wiley.com/cochrane/clsysrev/articles/CD008408/frame.html>; 2011 [accessed 28.04.14].

66 Bueno M, Yamada J, Harrison D, Khan S, Ohlsson A, Adams-Webber T et al. A systematic review and meta-analyses of nonsucrose sweet solutions for pain relief in neonates. Pain Res Manag 2013;18:153-61.

67 Austin D. The psychophysiological effects of music therapy in intensive care units. Paediatr Nurs 2010;22(3):14-20.

68 Spence K, Henderson-Smart D, New K, Evans C, Whitelaw J, Woolnough R. Evidenced-based clinical practice guideline for management of newborn pain. J Paediatr Child Health 2010;46:184-92.

69 Kang TM. Propofol infusion syndrome in critically ill patients. Annals Pharmacother 2002;36:1453-56.

70 Nolent P, Laudenbach V. Sedation and analgesia in the paediatric intensive care unit. Ann Fr Anesth Reanim 2008;27:623-32.

71 Vespasiano M, Finkelstein M, Kurachek S. Propofol sedation: intensivists' experience with 7304 cases in a children's hospital. Pediatrics 2007;120:e1411-17.

72 Phan H, Nahata MC. Clinical uses of dexmedetomidine in pediatric patients. Pediatr Drugs 2008;10:49-69.

73 Buck ML. Dexmedetomidine use in pediatric intensive care and procedural sedation. J Pediatr Pharmacol Ther 2010;15:17-29.

74 Playfor SD. Analgesia and sedation in critically ill children. Arch Dis Child 2008;93(3):87-92.

75 Tibballs J, Watson T. Symptoms and signs differentiating croup and epiglottitis. J Paediatr Child Health 2010;47(3):77-82.

76 Horeczko T, Enriquez B, McGrath NE, Gausche-Hill M, Lewis RJ. The Pediatric Assessment Triangle: accuracy of its application by nurses in the triage of children. J Emerg Nurs 2013;39:182-9.

77 Ayari S, Aubertino G, Girschig H, Van Den Abbeeled T, Denoyellee F, Couloignierf V et al. Management of laryngomalacia. Eur Ann Otorhinolaryngol Head Neck Dis 2013;130:15-21.

78 Dobbie AM, White DR. Laryngomalacia. Pediatr Clin North Am 2013;60:893-902.

79 Schmidt MH, Riley RH, Hee GY. Difficult double-lumen tube placement due to laryngeal web. Anaesth Intensive Care 2010;38:194-6.

80 Midyat J, Cakır E, Kut A. Upper airway abnormalities detected in children using flexible bronchoscopy. Int J Pediatr Otorhinolaryngol 2012;76:560-3.

81 Bryant J, Krishna SG, Tobias JD. The difficult airway in pediatrics. Adv Anesth 2013;31:31-60.

82 Endorf FW, Ahrenholz D. Burn management. Curr Opin Crit Care 2011;17:601-5.

83 Schramm C, Knop J, Jensen K, Plaschke K. Role of ultrasound compared to age-related formulas for uncuffed endotracheal intubation in a pediatric population. Pediatr Anesth 2012;22:781-6.

84 El-Orbany M, Connolly L. Rapid sequence induction and intubation: current controversy. Anesth Analg 2010;110:1318-25.

85 Neuhaus D, Schmitz A, Gerber A, Weiss M. Controlled rapid sequence induction and intubation – an analysis of 1001 children. Paediatr Anaesth 2013;23:734-40.

86 Byard RW. Diphtheria – 'The strangling angel' of children. J Forensic Leg Med 2013;20:65-8.

87 D'Agostino J. Pediatric airway nightmares. Emerg Med Clin North Am 2010;28:119-26.

88 Pfleger A, Eber E. Management of acute severe upper airway obstruction in children. Paediatr Respir Rev 2013;14:70-7.

89 Royal Children's Hospital. Clinical Practice Guideline – Laryngotracheobronchitis. Melbourne: Royal Children's Hospital; 2011.

90 Russell KF, Liang Y, O'Gorman K, Johnson DW, Klassen TP. Glucocorticoids for croup. Cochrane Database Syst Rev 2011;(1):CD001955.

91 Abdallah C. Acute epiglottitis: trends, diagnosis and management. Saudi J Anaesth 2012;6:279-81.

92 Australian Government Department of Health. Haemophilus influenza type b invasive infection. CDNA National Guidelines for Public Health Units. Canberra: Australian Government, <http://www.health.gov.au/internet/main/publishing.nsf/Content/cdna-song-hib.htm#contact>; 2014 [accessed 29.04.14].

93 Göktas O, Snidero S, Jahnke V, Passali D, Gregori D. Foreign body aspiration in children: field report of a German hospital. Pediatr Int 2010;52:100-3.

94 Australian Resuscitation Council. Management after resuscitation in paediatric advanced life support. Guideline 12.7. Melbourne, Australia: Australian Resuscitation Council; 2010.

95 Sodhi KS AS, Saxena AK, Singh M, Rao KLN, Khandelwal N. Utility of multidetector CT and virtual bronchoscopy in tracheobronchial obstruction in children. Acta Paediatr 2010;99:1011-5.

96 Myers TR. Guidelines for asthma management: a review and comparison of 5 current guidelines. Respir Care 2008;53:751-69.

97 The Global Initiative for Asthma. Global strategy for the diagnosis and management of asthma in children 5 years and younger. The Global Initiative for Asthma, <http://www.ginasthma.org/index.asp>; 2009 [accessed 10.05.14].

98 Ducharme FM, Tse SM, Chauhan B. Diagnosis, management, and prognosis of preschool wheeze. Lancet 2014;383(9928):1593-604.

99 Bardach A, Rey-Ares L, Cafferata ML, Cormick G, Romano M, Ruvinsky S et al. Systematic review and meta-analysis of respiratory syncytial virus infection epidemiology in Latin America. Rev Med Virol 2014;24(2):76-89.

100 Schroeder AR, Mansbach JM. Recent evidence on the management of bronchiolitis. Curr Opin Pediatr 2014;26(3):328-33.

101 Ranmuthugala G, Brown L, Lidbury BA. Respiratory syncytial virus – the unrecognised cause of health and economic burden among young children in Australia. Communicable Diseases Surveillance 2011;35:177-84.

102 Dede A, Isaacs D, Torzillo PJ, Wakerman J, Roseby R, Fahy R et al. Respiratory syncytial virus infections in Central Australia. J Paediatr Child Health 2010;46(1-2):35-39.

103 Bailey EJ, Maclennan C, Morris PS, Kruske SG, Brown N, Chang AB. Risks of severity and readmission of Indigenous and non-Indigenous children hospitalised for bronchiolitis. J Paediatr Child Health 2009;45:593-97.

104 Parker MJ, Allen U, Stephens D, Lalani A, Schuh S. Predictors of major intervention in infants with bronchiolitis. Pediatr Pulmonol 2009;44:358-63.

105 Eidelman AI, Megged O, Feldman R, Toker O. The burden of respiratory syncytial virus bronchiolitis on a pediatric inpatient service. Isr Med Assoc J 2009;11:533-36.

106 Vicencio AG. Susceptibility to bronchiolitis in infants. Curr Opin Pediatr 2010;22(3):302-6.

107 Abboud PA, Roth PJ, Skiles CL, Stolfi A, Rowin ME. Predictors of failure in infants with viral bronchiolitis treated with high-flow, high-humidity nasal cannula therapy. Pediatr Crit Care Med 2012;13:e343-49.

108 Carroll CL, Sala KA. Pediatric status asthmaticus. Crit Care Clin 2013;29:153-66.

109 Patel MM, Miller RL. Air pollution and childhood asthma: recent advances and future directions. Curr Opin Pediatr 2009;21:235-42.

110 Martel MJ, Rey E, Malo JL, Perreault S, Beauchesne MF, ForgetA et al. Determinants of the incidence of childhood asthma: a two-stage case-control study. Am J Epidemiol 2009;169:195-205.

111 Cornell A, Shaker M, Woodmansee DP. Update on the pathogenesis and management of childhood asthma. Curr Opin Pediatr 2008;20:597-604.

112 Delmas MC, Marguet C, Raherison C, Nicolau J, Fuhrman C. Les hospitalisations pour asthme chez l'enfant en France, 2002–2010. Arch Pediatr 2013;20:739-47.

113 Australian Institute of Health and Welfare. Asthma hospitalisation in Australia 2010–2011. Canberra: Australian Institute of Health and Welfare; 2013.

114 Anandan C, Nurmatov U, Van Schayck OCP, Sheikh A. Is the prevalence of asthma declining? Systematic review of epidemiological studies. Allergy 2010;65:152–67.

115 Centers for Disease Control and Prevention. FastStats. Asthma. Atlanta: Centers for Disease Control and Prevention, <http://www.cdc.gov/nchs/fastats/asthma.htm>; 2010 [accessed 28.09.14].

116 Watson L, Turk F, James P, Holgate ST. Factors associated with mortality after an asthma admission: a national United Kingdom database analysis. Respir Med 2007;101:1659-64.

117 Australian Centre for Asthma Monitoring. Asthma in Australia 2011. Canberra: Australian Institute of Health and Welfare, <http://www.aihw.gov.au/publication-detail/?id=10737420159>; 2011 [accessed 03.06.14].

118 Bloomberg GR. The exacerbation component of impairment and risk in pediatric asthma. Curr Opin Allergy Clin Immunol 2010;10:155-60.

119 Jackson DJ, Sykes A, Mallia P, Johnston SL. Asthma exacerbations: origin, effect, and prevention. J Allergy Clin Immunol 2011;128:1165-74.

120 Schramm CM, Carroll CL. Advances in treating acute asthma exacerbations in children. Curr Opin Pediatr 2009;21:326-32.

121 National Asthma Council Australia. Australian asthma handbook. National Asthma Council Australia Ltd, <http://www.asthmahandbook.org.au/uploads/AustralianAsthmaHandbookQuickReferenceGuide_Version1.0.pdf>; 2014.

122 Dehò A, Lutman D, Montgomery M, Petros A, Ramnarayan P. Emergency management of children with acute severe asthma requiring transfer to intensive care. Emerg Med J 2010;27:834-37.

123 Craske J, Dooley F, Griffiths L, McArthur L, White E, Cunliffe M. Introducing LAPPS (Liverpool Anticipatory Procedural Pain Score): the pragmatic development of an innovative approach to predicting and treating procedural pain and distress in children. J Child Health Care 2013;17:114-24.

124 Travers AH, Milan SJ, Jones AP, Camargo CA Jr, Rowe BH. Addition of intravenous beta(2)-agonists to inhaled beta(2)-agonists for acute asthma. Cochrane Database Syst Rev 2012;12:CD010179.

125 Powell C, Dwan K, Milan SJ, Beasley R, Hughes R, Knopp-Sihota JA et al. Inhaled magnesium sulfate in the treatment of acute asthma. Cochrane Database Syst Rev 2012;12:CD003898.

126 Travers AH, Jones AP, Camargo CA Jr, Milan SJ, Rowe BH. Intravenous beta(2)-agonists versus intravenous aminophylline for acute asthma. Cochrane Database Syst Rev 2012;12:CD010256.

127 Mayordomo-Colunga J, Medina A, Rey C, Diaz JJ, Concha A, Los Arcos M et al. Predictive factors of non-invasive ventilation failure in critically ill children: a prospective epidemiological study. Intensive Care Med 2009;35:527-36.

128 Papiris S, Manali E, Kolilekas L, Triantafillidou C, Tsangaris I. Acute severe asthma. Drugs 2009;69:2363-91.

129 Yang KD. Consensus, limitations and perspectives on pediatric asthma treatment. Pediatr Neonatol 2010;51:5-6.

130 Morrow BM, Argent AC. A comprehensive review of pediatric endotracheal suctioning: effects, indications, and clinical practice. Pediatr Crit Care Med 2008;9:465-77.

131 Kelly M, Gillies D, Todd DA, Lockwood C. Heated humidification versus heat and moisture exchangers for ventilated adults and children. Cochrane Database Syst Rev 2010;4:CD004711.

132 Nagaya K, Okamoto T, Nakamura E, Hayashi T, Fujieda K. Airway humidification with a heated wire humidifier during high-frequency ventilation using Babylog 8000 plus in neonates. Pediatr Pulmonol 2009;44:260-66.

133 Paratz JD, Stockton KA. Efficacy and safety of normal saline instillation: a systematic review. Physiotherapy 2009;95:241-50.

134 Copnell B, Tingay DG, Mills JF, Dargaville PA. Endotracheal suction techniques that effectively remove secretions do not preserve lung volume. Aust Crit Care 2009;22:61.

135 Jauncey-Cooke JI, Bogossian F, East CE. Lung protective ventilation strategies in paediatrics – a review. Aust Crit Care 2010;23:81-8.

136 Santschi M, Randolph AG, Rimensberger PC, Jouvet P. Mechanical ventilation strategies in children with acute lung injury: a survey on stated practice pattern. Pediatr Crit Care Med 2013;14:e332-37.

137 van Kaam AH, Rimensberger PC, Borensztajn D, De Jaegere AP. Ventilation practices in the neonatal intensive care unit: a cross-sectional study. J Pediatr 2010;157:767-71.

138 Shah PS, Ohlsson A, Shah JP. Continuous negative extrathoracic pressure or continuous positive airway pressure for acute hypoxemic respiratory failure in children. Cochrane Database Syst Rev 2008;1:CD003699.

139 Schönhofer B, Kuhlen R, Neumann P, Westhoff M, Berndt C, Sitter H. Clinical practice guideline: non-invasive mechanical ventilation as treatment of acute respiratory failure. Deutsches Ärzteblatt International (German) 2008;105:424-33.

140 Floret D. Non-invasive ventilation as primary ventilatory support for infants with severe bronchiolitis. Intensive Care Med 2008;34:1608-14.

141 Bancalari E, Claure N. The evidence for non-invasive ventilation in the preterm infant. Arch Dis Child 2013;98:F98-102.

142 Henderson-Smart DJ, Cools F, Bhuta T, Offringa M. Elective high frequency oscillatory ventilation versus conventional ventilation for acute pulmonary dysfunction in preterm infants. Cochrane Database Syst Rev 2009;3:CD000104.

143 Gupta P, Green JW, Tang X, Gall CM, Gossett JM, Rice TB et al. Comparison of high-frequency oscillatory ventilation and conventional mechanical ventilation in pediatric respiratory failure. JAMA 2014;168:243-9.

144 Brown KL, Ichord R, Marino BS, Thiagarajan RR. Outcomes following extracorporeal membrane oxygenation in children with cardiac disease. Pediatr Crit Care Med 2013;14(5 Suppl 1):S73-83.

145 MacLaren G, Dodge-Khatami A, Dalton HJ, MacLaren G, Dodge-Khatami A, Dalton HJ et al. Joint statement on mechanical circulatory support in children: a consensus review from the Pediatric Cardiac Intensive Care Society and Extracorporeal Life Support Organization. Pediatr Crit Care Med 2013;14(5 Suppl 1):S1-2.

146 Keckler SJ, Laituri CA, Ostlie DJ, St Peter SD. A review of venovenous and venoarterial extracorporeal membrane oxygenation in neonates and children. Eur J Pediatr Surg 2010;20(1):1-4.

147 Maslach-Hubbard A, Bratton SL. Extracorporeal membrane oxygenation for pediatric respiratory failure: history, development and current status. World J Crit Care Med 2013;2(4):29-39.

148 Maclaren G, Butt W, Best D, Donath S, Taylor A. Extracorporeal membrane oxygenation for refractory septic shock in children: one institution's experience. Pediatr Crit Care Med 2007;8:447-51.

149 Morini F, Goldman A, Pierro A. Extracorporeal membrane oxygenation in infants with congenital diaphragmatic hernia: a systematic review of the evidence. Eur J Pediatr Surg 2006;16:385-91.

150 Fisher JD, Nelson DG, Beyersdorf H, Satkowiak LJ. Clinical spectrum of shock in the pediatric emergency department. Pediatr Emerg Care 2010;26:622-25.

151 Black RE, Cousens S, Johnson HL, Lawn JE, Rudan I, Bassani DG et al, Child Health Epidemiology Reference Group of WHO and UNICEF. Global, regional, and national causes of child mortality in 2008: a systematic analysis. Lancet 2010;375(9730):1969-87.

152 Hartman ME, Linde-Zwirble WT, Angus DC, Watson RS. Trends in the epidemiology of pediatric severe sepsis. Pediatr Crit Care Med 2013;14(7):686-93.

153 Vila Pérez D, Cambra FJ, Jordan I, Esteban E, García-Soler P, Murga V et al. Prognostic factors in pediatric sepsis study from the Spanish Society of Pediatric Intensive Care. Pediatr Infect Dis J 2014;33:152-7.

154 Dellinger RP, Jaeschke R, Osborn TM, Nunnally ME, Townsend SR, Reinhart K et al, Surviving Sepsis Campaign Guidelines Committee including the Pediatric Subgroup. Surviving Sepsis Campaign: international guidelines for management of severe sepsis and septic shock, 2012. Intensive Care Med 2013;39:165-228.

155 Carcillo JA. Capillary refill time is a very useful clinical sign in early recognition and treatment of very sick children. Pediatr Crit Care Med. 2012;13:210-12.

156 Ackerman A. Meningococcal sepsis in children: persistent problem; new insights? Crit Care Med 2010;38:316-17.

157 Maitland K, Kiguli S, Opoka RO, Engoru C, Olupot-Olupot P, Akech SO et al. Mortality after fluid bolus in African children with severe infection. N Engl J Med 2011;364(26):2483-95.

158 Akech S, Ledermann H, Maitland K. Choice of fluids for resuscitation in children with severe infection and shock: systematic review. BMJ 2010;341:c4416.

159 Tobias JR, Ross AK. Intraosseous infusions: a review for the anesthesiologist with a focus on pediatric use. Anesth Analg 2010;110:391-401.

160 Luck R, Haines C, Mull C. Intraosseous access. J Emerg Med 2010;39(4):468-75.

161 Lampin ME, Rousseaux J, Botte A, Sadik A, Cremer R, Leclerc F. Noradrenaline use for septic shock in children: doses, routes of administration and complications. Acta Paediatr 2012;101:e426-30.

162 Menon K, McNally D, Choong K, Sampson M. A systematic review and meta-analysis on the effect of steroids in paediatric shock. Pediatr Crit Care Med 2013;14:474-80.

163 MacLaren G, Butt W, Best D, Donath S. Central extracorporeal membrane oxygenation for refractory pediatric septic shock. Pediatr Crit Care Med 2011;12:133-6.

164 Dash N, Al Khusaiby S, Behlim T, Mohammadi A, Mohammadi E, Al Awaidy S. Epidemiology of meningitis in Oman, 2000–2005. East Mediterr Health J 2009;15:1358-64.

165 Cherry JD. Recognition and management of encephalitis in children. Adv Exp Med Biol 2009;634:53-60.

166 Kawano G, Iwata O, Iwata S, Kawano K, Obu K, Kuki I et al. Determinants of outcomes following acute child encephalopathy and encephalitis: pivotal effect of early and delayed cooling. Arch Dis Child 2010;1-6.

167 Okanishi T, Maegaki Y, Ohno K, Togari H. Underlying neurologic disorders and recurrence rates of status epilepticus in childhood. Brain Dev 2008;30:624-28.

168 Newgard CD, Rudser K, Atkins DL, Berg R, Osmond MH, Bulger EM et al. The availability and use of out-of-hospital physiologic information to identify high-risk injured children in a multisite, population-based cohort. Prehosp Emerg Care 2009;13:420-31.

169 Van de Voorde P, Sabbe M, Rizopoulos D, Tsonaka R, De Jaeger A, Lesaffre E et al. Assessing the level of consciousness in children: a plea for the Glasgow Coma Motor subscore. Resuscitation 2008;76:175-79.

170 Cohen J. Interrater reliability and predictive validity of the FOUR score coma scale in a pediatric population. J Neurosci Nurs 2009;41:261-67.

171 Bonkowsky JL, Guenther E, Srivastava R, Filloux FM. Seizures in children following an apparent life-threatening event. J Child Neurol 2009;24:709-713.

172 Chen CY, Chang YJ, Wu HP. New-onset seizures in pediatric emergency. Pediatr Neonatol 2010;51:103-11.

173 American Academy of Pediatrics. Febrile seizures: guideline for the neurodiagnostic evaluation of the child with a simple febrile seizure. Pediatrics 2011;127:389-94.

174 Mastrangelo M, Midulla F, Moretti C. Actual insights into the clinical management of febrile seizures. Eur J Pediatr 2014;173(8):977-82.

175 Mirski MAA. Seizures and status epilepticus in the critically ill. Crit Care Clin 2007;24:115-47.

176 Abou Khaled KJ, Hirsch LJ. Updates in the management of seizures and status epilepticus in critically ill patients. Neurol Clin 2008;26:385-408.

177 Chin RFM, Neville BGR, Scott RC. Meningitis is a common cause of convulsive status epilepticus with fever. Arch Dis Child 2005;90:66-69.

178 Husain EH, Al-Shawaf F, Bahbahani E, El-Nabi MH, Al-Fotooh KA, Shafiq MH et al. Epidemiology of childhood meningitis in Kuwait. Med Sci Monit 2007;13(5):CR220-CR3.

179 March B, Eastwood K, Wright IM, Tilbrook L, Durrheim DN. Epidemiology of enteroviral meningoencephalitis in neonates and young infants. J Paediatr Child Health 2014;50:216-20.

180 National Notifiable Diseases Ssurveillance System Annual Report Writing Group. Australia's notifiable disease status 2010: annual report of the National Notifiable Diseases Surveillance System. Canberra: NNDSS; 2012.

181 Chang Q, Tzeng YL, Stephens DS. Meningococcal disease: changes in epidemiology and prevention. Clin Epidemiol 2012;4(1):237-45.

182 Baumer JH. Guideline review: management of invasive meningococcal disease, SIGN. Arch Dis Child 2009;94(2):46-49.

183 Branco RG, Amoretti CF, Tasker RC. Meningococcal disease and meningitis. Jornal de Pediatria (Rio de Janeiro) 2007;83(2 Supplement):S46-53.

184 Fowlkes AL, Honarmand S, Glaser C, Yagi S, Schnurr D, Oberste MS et al. Enterovirus-associated encephalitis in the California Encephalitis Project, 1998–2005. J Infect Dis 2008;198:1685-91.

185 Centers for Disease Control and Prevention. Pediatric bacterial meningitis surveillance – African region, 2002–2008. MMWR Morb Mortal Wkly Rep 2009;58:493-97.

186 Isaacman DJ, McIntosh ED, Reinert RR. Burden of invasive pneumococcal disease and serotype distribution among *Streptococcus pneumoniae* isolates in young children in Europe: impact of the 7-valent pneumococcal conjugate vaccine and considerations for future conjugate vaccines. Int J Infect Dis 2010;14:e197-209.

187 Menzies R, Turnour C, Chiu C, McIntyre P. Vaccine preventable diseases and vaccination coverage in Aboriginal and Torres Strait Islander people, Australia 2003 to 2006. Communicable Diseases Intelligence Quarterly Report 2008;32 Suppl:S2-67.

188 Jafri RZ, Ali A, Messonnier NE, Tevi-Benissan C, Durrheim D, Eskola J et al. Global epidemiology of invasive meningococcal disease. Popul Health Metr 2013;11(1):17.

189 Bargui F, D'Agostino I, Mariani-Kurkdjian P, Alberti C, Doit C, Bellier N et al. Factors influencing neurological outcome of children with bacterial meningitis at the emergency department. Eur J Pediatr 2012;171:1365-71.

190 Prasad K, Singh MB. Corticosteroids for managing tuberculous meningitis. Cochrane Database Syst Rev 2008;1:CD002244.

191 van de Beek D, de Gans J, McIntyre P, Prasad K. Corticosteroids for acute bacterial meningitis. Cochrane Database Syst Rev 2007;1:CD004405.

192 Thompson C, Kneen R, Riordan A, Kelly D, Pollard AJ. Encephalitis in children. Arch Dis Child 2012;97:150-61.

193 Fischer M, Lindsey N, Staples JE, Hills S. Japanese encephalitis vaccines: recommendations of the Advisory Committee on Immunization Practices (ACIP). MMWR Recomm Rep 2010;59(RR-1):1-27.

194 Fitch MT, Abrahamian FM, Moran GJ, Talan DA. Emergency department management of meningitis and encephalitis. Infect Dis Clin 2008;22(1):33-52.

195 Kneen R, Jakka S, Mithyantha R, Riordan A, Solomon T. The management of infants and children treated with aciclovir for suspected viral encephalitis. Arch Dis Child 2010;95:100-6.

196 Basu RK, Devarajan P, Wong H, Wheeler DS. An update and review of acute kidney injury in pediatrics. Pediatr Crit Care Med 2011;12:339-47.

197 Soler YA, Nieves-Plaza M, Prieto M, García-De Jesús R, Suárez-Rivera M. Pediatric risk, injury, failure, loss, end-stage renal disease score identifies acute kidney injury and predicts mortality in critically ill children: a prospective study. Pediatr Crit Care Med 2013;14:e189-95

198 Reveiz L, Guerrero-Lozano RC, Camacho A, Yara L, Mosquera PA. Stress ulcer, gastritis and gastrointestinal bleeding prophyllaxis in critically ill pediatric patients: a systematic review. Pediatr Crit Care Med 2010;11:124-32.

199 Mehta NM, Bechard LJ, Cahill N, Wang M, Day A, Duggan CP et al. Nutritional practices and their relationship to clinical outcomes in critically ill children – an international multicenter cohort study. Crit Care Med 2012;40:2204-11.

200 Botran M, Lopez-Herce J, Mencia S, Urbano J, Solana MJ, Garcia A. Enteral nutrition in the critically ill child: comparison of standard and protein-enriched diets. J Pediatr 2011;159:27-32.

201 Zamberlan P, Delgado AF, Leone C, Feferbaum R, Okay TS. Nutrition therapy in a pediatric intensive care unit: indications, monitoring and complications. J Parenter Enteral Nutr 2011;35:523-29.

202 Tume L, Latten L, Darbyshire A. An evaluation of enteral feeding practices in critically ill children. Nurs Crit Care 2010;15:291-99.

203 Botran M, Lopez-Herce J, Mencia S, Urbano J, Solana MJ, Garcia A et al. Relationship between energy expenditure, nutritional status and clinical severity before starting enteral nutrition in critically ill children. Br J Nutr 2011;105:731-37.

204 Wakeham M, Christensen M, Manzi J, Kuhn EM, Scanlon M, Goday PS et al. Registered dietitians making a difference: early medical record documentation of estimated energy requirement in critically ill children is associated with higher daily energy intake and with use of the enteral route. J Acad Nutr Diet 2013;113:1311-16.

205 Mehta NM, Bechard LJ, Dolan M, Ariagno K, Jiang H, Duggan C. Energy imbalance and the risk of overfeeding in critically ill children. Pediatr Crit Care Med 2011;12:398-405.

206 Eulmesekian PG, Perez A, Minces PG, Bohn D. Hospital-acquired hyponatraemia in postoperative pediatric patients: prospective observational study. Pedatr Crit Care Med 2010;11:479-83.

207 Carandang F, Anglemyer A, Longhurst CA, Krishnan G, Alexander SR, Kahana M et al. Association between maintenance fluid tonicity and hospital-acquired hyponatremia. J Pediatr 2013;163:1646-51.

208 Montanana PA, Alapont M, Ocon AP, Lopex PO, Prats JLL, Parreno JDT. The use of isotonic fluids as maintenance therapy prevents iatragenic hyponatraemia in pediatrics: a randomized, controlled open study. Pediatr Crit Care Med 2008;9:589-97.

209 Smith RL, Lin JC, Adelson PD, Kochanek PM, Fink EL, Wisniewski SR et al. Relationship between hyperglycemia and outcome in children with severe traumatic brain injury. Pediatr Crit Care Med 2012;13:85-91.

210 Macrae D, Grieve R, Allen E, Sadique Z, Morris K, Pappachan J et al. A randomized trial of hyperglycemic control in pediatric intensive care. N Engl J Med 2014;370(2):107-18.

211 Faustino EV, Bogue CW. Relationship between hypoglycaemia and mortality in critically ill children. Pediatr Crit Care Med 2010;11:690-98.

212 Kaur S, Kumar P, Kumar V, Sarin SK, Kumar A. Etiology and prognostic factors of acute liver failure in children. Indian Pediatr 2013;50:677-79.

213 Devictor D, Tissieres P, Afanetti M, Debray D. Acute liver failure in children. Clin Res Hepatol Gastroenterol 2011;35:430-37.

214 Faraj W, Dar F, Bartlett A, Melendez HV, Marangoni G, Mukherji D et al. Auxiliary liver transplantation for acute liver failure in children. Ann Surg 2010;251:351-56.

215 World Health Organization. World report on child injury prevention. Geneva: WHO; 2008.

216 Kreisfeld R. Hospitalised farm injury among children and young people, Australia 2000–01 to 2004–05. Adelaide: Australian Institute of Health and Welfare; 2008.

217 Tovell A, McKenna K, Bradley C, Pointer S. Hospital separations due to injury and poisoning, Australia 2009–10. Canberra: Australian Institute of Health and Welfare; 2012.

218 Australian Institute of Health and Welfare. A picture of Australia's children 2012. Canberra: Australian Government; 2012.

219 Kenefake ME, Swarm M, Walthall J. Nuances in pediatric trauma. Emerg Med Clin North Am 2013;31:627-52.

220 Royal Life Saving Society Australia. The national drowning report 2013. Sydney: Royal Life Saving Society Australia; 2014.

221 Austin S, Macintosh I. Management of drowning in children. Paediatr Child Health 2013;23:397-401.

222 Hynick NH, Brennan M, Schmit P, Noseworthy S, Yanchar NL. Identification of blunt abdominal injuries in children. J Trauma Acute Care Surg 2014;76(1):95-100.

223 Jakob H, Lustenberger T, Schneidmüller D, Sander AL, Walcher F, Marzi I. Pediatric polytrauma management. Eur J Trauma Emerg Surg 2010;36:325-38.

224 Fisher BM, Cowles S, Matulich JR, Evanson BG, Vega D, Dissanaike S. Is magnetic resonance imaging in addition to a computed tomographic scan necessary to identify clinically significant cervical spine injuries in obtunded blunt trauma patients? Am J Surg 2013;206:987-93; discussion 93-4.

225 Simpson JN, Teach SJ. Pediatric rapid fluid resuscitation. Curr Opin Pediatr 2011;23(3):286-92.

226 Puvanachandra P, Hyder AA. The burden of traumatic brain injury in Asia: a call for research. Pakistan Journal of Neurological Sciences 2009;4(1):27-32.

227 Sigurtà A, Zanaboni C, Canavesi K, Citerio G, Beretta L, Stocchetti N. Intensive care for pediatric traumatic brain injury. Intensive Care Med 2013;39(1):129-36.

228 Wing R, James C. Pediatric head injury and concussion. Emerg Med Clin North Am 2013;31:653-75.

229 Kochanek PM, Carney N, Adelson PD, Ashwal S, Bell MJ, Bratton S et al. Guidelines for the acute medical management of severe traumatic brain injury in infants, children and adolescents, second edition. Pediatr Crit Care Med 2012;13(Supplement):S1-S81.

230 Kamat P, Kunde S, Vos M, Vats A, Gupta N, Heffron T et al. Invasive intracranial pressure monitoring is a useful adjunct in the management of severe hepatic encephalopathy associated with pediatric acute liver failure. Pediatr Crit Care Med 2012;13:e33-38.

231 Stippler M, Ortiz V, Adelson PD, Chang Y-F, Tyler-Kabara EC, Wisniewski SR et al. Brain tissue oxygen monitoring after severe traumatic brain injury in children: relationship to outcome and association with other clinical parameters. J Neurosurg 2012;10:383-91.

232 Mahajan P, Jaffe DM, Olsen CS, Leonard JR, Nigrovic LE, Rogers AJ et al. Spinal cord injury without radiologic abnormality in children imaged with magnetic resonance imaging. J Trauma Acute Care Surg 2013;75:843-47.

233 Adelson PD, Wisniewski SR, Beca J, Brown SD, Bell M, Muizelaar JP et al, Paediatric Traumatic Brain Injury Consortium. Comparison of hypothermia and normothermia after severe traumatic brain injury in children (cool kids): a phase 3, randomised controlled trial. Lancet Neurol 2013;12(6):546-53.

234 Piedra MP, Thompson EM, Selden NR, Ragel BT, Guillaume DJ. Optimal timing of autologous cranioplasty after decompressive craniectomy in children. J Neurosurg Pediatr 2012;10:268-72.

235 Oluigbo CO, Wilkinson CC, Stence NV, Fenton LZ, McNatt SA, Handler MH. Comparison of outcomes following decompressive craniectomy in children with accidental and nonaccidental blunt cranial trauma. J Neurosurg Pediatr 2012;9:125-32.

236 Tovar JA, Vazquez JJ. Management of chest trauma in children. Paediatr Respir Rev 2013;14(2):86-91.

237 Aleman KB, Meyers MC. Mountain biking injuries in children and adolescents. Sports Med 2010;40:77-90.

238 Iqbal CW, St Peter SD, Tsao K, Cullinane DC, Gourlay DM, Ponsky TA et al. Operative vs nonoperative management for blunt pancreatic transection in children: multi-institutional outcomes. J Am Coll Surg 2014;218:157-62.

239 Sandler G, Leishman S, Branson H, Buchan C, Holland AJ. Body wall thickness in adults and children – relevance to penetrating trauma. Injury 2010 (41):506-9.

240 Scaife ER, Rollins MD, Barnhart DC, Downeya EC, Black RE, Meyers RL et al. The role of focused abdominal sonography for trauma (FAST) in pediatric trauma evaluation. J Pediatr Surg 2013;48:1377-83.

241 Sola JE, Cheung MC, Yang R, Koslow S, Lanuti E, Seaver C et al. Pediatric FAST and elevated liver transaminases: an effective screening tool in blunt abdominal trauma. J Surg Res 2009;157(1):103-7.

242 Dodgion CM, Gosain A, Rogers A, St Peter AD, Nichol PF, Ostlie DJ. National trends in pediatric blunt spleen and liver injury management and potential benefits of an abbreviated bed rest protocol. J Pediatr Surg 2014;49(6):1004-8.

243 Cavari Y, Pitfield AF, Kissoon N. Intravenous maintenance fluids revisited. Pediatr Emerg Care 2013;29:1225-31.

244 NSW Clinical Excellence Commission. Between the flags standard paediatric observation charts. 2nd ed. Sydney: NSW Health; 2013.

245 Fleming S, Thompson M, Stevens R, Heneghan C, Pluddermann A, Maconochie I et al. Supplement to: normal ranges of heart rate and respiratory rate in children from birth to 18 years of age: a systematic review of observational studies. Lancet [Internet]. 2011 [accessed 17.9.14]; 377.

246 Shann F. Drug doses. 15th ed. Parkville, Victoria: Royal Children's Hospital; 2010.

Chapter **28**

Pregnancy and postpartum considerations

Wendy Pollock, Emma Kingwell

Learning objectives

After reading this chapter, you should be able to:

- identify the core physiological adaptations of pregnancy pertinent to critical care nursing
- describe the antenatal assessment that would be required when caring for a woman 28 weeks pregnant in ICU
- describe the priorities of management for a postpartum woman admitted to ICU with preeclampsia
- outline the main causes of obstetric haemorrhage
- outline the standard postnatal care required by a woman in ICU, for the 48 hours following birth
- consider the resources and equipment available in your workplace that are specifically required for the care of pregnant and postpartum women.

Introduction

The admission of a pregnant or postpartum woman to ICU can extend ICU staff beyond their comfort zone. Pregnant and postpartum women undergo substantial physiological adaptations. Nursing staff also need to consider the fetus and be aware of, and manage, obstetric conditions. This chapter provides an overview of the epidemiology of critical illness in pregnancy, describes the physiological adaptations of pregnancy and the puerperium, outlines some key medical conditions and their interaction with pregnancy and describes the major obstetric conditions that are associated with critical illness. Additionally, we include guidance on specific practices related to caring for pregnant and postpartum women in ICU, for example assessment of fetal wellbeing and establishment of lactation. Further details on these topics can be found in textbooks that specifically deal with critical care obstetrics.[1-3] Research into critical care obstetrics is limited and at times the evidence being drawn on is dated, but still considered to be valid.

KEY WORDS

antenatal assessment

breastfeeding

critical illness in pregnancy

fetal wellbeing

medical disorders in pregnancy

postpartum care

severe maternal morbidity

severe obstetric haemorrhage

severe preeclampsia

Epidemiology of critical illness in pregnancy

Most women experience a healthy, normal pregnancy and the development of critical illness associated with pregnancy is usually sudden and unexpected. Approximately 1 in 370 births results in a maternal ICU admission, making up about 1% of the ICU population; more than three-quarters of admissions occur following the birth of the baby.[4,5] Admission of a pregnant woman to ICU is infrequent and more likely to be related to a non-obstetric diagnosis such as pneumonia or a motor vehicle crash. Conversely, in postpartum women, a condition directly associated with pregnancy is more common, usually preeclampsia or obstetric haemorrhage.[4] However, pregnant and postpartum women may be admitted to ICU with any diagnosis, which may or may not be associated with pregnancy.

Pregnant and postpartum admissions to ICU are usually short with most lengths of stay less than 24 hours. There is a vast variation in the threshold for admission to ICU. One European study of severe maternal morbidity reported ICU admission proportions of between 0 and 50% across different regions.[6] Additionally, many women when admitted to ICU do not receive any specific ICU intervention (Table 28.1), and their need for ICU admission has been questioned.[8] In general, about a third of women who experience severe maternal morbidity are admitted to ICU.[9] It is feasible that admission to ICU is preventable by upskilling midwifery services to provide an intermediate level of care[8] and, through early identification, treatment and management of severe illness.[8,10-13]

Practice tip

Any maternal death or death of a woman during pregnancy or within 42 days of having been pregnant should be reported to the relevant state authority in Australia and to the Perinatal and Maternal Mortality Review Committee in New Zealand, even if the pregnancy is not thought to have contributed to the cause of death.

In developed countries such as Australia, the mortality of pregnant and postpartum women admitted to ICU is relatively low at around 3% compared to the 15% mortality observed in the regular ICU population.[4]

Adapted physiology of pregnancy

Conception results in extensive physiological adaptations across most body systems (see Table 28.2). The physiological adaptations most relevant to critical care nursing include cardiovascular, respiratory, renal, gastrointestinal and coagulation and the role of the placenta as the maternal–fetal interface. The uterus and breasts obviously undergo major changes in pregnancy and any basic midwifery or obstetrics textbook, such as *Myles' textbook for midwives* or *Midwifery: preparation for practice* will describe these in detail.[14,15] The physiological adaptations described in this chapter refer to a singleton pregnancy only, as women with a multiple pregnancy (i.e. twins) may undergo further changes.[16] The physiological changes described refer to a non-labouring pregnant woman. Labour induces further changes to physiology, such as increased cardiac output.[17]

The puerperium, also referred to as the postpartum or postnatal period, is the 6 weeks following the end of pregnancy during which time the woman's body returns to the pre-pregnant state. The physiology of the puerperium is outlined below for the major body systems, with content specific to the uterus and breasts covered later in the section on postnatal assessment and lactation. Our knowledge of the timing and completeness of the reversal of the physiological adaptations in pregnancy is incomplete. Delivery of the placenta results in an abrupt reduction in all the placental hormonal levels, such as progesterone and oestrogens, and thus begins the physiological process for returning the woman's body to the non-pregnant state.

Cardiovascular system

The cardiovascular system undergoes a series of anatomical and physiological changes during pregnancy to support both the mother and fetus during this period.

TABLE 28.1

ICU interventions required by pregnant and postpartum women in ICU

ICU INTERVENTION	POLLOCK[13] (AUSTRALIA)[a] (*N* = 33)	PAXTON[7] (AUSTRALIA)[a] (*N* = 249)	HAZELGROVE[8] (UK)[b] (*N* = 210)	ZWART[9] (NETHERLANDS)[b] (*N* = 837)
Mechanical ventilation	67%	18%	45%	35%
Inotrope infusion	18%	4%	19%	9%
Pulmonary artery catheter	6%	NR	13%	3%
Renal replacement therapy	9%	1%	3%	2%

[a] Tertiary ICU level only.
[b] National/regional study, all ICU levels.

TABLE 28.2

Key physiological changes in pregnancy

PARAMETER	CHANGE DURING PREGNANCY
CARDIOVASCULAR SYSTEM	
Heart rate	↑ 10–15 beats/min
Blood pressure Systolic Diastolic	↓ 5–9 mmHg ↓ 6–17 mmHg
Cardiac output	↑ 30–50%
Systemic vascular resistance	↓ up to 35%
Central arterial and venous pressures	Unchanged
BLOOD AND ASSOCIATED COMPONENTS	
Blood volume	↑ 40–50%
Plasma volume	↑ 40–50%
Red blood cells	↑ 20–40%
White blood cells	↑ 100–300%
Platelets	Unchanged
Fibrinogen	↑ 100%
Serum albumin level	↓ 10–15%
RESPIRATORY SYSTEM	
Respiratory rate	Unchanged
Tidal volume	↑ 25–40%
Minute volume	↑ 40–50%
Oxygen consumption	↑ 15–20%
ARTERIAL BLOOD GAS ANALYSIS VALUES	
PaO_2	80–110 mmHg
$PaCO_2$	28–32 mmHg
pH	7.40–7.45
HCO_3^-	18–21
SaO_2	≥95%
Vital capacity	Unchanged
Functional reserve capacity	↓ 17–20%
Airway compliance and resistance	Unchanged
RENAL SYSTEM	
Glomerular filtration rate	↑ 40–50%
Serum urea and creatinine	↓
Urine output	Unknown
Proteinuria	<300 mg/day

Anatomical changes

The heart undergoes anatomical change during pregnancy including left ventricular hypertrophy and increases in the cross-sectional areas of the aortic, pulmonary and mitral valves of 12–14%. ECG changes include non-specific ST-segment changes, the development of a Q wave in lead III and a left-axis deviation pattern.[18] These are evident by the end of the first trimester and remain throughout the pregnancy.[19] As with the interpretation of any ECG, consider other information such as patient presentation (signs and symptoms) and blood test results to form a complete assessment of the woman's condition.

Blood volume

Very early in the pregnancy there is generalised vasodilation resulting in sodium and water retention. The causes of the vasodilation include hormonal factors (e.g. progesterone), peripheral vasodilators such as nitric oxide and, potentially, an as-yet unidentified pregnancy-specific vasodilatory substance.[20] The end result is a 40–50% increase in blood volume as well as a reduction in normal serum sodium level, from 140 to 136 mmol/L, and a reduction in plasma osmolality from 290 to 280 mosmol/kg. These changes persist throughout pregnancy.[21]

The red cell mass increases by 20–40% and plasma volume by 40–50% resulting in a relative haemodilutional anaemia. Venous haematocrit typically falls from a non-pregnant value of 40% to 34% near term.[22] The increase in blood volume is evident from 7 weeks' gestation peaking at around 30–32 weeks' gestation, and remaining stable until birth.[20,23] Women who do not experience this normal increase in blood volume are more prone to adverse outcomes such as preeclampsia.[24] This additional blood volume also prepares the woman for the normal blood loss associated with birth (<500 mL). Pregnant women are renowned for being able to maintain stable vital signs, with blood losses as much as 1500 mL, before acutely deteriorating.

Blood pressure

Blood pressure reduces in pregnancy; it begins dropping as early as 9 weeks' gestation, with the lowest levels recorded during the second trimester (16–28 weeks) and returns to pre-pregnancy measurements near term (see Table 28.2). If a woman does not experience the characteristic lowering of blood pressure, particularly during the second trimester, it is viewed as a potentially abnormal sign.

Heart rate, stroke volume and cardiac output

Maternal heart rate increases by 10–15 beats per minute during pregnancy as early as 5 weeks' gestation.[19,25] Tachycardia (>100 beats/min) is an abnormal sign that warrants further investigation.[26] Stroke volume is noted to increase between 18% and 32%, beginning as early as 8 weeks' gestation.[27,28] An increase in cardiac output is detectable from 5 weeks' gestation and continues to be 30–50% higher by 32 weeks' gestation.[20,28] A normal cardiac output in pregnancy may be as high as 8 L/min.

Systemic vascular resistance

The generalised vasodilation observed in early pregnancy reduces systemic vascular resistance by up to 35%, with some reduction already detectable by 8 weeks' gestation.[29]

Effect of posture on maternal haemodynamics

It is evident that from as early as 5–8 weeks' gestation, pregnancy is characterised by general vasodilation, increased blood volume and increased cardiac output. As the pregnancy advances, the bulk of the uterus begins to have an impact on maternal haemodynamics. After 20 weeks' gestation, a woman lying flat on her back may experience supine hypotension, secondary to aortocaval compression, with subsequent reduction in venous return, cardiac output and placental flow. A reduction in placental flow may occur even without a recorded drop in blood pressure. Consequently, it is inadvisable to nurse a pregnant woman of more than 20 weeks' gestation flat on her back. A left lateral lying position of at least 15° results in the best maternal cardiac output and may be achieved with the use of a wedge or pillows. Manual uterine displacement should be considered if supine positioning is required.[30,31]

Postpartum cardiovascular changes

Heart rate returns to pre-pregnancy levels by 10 days postpartum; blood pressure has normally returned to pre-pregnancy levels by term and does not change during the puerperium.[29,32] The first few days of the puerperium are associated with a profound diuresis, resulting in the haemoconcentration of blood. Therefore, the risk of thromboembolism is higher during the postpartum period than during pregnancy. Adequate measures should be implemented to prevent venous thromboembolism.[33]

Cardiac output increases briefly in the immediate postpartum period to compensate for blood losses and tends to increase by 50% of the pre-delivery value; at this point in the postpartum phase stroke volume is increased while the maternal heart rate is often slowed.[32] For most women, the immediate postpartum elevation in cardiac output only lasts for an hour or so. By 2 weeks postpartum, many haemodynamic parameters have returned to pre-pregnancy levels for the majority of women, although some have been recorded as remaining above pre-pregnancy levels at 12 months postpartum, including cardiac output.[17,29]

Respiratory system

The respiratory system undergoes widespread adaptation from early pregnancy with effects on the airway through to gaseous exchange at the alveolar level evident, including variation to 'normal' parameters when interpreting arterial blood gas results.

Changes to the upper airways and thorax

Normal physiological changes of pregnancy include generalised vasodilation of the upper airway vasculature, increased fat deposition around the neck and an increase in mucosal oedema. A combination of hormonal influences, likely progesterone and oestrogen, are at play. These physiological changes are thought to be responsible for the symptoms of rhinitis, nasal stuffiness and epistaxis that are common in pregnancy.[20]

Changes also occur to the chest wall with relaxation of ligaments resulting in an outwards flaring of the lower ribs and a 50% increase in the subcostal angle.[34] The diameter and the circumference of the thorax increase by 2 cm and 5–7 cm, respectively.[34,35] These physical changes are thought to cause the diaphragm to rise by 5 cm, well before there is any pressure from the advancing uterus.[35] Respiratory muscle function does not change significantly during pregnancy and rib cage compliance is unaltered.[34] The functional reserve capacity (the amount of air left in the lungs after expiration) is reduced by 17–20%, making the pregnant woman more vulnerable to hypoxaemia during any apnoeic period. Chest X-ray interpretation is unchanged during pregnancy.[32]

Changes to the physiology of breathing

From 5 weeks' gestation, multiple factors increase respiratory drive. Elevated progesterone levels are thought to lower the $PaCO_2$ threshold in the respiratory centre, resulting in hyperventilation.[18,36–38] Minute ventilation begins to increase soon after conception, peaking at 40–50% above pre-conception level at term.[18] The increase in minute ventilation is achieved by a 30–50% increase in tidal volume (e.g. an increase of 200 ± 50 mL at term), without any increase in respiratory rate.[18]

Consequently, normal arterial blood gas values are different in pregnancy (see Table 28.2). The reduced $PaCO_2$ level enables fetal CO_2 to passively cross the placenta for maternal excretion. PaO_2 normally increases by 10 mmHg, although the PaO_2 level is affected by posture, particularly as the pregnancy progresses.[39] Later in pregnancy the supine position can reduce PaO_2 by 10 mmHg when compared to the same woman in the sitting position.[40] The kidneys compensate for the lowered $PaCO_2$ by increasing bicarbonate excretion to maintain a normal pH.[39,41,42] Normal oxygen saturation in pregnancy has not been well investigated. It is likely to be 97–100% at sea level, with a healthy pregnant woman's saturation not dropping below 95% during moderate exercise.[43,44]

The notable hyperventilation of pregnancy is associated with a feeling of breathlessness in up to 75% of healthy pregnant women.[36] Distinguishing 'physiological dyspnoea' from 'pathological dyspnoea', for example developing cardiomyopathy, can present a challenge in pregnancy. Dyspnoea at rest is usually an abnormal sign in pregnancy.[45]

Postpartum respiratory changes

Complete resolution of the spirometry and arterial blood gas changes occurring in pregnancy is completed by 5 weeks postpartum,[39] although the daily transition of these parameters over the first week postpartum is not known. One very old study reported that CO_2 levels took between 2 and 5 days to return to normal non-pregnant values postpartum.[46] Regardless, with the fetus delivered, it is probable that no harm will be done to a woman by the titration of her ventilation requirements according to non-pregnant conventions and arterial blood gas values.

Renal system

All smooth muscle dilates in early pregnancy. This includes the renal tract, involving the renal pelvises, calyces, ureters and urethra. Each kidney lengthens by about 1 cm, which is explained by the dilation and associated mild hydro-nephrosis and increased vascularity of the kidneys, with no hypertrophy of renal tissue.[20] Another effect of widespread dilation is urinary stasis and an increased likelihood of urinary tract infection. Acute pyelonephritis is one of the most common renal complications of pregnancy and is associated with the onset of pre-term labour.[47]

The kidneys receive a 30% increase in blood flow. The glomerular filtration rate (GFR) increases 40–50% during the first trimester and then reduces slightly towards term.[21] The increase in GFR may result in both glycosuria and proteinuria in pregnancy. Glycosuria is not related to blood sugar levels and is unhelpful in monitoring diabetes. Proteinuria, up to 300 mg per 24 hours, is considered normal in pregnancy. Conversely, the high GFR results in lowered serum levels of both urea and creatinine. A plasma urea level exceeding 4.5 mmol/L and plasma creatinine level higher than 75 micromol/L should be viewed as abnormal and indicative of potential renal impairment.[21,48] There is conflicting information regarding normal urine output during pregnancy, with some studies suggesting no difference and others reporting an increase in 24-hour urine volume after 12 weeks' gestation.[47,49]

Postpartum renal changes

The most significant renal change is the diuresis that occurs in the first 1–3 days postpartum. This diuresis serves to offload the additional blood volume that the woman has had circulating for the duration of the pregnancy. There has been little examination of 'normal urine output' with the standard 0.5 mL/kg/h reported as a minimum acceptable level; however, a true 'normal' level is likely to be closer to 0.8 mL/kg/h.[50] Creatinine levels are within the normal non-pregnancy range within 24 hours postpartum, while the lower urea levels remain for at least 48 hours.[48] The bladder returns to the pelvis in the early postpartum period as the uterus and other organs resume their pre-pregnancy position.

Gastrointestinal system and liver

The uterus pushes abdominal organs aside as it advances, making assessment and diagnosis of an acute abdomen difficult. For example, the appendix is progressively displaced upwards and laterally from McBurney's point at the third month, reaching the level of the iliac crest by late pregnancy.[51] The bowel and other organs are generally displaced by the enlarging uterus; women with prior abdominal surgery and adhesions are predisposed to intestinal obstruction as a result.[52] There is an increase in intra-abdominal pressure that may contribute to another common pregnancy symptom, heartburn.

Generalised smooth muscle vasodilation occurs throughout the gastrointestinal tract. Thus there is delayed stomach emptying and a lax cardiac sphincter, leading to an increased risk of aspiration. Bowel peristalsis slows, commonly resulting in constipation and haemorrhoids.

Hepatobiliary changes in pregnancy

There is no significant increase in hepatic arterial blood flow during pregnancy. However, blood flow to the liver supplied by the portal vein doubles,[53] which may have an impact on oral medication metabolism. Changes in hepatic enzymes responsible for drug metabolism may alter the pharmacokinetics of some medications, e.g. higher plasma levels of midazolam. Serum albumin levels reduce to 30–40 g/L for the majority of pregnancy, with levels as low as 25 g/L normal during the second postpartum week.[48] This low albumin level reduces colloid osmotic pressure, contributing to the dependent oedema that is common in pregnancy.

The general smooth muscle vasodilation affects the hepatobiliary ducts, resulting in sluggish bile motility and delayed emptying of the gallbladder. These changes lead to an increased incidence of cholelithiasis and cholecystitis during pregnancy.

Haemostasis system

During pregnancy, the woman's body prepares for placental separation, and the resultant blood loss. Blood flow to the placental bed at term ranges from 600 to 800 mL/min. Both elements of the haemostasis system are activated during pregnancy (coagulation and fibrinolysis), with pregnancy, and particularly the postpartum period, associated with an increased risk of thrombus formation. Thromboembolic events remain a leading cause of maternal death in developed countries.[26,54] A number of changes to the haemostatic system occur during pregnancy (see Table 28.3).

Of note, gestational thrombocytopenia – a platelet level of $80–150 \times 10^9$/L – occurs in 6–8 % of women.[55,56] It generally has no negative impact on the woman or fetus

TABLE 28.3
Haemostatic changes during pregnancy[58–60]

HAEMOSTATIC COMPONENT	CHANGES DURING PREGNANCY
PLATELETS	
Count	Unchanged
Function and lifespan	Unchanged
CLOTTING FACTORS	
Factors VII, VIII and IX	Increased
Fibrinogen	Doubles by term
Other clotting factors	Mainly unchanged
FIBRINOLYSIS	
D-dimer level	Progressively increases throughout pregnancy By term, level >0.5 mg/L common

at these levels, as there is no pathology associated with the low platelet count.[57]

Changes in white blood cells and the immune system

There is continued debate on whether the pregnant state increases vulnerability to infection, secondary to some protective mechanism that prevents the woman's body from reacting to the fetus as a foreign body.[20] Pregnant women have increased innate immune system activity (non-specific response) and a lowered adaptive immune system (specific antibody response), with pregnant women more vulnerable to some infections such as malaria and varicella.[20,61,62] Pregnant women are often in contact with small children and potentially have an increased exposure to various infections. The white blood cell number increases throughout pregnancy, peaking around delivery when a normal level may be as high as 25×10^9/L.[48] The combined physiological changes in pregnancy result in features of systemic inflammatory response syndrome (SIRS) being present in normal pregnancy, and a modified SIRS definition may need to apply to the maternity population.[63]

The maternal–fetal interface

The junction of the maternal and fetal circulations is referred to as the maternal–fetal interface. Although under normal circumstances the circulations remain separated by layers of cells, the maternal–fetal interface is where the maternal and fetal systems interact.

Placenta

The placenta develops from the trophoblastic layer of the fertilised ovum and is completely formed and functioning 10 weeks following fertilisation.[64] The chorionic villi attach to the uterine wall via the decidua. The end result is an interface whereby maternal blood fills a space in which the nutritive villi float and are bathed in the maternal blood (Figure 28.1). The blood drains back into the maternal circulation via maternal sinuses and the endometrial veins. Approximately 150 mL of maternal blood, replenished three to four times per minute, bathes the villi in the intervillous space.[64] The chorionic villi maximise the available surface area to optimise the exchange of products across the maternal–placental interface. By term, this surface area is said to be as large as 13 m².[65] Initially, four layers of cells separate the maternal blood from the fetal blood, reducing to three after 20 weeks' gestation;

FIGURE 28.1 The maternal–placental interface.[14]

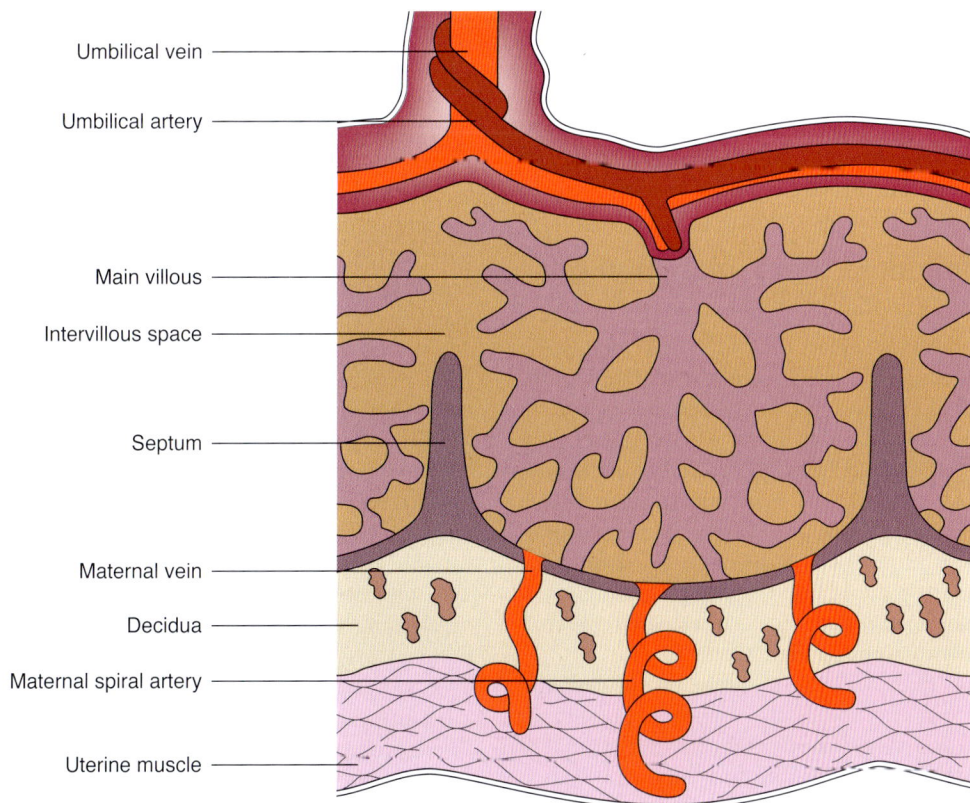

Adapted from Marshall J, Raynor M, eds. Myles' textbook for midwives. 16th ed. Oxford: Churchill Livingston/Elsevier; 2014, with permission.

these cell layers are collectively referred to as the 'placental membrane' or 'placental barrier'.[66] Damage to villi, such as a threatened abortion or blunt trauma, can enable fetal haemoglobin and squames to enter the maternal circulation, leading to rhesus isoimmunisation or, rarely, amniotic fluid embolism.

Role of the placenta

The placenta provides six major functions to sustain the pregnancy and fetus: respiration, nutrition, storage, excretion, protection and endocrine.[64] Fetal lungs are filled with fluid and all oxygenation and removal of carbon dioxide must be provided via the placenta. Fetal haemoglobin has a slightly different structure to adult haemoglobin and has a higher affinity for oxygen. Both oxygen and carbon dioxide cross the placental membrane by simple diffusion. Nutrients are actively transported across the placental membrane, with the placenta able to select the substances needed by the fetus, even at the expense of the mother if necessary.[64] The placenta is able to store glucose by converting it to glycogen and reconverting it to glucose as required and is also able to store iron and some fat-soluble vitamins.

The placental membrane operates as a barrier between the maternal and fetal circulations and provides a limited protective function. Generally, few bacteria can cross the placenta, although viruses can cross readily. The placenta produces large volumes of hormones including progesterone, oestrogens, placental lactogen, chorionic gonadotropin, growth factors, cytokine vasoactive substances, placental growth hormone, thyrotropin and corticotropin. The placenta does not have a nerve supply so all activities regulated by the placenta must be undertaken by other mechanisms, e.g. chemical, hormonal changes. Disorders of the placenta are thought to be a major contributor to preeclampsia and small-for-gestational-age neonates.

Impact of impaired utero–placental gas exchange

Effective gas exchange across the placental membrane depends on sufficient maternal blood pressure and adequate O_2 and CO_2 gradients for passive diffusion to occur. In response to hypoxaemia, a fetal brain-sparing mechanism goes into effect that increases fetal arterial pressure and redirects blood delivery to the main organs, namely the brain, heart and adrenal glands.[67] This centralisation of fetal blood flow is more apparent in response to maternal hypoxaemia than to reduced utero–placental blood flow. It appears that a less mature fetus (i.e. earlier gestation) may be less susceptible to asphyxia than a fetus at term.[67]

Whether the fetus will die in utero or survive, and the degree of any neurological compromise, depends on the degree and duration of asphyxia, the recurrent nature of asphyxia and the degree to which the fetus is able to compensate for the asphyxia. Antenatal asphyxia (asphyxia during pregnancy, not associated with labour) has been linked to the development of cerebral palsy, behavioural disorders and learning difficulties. The reasons for and extent of individual variation in fetal outcome are unknown.

Clinical implications of the physiological adaptations of pregnancy

The beginning point of any nursing practice is an understanding of normal anatomy and physiology. The normal physiological adaptations of pregnancy may be used to explain the so-called 'minor discomforts' of pregnancy, including constipation, varicose veins, indigestion, breathlessness and fatigue. For a critically ill pregnant woman being nursed in ICU, these normal physiological changes are highly relevant for her care. ICU nurses need to accommodate for, and take into account, the likely impact of the normal physiology of pregnancy on common ICU monitoring, interventions and care (see Table 28.4).

Diseases and conditions unique to pregnancy

There are a number of conditions unique to pregnancy that might cause a woman to become critically ill and result in admission to ICU, including preeclampsia, obstetric haemorrhage, amniotic fluid embolism and peripartum cardiomyopathy. These conditions are discussed in detail below.

Preeclampsia

The umbrella term 'hypertension in pregnancy' is used to describe a myriad of conditions in pregnancy where hypertension is a major feature, with the definition for hypertension unchanged during pregnancy: systolic BP ≥140 mmHg and/or diastolic BP ≥90 mmHg. These hypertensive conditions include gestational hypertension, pre-existing essential hypertension and preeclampsia, which incorporates eclampsia and haemolysis elevated liver enzymes and low platelets (HELLP) syndrome (Table 28.5). Comprehensive descriptions of these conditions and their management have been published by the UK's National Institute for Health and Clinical Excellence[68] and the Society of Obstetric Medicine Australia and New Zealand (SOMANZ).[69]

Preeclampsia is a condition unique to human pregnancy in that, while characterised by hypertension and proteinuria, it is a progressive, multisystem disorder consisting of variable clinical features related to widespread vasospasm. The indication for ICU admission is usually related to organ failure, caused by the widespread vasospasm and reduced organ perfusion that characterises the disease.[70] Preeclampsia can be a very serious condition and remains a leading cause of maternal death in both developed and developing countries.[71]

Aetiology

The placenta is strongly implicated in the cause of preeclampsia; its removal is the only definitive treatment for the condition. However, the exact mechanisms of the

TABLE 28.4

Clinical relevance of physiological adaptations in pregnancy

EFFECTS OF THE NORMAL PHYSIOLOGY OF PREGNANCY	CLINICAL IMPLICATIONS
CARDIOVASCULAR SYSTEM	
Increased likelihood of: • venous stasis • varicose veins • deep vein thrombosis Increased likelihood of: • haemorrhoids • swollen ankles	Consider use of thromboprophylaxis
Potential for aortocaval compression from about 20 weeks' gestation	Avoid nursing the woman flat on her back, e.g. tilt bed if unable to nurse woman on her side or use pillows/wedges to obtain a lateral tilt of at least 15° to maintain placental flow, full left lying is best CPR and haemodynamic measurements should be done with a left lateral tilt
Haemodynamic stability despite large blood loss Sudden deterioration	Be alert to subtle signs of haemodynamic compromise
RESPIRATORY SYSTEM	
Nasal passages more likely to bleed on instrumentation (e.g. nasal intubation, nasogastric insertion) More likely to bleed from the gums More prone to hypoxaemia during apnoea, e.g. when being intubated All pregnant women are considered to have a high-risk airway: • especially if the woman has preeclampsia • particularly if the woman is obese More likely to develop pulmonary oedema Diaphragm raised by about 5 cm	Nasal-tracheal intubation is not usually an option Have a doctor experienced with intubation on hand when a pregnant woman is being intubated Ensure that the artificial airway is protected and guard against accidental extubation Review the 'failed intubation' protocol in the ICU Pre-oxygenate with 100% O_2 prior to intubation or suctioning unless contraindicated Titrate fluid resuscitation carefully – especially in women with severe preeclampsia Check diaphragm location prior to ICC insertion for haemothorax/pleural effusion
GASTROINTESTINAL SYSTEM	
Pregnant woman is more likely to: • aspirate • develop constipation • present with advanced signs and symptoms of acute abdomen, e.g. appendicitis, bowel obstruction Pregnant women have additional and specific nutritional needs	Maintain cricoid pressure throughout CPR and intubation until the person obtaining an artificial airway instructs its release Chart bowel actions and ensure a bowel management strategy is implemented Early consideration of non-obstetric causes of an acute abdomen Consult with a dietician early to ensure that the woman receives adequate nutrition during ICU admission
RENAL SYSTEM	
Progesterone and relaxin causes relaxation and dilation of smooth muscles Renal calyces and renal pelvis become distended Ureters and urethra are elongated, dilated and have reduced peristalsis Stasis of urine and increased risk of ascending infection Acute pyelonephritis is associated with pre-term labour Bladder is displaced into the abdominal cavity after the first trimester	Minimise use of indwelling urinary catheter Renal impairment may be signified by lower serum urea and creatinine levels than in non-pregnancy Some glycosuria and proteinuria is normal in pregnancy The bladder is at risk of traumatic injury in the second and third trimesters

aetiology of the disease remain elusive and are likely to be complex and multifactorial. Theories explaining the pathophysiology of preeclampsia include immune malad–aptation, abnormal trophoblast embedding, endothelial activation and excessive inflammatory response, and a genetic susceptibility (see Box 28.1).[72] The contribution of each component and whether all components are relevant in all cases of preeclampsia are not known.

TABLE 28.5

Definitions of conditions characterised by hypertension in pregnancy

TERM	DEFINITION
Hypertension in pregnancy	Systolic BP ≥140 mmHg and/or a diastolic BP ≥90 mmHg[69]
Essential hypertension	Hypertension presenting in the first 20 weeks or that existed prior to the pregnancy without an apparent underlying cause[69]
Gestational hypertension	Hypertension arising after 20 weeks' gestation and resolving by 3 months postpartum No evidence of any other feature of the multisystem disorder preeclampsia[69]
Preeclampsia (also referred to as pregnancy-induced hypertension (PIH), toxaemia)	Hypertension arising after 20 weeks' gestation in combination with one or more of the following:[69] • Proteinuria >300 mg/24 h • Renal insufficiency: serum/plasma creatinine ≥0.09 mmol/L or oliguria • Liver disease: raised serum transaminases and/or severe epigastric/right upper quadrant pain • Neurological problems: convulsions (eclampsia), hyperreflexia with clonus, severe headaches with hyperreflexia, persistent visual disturbances • Haematological disturbances: thrombocytopenia, DIC, haemolysis • Fetal growth restriction
Eclampsia	Is a form of severe preeclampsia Generalised tonic–clonic seizures, not caused by epilepsy or other disease, and occurring ≥20 weeks' gestation, during labour or in the postpartum
HELLP syndrome	Is a form of severe preeclampsia, although hypertension may not be present Diagnosis of HELLP syndrome is made by the presence of the following three criteria: 1 Haemolysis: characteristic peripheral blood smear and serum lactate dehydrogenase (LDH) >600 U/L or serum total bilirubin ≥1.2 mg/dL 2 Elevated liver enzymes: serum aspartate aminotransferase ≥70 U/L 3 Low platelet count: <100 × 10^9/L

DIC = disseminated intravascular coagulopathy; HELLP = haemolysis, elevated liver enzymes and low platelets.

BOX 28.1

Theories on the pathophysiology of preeclampsia[72]

Placentation and the immune theory of preeclampsia:

• Maternal–fetal (paternal) immune maladaptation

• Superficial abnormal placentation

• Impaired spiral artery remodelling

Placental debris hypothesis: syncytiotrophoblast shedding:

• Increased syncytiotrophoblast shedding

• Placental ischaemia and reperfusion with subsequent oxidative stress

• Increased circulating levels of inflammatory cytokines, corticotropin-releasing hormone, free-radical species and activin A

Endothelial activation and inflammation:

• Enhanced vascular sensitivity to angiotensin II and noradrenaline with subsequent vasoconstriction and hypertension

• A fall in production and activity of vasodilator prostaglandins, especially prostacyclin and nitric oxide

Genes, the genetic-conflict hypothesis and genetic imprinting:

• Susceptibility genes, many of which interact with the maternal cardiovascular or haemostatic system, or with the regulation of maternal inflammatory responses

---

Preeclampsia is associated with impaired remodelling of the uterine spiral arteries and abnormal placental implantation. It is thought that maternal–fetal immune maladaptation could be the main cause for this superficial placentation.[72] Placental flow defects are detected as early as 12 weeks in some women who go on to develop preeclampsia.[73] Placental ischaemia and reperfusion with subsequent oxidative stress have been regarded as major pathogenetic drivers. It is likely that there is an excessive

or atypical maternal immune response to trophoblasts and the disease represents a failed interaction between the mother's and fetus' genetic make-up.[71] Further, two anti-angiogenic factors are considered centrally responsible for the endothelial dysfunction and maternal organ injury: soluble fms-like tyrosine kinase-1 (sFlt-1) and soluble endoglin.[74] The excessive systemic inflammatory response and associated endothelial dysfunction and enhanced vascular reactivity result in widespread vasospasm that precedes the onset of clinical signs, such as hypertension.[71] Other common clinical manifestations in preeclampsia include enhanced endothelial-cell permeability and platelet aggregation, explaining the increased likelihood of oedema and thrombosis.[72]

In summary, preeclampsia presents after 20 weeks' gestation, but the foundation for the disease relates to abnormal placentation early in the first trimester. Although a number of 'biomarkers' attempting to predict the onset of preeclampsia have been identified, there is no reliable predictive test in clinical use.[71]

Risk factors

A number of maternal characteristics are associated with an increased likelihood for the development of preeclampsia; these include:[72,75]

- nulliparity
- age ≥40 years
- pre-existing medical conditions including diabetes, chronic hypertension, chronic renal disease, antiphospholipid antibodies
- preeclampsia in a prior pregnancy, particularly if the previous preeclampsia presented prior to 34 weeks
- family history of preeclampsia, particularly on the maternal side of the family
- multiple pregnancy, e.g. twins
- body mass index >25 prior to pregnancy
- time between pregnancies (>10 years)
- achieving conception using assisted techniques, such as in vitro fertilisation.

Unfortunately, about half of the childbearing population has at least one risk factor. A high priority should be placed on early and accurate diagnosis of preeclampsia in a pregnant woman.

Incidence

The incidence of preeclampsia is reported to be 2–8%, with variations based on severity of the disease.[75] The incidence of eclampsia in developed countries has reduced since the routine use of magnesium sulfate has been adopted; in the UK, the rate is about three cases of eclampsia for every 10,000 births.[76] A prospective binational study on the incidence of eclampsia in Australia and New Zealand is underway, conducted by the Australasian Maternity Outcomes Surveillance System (AMOSS), and intends to document Australian and New Zealand population-based incidences for the first time.[77] The incidence of HELLP syndrome is reported to be between 0.11% and 0.67% of all pregnancies.[78,79] Preeclampsia is one of the most common indications for ICU admission at approximately one ICU admission for every 1000 deliveries.[4]

Clinical presentation and diagnosis

The clinical presentation of preeclampsia is often subtle, resulting in delayed diagnosis and treatment. Common

symptoms include feeling 'generally unwell', headache, heartburn, nausea and vomiting and oedema; all non-specific symptoms experienced by many pregnant women who do not have preeclampsia. Severe preeclampsia is associated with severe headache, hyperreflexia, visual disturbances, severe epigastric pain, right upper quadrant pain and even blindness. Diagnosis is made when the woman has hypertension (BP ≥140/90), in association with evidence of multisystem involvement (Box 28.2). Severe preeclampsia is diagnosed when the BP is ≥160/110, in association with multisystem involvement. Additionally, eclampsia and HELLP syndrome are considered severe variants of preeclampsia even if the woman is normotensive.

BOX 28.2

Diagnostic features of preeclampsia

Hypertension ≥140/90 accompanied by one or more of the following:

- Renal involvement:
  - Significant proteinuria: dipstick proteinuria subsequently confirmed by spot urine protein/creatinine ratio ≥30 mg/mmol or >300 mg protein in a 24-hour urine collection
  - Serum or plasma creatinine >90 micromol/L
  - Oliguria (<500 mL/24 h)
- Haematological involvement:
  - Thrombocytopenia (<100 × 10^9/L)
  - Haemolysis
  - Disseminated intravascular coagulation
- Liver involvement:
  - Raised serum transaminases
  - Severe epigastric or right upper quadrant pain
- Neurological involvement:
  - Convulsions (eclampsia)
  - Hyperreflexia with sustained clonus
  - Severe headache
  - Persistent visual disturbances (photopsia, scotomata, cortical blindness, retinal vasospasm)
- Stroke
- Pulmonary oedema
- Fetal growth restriction
- Placental abruption

Adapted from:

Lowe SA, Bowyer L, Lust K, McMahon L, Morton M, North R et al. The SOMANZ guideline for the management of hypertensive disorders of pregnancy 2014. Sydney: Society of Obstetric Medicine of Australia and New Zealand; 2014

Sibai B, Dekker G, Kupferminc M. Pre-eclampsia. Lancet 2005;365(9461):785–99.

This clinical diagnosis has replaced the traditional triad of signs of hypertension, proteinuria and oedema, in accordance with the increased understanding of the multisystem nature of the disease. Raised blood pressure is commonly, but not always, the first sign of the condition. Although proteinuria is the most commonly recognised additional feature after hypertension, it is not mandatory to make a clinical diagnosis. Oedema is no longer a specific sign of preeclampsia, though women who develop non-dependent oedema, such as facial oedema, should be investigated for evidence of preeclampsia.[69] Common investigations include urea, creatinine and electrolytes, full blood examination, liver function tests, serum uric acid, spot urine protein/creatinine ratio and 24-hour urine collection. Additional tests, such as coagulation studies, may be required as indicated by the clinical condition. Intrauterine fetal growth restriction is a sign of placental involvement (i.e. impairment) and investigation into fetal wellbeing, including an ultrasound for fetal growth estimation and amniotic fluid volume, and umbilical artery Doppler flow patterns should be performed routinely following a diagnosis of severe preeclampsia.

The presentation of preeclampsia is usually restricted to women ≥20 weeks' gestation unless they have a coexisting condition that is known to be associated with a <20 weeks presentation of preeclampsia including hydatidiform mole, multiple pregnancy, fetal triploidy, severe maternal renal disease or antiphospholipid antibody syndrome.[69] Importantly, preeclampsia should resolve within 3 months postpartum.

The UKOSS study found 45% of first eclamptic fits were during pregnancy, 19% during labour and 36% postpartum.[76] The majority of postpartum eclampsia occurs in the first 48 hours, although late-onset eclampsia may occur at 2 to 3 weeks postpartum. Despite the nomenclature, eclampsia can occur without any preceding signs and symptoms of preeclampsia. In the UKOSS eclampsia study, only 38% of women had established hypertension and proteinuria in the week preceding the eclamptic fit and 21% of women had no sign or symptom prior to the first eclamptic fit.[76] HELLP syndrome commonly presents during pregnancy with about 30% postpartum.[80]

Most women admitted to ICU with a diagnosis of preeclampsia have usually delivered prior to transfer, and require support for complications of preeclampsia, e.g. acute renal failure, disseminated intravascular coagulopathy (DIC), pulmonary oedema and fluid management. Once the placenta is delivered, most women improve within 24–48 hours; however, women with HELLP syndrome may experience a worsening of condition in the first 48 hours postpartum. Uncontrolled hypertension remains a major concern and is associated with cerebral haemorrhage, one of the dominant causes of death in women with preeclampsia.

Management priorities

Women with mild preeclampsia at term may be managed with induction of labour and delivery and experience few complications. The management of women with severe preeclampsia is focused on stablising the woman's condition, optimal timing of delivery of the baby (and placenta) and preventing complications of the condition. Women with eclampsia and HELLP syndrome require the same treatments as other women with severe preeclampsia, even though they may or may not have the same degree of hypertension.[69,81]

Prevention of eclampsia

Magnesium sulfate has received the most attention as an anticonvulsant in preeclampsia, with its mechanism of action thought to be connected to the release of prostacyclin from the endothelium, reversing the vasoconstriction that is the basis of the disease.[82,83] Magnesium is the anticonvulsant of choice to prevent and treat eclampsia.[84,85] Magnesium has been shown to halve the likelihood of eclampsia.[84] A common magnesium regimen is:[71,84]

- give a 4 g IV loading dose over 15–20 minutes
- administer an ongoing infusion of 1 g/h
- give an additional 2–4 g IV loading dose over 10 minutes to treat a recurrent eclamptic seizure
- continue infusion until 24 hours following delivery or 24 hours following the last eclamptic fit, whichever occurs later.

Elevated serum magnesium levels can depress deep tendon reflexes, urine output and respiratory rate. Although clinical assessment may identify potentially toxic magnesium levels,[71,84] there is no consensus as to the therapeutic serum magnesium required to prevent eclampsia. One author suggests a serum level of 2 mmol/L, but there is no rationale provided for this level.[86]

Control of hypertension

Obtaining control of high blood pressure remains a priority not only to improve organ perfusion but to minimise the risk of cerebral haemorrhage, a well-demonstrated hazard of hypertension in preeclampsia.[26] Both systolic and diastolic pressures are important and care should be taken to ensure a gradual lowering of blood pressure, as a rapid drop can compromise fetal wellbeing. There is no evidence for the superiority of any specific antihypertensive, although there is some evidence that diazoxide may result in a potentially harmful rapid drop in the woman's blood pressure and that ketanserin may not be as effective as hydralazine.[85] Intravenous labetolol has replaced IV hydralazine as the most common drug used to treat very high blood pressure in Australia, though both are commonly used. Refractory hypertension may be treated with IV glyceryl trinitrate (GTN) or nitroprusside. The target blood pressure is not well described, other than to avoid precipitous drops in BP and to maintain adequate placental perfusion. Research has used a target diastolic BP of 85–95 mmHg.[87]

Optimal fluid management

Despite being hypertensive, preeclamptic women are usually plasma-volume depleted.[88] In the past, intravenous fluid was administered in an attempt to restore the deficit, with no advantage noted between colloids and crystalloids. More recently, there has been a move towards conservative plasma volume expansion due to the risk of pulmonary oedema. In reviews of maternal deaths associated with preeclampsia, it was noticed that some women were dying from complications of fluid overload. Careful titration of intravenous fluid is required to optimise plasma volume and organ perfusion without the development of pulmonary oedema.[89] Central venous pressure is universally accepted as unhelpful to guide fluid management in preeclampsia. Transthoracic echocardiography (TTE) has demonstrated impaired systolic and diastolic function in women with preeclampsia and TTE is advocated by some to guide fluid management.[90] See also Box 28.3.

> ## BOX 28.3
>
> ### Management of women with HELLP syndrome using steroids
>
> The use of steroids has been evaluated in the management of HELLP syndrome in the belief that steroids may mitigate the severity of the disease. However, a *Cochrane Review* concluded that there was insufficient evidence to determine whether steroid use as a treatment for HELLP syndrome had a favourable outcome for mothers and babies, although steroids may be beneficial if an increase in platelet count was imperative.[91]

Thromboprophylaxis

Preeclampsia is an independent risk factor for thromboembolic disease and, when combined with prolonged bed rest as may occur with caesarean section, ICU admission, obesity and age ≥35 years, due consideration must be made of the need for thromboprophylaxis (in the absence of any contraindications). Thus women with severe preeclampsia admitted to ICU may meet the requirements for treatment with compression stockings and low-molecular-weight heparin for a minimum of 7 days.[33]

Betamethasone

When severe preeclampsia is diagnosed prior to 34 weeks' gestation, the woman is normally prescribed a single dose of betamethasone (11.4 mg IM) to promote fetal lung maturity and surfactant production. A second dose is recommended 24 hours after the first;[69] however, in reality, most women with severe preeclampsia have given birth within 24 hours. A Cochrane review has shown that treatment with antenatal corticosteroids reduces the risk of neonatal death, respiratory distress syndrome, cerebroventricular haemorrhage, necrotising enterocolitis, infectious morbidity, need for respiratory support and neonatal intensive care unit admission, with no adverse effects on the mother.[92]

Optimal timing of delivery

Women with severe preeclampsia can only be definitively cured by delivery, regardless of gestation. A number of studies have trialled 'temporising treatments' aimed at prolonging the pregnancy, especially when a woman develops early onset severe preeclampsia (<34 weeks' gestation). Although some have found that treatment with vasodilators and fluid administration prolong pregnancy with no adverse effect, prolonging the pregnancy is often associated with an increased chance of maternal complications, such as eclampsia, pulmonary oedema and cerebral haemorrhage.[71,93] Consequently, a woman with severe preeclampsia is usually stabilised (magnesium sulfate commenced and hypertension controlled) and arrangements made for delivery. Ideally, women <34 weeks' gestation should be transferred to a tertiary obstetric centre prior to delivery.

Subsequent pregnancy and long-term cardiovascular health

Women who have experienced preeclampsia are seven times more likely to experience preeclampsia again in a subsequent pregnancy than women who did not experience preeclampsia in their first pregnancy.[75] It seems that earlier onset preeclampsia and more severe disease are related to risk of recurrence. Some treatments, e.g. low dose aspirin, have shown benefit in reducing the likelihood of recurrence in select high risk groups. Importantly, women who have experienced preeclampsia are twice as likely to die from cardiovascular disease later in life, and thus preeclampsia is an important risk factor for cardiovascular disease development.[94]

> ### Practice tip
>
> Many maternity professionals abbreviate preeclampsia to PE. This can be very confusing given that, in other health care settings, the abbreviation PE usually stands for pulmonary embolism. Be clear in any notes that you make, and clarify when reading notes that have been given to you.

Obstetric haemorrhage

Obstetric haemorrhage is a generic term indicating that there is bleeding from the uterus or genital tract in a pregnant or postpartum woman. It may be used when a woman experiences early pregnancy bleeding, e.g. prior to 20 weeks' gestation, and also if she has experienced either antepartum (>20 weeks' gestation and prior to birth) or postpartum (after birth of the baby) haemorrhage. Of the estimated 289,000 maternal deaths each year, obstetric haemorrhage is a leading cause, directly accounting for 27% of all maternal deaths.[95] The past decade has seen an increase in both the incidence and severity of obstetric haemorrhage, with more women requiring a blood transfusion for postpartum haemorrhage than in the past.[96] Major obstetric haemorrhage is a common reason for postpartum women to be admitted to ICU at 0.7/1000 deliveries.[4] Scotland routinely gathered data on major obstetric haemorrhage, defined as an estimated blood loss ≥2500 mL and/or the transfusion of five or more units of blood and/or the administration of other blood products for coagulopathy. In 2012, one in every 170 women who gave birth in Scotland experienced a major obstetric haemorrhage.[97] Unfortunately, there is no agreed terminology for major obstetric haemorrhage, for example maternal/ obstetric, and massive/major/severe are often used interchangeably. Furthermore, definition of a 'major obstetric haemorrhage' is variable and may include >1500 mL blood loss, >2500mL blood loss, drop of >4 g/L Hb, >4 units of RBCs transfused within 4 hours, need for non-RBC blood products or >8 units of RBCs transfused within 24 hours. Regardless, major obstetric haemorrhage is often sudden and unexpected, and is frequently associated with an acute coagulopathy. Early recognition and treatment of major obstetric haemorrhage is vital to ensure the best outcome for mother and fetus. A repeated finding in maternal death reviews is a delay by obstetric providers in recognising the severity of haemorrhage and consequent deterioration in maternal condition.[26]

The common causes of antepartum and postpartum haemorrhage are described below with common management strategies presented at the end of the section. See also Box 28.4.

BOX 28.4

What about vaginal bleeding before the 20th week of gestation?

Vaginal bleeding before the 20th week of gestation (usually a type of miscarriage, e.g. threatened, incomplete) is considered 'early pregnancy bleeding' and is not categorised as antepartum haemorrhage. Septic abortion (or miscarriage) can cause profound bleeding in the days after the event when the infection has become established.

Antepartum haemorrhage

Antepartum haemorrhage (APH) is inconsistently defined throughout the world, with the most common definition as used in the UK: any bleeding from the genital tract occurring between the 24th week of gestation and the birth of the baby.[98] This is in contrast to the definition used in Australia where APH is defined as any bleeding from the genital tract occurring between the 20th week of gestation and the birth of the baby. APH occurs in 2–5% of all pregnancies.[99] Bleeding from the vagina prior to 20 weeks' gestation is referred to in terms of miscarriage (e.g. threatened) and is not classified as an APH. The two main causes of APH are placental abruption and placenta praevia.

Placental abruption (or abruptio placentae)

Placental abruption is premature separation (i.e. before the birth of the baby) of a normally-sited placenta from the uterine wall and is responsible for about 25% of APH.[99] Only a portion of the placenta separates with two-thirds separation considered severe. There are two relevant matters to consider with placental abruption: how much blood the woman has lost and how much placenta remains attached and functionally able to support the fetus. If the placenta partially separates along an edge of the placenta, blood loss is usually visible via the vagina. In some cases the centre part of the placenta detaches, leaving the rim attached all the way around (like the rim of a dinner plate) and, in these cases, the blood loss is usually not visible via the vagina (i.e. is concealed). However, the woman may have lost substantial blood volume and be in hypovolaemic shock. This type of placental abruption is usually accompanied by severe abdominal pain, and DIC commonly develops in response to blood being forced into uterine muscle tissue, referred to as a couvelaire uterus. Once half to two-thirds of the placenta is detached, the likelihood of fetal survival is low, especially if the woman is also hypotensive. In the majority of cases, only women with severe placental abruption are admitted to ICU and usually admission occurs following an emergency caesarean section. Understanding of the aetiology of placental abruption is not complete with approximately 20% of cases unexplained. For most women, placental abruption is associated with a known related factor such as preeclampsia, blunt trauma (e.g. car crash) or sudden reduction in uterine volume (e.g. after delivery of the first baby in a twin pregnancy).

Placenta praevia

Placenta praevia is when some or the entire placenta is abnormally sited in the lower segment of the uterus, often referred to as a low-lying placenta. Placenta praevia is graded as major, when placenta overlies the cervical os, and minor, when the placenta is not lying over the cervical os but is encroaching on the lower uterine segment.[99] A vaginal birth is not possible when the placenta blocks the cervix, necessitating a caesarean section. The lower uterine segment does not fully form until 28–32 weeks' gestation, and the shearing stress as the lower uterine segment forms may precipitate detachment of the placenta from the uterine wall causing maternal bleeding. Bleeding can occur at any time, is usually painless and may be massive. Placenta praevia is the main cause of APH, accounting for 30% of cases.[99] Management is dictated by the size of the blood loss and maternal condition, how much functioning placenta remains, fetal wellbeing and whether bleeding is ongoing. In severe cases, the woman is usually taken to theatre for an emergency caesarean section.

Placenta accreta is a serious complicating condition that may occur in conjunction with placenta praevia. The attachment of the placenta to the uterine wall is abnormal and is considered morbidly adherent. There are three levels of severity, although often all three are referred to as placenta accreta (see Box 28.5). Placenta accreta is strongly associated with prior caesarean section and a woman with an anterior placenta praevia and a prior caesarean section should be actively screened for placenta accreta (by ultrasound or MRI) prior to any elective caesarean section. Placental tissue can be very invasive and may infiltrate local structures such as the bladder. Many women with placenta accreta undergo emergency hysterectomy at the time of caesarean section, as a means to remove the placenta and control bleeding. An alternative management is to deliver the baby by caesarean section and leave the placenta in situ.[100] As long as a portion of the placenta does not detach, there will be no bleeding and, in most cases, the placenta will autolyse and be re-absorbed by the woman.

BOX 28.5

Types of placenta accreta

- Placenta accreta: the placenta is abnormally adherent to the uterine lining
- Placenta increta: the placenta invades the uterine muscle (myometrium)
- Placenta percreta: the placenta grows through the myometrium and into adjacent structures, such as the bladder and ureters

Adapted from Oyelese Y, Smulian JC. Placenta previa, placenta accreta, and vasa previa. Obstet Gynecol 2006;107(4):927–41, with permission.

Practice tip

Read a woman's operation report if she has a diagnosis of placenta accreta to identify the extent to which the placental tissue has invaded local structures, such as the bladder, ureters and bowel. For example, the bladder is often affected and a cystotomy may have been required to separate the placenta from the bladder.

Postpartum haemorrhage

Postpartum haemorrhage (PPH), a major cause of maternal death in developed and developing countries, is defined as ≥500 mL blood loss from the genital tract after the birth of the baby. The incidence and severity of PPH is increasing, in both caesarean and vaginal births.[96,101–103] PPH rates commonly sit at around 10% of all births although they may be as high as 25% in some jurisdictions.[104] Severe PPH lacks an agreed definition, with published definitions ranging from '≥1000 mL' to 'estimated blood loss ≥2500 mL or transfused ≥5 units of blood or received treatment for coagulopathy during the acute event'.[15,105] Consequently, the incidence of severe PPH varies depending on how it has been defined and ranges from 3.7/1000 deliveries to 4.6/1000 deliveries.[6,105] Additionally, PPH is classified according to the timing of the haemorrhage in relation to the birth. Primary PPH occurs within the first 24 hours after birth whereas secondary PPH occurs from

24 hours up to 6 weeks following birth. Primary PPH is often caused by uterine atony, while secondary PPH is more likely to be associated with retained products and associated infection.

The causes of PPH are varied and have been classified by the 'four Ts': tone, tissue, trauma and thrombin (Box 28.6). The cause of PPH should be identified and targeted with specific management, in conjunction with the general principles of haemorrhage management. See also Box 28.7.

BOX 28.6

Causes of postpartum haemorrhage characterised by the '4 Ts'[106]

Tone:
- Uterine atony
- Functional or anatomical distortion of the uterus (e.g. bi-cornuate uterus)

Tissue:
- Retained placental products
- Abnormal placenta

Trauma:
- Cervical and genital tract damage during delivery
- Uterine inversion

Thrombin:
- Coagulation disorders

Adapted from NSW Health. Maternity – prevention, early recognition and management of postpartum haemorrhage (PPH). Sydney: Department of Health, NSW; 2010.

BOX 28.7

Can PPH be prevented?

The most significant intervention shown to reduce the incidence of PPH is active management of the third stage of labour. This represents a group of interventions including controlled cord traction for placental delivery and prophylactic administration of a uterotonic at delivery: drugs that cause the uterus to contract. Active management of the third stage is associated with a lower incidence of PPH and a reduced need for a blood transfusion.

Severe obstetric haemorrhage management priorities

Whilst it is feasible for a pregnant woman in ICU to develop placental abruption, for example, the vast majority of women admitted to ICU with obstetric haemorrhage will be transferred following birth, and are thus postpartum on admission to ICU. These priorities focus on postpartum management. As with any major haemorrhage (see Chapter 21), the principles of treatment are:

- restore an adequate circulating volume and maintain oxygen and perfusion to vital organs
- obtain haemostasis and correct coagulopathy
- prevent complications.

See Box 28.8 for acute immediate treatment.

BOX 28.8

Summary of acute immediate treatment for PPH

Resuscitation and immediate management:

- ABC assess airway, breathing and circulation
- 'Rub up' the uterus
- 2 large bore cannulae and send bloods for rapid cross-match
- Administer oxytocics, e.g. syntocinon[107]
- Fluid resuscitation
- Determine the cause (4 Ts)
- Transfuse blood (O-negative in the first instance, then type specific)
- Prepare for transfer to theatre

Surgical treatment and other interventions:

- Delivery of placenta and uterine pathology, if applicable
- B-lynch suture
- Uterine tamponade, e.g. inflation of uterine balloon for local compression (Bakri balloon)
- Ligation of internal iliac or uterine arteries
- Hysterectomy
- Compression of the aorta
- Uterine replacement (if uterine inversion noted)
- Radiological arterial embolisation or balloon occlusion
- Consider systemic haemostatic agents
- Tranexamic acid

Maintaining circulating volume, oxygenation and perfusion

Haemodynamic instability following substantial blood loss is a frequent reason for admission to ICU.[108] Accurate estimation of blood loss is difficult as bleeding can be concealed, and blood loss may be mixed with amniotic fluid making accurate estimation a challenge, potentially leading to an underestimation of fluid resuscitation needs. Furthermore, peripartum women are at an increased risk of acute pulmonary oedema, which further complicates fluid resuscitation.[109,110] Standard resuscitation fluids, such as Hartmann's or normal saline, should be infused according to routine practice for the non-obstetric haemorrhage, remembering that large volumes of blood products may also be required.

Practice tip

Keep in mind the following:

- Serum albumin levels are decreased in normal pregnancy, with the lowest levels recorded in the postpartum period.[48]
- Cardiac output remains elevated postpartum for the first few days at least.
- Central venous pressure (CVP) and pulmonary artery pressure (PAP) can be interpreted the same as for non-obstetric patients.

Achieving haemostasis and correct coagulopathy

Specific interventions to control bleeding include radiological arterial embolisation or balloon occlusion of the internal iliac arteries, uterine compression suture (e.g. B-Lynch suture), use of an intrauterine balloon tamponade (e.g. Bakri balloon) and emergency hysterectomy. Women may need to return to theatre for abdominal packing for ongoing 'ooze' that may continue after a hysterectomy. Most women with severe obstetric haemorrhage in ICU have developed DIC that requires treatment with the appropriate blood products.[111] DIC is particularly common in these women, in part because of the normal changes in the clotting factors during pregnancy and in part due to the potential for an amniotic fluid embolism to have been the triggering event for the haemorrhage.[88,112,113]

Large volumes of blood products, such as packed red cells, fresh frozen plasma, platelets and cryoprecipitate are often required. Patient blood management guidelines have been developed by the National Blood Authority with module 1 (critical bleeding), module 4 (critical care) and module 5 (obstetrics and maternity) of most relevance.[114–116] Increasingly, it is thought that more aggressive use of fresh frozen plasma, cryoprecipitate and platelets in line with red blood cell usage is needed to prevent and/or correct haemorrhage coagulopathy. Hypofibrinogenaemia should be actively prevented and managed to maintain a level >2 g/L.[117] Fibrinogen is usually doubled by the end of pregnancy, and low fibrinogen levels are associated with increasing severity of PPH.[117] Fibrinogen concentrate for the treatment of PPH is of increasing interest and a study is underway: the FIB-PPH trial, fibrinogen concentrate as initial treatment for postpartum haemorrhage, which will examine whether fibrinogen concentrate reduces blood transfusion use in PPH.[118] Point-of-care devices that examine the quality of the clot, such as thromboelastography (TEG) and rotational thromboelastometry (ROTEM), are frequently used in tertiary centres to guide management of obstetric haemorrhage.

Recombinant factor VIIa has been used successfully in the management of severe obstetric haemorrhage and should be considered for use early in the management of the bleeding woman, with treatment more likely to be effective if administered before the woman becomes hypothermic and acidotic.[119] Tranexamic acid has shown some benefit in the management of PPH.[120] All maternity providers should have a 'massive transfusion protocol' that outlines action and escalation of care for massive bleeding.[116] Maternity adaptations from a standard massive transfusion protocol include: consideration for early triggering of the protocol given the common underestimation of blood loss and ability for the maternity patient to initially maintain haemodynamic stability despite large blood loss, aim to maintain a higher level of fibrinogen (>2.0 g/L) and avoidance of permissive hypotension while the uterus remains in situ.[116]

Preventing complications

Strategies to prevent the following complications should be implemented:

- Complications of major blood transfusion – these are similar in the obstetric patient as in the non-obstetric patient and include acid–base disturbance, transfusion-related acute lung injury (TRALI), hypocalcaemia, hyperkalaemia and hypothermia. Standard monitoring and treatment of these complications should be used.

- Increased risk of thrombosis – particularly in the early postpartum period as the risk is exacerbated by lengthy theatre procedures, bed rest associated with ICU admission and following major haemorrhage with an associated massive blood transfusion. Suitable thromboprophylaxis should be considered as soon as feasible and thromboembolic stockings and/or sequential compression devices should be applied.

- Acute kidney injury – irreversible renal failure has been reported as a sequela of acute kidney injury following severe postpartum haemorrhage.[121] Routine monitoring and management of renal impairment is required, keeping in mind that a pregnant patient has a lower urea and creatinine level than non-pregnant patients. Careful titration of fluid for renal purposes is needed due to the increased propensity for pulmonary oedema.

- Rh isoimmunisation – the potential to develop Rh isoimmunisation in Rh-negative women who have experienced antepartum haemorrhage should be considered.[122] A Kleihauer-Betke test should be done to quantify the amount of fetal cells in the maternal circulation and determine the dose of anti-D immunoglobulin required.

- Sheehan's syndrome – necrosis of the pituitary gland is a very rare complication of severe obstetric haemorrhage. The anterior lobe is most often affected due to physiological changes that occur during pregnancy. While the syndrome may go undetected for many years, one of the earliest symptoms is a failure to establish lactation, due to the absence of prolactin secretion. Sheehan's syndrome can be prevented by maintaining adequate circulating volume, oxygenation and perfusion.

Use of intraoperative cell salvage for obstetric haemorrhage

The introduction of cell salvage in obstetrics has been delayed compared to other surgeries for two key reasons: the theoretical risk of amniotic fluid embolism (AFE) and the risk of rhesus isoimmunisation.[123] The advent of new technologies, combined with an increasing obstetric haemorrhage rate, has seen cell salvage being introduced since the mid-1990s, and now becoming common practice.[123,124] Historical understanding of amniotic fluid embolism argued against the risk of infusing blood that potentially contained amniotic fluid. The more recent understanding that AFE is more aligned with an anaphylactic reaction has lessened these concerns as a woman has already been exposed to the contents of the fluid that are infused following cell salvage and, in practice, there has been no confirmed case of AFE following use of cell salvage infusion.[125] Regardless, it is common practice to use a different suction device from the time of amniotic membrane rupture until after delivery (which is not re-used) with blood aspirated from the surgical field collected by the cell salvage device.[124] A leukocyte depletion filter should always be used during the re-infusion of salvaged maternal blood to filter any remaining foreign proteins.[123] None of the currently available cell saver equipment is able to discern fetal from adult red blood cells and any present fetal cells are transfused to the woman. It is important for rhesus-negative women to have a post-infusion Kleihauer-Betke test to quantify the amount of fetal red cells in the maternal circulation to ensure that an adequate dose of anti-D immunoglobulin can be given to prevent isoimmunisation.

Amniotic fluid embolism

Amniotic fluid embolism (AFE) is a rare and incompletely understood obstetric emergency that usually occurs during labour or pregnancy termination, or shortly after delivery. Traditional understanding of the condition was based around the notion that amniotic fluid entered the maternal blood stream via the endocervical veins or placental bed, with amniotic fluid, fetal cells, hair or other fetal debris functioning as an embolus, and resulting in the dramatic cardiorespiratory collapse seen with the condition. However, not all women diagnosed with AFE have evidence of fetal squames/amniotic fluid substances in the pulmonary vasculature and many women who do not develop AFE have fetal cells found in the maternal circulation.[126]

More recently, improved understanding of the mechanics of labour and the interaction of amniotic fluid and maternal blood, as well as the striking similarities between clinical and haemodynamic findings in AFE and both anaphylaxis and septic shock, have led to a belief that a common pathophysiological mechanism is likely to be responsible for all these conditions.[127] As AFE resembles an anaphylactic reaction to fetal material rather than an embolic event, the term 'anaphylactoid syndrome of pregnancy', instead of AFE, has been proposed.[127]

AFE has also been likened to systemic inflammatory response syndrome, with the related inappropriate release of endogenous inflammatory mediators.[126] The trigger for AFE is not well understood, although it is thought to be a fetal antigen (which may arise from amniotic fluid). It is possible that all labouring women are exposed to the fetal antigen, with those affected by AFE exhibiting a rare and abnormal maternal immune response.[126] One of the difficulties blocking improved understanding of AFE is the lack of a diagnostic test.

Regardless of the level of understanding, the abnormal mediator release gives rise to acute lung injury, resulting in acute dyspnoea and hypoxia and often the development of acute respiratory distress syndrome. Within 30 minutes of the antigen insult, there is evidence of severe pulmonary hypertension with acute right ventricular failure.[128] It is thought that inflammatory mediators are a more likely cause of pulmonary vasoconstriction, with physical obstruction to the pulmonary vasculature (embolism) not the main mechanism.[126,129] The left ventricular failure seen in AFE is considered a secondary response due to poor left ventricular filling pressures. Concomitantly, substances in the amniotic fluid trigger a profound consumptive coagulopathy.

Incidence and risk factors

The incidence of AFE is thought to be in the range of 2–8 women per 100,000 deliveries making it a very rare event.[130] However, the lack of a diagnostic test is a serious limiting factor for accurate determination of incidence, with geographical variation reported. AFE is more common in North America (1 in 15,200 deliveries) than in Europe (1 in 53,800 deliveries);[129] this may represent a true difference in incidence or reflect differences in clinical diagnosis or methods of case identification.

Diagnosis remains one of exclusion and there is a long list of differential diagnoses, including air or thrombotic pulmonary emboli, septic shock, cardiomyopathy, acute myocardial infarction, anaphylaxis, transfusion reaction, aspiration, placental abruption, eclampsia, uterine rupture, local anaesthetic toxicity and primary postpartum haemorrhage.[127] Older obstetric literature quote mortality rates above 80%;[131] however, recent larger studies have shown that mortality in developed countries is more likely to be in the range of 13–30%.[129,130,132] Regardless, AFE remains a major contributor to maternal death, accounting for 5–15% of all maternal deaths in developed countries.[54,129]

Although controversy exists, the factors that have been proposed as contributing to an increased likelihood for AFE include:[126,127,129,130,132]

- induction of labour
- caesarean birth
- multiple pregnancy, e.g. twins
- maternal age ≥35 years
- forceps delivery
- placenta praevia, preeclampsia and placental abruption.

Given the rarity of AFE and the commonality of these potential risk factors, astute clinical assessment and early clinical suspicion based on the clinical presentation of the woman should be the focus for early identification and treatment.

Clinical presentation

The symptoms associated with AFE have been well described and usually comprise premonitory symptoms, such as restlessness, agitation and numbness/tingling prior to more severe maternal compromise such as sudden onset hypotension, dyspnoea, hypoxia, altered mental status and haemorrhage.[129] Collapse of the maternal cardiovascular system leads to fetal distress as the placenta is deprived of maternal oxygen, quickly leading to fetal demise unless the fetus is delivered swiftly. Premonitory symptoms, shortness of breath and fetal distress have been reported as the early signs in a UK study.[130] Overall, haemorrhage and associated coagulopathy, hypotension and shortness of breath were the most commonly recorded symptoms.[130] Cardiac arrest was documented in 40% of cases and seizure in 15%. Haemorrhage and coagulopathy may not be immediately apparent; some women die before it develops. However, these clinical features usually develop in women who survive the initial insult.

Patient management

There is no specific treatment for AFE; all therapy is supportive with the aim to maintain adequate oxygenation and perfusion, control haemorrhage and correct any coagulopathy. Common interventions include:[130]

- urgent delivery of the fetus
- emergency hysterectomy to control postpartum haemorrhage
- admission to ICU, with associated support such as mechanical ventilation, nitric oxide and extracorporeal membrane oxygenation (ECMO).

A full range of blood components, including fresh frozen plasma, platelets and cryoprecipitate may be required to correct the coagulopathy. Adjunct therapies such as recombinant factor VIIa have also been used with effect. Transoesophageal echocardiography may be very helpful to guide fluid and inotrope management to optimise preload and enhance cardiac output.

Although it is possible for a woman to experience an AFE in a subsequent pregnancy, repeat AFE is thought to be unlikely as the trigger for AFE is specific to each fetus the woman carries. There have been a number of published case reports of women having a successful subsequent pregnancy and none reporting repeat AFE in the same woman.

Peripartum cardiomyopathy

Peripartum cardiomyopathy, sometimes referred to as postpartum cardiomyopathy, is new onset heart failure in association with pregnancy. Diagnosis is usually dependent on all four of the following criteria: 1) the development of the disease in the last month of pregnancy or within 5 months of delivery; 2) absence of any other identifiable cause of heart failure; 3) absence of recognisable heart disease before the last month of pregnancy; and 4) left ventricle systolic dysfunction.[133] However, time of onset outside of the above criteria does occur occasionally. Peripartum cardiomyopathy is considered to be a dilated cardiomyopathy, resulting in a dilated left atrium and ventricle, and a reduced left ventricular ejection fraction (<45%).[134] Women commonly present with New York Heart Association class III or IV heart failure.[135] The incidence of peripartum cardiomyopathy varies widely from 1:100 in a small region of sub-Saharan Africa to 1:4000 in the USA, though many studies on peripartum cardiomyopathy were conducted on data that had been gathered retrospectively.[133,136] A prospective population-based study in the Netherlands found that 1 in 20,000 pregnancies required ICU admission for peripartum cardiomyopathy.[9]

The exact cause of peripartum cardiomyopathy is not well understood and a variety of factors have been implicated, including viral infection, autoimmune mechanisms, cytokine-mediated inflammation, increased myocyte apoptosis, increased oxidative stress, genetic disposition and/or cultural habits, and abnormal hormonal regulation.[135,137] More recently, it is postulated that oxidative stress cleaves the full-length, 23-kDa form of the hormone prolactin into an antiangiogenic, 16-kDa derivative.[138] Maternal mortality associated with peripartum cardiomyopathy is around 15%; however, it may be as low as 2% in developed countries.[139] Studies show that approximately 20–40% of women recover their left ventricular function, usually within 6 months though it may take up to 2 years.[134,140] Women who never fully recover their cardiac function require ongoing medical management; a small proportion of women go on to require a mechanical-assist device and heart transplantation.

Patient management

Women with peripartum cardiomyopathy present with varying degrees of left heart failure. Signs and symptoms of heart failure including dyspnoea, persistent cough, abdominal discomfort, palpitations and oedema may be mistaken for 'discomforts of pregnancy' and lead to a delay in diagnosis. The diagnosis of peripartum cardiomyopathy is one of exclusion requiring systematic investigation to exclude both cardiac and non-cardiac differential diagnoses such as pulmonary embolism, acute myocardial infarction, severe preeclampsia and pneumonia.[141] Echocardiography is a useful diagnostic tool with a left ventricular end-diastolic diameter >60 mm predictive of poor recovery, as is a LVEF <30%.[134] When available, a cardiac MRI allows for better chamber volume and functional assessment and is a more sensitive tool to identify a left ventricular thrombus.[134]

The principles of managing acute heart failure in women with peripartum cardiomyopathy are no different to the management of heart failure from any other cause, and aim to reduce preload and afterload and to increase cardiac contractility (see Chapter 10 for a full description). Unfortunately, ACE inhibitors and angiotensin antagonists are contraindicated in pregnancy.

Bromocriptine, a relatively new and novel treatment for peripartum cardiomyopathy, is still undergoing investigation. Recent advances in understanding the aetiology of peripartum cardiomyopathy have suggested that increased oxidative stress plays a significant role, and bromocriptine is directly able to reduce oxidative stress by blocking the release of prolactin.[142] Animal and early human studies show promise, with relapse of peripartum cardiomyopathy prevented in women in a subsequent pregnancy and rapid recovery in new-onset peripartum cardiomyopathy observed.[143–145] The addition of bromocriptine to a standard cardiac drug regimen to treat peripartum cardiomyopathy has resulted in improved outcomes.[146]

For women diagnosed with peripartum cardiomyopathy while pregnant, timing and mode of delivery are two other management decisions to be made. A multidisciplinary team, including cardiologist, obstetrician, anaesthetist and nursing/midwifery staff, should consider and plan for delivery dependent on maternal and fetal condition and the woman's known preferences. Ergometrine-containing drugs, used to contract the uterus post-delivery, are contraindicated because they cause vasoconstriction and the associated increase in afterload may be detrimental for maternal heart function. Synthetic preparations, such as oxytocin, are advised instead to prevent postpartum haemorrhage. Finally, given the postulated role of prolactin in the aetiology of peripartum cardiomyopathy, recent guidelines advise against breastfeeding in women who have been diagnosed with peripartum cardiomyopathy.[134]

Subsequent pregnancy

Family planning counselling is an important part of the care of women as they recover from peripartum cardiomyopathy. After a diagnosis of peripartum cardiomyopathy, women have a 30% risk of relapse in any subsequent pregnancy.[140,147] Peripartum cardiomyopathy remains an important cause of maternal death, and this may occur in association with subsequent pregnancies.

Exacerbation of medical disease associated with pregnancy

Women with pre-existing medical conditions pose additional challenges during pregnancy. In a population-based prospective study of all pregnant and postpartum admissions to ICU in the Netherlands, 28% of women had at least one chronic disease.[9] However, this pre-existing medical condition may not have been related to the need for ICU admission. For example, in an Australian study 39% of admissions to ICU had a medical history, but the pre-existing illness was related to the ICU admission in 24% of women.[13] Occasionally, pregnant and postpartum women are admitted to ICU with exacerbation of an underlying medical condition and two of the most common conditions, cardiac disease and asthma, are outlined in this section.

Cardiac disease

Cardiac disease in pregnancy consists of women who have congenital heart disease and women who have acquired heart disease, such as rheumatic heart disease.

Congenital heart disease

Congenital heart disease is a form of maternal cardiac disease that encompasses a broad spectrum of defects as outlined in Table 28.6. Congenital heart disease is one of the more common forms of congenital birth defects with the four most serious congenital cardiac defects having a combined rate in Australia of 12.4/10,000 births.[149] In Australia, more than 2000 babies are born with congenital heart disease annually;[150] worldwide, there are 1.35 million newborns diagnosed with congenital heart disease every year.[151] The etiology of congenital heart disease is complex, and often multifactorial arising from chromosomal anomalies (8–10%), DNA mutation (3–5%) and non-syndromal single gene disorders or teratogens.[150] Largely, the causes are unknown and attributed to factors within the maternal, fetal or placental environment. One recognised risk factor for the development of congenital heart disease in the fetus is maternal pregestational diabetes,[150] with the greatest period of fetal risk occurring before the seventh week of gestation.[152]

Increasing numbers of those affected with congenital heart disease are surviving into adulthood with the greatest increase in survival benefit seen in people with severe disease.[150] The number of adults living with congenital heart disease is predicted to continue growing, leading to clinicians being presented with the challenge of caring for women with significant heart disease reaching reproductive age and wishing to conceive and sustain a pregnancy through to term.[150] The risks that these women face in the pursuit of parenthood should not be overlooked[153] and are outlined in Table 28.7. A tool to predict the likelihood of a cardiac complication associated with pregnancy has been developed for women with pre-existing heart disease (Table 28.8). The combination of both cardiovascular

---

TABLE 28.6

Specific congenital cardiac conditions[148]

ACYANOTIC HEART DEFECT WITHOUT SHUNT	ACYANOTIC HEART DEFECT WITH SHUNT	CYANOTIC HEART DEFECTS	AORTIC DISEASES
Congenital aortic stenosis	Atrial septal defect	Tetralogy of Fallot	Marfan syndrome
Pulmonic stenosis	Ventricular septal defect	Complete transposition of great vessels	Ehlers-Danlos syndrome
Coarctation of aorta	Eisenmenger syndrome	Hypoplastic right heart	Loeys-Dietz syndrome
		Hypoplastic left heart	

Adapted from Harris IS. Management of pregnancy in patients with congenital heart disease. Progr Cardiovasc Dis 2011;53(4):305–11.

TABLE 28.7

Congenital heart disease and maternal risk in pregnancy[148]

HIGH RISK OF COMPLICATIONS OR DEATH (>15%)	MODERATE RISK OF COMPLICATIONS (5–15%)	LOW RISK OF COMPLICATIONS (<1%)
Pulmonary hypertension	Unrepaired cyanotic defects	Isolated aortic septal defect, repaired or unrepaired
Eisenmenger syndrome	Systemic right ventricle	Isolated ventricular septal defect, repaired or unrepaired
Coarctation of aorta, uncorrected with proximal aortic dilation	Well-functioning Fontan circulation	Coarctation repaired with normal proximal aortic size
Severe symptomatic aortic stenosis	Palliated Tetralogy of Fallot with severe pulmonic regurgitation and right ventricular dysfunction	Repaired Tetralogy of Fallot with normal right ventricular function and competent pulmonic valve
Single ventricle with poor systolic function – with or without Fontan		

Adapted from Harris IS. Management of pregnancy in patients with congenital heart disease. Progr Cardiovasc Dis 2011;53(4):305–11.

TABLE 28.8

Predictors of maternal risk for cardiac complications[154]

CRITERIA	EXAMPLE	POINTS[a]
Prior cardiac events	Heart failure, transient ischaemic attack, stroke before present pregnancy, arrhythmia (defined as symptomatic sustained tachyarrhythmia or bradyarrhythmia requiring treatment)	1
NYHA III/IV or cyanosis		1
Valvular and outflow tract obstruction	Aortic valve area <1.5 cm², mitral valve area <2 cm² or left ventricular outflow tract peak gradient >30 mm Hg	1
Myocardial dysfunction	LVEF <40% or restrictive cardiomyopathy or hypertrophic cardiomyopathy	1

LVEF = left ventricular ejection fraction; NYHA = New York Heart Association.

[a]Maternal cardiac event rates for 0, 1 and >1 points are 5%, 27% and 75%, respectively.

Adapted from Siu SC, Sermer M, Colman JM, Alvarez AN, Mercier L-A, Morton BC et al. Prospective multicenter study of pregnancy outcomes in women with heart disease. Circulation 2001;104:515–521.

and respiratory changes in pregnancy is poorly tolerated by some women, and cardiac disease in pregnancy still remains a leading cause of maternal death in Australia.[54]

Rheumatic heart disease

Rheumatic heart disease is the most frequently acquired heart disease and is a condition normally associated with developing countries.[155] In Australia, rheumatic heart disease is a significant concern in Aboriginal people and Torres Strait Islanders with rates in these communities in the Northern Territory noted to be the highest in the world, and over 30 times higher than those of non-Indigenous Australians.[155] Similarly, in New Zealand, Maori and Pacific Islanders have a much higher incidence of rheumatic heart disease than New Zealanders of European ancestry. Refugee and immigrant women who have migrated from developing countries such as in sub-Saharan Africa also have a higher risk for rheumatic heart disease in pregnancy. Rheumatic heart disease is a delayed complication of acute rheumatic fever, and results from an untreated group A streptococcus bacterial throat or skin infection.

Rheumatic heart disease is the progressive, structural heart damage that occurs after an initial episode of acute rheumatic fever. Rheumatic heart disease usually begins with generalised carditis; then, as the disease advances, mitral valve insufficiency develops though the aortic valve

may also be affected. Valvular pathology includes restricted leaflet mobility, valvular prolapse, focal or generalised valvular thickening and abnormal subvalvular thickening, chordae tendinae or papillary muscle rupture and scarring, resulting in regurgitation and, rarely, stenosis.

Serial echocardiography throughout pregnancy by a skilled provider is essential to monitor maternal cardiac function and, specifically, valvular dynamics in women with rheumatic heart disease. Imaging can be technically challenging during pregnancy, and cardiac indices need to be aligned with the normal echocardiography pregnancy reference range.[156]

Acute myocardial infarction

Acute myocardial infarction (AMI), once a rare condition not seen in pregnancy, is becoming more prevalent. The increasing incidence is thought to be related to the changing demographics of the pregnant population, which now includes higher proportions of older women and women who are obese.[157] AMI is the leading cardiac cause of maternal death in the UK, mostly related to undiagnosed ischaemic heart disease, which may not be considered as a diagnosis in pregnancy as women have traditionally been healthy and well.[24] Pregnancy has been reported to increase the risk of AMI 3–4 fold in same-age-matched non-pregnant women, with mortality rates ranging from 20% to 50% in some cases.[157] Diagnosis of AMI in pregnancy is the same as for the non-pregnant patient, with troponin levels considered both reliable and accurate.[158,159] Percutaneous coronary angiography is suggested as the treatment of choice for coronary reperfusion. There are limited data available to either support or refute the administration of thrombolytics such as tissue plasminogen activator in pregnancy.

Women with risk factors for heart disease (obesity, smoking, familial history and hyperlipidemia, hypertension and diabetes) should be screened and referred appropriately during pregnancy.[157] In the maternity setting, symptoms of acute myocardial infarction or heart failure, such as clamminess, sweating, tachycardia, fatigue, anxiety, breathlessness and chest pain should not be dismissed without adequate investigation. Although 'breathlessness' may be a common symptom experienced by pregnant women, nocturnal dyspnoea, or breathlessness at rest, is not normal even in the pregnant context. Similarly, heartburn, fatigue and dependent oedema may also indicate cardiovascular compromise. Undertaking a comprehensive health history and asking specific questions about the nature of symptoms, along with a physical assessment, are of crucial importance in obtaining an adequate assessment and accurate diagnosis in the complex maternity patient.

Other cardiac conditions

Rarely, spontaneous aortic dissection and coronary artery dissection may occur in pregnant women with no pre-existing cardiac disease.[160] Signs and symptoms of heart failure and complaints of chest pain must be investigated and not put down to the 'minor discomforts' of pregnancy.

Given that the cardiac output is expected to increase 40–50% in a normal pregnancy, any cardiac condition resulting in poor left ventricular function and/or restricted left ventricular outflow is particularly associated with poor outcomes in pregnancy.

Also relevant for the outcome of both mother and baby is whether any valvular disease has been repaired and whether a tissue or mechanical valve has been inserted. Use of anticoagulants is of particular concern during pregnancy, with warfarin contraindicated for use in pregnancy. However, the risk of thrombosis is relatively high in pregnant women and some women are advised to remain on warfarin despite the risk of associated congenital anomaly and the increased likelihood of miscarriage.[161]

> ### Practice tip
>
> Congenital and acquired cardiac disease can present for the first time during pregnancy, unmasked by the additional physiological requirements of pregnancy. Women with known pre-existing disease may experience unpredictable deterioration in cardiac function.

Patient management

All women with cardiac disease are considered to have a 'high risk' pregnancy and should receive maternity care by a multidisciplinary team including, as a minimum, obstetrician, midwife, cardiologist and anaesthetist.[162] The timing and location of delivery, choice of anaesthesia and delivery mode should each be discussed by the team with the woman, and planned well in advance. If a pregnant woman with cardiac disease is admitted to ICU, this multidisciplinary team should be consulted about her care. Priorities of care include:

- Pre-pregnancy counselling – this should allow a full and frank discussion about the likely risks of pregnancy for the individual and a discussion of treatment path. This is of particular importance for women who are on potentially teratogenic medication, such as warfarin or ACE inhibitors, and for women who may benefit from surgery or interventional treatment prior to conceiving. Additionally, women with congenital heart disease may require genetic counselling to determine the likelihood of congenital heart disease in any offspring.

- Diagnosis – standard investigations including chest X-ray, ECG, CT scan and MRI should be attended to as indicated by the clinical condition. In general, diagnostic imaging of a critically ill woman should not be withheld due to concerns about the fetus, with abdominal shielding used whenever possible.[163]

- Heart failure – as was outlined in the section on peripartum cardiomyopathy, the principles of treatment for heart failure in pregnancy are the same as for the non-pregnant population.

- Arrhythmias – commonly used drugs include digoxin, lignocaine, flecainide, verapamil, sotalol, propranolol, adenosine and amiodarone; although limited studies exist in the pregnant population, all have been used safely and effectively during pregnancy.[164] Transient neonatal hypothyroidism has been described in women on amiodarone and monitoring of neonatal thyroid function is recommended.[165]

- Cardiac surgery – interventions such as valvuloplasty may be required. Open-heart surgery is only performed during pregnancy when the maternal condition is critical, for example coronary artery dissection or severe dysfunctioning valve, because of the high probability of fetal loss associated with the woman going on bypass. Standard care should be provided to a pregnant woman, with care to nurse the woman ≥20 weeks' gestation with a 15° left lateral tilt if possible, to reduce the negative effects of aortocaval compression. Open-heart surgery and ECMO have been used successfully in pregnant women with good outcomes for mother and baby.[166,167]

- Thrombus prevention – this is a priority in women with valvular disease/prosthetic valves, atrial fibrillation or dilated heart chambers at risk of thrombus formation, especially because of the normal hypercoagulopathy associated with pregnancy. Warfarin embryopathy, a recognised collection of developmental anomalies such as nasal hypoplasia and epiphysis stippling, is associated with warfarin use in the first trimester; consequently, warfarin use is contraindicated. However, pregnant women with mechanical valves experience unacceptably high rates of valve thrombosis and embolism when switched to heparin, and so many cardiologists consider the risks associated with the continued use of warfarin in pregnancy to be lower than the risks of stopping it. Therefore, a regimen that balances the risk of thrombosis with that of fetal loss or malformation and risk of haemorrhage should be implemented, with some variation of: stopping warfarin for the whole first trimester or from 6–12 weeks' gestation and then resuming until close to delivery; replacing warfarin with unfractionated or low-molecular-weight heparin for the whole pregnancy or continuing warfarin throughout pregnancy and replacing it with heparin for delivery only. Appropriate dosing schedules for heparin have not been confirmed with low-dose heparin considered inadequate and high doses of unfractionated heparin not researched.[168]

- Secondary prevention of rheumatic heart disease – monthly IM penicillin, e.g. 1,200,000 units of benzyl penicillin, to minimise repeat acute rheumatic fever and associated further valve degeneration.[155]

Practice tip

When caring for a pregnant woman with cardiac disease or post-cardiac surgery, differences in normal haemodynamic and respiratory parameters in pregnancy must be considered.

Asthma

Asthma is the most common chronic health disease in pregnant women, affecting 4–8% of all pregnancies in the USA.[169] However, the incidence in Australia may be higher given the higher prevalence, 12–14%, of 'current asthma' in women of childbearing age.[170]

Course of asthma during pregnancy

The course of asthma during pregnancy is highly variable. Approximately one-third of women experience an improvement in asthma symptoms, one-third report no change and one-third experience exacerbation of asthma during pregnancy.[171] Very severe exacerbations of asthma during pregnancy requiring ICU admission are rare. A persisting problem in pregnant women with asthma is the potential for reluctance to treat (by doctors) and decreased medication compliance (by women), based on concerns about the safety of medication during pregnancy, with a substantial number of asthma exacerbations in pregnancy associated with non-adherence to prescribed drugs.[172,173] Studies comparing medication use have shown that pregnant women are also less likely to be prescribed systemic corticosteroids than non-pregnant asthmatics.[172,174] The second and third trimesters are commonly the time when a worsening of asthma symptoms will develop, although women may have an improvement in symptoms for the last 4 weeks of a term pregnancy.[172]

Effect of asthma on pregnancy

The relationship between asthma in pregnancy and adverse maternal and neonatal outcomes including preeclampsia, gestational diabetes, small-for-gestational-age neonates and pre-term birth is inconsistent. The general belief is that poor maternal and neonatal outcomes are associated with poor asthma management and not a result of the treatment itself.[175]

Patient management

A pregnant woman admitted to ICU with asthma may be experiencing new-onset asthma or an exacerbation of pre-existing asthma. Regardless, the management and treatment priorities are the same. Accurate diagnosis and evaluation of the disease is necessary and should involve the advice of a thoracic medicine specialist and an obstetrician, who will continue the care of the woman once discharged from ICU. Methacholine testing, used as a diagnostic tool for asthma, is contraindicated in pregnancy.[176] Treatment of severe asthma in pregnancy is no different to the treatment in non-pregnant patients (see Chapter 14), apart from the additional needs to monitor fetal wellbeing and consider the normal respiratory parameters in pregnancy (Figure 28.2). Severe hypoxaemia places the fetus at risk and should be avoided; maternal SaO_2 should remain ≥95%. Peak flow measures are recommended to be used during pregnancy to assess and monitor the woman's condition, with the normal values unchanged in pregnancy.[175] The risks associated with current asthma medication use in pregnancy are far less than the risks associated with uncontrolled asthma, and the regular schedule of asthma medications should be prescribed in pregnancy according to asthma symptom level.[176] Likewise, none of the common drug categories,

FIGURE 28.2 Acute management of exacerbation of asthma in pregnancy.

Initial treatment for acute asthma exacerbation	Assess patient response	Further evaluation and care
1) Give supplemental inhaled oxygen to keep O_2 saturation >95%. 2) Administration of inhaled salbuterol via nebuliser driven by oxygen every 20 minutes, up to three doses in the first hour. 3) If no improvement (or if severe exacerbation) give IV or oral corticosteroids. 4) Continuous external fetal monitoring for those > 24 weeks gestation.	**Good response:** PEFR 70% or more and sustained for 60 minutes. Normal exam, no distress, reassuring fetal status.	Discharge to home.
	Incomplete response: PEFR 50-69%. Continued mild or moderate symptoms.	Continue to monitor, add ipratropium bromide. Continue oxygen and inhaled salbuterol. Individualise plan for further observation or hospitalisation. Consider systemic steroids.
	Poor response: PEFR less than 50%, pCO_2 > 40-42 mmHg.	Continue fetal assessment. Consult intensive care unit for admission. IV corticosteroids.

Adapted from Hardy-Fairbanks AJ, Baker ER. Asthma in pregnancy: pathophysiology, diagnosis and management. Obstet Gynecol Clin North Am 2010;37(2):159–72, with permission.

such as inhaled corticosteroids, long-acting beta-agonists and leukotriene-receptor antagonists, is contraindicated during lactation.[176]

Special considerations

Any health condition resulting in ICU admission may occur in a pregnant woman. The more common of these include physical trauma, pneumonia and mental health disorders, and these are described in detail below. Drug and substance misuse in pregnancy can have harmful effects upon the woman, and her fetus. Substance misuse is complex, and may be interrelated with other factors such as domestic violence and mental health conditions, particularly in pregnancy. Obtaining a health history from a woman in the ICU setting may be challenging. If substance misuse is suspected, a toxicology screen may be useful to ensure the woman receives suitable care, management, support and referral to appropriate services for the remainder of the pregnancy.[177]

Trauma in pregnancy

The term 'trauma' refers to any accidental or intentional event resulting in injury, with motor vehicle accidents, falls and domestic violence most prevalent among the pregnant trauma population. Pregnancy is considered a period of low risk for traumatic injury. However, women who engage in risk-taking behaviour, such as misuse of alcohol and other substances, experience more injury.[178] Overall, the incidence of trauma in pregnancy is estimated to be in the range of 5–8% of all pregnancies, with motor vehicle accidents responsible for about half and falls and assaults accounting for roughly one-quarter each.[179,180]

Specific causes of injury in pregnant women include:

- Domestic violence – for women who experience domestic violence, 30% occurs for the first time during pregnancy; homicide during pregnancy and the postpartum period also occurs and intentional violence by an intimate partner is a relatively common reason for presentation to the emergency department.[26] The 'story' of the injury should be considered in relation to the presenting injury and likely mechanism of injury; another potential sign is when the woman appears evasive or reluctant to speak or disagree in front of her partner.[26] Pregnancy-related violence is associated with low-birth-weight babies, premature labour and fetal trauma.[181]

- Musculoskeletal injuries – pregnancy hormones affect joints and ligaments, making them more lax and pliable. This explains why pregnant women are more likely to experience joint injury, pelvic instability, back pain and strained and dislocated joints. The altered centre of gravity caused by the enlarged maternal abdomen explains why pregnant women readily fall off ladders, for example, when decorating the nursery.

- Motor vehicle trauma – is the most common reason for a pregnant woman to present to an emergency department with trauma. Unfortunately, some pregnant women believe there is no legal requirement to wear a seatbelt when pregnant and this places them and their fetus at increased risk.[182] Additionally, many pregnant women are not informed on the correct positioning of a seatbelt during pregnancy, and incorrect positioning can increase the likelihood of placental abruption in a crash (Figure 28.3).

Trauma in pregnancy presents a number of challenges; overwhelmingly, the single principle of management is to treat the mother.[183] Trauma assessment of the pregnant woman should include all the usual elements (see Chapter 24) with the following additional components.

Initial evaluation of the pregnant patient: the primary survey

Consideration should be given to all women of child-bearing age as to whether they may be pregnant.[184] If the woman is obviously pregnant, a rough estimate of gestation can be made by measuring the height of the fundus from the symphysis pubis. The height in cm roughly equates to the number of weeks' gestation, e.g. 22 cm = 22 weeks' gestation. The presence of fetal movement is a quick assessment of fetal wellbeing and, if the woman is conscious and over 18–20 weeks' gestation, she should be able to feel fetal movements. The physiological adaptations of pregnancy may initially mask serious injury, with vital signs and patient symptoms not reflective of the underlying injuries.[182] A pregnant woman's condition can rapidly deteriorate.

Use of imaging in pregnancy

All radiological investigations and imaging that are clinically indicated by the maternal condition should be attended to without delay over concerns for the fetus.[182]

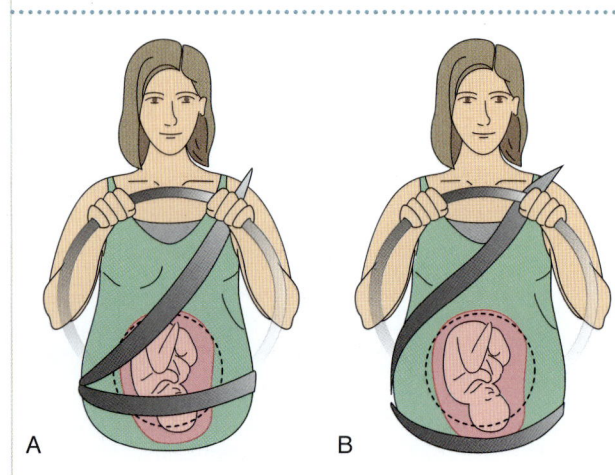

FIGURE 28.3 Positioning of a seatbelt during pregnancy. **A**, Incorrect positioning; **B**, correct positioning.

When possible and appropriate, a pelvic/abdominal lead shield may be used to protect the developing embryo/fetus. If a chest tube is necessary for a haemothorax, care should be taken to position the catheter 1–2 spaces higher than normal due to the raised diaphragm.

Obstetric assessment in trauma

If the woman's gestation is estimated to be 24 weeks or more, cardiotocography (CTG) should be conducted to assess fetal wellbeing (see the section on fetal assessment). If there has been any likelihood of blunt trauma to the abdomen (i.e. by the steering wheel or seatbelt position), a continuous 4-hour duration CTG should be done to identify any fetal distress resulting from a potential placental abruption.[184] An abdominal ultrasound is commonly done to assess fetal wellbeing and to identify any trauma to the fetus. Ultrasound is also useful in detecting free peritoneal fluid and maternal haemorrhage and may assist in the diagnosis of placental abruption.[182] The possibility of uterine rupture should also be considered even though it is rare (<1% of pregnant trauma patients).[182] Also remember that the bladder becomes an abdominal organ after 12 weeks' gestation and is more prone to traumatic injury.

Potential for perimortem caesarean section

If the woman is ≥20 weeks' gestation, perimortem caesarean section should be considered early if the woman requires resuscitation. If there is no response to effective CPR after 4 minutes, a perimortem caesarean section should be undertaken.[184] Preparations should be commenced (i.e. call the obstetric team) as soon as CPR commences.

Pneumonia

Pneumonia in pregnancy is one of the more common reasons why a pregnant woman may be admitted to ICU. Although studies have shown that pregnant women are not more likely to contract pneumonia, the severity of pneumonia experienced by women in these studies has not been well examined.[185] It is not known whether the ICU admission rate for pneumonia is higher in the pregnant population as opposed to the hospitalisation rate. Anecdotally, it is rare for a well woman of childbearing age to be admitted to ICU with community-acquired pneumonia; women living in disabled support accommodation and pregnant women are the exception. Varicella pneumonia is also more prominent in the pregnant population. It would appear from studies on pregnant admissions to ICU and maternal death reports that severe community-acquired pneumonia in previously well women is a persisting concern in the pregnant population.

It is not fully understood why pregnant women may be vulnerable to severe pneumonia though the adaptations to the mechanics of breathing and changes in the immune response may be contributing factors.[185] Additionally, it has been postulated that pregnant women are among

small children more often and may have an increased likelihood of exposure to infective agents. The treatment and management of pneumonia in pregnancy is no different to pneumonia in non-pregnant women: identify the causative organism and administer appropriate antibiotics/antiviral agents as indicated, maintain oxygenation and prevent complications (see Chapter 15). Assessment of fetal wellbeing and awareness of the changed respiratory parameters in pregnancy are the obvious additional requirements.

Pregnancy and influenza

WHO has recommended that all pregnant women receive the seasonal influenza vaccination since 2006, in recognition of the known increased risk that influenza poses during pregnancy and because vaccination during pregnancy is safe and confers immunity to the newborn for the first few vulnerable months. In developing countries, this policy has the potential to save the lives of many women and, in particular, their babies. In developed countries, maternal death caused by seasonal influenza is rare. However, the pandemic influenza, H1N1 09 (referred to as 'swine flu'), which swept across the world in 2009, demonstrated how vulnerable pregnant women are to influenza and emphasised the importance of influenza vaccination to prevent severe disease.

The H1N1 2009 flu epidemic killed seven pregnant/postpartum women in Australia and New Zealand in 3 months.[186] Over 60 women were admitted to ICU and a number of their babies died. Women in the second half of pregnancy were over 13 times more likely to be admitted to ICU with H1N1 influenza than non-pregnant women of child-bearing age. Pregnant and postpartum women admitted to ICU with H1N1 influenza were particularly unwell, with 14% of women requiring ECMO.[187]

Mental health disorders

Mental health disorders during pregnancy and the postpartum consist of women with pre-existing disease and women who develop signs and symptoms of mental health disease for the first time. The mental health disorder may be separate from the pregnancy or there may be a relationship between the pregnancy and the development of the disorder, such as postnatal depression.

Pre-existing mental health disorders

The underlying principles of management of pregnant women with a pre-existing mental health disorder are the same as for non-pregnant women: safety of the woman, stabilisation of the mental illness and empowerment of, and support for, the woman to make her own choices. A considerable additional challenge is maintaining stability of the mental health disorder if changes to medication are required due to potential teratogenesis or contraindication for use during pregnancy. Generally speaking, if the indication for treatment is unchanged, treatment should be continued during pregnancy.[188]

Pregnant women with pre-existing mental health disorders may require admission to ICU due to acute deterioration in their mental health. This is most likely to be as a result of cessation or alteration of their regular medications.[189,190] Most relapses occur in the first trimester and many women who initially stop their medication recommence it during the pregnancy.[189] Routine care should be provided as clinically indicated, keeping in mind the additional requirements to monitor fetal wellbeing, conduct standard antenatal assessment and consider the impact of the physiological adaptations on treatments.

Mental health disorders related to pregnancy

Suicide related to unwanted pregnancy remains a cause of maternal death in developed countries, especially in adolescents and in women from cultures where childbirth outside of marriage is unacceptable.[54] Depression may arise during pregnancy (antenatal depression) although it is more likely to present during the postpartum (postpartum depression). The most severe mental health disorder related to pregnancy is puerperal psychosis.

Puerperal psychosis

Puerperal psychosis is a rare mental health complication of pregnancy, said to occur in 1/1000 births, though the incidence seems to be falling with a recent incidence of 0.19/1000 deliveries reported.[191,192] The majority of cases occur in women with pre-existing mental illness, such as bipolar disorder, with just 0.03/1000 deliveries occurring in women with no pre-existing mental health disorder.[192] It usually presents within 2 weeks postpartum and is associated with an increased risk of suicide and infanticide.[193] Women with puerperal psychosis are frequently delusional, suffer hallucinations and require acute hospitalisation for treatment.

Postpartum depression

Postnatal depression is defined as a non-psychotic depressive illness; most definitions specify occurrence within 3 months postpartum although some specify a shorter period of only 1 month.[194,195] Risk factors include prior mental illness, poor social supports, relationship disharmony and recent life events.[194] Depression in the postpartum period raises treatment issues for the nursing mother and the developing infant.[194]

Early diagnosis and effective treatment is indicated. Self-harm in the first 12 months postpartum is a severe concern for women with serious depression. Care in the ICU is no different to that provided to other patients admitted with severe depression. Postnatal depression is not a contraindication to lactation, although some medication may be contraindicated. Medication should be prescribed as warranted on clinical grounds and may include antidepressants, hormonal treatment and psychological treatments.

Caring for pregnant women in ICU

Any pregnant woman in ICU is considered to be carrying an 'at-risk' fetus. This means that fetal wellbeing may be compromised and that he/she is at risk of sustaining injury/suboptimal growth and development or death in utero. There are circumstances when the woman's clinical status would improve by delivery of the fetus, and times when the fetus needs to be delivered to increase the likelihood of its own survival. Consideration of both the maternal condition and fetal wellbeing contributes to the decision on when to deliver a fetus. Delivery prior to 24 weeks' gestation is only an option if the maternal condition is very critical and considered necessary to potentially save the woman's life; it is likely that the neonate's care in this instance would be palliative. Even though about half of babies born <24 weeks survive, they do so with a far higher risk of permanent disability.[196] Once gestation reaches 28 weeks, the neonate has more than a 90% chance of survival when cared for in a neonatal intensive care unit.[196]

Childbirth is a highly significant event in many cultures with associated specific practices and beliefs. These practices vary widely and, in particular, may relate to the pregnant woman, the birth event, the placenta, breastfeeding and the postpartum period.[197] For general principles on culturally sensitive care see Chapter 8.

Obesity in pregnancy is associated with adverse outcomes for both the mother and the baby, with a dose-dependent relationship: the higher the BMI, the higher the likelihood of adverse outcomes.[198] This includes a nearly four-fold increased likelihood of admission to ICU for women with a BMI >50.[199] See Chapter 6 for general principles of caring for bariatric patients. From the maternity perspective, obesity in pregnancy poses difficulties in caring for women including: determining fetal wellbeing, assessment of gestation and monitoring the progress of labour and increased incidences of preeclampsia and gestational diabetes.[198] Additionally, thromboprophylaxis should be considered early given the increased risk of thrombosis in pregnancy/postpartum, which is magnified further in obese women.

Mechanical ventilation of the pregnant woman

The provision of mechanical ventilation to a pregnant woman occurs rarely and there is very little evidence to guide practice. Pregnancy is considered a 'high risk airway' with the reported 'failure to intubate' rate about 1 in 250,[200] approximately eight times more likely than in the non-pregnant population. The physiological changes of pregnancy that contribute to the increased difficulty in intubation have already been described. Nasal intubation is not usually an option for pregnant women due to the risk of epistaxis. Women with preeclampsia may also have substantial pharyngeal oedema.

The principles of mechanical ventilation in pregnancy are the same as those for the non-obstetric population (see Chapter 15) with additional considerations as follows:

- Ensure target end points reflect the normal ABGs for pregnancy.
- A small reduction in maternal oxygenation can severely impact on fetal oxygenation because of the left shift in the oxyhaemoglobin dissociation curve associated with fetal haemoglobin.[201]
- Permissive hypercapnia has not been evaluated in pregnancy (remember that fetal carbon dioxide is higher than the maternal level, given the gradient across the placental membrane).
- Normal tidal volumes in pregnancy are increased by up to 40–50% of non-pregnant values, although the mechanical provision of these larger tidal volumes with respect to volutrauma has not been examined; in practice, often respiratory rate is increased first and then increases in tidal volume are only used when necessary.[109]
- A nurse caring for a ventilated pregnant patient should be alert to any patient restlessness or increasing sedation requirements and ask for midwifery assistance to assess for the onset of labour.

Other, less common, methods to support gas exchange have been reported in the literature in the form of case studies. Of note, nitrous oxide, hyperbaric oxygen treatment and extracorporeal membrane oxygenators have all been used successfully to treat acute conditions, such as pulmonary embolism, in pregnant women.[202–204]

Practice tip

Remember that pregnancy is associated with a poor tolerance of short-term apnoea, for example during induction of anaesthesia and/or intubation, and pre-oxygenation is important.

Practice tip

Medical staff with experience in the management of a pregnant or difficult airway should be present when a pregnant woman is intubated.

Fetal assessment

Assessment of fetal wellbeing in ICU presents a number of challenges. Most notable is that many pregnant women in ICU receive sedative medication that has the effect of sedating the fetus. The standard methods for monitoring and assessing fetal wellbeing include presence of fetal movements, continuous CTG monitoring, intermittent auscultation of the fetal heart rate, ultrasounds and fetal biophysical profiles. These assessments are based on the pattern and rate of the fetal heartbeat, the breathing and swallowing action of the fetus in utero, the volume of amniotic fluid and on fetal movements.[205] Uterine artery Doppler flow measurements have also proven useful.[206,207] Critical illness and its treatment induce circumstances that make it difficult to interpret these tests of fetal wellbeing with any certainty; for example, morphine decreases the biophysical profile of the fetus.[208] With fetal mortality in pregnant women admitted to ICU as high as 20%,[8,13] the assessment of fetal wellbeing during maternal critical illness is of prime importance, in part to optimise timing of delivery.

FIGURE 28.4 Normal CTG trace. FHR = fetal heart rate; UA = uterine activity.

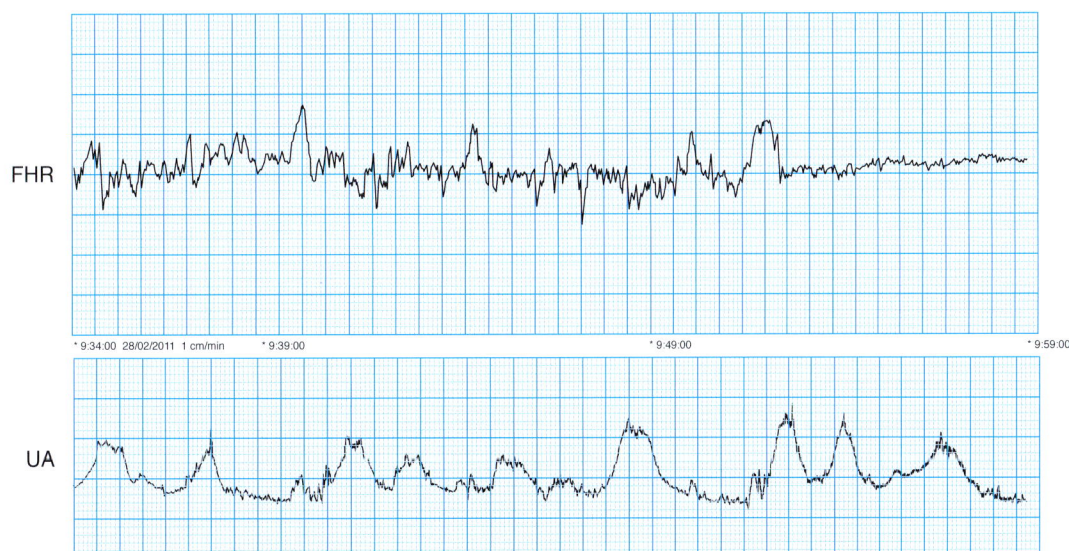

Cardiotocograph

Cardiotocographs (CTGs) consist of two pieces of information: a Doppler recording fetal heart rate pattern and a pressure transducer detecting uterine muscle contraction. Both elements are recorded on a timed graph so that one may consider the fetal response to uterine contraction (Figure 28.4). Thus, CTGs provide information about the fetal heart rate and whether there is any uterine contraction. A normal fetal heart rate is 110–160 beats/min with variability in the rate. Details of the patient's condition and treatment and the date and time the recording was taken should be documented on the trace. Many tertiary obstetric hospitals offer a CTG interpretation service for general hospitals without maternity staff to assist with interpretation of CTGs. A CTG provides superior information to an intermittent fetal heart rate (by stethoscope or Doppler) and should be used when possible. The required frequency and duration of a CTG recording will vary according to clinical condition. For example, suspected placental abruption following blunt trauma may require 4 hours of continuous monitoring. A CTG is recommended during and following elective cardioversion and any other major procedure. CTGs are usually only indicated if the fetus is >24 weeks' gestation and there is the potential to act on adverse findings, such as emergency delivery. The CTG is an indication of fetal wellbeing at the time the trace is recorded and the fetal condition can change rapidly according to changes in maternal condition.

Ultrasound

An ultrasound is able to measure core components of fetal anatomy, such as head circumference and femur length, to determine fetal size as well as quantify adequacy of amniotic fluid volume. Thus, ultrasound is used to consider adequacy of fetal growth in relation to the gestation and is a component of the biophysical profile regarding fetal movement and swallowing patterns. Serial ultrasounds, e.g. weekly, are used to monitor adequate fetal growth and would be a helpful adjunct to the care of a pregnant woman in ICU with a long-term problem, such as Guillain–Barré syndrome.

Practice tip

There is a legal requirement in both Australia and New Zealand for all births to be registered with the Registry of Births, Deaths and Marriages. A birth in both countries is defined as the delivery of a baby of at least 20 weeks' gestation or, if gestation is unknown, weighing at least 400 g, who is either live born or stillborn.[209,210]

Adapted with permission from:

New Zealand Health Information Service. Report on Maternity 2010. Wellington: Ministry of Health; 2012

Li Z, Zeki R, Hilder L, Sullivan EA. Australia's mothers and babies 2011. Perinatal statistics series no. 28. Cat. no. PER 59. Canberra: AIHW National Perinatal Epidemiology and Statistics Unit; 2013.

Preparation for pre-term birth

If it becomes apparent that the woman is likely to give birth, i.e. has gone into pre-term labour or the maternal condition deteriorates and the decision is made to deliver the baby pre-term, pre-planning is required to improve neonatal outcome.

Enhancement of newborn lung function

Women likely to give birth prior to 35 weeks' gestation are normally prescribed two doses of betamethasone (11.4 mg IM), 24 hours apart, to promote fetal lung maturity and surfactant production.[211] A significant reduction in rates of neonatal death, respiratory distress syndrome and intraventricular haemorrhage results from antenatal corticosteroid administration with the best effects seen when birth occurs more than 24 hours but less than 7 days after the second dose.[211] However, birth should not be delayed to fulfill any time requirement related to steroid administration if the birth circumstances are urgent. Some benefit is seen even if birth occurs < 24 hours after a single dose.[211]

Fetal neuroprotection

Magnesium sulfate administration to a woman <30–32 weeks' gestation with a viable fetus, who is considered likely to give birth in the following 24 hours, has been shown to reduce the likelihood of cerebral palsy developing in the infant.[212] A common regimen is 4 g IV loading dose over 20–30 minutes followed by a continuous infusion at 1 g/h for 24 hours or until birth (whichever is sooner).[212] However, the 'best' dosage regimen has not been determined.[213] Magnesium sulfate for neuroprotection has been adopted as standard practice[214] though it is important not to delay emergency birth in order to facilitate magnesium treatment.

Modifications to basic and advanced life support

Generally speaking, all standard basic and advanced life support algorithms can be used with only minor adaptations for the pregnant and postpartum woman (see Box 28.9).[215] For women over 20 weeks' gestation, the sheer bulk of the uterus and contents impairs any ability to obtain adequate circulation using cardiac compressions; therefore left lateral displacement of the uterus is necessary. Regardless, it is very difficult to obtain adequate perfusion during CPR of an obviously pregnant woman and arrangements should be made for an emergency caesarean section, as soon as resuscitation commences. A caesarean section should proceed if there is no response to 4 minutes of CPR. Expect a difficult intubation and try to have an experienced person intubate the trachea. Finally, consider the list of obstetric conditions that may have precipitated the arrest and provide any specific appropriate treatment. Cardiac arrest in pregnancy is a rare event and the chance of a successful resuscitation is about the same as a non-pregnant arrest.

BOX 28.9

Maternal cardiac arrest algorithm[215]

First responder:

- Activate cardiac arrest team, e.g. Code Blue and note time.
- Place the woman supine.
- Commence chest compressions as per standard BLS algorithm. Place hands slightly higher on the sternum than usual due to raised diaphragm.

Subsequent responders:

- Apply standard BLS and ALS algorithms.
- Commence documentation of cardiac arrest management, e.g. time of onset.
- Do not delay defibrillation.
- Give standard ALS drugs and doses.
- Use 100% oxygen.
- Monitor effectiveness of ventilation and CPR quality.
- Provide the standard post-arrest care.

Maternal modifications:

- Start IV above the diaphragm.
- Assess for hypovolaemia and treat appropriately but cautiously.
- Anticipate a difficult airway.
- If the woman is on a magnesium infusion, cease and consider administration of calcium chloride 10 mL in 10% solution or calcium gluconate 30 mL in 10% solution to treat hypermagnesaemia.

- Continue all elements of resuscitation effort during and after caesarean section.

Women with an obviously gravid uterus, e.g. >20 weeks' gestation:

- To relieve aortocaval compression and enable more effective CPR, manually displace the uterus towards the left.
  - Alternatively, use a wedge to position the woman in a left lateral tilt.
- Remove any internal or external fetal monitors if present.
- Prepare for a potential emergency caesarean section.
- Call for immediate obstetrician attendance when the arrest is activated.
- Aim for delivery within 5 minutes of onset of resuscitative efforts.

Consider and treat any possible contributing factors:

- Haemorrhage with or without DIC.
- Assess for placental abruption/praevia and uterine atony if the woman is postpartum.
- Embolism, e.g. pulmonary, amniotic fluid.
- Anaesthetic complications, e.g. high spinal block.
- Cardiac disease, e.g. pre-existing or new.
- Preeclampsia.
- Sepsis.

Adapted from Vanden Hoek TL, Morrison, LJ, Shuster M, Donnino M, Sinz E, Lavonas EJ et al. Part 12: Cardiac arrest in special situations: 2010 American Heart Association guidelines for cardiopulmonary resuscitation and emergency cardiovascular care. Circulation 2010;122(18 Suppl 3):S829–61.

Prevention of rhesus disease

During pregnancy, a small amount of fetal blood can enter the maternal circulation. If the mother is Rh-negative and the fetus is Rh-positive, the mother produces antibodies against the rhesus D antigen on her baby's red blood cells. During this, and subsequent, pregnancies the anti-D antibodies are able to pass across the placenta to the fetus and, if the level is sufficient, cause destruction of rhesus D-positive fetal red blood cells, leading to the development of rhesus disease. The disease ranges from mild to severe, and the consequences for the fetus can include varying degrees of anaemia, hydrops fetalis or ultimately stillbirth. Management of rhesus disease is outlined in Table 28.9.

Most rhesus disease can be prevented by treating the Rh-negative mother during pregnancy or promptly (within 72 hours) post childbirth.[216] The mother is given an intramuscular injection of 500 IU of anti-D immunoglobulin,

which destroys any Rh D-positive fetal red blood cells in her circulation before the maternal immune system can discover them and produce antibodies. This is passive immunity and the effect of the immunity will diminish post injection at around 4 to 6 weeks. Anti-D immunoglobulin is used to prevent the development of anti-D antibodies and is of no use once the antibodies are present. Administration of 625 IU of anti-D immunoglobulin to all rhesus D-negative pregnant women at 28 and 34 weeks is now routine care, even in the absence of any vaginal bleeding, and also within 72 hours following birth.[216]

Practice tip

The dose of anti-D immunoglobulin depends on the amount of fetal blood cells detected in the maternal blood using the Kleihauer-Betke test. The more fetal cells present, the higher the dose of anti-D required.

TABLE 28.9

Management of rhesus disease

BLOOD TESTS AND MANAGEMENT	RATIONALE
Kleihauer-Betke test or flow cytometry	Confirms that fetal blood has passed into the maternal circulation, also estimates the amount of fetal blood that has passed into the maternal circulation
Indirect Coombs test	Screens maternal blood for anti-D antibodies that may pass through the placenta and cause haemolytic disease of the newborn
FETAL BLOOD (OR UMBILICAL CORD BLOOD) TESTS	
Direct Coombs test	Confirms that maternal anti-D antibodies are present in the fetal/newborn circulation
Full blood count	Specifically, the haemoglobin level and platelet count to assess for anaemia
Bilirubin	Both total and indirect
ANTENATAL CARE	
Serial ultrasound and Doppler examinations	Detect signs of fetal anaemia such as increased blood flow velocities and monitor hydrops fetalis
Quantitative analysis of maternal anti-Rh D antibodies	An increasing titre level suggests fetal rhesus disease
Intrauterine blood transfusion	Blood transfused into fetal umbilical vein, method of choice since the late 1980s, more effective than intraperitoneal transfusion
Early delivery	Usually post 36 weeks' gestation
POSTNATAL CARE	
Phototherapy for neonatal jaundice in mild disease	Converts fat-soluble unconjugated bilirubin to water-soluble bilirubin that can be excreted by the newborn
Newborn exchange transfusion	Used if the neonate has moderate or severe disease; the blood for transfusion must be less than a week old, Rh negative, ABO compatible with both the fetus and the mother and be cross-matched against the mother's serum

Glucose management in pregnancy

Pregnancy is associated with changes to carbohydrate and fat metabolism in order to provide adequate nutrients to the fetus during pregnancy. Some of the pregnancy hormones, such as human placental lactogen, contribute to a progressive insulin resistance as the hormone levels increase throughout the pregnancy. Of practical importance, glucose readily crosses the placenta while insulin does not. If the mother has persistently high glucose levels, from either pre-existing diabetes or gestational diabetes, the fetus may be large for gestational age (macrosomic) and the fetus may develop hyperinsulinaemia. Additionally, hyperglycaemia is associated with poor obstetric and neonatal outcomes including birth trauma, caesarean birth, preeclampsia, newborn respiratory distress syndrome and stillbirth.[217] Recommended capillary blood glucose level targets for women with diabetes are <5.0 mmol/L fasting and <6.7 mmol/L 2 hours after a meal.[218] Although hyperglycaemia is associated with adverse obstetric and neonatal outcomes, hypoglycaemia should also be avoided.

Sepsis associated with pregnancy

Maternal sepsis can occur at any time during pregnancy and postpartum and from any cause. Common obstetric-related events include termination of pregnancy, spontaneous miscarriage, prolonged rupture of membranes, caesarean and vaginal birth and mastitis, and non-obstetric-related events include urinary tract infection and pyelonephritis, and respiratory tract infection. The most common organism responsible for maternal sepsis resulting in death is Lancefield group A *Streptococcus* (also known as *Streptococcus pyogenes*).[26] Notable in the review of maternal deaths from sepsis is the rapidity with which some women succumbed. The septic course is often insidious and women may appear deceptively well before suddenly collapsing, often with little or no warning.[26] Although there is no research evaluating the Surviving Sepsis Campaign guidelines in the maternity setting, they are recommended for use.[26,219] Management of sepsis is described in Chapter 21.

Medication administration in pregnancy

Many drugs used in the critical care environment have not been researched for safe use in pregnant or lactating mothers. There are two key periods when consideration of drug therapy is paramount: during the first trimester when embryo/fetal malformations may occur and immediately prior to delivery as the newborn baby may be adversely affected, e.g. sedated and unable to spontaneously breathe. The decision to administer various medications is often a balance between the benefit of administering the drug to the pregnant woman and the risk of not administering the drug.

There are a number of anatomical, physiological, cellular and molecular changes in pregnancy that affect the pharmacokinetic and pharmacodynamic mechanisms of drugs administered during pregnancy.[220] These include reduced serum protein levels (reduced protein binding capacity), increased circulating volume (potential for dilution), delayed gut motility (potential for increased gut absorption), increased glomerular filtration rate (potential for increased excretion) and changes to maternal drug-metabolising enzymes (difficult to predict metabolism pattern of regular drugs).[221] Medication may be classified according to the likelihood for teratogenesis; however, there may be little understanding about efficacy in pregnancy. Standard adult doses may be inadequate or toxic during pregnancy due to the adapted physiology of pregnancy.[220]

Potential for teratogenesis

A teratogen is any agent that increases the incidence of a congenital anomaly.[14] The major organs are developed by 10 weeks' gestation; however, the recommendation is to avoid any teratogenic drug throughout the first trimester (14 weeks).[14] Some medications exert an adverse effect in the second or third trimesters of pregnancy, such as ACE inhibitors (fetal anuria and stillbirth), indomethacin (potential premature closure of the ductus arteriosus) and selective serotonin uptake inhibitors (neonatal withdrawal syndrome).[14] Medical staff prescribing drugs and nursing staff administering them should each check the potential impact of the medication in pregnancy, and consult a pharmacist when possible.

Immediately prior to delivery

Apart from effects on the structural development of the fetus in the first trimester, the other key time for consideration of drug administration is immediately prior to delivery. Common sedative agents such as midazolam, morphine, fentanyl and propofol cross the placenta readily and exert an action on the fetus.[222–224] Consequently, even mature term babies may be born sedated and require assistance with breathing. Planning for delivery of a pregnant woman in ICU should include the involvement of a paediatrician/neonatologist or the local newborn emergency transport service (NETS) if no paediatricians are on site.

Therapeutic routine drug therapy in pregnancy

For women admitted to ICU for prolonged periods of time, for example those with Guillain–Barré syndrome, consideration may be given to routine therapeutic medication in pregnancy. For example, folic acid (400 mcg daily) is recommended pre-conception and throughout the first trimester to prevent neural tube defects.[14] Similarly, iron and vitamin D supplementation may be indicated dependent on blood levels. Vitamin D deficiency is common, yet often unrecognised in critically ill patients.[225] Maternal vitamin D deficiency is associated with childhood asthma and increased risk of osteoporotic fracture in their offspring.[226,227] Due attention should be paid to a pregnant woman's nutritional status in ICU as poor nutrition during pregnancy is associated with many poor birth outcomes and pregnancy is associated with increased nutritional requirements.[228]

Caring for postpartum women in ICU

Women admitted to ICU during the postpartum phase are often separated from their newborn, possibly even transferred to another hospital, and may not even set eyes on their child for days, until they are discharged from ICU.[4] Specific care that should be provided to the postpartum woman includes observations, assistance to establish lactation as required and support for the mother by early nurturing of a mother–infant bond. Finally, attention to the psychological needs of both the woman and her partner is an important part of care.

Routine postpartum observations

Ongoing surveillance of a postpartum woman is essential in addition to any ad hoc visits provided by a midwife. Routine maternity observations include assessment of the fundus, PV loss and perineum, assessment of the breasts and nipples, consideration of deep vein thrombosis and thromboprophylaxis and evaluation of her psychological wellbeing and transition to motherhood (see Box 28.10).

Uterine involution

The term 'involution' means the return of the uterus to its normal size, tone and position. The vagina, ligaments of the uterus and muscles of the pelvic floor also return to their pre-pregnant state during the involution process. During this process, the lining of the uterus is cast off in the lochia, more commonly referred to as PV loss, and is later replaced by the new endometrium. Following birth, and post expulsion of the placenta, the muscles of the uterus

---

BOX 28.10

Routine postnatal observations

- Examination of breasts, looking for signs of engorgement, mastitis, cracked nipples
- Height, depth and texture of fundus, to ensure involution is happening
- Lochia, inspection of PV loss
- Examination of perineum/wound for signs of healing
- Examination for signs of deep vein thrombosis; thromboprophylaxis is often indicated in a postpartum ICU woman
- Micturition and bowels; to ensure bowel and urinary pattern returning to normal

constrict the blood vessels, so the blood circulating within the uterus is dramatically decreased. Redundant muscle, fibrous and elastic tissue is disposed of – the phagocytes of the blood stream deal with this – but the process is usually incomplete and some elastic tissue remains. So a uterus that has once been pregnant will never return fully to its pre-pregnant state.

The rate of involution is measured by the rate of descent of the uterine fundus (the top of the uterus) in relation to either the belly button or the symphysis pubis. Important markers include:

- At day 1 postnatal, the height of the fundus is usually at the belly button.
- There is a steady decrease in size of around 1 cm per day.
- As the uterus reduces, it also recedes and is deeper to palpate.
- By postnatal day 7, the fundal height is often only 2–3 cm above the symphysis pubis and by day 10 it is usually not palpable at the symphysis pubis.
- The rate of involution is slower in multiparity women or if there is an infection present or retained placental tissue/clots.

A normally contracted uterus is very hard; as you palpate the fundus to locate the top and feel the texture of the uterus, you cannot push your fingertip into the tissue of the uterus. A so-called boggy uterus is one that is not contracted properly and the fundus does not feel very hard on palpation. Reasons for a 'boggy uterus' include uterine atony, retained tissue/membrane/clot or a full bladder that is impeding the uterine nerve stimulus to contract. The uterus responds well to tactile stimulation, and the first treatment for a 'boggy uterus' is to 'rub-up' the fundus. This involves palpating the top of the uterus and literally giving it a rub. The uterus will usually respond and you will feel it tighten and become harder. Such an action may result in a small gush of PV loss. On some occasions, an uterotonic, a drug that causes the uterus to contract, may be needed to ensure the uterus is contracting properly. If the uterus does not contract properly, the vessels that fed the placental bed will not be closed off by the uterine muscle contraction (called the living ligature) and the woman will continue to bleed.

Practice tip

Uterotonics, drugs that cause the uterus to contract, are usually stored in the refrigerator. For example, syntocinon, syntometrine.

Practice tip

Many midwives document fundal height by finger widths in relation to the belly button. For example, two finger widths below the belly button would be notated by 2F ↓⊙.

Lochia and perineal care

The changes in the appearance of the lochia are described in three stages: lochia rubra, lochia serosa and lochia alba.[229] Lochia rubra consists of blood coming chiefly from the placental site. Three or 4 days post-delivery the lochia changes to a brownish colour and is called lochia serosa. Seven days post-delivery the lochia again changes to yellowish in appearance; this is called lochia alba. Normal lochia is not offensive in odour. Offensive lochia with or without maternal pyrexia may indicate a uterine infection. High and low vaginal swabs for culture and sensitivity, and the commencement of antibiotic cover, should be initiated. Offensive lochia coupled with a high non-involuting (and boggy) uterus may require ultrasound to exclude retained placental tissue. An infected placental site may result in a secondary postpartum haemorrhage.

Regular assessment of the PV loss is required in the early postpartum phase. Generally, this includes 1–2-hourly checks if the PV loss is relatively heavy (pad soaked within 1–2 hours) for the first day, progressing to 4-hourly checks on day 2, with further reductions in observation frequency based on clinical condition. Check the fundus and PV loss regularly enough to detect any excessive blood loss or loss of uterine tone. The colour and volume of PV loss is usually documented along with any pad changes. Weighing pads to determine PV loss is preferable to describing the loss as 'mild', 'moderate' or 'severe'.

The perineum should also be examined twice a day, even for women that have had a caesarean birth. A vulval haematoma or varicosities may have formed and require attention. For women that have had a vaginal birth, check the perineum to see if there was any tear or episiotomy at delivery. If there is a tear or any sutures, make sure to keep the region clean and observe for signs of infection or wound dehiscence. Ice packs applied to the perineum may help with any swelling and discomfort.

Increased potential for deep vein thrombosis

All postpartum women have an increased likelihood for deep vein thrombosis (DVT). Most postpartum women admitted to ICU would fulfil the criteria that recommend medical thromboprophylaxis. Routine postpartum care involves examining the legs for signs of DVT and appropriate use of thromboembolic stockings, sequential compression devices and thromboprophylaxis as required (see www.rcog.org.uk for more details).[33]

Breast care and breastfeeding

A woman's breasts and nipples should be assessed once a shift to assess their condition and identify signs of complications, such as mastitis. Assess all women, regardless of whether they intend to breastfeed or not. The breasts are usually soft although, as the milk comes in, they may become engorged; hot, hard or lumpy in places; and tender to touch. A reddened localised region may be indicative of mastitis and require treatment with antibiotics. The nipples should be inspected for damage if the woman is using a breast pump or breastfeeding. Hand expressing should not damage or crack the nipples whereas uneven or strong machine suction pressure can cause trauma. Colostrum (or milk once it has come in) may leak from the nipples and can be rubbed gently over the nipples to promote healthy tissue.

Initiation and establishment of lactation

The establishment and maintenance of lactation is a hormone-mediated process. The physiological trigger for the establishment of lactation is a fall in progesterone combined with maintained levels of prolactin and cortisol.[230] In the initial postnatal period colostrum is produced. The normal timing for milk to 'come in' is between 3 and 4 days post-delivery,[231] although establishment and 'coming in' of breast milk may be delayed in critically ill women. Additionally, the drug dopamine may hinder lactation, as it inhibits prolactin secretion.[232] It is not likely that the severity of maternal illness plays much of a role in the initial capacity to produce milk; anecdotally, 100 mL of breast milk has been expressed 4-hourly from a postpartum woman on ECMO. The initial regularity of hand expression and milk removal provide the stimulus to produce milk.

For women who prefer to breastfeed the infant, reasonable attempts to support this decision should be made. Most women make a decision regarding infant feeding either before becoming pregnant or during the first trimester and, in all pregnant women, the breasts have developed and are capable of producing milk from 22 weeks onwards.[233,234]

There is some debate regarding how crucial the first 24–48 hours are for the successful establishment of lactation.[235,236] In many cultures, colostrum is considered poisonous and breastfeeding is withheld until after 48 hours, and so clearly the absence of breast stimulation in the first 48 hours does not prohibit the establishment of lactation.[237] Hand expressing is recommended for the first few days until the milk 'comes in', and then to start and finish each expressing episode along with the use of a breast pump (see Box 28.11 for principles and Figure 28.5 for process). It is not uncommon for only a few drops of colostrum to be expressed each time in the first couple of days.[238] It is believed that even a small total expressed volume of 5–10 mL per day of colostrum may be of value to stimulate the 'coming in' of full milk production.[230] The two key factors that support the establishment of lactation are breast stimulation (infant suckling, hand expression) and milk removal. The more often you express and remove milk, the positive feedback mechanisms ensure that more milk is produced. Frequent, short expression of the breasts is more effective than prolonged infrequent expressing. Overnight expression is also important.

If the mother's intention was to formula feed, or if the baby has died, then the lactation process may be suppressed. In practice, this means providing no stimulation to the breasts (i.e. no hand expression). Although used in the past,

> ### BOX 28.11
>
> #### Principles of expressing breast milk
>
> **How often should I express?**
>
> Generally speaking, women are recommended to express 2–3-hourly. This may be difficult to achieve in the ICU environment. Clinicians should aim for at least 6 times per 24 hours including at least once overnight.
>
> **Hand express or machine express?**
>
> It is recommended to use hand expression only in the first few days with use of a machine reserved for when the milk has come in. Always start and finish the expression by hand, as hand expression provides a better stimulus for milk production than the machine does, and promotes release of the 'let-down' reflex which will assist with milk flow and removal. Expressing by hand or machine should not be painful.
>
> **Storage and transport of expressed milk**
>
> The most useful container for collection of expressed colostrum is a 2- or 5-mL syringe and a specimen M&C container for small volumes of milk. Always label the container with the woman's name, and the date and time of the expression. Use a new collection container for each expression. Breast milk must be stored in a refrigerator and may be frozen. A 'cooler bag' with ice packs should be used to transport the milk from ICU to where the baby is being cared for.

FIGURE 28.5 How to hand express.

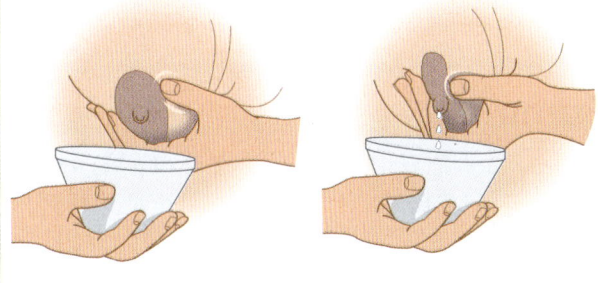

medications are rarely used to influence this process. With no breast expression, some women may still experience milk 'coming in' at or after day 4 postpartum and comfort measures may assist if the breasts become very uncomfortable. Cold compresses may be of use and it is important for the critical care nurse to observe for signs like reddened hot areas on the breast that may be an indication of mastitis.

Medication administration and lactation

Many drugs are safe to use in breastfeeding, although most common critical care drugs have not been well evaluated.[239] Even if the woman is receiving a medication that is contraindicated during breastfeeding, you can still express (and discard) the milk to establish the process of lactation, unless the woman is likely to stay on the medication long term.

The safety of the expressed milk for the baby depends on three factors: the amount of the medication in the milk, the oral bioavailability of the medication and the ability of the infant to metabolise the medication.[240] The gestation and condition of the infant are relevant as the function of the gut, liver and kidney varies with maturity and illness. Consequently, advice from the baby's neonatologist or paediatrician can help determine whether the neonate can receive the expressed breast milk, or whether it should be discarded.

Psychology of the puerperium

Major emotional changes take place in the majority of women during the puerperium, but there is a wide variation in the amount of distress caused by these changes. The first 3 days post-delivery are known as the latent period because functional mental illness is very unlikely to occur during this time interval. The woman is usually in a state of euphoria, excitement and restlessness; extreme tiredness is also present. Days 3–10 are often referred to as the 'baby blues' and are characterised by emotional lability (mood swings).[241] The 'baby blues' are usually characterised by thoughts of inadequacy and generalised panic that there is something wrong with either their baby or themselves. A very severe 'baby blues' response may herald the onset of postnatal depression.

The family unit

Maternal admission to ICU often separates the mother from her newborn and may also be associated with a period of heavy sedation/loss of consciousness. Thus the woman may not be able to recollect the birth process and will often not have seen her baby before being transferred to ICU.

Promoting maternal–infant attachment

Promoting maternal–infant attachment depends on the condition of both the mother and her baby, and their physical locations. The best case scenario is that the baby is able to 'room in' with the mother for periods of time in ICU. Skin to skin contact is usually recommended to promote bonding.[242] Alternatively, the baby may be able to visit the mother in ICU or the mother may be able to visit the baby in NICU. Physically seeing and touching the baby may be an important step for the mother. Newer technologies, like Skype, have been used by some ICUs to enable the mother to see her baby in a different hospital and to watch significant events, such as the first bath.

The use of diaries, one about the mother's condition and one about the baby's progress, complete with photos, visitor and clinician entries, is another strategy that may be useful to promote maternal–infant attachment. The first few days following birth are often a blur for the mother with little recollection of events. It is also common to have photographs of the baby for the mother to look at, and clinicians keep in touch with the nursery where the baby is being cared for and give the mother regular updates on the baby's condition.

Caring for the partner and other family members

The partner is similarly 'bowled over' by the sudden and severe illness of the mother. The partner is often torn between two ICUs, with the newborn admitted to NICU in one hospital and the mother in ICU in another hospital. This situation is further compounded if there are other children to consider. Usual strategies such as explanation, open visiting and social work support are important.

Summary

Intensive care management of pregnant and postpartum women is challenging for a variety of reasons including, but not limited to, the presence of the fetus, physiological adaptations of pregnancy and due to clinical conditions that are unique to the obstetric population. ICU staff are often not educationally prepared to provide midwifery care and there may be difficulty in obtaining midwifery and obstetric consultation. Importantly, childbirth is viewed as a normal, healthy event in our society and is usually a cause of celebration. A life-threatening event associated with childbirth may seem more overwhelming due to this context. The best outcomes for both the mother and her baby will result from collaborative and coordinated care between maternity and critical care service providers.

Case study

Daisy is a 29-year-old nulliparous Aboriginal woman with type 2 diabetes, asthma and pre-existing rheumatic heart disease. She was admitted to the antenatal ward of a tertiary maternity hospital with increasing shortness of breath, dull, heavy left-sided chest pain and a productive cough following an antenatal outpatient appointment at 29 weeks' gestation. Daisy had been undergoing regular antenatal visits at a tertiary maternity centre from 15 weeks' gestation due to the high-risk nature of her pregnancy.

Daisy's medical history was complex and presented many challenges to the multidisciplinary team providing her care. The most significant of her health problems was her rheumatic heart disease, which required an aortic valve replacement and then re-do aortic (25 mm) and mitral (29 mm) valve replacements when she was 19 years and 23 years, with mosaic tissue valves. Daisy suffered from obesity, with suboptimal glycaemic control of her type 2 diabetes diagnosed when she was 22 years as well as mild asthma. She was an occasional marijuana and cigarette smoker. Daisy suffered from vitamin D and iron deficiency requiring supplementation. Daisy's blood group is O negative.

At 29 weeks' gestation, physical assessment in the antenatal clinic revealed an elevated jugular venous pressure (JVP), bilateral respiratory wheeze and crepitus upon auscultation, a persistent moist cough coupled with an exercise tolerance of 50 metres and the inability to climb stairs. Her vital signs were unremarkable with oxygen saturations of 99% on room air, a heart rate of 80 bpm and blood pressure of 112/66 mmHg. The fetus was active, with a regular fetal heart rate documented at 146 bpm. Daisy had a chest X-ray and was subsequently admitted to the antenatal ward with mild congestive cardiac failure requiring 20 mg oral frusemide daily, 25 mg bd metoprolol and adequate rest.

Three days later, at 30 weeks' gestation, a formal transthoracic echocardiograph (TTE) was performed. It demonstrated moderate pulmonary hypertension at 62/37 mmHg with moderate pulmonic regurgitation and mild-moderate tricuspid regurgitation. Severe left atrial dilation and mitral stenosis was also detected. Sildenafil 50 mg TDS was commenced to combat the pulmonary hypertension. Metoprolol was increased to 50 mg bd and 50 mg daily spiralactone commenced. Daisy was commenced on daily 1.5-L fluid restriction.

Throughout Daisy's antenatal stay, her vital signs remained within the normal parameters of pregnancy. Her glycaemic control was good and her fetus was active and growing appropriately. However, at 31^{+3} weeks of gestation, Daisy developed acute, sudden onset pulmonary oedema and congestive cardiac failure, with SaO_2 <75% and was admitted to a tertiary general adult hospital. An emergency caesarean section was performed and a live baby girl was born weighing 1500 g. Daisy was admitted to ICU immediately postpartum and placed on extracorporeal membrane oxygenation (ECMO) and continuous renal replacement therapy (CRRT) for multiple organ failure.

The greatest challenges in the first 5 days of her admission were managing cardiogenic shock, oxygenation status and sepsis. She required high levels of oxygenation (FiO_2 0.8), and was unable to be re-positioned due to poor cardiac function with a left ventricular ejection fraction (LVEF) of 22%. She was initially cared for by two nurses, and had daily midwifery visits to assess PV loss, wound healing, breast milk production and to discuss the progress of her baby.

Daisy's ECMO was discontinued after 3 days though she remained on high doses of adrenaline, noradrenaline and dobutamine. She was persistently anaemic with Hb <75 g/dL and initially required daily TTE. A tracheostomy was performed on day 8. Daisy developed pneumonia (grown on culture), requiring frequent suctioning, position changes and antibiotics.

By day 11, Daisy's oxygen requirements had reduced to FiO_2 0.5. Her inotropes had been weaned as her cardiac function had improved significantly with an LVEF of 38%. Daisy's renal function remained poor, and she continued CRRT for another 4 days. After 15 days of ventilation, Daisy was able to be weaned onto the Swedish nose for 2-hourly intervals interchanged with pressure support ventilation throughout the day. She had established a regular milk supply, and PV loss had stopped and her caesarean section wound was healing well. On day 18, Daisy's tracheostomy was removed and she was discharged from the ICU to the medical high dependency unit for further care and a plan to re-do her faulty aortic and mitral valves.

CASE STUDY QUESTIONS

1. You are assigned to care for Daisy when she is admitted to ICU. Outline the key elements of your admission assessment that relate to her midwifery care.

2. Outline what is required to prevent Rh D isoimmunisation in Daisy.

3. Daisy's partner visits the unit and explains that she was very determined to breastfeed her baby. How could you support Daisy's wishes while she is in ICU to breastfeed her baby? How should expressed breast milk be stored in the ICU? How much breast milk should Daisy produce in the first 48 hours postpartum? Is Daisy's milk safe to feed to her pre-term baby?

4. Is it safe for Daisy's baby to visit her in the ICU? How could bonding between mother and baby be facilitated in this environment?

5 Following birth and commencement of ECMO and CRRT, discuss the postpartum care that would routinely be required by Daisy and how her critical illness may impact on that care and on her postpartum wellbeing.

6 Daisy requires valvular replacement surgery. Her partner and family live in a remote Aboriginal community, a 15-hour drive from the city. What support services and resources will her partner and baby need in order to adjust as a family with Daisy requiring a long hospital stay in the city as an inpatient?

RESEARCH VIGNETTE

Austin DM, Sadler L, McLintock C, McArthur C, Masson V, Farquhar C et al. Early detection of severe maternal morbidity: a retrospective assessment of the role of an Early Warning Score System. Aust N Z J Obstet Gynaecol 2014;54:152–5

Abstract

Background: The Early Warning Scoring (EWS) surveillance system is used to identify deteriorating patients and enable appropriate staff to be called promptly. However, there is a lack of evidence that EWS surveillance systems lead to a reduction in severe morbidity.

Aims: To determine whether EWS may have improved the detection of severe maternal morbidity or lessened the severity of illness among women with severe morbidity at a large tertiary maternity unit at Auckland City Hospital (ACH), New Zealand.

Methods: Admissions to intensive care, cardiothoracic and vascular intensive care, or an obstetric high-dependency unit (HDU) were identified from clinical and hospital administrative databases. Case reviews and transcribed observation charts were presented to a multidisciplinary review group who, through group consensus, determined whether an EWS might have hastened recognition and/or escalation and effective treatment.

Results: The multidisciplinary review team determined that an EWS might have reduced the seriousness of maternal morbidity in five cases (7.6%), including three admissions for obstetric sepsis to intensive care unit and two to obstetric HDU for post-partum haemorrhage. No patient had a complete set of respiratory rate, heart rate, blood pressure and temperature recordings at every time period.

Conclusions: These findings have been used to support introduction of an EWS to the maternity unit at ACH.

Critique

The United Kingdom Confidential Enquiry into Maternal Death (UKCEMD) has recommended the use of a Modified Early Obstetric Warning Scoring system (MEOWS) since 2007 to facilitate early recognition of clinical deterioration in an effort to avoid adverse outcomes.[26] In comparison, the maternity sectors in Australia and New Zealand have been slow to adopt track and trigger observation and response charts. The study examined whether the use of an Early Warning Score (EWS) chart would have improved the detection of severe maternal morbidity or lessened the severity of illness, in a retrospective cohort, prior to the implementation of the EWS in the maternity population.[243]

This is a single centre study that examined two years' of obstetric admissions to ICU/HDU. The researchers identify the lack of data on the relationship between EWS and any potential reduction in severe maternal morbidity as the rationale for their study. The clinical setting, context of the study and inclusion and exclusion criteria were clearly described. A random sample of the women admitted to the obstetric HDU was included although no explanation was given regarding the sample size selected. Potential cases were identified using the maternity clinical database, the clinical management system and the ICU clinical database, so it is unlikely that many women will have been missed unknowingly.

Two members of the research team prepared case note summaries and plotted the EWS for each case using the clinical records available at the time. The EWS (and associated parameters) adopted for this project was the standard EWS used across the hospital, without any modification for maternity patients. The rationale provided was that the hospital EWS team thought there was more benefit in using a standard chart across the hospital rather than having two charts – one modified for maternity.

A multidisciplinary team, consisting of midwifery, obstetric, anaesthetic, medical and ICU staff, reviewed the case summaries and EWS score charts; there was no blinding the team to the outcome of the women and, by definition, all women were admitted to ICU or HDU. The team determined 'by consensus' whether an EWS might have triggered earlier detection and escalation, and 'potentially avoided' severe maternal morbidity. There is no detail on what this actually meant or how it was done, e.g. did consensus mean 'discussed until all agreed' or only until the 'majority agreed'? Ethics approval from the relevant authority was noted.

The results are clearly reported. All potential cases are accounted for, with 24 ICU admissions and 40 HDU admissions – 64 women in total – included. The researchers felt that five women (7.6%) would have potentially benefited from an EWS if appropriate escalation had occurred based on the physiological derangement. Notably, no woman had a full set of observations documented at each time point when observations were taken. The most common missing vital sign was respiratory rate – however, only one of the seven charts in use in the maternity services at this time had a space to record respiratory rate. The researchers discuss this limitation and refer to research that has consistently found respiratory rate to be of use in the early detection of clinical deterioration in other clinical settings. The tables display useful information in a way that is easy to understand.

The decision to use a 'standard EWS' rather than one modified for maternity may have been rather shortsighted given that the purpose of the study was to examine any 'benefit' of an EWS in the maternity setting. While the researchers argue that the study by Carle et al[244] demonstrated no benefit in maternity modified trigger parameters, the limitations of Carle's study (data used after admission to ICU only and mortality as outcome) plus the lack of any clinical application/external validity did not equate with a recommendation to adopt a non-obstetric EWS. Carle et al note that 'it is important that the score meets with the expectations of the clinicians who will be implementing the score' (p 363), that 'obstetric-specific conditions need to be considered' (p 365) and they advocate for a maternity modified EWS.[244] The reviewed study by Austin et al[243] was a missed opportunity to compare the clinical application of a maternity modified EWS with a standard EWS. No maternity staff would consider it reasonable for a woman with a systolic BP of 170 to attract 0 points in an EWS, which would have been the case with the standard EWS used in the study. It is well accepted that maternity patients have great physiological reserve (e.g. ↑ cardiac output, ↑ circulating volume) and may experience sudden, acute deterioration. Further, blood pressure is of particular relevance in maternity patients, with a lowering of BP normal in pregnancy, and using non-maternity systolic BP parameters to trigger a response seems unhelpful. It was disappointing that there was not more discussion about their use of a standard EWS and if there would have been potential further benefit with a maternity modified EWS once they were reviewing the cases. For example, sixteen of the women (25%) had a hypertensive disorder and it is well recognised that effective treatment of systolic hypertension may prevent cerebral haemorrhage, the leading cause of death related to preeclampsia.[26]

Overall, this study found that the application of a general EWS would have potentially prevented 8% of severe maternal morbidity. The researchers correctly assert that the adoption of an EWS may help with more regular documenting of respiratory rate, which may be of use in detecting clinical deterioration early. Despite the limitations outlined above, this study adds to the small and building literature on the use of EWS in the maternity population.

Learning activities

1   List the key physiological adaptations of the cardiovascular and respiratory systems during pregnancy.

2   Outline the key causes of antenatal haemorrhage and postpartum haemorrhage.

3   Explain why a magnesium sulfate infusion is used for the management of severe preeclampsia in the postpartum period, and outline the typical loading and maintenance doses recommended for magnesium sulfate therapy.

4   Identify the maternity-specific resources and equipment in your workplace. For example, are their maternity-specific modifications in your ALS protocol, do you have a wedge on your resuscitation trolley, what policies and procedures do you have in place to support the care of a maternity patient?

Online resources

3 Centres collaboration, http://3centres.com.au

Australasian Maternity Outcomes Surveillance System (AMOSS), www.amoss.com.au and www.amoss.com.nz

British Thoracic Society British guideline on asthma management, www.brit-thoracic.org.uk/clinical-information/asthma/asthma-guidelines.aspx

National Heart Foundation of Australia and the Cardiac Society of Australia and New Zealand, www.heartfoundation.org.au/information-for-professionals/Clinical-Information/Pages/arf-rhd.aspx

National Perinatal Statistics Unit, www.preru.unsw.edu.au/PRERUWeb.nsf/page/AIHW+National+Perinatal+Statistics+Unit

Perinatal and Maternal Mortality Review Committee (PMMRC), www.pmmrc.health.govt.nz

Royal College of Obstetricians and Gynaecologists, www.rcog.org.uk/files/rcog-corp/GT37ReducingRiskThrombo.pdf

Society of Obstetric Medicine of Australia and New Zealand (SOMANZ), The SOMANZ guideline for the management of hypertensive disorders of pregnancy (2014), www.somanz.org

UK Confidential Enquiry into Maternal Death, www.npeu.ox.ac.uk/mbrrace-uk/programme-of-work

United Kingdom Obstetric Surveillance System (UKOSS), www.npeu.ox.ac.uk/ukoss

Further reading

Belfort MA, Saade GR, Foley MR, Phelan JP, Dildy GA, eds. Critical care obstetrics. 5th ed. Hoboken: Wiley-Blackwell; 2010.

Coad J, Dunstall M. Anatomy and physiology for midwives. 3rd ed. Edinburgh: Churchill Livingston/Elsevier; 2011.

Foley M, Strong T, Garite T, eds. Obstetric intensive care manual. 3rd ed. Columbus: McGraw-Hill; 2010.

Marshall J, Raynor M, eds. Myles' textbook for midwives. 16th ed. Oxford: Churchill Livingston/Elsevier; 2014.

Pairman S, Pincombe J, Thorogood P, Tracy S, eds. Midwifery preparation for practice. 3rd ed. Chatswood: Churchill Livingstone, 2014.

Pearlman M, Tintinalli J, Dyne P, eds. Obstetric and gynecologic emergencies: diagnosis and management. Chicago: McGraw-Hill Professional Publishing; 2004.

Van de Velde M, Scholefield H, Plante L, eds. Maternal critical care: A multidisciplinary approach. New York: Cambridge University Press; 2013.

References

1 Belfort MA, Saade GR, Foley MR, Phelan JP, Dildy GA, eds. Critical care obstetrics. 5th ed. Hoboken: Wiley-Blackwell; 2010.
2 Foley M, Strong T, Garite T, eds. Obstetric intensive care manual. 3rd ed. Columbus: McGraw-Hill; 2010.
3 Van de Velde M, Scholefield H, Plante L, eds. Maternal critical care: A multidisciplinary approach. New York: Cambridge University Press; 2013.
4 Pollock W, Rose L, Dennis CL. Pregnant and postpartum admissions to the intensive care unit: a systematic review. Intens Care Med 2010;36(9):1465–74.
5 Harrison DA, Penny JA, Yentis SM, Fayek S, Brady AR. Case mix, outcome and activity for obstetric admissions to adult, general critical care units: a secondary analysis of the ICNARC Case Mix Programme Database. Crit Care 2005;9(Suppl 3):S25–37.
6 Zhang WH, Alexander S, Bouvier-Colle MH, Macfarlane A; MOMS-B Group. Incidence of severe pre-eclampsia, postpartum haemorrhage and sepsis as a surrogate marker for severe maternal morbidity in a European population-based study: the MOMS-B survey. BJOG 2005;112(1):89–96.
7 Paxton JL, Presneill J, Aitken L. Characteristics of obstetric patients referred to intensive care in an Australian tertiary hospital. Aust N Z J Obstet Gynaecol 2014;54(5):445-9.
8 Hazelgrove JF, Price C, Pappachan VJ, Smith GB. Multicenter study of obstetric admissions to 14 intensive care units in southern England. Crit Care Med 2001;29(4):770–75.
9 Zwart J, Dupuis J, Richters A, Ory F, van Roosmalen J. Obstetric intensive care unit admission: a 2-year nationwide population-based cohort study. Intensive Care Med 2010;36(2):256–63.
10 Lawton B, Wilson L, Dinsdale R, Rose S, Brown S, Tait J et al. Audit of severe acute maternal morbidity describing reasons for transfer and potential preventability of admissions to ICU. Aust N Z J Obstet Gynaecol 2010;50(4):346–51.
11 Geller SEM, Adams G, Kominiarek MA, Hibbard JU, Endres LK, Cox SM et al. Reliability of a preventability model in maternal death and morbidity. Am J Obstet Gynecol 2007;196(1):57.e1–57.e6.
12 Sadler LC, Austin DM, Masson VL, McArthur CJ, McLintock C, Rhodes SP et al. Review of contributory factors in maternity admissions to intensive care at a New Zealand tertiary hospital. Am J Obstet Gynecol 2013;209(6):e1-7.

13 Pollock W. Critically ill pregnant and postpartum women in Victoria: characteristics, severity of illness and the provision of acute health services. PhD thesis. Melbourne: The University of Melbourne; 2007.

14 Marshall J, Raynor M, eds. Myles' textbook for midwives. 16th ed. Oxford: Churchill Livingston/Elsevier; 2014.

15 Pairman S, Pincombe J, Thorogood P, Tracy S, eds. Midwifery preparation for practice. 3rd ed. Chatswood: Churchill Livingstone; 2014.

16 Norwitz, ER, Edusa V, Park JS. Maternal physiology and complications of multiple pregnancy. Semin Perinatol 2005;29(5):338–48.

17 Robson SC, Dunlop W, Moore M, Hunter S. Haemodynamic changes during the puerperium: a Doppler and M-mode echocardiographic study. BJOG 1987;94(11):1028–39.

18 Crapo, RO. Normal cardiopulmonary physiology during pregnancy. Clin Obstet Gynecol 1996;39(1):3–16.

19 Hunter S, Robson S. Adaptation of the maternal heart in pregnancy. Br Heart J 1992;68(6):540–43.

20 Norwitz E, Robinson J, Malone F. Pregnancy-induced physiologic alterations. In: Dildy GA, Belfort MA, Saade GR et al, eds. Critical care obstetrics. 4th ed. Massachusetts: Blackwell Science; 2004, p 19–42.

21 Davison JM. The kidney in pregnancy: a review. J Royal Soc Med 1983;76(6):485–501.

22 Hytten F. Blood volume changes in normal pregnancy. Clin Haematol 1985;14(3):601–12.

23 Duvekot JJ, Peeters L. Renal hemodynamics and volume homeostasis in pregnancy. Obstet Gynecol Surv 1994;49(12):830–39.

24 Salas SP, Marshall G, Gutierrez BL, Rosso P. Time course of maternal plasma volume and hormonal changes in women with preeclampsia or fetal growth restriction. Hypertension 2006;47(2):203–8.

25 Nevo O, Soustiel JF, Thaler I. Maternal cerebral blood flow during normal pregnancy: a cross-sectional study. Am J Obstet Gynecol 2010;203(5):e471–6.

26 Centre for Maternal and Child Enquiries (CMACE). Saving Mothers' Lives: reviewing maternal deaths to make motherhood safer: 2006–08. The Eighth Report on Confidential Enquiries into Maternal Deaths in the United Kingdom. BJOG 2011;118(Suppl 1):1–203.

27 Mabie WC, DiSessa TG, Crocker LG, Sibai BM, Arheart KL. A longitudinal study of cardiac output in normal human pregnancy. Am J Obstet Gynecol 1994;170(3):849–56.

28 Robson SC, Hunter S, Boys RJ, Dunlop W. Serial study of factors influencing changes in cardiac output during human pregnancy. Am J Physiol Heart Circ Physiol 1989;256(4):H1060–65.

29 Clapp JF, Capeless E. Cardiovascular function before, during, and after the first and subsequent pregnancies. Am J Cardiol 1997;80(11):1469–73.

30 Bamber JH, Dresner M. Aortocaval compression in pregnancy: the effect of changing the degree and direction of lateral tilt on maternal cardiac output. Anesth Analg 2003;97(1):256–8.

31 Kinsella SM. Lateral tilt for pregnant women: why 15 degrees? Anaesth 2003;58(9):835–6.

32 Duvekot JJ, Peeters L. Maternal cardiovascular hemodynamic adaptation to pregnancy. Obstet Gynecol Surv 1994;48(12):S1-14.

33 Royal College of Obstetricians and Gynaecologists (RCOG). Reducing the risk of thrombosis and embolism during pregnancy and the puerperium. Green-top Guideline no. 37. London: RCOG; 2009.

34 Contreras G, Gutiérrez M, Beroíza T, Fantín A, Oddó L, Villarroel L et al. Ventilatory drive and respiratory muscle function in pregnancy. Am Rev Respir Dis 1991;144(4):837–41.

35 Weinberger SE, Weiss ST, Cohen WR, Weiss JW, Johnson TS. Pregnancy and the lung. Am Rev Respir Dis 1980;121(3):559–81.

36 Jensen D, Webb KA, O'Donnell DE. Chemical and mechanical adaptations of the respiratory system at rest and during exercise in human pregnancy. Appl Physiol Nutr Metab 2007;32(6):1239–50.

37 Jensen D, Duffin J, Lam YM, Webb KA, Simpson JA, Davies GA et al. Physiological mechanisms of hyperventilation during human pregnancy. Respir Physiol Neurobiol 2008;161(1):76–86.

38 Weissgerber TL, Wolfe LA, Hopkins WG, Davies GAL. Serial respiratory adaptations and an alternate hypothesis of respiratory control in human pregnancy. Respir Physiol Neurobiol 2006;153(1):39–53.

39 Templeton A, Kelman GR. Maternal blood-gases, (PAO_2-PaO_2): physiological shunt and VD/VT in normal pregnancy. Brit J Anaesth 1976; 48(10):1001–4.

40 Prodromakis E, Trakada G, Tsapanos V, Spiropoulos K. Arterial oxygen tension during sleep in the third trimester of pregnancy. Acta Obstetricia et Gynecologica Scandinavica 2004;83(2):159–64.

41 MacRae DJ, Palavradji D. Maternal acid–base changes in pregnancy. BJOG 1967;74(1):11–16.

42 Andersen GJ, James GB, Mathers NP, Smith EL, Walker J. The maternal oxygen tension and acid–base status during pregnancy. BJOG 1969;76(1):16–19.

43 Richlin S, Cusick W, Sullivan C, Dildy G, Belfort M. Normative oxygen saturation values for pregnant women at sea level. Primary Care Update for OB/GYNS 1998;5(4):154–5.

44 Langford E, Khwanda A, Langford K. Oxygen saturation response to exercise in healthy pregnant women: a simple protocol and normal range. Obstet Med 2010;3(2):65–8.

45 Zeldis SM. Dyspnea during pregnancy: distinguishing cardiac from pulmonary causes. Clin Chest Med 1992;13(4):567–85.

46 Boutourline-Young H, Boutourline-Young E. Alveolar carbon dioxide levels in pregnant, parturient and lactating subjects. BJOG 1956;63(4):509–28.

47 Davison J M, Vallotton MB, Lindheimer MD. Plasma osmolality and urinary concentration and dilution during and after pregnancy: evidence that lateral recumbency inhibits maximal urinary concentrating ability. BJOG 1981;88(5):472–9.

48 Klajnbard A, Szecsi PB, Colov NP, Andersen MR, Jørgensen M, Bjørngaard B et al. Laboratory reference intervals during pregnancy, delivery and the early postpartum period. Clin Chem Lab Med 2010;48(2):237–48.

49 Lindheimer M. Polyuria and pregnancy: its cause, its danger [Editorial]. Obstet Gynecol 2005;105(5, Part 2):1171–2.

50 Mackenzie MJ, Woolnough MJ, Barrett N, Johnson MR, Yentis SM. Normal urine output after elective caesarean section: an observational study. Int J Obstet Anesth 2010;19(4):379–83.

51 Baer J, Reis R, Arens R. Appendicitis in pregnancy: with changes in position and axis of the normal appendix in pregnancy. JAMA 1932;98(16):1359–64.

52 Augustin G, Majerovic M. Non-obstetrical acute abdomen during pregnancy. Euro J Obstet Gynecol Reprod Biol 2007;131(1):4–12.

53 Nakai A, Sekiya I, Oya A, Koshino T, Araki T. Assessment of the hepatic arterial and portal venous blood flows during pregnancy with Doppler ultrasonography. Arch Gynecol Obstet 2002;266(1):25–9.

54 Johnson S, Bonello MR, Li Z, Hilder L, Sullivan EA. Maternal deaths in Australia 2006–2010, Maternal deaths series no. 4. Cat. no. PER 61. Canberra: AIHW; 2014.

55 Salnlo S, Kekomaki R, Rllkonen S, Teramo K. Maternal thrombocytopenia at term: a population-based study. Acta Obstetricia et Gynecologica Scandinavica 2000;79(9):744.

56 Burrows RF, Kelton JG. Incidentally detected thrombocytopenia in healthy mothers and their infants. N Engl J Med 1988;319(3):142–5.

57 Hellgren M. Hemostasis during normal pregnancy and puerperium. Semin Thromb Hemost 2003;29(2):125,130.

58 Szecsi PB, Jorgensen M, Klajnbard A, Andersen MR, Colov NP, Stender S. Haemostatic reference intervals in pregnancy. Thromb Haemost 2010;103(4):718–27.

59 Paniccia R, Prisco D, Bandinelli B, Fedi S, Giusti B, Pepe G et al. Plasma and serum levels of D-dimer and their correlations with other hemostatic parameters in pregnancy. Thromb Res 2002;105(3):257–62.

60 Uchikova EH, Ledjev II. Changes in haemostasis during normal pregnancy. Euro J Obstet Gynecol Reprod Biol 2005;119(2):185–8.

61 Miller EM. Changes in serum immunity during pregnancy. Am J Human Biol 2009;21(3):401–3.

62 Rogerson SJ, Hviid L, Duffy PE, Leke RFG, Taylor DW. Malaria in pregnancy: pathogenesis and immunity. Lancet Infect Dis 2007;7(2):105–17.

63 Albright CM, Ali TN, Lopes V, Rouse DJ, Anderson BL. The Sepsis in Obstetrics Score: a model to identify risk of morbidity from sepsis in pregnancy. Am J Obstet Gynecol 2014;211(1):39.e1-.e8.

64 Vance M. The placenta. In: Fraser D, Cooper M, eds. Myles' textbook for midwives. 15th ed. Oxford: Churchill Livingstone/Elsevier; 2009, pp 147–56.

65 Kingdom J, Huppertz B, Seaward G, Kaufmann P. Development of the placental villous tree and its consequences for fetal growth. Eur J Obstet Gynecol Reprod Biol 2000;92(1):35–43.

66 Gude NM, Roberts CT, Kalionis B, King RG. Growth and function of the normal human placenta. Thromb Res 2004;114(5–6):397–407.

67 Low J. Fetal asphyxia and brain damage. Fetal and Maternal Medicine Review 2001;12(2):139–58.

68 National Collaborating Centre for Women's and Children's Health. Hypertension in pregnancy: the management of hypertensive disorders in pregnancy. NICE Clinical Guideline. London: RCOG; 2011.

69 Lowe SA, Bowyer L, Lust K, McMahon L, Morton M, North R et al. The SOMANZ guideline for the management of hypertensive disorders of pregnancy 2014. Sydney: Society of Obstetric Medicine of Australia and New Zealand; 2014.

70 Roberts JM, Redman CWG. Pre-eclampsia: more than pregnancy-induced hypertension. Lancet 1993;341(8858):1447–51.

71 Steegers EAP, von Dadelszen P, Duvekot JJ, Pijnenborg R. Pre-eclampsia. Lancet 2010;376(9741):631–44.

72 Sibai B, Dekker G, Kupferminc M. Pre-eclampsia. Lancet 2005;365(9461):785–99.

73 Plasencia W, Maiz N, Bonino S, Kaihura C, Nicolaides KH. Uterine artery Doppler at 11 + 0 to 13 + 6 weeks in the prediction of pre-eclampsia. Ultrasound Obstet Gynecol 2007;30(5):742–9.

74 Kaitu'u-Lino TJ, Tuohey L, Ye L, Palmer K, Skubisz M, Tong S. MT-MMPs in pre-eclamptic placenta: relationship to soluble endoglin production. Placenta 2013;34:168-73.

75 Duckitt K, Harrington D. Risk factors for pre-eclampsia at antenatal booking: systematic review of controlled studies. BMJ 2005;330(7491):565–72.

76 Knight M. Eclampsia in the United Kingdom 2005. BJOG 2007;114(9):1072–8.

77 Australasian Maternity Outcomes Surveillance System Project website, <http://www.amoss.com.au> [accessed 12.10].

78 Abraham KA, Connolly G, Farrell J, Walshe JJ. The HELLP syndrome, a prospective study1. Ren Fail 2001;23(5):705–13.

79 Weinstein L. Preeclampsia/eclampsia with hemolysis, elevated liver enzymes and thrombocytopenia. Obstet Gynecol 1985;66(5):657–60.

80 Haram K, Svendsen E, Abildgaard U. The HELLP syndrome: Clinical issues and management. A Review. BMC Pregnancy Childbirth 2009;9(1):8.

81 Vigil-De Gracia P. Pregnancy complicated by pre-eclampsia-eclampsia with HELLP syndrome. Int J Gynecol Obstet 2001;72(1):17–23.

82 Young BC, Levine RJ, Karumanchi SA. Pathogenesis of preeclampsia. Annual Review of Pathology: Mechanisms of Disease 2010;5(1):173–92.

83 Sontia B, Touyz RM. Role of magnesium in hypertension. Arch Biochem Biophys 2007;458(1):33–9.

84 The Magpie Trial Group. Do women with pre-eclampsia, and their babies, benefit from magnesium sulphate? The Magpie Trial: a randomised placebo-controlled trial. Lancet 2002;359(9321):1877–90.

85 Duley L, Henderson-Smart DJ, Meher S. Drugs for treatment of very high blood pressure during pregnancy. Cochrane Database Syst Rev 2006:CD001449.

86 Rugarn O, Moen S, Berg G. Eclampsia at a tertiary hospital 1973–99. Acta Obstetricia et Gynecologica Scandinavica 2004;83(3):240–45.

87 Ganzevoort W, Rep A, Bonsel GJ, Fetter WPF, van Sonderen L et al. A randomised controlled trial comparing two temporising management strategies, one with and one without plasma volume expansion, for severe and early onset pre-eclampsia. BJOG 2005;112(10):1358–68.

88 Dildy GA, Belfort MA, Saade GR, Phelan JP, Hankins GD, Clark SL, eds. Critical care obstetrics. 4th ed. Massachusetts: Blackwell Science; 2004.

89 Smith CV, Phelan JP. Determinants for invasive monitoring in severe preeclampsia. Contemporary Obstetrics and Gynaecology 1986;109–124.

90 Dennis AT, Castro JM. Transthoracic echocardiography in women with treated severe pre-eclampsia. Anaesth 2014;69(5):436-44.

91 Woudstra DM, Chandra S, Hofmeyr GJ, Dowswell T. Corticosteroids for HELLP (hemolysis, elevated liver enzymes, low platelets) syndrome in pregnancy. Cochrane Database Syst Rev 2010:CD008148.

92 Roberts D, Dalziel SR. Antenatal corticosteroids for accelerating fetal lung maturation for women at risk of preterm birth. Cochrane Database Syst Rev 2006:CD004454.

93 Visser W, Wallenburg HCS. Maternal and perinatal outcome of temporizing management in 254 consecutive patients with severe pre-eclampsia remote from term. Eur J Obstet Gynecol Reprod Biol 1995;63(2):147–54.

94 Brown M, Best K, Pearce M, Waugh J, Robson S, Bell R. Cardiovascular disease risk in women with pre-eclampsia: systematic review and meta-analysis. Eur J Epidemiol 2013;28:1-19.

95 World Health Organization. Maternal mortality infographic, <http://www.who.int/reproductivehealth/publications/monitoring/maternal-mortality-infographic.pdf>; 2014 [accessed 23.09.14].

96 Cameron CA, Roberts CL, Olive EC, Ford JB, Fischer WE. Trends in postpartum haemorrhage. Aust N Z J Public Health 2006;30(2):151–6.

97 Health Improvement Scotland. Scottish confidential audit of severe maternal morbidity: reducing avoidable harm. 10th Annual Report. Edinburgh: Health Improvement Scotland, <http://www.healthcareimprovementscotland.org>; 2014 [accessed 23.09.14].

98 Royal College of Obstetricians and Gynaecologists. Green-top guideline no. 63. Antepartum haemorrhage. London: Royal College of Obstetricians and Gynaecologists; 2011.

99 3 Centres Collaboration. Antepartum haemorrhage clinical practice guidelines, <http://3centres.com.au/library/public/file/guidelines/Complications_in_Pregnancy_and_Birth/Antepartum_Haemorrhage.pdf>; 2010 [accessed 12.10].

100 Bretelle F, Courbiere B, Mazouni C, Agostini A, Cravello L, Boubli L et al. Management of placenta accreta: morbidity and outcome. Eur J Obstet Gynecol Reprod Biol 2007;133(1):34–9.

101 Ford JB, Roberts CL, Simpson JM, Vaughan J, Cameron CA. Increased postpartum hemorrhage rates in Australia. Int J Gynecol Obstet 2007;98(3):237–43.

102 Henry A, Birch MR, Sullivan EA, Katz S, Wang YPA. Primary postpartum haemorrhage in an Australian tertiary hospital: a case-control study. Aust N Z J Obstet Gynaecol 2005;45(3):233–6.

103 Roberts CL, Ford J, Algert CS, Bell J, Simpson JM, Morris JM. Trends in adverse maternal outcomes during childbirth: a population-based study of severe maternal morbidity. BMC Pregnancy Childbirth 2009;9(1):7.

104 Consultative Council on Obstetric and Paediatric Mortality and Morbidity. 2010/2011 Victoria's mothers and babies. Victoria's maternal, perinatal, child and adolescent mortality. Melbourne: Department of Health; 2014.

105 Brace V, Kernaghan D, Penney G. Learning from adverse clinical outcomes: major obstetric haemorrhage in Scotland, 2003–05. BJOG 2007;114(11):1388–96.

106 NSW Health. Maternity – prevention, early recognition and management of postpartum haemorrhage (PPH). Sydney: Department of Health, NSW; 2010.

107 Mousa HA, Alfirevic Z. Treatment for primary postpartum haemorrhage. Cochrane Database Syst Rev 2007:CD003249.

108 Lapinsky S, Kruczynski K, Seaward G, Farine D, Grossman R. Critical care management of the obstetric patient. Can J Anaesth 1997; 44(3):3259.

109 Campbell L, Klocke R. Implications for the pregnant patient. Am J Respir Crit Care Med 2001;163(5):1051–4.

110 Huang WC, Chen CP. Pulmonary edema in pregnancy. Int J Gynecol Obstet 2002;78(3):241–3.

111 Chamberlain G, Steer P. ABC of labour care: obstetric emergencies. BMJ 1999;318(7194):1342–5.

112 Letsky E. Coagulation defects. In: de Swiet M, ed. Medical disorders in obstetric practice. 4th ed. Oxford: Blackwell Publishing; 2002, pp 61–96.

113 Slaytor EK, Sullivan EA, King JF. Maternal deaths in Australia 1997–1999. Sydney: AIHW National Perinatal Statistics Unit (Maternal Deaths Series No 1); 2004.

114 National Blood Authority. Patient blood management guidelines. Module 1: Critical bleeding/massive transfusion. Canberra: National Blood Authority, <htttp://www.nba.gov.au>; 2011.

115 National Blood Authority. Patient blood management guidelines. Module 4: Critical care. Canberra: National Blood Authority; 2013.

116 National Blood Authority. Patient blood management guidelines. Module 5: Obstetrics and maternity. Canberra: National Blood Authority; 2015.

117 Cortet M, Deneux-Tharaux C, Dupont C, Colin C, Rudigoz R-C, Bouvier-Colle M-H et al. Association between fibrinogen level and severity of postpartum haemorrhage: secondary analysis of a prospective trial. Br J Anaesth 2012;108(6):984-9.

118 Wikkelsoe AJ, Afshari A, Stensballe J, Langhoff-Roos J, Albrechtsen C, Ekelund K et al. The FIB-PPH trial: fibrinogen concentrate as initial treatment for postpartum haemorrhage: study protocol for a randomised controlled trial. Trials 2012;13(1):110.

119 Phillips L, McLintock C, Pollock W, Gatt S, Popham P, Jankelowitz G et al. Recombinant activated Factor VII in obstetric hemorrhage: experiences from the Australian and New Zealand haemostasis registry. Anesth Analg 2009;109(6):1908–15.

120 Novikova N, Hofmeyr GJ. Tranexamic acid for preventing postpartum haemorrhage. Cochrane Database Syst Rev 2010;7:CD007872.

121 Wang HY, Chang CT, Wu MS. Postpartum hemorrhage complicated with irreversible renal failure and central diabetes insipidus. Ren Fail 2002;24(6):849–52.

122 Fung Kee Fung K, Eason E, Crane J, Armson A, De La Ronde S, Farine D et al. Prevention of Rh alloimmunization. J Obstet Gynaecol Canada 2003;25(9):765–73.

123 Allam J, Cox M, Yentis SM. Cell salvage in obstetrics. Int J Obstet Anesth 2008;17(1):37–45.

124 King M, Wrench I, Galimberti A, Spray R. Introduction of cell salvage to a large obstetric unit: the first six months. Int J Obstet Anesth 2009;18(2):111–17.

125 Catling S. Blood conservation techniques in obstetrics: a UK perspective. Int J Obstet Anesth 2007;16(3):241–9.

126 Clark SL. Amniotic fluid embolism. Obstet Gynecol 2014;123(2, Part 1):337-48.

127 Tuffnell DJ, Slemeck E. Amniotic fluid embolism. Obstet Gynaecol Reprod Med 2014;24(5):148-52.

128 Shechtman M, Ziser A, Markovits R, Rozenberg B. Amniotic fluid embolism: early findings of transesophageal echocardiography. Anesth Analg 1999; 89(6):1456–8.

129 Conde-Agudelo A, Romero R. Amniotic fluid embolism: an evidence-based review. Am J Obstet Gynecol 2009;201(445):e1–13.

130 Knight M, Tuffnell D, Brocklehurst P, Spark P, Kurinczuk JJ on behalf of the UKOSS. Incidence and risk factors for amniotic-fluid embolism. Obstet Gynecol 2010;115(5):910–17.

131 Aguillon A, Andjus T, Grayson A, Race GJ. Amniotic fluid embolism: a review. Obstet Gynecol Surv 1962;17(5):619–36.

132 Abenhaim HA, Azoulay L, Kramer MS, Leduc L. Incidence and risk factors of amniotic fluid embolisms: a population-based study on 3 million births in the United States. Am J Obstet Gynecol 2008;199(1):e41–49.

133 Pearson GD, Veille JC, Rahimtoola S, Hsia J, Oakley CM, Hosenpud JD et al. Peripartum cardiomyopathy: National Heart, Lung, and Blood Institute and Office of Rare Diseases (National Institutes of Health) Workshop Recommendations and Review. JAMA 2000;283(9):1183–8.

134 Sliwa K, Hilfiker-Kleiner D, Petrie MC, Mebazaa A, Pieske B, Buchmann E et al. Current state of knowledge on aetiology, diagnosis, management, and therapy of peripartum cardiomyopathy: a position statement from the Heart Failure Association of the European Society of Cardiology Working Group on peripartum cardiomyopathy. Eur J Heart Fail 2010;12(8):767–78.

135 Sliwa K, Fett J, Elkayam U. Peripartum cardiomyopathy. Lancet 2006;368(9536):687–93.

136 Ntusi N, Mayosi B. Aetiology and risk factors of peripartum cardiomyopathy: a systematic review. Int J Cardiol 2009;131(2):168–79.

137 Cruz M, Briller M, Hibbard J. Update on peripartum cardiomyopathy. Obstet Gynecol Clin N Am 2010;37(2):283–303.

138 Hilfiker-Kleiner D, Struman I, Hoch M, Podewski E, Sliwa K. 16-kDa prolactin and bromocriptine in postpartum cardiomyopathy. Curr Heart Fail Rep 2012;9:174-182.

139 Mielniczuk LM, Williams K, Davis DR, Tang ASL, Lemery R, Green MS et al. Frequency of peripartum cardiomyopathy. Am J of Cardiol 2006;97(12):1765–8.

140 Fett JD, Sannon H, Thélisma E, Sprunger T, Suresh V. Recovery from severe heart failure following peripartum cardiomyopathy. Int J Gynecol Obstet 2009;104(2):125–7.

141 Egan DJ, Bisanzo MC, Hutson HR. Emergency department dvaluation and management of peripartum cardiomyopathy. Emerg Med 2009;36(2):141–7.

142 Hilfiker-Kleiner D, Sliwa K. Pathophysiology and epidemiology of peripartum cardiomyopathy. Nat Rev Cardiol 2014;11(6):364-70.

143 Ichida M, Katsurada K, Komori T, Matsumoto J, Ohkuchi A, Izumi A et al. Effectiveness of bromocriptine treatment in a patient with peripartum cardiomyopathy. J Cardiol Cases 2010;2(1):e28–31.

144 Hilfiker-Kleiner D, Kaminski K, Podewski E, Bonda T, Schaefer A, Sliwa K et al. A cathepsin D-cleaved 16-kDa form of prolactin mediates postpartum cardiomyopathy. Cell 2007;128(3):589–600.

145 Hilfiker-Kleiner D, Meyer GP, Schieffer E, Goldmann B, Podewski E, Struman I et al. Recovery from postpartum cardiomyopathy in 2 patients by blocking prolactin release with bromocriptine. J Am Coll Cardiol 2007;50(24):2354–5.

146 Haghikia A, Podewski E, Libhaber E, Labidi S, Fischer D, Roentgen P et al. Phenotyping and outcome on contemporary management in a German cohort of patients with peripartum cardiomyopathy. Basic Res Cardiol 2013;108(4):1-13.

147 Elkayam U, Tummala PP, Rao K, Akhter MW, Karaalp IS, Wani OR et al. Maternal and fetal outcomes of subsequent pregnancies in women with peripartum cardiomyopathy. N Engl J Med 2001;344(21):1567–71.

148 Harris IS. Management of pregnancy in patients with congenital heart disease. Progr Cardiovasc Dis 2011;53(4):305-11.

149 Abeywardana S, Sullivan EA Congenital anomalies in Australia 2002–2003. Birth anomalies series no. 3. Sydney: Australian Institute of Health and Welfare National Perinatal Statistics Unit; 2008.

150 Silversides CK, Marelli A, Beauchesne L, Dore A, Kiess M, Salehian O et al. Canadian Cardiovascular Society 2009 Consensus Conference on the management of adults with congenital heart disease: executive summary. Can J Cardiol 2010;26(3):143–50.

151 van der Linde D, Konings EEM, Slager MA, Witsenburg M, Helbing WA, Takkenberg JJM et al. Birth prevalence of congenital heart disease worldwide: a systematic review and meta-Analysis. J Am Coll Cardiol 2011;58(21):2241-7.

152 Coad J, Dunstall M. Anatomy and physiology for midwives. 3rd ed. Edinburgh: Churchill Livingston/Elsevier; 2011.

153 Rao S, Ginns JN. Adult congenital heart disease and pregnancy. Semin Perinatol 2014;38(5):260-72.

154 Siu SC, Sermer M, Colman JM, Alvarez AN, Mercier L-A, Morton BC et al. Prospective multicenter study of pregnancy outcomes in women with heart disease. Circulation 2001;104:515-521.

155 RHD Australia (ARF/RHD writing group), National Heart Foundation of Australia and the Cardiac Society of Australia and New Zealand. Australian guideline for prevention, diagnosis and management of acute rheumatic fever and rheumatic heart disease. 2nd ed. Darwin: Menzies School of Health Research; 2012.

156 Mesa A, Jessurun C, Hernandez A, Adam K, Brown D, Vaughn WK et al. Left ventricular diastolic function in normal human pregnancy. Circulation 1999;99(4):511-7.

157 Merrigan O. Diagnosing and treating acute myocardial infarction in pregnancy. Br J Nurs 2009;18(21):1300-4.

158 Firoz T, Magee LA. Acute myocardial infarction in the obstetric patient. Obstet Med 2012;5(2):50-7.

159 Bush N, Nelson-Piercy C, Spark P, Kurinczuk JJ, Brocklehurst P, Knight M. Myocardial infarction in pregnancy and postpartum in the UK. Eur J Prev Cardiol 2013;20(1):12-20.

160 Koul AK, Hollander G, Moskovits N, Frankel R, Herrera L, Shani J. Coronary artery dissection during pregnancy and the postpartum period: two case reports and review of literature. Catheter Cardiovasc Interv 2001;52(1):88–94.

161 Sadler L, McCowan L, White H, Stewart A, Bracken M, North R. Pregnancy outcomes and cardiac complications in women with mechanical, bioprosthetic and homograft valves. Br J Obstet Gynaecol 2000;107(2):245–53.

162 Bowater SE, Thorne SA Management of pregnancy in women with acquired and congenital heart disease. Postgraduate Med J 2010;86(1012):100–5.

163 Cusick SS, Tibbles CD. Trauma in pregnancy. Emerg Med Clin N Am 2007;25(3):861–72.

164 Yankowitz J. Fetal effects of drugs commonly used in critical care. In: Dildy GA, Belfort MA, Saade GR, Phelan JP, Hankins GDV, Clark SL eds. Critical care obstetrics. 4th ed. Massachusetts: Blackwell Science; 2004, pp 612–19.

165 Bartalena L, Bogazzi F, Braverman LE, Martino E. Effects of amiodarone administration during pregnancy on neonatal thyroid function and subsequent neurodevelopment. J Endocrinol Invest 2001;24(2):116–30.

166 Arnoni RT, Arnoni AS, Bonini RCA, de Almeida AFS, Neto CA, Dinkhuysen JJ et al. Risk factors associated with cardiac surgery during pregnancy. Ann Thorac Surg 2003;76(5):1605–8.

167 King P, Rosalion A, McMillan J, Buist M, Holmes P. Extracorporeal membrane oxygenation in pregnancy. Lancet 2000;356(9223):45–6.

168 Chan WS, Anand S, Ginsberg JS. Anticoagulation of pregnant women with mechanical heart valves: a systematic review of the literature. Arch Intern Med 2000;160(2):191–6.

169 Kwon H, Belanger K, Bracken M. Asthma prevalence among pregnant and childbearing-aged women in the United States: estimates from National Health Surveys. Ann Epidemiol 2003;13(5):317–24.

170 Australian Centre for Asthma Monitoring. Asthma in Australia 2008. AIHW Asthma Series no. 3. Canberra: Australian Institute of Health and Welfare; 2008.

171 Juniper E, Newhouse M. Effect of pregnancy on asthma: a critical appraisal of the literature. In: Schatz M, Zeiger RS, eds. Asthma and allergy in pregnancy and early infancy. New York: Marcel Dekker; 1993, pp 223–49.

172 Hardy-Fairbanks AJ, Baker ER. Asthma in pregnancy: pathophysiology, diagnosis and management. Obstet Gynecol Clin North Am 2010;37(2):159–72.

173 Gluck JC, Gluck PA. The effect of pregnancy on the course of asthma. Immunol Allergy Clin N Am 2006;26(1):63–80.

174 Murphy VE, Gibson P, Talbot PL, Clifton VL. Severe asthma exacerbations during pregnancy. Obstet Gynecol 2005;106(5):1046–54.

175 Cydulka RK, Emerman CL, Schreiber D, Molander KH, Woodruff PG, Camargo CA Jr. Acute asthma among pregnant women presenting to the emergency department. Am J Respir Crit Care Med 1999;160(3):887–92.

176 Schatz M, Dombrowski M P. Asthma in pregnancy. N Engl J Med 2009;360(18):1862–9.

177 Steven G, Whitworth, MK, Cox S. Substance misuse in pregnancy. Obstet Gynaecol Reprod Med 2014;24(10):309-314.

178 Patteson SK, Snider CC, Meyer DS, Enderson BL, Armstrong JE, Whitaker GL et al. The consequences of high-risk behaviors: trauma during pregnancy. Trauma 2007;62(4):1015–20.

179 Mattox KL, Goetzl L. Trauma in pregnancy. Crit Care Med 2005;33(10):S385–9.

180 Connolly AM, Katz VL, Bash KL, McMahon MJ, Hansen WF. Trauma and pregnancy. Amer J Perinatol 1997;14(6):331,336.

181 Jasinski J. Pregnancy and domestic violence: a review of the literature. Trauma Violence Abuse 2004;5(1):47–64.

182 Brown HL. Trauma in pregnancy. Obstet Gynecol 2009;114(1):147–60.

183 Einav S, Sela HY, Weiniger CF. Management and outcomes of trauma during pregnancy. Anesthes Clin 2013;31:141-156.

184 Queensland Clinical Guidelines: Trauma in pregnancy. Brisbane: Queensland Health, <http://www.health.qld.gov.au/qcg/documents/g-trauma.pdf>; 2014.

185 Goodnight WH, Soper DE. Pneumonia in pregnancy. Crit Care Med 2005;33(10):S390–97.

186 The ANZIC Influenza Investigators and Australasian Maternity Outcomes Surveillance System. Critical illness due to 2009 A/H1N1 influenza in pregnant and postpartum women: population based cohort study. BMJ 2010;340:c1279.

187 The ANZIC Influenza Investigators. Critical care services and 2009 H1N1 influenza in Australia and New Zealand. N Engl J Med 2009;361(20):1925–34.

188 Klinger G, Merlob P. Selective serotonin reuptake inhibitor induced neonatal abstinence syndrome. Isr J Psychiatry Relat Sci 2008;45(2):107–13.

189 Cohen LS, Altshuler LL, Harlow BL, Nonacs R, Newport DJ, Viguera AC et al. Relapse of major depression during pregnancy in women who maintain or discontinue antidepressant treatment. JAMA 2006;295(5):499–507.

190 Kulkarni J. Special issues in managing long-term mental illness in women. Int Rev Psychiatry 2010;22(2):183–90.

191 Brockington I. Postpartum psychiatric disorders. Lancet 2004;363(9405):303–10.

192 Tschinkel S, Harris M, Le Noury J, Healy D. Postpartum psychosis: two cohorts compared, 1875–1924 and 1994–2005. Psychol Med 2007;37(4):529–36.

193 Sharma V, Mazmanian D. Sleep loss and postpartum psychosis. Bipolar Disord 2003;5(2):98–105.

194 Craig C, Howard L. Postnatal depression. BMJ Clin Evid 2009;1:1407.

195 Wylie L, Hollins Martin CJ, Marland G, Martin CR, Rankin J. The enigma of post-natal depression: an update. J Psychiatr Ment Health Nurs 2010;18(1):48–58.

196 Chow SSW. Report of the Australian and New Zealand Neonatal Network 2011. Sydney: Australian and New Zealand Neonatal Network; 2013.

197 Selin H, Stone PK, eds. Childbirth across cultures: Ideas and practices of pregnancy, childbirth and the postpartum. London, New York: Springer; 2009.

198 Martin A, Krishna I, Ellis J, Paccione R, Badell M. Super obesity in pregnancy: difficulties in clinical management. J Perinatol 2014;34:495-502.

199 Knight M, Kurinczuk JJ, Spark P, Brocklehurst P, on behalf of the UK Obstetric Surveillance System. Extreme obesity in pregnancy in the United Kingdom. Obstet Gynecol 2010;115:989-97.

200 McDonnell NJ, Paech MJ, Clavisi OM, Scott KL. Difficult and failed intubation in obstetric anaesthesia: an observational study of airway management and complications associated with general anaesthesia for caesarean section. Int J Obstet Anesth 2008;17(4):292-7.

201 Cousins L. Fetal oxygenation, assessment of fetal well-being, and obstetric management of the pregnant patient with asthma. J Allergy Clin Immunol 1999;103(2, Suppl 1): S343–9.

202 Bugge JF, Tanbo T. Nitric oxide in the treatment of fulminant pulmonary failure in a young pregnant woman with varicella pneumonia. Eur J Anaesthesiol 2000;17(4):269–72.

203 Silverman RK, Montano J. Hyperbaric oxygen treatment during pregnancy in acute carbon monoxide poisoning. A case report. J Reprod Med 1997;42(5):309–11.

204 Plotkin JS, Shah JB, Lofland GK, DeWolf AM. Extracorporeal membrane oxygenation in the successful treatment of traumatic adult respiratory distress syndrome: case report and review. Trauma 1994;37(1):127–30.

205 Manning FA. Fetal biophysical profile. Obstet Gynecol Clin North Am 1999;26(4):557–77.

206 Bobby P. Multiple assessment techniques evaluate antepartum fetal risks. Pediatr Ann 2003;32(9):609–16.

207 Harman CR, Baschat AA. Comprehensive assessment of fetal wellbeing: which Doppler tests should be performed? Curr Opin Obstet Gynecol 2003;15(2):147–57.

208 Kopecky EA, Simone C, Knie B, Koren G. Transfer of morphine across the human placenta and its interaction with naloxone. Life Sci 1999;65(22):2359–71.

209 New Zealand Health Information Service. Report on Maternity 2010. Wellington: Ministry of Health; 2012.

210 Li Z, Zeki R, Hilder L, Sullivan EA. Australia's mothers and babies 2011. Perinatal statistics series no. 28. Cat. no. PER 59. Canberra: AIHW National Perinatal Epidemiology and Statistics Unit; 2013.

211 Royal College of Obstetricians and Gynaecologists. Greentop Guideline No 7. Antenatal corticosteroids to reduce neonatal morbidity and mortality. 2010. London: Royal College of Obstetricians and Gynaecologists; 2010.

212 The Antenatal Magnesium Sulphate for Neuroprotection Guideline Development Panel. Antenatal magnesium sulphate prior to preterm birth for neuroprotection of the fetus, infant and child: National clinical practice guidelines. Adelaide: The University of Adelaide; 2010.

213 Bain E, Middleton P, Crowther CA. Different magnesium sulphate regimens for neuroprotection of the fetus for women at risk of preterm birth. Cochrane Database Syst Rev 2012;2:CD009302. doi: 10.1002/14651858.CD009302.pub2.

214 Ow LL, Kennedy A, McCarthy EA, Walker SP. Feasibility of implementing magnesium sulphate for neuroprotection in a tertiary obstetric unit. Aust N Z J Obstet Gynaecol 2012;52(4):356-60.

215 Vanden Hoek TL, Morrison, LJ, Shuster M, Donnino M, Sinz E, Lavonas EJ et al. Part 12: Cardiac arrest in special situations: 2010 American Heart Association guidelines for cardiopulmonary resuscitation and emergency cardiovascular care. Circulation 2010;122(18 Suppl 3):S829–61.

216 Royal Australian and New Zealand College of Obstetricians and Gynaecologists. College Statement: C-Obs 6. Guidelines for the use of Rh (D) immunoglobulin (Anti-D) in obstetrics in Australia. 2011. Melbourne: RANZCOG; 2011.

217 Pridjian G, Benjamin TD. Update on gestational diabetes. Obstet Gynecol Clin North Am 2010;37:255-67.

218 Nankervis A, McIntyre HD, Moses R, Ross GP, Callaway L, Porter C et al, for the Australasian Diabetes in Pregnancy Society. ADIPS consensus guidelines for the testing and diagnosis of hyperglycaemia in pregnancy in Australia and New Zealand (2014). Australian Diabetes in Pregnancy Society. Sydney, <http://adips.org/information-for-health-care-providers-approved.asp> [accessed 30.11.14].

219 Bamfo J. Managing the risks of sepsis in pregnancy. Best Pract Res Clin Obstet Gynaecol 2013;27:583–95.

220 Malek A, Mattison DR. Drug development for use during pregnancy: impact of the placenta. Expert Rev Obstet Gynecol 2010;5(4):437–54.

221 Hodge LS, Tracy TS. Alterations in drug disposition during pregnancy. Expert Opin Drug Metab Toxicol 2007;3(4):557–71.

222 Bacon RC, Razis PA. The effect of propofol sedation in pregnancy on neonatal condition. Anaesthesia 1994;49(12):1058–60.

223 Kopecky EA, Ryan ML, Barrett JFR, Seaward PGR, Ryan G, Koren G et al. Fetal response to maternally administered morphine. Am J Obstet Gynecol 2000;183(2):424–30.

224 Littleford, J. Effects on the fetus and newborn of maternal analgesia and anesthesia: a review. Can J Anaesth 2004;51(6):586–609.

225 Lee P, Eisman J, Center J. Vitamin D deficiency in critically ill patients. N Engl J Med 2009;360(18):1912–14.

226 Camargo C, Rifas-Shiman S, Litonjua A, Rich-Edwards J, Weiss S, Gold DR et al. Maternal intake of vitamin D during pregnancy and risk of recurrent wheeze in children at 3 y of age. Am J Clin Nutr 2007;85(3):788–95.

227 Javaid MK, Crozier SR, Harvey NC, Gale CR, Dennison EM, Boucher BJ et al. Maternal vitamin D status during pregnancy and childhood bone mass at age 9 years: a longitudinal study. Lancet 2006;367(9504):36–43.

228 Abu-Saad K, Fraser D. Maternal nutrition and birth outcomes. Epidemiol Rev 2010;32(1):5–25.

229 Sherman D, Lurie S, Frenckle E, Kurzweil Y, Bukovsky I, Arieli S. Characteristics of normal lochia. Am J Perinatol 1999;16(8):399–402.

230 Neville MC, Morton J. Physiology and endocrine changes underlying human lactogenesis II. J Nutrition 2001;131(11):S3005–8.

231 Neville MC, Keller RP, Seacat J, Lutes V, Neifert M, Casey C et al. Studies in human lactation: milk volumes in lactating women during the onset of lactation and full lactation. Am J Clin Nutr 1988;48(6):1375–86.

232 Grattan DR. Behavioural significance of prolactin signalling in the central nervous system during pregnancy and lactation. Reproduction 2002;123(4):497–506.

233 Arora S, McJunkin C, Wehrer J, Kuhn P. Major factors influencing breastfeeding rates: mother's perception of father's attitude and milk supply. Pediatrics 2000;106(5):E67.

234 Hartmann P, Cregan M, Ramsay DT, Simmer K, Kent JC. Physiology of lactation in preterm mothers: initiation and maintenance. Pediatr Ann 2003;32(5):351–5.

235 Sozmen M. Effects of early suckling of cesarean-born babies on lactation. Biol Neonate 1992;62(1):67–8.

236 Woolridge M, Greasley V, Silpisornkosol S. The initiation of lactation: the effect of early versus delayed contact for suckling on milk intake in the first week post-partum: a study in Chiang Mai, Northern Thailand. Early Hum Dev 1985;12(3):269–78.

237 Morse JM, Jehle C, Gamble D. Initiating breastfeeding: a world survey of the timing of postpartum breastfeeding. Int J Nurs Stud 1990;27(3):303–13.

238 Meier PP. Breastfeeding in the special care nursery. Prematures and infants with medical problems. Pediatr Clin North Am 2001;48(2):425–42.

239 Hale T. Breastfeeding pharmacology, <http://www.infantrisk.com> [accessed 02.11].

240 Hale TW. Medications in breastfeeding mothers of preterm infants. Pediatr Ann 2003;32(5):337–47.

241 Swyer G. Postpartum mental disturbances and hormone changes. BMJ 1985;290(6477):1232–3.

242 Christensson K, Cabrera T, Christensson E, Uvnäs-Moberg K, Winberg J. Separation distress call in the human neonate in the absence of maternal body contact. Acta Paediatr 1995;84(5):468–73.

243 Austin DM, Sadler L, McLintock C, McArthur C, Masson V, Farquhar C et al. Early detection of severe maternal morbidity: a retrospective assessment of the role of an Early Warning Score System. Aust N Z J Obstet Gynaecol 2014;54(2):152-5.

244 Carle C, Alexander P, Columb M, Johal J. Design and internal validation of an obstetric early warning score: secondary analysis of the Intensive Care National Audit and Research Centre Case Mix Programme database. Anaesthesia 2013;68(4):354-67.

Chapter **29**

Organ donation and transplantation

Debbie Friel

Learning objectives

After reading this chapter, you should be able to:

- differentiate between coma and brain death
- understand the process of donor identification and referral
- be aware of best practice for the consent-seeking process
- understand the principles of donor management.

Introduction

Transplantation is a life-saving and cost-effective form of treatment that enhances the quality of life, often completely transforming the lives of people with end-stage chronic diseases. Allografts are transplanted organs or tissues from one person (living or cadaveric) to another person. Transplantation surgery commenced in Australia in 1911, with a pancreas transplant in Launceston General Hospital, Tasmania. Other tissue and solid organ transplantations followed, retrieved from donors without cardiac function: the first cornea in 1941; kidney in 1956; and livers and hearts in 1968. Transplantation in New Zealand began in the 1940s with corneal grafting, and the first organ transplants were kidney and heart valve transplantation in the 1960s.[1] This chapter outlines contemporary practice in human organ transplantation in Australia and New Zealand outlining the legislation that governs the types of transplants performed and the role of the critical nurse as part of a multidisciplinary team in the management and care of the donor and the family.

The first successful human-to-human transplant of any kind was a corneal transplant performed in Moravia (now the Czech Republic) in 1905.[1] It took many decades to progress to solid organ transplantation. In 1968 Harvard Medical School produced a report on the 'hopelessly unconscious patient'. This report noted that life support could be withdrawn from patients diagnosed with 'irreversible coma' or 'brain death' (terms they used interchangeably) and that, with appropriate consent, the organs could be removed for transplantation.[2] The committee's primary concern was to provide an acceptable course of action to permit withdrawal of mechanical ventilator support for the purpose of organ donation for human transplantation. In 1981, a USA President's Commission

KEY WORDS
....

brain death

consent

coroner

designated officer

DonateLife

next of kin

organ donation

organ donor

organ recipient

organ retrieval

transplant

declared that individual death depended on either irreversible cessation of circulatory and respiratory functions or irreversible cessation of all functions of the entire brain. The consequent *Uniform Determination of Death Act* referred to 'whole brain death' as a requirement for the determination of brain death.[2]

Legislation that defined brain death and enabled beating-heart retrieval was enacted in New Zealand in 1964 and in Australia from 1982, and in most European countries it was occurring during similar time periods. This legislation heralded the establishment of formal transplant programs.[3] In Australia, the first heart and lung program commenced in 1983, a liver transplant program in 1985, combined heart–lung transplant in 1986, combined kidney and pancreas in 1987, single lung in 1990[2] and small bowel in 2010. In New Zealand, bone was first transplanted in the early 1980s and the first heart transplant occurred in 1987. Skin transplantation occurred in 1991, lung transplantation in 1993 and liver and pancreas transplantation in 1998.[4] The success of transplantation in the current era as a viable option for end-stage organ failure is primarily due to the discovery of the immunosuppression agent cyclosporin A.[5] This chapter discusses the processes and clinical implications of cadaveric organ and tissue donation, within a critical care nursing context.

Donation systems

There are currently two general systems of approach to seeking consent for cadaveric organ and tissue donation in operation around the world. Some countries (e.g. Spain, Singapore and Austria) have legislated an 'opt out', or presumed consent, system where eligible persons are considered for organ retrieval at the time of their death if they have not previously indicated their explicit objection[6] (see Table 29.1). In Australia, New Zealand, the USA, the UK and most other common-law countries, the approach is to 'opt in', with specific consent required from the potential donor's next of kin.[1] In some states of Australia (for example, New South Wales and South Australia) and in New Zealand people can indicate an intent for consent to organ donation on their driver's licence, and in all Australian states on the Australian Organ Donor Register (AODR).[7,8] In Singapore, the *Human Organ Transplant Act* of 1987 combines a presumed consent system with a required consent system for the Muslim population. The informed consent legislations of Japan and Korea are two of the most recent to come into force, in 1997 and 2000 respectively; before then, only living donation and donation after cardiac death were possible.[8]

Types of donations

Organ and tissue donation includes retrieval of organs and tissues both after death and from a living person. Donations from a living person include regenerative tissue (blood and bone marrow) and non-regenerative tissue (cord blood, kidneys, liver (lobe/s), lungs (lobe/s), femoral heads). The implications of consent are different for each type of requested tissue. For example, the collection of bone marrow and the retrieval of a kidney, the lobe of a liver or lung are invasive procedures that could potentially risk the health and wellbeing of the donor.[9] In contrast, donation of a femoral head could be the end-product of a total hip replacement, where the bone is otherwise discarded. Similarly, cord blood from the umbilical cord is discarded if not retrieved immediately after birth.

After cardiac death, many people can still be donors for eyes, heart valves and cardiac tissue, long bones, pelvis, tendons, ligaments and skin.[10] It is after confirmation of brain death that the 'traditional' organs of the heart, lungs, liver, kidneys, pancreas, intestine and tissues can be retrieved, as well as tissues, including eyes. In Australia in 2010 a national protocol for the reintroduction of Donation after Cardiac Death (sometimes referred to as non-beating heart donation or donation after circulatory death) was introduced. This enables the potential donation of lungs, kidneys, liver and sometimes pancreas, along with tissues and eyes.[1]

Organ donation and transplant networks

The donation and transplantation process in many countries including Australia and New Zealand is a nationally coordinated process in the healthcare system, a unique arrangement given the disparity between state health departments and funding arrangements between federal and state health departments.

The Organ and Tissue Authority in Australia

Legislation governing organ and tissue donation in Australia is based in state and territory jurisdictions. The national network of organ and tissue donation agencies is known in Australia as the Australian Organ and Tissue Authority (AOTA). Solid organ donation agencies are based in New South Wales (in partnership with the Australian Capital Territory), Victoria (with Tasmania), South Australia, Northern Territory, Queensland and Western Australia. Separate state-based tissue banks facilitate tissue retrieval around Australia apart from Western Australia, where the organ donation agency coordinates all organ and tissue retrieval. Other countries use similar models of governance using the multidisciplinary approach to donor care and use of designated requestor.[1]

The Australian Organ and Tissue Authority (AOTA) is Australia's peak body that works with all jurisdictions and sectors to provide a nationally coordinated approach to organ and tissue donation for transplantation. The Authority was established in 2009 under the *Australian Organ and Tissue Donation and Transplantation Authority Act 2008* as an independent statutory authority within the

TABLE 29.1

Type of legislation by country[1]

COUNTRY	TYPE OF LEGISLATION	YEAR AND DESCRIPTION OF LEGISLATION
Australia	Informed consent	1982, donor registry since 2000
Austria	Presumed consent	1982, non-donor register since 1995
Belgium	Presumed consent	1986, combined register since 1987, families informed and can object to organ donation
Bulgaria	Presumed consent	1996, in practice, consent from family required
Canada	Informed consent	1980
Croatia	Presumed consent	2000, family consent always requested
Cyprus	Presumed consent	1987
Czech Republic	Presumed consent	1984
Denmark	Informed consent	1990, combined register since 1990, previously presumed consent
Estonia	Presumed consent	No date identified
Finland	Presumed consent	1985
France	Presumed consent	1976, non-donor register since 1990; families can override the wishes of the deceased
Germany	Informed consent	1997
Greece	Presumed consent	1978
Hungary	Presumed consent	1972
India	Informed consent	1994
Ireland	Informed consent	Follows UK legislation
Israel	Presumed consent	1953
Italy	Presumed consent	1967, combined register since 2000, families consulted before retrieval
Japan	Informed consent	1997
Korea	Informed consent	2000
Latvia	Presumed consent	No date identified
Lithuania	Informed consent	No date identified
Luxemburg	Presumed consent	1982
The Netherlands	Informed consent	1996, combined register since 1998
New Zealand	Informed consent	1964
Norway	Presumed consent	1973, families consulted and can refuse
Poland	Presumed consent	1990, non-donor register since 1996
Portugal	Presumed consent	1993, non-donor register since 1994
Romania	Informed consent	1998, combined register since 1996
Singapore	Presumed consent	1987, informed consent for Muslim population
Slovak Republic	Presumed consent	1994
Slovenia	Presumed consent	1996
Spain	Presumed consent	1979, in practice, consent required from families
Sweden	Presumed consent	1996, families can veto consent if wishes of the deceased are not known; previously informed consent
Switzerland	Informed consent	1996, some Cantons have presumed consent laws
Turkey	Presumed consent	1979, in practice, written consent required from family
United Kingdom	Informed consent	1961, donor register since 1994
United States of America	Informed consent	1968, donor registers in some states

Note: A combined register is a register of consent and refusal.

Australian Government Health and Ageing portfolio to maximise rates of donation, and achieve the nine national reform agenda measures:

1 a national approach and system: a national authority and network of DonateLife agencies
2 specialist hospital staff and systems dedicated to organ donation
3 activity funding for hospitals
4 national professional awareness and education
5 coordinated ongoing community awareness and education
6 support for donor families
7 safe, equitable and transparent national transplantation processes
8 a national eye and tissue donation and transplantation network
9 other national initiatives, including living donation programs.

This initial aim of the Australian Organ and Tissue Authority (AOTA) was to 'spearhead and be accountable for a new world's best practice national approach and system to achieve a significant and lasting increase in the number of life-saving and life-transforming transplants for Australians'. The DonateLife Network, under the Australian Organ and Tissue Authority (AOTA), includes DonateLife agencies and hospital-based staff across Australia dedicated to organ and tissue donation. DonateLife agencies were re-formed and re-named as part of the nationally integrated network to manage and deliver the organ donation process according to national protocols and systems and in collaboration with their hospital-based colleagues.[1] Legislation in New Zealand is national, with Organ Donation New Zealand coordinating all organ and tissue retrieval from deceased donors.[4]

Regulation and management

In Australia, quality processes involved in organ and tissue retrieval and transplant are governed by the Therapeutic Goods Administration.[11] In New Zealand there is currently an unregulated market for medical devices and complementary medicines, although an agreement to establish a *Joint Scheme for the Regulation of Therapeutic Products* between the Governments of Australia and New Zealand is in place.[9] Other countries have similar agencies that regulate the standards for healthcare products including organ and tissue donation.[10]

In Australia, the process of potential donor identification and management in critical care is directed by the Australian and New Zealand Intensive Care Society (ANZICS).[2] Education of health professionals is facilitated by DonateLife agencies, and offers a suite of training resources, encompassing three units in their professional education package titled ADAPT (Australian Donor Awareness Program). Nationally, ADAPT remains the core training module for critical care nurses, in association with the Australian College of Critical Care Nurses

(ACCCN) and the College of Intensive Care Medicine (CICM). Internationally, the European Training Program on Organ Donation is a partnership of European centres, which provides professional education for different professional profiles in a blended learning environment; and India offers online learning for medical staff endorsed by several societies in Europe.[6] The United Network for Organ Sharing in the USA offers a range of education and resource access to professionals in the organ donation and transplant networks.

Donor criteria and organ allocation is regulated by the Transplantation Society of Australia and New Zealand (TSANZ). Donor and recipient data are collated by the Australia and New Zealand Organ Donation Registry (ANZOD Registry) and published on an annual basis. Professional groups related to this specialty area also cover both countries. The Australasian Transplant Coordinators Association (ATCA) is composed of clinicians working as donor and/or transplant coordinators, and the Transplant Nurses Association (TNA) is a specialty group for nurses working with transplant recipients (see *Online resources*).

Legislation governing organ donation in New Zealand and Australia takes the form of legislated Acts covering the use of human tissue both before and after death. These legislations enable a person to choose to be a donor, and organ donation can proceed unless that wish is reversed or the family does not consent. If the deceased's wishes are not apparent, consent for organ donation rests with the next of kin.

In Australia the legislation defines death as the:

- irreversible cessation of all function of the brain of the person
  or
- irreversible cessation of circulation of blood in the body of the person.[2]

Tissue donation is also very tightly regulated in all of Australia and New Zealand. In Australia, the Commonwealth statutory body is the Therapeutic Goods Administration (TGA)[11] and in New Zealand, the statutory body is the Medicines and Medical Devices Safety Authority (MEDSAFE).

Identification of organ and tissue donors

The four main factors that directly influence the number of multi-organ donations are:

1 incidence of brain death
2 identification of potential donors (both cardiac death and brain death donors)
3 brain death confirmation and informed consent for donation
4 donor management after brain death.

Brain death

The incidence of brain death has traditionally determined the size of the potential organ donor pool. Diagnosis of brain death is now widely accepted, and most developed countries have legislation governing the definition of death and the retrieval of organs for transplant.[12] In Australia and New Zealand the most common cause of brain death has changed from traumatic head injury to cerebrovascular accident, which has implications for the organs and tissues retrieved. Donors are older and often have cardiovascular and other comorbidities.[13] If organs and tissues are not going to be retrieved for transplantation, there is no legal requirement to confirm brain death if treatment is deemed futile.[2]

Two medical practitioners participate in determining brain death; in Australia one must be a designated specialist (described later). Brain death is observed clinically only when the patient is supported with artificial ventilation, as the respiratory reflex lost due to cerebral ischaemia will result in respiratory and cardiac arrest. Artificial (mechanical) ventilation maintains oxygen supply to the natural pacemaker (SA node) of the heart, which functions independently of the central nervous system. Brain death results in hypotension due to loss of vasomotor control of the autonomic nervous system, loss of temperature regulation, reduction in hormone activity and loss of all cranial nerve reflexes. Table 29.2 lists the conditions commonly associated with brain death, but not all people who have progressed to brain death exhibit all of the conditions. Irrespective of the degree of external support, cardiac standstill will occur in a matter of hours to days once brain death has occurred.[15,16]

TABLE 29.2
Conditions associated with brain death[2,13]

CONDITION	INCIDENCE
Hypotension	81%
Diabetes insipidus	53%
Disseminated intravascular coagulation	28%
Arrhythmias	27%
Cardiac arrest	25%
Pulmonary oedema	19%
Hypoxia	11%
Acidosis	11%

Testing methods

The aim of testing for brain death is to determine irreversible cessation of brain function. Testing does not demonstrate that every brain cell has died but that a point of irreversible ischaemic damage involving cessation of the vital functions of the brainstem has been reached. There are a number of steps in the process, the first being the observation period. With the exception of a hypoxia-ischaemic brain injury that has been treated with therapeutic hypothermia, where an observation period of 24 hours is required following rewarming to

BOX 29.1
Preconditions of brain death testing[2]
- Known diagnosis of injury and coma is consistent with progression to brain death.
- Exclude involvement of drugs.
- Exclude metabolic causes for coma (e.g. severe electrolyte or endocrine abnormalities).
- Exclude hypothermia (core temperature greater than 35°C).
- Systolic BP >80 mmHg.
- Confirm neuromuscular conduction.

35°C,[2] an observation period of at least 4 hours from onset of observed no response is required. This must be documented before the first set of testing commences, in the context of a patient being mechanically ventilated with a Glasgow Coma Scale score of 3, non-reacting pupils, absent cough and gag reflexes and no spontaneous respiratory effort.[2] The second step is to consider the preconditions (see Box 29.1). Once the observation period has passed (during which the patient receives ongoing treatment) and the preconditions have been met, formal testing can occur.

Practice tip

When testing for corneal reflex, take care not to cause corneal abrasion, which might preclude the cornea from being transplanted if the patient is a potential eye/corneal donor.

If it is possible, inviting the next of kin to observe the second set of clinical tests may assist their comprehension of brain death. If this is possible, assign a support person to be with the family to assist in explaining and interpreting the testing process.

Adapted from Siminoff LA, Mercer MB, Arnold R. Families' understanding of brain death. Prog Transplant 2003;13(3): 218–24, with permission.

Formal testing for brain death is undertaken using either clinical assessment or cerebral blood flow studies.[2] Clinical assessment of the brainstem involves assessment of the cranial nerves and the respiratory centre. The most common approaches to testing are described in Table 29.3. Brain death is confirmed if there is no reaction to stimulation of these reflexes, with the respiratory centre tested last and only if the other reflexes are absent. The tests may be done consecutively, but not simultaneously, with no fixed interval between the two sets of clinical tests required, except in specific age-related criteria.[2]

If the preconditions outlined in Box 29.1 are unable to be verified, brain death can be confirmed using cerebral blood flow imaging to demonstrate absent blood flow to

TABLE 29.3

Clinical brain death testing[2,17]

TEST	CRANIAL NERVES/ NEUROLOGICAL FUNCTION	TEST TECHNIQUE	OUTCOME
1 Response to painful stimuli	Trigeminal V (sensory), facial VII (motor)	Stimulus within the cranial nerve distribution (e.g. firm pressure over supraorbital region)	If reflex is absent, the patient will not grimace or react
2 Pupillary response to light	Optic II, oculomotor III	Using torch	If reflex is absent, the pupils are fixed: may or may not be dilated
3 Corneal reflex	Trigeminal V (sensory), facial VII (motor)	Using wisp of cotton wool to touch the cornea	If reflex is absent, the eyes will not react or blink
4 Gag reflex	Glossopharyngeal IX, vagus X	Using a tongue depressor on the oropharynx or moving ETT	If reflex is absent, there is no gag or pharyngeal response
5 Cough reflex	Glossopharyngeal IX, vagus X	Using suction catheter down ETT to deliberately stimulate the carina	If reflex is absent, there is no cough response
6 Oculovestibular reflex	Vestibulocochlear VII, oculomotor III, abducens VI	Checking first that both tympanic membranes are intact or not obstructed; then slowly irrigating both ears with 50 mL iced water while eyes are held open	If reflex is absent, the eyes remain fixed rather than deviating towards the stimulus
7 Apnoea test	Medullar respiratory centre	Last test to be performed when all other reflexes have proven to be absent. The patient is preoxygenated on 100% O_2, an ABG analysis is performed to ascertain the baseline CO_2, then the patient is disconnected from mechanical ventilation but supplied with oxygen via catheter or T piece; the patient is observed for signs of respiratory effort	The period of time disconnected from the ventilator must be long enough for the arterial CO_2 level to rise to a threshold high enough to normally stimulate respiration, i.e. an arterial CO_2 >60 mmHg and an arterial pH of <7.30
8 Oculocephalic reflex (doll's eyes)	Ocular function and internuclear pathway in brainstem for cranial nerves III, IV, VI; labyrinthine semicircular canals, otoliths and neck muscle proprioceptors	Although not a formal component of brain death testing, this reflex may be tested as routine practice. The test must not be performed if an unstable cervical spine is suspected. Holding the eyes open, rotate the head from side to side, observing the position of the eyes	If the reflex is absent, the eyes will move with the head and do not move within their orbit, indicating significant brainstem injury

ABG = arterial blood gas; CO_2 = carbon dioxide; ETT = endotracheal tube.

the brain. Both contrast angiography and radionuclide scanning can be used to confirm brain death. Contrast angiography can be performed by direct injection of contrast into both carotid arteries and one or both of the vertebral arteries, or via the vena cava or aortic arch. Brain death is confirmed when there is no blood flow above the carotid siphon. A radionuclide scan is performed by administering a bolus of short-acting isotope intravenously or by nebuliser while imaging the head using a gamma camera for 15 minutes. No intracranial uptake of isotope confirms absent blood flow to the brain.[18]

If brain death is confirmed, the time of death is recorded as the time of certification of the testing result (i.e. at the completion of the second set of clinical tests, or the documentation of the results of the cerebral blood flow scan).[2]

Identification of a potential multi-organ donor

The second factor influencing the number of actual organ donors is identification of a potential donor. A potential donor is defined in this situation as a patient who is suspected of, or is confirmed as, being brain dead. Inclusion and exclusion criteria for organ and tissue donation are constantly being reviewed and refined, and may also be dependent on the critical waiting list patients.[19] When considering the medical suitability of potential organ donors, advice can be sought 24 hours a day, 7 days a week, from respective state and territory organ donation agencies in Australia (see *Online resources*).

Seeking consent

The third factor influencing the number of donors is brain death confirmation and informed consent for donation. In line with the various state human tissue acts and Therapeutic Goods Administration guidelines in Australia, consent is sought for individual organs and tissues, rather than making a 'global' approach. If granted, the individual tissues are recorded on the consent form or named if the consent is being recorded over the telephone; only those tissues granted will be retrieved.

Common practice in Australia and New Zealand is for the treating medical staff either to initiate or at least to be involved in approaching the next of kin after death has been confirmed.[2] Approaching the next of kin to seek consent is part of the duty of care to patients who may have indicated their wish to be a donor at the time of their death.[2] Offering the option of organ donation is also considered part of the duty of care to the family.[2] This view is supported by a survey of donor families, who all indicated that they were grateful to have been provided with the option.[20] Three elements are involved when approaching a family regarding the option of organ donation:

1 their knowledge, beliefs and attitudes
2 their in-hospital experience
3 any beliefs and biases of health professional/s conducting the approach.[21]

The outcome of an approach cannot be predicted or anticipated, as it may affect the 'spirit' in which the approach is made. A large USA study demonstrated that clinical staff were incorrect 50% of the time when asked to predict the response of next of kin.[22]

Attitudes to organ donation are influenced by spiritual beliefs, cultural background, prior knowledge about organ donation, views on altruism and prior health experiences.[21] Next of kin consider two aspects associated with existing attitudes and knowledge: the decision maker(s)' own thoughts and feelings and the previous wishes and beliefs of the person on whose behalf they are making the decision.[23] There is evidence of a link between consent rates and prior knowledge of the positive outcomes of organ donation.[21,24] A large USA study found that consent rates improved when conversations about brain death and organ donation were separated, were held in a private setting and when an organ donation professional/trained requestor was involved.[21]

Delivery of relevant information

An important consideration for all health professionals is that family members may have a diminished ability to receive and understand information because of their stress and psychological responses at this time of family crisis.[20, 21,25] As interviews held with the family are the foundation of the entire organ donation and transplant process, the discussion about brain death must be clear and emphatic, using language free of medical terminology, and include an explanation of the physical implications.[26] Diagrams, analogies, scans and written materials have been suggested as useful aids for enhancing understanding by next of kin.[27] One approach is to describe brain death as like a jigsaw puzzle with a piece missing, to illustrate the relationship of the brain to the rest of the body.[27] Opportunities for staff to train and role-play this scenario with programs like ADAPT in Australia and the European Training Program on Organ Donation in Europe (see *Online resources*) improve the likelihood of meeting the needs of families.[1,27,28]

As the time of confirmation of brain death is the person's legal time of death, multiple family conversations may occur with the family to discuss their options and associated implications. Options are to: 1) cease ventilation and allow cardiac standstill to occur; or 2) maintain ventilation and haemodynamic support to explore and potentially facilitate viable organ and tissue donation. The retrieval process must be fully explained to ensure an informed decision, but not to overload the next of kin.[21] Table 29.4 lists some aspects of the organ donation process that ought to be included in such a discussion. As information given to a family contains both good news and bad news it is suggested to start with the positive news – the benefits of donation, the right of the family to refuse consent and the lack of cost – and then move to the less positive news – the reality of the surgical intervention and the lack of guarantee that the organs will be transplanted.[1] Families frequently gain solace from the positive aspects of donation, of helping or reducing the suffering of other families. Of note, a best practice approach aims to assist the family to make the decision that is 'right' for them and does not necessarily result in gaining consent.

Meetings with the family

Identifying who the appropriate family members are to meet with in relation to organ donation is a first consideration, and then the process by which the discussions will be held needs to be considered. In Australia the definition of next of kin for adults and children is listed in strict order (see Table 29.5). In New Zealand there is no hierarchy of next of kin, with the definition including a surviving spouse or relative.[2] In both countries, the next of kin can override the known wishes of the deceased regarding consent, but experience shows that the family rarely disagree if the wishes of the deceased are known, regardless of their own personal beliefs.[2]

The timing, location, content and process of discussions with the family are all important considerations. An effective protocol for communicating with the family of a potential donor must include: 1) frequent and honest updates on the patient's prognosis; 2) clear explanation of brain death; 3) the decoupling of the brain death and organ donation conversations[21,29] until the family accepts that the patient is dead; 4) conversations held in a private and quiet setting;[21,22,29] and 5) involvement of an organ donation professional with a clear definition of roles.[22]

There is compelling evidence that the meeting confirming diagnosis of brain death should be held separately or decoupled from the conversation about the option of organ and tissue donation.[29] In reality, the pace and flow of discussions should be assessed on a case-by-case basis, as there may be circumstances when the discussion about organ donation is appropriately held prior to the confirmation of death.[2,30]

Three other influential components of this process come from surveys completed with donor and non-donor families:

1 use of inappropriate terms such as 'harvest' to name the organ retrieval surgery (this is considered harsh and undignified) and 'life support' to name the ventilator (this could perpetuate the hope of a chance of survival or recovery)[2]

TABLE 29.4

Information about the organ donation process and retrieval to assist in informed decision making[1,21]

DECISION	ISSUES
Ensure that the next of kin (NOK) have understanding of:	• Brain death • Time of death • Eventual organ failure if kept ventilated in critical care • The two options: to immediately cease ventilation or organ donation
If they choose to donate:	• They will not be with the donor at time of cardiac arrest • Donor will remain in critical care, monitored and ventilated until going to theatre for retrieval • Explain the organ retrieval surgery, including the presence of an anaesthetist to monitor the haemodynamics and ventilation • Explain to the family that the person no longer feels any pain, so an anaesthetic is not given • Discuss which organs and tissue would be potentially medically suitable for retrieval for transplant • Next of kin can give specific consent; they are not obliged to grant global consent • Only named organs and tissues with consent are retrieved • Advise expected length of process • Explain reason for bloods being taken and stored • Advise that a coordinator will be present through the entire process • Explain how the donor will look after the retrieval • Organ donation will not delay funeral plans • Explain consent form • Provide copy of consent form • Explain privacy implications of *Human Tissue Act*, for donor family and transplant recipients • Explain reasons why donation may not proceed • Explain that organs may be transplanted interstate • In the event of an abnormality/diseases, organs will not be retrieved • Explain consent for research: offer copy of research page • The site designated officer will also sign the consent form
If coroner's case:	• Coroner's consent required • Police identification required • Autopsy? Brain retrieval? • Deceased will go to the coroner's mortuary after retrieval • Explain contact with coroner's court
If organs are retrieved and not able to be transplanted:	• Offer options. Will be returned and placed with donor, or disposed of as medical waste
Support services:	• Offer viewing of patient or a telephone call after the retrieval • Offer lock of hair and/or handprint • Provide contact details of coordinator • Provide printed information • Explain other support services available
Follow-up information:	• Outcome of retrieval • Recipient outcomes • Written material and letters • Counselling services • Availability of transplant coordinator to answer questions

2 attire of the personnel involved – staff wearing surgical scrubs or plastic aprons made families wonder what was being done to their relatives that required health professionals to be wearing such clothing, and donor coordinators not wearing uniforms were easier to speak to[21]

3 timing or use of the information from consent indicator sources such as organ donor registers and driver's licence was thought to be coercive and disrespectful.[21] Current clinical practice in Australia involves checking of the Australian Organ Donor Register (AODR) and informing the family to assist them in making an informed decision about their loved one's wishes.

TABLE 29.5

Definition of next of kin for children and adults in Australian legislation[2]

DONOR	ORDER OF SENIORITY	RELATIONSHIP
Child	1	Parent
	2	Adult sibling (over 18 years)
	3	Guardian (immediately before death)
Adult	1	Spouse or de facto (at time of death)
	2	Adult offspring (over 18 years)
	3	Parent
	4	Adult sibling (over 18 years)

Staff roles, delineation and involvement

Staff involved in the explanation of brain death must have a clear understanding of brain death, and have practised explaining it themselves before attempting to explain it to a family.[21] Ideally, requestors are specifically trained in the approach of requesting organ and tissue donation and have completed the ADAPT course. Additionally, having the organ donor coordinator present to answer specific questions raised by the family assists in the process.[2] The process of organ and tissue donation in critical care is significant for all concerned. When death is confirmed it marks the end of an episode that has been catastrophic for both patient and loved ones, and a potentially stressful and exhausting experience for staff.[1,25,31] Approaching a potential donor family is a multidisciplinary team effort, and guidelines encourage treating medical staff to continue their involvement with patient and family after brain death is confirmed, for continuity of care.[2] Nursing staff involvement in the process of organ and tissue donation is central and intrinsic, including the practicalities of the process, and care of the potential donor and family during the decision-making process.[21] Donor families have identified nurses as being the most helpful health professionals in providing information and emotional support.[2,11]

A holistic approach to supporting families in critical care also includes involvement of social workers and pastoral care workers and other allied health professionals. Often these health professionals have been working with the family for a number of days and act as confidants and a resource for information on issues such as implications of a coronial enquiry and a religious denomination's stance on organ donation. Most major religions are supportive of organ and tissue donation for transplant and would instruct the family to make the decision that they felt was correct.[1,32]

In many countries there are organ donation coordinators that act as a resource and are invited into critical care when appropriate.[1,32] A professional who is an expert in

---

Practice tip

The multidisciplinary team involved in the process of organ donation is not limited to staff within the ICU. In order for the donor's wishes to become a reality and provide organ and tissues for transplantation the following disciplines are involved:[1]

- medical
- nursing
- allied health
- pastoral care
- operational services
- administration
- police service
- coroner's and magistrate's office
- designated officer.

Adapted with permission from the DonateLife website, <http://www.donatelife.gov.au>.

---

donation and has the time to spend with the family may be the best person to undertake an approach to a potential donor family.[21,33]

Role of designated specialists

In most countries, senior medical staff eligible to certify brain death using brain death criteria must be appointed by the governing body of their health institution, have relevant and recent experience and not be involved with transplant recipient selection.[34] In Australia, the most common medical specialties appointed to the role are intensivists, neurologists and neurosurgeons in metropolitan centres, and general surgeons or physicians in rural settings.[34]

In New Zealand the role is not appointed although medical staff confirming brain death must also act independently; neither can be members of the transplant team, and both must be appropriately qualified and suitably experienced in the care of such patients.[2] The New Zealand Code of Practice for Transplantation[35] also recommends that the medical staff not be involved in treating the recipient of the organ to be removed, and one of the doctors should be a specialist in charge of the clinical care of the patient.

Role of designated officers

Under Australian law, a 'designated officer' is appointed by the governing body of the institution to authorise a non-coronial postmortem and the removal of tissue from a deceased person for transplant or other therapeutic, medical or scientific purposes.[2] The designated officer must be satisfied that all necessary inquiries have been made and any necessary consent has been obtained before granting authority. Medical, nursing and administrative staff can be appointed to the role, but they must not act in a case if they have had clinical or personal involvement in the donor's case.[2]

The term 'designated officer' is not used in New Zealand legislation. A person with equivalent authority under the *Human Tissue Act 2008* is the person lawfully in possession of the body.[35] In the case of a hospital, this person is specified as the medical officer in charge.[2] In practice, the treating clinician undertakes this consultation with the family.

Role of coroner and forensic pathologists

Because of the nature of their death, many donors are subject to coronial inquiry. In this case, permission to undertake organ and tissue retrieval is sought from the respective forensic pathologist and coroner according to local policy and procedure as part of the consent-seeking process. The coronial system is very supportive of donation for transplant and, in 2012, 43% of the Australian and 50% of New Zealand multi-organ donors were coroner's cases.[34]

Consent indicator databases

The most influential variable that an individual may use to affect family unit decision making is the existence of an advance care directive or prior indication of consent, as this information has made decision making 'easier'[36] and preserved patient autonomy,[28,36] enabling wishes of the

TABLE 29.6

Consent indicator databases in Australia and New Zealand[7,12,39]

COUNTRY	DATABASE NAME	HOST	ACCESS TO DATABASE INFORMATION	AVAILABILITY TO JOIN
Australia	Australian Organ Donor Register	Medicare Australia	Limited to coordinators nominated by state DonateLife agencies and tissue banks	Via Medicare offices, internet or phone (1800 777 203)
	Driver's licence	State roads and transport authorities (varies by state)	Limited to coordinators nominated by state donation agencies and tissue banks	Driver's licence application and renewal form
New Zealand	Driver's licence	Land Transport New Zealand database	Limited to coordinators nominated by the National Transplant Donor Coordination Office	Driver's licence application and renewal form

patient to be followed even when family decision makers would have made the opposite decision. Conversely, if the family members were opposed to donation despite the presence of an indication of consent from the potential donor, the retrieval would not occur on ethical grounds.[1] Table 29.6 lists prospective donation databases available in Australia and New Zealand.

Cultural competence

With large cultural mixes in many countries including Australia and New Zealand, best practice for approaching a family includes openness and awareness of what information the family member(s) may need to make their decision. As significant differences also exist within various cultural groups, expectations of responses cannot be stereotyped. When healthcare professionals are unsure of how a family may perceive a situation it is best to ask, as acknowledgment of expectations and needs can lead to improved communication.[21,22] Importantly, the most significant differences between potential donor families are socioeconomic and educational factors, rather than cultural or racial background.[37,38,39] Therefore, individual assessment must guide the approach by health professionals. Cultural aspects of critical care nursing practice are discussed in Chapter 8.

Organ donor care

Understanding the brain death physiology and the importance of time management is critical in the management of a potential organ donor. Those patients who have sustained traumatic brain injuries can deteriorate rapidly following brain death, exhibiting severe physiological instability requiring vigilant monitoring and specialised treatment to stabalise and maintain organ perfusion. This is a time of great distress for families with the patient's death usually the result of a sudden, unexpected illness or injury, and therefore discussion surrounding organ and tissue donation must be undertaken in a sensitive manner by skilled requestors who possess a strong professional commitment to the quality of the process.[2,37,40]

Ideally, the time between brain death and organ retrieval should be minimised to ensure an optimal outcome for transplant recipients. Therefore, the focus of medical management changes from ensuring brain perfusion to maintaining good organ perfusion for transplantation.[37] Early referral, application of recognised management protocols and collaboration between the donation centre and retrieval teams are paramount. Donor family care forms a crucial part of the process, with up-to-date and accurate information essential to ensure the bereavement process is managed appropriately.

Referral of potential donor

If consent is granted, the donor referral process usually commences immediately. The longer the time delay, the more likely that organ failure-related complications will occur.[12] In 2012, the median time from brain death confirmation to the commencement of organ retrieval was 18.5 hours in Australia and 14.2 hours in New Zealand.[35]

The referral process begins with hospital-based specialists and donor coordinators collating the past and present medical, surgical and social history of the potential donor, and relaying this information to the relevant transplant units (see Table 29.7). In Australia, a National Electronic Donor Record was introduced in 2014, enabling secure and rapid relay of information to transplant units as opposed to individual transplant unit telephone calls to relay information. Using this information, transplant teams allocate the organs to the most suitable and appropriate recipient/s. If the transplant team does not have a suitable recipient, the offer is extended to another team in Australia or New Zealand on rotation using Transplant Society of Australia and New Zealand (TSANZ) guidelines.[19,41]

Practice tip

All brain dead patients should be referred to the relevant state DonateLife agency for advice regarding medical suitability. Contacting the state DonateLife agency for advice does not constitute an obligation or formal referral for organ donation.

Adapted with permission from Australasian Transplant Coordinators Association. National guidelines for organ and tissue donation, 4th ed. Sydney: ATCA; 2008.

TABLE 29.7

Australasian Transplant Coordinators Association (ATCA) referral information[32,37,40]

SECTION	DETAILS
Personal details	Address, phone number, sex, age, height, weight, race, religion, build, occupation
Current admission details	Dates and time of hospital admission, intubation, critical care admission Other trauma or significant event
Declaration of brain death	Cause of death, time, date, method of testing
Consent details	Which organs, designated officer details, coroner's details, police details, who gave consent, which databases accessed
Donor history	Family, medical, surgical, travel, social and sexual history
Blood results	Blood group, biochemistry and haematology on admission and within past 12 hours, microbiology, gas exchange
Test results	Chest X-ray including lung field measurements, ECG, echocardiogram, bronchoscopy, sputum
Haemodynamics	BP, MAP, HR, CVP, temperature
Admission history	Cardiac arrest, temperature, renal function, nutrition, drug and fluid administration
Physical examination	Scars, trauma, needle marks etc

BP = blood pressure; CVP = central venous pressure; ECG = electrocardiogram; HR = heart rate; MAP = mean arterial pressure.

Tissue typing and cross-matching

A vital component of the assessment and referral process is tissue typing, cross-matching and virology testing of the potential donor's blood. Blood is taken from an arterial or central line of the potential donor and sent to the relevant accredited laboratory (see Table 29.8). Tissue typing identifies the human leucocyte antigen (HLA)

phenotype from the genes on chromosome 6. The HLA molecules control actions of the immune system to differentiate between 'self' and foreign tissue, and initiate an immune response to foreign matter. As a transplanted organ will always be identified as foreign tissue by the recipient's body, immunosuppressive drugs are used to suppress the immune response. A cross-match is routinely

TABLE 29.8

Blood tests required for organ donation[2,40,42]

MEASUREMENT REQUIRED	TEST
Serology	• HIV I and II • HTLV 1 antibody • Hepatitis B sAg • Hepatitis B sAb • Hepatitis B core Ab • Hepatitis C sAb • CMV (IgG) • EBV (excluding NSW) • Syphilis (excluding SA) • Toxoplasma IgG and IgM (SA, NT and WA only) • HSV (WA only)
NAT screen (nucleic acid test)	• This is not routinely performed on all donors. Testing is currently only available through the Australian Red Cross Blood Service. The State DonateLife Coordinator facilitates the process • HIV NAT Screen (Vic and NSW routinely test) • HCV NAT Screen (Vic and NSW routinely test)
Tissue typing	• Cross-matching with the blood of potential recipients of relevant ABO

Ab = antibody; CMV = cytomegalovirus; EBV = Epstein–Barr virus; HCV = hepatitis C virus; HIV = human immunodeficiency virus; HSV = herpes simplex virus; HTLV = human T-lymphotropic virus; IgG = immunoglobulin G; IgM = immunoglobulin M; NAT = nucleic acid testing; sAb = surface antibody; sAg = surface antigen.

used to predict the level of this response. Lymphocytes from the potential donor are added to the potential recipient's serum to test whether the recipient has an antibody that is specific to the donor's HLA antigens. A positive cross-match reaction, where the recipient's serum destroys the donor's cells, is a contraindication for transplantation.[32,41]

Donor management

The fourth factor influencing the number of actual organ donors is the clinical management that the donor and family receive after confirmation of death. The aim of donor management is to support and optimise organ function until organ retrieval commences, while maintaining dignity and respect for the donor and support for the family. All aspects of ICU treatment, apart from brain-oriented therapy, should continue until it is certain that organ donation will not occur.[2] Ideal parameters for biochemistry, vital signs and urine output and clinical management are detailed in Box 29.2.

Retrieval surgery

Organ retrieval surgery occurs in the hospital where the donor has been managed in the ICU (often following transfer from a regional or rural hospital), with the local operating theatre staff integral to the process. The donor is transferred to theatre after routine preoperative checks and documentation is completed, including death certification and consent for organ and tissue retrieval. All

documentation, particularly consent, is viewed by all members of the retrieval surgical team before surgery commences. Depending on which organs are to be retrieved, the retrieval teams will be tasked to abdominal organs and thoracic organs, and will bring most of their specialised equipment with them. An anaesthetist monitors haemodynamics, ventilation and administers medications, which may include a long-acting muscle relaxant given prior to the surgical procedure, to prevent interference in the surgical process by spinal reflexes, only after consultation with the retrieval team.[32] No other anaesthetic agents are administered. The local scrub staff will work with the visiting surgical teams, and the DonateLife donor coordinator will be present to document the procedure and outcomes, fulfill any family wishes in regard to theatre and act as a resource for all staff present.

Surgery may take 4 to 5 hours depending on the extent of the retrieval; cross-clamp will occur once the surgeons have identified all the various anatomical points. The aorta is cross-clamped with vascular clamps below the diaphragm and at the aortic arch, the heart is stopped and ventilation is ceased. Retrieval teams administer a cold perfusion fluid with an electrolyte mix specific to the organs being retrieved, and remove the organs. Organs are bagged with sterile ice and perfusion fluid and transported by the retrieval teams to the transplanting hospitals. The donor's surgical wound, from the sternal notch to the pubis, is closed by the surgeons in

---

BOX 29.2

Medical management of the potential donor[2,25]

Referral

- Refer all potential organ donors to the local State DonateLife agency, even if uncertain of medical suitability. Criteria for suitability change over time and may vary according to recipient circumstances (i.e. if someone is on the critical list).

Medical management

- Maintain MAP >70 mmHg: maintain euvolaemia, if required administer vasopressor agents (e.g. noradrenaline and/or vasopressin 5–2.5 U/h).

- Maintain adequate organ perfusion (monitor urine output, lactate), consider invasive haemodynamic monitoring.

- Monitor electrolytes (Na⁺, K⁺) every 2 to 4 hours and correct to normal range

- Suspected diabetes insipidus (UO >200 mL/h, rising serum sodium): administer desmopressin (DDAVP) (e.g. 4 mcg IV in adults) and replace volume loss with 5% dextrose or sterile water for infusion (via CVAD only, observing closely for signs of haemolysis).

- Treat hyperglycaemia (actrapid infusion): aim for blood glucose 5–8 mmol/L.

- Keep temp >35°C. Pre-emptive use of warming blankets is advised as hypothermia may be difficult to reverse once it has developed.

- Provide ongoing respiratory care (frequent suctioning, positioning/turning, PEEP, recruitment manoeuvres).

- Maintain haemoglobin >80 g/L.

Hormone replacement therapy

The use of hormonal replacement therapy remains controversial and it is infrequently used in Australia. Some centres use it in the setting of persistent haemodynamic instability (despite volume resuscitation and low-dose inotropes) and/or if cardiac ejection fraction <45%. Typical regimens include:

- triiodothyronine (T3) – 4 mcg IV bolus, then 3 mcg/h by IV infusion

- arginine vasopressin (AVP) – 0.5 to 4.0 U/h to maintain MAP 70 mmHg

- methylprednisolone – 15 mg/kg IV single bolus.

a routine manner and dressed with a surgical dressing. If the donor is not a coroner's case, the remaining lines, catheter and drains are removed according to local policy, the patient is washed and arrangements are made to transfer the patient to a location for family viewing or to the mortuary. Musculoskeletal tissue and retinal retrieval can occur after the solid organ retrieval in theatre or later in the mortuary.[42]

Donor family care

Supportive care of a donor family begins from the time their family member is admitted to hospital and continues beyond organ retrieval. In addition to personal factors such as cultural background, family dynamics, coping skills and prior experiences with loss that may influence the grieving process, the family of an organ and tissue donor will be dealing with a number of unique factors. Death of their family member was possibly sudden and unexpected; brain death can be difficult to understand when people look as if they are asleep rather than dead; having the option of organ donation may mean making a decision on behalf of the person if his/her wishes were not known; and the process of organ donation means they will not be with the person when their heart stops.[21] Further information about specific cultural groups and general considerations for tailoring discussions to the family's background can be found in Chapter 8.

Practice tip

Prior to family meetings regarding organ donation it is beneficial for staff to go over their roles and the potential conversation that might occur. Providing an opportunity for staff debriefing or operational reviews of the donation and retrieval process is also important, particularly in regional or rural settings where cases may be infrequent and the community is smaller. The donor coordinator will record the names of all personnel involved in the process to be included in the follow-up correspondence of thanks and to notify the outcome of the donation and subsequent transplantations.

Donor families benefit from emotional and physical support throughout and after the organ donation process. In critical care units, this support can include open visiting times, privacy for meetings, clear and precise information and regular contact with the attending clinical team, support personnel and the DonateLife donor coordinator. After organ retrieval, ongoing care can include contact with a bereavement specialist, written material, telephone support, private or group counselling and correspondence from recipients.[1] Most Australian and New Zealand organ donation agencies have cost-free structured aftercare and follow-up programs with these features (see *Online resources*). Involvement of trained personnel with a donor family through this process can positively influence the family's grief journey.[1,32]

The National Donor Family Support Service operates through the DonateLife Network and is a nationally consistent program of support provided to cadaveric organ and/or tissue donor families. All families whose next of kin are identified as possible donors are offered end-of-life support including bereavement counselling at the time, whether or not the potential donor proceeds to donation.[1]

Donation after cardiac death

Donation after cardiac death (DCD), also known as non-heart-beating donor (NHBD) and in some instances as donation after circulatory death, provides a solid organ donation option for a patient who has not progressed and is not likely to progress to brain death. Prior to brain death legislation, donation after cardiac death was the source of cadaveric kidneys for transplant.[43,44] Four categories of potential DCD donors, known as the Holland–Maastricht categories, have been identified:

1 dead on arrival (uncontrolled)
2 failed resuscitation (uncontrolled)
3 withdrawal of support (controlled)
4 arrest following brain death (uncontrolled).[40]

DCD programs around the world are being re-established, with successful retrieval and transplant of kidneys, livers and lungs.[43] The Australian Organ and Tissue Authority has developed a national DCD protocol that outlines an ethical process that respects the rights of the patient and ensures clinical consistency, effectiveness and safety for both donors and recipients.[1]

Identification of a potential DCD donor

Using lessons learnt from multi-organ donor programs, the aims of a successful DCD program are to maintain dignity for the donor at all times, provide the donor family with support and information and limit warm ischaemia time (time from withdrawal of ventilation and treatment to confirmation of death to commencement of infusion of cold perfusion fluid and/or organ retrieval). Longer warm ischaemia time potentiates the risk of irreparable hypoxic damage to the organ.[32] As noted above, Holland–Maastricht category 3 is the only option that can be controlled and possibly regulate warm ischaemia time. A potential category 3 DCD donor is a person ventilated and monitored in critical care about whom a decision has already been made that further treatment is futile, and current interventions are to be withdrawn. Clinical suitability assessment for organ retrieval replicates a multi-organ donor, with medical, surgical and social history, virology and organ function information collected. Legal requirements of the consent-seeking process also reflect those of a multi-organ donor. Potential donor families are informed that retrieval may not occur due to a number of factors, including the length of time from treatment withdrawal to cardiac standstill.[32]

Retrieval process alternatives

Withdrawal of treatment for a potential category 3 DCD patient can occur in critical care or in the operating theatre, depending on which organs are planned for retrieval. Death is determined by cessation of circulation, with recommendations that the ECG is not monitored (electrical activity can persist for many minutes following cessation of circulation), but an arterial line is used to determine the time of cessation of circulation.[2] If withdrawal occurs in critical care, an intra–abdominal catheter may be inserted via the femoral artery after cardiac standstill to infuse cold perfusion fluid into the abdominal cavity. If the lungs are to be retrieved, perfusion fluid may be infused via bilateral intercostal catheters.[43] The patient is then transferred to theatre for organ retrieval. When withdrawal of treatment occurs in theatre, a catheter is not required and retrieval may commence after the patient is declared deceased (cessation of circulation for greater than 2 minutes). If the patient does not die during the window of time available for organ retrieval, they are transferred back to ICU.[1]

Tissue-only donor

People confirmed as dead using cardiac criteria can be tissue donors. Eyes (whole and corneal button) are retrieved for cornea and sclera transplant. Musculoskeletal tissue is used for bone grafting (long bones of arms and legs, hemipelvis), urology procedures and treatment of sport injuries (ligaments, tendons, fascia and meniscus). Heart valves (bicuspid, tricuspid valves, aortic and pulmonary tissue) are used for heart valve replacement and cardiac reconstruction. Skin (retrieved from the lower back and buttocks) is used for the treatment of burns.[1]

Identification of a potential tissue-only donor

The most influential aspect for tissue donation is early notification of the potential donor's death to the relevant tissue bank, ideally within hours of the person's death. All deceased persons can be considered potential donors, with assessment for clinical suitability on a case-by-case basis. As noted earlier, there is no expectation that treating clinicians will be required to make that decision or make the approach to the next of kin. In general, once the death notification has been received, the determining factors are age, cause of death, time elapsed since death, virology results and presence of infection. The legal requirements of the consent-seeking process mirror those of the multi-organ donor.

After checking medical suitability and the relevant consent indicator database, a coordinator from the tissue bank or other trained personnel approach the next of kin with the option of tissue retrieval. Eyes can be retrieved up to 12 hours, and heart valves, skin and bone up to 24 hours after death. Of note, eye and heart valve donors can be up to 60 years old, and musculoskeletal donors up to 55 years of age.[43] After tissue retrieval, every effort is made to restore anatomical appearance. Wounds are sutured closed and covered with surgical dressings, limbs given back their form, and eye shape is restored with the lids kept closed with eye caps.[1,32] Support requirements for families of tissue-only donors share many aspects of programs provided for families of multi-organ donors. A sensitive approach, provision of adequate information to assist informed decision making, offers of bereavement counselling and follow-up information of recipient outcomes are evidence-based strategies of successful programs.[1,21]

Summary

This chapter provided an overview of organ donation. In several countries, including Australia and New Zealand, opt-in systems of giving consent for organ and tissue donation are in place but in other countries, such as Singapore and Spain, opt-out systems are used. After death has been confirmed or is impending in the case of DCD, the option of organ and tissue donation is given to the next of kin and information from a consent indicator database is sought to determine the wishes of the person. Each person is assessed on a case-by-case basis to determine medical suitability for organ and tissue retrieval for transplant. The treating clinicians are not expected to make this decision but their involvement and care are vital. Support and information are available around the clock from the respective donor agencies and tissue banks. Donor family care commences at the time of the family member's admission and continues as required with structured bereavement programs specific to donor family care. In Australia and New Zealand, intent to be an organ and tissue donor can be indicated by people when alive or by the next of kin after death.

Three 'types' of organ or tissue donor are identified including the multi-organ and tissue donor (after brain death has been confirmed), the donor after cardiac death and the tissue-only donor (after cardiac death).

Four factors have been identified that directly influence the number of multi-organ donations internationally and include the incidence of brain death, the identification of potential donors, brain death confirmation and gaining informed consent for donation and, finally, the management of the donor following the confirmation of brain death.

There is evidence to address each factor, but each case needs to be approached on a case-by-case basis. The medical suitability for every potential donor is assessed individually at the time of the person's death, and support and guidance from donor agencies and tissue banks are available at all times. Internationally, priority is given to providing care and support of the potential and actual donor family and, as part of this, regular routine follow-up and debriefing opportunities for all staff involved are important to manage stress reactions or other concerns.

Case study

DAY 1

An unidentified man, estimated to be in his 40s, collapsed while jogging on a major road at 0650 hours, which was witnessed by several people. He was unrousable at the scene, and an ambulance was immediately called, arriving in less than 3 minutes. He was immediately intubated and placed on a portable ventilator, cannulated and transported to the local hospital. He arrived at the hospital 22 minutes later. On arrival to the emergency department at 0712, his vital signs included: Glasgow Coma Score (GCS) 3, BP 180/110 mmHg, heart rate (HR) 50, SaO$_2$ 96%, intubated with no respiratory effort, absent limb reflexes including pain response. His weight was estimated at 85 kg. Following assessment by the emergency department team, he was ventilated, additional IV access gained and transferred for urgent cerebral computerised tomography (CT), which revealed a grade V subarachnoid haemorrhage (SAH). The patient carried no formal identification, but had been using an iPhone with earphones, and police were notified to help identify the man and locate next of kin.

At 0950 further assessment by the emergency department team revealed: unresponsive pupils, sinus rhythm, normotensive, GCS 3, with no sedative agents required. Following consultation with the intensive care team, the patient was transferred to ICU pending formal identification and discussion with the next of kin. In line with hospital policy, the executive director of medical services was notified, who also acted as the designated officer. The regional donor coordinator (RDC) who worked within the ICU was also notified, as the patient's prognosis was deemed to be very poor with treatment futile.

At 1100 he was admitted to critical care: haemodynamic status remained unchanged, pupils unequal, fully ventilated (synchronised intermittent mandatory ventilation [SIMV], respiratory rate 20, tidal volume 400 mL, positive end-expiratory pressure [PEEP] 5), with no sedation or paralysing agents, afebrile 35.5°C. The donor coordinator attended and outlined to staff the process of potential donor management. The hospital's donor kit was accessed, which contains all referral information, access to documentation for both staff and family, blood tubes and mailing packs.

By 1330 police notified staff in ICU of the man's identity: Mark Antonelli, aged 42, a local teacher, married to Kate with two children aged 9 and 11. He been out for his regular jog and had not returned home by the time Kate had returned from the school run. Kate had been notified by the police through accessing Mark's phone contacts, and the police advised they would bring Kate to the hospital at 1400 hours.

The family conference involving Mark's wife, two children, his parents, the intensivist, senior registrar, social worker and nursing staff started at 1400 hours and, at this point, Mark's family were informed that his haemorrhage was life-threatening and irreversible with prognosis noted as extremely poor, suboptimal neurological state with residual impairment at best and progression to brain death a likelihood within 12 hours.

At 1445, with no sedative agents having been administered during Mark's admission, the first set of brain stem death tests was performed by the intensivist and registrar, revealing fixed dilated pupils, complete absence of all reflexes and PCO$_2$ 66 with apnoea. Documentation of these parameters was completed by both the intensivist and registrar in the DonateLife form and progress notes.

A follow-up conference with the family was held at 1510 to inform them of the results and the wife asked if she could be present for the second set of tests to affirm that her husband will not recover. The team agreed to this and at 1630 a second set of tests was completed by a second team, confirming brain death. Mark's wife, a social worker, the bedside nurse, a student nurse and a donor coordinator were present for this set of testing. Absent reflexes, fixed dilated pupils and apnoea with elevated PCO$_2$ 68 mmHg were noted and documented.

The RDC who had been present in ICU notified the state donor coordinator and liaised with the ICU team for an interdisciplinary family meeting to discuss the option of organ donation.

At 1700 a family conference with the intensivist, bedside nurse, social worker, regional donor coordinator and Mark's family, including children, was held. The discussion centred around confirmation of brain death. Mark's wife asked what the next step might be and whether Mark might be able to donate his kidney to her best friend who is waiting for a kidney transplant. The RDC explained the process of donation as a gift and honouring Mark's wishes and the inability to direct donations. Mark's family consented to donate all organs and tissues and reflected on discussions he had had with them just a few months ago when they had seen an article in the paper about a transplant recipient.

The RDC contacted the state agency at 1725 to begin the referral process and explained to the ICU staff events over the next 24 hours in the management of Mark's physiological status, referral documentation and formal identification processes. The coroner was then contacted for permission for organ and tissue retrieval and blood collected and sent for virology, tissue typing and cross-matching. Patient history and current status information were collected for referral. Written material was provided to the family by the RDC that outlined the process of donation, support and counselling options and grief and bereavement information. Contact details of family members were confirmed for follow-up by the RDC.

A rapid sequence of events followed at this point with the state DonateLife organ donor coordinator undertaking referral to transplant teams at 1945. The police returned to ICU to undertake formal identification of Mark with his family at 2015; and by 2300 transplant teams confirmed acceptance of the referral with identification of potential recipients for heart, lungs, liver, kidneys and pancreas.

Mark's family left the hospital to go home just after 2300 hours knowing that the retrieval would commence in the early morning. They agreed to the offer by the state DonateLife donor coordinator to phone them in the morning to confirm the outcome. Ongoing monitoring of ventilation and haemodynamics, and care including physiotherapy treatments continued throughout the evening.

DAY 2

At 0500, retrieval teams arrived from interstate coordinated by the state donor coordinator and were escorted to the operating theatre by the hospital nursing supervisor. All equipment and instrumentation was provided by the teams and set-up commenced immediately with the retrieval commencing 45 minutes later. Retrieval of the heart, lungs, liver, kidneys and pancreas took place within 4 hours with the liver split intraoperatively for two recipients.

The RDC rang Mark's family at 0830 to inform them that the retrieval had gone according to plan and advised that she would call again the following day with updates on the recipients' progress. The family advised they would attend shortly for viewing as discussed at the family meeting the previous evening.

At 1000 Mark's body was returned to ICU where Kate and her children, as well as Mark's parents, returned to view his body following the retrieval. A private room with minimal equipment and chairs was prepared by the staff and the family was assisted by the social worker, the same bedside nurse and student nurse from the previous day and the RDC. After the viewing, Mark's body was transported to the mortuary, escorted by the bedside nurse, student nurse and police officers; and immediately following the RDC provided a debrief session in the meeting room attached to ICU together with the social worker for all staff that had been involved in the case from all departments to capture staff.

The following day (day 3), the state donor coordinator contacted the transplant teams to find out recipients' progress and then contacted the donor family and the staff of the hospital to inform them of the outcomes. Letters detailing this information were sent to the family and the staff of the hospital within days of the retrieval.

CASE STUDY QUESTIONS

1 What constitutes eligibility for organ donation?
2 What methods are used to confirm brain death in Australia and New Zealand?
3 Who is the legal next of kin in the consent process?
4 Under which circumstances does the coroner need to be involved?

RESEARCH VIGNETTE

Orøya A, Strømskag K, Gjengedala E. Approaching families on the subject of organ donation: a phenomenological study of the experience of healthcare professionals. Intensive Crit Care Nurs 2013;29(4):202–211

Abstract

The aim of this study was to explore healthcare professionals' experiences and gain a deeper understanding of interactions with families when approaching the subject of organ donation. A hermeneutic phenomenological approach was used to explore the participants' experiences. Data were collected through a combination of observation and in-depth interviews with nurses, physicians and hospital chaplains recruited from two intensive care units (ICUs) in a Norwegian university hospital. A thematic analysis was used to analyse the data, and three main themes emerged from this analysis: crucial timing, challenging conversations and conflicting expectations. The results revealed that the situation was of a sensitive nature and that finding the best possible time to address the issue in a meaningful manner was a challenge. Respect for the patients' wishes and the families' decisions was an expressed value among the participants, but conflicting expectations about bringing up the subject were also present. This study contributes to the understanding of healthcare professionals' challenges when they are facing brain death as an inevitable outcome of a patient's clinical condition and must approach families on the subject of organ donation.

Critique

This small Norwegian qualitative observation and interview study was undertaken in 2006. The sample comprised healthcare professionals who had interaction with families of critically ill patients diagnosed with severe brain injuries and were likely to proceed to a state of brain death. A hermeneutic phenomenological approach was used, and accurately described as being 'based on the Heideggarian view that understanding is based on our pre-understanding' (p 203), with the researcher also identified as having prior experience in critical care.

Participant selection occurred across two ICU sites in Norway with a combined average donation rate of 19 per year. Thirty-two participants were selected for in-depth interviews (with a breakdown of professional disciplines) consistent with methodology chosen by the researchers. The interview process occurred across 2006 and 2007 with interviews lasting up to 150 minutes and transcribed verbatim for thematic analysis, to reveal three main themes, each with subsets of themes. The article does not elaborate on whether the transcripts and interpretation were returned to participants for accuracy of transcription and analysis.

The analysis described three clearly identified themes: 'crucial timing', 'challenging conversations' and 'conflicting expectations'. The findings were clearly articulated, with illustrations and participant quotes used to elaborate the identified issues and subthemes. The researchers identified that within interpretive phenomenology there is no clear end point for the interpretive process, and described this as allowing for future exploration of the themes and subthemes to occur.

Limitations were clearly identified by the researcher as being the inability to attend all the family meetings that led to health professionals being identified for the study; and that not all health professionals who were involved were able to be interviewed. Site limitations were also identified, with the focus on two Norwegian centres and further considerations of national policy and cultural influences further limiting the transferability to other countries.

Overall, this paper acknowledged the need of caring for the families of potential organ donors through the interview process, and outlined the need for healthcare professionals to maintain awareness of the power imbalance in the consent process to ensure 'informed' consent is given, not just 'obtaining presumed consent'.

Learning activities

1   Will organ retrieval mutilate the body of the person?

2   What follow-up is provided to the family of the donor?

3   What is the role of the designated officer?

Online resources

Achieving Comprehensive Coordination in Organ Donation throughout the European Union (ACCORD), www.accord-ja.eu

Australasian Donor Awareness Program (ADAPT), www.donatelife.gov.au/professional-education-package

Australasian Transplant Coordinators Association (ATCA), www.atca.org.au

Australia and New Zealand Cardiothoracic Organ Transplant Registry, www.anzcotr.org.au

Australia and New Zealand Dialysis and Transplant Registry (ANZDATA), www.anzdata.org.au

Australia and New Zealand Liver Transplant Registry, www.anzltr.org

Australia and New Zealand Organ Donation Registry (ANZOD), www.anzdata.org.au/anzod/v1/indexanzod.html

Australian and New Zealand Intensive Care Society (ANZICS), www.anzics.com.au

Australian Bone Marrow Registry, www.abmdr.org.au/

Australian College of Critical Care Nurses (ACCCN), www.acccn.com.au

Australian Corneal Graft Registry, www.flinders.edu.au/medicine/sites/ophthalmology/clinical/the-australian-corneal-graft-registry.cfm

Australian Organ Donor Register (AODR), www.medicareaustralia.gov.au/organ

British Organ Donor Society, http://body.orpheusweb.co.uk

Coalition on Donation, www.shareyourlife.org

DonateLife, www.donatelife.gov.au

Donor Tissue Bank of Victoria, www.vifm.org/forensics/donor-tissue-bank-of-victoria

European Training Program on Organ Donation (ETPOD), etpod.il3.ub.edu

Eye Bank of South Australia, www.flinders.edu.au/medicine/sites/ophthalmology/clinical/#eye

Gift of Life, www.giftoflife.on.ca

Global Observatory on Donation and Transplantation (GODT), www.transplant-observatory.org/Pages/home.aspx

International Registry in Organ Donation and Transplantation (IRODaT), www.irodat.org

Japan Organ Transplant Network, www.jotnw.or.jp

Lions Corneal Donation Service, cera.clientstage.com.au/our-work/lions-eye-donation-service

Lions Eye Bank (WA), www.lei.org.au/go/lions-eye-bank

Lions NSW Eye Bank, www.eye.usyd.edu.au/eyebank

MESOT: The Middle East Society for Organ Transplantation, www.mesot-tx.org

Multi Organ Harvesting Aid Network Foundation, www.mohanfoundation.org

National Organ Donation Collaborative (NODC), www.nhmrc.gov.au/nics/programs/nodc/index.htm#trans

New Zealand National Eye Bank, www.eyebank.org.nz

New Zealand National Transplant Donor Coordination Office, www.donor.co.nz

Organ Procurement and Transplantation Network, optn.transplant.hrsa.gov

Perth Bone and Tissue Bank, www.perthbonebank.com

Queensland Bone Bank, http://temp.donatelife.gov.au/the-network/donatelife-in-qld/queensland-bone-bank

Queensland Eye Bank, http://temp.donatelife.gov.au/the-network/donatelife-in-qld/queensland-eye-bank

Queensland Heart Valve Bank, http://temp.donatelife.gov.au/the-network/donatelife-in-qld/queensland-heart-valve-bank

Queensland Skin Bank, http://temp.donatelife.gov.au/the-network/donatelife-in-qld/queensland-skin-bank

Transplant News Network, www.centerspan.org

Transplant Nurses' Association (TNA), www.tna.asn.au

Transplantation Society of Australia and New Zealand (TSANZ), www.tsanz.com.au

United Network for Organ Sharing (UNOS), www.unos.org

World Health Organization, www.who.int/transplantation/en

Further reading

Australian and New Zealand Intensive Care Society (ANZICS). The ANZICS statement on death and organ donation (edition 3.2). Melbourne: ANZICS; 2013.

Australian College of Critical Care Nurses. ACCCN position statement on organ and tissue donation and transplantation, <https://www.acccn.com.au/about-us/position-statements>; 2009.

European Commission. Organ donation and transplantation. Special Eurobarometer 333a. Belgium: European Commission, <ec.europa.ed/public_opinion/archives/ebs/ebs_333a_en.pdf>; 2010.

National Health and Medical Research Council (NHMRC). National protocol for donation after cardiac death, <http://www.donatelife.gov.au>; 2010.

Rudge C, Mateasanz R, Delmenica FL, Chapman J. International practices of organ donation. Br J Anaesth 2012;108:48–55.

Russ GR. Organ donation in Australia: international comparisons, <http://www.donatelife.gov.au>.

Snell GI, Levvey BJ, Williams TJ. Non-heart beating organ donation. Intern Med J 2004:34:501–3.

World Health Organization. Global glossary on organ donation, <http://www.who.int/transplantation/activities/GlobalGlossaryonDonation Transplantation.pdf?ua=1>.

References

1 DonateLife website, <http://www.donatelife.gov.au> [accessed June 2014].
2 Australian and New Zealand Intensive Care Society (ANZICS). The ANZICS statement on death and organ donation (edition 3.2). Melbourne: ANZICS; 2013.
3 Chapman JR. Transplantation in Australia – 50 years in progress. Med J Aust 1992;157(1):46–50.
4 Organ Donation New Zealand website, <www.donor.co.nz/donor/transplants/history.php>, [accessed 06.14].
5 Borel JF, Feurer C, Gubler HU, Stähelin H. Biological effects of cyclosporin-A: a new antilymphocytic agent. Agents Actions 1976;6:468–75.
6 Multi Organ Harvesting Aid Network (MOHAN). Foundation website, <http://www.mohanfoundation.org>; [accessed 07.14].
7 Medicare Australia. Australian Organ Donor Register, <http://www.medicareaustralia.gov.au/organ>; [accessed 08.14].
8 Kim JR, Elliott D, Hyde C. The influence of sociocultural factors on organ donation and transplantation in Korea: findings from key informant interviews. J Transcult Nurs 2004;15(2):147–54.
9 Gleeson G. Organ transplantation from living donors. Bioethics Outlook; 2000;11(1):5.
10 Suguitan GA, Cabanayan-Casasola RA, Danguilan RA, Jaro JMA. Outcomes of referrals for deceased organ sonation to the government organ procurement organisation. Transplant Proc 2014;46:1074-6.
11 Haupt WF, Rudolf J. European brain death codes: a comparison of national guidelines. J Neurol 1999;246:432-7.
12 Therapeutic Goods Administration website, <http://www.tga.gov.au>; [accessed 07.14].
13 Arbour RB. Brain death: assessment, controversy and confounding factors. Crit Care Nurs 2013;33(6):27-46.
14 Scheinkestel CD, Tuxen DV, Cooper DJ, Butt W. Medical management of the (potential) organ donor. Anaesth Intensive Care 1995;23(1):51-9.
15 Bugge JF. Brain death and its implications for management of the potential organ donor. Acta Anaesthesiol Scand 2009;53:1239-50.
16 Siminoff LA, Gordon N, Hewlett J, Arnold RM. Factors influencing families consent for donation of solid organs for transplantation. JAMA 2001;286(1):71-7.
17 Dobb GJ, Weekes JW. Clinical confirmation of brain death. Anaesth Intensive Care 1995;23(1):37–43.
18 Zuckier LS, Kolano J. Radionuclide studies in the determination of brain death: criteria, concepts, and controversies. Semin Nucl Med 2008;38(Neuronuclear Imaging):262–273.
19 The Transplantation Society of Australia and New Zealand Inc (TSANZ) website, <http://www.tsanz.com.au>; [accessed 11.14].
20 Australasian Transplant Coordinators Association (ATCA). National donor family study: 2004 report. Melbourne: ATCA; 2004.
21 Yousefi H, Roshani A, Nazari F. Experiences of the families concerning organ donation of a family member with brain death. Iran J Nurs Midwifery Res 2014;19(3):323-9.
22 Verble M, Worth J. Fears and concerns expressed by families in the donation discussion. Prog Transplant 2000;10(1):48–55.
23 Verble M, Worth J. Biases among hospital personnel concerning donation of specific organs and tissues: implication for the donation discussion and education. Journal of Transplant Coordinators 1997;7(2):72–7.
24 DeJong W, Franz HG, Wolfe SM, Nathan H, Payne D, Reitsma W et al. Requesting organ donation: an interview study of donor and non-donor families. Am J Crit Care 1998;7(1):13–23.
25 Australasian Transplant Coordinators Association (ATCA). National guidelines for organ and tissue donation. 4th ed. Sydney: ATCA; 2008.
26 Coyle MA. Meeting the needs of the family: the role of the specialist nurse in the management of brain death. Intensive Crit Care Nurs 2000;16(1):45–50.

27 Haddow G. Donor and nondonor families' accounts of communication and relations with healthcare professionals. Prog Transplant 2004;14(1):41–8.

28 Morton J, Blok GA, Reid C, Van Dalen J, Morley M. The European Donor Hospital Education Programme (EDHEP): enhancing communication skill with bereaved relatives. Anaesth Intensive Care 2000;28(2):184–90.

29 Streat S, Silvester W. Organ donation in Australia and New Zealand – ICU perspectives. Crit Care Resusc 2001;3(1):48–51.

30 Pearson A, Robertson-Malt S, Walsh K, Fitzgerald M. Intensive care nurses' experiences of caring for brain dead organ donor patients. J Clin Nurs 2001;10(1):132–9.

31 Oroy A, Stromskag KE, Gjengedal E. Approaching families on the subject of organ donation: a phenomenological study of the experience of healthcare professionals. Intensive Crit Care Nurs 2013;29:202-11.

32 Mercer L. Improving the rates of organ donation for transplantation. Nurs Stand 2013;27(26):35-40.

33 Gomez MP, Perez B, Manyalich M. International Registry in Organ Donation and Transplantation – 2013. Transplant Proc 2014;46:1044-48.

34 Australia and New Zealand Organ Donation Registry (ANZOD). Registry report 2013. Adelaide: ANZOD; 2013.

35 *New Zealand Human Tissue Act 2008*. Section 2, <http://www.health.govt.nz/search/results/tissue%20act>; [accessed 11.14].

36 Thompson TL, Robinson JD, Kenny RW. Family conversations about organ donation. Prog Transplant 2004;14(1):49–55.

37 Irving MJ, Tong A, Jan S, Cass A, Rose J, Chadban S et al. Factors that influence the decision to be an organ donor: a systematic review of the qualitative literature. Nephrol Dial Transplant 2012;27(6):2526-33.

38 Wong LP. Factors limiting deceased organ donation: focus groups' perspective from culturally diverse community. Transplant Proc 2010;42:1439-44.

39 Australasian Transplant Coordinators Association (ATCA). National donor family study: 2000 report. Melbourne: ATCA; 2000.

40 Brook NR, Waller JR, Nicholson ML. Nonheart-beating kidney donation: current practice and future developments. Kidney Int 2003;63(4):1516–29.

41 Australasian Transplant Coordinators Association (ATCA). Confidential donor referral form. Sydney: ATCA; 2010. Same as ref 39?

42 Regehr C, Kjerulf M, Popova S, Baker A. Trauma and tribulation: the experience and attitudes of operating room nurses working with organ donors. J Clin Nurs 2004;13(4):430–7.

43 Levvey B, Griffiths A, Snell G. Non-heart beating organ donors: a realistic opportunity to expand the donor pool. Transplant Nurs J 2004;13(3):8–12.

44 Lewis J, Peltier J, Nelson H, Snyder W, Schneider K et al. Development of the University of Wisconsin Donation after Cardiac Death evaluation tool. Prog Transplant 2003;13(4):265–73.

Appendix A

Practice standards for specialist critical care nurses

DOMAIN	NO.	STANDARD	NO.	ELEMENT
Professional practice The standards in this domain relate to the professional, legal and ethical responsibilities of critical care nurses and include knowledge of the legal implications of critical care nursing practice, accountability for practice and the ability to interpret unfamiliar situations in a legal and ethical sense. The standards also include awareness and protection of the rights of patients and their families	1	Functions within professional and legal parameters of critical care nursing practice	1.1	Applies a knowledge of relevant legislation, professional standards, policies and procedures to critical care nursing practice
			1.2	Observant of the legal implications of actions taken within the critical care team and fulfils the duty of care in clinical practice
			1.3	Recognises and responds to unsafe or unprofessional practices by reporting appropriately
			1.4	Applies the required legal and ethical framework of recording information in the critical care setting
			1.5	Contributes to formation of policies and protocols to ensure safe patient outcomes
	2	Protects the rights of patients and their families	2.1	Applies knowledge of, and advocates for, the rights of patients and their families in critical care settings
	3	Demonstrates accountability for nursing practice	3.1	Accepts responsibility for own actions
			3.2	Makes complex and informed independent decisions within own level of competence and scope of practice
	4	Demonstrates and contributes to ethical decision making	4.1	Demonstrates an accurate knowledge of contemporary ethical issues underpinning critical care nursing practice and complies with the profession's code of ethics and code of conduct
			4.2	Contributes to multidisciplinary ethical discussion and decision-making processes/framework within the critical care setting

DOMAIN	NO.	STANDARD	NO.	ELEMENT
Provision and coordination of care This domain relates to essential nursing practices that establish and sustain a holistic nurse–patient–family relationship that optimises the wellbeing of the patient and family. The standards include an ability to address the physiological, psychological, physical, emotional and spiritual needs of the patient and family, as well as to optimise the physical and non-physical environment	5	Provides patient- and family-centred critical care	5.1	Involves the patient and family as active participants in the process of care
			5.2	Practises with cultural sensitivity and awareness of social factors to enhance patient and family wellbeing
			5.3	Personalises the patient care environment
			5.4	Meets the comfort needs of patients and their families
			5.5	Establishes, maintains and concludes therapeutic interpersonal relationships with patients and their families
	6	Promotes optimal comfort, wellbeing and safety in a highly technological environment that is often unfamiliar to patients and families	6.1	Ensures a safe environment for patients, families and staff by identifying, minimising or eliminating risks
	7	Manages and coordinates the care of a variety of patients	7.1	Organises workload to meet planned and unplanned patient care needs to ensure optimal patient outcomes
			7.2	Negotiates and delegates care to optimise matching between nurses' scope of practice and the complexity of care for individual patients
			7.3	Optimises delivery of care through the effective use of human and physical resource management
	8	Manages therapeutic interventions	8.1	Acts on assessment findings to appropriately initiate, monitor and manage therapeutic interventions
			8.2	Applies specialised knowledge in the use of critical care technologies
Critical thinking and analysis This domain relates to applying specialised knowledge for clinical problem solving. Integrated clinical decision making provides a foundation for the application of research evidence to practice. The domain reflects the capacity of the critical care nurse to respond to planned and unanticipated changes in patient care and to recognise the need for advanced assessment, planning and application of specialised knowledge to deliver evidence-based care	9	Applies integrated patient assessment and interpretive skills to achieve optimal patient outcomes	9.1	Gathers, analyses and integrates data from a variety of sources and acts on the significance of findings to formulate an individualised plan of care
	10	Develops and manages a plan of care to achieve desired outcomes	10.1	Formulates and implements an integrated plan of care incorporating specialised knowledge to achieve desired patient outcomes
			10.2	Assesses effectiveness of nursing care to achieve desired outcomes and reviews plan accordingly
			10.3	Enables continuity of care in collaboration with other members of the healthcare team

DOMAIN	NO.	STANDARD	NO.	ELEMENT
	11	Evaluates and responds effectively to changing situations	11.1	Initiates pre-emptive interventions in order to avoid complications
			11.2	Analyses alterations in physiological parameters and intervenes appropriately
			11.3	Anticipates, evaluates and responds effectively to physiological deterioration and emergency situations
	12	Engages in and contributes to evidence-based critical care nursing practice	12.1	Maintains an informed position in relation to current research studies and incorporates evidence-informed practice into critical care setting
			12.2	Promotes and participates in quality activities to improve critical care patient outcomes
Collaboration and leadership The standards in this domain relate to the leadership and education role displayed by the specialist critical care nurse and integral part played by experienced critical care nurses in the professional development of peers, students and less experienced staff	13	Collaborates with the critical care team and other health professionals to achieve desired outcomes	13.1	Establishes and maintains collaborative and constructive relationships with colleagues in critical care and the broader healthcare team
			13.2	Acts as an advisor beyond the walls of the critical care environment
	14	Acts to enhance the professional development of self and others	14.1	Assesses own abilities and engages in activities to enhance personal and professional development
			14.2	Identifies and assists in meeting the learning needs of others
			14.3	Actively participates in promoting the profession of critical care
	15	Contributes toward a supportive environment for all members of the healthcare team	15.1	Initiates strategies to support colleagues and facilitates resolution of situations that may impact on the wellbeing of others

Normal laboratory values

Blood analysis: parameters, applications and normal ranges

PARAMETER	APPLICATION	NORMAL RANGE
Adrenocorticotrophic hormone (ACTH)	Aetiology of corticosteroid abnormality	<10 pmol/L
Albumin	Hydration, nutrition status, protein-related disorders and liver disease	32–45 g/L
Alkaline phosphatase (ALP)	Hepatobiliary or bone disease	Neonates/paediatrics: 0 days to <1 week (80–380) U/L 1 week to <4 weeks (120–550) U/L 4 weeks to <26 weeks (120–650) U/L 26 weeks to <2 years (120–450) U/L 2 years to <6 years (120–370) U/L 6 years to <10 years (120–440) U/L Males: 10 years to <14 years (130–530) U/L 14 years to <15 years (105–480) U/L 15 years to <17 years (80–380) U/L 17 years to <19 years (50–220) U/L 19 years to <22 years (45–150) U/L 22 years to <120 years (30–110) U/L Females: 10 years to <13 years (100–460) U/L 13 years to <14 years (70–330) U/L 14 years to <15 years (50–280) U/L 15 years to <16 years (45–170) U/L 16 years to <22 years (35–140) U/L 22 years to <120 years (30–110) U/L
Alanine aminotransferase (ALT)	Liver damage	Neonate: <50 U/L Adult: <35 U/L
Amylase	Acute pancreatitis	Varies based on laboratory method (25–130 U/L) GCUH[1]
Anion gap	Aetiology of metabolic acidosis	8–16 mmol/L (4–13 mmol/L if K not included)
Aspartate aminotransferase (AST)	Liver damage	Neonates: <80 U/L Adults: <40 U/L

PARAMETER	APPLICATION	NORMAL RANGE
Base excess (arterial blood)	Metabolic component of acid–base disorders	(−3) to (+3) mmol/L
Bicarbonate (HCO$_3^-$)	Acid–base disorders, particularly metabolic component	Neonates/paediatrics: 0 days to <1 week (15–28) mmol/L 1 week to <2 years (16–29) mmol/L 2 years to <10 years (17–30) mmol/L 10 years to <18 years (20–32) mmol/L Adults: 18 years to <120 years (22–32) mmol/L
Bilirubin	Hepatobiliary disease and haemolysis	Total: <20 micromol/L Direct: <7 micromol/L
Calcium (Ca^{2+})	Hyper/hypocalcaemia	Neonates/paediatrics: 0 days to <1 week (1.85–2.80) mmol/L 1 week to <26 weeks (2.20–2.80) mmol/L 26 weeks to <2 years (2.20–2.70) mmol/L 2 years to <18 years (2.20–2.65) mmol/L Adults: 18 years to <120 years (2.10–2.60) mmol/L Calcium corrected for albumin: 18 years to <120 years (2.10–2.60) mmol/L Ionised calcium: 18 years to <120 years (1.16–1.30) mmol/L
Carboxyhaemoglobin	Carbon monoxide exposure	0.2–2.0% of total haemoglobin normally, up to 8.5% in heavy smokers
Chloride (Cl$^-$)	Causes of acid–base disturbance	Neonates/paediatrics: 0 days to <1 week (98–115) mmol/L 1 week to <18 years (97–110) mmol/L Adults: 18 years to <120 years (95–110) mmol/L
Cholesterol	Lipid status	Total: ≤4.0 mmol/L (recommended by NHF) HDL: 1.0–2.2 mmol/L (females) 0.9–2.0 mmol/L (males) Therapeutic targets: >1.0 mmol/L LDL: 2.0–3.4 mmol/L Therapeutic targets: <2.5 mmol/L
Creatinine kinase (CK)	Diagnosis of myocardial damage	Neonate: 70–380 U/L Adult female: 30–180 U/L Adult male: 60–220 U/L
Creatine kinase MB isoenzyme (CKMB)	Diagnosis of myocardial damage	CKMB 0–10 U/L; 0-5% of the total CK
Creatinine (Cr)	Renal function, particularly glomerular filtration	Neonates/paediatrics: 0 days to <1 week (22–93) micromol/L 1 week to <4 weeks (17–50) micromol/L 4 weeks to <2 years (11–36) micromol/L 2 years to <6 years (20–44) micromol/L 6 years to <12 years (27–58) micromol/L Adult males: 12 years to <15 years (35–83) umol/L 15 years to <19 years (50–100) umol/L 19 years to <60 years (60–110) umol/L Adult females: 12 years to <15 years (35–74) umol/L 15 years to <19 years (38–82) umol/L 19 years to <60 years (45–90) umol/L

PARAMETER	APPLICATION	NORMAL RANGE
Glucose	Hyper/hypoglycaemia	Fasting: 3.0–5.4 mmol/L Random: 3.0–7.7 mmol/L
Iron	Iron deficiency or overload	Varies according to laboratory method
L-lactate	Metabolic acidosis	Fasting arterial blood: 0.3–0.8 mmol/L. Fasting venous blood: 0.3–1.3 mmol/L
Lactate dehydrogenase (LDH)	Assessment of liver disease	120–250 U/L (method and age dependent). Normal range for adults
Magnesium (Mg)	Hypomagnesaemia	Neonates/paediatrics: 0 days to <1 week (0.60–1.00) mmol/L 1 week to <18 years (0.65–1.10) mmol/L Adults: 18 years to <120 years (0.70–1.10) mmol/L
Myoglobin (serum)	Detection of muscle damage	<55 mcg/L
Osmolality	Suspected poisoning with some substances, e.g. alcohol, methanol	Neonates: 270–290 mmol/kg Adults: 275–295 mmol/kg
Phosphate (PO_4)	Renal failure, hyper-/hypoparathyroidism metabolic bone disease	Neonate/paediatrics: 0 days to <1 week (1.25–2.85) mmol/L 1 week to <4 weeks (1.50–2.75) mmol/L 4 weeks to <26 weeks (1.45–2.50) mmol/L 26 weeks to <1 year (1.30–2.30) mmol/L 1 year to <4 years (1.10–2.20) mmol/L 4 years to <15 years (0.90–2.00) mmol/L 15 years to <18 years (0.80–1.85) mmol/L Adults: 18 years to <20 years (0.75–1.65) mmol/L 20 years to <120 years (0.75–1.50) mmol/L
Potassium (K^+)	Hyper/hypokalaemia	Neonates/paediatrics: 0 days to <1 week (3.8–6.5) mmol/L 1 week to <26 weeks (4.2–6.7) mmol/L 26 weeks to <2 years (3.9–5.6) mmol/L 2 years to <18 years (3.6–5.3) mmol/L Adults: 18 years to <120 years (3.5–5.2) mmol/L
Protein	Used in conjunction with albumin to calculate globulin, diagnosis of protein- and nutrition-related disorders	Neonate: 40–75 g/L Child <2 years: 50–75 g/L Adults: 60–80 g/L
Sodium (Na^+)	Fluid and electrolyte status	Neonates/paediatrics: 0 days to <1 week (132–147) mmol/L 1 week to <18 years (133–144) mmol/L Adults: 18 years to <120 years (135–145) mmol/L
Triglyceride	Lipid status	<1.7 mmol/L (fasting)
Troponin I or troponin T	Myocardial infarction	Normally not detected
Urea	Renal function	Neonates: 1.0–4.0 mmol/L Adults: 3.0–8.0 mmol/L

Haematology: parameters, applications and normal values

PARAMETER	APPLICATION	NORMAL VALUE
Activated clotting time (ACT)	Heparin therapy	Varies based on product in use
Activated partial thromboplastin time (APTT)	Coagulopathy and monitoring of heparin therapy	Varies based on laboratory methods, usually 25–35 seconds
Antithrombin III (AT III)	Investigation of venous thromboembolism	Varies based on laboratory method Functional (guide only): 80–120% of activity in pooled normal plasma Immunoassay (guide only): 0.2–0.4 g/L
Bleeding time	Assessment in some bleeding disorders, e.g. von Willebrand's disease	For investigation of bleeding risk, please refer to Coagulation profile, Platelet function analyser (PFA), Platelet aggregometry
D-dimers	Indication of recent or ongoing fibrinolysis, possibly indicating disseminated intravascular coagulation (DIC)	Varies based on laboratory method
Haemoglobin (Hb)	Anaemia	Children 6–59 months: ≥ 110 g/L Children 5–11 years: ≥ 115 g/L Children 12–14 years: ≥ 120 g/L Non-pregnant women (≥ 15 years): ≥ 120 g/L Pregnant women: ≥ 110 g/L Men (≥ 15 years): ≥ 130 g/L
International normalised ratio (INR)	Oral anticoagulant therapy	Varies according to clinical indication. Typically 2.0–3.0, although a target of up to 4.5 may be used in those with a mechanical heart value
Packed cell volume (PCV) (also referred to as haematocrit)	Anaemia	Infant (3 months): 0.32–0.44 Child (3–6 years): 0.36–0.44 Child (10–12 years): 0.37–0.45 Adult (female): 0.37–0.47 Adult (male): 0.40–0.54
Plasminogen	Investigation of tendency towards clotting, e.g. venous thromboembolism	50–150%
Platelet count	Excessive or inappropriate bleeding	$150–400 \times 10^9$/L
Prothrombin time (PT)	Detection of coagulation factor deficiencies due to vitamin K deficiency	Varies based on laboratory Reagent dependent; prothrombin time generally 11–15 seconds
Red cell count (RCC)	Anaemia	Neonate/paediatrics: Term cord blood: $4.0–6.0 \times 10^{12}$/L 3 months: $3.2–4.8 \times 10^{12}$/L 1 year: $3.6–5.2 \times 10^{12}$/L 3–6 years: $4.1–5.5 \times 10^{12}$/L 10–12 years: $4.0–5.4 \times 10^{12}$/L Adults: Female: $3.8–5.8 \times 10^{12}$/L Male: $4.5–6.5 \times 10^{12}$/L
Thrombin time (TT)	Acquired or inherited disorders of haemostasis	Varies based on laboratory method, but usually 14–16 seconds
White cell count (WCC)	Infection or inflammatory disease	Neonate: $6.0–22.0 \times 10^9$/L Child (1 year): $6.0–18.0 \times 10^9$/L Child (4–7 years): $5.0–15.0 \times 10^9$/L Child (8–12 years): $4.5–13.5 \times 10^9$/L Adult: $4.0–10.0 \times 10^9$/L

Urine analysis: parameters, applications and normal values

PARAMETER	APPLICATION	NORMAL VALUE
Albumin	Diabetic nephropathy, renal disease	Normal: <30 mg albumin/g creatinine Microalbuminuria: 30–300 mg albumin/g creatinine Macroalbuminuria: >300 mg albumin/g creatinine
Calcium	Renal calculi	2.5–7.5 mmol/24 hours Fasting spot urine: Males: 0.04–0.45 mol/mol creatinine Females: 0.10–0.58 mol/mol creatinine
Chloride	Identification of site of chloride loss in electrolyte disturbance	Dependent on intake, but usually 100–250 mmol/24 hours
Cortisol (free)	Adrenocortical hyperfunction	100–300 nmol/24 hours
Creatinine clearance	Glomerular filtration rate	>70 mL/min in a young adult, typically falling approx. 0.5 mL/min per year at ages over 30 years
Magnesium	Urinary magnesium loss	2.5–8.0 mmol/24 hours (related to daily intake)
Myoglobin	Suspected rhabdomyolysis	Not normally detected
Osmolality	Renal disease, syndrome of inappropriate antidiuretic hormone, polyuric syndromes	50–1200 mmol/kg
Potassium	Differentiation of renal potassium loss from other causes of hypokalaemia	40–100 mmol/24 hours (related to daily intake)
Protein	Renal disease	<150 mg/24 hours During pregnancy: <250 mg/24 hours
Sodium	Causes of hyponatraemia	In hyponatraemia or hypovolaemic shock without acute tubular necrosis, urine sodium should be <20 mmol/L and fractional excretion of sodium should be <1.5% If extracellular fluid volume and plasma sodium are normal, urine sodium should equal intake minus non-renal losses, typically 75–300 mmol/24 hours
Urea	Renal function, occasionally assessment of nitrogen balance in patients receiving parenteral nutrition	420–720 mmol/24 hours

Blood gases: parameters and normal values

PARAMETER	NORMAL VALUE
ARTERIAL	
pH	7.35–7.45 (35–45 nmol/L)
Partial pressure of oxygen (PaO$_2$)	11.0–13.5 kPa (80–100 mmHg) (varies with age)
Partial pressure of carbon dioxide (PaCO$_2$)	4.6–6.0 kPa (35–45 mmHg)
Oxygen saturation (SaO$_2$)	>94%
VENOUS	
pH	7.34–7.42
Partial pressure of oxygen (PvO$_2$)	37–42 mm Hg
Partial pressure of carbon dioxide (PvCO$_2$)	42–50 mm Hg
Oxygen saturation (SvO$_2$)	>70%

Reference

1   The Royal College of Pathologists of Australasia. RCPA manual. 7th ed. ISSN 1449-8219. <http://www.rcpa.edu.au/Library/Practising-Pathology/RCPA-Manual/Home>; 2015 [accessed 02.03.15].

Glossary of terms

ablation. Therapy designed to destroy tissues that generate or sustain arrhythmias.

Aboriginal. Refers to both Aboriginal and Torres Strait Islander peoples.

actigraph. Used for measuring movement, in particular to measure the quantity of sleep.

action potential. The electrical activity developed in a muscle or nerve cell during activity.

acute coronary syndrome (ACS). A broad spectrum of clinical presentations, spanning ST-segment elevation myocardial infarction through to an accelerated pattern of angina without evidence of myonecrosis.

acute respiratory distress syndrome. An acute syndrome of rapid onset in which the patient has evidence of hypoxia and non-cardiogenic pulmonary oedema.

acute respiratory failure. Occurs when there is a reduction in the body's ability to maintain either oxygenation or ventilation, or both.

advance directives. A method to document preferences about an individual's future health care should situations arise where they are no longer competent to make decisions.

advanced life support. The provision of effective airway management, ventilation of the lungs and production of circulation by means of techniques additional to those of basic life support. These techniques may include, but not be limited to, advanced airway management, tracheal intubation, intravenous access/drug therapy and defibrillation.

adverse event. An injury or event that is due to healthcare management and results in temporary or permanent harm to patients.

afterload. The load imposed on the muscle during contraction, and translates to systolic myocardial wall tension.

allograft. A tissue graft from a donor of the same species as the recipient but not genetically identical.

anabolism. The chemical process by which complex molecules, such as peptides, proteins, polysaccharides, lipids and nucleic acids, are synthesised from simpler molecules.

anastomosis. A surgical connection between two structures.

anhidrosis. Absence of sweating.

antepartum haemorrhage. Any bleeding from the genital tract after 20 weeks' gestation and before the birth of the baby.

anterior cord syndrome. Spinal cord injury to the motor and sensory pathways in the anterior parts of the spine; thus patients are able to feel crude sensation, but movement and detailed sensation are lost in the posterior part of the spinal cord.

anxiety. A disorder characterised by excessive concern or worry with difficulty controlling the level of concern, and with irritability, restlessness and disturbed sleep.

arterial blood gas. An arterial blood sample taken to assess pH, bicarbonate, oxygen and carbon dioxide levels, and other electrolytes.

asterixis. Abnormal tremor, especially in the hands.

asthma. A lower respiratory tract disease characterised by mucosal and immune system dysfunction. The chronic inflammatory process causes narrowing of bronchial airways, obstructing airflow leading to episodes of wheezing, breathlessness and chest tightening.

auscultation. The action of listening to sounds from the heart, lungs or other organs, typically with a stethoscope.

automatic tube compensation. A feature available on some ventilators in which the ventilator employs an algorithm to increase airway pressure to overcome the resistance of the artificial airway during inspiration.

autonomic dysreflexia. Dysfunctions of the autonomic nervous system characterised by abnormalities in heart rate, respiratory rate, systolic blood pressure and increased muscle tone and temperature. Other characteristics include decerebrate (extensor) or decorticate (flexor) posturing, and profuse sweating.

axon. Part of the neuron that transmits information to other neurons.

backwards upwards right pressure manoeuvre. A technique where pressure is applied to mobilise the thyroid cartilage in the sequence backwards (towards the spine) and to the right side in order to help visualise the vocal cords and assist with intubation.

beneficence. To do good; promoting the wellbeing of another person.

best interests. Acting in a way that optimally promotes good for the individual and is a principle for making decisions about health care.

biphasic. Pattern of electrical flow where the current reverses direction in the middle of the waveform, flowing first from one electrode pad, through the heart, to the second electrode pad, and then from the second pad through the heart to the first.

birth. The complete expulsion or extraction from its mother of a baby of at least 20 weeks' gestation or, if gestation is unknown, weighing at least 400 g, who is either born alive or stillborn.

birth weight. The first weight of the baby (stillborn or live born) obtained after birth.

bronchiolitis. Obstruction of the small airways, resulting in air trapping and respiratory distress, generally seen in infants less than 12 months of age.

Brown–Séquard syndrome. Injury to the left or right side of the spinal cord. Movements are lost below the level of injury on the injured side, but pain and temperature sensation are lost on the opposite side of injury.

business case. A management tool used to outline the clinical needs (who, what, when, where and how) and their implications, such as the expected financial return on investment.

caesarean section/birth. Operative birth through an abdominal incision.

capnography. Monitoring of expired carbon dioxide.

caput medusa. The appearance of distended and engorged paraumbilical veins that radiate from the umbilicus across the abdomen.

cardiac arrest. Cessation of heart action recognised by the absence of response, absence of normal breathing and absence of movement.

cardiac pacing. The delivery of an electrical impulse to either or both the atria and ventricles to initiate or maintain normal cardiac electrical activity.

cardiopulmonary resuscitation. Comprises those techniques used to minimise the effects of circulatory arrest and to assist the return of spontaneous circulation, including the technique of rescue breathing combined with external chest compressions.

care bundle. A set of evidence-based interventions or processes of care, applied to selected patients in order to ensure appropriate, standardised care.

catabolism. The convergent process, in which many different types of molecules are broken down into relatively few types of end products.

central cord syndrome. Injury to the centre of the cervical spinal cord, producing weakness, paralysis and sensory deficits in the arms but not the legs.

cerebral microdialysis. A tool for investigating the metabolic status of the injured brain. The microdialysis probe is inserted into the cerebral tissue where substances in the extracellular fluid surround the semipermeable membrane at the tip of the catheter. Following equilibration of the tissue metabolites with the perfusion fluid, the dialysate can be analysed for concentrations of products of energy metabolism (glucose, lactate, pyruvate) as indicators of hypoxia and ischaemia.

cerebral oedema. Increased brain water content.

cerebral spinal fluid. An ultrafiltrate of blood plasma composed of 99% water, making it close to the composition of the brain extracellular fluid.

cerebrovascular resistance. The amount of resistance created by the cerebral vessels, which is controlled by the autoregulatory mechanisms of the brain.

checklist. A list of action items or criteria arranged in a systematic way, allowing the person completing it to record the presence or absence of individual items having been undertaken.

chemoreceptor. A sensor that responds to change in chemical composition in the blood.

chemosis. Conjunctival oedema, often associated with positive pressure ventilation, positive end-expiratory pressure or prone positioning.

child. 'Young child' is aged between 1 and 8 years and 'older child' is aged between 9 and 14 years inclusive.

chronic heart failure (CHF). Refers to a complex syndrome distinguished by a number of characteristics, particularly shortness of breath or fatigue, that occur at rest or on exertion. It is also characterised by objective evidence of cardiac dysfunction or structured cardiac abnormalities that impair the left ventricle from filling with or ejecting blood to meet the body's demands.

clinical decision making. The cognitive processes and strategies that nurses use when utilising data to make clinical decisions regarding patient assessment and care.

clinical practice guideline. Statements about appropriate health care for specific clinical circumstances.

coagulopathy. Disorder of the clotting mechanism of the blood, which can be caused by pre-existing disease, medications, pathophysiological conditions such as hypothermia and acidosis or current treatment such as massive blood transfusion.

coma. A state of unresponsiveness from which the patient cannot be aroused by verbal and physical stimuli to produce any meaningful response; therefore, coma implies the absence of both arousal and content of consciousness.

complementary therapies. Treatments that have not been considered part of standard Western medicine but that are increasingly being used in combination with standard medical treatments. These may include therapies for pain, such as massage and relaxation techniques, and some nutritional therapies.

conduction. The process by which electrical activity is directly transmitted through cells when there is a difference of electrical potential between adjoining regions, without movement of the tissue.

contact activation pathway. Previously termed the 'intrinsic' coagulation pathway.

continuous lateral rotation therapy. An intervention in which the patient is rotated continually, on a specialised bed, through a set number of degrees; it helps to relieve pressure areas and can significantly improve oxygenation. It is also known as kinetic bed therapy.

contractility. The force of ventricular ejection, or the inherent ability of the ventricle to perform external work, independent of afterload or preload.

coronary heart disease or coronary artery disease. A narrowing of the small blood vessels that supply blood and oxygen to the heart.

counterpulsation. Rapid inflation of the intra-aortic balloon catheter at the onset of diastole of each cardiac cycle and then deflation immediately before the onset of the next systole.

critical care nursing. Specialised nursing care of critically ill patients who have an immediate life-threatening or potentially life-threatening illness or injury.

critically ill patients. Patients who have an immediate life-threatening or potentially life-threatening illness or injury causing compromise to the function of one or more organs.

cross-clamp. The act of clamping the aorta to achieve a controlled arrest of the heart, ceasing blood flow to all organs, and commencement of infusion of cold perfusion fluid during organ retrieval surgery. Marks the beginning of cold ischaemic time.

croup (laryngotracheobronchitis). A set of symptoms caused by acute swelling causing obstruction in the upper airway (larynx, trachea and bronchi) from inflammation and oedema and is most commonly seen in winter months.

cultural safety. Involves effective nursing practice whereby patients and their families determine that their cultural needs have been met and that they feel safe. Effective nursing practice requires nurses to reflect on their own cultural location and how this may influence the way in which they interact with patients from another culture. In addition to ethnically related culture, culture is defined broadly to include age, generation, gender, sexual orientation, socioeconomic status, migrant experience, occupation, religious or spiritual beliefs and disability.

cytotoxic/histotoxic anoxia. The inability to use oxygen, even when available.

cytotoxic oedema. Cellular swelling, usually of astrocytes in the grey matter, which is generally seen after cerebral ischaemia caused by cardiac arrest or minor head injury.

damage-control surgery. A four-stage surgical approach that involves rapid initial control of haemorrhage and contamination, usually with packing and temporary closure, followed by ongoing resuscitation in the ICU and reoperation for definitive repair and reconstruction.

dendrite. Part of the neuron that receives positive or negative charges from other neurons.

donation after cardiac death. A solid organ donation option for a patient who has not progressed and is not likely to progress to brain death. It is also known as non-heart-beating donor and donation after circulatory death.

depolarisation. The electrical state in an excitable cell where the inside of the cell becomes less negative relative to the outside.

eclampsia. A severe variant of preeclampsia, characterised by tonic–clonic seizures that are not caused by any pre-existing disease or other identifiable causes, e.g. epilepsy, cerebral haemorrhage.

electroencephalography. The recording of electrical activity by sensors along the scalp produced by the firing of neurons within the brain.

embolism. Obstruction of an artery, typically by a blood clot or an air bubble.

encephalitis. Inflammation of the brain substance.

endotracheal tube. An artificial airway used in critical care settings to enable delivery of mechanical ventilation and clearance of airway secretions.

enzyme. Substance produced by a living organism that acts as a catalyst to bring about a specific biochemical reaction.

epiglottitis. Inflammation of the epiglottis, frequently involving surrounding structures, with the classic description of a swollen, cherry-red, softened and floppy epiglottis, which tends to fall backwards, obstructing the airway.

ethics. The study of rational processes to inform a course of action in response to a particular situation where conflicting options exist.

evidence-based nursing. The conscientious, explicit and judicious use of research-based information in making decisions about care delivery to individuals or groups of patients.

extracorporeal membrane oxygenation. Therapy in which blood is removed from the patient and oxygenated in an artificial membrane before being returned to the patient, i.e. circulation of blood outside the body provides total artificial support of cardiac and pulmonary function.

family. Those closest to the person in knowledge, care and affection, including the immediate biological family; the family of acquisition (related by marriage or contract); and the family of choice and friends (not related biologically or by marriage or contract).

family-centred care. Incorporates planning, delivery and evaluation of health care that is governed by mutually beneficial partnerships among healthcare providers, patients and families.

fidelity. Keeping promises; honouring contracts and commitments.

flaccid areflexic paralysis. Paralysis that is characterised by an absence of reflexes and lack of muscle tone.

general anaesthesia. A drug-induced state where the patient will not respond to stimuli, including pain.

gestation. The estimated gestational age of the baby in completed weeks using all available obstetric information (clinical estimation, ultrasound, cycle length etc), counting from the first day of the woman's last menstrual period. Commonly recorded as $35^{+2}/40$, indicating that the gestation is 35 weeks and 2 days.

gravidity. The total number of pregnancies a woman has had, including the index pregnancy, regardless of the outcome (therefore including spontaneous and induced abortions and any stillborn or live born infants).

Guillain–Barré syndrome. An immune-mediated disorder resulting from generation of autoimmune antibodies and/or inflammatory cells that cross-react with epitopes on peripheral nerves and roots, leading to demyelination or axonal damage or both, and autoimmune insult to the peripheral nerve myelin.

gynaecomastia. Benign enlargement of the breast tissue in males.

haemodynamic monitoring. The measurement of pressure, flow and oxygenation within the cardiovascular system.

heart failure with preserved ejection fraction (HFpEF). Refers to impaired diastolic filling of the left ventricle. There may or may not be impaired systolic dysfunction.

heart failure with reduced ejection fraction (HFrEF). Refers to inability of the heart to contract in systole.

HELLP syndrome. A severe variant of preeclampsia characterised by **H**aemolysis, **E**levated **L**iver enzymes and **L**ow **P**latelets.

high-frequency oscillatory ventilation. The use of supra-physiological ventilatory rates and tidal volumes less than anatomical dead space by specialised ventilators to accomplish gas exchange. Typical ventilator rates are 3–15 Hz or 180–600 breaths/min (1 Hz = 60 breaths).

homeostatic. The tendency of the body to seek and maintain a condition of balance or equilibrium within its internal environment.

hypercapnoeic respiratory failure. Also known as type II respiratory failure (or failure to ventilate), presents with a high $PaCO_2$ as well as a low PaO_2.

hypoxaemic respiratory failure. Also known as type I respiratory failure (or failure to oxygenate), presents with a low PaO_2 and a normal or low $PaCO_2$.

icterus. Jaundice.

Indigenous person. Aboriginal or Torres Strait Islander person of Australia or Maori person of New Zealand.

induction of labour. Procedure performed for the purpose of initiating and stimulating the process of labour. This may include the artificial rupture of the membranes and/or the use of uterine stimulating medication.

infant. A person less than approximately 1 year of age.

infant death. The death of an infant occurring within 1 year of birth.

intra-aortic balloon pump (IABP). Mechanical assistance for a failing heart based on the principles of diastolic augmentation and systolic unloading by counterpulsation of a balloon in the aorta.

intracranial hypertension. A sustained intracranial pressure of >15 mmHg.

intracranial pressure. The pressure exerted by the contents of the brain within the confines of the skull. Normal ICP is 0–10 mmHg.

jugular venous oximetry. Jugular venous catheterisation used to collect data on oxygen-based variables such as jugular venous oxygenation, cerebral oxygen extraction and arteriovenous difference in oxygen, which can indicate changes in cerebral metabolism and blood flow.

justice. Fair, equitable and appropriate treatment in light of what is due or owed to an individual.

laryngotracheobronchitis. Also known as croup; a set of symptoms caused by acute swelling causing obstruction in the upper airway (larynx, trachea and bronchi) from inflammation and oedema and is most commonly seen in winter months.

live birth. The birth of an infant, regardless of maturity or birth weight, who breathes or shows any other signs of life after being born.

magnetic resonance imaging. An imaging technique that uses the characteristic of hydrogen protons, which function like tiny spinning magnets, to generate images of the brain and body.

malignant hyperthermia. An acute pharmacogenetic disorder, which develops during or after the application of general anaesthesia involving volatile agents and/or depolarising muscle relaxants. The autosomal dominant disorder likely occurs because of a defect in calcium channel regulation in the muscle cell. Malignant hyperthermia is a hyper-metabolic state caused primarily by continued contraction of the skeletal muscles. This results in increased carbon dioxide production, skeletal muscle rigidity, tachyarrhythmias, unstable haemodynamics, respiratory acidosis, cyanosis, hyperkalaemia, lactic acidosis, fever and eventually (if untreated) death.

mechanical circulatory support. Partial or total cardiovascular support devices such as IABP, ventricular assist devices and total artificial hearts.

medical futility. Treatment with no apparent benefit to the patient.

meningitis. Inflammation of the pia and arachnoid layers of the meninges.

monophasic. Pattern of electrical flow where the current, throughout the pulse, flows in one direction, from one electrode pad through the heart to the other electrode pad.

morality. The norms widely shared by a community or among members of a professional group about what is 'right' or 'wrong' about human conduct, the widely held views then forming stable social consensus.

multigravida. A woman who is pregnant for the second or subsequent time.

multipara. A woman who has had more than one pregnancy resulting in a live birth or stillbirth.

murmur. A low continuous background noise.

myasthenia gravis. An autoimmune disorder caused by autoantibodies against the nicotinic acetylcholine receptor on the postsynaptic membrane at the neuromuscular junction, which is characterised by weakness and fatigue in voluntary muscles.

myelin sheath. A lipid–protein casing that covers the neuron and provides protection to the axon, speeding the transmission of impulses along the nerve cells.

myocardial infarction. Myocardial cell death due to prolonged ischaemia.

near-infrared spectroscopy. A non-invasive method of monitoring continuous trends of cerebral oxygenated and deoxygenated haemoglobin by utilising an infrared light beam transmitted through the skull.

negligence. A legal term where the provider owed a duty of care to the recipient; they failed to meet that duty; the recipient sustained damages as a result; and the provider should have reasonably foreseen that these damages would occur.

neonatal death. The death of a live born infant, within 28 days of birth, whose birth weight was at least 400 g or of at least 20 weeks' gestation.

neonate. An infant in the first minutes to hours following birth.

neuroglia. The non-neuronal cells of the nervous system that are 10–50 times more prevalent than the number of neurons.

neuron. A specialised cell in the nervous system comprised of a dendrite, cell body (also known as soma) and axon.

neurotransmitter. A chemical messenger used by neurons to communicate in one direction with other neurons.

neutrally adjusted ventilatory assistance. A type of ventilation that uses diaphragmatic movement to trigger gas flow and breath delivery.

non-maleficence. Doing no harm and maximising possible benefits while minimising possible harm.

non-technical skills. Cognitive, social and personal skills that complement technical skills and contribute to safe and efficient task performance.

nullipara. A pregnant woman who has not had a prior birth of an infant of 20 weeks' gestation or more.

open disclosure. Telling the truth to the patient or family about what and how an adverse event has occurred.

palmar erythema. Reddening of the skin on the palmar aspects of the hands.

parity. Number of previous pregnancies resulting in live birth or stillbirth.

partogram. Birth suite chart that records maternal and fetal monitoring during labour, and the progress of labour, e.g. strength and frequency of contractions, fetal descent.

parturient. Pregnant woman; of or relating to giving birth.

patient dependency. An approach to quantify the care needs of individual patients, classifying patients into groups requiring similar nursing care.

patient safety. Reduction of the risk of unnecessary harm to patients to an acceptable level.

perinatal death. A stillbirth or neonatal death.

person-centred care. Emphasis on the individual nature of the person with the illness that promotes the perception (and reality) of equal power and a shared partnership between the person and healthcare provider/s.

placenta accreta. Abnormal adherence of the placenta to the uterine wall.

placenta praevia. The placenta is partially or wholly implanted in the lower uterine segment on either the anterior or posterior wall.

polysomnography. The continuous recording of various physiological variables during sleep; these variables typically include brain wave activity, eye movement and muscle tone.

postpartum. After birth. The postpartum period is normally classified as the 6 weeks following birth, when the woman's body returns to the pre-pregnancy state.

postpartum haemorrhage. ≥500 mL blood loss from the genital tract following birth. It is categorised as primary, within the first 24 hours following birth, or secondary, from 24 hours to 6 weeks postpartum.

post-traumatic amnesia. A disorder after brain injury reflecting the time elapsed from injury until recovery of full consciousness and the return of ongoing memory.

preeclampsia. A multisystem pregnancy disorder resulting from widespread vasospasm that is often characterised by hypertension and proteinuria.

preload. The load imposed by the initial fibre length of the cardiac muscle before contraction (i.e. at the end of diastole).

primigravida. A woman pregnant for the first time.

primipara. A woman who has had one pregnancy resulting in a live birth or stillbirth.

pseudocholinesterase deficiency. An inherited abnormality in the pseudocholinesterase enzyme that results in slower metabolic degradation of the depolarising neuromuscular blocking agent suxamethonium (succinylcholine).

pulse oximetry. The measurement of peripheral arterial oxygen saturation.

quality monitoring. Measurement of and responses to the incidence and patterns of adverse events.

rapid response system. System developed to recognise and provide emergency response to patients who experience acute deterioration.

regional anaesthesia. An umbrella term used to describe injection of local anaesthetic in the vicinity of major nerve bundles supplying specific body areas to produce nerve blocks, epidural and spinal blocks.

repolarisation. The process by which the membrane potential of a neuron or muscle cell is restored to the cell's resting potential.

research participant. Individual (or group of living individuals) about whom a researcher conducting research obtains data through intervention or interaction with that person or their identifiable private information.

resuscitation. Preservation or restoration of life by the establishment and/or maintenance of airway, breathing and circulation, and related emergency care.

return of spontaneous circulation (ROSC). Resumption of sustained perfusing cardiac activity associated with significant respiratory effort after cardiac arrest.

root cause analysis. A detailed method to investigate an adverse event whereby the system and processes that contributed to the event are examined in an effort to identify system or process improvements to prevent the event from reoccurring.

safety culture. The product of individual and group values, attitudes, perceptions, competencies and patterns of behaviour that determine the commitment to, and the style and proficiency of, an organisation's health and safety management.

seizure. An abrupt discharge of ions from a group of neurons resulting in epileptic activity. Seizures are classified depending on how they start: as partial or focal seizures; generalised or full body seizures involving both cerebral hemispheres; or partial seizures with secondary generalisation.

sensory overload. A prolonged overstimulus of the senses that can result from excessive or prolonged periods of noise, light, odours and touch from both equipment and personnel.

situational awareness. An individual's awareness and understanding of information that is relevant to their current environment and task.

skill mix. The ratio of caregivers with various skills, training and experience in a clinical unit.

somnolence. A state of unconsciousness from which the patient can be fully awakened.

spider angiomata. Swollen blood vessels slightly beneath the surface of the skin. There is usually a central red spot with extensions moving outward like a spider web.

spontaneous breathing trial. A technique in which the patient is removed from the ventilator to see if they are able to breath unassisted by the mechanical ventilator.

spontaneous vaginal birth. Birth without intervention in which the baby's head is the presenting part.

status epilepticus. Enduring seizure activity that is not likely to stop spontaneously. Traditionally defined as 30 minutes of continuous seizure activity, it has been changed to 5 minutes or 2 or more seizures without full recovery of consciousness between the seizures.

status epilepticus. Enduring seizure activity that is not likely to stop spontaneously. Traditionally defined as 30 minutes of continuous seizure activity, it has been changed to 5 minutes or 2 or more seizures without full recovery of consciousness between the seizures.

stillbirth. The birth of an infant weighing at least 400 g or of at least 20 weeks' gestation, which shows no signs of life after birth.

stress. A state of mental or emotional strain or suspense.

stupor. A state of unconsciousness from which the patient can be awakened to produce inadequate responses to verbal and physical stimuli.

tissue factor pathway. Previously termed the 'extrinsic' coagulation pathway.

transcranial Doppler. A safe and reliable ultrasound technology for measuring cerebrovascular blood velocities and evaluating cerebral circulation and haemodynamics.

transformational leadership. A style of leadership characterised by developing a shared vision, inspiring and communicating, valuing others, challenging and stimulating, developing trust and enabling others.

traumatic brain injury. Heterogeneous pathophysiological process from a mixture of diffuse and focal lesions on the brain because of the mechanism of injury. It can range in severity from concussion through to post-coma unresponsiveness.

values. The beliefs and attitudes that individuals hold about what is important and that therefore influence individual actions and decision making.

vasogenic oedema. Extracellular brain oedema from increased capillary permeability.

venous thromboembolism. A term used to reflect both deep vein thrombosis and pulmonary embolism.

ventilator-associated pneumonia. A form of hospital-acquired pneumonia that occurs in patients who are mechanically ventilated.

ventricular assist device (VAD). Full or partial ventricular assistance provided by an implanted device.

veracity. Telling the truth; full and honest disclosure so that individuals can weigh up the risks and benefits of treatments.

warm ischaemia. Time taken from withdrawal of ventilation and treatment to the confirmation of death of a donation after cardiac death (DCD) donor to the commencement of infusion of cold perfusion fluid and/or organ retrieval.

Index